D.H.W

PRINCIPLES OF MOLECULAR MEDICINE

Section Editors

Dennis Ausiello, MD
Department of Medicine
Massachusetts General Hospital
Boston, MA

Andrea Ballabio, MD
Telethon Institute of Genetics and Medicine (TIGEM)
Milano, Italy

Michael J. Holtzman, MD
Division of Pulmonary and Critical Care Medicine
St. Louis, MO

Ethylin Wang Jabs, MD
Center for Medical Genetics
Johns Hopkins University School of Medicine
Baltimore, MD

Laurence Kedes, MD
Institute for Genetic Medicine and Program for Gene Therapy
University of Southern California School of Medicine
Los Angeles, CA

Thomas S. Kupper, MD
Dermatology Division
Brigham and Women's Hospital
Boston, MA

Joseph B. Martin, MD, PhD
Faculty of Medicine
Harvard Medical School
Boston, MA

Michael J. McPhaul, MD
Department of Internal Medicine
University of Texas Southwestern Medical Center
Dallas, TX

Charles B. Nemeroff, MD, PhD
Department of Psychiatry and Behavioral Medicine
Emory University School of Medicine
Atlanta, GA

James C. Reynolds, MD
Division of Gastroenterology and Hepatology
Allegheny University of the Health Sciences
Philadelphia, PA

Anthony Rosenzweig, MD
Cardiac Unit and Cardiovascular Research Institute
Massachusetts General Hospital
Boston, MA

Swee Lay Thein, MRCP, FRCPath
MRC Molecular Haemotology Unit
Institute of Molecular Medicine
John Radcliff Hospital, Headington
Oxford, UK

Ralph C. Williams, Jr., MD
Division of Rheumatology
Department of Medicine
University of Florida
Gainesville, FL

Principles of Molecular Medicine

Edited by

J. Larry Jameson, MD, PhD

Northwestern University Medical School
Chicago, IL

Foreword by

Francis S. Collins, MD, PhD

National Human Genome Research Institute
Bethesda, MD

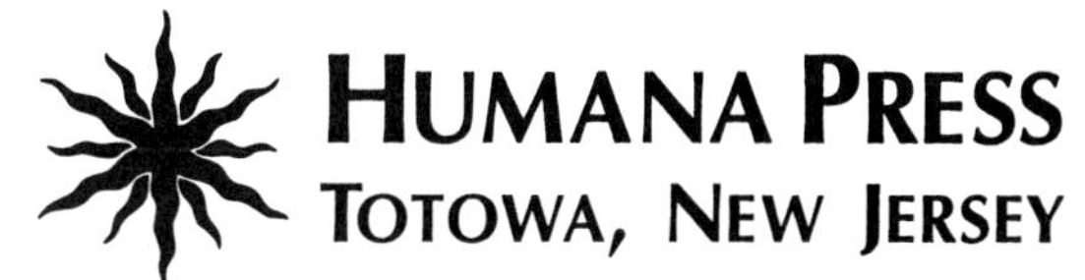

999 Riverview Drive, Suite 208
Totowa, New Jersey 07512

For additional copies, pricing for bulk purchases, and/or information about other Humana titles, contact Humana at the above address or at any of the following numbers: Tel: 973-256-1699; Fax: 973-256-8341; E-mail: humana@humanapr.com

Due diligence has been taken by the publishers, editors, and authors of this book to assure the accuracy of the information published and to describe generally accepted practices. The contributors herein have carefully checked to ensure that the drug selections and dosages set forth in this text are accurate and in accord with the standards accepted at the time of publication. Notwithstanding, as new research, changes in government regulations, and knowledge from clinical experience relating to drug therapy and drug reactions constantly occurs, the reader is advised to check the product information provided by the manufacturer of each drug for any change in dosages or for additional warnings and contraindications. This is of utmost importance when the recommended drug herein is a new or infrequently used drug. It is the responsibility of the treating physician to determine dosages and treatment strategies for individual patients. Further it is the responsibility of the health care provider to ascertain the Food and Drug Administration status of each drug or device used in their clinical practice. The publisher, editors, and authors are not responsible for errors or omissions or for any consequences from the application of the information presented in this book and make no warranty, express or implied, with respect to the contents in this publication.

Cover design by Thomas B. Lanigan and Patricia F. Cleary.

This publication is printed on acid-free paper. ∞
ANSI Z39.48-1984 (American National Standards Institute) Permanence of Paper for Printed Library Materials.

Printed in the United States of America. 10 9 8 7 6 5 4 3 2 1

Library of Congress Cataloging-in-Publication Data

Principles of molecular medicine / edited by J. Larry Jameson
foreword by Francis S. Collins.
p. cm.
Includes index.
ISBN 0-89603-529-8 (alk. paper)
1. Medical genetics. 2. Pathology, Molecular. 3. Molecular biology.
I. Jameson, J. Larry.
[DNLM: 1. Genetics, Medical. 2. Molecular Biology. QZ 50 P9573
1998]
RB155.P695 1998
616'.042—dc21
DNLM/DLC
for Library of Congress 98-17729
CIP

Foreword

Until recently, medical genetics and molecular medicine were considered the exclusive province of academic specialists in tertiary-care medical centers. Queried about their familiarity with molecular genetic aspects of clinical medicine, most primary-care providers only a few years ago would have responded that such matters were irrelevant to their daily practice.

Yet few could say that today. Few internists or general practitioners have not prescribed recombinant insulin, tPA, or erythropoetin; few pediatricians have not gone through the molecular evaluation of a child with dysmorphology or learning disability; few obstetricians have not performed amniocentesis or CVS for couples at increased genetic risk; and few general surgeons have not faced penetrating questions about the role of genetic testing or prophylactic surgery from women with a strong family history of breast or ovarian cancer.

This level of emergence of molecular genetics into clinical medicine is still quite modest, however, compared to what is coming. As the human genome project hurtles toward completion of the sequence of a reference human genome, and the identification of all human genes, by 2005, the pace of revelations about human illness will continue to accelerate. Until recently, most disease-gene discoveries have related to single-gene disorders (cystic fibrosis, fragile X syndrome, and so on) or to Mendelian subsets of more common illnesses (BRCA1 and BRCA2, the hereditary nonpolyposis colon cancer syndromes, and so on). But with the initiation in 1998 of an aggressive new genome project goal, cataloging all common human sequence variations, it is expected that the weaker polygenic contributors to virtually all diseases will begin to be discerned. Many consequences will result. Individualized preventive medicine strategies, rooted in the gene-based determination of future risk of illness, will become part of the regular practice of medicine. New designer drugs, based not on empiricism but on a detailed understanding of the molecular pathogenesis of disease, will appear. Pharmacogenomics, wherein the efficacy and toxicity of a particular drug regimen can be predicted based on patient genotype, will become a standard component of designing optimum therapy for the individual. And gene therapy, fed by a wealth of disease-gene discoveries, will mature into a significant part of the physician's armamentarium against disease.

As we watch this train coming down the track, this is an ideal time to collect information about molecular medicine into one authoritative text. *Principles of Molecular Medicine* aims to do just that, bridging the current gap between basic science and the bedside. It will thus be useful to researchers and clinicians alike. With more than 100 chapters covering a wide variety of topics, its distinguished cohort of section editors, and its abundant tables and illustrations, it provides an accessible and much needed manual to the present and the future of molecular genetics and medicine.

Francis S. Collins

Preface

For most physicians, molecular medicine and genetics have not traditionally played a major role in day-to-day clinical practice. However, new insights into the molecular basis of disease are being generated at an ever-increasing rate, resulting in a transformation in our understanding and management of diseases. This explosion of information has been ignited by a variety of technological advances, and has been fueled by the rapid progress of the human genome project. It is widely recognized that molecular biology is now causing a paradigm shift in the teaching and practice of medicine. The promise of molecular medicine is exciting, but there are also great challenges in the integration of this rapidly advancing field into our understanding and treatment of disease. *Principles of Molecular Medicine* attempts to close the gap between traditional textbooks of medicine and the burgeoning database of new knowledge that has been generated by molecular biology.

The book's title, *Principles of Molecular Medicine*, reflects our effort to translate the advances provided by genetics and molecular biology into each of the major specialties of medicine. By analogy with traditional textbooks of medicine, the book is organized according to major organ systems. This format is familiar to most medical readers and thus conforms to the specialty areas of many authors and readers. We believe that this book will be of value to a broad audience that includes sophisticated students, specialists who are seeking updates in their own areas or on topics that they have not followed closely, and practicing physicians who remain vitally interested in learning about the remarkable changes in molecular medicine.

Each of the various specialty sections of *Principles of Molecular Medicine* have been edited by experts in their respective fields. The book opens with a series of introductory chapters, and each specialty section contains additional background overview chapters that address issues of molecular pathophysiology specific to their respective organ systems. Even though the field of molecular medicine is evolving quickly, the book contains up-to-date reviews of the genetic basis of diseases, with an emphasis on principles that should allow the reader to integrate basic knowledge with all the latest breakthroughs. Our authors have aspired to clarify complex topics with many lucid figures that depict cellular and genetic pathways. And we have placed particular emphasis on the molecular mechanisms of disease and on those new concepts resulting from application of the tools of molecular biology. An especially exciting dimension of the book is the translation of the many recent advances in research into clinically useful information; each of our authors has attempted to project the future implications of recent developments in their specialty areas.

Beyond the insights afforded into the pathophysiology of disease, it can be argued that genetics plays a role in virtually every medical condition. It has been estimated that the human genome contains between 50,000 and 80,000 genes. Though many diseases are caused by mutations in critical genes, it is becoming increasingly evident that one's "genetic background" can result in predisposition to many diseases or can modify the host response to environmental events. In some cases, such as hypertension and cardiovascular disease, the genetic contributions are polygenic, and we are still in the early stages of identifying the many genes that contribute to these conditions. In other instances, such as hemophilia, cystic fibrosis, and hundreds of other disorders, the responsible genes have already been well-characterized.

From one perspective, the onslaught of new information can seem daunting and difficult to assimilate, particularly because much of the technology and terminology is new. Ironically, the new insights provided can in fact greatly simplify areas that were previously mysterious. For example, several different genetic defects can cause peripheral neuropathies, but disruption of the normal folding of myelin sheaths appears to represent a common final pathway. Likewise, several genetically distinct forms of Alzheimer disease appear to share a common final pathway that involves the formation of neurofibrillary tangles. Identification of the nature of the defective genes (e.g., dystrophin, CFTR, FGF-receptor) can pinpoint the pathway that is involved in key physiologic processes. Similarly, transgenic and gene "knockout" models can reveal the physiologic function of genes.

One of the surprises in this new field of molecular medicine is its already pervasive impact in every specialty of medicine. For example, cardiologists are unraveling the molecular basis of inherited cardiomyopathies and ion channel defects that predispose to arrhythmias. Neurologists have identified a startling number of genes in which mutations lead to neurodegenerative disorders. Not surprisingly, hematology has progressed rapidly from the classic genetic descriptions of hemoglobinopathies to define the molecular basis of other disorders, including red cell membrane defects, clotting disorders, and thrombotic disorders. The genetic causes of leukemias and lymphomas have created important paradigms for understanding mechanisms of neoplasia. The identification of the cystic fibrosis transporter allows molecular diagnosis of this disease, and gene therapy protocols are underway at several centers. Inherited variations in the immune system impact upon susceptibility to infectious agents, as well as an array of inflammatory and autoimmune disorders. Our understanding of such viral infections as hepatitis and HIV has been aided greatly by the use of recombinant DNA technology. In endocrinology, new insights into hormone action, sexual differentiation, and mechanisms of endocrine neoplasia have been gained by elucidating the nature of genetic defects. Moreover, the field of hormone and signal transduction has revealed a remarkably intricate network of interacting pathways that mediate cellular responses to external signals. In nephrology, a cause of polycystic kidney disease has been identified and the molecular pathogenesis of ischemic and inflammatory disorders are becoming clearer. In dermatology, there has been remarkable progress in mechanisms of neoplasia, the molecular pathogenesis of pemphigoid diseases, and a variety of other autoimmune disorders. Psychiatry too is an area in which the role of genetics is rapidly emerging as highly important; the foundations for this development are outlined in our chapters on behavior, schizophrenia, affective disorders, and alcoholism. Molecular mechanisms have also now been elucidated for many "classic" genetic disorders. Studies of Prader-Willi, Angelman, and Beckwith-Wiedemann syndromes have revealed a critical role for imprinting. The impact of nucleotide repeat disorders has been documented in the fragile X syndrome, as well as for such neurologic disorders as Huntington disease. In most cases, our new knowledge of these disorders has improved the feasibility and accuracy of diagnostic testing, enhanced our understanding of pathophysiology, and is beginning to unmask new avenues for therapy, including gene therapy.

We have been fortunate to enlist the expertise of a renowned international group of section editors and authors for *Principles of Molecular Medicine*. They have generously taken time from their full palette of research, teaching, and clinical activities to prepare chapters in a manner that is useful to individuals both within and outside of their specialty areas. Although the book contains more than 120 chapters, it is not all-inclusive. Rather, we have focused on disorders in which there has been substantial recent progress and for which there appear to be gaps in coverage elsewhere. The reader is encouraged to seek out further sources for additional information. A particularly valuable resource is the on-line version of Mendelian Inheritance of Man (OMIM), which can be accessed at www3.ncbi.nlm.hih.gov./OMIM. The molecular basis of metabolic disorders has been well-covered in textbooks of internal medicine and in Scriver's, *The Metabolic and Molecular Basis of Inherited Disease*. We anticipate that *Principles of Molecular Medicine* will evolve with the field, retaining an emphasis on clinical molecular medicine.

In addition to the dedication and scholarship of our section editors and authors, a great many individuals have contributed to the success of this book. The idea for the text was conceived in discussions with Victoria Reeders. Mary Kay McMahon provided enormous effort toward the timely completion of this project, superimposed upon her many other responsibilities. Kristina Stanfield, Patty Kalan, Joanne McAndrews, and William Lowe helped to ensure that last-minute updates were included. I am also grateful to the many colleagues who took the time to proofread and critique chapters. Many thanks are owed to Thomas Lanigan at Humana Press for his enthusiastic support and for ushering this concept to completion. I am grateful to many mentors and students for stimulating my interest in molecular medicine. Among these individuals, I especially acknowledge Joel Habener and William Crowley, with whom I have shared the excitement that comes with new insight and discovery. On a personal note, my wife, Michele, and my children, Ryan, Christina, and Jimmy, provided the encouragement that has allowed me to work in the mode of a perpetual student.

J. Larry Jameson

Contents

Contributors

D. Craig Allred, MD, *Department of Pathology, University of Texas Health Science Center, San Antonio, TX*
Grant J. Anhalt, MD, *Department of Dermatology, Johns Hopkins University, Baltimore, MD*
Stylianos E. Antonarakis, MD, *Division of Medical Genetics, University of Geneva Medical School, Geneve, Switzerland*
Amin Arnaout, MD, *Massachusetts General Hospital, Renal Unit, Charlestown, MA*
Andrew Arnold, MD, *Center for Molecular Medicine; Division of Endocrinology and Metabolism, University of Connecticut Health Center, Farmington, CT*
Dennis A. Ausiello, MD, *Department of Medicine, Massachusetts General Hospital, Boston, MA*
Sherri J. Bale, PhD, *Genetic Studies Section, Laboratory of Skin Biology, NIAMS, National Institutes of Health, Bethesda, MD*
Melora D. Berardo, MD, *Cytopathology Center, Johnson City, TN*
Susan H. Blanton, MD, *Department of Pediatrics, University of Virginia, Charlottesville, VA*
Jean L. Bolognia, MD, *Department of Dermatology, Yale Medical School, New Haven, CT*
Joseph V. Bonventre, MD, PhD, *Massachusetts General Hospital, Renal Unit, Charlestown, MA*
Larry Borish, *Department of Pediatrics, National Jewish Hospital, Denver, CO*
Karen D. Bradshaw, MD, *Department of Obstetrics and Gynecology, University of Texas Southwestern Medical Center, Dallas, TX*
Beverley A. Britt, *Department of Anesthesia, University of Toronto, Toronto General Hospital, Toronto, Ontario, Canada*
Steven L. Brody, MD, *Washington University School of Medicine, Division of Pulmonary and Critical Care Medicine, St. Louis, MO*
Dennis Brown, MD, *Renal Unit, Massachusetts General Hospital, Charlestown, MA*
Robert H. Brown, Jr., MD, *Day Neuromuscular Laboratory, Massachusetts General Hospital, East, Charlestown, MA*
Mario Castro, *Division of Pulmonary and Critical Care Medicine, Washington University School of Medicine, St. Louis, MO*
Nicholas A. Cataldo, *Department of Ob/Gyn, Stanford University, Stanford, CA*
Yiu-mo Chan, *Genetics Division, Children's Hospital, Boston, MA*
Alvin J. Chin MD, *Cardiology Division, Children's Hospital of Philadelphia, PA*
Angela M. Christiano, PhD, *Department of Dermatology, Columbia University, New York, NY*
George P. Chrousos, MD, FAAP, FACP, *NIH Clinical Center, Bethesda, MD*
Jaime O. Claudio, MSC, *Center for Research in Neuroscience, McGill University and Montreal General Hospital, Montreal, Quebec, Canada*
Joy D. Cogan, *Department of Pediatrics, Division of Genetics, Vanderbilt University School of Medicine, Nashville, TN*
M. Michael Cohen, Jr., DMD, PhD, *Dalhousie University, Halifax, Nova Scotia, Canada*
Jonathan Cohn, MD, *Department of Medicine, Duke University, Durham, NC*
Gilbert Cote, PhD, *University of Texas, MD Anderson Cancer Center, Houston, TX*
Finbarr E. Cotter, *Molecular Haematology Unit, LRF Centre for Childhood Leukemia, Institute of Child Health, London, UK*
Meret E. Cudkowicz, MD, *Day Neuromuscular Laboratory, Neurology Service, Massachusetts General Hospital, Charlestown, MA*
Martina Daly, PhD, *Division of Molecular and Genetic Medicine, Royal Hallamshire Hospital, Sheffield, UK*
Douglas C. Dean, *Division of Pulmonary and Critical Care Medicine Washington University School of Medicine, St. Louis, MO*
Michael R. DeBaun, *Genetic Epidemiology Branch, National Cancer Institute, Bethesda, MD; Present Address: Department of Pediatrics, Division of Hematology and Oncology, Washington University School of Medicine, St. Louis, MO*
Jean Delaunay, MD, PhD, *Department of Biochemistry and Molecular Biology, Faculte de Medicine Grange-Blanche, Genetique Moleculaire Humaine, Institute Pasteur de Lyon, France*
J. Raymond DePaulo, Jr., MD, *Department of Psychiatry and Behavioral Sciences, Johns Hopkins University School of Medicine, Baltimore, MD*
Eric J. Devor, PhD, *Department of Psychiatric Research, University of Iowa College of Medicine, Iowa City, IA*

LUIS A. DIAZ, MD, *Dermatology Department, Medical College of Wisconsin, Milwaukee, WI*

DAVID A. DICHEK, MD, *Gladstone Institute of Cardiovascular Disease, University of California, San Francisco, CA*

JOHN J. DIGIOVANNA, MD, *Division of Dermatopharmacology, Department of Dermatology Brown University School of Medicine, Rhode Island Hospital, Providence, RI*

XIANG DING, PhD, *Department of Dermatology, Medical College of Wisconsin, Milwaukee, WI*

DEBORAH A. DRISCOLL, MD, *Children's Hospital of Philadelphia, PA*

DANIEL B. DUBIN, MD, *Division of Dermatology, Brigham and Women's Hospital, Boston, MA*

N. LAWRENCE EDWARDS, MD, *Department of Medicine, University of Florida, Gainesville, FL*

JAMES T. ELDER, MD, PhD, *Dermatology and Radiation Oncology (Cancer Biology), Department of Dermatology, University of Michigan Medical Center, Ann Arbor, MI*

ELLEN R. ELIAS, *New England Medical Center Hospitals, Boston, MA; Present Address: Children's Hospital, Boston, MA*

SARAH H. ELSEA, PhD, *Department of Neurology, Baylor College of Medicine, Houston, TX*

BEVERLY S. EMANUEL, PhD, *Children's Hospital of Philadelphia, PA*

ERVIN EPSTEIN, JR., MD, *Department of Dermatology, San Francisco General Hospital, San Francisco, CA*

HENRY F. EPSTEIN, MD, *Baylor College of Medicine, Houston, TX*

JANET A. FAIRLEY, MD, *Department of Dermatology, Medical College of Wisconsin, Milwaukee, WI*

ARTHUR FALEK, PhD, *Department of Psychiatry and Behavioral Science, Emory University School of Medicine, Atlanta, GA*

STEPHEN V. FARAONE, PhD, *Department of Psychiatry, Massachusetts Mental Health Center, Boston, MA*

ANDREW P. FEINBERG, MD, MPH, *Johns Hopkins University School of Medicine, Baltimore, MD*

BETH A. FINE, MS, *Graduate Program in Genetic Counseling; Obstetrics & Gynecology, Northwestern University Medical School, Chicago, IL*

CLAIR A. FRANCOMANO, MD, *Medical Genetics Branch, National Human Genome Research Institute, National Institutes of Health, Bethesda, MD*

ELAINE FUCHS, PhD, *Department of Molecular Genetics and Cell Biology, Howard Hughes Medical Institute, University of Chicago, IL*

ROBERT F. GAGEL, MD, *Section of Neoplasia and Hormonal Disorders, University of Texas MD Anderson Cancer Center, Houston, TX*

GREGORY G. GERMINO, MD, *Division of Nephrology, Johns Hopkins University School of Medicine, Baltimore, MD*

ROBERT E. GERSZTEN, MD, *Cardiac Unit and Cardiovascular Research Institute, Massachusetts General Hospital, Charlestown, MA*

SOOSAN GHAZIZADEH, *Department of Oral Biology and Pathology, SUNY at Stony Brook, NY*

GEORGE J. GIUDICE, PhD, *Department of Dermatology, Medical College of Wisconsin, Milwaukee, WI*

LOWELL A. GOLDSMITH, MD, *University of Rochester School of Medicine and Dentistry, Rochester, NY*

MAUREEN M. GOODENOW, *Department of Pediatrics, University of Florida College of Medicine, Gainesville, FL*

ANNE GOODEVE, PhD, *Division of Molecular and Genetic Medicine, Royal Hallamshire Hospital, Sheffield, UK*

JEROME L. GORSKI, MD, *University of Michigan Medical School, Ann Arbor, MI*

PIET C. DE GROEN, MD, *Center for Basic Research in Digestive Diseases, Mayo Medical School, Clinic, and Foundation, Rochester, MN*

MARCUS GROMPE, MD, *Department of Molecular and Medical Genetics, Oregon Health Sciences University, Portland, OR*

KARL-HEINZ GRZESCHIK, PhD, *Institute for Humangenetik und Humangenetik Polikinik, Bahnhofstrasse, Marburg, Germany*

SANJEEV GUPTA, MBBS, MD, MRCP, *Liver Research Center, Albert Einstein College of Medicine, Bronx, NY*

DANIEL A. HABER, MD, PhD, *Massachusetts General Hospital Cancer Center, Charlestown, MA*

ANDREW HAYNES, DM, MRCP, MRCPath, *Department of Haematology, Nottingham City Hospital and University of Nottingham, UK*

STEVEN C. HEBERT, MD, *Renal Division, Department of Medicine, Brigham and Women's Hospital, Boston, MA; Present Address: Division of Nephrology, Vanderbilt University Medical Center, Nashville, TN*

JACQUELINE T. HECHT, PhD, *Department of Pediatrics, University of Texas Medical School, Houston, TX*

PIRKKO HEIKKILÄ, MSc, *Division of Matrix Biology, Department of Medical Biochemistry and Biophysics, Karolinska Institute, Stockholm, Sweden*

ERIC P. HOFFMAN, PhD, *Department of Molecular Genetics, University of Pittsburgh School of Medicine, Pittsburgh, PA*

MICHAEL J. HOLTZMAN, MD, *Division of Pulmonary and Critical Care Medicine, Washington University School of Medicine, St. Louis, MO*

RICHARD HONG, MD, *Genetics Laboratory, University of Vermont, Burlington, VT*

MICHAEL F. IADEMARCO, *Division of Pulmonary and Critical Care Medicine, Washington University School of Medicine, St. Louis, MO*

MARK A. ISRAEL, MD, *Department of Neurological Surgery, Preuss Laboratory for Molecular Neuro-oncology, Brain Tumor Research Center, University of California, San Francisco, CA*

HOWARD J. JACOB, PhD, *Department of Physiology, Medical College of Wisconsin, Milwaukee, WI*

J. LARRY JAMESON, MD, PhD, *Division of Endocrinology, Metabolism, and Molecular Medicine, Northwestern University Medical School, Chicago, IL*

DONALD R. JOHNS, MD, *Division of Neuromuscular Disease, Beth Israel Hospital, Harvard Medical School, Boston, MA*

WADE JOHNSON, *Division of Endocrinology, Metabolism, and Molecular Medicine, Northwestern University Medical School, Chicago, IL*

ROBERT W. KARR, MD, *Searle Discovery Research, Monsanto, St. Louis, MO*

WILLIAM J. KIMBERLING, PhD, *Boys Town National Research Hospital, Omaha, NE*

GEORGE KOIKE, *Medical College of Wisconsin, Department of Physiology, Milwaukee, WI*
TADEUSZ M. KOLODKA, *Department of Oral Biology and Pathology, SUNY at Stony Brook, NY*
PETER KOPP, MD, *Division of Endocrinology, Metabolism, and Molecular Medicine, Northwestern University Medical School, Chicago, IL*
T. RAJENDRA KUMAR, PhD, *Department of Pathology, Baylor College of Medicine, Houston, TX*
HON-REEN KUO, PhD, *New Jersey Medical School, Newark, NJ*
THOMAS S. KUPPER, MD, *Dermatology Division, Brigham and Women's Hospital, Boston, MA*
SANTIAGO LAMAS, MD, PhD, *Department of Protein Structure and Function, Center for Biological Investigation, Madrid, Spain*
MURIEL W. LAMBERT, *New Jersey Medical School, Newark, NJ*
W. CLARK LAMBERT, MD, PhD, *New Jersey Medical School, Newark, NJ*
DAVID A. LANE, *Department of Haematology, Charing Cross & Westminster Medical School, London, UK*
NICHOLAS F. LARUSSO, MD, *Center for Basic Research in Digestive Diseases, Mayo Medical School, Clinic, and Foundation, Rochester, MN*
E. CARWILE LEROY, MD, *Chairman, Department of Microbiology and Immunology, Medical University of South Carolina, Charleston, SC*
DONALD Y. M. LEUNG, MD, *Department of Pediatrics, National Jewish Hospital, Denver, CO*
BARRY LONDON, MD, PhD, *Division of Cardiology, University of Pittsburgh Medical Center, Pittsburgh, PA*
FRANK M. LONGO, MD, PhD, *Veterans Affairs Medical Center, San Francisco, CA*
DWIGHT C. LOOK, *Division of Pulmonary and Critical Care Medicine, Washington University School of Medicine, St. Louis, MO*
WILLIAM L. LOWE, JR., MD, *Division of Endocrinology, Metabolism, and Molecular Medicine, Northwestern University Medical School, Chicago, IL*
JAMES R. LUPSKI, MD, PhD, *Molecular and Human Genetics; Pediatrics Department of Molecular and Human Genetics, Baylor College of Medicine, Houston, TX*
LUCIO LUZZATTO, *Department of Human Genetics, Memorial Sloan Kettering Cancer Center, New York, NY*
SUSAN M. MACDONALD, *Department of Medicine, Johns Hopkins Asthma and Allergy Center, Baltimore, MD*
DAVID H. MACLENNAN, PhD, FRS, *Banting and Best Department of Medical Research, University of Toronto, Charles H. Best Institute, Toronto, Ontario, Canada*
CALUM MACRAE, *Brigham and Women's Hospital, Boston, MA*
LAIRD D. MADISON, MD, PhD, *Division of Endocrinology, Metabolism, and Molecular Medicine, Northwestern University Medical School, Chicago, IL*
MARCO MARCELLI, MD, *Veteran Administration Medical Center, Houston, TX*
JOSEPH B. MARTIN, MD, PhD, *Dean, Faculty of Medicine, Boston, MA*
MARTIN M. MATZUK, *Departments of Pathology, Cell Biology, and Molecular and Human Genetics, Baylor College of Medicine, Houston, TX*
MARCY MCDONALD, PhD, *Molecular Neurogenetics Unit, Massachusetts General Hospital, Charlestown, MA*
ELIZABETH A. MCGEE, MD, *Department of OB/GYN, University of Texas Southwestern Medical Center, Dallas, TX; Present Address: Department of OB/GYN, Stanford University Medical Center, Stanford, CA*
FRANCIS J. MCMAHON, MD, *The Johns Hopkins University School of Medicine, Baltimore, MD*
MICHAEL J. MCPHAUL, MD, *Department of Internal Medicine, University of Texas Southwestern Medical Center, Dallas, TX*
SHLOMO MELMED, MD, *Cedars Sinai Medical Center, Los Angeles, CA*
THOMAS MICHEL, MD, PhD, *Brigham and Women's Hospital, Harvard Medical School, Boston, MA*
MAXIMILIAN MUENKE, MD, *Division of Human Genetics and Molecular Biology, Children's Hospital of Philadelphia, PA; Present Address: Medical Genetics Branch, National Human Genome Research Institute, National Institutes of Health, Bethesda, MD*
DIYA F. MUTASIM, MD, *Department of Dermatology, University of Cincinnati College of Medicine, Cincinnati, OH*
KHEDOUDJA NAFA, *Department of Human Genetics, Memorial Sloan Kettering Cancer Center, Memorial Hospital, Sloan Kettering Institute, New York, NY*
DAVID L. NELSON, PhD, *Baylor College of Medicine, Houston, TX*
CHARLES B. NEMEROFF, MD, PhD, *Department of Psychiatry and Behavioral Medicine, Emory University School of Medicine, Atlanta, GA*
MARIA I. NEW, MD, *Department of Pediatrics, The New York Hospital, Cornell Medical Center, New York, NY*
PAUL NGHIEM, MD, PhD, *Dermatology, Brigham and Women's Hospital, Boston, MA*
LYNDA Q. NGUYEN, *Division of Endocrinology, Metabolism, and Molecular Medicine, Northwestern University Medical School, Chicago, IL*
ROBERT D. NICHOLLS, DPhil, *Department of Genetics, Case Western Reserve University, Cleveland, OH*
KIM E. NICHOLS, MD, *Massachusetts General Hospital Cancer Center, Charlestown, MA*
ROSARIO NOTARO, *Department of Human Genetics, Memorial Sloan Kettering Cancer Center, New York, NY*
JOAN M. O'BRIEN, MD, *Department of Ophthalmology, University of California, San Francisco, CA*
PETER O'CONNELL, MD, *Department of Pathology, University of Texas Health Sciences Center, San Antonio, TX*
ROBIN OLDS, *Department of Pathology, University of Otago, Dunedin, New Zealand*
ERIC N. OLSON, PhD, *Department of Biochemistry/Molecular Biology, MD Anderson Cancer Center, University of Texas, Houston, TX*
LUIZ F. ONUCHIC, MD, PhD, *Division of Nephrology, Johns Hopkins University School of Medicine, Baltimore, MD*

Michael Ott, MD, *Albert Einstein College of Medicine, Bronx, NY*

Amy S. Paller, MD, *Children's Memorial Hospital, Chicago, IL*

Pragna I. Patel, PhD, *Department of Neurology, Baylor College of Medicine, Houston, TX*

Ian Peake, *Division of Molecular and Genetic Medicine, Royal Hallamshire Hospital, Sheffield, UK*

Richard G. Pestell, MD, FRACP, PhD, *Department of Medicine and Developmental and Molecular Biology, The Albert Einstein Cancer Center, Albert Einstein College of Medicine, Bronx, NY*

John A. Phillips, MD, *Pediatrics & Biochemistry, Vanderbilt University School of Medicine, Nashville, TN*

Paul M. Plotsky, PhD, *Department of Psychiatry and Behavioral Sciences, Emory University School of Medicine, Atlanta, GA*

Stanley B. Prusiner, MD, *Departments of Neurology and of Biochemistry and Biophysics, University of California, San Francisco, CA*

Ching-Hon Pui, *St. Jude's Children's Research Hospital, Memphis, TN*

Charmian A. Quigley, MBBS, *Riley Children's Hospital, Indianapolis, IN*

Andrew P. Read, MA, PhD, *Department of Medical Genetics, St. Mary's Hospital, Manchester, UK*

James C. Reynolds, MD, *Division of Gastroenterology and Hepatology, Allegheny University of the Health Sciences, Philadelphia, PA*

C. Sue Richards, PhD, *Department of Molecular and Human Genetics, Baylor DNA Diagnostic Laboratory, Baylor College of Medicine, Houston, TX*

Jacques Rochette, BM, DPharm, DSc, *MRC Molecular Haemotology Unit, Institute of Molecular Medicine, John Radcliff Hospital, Headington, Oxford, UK; Present Address: Medical Genetics, Faculte de Medecine, Universite Jules Verne, Amiens, France*

Daniel B. Rosenbluth, MD, *Division of Pulmonary and Critical Care Medicine, Washington University School of Medicine; Adult Cystic Fibrosis Clinic, Barnes-Jewish Hospital, St. Louis, MO*

Anthony Rosenzweig, MD, *Cardiac Unit and Cardiovascular Research Institute, Massachusetts General Hospital, Charlestown, MA*

Bruno Rotoli, *Hematology, Federico II University Medical School, Napoli, ITALY*

Guy A. Rouleau, MD, PhD, *Montreal General Hospital, Montreal, Quebec, Canada*

Deborah C. Rubin, MD, *Division of Gastroenterology, Washington University School of Medicine, St. Louis, MO*

Jeffrey E. Rubnitz, *St. Jude's Children's Research Hospital, Memphis, TN*

Juan Ruiz, MD, PhD, *Centro de Investigaciones Biomedicas, Facultidad de Medicina, Universidad de Navaria, Pamplona, Spain*

Nigel Russell, MD, FRCP, FRCPath, *Department of Hematology, Nottingham City Hospital and University of Nottingham, UK*

Deepak Sampath, *Division of Pulmonary and Critical Care Medicine, Washington University School of Medicine, St. Louis, MO*

Saumyen Sarkar, PhD, *Brigham and Women's Hospital, Boston, MA*

Christine E. Seidman, MD, *Department of Genetics, Harvard Medical School, Boston, MA*

J. G. Seidman, PhD, *Brigham and Women's Hospital, Boston, MA*

Robert M. Senior, MD, *Pulmonary and Critical Care Medicine, Washington University School of Medicine, St. Louis, MO*

Steven D. Shapiro, MD, *Washington University School of Medicine, St. Louis, MO*

Sarah Shefelbine, *University of Texas, MD Anderson Cancer Center, Houston, TX*

Barbara A. da Silva, MD, *Endocrinology, Metabolism, and Molecular Medicine, Northwestern University Medical School, Chicago, IL*

John W. Sleasman, *Department of Pediatrics, University of Florida, Gainesville, FL*

Edwin A. Smith, MD, *Division of Rheumatology and Immunology, Department of Medicine, Medical University of South Carolina, Charleston, SC*

Eric Sobel, MD, *Division of Rheumatology, Department of Medicine, University of Florida, Gainesville, FL*

Richard D. Sontheimer, MD, *Department of Dermatology, University of Texas Southwestern Medical Center, Dallas, TX*

Andrew F. Stewart, MD, *Division of Endocrinology and Metabolism, West Haven VA Medical Center, West Haven, CT; Present Address: Division of Endocrinology, University of Pittsburgh Medical Center, Pittsburgh, PA*

P. H. St. George-Hyslop, MD, FRCP, *Centre for Research in Neurodegenerative Diseases, University of Toronto, Ontario, Canada*

Peter M. Steinert, PhD, *Laboratory of Skin Disease, National Institutes of Health, Bethesda, MD*

Constantine A. Stratakis, *Section on Pediatric Endocrinology, National Institutes of Health, Bethesda, MD*

Vikas P. Sukhatme, MD, PhD, *Renal Division, Beth Israel Deaconess Medical Center, Boston, MA*

Lorne B. Taichman, PhD, *Department of Oral Biology and Pathology, SUNY at Stony Brook, NY*

Stephen J. Tapscott, MD, PhD, *Fred Hutshinson Cancer Center, Seattle, WA*

Swee Lay Thein, MRCP, FRCPath, *MRC Molecular Haematology Unit, Institute of Molecular Medicine, John Radcliffe Hospital, Headington, Oxford, UK*

Pamela M. Thomas, MD, *University of Michigan Medical Center, Ann Arbor, MI*

Karl Tryggvason, MD, PhD, *Division of Matrix Biology, Department of Medical Biochemistry and Biophysics, Karolinska Institute, Stockholm, Sweden*

Ming T. Tsuang, MD, PhD, DSc, *Department of Psychiatry, Massachusetts Mental Health Center, Boston, MA*

Jouni Uitto, MD, PhD, *Department of Dermatology and Cutaneous Biology, Thomas Jefferson University, Philadelphia, PA*

Giuseppe Vassalli, *Gladstone Institute of Cardiovascular Disease, University of California, San Francisco, CA*

John J. Voorhees, MD, *Dermatology Department, University of Michigan Medical Center, A. Alfred Taubman Health Center, Ann Arbor, MI*

Patricia A. Ward, MS, *Department of Molecular and Human Genetics, Baylor College of Medicine, Houston, TX*

Ethylin Wang Jabs, MD, *Center for Medical Genetics, Johns Hopkins Hospital, Baltimore, MD*

Timothy E. Weaver, *Division of Pulmonary Biology, Children's Hospital Medical Center, Cincinnati, OH*

Steven Jay Weintraub, MD, *Departments of Internal Medicine and Cell Biology and Physiology, Washington University School of Medicine, St. Louis, MO*

David Whitcomb, MD, PhD, *University of Pittsburgh, PA*

Jeffrey A. Whitsett, MD, *Division of Pulmonary Biology, Children's Hospital Medical Center, Cincinnati, OH*

Ralph C. Williams, Jr., MD, *Division of Rheumatology, Department of Medicine, University of Florida, Gainesville, FL*

Robert C. Wilson, PhD, *Department of Pediatrics, Cornell University Medical College, New York, NY*

Peter Winship, DPhil, *Division of Molecular and Genetic Medicine, Royal Hallamshire Hospital, Sheffield, UK*

George Y. Wu, MD, PhD, *GI Division, University of Connecticut School of Medicine, University of Connecticut Health Center, Farmington, CT*

Andrew R. Zinn, MD, PhD, *McDermott Center, University of Texas Southwestern Medical Center, Dallas, TX*

Huda Zoghbi, MD, *Howard Hughes Medical Institute, Department of Pediatrics, Molecular and Human Genetics, and Neurology, Baylor College of Medicine, Houston, TX*

Color Plates

Color plates appear as an insert following p. 684.

Plate 1 (Fig. 4 from Chapter 68). Expression of β-galactosidase in porcine kidneys following in vivo perfusion with an adenovirus containing the β-galactosidase reporter gene under the cytomegalovirus promoter.

Plate 2 (Fig. 2B from Chapter 75). Lesional skin from the epidermal nevus, showing normal basal cells, but hyperkeratosis and cytolysis in suprabasal cells.

Plate 3 (Fig. 1 from Chapter 12). Fetal circulation in the human; neonatal circulation in the human.

Plate 4 (Fig. 3 from Chapter 14). Expression of VCAM-1 at sites of atherogenesis.

Plate 5 (Fig. 2 from Chapter 29). The "open ends" of class II molecule.

Plate 6 (Figs. 1–4 from Chapter 76). Fig. 1. Hyperkeratotic irregular papules in Darier's disease on sun-exposed sites. Fig. 2. Hemorrhagic vesicle-papules in kindred with Darier's disease. Fig. 3. Red and white linear longitudinal bands in nails of patient with Darier's disease. Fig. 4. Papules and erosions characterizing Hailey-Hailey disease.

Plate 7 (Fig. 1A–C from Chapter 73). Clinical pictures of EBS patients.

Plate 8 (Fig. 7 from Chapter 92). Expression pattern of a *myogenin-lacZ* transgene in an 11.5-day mouse embryo.

Plate 9 (Fig. 2 from Chapter 92). Activation of MHC expression in fibroblasts expressing exogenous MyoD.

Plate 10 (Fig. 3 from Chapter 92). Schematic representation of a MyoD/E12 heterodimer.

INTRODUCTION TO MOLECULAR MEDICINE

I

SECTION EDITORS:

ANDREA BALLABIO AND J. LARRY JAMESON

1 Organization of the Human Genome, Chromosomes, and Genes

Sarah H. Elsea and Pragna I. Patel

INTRODUCTION

DNA is the chemical basis of heredity. Within its sequence is the information necessary for cells to live, grow, differentiate, and replicate. It is the DNA that provides both consistency (all humans generally look the same) and variability (height, eye, and hair color) among organisms. While the human genome is extremely polymorphic and the majority of deviations in DNA sequence are thought to be benign, variations in its sequence can and do lead to genetic disorders. Although we currently understand the roles of only a small percentage of the total number of genes, great strides are being made toward elucidating the physical and molecular structure and function of the human genome. Through this knowledge we can more fully appreciate the complex physiology of the human organism.

With the evergrowing number of diseases thought to have a genetic basis, it is important to understand the structure and function of DNA and chromosomes, as well as the genes they encode. This knowledge will enhance determination of the gene(s) underlying a particular disease as well as design of potential treatments and cures for the disease. This chapter will provide a basis for general understanding of the principles behind the field of molecular genetics.

GENOME ORGANIZATION

Human DNA is packaged in 23 pairs of chromosomes, specifically 22 homologous pairs of chromosomes (autosomes numbered 1–22) and two sex chromosomes, XX in females and XY in males; this represents the diploid genome. The human genome consists of approximately 6 billion bp of DNA and is estimated to contain 50,000–100,000 genes. For a chromosome to function properly, it must be able to replicate, segregate, and maintain itself from one generation to the next. These fundamental processes require that a chromosome contain at least one origin of replication, a centromere for proper segregation of daughter chromosomes, and a telomere for complete replication and maintenance of the DNA (Fig. 1-1).

Each chromosome is comprised of a single linear duplex DNA molecule that is complexed with numerous proteins. This DNA–protein complex is termed chromatin during interphase of the cell cycle (Fig. 1-2). If the DNA contained in a single cell were stretched from end to end, it would measure about two meters in length. One can imagine that such an enormous amount of DNA would be difficult to contain in the nucleus of a single human cell. Indeed, an elaborate system of packaging/folding (or supercoiling) is necessary for replication, transcription, recombination, and maintenance of the DNA from one generation to the next. As illustrated in Fig. 1-1, during this very orderly process, basic proteins (called histones) provide a core around which the DNA is wrapped, forming nucleosomes. Nucleosomes are not formed randomly but rather are phased along the DNA such that the position of a nucleosome along any given stretch of DNA is the same from cell to cell. These nucleosomes are further organized into higher order solenoid structures, which are packed into loops attached to a nonhistone protein scaffold. As the cell cycle progresses into prophase, the loops thicken into chromomeres, which can be seen as densely staining regions of the chromosomes. This thickening process continues and eventually the DNA condenses into the highly organized ultrastructure of mitotic chromosomes, thus compacting the DNA ~8000-fold at metaphase (Figs. 1-1 and 1-2). This higher order packaging process not only compacts the DNA within the nucleus but is also important for gene regulation and protection of the DNA from nucleases. The higher order structure of the chromatin is fluid and dynamic, with condensation/decondensation of the DNA occurring throughout the cell cycle (Fig. 1-2).

There are several classes of DNA within the human genome. In general, less than 10% of the genome actually encodes genes. The more densely packed regions of the chromosomes, particularly near the centromeres, are termed heterochromatin and are not transcribed, whereas transcriptionally active sequences are located within less densely packed regions termed euchromatin. Approximately 75% of the genome is made of unique or single-copy DNA, whose sequences are represented only once per haploid genome (haploid refers to half the complement of chromosomes; in other words, the DNA donated by either a sperm or an egg). In contrast, the remaining portion of the genome consists of several classes of repetitive DNA, whose sequences are present anywhere from two to as high as 10^7 copies per haploid genome. While it is not known what role repetitive DNA plays in the cell, it is thought to either function in maintenance of chromosome structure or gene regulation, or, in fact, it may have no function at all.

Even though unique DNA makes up the majority of the sequences in the genome, only a small proportion of this DNA actually codes for proteins (coding regions of genes). Some of the

From: *Principles of Molecular Medicine* (J. L. Jameson, ed.), ©1998 Humana Press Inc., Totowa, NJ.

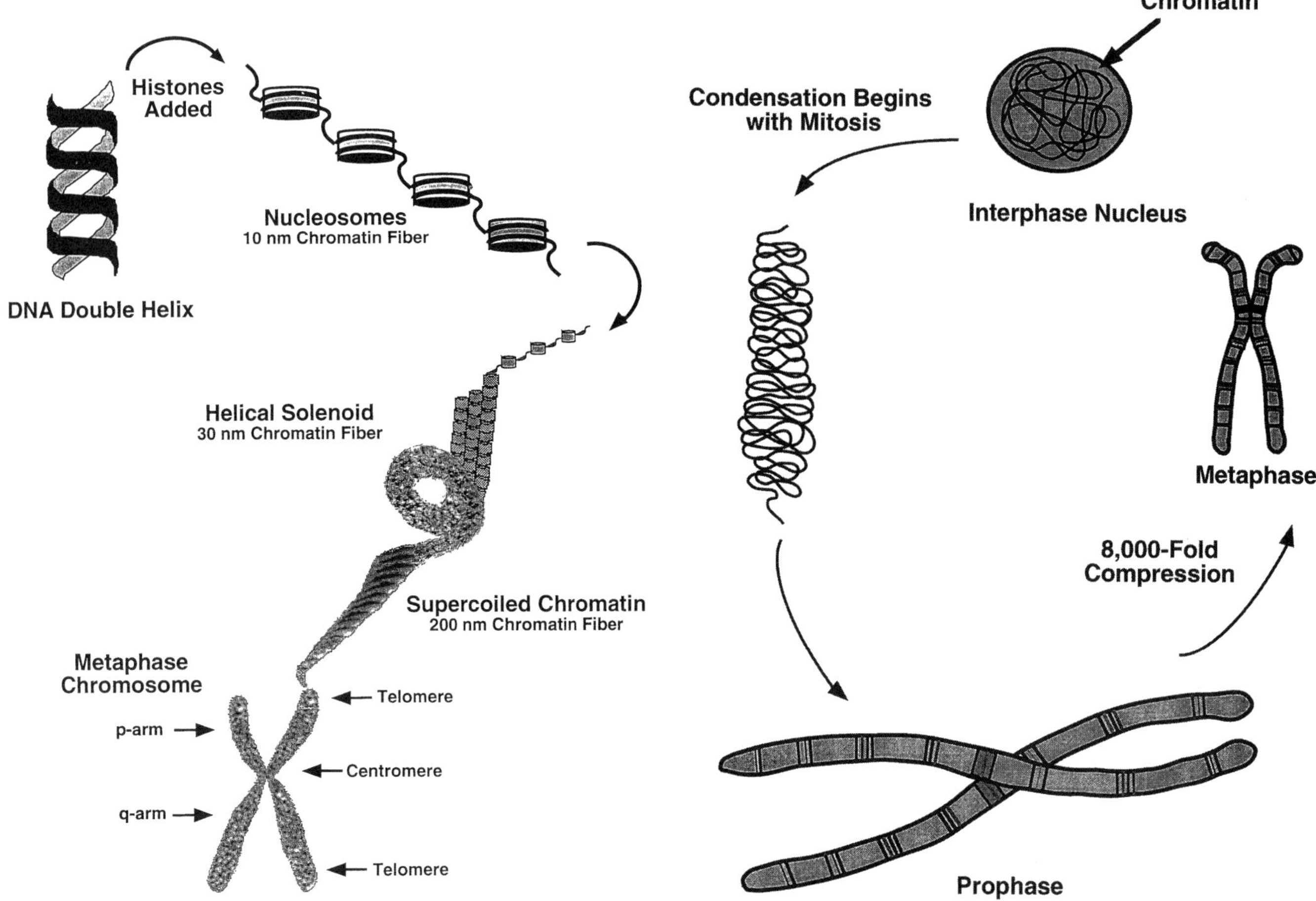

Figure 1-1 Chromatin structure. Chromatin is a complex of DNA and proteins. DNA is wrapped around histones and other nonhistone proteins in an orderly fashion to form nucleosomes, which are then further organized into solenoid structures and finally form the highly condensed metaphase chromosome.

Figure 1-2 Condensation/decondensation of DNA in the cell cycle. The interphase nucleus contains chromatin that is dispersed throughout the nucleus. In prophase, the replicated chromosomes begin to condense, and, by metaphase, the chromatin has condensed ~8000-fold.

DNA functions in the regulation of these genes (noncoding sequences within the gene). Long stretches (>25 kb) of unique DNA are rare, and these single-copy sequences are often found interspersed between stretches of repetitive sequences.

Repetitive DNA can either be clustered within or dispersed throughout the genome. Clustered repeat sequences comprise 10–15% of the genome and comprise arrays of short repeats organized in a head-to-tail fashion. These tandem repeats are collectively called satellite DNAs. These repeats can vary in length from a few nucleotides to several million. Their location varies as well, with some repeats found only in the heterochromatin of the centromeres or telomeres and some found only on particular chromosomes. Minisatellite DNA repeats are generally 15–465 bp in length but can run up to ~20 kb. These repeats are typically found along the length of each chromosome and are used as DNA markers for mapping of the genome as well as for chromosome analysis.

Another class of repeat sequences includes related sequences that are dispersed throughout the genome (sometimes within genes), constituting approximately 15% of the total DNA. While several subclasses of these repeats exist, two are of particular importance. SINES are short interspersed sequences. The best characterized of these elements are those belonging to the Alu family, so named because these repeats contain an *Alu*I restriction site near the middle of the sequence. SINES, while not precisely conserved, are of similar sequence, ~300 bp in length, and are present in about 300,000–500,000 copies per haploid genome, accounting for ~3–6% of the genome. Although the function of these repeats is not known, the sequence is related to that of 7SL RNA. In addition, Alu sequences are of medical importance because these repeats may act as transposable elements, causing aberrant recombination between different Alu family members resulting in mutations that may lead to genetic disease.

A second major class of repetitive DNA is termed LINES, or long interspersed sequences of DNA. A well-represented member of this family is L1, which is found in ~20,000–50,000 copies per human genome, runs about 6 kb in length, and makes up ~3–4% of the total DNA in a cell. A portion of the L1 sequence is similar to the viral enzyme reverse transcriptase. These sequences have also been implicated in the cause of several mutations in hereditary disease due to their potential function as transposable elements.

GENE STRUCTURE AND ORGANIZATION

As discussed, DNA is the hereditary material of the cell. Its sequence encodes genes which, in turn, code for RNAs and ultimately, proteins. Basically, DNA is transcribed into RNA, which is then processed and translated into protein (Fig. 1-3A).

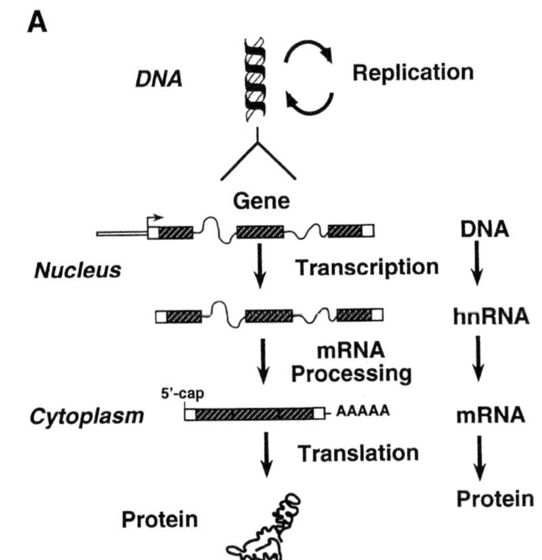

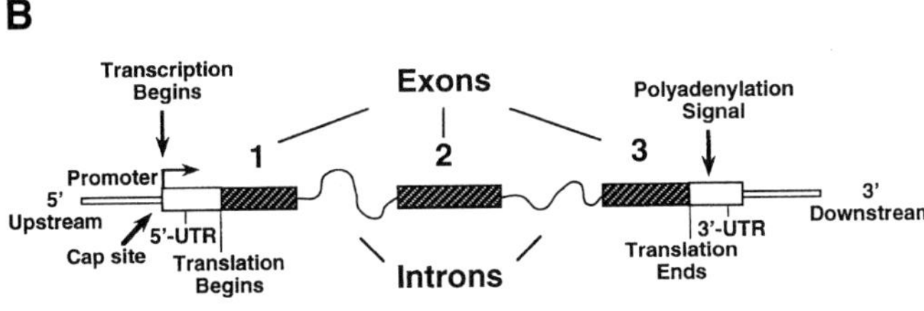

Figure 1-3 How does a gene work? **(A)** DNA is replicated and transcribed into RNA, which is then processed to remove introns. Translation then produces a functional protein. **(B)** Diagram of the basic aspects of a gene necessary for proper transcription and translation of the DNA.

Proteins were originally thought to be encoded by continuous segments of DNA, but actually very few genes contain uninterrupted coding regions. The vast majority of genes are interrupted by one or, typically, several noncoding regions called intervening sequences or introns (Fig. 1-3B). Introns are transcribed into RNA but are removed when it is processed into its mature form (mRNA); therefore, the sequences contained in the intron are not represented in the translated product. The coding sequences, called exons, actually dictate the protein sequence.

A schematic representing the features of a typical gene are shown in Fig. 1-3. Genes have been found that range in size from ~100 bp to ~2.3 Mb, but most genes are thought to range between 1 and 200 kb. As illustrated in Fig. 1-3, genes not only include the coding region but also include surrounding sequences that may help in regulation of that gene's expression. These sequences include: "start" and "stop" signals for both transcription and translation; the promoter region, which lies 5' to the coding region and helps regulate transcription; the 5'-untranslated region (5'-UTR), which may function in regulation; and the 3'-untranslated region (3'-UTR), which contains the polyadenylation signal important for maturation of mRNA and also may be involved in other aspects of RNA processing, transport, degradation, and translation.

New genes arise during evolution as a consequence of duplication, divergence, recombination, and mutations in old or existing genes. As a result, many genes are related to others and belong to a larger family of genes with related sequence, structure, and/or function. There are several examples of gene families found either dispersed throughout or sometimes in gene clusters in the human genome. These include genes for globin, myosin, visual pigment, seven-transmembrane-spanning receptors, small nuclear RNAs, and immunoglobulins.

Just as functional genes are found in the genome, so are related genes that either have lost their function or were not fully functional from the start. These sequences, referred to as pseudogenes, are thought to be byproducts of evolution and can arise as a result of incomplete duplication events, mutations, or from processed or unprocessed transcripts becoming incorporated into the DNA. They are abundant throughout the genome.

CYTOGENETICS

While the distribution of genes and repetitive sequences across the genome is not uniform, chromosomes do form consistent and interesting patterns in their organization. Chromosomes can be stained and examined microscopically to reveal distinct light and dark banding patterns. For example, it is thought that metaphase bands that stain lightly with Giemsa (termed G-banding) harbor more housekeeping and tissue-specific genes, SINES, and GC-rich regions of DNA, whereas the darker-staining Giemsa bands tend to contain fewer genes, more LINES, and have a lower GC content.

Chromosomal abnormalities contribute significantly toward congenital malformations and are responsible for >50% of all spontaneous abortions/miscarriages. In addition, ~0.7% of newborns (and ~2% of live births in women over 35 years of age) have significant chromosomal abnormalities. Furthermore, many cancers result from these types of aberrations as well. Chromosome analysis is indicated under several circumstances, including multiple miscarriages, fertility problems, hematological malignancies, multiple congenital anomalies, sexual differentiation disorders, and/or if there is a known or suspected abnormality, such as a family history of mental retardation in males.

Cytogenetic analysis of chromosomes in peripheral blood lymphocytes has facilitated the identification of many chromosomal abnormalities. In these analyses, the lymphocytes are blocked at metaphase and stained with Giemsa. This process results in the light and dark staining mentioned above. G-banding gives ~350–550 bands per haploid set, where 1 band is equal to ~5–10 million bp, representing a few to many genes. Alternatively, a prophase block can give a higher resolution of ~850 bands.

Basic chromosome morphology is illustrated in Figs. 1-4 and 1-5. The short arm is termed "p" for petite and the long arm is designated "q." Chromosomes are acrocentric if the centromere lies near the end of the chromosome, metacentric if the centromere lies near the middle, and submetacentric if the centromere is located between the center and the end of the chromosome. The numbering of the bands on each chromosome is from the centromere to the telomere on each the short and the long arms. The chromosomes in a single cell are arranged by number into karyotypes, which provide a visual representation of an individual's chromosomes (Fig. 1-4). Karyotypes may reveal deletions, duplications, and/or rearrangements and can help to localize the region of DNA responsible for the genetic disorder in question. The nomenclature used for describing chromosome morphology is detailed in Table 1-1.

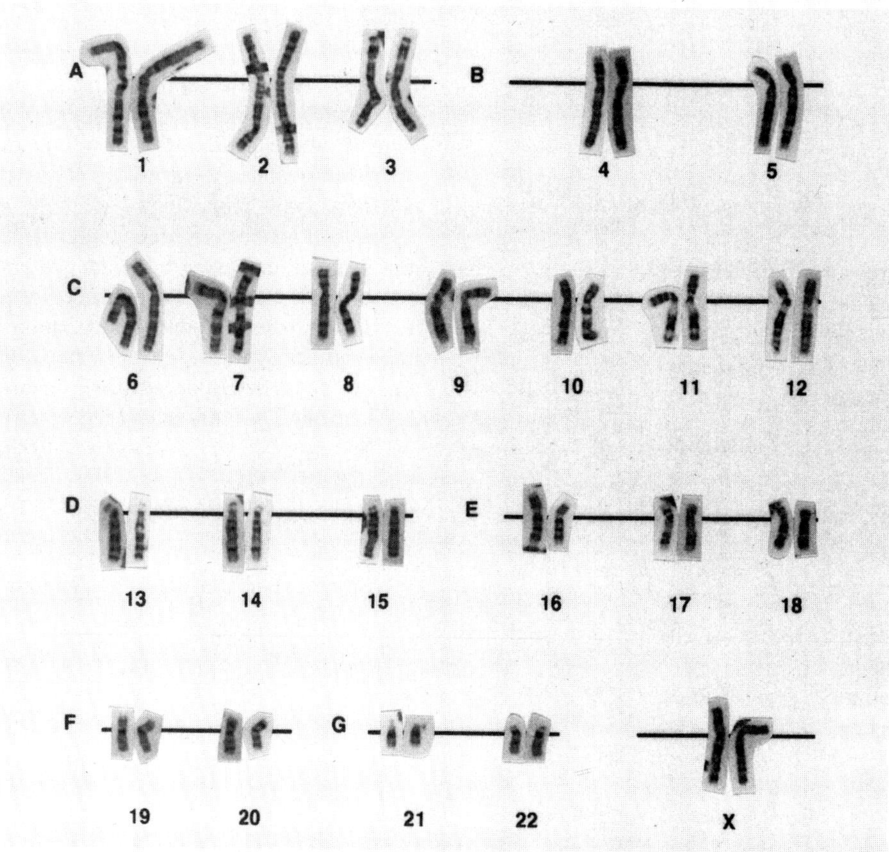

Figure 1-4 A human karyotype of G-banded chromosomes. A normal female (46, XX) karyotype is shown. Chromosomes are placed in groups based on their size and structure. (Karyotype kindly provided by Lisa Shaffer, PhD.)

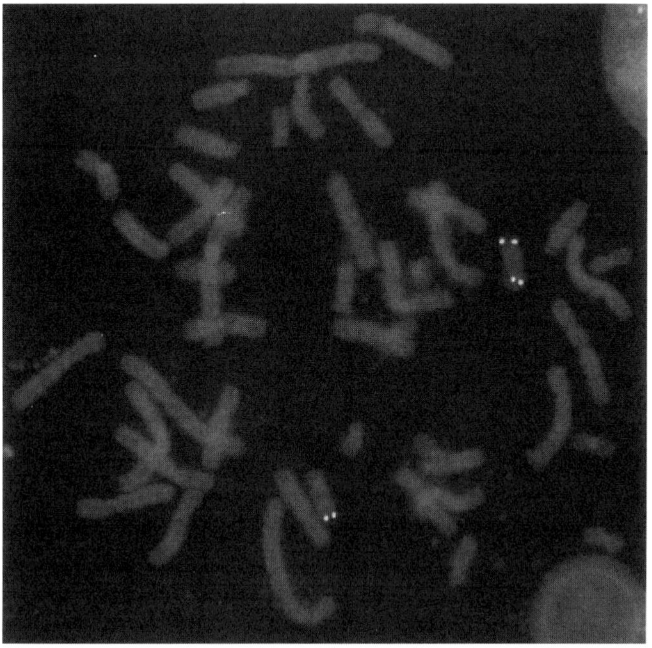

Figure 1-5 Fluorescence *in situ* hybridization to metaphase chromosomes. Pictured is a metaphase spread of a patient with Smith-Magenis syndrome. This syndrome results from an interstitial deletion on chromosome 17p11.2. Controls probes for 17q are present on each chromosome 17, while the diagnostic probe for Smith-Magenis syndrome is present on only one chromosome at 17p11.2.

Table 1-1
Karyotype Terminology

1–22	Autosome numbers
X,Y	Sex chromosomes
cen	Centromere
del	Deletion
dcr	Derivative of a chromosome
dic	Dicentric chromosome
du	Duplication
fra	Fragile site
i	Isochromosome
ins	Insertion
inv	Inversion
mar	Marker chromosome
mat	Maternal origin
p	Short arm of chromosome
pat	Paternal origin
q	Long arm of chromosome
r	Ring chromosome
rcp	Reciprocal translocation
t	Translocation
ter	Terminus (i.e., pter or qter)
+ or –	Placed before a chromosome number, indicates addition or loss of entire chromosome, as in +21 for Down syndrome. Placed after the chromosome number, indicates gain or loss of a part of that chromosome, as in 5q- for Cri-du-Chat.
:	Breakage
::	Breakage and reunion
/	Mosaicism (i.e., 46/47 indicates a mixed cell population in which some cells have 46 and others have 47 chromosomes)

There are several relatively common types of chromosomal abnormalities. The most common aberration is aneuploidy, which can mean either an extra chromosome or a deleted chromosome. Normal human genotypes have 46 chromosomes, including two sex chromosomes (46, XX for females; 46, XY for males). Down syndrome (47, XX, +21) would be an example of aneuploidy or trisomy 21, while Turner syndrome (45, X) is an example of monosomy. Other gross abnormalities include uniparental disomy (both chromosomes in a pair come from a single parent), marker chromosomes (extra chromosomal pieces or supernumerary chromosomes), ring chromosomes (partial chromosomes containing centromeres resulting from the deletion of the telomeric ends of the p and q arms), and mosaicism (where a fraction of the cells in the body have normal chromosomes, while the remaining cells carry an aberration; this may or may not produce a phenotype). Structural problems can also result from deletions, duplications, translocations, inversions, and unequal crossing-over.

MOLECULAR CYTOGENETICS

Preparations of intact chromosomes can also be used for molecular genetic diagnosis, analysis of gene deletions and duplications, and mapping of genes within the genome. Fluorescence *in situ* hybridization (FISH) uses fluorescently tagged DNA probes and fluorescence microscopy to determine the relative location of that particular DNA sequence (Fig. 1-5). This allows for localization of the DNA probe to subchromosomal regions of the genome that G-banding cannot determine. Standard FISH analysis with metaphase chromosomes provides resolution to within 5–10 Mb and serves to bridge the gap between standard cytogenetic analysis and detailed molecular analysis using purified DNA. This technique is rapidly improving. With the use of multicolor probes and interphase chromosomes (where the DNA is less compact), resolution of probes can be obtained to within 100 kb. Additionally, sets of markers can be applied that effectively "paint" the chromosomes so that it can be determined if small segments of DNA have been rearranged and to diagnose aneuploidies. FISH is fast becoming important for long-range genome mapping and ordering of markers within a segment of DNA.

SELECTED REFERENCES

Alberts B, Bray D, Lewis J, Raff M, Roberts K, Watson JD. Molecular Biology of the Cell. 2nd ed. New York: Garland, 1989.

Dracopoli NC, Haines JL, Korf BR, et al. Current Protocols in Human Genetics. New York: Wiley, 1995.

Lewin B. Genes VI. New York: Oxford University Press, 1996.

Scriver CR, Beaudet A, Sly WS, Valle D. In: Metabolic and Molecular Bases of Inherited Disease. 7th ed. New York: McGraw-Hill, 1995.

2 Recombinant DNA and Genetic Techniques

MARCUS GROMPE, WADE JOHNSON, AND J. LARRY JAMESON

INTRODUCTION

Although DNA was recognized as the chemical substrate of heredity in the early 1940s, studies to examine its structure and function were historically quite difficult because of the lack of tools for its isolation and experimental manipulation. In the early 1970s, a series of technological breakthroughs began that dramatically changed our ability to study the role of DNA in biology and genetics. The impact of methodologic advances in the fields of molecular biology and genetics cannot be overemphasized. Since the mid-1970s, eight Nobel prizes have been awarded for research that led directly or indirectly to major methodological advances in addition to their profound new insights into biology and chemistry. Examples include the discovery of reverse transcriptase, restriction enzymes, plasmid cloning vectors, DNA sequencing, PCR, and others (Table 2-1).

The methods available for research in molecular biology and genetics continue to increase rapidly. Although many of these techniques are relatively complex, a basic knowledge of a limited number of basic procedures will be sufficient for the general reader of this book. In practical terms, many common laboratory protocols are now available as "kits" that are provided by biotechnology companies. These kits typically provide detailed instructions as well as relevant controls. Despite the ready availability of such reagents, it is still important to understand the biochemistry of the reactions and the limitations of protocols if success is to be achieved. A number of excellent molecular biology manuals have been published, many devoting several hundred pages to individual protocols (*see* Selected References). The methods have been divided into six general groups:

1. Important chemical and enzymatic manipulations of DNA and RNA.
2. Methods for the production of DNA and RNA for various applications.
3. Techniques for analysis of DNA and RNA.
4. Expression of recombinant proteins.
5. Determination of protein–DNA interactions.
6. Identification of protein–protein interactions.

ENZYMATIC MANIPULATIONS OF DNA AND RNA

RESTRICTION ENDONUCLEASES Restriction endonucleases are bacterial enzymes that cut double-stranded DNA in a sequence-specific manner. Biologically, the function of these enzymes is to "restrict" the entry of foreign DNA by cleaving it at recognition sites that do not exist in the host bacterium. Each enzyme has a specific sequence that it recognizes, binds, and cuts. These recognition sites usually consist of a code of 4–8 bp, and the restriction endonucleases will only cut sequences that perfectly match this code. For example, the recognition sequence for the enzyme *Eco*RI is GAATTC. All sites with this sequence will be cleaved by the enzyme (Fig. 2-1), but even a single base mismatch, such as CAATTC, will prevent DNA digestion. The chance of finding a specific restriction site in a given piece of DNA is largely dependent on the number of bases in the recognition site. Based on the probability that the four nucleotides (GATC) will create a characteristic restriction site, a 4-base cutter should cut human genomic DNA every 2.5×10^2 bp, whereas an 8-base cutter would cut on average of every 1.0×10^6 bp.

Restriction enzymes can cut DNA in three basic ways: they can cut the recognition site asymmetrically to leave ends with 5' or 3' overhangs, or they can cut symmetrically to leave blunt ends (Fig. 2-1). Restriction enzymes are named according to the bacteria from which they were isolated (e.g., *Eco*RI from *Escherichia coli*). Hundreds of different restriction endonucleases are commercially available today.

In practical terms, the restriction enzyme is incubated with DNA in a compatible buffer solution and cuts the DNA into pieces of a defined size. Because the cleavage is sequence-specific, different DNAs will produce a characteristic digestion pattern (Fig. 2-2). These unique DNA fingerprints can be recognized after separation of the different size fragments by gel electrophoresis. The production of such restriction maps represents one of the major uses of these enzymes. A second major use of restriction endonucleases is to "cut and paste" DNA in order to generate novel DNA sequences that are used in a variety of methods.

DNA LIGASES DNA ligases are enzymes that attach two pieces of DNA covalently to one another. T4 DNA ligase is the most commonly used enzyme. The reaction occurs between the 3' hydroxy group of one DNA strand and the phosphate group of the partner strand (Fig. 2-3). ATP provides the energy for the reaction. DNA ligation can occur efficiently only between compatible ends of DNA fragments, and this specificity gives the investigator some control over how different DNA fragments ligate together in a reaction mix. The most common use of ligation is to incorporate a piece of DNA into a cloning vector.

From: *Principles of Molecular Medicine* (J. L. Jameson, ed.), ©1998 Humana Press Inc., Totowa, NJ.

Table 1-1
Recent Nobel Prizes and Molecular Genetic Technology

Year	*Scientist(s)*	*Discovery*	*Technique derived*
1975	D Baltimore R Dulbecco HM Temin	The interaction between tumor viruses and the genetic material	Reverse transcriptase
1978	W Arber D Nathans HO Smith	Restriction enzymes and their application to molecular genetics	Restriction enzymes
1980	P Berg	Biochemistry of nucleic acids	Plasmids
1980	W Gilbert F Sanger	Determination of base sequences in nucleic acids	DNA sequencing
1984	NJ Jerne GJF Kohler C Milstein	Principles for the production of monoclonal antibodies	Monoclonal antibodies
1989	JM Bishop HE Varmus	The cellular origin of retroviruses	Reverse transcriptase
1993	R Roberts P Sharp	Genes are split into exons	Structure of genes
1993	M Smith KB Mullis	PCR and oligonucleotide-directed mutagenesis	PCR Site-directed mutagenesis

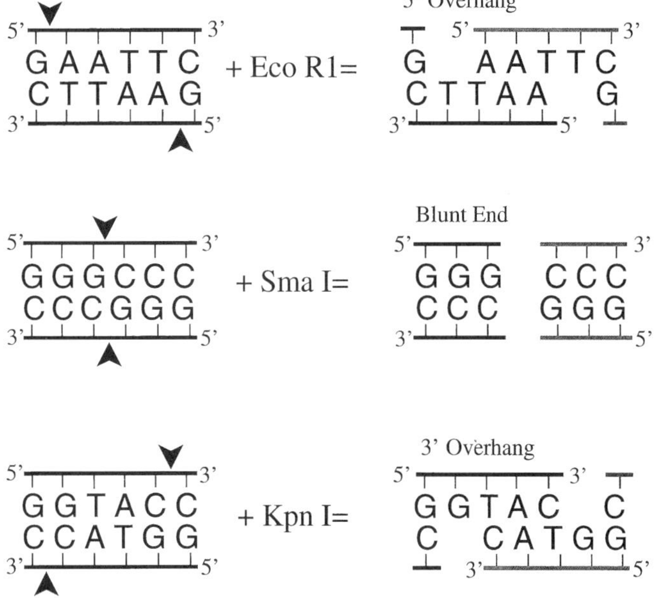

Figure 2-1 Restriction enzyme cleavage. Three enzymes are shown which digest DNA in three separate ways. *Eco*RI, 5' overhang; *Sma*I, blunt end; *Kpn*I, 3' overhang. Arrowheads indicate the site of cleavage within the restriction site for each enzyme.

DNA POLYMERASES DNA polymerases are enzymes that use a single strand of DNA as a template for the synthesis of a second strand. All DNA polymerases require a primer, and all DNA polymerases synthesize new DNA in a 5' to 3' direction. A primer is a small piece of DNA that is complementary to the strand to be copied. Polymerases attach to the primer sites and then extend the primer in a 5' $\rightarrow$ 3' direction using individual deoxynucleotides as building blocks (Fig. 2-4). DNA polymerases have multiple uses. Among these are the production of radioactively labeled DNA, the polymerase chain reaction, and DNA sequencing.

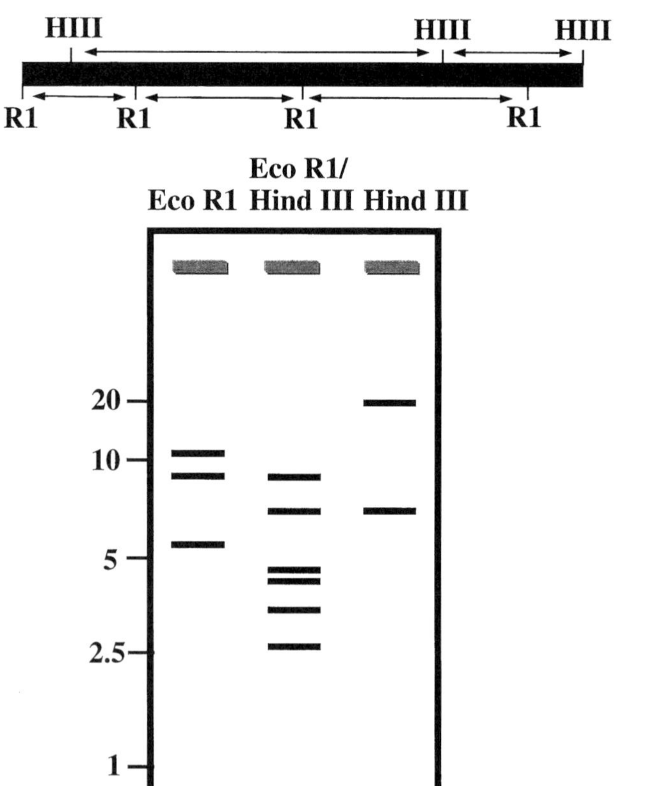

Figure 2-2 DNA digestion pattern. Restriction digestion pattern of DNA with *Eco*RI and *Hin*dIII as well as the two enzymes combined. After electrophoresis, the DNA smaller fragments migrate through the gel faster than larger fragments. Basepair sizes are indicated on the left side of the gel.

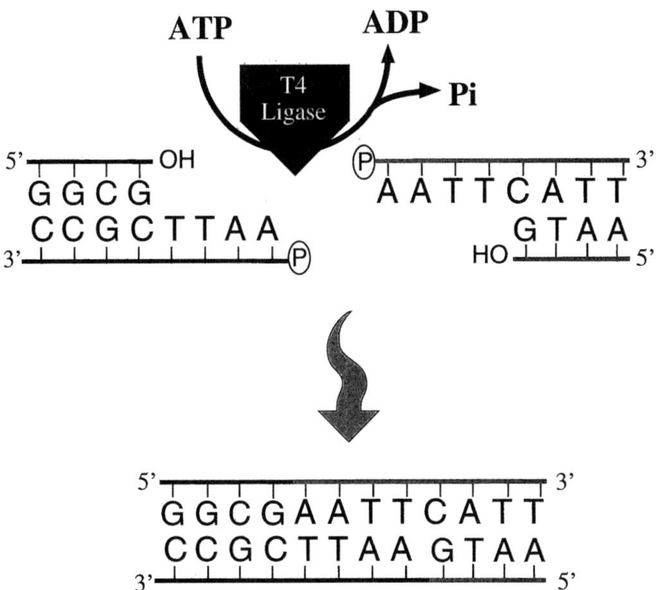

Figure 2-3 Ligase reaction. T4 DNA ligase will catalyze the joining of complementary ends of DNA by joining the 5' phosphate group to the 3' OH group of two strands of DNA. This reaction requires ATP as well as compatible ends of DNA.

REVERSE TRANSCRIPTASE Reverse transcriptase (RT) enzymes are a subtype of DNA polymerase that utilize RNA as a template to produce DNA. They also require a primer and synthesize in the 5' → 3' direction. Reverse transcriptases are isolated from retroviruses, which have the ability to reverse copy their RNA genome for their life cycle in mammalian cells. The major use of RT is to copy mRNA into DNA, which is then called "complementary DNA" or cDNA. The reaction of RT on an RNA template produces a hybrid RNA-DNA molecule. The DNA in this hybrid is called "first-strand cDNA" and can be used to generate another complementary copy of DNA to create double-stranded DNA (dsDNA). In this manner, cDNA is used to generate libraries representing the expressed genes of a tissue *(see below)* and as a substrate for polymerase chain reaction (PCR) in the sequence analysis of RNA species.

RADIOLABELING Radioactive DNA is an important reagent in molecular biology, as it serves as a valuable hybridization probe. There are two basic ways to incorporate radioactivity into DNA: internal labeling and end-labeling. For internal labeling, DNA is denatured into single strands by boiling, and DNA polymerase is used to copy the strand in the presence of a radioactively labeled nucleotide (most commonly ^{32}P-dCTP). The newly synthesized strand is therefore highly radioactive. Polynucleotide kinase is used for end-labeling. This enzyme transfers the radioactivity from an ATP molecule to the 5' end of single-stranded DNA. Only the most 5' base is labeled, and no radioactivity is incorporated internally in the DNA molecule. Several nonradioactive methods are also available for "labeling" DNA. For example, biotinylation allows detection with avidin-based systems, and digoxygenin can be detected with enzyme-linked assays.

ISOLATION OF GENOMIC DNA, TOTAL RNA, AND POLY(A) RNA

In order to be accessible for manipulation, diagnostic studies, and therapeutic uses, DNA and RNA must be isolated in suitable form and quantity. The best method of DNA or RNA isolation, and propagation depends on the intended use. Although most techniques are labor-intensive and require large amounts of starting material, the use of isolation kits from a variety of biotechnology companies have made the isolation of DNA and RNA a relatively simple matter. Both classical isolation and kit isolation methods utilize the basic principles outlined below.

ISOLATION OF TOTAL GENOMIC DNA Genomic DNA is double-stranded and can be isolated from any kind of cell, including bacteria, yeast, plants, and animal cells. For most uses, it is desirable that the DNA remain as undamaged and the highest molecular weight as possible. The process of purifying DNA tends to introduce strand breaks and to reduce its molecular weight, but proper precautions can minimize shearing. There are many variations in the details of DNA isolation protocols, but all involve lysis of the cell and nucleus (if the cell has a nucleus) as a first step. A suspension of the DNA-containing cells is incubated with detergents and/or lytic enzymes for this purpose. The next step involves dissociation of the DNA from any attached proteins (such as histones). Most protocols utilize a strong protein degrading enzyme (proteinase K) for this purpose. This step also inactivates any DNA degrading cellular enzymes (nucleases). The partially degraded proteins are removed from the solution by phenol/chloroform extraction, salt precipitation, or the solution being passed over a column, which retains the DNA. DNA is precipitated from the remaining solution by ethanol precipitation. High-molecular-weight DNA (such as human genomic DNA) will form threads when precipitated in this way and can then be "spooled" from the solution with a glass rod. The DNA is then dried and redissolved in an aqueous buffer for further use and is stable in this form for several years.

ISOLATION OF TOTAL CELLULAR RNA Several different forms of RNA exist in cells, including messenger RNAs (mRNA), ribosomal RNAs (rRNA), transfer RNAs (tRNA), and others. For many types of studies (Northern blots, RT-PCR), the isolation of total cellular RNA species is acceptable. In contrast to DNA, RNA is single-stranded and relatively unstable. During RNA isolation and storage, constant caution should be taken to avoid degradation by RNase enzymes, which are ubiquitous. For RNA isolation, cells, or tissues are homogenized in a solution that contains RNase-inhibiting compounds, such as the chaotropic chemical guanidinium isothiocyanate. Many different methods are available for the next step, which involves separating the RNA from genomic DNA. As in DNA isolation, the purified RNA is precipitated with ethanol during the final step of all procedures. Aqueous RNA solutions should be stored frozen.

ISOLATION OF mRNA For certain applications, total cellular RNA is inadequate. Ribosomal RNA represents the bulk of total cellular RNA and only 1–3% of all RNA is mRNA. In order to make libraries of expressed sequences or to detect rare mRNA species on Northern blots, it is important to isolate mRNA as the starting material. Most mRNAs are poly-adenylated (poly[A]RNA), and this feature can be exploited for their capture. Total cellular RNA is passed over a column or resin of polydeoxythymine (oligo d/T column, poly-dT) bound to a solid phase. Poly(A) RNA binds to the poly-dT and is immobilized on the solid phase. The remaining unbound RNA is then washed off, and the poly(A) RNA is eluted in a subsequent step.

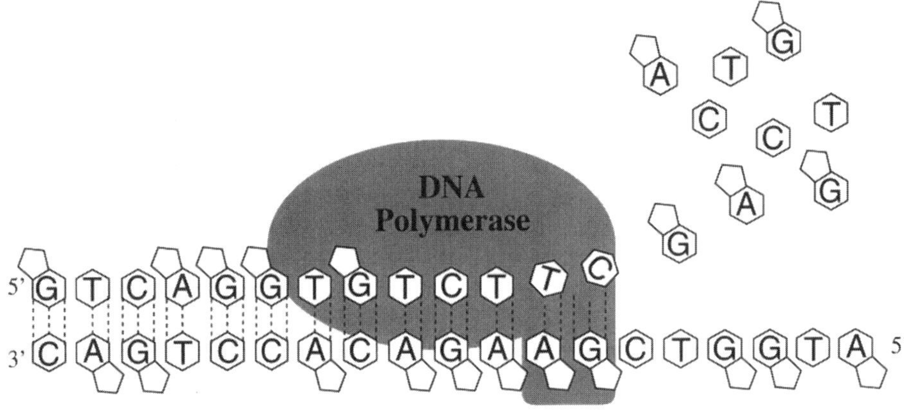

Figure 2-4 DNA polymerase-mediated synthesis of DNA. DNA polymerase will attach free nucleotides to an existing primer in the 5' to 3' direction in a complementary fashion. The dashed line indicates the complementary bases.

CLONING DNA

In the DNA isolation method described above, the genome of cells is the source of DNA; therefore, all sequences will be represented in the same abundance as they exist in the cell. Depending on the genome size of the organism, individual genes of interest represent only a minute fraction of the total DNA in a cell. For example, the average single gene in humans (~100,000-bp size) represents only 0.003% of the total genome. Thus, individual genes are much too dilute in such samples to be useful for detailed studies (such as DNA sequencing).

This problem is solved by the cloning of DNA, which allows the preparation of large and pure quantities of a single DNA species. All methods of DNA cloning involve the ligation of a sequence of interest (such as a human gene) into a cloning vector. Cloning vectors are DNA sequences that exist inside a cell (in most cases the bacterium *E. coli*) but are not part of the genome of that cell. The cloning vehicle (and the cloned DNA within it) replicates inside the host cell, producing large quantities of a specific DNA sequence that can be isolated for further study.

E. Coli PLASMIDS Cloning into *E. coli* plasmids remains the most important method for preparing large quantities of pure DNA. Plasmids are small circles of double-stranded DNA (2000–5000 bp) that replicate inside bacterial cells (Fig. 2-5). Plasmids have their own origin of replication and can propagate themselves with the help of the endogenous cellular machinery. Cloning plasmids contain a selectable marker, usually a gene that confers resistance to an antibiotic. *E. coli* cells containing this antibiotic-selectable plasmid are then able to grow in media containing the respective antimicrobial agent. Many plasmids contain the β-lactamase gene, allowing growth in ampicillin. Low- and high-copy-number plasmids are distinguished. Pure plasmid DNA can be isolated from *E. coli* genomic DNA, because plasmid DNA is much smaller in size than *E. coli* genomic DNA (the *E. coli* genome is ~1×10^6 bp). The plasmid-containing *E. coli* cells are grown in a large volume of liquid culture media containing the antibiotic of choice. The cells are then pelleted by centrifugation and lysed, either with alkali, or using detergents. All plasmid preparation methods use size selection to remove the high-molecular-weight genomic DNA and RNA leaving only the small circular plasmid DNA. Milligram quantities of pure plasmid DNA can be prepared from a 1-L culture of *E. coli* cells containing a high-copy-number plasmid.

Modern *E. coli* plasmids have been engineered to contain a region with multiple useful restriction endonuclease sites (polylinker sites). In order to clone a gene of interest, the following procedure is followed (Fig. 2-5): DNA from the parental plasmid is cut with a restriction endonuclease, thus opening the ring and converting it to a linear molecule. A linear double-stranded DNA sequence of interest is generated with matching ends and is then ligated into the gap to regenerate a circular plasmid. The ligated plasmid is introduced by a process called transformation into a strain of *E. coli* that is sensitive to the antibiotic resistance marker carried by the plasmid. Transformation of bacteria can be accomplished by either heating the DNA-bacteria mix at 42°C for 1 min or by a quick pulse of electricity (electroporation). Both methods move the plasmid DNA through the bacterial wall and into the bacterial cell. After transformation, the bacteria are grown on antibiotic-containing plates. Only cells that have taken up a circular plasmid are able to survive and form colonies in the presence of the antibiotic. Individual bacterial colonies are also called "clones," because every cell in the colony is genetically identical. Individual clones can be expanded in liquid media for the preparation of large amounts of plasmid DNA. Since bacterial cells are immortal and can continue to divide without limit, plasmid-containing clones represent a permanent source of DNA. The cells can be stored frozen indefinitely, and clones can be mailed and shared with other laboratories.

Modern high-copy-number plasmids are about 3 kb in size and can accommodate inserts of up to 15 kb. Most DNA cloned in plasmids, however, is less than 10 kb in size and larger sequences are frequently unstable. Thus, only relatively small pieces of DNA can be cloned in plasmid vectors. For this reason, multiple cloning vectors capable of harboring larger DNA sequences have been developed. The most important of these will be briefly described below.

PHAGE CLONING VECTORS Bacteriophage λ is a virus that infects *E. coli* cells and has been used extensively for cloning. Its structure is very different from plasmids. Virus particles consist of a protein envelope and core and a linear double-stranded DNA genome. For cloning purposes, much of the wild-type genome has been removed to allow replacement by exogenous DNA. In contrast to plasmids, inserts of up to 23 kb in size are stable in phage.

Cloning in phage (Fig. 2-6) is performed in the following way: A large internal portion of the wild-type phage genome is removed by restriction digestion leaving a long (or left) and short (or right)

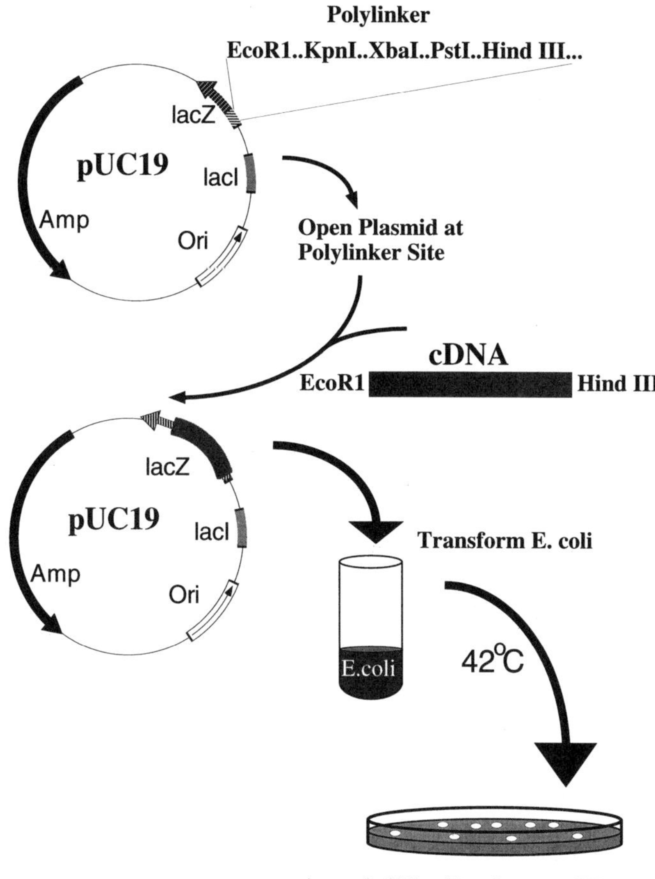

Figure 2-5 Subcloning in bacteria. pUC 19 cloning vector is used to propagate cDNA. The plasmid carries a bacterial origin of replication (ORI). Also, a resistance gene for selection in ampicillin media (Amp), as well as a gene that can be used to detect for insertion of cDNA (*lac*Z). After opening the plasmid and introduction of the cDNA through restriction enzyme digestion and ligation, the construct is transformed into bacteria *(E. coli)* through either heat shock or electroporation. After transformation, bacteria are plated on resistant media, allowing the bacteria to grow only if they have taken up the plasmid containing the resistance gene. Growing the colonies with X-gal, a substrate for B galactosidase, clones that have been inserted into the *lac*Z gene and disrupted its reading frame, will no longer be able to metabolize X-gal and will appear white on the media plate. However, those colonies that may have religated and still contain a functional *lac*Z gene will metabolize X-gal and have a blue appearance.

arm. Neither of these two arms alone contains enough sequence to produce an infectious phage nor are the arms large enough to be packaged. The DNA sequence of interest is then ligated between the two arms, restoring a single large DNA genome. A "packaging extract" containing viral structural proteins isolated from wild-type phage is then used to package the recombinant phage and to infect *E. coli* cells.

After infection of a bacterial cell, λ phage replicates to high copy numbers within the cell and then lyses it. Phage particles are released and can infect other *E. coli* cells. When propagated on agar plates, phage will then lyse bacterial cells and leave a hole or "plaque" in the lawn of bacteria. Each plaque represents a clone of DNA, because all the phage in a plaque are genetically identical. When a liquid culture of *E. coli* is infected with phage, most of the cells will lyse and a high density of phage particles is attained. Phage particles can then be purified and their DNA isolated in large quantities.

Recently, one other *E. coli* bacteriophage has become an important cloning vehicle. Phage P1 can stably harbor DNA inserts of up to 100 kb and is therefore used to clone long stretches of genomic DNA.

COSMIDS Cosmids harbor inserts of ~40 kb and are very useful cloning vectors. Their properties are similar to plasmids in many aspects. Cosmids can propagate in *E. coli* and do not lyse their host cell. Antibiotic resistance genes (usually ampicillin) are used to select for cosmid-containing cells, which form colonies on plates. Inserts are ligated into convenient restriction sites.

BACTERIAL ARTIFICIAL CHROMOSOMES Bacterial artificial chromosomes (BACs) are a special *E. coli* plasmid that can stably replicate very large inserts of genomic DNA. BAC inserts can be as large as 180 kb, and complete libraries of the human genome are now available in BACs. In contrast to YACs *(see below)*, BAC inserts are usually pure (nonchimeric), and the BAC DNA is very easy to isolate.

YEAST ARTIFICIAL CHROMOSOMES Yeast artificial chromosomes (YACs) have become very important in the human genome project, because they can harbor by far the largest inserts (up to 2000 kb). Because of this, a single YAC can cover a relatively large genomic region. In contrast to all other cloning vehicles described here, YACs are not grown in bacteria, but in the yeast *Saccharomyces cerevisiae*. YACs consist of a artificial centromere, the insert, and an artificial telomere, thus literally representing an artificial chromosome. Both the artificial centromere and the telomere contain different selectable marker genes. In order to generate a YAC, large pieces of DNA are ligated to the centromere on one end and the telomere on the other. This construct is then introduced into yeast, which is incubated on selective media plates. Only those yeast cells that contain both the telomere and centromere (and therefore both selectable marker genes) will survive and form colonies. Individual colonies (clones) can then be picked, grown in liquid culture, and YAC DNA can be isolated from the yeast cells.

YACs have the advantage of containing very large inserts, but they have the disadvantage of frequently being chimeric. Chimeric YACs contain inserts from more than one region of the genome, which can limit their experimental utility. For example, a chimeric YAC may contain an insert from chromosome 3p fused to a portion of chromosome 15.

LIBRARIES Cloning vectors such as those described above can be used to replicate a DNA sequence of interest and purify large quantities. But how are genes of interest found in the first place? The process by which gene(s) are isolated from the complex mix of DNA sequences found in cells of higher organisms will be described briefly.

Most gene-isolation strategies have traditionally involved the generation of a library of DNA or RNA sequences. The beginning material for the library is a complex mix of DNA known to contain the sequence of interest. For example, the starting material for the isolation of a human gene would be total genomic DNA isolated from human cells. This DNA is then broken down into fragments of the appropriate size by mechanical shearing or by restriction endonuclease digestion. The appropriate size depends on the cloning vector to be used. For λ phage libraries, the average fragment

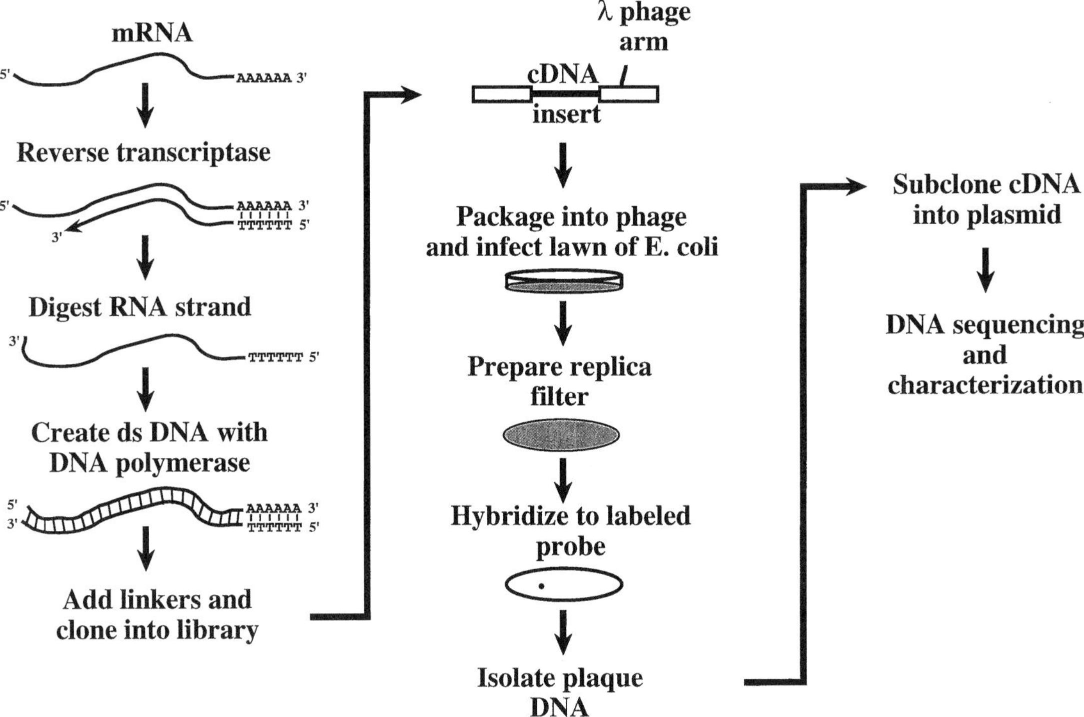

Figure 2-6 Construction of a cDNA library. mRNA is isolated and reverse-transcribed by reverse transcriptase. The RNA strand is digested away leaving single-stranded DNA to which oligo d/T primers and DNA polymerase are added. These primers will anneal to the poly (A) tail of the cDNA and are extended by DNA polymerase. The double-stranded cDNA is ligated into λ phage arms, and bacteria are infected. Filter lifts are performed on the lysed bacteria and hybridized with the appropriate probe. Following hybridization and autoradiography, the appropriate plaques may be isolated and the corresponding phage purified and characterized. Adapted with permission. (Jameson JL. Applications of molecular biology in endocrinology. In: DeGroot LJ, ed. Endocrinology, 3rd ed., Philadelphia, PA: WB Saunders, 1995; pp. 119-147.)

size should be 8–25 kb. This mixture of fragments is ligated into a cloning vector and the ligation reaction is used to infect or transform *E. coli* bacteria. The biology of cloning vectors assures that each individual bacterium will contain only one cloning vector with an insert. Thus, this procedure divides the initial complex mix of DNA into millions of individual clones, each of which contains only a single DNA sequence, a library. Libraries can be produced from any source of double-stranded DNA.

In order to identify the protein-coding regions of genes, however, it is necessary to generate libraries from expressed sequences. This type of library is called cDNA library and the starting material is messenger RNA (Fig. 2-6). To isolate the gene for a liver metabolic enzyme, for example, mRNA would be purified from homogenized liver. This material contains all mRNAs that are present in the liver. Some mRNAs will be very abundant, because they encode proteins present in high amounts in liver. Others transcripts will be rare. Reverse transcription is then used to copy the mix of mRNAs into first-strand cDNA. The cDNAs are then converted to double-stranded DNA and ligated into a cloning vector to produce the cDNA library. It is important to note that cDNA libraries are tissue-specific, because each tissue expresses a different set of genes. Similarly, cDNA libraries are specific for a developmental stage of the organism.

Once a library of clones has been generated from the nucleic acid source of interest, the challenge is to find the specific individual clone with the gene among the millions of clones in the library. This is achieved by library screening. The bacteria containing the library are spread on agar plates at a defined density, which is low enough to permit the isolation of individual clones. A phage library produced from human genomic DNA, for example, would be plated a density of 50,000 plaques per plate. At this density, 20 plates represent about 1,000,000 individual clones. Part of each colony/plaque on a plate is then transferred, as an exact copy, onto a nitrocellulose or nylon filter in a procedure termed "filter lift." These filters are then processed to covalently bind either the DNA or the expressed proteins of the transferred plaques/colonies. The filters are incubated with a radioactively labeled DNA probe or specific antibodies, which will bind to the position on the filter occupied by a individual clone containing the desired DNA or expressing the sought-after protein. The corresponding clone is then picked from the original plate based on the position marked on the filter. DNA in the clone can then by amplified and isolated as described above, usually by subcloning it into plasmid vectors.

CHEMICAL PROPAGATION OF DNA

Large amounts of pure double-stranded DNA can be produced chemically by a method called the polymerase chain reaction (PCR) rather than by propagating cloning vectors inside living cells. Relatively small quantities of single-stranded DNA can be synthesized from individual nucleotides by oligonucleotide synthesis.

OLIGONUCLEOTIDES A prerequisite for the advent of the now ubiquitously used polymerase chain reaction was the ability to chemically synthesize short pieces of DNA of defined sequence (oligonucleotides). This process begins with the attachment of the most 5' base in the oligonucleotide sequence to a solid polymer support. Each new base in the sequence is then added to the 3' OH-group of the attached bases in a stepwise fashion until the entire desired sequence has been synthesized. During each cycle of syn-

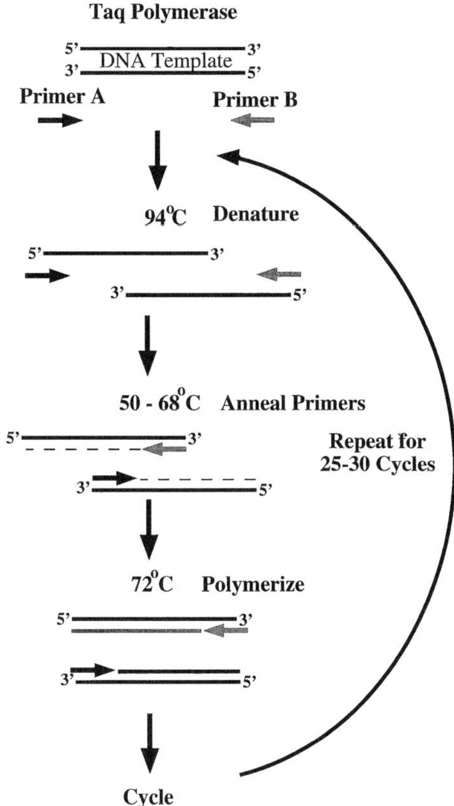

Figure 2-7 PCR reaction. DNA template, primers A and B, and DNA polymerase *(Taq)* are combined in a reaction that will cycle through denaturation, annealing, and extension temperatures, allowing the amplification of DNA between the primer pairs.

thesis, only one new base is added, providing strict control over the sequence of the completed oligonucleotide. Conventional oligonucleotides contain one of the four bases contained in DNA at each position. However, it is also possible to customize the procedure and to utilize unusual nucleotides (e.g., inosine), modified nucleotides (tagged with fluorescent dyes or digoxygenin), or more than one base in a single position (degenerate oligonucleotides).

POLYMERASE CHAIN REACTION PCR permits the investigator to generate large quantities of a specific DNA sequence from a complex mix of DNA within a very short period of time and without cloning. The procedure uses a thermostable DNA polymerase and two synthetic oligonucleotides (Fig. 2-7). The DNA sequence of the gene to be amplified needs to be partially known, so that two oligonucleotide primers corresponding to the ends of this target can be synthesized. The procedure then consists of repeated cycles of three steps: (1) denaturation of dsDNA, (2) primer annealing to DNA, and (3) primer extension. During denaturation, heat (94–98°C) is used to separate the two strands of the target DNA into single strands. These single strands are then available to hybridize to the matching oligonucleotide during the annealing step if the temperature of the reaction is lowered below the melting point for the oligonucleotide-DNA hybrid (usually 50–68°C). Once a primer has annealed, the DNA polymerase (*Taq* polymerase from the bacterium *Thermophilus aquaticus*) can copy the remainder of the single strand at 72°C, if the required deoxynucleotide triphosphates (dNTPs) are provided. Each of the originally present strands of the target DNA is copied and the amount of DNA is doubled with each cycle. Thus, after 25–30 cycles, the desired sequence can be enriched over a millionfold. This allows direct visualization as a distinct band in an agarose gel, and this amount of DNA is more than adequate for cloning or DNA sequencing. The sequential temperature changes required for PCR are performed by machines called thermocyclers. A complete PCR typically takes about 1–3 h and is therefore the most rapid method to produce a specific DNA sequence for further study. Limitations of PCR include misincorporation of nucleotides by the *Taq* polymerase (*Taq* errors) and the inability to amplify relatively large lengths of DNA (several kilobases). Modified versions of *Taq* polymerase with higher fidelity can reduce the rate of PCR errors and increase the length of fragments that can be amplified.

PCR has numerous uses that are reviewed in detail in the attached references. As examples, PCR is used to: (1) amplify specific regions of DNA for genetic engineering strategies that do not depend on the presence of restriction enzymes; (2) amplify genomic DNA for diagnostic studies; (3) amplify DNA for sequencing protocols; (4) to insert site-directed mutations; and (5) in combination with reverse transcriptase, to quantify to the amount of starting mRNA (RT-PCR).

SITE-DIRECTED MUTAGENESIS

PCR has greatly enhanced the ease with which site-directed mutagenesis can be performed (although other procedures are also available for mutagenesis). Site-directed mutations have many valuable applications, including structure-function studies of receptors, transcription factors, enzymes, and other transcription factors. Site-directed mutations are also introduced into the regulatory elements of genes to alter transcription factor binding sites and assess the effects on promoter function. Site-directed mutations also facilitate genetic engineering by allowing the introduction of new restriction sites.

Mutagenesis typically involves a single nucleotide substitution, although it is also possible to change several basepairs at once (including small deletions or insertions). One commonly used protocol is referred to as overlap extension mutagenesis (Fig. 2-8). In this procedure, mutagenesis is performed by creating an oligonucleotide primer that is complementary to the normal DNA sequence except for the mutant base, which is generally positioned near the 5' end of the oligonucleotide to assure adequate priming. Using PCR, the mutant primer is incorporated into the newly synthesized DNA. Subsequently, the DNA products of this first PCR (now containing the mutation) are used to prime a second PCR in conjunction with a new oligonucleotide primer. After a few PCR cycles, a long mutant template is created that can be amplified further by using traditional PCR. Several variations of this strategy are reviewed in the listed references.

ANALYSIS OF DNA AND RNA

GEL SEPARATION The size-based separation of DNA and RNA fragments by electrophoresis in various gels systems is a very important basic technique in molecular biology and is outlined briefly. At neutral pH, DNA and RNA are negatively charged and will migrate toward the anode in an electrical field. If this migration takes place within a polymer matrix (gel), small fragments move more rapidly than larger fragments (Fig. 2-2). Thus, electrophoretic migration through a gel gradually separates a mixture of DNA fragments of different sizes into distinct bands. Many

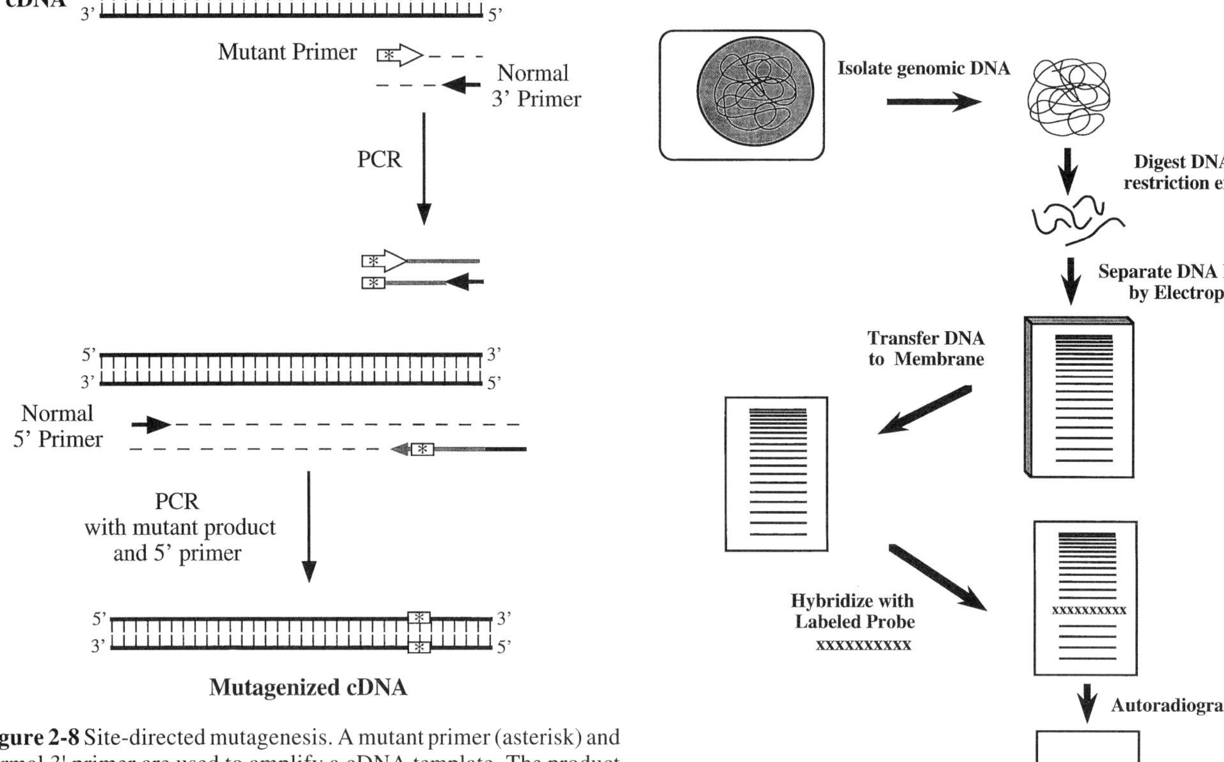

Figure 2-8 Site-directed mutagenesis. A mutant primer (asterisk) and normal 3' primer are used to amplify a cDNA template. The product of this reaction is used to amplify the template in conjunction with a normal 5' primer. This reaction results in a mutagenized cDNA that can be amplified further using normal primers.

Figure 2-9 Southern blot. Genomic DNA is isolated and digested with the appropriate restriction enzymes. DNA is then run on an agarose gel and transferred to a membrane support to which the DNA is covalently attached. Following transfer, the DNA is hybridized to the appropriate ^{32}P-labeled probe. Specific interactions between the DNA and labeled probe are detected by exposing the membrane-DNA to autoradiographic film. Adapted with permission. (Jameson JL. Applications of molecular biology in endocrinology. In: DeGroot LJ, ed. Endocrinology, 3rd ed., Philadelphia, PA: WB Saunders, 1995; pp. 119–147.)

different gel matrices can be used for nucleic acid separations, but agarose and polyacrylamide gels are used most commonly. Agarose gels are suitable for the separation of DNA fragments in the 0.1- to 20-kb range, whereas polyacrylamide are used to separate small DNA fragments in the 0.025- to 2-kb range. The inclusion of denaturants such as urea allows single-base resolution in polyacrylamide gels (e.g., for DNA sequencing). A specialized kind of agarose gel electrophoresis termed pulsed field gel electrophoresis (PFGE) is used for the separation of very large fragments (up to 1000 kb). Different techniques are used to visualize the DNA fragments after separation by gel electrophoresis. If the fragment is relatively abundant, gels can be stained during or after electrophoresis, and the DNA can be directly visualized. Ethidium bromide will bind to DNA and lead to red fluorescence under UV light. If there is too little DNA for direct visualization, radioactivity is used for detection (*see* hybridization, *below*).

NUCLEIC ACID HYBRIDIZATION One of the most commonly used analytical methods is nucleic acid hybridization. This technique is used for Southern blotting, Northern blotting, and for screening libraries. The goal of this method is to visualize a specific nucleic acid (DNA or RNA) sequence in the background of a complex mixture of other sequences. The technique takes advantage of the fact that the two complementary strands of nucleic acids will bind to each other (hybridize) with very high specificity. In contrast, noncomplementary nucleic acid sequences do not bind very efficiently, because nucleotide mismatches lower the melting temperature. To detect a particular species of DNA or RNA in a complex mixture, the constituents are first immobilized on a membrane and converted into a single-stranded form (*see* Southern and Northern blotting, *below*). A hybridization solution containing radioactively labeled single-stranded probe is added and the radiolabeled probe allowed to hybridize under defined conditions. The temperature and salt concentration of the hybridization fluid determine the specificity of binding. At high temperature and low salt concentration, the probe will bind only to a perfectly complementary target sequence. After hybridization, the excess nonbound radioactivity is washed off, leaving a radioactive signal to be detected only at the location of the specific target sequence. The radioactive signal is visualized by exposure to an X-ray film yielding a black spot or band at the site of the radioactivity.

SOUTHERN BLOTTING When genomic DNA is digested with restriction endonucleases and separated by gel electrophoresis, individual fragments cannot be visualized, even if large quantities of DNA are used. Because of the complexity of genomic DNA, restriction digests will invariably result in a "smear" of thousands of DNA fragments when visualized with ethidium bromide staining. In order to detect specific fragments within this smear, hybridization with radioactive probes is used in a procedure termed Southern blotting (after Ed Southern) (Fig. 2-9). Southern blotting begins with the separation of restriction-digested

Table 2-2
Summary of Blotting Procedures

Procedure	*Substance detected*	*Probe*	*Major application*
Southern blot	DNA	Nucleic acid	Gene structure
Northern blot	RNA	Nucleic acid	Gene expression
Western blot	Protein	Antibody	Protein levels
Southwestern blot	Protein	DNA	DNA–protein interactions
Farwestern blot	Protein	Protein	Protein–Protein interactions

Adapted with permission. (Jameson JL. Applications of molecular biology in endocrinology. In: DeGroot LJ, ed. Endocrinology, 3rd ed., Philadelphia, PA: WB Saunders, 1995; pp. 119–147.)

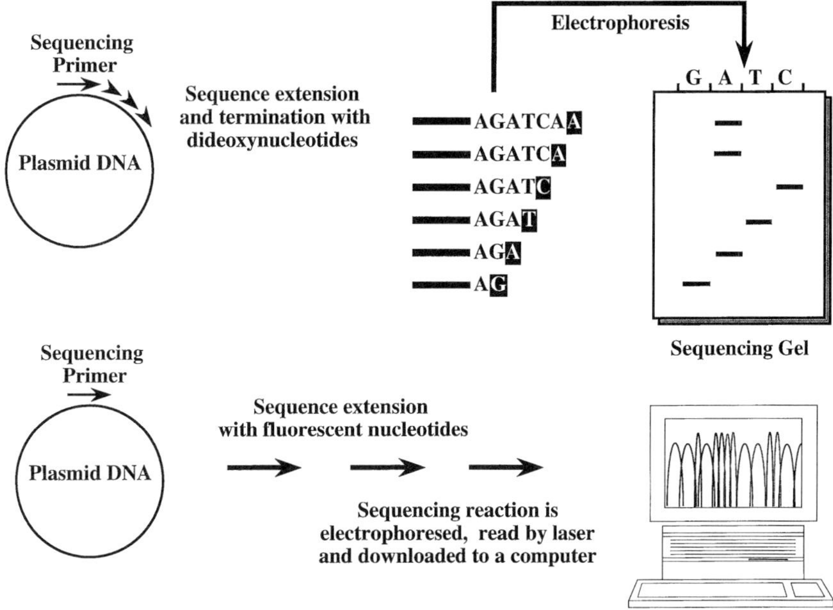

Figure 2-10 Sequencing of DNA. Template, primer, and polymerase are added to a reaction in which both dideoxy and deoxynucleotides are present. Four separate reactions are used in which ddATP, ddTTP, ddCTP, and ddGTP are used individually. Each of these reactions is run on a polyacrylamide gel. Alternatively, the sequencing reactions can be carried out using fluorescently labeled nucleotides (or primers) to allow detection by a laser. The DNA sequence is then downloaded into a computer. Adapted with permission. (Jameson JL. Applications of molecular biology in endocrinology. In: DeGroot LJ, ed. Endocrinology, 3rd ed., Philadelphia, PA: WB Saunders, 1995; pp. 119–147.)

DNA by gel electrophoresis. After the separation, the DNA is denatured (separated into two single strands) by treatment with alkali, and the single strands are transferred onto a membrane by capillary transfer. The DNA binds covalently to the membrane and is immobilized on this solid phase, creating a replica of the fragments in the gel. Specific DNA fragments can then be identified on the membrane using hybridization probes that are specific for the gene fragment of interest.

NORTHERN BLOTTING Gel separation and nucleic acid hybridization can also be used to analyze RNA in a procedure termed Northern blotting (Table 2-2). There are several important differences in comparison with Southern blotting. First, RNA is more susceptible to degradation than DNA. Electrophoresis is therefore carried out in a buffer that contains protective chemicals (usually formaldehyde). Second, RNA is already single-stranded and requires milder denaturation. Third, specific RNA species already have a defined size, and therefore enzymatic digestion is not needed in order to obtain a band pattern. The two procedures are similar, however, in that the RNA is transferred onto a membrane via capillary diffusion after electrophoresis. Usually ultraviolet light is used to crosslink the RNA onto the membrane to immobilize it.

DNA SEQUENCING

The determination of the actual nucleotide sequence represents the most detailed level of DNA analysis. Several different techniques are available for DNA sequencing, but the dideoxy chain termination method originally developed by Sanger is now used the most widely (Fig. 2-10). DNA must first be denatured and separated into single strands by heating. A single radioactively labeled oligonucleotide primer is then added to the reaction and anneals to its matching sequence on the target DNA. DNA polymerase is then used to copy the single-stranded DNA. In the presence of saturating quantities of all four deoxynucleotide triphosphates (dATP + dTTP + dGTP + dCTP = dNTPs), a large extension product radioactively labeled at its end would be generated, whereas no sequence information would be generated. The addition of small quantities of dideoxy nucleotide triphosphates (ddNTPs) to the dNTP mix, however, leads to sequence information. Dideoxynucleotides are incorporated into the 3' end of the newly synthesized strand, but the DNA polymerase cannot add new bases onto the ddNTP. Thus, the incorporation of a ddNTP leads to chain termination. By adding appropriate ratios of dNTP and ddNTPs, it is possible to achieve conditions in which chain termination occurs randomly at each nucleotide position. For example, if a primer extension was performed in the presence of dATP, dTTP, dGTP, and ddCTP, the polymerase will synthesize a new strand of DNA until it has to use ddCTP (e.g., when the complementary base is G). The ddCTP will be incorporated, but the polymerase cannot extend beyond this point. The length of the radioactive extension product therefore defines the position of the first G in the strand that is being copied. In order to determine the position of not only the first G, but additional Gs in the DNA, real sequencing reactions would be performed in the presence of a mix of dCTP and ddCTP at a molar ratio of ~200:1. In this setting there is a ~1:200 chance for a chain termination to occur when a G is present in the strand being sequenced. Extension products of multiple lengths will be generated and can be visualized after electrophoresis in a polyacrylamide gel. Based on its length, each fragment precisely defines the position of a G. In order to determine the positions of all four bases, four separate sequencing reactions are performed for each sample. In each case, a mixture of a given dNTP and its corresponding ddNTP is used in combination with saturating amounts of the three other dNTPs. The four reactions are then electrophoresed in adjacent lanes in a sequencing (denaturing polyacrylamide) gel, thereby permitting direct reading of the DNA sequence. Despite the relative complexity of chain termination theory, DNA sequencing in practice is relatively straightforward.

Modern technology has allowed partial automation of DNA sequencing. For large-scale projects, robotics can be used to prepare sequencing reactions. Perhaps more importantly, instrumentation allows real-time "reading" of DNA sequencing gels and automated entry into computer databases. In addition to the reduction in human effort, such automation reduces errors inherent in reading and entering DNA sequence manually. Currently, most automated sequencers use fluorescent dyes rather than radioactivity. The dyes can be incorporated into either the sequencing primers or into the incorporated nucleotides. As with manual sequencing, gel electrophoresis (or capillary electrophoresis) is used to separate DNA fragments by size. However, with automated sequencers, detection of the fluorescent DNA fragments occurs via a laser beam, and the signal is processed by a computer. Other methods of automated sequencing are in development, including the use of DNA chips. In this strategy, a large ordered array of oligonucleotides are attached to DNA chips. Hybridization of DNA fragments to the chips allows the detection of overlapping sequences that can be converted into a contiguous sequence of DNA. This technology is particularly promising for the detection of polymorphisms and mutations, because a known sequence can be applied to the chips with specific variations at each nucleotide.

DETECTION OF DNA SEQUENCE POLYMORPHISMS

DNA sequence polymorphisms play an important role in molecular genetics. A DNA polymorphism is a DNA sequence alteration that is found at a frequency of >1% in a given population. In contrast to mutations, these sequence alterations do not adversely affect the function of genes. They can be thought of as neutral variations in DNA sequence. Polymorphisms are important, because they permit the tracking of gene loci and attached regions in pedigrees. Many different classes of DNA polymorphisms and methods for their detection exist. The most important of these will be reviewed here.

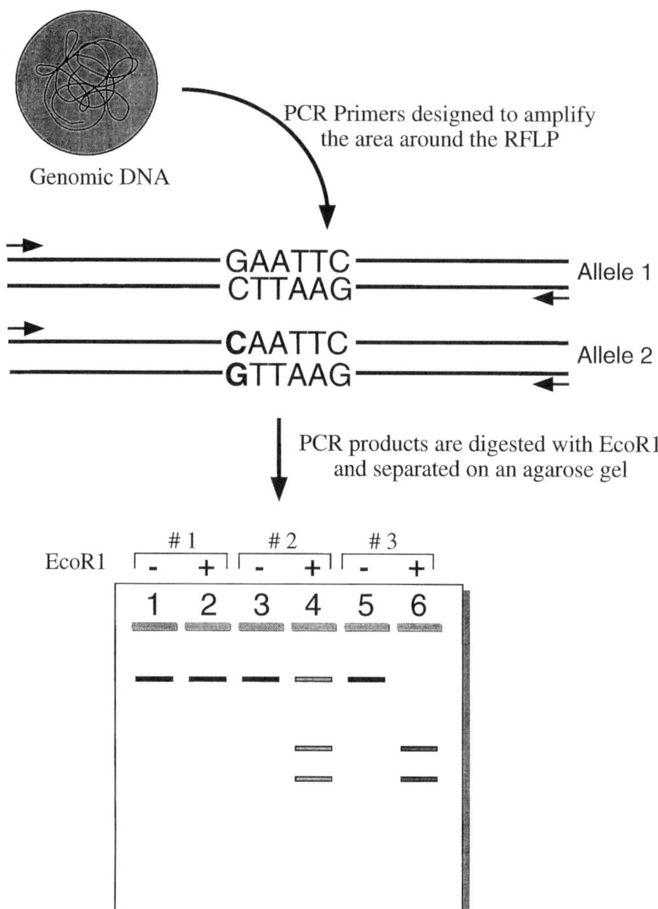

Figure 2-11 Restriction fragment length polymorphism (RFLP). Genomic DNA is isolated and primers are added with DNA polymerase to amplify the targeted region of DNA. The two alleles differ in a *Eco*RI restriction site, the first allele having a *Eco*RI site (GAATTC), the second allele having a C for a G base change (CAATTC). Following amplification and digestion with *Eco*RI, the products are run on an agarose gel along with uncut samples. Individual 1 is homozygous for allele 1, individual 2 is heterozygous for the alleles, and individual 3 is homozygous for allele 2.

RESTRICTION FRAGMENT-LENGTH POLYMORPHISMS

The simplest kind of DNA polymorphism is a single-base change. If the altered base lies within a recognition site for a restriction endonuclease, it may destroy the recognition sequence of this enzyme and abolish the site (Fig. 2-11). Alternatively, the polymorphism may create a new site. Single-base polymorphisms of this nature will alter the size of DNA fragments resulting from a digestion with this enzyme. The altered size bands can be detected after agarose gel electrophoresis and Southern blotting. If a restriction site was destroyed, the polymorphic band will be larger, and if a new site was generated, it will be smaller than the prevalent band in the general population. Single-base polymorphisms have been estimated to be present approximately every 1 kb in the human genome. About 1/6 of these changes will be detectable as a restriction fragment-length polymorphism (RFLP). Although RFLPs are relatively abundant in the genome, their use is limited by the fact that there are only two possible alleles for each polymorphism. The restriction site is either present or absent. In addition, Southern blotting requires relatively large amounts of DNA for analyses (5–10 μg).

Table 2-3
Techniques Used for the Detection of Mutations

Method	*Gene deletions*	*Gene rearrangements*	*Loss of heterozygosity*	*Linkage*	*Point mutations*
Cytogenetics (FISH)			+		
Southern blot	+	+			
RFLP			+	+	
VNTR			+	+	
PCR	+	+	+	+	+
DNA sequencing					+
Mismatch cleavage					+
OSH					+
DGGE					+
SSCP					+
PTT					+

FISH, fluorescent *in situ* hybridization; RFLP, restriction fragment length polymorphism; VNTR, variable number tandem repeat; PCR, polymerase chain reaction; OSH, oligonucleotide specific hybridization; DGGE, denaturing gradient gel electrophoresis; SSCP, single-stranded conformational polymorphism; PTT, protein truncation test. Adapted with permission. (Jameson JL. Applications of molecular biology in endocrinology. In: DeGroot LJ, ed. Endocrinology, 3rd ed. Philadelphia: WB Saunders, 1995; pp. 119–147.)

VARIABLE NUMBER TANDEM REPEATS Another important class of polymorphisms are the variable number tandem repeats (VNTRs) (minisatellites), used for forensic applications and paternity testing. VNTRs consist of reiterated repeats of small DNA sequences (0.1–10 kb) in multiple copies. The number of repeats in a VNTR is highly polymorphic (e.g., very variable between individuals in a population). To detect the polymorphism, a restriction endonuclease is used, which cuts outside of the repeat. The fragments obtained from such a digest will vary depending on the number of repeats and are readily distinguished by agarose gel electrophoresis and Southern blotting. In contrast to RFLPs, VNTR polymorphisms can have many different alleles (in some cases over 100), resulting in many different fragment sizes. However, VNTRs are relatively rare polymorphisms, and their density in the human genome is insufficient to permit linkage analysis for all human chromosomes.

MICROSATELLITES Microsatellite repeats are similar to VNTRs in that a simple sequence is reiterated in multiple copies, and the alleles are distinguished by their sizes. However, the repeats in microsatellites are much more simple. The most commonly used repeat sequences are dinucleotide, trinucleotide, and tetranucleotide repeats. Dinucleotide repeats are common in mammalian genomes, particularly the dinucleotide CA. Microsatellite repeats are detected by PCR. Two primers flanking the repeat are used to amplify the region, and the products of the PCR reaction are then analyzed in a denaturing polyacrylamide gel (*see* Chapter 5). If a dinucleotide repeat differs from the population by a single repeat unit, this will give rise to a PCR product that is differs in size by 2 bp. Differences of this magnitude, however, are detectable in polyacrylamide gels. Similar to VNTRs, microsatellite repeats usually have many different alleles (repeat sizes). Because their detection is PCR-based, and because they are common in the genome, this class of polymorphisms has become the most important for gene mapping and diagnostic linkage analysis (*see* Chapters 4 and 5).

DETECTION OF MUTATIONS

Mutations are DNA sequence alterations that change the function of a gene or the protein encoded by the DNA sequence. Many different kinds of changes can disrupt gene function. These include: gene rearrangements, deletions of DNA (large and small), insertions, and single-base changes. The optimal technique for the detecting mutations is dependent on the nature of the mutation (Table 2-3). Large chromosomal rearrangements, insertions, and deletions (megabases in size) are best analyzed by cytogenetic techniques, including fluorescent *in situ* hybridization (FISH). FISH uses fluorescently labeled probes to hybridize to chromosomes. A catalog of fluorescent probes is available for mapping each chromosome as well as typical inversions and deletions. Southern blotting is used to detect sequence changes that involve hundreds to thousands of bases.

More subtle mutations, including insertions and deletions of a few base pairs, and single-base changes, require specialized techniques for screening and characterizing mutations. There are two basic starting materials for mutation analyses: mRNA and genomic DNA. In comparison to genomic DNA, the analysis of mRNA has the advantage that the entire transcript can be analyzed in one piece (the introns have been spliced out). The disadvantage of mRNA analysis is that the gene of interest has to be expressed in accessible tissue. For example, a gene responsible for a brain disorder may not be expressed in skin or blood cells. On the other hand, it is sometimes possible to extract mRNA from leukocytes to characterize a gene that is expressed predominantly in another tissue (e.g., thyroid-stimulating hormone receptor mRNA). In order to analyze mRNA for mutations, reverse transcriptase is used to produce first-strand cDNA. This cDNA is then specifically amplified by PCR. This procedure is termed reverse transcriptase-PCR (RT-PCR). Genomic DNA is present in all cells regardless of whether or not the gene is expressed. However, the "interesting" protein coding sequences of the gene are dispersed on multiple exons, which can be thousands of base pairs apart (*see* Chapter 1). Therefore, in order to analyze genomic DNA for mutations, individual exons are amplified by PCR for analysis. Several methods exist to detect mutations on PCR products derived from mRNA or genomic DNA. These include a variety of screening methods that detect altered DNA secondary structure including denaturing gradient gel electrophoresis (DGGE), single-stranded conformational polymorphism (SSCP), and several mismatch cleavage techniques. These techniques are most useful for screening large genes in which mutations occur in a widely distributed manner. The protein truncation test (PTT) is also useful for detecting frameshift or premature stop mutations in large genes. In this case, the mRNA

Table 2-4
Selected Uses of Recombinant Proteins

Purpose of recombinant protein expression	*Examples*
Unlimited amount of biologically active drug	Insulin, growth hormone, erythropoietin
Abundant source of pure enzyme	Restriction endonucleases, *Taq* polymerase
Protein structural studies	X-ray crystallography, NMR
Structure–function studies	Transcription factors, enzymes
Drug screening	Receptors, enzymes
Raise antibodies	Protein antigen
Detect protein–protein interactions	Yeast two-hybrid assays, farwestern screening

is converted to cDNA, transcribed, and translated in vitro, allowing the detection of mutations that truncate the protein. For genes that have "hot spots" for recurring mutations, oligonucleotide-specific hybridization (OSH) can be used to detect specific mutations that allow mutant oligonucleotides to hybridize to mutated genomic DNA. As noted above, DNA chip technology is likely to play an analogous role in mutation detection in the future. DNA sequencing is the most definitive technique for detecting mutations and will determine the exact nature of the genetic change. Using a combination of PCR and direct DNA sequencing, it is practical to screen many small genes for mutations. Improvements in the protocols for automated DNA sequencing now allow reliable detection of heterozygous mutations (dominant or compound heterozygotes). These protocols allow about 500 bp to be sequenced reliably in a single run.

EXPRESSION OF RECOMBINANT PROTEINS

The ability to express large quantities of functional recombinant proteins is one of the many advantages conferred by the cloning of cDNAs. There are many practical uses for recombinant proteins (Table 2-4). They provide unlimited sources for reagents such as restriction enzymes and represent an invaluable source for hormones and growth factors, such as human insulin and erythropoietin, that are difficult to isolate in abundance from natural sources. The availability of abundant amounts of recombinant proteins has greatly facilitated biophysical studies and structure-function analyses of proteins.

IN VITRO TRANSLATION OF RECOMBINANT PROTEINS There are now numerous methods and hosts for expressing recombinant proteins, only some of which will be reviewed here. The simplest form of expression involves in vitro translation using reticulocyte lysates. In this method, mRNA (usually transcribed in vitro from a cDNA cloned into a plasmid) is translated using crude preparations of ribosomes present in reticulocyte lysates. Although the amount of protein is not large, it is possible to label it by including radioactive amino acids (e.g., ^{35}S-methionine). In vitro translated proteins can be used as substrates for enzymes, in catalytic reactions, immunoprecipitations, DNA–protein interaction assays, and so on.

***E. Coli* EXPRESSION OF RECOMBINANT PROTEINS** *E. coli* were an early host for expression and continue to represent an important source for producing recombinant proteins. Expression in *E. coli* works best for relatively small, intracellular proteins that do not require extensive posttranslational modification for function. Proteins are expressed using plasmid expression vectors, many of which can be induced by treatment with reagents such as IPTG (relieves promoter repression), to cause high-level expression before purification. Attaching proteins of interest to other molecules such as β galactosidase can sometimes stabilize a protein that is otherwise subject to degradation in *E. coli*. It is also common to add a purification tag to the expressed protein to facilitate its recovery after expression. Common tags include glutathione-*S*-transferase (GST) for isolation on glutathione columns or a polyhistidine tag for isolation on nickel columns. Advantages of *E. coli* expression include the relative ease of the recombinant DNA manipulations (similar to plasmid cloning) and the rapid selection and expression process. Disadvantages include its inability to perform complex processing like glycosylation, and the fact that some proteins are labile (or toxic) in this host. Also, large proteins are not usually produced or folded efficiently.

BACULOVIRUS-MEDIATED EXPRESSION OF RECOMBINANT PROTEINS Baculovirus-driven expression in insect cells is another very common strategy for recombinant protein expression. Using transfer plasmids containing the cDNA of interest, recombination occurs with the baculoviral DNA in Sf9 cells such that the DNA sequence encoding a major viral coat protein, polyhedrin, is replaced with the protein of interest. This results in very high expression of the recombinant protein. Sf9 cells can carry out glycosylation (although structurally distinct from mammalian cells), and it is also possible to coexpress more than one protein subunit (e.g., immunoglobulins). The recombinant protein often assumes a relatively normal cellular localization (e.g., receptors on the membrane; transcription factors in the nucleus), although the high level of overexpression ultimately distorts this pattern. The high level of expression facilitates purification unless aggregation occurs. However, the requirements of recombination and selection make this system somewhat cumbersome if a large array of mutant proteins need to be investigated.

EXPRESSION IN MAMMALIAN CELL LINES For many proteins, it is desirable to perform expression in mammalian cell lines. These systems, while they rarely produce proteins as efficiently as *E. coli* or Baculovirus, have the advantage of processing complex polypeptides using intracellular machinery adapted for this purpose. In addition to requirements for precise peptide processing, folding, or glycosylation, the purpose of producing many recombinant proteins requires their expression in an homologous or tissue-specific system. For example, studies of certain receptors or transcription factors require their expression in cells that contain appropriate cofactors or targets. In the case of mammalian cell lines, expression of a cDNA is usually driven by a strong viral promoter. Alternatively, inducible expression vectors have been developed that allow selection of a clonal cell line followed by induction of the promoter by the addition (or removal) of reagents (e.g., tetracycline) that modulate promoter activity. Proteins with appropriate leader sequences may be secreted into the media. Although this results in dilution, there are many fewer contaminants in the extracellular media compared to the intracellular contents.

EXPRESSION BY ADENOVIRAL VECTORS A variety of viruses have been used for expression in mammalian cells, taking advantage of the natural tropism of viruses and their ability to induce alterations in the intracellular protein synthesis machinery that results in high-level expression. Adenoviral vectors have been of interest because they infect a wide spectrum of mammalian cells and because the adenoviral genome has been successfully altered to create replication-deficient viruses that can harbor mammalian gene sequences. Adenoviruses have been used to express recombinant proteins in cell lines and tissues that are otherwise difficult to transfect with high efficiency. However, their use as vectors for gene therapy has made them a particularly attractive system for gene expression.

By deleting key adenoviral genes, the modified virus can function as a carrier of mammalian genes. Introduction of the viral vector containing the gene of interest into E1a-expressing 293 cells allows the virus to be packaged and harvested, but it does not replicate in other cells. Adenovirus vectors have been used to express normal genes in defective organs (e.g., expression of CFTR in the lungs of patients with cystic fibrosis), to express toxic genes in tumors (e.g., *thymidine kinase* in brain tumors), and to target cell-cycle arrest genes in proliferating vascular cells. Limitations of adenovirus include an inability to accept foreign DNA greater than about 10 kb, relatively short-term expression in vivo (weeks to months), cytotoxicity, and induction of immune responses. Several other viral delivery systems are under investigation including Adeno-associated virus, Herpes virus, and retroviruses (which integrate in the host genome). Vaccinia viruses have also been used to express recombinant proteins in cell lines, such as HeLa cells, and provide an efficient mechanism for high-level expression of genes in mammalian cell lines.

OTHER SYSTEMS FOR RECOMBINANT PROTEIN EXPRESSION Although some of the guidelines noted above can help to direct the choice of an expression system, often this requires empiric trials of different systems to determine which one yields the highest levels of expression, the best bioactivity, or is most cost-effective in terms of reagents or labor. Thus, it is valuable to have an array of other alternative expression systems. Discussion of each of these is beyond the scope of this chapter, but they are described in the references. Other expression systems are as diverse as production in animal milk, *Drosophila*, yeast, and plants.

PROTEIN INTERACTIONS WITH DNA

Studies of protein–DNA interactions usually involve transcription factors that bind to regulatory elements in the promoters of genes (*see* Chapter 3). Characterization of these interactions can be accomplished by a variety of footprinting assays and more direct studies of protein binding to DNA, such as electrophoretic mobility shift assays. The goal of these studies is to identify the protein binding region of a gene, to characterize the transcription factor, and to correlate these results with functional studies of the promoter regulation.

DNA FOOTPRINTING Footprinting techniques refer to the fact that proteins can protect DNA from digestion by a nuclease, thereby leaving a footprint in the position where the protein was bound (Fig. 2-12). Footprinting assays can be performed in vivo and in vitro, and these approaches often give different results, suggesting that the interactions (or proteins involved) may be different in the intact cell in comparison to naked DNA that has been mixed with nuclear protein extracts.

For in vitro footprinting, DNA is labeled on one of the two strands and mixed with nuclear proteins. After allowing the sequence-specific proteins to bind to DNA, the nuclease DNase I is added at a concentration that will digest the DNA in a nearly random manner. The DNase I concentration used should cause somewhat less than one digestion per template to produce a ladder of labeled fragments. Where protein is bound to DNA, there will be an area that is protected from DNase I digestion. As a control, digestion of the same DNA fragment is carried out in the absence of nuclear proteins, or better still, using extracts that lack specific transcription factors. Digestion reactions are run on a DNA sequencing gel, such that a ladder of fragments is obtained. The areas that were protected by proteins are undigested compared to control DNA and appear as gaps. In vivo footprinting is similar except that permeabilized cells, or intact nuclei, are exposed to DNase I before isolation of DNA. The pattern of protection and digestion can be determined by using ligation-mediated PCR. Some footprinting procedures detect the ability of chemical modifications of specific residues (e.g., methylation) to modify access to DNA. For example, cells can be treated with dimethyl sulfate (DMS), which methylates guanine residues on the N7 position. DMS moves freely into the cell and methylates about 1 in 50 guanine residues. If a protein contacts a specific guanine residue, it will protect it from methylation and subsequent cleavage by piperidine. In addition, DMS treatment and piperidine cleavage can be combined when ligation-mediated PCR with gene-specific primers is used to amplify the gene of interest.

Although they are valuable for defining protein-binding regions, footprinting assays have several shortcomings. It is only possible to analyze about 150–200 bp at a time. Although one may identify a protected region of a gene, little information is gained concerning the number or nature of the bound proteins. The sensitivity of the assay is relatively low and detects primarily abundant, high-affinity proteins, since any free DNA in the reaction will partially obscure a footprint. The resolution of the binding site is relatively low, as DNase I cleavage may occur several basepairs away from a binding site and is somewhat sequence-specific. Last, it is relatively difficult to carry out detailed mutagenesis studies of the protein interaction site. For these reasons, other procedures such as the electrophoretic mobility shift assay (EMSA) have gained favor.

ELECTROPHORETIC MOBILITY SHIFT ASSAYS (EMSA) The EMSA is based on the fact that proteins bound to DNA shift its mobility during gel electrophoresis, forming new low-mobility complexes (Fig. 2-12). Whereas footprint analyses provide information about a broad region of interaction (150–200 bp), the labeled DNA used for EMSA is generally 10–50 bp in length. EMSA is highly sensitive and, because mutant oligonucleotides can be readily synthesized, the assay is particularly useful for determining the exact nucleotides necessary for protein binding. The changes in mobility of the DNA-protein complexes are somewhat proportional to the molecular mass of the protein complexes. For this reason, EMSA is useful for studies of protein dimerization and for resolving oligomeric protein complexes. EMSA also allows further characterization of the protein of interest by performing competition studies with unlabeled oligonucleotide and by using antibodies to supershift specific proteins.

The assay is performed by labeling an oligonucleotide with ^{32}P and performing incubations with proteins in nuclear or whole-cell extracts. It is usually necessary to include nonspecific oligonucleotides or carrier DNA to reduce the nonspecific binding to the labeled probe. The reactions are then subjected to nondenaturing polyacrylamide gel electrophoresis and exposed to autoradiographic film. The unbound DNA and DNA–protein complexes appear as distinct bands, reflecting their original mobility in the gel. Excess unlabeled oligonucleotide can be used as a

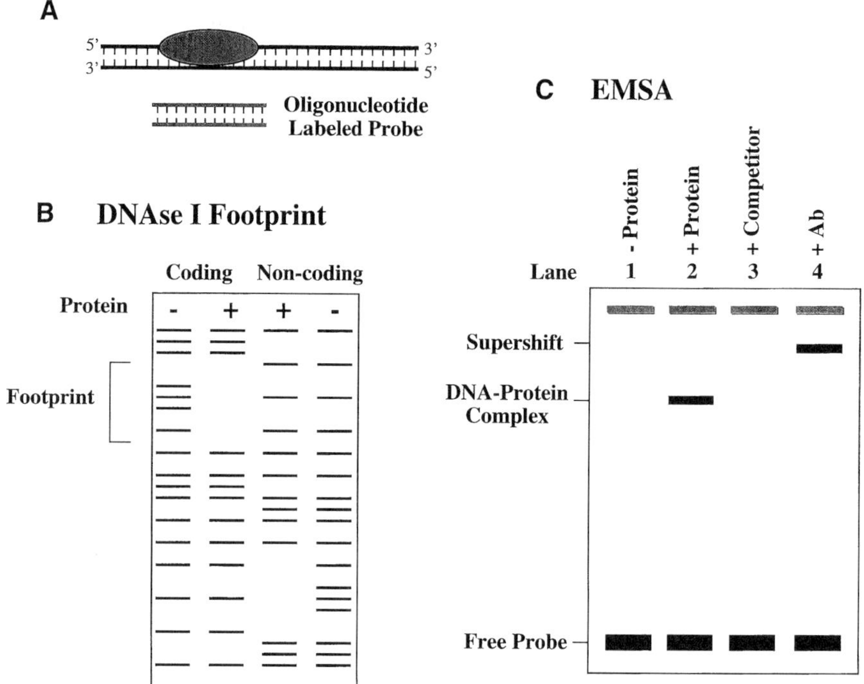

Figure 2-12 DNase I footprinting and electrophoretic mobility shift assays (EMSA). A variety of techniques can be used to detect DNA–protein interactions. **(A)** Schematic illustration of a transcription factor bound to DNA. **(B)** DNase I digestion of labeled DNA generates a ladder of labeled fragments. Protein bound to DNA protects it from digestion with DNase I, creating the appearance of a footprint. **(C)** EMSA refers to a delayed migration of labeled DNA caused by the binding of protein to DNA. The mobility shift of labeled DNA in the presence of protein is depicted in lane 2. Addition of unlabeled competitor DNA displaces bound protein (lane 3). Addition of an antibody (Ab) against the protein causes a supershift of the complex (lane 4).

competitor to establish the specificity of binding to the labeled probe. By using distinct oligonucleotide sequences that are known to bind particular proteins, it is possible to provide evidence for the nature of the bound proteins. As noted above, it is possible to further define the identity of binding proteins by using antibodies against candidate proteins. Antibodies can cause two different outcomes. If the antibody recognizes the protein in such a way that it alters DNA binding (e.g., recognizes the DNA binding domain), it may inhibit binding. Alternatively, an antibody may interact with the protein while it is bound to DNA, causing a supershift because of the addition of the high-molecular-mass antibody.

DNA AFFINITY COLUMN Isolation of unknown proteins can sometimes be accomplished by the use of an oligonucleotide affinity column. Using the methodologies described above, specific protein-binding DNA sequences can be identified along with mutations that disrupt protein binding. These oligonucleotides (usually multimerized) are biotinylated and attached to an avidin-containing column matrix. After partial purification, relatively crude protein extracts can be passed over the DNA affinity column that will retain specific binding proteins. It is sometimes useful to apply the eluted proteins to a mutant oligonucleotide column to eliminate nonspecific binding proteins. Several cycles of affinity chromatography can greatly enrich the specific activity of binding proteins. A common goal in this procedure is to obtain enough protein with sufficient purity for peptide sequencing to allow identification and cloning (using degenerate oligonucleotides) of the cognate transcription factor. Other uses include partial purification of transcription factors for in vitro transcription assays.

PROTEIN–PROTEIN INTERACTIONS

Protein–protein interactions can be identified by a variety of methods. Three methods will be discussed below: farwestern, immunoprecipitation, and yeast two-hybrid analyses.

FARWESTERN In a farwestern analysis, a protein is labeled and used to detect interacting proteins in a manner somewhat analogous to the use of antibodies in a Western blot (Table 2-2). The protein of interest must be expressed and labeled. If the protein is a phosphoprotein, in vitro phosphorylation with labeled ^{32}P-ATP and an appropriate kinase can be used. Alternatively, a protein kinase A tag may be added to the cDNA, allowing in vitro phosphorylation of the protein with protein kinase A. In vitro translation with radioactive amino acids such as ^{35}S-Met can also be used to label proteins that are to be used as probes. The assay is performed by subjecting whole cell extracts or nuclear extracts (or known proteins) to denaturing gel electrophoresis and allowing the proteins to renature during the transfer to a membrane. The labeled protein is then used to detect specific proteins on the membrane, providing an indication of the number of protein interactions and the approximate molecular weights of interacting proteins.

An analogous procedure can be used to screen expression cDNA libraries. Usually, farwestern blots of protein extracts are used to demonstrate that the protein probe works well and to establish specificity before a library is screened. This strategy was used, for example, to clone CREB binding protein (CBP) using ^{32}P-labeled CREB (cAMP response element-binding protein).

IMMUNOPRECIPITATION Immunoprecipitation involves the use of a specific antibody directed against a protein to precipitate it (along with other interacting proteins) from crude extracts. Currently, many antibodies (either polyclonal or monoclonal) are raised against recombinant proteins. Alternatively, if an antibody is unavailable, an epitope tag can be added to a cDNA to allow immunoprecipitation of the expressed protein.

In many cases, immunoprecipitation is carried out using cells that have been metabolically labeled with ^{35}S-methionine to allow detection of relatively small amounts of protein. After metabolic labeling, cells are lysed and incubated with the antibody to a specific protein. Precipitation is often performed using Staph A to recognize antibody complexes. After denaturing gel electrophoresis, precipitated proteins can be visualized by autoradiography. As noted above, in addition to the protein that the antibody is directed against, immunoprecipitation may also bring down proteins that are associated with the protein of interest. It is important to distinguish candidate-associated proteins from proteins that are precipitated nonspecifically.

YEAST TWO-HYBRID The yeast two-hybrid method takes advantage of the modularity of proteins. Construction of a hybrid molecule between the DNA-binding domain of a yeast transcription factor, Gal 4, and the protein of interest, creates a "bait" with which one can search for protein–protein interactions. The other construct is created by fusing a candidate-interacting protein to the transcription-activating domain, VP16. In this manner, a successful protein–protein interaction will bring the VP16 transactivation domain to the Gal 4 DNA binding domain, inducing transcription of genes that contain Gal 4 target sequences (Fig. 2-13). A variation of this procedure inserts a library of cDNA sequences into the VP16-containing construct to test for clones that interact with the bait protein, thereby inducing the transcription of selectable genes in yeast.

In a common version of this procedure, yeast cells are transformed with the cDNA-VP 16 fusion genes and transferred to restricted media. The gene necessary for growth on the restricted media is under the control of the Gal 4 transcription factor. The Gal 4 is fused with the protein-interaction domain of interest and should be designed to lack a transactivation domain. In this manner, for the yeast to grow on restricted media, protein–protein interactions must occur that bring the VP16 activation domain to the Gal 4 DNA-binding domain. From yeasts that are selected, clones of the VP16 fusion proteins can be isolated and analyzed further.

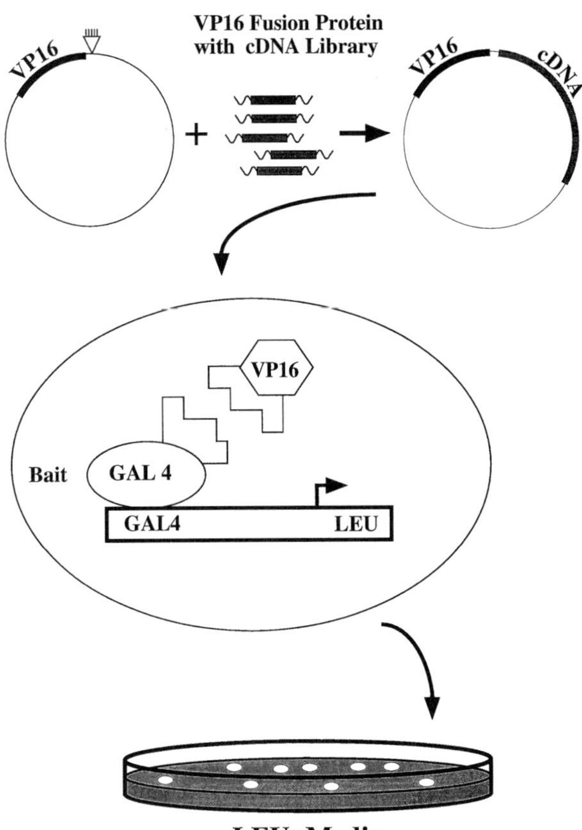

Figure 2-13 Yeast two-hybrid assay. A cDNA library is inserted into the VP16 fusion construct and introduced into yeast cells carrying the Gal 4 fusion construct, bait. A Gal 4 construct is created by fusing the Gal 4 DNA binding domain and the gene of interest. If protein–protein interactions take place between the gene of interest and the random cDNA-VP16 fusion, expression of the *leucine* gene will allow for the growth of yeast on leucine minus media.

ASSAYS OF GENE TRANSCRIPTION

Transcription assays are used to identify pathways that induce gene expression at the level of transcriptional initiation. In this manner, they extend the information gained by studies of steady-state mRNA levels, which are usually determined by techniques such as Northern blots, RNase protection assays, or RT-PCR. Using reporter genes as a reflection of the activity of transfected promoter–reporter fusion genes, it is possible to dissect the DNA regulatory elements within the promoter. An overview of nuclear run-on transcription assays and reporter gene assays will be presented in this section.

NUCLEAR RUN-ON ASSAYS Having demonstrated regulation of a mRNA by Northern blot or alternative methods, it is often important to know whether alterations in steady-state mRNA levels are because of changes in transcription of the gene or changes in mRNA stability. The nuclear "run-on assay" is classic approach for studies of transcriptional regulation. In this procedure, nuclei are isolated after a specific stimulus and allowed to carry out mRNA synthesis in vitro, because the amount of mRNA synthesis under these conditions reflects the number of transcripts initiated prior to isolation of nuclei. The initiated transcripts are elongated in the presence of radiolabeled ribonucleotides, and the labeled mRNA is hybridized to specific clones of immobilized DNA to allow quantitation.

TRANSIENT GENE EXPRESSION AND REPORTER GENE ASSAYS IN TRANSFECTED CELLS Transient gene expression studies provide an alternative technique for examining transcriptional control (Fig. 2-14). This method also allows detailed mutagenesis of cloned promoter sequences prior to their introduction into cells. In this procedure, the promoter sequences of genes are fused to a reporter gene that can be assayed readily. Common reporter genes include *chloramphenicol acetyltransferase* (CAT) and *luciferase* (LUC). In each case, these reporter genes represent enzyme activities that are not normally found in eukaryotic cells. Thus, in the absence of gene transfer, the background activity of these reporter enzymes is negligible. A host of commercial vectors are now available to allow the insertion of promoter or enhancer elements into various reporter gene constructs.

CAT assays catalyze the transfer of the acetyl group from acetyl-CoA to the substrate, chloramphenicol, and can be monitored by thin-layer chromatography, enzyme-linked immunosorbent assay (ELISA), or by liquid scintillation counting.

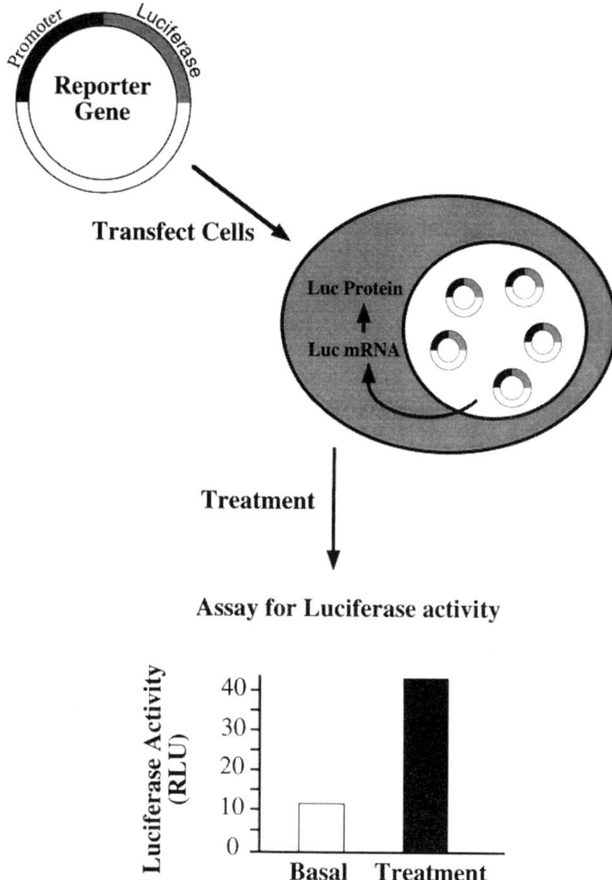

Figure 2-14 Luciferase reporter assay. Reporter plasmid is transfected into cells. Reporter plasmids mediate the transcription of the *luciferase* gene, which is then translated into luciferase protein. Six to forty-eight hours later the cells are lysed and assayed for luciferase activity. Adapted with permission. (Jameson JL. Applications of molecular biology in endocrinology. In: DeGroot LJ, ed. Endocrinology, 3rd ed., Philadelphia, PA: WB Saunders, 1995; pp. 119–147.)

Luciferase assays use the *luc* gene from the firefly, *Photinus pyralis*, which catalyzes the reaction of D-luciferin and ATP in the presence of O_2 and Mg^{+2}, to result in light emissions than can be measured using a luminometer. For both assays, the amount of enzyme activity is proportional to the amount of mRNA expressed, which, in turn, reflects the activity of the promoter being used. Luciferase assays are 30–100 times more sensitive than CAT assays. A variety of other reporter genes are also used, including β *galactosidase*, *growth hormone*, *alkaline phosphatase*, and *green fluorescent* protein genes.

The promoter–reporter fusion gene constructs are introduced into cells using a process referred to as transfection. Common transfection protocols include $Ca^{2+}PO_4$, DEAE-dextran, lipid-based, and electroporation. Transfected genes are transcriptionally active over 24–72 h, allowing relatively rapid analyses of promoter function. Alternatively, transfected genes can be stably introduced into cells by selecting for a resistance marker such as neomycin or dihydrofolate reductase. The principal goal of transfection experiments is to define DNA sequences that are required for promoter function or that respond to a specific extracellular signal or second messenger pathway. A variety of methods are now available to allow deletion or site-directed mutagenesis of promoter elements (Fig. 2-8). This approach has been critical for defining DNA sequences that regulate tissue-specific expression, basal promoter activity, and responses to intracellular signaling pathways.

SELECTED REFERENCES

Adams MD, Fields C, Venter JC. Automated DNA Sequencing and Analysis. New York: Academic, 1994.

Ausubel FM, Brent R, Kingston RE, et al. Short Protocols in Molecular Biology, 3rd ed. New York: Wiley, 1995.

Boultwood J. Gene Regulation: A Eukaryotic Perspective, 2nd ed. Totowa, NJ: Humana, 1997.

Harwood AJ. Basic DNA and RNA Protocols. Totowa, NJ: Humana, 1996.

Innis M, Gelfand DH, Sninsky JJ. PCR Strategies. New York: Academic, 1995.

Kneale GG. DNA-Protein Interactions: Principles and Protocols. Totowa, NJ: Humana, 1994.

Landegren U. Laboratory Protocols for Mutation Detection. Oxford, UK: Oxford University Press, 1996.

Latchman DS. Transcription Factors: A Practical Approach. Oxford, UK: IRL/Oxford University Press, 1993.

Leitch AR, Shwarzacher T, Jackson D, Leitch IJ. *In Situ* Hybridization. Oxford, UK: BIOS Scientific, 1994.

Lewin B. The extraordinary power of DNA technology. In: Genes V. Oxford, UK: Oxford University Press, 1994; pp. 633-656.

Tijssen P. Hybridization with Nucleic Acid Probes (Parts I and II). Amsterdam, North Holland: Elsevier, 1993.

Trower MK. In Vitro Mutagenesis Protocols. In: Methods in Molecular Biology, vol. 57, Totowa, NJ: Humana, 1996.

Tuan RS, Recombinant Gene Expression Protocols. Totowa, NJ: Humana, 1996.

Watson JD, Gilman M, Witkowski, Zoller M. Recombinant DNA, 2nd ed. New York: WH Freeman, 1992.

White BA. PCR Cloning Protocols: From Molecular Cloning to Genetic Engineering. Totowa, NJ: Humana, 1997.

Wu R. Recombinant DNA Methodology II. New York: Academic, 1995.

3 Transcriptional Control of Gene Expression

WADE JOHNSON AND J. LARRY JAMESON

INTRODUCTION

The concepts of gene function and transcriptional control are intimately intertwined. Early ideas about genes were based on specific traits that could be transmitted in a predictable manner through generations. From Gregor Mendel's studies of peas, the principle of using statistical approaches to understand genetics was established. His studies revealed the ability to predict the proportions of peas that would be yellow or green or exhibit smooth or wrinkled traits. The notion that these or other transmissible features were conveyed by genes was made more concrete by the studies of T. H. Morgan, who studied genetic transmission in Drosophila. Morgan demonstrated that certain traits were inherited together (or linked), reflecting their locations on the same chromosome. He also found that genes underwent recombination in a manner that reflected their distance from one another on a chromosome. Thus, genes that are widely separated have a greater statistical chance to undergo recombination than do genes that are immediately adjacent. These concepts of genes predated, of course, any understanding of the physical structure of a gene.

Pivotal concepts in the field of gene expression were articulated by Francois Jacob and Jacques Monod. They formulated the idea of a "messenger," now known to be mRNA, that linked genes to their biochemical effectors, such as enzymes and structural proteins. Inherent in the proposal of a messenger is the need to control gene expression. Thus, Jacob and Monod postulated an "operator," which would serve as a control switch for gene expression. This model proposed that repressors acted on the operator element and that expression could be activated by blocking the repressor.

The idea that gene expression (mRNA synthesis) is a regulated event is linked to the genetic concepts of alleles that act in *cis* and *trans*. Initially, these terms described the results of genetic complementation tests that were designed to determine whether recessive mutations reside in the same (*cis*) gene or in different (*trans*) genes. More recently, these terms have been adapted to describe other features of gene expression. Specifically, it has been convenient to conceptualize the promoter regions of genes in terms of *cis* and *trans*. For example, *cis*-acting mutations in an operator, normally controlled by a repressor protein, result in constitutive activation. Such a mutation affects only the genes that are directly linked to, and regulated by, the operon. Thus, the *cis*-acting sequences often refer to the regulatory DNA elements that control a gene. In contrast, *trans*-acting mutations refer to a diffusible factor, often a transcription factor. The conceptualization of *trans*-acting factors interacting with *cis*-elements in target genes helps to transfer genetic concepts into biochemical terms.

The field of gene regulation has a long history of creating models that predate detailed biochemical explanations. The idea of regulatory cascades required accepting the notion of diffusible factors before there was direct evidence for their existence. The *cis*-acting regulatory elements in promoters have often been characterized by mutagenesis before obtaining direct evidence that they bind a transcription factor. In practice, this is almost always true. Now that transcription factor interactions with DNA can be demonstrated more readily using sensitive techniques such as DNA-protein mobility shift assays, a new set of questions has arisen concerning how these DNA-bound proteins interact with the basal transcription apparatus. There is now a large body of evidence for the presence of adaptor or coactivator proteins, and the ability to use transcription factors to clone interacting coactivator proteins has greatly expanded our understanding of this family.

This chapter will focus largely on the principles of transcriptional control in higher eukaryotes. We acknowledge that many lines of thinking have arisen from studies of prokaryotes, yeast, and viruses. Indeed, the conservation of protein structure and regulatory pathways is very useful. Reflecting this conservation, many mammalian transcription factors are functional in yeast and vice versa. Nevertheless, space limitations necessitate a more limited review. Although the major focus is on transcriptional regulation, gene expression ultimately integrates many distinct regulatory steps, including transcription termination, mRNA stability, and the control of mRNA translation. Discussion of these other topics can be found in the listed references. We also hope to link information on transcriptional regulation to other topics covered in this book, including disease states that involve mutations in transcription factors.

The function of normal and mutant genes is influenced by their levels and patterns of expression as well as by the properties of the expressed proteins. Some disorders are caused by mutations in the regulatory regions of genes (e.g., some thalassemias) or more commonly because of mutations in transcription factors *(see below)*. In disorders that involve imprinting, the clinical manifestations largely reflect diminished gene expression from one of the parental alleles (e.g., Prader-Willi Syndrome). At least 20% of expressed genes are involved in gene and protein expression. By

From: *Principles of Molecular Medicine* (J. L. Jameson, ed.), ©1998 Humana Press Inc., Totowa, NJ.

comparison, it has been estimated, based on the composition of expressed sequence tagged (EST) genes from many different tissues, that cell structure and motility involve 8%, cell signaling involves 12%, and cell division involves 4% of the expressed genes. Although these results are preliminary (based on 7000 of an estimated 50,000–80,000 expressed genes), and the categorization is somewhat arbitrary, it is clear that a major fraction of genes are devoted to the control of gene expression. In addition to severe mutations in transcription factors, it is likely that many polygenic disorders will involve alterations in the levels of expression of certain genes or the sensitivity of a promoter to environmental effects.

STRUCTURE OF GENES

STRUCTURE AND FUNCTION OF THE NUCLEOSOME The formation of chromatin is a characteristic feature of eukaryotic DNA (*see* Chapter 1). Chromatin is composed of histones, nonhistone proteins, and DNA. The histones are highly conserved proteins involved in the packaging of DNA into nucleosomes (Fig. 3-1). Most DNA (~ 95%) is associated with nucleosomes. The nucleosomes function at several levels to provide hierarcheal organization of DNA. The first order of organization consists of 10-nm "beads on a string" in which nucleosomes and DNA are arranged in a linear fashion. The second order (30-nm fiber) arises when the nucleosomes are compacted into an helical array in a process that requires nonhistone proteins. The third order occurs when the fibers are packed on themselves to form euchromatin (low packaging) or heterochromatin (high packaging).

Histones 2A, 2B, 3, and 4 (H2A, H2B, H3, and H4) form the core nucleosome. Two molecules of H2A, H2B, H3, and H4 form the octameric core of the nucleosome. Histone 1 (H1) protein is probably not involved in the formation of the core nucleosome, as 10-nm fibers can be constructed without H1. However, second-order packing into the 30-nm fiber requires H1, which resides on the outside of the DNA-nucleosome complex and stabilizes the higher order structure. Based on digestion patterns generated by monococcal nuclease, it has been established that approximately 200 bp of DNA are associated with each nucleosome. DNA (80 bp) wraps around each core nucleosome twice like thread around a spool. A spacer (40 bp of DNA) links nucleosomes together to create the "beads on a string" appearance seen using electron microscopy.

In addition to playing a structural role in DNA packaging, it is likely that nucleosomes also participate in gene regulation. During the cell cycle, the structure of nucleosomes changes. In S phase, when DNA replication occurs, nucleosomes are acetylated. Acetylation occurs on lysine residues at the carboxyterminus of histone proteins and may alter their interactions with DNA. During G2 and mitosis, the nucleosomes are deacetylated and highly condensed.

Transcription factors have been shown to modulate the acetylation of histones, potentially modifying nucleosome structure as a mechanism of controlling gene transcription. For example, histone acetylation may create a more open chromatin configuration that allows other transcription factors to gain access to the regulatory regions of a gene. The transcriptional coactivator, CREB-binding protein (CBP), possesses intrinsic histone acetyltransferase (HAT) activity. CBP also recruits other HAT proteins such as P/CAF. It has been speculated that histone acetylation may be an important mechanism by which CBP increases gene transcription. Other transcription factors (often repressors) recruit histone deacetylases. MAD/MAX and Mxi1/MAX heterodimers bind Sin3, which acts as a scaffold protein to bind histone deacetylases 1 or 2 (HDAC 1, 2). Myc transformation of tissue culture cells can be blocked by MAX/Sin3 fusion proteins, but this inhibition is not seen using Sin3 proteins that do not bind to HDAC 1 or 2. Nuclear receptor co-repressors such as NCoR and SMRT also bind Sin3 and HDAC1 and 2 *(see below)*.

STRUCTURE OF THE TRANSCRIPTION UNIT A gene refers to an individual transcription unit that encodes either a single protein or a protein subunit. Genes are divided structurally into 5' and 3' regulatory regions that flank either side of the exons and introns (*see* Chapter 1). Exons refer to the portion of genes that are eventually spliced together to form messenger RNA. Introns refer to the spacing regions between the exons that are spliced out of precursor RNAs during RNA processing. The upstream 5' flanking regions of genes typically contain hormone response elements and other regulatory regions, including sequences involved in the initiation of transcription *(see below)*. This regulatory region of the gene is also referred to as the promoter, although this term is generally reserved for the proximal 100–300 bp upstream from the transcriptional start site. The minimal core promoter consists of a TATA box (which binds TBP, TATA-binding protein) and initiator sequences that enhance the formation of an active transcription complex. Transcriptional termination signals reside at the 3' end of the gene. In some instances, regulatory elements also reside downstream of the gene or in introns. Specific signals such as the AAUAAA sequence at the 3' end of the mRNA are involved in designating the site for polyadenylation (poly[A] tail).

With the exceptions noted above, the regulatory regions of genes generally reside in the 5' flanking DNA sequence of the gene. There is, however, great variation in the amount of DNA sequence that is required for normal expression of a gene. Almost all genes contain numerous (10–20) regulatory elements within the first 300 bp of the promoter (although comprehensive studies may be required to identify all elements). Most genes also contain several enhancer elements that are located further upstream. In some cases, such as the globins and the immunoglobulin genes, enhancers are located at great distances (>5 kb) from the remainder of the gene. An enhancer element was traditionally defined as a regulatory element that could operate over great distances and in an orientation-independent manner. However, further characterization of these elements, and the transcription factors that they bind, reveals considerable functional overlap with other promoter regulatory elements. Therefore, the distinction between enhancers and promoter regulatory elements has become blurred. The properties of these regulatory elements are strongly influenced by their locations in the gene and by the nature of surrounding DNA sequences.

The organization of a prototypical promoter is depicted in Fig. 3-2. The promoter contains a TATA box located about 30 bp upstream from the site of transcriptional initiation. Initiator sequences typically surround the transcriptional start site. The initiation of translation starts at the first ATG triplet codon within eukaryotic mRNA. The sequences prior to this ATG comprise the 5' untranslated region (5' UTR) and the most 5' base within the 5' UTR constitutes the transcriptional start site (designated as +1). The 5' UTR varies greatly in length in different genes, and it may contain several exons. For this reason, it can be challenging to identify the location of the promoter, even when the coding region of the gene has been found.

Several techniques are used to characterize the transcriptional start site(s) and, thereby, the location of the promoter. The S1 nuclease protection assay uses a single-stranded radio-

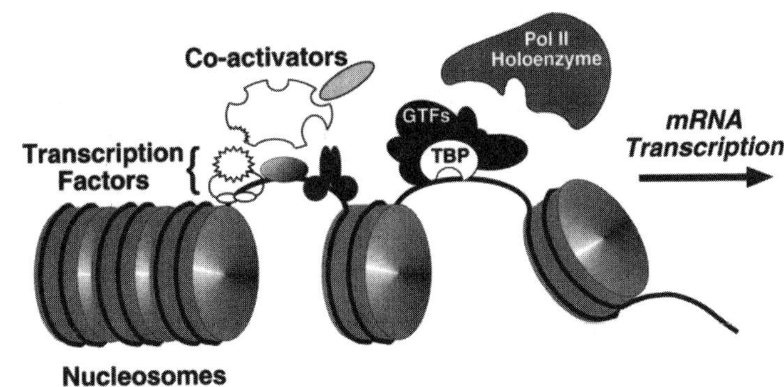

Figure 3-1 Role of nucleosomes in gene transcription. DNA is wrapped around nucleosomes, resembling thread on a spool. Actively transcribed genes exhibit an open chromatin structure in which nucleosomes have been disrupted or shifted to a different location along DNA. Altered nucleosome positioning allows the binding of transcription factors which, in turn, recruit coactivators and other components of the basal transcription apparatus (TBP, GTFs, Pol II). GTFs, General Transcription Factors; TBP, TATA-binding protein; Pol II, RNA Polymerase II.

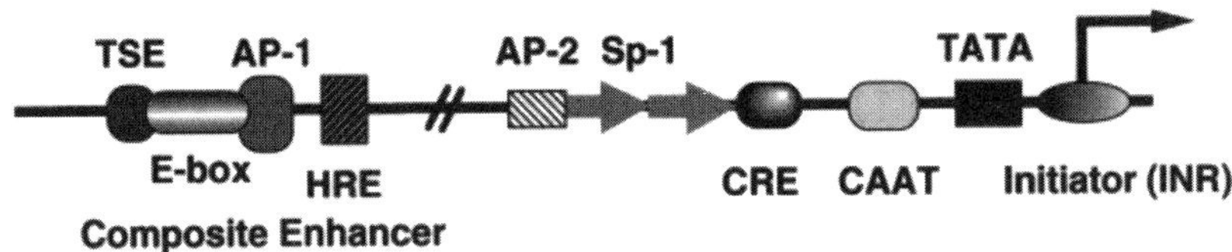

Figure 3-2 Structure of the regulatory region of a gene. A prototypical gene is depicted with an array of DNA regulatory elements. The core promoter includes the TATA-box that binds TATA-binding protein (TBP) and an initiator (INR) at the site of transcriptional initiation. The proximal promoter contains a CAAT-box that can bind several different transcription factors including CAAT-box/enhancer-binding protein (C/EBP), a cAMP response element (CRE) that binds members of the CREB/AP-1 family, an Sp-1 site (binds Sp-1), and an AP-2 site (binds AP-2). A composite enhancer is shown in the more distal 5'-flanking region of the promoter. It contains several closely spaced regulatory elements including a tissue-specific element (TSE), an E box (binds members of the bHLH family), and an AP-1 (c-Jun/c-Fos heterodimer) site. The composite nature of the enhancer allows combinatorial interactions of several different transcription factors to result in highly specific regulation. An adjacent hormone response element (HRE) is a binding site for members of the nuclear receptor family. Note that some regulatory elements, such as the AP-1 site, might reside in either enhancer or proximal promoter (e.g., CRE) locations.

labeled DNA probe that spans the 5' UTR and the transcription start site. S1 nuclease digests single-stranded RNA and DNA, leaving the protected DNA-RNA hybrid undigested. The length of the protected fragment allows the position of the start site to be deduced. An alternative approach uses primer extension in which a radiolabeled primer and reverse transcriptase are used to extend the mRNA to its 5' end. The promoter sequence adjacent to the identified transcriptional start site often contains characteristic sequences such as a TATA box and other DNA regulatory elements.

The TATA box is the site of binding for TATA-binding protein (TBP), which is a key component of transcription factor II D ($TF_{II}D$). The proximal region of the promoter is generally densely packed with transcription factor binding sites, only some of which are shown. This region often contains sites for ubiquitous proteins such as Sp-1, CAAT box/enhancer-binding protein (C/EBP), cAMP response element-binding protein (cAMP), or Activator Protein-1 (AP-1). However, factors involved in cell-specific expression may also bind to these sequences. Examples include interactions of bHLH proteins with E boxes in the myogenic genes (*see* Chapter 92), steroidogenic factor-1A (SF-1) for the steroidogenic enzyme promoters (*see* Chapter 57), or Pit-1 for the growth hormone promoter (*see* Chapter 49). At greater distances from the promoter, additional regulatory elements are often clustered in such a way that they form composite enhancers. These elements may be small, or they may contain several repeats of different transcription factor-binding sites dispersed over several hundred basepairs. In some cases, these distant enhancers are important for developmental expression (e.g., globins), cell-specific expression (e.g., immunoglobulins), or hormonal regulation (e.g., glucocorticoid response elements [GREs]). Although enhancer and promoter elements are usually depicted in a linear manner along DNA, it is likely that DNA looping occurs to allow interactions of enhancer-bound transcription factors with components of the basal promoter (Fig. 3-3). When active, these enhancer sites may confer DNase I sensitivity, reflecting the absence of nucleosomes, and an open configuration that allows increased access of DNase I (and other transcription factors).

The anatomy of a promoter is usually defined by a combination of gene transfer experiments to assess the effects of promoter mutants and studies of protein–DNA interactions *(see above)*. In the gene transfer experiments, various promoter regions are linked to a reporter gene, such as the gene encoding luciferase. Sequential deletions of the promoter provide a gross delineation of the locations of regulatory elements, but this strategy may miss functional elements that act in combination with sequences that have been deleted. Ideally, point mutations are introduced into candidate regulatory elements to assess their role in the context of the native promoter. It is advantageous to simultaneously search for transcription factor binding sites, either using DNase I footprinting or gel shift assays. DNase I footprinting is most useful for screening 100- to 300-bp regions of DNA for the locations of protein-bind-

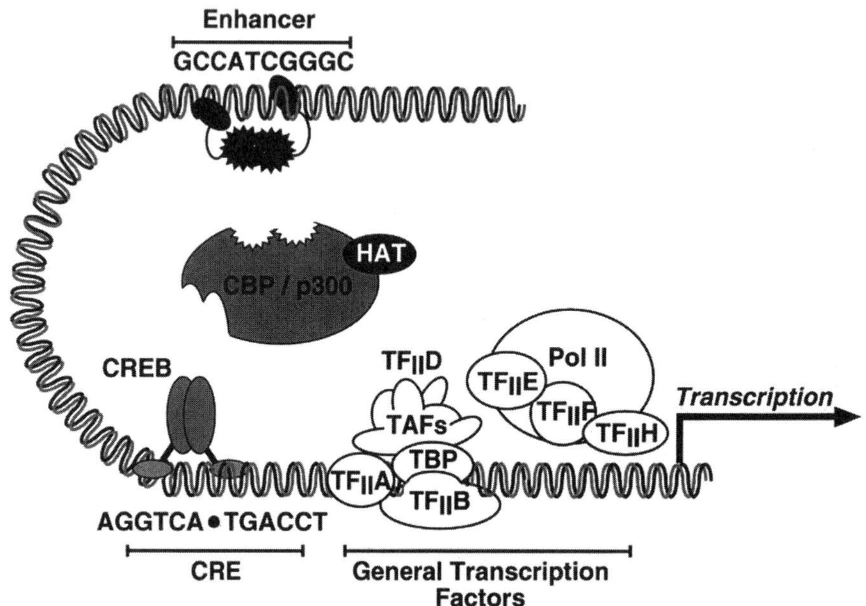

Figure 3-3 Enhancer interactions with proximal promoter elements. Many enhancers reside a great distance from the site of transcriptional initiation. DNA bending, or looping, has been proposed to allow protein–protein interactions. In the model shown, an enhancer binds a dimeric transcription factor that interacts with the coactivator protein, CREB-binding protein (CBP). CBP integrates the actions of many different transcription factors, including phosphorylated cAMP response element-binding protein (CREB). CBP, or its homolog, p300, interacts with other proteins including histone acetyltransferase (HAT) and general transcription factors (GTFs) such as $TF_{II}B$, and so on to induce transcription by RNA Polymerase II (Pol II).

ing sites. After the identification of protein binding sites by footprinting, the electrophoretic gel mobility shift assay (EMSA) is useful for more detailed analyses of protein–DNA interactions. EMSA is a very sensitive measure of protein–DNA interactions and is relatively simple to perform from a technical perspective. Competition studies using unlabeled DNA or supershift studies using antibodies directed against candidate transcription factors can help to verify the nature of the bound transcription factor.

CLASSIFICATION AND FUNCTION OF TRANSCRIPTION FACTORS

Because of the large number and diverse functions of transcription factors, it is helpful to group them into several classes based on their roles in gene transcription. In this chapter, transcription factors are divided into general transcription factors (GTFs), DNA sequence-specific transcription factors, and transcriptional coactivators and corepressors. The general transcription factors include a large number of proteins that are involved in the assembly of the basal transcription apparatus. As their name implies, the sequence-specific transcription factors include proteins that bind to DNA regulatory elements in the enhancers or promoters of genes. Coactivators and corepressors bind to other transcription factors through protein–protein interactions and regulate transcription by altering chromatin structure or by making contacts with the basal transcriptional machinery.

GENERAL TRANSCRIPTION FACTORS Eukaryotic cells contain three RNA polymerases that catalyze the transcription of DNA into RNA. Polymerase I transcribes ribosomal RNAs (rRNA), polymerase II transcribes protein coding genes (mRNAs), and polymerase III transcribes tRNAs. Although RNA polymerase II and its core proteins are able to catalyze RNA synthesis, they are insufficient for regulating gene-specific transcription. A large number of proteins are required for polymerase II (Pol II)-mediated transcription. Sequences associated with the core promoter (TATA box, Initiator) and gene-specific enhancers each serve to bind additional general transcription factors (GTFs) including TF_{II} A, B, D, E, F, and H, as well as RNA polymerase II and associated proteins such as suppressor of RNA polymerase B (II) (SRB). Purification of the RNA polymerase holoenzyme, which is transcriptionally inactive, with TF_{II} B, E, F, and H already bound, suggests that two major complexes of GTFs may be present in the cell: RNA polymerase holoenzyme and $TF_{II}D$.

$TF_{II}D$ refers to a protein complex composed of TBP and several TBP-associated factors (TAF_{II}'s). TBP is highly conserved through evolution. Drosophila TBP and mammalian TBP can be substituted for one another in vitro transcription assays. TBP binds specifically to the TATA box, binding in the minor groove of DNA, creating a 90° bend in the DNA. Some promoters do not contain a consensus TATA box, but TBP is still necessary for transcription. In the case of these TATA-less promoters, other GTFs apparently tether TBP and $TF_{II}D$ to the promoter. Many of the TATA-less promoters are characterized by multiple transcriptional start sites, suggesting that one role of the TATA box is to specify a precise position for transcriptional initiation. In addition to TBP, $TF_{II}D$ contains at least eight TAF_{II}s that recognize various promoters and establish contacts with other transcription factors. $TF_{II}A$ contacts TBP and stabilizes the TATA box interaction. $TF_{II}B$ contacts DNA on both the 5' and 3' side of the TATA box, specifies the transcriptional start site, and it is important for enhancer-mediated stimulation of transcription in vitro. $TF_{II}H$ contains helicase and kinase activities that are necessary for the initiation of transcription. As noted later, mutations in $TF_{II}H$ are one cause

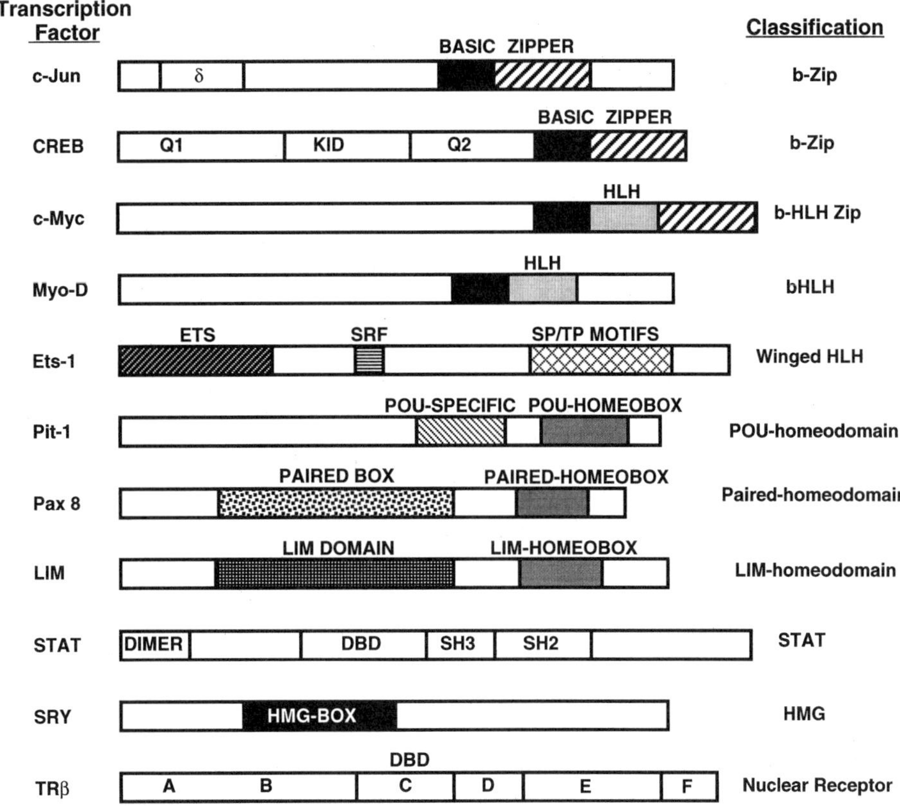

Figure 3-4 Classes of transcription factors. The structures of selected classes of transcription factors are depicted schematically. In general, the factors are classified according to their DNA-binding domains. Examples of transcription factors are shown at the left and the class of transcription factor is shown at the right. Some of the identified functional domains are shown. Q1 and Q2, represent activation domains; KID, kinase inhibitory domain; HLH, helix loop helix; SRF, serum response factor; SP/TP, serine, threonine phosphorylation; HMG, high mobility group; POU, Pit-1/Oct-1/Unc.

of xeroderma pigmentosa, which is characterized by DNA repair defects in response to UV irradiation. $TF_{II}E$ recruits $TF_{II}H$ to the preinitiation complex, and modulates the activity of $TF_{II}H$. $TF_{II}F$ recruits RNA polymerase II to the preinitiation complex.

In higher eukaryotes, the role that TAFs play in transcription is only partially understood. The composition of TAF_{II}s associated with the $TF_{II}D$-TBP complex provides a degree of specificity for RNA polymerase II. TAF function has been examined for a few transcription factors such as Sp1, which interacts with $dTAF_{110}$ in vitro. Transcription factor-TAF interactions likely serve as a bridge between enhancer regions and the basal transcription apparatus. Transcriptional activation via TAFs is influenced by the DNA sequence surrounding the TATA box and the Initiator. Hence, the core promoter architecture plays an important role in gene-specific regulation by recruiting the appropriate basal transcription factors.

DNA SEQUENCE-SPECIFIC TRANSCRIPTION FACTORS The ability of the basal transcriptional apparatus to respond to cell-specific and environmental signals is accomplished through DNA sequences that are specific to a given gene. These DNA regulatory sequences often reside in enhancer elements that are capable of conferring functions to a broad array of minimal promoters. Transcription factors that bind to enhancer regions are usually modular in structure and contain a DNA-binding domain and one or more activation domains. A partial compilation of various classes of sequence-specific transcription factors is shown in Fig. 3-4. This classification is based on the domain that binds to DNA and includes bZip, bHLH, homeodomain, and zinc-finger-containing classes of transcription factors. This classification is somewhat arbitrary, because some factors contain more than one type of domain or DNA-binding regions that are poorly defined. Examples of the functional roles of some of these sequence-specific factors are discussed later in this chapter.

It is striking that a relatively small number of DNA-binding structures have been used to generate tremendous diversity among the thousands of sequence-specific transcription factors. A transcription factor database on the Internet (http://transfac.gbf.de/) contains hundreds of different transcription factors and allows a promoter region to be searched for recognition sites for sequence-specific transcription factors. However, empirical determination of factor binding and function is ultimately necessary, because many consensus sequences are not particularly selective and transcription factor interactions can be dramatically influenced by surrounding DNA sequences or DNA-bound proteins.

TRANSCRIPTIONAL COACTIVATORS AND COREPRESSORS This class of transcription factors has been identified relatively recently. Because these proteins do not interact directly with DNA, it has been challenging to isolate these factors. However, largely based on techniques that detect protein–protein interactions (e.g., yeast two-hybrid, farwestern techniques), the list of identified members of this family is growing rapidly (Table 3-1).

Table 3-1
Transcriptional Coactivators and Corepressors

Cointegrators	**Interacting proteins**
CBP/p300	Nuclear Receptors[a]: (RAR, RXR, ER, TR, PR, GR) CREB, c-Fos, c-Jun, JunB, YY1, E1a, SV40 Tag, c-Myb, SRC-1, Sap 1a, STAT2, MyoD, E2F-1, TBP, $TF_{II}B$, p/CAF, $pp90^{RSK}$, Tax, SREBP-2, p53
Coactivators	**Nuclear receptors**
ARA_{70}	AR
GRIP 95, GRIP 120, GRIP 170	GR
p140 (ERAP 140, RIP 140)	ER, RAR
p160 (ERAP 160, RIP 160)	ER, RAR
SRC-1/ Nco-A1	PR, ER, RAR, RXR, TR, GR
Sug 1/Trip 1	TR, RAR, RXR
TIF 1	ER, RAR, RXR
TIF 2/GRIP 1	PR, ER, RAR, RXR
Corepressors	**Nuclear receptors**
NCoR 1	TR, RAR
SMRT	TR, RAR

[a]*See* Fig. 3-9 for abbreviations.

Coactivators have been identified primarily by using yeast two-hybrid screening assays. This assay takes advantage of the modularity of proteins. A yeast transcription factor, Gal 4, is fused to the protein of interest to create a "bait" with which to test for protein–protein interactions. By introducing a library of expressed cDNAs linked to a known transactivation domain (e.g., VP16), it is possible to select (by transcription of selectable genes) for interactions between the bait and proteins expressed from the cDNA library. An alternative to the yeast two-hybrid approach is to use farwestern analysis to screen for direct protein–protein interactions. The protein of interest is expressed, radiolabeled, and used to detect interacting proteins either from cell extracts (analogous to a Western blot) or from expression libraries. This method allowed phosphoCREB to be used to isolate clones for CBP.

It is likely that most sequence-specific transcription factors will be shown to interact with transcriptional coregulators. These proteins provide a mechanism for integrating the effects of several different transcription factors, and they also provide a linkage between enhancer-binding proteins and general transcription factors. Examples of regulation by coactivators are discussed later in this chapter using CBP/p300 as an example of an activator and the interaction of the thyroid hormone receptor with NCoR (nuclear receptor corepressor) as an example of a repressor.

OVERVIEW OF MODELS FOR TRANSCRIPTIONAL CONTROL

There is enormous variability in mechanisms of transcriptional control. In fact, every gene is controlled uniquely, whether in its spatial or temporal pattern of expression, or in its response to extracellular signals. Examples of signaling pathways that activate transcription factors are depicted in Fig. 3-5 (*see* Chapter 46). Thus, in addition to the diversity of transcription factors that are available, there is substantial diversity in the pathways that can activate transcription factors. Despite the myriad pathways and mechanisms for transcriptional activation (and repression), it is useful to consider fundamental models that recur for different genes.

TRANSCRIPTIONAL ACTIVATION Transcriptional activation can be divided into three main mechanisms (Fig. 3-6): (1) altered chromatin structure, (2) posttranslational modifications such as phosphorylation, (3) displacement of a repressor protein. These models are not mutually exclusive and some transcription factors participate in several different types of regulation.

The topic of chromatin reorganization was discussed above. Regulation of the *MMTV* promoter by the glucocorticoid receptor appears to involve alterations in chromatin structure. In this case, the glucocorticoid receptor is proposed to displace nucleosomes in a manner that allows the binding of additional transcription factors such as NF-1. CBP, which transduces the actions of many transcription factors *(see below)*, may also function in part through alterations in chromatin as several of the proteins that it recruits possess histone acetyltransferase activity.

Phosphorylation and dephosphorylation are key steps in the covalent modification of many transcription factors. Phosphorylation of the aminoterminal δ domain of c-Jun by Jun N-terminal kinase (JNK) stimulates the transcriptional activity of c-Jun. However, phosphorylation by mitogen-activated protein kinase (MAPK) near DNA binding domain of c-Jun inhibits transactivation. Hence, for maximal activation of c-Jun, both phosphorylation and dephosphorylation must occur in different regions of the protein. The role of phosphorylation in the control of CREB transcription has also been studied extensively. In this case, phosphorylation of a key serine residue (Ser 133) by one of several different kinases is required for transcriptional activation. Phosphorylation induces conformational changes in CREB that are necessary for interactions with CBP.

Ets-1 is phosphorylated by MAPK. When binding to its consensus DNA sequence, Ets-1 undergoes a conformational change, which induces its full activation. However, Ets-1 must interact with another factor to stabilize its interactions with the DNA. This type of synergism is exemplified by the c-*fos* promoter, where the binding of serum response factor (SRF) to the serum response element (SRE) recruits ternary complex factors (Ets-1). The synergistic interaction between SRF and Ets-1 accounts in part for rapid induction of the c-*fos* promoter in response to serum.

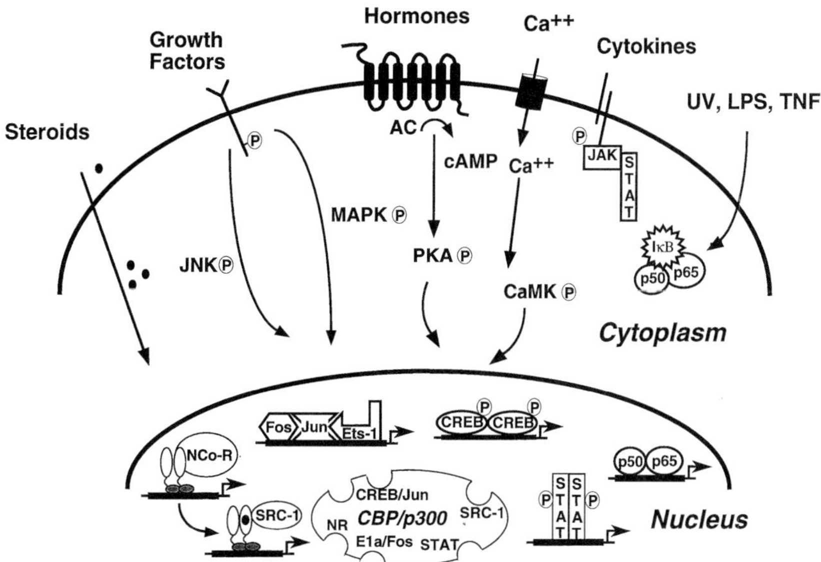

Figure 3-5 Signal transduction and transcriptional control. A diverse array of signaling pathways activate transcription (*see* Chapter 46). A highly simplified schema is shown to illustrate some of these pathways. Steroids (or other nuclear receptor ligands) diffuse through the cell membrane to act on nuclear receptors. For some of these receptors (e.g., RAR, TR), the ligand displaces a nuclear corepressor (NCoR) and allows interactions with a steroid receptor coactivator, SRC-1. Growth factors activate a variety of tyrosine kinase receptors that stimulate kinase cascades including mitogen-activated kinase (MAPK) and c-Jun kinase (JNK). These kinases activate transcription factors such as AP-1 (c-Jun/c-Fos) and Ets-1. Hormones (e.g., catecholamines, peptide hormones) can interact with seven transmembrane G-protein-coupled receptors to activate adenylyl cyclase (AC), resulting in cAMP production and stimulation of protein kinase A (PKA). This pathway activates transcription factor CREB, which can also be stimulated by other kinase pathways, including Ca^{2+}-mediated activation of CaMK (Ca^{2+}-mediated kinases). Cytokines stimulate the Janus kinases-signal transducers and activators of transcription (JAK-STAT) pathway, resulting in translocation of phosphorylated STAT transcription factors to the nucleus. Several cellular stress pathways (UV, ultraviolet light; LPS, lipopolysaccharide; TNF, tumor necrosis factor) activate NFκB (p50/p65) by dissociating the inhibitor, IκB. CREB-binding protein (CBP) binds to many different transcription factors, providing a mechanism for integration (or competition) among transcription factors.

In other cases, posttranscriptional modifications influence the cellular localization of a transcription factor (Fig. 3-5). NFκB is found in a cytoplasmic complex that consists of two subunits, p50 and p65, along with IκB. IκB binds to the two subunits and prevents their nuclear localization by masking the nuclear localization signal (NLS) within NFκB. Activation of NFκB requires the ubiquination and subsequent degradation of IκB, which allows translocation of NFκB to the nucleus. Signal transducers and activators of transcription (STAT) proteins are also found in an dormant state in the cytoplasm. Activation of cytokine receptors stimulates Janus Kinase (JAK), which phosphorylates the receptors, allowing recruitment of the STAT proteins (*see* Chapter 46). Once localized to the cytokine receptors, the STATs are phosphorylated, inducing dimerization and translocation to target genes in the nucleus.

Figure 3-6 *(right)* Mechanisms of transcriptional activation. Several models of transcriptional activation are shown (*see text* for details). **(A)** An activator protein induces an alteration in nucleosomes, thereby changing chromatin structure and allowing the recruitment of additional activators to DNA. **(B)** An activator is stimulated by a posttranslational modification such as phosphorylation, leading to the recruitment of additional activator proteins. **(C)** An activator displaces a repressor protein that binds to the same, or to an overlapping, site.

Mechanisms of Transcriptional Activation

A

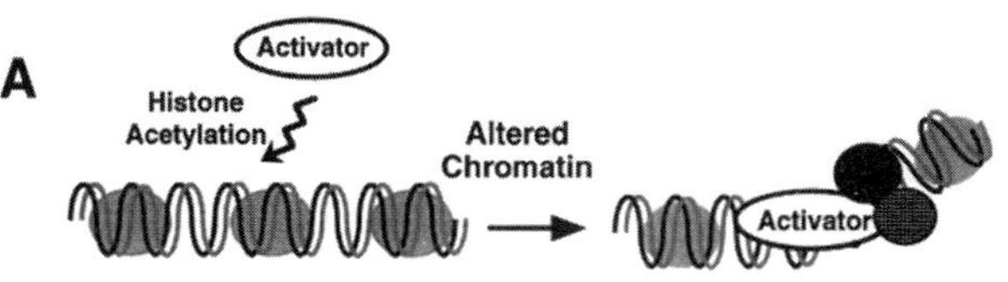

B

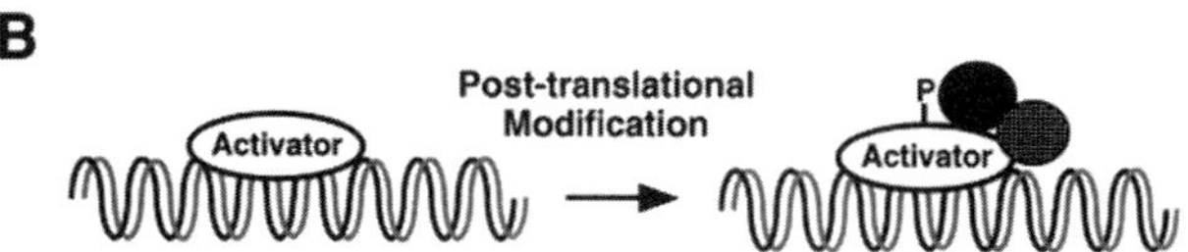

C

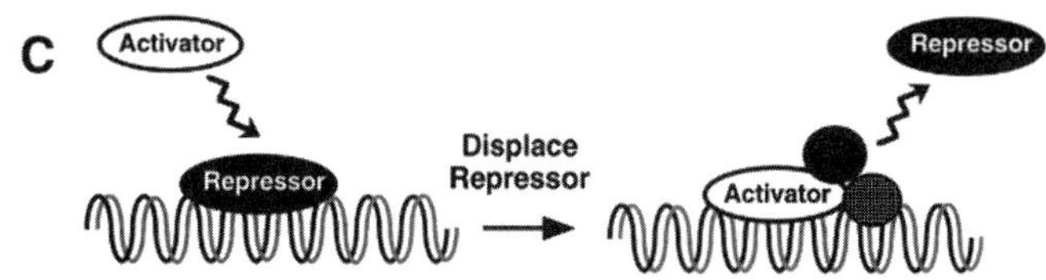

Figure 3-6

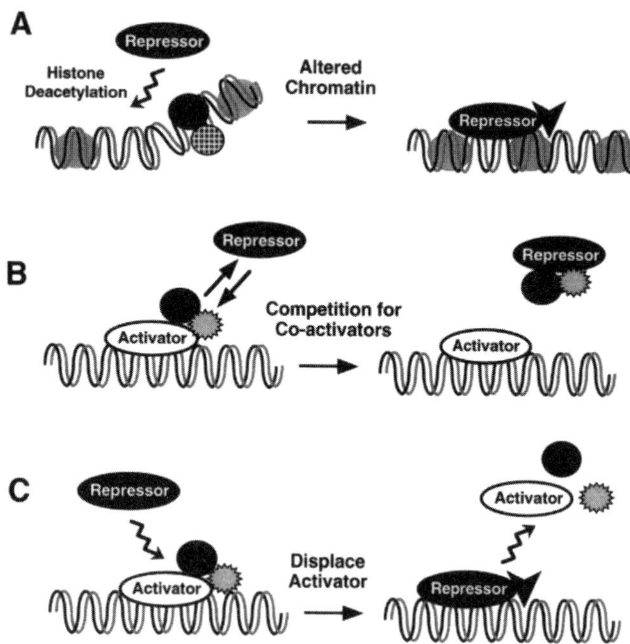

Figure 3-7 Mechanisms of transcriptional repression. Several models of transcriptional activation are shown (*see text* for details). **(A)** A repressor protein induces an alteration in nucleosomes, allowing the recruitment of additional proteins that silence transcription. **(B)** A repressor protein competes for coactivator proteins. This mechanism is sometimes referred to as transcriptional "squelching." **(C)** A repressor protein displaces an activator that binds to the same, or an overlapping, site.

Another model for transcriptional activation involves displacement of a repressor by an activator. This model applies in particular to developmental cascades, in which the induction of a new transcription factor may be sufficient to stimulate transcription, or it may displace a pre-existing repressor. The orphan nuclear receptor, COUP-TF, acts as a repressor of many genes that contain nuclear receptor binding sites. Under circumstances in which other nuclear receptors are induced or activated, they can displace COUP-TF and activate transcription.

TRANSCRIPTIONAL REPRESSION In general, mechanisms of transcriptional repression have not been studied to the same extent as mechanisms of transcriptional activation. In part, this reflects the technical challenges involved in measuring inhibition from a basal state of transcription. In certain respects, models for transcriptional repression are the reciprocal of activation, but there are also differences.

As shown in Fig. 3-7, some repressors act by causing histone deacetylation (as opposed to acetylation in activation). As described, this pathway has been investigated recently for the MAD/MAX proteins and nuclear receptors (RAR, TR). In these cases, the transcription factors bind Sin3 and recruit histone deacetylases. For nuclear receptors, transcriptional silencing is seen in the absence of ligand, and this is reversed at ligand binding *(see below)*.

Also analogous to mechanisms of activation is the possibility that repressors can act by displacing activators. A good example of this pathway involves expression of inducible cAMP early repressor (ICER), which can compete for the binding of CREB or CREM to cAMP response elements. ICER contains the bZip DNA binding domain of CREM, but does not contain the transactivation domains. Thus, when it occupies the DNA binding site, it is inactive and blocks access of other transactivators. The functional role of ICER is discussed later as a model for autoregulation of gene expression.

A distinct mechanism for transcriptional repression involves the inhibition of transcriptional activators, either by direct interactions between the repressor and an activator or by competition for a coactivator. An example of direct inhibition involves Id inhibition of bHLH factors. In this case, Id lacks a DNA binding domain, but it retains a dimerization domain, allowing interactions with bHLH proteins such as Myo D, E12, and E47. Dimerization of these proteins with Id forms an inactive complex and blocks the action of these transcription factors. Another example of direct interactions is illustrated by inhibition of NFκB or c-Jun by the glucocorticoid receptor. The glucocorticoid receptor has been shown to interact directly with these transcription factors to inhibit their action. However, it has also been suggested that the activated form of the glucocorticoid receptor may compete for the coactivator, CBP, which is also shared by c-Jun. Thus, negative regulation by the glucocorticoid receptor may occur by direct interactions and by competition for coactivators. Competition for rate-limiting coactivators may prove to be a relatively common model for transcriptional repression. For example, most cases of transcriptional squelching likely involve competition for limiting amounts of transcriptional coactivators.

PRINCIPLES OF TRANSCRIPTIONAL CONTROL

TRANSCRIPTION FACTORS ARE COMPOSED OF MODULAR FUNCTIONAL DOMAINS Soon after transcription factors were cloned, structure–function studies revealed a remarkable property: The functional domains of transcription factors are often separable and transferable. For example, domains involved in DNA binding can be localized to a relatively limited region of the protein and even swapped or exchanged into other transcription factors. Similarly, domains involved in dimerization, nuclear localization, phosphorylation, ligand binding, and transcriptional activation can also be localized and transferred to other proteins. These features suggest that for many transcription factors, functional domains are localized and are not created by complex three-dimensional interactions between distant parts of the protein. Another implication of this finding is that functional domains are often conserved during evolution. These "evolutionary modules" diverge, but retain enough similarity that homology is readily detected. Homeodomains provide an example of a conserved functional region that has become greatly diversified during evolution. The homeodomain proteins are typically involved in developmental events such as segmentation or cell lineage. The homeodomain itself is involved in DNA sequence recognition.

Two examples of transcription factors with well-characterized modular domains are shown in Fig. 3-4. The transcription factor, CREB, is representative of the basic leucine zipper (b-Zip) family of transcription factors. The carboxyterminal end of CREB contains a highly basic region adjacent to a series of repeated hydrophobic residues (primarily leucines) that are part of an amphipathic α-helix. The rotation of the α-helix positions the hydrophobic residues on the same surface of the protein. This feature has led to

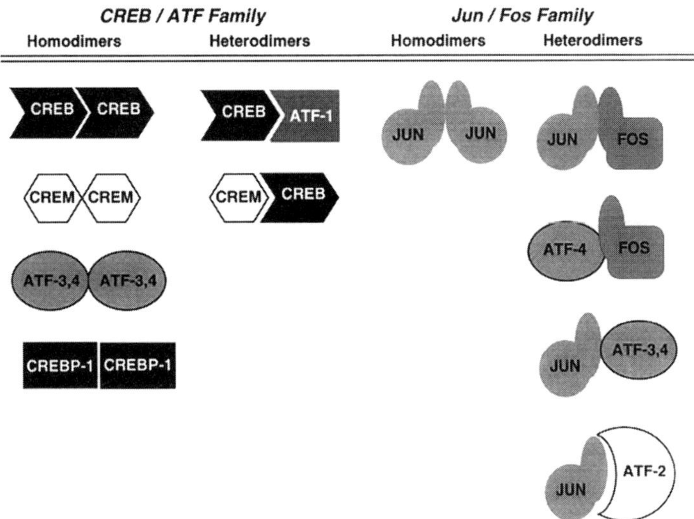

Figure 3-8 b-Zip family of transcription factors. b-Zip transcription factors are characterized by a domain comprised of a basic region adjacent to a leucine zipper. This domain mediates dimerization and DNA binding. The family can be subdivided into the CREB/ATF and Jun/Fos family. Different members of the family preferentially form homodimers or heterodimers. CREB, cAMP response element binding; CREM, cAMP response element modulator; ATF, activating transcription factor; CREBP, cAMP response element-binding protein.

the description of a "leucine zipper," in which a series of leucines (or other hydrophobic amino acids) are aligned with their hydrophobic side chains protruding from the protein. The hydrophobic amino acids create a dimerization interface that results in a coiled-coil of the two α helices. The adjacent basic residues are available to make contacts with negatively charged DNA. The DNA-sequence recognition sites for this family of transcription factors are palindromic in nature. Thus, there is twofold symmetry (e.g., TGAC • GTCA) in the DNA sequence, and the structure of the DNA element reflects in the symmetry of the transcription factor dimer. The binding affinity of the dimer is much greater than the protein monomers. This probably reflects conformational changes that occur after protein dimerization, as well as the additional interactions with DNA that are conferred by having two proteins make contacts with DNA. Members of the b-Zip family can form homodimers (e.g., CREB-CREB) or heterodimers (e.g., Jun-Fos), providing a mechanism for diverse interactions (Fig. 3-8). Subtle variations in the DNA recognition site provide specificity for the binding of different dimers.

In addition to its DNA-binding and dimerization domains, CREB also contains well-characterized transcriptional activation domains in its central and aminoterminal regions. These regions contain numerous sites for phosphorylation by enzymes such as protein kinase A and Ca^{2+}-dependent kinases. These phosphorylation events alter protein conformation and result in transcriptional activation. The modularity of this domain has been revealed by its ability to transfer transcriptional activation to the DNA binding domain of GAL4. The GAL4-CREB fusion protein recognizes a GAL4 target gene, but it is transcriptionally activated by protein kinase A. In this experimental paradigm, it has been possible to mutate specific serine residues in CREB to demonstrate that they are involved in phosphorylation-dependent transcription. As described below, phosphorylation of CREB allows the recruitment of a transcriptional coactivator, CBP.

The modular structure of the TR is also shown in Fig. 3-4. This receptor is representative of other nuclear receptors such as the glucocorticoid receptor, estrogen receptor, and retinoic acid receptor (Fig. 3-9). This nuclear receptor superfamily also includes a number of so-called orphan nuclear receptors for which a specific ligand has not been identified. Each member of this family contains a centrally located DNA-binding domain that is formed by two zinc fingers. The modular properties of this domain have been demonstrated in swapping experiments. For example, exchanging the DNA-binding domains of the thyroid hormone and glucocorticoid receptors switches their DNA recognition properties. Thus, a gene that is normally a target for the thyroid hormone receptor can be activated by glucocorticoids when the DNA binding domain from the thyroid hormone receptor is inserted into the glucocorticoid receptor. DNA-binding specificity is provided primarily by a stretch of amino acids (P-box) at the carboxy-terminal base of the first zinc finger. This region was identified because, in evolutionary comparisons of the zinc fingers in different receptors, it represented an area of hypervariability. Thus, substitution of this motif in the glucocorticoid receptor with that from the estrogen receptor switches its DNA-binding specificity to that of the estrogen receptor.

The carboxy-terminal region of the nuclear receptors contains several functional domains, including nuclear localization, dimerization, ligand binding, repression, and activation domains. The locations of these domains have been demonstrated by swapping protein region experiments to create chimeric nuclear receptors as well as by performing site-directed mutagenesis. The ligand-binding properties of these receptors require most of the carboxy-terminus. Consistent with this, the X-ray crystal structures demonstrate that the ligands bind deep in a pocket formed by several α-helical loops. During ligand binding, the receptor undergoes conformational changes, including repositioning of the transcriptional activation domains that contact coactivators.

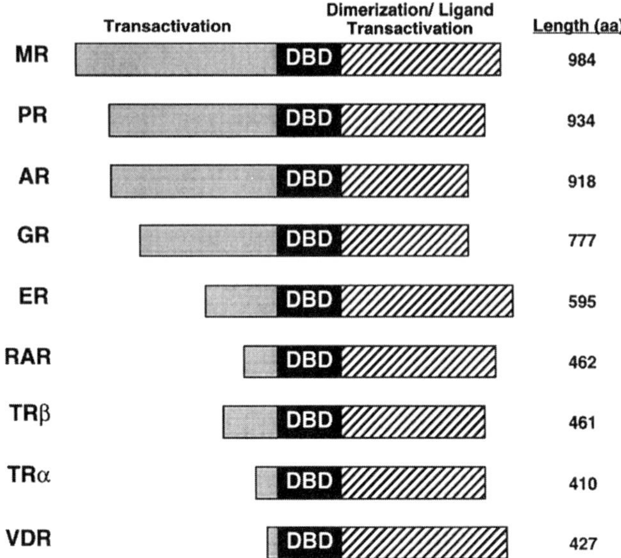

Figure 3-9 Comparison of nuclear receptors. Nuclear receptors share a highly conserved central DNA-binding domain (DBD) that consists of two (C2H2) zinc fingers. The carboxy-terminal region contains several functional domains including ligand binding, dimerization, transcriptional repression, and transcriptional activation. The amino-terminal domain is highly variable in length and contains additional transactivation domains. The lengths (in amino acids) are shown at the right side of the figure. MR, mineralocorticoid receptor; PR, progesterone receptor; AR, androgen receptor; GR, glucocorticoid receptor; ER, estrogen receptor; RAR, retinoic acid receptor; TR, thyroid hormone heceptor; VDR, vitamin D receptor.

Somewhat analogous to the b-Zip family of transcription factors, the nuclear receptors also form dimers. In this case, the dimerization domain is less clearly defined than the leucine zipper, but probably also involves hydrophobic interactions. In many cases, the nuclear receptors form heterodimers as well as homodimers. For example, the thyroid hormone receptor can homodimerize, but it also forms a heterodimer in combination with the retinoid X receptor (RXR). A second dimerization interface exists in the zinc-finger DNA-binding domain. The zinc fingers thereby orient the two monomers by interacting with specific DNA sequences. Thus, the target DNA site participates in a ternary complex of DNA and two protein subunits. In the case of the thyroid hormone receptor, the DNA recognition sites are surprisingly complex. Although most sites conform to a conserved half-site (AGGTCA) that interacts with one of the receptor monomers, the orientation of the two half-sites relative to one another is quite variable. For example, the half-sites can be arranged head-to-head (as a palindrome), head-to-tail (direct repeat), or tail-to-tail. These distinct orientations would predict that the carboxy-terminal dimerization domains would be positioned very differently or even on opposite sides of the DNA. However, these receptors appear to have a remarkably flexible hinge domain between the DNA binding domain and the carboxy-terminal dimerization domain. This hinge allows dimerization to occur irrespective of the alignment of the zinc-finger domains. In this way, the hinge has preserved the modularity of functional domains, while allowing great diversity in the DNA target sequences.

Transcriptional activation domains in the nuclear receptors have been localized in the carboxy-terminus, but also in the amino-terminus. The amino-terminal activation domains are constitutive or ligand-independent. This region of the nuclear receptors varies greatly in length and in sequence (Fig. 3-9). The activation domain in the carboxy-terminus is usually located near the extreme end of the protein. For many nuclear receptors, this function localizes to an amphipathic α helix that undergoes a marked conformational change during ligand binding. This region of the receptor contains a signature motif, LXXLL, that appears to be involved in interactions with coactivators (Table 3-1). The coactivators interact with the carboxy-terminal domain in a ligand-dependent manner, and it is thought that the recruitment of coactivators leads to interactions with the basal transcription apparatus, resulting in increased transcription.

The nuclear receptor carboxyterminal domain also interacts with corepressors such as NCoR and SMRT (Table 3-1). The corepressors bind close to the nuclear receptor hinge domain. In the case of the thyroid hormone receptor, the corepressors interact only in the absence of ligand. Thus, the ligand acts as a transcriptional switch (Fig. 3-10). In its absence, corepressors bind to the receptor and suppress transcription. Addition of the ligand dissociates the corepressor and allows the recruitment of coactivators. In physiologic terms, these properties allow thyroid hormone to induce a dynamic range of responses in its target genes.

DIMERIZATION PROVIDES A MECHANISM FOR DIVERSITY USING A LIMITED REPERTOIRE OF TRANSCRIPTION FACTORS Dimerization is common for many classes of transcription factors. The ability to dimerize accomplishes several goals:

1. Dimers allow the generation of diverse combinations of related factors.
2. Dimers provide the opportunity for variations in DNA sequence to specify interactions with different combinations of related factors.
3. Dimers can increase the affinity of transcription factor binding to DNA by contributing the energy (and conformational changes) induced by protein–protein interactions as well as by making additional contacts with DNA.
4. Dimers create an opportunity for pivotal transcriptional switches if some partners activate, whereas others inhibit it.

Many of these principles of dimerization have already been illustrated in the discussions of the modular domain of the b-Zip and nuclear receptor families of transcription factors. The basic helix-loop-helix (bHLH) family of transcription factors also emphasize the important role of dimerization. The helix-loop-helix motif was first identified as a DNA binding domain in λ-phage repressors. Variations of this structure are also found in homeodomain proteins and in the bHLH proteins. In the latter group, amphipathic helices that are connected by the loop create a dimerization surface and the basic regions of the protein partners make contacts with DNA. The DNA consensus sequence is typically an imperfect palindrome (CANNTG), reflecting the symmetry of the dimer. This family of transcription factors is often involved in cell lineage and growth regulation. Some of the factors such as E12 and E47 are expressed ubiquitously, whereas other factors (e.g., MyoD) are expressed in a tissue-specific manner (*see* Chapter 92). The ability to form homodimers and heterodimers is variable. For

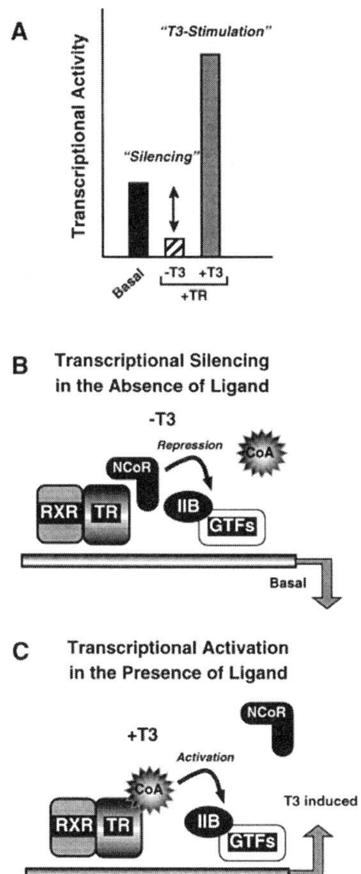

Figure 3-10 Transcriptional silencing and activation by the thyroid hormone receptor. **(A)** The thyroid hormone receptor (TR) silences transcription in the absence of its ligand, T3. Addition of the ligand reverses transcriptional silencing and induces transcription above the initial basal level of transcription. **(B)** Schematic depiction of transcriptional silencing based on the ability of TR to recruit a nuclear corepressor, NCoR. NCoR, in turn, recruits additional proteins (not shown) such as Sin3 and histone deacetylases, which may function to alter chromatin structure. **(C)** Depiction of transcriptional activation. T3 dissociates NCoRs and allows the recruitment of coactivators such as SRC (steroid receptor coactivator) to induce transcriptional activation.

example, E47 forms homodimers efficiently, but MyoD does not, and it preferentially forms heterodimers with one of the ubiquitous factors (e.g., E12/MyoD). The array of ubiquitous and cell-specific factors creates a combinatorial code that leads to selective gene expression. The bHLH family of dimers is also notable for the presence of a class of inhibitory domain partners, (Id). The Id proteins retain dimerization but lack DNA binding, thereby blocking the action of their protein partners. The availability of proteins such as Id provides an alternate mechanism for controlling target genes. For example, overexpression of Id can prevent MyoD-directed myogenesis. An analogous inhibitory pathway may also exist in the b-Zip proteins. In this case, inhibitory proteins such as CHOP or CREM (isoforms α, β, γ), can form inhibitory complexes with selected other members of the b-Zip family. In the nuclear receptor family, proteins such as COUP-TF dimers usually function to block target DNA sites, and a splicing variant (lacking the transactivation domain) of the thyroid hormone receptor, TRα2, binds RXR to form an inactive heterodimer.

UNIQUE COMBINATIONS OF TRANSCRIPTION FACTORS PROVIDE MECHANISMS FOR TISSUE-SPECIFIC EXPRESSION The issue of cell-specific expression has fascinated molecular biologists since the first Northern blots revealed that some genes are only expressed in one or a limited number of cell types. Among some of the early human cDNAs that were cloned, several exhibited highly restricted patterns of expression (e.g., globin, growth hormone, insulin, chorionic gonadotropin). Initially, investigators analyzed the promoter regions of these genes in search of cell-specific transcription factors in order to account for this property. Although such factors exist, it has been discovered repeatedly that the expression and function of many promoters are controlled by multiple regulatory elements and their cognate transcription factors. In the case of growth hormone, for example, the tissue-specific transcription factor, Pit-1, has been identified. Pit-1 is a member of the POU-homeodomain family, expressed specifically in the pituitary gland. The growth hormone promoter contains multiple binding sites for Pit-1. When coexpressed with the growth hormone promoter in nonpituitary cells, Pit-1 enhances growth hormone expression in the "ectopic" locus. However, in the absence of other enhancer binding factors, Pit-1 activates the growth hormone promoter rather weakly. When combined with other ubiquitous factors such as the thyroid hormone receptor, there is synergistic stimulation of the promoter. Synergistic interactions of transcription factors are commonly observed, particularly when an element contains adjacent cell-specific and ubiquitous factor-binding sites.

Mechanisms of cell-specific expression have expanded to embrace the concept of a "combinatorial code." This model holds that combinations of several different transcription factors allow unique patterns of transcription, including cell-specific expression. This idea is illustrated for several genes that are uniquely expressed in the thyroid gland, such as *thyroglobulin* and *thyroid peroxidase*. An array of transcription factors that bind to these promoters have been identified. TTF-1 (thyroid transcription factor-1) is highly expressed in the thyroid, but it is also expressed in the lung and brain. Another factor, PAX-8 (a paired box member), is expressed in thyroid, but also in the kidney. Although each of these factors are expressed selectively in the thyroid, they are also expressed in other tissues. However, their combined expression is unique to the thyroid gland. The absence of expression of thyroglobulin in other locations such as lung or kidney emphasizes the need for the combinations of transcription factors to achieve high-level tissue-specific expression.

Transgenic studies provide additional evidence that highly stringent mechanisms control gene transcription. Although transient expression studies often suggest that a limited region of a promoter is sufficient for high-level expression in a cell-type specific manner, transgenic studies frequently show different results. It is not uncommon to find that the proximal promoter sequence alone results in relatively low expression in the expected target tissue, or that leaky expression occurs in other cell types. In many cases, additional 5'-flanking sequences, or the inclusion of other regions of the gene (exons, introns, 3'-flanking sequences), allow recapitulation of the native pattern of expression (e.g., *proopiomelanocortin*, *vasopressin*). Presumably, control elements that either enhance cell-specific expression or suppress ectopic expression reside in these other regions of the gene.

Studies of c-*fos* promoter elements dramatically demonstrate the importance of combinatorial regulatory elements for normal function of the promoter in vivo. Transfection studies delineated a number of c-*fos* promoter elements including a sis-inducible element (SIE), SRE, an AP-1 site, and a Ca^{2+}-cAMP response element (CARE). Each of these elements functioned independently in transfection assays and only partially decreased c-*fos* promoter activity when mutated. In contrast, a mutation in any one of these elements was sufficient to preclude c-*fos* expression in transgenic mice, indicating strong interdependence in vivo.

TRANSCRIPTION FACTORS THAT INTERACT DIRECTLY WITH DNA SERVE TO RECRUIT ADDITIONAL REGULATORS THROUGH PROTEIN–PROTEIN INTERACTIONS The methods used to identify transcription factors have generally relied on interactions with DNA. For example, proteins that interact with enhancer elements can be identified by DNase I footprinting or gel shift assays. Using these and other strategies for transcription factor isolation, a large array of sequence-specific DNA-binding transcription factors have now been identified (Fig. 3-4). Although identification of these transcription factors represents a major advance, important questions remain concerning how the DNA-bound transcription factors act to initiate transcription.

Several lines of evidence have suggested that additional proteins serve as intermediates between enhancer binding factors and components of the basal transcription machinery. Genetic studies in yeast have identified a set of genes *(SWI1, SWI2/SNF2, SWI3, SNF5, SNF6)* that are involved in transcriptional activation and analogous proteins have been identified in *Drosophila*. Some of these proteins, such as SWI2/SNF2, appear to function by converting chromatin into a transcriptionally active, open form. A variety of viral proteins also appear to function as coactivators. For example, the adenovirus E1a protein can activate or repress transcription that is mediated by a variety of cellular genes, even though E1a does not bind directly to DNA.

Attempts to reconstitute transcription systems in vitro also supports the existence of non–DNA-binding coactivators. Early studies were able to reconstitute basal transcription in vitro using proximal promoter regions and initiator elements. However, the addition of upstream regulatory elements that have major effects on transcription in transfected cells, or in transgenic models, rarely induces marked activation, even when cognate transcription factors are added. Although there have been some success in the reconstitution of enhancer-mediated transcription (e.g., progesterone receptor), most such experiments still employ relatively unpurified nuclear extracts. The presence of coactivators in these systems is suggested by the loss of transcriptional activation with additional purification steps and by the ability to inhibit transcription by including excess amounts of transcription factors. Alternatively, it has been possible to demonstrate potentiation of in vitro transcription by supplementing the reaction with rate-limiting factors. Complementation of HeLa cell extracts with fractionated proteins from B cells was shown to enhance the activity of Oct-dependent transcription from the *immunoglobulin* promoter. An additional line of evidence suggesting the presence of coactivators involves overexpression experiments in transfected cells. In this paradigm, overexpression of many DNA-binding transcription factors is inhibitory. This "squelching" phenomenon has been proposed to involve the titration of rate-limiting coactivators (Fig. 3-7B). Moreover, when different transcription factors are used, there is often crosstalk of the squelching effect, suggesting that some coactivators are shared by several different transcription factors. For example, overexpression of an estrogen receptor can inhibit transcription by the glucocorticoid receptor, suggesting that they share a common coactivator (this is now known to be SRC-1, among others). In other cases, the squelching phenomenon appears to be less specific. For example, overexpression of a strong transactivator, such as the viral protein, VP16, can inhibit transcription by most genes. A key issue has been to elucidate whether these effects are nonspecific or actually serve as a bioassay for coactivators.

Several experimental approaches now provide direct evidence for coactivators. Using a yeast one-hydrid approach, a B-cell coactivator, Bob-1, that interacts with the octamer-binding protein, was isolated. This factor contains an interaction domain that contacts the POU domain of Oct-1 or Oct-2 and can modify its DNA binding specificity as well as enhancing transcriptional activation. As noted, a number of coactivators for the nuclear receptors have been isolated (Table 3-1), primarily by using a yeast two-hybrid strategy, in which the activation domain of the receptor is used as bait. The coactivators interact directly with the nuclear receptors without making contacts with DNA. They interact with the receptor in a ligand-dependent manner, implying a conformational change in the receptor. One class of the steroid receptor coactivators, SRC, interacts with the carboxy-terminal activation domain through a hydrophobic motif, LXXLL. The coactivator contains additional sequences that are involved in transactivation. Exactly how the coactivators facilitate transactivation remains unclear, but it is likely that additional intermediates connect these factors with the basal transcription machinery.

The CREB-binding protein (CBP), was identified based on direct protein–protein interactions. CREB was shown to detect a high molecular weight protein in farwestern blot assays, but only after phosphorylation of CREB at a residue (Ser 133) known to be required for transactivation. Based on this observation, radiolabeled phosphorylated CREB was used to screen cDNA expression libraries, allowing identification and cloning of CBP. CBP is postulated to function as an integrator of transcription, because in addition to CREB, it appears to mediate the actions of a large array of transcription factors and other coactivators (Fig. 3-11). A homolog of CBP, referred to as p300, was identified initially as target of adenovirus E1a protein. CBP contains distinct interaction domains for various classes of transcription factors. For example, the nuclear receptors interact with the aminoterminal region of CBP, whereas CREB interacts with a more central motif. CBP has been shown to enhance nuclear receptor transcription, particularly when combined with other coactivators such as SRC. Some experiments suggest that limiting amounts of CBP may provide a mechanism for transcriptional crosstalk between pathways. For example, AP-1-mediated transcription is inhibited by the activated glucocorticoid receptor, but this inhibition is reversed by the addition of excess CBP. CBP contains endogenous histone acetyltransferase (HAT) activity, and it also recruits a histone acetyltransferase to the promoter. One mechanism by which CBP may function is by altering histone acetylation and nucleosome structure.

As noted at the beginning of this chapter, initial concepts of gene regulation were based on models of repressors. In addition to repressors that bind directly to DNA, there is now good evidence for corepressors that act to silence gene transcription through interactions with DNA-bound proteins. This group of factors is exemplified by the nuclear receptor corepressors, silencing

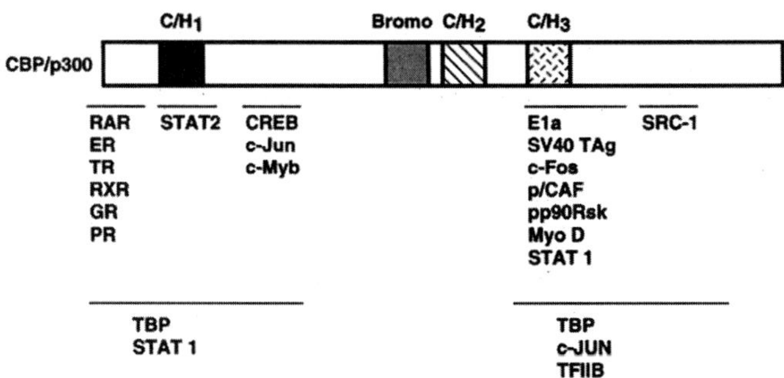

Figure 3-11 Domains of CBP. CREB-binding protein (CBP) is a large (270 kDa) protein that interacts with a many different transcription factors. Its domains are shown above the figure and interacting transcription factors are shown below the figure. RAR, retinoic acid receptor; ER, estrogen receptor; TR, thyroid Hormone receptor; RXR, retinoid X receptor; GR, glucocorticoid receptor; PR, progesterone receptor; STAT2, signal transducers and activators of transcription; CREB, cAMP response element binding; SV40 TAg, Simian virus 40 large T antigen; TBP, TATA-binding protein; TFIIB, transcription factor IIB; SRC-1, steroid receptor coactivator.

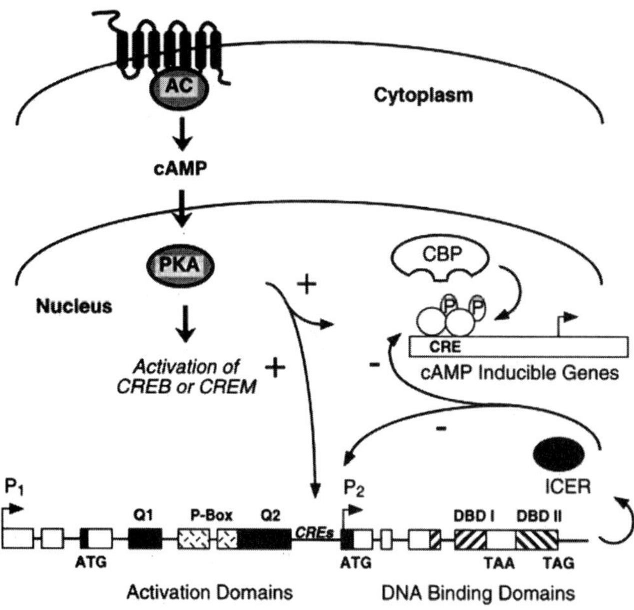

Figure 3-12 Autoregulation of transcription. Control of *cAMP response element modulator (CREM)* gene expression is shown as an example of autoregulation. The *CREM* gene contains two promoters, P1 and P2. The P1 promoter drives expression of a full-length protein that contains both activation domains (Q1, P-Box, Q2) and DNA-binding domains (DBD). The P2 promoter is located within an intron and drives expression of a small protein that only contains the CREM dimerization and DNA-binding domains. The P2 promoter contains a series of cAMP response elements (CREs) that are activated by the adenylyl cyclase (AC)-cAMP-protein kinase A (PKA) cascade. This pathway stimulates CREB and CREM, which induce the activity of the P2 promoter as well as other cAMP-responsive genes. Activation of the P2 promoter results in expression of *inducible* cAMP early repressor (ICER), which functions as repressor of CREs. Thus, ICER terminates its own production from the CREM gene and also inhibits a subset of other cAMP-responsive genes.

mediator of retinoid and thyroid receptors (SMRT) and nuclear receptor corepressor (N-CoR). These proteins were also cloned by a yeast two-hybrid approach. However, rather than binding to the receptors in the presence of ligand, they only interact in the absence of ligand. In addition to transfection studies, the ability of these factors to silence transcription has also been demonstrated using in vitro transcription assays, in which relief of silencing can be demonstrated by the addition of excess unliganded receptor (opposite of squelching). The mechanism of transcriptional silencing appears to involve Sin3A, which is a homolog of the yeast transcriptional repressor, Sin3p. In addition, a histone deacetylase interacts with Sin3A to form a multisubunit repressor complex. Thus, modifications of the state of histone acetylation, and the nature of nucleosome phasing near the regulatory region of genes, may represent a common pathway for control by transcriptional repressors and activators.

FEEDBACK MECHANISMS CONTROL THE TRANSCRIPTION OF MANY GENES

Although much work has focused on mechanisms of transcriptional activation, it is also important to switch genes off in a controlled manner. In some cases, this is a matter of reversing the step that leads to activation. For example, transcription factors that are activated by phosphorylation can be dephosphorylated by specific phosphatases. For a few genes, a pathway of autoregulation has been identified in which the product of a gene acts to regulate its own promoter. Autoregulation can be positive to result in rapid induction, or it can be negative to inhibit transcription once a certain level of the gene product has been achieved.

An example of both positive and negative feedback control occurs for the *Pit*-1 gene. The *Pit*-1 promoter contains regulatory elements that bind Pit-1, resulting in a positive feedback loop. However, high levels of Pit-1 are inhibitory, apparently because they bind to low-affinity sites downstream of the transcriptional start site. Thus, low levels of Pit-1 act positively, but high levels are inhibitory.

Another type of feedback inhibition is illustrated by control of *CREM* gene expression (Fig. 3-12). Like CREB, CREM is a phosphoprotein that regulates cAMP-responsive genes. However, CREM has multiple isoforms that act as either activators or repressors of transcription. CREM isoforms α, β, and γ are repressors, whereas isoforms τ, τ1, τ2, and τα are activators. Each of these isoforms are splicing variants derived from the P_1 promoter. The *CREM* gene also contains an intronic promoter, P_2, which transcribes ICER. The P_2 promoter contains several cAMP response elements. Thus, activation of the cAMP pathway and CREM expression results in rapid induction of ICER. ICER is a 120-amino acid (13.4-kDa protein) that contains only the DNA binding and dimerization domains of CREM. Because it binds to DNA, but lacks transactivation domains, ICER functions as a powerful repressor of cAMP-induced transcription. ICER may also inhibit CREB and CREM by forming inactive heterodimers.

Physiologically, the induction of ICER appears to terminate or dampen activation by the cAMP pathway. During spermatogenesis, CREMτ is initially induced in mature germ cells in response to stimulation by follicle-stimulating hormone (FSH). CREMτ expression leads to an increase in CRE-driven promoters, including the P_2 promoter that expresses ICER. Increasing levels of ICER feed back to attenuate the duration and amplitude of cAMP-responsive gene transcription. Hence, the increase in ICER protein downregulates its own transcription to terminate the cycle. This pathway also plays a role in the control of circadian rhythms. In the pineal gland, ICER levels vary dramatically during the 24-h cycle, with peak levels occurring at night. The enzyme serotonin *N*-acetyltransferase (NAT), which is involved in melatonin synthesis, is increased in CREM-deficient mice. Characterization of the NAT promoter revealed an ICER binding site, suggesting that increased expression results from the absence of ICER inhibition in the CREM-deficient mice.

ROLE OF TRANSCRIPTION FACTORS IN GENETIC AND ACQUIRED DISORDERS

As noted, a substantial fraction of expressed genes encode transcription factors. It is therefore not surprising that transcription factors have been associated with a number of different genetic disorders (Table 3-2). Transcription factors are obvious candidates to cause genetic and neoplastic disorders because of their roles as regulators of developmental pathways and as switches that respond to environmental signals. Therefore, it is possible to eliminate the expression of a gene, not only by a direct mutation in that gene, but also as a result of a mutation in a transcription factor that controls expression of the gene *(in trans)* or by preventing the development of the cell lineage in which the gene is expressed. Pit-1 mutations illustrate these points. Pit-1 is a POU-homeodomain protein that is selectively expressed in certain pituitary gland cell types. Pit-1 directly regulates the expression of pituitary genes including the *growth hormone* and *prolactin* genes (*see* Chapter 49). Mutations in Pit-1 cause deficiencies in growth hormone and prolactin and also impair the development of the somatomammotrope cell lineage that produces these hormones. In this manner, the transcription factor mutation results in clinical manifestations that resemble mutations in the target genes *(growth hormone, prolactin)*. However, in this case, the phenotype is broadened (includes thyroid-stimulating hormone) because the transcription factor participates in a cascade that controls the development of cell lineage in the pituitary.

Several other examples of transcription factors that control developmental cascades are summarized in Table 3-2. Genes in the paired box homeotic (PAX) family cause a wide variety of development disorders, which reflect their restricted patterns of distribution (*see* Chapter 112). The bHLH (basic helix-loop-helix) group of transcription factors have also been identified in many genetic disorders (e.g., Twist, MITF, MXI-1). This family of factors, which typically bind to DNA as heterodimers, are frequently involved in cell lineage development and tissue-specific expression (*see* Chapter 92). In addition to disorders that have already been identified, gene knockout experiments in mice predict an important role for these factors in other developmental disorders. The high-mobility group (HMG) proteins, SRY and SOX-9, comprise part of a pathway that leads to normal male sexual differentiation (*see* Chapters 57 and 58). Mutations in SRY cause XY sex reversal, and mutations in SOX-9 cause sex reversal in addition to skeletal abnormalities. The exact function of the HMG proteins remains unclear, but they are thought to induce DNA bending, which may facilitate the transcription of target genes. The homeodomain proteins, HNF-4α, HNF-1α, and IPF-1, participate in a pathway that leads to normal pancreatic islet cell development and function (*see* Chapter 47). Mutations in HNF-4α and HNF-1α cause a form of late-onset diabetes mellitus referred to as maturity onset diabetes of the young (MODY). Homozygous mutations in IPF-1 cause pancreatic agenesis, whereas heterozygous mutations appear to cause another form of MODY. These genes illustrate how mutations in several different steps in the same developmental pathway can result in phenotypically similar disorders (nonallelic genetic heterogeneity).

Mutations in the steroid hormone superfamily of nuclear receptors cause hormone resistance syndromes. For example, androgen receptor mutations (X-linked) cause androgen insensitivity. Severe mutations result in a syndrome referred to as testicular feminization, in which there is absolute resistance to androgen action, and the sexual phenotype appears female, even though inguinal testes are present and high levels of testosterone are produced (*see* Chapter 60). Similarly, estrogen, glucocorticoid, and vitamin D resistance syndromes result from mutations in their respective nuclear hormone receptors. Although these phenotypes can be predicted in part, the naturally occurring mutations have helped to elucidate the functional roles of the hormones and their receptors. For example, the estrogen receptor mutation prevented epiphyseal closure in the long bones, revealing that estrogen action is required (and cannot be substituted by androgens) for this event. In contrast to the other nuclear receptors, mutations in the thyroid hormone receptor illustrate a distinct property of some transcription factor mutations: the ability to function in a dominant negative manner. Thyroid hormone receptor mutations are transmitted in an autosomal dominant manner and cause partial end organ resistance to thyroid hormones (*see* Chapter 50). The basis for dominant transmission has been shown to involve the binding of mutant thyroid hormone receptors to target genes to block the function of the receptor from the normal allele. Consistent with this model, these receptor mutants retain the ability to form dimers and to bind to DNA, but they lack the ability to bind hormone or to initiate transcription. Analogous dominant negative mutations have been described for Pit-1, and are likely to be relatively common among transcription factor disorders, because they are manifest in the heterozygous state, and the modular nature of transcription factors lends itself to mutations that selectively inactivate one functional domain while preserving other features such as dimerization or DNA binding.

The relevance of modular functional domains in transcription factors in disease is also illustrated by the formation of chimeric factors in neoplasia (*see* Chapter 7). Particularly in leukemias and lymphomas (*see* Chapters 26 and 27), but also in soft tissue tumors (*see* Chapter 95), translocations combine different transcription factor domains or bring a transcriptional activation region under the control of a heterologous gene. Several examples of such translocations are listed in Table 3-2. In one case, the t(1;19)(q23; p13) translocation in pre–B-cell acute lymphoblastic leukemia fuses the PBX homeodomain gene to the transactivation domain of the E2A transcription factor gene. Similarly, in promyelocytic leukemia, a translocation t(15;17)(q22;q21) combines a zinc finger ring domain (PML) with the ligand binding and transactivation domain of the retinoic acid receptor. In this case, the chimeric receptor retains responsiveness to retinoic acid, which has been shown to induce differentiation of leukemic cells. The FUS-CHOP translocation (12;16)(q13;p11) may combine features of chimeric proteins and dominant negative activity and is associated with myxoid

Table 3-2

Examples of Transcription Factor Mutations and Rearrangements That Cause Disease

Transcription factor	*Class of factor*	*Disorder*
Developmental/multi-organ		
Brn-4[a]	POU domain	X-linked deafness; stapes fusion
PAX-2	Paired box homeotic	Colobomas optic nerve/ renal hypoplasia
PAX-3	Paired box homeotic	Waardenburg syndrome type 1
PAX-6	Paired box homeotic	Aniridia; Peter's anomaly
Ptx-1	Bicoid homeodomain	Rieg syndrome
Twist	bHLH	Saethre-Chotzen syndrome
MITF	bHLH	Microphthalmia; Waardenburg 2A
CBFα1	Runt domain	Cleidocranial dysplasia
GLI-3	Kruppel	Greig cephalopolysyndactyly
CBP	Bromodomain coactivator	Rubenstein-Taybi syndrome
Endocrine		
Pit-1	POU-homeodomain	Pituitary insufficiency
SRY	HMG	Sex reversal
SOX-9	HMG	Campomelic dysplasia; sex reversal
HNF-4	Nuclear receptor	MODY1
HNF-1α	Homeodomain	MODY3
IPF-1	Homeodomain	Pancreatic agenesis; MODY 4
TRβ	Zinc finger nuclear receptor	Resistance to thyroid hormone
AR	Zinc finger nuclear receptor	Androgen insensitivity
ERα	Zinc finger nuclear receptor	Estrogen resistance
GR	Zinc finger nuclear receptor	Glucocorticoid resistance
VDR	Zinc finger nuclear receptor	Vitamin D-resistant rickets type IIA
DAX-1	Nuclear receptor-like	Adrenal hypoplasia congenita
Cancer/hematology		
Rb	Cell cycle	Retinoblastoma; other cancers
p53	HLH-like; cell cycle	Li-Fraumeni syndrome; other cancers
WT1	Zinc finger	Wilm's tumor; Denys-Drash syndrome
MXI-1	bHLH	Prostate cancer
TFIIH	General transcription factor	Xeroderma pigmentosa; Cockayne syndrome
VHL	Transcription elongation	Von-Hippel-Lindau syndrome; Renal Ca
XH2	Chromatin remodeling	Mental retardation; α thalassemia
HMGI-C	HMG	Benign mesenchymal tumors
PTH-Cyclin D1	Translocation; cell cycle	Parathyroid adenoma
FUS-CHOP	Trans. factor-b-Zip	Mixed liposarcomas
Pax-3,7-FKHR	Paired box homeotic-forkhead	Alveolar rhabdomyosarcoma
EWS-ATF-1	Translocation; b-Zip	Ewing's sarcoma
E2A-PBX	Transc. factor-Homeodomain	Acute lymphoblastic leukemia
MLL-ELL	Translocation; elongation	Acute myeloid leukemia
CBFβ-MYHII	Translocation; MYHII	Acute myeloid leukemia
MLL-AF9	Translocation; AF9	Acute myeloid leukemia
PML-RAR	Translocation; Retinoid action	Acute promyelocytic leukemia
PDGFR-ETS	Translocation; ETS	Chronic myelogenous leukemia
TCR-Hox-11	Translocation; Homeodomain	T-cell leukemia
TCR-TTG-1,2	Translocation; LIM	T-cell leukemia
TCR-TAL-1,2	Translocation; Twist	T-cell leukemia
MLL-AF4	Translocation; AF4	Leukemia
TEL-AML1	Translocation; AML1	Leukemia
E2A-HLF	Translocation; b-Zip	Leukemia
Ig-MYC	Translocation; bHLH	Lymphoma; leukemia
RFX-A	RFX	Bare lymphocytes; MHC class II deficiency

[a]Many transcription factor abbreviations are now standard nomenclature. Selected abbreviations include: Brn-4, Brain-4; PAX, paired box homeotic gene; Ptx, pituitary homeo box; MITF, microphthalmia associated transcription factor; CBF, core-binding factor; GLI, amplified in Glioblastoma; CBP, CREB (cAMP responsive element binding)-binding protein; Pit, pituitary specific transcription factor; SRY, sex determining region Y; SOX, SRY box; HNF, hepatocyte nuclear factor; IPF, insulin promoter factor; TR, thyroid hormone receptor; AR, androgen receptor; ER, estrogen receptor; GR, glucocorticoid receptor; VDR, vitamin D receptor; DAX, dosage-sensitive sex-reversal-adrenal hypoplasia congenita critical region on the X-chromosome; Rb, retinoblastoma; WT, Wilm's tumor; MXI, MAX-interacting protein; VHL, Von Hippel-Lindau; HMG, high-mobility group; PTH, parathyroid hormone; FUS, fusion; EWS, Ewing's sarcoma; ATF, activating transcription factor; CHOP, C/EBP homologous protein; FKHR, Forkhead related; PBX, pre–B-cell leukemia; MLL, mixed lineage leukemia; ELL, elongation factor homologous to MLL; MYH, myosin heavy-chain polypeptide; PML, promyelocytic leukemia; RAR, retinoic acid receptor; PDGFR, platelet-derived growth factor receptor; HOX, homeobox; TCR, T-cell receptor; TAL, T-cell acute leukemia; TEL, translocation ETS leukemia; RFX-A, regulatory factor associated.

liposarcomas. The CHOP protein is normally a dominant inhibitor of members of the b-Zip family of transcription factors. However, in combination with FUS, which contains a transactivation domain, its inhibitory properties may be converted to activation. In other cases, the translocation results in ectopic expression of a transcription factor. This property is illustrated by translocations such as TCR-TAL, in which the T-cell receptor gene results in targeted overexpression of the twist-like protein, TAL. Similarly, the fusion of the *Ig* promoters to *Myc* causes overexpression of Myc in certain lymphomas and leukemias, and the *PTH* promoter has been shown to drive expression of cyclin D1 in a subset of parathyroid adenomas (*see* Chapter 51).

Transcription factors that are linked to cell-cycle control, such as Rb and p53, play major roles in neoplasia (*see* Chapter 7). Rb was discovered as a result of mapping the locus for the childhood disorder, retinoblastoma (*see* Chapter 105). This disorder established the principle of the so-called two-hit model for certain dominantly transmitted cancer syndromes. In this case, an inherited mutation in one copy of Rb creates a circumstance in which a second somatic mutation results in the inactivation of both alleles, leading to clonal expansion of neoplastic cell. Subsequent studies have shown that somatic Rb mutations occur in many different kinds of cancers (e.g., osteosarcoma, brain tumors, breast, genitourinary), some of which overlap with the tumors that develop in patients with germline mutations in Rb. The principle of the two-hit model for germline mutations is also illustrated by p53, which causes Li-Fraumeni syndrome (early breast cancer, soft tissue sarcomas, brain tumors, adrenal tumors, and so on). p53 activates a number of genes involved in cell cycle control including p21. p53 acts at the G1/S checkpoint and also governs the ability to arrest cell growth and to permit cells to undergo apoptosis (*see* Chapter 6). In addition to germline mutations in p53 in Li-Fraumeni syndrome, somatic mutations in p53 are among the most common tumor suppressor gene mutations in cancer (*see* Chapter 40).

It is surprising that mutations in factors such as the RARs do not have even more severe effects on cellular function. The phenotypes of the mice with knockouts of individual RAR isoforms (e.g., α, β, γ) are relatively subtle (occasional skeletal defects). The absence of a more severe phenotype has been attributed to the possibility of redundant function by the other isoforms. Other examples are emerging in which mutations in factors presumed to play a fundamental role in the function of the cell (and therefore assumed to be embryonic lethal) actually cause relatively specific postnatal syndromes. For example, a mutation in a component of the general transcription factor, $TF_{II}H$, is one cause of xeroderma pigmentosa. Similarly, the Von Hippel-Lindau gene product, which is involved in the control of transcriptional elongation, causes a syndrome consisting of predisposition to renal cancers, pheochromocytomas, retinal angiomas, and hemangiomas of the central nervous system (*see* Chapter 71). Another example is provided by the protein, CBP, which serves as a transcriptional integrator that links other transcription factors to the basal transcription factors. CBP is a coactivator for an enormous number of transcription factors including CREB and AP-1, nuclear receptors, c-myb, and STAT proteins (Fig. 3-11). Haploinsufficiency of CBP causes a severe, and characteristic, syndrome referred to as Rubenstein-Taybi. These patients have mental retardation, characteristic facies, broad thumbs, and great toes. In addition to its remaining normal allele, CBP function may be complemented to some degree by a homologous protein, p300. In view of the fraction of the genome that is dedicated to expression of transcription factors, we can expect the list of disorders caused by transcription factor mutations to grow further.

SELECTED REFERENCES

Alland L, Muhle R, Hou H. Role for N-CoR and histone deacetylase in Sin3-mediated transcriptional repression. Nature 1997;387:49–55.

Aso T, Shilatifard A, Conaway JW, Conaway RC. Transcription syndromes and the role of RNA polymerase II general transcription factors in human disease. J Clin Invest 1996;97:1561–1569.

Bannister AJ, Kouzarides T. The CBP co-activator is a histone acetyltransferase. Nature 1996;384:641–643.

Baron MH. Transcriptional control of globin gene switching during vertebrate development. Biochim Biophys Acta 1997;1351:51–72.

Chiba H, Muramatsu M, Nomoto A, Kato H. Two human homologues of Saccharomyces cerevisiae SWI2/SNF2 and Drosophila brahma are transcriptional coactivators cooperating with the estrogen receptor and the retinoic acid receptor. Nucleic Acids Res 1994; 22:1815–1820.

Choy B, Green MR. Eukaryotic activators function during multiple steps of preinitiation complex assembly. Nature 1993;366:531–536.

Glass CK, Rose DW, Rosenfeld MG. Nuclear receptor coactivators. Curr Opin Cell Biol 1997;9:222–232.

Gstaiger M, Knoepfel L, Georgiev O, Schaffner W, Hovens CM. A B-cell coactivator of octamer-binding transcription factors. Nature 1995;373:360–362.

Guarente L. Transcriptional coactivators in yeast and beyond. Trends Biochem Sci 1995;20:517–521.

Heinzel T, Lavinsky RM, Mullen TM, et al. A complex containing N-CoR, mSin3 and histone deacetylase mediates transcriptional repression. Nature 1997;387:43–48.

Hill CS, Treisman R. Transcriptional Regulation by Extracellular Signals: Mechanisms and Specificity. Cell 1995;80:199–211.

Judson HF. The Eighth Day of Creation: Makers of the Revolution in Biology. New York: Simon and Schuster, 1979; pp. 1–686.

Kamei Y, Xu L, Heinzel T, Torchia J, Kurokawa R, Gloss B, et al. A CBP integrator complex mediates transcriptional activation and AP-1 inhibition by nuclear receptors. Cell 1996;85:403–414.

Kingston RE, Green MR. Modeling eukaryotic transcriptional activation. Curr Biol 1994;4:325–332.

Kwok RP, Lundblad JR, Chrivia JC, et al. Nuclear protein CBP is a coactivator for the transcription factor CREB. Nature 1994;370:223–226.

Laherty CD, Yang WM, Sun JM, Davie JR, Seto E, Eisenman RN. Histone deacetylases associated with the mSin3 corepressor mediate mad transcriptional repression. Cell 1997;89:349–356.

Latchman DS. Transcription-factor mutations and disease. N Engl J Med 1996;334:28–33.

Lewin B. Genes V. Oxford; Oxford University Press, 1994; pp. 1–1272.

Liu F, Green MR. Promoter targeting by adenovirus E1a through interaction with different cellular DNA-binding domains. Nature 1994;368: 520–525.

Paranjape SM, Kamakaka RT, Kadonaga JT. Role of chromatin structure in the regulation of transcription by RNA polymerase II. Annu Rev Biochem 1994;63:265–297.

Ptashne M, Gann A. Transcriptional activation by recruitment. Nature 1997;386:569–577.

Rabbitts TH. Chromosomal translocations in human cancer. Nature 1994;372:143–149.

Rhodes SJ, Chen R, DeMattia GE, et al. A tissue-specific enhancer confers Pit-1-dependent morphogen inducibility and autoregulation on the pit-1 gene. Genes Dev 1993;7:913–932.

Robertson LM, Kerppola TK, Vendrell M, et al. Regulation of c-fos expression in transgenic mice requires multiple interdependent transcription control elements. Neuron 1995;14:241–252.

Roeder RG. The role of general initiation factors in transcription by RNA polymerase II. Trends in Biochem Sci 1996;21:327–335.

Sassone-Corsi P. Transcription factors responsive to cAMP. Annu Rev Cell Dev Biol 1995;11:355–377.

Sauer F, Hansen SK, Tjian R. DNA template and activator-coactivator requirements for transcriptional synergism by Drosophila bicoid. Science 1995;270:1825–1828.

Shikama N, Lyon J, La Thangue NB. The p300/CBP family: integrating signals with transcription factors nad chromatin. Trends in Cell Biology 1997;6:230–236.

Smale ST. Transcription initiation from TATA-less promoters within eukaryotic protein-coding genes. Biochim Biophys Acta 1997;1351:73–88.

Smith CL, Onate SA, Tsai MJ, O'Malley BW. CREB binding protein acts synergistically with steroid receptor coactivator-1 to enhance steroid receptor-dependent transcription. Proc Natl Acad Sci USA 1996;93:8884–8888.

Tjian R, Maniatis T. Transcriptional activation: a complex puzzle with few easy pieces. Cell 1994;77:5–8.

Torchia J, Rose DW, Inostroza J, et al. The transcriptional co-activator p/CIP binds CBP and mediates nuclear- receptor function. Nature 1997;387:677–684.

Wade PA, Wolffe AP. Chromatin: histone acetyltransferases in control. Curr Biol 1997;7:R82–R84.

Wolffe AP. Transcription: in tune with the histones. Cell 1994;77:13–16.

Wolffe AP. Transcriptional control. Sinful repression. Nature 1997;387:16, 17.

Zwicker J, Muller R. Cell-cycle regulation of gene expression by transcriptional repression. Trends Genet 1997;13:3–6.

4 Transmission of Human Genetic Disease

PETER KOPP AND J. LARRY JAMESON

INTRODUCTION

Molecular DNA analysis has become an integral part of all medical specialties. Although the immense size and complexity of the human genome is daunting, recent progress in the Human Genome Project has greatly increased our knowledge of the genetic basis of many human diseases (*see* Chapter 5). The impact of molecular DNA analysis and genetics in clinical medicine includes new approaches for the diagnosis of diseases, the detection of pathogens, screening for disease predisposition, genetic counseling, drug development, pharmacotherapy, and, in selected cases, gene therapy.

More than 3000 human diseases are known to be caused by defects in single genes and to follow a Mendelian mode of inheritance. Moreover, many disease processes are influenced by the genetic background of the affected individual. There is often a complex interaction between environmental factors and genetic predisposition. Many of these disorders (e.g., hypertension, coronary artery disease, asthma, diabetes) represent major public health problems and the elucidation of their pathogenesis remains an extraordinary challenge. Other genetically determined forms of disease include the syndromes caused by chromosomal aberrations and inherited cancer syndromes, as well as nonhereditary somatic cell DNA defects that occur in cancer.

DNA AND THE TRANSMISSION OF GENETIC INFORMATION The double-stranded macromolecule DNA contains the genetic information. It consists of two complementary strands that wrap around one another to form a double helix. Each strand is a linear arrangement of four different bases: adenine (A), thymine (T), cytosine (C), and guanine (G). The order of the bases forms the DNA sequence. The two DNA strands are held together by hydrogen bonds formed between the complementary bases G and C, or A and T. Because the nucleotide chains within the double-stranded DNA are strictly complementary, each can serve as template for the formation of a new strand. This semiconservative form of replication ensures that each dividing cell receives an identical copy of DNA (*see* Chapter 6).

In the coding sequence of a gene, each set of three DNA bases forms a codon, the genetic code for the incorporation of one of the 20 amino acids found in proteins (Fig. 4-1). A series of codons thus defines which amino acids will be synthesized into a given polypeptide. The protein-coding instructions found in the DNA sequence of a gene are first transcribed into mRNA. The mRNA is translocated from the nucleus into the cytoplasm, where it is translated by ribosomes into a string of amino acids (protein synthesis).

From: *Principles of Molecular Medicine* (J. L. Jameson, ed.), ©1998 Humana Press Inc., Totowa, NJ.

CHROMOSOMES, GENES, AND DNA

A detailed description of molecular genetic techniques is beyond the scope of this chapter, but it is useful to present some of the key concepts and techniques that are essential for the analysis of the genome and genetic diseases (*see* Chapters 1 and 2). Aspects of gene manipulation are also covered in chapters on transgenic models (*see* Chapter 10) and gene therapy (*see* Chapter 18).

SIZE AND ORGANIZATION OF THE HUMAN GENOME The genome is encoded by a coiled polymer of deoxyribonucleic acid (DNA) that is separated into several segments, the chromosomes (*see* Chapter 1). In humans, every somatic cell is diploid and contains two sets of 23 chromosomes. A child receives one copy of every chromosome from its mother, and one copy from its father. The 22 autosomal chromosomes are present in two copies, and are similar in females and males. The sex chromosomes, X and Y, are dissimilar. Only a small segment of the short arm of both the X and Y chromosomes, the pseudoautosomal region (PAR), shares homology. Females have two X chromosomes (XX), while males are heterogametic (XY). The DNA of a single or haploid set of chromosomes consists of approximately 3×10^9 bp (3000 Mb), with the smallest chromosome containing ~50 Mb (chromosome 21) and the largest ~263 Mb (chromosome 1).

A gene consists of regulatory DNA sequences, coding sequences (exons), and intervening noncoding sequences (introns). The sequences of a gene that encode a protein are located in exons, which are spliced together to form the messenger ribonucleic acid (mRNA). Based on the number of expressed mRNAs, it has been estimated that the human genome contains about 70,000 to 100,000 genes. The size and structure of genes is highly variable. Some small genes consist of a few hundred basepairs, while the largest gene known to date, the X-chromosomal gene encoding the protein dystrophin, contains about 2×10^6 bp with more than 100 introns. Mutations in this gene lead to two distinct clinical conditions, Duchenne Muscular Dystrophy (DMD) and Becker Muscular Dystrophy (BMD). Some chromosomal regions, particularly near the centromeres, do not contain genes, while others display a high gene density. Occasionally, genes are grouped into clusters in which several copies of genes with similar function are located near one another. Examples of gene clusters are the growth hormone genes, or the genes encoding α and β globin. In other

First Base	Second Base U	Second Base C	Second Base A	Second Base G	Third Base
U	Phe	Ser	Tyr	Cys	U
	Phe	Ser	Tyr	Cys	C
	Leu	Ser	Stop	Stop	A
	Leu	Ser	Stop	Trp	G
C	Leu	Pro	His	Arg	U
	Leu	Pro	His	Arg	C
	Leu	Pro	Gln	Arg	A
	Leu	Pro	Gln	Arg	G
A	Ile	Thr	Asn	Ser	U
	Ile	Thr	Asn	Ser	C
	Ile	Thr	Lys	Arg	A
	Met	Thr	Lys	Arg	G
G	Val	Ala	Asp	Gly	U
	Val	Ala	Asp	Gly	C
	Val	Ala	Glu	Gly	A
	Val	Ala	Glu	Gly	G

Figure 4-1 Genetic code. A codon for an amino acid consists of three nucleotides (triplet). One amino acid may be encoded by several different codons (degeneracy of the genetic code). The code includes sequences for the start codon and the stop codon.

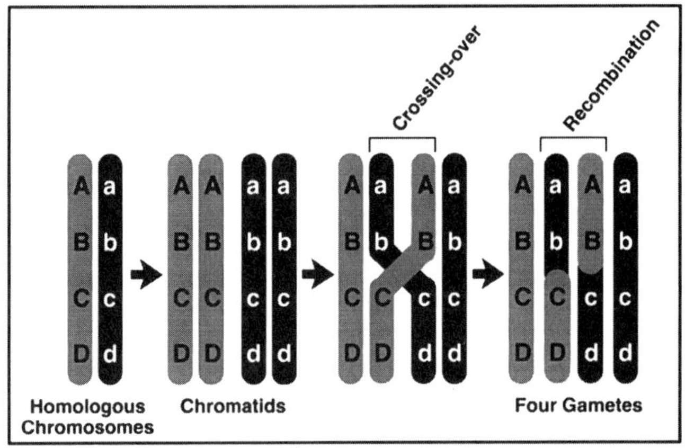

Figure 4-2 Crossing-over and recombination. During chiasma formation, either of the two chromatids on one chromosome pairs with one of the chromatids of the homologous chromosome. Genetic recombination through crossing-over results in recombinant and nonrecombinant chromosome segments in the gametes. Such recombination events occur frequently and, together with the random segregation of maternal and paternal chromosomes, generates genetic diversity in gametes.

instances, functionally related genes are located on different chromosomes.

Expressed genes encompass only about 20% of the total genome. A large amount of genomic DNA is not formed of single-copy sequences, but consists of repetitive sequences of various types. Short interspersed repetitive elements (SINE; 100–500 bp) and long interspersed repetitive elements (LINE; 6000–7000 bp) are spread throughout the genome. Another form of repetitive sequences, microsatellites, consist of 10–50 copies of simple sequence repetitions. Their functional role is not well defined, but they provide an important tool for establishing genetic maps and performing linkage studies *(see below)*.

MITOSIS AND MEIOSIS For tissue development and growth, eukaryotic cells progress through cycles of cell division and differentiation (*see* Chapter 6). Each cell division (mitosis) results in two genetically identical diploid (2n chromosome sets) daughter cells that are derived from the precursor cell. The first step in mitosis is the duplication of each parental chromosome, yielding two pairs of sister chromatids (2n → 4n). The chromosomes then condense and the nuclear membrane disappears. Subsequently, the chromosomes are arranged along the equatorial plate at metaphase. The two identical sister chromatids, held together at the centromere, are attached to the mitotic spindles. They then divide and migrate to opposite poles of the cell. After formation of a nuclear membrane around the two separated sets of chromatids, the cell divides and two diploid daughter cells are formed.

The gametes, oocytes or sperm, contain a single copy of each chromosome, a haploid (1n) chromosome set. When a sperm fertilizes an egg, the two haploid sets are combined, resulting in a new zygote containing two copies of each chromosome (diploid or 2n). The generation of the haploid gametes from diploid germ cells (oogonia, spermatogonia) occurs through meiosis, which consists of two cell divisions. During the first mitotic cell division, there is an exchange between homologous chromosomes generating genetically unique gametes. After formation of the two sister chromatids (2n → 4n), homologous chromosomes pair and form chiasmata (Fig. 4-2). Either of the two chromatids can pair with the homologous chromosome and undergo a process called crossing-over, in which segments of the maternal homolog recombine with the paternal homolog to form hybrid chromosomes in the place of the original ones. Such recombination events occur frequently, and it appears that at least one chiasma occurs on each chromosome arm. After these exchanges have been completed, the chromosomes segregate randomly. Because there are 23 chromosomes, there are 2^{23} (>8 million) possible combinations of chromosomes. Together with the exchanges that occur during recombination, chromosomal segregation generates great genetic diversity in gametes. After the first meiotic division, which gives rise to two daughter cells (2n), the two chromatids of each chromosome are separated during the second meiotic division and this results in four gametes with one chromatid (1n).

GENOTYPE AND PHENOTYPE A segment of DNA that is inherited in a Mendelian fashion (e.g., a gene) is called a locus. The genetic information at a given gene locus is defined as a genotype. Differences in the DNA sequence, and thus the genotype, are defined as alleles. If two alleles are present at a given locus, there are three possible genotypes. The genotype can be identical (homozygous) for one or the other allele, or it can consist of the combination of the two alleles (heterozygous). If there are more than two alleles, the number of possible genotypes increases accordingly.

The phenotype defines the visible or measurable characteristics of an individual. The term wild type describes the normal gene, including different allelic variants. A mutant genotype may or may not change the phenotype. If the phenotype of a mutant allele can be recognized in the heterozygous state, it is dominant. If alleles can only be recognized in the homozygous state, they are recessive. If both alleles can be recognized in the heterozygous state, they are codominant (e.g., the alleles A and B in the ABO blood system).

The widespread nature of genetic diversity is illustrated by subtle phenotypic variations between, and within, different ethnic groups. Biochemical polymorphisms, not readily perceptible by phenotype, can also be detected in many normal proteins that exist in various forms in a population. These variants are explained by the existence of multiple alleles at the level of the gene. The first such polymorphism to be clearly defined was the ABO blood group system. Molecular genetic analyses have revealed a surprisingly great degree of genetic variation. About 1 in 200 bp in the human genome is polymorphic. They are particularly frequent in noncoding regions of the genome and include single-basepair changes and variations in repetitive sequences. A polymorphism may change the protein sequence when it is located in coding regions and the substitution changes the amino acid specified by a codon. Polymorphisms are inherited according to Mendelian laws, a feature that is used in linkage studies or forensic applications.

Polymorphisms may have no impact on phenotype, or they may contribute to population diversity without being associated with disease. Alternatively, they may contribute to the susceptibility to, or expression of, certain diseases. A high degree of genetic diversity increases the ability of a population to adapt to changing environmental conditions, and it decreases the risk of recessive diseases.

GENETIC HETEROGENEITY Genetic heterogeneity refers to a similar phenotypic alteration that results from defects in different genes. For example, genetic heterogeneity occurs in Maturity-Onset Diabetes of the Young (MODY), which can result from defects in the glucokinase gene, as well as the genes encoding HNF-1α (Hepatocyte nuclear factor-1α) or HNF-4α (*see* Chapter 47).

Allelic or intragenic heterogeneity refers to alternate genotypes at the same locus that result in the same or similar phenotype. In cystic fibrosis, more than 600 mutations have been identified in the gene encoding the cystic fibrosis transmembrane conductance regulator protein (*see* Chapter 37). In allelic heterogeneity, linkage studies will identify the same locus. In contrast, genetic heterogeneity results in a similar phenotype, but linkage analyses identify distinct loci in different families.

TECHNIQUES USED IN GENETICS

RESTRICTION ENDONUCLEASES Restriction endonucleases are bacterial enzymes that recognize and cleave DNA at specific nucleotide sequences, called restriction sites (*see* Chapter 2). The most common restriction sites are sequences of 4–6 bp. Many of these sequences are palindromic (twofold axis of symmetry). A restriction enzyme recognizing a four-base sequence will find a target sequence every 4^4 (256) bases, a six-base cutter every 4^6 (4036) bases in a randomly composed DNA fragment. Cleavage can result in blunt ends of DNA or short single-stranded ends known as cohesive or sticky ends. The ability to manipulate DNA with restriction enzymes is of fundamental importance and includes applications like Southern analysis *(see below)* and the cloning of DNA fragments. If a sequence variation leads to loss or introduction of restriction sites, it is called a restriction fragment length polymorphism (RFLP). These polymorphic markers can be used for linkage studies.

PCR The polymerase chain reaction (PCR), introduced in 1985, has profoundly changed the way DNA analyses are performed, and it has become a cornerstone of molecular biology and genetic analysis. PCR allows the amplification of a defined DNA segment several millionfold. In the first step, the double stranded (ds) template DNA is denatured by heating (Fig. 4-3). Second, specific synthetic oligonucleotides primers of about 20 bp are annealed on either side of the segment of interest. The complementary strand located between the primers is then synthesized by a DNA polymerase. This procedure is usually repeated for about 30 cycles using automated heating blocks. After each cycle, all the dsDNA present from the preceding cycle serves as template. The DNA is therefore doubled after every cycle, resulting in an exponential increase in the amount of replicated DNA.

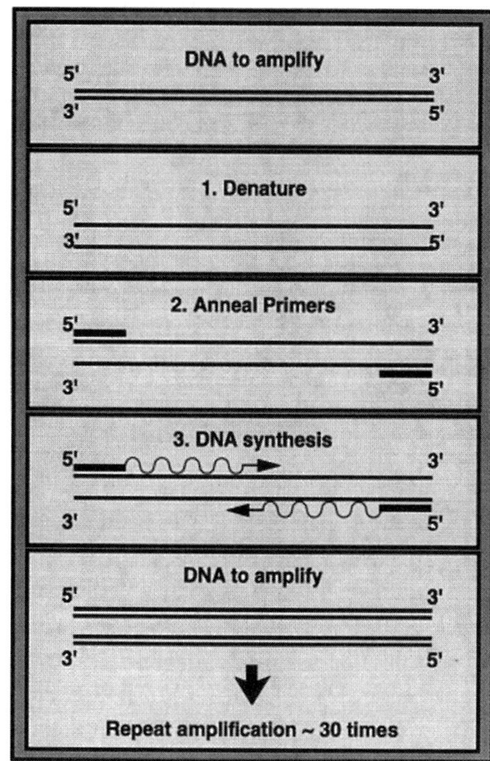

Figure 4-3 Polymerase chain reaction. The polymerase chain reaction (PCR) generates multiple copies of a DNA segment. The double stranded (ds) template DNA is denatured, specific synthetic oligonucleotides primers of about 20 bp are annealed on each side of the segment of interest, and the complementary strand is then synthesized by a heat-stable DNA polymerase. After each cycle, the dsDNA from the preceding cycle serves as template. The amount of DNA is therefore doubled after every cycle, resulting in an exponential increase.

Reverse transcriptase-PCR (RT-PCR) is another important strategy for molecular analysis. The starting material in this case is mRNA. The mRNA is reverse-transcribed into cDNA by the enzyme reverse transcriptase (first-strand synthesis). Subsequently, cDNA segment(s) can be amplified by PCR as described above.

DNA SEQUENCING Several protocols have been developed for the determination of DNA nucleotide sequence. In both traditional methods (Maxam-Gilbert or Sanger), the template DNA is used to generate fragments of DNA, which differ in size. Using high-resolution gel electrophoresis, these DNA molecules are separated at single-base resolution, allowing the sequence of the template DNA to be deduced. Maxam-Gilbert sequencing takes advantage of chemicals that cleave DNA at specific bases, thus resulting in fragments of different lengths. In the Sanger sequenc-

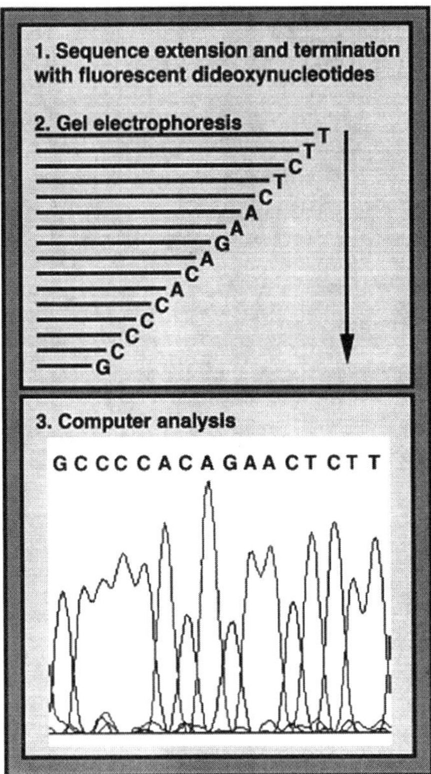

Figure 4-4 Automated DNA sequencing using fluorescently labeled dideoxynucleotides. Among the many methods in use for DNA sequencing, the chain termination methodology is widespread, and automated procedures are now used with increasing frequency. Automated procedures use fluorescently labeled dideoxynucleotides (or primers) and direct computer analysis of the sequence. A sequencing primer is bound to the template DNA. Dideoxynucleotides carrying different fluorescent labels are included in these reactions to terminate DNA polymerization when they are incorporated instead of the normal nucleotide. Electrophoresis of these reactions allows separation of the elongation products, which are directly analyzed by a computer.

ing method, DNA chains of varying length are generated by using dideoxynucleotides to terminate extension of the sequence by a DNA polymerase (chain termination method). By running four reactions in parallel (one for each dideoxynucleotide) and separating the products by electrophoresis on polyacrylamide gels, it is possible to determine the sequence of the template. Automated procedures are now used with increasing frequency to analyze DNA sequences. These procedures are usually based on the chain termination method and employ fluorescently labeled dideoxynucleotides or primers followed by direct computer analysis of the sequence. A typical example is shown in Fig. 4-4. These methods are, however, still relatively labor- and cost-intensive. For example, it has been estimated that sequencing the whole human genome by such an approach would result in costs of at least $3 billion at $1–$2 per base, and that it would require 30,000 work-years.

Currently, efforts are underway to develop new DNA sequencing technologies that are faster, more sensitive, and more cost-effective. Methodologies that are being explored include detection of fluorescently labeled bases in flow cytometry, direct reading of the base sequence on a DNA strand with the use of scanning, tunneling, or atomic force microscopies, mass spectrometric analysis of DNA sequence, and sequence analysis with DNA chips consisting of large arrays of oligonucleotides to which the DNA can be hybridized.

CYTOGENETICS AND FLUORESCENT *in situ* HYBRIDIZATION (FISH) Chromosomes can be stained and visualized under a light microscope. They display a characteristic pattern of light and dark bands reflecting regional variations in DNA composition. Differences in size and banding patterns allows one to distinguish the 22 autosomes and sex chromosomes to determine the karyotype of an individual. This type of cytogenetic analysis reveals the presence of major chromosomal abnormalities, including missing or extra copies of a chromosome, gross deletions, insertions, or translocations.

Fluorescent *in situ* hybridization (FISH) combines conventional cytogenetics with DNA hybridization. Chromosomes are prepared from nucleated cells and hybridized with fluorochrome-labeled DNA probes specific for various loci. Numerical and structural aberrations can then be detected by analysis of the fluorescence pattern. FISH is gradually replacing conventional cytogenetic analyses. The high resolution of FISH is useful for diagnostic purposes, and it is also helpful in the construction of chromosomal maps. Using interphase chromosomes, such probes can improve map resolution to about 100,000 bp.

GENE MAPPING Given the size and complexity of the human genome, the identification and location of genes is not trivial. Maps of the entire genome have now been developed to facilitate the localization of a gene of interest. Different types of maps (genetic or physical) describe the order of markers and the distances between them on each chromosome. One of the primary goals of the Human Genome Project is to increase the resolution of these maps until the exact location of every gene is known (*see* Chapter 5).

A genetic map determines the relative position of a gene or locus based on the recombination frequencies relative to other loci on the same chromosome. It is expressed in recombination units or centiMorgans (cM). The genetic map is up to 40% longer in chromosomes derived from females because of a higher frequency of recombination during the formation of oocytes. Any polymorphic sequence whose inheritance pattern can be followed is useful for mapping purposes. Examples of useful markers include RFLPs and microsatellite repeats. The genetic map is then constructed by assessing how frequently two markers are inherited together by linkage studies. The chromosomal location of a gene responsible for an inherited disease can be determined by tracking the inheritance of DNA markers *(see below)*.

Physical maps indicate the position of loci in absolute values. The various types of physical maps differ in their degree of resolution. A cytogenetic or chromosomal map determines the position of genetic loci relative to characteristic chromosomal bands observed under light microscopy. cDNA maps are of particular interest because they allow analyses of expressed genomic regions. After synthesis of cDNA from mRNA using reverse transcriptase, the origin of the cDNA can be mapped to particular chromosomal regions by hybridization. Sequence-tagged sites (STS) are short DNA segments with known locations on the genetic map (*see* Chapter 5). They can be used to array DNA fragments that have been cloned into yeast artificial chromosomes (YACs). The presence or absence of a given STS in a cloned fragment of DNA can then be compared in different YACs to identify overlapping clones. This leads to the characterization of contiguous DNA

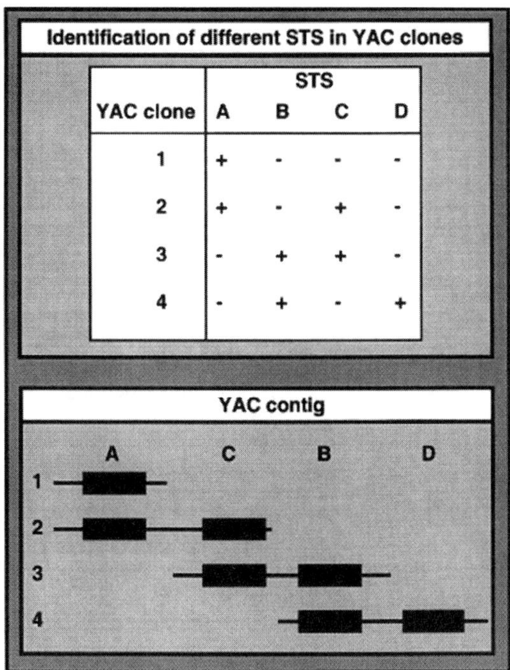

Figure 4-5 STS content map. The presence or absence of sequence tagged sites, short DNA segments of known sequence, can be determined in various clones of yeast artificial chromosomes (YAC). The comparison of STS sequences in different YAC clones allows their order to be determined.

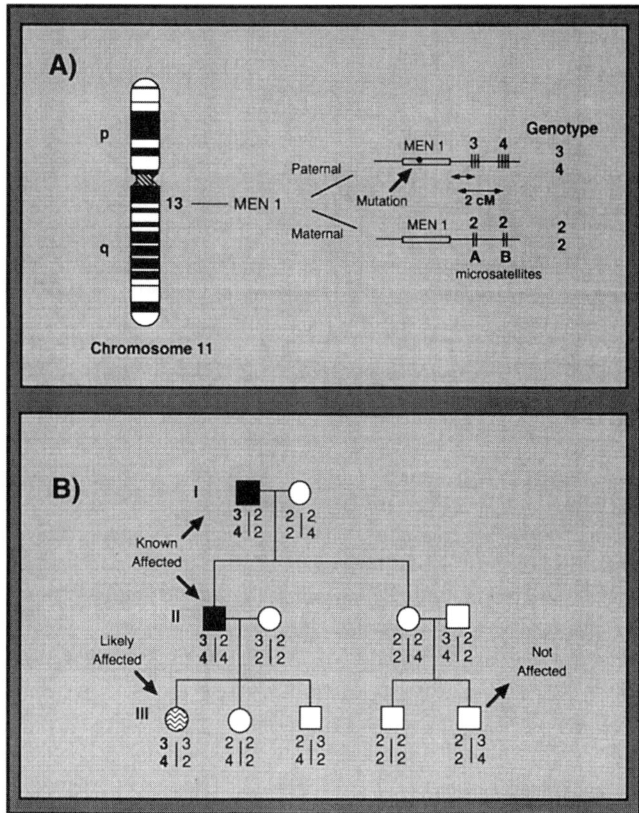

Figure 4-6 Linkage analysis in multiple endocrine neoplasia type 1 (MEN-1). **(A)** Schematic representation of human chromosome 11 depicting the position of the MEN 1 gene at band q13. In any individual, there is a paternal and a maternal allele for MEN 1. Hypothetical microsatellite markers A and B are shown near the MEN 1 locus. The A marker is closer to the MEN-1 gene. Based on the number of repeats in the microsatellites, genotypes are defined such that the paternal allele is "3-4" and the maternal allele is "2-2." Based on the pedigree (or DNA sequencing if available), the "3-4" genotype is shown to be linked to the MEN 1 gene. **(B)** Pedigree of a family with MEN 1. Alleles of family members are denoted by the genotypes based on microsatellites at A and B. Within the affected family, the disease is carried on the "3-4" allele (bold). Those affected or carrying the disease are shaded. Note that the male in generation II, who is not part of the original family, also possesses the "3-4" allele, but is not affected, indicating that a specific genotype is linked only within a family, not in the general population.

sequences, commonly referred to as contigs (Fig. 4-5). The highest resolution physical map will provide the complete DNA sequence of each chromosome in the human genome.

LINKAGE Genetic linkage provides the basis for the development of genetic maps, and it is used for the detection of new genes by positional cloning *(see below)*. Linkage is also used diagnostically to predict transmission of a disease gene. A prerequisite for linkage analyses are various types of sequence polymorphisms, like RFLPs, variable number of tandem repeats (VNTR), or microsatellites, which are used to distinguish the parental origin of alleles. Gene loci in the parental chromosomes may undergo recombination or remain nonrecombinant. The observed frequency of recombination between two loci is a function of their distance and is expressed in centiMorgans (cM). If the recombination frequency between two loci is 1%, the two loci are said to be 1 cM apart (1 cM corresponds to about 1 Mb of DNA). Because recombination frequency increases as a function of genetic distance, the closer together two loci are, the higher the likelihood that they will be inherited together (genetic linkage). A set of closely linked markers that are inherited together define a haplotype. DNA loci are identified by a specific nomenclature. For example, the locus D7S525 refers to human chromosome 7, segment 525, and is found on the short arm of chromosome 7.

In order to identify a chromosomal locus that segregates with a disease, it is necessary to determine the genotype of DNA samples from one or several pedigrees. Subsequently, one can determine whether certain marker alleles cosegregate with the disease. When a series of genetic markers are used to establish linkage to a disease phenotype in large informative kindreds, markers that are closest to the disease gene are less likely to undergo recombination events and will attain a higher linkage score. The data resulting from the characterization of multiple loci are then analyzed by computer programs. Linkage is usually expressed as a Lod (logarithm of odds) score, which is a ratio of the probability that the disease and marker loci are linked rather than unlinked. Lod scores are expressed as the logarithm to the base 10 such that positive numbers favor linkage and negative scores support nonlinkage. Lod scores of +3 (1000:1) are generally accepted as supporting linkage, whereas a score of –2 is consistent with the absence of linkage.

An example of the use of linkage analysis is shown in Fig. 4-6. In this case, the gene for the autosomal dominant disorder, multiple endocrine neoplasia type 1 (MEN-1), is known to be located on chromosome 11q13. Hypothetical polymorphic microsatellite markers are close to the MEN-1 gene, which encodes a protein, menin (currently of unknown function). In the pedigree shown, the affected grandfather in generation I carries alleles 3 and 4 on the chromosome with the mutated MEN-1 gene and alleles 2 and 2 on his other chromosome 11. Consistent with the linkage of the 3/4 genotype to the MEN-1 locus, his son in generation 2 is affected, whereas his daughter (who inherits the 2/2 genotype from her father) is unaffected. In the third generation, transmission of the 3/4 genotype indicates risk of developing MEN-1, assuming no genetic recombination between the 3/4 alleles and the MEN-1 gene. If a specific mutation in the MEN-1 gene is identified within a family, it is possible to track transmission of the mutation itself, thereby eliminating uncertainty caused by recombination.

CLONING OF GENES DNA may be amplified by cloning DNA fragments into suitable vectors that can be propagated in host cells. Vectors include DNA molecules derived from viruses, bacteria, or yeast that replicate independent of the genome of the host cell. After digestion of both the vector and the DNA to be inserted with restriction enzymes, they can be joined using DNA ligase. The vector carrying the fragment is then transferred into host cells (bacteria, yeast, or eukaryotic cells) where it is replicated. These manipulations allow the generation of large amounts of DNA for further experimental studies (*see* Chapter 2).

This type of manipulation can be performed with a single DNA fragment to be amplified, or one can create libraries in which all fragments derived from genomic DNA are represented in the final collection of colonies. In principle, a genomic library represents multiple cloned fragments of the entire genome. Genomic libraries can also be generated from single chromosomes after selection with fluorescence-activated cell sorters (FACS). cDNA libraries can also be created, using the mRNA of a selected tissue, and several modifications allow enrichment for certain mRNAs (e.g., poly[A] or size-selected), thus increasing the chance to find clones of interest.

After the preparation of libraries, the next step consists of isolating the recombinant clone containing the genomic or coding sequence of a gene. If there is some information on the protein encoded by this gene, microsequencing of a partial amino acid sequence allows synthesis of oligonucleotides based on the genetic code. Because of the degeneracy in the genetic code, this strategy employs a group of oligonucleotides. The oligonucleotides are radiolabeled and hybridized to clones within the library. Clones with a positive signal are isolated and propagated. Sequencing the DNA fragment inserted in the vector will provide information on at least a part of the gene of interest.

It is also possible to clone genes without having prior information on the protein. This strategy is referred to as positional cloning or reverse genetics (Fig. 4-7). This approach was introduced in the late 1980s has been successful for the identification of many genes, including those causing cystic fibrosis, Duchenne muscular dystrophy, polycystic kidney disease, and the MEN syndromes. The first step consists of establishing genetic linkage between a disease phenotype and DNA markers. This allows determination of the chromosomal region where the candidate gene is located. The identification of markers residing close to a gene provides the starting point for chromosome walking or jumping, which can be used to move progressively closer to the gene of interest. These methods allow one to screen sequences between the markers for the presence of functional genes. If one or several candidate genes are identified, they can be cloned and sequenced. The final step involves the demonstration that the isolated gene harbors a mutation that segregates with the disease.

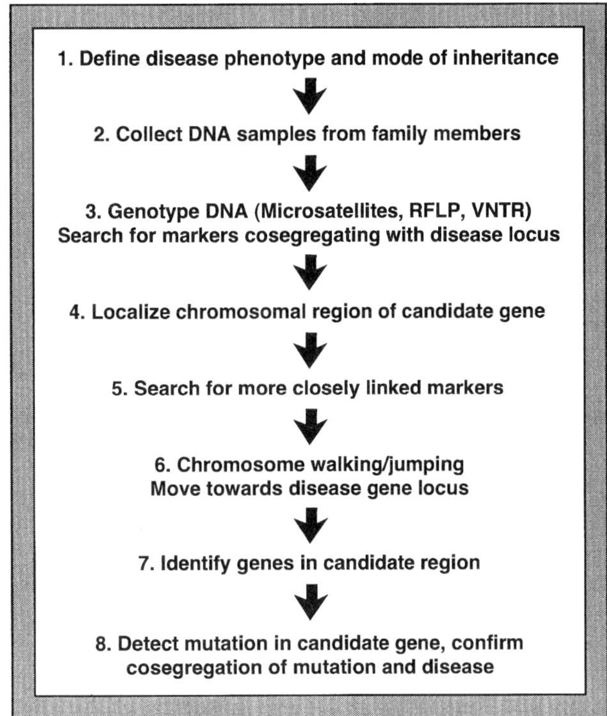

Figure 4-7 Positional cloning. A schematic outline is presented for the typical steps involved in the identification of a disease gene by positional cloning.

MUTATIONS In a broad sense, a mutation can be defined as any change in the primary nucleotide sequence of DNA, regardless of its functional consequences. A mutation in germ cells will lead to its presence in every cell of an organism, and it will be transmitted to the offspring. Some mutations may be lethal, while others are less deleterious, and some confer an evolutionary advantage. Somatic mutations, limited to a clone of cells in a given tissue, play an important role in the development of neoplasms. With the exception of triplet repeats which can expand (*see below*), mutations usually remain stable.

Structurally, mutations are very diverse. They can involve the entire genome as in triploidy, as well as gross numerical or structural alterations in chromosomes (Table 4-1). Large deletions may affect a portion of a gene, an entire gene, or if several genes are involved, they may lead to a contiguous gene syndrome. Unequal crossing-over between homologous genes can result in fusion gene mutations, well-illustrated by color blindness. Mutations can also involve changes in only a few or a single basepair. Mutations involving single nucleotides are referred to as point mutations. Analogous to gross chromosomal changes, point mutations may consist of substitutions, deletions, or insertions. Substitutions may be silent or change the respective codon. If the change occurs in a coding region, it is called a missense mutation. Substitutions are called transitions if a purine is replaced by another purine base (A↔G) or a pyrimidine is replaced by another pyrimidine (C↔T). Changes from a purine to a pyrimidine or vice versa are referred to as transversions. Deletions or insertions cause a shift of the translational reading frame, typically resulting in a premature stop (nonsense mutation). Mutations in intronic sequences may eliminate or create splice donor or splice acceptor sites, resulting in an abnormally spliced mRNA from the mutated gene. Mutations may

Table 4-1
Examples of Different Types of Mutations

Type of mutations	*Example*
Genome	
Abnormal chromosome set	Triploidy, tetraploidy
Chromosome	
Abnormal number of autosomal chromosomes	Trisomy 21, 18, 13
Abnormal number of sex chromosomes	Klinefelter syndrome, Turner syndrome
Translocation	Acute myeloid leukemia t(9;22)(q34:q11) "Philadelphia chromosome"
Deletion	Cri du chat syndrome 5p-
Duplication	Dosage-sensitive sex reversal (Xp dup)
Inversion	Ret oncogene inv (10)(q11.2q21) in papillary thyroid carcinoma (PTC)
Gene	
Deletion	Duchenne muscular dystrophy, Thalassemia
Duplication, insertion	Charcot-Marie-Tooth Type I
Fusion	Glucocorticoid-remediable aldosteronism
Inversion	Hemophilia A
Triplet expansion	Fragile X syndrome, Huntington disease
Missense point mutation	Cystic fibrosis
Nonsense point mutation	Cystic fibrosis
Frameshift	Cystic fibrosis
Splicing mutation	β Globin

also be found in the regulatory sequences of genes and can cause reduced or absent transcription of genes.

In some cancer syndromes, there is an inherited predisposition to tumor formation (*see* Chapter 7). In retinoblastoma, the tumor develops when both copies of the retinoblastoma gene become defective through two somatic events (sporadic retinoblastoma) or through a somatic loss of the normal allele in an individual with an hereditary defect in the other allele (hereditary retinoblastoma) (*see* Chapter 105). This "two-hit model," initially proposed by Knudson, applies to several other inherited cancer syndromes. The defective allele is inherited in a Mendelian fashion and follows a dominant pattern, but tumorigenesis results from a recessive loss of the tumor suppressor gene in an affected tissue. In other instances, the development of cancer typically requires defects in multiple genes, a process termed multistep carcinogenesis (*see* Chapter 7).

Testing for DNA mutations has several advantages in comparison to analyses at the protein level. DNA is easy to isolate and, in contrast to proteins, it is not differentially regulated in various tissues. DNA can be isolated from many sources, including white blood cells, tissue samples, exfoliated cells, and hair roots. A variety of methods have been developed for mutational analyses (Table 4-2). Large mutations, deletions, insertions, rearrangements, or expansions of triplet repeats can be detected by Southern blotting or PCR. In Southern analysis, high molecular DNA is digested with restriction enzymes. This results in multiple DNA fragments that can be separated by gel electrophoresis. After transfer of DNA to a membrane, the DNA can be denatured and hybridized with radioactive probes that detect a particular sequence among the countless other fragments. Differences in the hybridization patterns obtained by Southern blotting can indicate deletions or insertions in the genomic DNA (Fig. 4-8). For example, Southern blotting can be used in the diagnosis of the α-thalassemia variant found in Southeast Asia (*see* Chapter 20). In some cases of this autosomal recessive disorder, there is a large deletion of both α-globin genes from the 30 kb gene cluster on chromosome 1. Because the deletion encompasses the ζ-globin gene, it leads to hydrops fetalis and intrauterine death.

RT-PCR can be useful for detecting absent or reduced levels of expression of an mRNA resulting from a mutated allele. Screening for point mutations can be performed by numerous methods (Table 4-2). They are based on the recognition of mismatches between nucleic acid duplexes, electrophoretic separation of single or double-stranded DNA, or sequencing of DNA fragments amplified by PCR. DNA sequencing can be performed directly on PCR products or by using fragments cloned into plasmid vectors. The sensitivity of these methods varies between 80 and 100%. Protein truncation tests (PTT) can be used to detect mutations resulting in premature termination of a polypeptide during its synthesis. The isolated cDNA is transcribed and translated *in vitro* and the proteins are analyzed by gel electrophoresis. Comparison with the wild-type protein allows detection of truncated mutants. This approach is particularly helpful for the detection of loss of function mutations in large genes.

GENETIC DISEASES

CATEGORIES OF GENETIC DISEASE Taken together, genetic diseases form a substantial group of human disease. More than one-third of all pediatric hospital admissions are because of disorders that are caused, at least in part, by genetic factors. About 6–8% consist of single-gene defects, 0.4–2.5% are from chromosomal disorders, and the remaining group are genetically influenced. Overall, 3–5% of diseases in the general population are estimated to be genetically determined. Accurate estimates are difficult because different genetic defects can lead to the same phenotype (genetic heterogeneity), and a large number of genetic diseases are relatively rare. These difficulties should be kept in mind when assessing genetic risk. If one includes disorders with a strong polygenic predisposition, such as Type 2 diabetes mellitus, hypertension, or hyperlipidemias, then the role of genetics in common disorders is even greater.

Every classification of genetic diseases harbors some degree of oversimplification because of overlaps between the different cat-

Table 4-2
Methods Used for the Detection of Mutations

Method	*Principle*	*Type of mutation detected*
Cytogenetic analysis	Numerical and structural analysis of chromosomes	Numerical or structural abnormalities in chromosomes
FISH (fluorescent *in situ* hybridization)	Hybridization to chromosomes with fluorescently labeled probes	
Southern blot	Hybridization with DNA probe after digestion of high molecular DNA	Large deletions, insertions, rearrangements, expansions of triplet repeats, amplifications
PCR (polymerase chain reaction)	Amplification of DNA segment	Expansion of triplet repeats, variable number of tandem repeats (VNTR), gene rearrangements, translocations
Sequencing	Direct sequencing of PCR products Sequencing of DNA segments cloned into plasmids	Point mutations, small deletions, and insertions
SSCP (single-strand conformational polymorphism)	PCR of DNA segment: mutations result in conformational change and altered mobility	Point mutations, small deletions, and insertions
DGGE (denaturing gradient gel electrophoresis)	PCR, altered mobility of amplified segment harboring a mutation	Point mutations, small deletions, and insertions
OSH (oligonucleotide specific hybridization)	Hybridization of oligonucleotides ± altered sequence to amplified genomic DNA	Point mutations, small deletions, and insertions
RNase cleavage	Cleavage of mismatch between mutated and wild-type sequence	Point mutations, small deletions, and insertions
RFLP (restriction fragment length polymorphism)	Detection of altered restriction pattern of genomic DNA (Southern blot) or PCR products	Point mutations, small deletions, and insertions
RT-PCR (reverse transcriptase-PCR)	Reverse transcription, amplification of DNA segment → absence or reduction of mRNA	Indirect evidence for presence of mutation, cDNA cloning for sequencing
PTT (protein truncation tests)	Transcription/translation of cDNA isolated from tissue sample	Mutations leading to premature truncations

egories. Genetic diseases can be classified generally into the following major categories:

1. Chromosomal disorders with numerical or structural abnormalities in one or several chromosomes.
2. Mendelian or monogenic disorders, characterized by a single mutant gene inherited according to Mendelian rules.
3. Multifactorial diseases or complex disease traits, defined by the interaction of multiple genes and one or multiple environmental factors.
4. Nonclassical forms of genetic disease, a heterogeneous group that includes disorders influenced by genomic imprinting, or caused by uniparental disomy, trinucleotide repeats, and various forms of mosaicism.
5. Mitochondrial disorders resulting from mutations in the mitochondrial genome. Because mitochondrial DNA is transmitted through the maternal line, the pattern of inheritance differs from Mendelian disorders.
6. Mutations arising in differentiated somatic cells, which are of particular importance in the development of neoplasms. Although they are not inherited, they may occur in individuals with an inherited predisposition.

CHROMOSOMAL DISORDERS Chromosomal or cytogenetic disorders are defined by numerical or structural aberrations in chromosomes. They are frequent causes of abortions, developmental disorders, malformations, and malignancies. In humans, numerical chromosome aberrations occur in approximately 1 of 400 neonates. Triploidy and tetraploidy refer to circumstances in which each chromosome is present threefold or fourfold, respectively, instead of the usual diploid set. Triploidy is one of the most frequent chromosomal aberrations in humans and is found in about 15% of spontaneous abortions and severe malformations. The additional set of chromosomes may be of paternal or maternal origin. Aneuploidy describes a deviation from the normal chromosome number in a single pair of chromosomes. In a trisomy, three copies of a chromosome are present, and in a monosomy, one of the chromosomes is missing. Trisomies and monosomies are caused by nondisjunction in the first or second meiotic division and may be of paternal or maternal origin. Some of the most frequent abnormalities of chromosome number are listed in Table 4-3.

Structural defects in chromosomes arise from translocations, deletions, inversions, insertions, isochromosomes, dicentric chromosomes, and ring chromosomes. If no chromosomal material has been lost or gained, the rearrangement is referred to as balanced. If it is unbalanced, there is either a loss or gain of chromosomal DNA. A large number of congenital syndromes caused by structural changes in chromosomes can be recognized based on their characteristic clinical phenotype. Furthermore, chromosomal translocations play an important role in certain malignancies, such as leukemias and lymphomas (*see* Chapters 26 and 27).

MENDELIAN OR MONOGENIC DISORDERS Because most traits examined by Mendel were caused by single genes, monogenic human diseases are frequently referred to as Mendelian disorders. Information about many of these genetic disorders

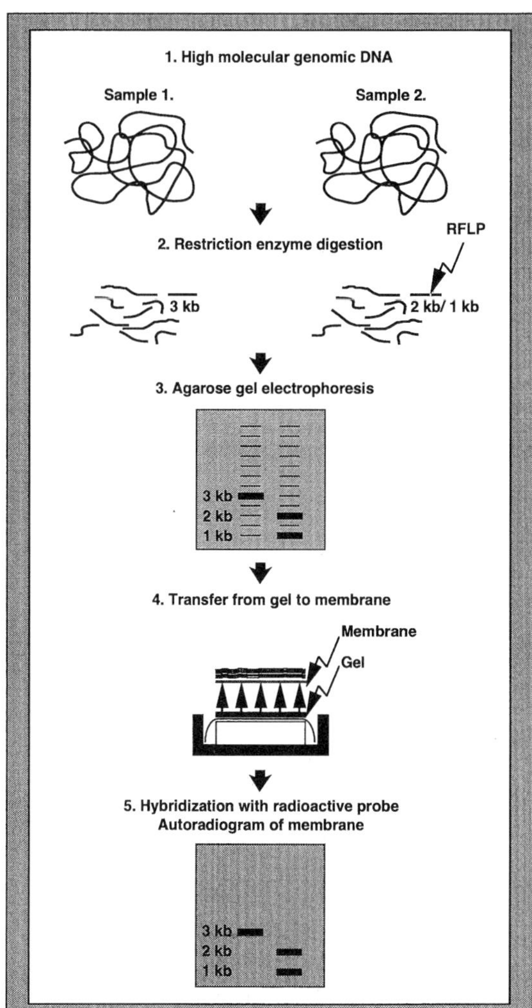

Figure 4-8 Southern blot. A Southern blot can be used to detect alterations in gene structure (e.g., deletions, insertions, variable number tandem repeat [VNTR], or restriction fragment length polymorphism [RFLP]). Genomic DNA is digested with one or several restriction enzymes. The digestion products are separated on an agarose gel and transferred to a membrane. Hybridization of the immobilized DNA with a radiolabeled probe allows detection of specific fragments by autoradiography. As illustrated, an RFLP can lead to differences in the length of the detected fragments. Such polymorphisms are used in linkage studies to assess whether a disease cosegregates with a genetic marker.

can be found in a large, continuously evolving compendium, Mendelian Inheritance in Man (MIM), initiated by V. A. McKusick. It is also accessible on-line (OMIM: On-line Mendelian Inheritance in Man, http://www3.ncbi.nlm.nih.gov/Omim).

The Mendelian laws predict the transmission of alleles within a family, and these are depicted graphically in family trees or pedigrees. Standard symbols used for describing pedigrees are shown in Fig. 4-9. As an example, the segregation of genotypes in the offspring of parents with two distinct alleles, one dominant and one recessive, is illustrated in Fig. 4-10. Some relatively common Mendelian disorders are listed in Table 4-4, and the characteristic modes of inheritance are shown in Fig. 4-11. A dominant allele, *A*, and a recessive allele, *a*, can display three Mendelian modes of inheritance: autosomal dominant, autosomal recessive, and X-linked. The mode of inheritance for a phenotypic trait or disease is determined by pedigree analysis. In autosomal dominant disorders, individuals can be affected in each generation. The disease does not occur in the offspring of unaffected individuals. Males and females are affected with equal frequency (Fig. 4-11A). The child of an affected individual has a 50% risk of inheriting the mutated gene. In an autosomal recessive disease, both parents of an affected individual are obligate heterozygotes (Fig. 4-11B). The affected individual, who can be of either sex, can be a homozygote or compound heterozygote (distinct mutations in each copy of the gene) for a gene defect. Normally, heterozygous carriers of a defective gene are clinically normal. There is a 25% chance that an offspring will be affected. Many autosomal recessive diseases are rare and often occur in cases of parental consanguinity. X-chromosomal inheritance refers to the transmission of genes located on the X chromosome (Fig. 4-11C). A daughter always inherits her father's X chromosome together with one of the two maternal X chromosomes. A son inherits the Y chromosome from his father and one of the maternal X chromosomes. Thus, there is no father-to-son transmission in X-linked inheritance, and all daughters of an affected male are obligate carriers of the mutant allele. Since males have only one X chromosome, they are hemizygous for a mutant allele and are therefore more likely to develop the mutant phenotype, regardless of whether the mutation is dominant or recessive. A female may be either heterozygous or homozygous for a mutant allele, which may be dominant or recessive. In addition, the expression of X-chromosomal genes is influenced by X chromosome inactivation *(see below)*.

The frequency of Mendelian disorders varies substantially in different populations. For example, the autosomal recessive disorder sickle-cell anemia occurs with the highest frequency in populations originating from West Africa, β thalassemia is frequently found in Asians, and cystic fibrosis occurs most often in individuals of European descent. In many of the more prevalent disorders, a selective advantage has been proposed for heterozygous gene carriers and may provide an explanation for the high frequency of the mutated allele. In disorders with a low prevalence, but a relatively high frequency within a defined population, a founder effect is more likely.

PHENOTYPIC VARIABILITY IN MENDELIAN DISORDERS

The phenotype associated with certain mutations can vary in the degree of penetrance. For example, in hypertrophic obstructive cardiomyopathy (HOCM), an autosomal dominant disorder characterized by obstruction of left ventricular outflow resulting from ventricular hypertrophy, some mutations in the myosin heavy-chain β gene exhibit 100% penetrance in adults. In other words, all carriers of the mutation will develop the disease (*see* Chapter 13). Other mutations in the same gene display a penetrance of about 50%, such that an individual carrying the mutant genotype may not manifest the disease phenotype. In this situation, the mutant gene is called nonpenetrant. Although a carrier of the mutant gene may not develop the disease, it will still be transmitted to the next generation where it may be penetrant or nonpenetrant. In addition, the HOCM phenotype may be caused by molecular alterations in other genes, a phenomenon referred to as genetic heterogeneity *(see above)*. Determination of penetrance may be dependent on the sensitivity of the methodology used for the assessment of the phenotype. Penetrance can also be dependent on the presence or absence of environmental factors: If there is no exposure to disease-causing agents, some genetic defects may not become apparent. This is illustrated by hyperlipidemias, hemochromatosis, or porphyrias, all disorders that are significantly modulated by diet.

Table 4-3
Frequent Chromosome Abnormalities

Disorder	*Chromosomal genotype*	*Frequency*
Abnormal no. of chromosome sets		
Triploidy	69XX, 69XY	Frequent in miscarriage
Tetraploidy	92XX, 92XY	Frequent in miscarriage
Abnormal no. of autosomes		
Trisomy 21		1/600
Trisomy 18		1/5000
Trisomy 13		1/15,000
Abnormal no. of sex chromosomes		
Klinefelter syndrome	47XXY	1/1000 males
XYY-syndrome	47XYY	1/1000
Turner syndrome	45X0, 45X/46X0, 45X/46XY (mosaicism)	1/10,000 females
Triple-X syndrome	XXX	1/1000

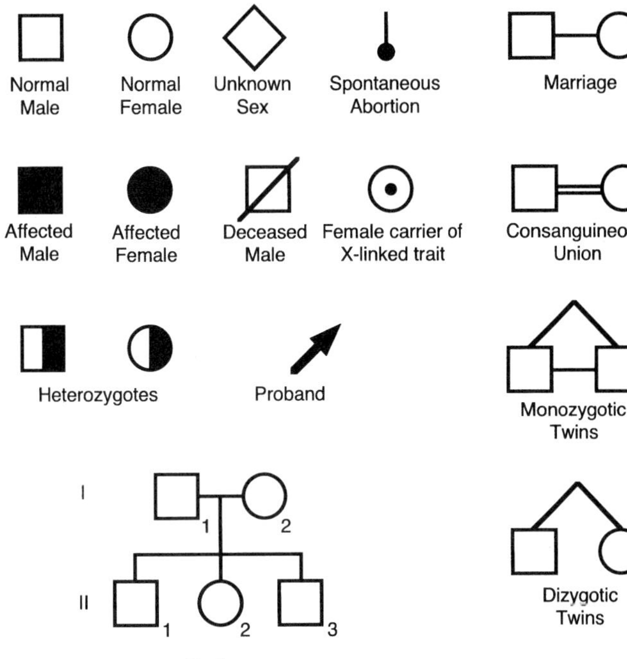

Figure 4-9 Symbols used in pedigree analyses.

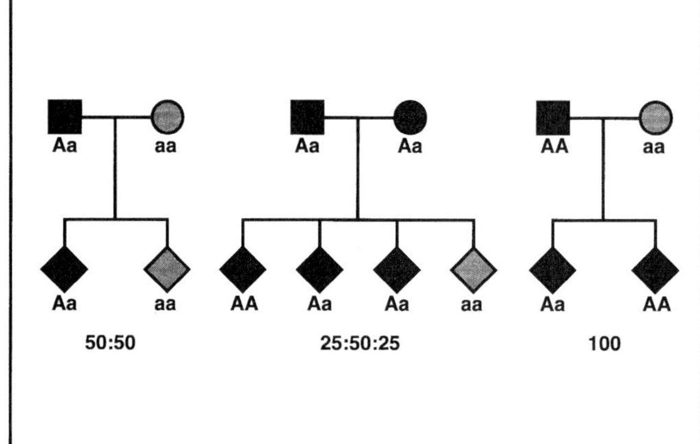

Figure 4-10 Segregation of alleles. Segregation of genotypes in the offspring of parents with a dominant (A) and a recessive (a) allele. The distribution or segregation of the parental genotypes to their children depends on the combination of the alleles in the parents. The Mendelian laws predict the combinations and frequencies in the offspring *(see text)*.

Variability in clinical expressivity characterizes the spectrum of phenotypic changes among different individuals with a given genotype. It includes differences in the type and severity of symptoms, as well as the age of onset of a disease. A classical example is the multiple endocrine neoplasia syndrome type 1 (MEN-1), an autosomal dominant syndrome characterized by tumors of the parathyroid glands, the anterior pituitary, and the endocrine pancreas. By age 50, almost 100% of the gene carriers develop parathyroid tumors (*see* Chapter 51). In contrast, there is a great variability in the development of other manifestations of MEN-1 among siblings carrying the mutated gene.

AUTOSOMAL DOMINANT DISORDERS Diseases inherited in an autosomal dominant manner result from one mutant allele and a normal allele on the other chromosome. Unless it is a new germline mutation, each affected child has an affected parent. The probability that an offspring will be affected is 50% because the alleles segregate at meiosis. Children with a normal genotype will have only unaffected offspring (Fig. 4-11A). Both males and females can be affected, since the defective gene is on one of the 22 autosomes. Autosomal dominant disorders can, however, manifest themselves in a sex-limited pattern as exemplified by familial male-limited precocious puberty, which is caused by activating mutations in the gene encoding the LH-receptor (Chapter 57). The clinical manifestations of autosomal dominant disorders may be variable because of differences in penetrance or expressivity *(see above)*. In certain cases, a mutant gene may be nonpenetrant. These variations can lead to difficulties in the recognition that a disorder is inherited.

Approximately 1 in 100,000 newborns will harbor a new mutation at a given locus, and in the case of a dominant allele, this may result in phenotypic changes. *De novo* germline mutations are thought to occur more frequently during later cell divisions in gametogenesis, which explains why siblings are rarely affected. In some cases, however, the mutation may occur early in gametogenesis, resulting in gonadal mosaicism, which can lead to multiple affected sibs, despite the fact that somatic cells of the parents do not harbor the mutation. Gonadal mosaicism is, for example, found in Duchenne muscular dystrophy and osteogenesis imperfecta.

Table 4-4
Selected Monogenic Disorders

Autosomal dominant disorders
Familial hyperlipidemia
Familial hypercholesterolemia
Huntington disease
Polycystic kidney disease
Spherocytosis
Marfan syndrome
Neurofibromatosis
Hereditary nonpolyposis colon cancer
Polyposis of the colon
Familial breast cancer
Willebrand disease
Hypertrophic obstructive cardiomyopathy (HOCM)
Myotonic dystrophy
Otosclerosis
Autosomal recessive disorders
Cystic fibrosis
Sickle-cell anemia
β-Thalassemia
α1-antitrypsin deficiency
Congenital adrenal hyperplasia
Phenylketonuria
Hemochromatosis
Tay-Sachs disease
X-linked disorders
Color blindness
Hemophilia A
Hemophilia B
Glucose-6-phosphate dehydrogenase deficiency
Duchenne muscular dystrophy
Becker muscular dystrophy
Fragile X syndrome
X-linked ichthyosis

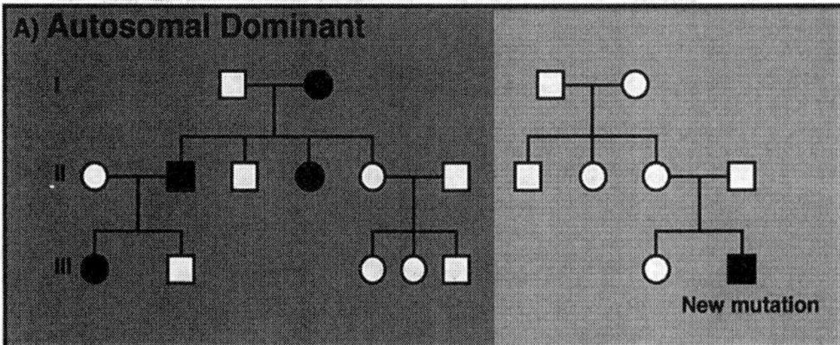

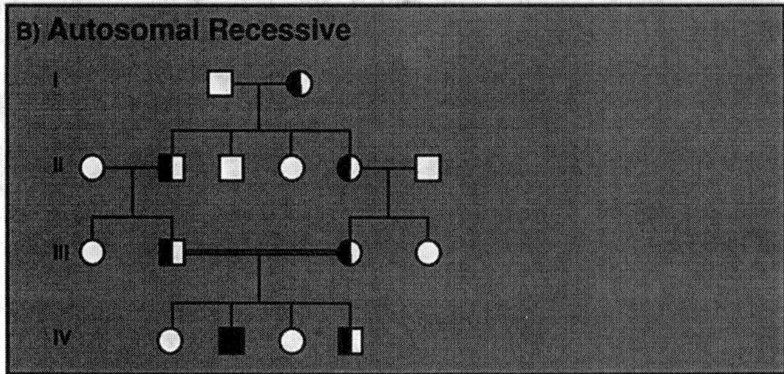

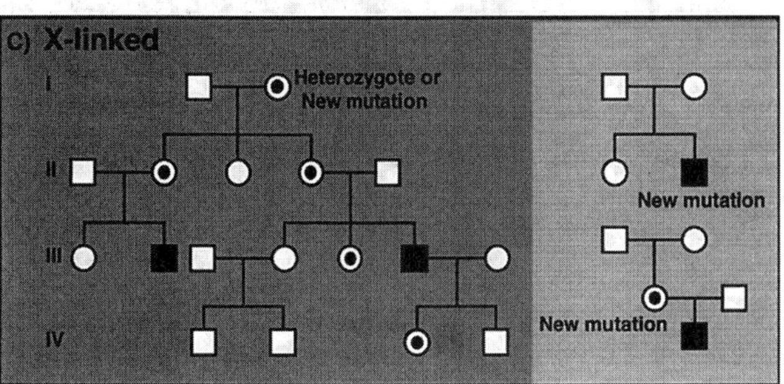

Figure 4-11 Mendelian inheritance. Pairs of alleles can display three Mendelian modes of inheritance: autosomal dominant, autosomal recessive, and X-chromosomal. The mode of inheritance for a given phenotypic trait or disease is determined by pedigree analysis. **(A)** In autosomal dominant disorders, affected individuals are found in successive generations. The disease does not occur in the offspring of unaffected individuals. Both males and females can be affected. The offspring of an affected individual have a 50% risk of inheriting the mutated gene. New mutations in one allele may lead to disease. **(B)** In an autosomal recessive disease, both parents of an affected individual are usually heterozygotes for a defective allele. The affected individual, who can be of either sex, is a homozygote or compound heterozygote. Generally, heterozygous carriers of a defective allele are clinically normal. There is a 25% chance that an offspring will be affected (homozygous recessive). Many autosomal recessive diseases occur in cases of parental consanguinity. **(C)** Characteristic features of X-linked inheritance are that there is no father-to-son transmission, and all daughters of an affected male are obligate carriers of the mutant allele. Males are hemizygous for the mutant allele, and they are more likely to develop the mutant phenotype, regardless of whether the mutation is dominant or recessive. A female may be either heterozygous or homozygous for the mutant allele, which may be dominant or recessive. *De novo* mutations in males may result in disease.

New germline mutations occur more frequently in fathers of advanced age. The average age of fathers with new germline mutations causing Marfan syndrome is 37 years, whereas fathers who transmit the disease by inheritance have an average age of 30 years. The ability to reproduce may be affected by autosomal dominant disorders, and the frequency of the disease will then reflect the occurrence of new mutations during gametogenesis.

A mutant dominant allele may result in an abnormal phenotype because of several pathogenic mechanisms. Haploinsufficiency refers to the fact that half of the normal gene product may not be sufficient to result in a normal phenotype. This applies, for example, to rate-limiting enzymes in heme synthesis causing porphyrias (*see* Chapter 42). An increase in dosage of a gene product may also result in disease. In Charcot-Marie-Tooth type 1a, a duplication of the *PMP22* gene results in high levels of expression of peripheral myelin protein 22, and this dosage effect underlies the demyelinating neuropathy (*see* Chapter 101). A mutant protein may also interfere with the function of the normal protein and act as a dominant negative. This is illustrated by mutations in the thyroid hormone receptor β in the syndrome of resistance to thyroid hormones (*see* Chapter 50).

AUTOSOMAL RECESSIVE DISORDERS Autosomal recessive disorders are clinically manifest only if the patient is a homozygote or compound heterozygote (distinct mutations in the gene from the two different chromosomes) for a defect in a single gene. Heterozygous carriers of a defective allele are clinically normal. Although many recessive disorders appear to be truly recessive, it should be emphasized that heterozygotes may display subtle differences in phenotype that only become apparent with more precise testing or in the context of certain environmental influences. For example, in sickle-cell anemia, heterozygotes are normally asymptomatic. In situations of dehydration or diminished oxygen pressure, they can occasionally experience sickle-cell crises.

In most cases of a recessive disorder, an affected individual is the offspring of two heterozygotes. In this situation, there is a 25% chance of a normal genotype, a 50% probability of a heterozygous state, and a 25% risk of disease. If a heterozygote mates with a homozygote, the probability of disease increases to 50% for each child and the pedigree analysis may mimic an autosomal dominant mode of inheritance. If a mutant recessive allele is rare in a population, affected individuals are often the offspring of consanguineous parents. In contrast to autosomal dominant disorders, new mutations for recessive alleles rarely manifest themselves, because they result in an asymptomatic carrier. Males and females are affected with the same frequency unless the mutation has a sex-specific effect (e.g., steroid 5α-reductase type II deficiency, which affects only males; *see* Chapter 59).

The clinical expression of autosomal recessive disorders is usually more uniform than in autosomal dominant disorders. Most mutated alleles lead to a complete or partial loss of function. They frequently involve enzymes in metabolic pathways, receptors, or components of signaling cascades. Recessive disorders are generally rare because of the fact that homozygotes may have reduced biological fitness. The high frequency of certain autosomal recessive disorders such as sickle-cell anemia, cystic fibrosis, and thalassemia has been proposed to reflect a biological advantage for heterozygotes.

X-LINKED DISORDERS The characteristic pattern of inheritance of X-linked disorders is shown in Fig. 4-11C. In X-linked inheritance, there is no father-to-son transmission, and all daughters of an affected male are obligate carriers of the mutant allele. The risk of developing a disease resulting from a mutant X-chromosomal gene is thus different in males and females. While males hemizygous for the mutant allele are always affected, the heterozygous females may be asymptomatic (X-linked recessive) or affected (X-linked dominant). New mutations can result in affected males or heterozygous females. As described below, X chromosome inactivation may influence the expression of an X-linked disease in a heterozygous female. Some X-linked disorders are listed in Table 4-4. In some cases (e.g., incontinentia pigmenti), the mutated allele is lethal in the hemizygous males, and affected women have an increased frequency of spontaneous abortions of male fetuses.

Y-LINKED DISORDERS Only a few genes are known on the Y chromosome. One of these, the sex-region determining Y factor (SRY) or testis determining factor (TDF), is crucial for the development of the normal male phenotype. Since the SRY region is close to the pseudoautosomal region of the sex chromosomes, crossing-over occasionally occurs between the X and Y chromosomes. Translocations between the X and Y chromosome can subsequently result in XY females with the Y chromosome lacking the SRY gene or XX males harboring the SRY factor on one of the X chromosomes (*see* Chapter 58). Point mutations in the SRY gene may also result in individuals with an XY genotype and an incomplete female phenotype. Most of these mutations occur *de novo*. Men with oligospermia/azoospermia frequently have microdeletions on the long arm of the Y chromosome that involve the azoospermia factor (AZF).

MULTIFACTORIAL DISEASES OR COMPLEX DISEASE TRAITS In many diseases that appear to have some genetic component, there is no clear evidence for classical Mendelian inheritance. However, many common diseases such as asthma (*see* Chapters 35 and 36), rheumatoid arthritis (*see* Chapter 34), diabetes mellitus (*see* Chapter 47), schizophrenia (*see* Chapter 109), hypertension (*see* Chapter 16), and many others exhibit familial predisposition. In many of these cases, interactions between genetic factors and the environment may be involved in the pathogenesis of the disease.

Several lines of evidence point towards polygenic (multiple genes) inheritance. A role for genetics is supported if a disorder occurs at a higher frequency in certain ethnic groups. Since environmental factors may have an important influence, it is important to assess whether the disease frequency is modulated if members of such a population move to a different environment. A genetic component in a multifactorial disease is also suggested if the disorder occurs at a higher frequency in the immediate relatives of an index case in comparison to the general population. Finally, the concordance in monozygotic and dizygotic twins may give important clues for the presence or absence of complex traits. If the concordance rate is high in monozygotic twins in comparison to dizygotic twins, genetic factors are likely to be important.

X-CHROMOSOME INACTIVATION, GENOMIC IMPRINTING, AND UNIPARENTAL DISOMY Although females contain two X chromosomes, the expression of many X-chromosomal genes is not greater in females than in males. This is because of random inactivation of either the paternal or the maternal X chromosome in each somatic cell of a female during early embryogenesis, a phenomenon also referred to as lyonization. X-inactivation is caused by differential methylation of cytosine nucleotides. Methylation of the inactive copy of the X chromosome results in formation of the X chromatin, which is visible as a Barr body. X-inactivation is not reversible, and the same chromosome is inactivated in daughter cells.

Methylation is not only involved in X-chromosome inactivation, but also plays an important role in the regulation of gene expression. Active genes often display diminished or absent methylation, whereas inactive genes are hypermethylated. Methylation occurs at the 5' position in the cytosine of cytosine-guanine (CpG) dinucleotides. Unmethylated or hypomethylated CpG (cytosine-phosphate-guanine) clusters often indicate the beginning of a structural gene that is being expressed, and they are sometimes used in positional cloning for the identification of genes. The mechanism by which methylation leads to inactivation of gene expression is not well-understood. It could alter chromatin structure or interfere with the binding of transcription factors to regulatory DNA sequences. Alternatively, methylation might be an epiphenomenon that occurs following the inactivation of a gene by other mechanisms. The complex control of gene expression at the transcriptional level is discussed in Chapter 3.

According to Mendelian principles, the parental origin of a mutant gene is irrelevant for the expression of a phenotype. As described above in the context of X-chromosome inactivation, there are some important exceptions to this rule. Inactivation of genes or chromosomal regions on one of the two chromosomes also occurs on autosomes. This phenomenon, referred to as genomic imprinting, leads to preferential expression of an allele, depending on its parental origin, resulting in transmission of disease in a manner that is dependent on the sex of the transmitting parent. The fact that identical regions can differ in their functional activity depending on whether they are of maternal or paternal origin is also illustrated by zygotes with two maternal or two paternal sets of chromosomes. Cells with two copies of maternal chromosomes develop into the inner cell mass of the embryo, whereas cells with two sets of paternal chromosomes almost exclusively form the extraembryonal cells of the trophoectoderm. These observations indicate that some genes are differentially expressed from paternal and maternal chromosomes.

The principle of genomic imprinting has important implications for a subset of human disorders. Classical examples are the Prader-Willi-Syndrome and the Angelman Syndrome (Chapter 117). The Prader-Willi-Syndrome, characterized by diminished fetal activity, obesity, hypotonia, mental retardation, short stature, and hypogonadotropic hypogonadism, is caused in most cases by deletions on the short arm of chromosome 15. The deletions in the Prader-Willi-Syndrome occur exclusively on the paternally derived chromosome. In contrast, patients with Angelman syndrome (which is characterized by mental retardation, seizures, ataxia, and hypotonia) have deletions at the same site of chromosome 15, but they occur only on the maternally derived chromosome (Fig. 4-12A). The two syndromes may also result from uniparental disomy (Fig. 4-12B). In this case, the syndromes are not caused by deletions on chromosome 15, but by inheritance of either two maternal chromosomes (resulting in Prader-Willi syndrome) or of two paternal chromosomes (causing Angelman syndrome).

Genomic imprinting, or uniparental disomy, is involved in the pathogenesis of several other disorders and malignancies. Hydatiform mole contains a normal number of diploid chromosomes, but they are all of paternal origin. The opposite occurs in ovarian teratomata with 46 chromosomes of maternal origin. Overexpression of the imprinted gene for insulin-like growth factor II (IGF-II) is involved in the pathogenesis of the cancer-predisposing Beckwith-Wiedemann syndrome (BWS) (*see* Chapter 116). These children show somatic overgrowth with organomegaly and hemihypertrophy, and they have an increased risk of developing embryonal malignancies such as Wilm's tumor (*see* Chapter 71). Normally, only the paternally derived copy of the IGF-II gene is active. Imprinting of the IGF-II gene is regulated by H19, an RNA transcript that is not translated into protein. Disruption or lack of methylation of H19 leads to a relaxation of IGF-II imprinting which subsequently results in overgrowth.

TRINUCLEOTIDE REPEATS Trinucleotide repeats are found in several genes and their number can vary among healthy individuals (*see* Chapter 100). For example, the number of CAG repeats in the first exon of the androgen receptor (AR) gene is lowest in African Americans, intermediate in Caucasians, and highest in Asians (Chapter 60). Of note, the frequency of prostatic cancer is inversely proportional to the length of the repeats.

An increase in the number of repeats above a certain critical threshold is associated with several diseases (Table 4-5). The repeats can be located within the coding region as in Huntington disease (*see* Chapter 97) or the X-linked form of spinal and bulbar muscular atrophy (SBMA, Kennedy syndrome), which is caused by an expansion in the polyglutamine tract encoded by CAG repeats in the first exon of the androgen receptor. In other instances (e.g., in myotonic dystrophy and in the fragile X syndrome), the repeats are not located in coding regions of genes. If an expansion is present, the DNA fragment is unstable and generally tends to expand further with additional cell divisions.

The length of the expansion and the age of onset, or the severity of a disease, often correlate. Since the repeat length tends to increase from generation to generation, the manifestations of the disease are observed at an earlier age, a phenomenon called anticipation. In addition, the repeat number may vary in some disorders within an individual in a tissue-specific manner. In myotonic dystrophy, the CTG repeat can be tenfold higher in muscular tissue compared to lymphocytes (Chapter 94). The mechanism by which the expansion of such repeats occurs is still debated. Moreover, the molecular mechanisms leading to the respective diseases are poorly defined.

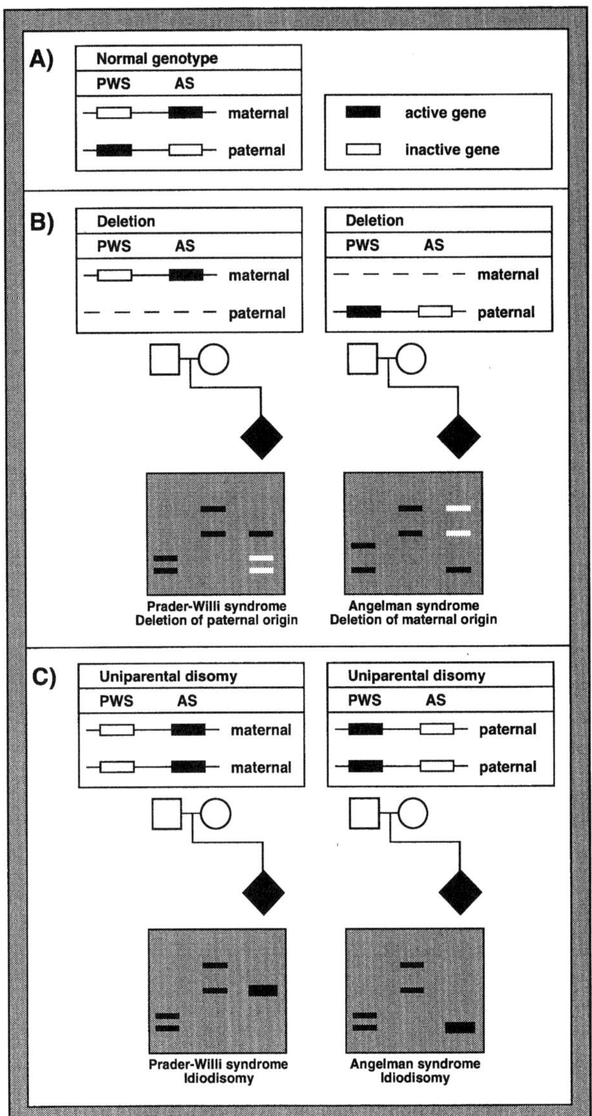

Figure 4-12 Genomic imprinting and uniparental disomy. Model for Prader-Willi syndrome and Angelman syndrome. The two distinct disorders are caused by loss of function of two closely adjacent loci on chromosome 15, which undergoes genomic imprinting. **(A)** Normal situation. The maternal PWS locus and the paternal AS locus are inactivated. **(B)** PWS and AS caused by deletions of the paternal and the maternal alleles, respectively, of chromosome 15q11-13. Southern blots with the marker D15S11 illustrate the absence of a positive hybridization for the paternal (PWS) or maternal (AS) alleles. **(C)** Uniparental disomy, the inheritance of two maternal copies (PWS) or two paternal copies (AS) can lead to the same phenotypes. In this case, a Southern blot with the probe D15S11 shows an increased intensity for one of the maternal (PWS) or paternal alleles (AS).

Table 4-5
Selected Disorders Caused by Nucleotide Repeats

Disease	*Locus*	*Repeat*	*Triplet length*	*Gene product*	*MIM no.*
Spinobulbar muscular atrophy (SBMA)	X	CAG	Normal: 11-34 Disease: 40-62	Androgen receptor	313200
Fragile X-syndrome FRAXA	Xq27.3	CGG	Normal: 6–50 Disease: 200–300	FMR-1 protein	309550
Fragile X-syndrome FRAXE	Xq28	GCC	Normal: 6–25 Disease: >200	FMR-2 protein	309548
Myotonic dystrophy	19q13.3	CTG	Normal: 5–30 Disease: 200–1000	Myotonin protein kinase	160900
Huntington disease	4p16.3	CAG	Normal: 11–34 Disease: 37–121	Huntingtin	143100
Spinocerebellar atrophy type 1	6p21.3-21.2	CAG	Normal: 19–36 Disease: 43–81	Ataxin 1	164400
Dentatorubral pallidoluysian atrophy	12p	CAG	Normal: 7–23 Disease: 49–75	Atrophin	125370
Machado Joseph	14q24.3-32	CAG	Normal: 13–36 Disease: 68–79	MJDI	109150
Friedreich ataxia	9q13	GAA	Normal: 7–22 Disease: 200–900	Frataxin	229300

MOSAICISM Mosaicism refers to the presence of two or more cell lines in an individual that differ in their genotype. Cell mosaicism can result from a mutation that occurs during embryonic, fetal, or extrauterine development. The developmental stage at which the defect arises will determine whether germ cells or only somatic cells are involved. Chromosomal mosaicism results from nondisjunction at an early embryonic mitotic division, leading to the persistence of more than one cell line.

Somatic mosaicism is characterized by a patchy distribution of somatic cells containing a mutation. For example, the McCune-Albright syndrome is caused by activating mutations in the stimulatory G protein, Gsα, that occur early in development. The clinical phenotype varies depending on the tissue distribution of the mutation. The manifestations can include ovarian cysts that secrete sex steroids and cause precocious puberty, polyostotic fibrous dysplasia, *café au lait* skin pigmentation, pituitary adenomas, and hypersecreting autonomous thyroid nodules. Germ cell mosaicism or gonadal mosaicism should be suspected when parents seem to be normal on genetic testing, but have several affected offspring with a dominant or X-linked disorder. In these instances, the mutation may have occurred early in gametogenesis.

MITOCHONDRIAL INHERITANCE Several diseases arising from mutations in the mitochondrial genome are known in humans (*see* Chapter 103). Each mitochondrion has several copies of a circular chromosome. This DNA predominantly encodes proteins that are components of the respiratory chain. They are transmitted through the maternal line because sperm do not contribute cytoplasmic components to the zygote. The disease will therefore not be transmitted from an affected man to his children, but all the children from an affected mother will be affected.

In contrast to the nuclear chromosomes, the mitochondrial chromosome is present in numerous copies in the cell, and variable numbers of mitochondria are present in cells of different tissues. Different offspring may inherit various ratios of mutant and wild-type mitochondrial genomes (heteroplasmy) that lead to phenotypic variability. During cell replication, the genotype may also shift in the direction of the wild type or mutant chromosomes. Examples of mitochondrial diseases are listed in Table 4-6.

SOMATIC MUTATIONS Mutations that occur during embryogenesis, or later in development, are referred to as somatic mutations. Because these mutations do not involve the germline, they are not transmitted to the offspring. Somatic mutations have their most important role in various forms of neoplasia (*see* Chapter 7). Undoubtedly, many mutations occur that are silent, because they fail to alter the expression or function of genes. Another large group of somatic mutations may be deleterious to cellular function, but they result in apoptosis or programmed cell death, and are therefore not discovered (*see* Chapter 6). Rarely, mutations will enhance cell proliferation or prolong cell survival, and this group is associated with the development of tumors. These mutations can be identified because they confer a selective survival advantage, resulting in clonal expansion of cell population harboring the mutation.

Activating mutations have been described in many oncogenes. Some of these mutations activate growth factor receptors (e.g., *ret*), whereas others stimulate growth factor signaling pathways (e.g., *ras*). Another group of somatic mutations inactivate tumor suppressor genes such as *retinoblastoma* (*Rb*). Somatic "second hits" in tumor suppressor genes occur in several inherited cancer syndromes in which the "first hit" has already been transmitted in the germline. Examples of these syndromes include retinoblastoma (*Rb*), Li-Fraumeni (*p53*), and multiple endocrine neoplasia type I (*MEN-I*). Many models of tumorigenesis invoke the concept of multistep carcinogenesis. In this scenario, an individual may inherit certain mutations or a predisposition to errors in DNA repair. However, these features alone are not usually sufficient for neoplasia in the absence of additional, somatic mutations. Multistep carcinogenesis proposes an accumulation of mutations, some of which may involve the activation of oncogenes, others inactivate tumor suppressor genes, and another group may impair apoptosis (e.g., *p53*). The characterization of these types of somatic mutations is used increasingly to classify tumors for the purpose of prognosis and may eventually provide new strategies for treatment.

SCREENING FOR GENETIC DISORDERS

The detection of genetic disorders by means of DNA testing is playing an increasing role in prenatal diagnosis, newborn, and

Table 4-6
Selected Mitochondrial Diseases

Disease/syndrome	*MIM no.*
MELAS syndrome: mitochondrial myopathy with encephalopathy, lactic acidosis, and stroke	540000
Leber optic atrophy: hereditary optical neuropathy	535000
Kearns-Sayre syndrome (KSS): ophthalmoplegia, retinal pigment degeneration, cardiomyopathy	530000
MERRF syndrome: myoclonic epilepsy and ragged red fibers	545030
Maternally inherited myopathy and cardiomyopathy (MMC)	590050
Neurogenic muscular weakness with ataxia and retinitis pigmentosa (NARP)	551500
Progressive external ophthalmoplegia (CEOP)	258470
Pearson syndrome (PEAR): bone marrow and pancreatic failure	557000
Autosomal dominant inherited mitochondrial myopathy with mitochondrial deletion	157640

population screening, as well as predictive testing (*see* Chapter 9). Although these tests are extremely helpful in some instances, they are associated with difficult ethical questions, some of which are briefly addressed at the end of this chapter.

Chorionic villus sampling (CVS) and ultrasound-guided umbilical vein puncture allow analyses of fetal DNA during the first trimester, and amniocentesis is used to test for genetic diseases during the second trimester. Generally accepted indications to perform such analyses include the presence of a known familial genetic disease and advanced maternal age. Disorders for which prenatal diagnosis is routinely available include the thalassemias, hemophilias A and B, cystic fibrosis, and chromosomal abnormalities that can be identified by fluorescent *in situ* hybridization (FISH). Determination of the sex has major implications in X-linked disorders (e.g., Duchenne muscular dystrophy or hemophilia). Other applications of prenatal DNA testing include the diagnosis of congenital infections and Rhesus blood group incompatibility.

Newborn screening for frequent diseases is well-established for disorders that can be altered by early treatment, such as congenital hypothyroidism, phenylketonuria, and galactosemia. In some countries, these newborn screening programs have been expanded, and the application of PCR to newborn blood spots opens the door for further testing, as exemplified by screening for cystic fibrosis, sickle-cell disease, or congenital adrenal hyperplasia. Issues that have to be addressed before accepting new screening programs include cost-effectiveness, adequate counseling, and therapeutic consequences.

Population screening strategies are also becoming more practical because PCR allows testing of a large number of samples relatively rapidly and economically. Population screening can be performed using different strategies. In selective screening programs, DNA testing is performed by mutational analysis or linkage studies in individuals at risk for a genetic disorder known to be present in a family (e.g., Tay-Sachs disease). Mass screening programs require tests of high sensitivity and specificity in order to be cost-effective. In epidemiological surveys, this type of screening program allows determination of the prevalence of certain disorders. Prerequisites for their success are that the disorders be potentially serious, that they can be influenced at a presymptomatic stage by changes in behavior, diet and/or pharmaceutical manipulations, and that the screening does not result in any harm or discrimination ("primum nil nocere"). Screening for the autosomal recessive neurodegenerative storage disease, Tay-Sachs, in Jewish populations resulted in a reduction of the number of affected individuals. In contrast, the screening for sickle-cell trait and disease in African Americans led to unanticipated problems of discrimination by health insurers and employers. Mass screening programs harbor further potential problems. Although screening for the most common genetic alteration in cystic fibrosis (ΔF508 mutation), with a frequency of ~70% in Northern Europe, is feasible and seems to be effective, it is important to keep in mind that the disease can be caused by more than 600 other mutations. The search for these less common mutations would substantially increase the costs and workload, but result in little impact on the effectiveness of the screening program as a whole.

Population screening is also performed as a part of occupational screening programs that aim to detect increased risk for certain activities (e.g., α1-antitrypsin deficiency and smoke or dust exposure). Detection and exclusion of individuals with increased risk should not replace or diminish efforts to increase the safety of the working environment.

ETHICAL CONSIDERATIONS

Ethical issues surrounding genetics and genetic testing continue to be a topic of considerable debate. The sequencing of the human genome, the identification of its genes, and the association of genetic defects with disease raise many issues concerning the implications for the individual and mankind. The recent cloning of mammals underlines the relevance of these issues.

Ethical discussions are influenced by education, cultural traditions, religion, attitudes toward human values, and also political structures and historical context. Progress and the advantages of genetic medicine have to be balanced against their potential risks. Although the magnitude of benefits is difficult to predict, it is essential that genetic testing does not result in harm for individuals or groups within a society. Modern genetics has demonstrated that the concept of eugenics as a strategy for the elimination of human disease cannot be effective. The fact that this approach has been misused in the past must not be forgotten.

Testing for disease predisposition may lead to a profound change in the way we screen and treat disease, and it opens the possibility for early recognition. However, it also entails a risk of discrimination and loss of privacy, health benefits, and employment. In many countries, lawmakers are therefore establishing legislation that will prevent health plans from discriminating against people on the basis of their genetic inheritance, or using genetic screening to deny coverage or to establish premiums.

Prenatal diagnosis of a disorder may lead to ethical dilemmas for parents (*see* Chapter 9). The ethical implications of terminating a pregnancy continue to be controversial in many societies. In all these situations, adequate counseling is therefore paramount.

Other difficult situations may arise if DNA testing results in detection of nonpaternity, which occurs in 3–5% of randomly studied children in many cultures. Particular problems may arise when healthy children are tested. Testing may be acceptable in the context of a disorder for which early intervention will improve prognosis, but it is more problematic when this is not the case. This leads to the question of when or whether tests for these types of inherited disorders should be performed. For example, in Huntington disease, which cannot currently be influenced by any form of treatment, individuals are not tested before they are able to give informed consent (*see* Chapter 97). The complexity of these issues will probably increase further as multifactorial disorders are characterized more thoroughly at the genetic level.

The hope that molecular medicine will contribute significantly to diminish the burden of disease in the long term seems, however, realistic. For molecular medicine to be successful, it is essential that the ethical principles of social justice, equality of treatment, confidentiality of test results, and the absence of discrimination based on genetic screening are fully respected.

SELECTED REFERENCES

Alberts B, Bray D, Lewis J, Ruff M, Roberts K, Watson JD. Molecular Biology of the Cell, 3rd ed. New York: Garland, 1994.

Beaudet AL. Genetics and disease. In: Fauci AS, Braunwald E, Isselbacher KJ, et al., eds. Harrison's Principles of Internal Medicine, 14th ed. New York: McGraw-Hill, 1997; pp. 365–395.

Brock DJH. Molecular Genetics for the Clinician, 1st ed. Cambridge, U.K.: Cambridge University Press, 1993.

Collins FS. Positional cloning moves from perditional to traditional. Nat Genet 1995;9:347–350.

Dracopoli NC, Haines JL, Korf BR, et al., eds. Current Protocols in Human Genetics. New York: Wiley, 1994.

Gelehrter TD, Collins FS. Principles of Medical Genetics. Baltimore, MD: Williams & Wilkins, 1990.

Lewin B. Genes V. Oxford, UK: Oxford University Press, 1994.

McKusick VA. Mendelian Inheritance in Man: A Catalog of Human Genes and Genetic Disorders, 11th ed. Baltimore, MD: Johns Hopkins University Press, 1994.

Ott J. Human Genetic Linkage, 2nd ed. Baltimore, MD: Johns Hopkins University Press, 1992.

Passarge E. Color Atlas of Genetics. New York: Thieme, 1995.

Pembrey ME. Genetic factors in disease. In: Weatherall DJ, Ledingham JGG, Warrell DA, eds. Oxford Textbook of Medicine, Oxford, UK: Oxford University Press, 1996; pp. 100–138.

Reilly PR, Boshar MF, Holtzman SH. Ethical issues in genetic research: disclosure and informed consent. Nat Genet 1997;15:16–20.

Rimoin DL, Conner JM, Pyeritz RE, Emery AEH. Emery and Rimoin's Principles and Practice of Medical Genetics, 3rd ed. New York: Churchill Livingstone, 1996.

Scriver CR, Beaudet CR, Sly WS, Valle D, eds. The Metabolic and Molecular Bases of Inherited Disease, 7th ed. New York: McGraw-Hill, 1995.

Thompson MW, McInnes RR, Willard HF, eds. Genetics in Medicine, 5th ed. Philadelphia, PA: WB Saunders, 1991.

Weatherall DJ. The New Genetics in Clinical Practice, 3rd ed. Oxford, U.K.: Oxford University Press, 1992.

5 The Human Genome Project

J. LARRY JAMESON

INTRODUCTION

The Human Genome Project (HGP) was conceived in the mid-1980s as an ambitious effort to characterize the human genome, ultimately culminating with a complete DNA sequence by the year 2005. The accomplishment of this goal would locate the ~80,000 genes and provide the DNA sequence (~3×10^9 bp) for the entire genome at an estimated cost of $3 billion over 15 years. The project has evolved as an international effort, driven forward by numerous scientific groups and funding agencies. Exchange of information and biological materials has been facilitated by the Human Genome Organization (HUGO). In the United States, the genome project was officially launched in 1990 by the National Institutes of Health (NIH) and the Department of Energy (DOE). The goals, as initially conceived were (1) creation of genetic maps, (2) development of physical maps, and (3) determination of complete sequence of human DNA.

INITIATION OF THE GENOME PROJECT AS "BIG SCIENCE"

From its inception, the goals of the HGP seemed daunting, and some considered it unrealistic, if not foolhardy. In addition to issues of cost, there was much debate concerning the goals of the genome project, its organization and timetable, and whether it would raise insurmountable ethical issues. There was particular concern that resources committed to the genome project would detract from traditional investigator-initiated research. On the other hand, proponents emphasized that analyses of the genome were inevitable and that, in the absence of a systematic approach, genetic studies would be inefficient and even more costly. In terms of its potential impact, analogies were drawn to the space program and to attempts to unravel the periodic table of elements. Most anticipated that the genome project would spin off new technologies in parallel with completion of its scientific goals. Moreover, it was expected that progress in the genome project would provide even more opportunities for hypothesis-driven research and for applications to clinical medicine. As described below, the genome project appears to be living up to the expectations of its proponents.

SCOPE OF THE PROJECT

A few facts help to appreciate the scope of the human genome project. The 23 pairs of human chromosomes are thought to encode approximately 50,000–80,000 genes. It is estimated that only about 5–10% of the human genome encodes protein-coding regions of genes. The remainder of the genome comprises regulatory regions, introns, and repetitive sequences. Thus, only a minority of the genome is expressed in the form of mRNA, which is subsequently translated into protein. It is for this reason that analyses of expressed sequence tags (ESTs), short fragments of cDNA sequence from a particular tissue, provide a powerful approach for identifying gene sequences that encode proteins. The total length of DNA is about 3 billion bp, nearly 1000-fold greater than the *Escherichia coli* genome. At the outset of the HGP, most molecular biologists might be able to sequence and analyze a 30,000-kb locus over the course of a year. Thus, in the absence of technological advances, 100 years would be required for 1000 such individuals to complete DNA sequencing. For this reason, initial emphasis was placed on mapping and on the development of new sequencing and computer database technologies.

An analogy that has been used to illustrate the complexity of the human genome is to compare it with the amount of information in an encyclopedia that is written in the four-letter code of DNA (A, G, T, and C). Thus, the chromosomes might be analogous to volumes of the encyclopedia, with genes corresponding to paragraphs. This analogy emphasizes the challenge of identifying single nucleotide changes that might cause a disorder such as cystic fibrosis or sickle-cell anemia. In this case, the mutation would consist of a single letter change on one of the pages of the encyclopedia. In addition to identifying disease-causing genes, a critical first step is to create a table of contents and an index for the book, which allows one to find the relevant genes. This is the goal of genetic and physical mapping stages of the genome project.

GENETIC MAPS

The complexity of the human genome emphasizes the importance of first establishing a genetic and a physical map. In this manner, the locations of genes can be described. In addition, it allows genetic linkage to be determined. That is, genes that are physically close to one another on a chromosome will be transmitted together, except when a recombination event has occurred during meiosis to exchange homologous regions of DNA. The genetic and physical maps differ in the following manner. A genetic map is measured in centiMorgans (cM) and is based on distances between genes that are estimated by recombination frequency. The physical map is the actual distance (in bp of DNA sequence) between genes.

From: *Principles of Molecular Medicine* (J. L. Jameson, ed.), ©1998 Humana Press Inc., Totowa, NJ.

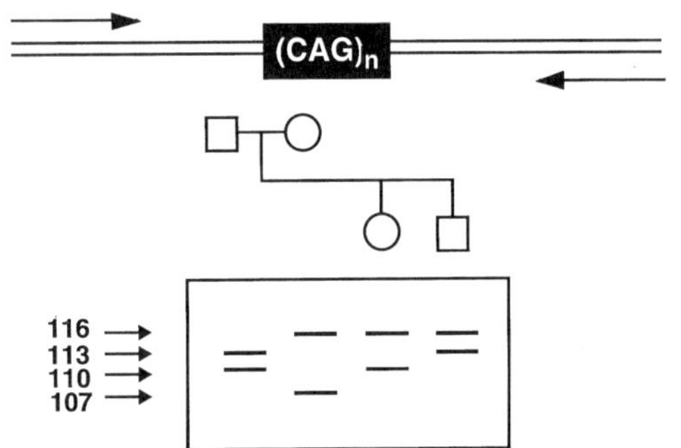

Figure 5-1 Detection of allelic variants using microsatellite markers. An example of a microsatellite consisting of a triplet nucleotide repeat (CAG) is shown. PCR primers on either side of the repeat results in PCR products of varying length, depending on the number of triplet repeats. In this example, the father has alleles of 110 and 113 and the mother has alleles of 107 and 116. The children each inherited the 116 allele from their mother and distinct alleles from their father. In this manner, microsatellites allow determination of chromosomal transmission within a family.

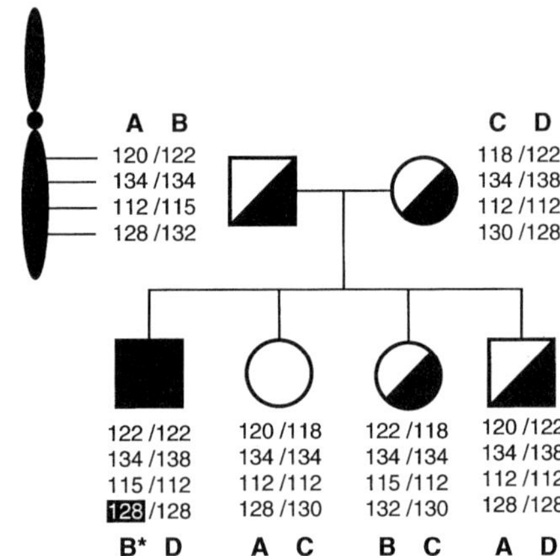

Figure 5-2 Genotype analysis using microsatellite markers. The pedigree illustrates autosomal recessive transmission. An array of microsatellite markers are shown along the long arm of one of the chromosomes. Note that some markers are dinucleotide repeats whereas others are trinucleotide repeats. The parents are heterozygous for most of the markers, which have been selected based on their high degree of heterozygosity within the population. Thus, when several markers are combined, it is relatively easy to document chromosomal transmission within the pedigree. One can assign letters (A–D) that correspond to the various chromosomes, reflecting the transmission of linked alleles. In this case, a putative disease gene is carried by each parent. The mutation resides on chromosome B in the father and chromosome D in the mother. Thus, a son with the BD genotype is affected, a daughter with genotype AC is unaffected, and the children with genotypes BC and AD are each carriers even though they inherited the disease gene from different parents. An example of recombination is illustrated in the affected son. In this case, the chromosome labeled B* received the 128 (black shading) microsatellite marker, which must be derived from the father's chromosome A. Because this son is affected, this crossover event indicates that the disease-causing gene resides centromeric to this microsatellite.

The unit of genetic distance, centiMorgans, is named after Thomas H. Morgan, a geneticist who provided early evidence for genetic linkage and established the concept that recombination frequency varies as a function of the distance between two genetic loci. By definition, 1 cM corresponds to a recombination frequency of 1%. For example, consider two polymorphic markers (A, B) on chromosome 11 that are linked to the gene causing multiple endocrine neoplasia type 1 (MEN-1). If sufficient pedigrees are examined, it is possible to determine which marker is closer to the disease locus by determining the frequency with which each marker undergoes recombination relative to the disease phenotype. If marker A undergoes recombination at a rate of 0.2, whereas marker B exhibits a lower recombination frequency (0.1), it can be concluded that marker B lies between marker A and the MEN-1 gene as long as there is data that neither marker is on the other side of MEN-1.

There are several reasons why there might be discrepancies between a genetic and a physical map. For example, some genomic regions may exhibit relatively high recombination frequencies. This would result in a greater genetic distance relative to a physical map. Recombination appears to be about twice as common during meiosis in females. Thus, most of genetic distances are "sex-averaged" distances.

Rapid progress in the creation of a genetic map reflects synergistic interactions among investigators from many countries. In addition, there have been important technical advances, particularly involving the use of highly polymorphic microsatellite markers. Microsatellites consist of di-, tri-, or tetranucleotide repeats. Within any given microsatellite marker, the number of repeats is highly variable in the population (Fig. 5-1). This makes it probable (~70% chance) that an individual will be heterozygous for the marker. In addition, their spouse is also likely to be heterozygous, or may even have a distinct set of repeats, greatly enhancing the power of linkage studies (Fig. 5-2). In the example shown, the array of microsatellite markers makes it possible to determine genetic transmission within a family with great certainty. A large array of these markers have now been identified and have been ordered throughout the genome.

The Genethon human linkage map was updated in 1996. At that point, the map consisted of more than 5000 microsatellite repeat polymorphisms with a mean heterozygosity of 70%. Genotyping with the microsatellite markers was performed using the CEPH (Centre d'Etudes du Polymorphisme Humaine) families. The estimated length of the map is 3699 cM, with an average interval size of about 1.6 cM. In combination with other genetic maps and markers, most regions of the genome can now be analyzed at the cM level. In the future, it may be possible to develop an array of single nucleotide polymorphisms that could be used in conjunction with DNA chip technology. In addition to increasing the density of markers, chip technology would be amenable to begin high throughput screening of genetic loci.

CONSTRUCTION OF PHYSICAL MAPS AND CLONING OF THE ENTIRE GENOME

In physical terms, 1 cM is roughly 1 million bp (1 Mb). The physical map reflects the arrangement and distances between genes and exists at several levels of resolution. A low-resolution map would reveal which chromosome carries a particular gene. The use of such techniques as fluorescence *in situ* hybridization (FISH) allows determination of the location of a particular gene on a chromosome. By using different fluorescent tags, it is possible to "paint" chromosomes and demonstrate the relative locations of genes, but still at a relatively low resolution. A higher level of

Table 5-1
Size of DNA Inserts in Various Vectors

Vector	*DNA insert, kb*
Yeast artificial chromosome (YAC)	1000
Bacterial artificial chromosome (BAC)	250
Cosmid	35
λ Phage	15
Plasmid	10

resolution can be achieved after cloning large DNA fragments and estimating distances using empiric methods such as gels to determine the sizes of an array of overlapping fragments, or DNA sequencing to determine the actual length between genes. As noted below, a parallel goal of the genome project is to insert large segments of the human genome into cloning vectors such as yeast artificial chromosomes (YACs) (Table 5-1). Additional mapping often involves the use of BACs (bacterial artificial chromosomes) and traditional cloning vectors such as lambda phage. Although YACs allow insertion of large fragments of DNA, BACs are gaining favor because of less frequent recombination. The isolation and physical separation of chromosomes has also allowed the preparation of chromosome-specific libraries.

The cloning of large segments of genomic DNA into YACS and cosmids greatly facilitates high-resolution gene mapping, particularly using "contigs," in which an ordered array of overlapping clones can be established (Fig. 5-3). An example of this approach on chromosome 21 is described further in Chapter 117. The goal of achieving a high-resolution physical map of the human genome has now been achieved and greater than 95% of the genome has been cloned into overlapping fragments. A major advance has been the use of sequence tagged sites (STSs) as a standard unit for physical mapping. The STSs serve as landmarks that allow overlapping cloned fragments to be arranged in the same order in which they occur in the genome. The STSs consist of 200–500 bp, which can be retrieved from computer databases as opposed to having to use stored clones. Thus, using PCR, investigators can amplify an STS to gain ready access to map locations.

The Whitehead group has now described the locations of more than 15,000 STS markers, which were screened against about 30,000 YAC clones from the CEPH-Genethon libraries. As of 1995, this map had an average distance of about 200 kb between markers. Ideally STSs would be available at intervals between 50 and 100 kb, which would allow the rapid localization of most disease genes. This will require at least 30,000 STSs. The feasibility of this approach has been enhanced by automation using a "genomatron" that performs 150,000 PCR reactions per run.

DNA SEQUENCING

A long-term goal of the genome project is to obtain DNA sequences for the entire human genome as well as model organisms, such as *Saccharomyces cerevisiae* (now completed, 12.4 million bp), *Caenorhabditis elegans*, and the mouse. At present, only a few percent of the human genome have been sequenced. The amount of DNA sequencing required is daunting for several reasons. Currently available technology is relatively expensive (0.20–0.30 dollars/base) and slow. Sequence accuracy and information management must be assured in parallel with technical advances. A current goal is to achieve 99.99% (1 error in 10,000 bp) accuracy. The issue of polymorphic variants in human sequence will only be addressed in the long term. There are probably polymorphic sequence variants approximately 1 out of every 1000 bp. Although this variation is low (99.9% identical), it suggests as many as 3 million sequence differences between any two unrelated individuals.

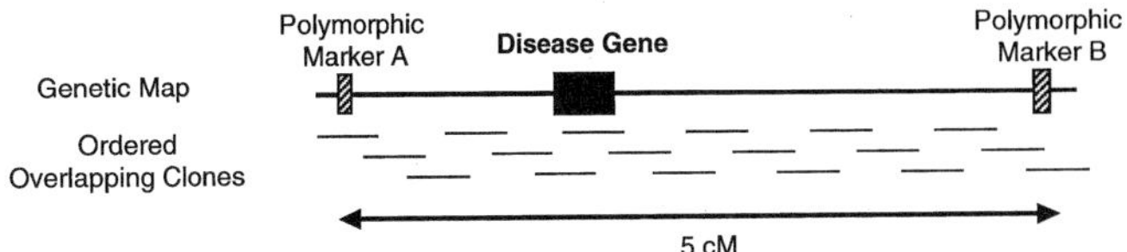

Figure 5-3 A physical genomic map with an ordered array of "contigs." A genetic map is shown with polymorphic markers A and B, shown on either side of a disease gene. Below the genetic map, a physical map consisting of overlapping clones is shown. The group of clones are referred to as a contig and can be ordered based on shared sequences, usually a sequence-tagged site (STS).

Despite these challenges, there have been remarkable advances in sequencing capabilities. A decade ago, most DNA sequencing was performed manually. Radioactive sequences had to be developed onto film and the nucleotide sequence was entered into databases manually. Automated DNA sequencing has made a major impact on throughput, particularly because the fluorescently labeled sequence can be read directly into computer systems. A goal is to develop sequencing capability of approximately 50–80 Mb per year. This will require the combined use of robotics and automation in conjunction with informatics. It is presently unclear whether the DNA sequence of the entire genome will be completed by the year 2005. However, several aspects of the genome project have progressed at an accelerated rate because of unanticipated technological advances. At present, most sequencing efforts remain based on gels that resolve DNA sequence at a single nucleotide level. There are efforts to develop new sequencing technologies, including the use of DNA chips. This technology, based on the use of arrays of oligonucleotides that are applied to DNA chips, is particularly promising for detecting variations and mutations in known DNA sequences.

MAJOR ADVANCES AND FUTURE CHALLENGES

Considering its controversial inception, the human genome project has progressed remarkably well. The genome project has already catalyzed many advances in human genetics. The development of a high-resolution genetic and physical map makes it possible to more rapidly identify disease-causing genes by positional cloning. These efforts in turn provide additional sequence and physical map information about specific regions of the genome. As depicted in Fig. 5-4, the number of disorders identified by positional cloning has increased markedly in recent years; this trend can be expected to continue. The identification of the cystic fibrosis gene in 1989 represented a landmark example of positional cloning. In 1996, examples of positional cloning included Friedrich's ataxia, long QT syndrome, basal cell nevus syndrome, hemochromatosis, a form of Maturity Onset Diabetes of the Young (MODY), and Treacher Collins syndrome, among many others.

The genome project has stimulated interest in the private sector in the applications of genetics. Characterization of expressed sequence tags (ESTs) has greatly enhanced the database of known

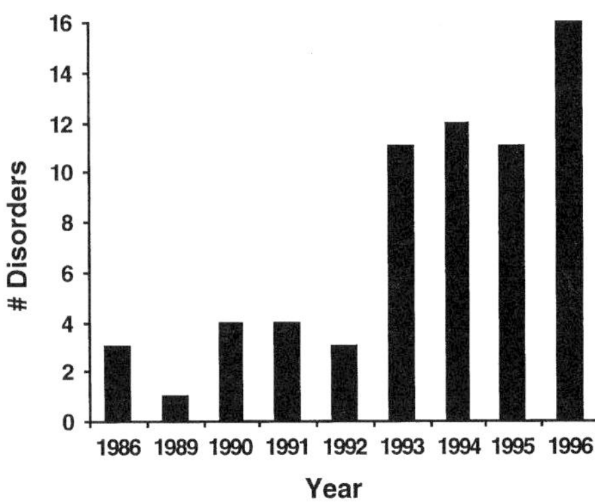

Figure 5-4 Number of genes that cause inherited disorders identified by positional cloning.

expressed genes. In the future, we can expect these databases to be merged with physical maps such that expressed genes can be superimposed onto physical maps. We can also expect increasing interest in changes in pattern of gene expression in disease states, including cancer.

Implicit in the human genome project is the idea that identifying disease-causing genes can lead to improvements in diagnosis, prognosis, and treatment. It is estimated that most individuals harbor several serious recessive genes. Because the frequency of mutations in most of these genes is low, it is unlikely that both members of a couple would carry mutations in the same gene, unless there is consanguinity or a restricted gene pool. However, the polymorphic variation in DNA also confers risk to a large number of less serious susceptibility genes. Most polygenic disorder reflect the cumulative risk of several different susceptibility genes. The ability to test for disease genes, whether serious mutations with relative high gene frequencies or various susceptibility genes, is already a reality and can be expected to expand rapidly with improvements in technology. The diagnosis of most disorders is currently made on clinical grounds in conjunction with radiographic or laboratory tests. Nevertheless, there is often some degree of uncertainty, resulting in a "differential diagnosis." The ability to add genetic tests will not always remove uncertainty, but it adds a powerful new dimension. For example, a patient with medullary thyroid cancer and a germline mutation in the ret oncogene can be diagnosed with multiple endocrine neoplasia type II. Molecular genetics also improves the categorization of disease. For example, Duchenne's and Becker's muscular dystrophies are now known to involve the same genetic locus (dystrophin), but the mutations differ in their impact on the encoded protein. Similarly, the "classic" and "adult-onset" forms of congenital adrenal hyperplasia are now known to represent mutations in the 21-hydroxylase gene that vary in severity. In general, the diagnostic capability of molecular diagnostics is much greater than the prognostic information that results. In part, this reflects still-limited genotype–phenotype correlations. In addition, genetic background and environmental influences can greatly modify the course of many genetic diseases. For example, individuals with lipoprotein abnormalities can have a highly variable clinical course, depending on other genes that act on lipid metabolism as well as environmental influences such as diet composition and weight gain.

An ultimate goal is to use the results of the genome project to improve the therapy of diseases. Success in this area might result from several venues. Perhaps the first advance will come from screening and prevention. Thus, patients known to carry a risk factor gene could be screened selectively for certain diseases or treated prospectively. For example, individuals known to carry genes that predispose to colon cancer would undergo earlier and more intensive screening. Individuals with genes that predispose to non–insulin-dependent diabetes mellitus could receive counseling about diet and weight gain, and may be treated early to prevent metabolic decompensation. Gene discovery will provide targets for screening for new drugs. The availability of recombinant hormones such as growth hormone, insulin, and erythropoietin has already had a major impact on clinical medicine. The potential role of gene therapy has received much attention. For certain enzyme deficiency disorders, such as adenosine deaminase deficiency, the technique has great promise. Its role for many other diseases, such as cystic fibrosis or sickle-cell anemia, remains to be established. In addition to classic genetic disorders, gene therapy may have an adjunctive role in the management of atherosclerotic lesions or the treatment of cancers. Currently, major issues that face gene therapy include the need to target therapy to specific tissues (e.g., cancers), the need to regulate gene expression (e.g., insulin in diabetes), and the need to sustain long-term expression (e.g., cystic fibrosis).

The genome project raises many ethical issues, which have been addressed in parallel with the other major goals of the project. Advances in such areas as the predisposition to cancer, atherosclerosis, or degenerative neurologic diseases such as Huntington's or Alzheimer's disease raise important questions concerning genetic counseling, privacy, and genetic discrimination in the workplace or by insurance companies. In addition, the scientific advances of the genome project require ongoing public and professional education, and there is the potential for unrealistic fears or expectations. The US federal government has established the "Ethical, Legal, and Social Implications" (ELSI) working group to help address ethical issues that arise from the genome project. Analogous groups exist in several other countries.

Many issues raised by the genome project are familiar in principle to medical practitioners. For example, a patient with increased LDL cholesterol, high blood pressure, or a strong family history of early myocardial infarction, is known to be at increased risk of coronary heart disease. Likewise, patients with phenylketonuria, cystic fibrosis, or sickle-cell anemia are often identified as having a genetic disease early in life. These precedents can be helpful for adapting policies that relate to genetic information. The genome project is, nevertheless, accelerating the rate of new information. In addition, the new information is greatly expanding the repertoire of diseases that can be characterized at the genetic level. One confounding aspect of the rapid expansion of information is that the ability to make clinical predictions often lags behind the genetic advances. For example, when genes that predispose the breast cancer, such as BRCA1, are described, there is tremendous public interest in the potential to predict disease; but many years of clinical research are required to rigorously establish genotype and phenotype correlations.

In the future, increased education will be required to adequately address many of the issues related to advances in molecular medicine. Whether related to informed consent, participation in research, or the management of a genetic disorder that affects an individual or their families, there is great need for more information on the fundamental principles of genetics. The lay press has glorified many aspects of genetics and, in such cases as gene therapy, expectations have been raised to unrealistic levels. The pervasive nature of molecular medicine also makes it imperative for physicians and other health care professionals to become more informed about genetics and to provide advice and counseling in conjunction with trained genetic counselors (*see* Chapter 9).

SELECTED REFERENCES

Collins F, Galas D. A new five-year plan for the U.S. Human Genome Project. Science 1993;262:43–46.

Haseltine WA. Discovering genes for new medicines. Sci Am 1997; 276:92–97.

Hudson KL, Rothenberg KH, Andrews LB, Kahn MJ, Collins FS. Genetic discrimination and health insurance: an urgent need for reform. Science 1995;270:391–393.

Jordan E, Collins FS. A march of genetic maps. Nature 1996;380: 111,112.

Schuler GD, Boguski MS, Stewart EA, Stein LD, Gyapay G, Rice K, et al. A gene map of the human genome. Science 1996;274: 540–546.

Venter JC, Smith HO, Hood L. A new strategy for genome sequencing. Nature 1996;381:364–366.

Watson JD. The human genome project: past, present, and future. Science 1990;248:44–49.

Weissenbach J. Landing on the genome. Science 1996;274:479.

6 The Cell Cycle

LYNDA Q. NGUYEN AND J. LARRY JAMESON

INTRODUCTION

The cell cycle consists of a set of highly ordered events that result in the duplication and division of a cell. This process requires the synthesis of a new copy of DNA, segregation of chromosomes, mitosis, and apportionment of the cellular contents. Multiple extracellular signals control entry and exit from the cell cycle to coordinate normal cell growth and to avoid uncontrolled cell proliferation. Various steps in the progression of the cell cycle are regulated rigorously to allow surveillance of the cycle and to avoid errors in DNA replication. This chapter reviews the molecular basis for control of the cell cycle. Much progress has come from studies of yeast, clams, and other model systems. These mechanisms are largely conserved in mammalian systems, which are the main focus of this chapter.

GENERAL MECHANISMS

Early studies using light microscopy allowed some of the events the cell cycle, such as mitosis, to be observed. When DNA was radiolabeled with ^{3}H-thymidine, it was possible to visualize the segregation of chromosomes. From these experiments, it was learned that newly replicated DNA becomes condensed and aligned at the mitotic spindle, and that sister chromatids segregate to opposite poles of the cell before the actual division of the cell. There are few visible changes during the interval between cell divisions (interphase) except for the increase in cell volume and mass. For this reason, molecular and genetic approaches have been essential for understanding the processes that control the cell cycle.

Cellular replication can be divided into several distinct phases. Mitosis (M phase) refers to the process of chromosomal segregation and actual cell division. Mitosis results in the division of one cell into two identical daughter cells, each bearing a complete diploid (2n) complement of chromosomes. Mitosis is divided into prophase, metaphase, anaphase, and telophase. These stages, along with several additional subdivisions, are based on characteristic features associated with chromosomal segregation, mitotic spindle formation, and cell division (Fig. 6-1). The cell cycle may also lead to meiosis, producing gametes with a haploid (1n) number of chromosomes. Although the mechanisms controlling mitosis and meiosis have some similarities, this chapter will focus on the mitotic cycle of the somatic cell. The interval between cell divisions is referred to as interphase, which is classically divided into three stages: G1, S, and G2 (Fig. 6-2). In addition, G0 refers to a resting state when cells have exited from the active cell cycle and have not committed to reenter the process of cell division. During G1, the effects of extracellular nutrients, mitogens, and growth factors induce the transcription of genes that are necessary for DNA synthesis, and the cell transitions into a committed state that will ultimately lead to the replication of DNA during the S (synthetic) phase. During G2, there is additional cellular growth and repair of DNA replication errors before the cell enters mitosis (M phase). After mitosis, cytokinesis, the actual process of cell division, occurs. If conditions are not appropriate for another round of cell division, G0 can be entered for an indefinite period of time before the cell makes the transition back into G1.

In a rapidly proliferating somatic cell, the entire cycle requires about 18–24 h. G1 occupies the longest time and may require up to 12 h. DNA replication during S phase may last from 6 to 8 h, depending on the size of the genome and the number of replication origins that are initiated simultaneously. G2 requires approximately 3–4 h, and mitosis can occur within an hour.

THE CYCLINS AND THEIR CYCLIN-DEPENDENT KINASES

The cyclin-dependent kinases (CDKs) coordinate specific transitions that occur at defined times during the cycle. Originally described by Hartwell in his studies of the budding yeast *Saccharomyces cerevisiae*, the genes encoding these proteins were named cell-division cycle or *cdc* genes. Mutations in the *cdc* genes caused an arrest at specific points in the cell division cycle. One of the first *cdc* genes to be isolated was *cdc2*, which was found by Nurse during studies of the fission yeast, *Schizosaccharomyces pombe*. Mutations in *cdc2* caused arrest at two points in the cell cycle; either before "start," where the yeast cell becomes committed to DNA replication, or just before mitosis. The *cdc2* gene encodes a 287 amino acid protein with high homology to protein kinases. As opposed to the yeast *S. cerevisiae*, which contains a single cell cycle CDK (cdc28), and *S. pombe* (cdc2), mammalian cells have several: Cdc2, CDK2, CDK3, CDK4, CDK6, and CDK7, which act at different transitions in the cell cycle.

Activation of CDK activity requires their association with another group of proteins known as the cyclins (cyclin D, H, E, A, and B). Cyclins were initially identified by Hunt in developing sea urchin and clam eggs. The levels of the various cyclins fluctuate during the cell cycle in a characteristic manner (Fig. 6-3). Cyclin D is induced during G1 and remains elevated throughout the cell

From: *Principles of Molecular Medicine* (J. L. Jameson, ed.), ©1998 Humana Press Inc., Totowa, NJ.

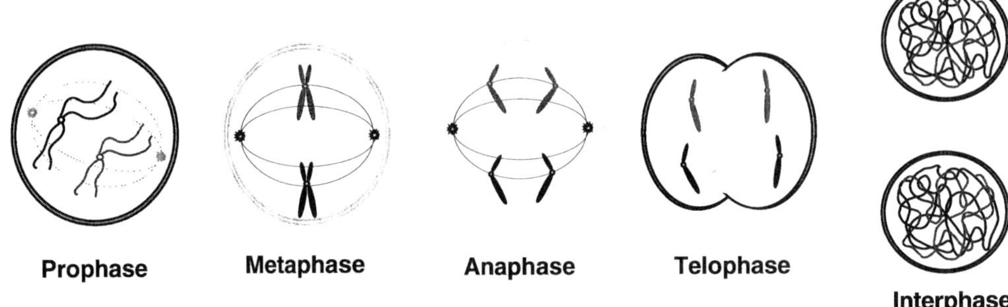

Figure 6-1 Stages of mitosis. For simplicity, only the nucleus is shown, and only two chromosomes are illustrated. Although mitosis is a continuous process, it is useful to divide it into several distinct stages. Prophase refers to the initial stage of mitosis during which chromosomes begin to condense, centrioles appear and initiate the formation of the mitotic spindle, and the nucleus begins to disintegrate. Metaphase is characterized by the alignment of chromosomes along the equitorial plate of the cell. The chromosomes are highly contracted at this stage and are attached to the microtubules via kinetochores. Anaphase begins with the separation of the two chromatids of each chromosome. Telophase is characterized by reformation of the nuclear envelope around the dividing nuclei and by the decondensation of chromatids as the cells are restored to the interphase state. Several of these stages of mitosis that can be subdivided into intermediate events are not shown.

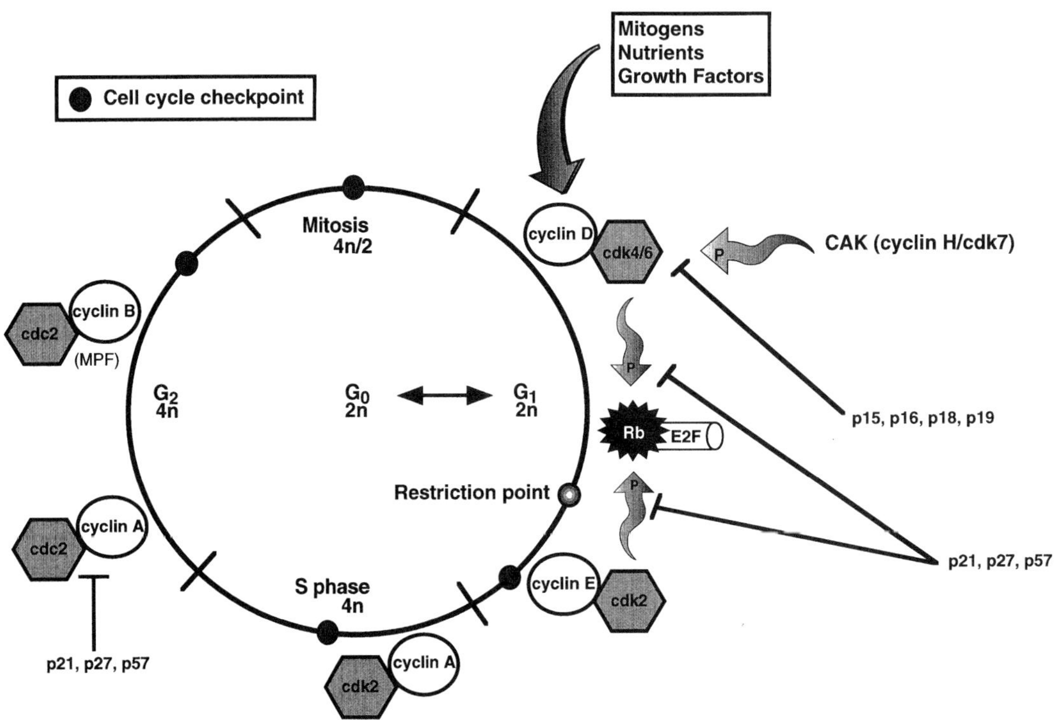

Figure 6-2 Overview of the cell cycle. A schematic representation of various changes in cyclin/CDK activity during the cell cycle is depicted. Growth factors induce the synthesis of D-type cyclins, thereby causing an association with CDK4 and CDK6 in early G1. Additional phosphorylation of CDK4/CDK6 by CAK is required for CDK activation. Phosphorylation of Rb by cyclin D/CDK4/CDK6 is required to drive the cell past the restriction point, where mitogenic stimulation is no longer needed, and signals the entry into S phase. Cyclin E/CDK2 kinase activity is subsequently needed to maintain Rb in its hyperphosphorylated state. Although cyclin A is synthesized in late G1, it associates with CDK2 throughout S phase and later with cdc2 in late S phase and early G2. Cyclin B complexes with cdc2 during G2; this complex was originally known as MPF. CDK inhibitors either block cyclin/CDK assembly and/or inhibit CDK activities, serving to arrest cells at specific points until conditions are optimal to reenter the cell cycle. Cells emerging from quiescence in G0 or from mitosis may reenter G1 and continue with the division process.

cycle. Cyclin E is produced transiently in late G1 and declines before S phase. Cyclins A and B are also known as the mitotic cyclins. Cyclin A is synthesized in late G1 and throughout S phase. It activates CDK2 during S phase and cdc2 during G2. Cyclin B is produced during G2 and also activates cdc2. Both cyclins A and B are degraded during M phase. All cyclins contain a characteristic 100-amino acid "cyclin box" which is located in the amino-terminal region. Proteolysis of the mitotic cyclins is conferred by a 9-amino acid motif referred to as the destruction box (D box), which is also located at the amino-terminal region of the proteins. The D box is necessary for ubiquitination and subsequent proteolytic degradation. Proteolysis of cyclins A and B triggers exit

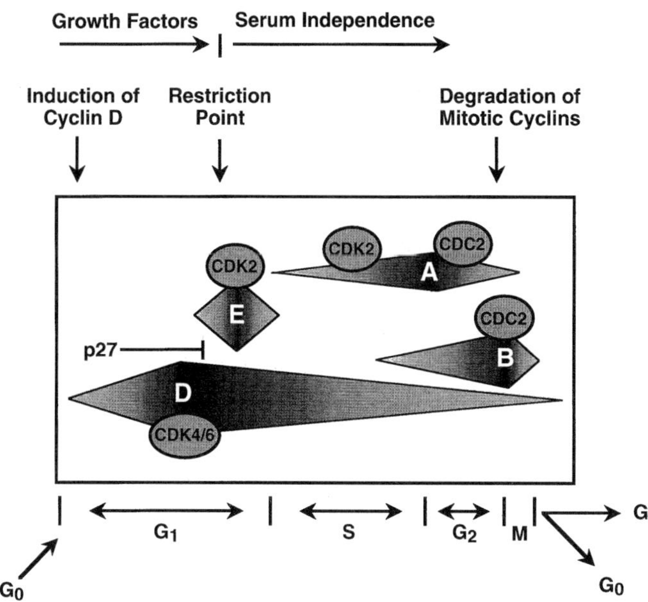

Figure 6-3 Changes in cyclins during the cell cycle. The levels of different cyclins are depicted schematically. Early in G1, growth factors and mitogens induce the transcription of the D-type cyclins (D1, D2, D3) that accumulate and persist through most of the cell cycle. After G1, cyclin D is translocated from the nucleus to the cytoplasm. Cyclin associates with several CDKs (CDK 2, CDK 4, CDK 6). Cyclin E accumulates in late G1, associates with CDK2, and is destroyed rapidly as cells enter S phase. The mitotic cyclins, cyclin A and cyclin B, increase in S phase and G2, and are degraded by the anaphase promoting complex (APC) before the end of mitosis. Cyclin A associates with CDK 2 during S phase and with cdc 2 during G2. cdc2-cyclin B complexes are restricted to M phase.

from mitosis. As described below, proteolysis also occurs at other phases of the cell cycle to enable specific transitions (e.g., proteolysis of CDK inhibitors during G1; proteolysis of inhibitors to allow transition from metaphase to anaphase).

The cyclin-CDK complexes are subject to input from multiple pathways. The kinase activity of the CDKs is regulated by phosphorylation (both positively and negatively) and by dephosphorylation. The cyclin/CDK complexes are also negatively controlled by several groups of inhibitors (Fig. 6-2). Proteins such as p21$^{WAF1/CIP1}$ act by directly inhibiting CDK kinase activity, whereas proteins such as Suc1 modify the specificity or accessibility of CDKs for regulatory proteins. Cyclins also contribute to CDK substrate specificity. The phosphorylation of substrates (e.g., Rb) by specific cyclin/CDK complexes induces the transcription of genes, whose products are needed to drive the cell through each transition of the cell cycle. It can be speculated that each of these regulatory proteins, in addition to the cyclins and their associated kinases, are potential targets for dysregulation of cell cycle control.

RESTRICTION POINT CONTROL AND G1 TO S PROGRESSION

Mitogenic signals, such as growth factors, induce cells to enter and progress through G1. The D-type cyclins (D1, D2, and D3) serve as growth factor sensors and are transcribed in response to growth factor stimulation (Fig. 6-3). Cyclin synthesis, and interaction with their CDK partners (CDK4 and CDK6), also depends on mitogenic stimulation. As long as nutrient and growth factor availability is sustained, cyclin synthesis and the assembly of cyclin D/CDK4 and cyclin D/CDK6 complexes continue to occur. After a cell reaches the restriction point (R) in late G1, it is committed to DNA replication and subsequently enters S phase, where mitogenic stimulation is no longer required for cell cycle progression.

Cyclin D/CDK4/CDK6 complexes are activated through phosphorylation by a CDK-activating enzyme known as CAK, which is now recognized to be a complex between cyclin H and CDK7. The kinase activities of these cyclin/CDK complexes are crucial in the activation of substrates that play a vital role in the G1 to S phase transition. A primary target of the cyclin/CDK complex is the protein product of the *retinoblastoma* (*Rb*) tumor suppressor gene. Phosphorylation of Rb results in the dissociation of E2F transcription factors and is necessary for passage through the restriction point *(see below)*.

A family of inhibitors known as the Inhibitors of CDK4 (INK4) proteins block the activities of the cyclin D/CDK4/CDK6 complexes. These inhibitors, which include p16^{Ink4}, p15^{Ink4B}, p18^{Ink4C}, and p19^{Ink4D}, can induce G1 arrest (Fig. 6-2). Inactivation of these inhibitors allow uncontrolled cell proliferation and increased genomic instability, and p15 and p16 are targets for mutations in certain malignancies (*see* Chapters 7 and 85). Inactivation of the *Rb* gene shortens the G1 phase, reduces cell size, and decreases the dependence on mitogenic stimulation. Disruption of the Rb pathway occurs in several forms of cancer (*see* Chapters 7 and 105). In cultured cells that lack Rb, the ectopic expression of INK4 proteins no longer arrests cells, confirming that Rb is an important target for these inhibitors.

In late G1, the synthesis of cyclin E is upregulated, presumably through E2F, since the *cyclin E* gene has been shown to contain an E2F-response element. Cyclin E/CDK2 activity may therefore be regulated by a positive feedback mechanism. Entry into S phase is highly dependent on the proteolytic degradation of cyclin E by ubiquitin-dependent pathways. Phosphorylation by its catalytic partner, CDK2, targets cyclin E for destruction. As cyclin E/CDK2 activity decreases, cyclin A synthesis is induced. Accumulation of the cyclin A/CDK2 complexes signals entry into S phase. Cyclin D/CDK2 and cyclin A/CDK2 complexes may interact with the DNA replication origins. Cyclin A/CDK2 also binds E2F/DP-1 dimers, phosphorylating a regulatory residue on DP-1, thereby preventing DNA binding of the E2F/DP-1 complex. Inactivation of E2F helps to ensure cell cycle progression into S phase and prevents reversion back to G1.

The cyclin D/CDK4/CDK6, cyclin E/CDK2, and cyclin A/CDK2 kinase activities are inhibited by another group of proteins that includes p21$^{WAF1/CIP1}$, p27^{KIP1}, and p57^{KIP2} (Fig. 6-2). These CDK inhibitors (CDKIs) also impair CAK activity. The *p27* gene product may be one the most important proteins involved in restriction point control; p27 represses the activity of cyclin E/CDK2 and cyclin A/CDK2 until entry into S phase. Depriving proliferating fibroblasts of serum mitogens increases p27, thereby causing an immediate arrest at G1. The tumor suppressor gene, *p53*, also induces p27. In addition, p15 and p27 may provide a pathway for TGF-β-mediated growth suppression. The *p15* gene is activated in response to TGF-β, a growth factor that suppresses the proliferation of several cell types, including colon and prostate epithelial cells; p15 binds cyclin D/CDK4 and cyclin D/CDK6 complexes to displace p27, allowing it to bind cyclin E/CDK2 and block cell cycle progression.

S PHASE

Once a cell is committed to the initiation of DNA replication, the process continues until duplication of the entire genome is complete. In the human genome, this entails the accurate duplication of approximately 3 billion bp of DNA. An enormous level of replication fidelity is required to accurately synthesize this amount of DNA. In addition to a highly regulated and well-conserved replication system, the existence of a proofreading mechanism (3' to 5' exonuclease) that detects misincorporated nucleotides, and a mismatch-repair system, helps to assure replication fidelity. In eukaryotes, an intricate network of DNA repair systems can delay the cell cycle to allow polymerase errors to be recognized and repaired. These systems also repair DNA damage that is induced by mutagens, such as oxidation products, spontaneous depurination or depyrimidination, chemical adducts, and the effects of ultraviolet (UV) radiation and ionizing radiation.

Defects in the DNA repair process predispose to several forms of cancer. The cancer-prone disorder, xeroderma pigmentosum (XP), results in deficient repair of UV-induced and oxidation-induced lesions (*see* Chapter 81). DNA repair defects and hypersensitivity to DNA damage are also associated with several other autosomal recessive syndromes, including Bloom's syndrome (BS), Fanconi's anemia (FA) and ataxia telangiectasia (AT).

The search for the human homologs of yeast mismatch-repair genes allowed the identification of *MSH2*. Soon thereafter, defects in this gene were shown to cause hereditary nonpolyposis colon cancer (HNPCC). In addition, *MSH2*-deficient mice have been shown to be highly susceptible to lymphoid tumors. Several other genes, including *MLH1* and *PMS2*, whose products are also involved in mismatch repair, are additional causes of HNPCC. Another form of DNA repair, called transcription-coupled repair, occurs during the transcription of DNA into RNA. Long strands of DNA that are unwound during transcription must be mended to reform the double strands. Patients with Cockayne syndrome (CS) exhibit defective mechanisms in transcription-coupled repair.

One of the important roles of the p53 tumor suppressor occurs during times of damage to DNA. DNA strand breaks induced by UV or ionizing radiation induce production of the p53 protein; this in turn stimulates the expression of genes (e.g., *p21*) that cause cell cycle arrest. p21 prevents DNA synthesis by binding proliferating cell nuclear antigen (PCNA), a subunit of the DNA polymerase δ enzyme complex involved in both DNA replication and repair. p53 also induces GADD45 and cyclin G, both of which contribute to G1 cell cycle arrest, allowing time for DNA repair. Germline mutations in *p53* cause Li-Fraumeni syndrome (LFS), which is associated with a high incidence of multiple cancers, including breast, ovary, and brain tumors (*see* Chapter 7). Inactivating p53 mutations are also among the most common somatic mutations in malignancies, emphasizing its importance in the maintenance of normal cell growth.

MECHANISMS CONTROLLING DNA REPLICATION

Important insight into mechanisms controlling DNA replication initially came from a series of cell fusion experiments. When a cell in G1 was fused to a cell in S phase, the nucleus of the G1 cell began to replicate its DNA prematurely, indicating that the G1 nucleus is competent for replication and that the S phase cell contains an activator. However, when G2 cells were fused with G1 cells, the G2 nuclei failed to reinitiate DNA replication, whereas the G1 nuclei replicate normally, indicating that G2 nuclei cannot rereplicate DNA until passage through mitosis. The same held true when G2 nuclei were fused with cells in S phase. Several conclusions were drawn from the above experiments. First, only chromosomes from the G1 phase of the cell cycle are competent for DNA replication. Second, cells in S phase contain an activator that initiates DNA replication from G1 chromosomes. Third, G2 cells do not contain repressors and their nuclei must progress through mitosis before DNA replication can occur.

The control of DNA replication relies on the ordered assembly of specific proteins at the origins of replication. These proteins are necessary to form a competent, prereplicative chromosomal state. In eukaryotes, the origins of replication are determined by *cis*-acting sequences called replicator elements, and *trans*-acting proteins (initiator proteins) bind to the replicators. Because of the large amount of DNA that must be duplicated in eukaryotic genomes, multiple origins of replication are formed to accommodate the constraints of size and time. In the eukaryotic genome, approximately 10^3 to 10^5 replication initiation events occur during each cell cycle.

Recent discoveries in yeast have further elucidated this process. In *S. cerevisiae*, a multisubunit complex known as the origin recognition complex (ORC) has been shown to bind the initiator elements A and B. Consisting of six proteins, the ORC serves as a docking site for protein–protein interactions that regulate the initiation of replication. Other proteins, including cdc6p from budding yeast, and $cdc18^+$ from fission yeast, are also needed to form the prereplication complex. The proper assembly of this multisubunit complex defines the prereplicative state of the chromosomes in G1.

Studies using *Xenopus* egg extracts have provided evidence for activators of DNA replication. G1 nuclei from human HeLa cells are able to initiate DNA replication in the presence of egg extracts, but G2 nuclei are not. When the G2 nuclei are permeabilized and then repaired, DNA replication occurs. This finding led to the idea that G1 nuclei are competent, because factors sequestered in the cytoplasm are able to interact with chromatin when the nuclear envelope is disassembled during mitosis. However, once initiation of DNA replication occurs, the factor is destroyed, thereby preventing rereplication of the DNA.

Using yeast genetics, the mini-chromosome maintenance (MCM) family of proteins have been identified as factors that confer the replication-competent state of chromatin in G1. The MCM proteins include MCM2, MCM3, MCM4/cdc54, MCM5/cdc46, and MCM7/cdc47, and mutations in their genes cause a high rate of mini-chromosome loss. MCM proteins that are bound to chromatin are degraded as S phase progresses.

The formation of a prereplication complex therefore consists of the ORC, proteins such as Cdc6p, and the MCM complex. The activity of cyclins and their associated CDKs is important for activating DNA replication as well as blocking the reassembly of the prereplication complex once DNA synthesis is complete. During S phase, this requires the association between cyclin A and CDK 2, and in M phase, cyclin A/cdc2 and cyclin B/cdc2.

The mechanisms involved in the actual process of DNA replication are reasonably well-understood. As described above, DNA synthesis is initiated from multiple independent replicons. Because DNA is double-stranded, it is necessary to copy both strands simultaneously (Fig. 6-4). This can occur in either a unidirectional

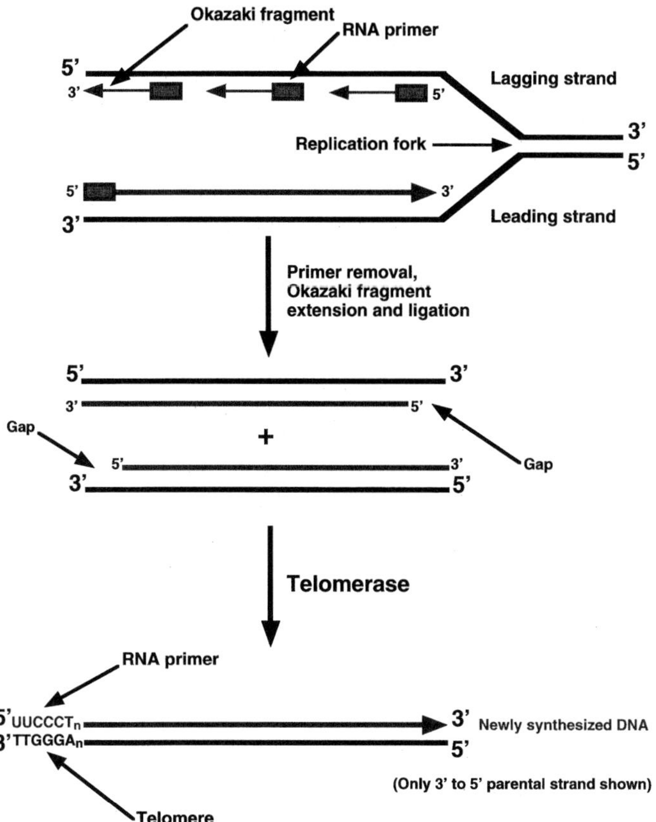

Figure 6-4 Replication of DNA. A replication fork is illustrated. After separation and unwinding of the DNA double helix, DNA replication proceeds in the 5' to 3' direction on opposite strands. The leading strand is synthesized continuously towards the replication fork. Synthesis of the lagging strand is initiated discontinuously as the fork unwinds, resulting in Okazaki fragments that are subsequently ligated together. At the end of chromosomes, telomeres exist to allow repair of the ends of DNA. The enzyme, telomerase, extends the 3' end of the parental strand, providing an elongated template.

(one replication fork) or bidirectional (two replication forks) manner. An RNA fragment that is complementary to the single-stranded region exposed by the replication fork serves as a primer for DNA synthesis, which occurs in a 5' to 3' direction. On the "leading" strand, DNA synthesis occurs continuously, whereas it is discontinuous on the opposite "lagging" strand, which is made available as the fork unwinds. The discontinuous Okazaki fragments on the lagging strand are subsequently ligated together.

A unique circumstance arises for DNA replication at the ends of the chromosomes. Since DNA polymerase requires a labile RNA primer to initiate synthesis, some bases at the 3' end of each template are not copied. Thus, the DNA strands would become progressively shorter with each cycle of replication in the absence of a mechanism to repair the ends. The identification of repeated GC-rich fragments at the ends of chromosomes, referred to as telomeres, provides a compensating mechanism for this process. Telomeres act as a template for the enzyme, telomerase, which extends the repeats (in the 3' direction) with each cycle of division. The presence of telomerase is required for ongoing cell division, and the loss of telomerase activity may represent a mechanism of cellular senescence.

G2 TO M PHASE TRANSITION

During G2, there are checkpoints to assure that DNA has been faithfully copied before entry into mitosis. DNA repair systems can be activated to correct errors that may have occurred during the replication process. In addition, cellular proteins involved in the assembly of the mitotic spindle and cell division are produced.

The cyclin/CDK complex involved in M phase was first identified through use of the *Xenopus* oocyte assay. When meiotic oocytes arrested in G2 are injected with M-phase cytoplasm from a mature unfertilized egg, the recipient oocyte is driven into M phase. These experiments led to the conclusion that a maturation promoting factor (MPF) in the cytoplasm of the egg caused the oocyte to complete cell division. MPF is now known to be a complex between the mitotic cyclin B and cdc2. Cyclin B, which is synthesized in late S phase, complexes with unphosphorylated cdc2. In *S. cerevisiae*, an additional level of regulation is provided by the competing actions of the tyrosine kinase Wee1 and the phosphatase cdc25. Phosphorylation by Wee1 on tyrosine 15 inactivates cdc2 kinase activity, whereas dephosphorylation of the same residue by cdc25 reactivates the complex. It is likely that mammalian homologs of these proteins also exist. Targets for MPF are not well-characterized, but both mitogen activated kinase (MAPK) and MPM2 kinase are potential substrates.

PROTEOLYSIS AND THE M TO G1 TRANSITION

Protein degradation is required for the preparatory events that occur before DNA replication and for entry into and exit from mitosis. Two major ubiquitin-dependent pathways mediate proteolysis at distinct points in the cell cycle (Fig. 6-5). The first pathway, involving a protein called cdc34, initiates DNA replication by degrading the CDK inhibitor SIC1. Using temperature-sensitive *cdc34* mutants in budding yeast, it was discovered that *cdc34* encodes a ubiquitin-conjugating enzyme, E2. Following activation by the E1 ubiquitin-activating enzyme, ubiquitin is transferred to the target protein, SIC1, by cdc34 (E2) through a transesterification reaction. Subsequent multiubiquitination by the ubiquitin-ligating enzyme E3 targets SIC1 to the 26S proteasome for degradation; cdc34 also participates in the destruction of the G1 cyclins, CLN2 and CLN3, in yeast. Ubiquitin-dependent degradation of a CDK-inhibitor represents a crucial event needed for entry into S phase.

The second pathway involves a multiprotein complex called the anaphase-promoting complex (APC). This complex mediates the entry and exit from mitosis by targeting anaphase inhibitors (PDS1 and CUT2) and mitotic cyclins A and B for destruction, also via the ubiquitin-proteasome pathway (Fig. 6-5). Although APC appears to be a large E3, it acts primarily by bringing together ubiquitin-charged E2s and D-box-containing substrates. As discussed previously, the D-box is a 9-amino acid motif in the aminoterminal domain of mitotic cyclins, which is necessary for degradation via the ubiquitin pathway. This degradation represents an irreversible step that assures exit from mitosis.

CELL-CYCLE CHECKPOINTS

The empirical definition of a cell-cycle checkpoint was provided by Hartwell and Weinert as an event B that is dependent on the completion of a prior event A. A checkpoint occurs if a loss-of-function mutation relieves the dependence. In biochemical terms, a checkpoint represents a surveillance system that allows the detection of an incomplete previous step in the cell cycle or

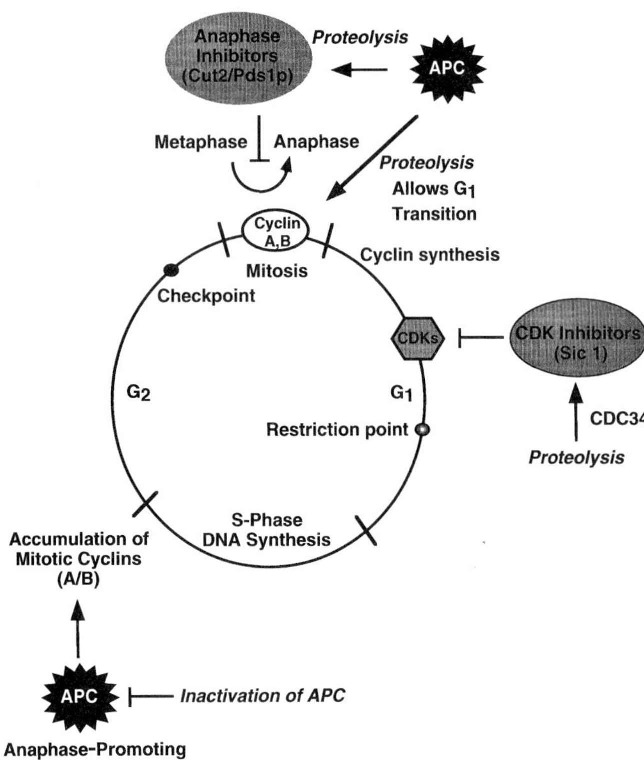

Figure 6-5 Role of proteolysis in cell cycle control. Proteolysis plays a critical role in several transitions during the cell cycle (*see* review by Kirschner and colleagues for details). Degradation of the mitotic cyclins (cyclin A and B) is mediated by the APC and is required for exit from mitosis. During G1, the cdc34 pathway degrades inhibitors of G1 CDKs (e.g., CDK2, CDK4), allowing passage into S phase. Inactivation of the APC allows the accumulation of mitotic cyclins that are involved in S-phase as well as the transition into mitosis. The APC also mediates proteolysis of anaphase inhibitors, permitting a transition from metaphase to anaphase.

damage to the genome or mitotic spindle. When cell-cycle checkpoint pathways are functioning correctly, cells arrest at specific phases, depending on when damage is sensed, to allow time for repair and to activate genes involved in the repair process.

Checkpoint regulatory pathways have been elucidated primarily based on analyses of *cdc* mutants in budding and fission yeast. Checkpoints exist for DNA damage, DNA replication blocks, and improper spindle assembly. The DNA damage checkpoint can be implemented at three times during the cell cycle: G1/S transition, progression through S phase, and at the G2/M transition. Four genes in *S. cerevisiae*, *RAD9*, *RAD17*, *RAD24*, and *MEC3*, serve as sensors of single-strand DNA, and they are required for G1 and G2 arrest in response to DNA damage.

Three genes act at the replication checkpoint in budding yeast: *POL2*, *DPB11*, and *RFC5*. They are all candidate sensors of DNA replication. DPB11 is required for replication arrest in response to hydroxyurea, an inhibitor of ribonucleotide reductase. DNA damage occurring during S phase is sensed by POL2, whereas DNA damage incurred during G1 and G2 is sensed by RAD9. RCF5 is a component of the replication factor C that binds to gapped DNA (e.g., during lagging-strand DNA synthesis). RCF5 recruits PCNA and DNA polymerase δ for repair. Two proteins, MEC1, a member of the phosphoinositide kinase family, and RAD53, a protein kinase, transduce the DNA damage signals to the repair systems. The sensors of spindle assembly are less well characterized. However, several yeast genes—*MAD1*, *MAD2*, and *MAD3* (mitotic arrest defective), and *BUB1*, *BUB2*, and *BUB3* (budding uninhibited by benzimidazole)—have been implicated in the spindle assembly checkpoint.

Similar checkpoint control pathways exist in mammalian cells, although fewer of the proteins have been identified. Three proteins controlling the DNA damage checkpoint include ATM (mutated in ataxia telangiectasia), the tumor suppressor p53, and the CDK inhibitor p21. p53 is a transcription factor that is induced in response to DNA damage, although how it is activated remains unknown. As noted above, p53-mediated G1 arrest results from activation of the *p21* gene. p21 directly inhibits the activity of CDKs needed for entry into S phase, and p21 knockout mice exhibit a partial failure to arrest at G1. Inactivation of p53 (e.g., by SV40 large t-antigen) may extend the life of cells that are of late passage, thereby inplicating p53 in cellular senescence. Cells from p53 nullizygous mice are able to escape cellular senescence and produce aneuploid immortalized cell lines.

p53 appears to be at least partially regulated by ATM, as cells lacking ATM show reduced and delayed activation of the *p53* gene in response to DNA damage. However, independent regulatory mechanisms must exist, as ATM mutant cells can still undergo p53-dependent apoptosis. Apoptosis can be considered a type of cell-cycle checkpoint. In the intact organism, destruction of damaged cells by apoptosis provides an important control against the accumulation of genetic damage. The *p53* gene is one of the most frequent mutations in human cancers. The *ATM* gene is a target of mutations as well; cells from patients with the cancer-prone syndrome ataxia telangiectasia exhibit defects in all three DNA damage-induced checkpoints.

Cellular senescence may also be considered as a cell-cycle checkpoint. This phenomenon is especially evident in culture, where normal cells undergo a limited number of divisions before reaching senescence. As noted above, shortened chromosomal telomeres and suppression of telomerase activity may be a mechanism for cell senescence. The re-expression of telomerase activity often occurs in tumorigenesis, resulting in the development of immortal cells.

CONTROL OF CELLULAR PROLIFERATION AND DIFFERENTIATION

A multitude of factors influence the ability of a cell to proceed through the cell cycle, to advance into a more differentiated state, or to undergo apoptosis. Factors such as cell-to-cell contact, viral infection, and mitogenic or inhibitory signals (or their withdrawal) initiate intracellular cascades that communicate signals to the molecular machinery in the nucleus. Many of these pathways, including their respective receptors and corresponding intracellular signaling molecules (second messengers and protein kinases), have been identified, and some have been implicated in tumorigenesis (*see* Chapters 7 and 46).

Although remarkable progress has been made in our understanding of the complex signaling pathways for growth factors, the mechanisms by which they induce cell division remain unclear. Terminally differentiated cells do not reenter the cell cycle. However, many growth factors induce both cell proliferation and differentiation, presumably by acting on progenitor cells that have not progressed beyond an irreversible stage of differentiation. For example, insulin stimulates the division of many cells, but it also induces differentiation (e.g., 3T3-L1 fibroblasts into differentiated adipocytes). In the case of hematopoietic cells, various cytokines stimulate the division of progenitor cells, but also move cells along a differentiation pathway. One explanation for these dual effects of growth factors involves their ability to activate parallel signaling cascades that ultimately have distinct cellular effects. It is also important to view the effects of a growth factor in the context of other extracellular stimuli that may act synergistically or antagonistically. Thus, the convergence of signaling pathways from different growth factors can elicit selective cellular responses. The pattern and timing of growth factor exposure is also important in determining cellular responses. For example, brief exposure to nerve growth factor (NGF) may induce cell division, whereas prolonged exposure favors neuronal differentiation.

Extracellular signals exert their strongest influence on the cell cycle during a narrow window of time in G1. Signals from growth factors such as epidermal growth factor (EGF) and insulin-like growth factor-1 (IGF-1) are integrated along with those from inhibitory factors such as transforming growth factor-β (TGF-β). An example of growth factor signaling is illustrated by EGF, which is a potent stimulator of cell proliferation. EGF binds to its membrane-bound tyrosine kinase receptor, resulting in receptor dimerization and autophosphorylation of specific tyrosine residues. These phosphorylated tyrosines induce the recruitment of Grb2 through its SH2 domain and the Sos protein through its SH3 domain. This complex activates the Ras signaling pathway (*see* Chapter 46). GTP-bound Ras stimulates the serine-threonine kinase Raf, which phosphorylates the mitogen-activated protein kinase (MAPKK or MEK). MAPKK phosphorylates the mitogen-activated protein kinase MAPK (or extracellular signal-related kinase; ERK). MAPK acts in the nucleus to phosphorylate and regulate the activity of oncogene products involved in cell cycle progression and growth, including c-*fos*, c-*jun*, and c-*myc*. In addition, cyclin D is upregulated in response to mitogens, leading to the activation of cyclin-dependent kinase activity.

Interactions mediated by cadherins provide an additional means of cell–cell as well as intracellular signaling. Cadherins are transmembrane Ca^{2+}-dependent adhesion receptors that play important roles in cell recognition and sorting during development and in the maintenance of solid tissue. Cadherins form complexes with cytoplasmic proteins known as catenins (α and β catenin). The association of cadherins with catenins is important for cytoskeletal alterations associated with cell recognition and morphogenesis. The intracellular domain of several cadherins (e.g., E cadherin) interacts with cytoskeletal-related proteins, such as globular actin, α actinin, vinculin, and ankyrin. The cadherins can also associate with signaling molecules such as the protein tyrosine kinases, Src, and Yes. β catenin is a substrate for Src, and its phosphorylation perturbs cadherin-mediated cell–cell adhesion. Intracellular signaling by cadherins can influence the availability of free β catenin, which serves as a substrate in the Wnt signaling pathway that regulates early development and cell fate in *Drosophila*. Defects or downregulation in cadherin or β-catenin function has been implicated in tumorigenesis (e.g., APC [adenomatous polyposis coli], DCC [deleted in colorectal cancer]), as loss of cell adhesion is associated with increased invasiveness of tumor cells.

Other proteins activated by less direct mechanisms also contribute to the control of cell-cycle progression. Several growth factors activate phospholipase C, which hydrolyzes phosphatidylinositol-4, 5-*bis*-phosphate (PIP_2) into two second messengers: diacylglycerol (DAG) and inositol 1, 4, 5-*tris*-phosphate (IP_3). DAG is able to activate protein kinase C, thereby stimulating gene transcription and cell proliferation. IP_3 releases calcium ions from intracellular stores and calmodulin, a calcium-binding protein, can also regulate the activities of other kinases in the cell.

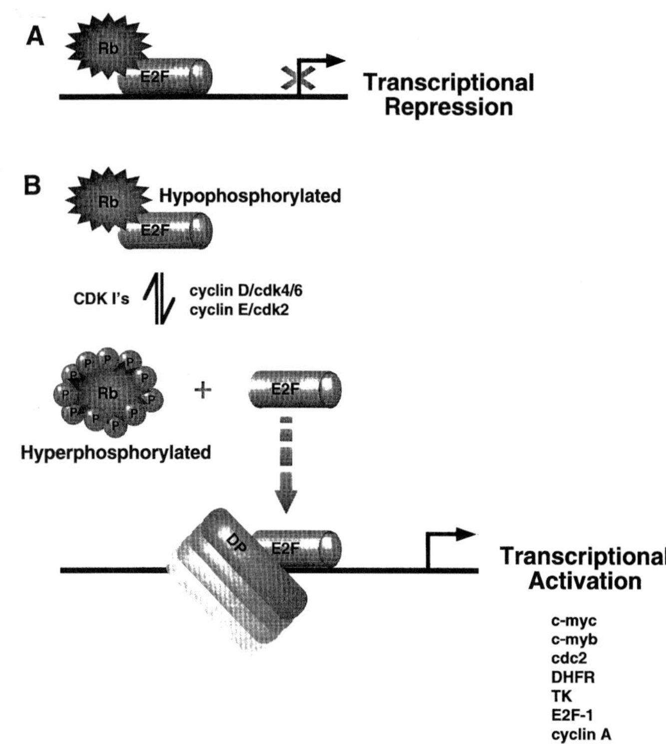

Figure 6-6 Control of Rb activity during G1 to S progression. **(A)** In its hypophosphorylated form, Rb is capable of binding E2F, preventing E2F-mediated transcriptional activation. **(B)** Phosphorylation of Rb by the active cyclin/CDK complexes during mid-to-late G1 causes the release of E2F from Rb, allowing E2F to heterodimerize with members of the DP family of transcription factors. As long as Rb is maintained in its hyperphosphorylated state, E2F/DP-mediated transcription of genes required for G1 to S phase progression continues. Factors favoring mitogenesis can regulate transcriptional activity by modulating Rb phosphorylation. In turn, growth inhibitory factors acting through CDKIs can reverse the hyperphosphorylated state of Rb.

Accumulating evidence suggests that Rb is a central target for the convergence of many of these signaling pathways (Fig. 6-6). Cells emerging from mitosis require prolonged and continuous growth factor stimulation until the restriction point is reached during mid to late G1. After the restriction point, serum is no longer required, and the cell can progress through S phase and the remainder of the cell cycle.

Regulation of the activity of Rb occurs largely as a result of phosphorylation. In its hypophosphorylated form, Rb associates with the E2F family of transcription factors (E2F1–E2F5). E2F-1 through E2F-3 associate with Rb (p105), whereas E2F-4 and E2F-5 associate preferentially with the Rb-related proteins, p107 and p130. The association with Rb can occur while the E2Fs are bound to the promoters of various genes and may account for the ability of hypophosphorylated Rb to actively repress gene transcription. Cyclin D/CDK4/CDK6 mediate the phosphorylation of Rb, and cyclin E/CDK2 is required to maintain Rb in a hyperphosphorylated state. When Rb is hyperphosphorylated, E2Fs dissociate and heterodimerize with the DP family of transcription factors (DP-1, DP-2, DP-3). These heterodimeric transcription factors bind to sequences in the regulatory regions of genes important in the control of cell growth, including c-*myc*, B-*myb*, *cdc2*, *DHFR*, *thymidine kinase*, and *E2F-1* itself.

Growth inhibitory factors prevent Rb phosphorylation through modulation of the CDKs that phosphorylate Rb. These signals block Rb phosphorylation by activating various CDK inhibitor proteins. Three signals have been identified that block Rb phosphorylation in this manner: TGF-β, cyclic AMP (cAMP), and contact inhibition. As described previously, TGF-β prevents Rb phosphorylation by inducing the expression of p15, which competes with D cyclins for binding to CDK4/CDK6. In addition, TGF-β has been shown to decrease levels of CDK4 in certain cell types. cAMP activates the protein kinase A (PKA) signaling cascade, which can inhibit Rb phosphorylation. cAMP also results in the phosphorylation of transcription factors, such as the cAMP response element-binding protein (CREB). Phosphorylated CREB recruits the coactivator CBP (CREB-binding protein), which links CREB to the basal transcription machinery, promoting the induction of gene transcription (*see* Chapter 3). In some cell types, activation of cAMP-responsive genes in combination with the inhibition of Rb phosphorylation leads to cellular differentiation.

It is important to note that a variety of other Rb-binding proteins have been identified. Among these are Elf-1, MyoD, PU.1, ATF-2, and c-Abl, although the effector functions of these proteins are largely unknown. Hypophosphorylated Rb has been shown to bind the catalytic domain of the nuclear tyrosine kinase c-Abl. This interaction blocks the kinase function of the proto-oncogene; phosphorylation of Rb releases c-Abl and allows it to phosphorylate nuclear substrates, some of which may be involved in cell growth.

APOPTOSIS

Apoptosis, or programmed cell death, is a normal cellular process that occurs in response to many different stimuli, including UV and ionizing radiation, chemotherapy, hypoxia, viral agents (E1A and E7), proto-oncogene expression (*E2F-1* and c-*myc*), and growth factor or hormone withdrawal. As opposed to cellular senescence, apoptosis is an energy-dependent process that results in distinct morphological changes in the cell. Nuclei become condensed and fragmented, DNA is degraded, and cells shrink and are eventually degraded by a lysosome-mediated pathway. Apoptosis plays a critical role in development and homeostatic processes, including development of the nervous system and in the lymphoid selection process of the immune system.

The apoptotic response can vary depending on the cell type and the nature of the stimulus. A number of gene products involved in cell cycle control mediate this response, including *Rb* and c-*myc*, although most work has centered around the actions of p53. p53-mediated apoptosis occurs primarily in response to DNA damage induced by UV radiation, hypoxia, or viral infection. A growing body of evidence points toward a cooperative interaction between the p53 and Rb/E2F pathways. The adenovirus E1A and the human papilloma virus (HPV) E7 proteins stabilize and activate p53, thereby inducing p53-dependent apoptosis. In response to p53 actions, viral proteins such as the HPV E6 protein and E1A can bind the tumor suppressor Rb and inactivate it. This relieves Rb-mediated repression of E2F-DP-1 complexes. If p53 is absent, free E2F can promote uncontrolled progression through the cell cycle. In fact, overexpression of E2F results in failure of cells to arrest in G1 or to exhibit apoptosis. Similar effects have been seen with the loss of Rb.

The apoptotic response appears to be induced by separate p53 transcription-dependent and transcription-independent pathways. The *bax* and *insulin-like growth factor-binding protein 3* (IGF-BP3) genes are both regulated by p53. The *bax* gene encodes a protein with homology to the survival factor Bcl-2. Heterodimerization with Bax inactivates Bcl-2, thereby promoting cell death. p53 regulation of IGF-BP3 can block the mitogenic response of cells to IGF-1 by inhibiting IGF-1 interaction with its receptor.

Although programmed cell death can occur by pathways independent of p53 (e.g., glucocorticoids), the p53-mediated pathways prevail in most circumstances. In situations in which DNA damage has occurred, or when the supply of survival factors is low, the p53-dependent apoptotic response becomes engaged. This response is important to preclude the development of tumors, and it also appears to play a role in effective responses to cancer therapy, including chemotherapy and radiation treatments.

SELECTED REFERENCES

Baserga R. Oncogenes and the strategy of growth factors. Cell 1994;79: 927–930.

Chiu CP, Harley CB. Replicative senescence and cell immortality: the role of telomeres and telomerase. Proc Soc Exp Biol Med 1997; 214:99–106.

Collins K, Jacks T, Pavletich NP. The cell cycle and cancer. Proc Natl Acad Sci USA 1997;94: 2776–2778.

Elledge S. Cell cycle checkpoints: preventing an identity crisis. Science 1996;274:1664–1672.

Evans T, Rosenthal ET, Youngblom J, Distel D, Hunt T. Cyclin: a protein specified by maternal mRNA in sea urchin eggs that is destroyed at each cleavage division. Cell 1983;33:389–396.

Hartwell LH. Cell division from a genetic perspective. J Cell Biol 1978;77:627–637.

Hartwell LH, Weinert T. Checkpoints: controls that ensure the order of cell cycle events. Science 1989;246:629–634.

Holzman D. Mismatch repair genes matched to several new roles in cancer. J Natl Can Inst 1996;88:950,951.

Hunter T. Oncoprotein networks. Cell 1997;88:333–346.

Kastan MB. Molecular biology of cancer: the cell cycle. In: DeVita VT, Hellman S, Rosenberg, SA, eds. Principles and Practice of Oncology. Philadelphia, PA: Lippincott-Raven, Philadelphia, 1997; pp. 121–134.

King RW, Deshaies RJ, Peters J-M, Kirschner MW. How proteolysis drives the cell cycle. Science 1996;274:1652–1659.

Ko LJ, Prives C. p53: puzzle and paradigm. Gen Dev 1996;10:1054–1072.

Levine AJ. p53, the cellular gatekeeper for growth and division. Cell 1997;88:323–331.

Lewin B. Genes V. Oxford, UK: Oxford University Press, 1994.

McIntosh JR, Koonce MP. Mitosis. Science 1989;246:622–628.

Nasmyth K. Viewpoint: putting the cell cycle in order. Science 1996;274: 1643–1645.

Nurse P, Bisset Y. Gene required in G1 for commitment to cell cycle and in G2 for control of mitosis in fission yeast. Nature 1981;292:558–560.

Paulovich AG, Toczyski DP, Hartwell LH. When checkpoints fail. Cell 1997;88:315–321.

Pines J. Cyclins and their associated cyclin-dependent kinases in the human cell cycle. Signaling from the plasma membrane to the nucleus. Biochem Soc Trans 1993;21:921–925.

Sherr CJ. Cancer cell cycles. Science. 1996;274:1672–1677.

Stillman B. Cell cycle control of DNA replication. Science. 1996;274: 1659–1664.

Weinberg RA. The retinoblastoma protein and cell cycle control. Cell 1996;81:323–330.

7 Oncogenes and Tumor Suppressor Genes

J. LARRY JAMESON

DEFINITION AND DISCOVERY OF ONCOGENES AND TUMOR SUPPRESSOR GENES

Cancer is caused by an accumulation of genetic alterations that confer a survival advantage to the neoplastic cell. These genetic changes can affect multiple facets of cellular function, including an increased rate of cell proliferation, resistance to apoptosis, altered tissue invasiveness, production of growth and angiogenic factors, and the ability to escape immune surveillance. Different cancers reflect these features to varying degrees, depending on the nature of their cellular functions and genetic changes.

The genetic basis for cancer is reflected in the clonal nature of neoplastic cells. As depicted in Fig. 7-1, cell proliferation can involve either polyclonal or monoclonal expansion of the cell population. Polyclonal growth or hyperplasia reflects the response to an extrinsic growth factor or to an intrinsic genetic alteration that is shared by all (e.g, MEN-2, germline ret mutation) or some (e.g., McCune-Albright, postzygotic somatic Gsα mutation) of the cells. Hyperplastic cells may subsequently acquire one or more somatic mutations and develop clonal derivatives. Monoclonal growth reflects the acquisition of somatic mutations that confer a survival advantage. Multistep models of tumorigenesis *(see below)* postulate that multiple different mutations are acquired over time. Thus, an initial clone would give rise to additional clonal variants as they acquire distinct mutations, some of which may foster tumor growth and expansion by favoring tissue invasion or metastasis.

The recognition that cancer is a genetic disease has led to an intensive effort to characterize genetic alterations in tumors and to understand how these genes function in the context of the normal and neoplastic cell. The idea that cancer might be caused by genetic changes has long been suspected by clinicians who noted that certain cancers tend to "run in families." Several landmark advances in virology, cytogenetics, and molecular biology have converted this intuitive assessment into a firm scientific foundation. In the early 1900s, Rous demonstrated transmission of sarcoma in chickens by using cell-free filtrates that contained a virus now known to be a retrovirus, Rous sarcoma virus (RSV). Identification of the transforming principle in the virus revealed that it harbored an altered form a normal cellular gene, *src*. The viral gene product was referred to as an oncogene, derived from the Greek, *onkos*, which refers to a mass or tumor. Subsequent studies have shown that many viral oncogenes correspond to altered versions of normal cellular genes, which are referred to as proto-oncogenes. The ability of retroviruses to "reverse transcribe" mRNA accounts for their ability to capture cellular gene products. Analyses of such viral oncogenes has helped to identify many critical cellular genes including *src*, *ras*, *raf*, *kit*, *jun*, *fos*, *ets*, and others.

DNA tumor viruses have also played an important role in our current understanding of neoplasia. In this case, the viruses produce proteins that target key cellular regulatory proteins, such as retinoblastoma (Rb) and p53. For example, the SV40 large T antigen associates with, and inactivates, Rb. Remarkably, other viral products including adenovirus E1A and papilloma virus protein E7 also target Rb. Although these viral proteins are structurally unrelated, they each appear to associate with the so-called pocket of Rb to prevent interactions with cellular transcription factors like E2Fs, which are involved in control of S-phase genes (Fig. 7-2). These cellular targets of DNA tumor viruses are now known to be tumor suppressor genes.

Historically, the presence of tumor suppressor genes was suspected, based on several lines of evidence. The malignant phenotype of certain tumors could be suppressed by fusion with normal cells, implying the presence of a suppressor gene in the normal cell. Chromosomal losses in the hybrids eventually resulted in reversion back to the malignant phenotype. Ultimately, it was possible to observe partial alterations in tumorigenicity by the introduction of single chromosomes into the malignant cells. For example, insertion of chromosome 11 (now known to harbor the *WT-1* gene) was sufficient to suppress tumorigenicity in a Wilm's tumor cell line.

These laboratory experiments were paralleled by observations in humans that certain hereditary forms of cancer are transmitted in an autosomal dominant manner *(see below)*. Based on the age-dependent appearance of retinoblastoma, Knudson postulated a "two-hit" model for the disorder (Fig. 7-3). In this model, the first "hit" or mutation is inherited in the germline and the second mutation is acquired as a somatic event involving either the remaining normal allele or another gene. As described below, the second hit typically involves the remaining normal allele. This model, which has proven to explain a number of hereditary cancer syndromes, implied a loss of function, and was in a sense, recessive.

The identification and characterization of the *Rb* gene has converted this statistical model into concrete mechanisms (*see* Chapter 105). Cytogenetic studies in patients with inherited forms of retinoblastoma revealed deletions of chromosome 13q14. Additional studies showed that tumors from patients with retinoblas-

From: *Principles of Molecular Medicine* (J. L. Jameson, ed.), ©1998 Humana Press Inc., Totowa, NJ.

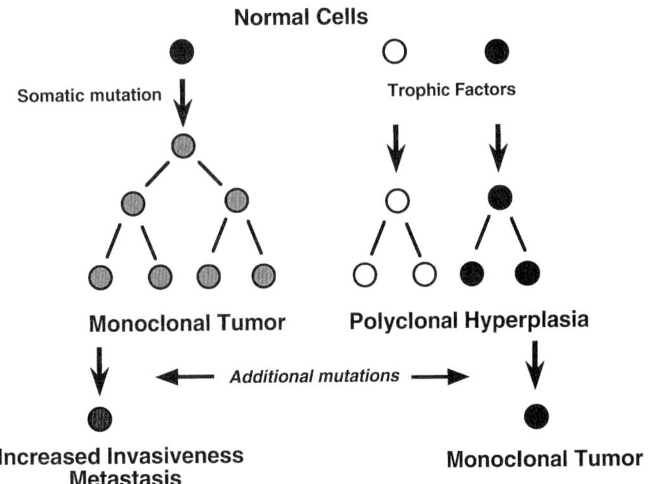

Figure 7-1 Clonal expansion of cancer cells. Growth responses can be divided into hyperplasic (polyclonal) or monoclonal expansion of cells. Hyperplasia reflects the actions of growth factors that increase the proliferation of a population of cells. In contrast, monoclonal expansion reflects increased proliferation from a single ancestral cell, reflecting a growth advantage conferred by a somatic mutation. Monoclonal and polyclonal tumors can be distinguished based on patterns of X-chromosomal inactivation (in females) or based on the presence of a characteristic somatic mutation in a monoclonal tumor. Hyperplasia may predispose cells to develop somatic mutations, allowing a monoclonal population to emerge. Additional mutations in monoclonal tumors allows new clonal populations with increased rates of growth or invasiveness to emerge. Adapted with permission. (Jameson JL. Principles of hormone action. In: Weatherall DJ, Ledingham JGG, Warrell DA, eds. Oxford Textbook of Medicine, 3rd ed. Oxford, U.K.: Oxford Medical, 1996; pp.1553–1573.)

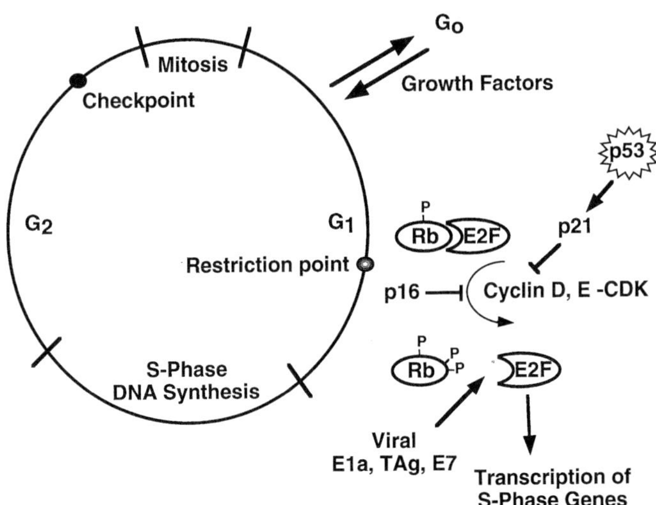

Figure 7-2 The pivotal role of the Rb tumor suppressor gene in control of the cell cycle. The cell cycle is depicted schematically with its characteristic stages (G_0, M, G_1, G_2, S). G_0 represents a quiescent state in which cells exit or enter the cell cycle. A key restriction point is noted in G_1. After passage through this point, cell are committed to progress into the S phase. An additional checkpoint is noted in G_2 before cells initiate mitosis. The Rb gene product plays a key role in progression through the restriction point. In its hypophosphorylated state, Rb binds E2F transcription factors, making them inaccessible for transcription of S-phase genes. Increasing amounts of cyclin D1 in association with cdk4 or cdk6 result in hyperphosphorylation of Rb. Cyclin E, in association with cdk2, also contributes to Rb phosphorylation. Phosphorylated Rb no longer associates with E2Fs, freeing them to interact with target genes (e.g., DNA polymerase, thymidine kinase, dihydrofolate reductase) that are involved in S phase. p16 is capable of blocking the actions of Cyclin D1/cdk 4,6, and this may account for its role as a tumor suppressor in some malignancies, as the absence of p16 would favor unrestricted progression through the cell cycle. A possible role for p53 is also shown. Cell injury can stimulate p53 levels leading to increased p21, a probable inhibitor of the actions of Cyclins D and E. Thus, the absence of p53 might prevent restriction of cell division in damaged cells. Viral gene products (E1a, large TAg, E7) bind Rb and dissociate E2Fs, therefore having similar effects as Rb hyperphosphorylation.

toma frequently showed loss of heterozygosity (LOH) in this region of chromosome 13, and that the remaining abnormal allele was transmitted from the affected parent. These experiments confirmed the loss of function hypothesis and established the importance of using loss of heterozygosity as a means for detecting tumor suppressor genes. The cloning of the *Rb* gene allowed demonstration of germline mutations in patients who did not have deletions. In addition, it was shown that patients with sporadic forms of retinoblastoma had acquired two somatic hits in which each allele received an independent mutation.

The Rb protein plays a pivotal role in control of the cell cycle. As depicted in Fig. 7-2, Rb helps to govern the restriction point between G1 and S phase (*see* Chapter 6). Hypophosphorylated Rb binds transcription factors, including E2Fs. Upon Rb phosphorylation by Cyclin-CDK complexes, E2Fs (particularly E2Fs 1–3) dissociate from Rb to stimulate the transcription of genes that are involved in DNA synthesis. The loss of both *Rb* genes is therefore predicted to enhance cell proliferation. Because *Rb* is expressed ubiquitously, it is unclear why only certain tumors (retinoblastomas, osteosarcomas, soft tissue sarcomas, melanomas) develop with increased frequency in patients with germline *Rb* mutations.

Cytogenetics have played an important role in the characterization of genetic alterations, particularly in hematologic malignancies (*see* Chapters 26 and 27). Characteristic chromosomal rearrangements suggested the presence of an oncogene. For example, in chronic myelogenous leukemia (CML), the description of the Philadelphia chromosome t(9;22)(q34;q11) was recognized early as a characteristic cytogenetic abnormality. This translocation is now known to fuse the *bcr* gene on chromosome 22 with the c-*abl* gene on chromosome 9. The fusion protein combines the tyrosine kinase activity of c-*abl* with abnormal regulation and cellular localization conferred by *bcr*. Another striking example involves a translocation t(8;14)(q24;q32) of the IgH chain gene with c-*myc* in Burkitt's lymphoma. In this case, the regulatory regions of the immunoglobulin gene result in the overexpression of c-*myc* in lymphoid cells, causing increased cell proliferation. A number of such translocations and chromosomal inversions have now been described (Table 7-1). In general, they involve either abnormal expression of a cellular kinase or transcription factor or, the production of a fusion protein with altered functional properties.

CLASSES AND FUNCTIONS OF ONCOGENES

GROWTH FACTORS Oncogenes can be categorized according to their cellular functions (Fig. 7-4). A few oncogenes function as growth factors (Table 7-2). For example, v-sis is structurally related to β chain of platelet-derived growth factor (PDGF), and int-2 corresponds to members of the fibroblast growth factor (FGF) family. Although these oncogenes do not play major roles

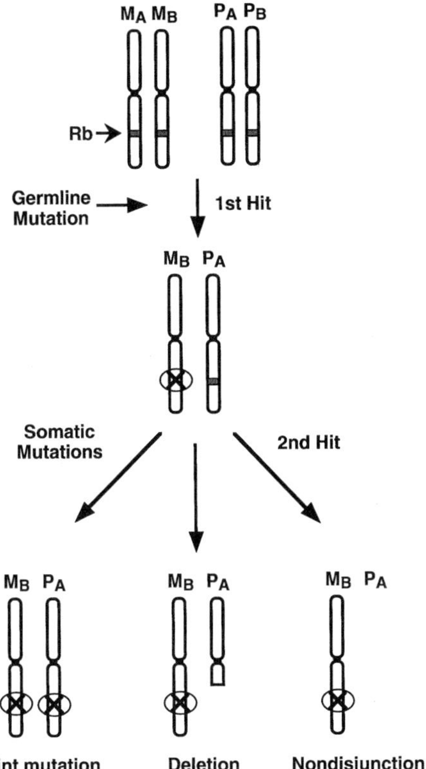

Figure 7-3 Two-hit model for retinoblastoma inactivation. The principles involved in the "two-hit" model are illustrated schematically. The *Rb* gene is located on chromosome 13q14. The Maternal (M) and Paternal (P) chromosomes are denoted as A or B. The first hit involves a germline mutation (depicted by an **X**) on chromosome M_B. Subsequently, several different types of somatic second hits can occur. A second point mutation can inactivate the normal allele inherited from the father (P_A). Deletions of part of chromosome 13, internal deletions, or translocations can also lead to inactivation of the normal *Rb* gene. Nondisjunction with loss of the normal chromosome 13 can cause loss of the normal *Rb* gene. The germline mutation causes a predisposition to retinoblastoma, as any inactivating second hit will be selected because of clonal proliferation. An analogous series of events can occur in sporadic tumors. In this case, both the first and second hits occur somatically.

Table 7-1
Examples of Oncogene Rearrangements and Fusions

Type of rearrangement	*Rearranged oncogene(s)*	*Disorder*
Gene activation	IgH-c-MYC	Burkitt's lymphoma
	IgH-Cyclin D1	Mantle cell lymphoma
	TCR-β-TAL-2	T-cell acute lymphoblastic leukemia
	TCR-α-HOX11	T-cell acute lymphoblastic leukemia
	PTH-Cyclin D1	Parathyroid adenomas
	ELE1-RET	Papillary thyroid cancer
Gene fusions		
	BCR-ABL	Chronic myelogenous leukemia
	AML-1-CBFα	Acute myelogenous leukemia
	FUS-CHOP	Myxoid liposarcomas
	EWS-FLI-1	Ewing's sarcoma
	PML-RARα	Promyelocytic leukemia

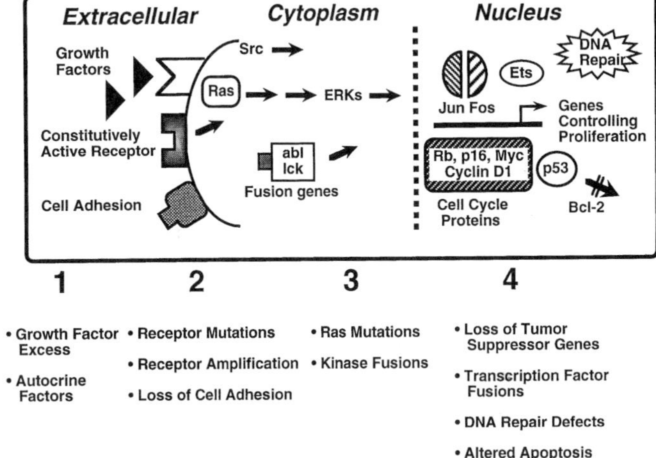

Figure 7-4 Sites of cellular actions of oncogenes and tumor suppressor genes. Oncogenes act at multiple sites of cellular function. (1) The extracellular environment can influence cell function by the overproduction of various growth factors. Not shown are important extracellular effects of angiogenic factors and proteolytic enzymes. (2) At the level of the cell membrane, adhesion molecules such as DCC and APC influence tumor invasiveness. Membrane receptors can be constitutively activated (e.g., Ret, TSH-R) or the receptors can be amplified (e.g., ErbB-2). (3) Ras is a prototypical example of signal transduction molecule that stimulates proliferation when activated. (4) Nuclear proteins include a number of targets for oncogenesis. Proteins such as AP-1 (Jun/Fos) and Ets are targets for several of the transducing signal transduction cascades, including Src, Ras, and ERKs. Some nuclear proteins, such as Myc, are amplified or overexpressed (Cyclin D1) in certain tumors. p53 plays a role in controlling the cellular response to injury (inhibits G_1/S) and helps to direct apoptosis. Several DNA repair enzymes cause familial adenomatous polyposis when mutated. Adapted with permission. (Jameson JL. Principles of hormone action. In: Weatherall DJ, Ledingham JGG, Warrell DA, eds. Oxford Textbook of Medicine, 3rd ed. Oxford, U.K.: Oxford Medical, Oxford, 1996; pp.1553–1573.)

in human cancer, they illustrate the importance of growth factors and their signaling pathways for the growth of tumors.

A more prominent functional role for growth factors stems from their overproduction as a consequence of the actions of other oncogenes. Many tumors produce growth factors, such as insulin-like growth factor-1 (IGF-1), IGF-2, epidermal growth factor (EGF), and tumor growth factor-α (TGF-α), which stimulate cell growth in an autocrine manner. The mechanisms that lead to growth factor overexpression are relatively obscure, but account in part for the ability of transformed cells to grow in the presence of reduced serum and for the ability of conditioned media from transformed cells to foster the growth of other cell lines. As depicted in Fig. 7-2, growth factors act in the cell cycle to enhance the entry from the quiescent state (G_0) and they stimulate progression to the restriction point in G_1. Other growth factors, such as TGF-β, can oppose entry into the cell cycle, in part by increasing levels of cyclin dependent (cdk) inhibitors. Thus, the balance of growth factors and the activity of their receptors can have profound effects on cell proliferation. Growth factors also influence the initiation of apoptosis (programmed cell death). Withdrawal of growth factors (or other nutrients) favors apoptosis, and their presence helps to prevent it.

Table 7-2
Functional Classes of Oncogenes and Tumor Suppressor Genes

Class	*Oncogene*	*Function*
Growth factors	sis	Homologous to the β chain of platelet-derived growth factor (PDGF)
	int-2	Integration site for MMTV; fibroblast growth factor-3,4 (FGF-3,4) genes
Receptor tyrosine kinases	erbB-2	Orphan receptor related to the epidermal growth factor receptor (EGF-R)
	ret	Activated form of tyrosine kinase; binds glial derived nerve growth factor
Non-receptor tyrosine kinases	abl	Translocates to bcr; interacts with cell cycle proteins
	src	Membrane associated tyrosine kinase; activates mitogenic signaling cascades
Cell surface proteins	DCC	Deleted in colorectal cancer gene involved in cell adhesion
	APC	Adenomatous polyposis gene that interacts with β-catenin and E-cadherin
GTPases	ras	Activates signaling cascades including MAPKs/ERKs
	Gsα	Activates adenylyl cyclase
Protein kinases	mos	A MEK-like enzyme
	raf	Serine kinase in the ras pathway
Transcription factors	jun	B-Zip protein that complexes with fos to form AP-1
	myc	bHLH protein that regulates cell cycle factors
Cell-cycle factors	Rb	Retinoblastoma undergoes phosphorylation to regulate cell cycle progression
	p53	Transcription factor that regulates cell-cycle genes and apoptosis
DNA repair	ATM	Ataxia-telangiectasia gene involved in cell-cycle checkpoints and p53 directed apoptosis
	hMSH2	Human mutS homolog involved in DNA mis-match repair
Programmed cell death	Bcl-2	Blocks apoptosis; interacts with other cell proteins such as Bax to control apoptosis

The functional effects of growth factors on tumor development are emphasized by several transgenic models. Disruption of the inhibin α-subunit gene results in ovarian granulosa cell tumors with nearly complete penetrance (*see* Chapter 10). Inhibin normally combines with a β-subunit of activin and antagonizes the action of the activin homodimer. Activin is a member of the TGF-β family of growth factors that exerts pleomorphic growth effects in various tissues, including the ovary. In this model, the loss of inhibin is thought to result in unopposed actions of activin, which induce ovarian and adrenal tumors. Crossbreeding the inhibin-deficient mice with p53-deficient mice greatly accelerates the development of tumors. This model illustrates the profound effect of unbalanced growth factor action and its ability to act in a tissue-selective manner. Another informative model involves disruption of the gene encoding the IGF-1 receptor. Fibroblast cells derived from these mice are resistant to transformation by SV40 large T antigen and/or activated *ras*. Reintroduction of the receptor confers the ability to undergo transformation, emphasizing the role of the IGF-1 pathway in cell proliferation and transformation.

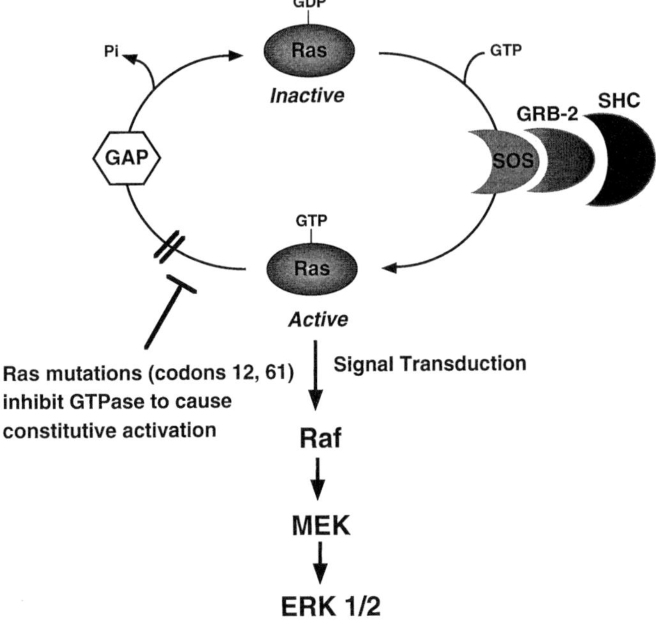

Figure 7-5 The cycle of ras activation and effect of mutations. Ras is a guanine-nucleotide protein. When GTP is bound, Ras is active, and it is normally inactivated by hydrolysis of GTP to GDP, resulting in an inactive state. SOS (son of sevenless), also called guanine-nucleotide releasing protein (GNRP), regulates Ras activity and responds to input from the SH2 domain proteins, GRB-2 and SHC. The catalytic activity of Ras is also modulated by GAP (GTPase activating protein). The *NF-1* gene (causes Von Recklinghausen's neurofibromatosis) is homologous to *gap*. Mutations in *ras* prevent GTP hydrolysis, resulting in constitutive activation. Ras participates in several signaling pathways, including activation of Raf, MEK, and ERKs, which stimulate mitogenesis.

Growth factors act by initiating a variety of signaling cascades that involve other oncogenes. These signal transduction pathways are discussed further in Chapter 46. EGF, for example, activates a tyrosine kinase receptor. Ligand-induced homodimerization of the EGF-receptor results in autophosphorylation that allows the recruitment of SH2 domain-containing adaptor proteins such as Grb-2. Grb-2, in turn, associates with the guanine-nucleotide exchange protein, son of sevenless (SOS), through an SH3 domain to enhance the activation of Ras (Fig. 7-5). Ras plays a pivotal role in growth factor signaling. It can also be activated by mitogenic Giα-coupled seven transmembrane receptors, probably through the release of βγ-subunits and by activation of *src* kinase. Activation of focal adhesion kinase (FAK) by integrins can also lead to

Ras activation. Ras initiates a mitogen-activated kinase (MAPK) cascade that includes Raf, MEK, and ERKs (extracellular regulated kinases). These kinases act on numerous cellular targets including the cytoskeleton and activation of transcription factors such as AP-1 (c-Jun/c-Fos) and Ets-1. c-*jun* and c-*fos*, which are themselves early response genes, form the AP-1 complex that activates a variety of genes involved in cell growth control.

RECEPTOR TYROSINE KINASES Growth factor receptors not only serve to transduce the signals of extracellular growth factors, but they are also important targets of mutations or altered expression that contribute to tumorigenesis. The tyrosine kinase class of receptors includes oncogenes such as *ret* (a receptor tyrosine kinase that binds glial derived nerve growth factor), *trk* (nerve growth factor class), kit (steel receptor), *fms* (colony stimulating 1 receptor), *erbB* (epidermal growth factor, EGF, receptor), and *erbB-2/neu* (EGF-related receptor). As noted above, this group of receptors are thought to act primarily by signaling through the *ras*-MAPK cascade.

In some cases, such as *erbB* and *erbB-2/neu*, receptor amplification leads to marked overexpression. When amplification involves deletion of the ligand binding domain, constitutive activation can result. Amplification of these receptors is particularly common in head and neck cancers, esophageal and gastric cancers, and in breast cancer.

Point mutations can also activate tyrosine kinase receptors. The *ret* receptor is a prototype for activation by point mutations that cause constitutive activation of the receptor. Mutations in *ret* cause multiple endocrine neoplasia type 2 (MEN-2) (*see* Chapter 54). The MEN-2 mutations are clustered in a group of cysteines that are thought to form disulfide bonds in the extracellular ligand-binding domain of the receptor. MEN-2 is transmitted in an autosomal dominant manner. Individuals who inherit a mutant *ret* receptor exhibit hyperplasia of the calcitonin-producing medullary thyroid cells at a very early age. Subsequently, they have a high incidence of developing medullary thyroid cancer. Presumably, the development of medullary thyroid cancer involves a second hit, although the target(s) of subsequent mutations are not known. In practical terms, it is now recommended that patients who inherit *ret* mutations undergo prophylactic thyroidectomy and receive screening for additional features of MEN-2 (pheochromocytoma and hyperparathyroidism).

It is notable that the action of the *ret* oncogene is conceptually distinct from that described above for *Rb*, even though both are transmitted in an autosomal dominant manner. As a tumor suppressor gene, *Rb* requires inactivation of both alleles, whereas the mutant form of *ret* initiates the process of tumorigenesis directly. Interestingly, mutations in the tyrosine kinase domain of *ret* cause a phenotypically distinct disorder, MEN-2b, which differs by including mucosal neuromas. *Ret* also plays a role in papillary cancer of the thyroid. In this case, chromosomal inversions (inv[10]) bring the tyrosine kinase domain of *ret* under the control of one of several fusion genes (e.g., *ELE-1*). This recombination leads to overexpression of the activated form of *ret* in the thyroid cell (where it is not normally expressed). Further expanding the role of *ret* in human disease is the observation that inactivating mutations cause Hirschprung's disease.

SIGNAL TRANSDUCTION The role of signal transduction molecules as oncogenes is exemplified by *ras*. There are three *ras* genes (*N-ras*, *H-ras*, *K-ras*) that were initially identified as transforming rodent sarcoma viruses. Mutant forms of *ras* were later identified as the transforming principle in DNA derived from several types of human tumors. *Ras* is now recognized as one of the most common genetic alterations in human cancers. Ras mutations occur in 90% of certain cancers (e.g., pancreatic) and in 10–30% many other types of cancer including leukemias, melanomas, thyroid cancer, colon cancer, and lung cancer. Although the *ras* gene is amplified in some tumors, more commonly it is activated by point mutations.

The biochemical basis of *ras* mutations is now well understood in terms of protein structure and activity. Ras activity is controlled by the binding and hydrolysis of GTP. The cycle of Ras activation and inactivation is depicted in Fig. 7-5. When GTP is bound, Ras is active, and it is inactivated by hydrolysis of GTP to GDP. Extensive structural, mutagenesis, and biochemical analyses have revealed that *ras* mutations act by preventing GTP hydrolysis, retaining the protein in an active state. The locations of *ras* mutations are clustered in amino acids 12, 13, and 61, each of which has been shown to play a critical role in nucleotide binding and/or hydrolysis. The inability to inactivate Ras leads to stimulation of the MAP kinase signal transduction cascade and uncontrolled cell proliferation.

Ras catalysis of GTP is regulated by SOS, also called guanine-nucleotide releasing protein (GNRP), which responds to input from the SH2 domain-containing proteins, GRB-2 and SHC. In this manner, Ras activity can be activated by numerous growth factor pathways (Fig. 7-6). The catalytic activity of Ras is also modulated by GAP (GTPase activating protein). The *NF-1* gene (which causes Von Recklinghausen's neurofibromatosis type 1) is homologous to GAP. Inactivating mutations of both *NF-1* alleles are predicted to result in diminished GTPase activity and increased activity of Ras or other related proteins. Thus, *NF-1* functions like a tumor suppressor gene.

Ras is tethered to the cytoplasmic side of the cell membrane by farnesylation. Mutations that eliminate the farnesylation site in the carboxyterminus of Ras eliminate its signaling function, presumably because of a requirement for subcellular localization to contact other components of the signal transduction cascade. Efforts to inhibit Ras farnesylation represent a promising therapeutic strategy for blocking the actions of activated forms of *ras*.

The guanine nucleotide-binding G proteins are structurally related to Ras. Moreover, homologous mutations have been described in Gsα, Giα2, and Giα3. In the case of Gsα, the mutations occur in codons 201 and 227, and also prevent GTP hydrolysis, resulting in constitutive activation of the adenylyl cyclase pathway. Gsα mutations that develop postzygotically cause McCune-Albright syndrome, which is characterized by polyostotic fibrous dysplasia, *café au lait* spots, hyperfunctioning ovarian cysts, and autonomous function in other glands, including the thyroid and pituitary glands (*see* Chapters 46 and 59). The development of these lesions reveals tissues in which the cAMP pathway is mitogenic. Somatic mutations in Gsα occur in about 30% of GH-secreting pituitary tumors (*see* Chapter 48) and can cause autonomously functioning thyroid nodules. It is notable that mutations have also been identified at other steps in the cAMP signaling pathway. Activating mutations have been described in the thyroid-stimulating hormone (TSH) receptor. These mutations, which appear to cause hormone-independent coupling to Gsα, cause congenital hyperthyroidism and nodular goiter when transmitted in the germline or autonomous nodules when acquired as somatic mutations (*see* Chapter 50).

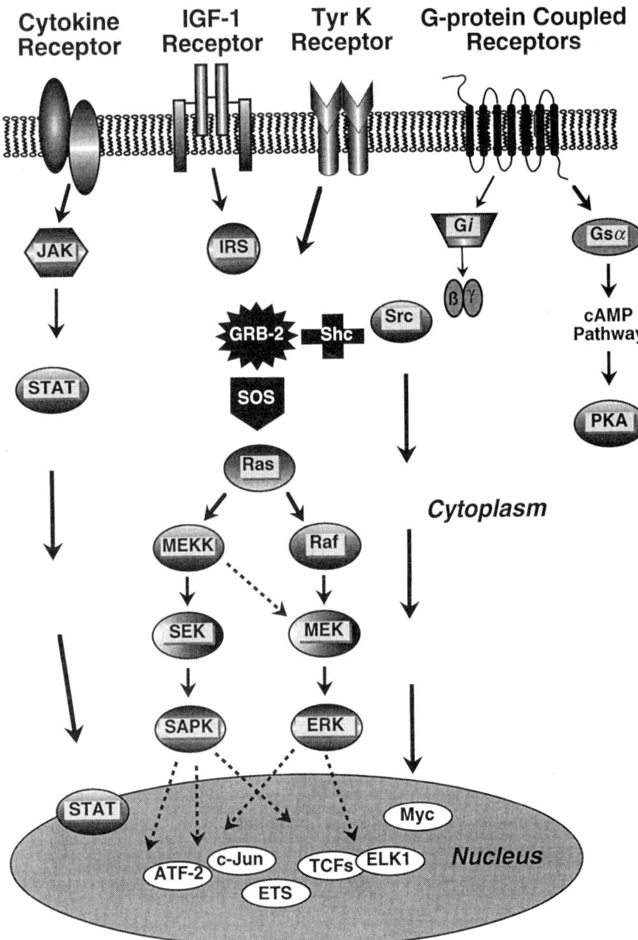

Figure 7-6 Growth factor signaling pathways. Representative growth factor receptors are shown including a cytokine receptor, the insulin-like growth factor-1 (IGF-1) receptor, a tyrosine kinase receptor (e.g., EGF), and a G-protein-coupled receptor (different members can signal via Giα or Gsα). Each of these receptors can activate an array of signaling pathways, not all of which are shown, and the central role of ras is emphasized. Cytokine receptor signaling may also interface with the Ras cascade, but most prominently activates the STAT (signal transducers and activators of transcription) proteins, which, during phosphorylation by Janus kinase (JAK), translocate to the nucleus to activate transcription of target genes. Tyrosine kinases induce the binding of an SH2 domain protein Grb2, which binds to guanine nucleotide exchange factor, SOS. This pathway can also be activated by the IGF-I receptor via insulin related substrate (IRS). Gsα-coupled receptors act primarily through the cAMP-PKA (protein kinase A) pathway, which is mitogenic in some cell types. Giα-coupled receptors can activate the Ras pathway through βγ-subunits, likely through src kinase. Ras activates several downstream kinases in a cell type specific manner. The preferential activation of a particular mitogen activated protein kinase (MAPK) module, such as activation of the extracellular-regulated kinase (ERK) rather than the stress-activated protein kinase (SAPK) pathway provides a mechanism for specific responses. There are many targets of these kinases, including a variety of transcription factors that are involved in cellular growth responses.

TRANSCRIPTION FACTORS Several of the oncogenic transcription factors were initially identified based on their association with transforming viruses (e.g., Jun, Fos, Ets, Myb, Rel, Erb-A). Others were recognized because of their presence as fusion products that result from translocations, inversions, or retroviral insertions (Table 7-1). These rearrangements can activate transcription factors in inappropriate tissues, at the wrong stage of cellular development, or at increased levels (*see* Chapter 3). In some cases (e.g., PML-RARα), the transcription factor prevents normal cellular differentiation and allows cells to retain responsiveness to proliferative signals. In other cases (e.g., IgH-Myc), overexpression of Myc favors cell proliferation by enhancing entry into the cell cycle.

A number of the signal transduction pathways discussed above converge on the transcription factor proto-oncogenes. c-Jun and c-Fos form the transcription factor, AP-1, which is a member of the B-Zip family of transcription factors that dimerize via a leucine zipper motif. Reflecting its dimeric structure, AP-1 recognizes variations of a palindromic DNA element, TGAGTCA, that resides in the regulatory regions of target genes. Numerous genes contain AP-1 sites, although the genes involved in v-Jun-mediated transformation remain unknown. Jun is one of the transcription factor targets for the Ras signaling pathway. Amino-terminal phosphorylation of Jun by Jun N-terminal kinases (JNKs) and stress-activated protein kinases (SAPKs) enhances its ability to transactivate genes.

CLASSES AND FUNCTIONS OF TUMOR SUPPRESSOR GENES

Tumor suppressor genes are defined as genes that sustain loss of function in the development or progression of neoplasms. Thus, tumor suppressor genes are characterized by inactivating mutations, whether inherited in the germline or acquired by somatic mutation. Although the initial tumor suppressor genes like *Rb* are involved in cell-cycle control, the class of tumor suppressors has broadened to include genes with a variety of cellular functions. As described below, the products of tumor suppressor genes include proteins involved in transcriptional regulation (e.g., WT-1), cell-cycle progression (e.g., p53, p16), RNA elongation, (e.g., VHL), signaling pathways (e.g., NF-1, DPC-4, Patched), and DNA repair (e.g., MSH-2). As a group, tumor suppressor genes function at key junctures in the control of cell proliferation, differentiation, apoptosis, and response to genetic damage.

CELL-SURFACE PROTEINS Cell-surface proteins other than receptors are now recognized as important sites for oncogenesis. These factors function like tumor-suppressor genes in the sense that loss of function (by mutation or deletion) contributes to tumorigenesis. Examples in this class include *DCC* (deleted in colorectal cancer) and adenomatous polyposis coli (*APC*). *DCC* was recognized because of localization to a region of chromosome 18q that was frequently deleted in colorectal cancer (~70% of cases). The *DCC* gene encodes a large protein that is involved in cell adhesion. Loss of *DCC* also occurs in other types of tumors including brain, breast, and pancreatic cancers.

The *APC* gene causes familial adenomatous polyposis (FAP) with a prevalence of about 1 in 7000 individuals. It was localized to chromosome 5q21 based on cytogenetic and linkage studies. The *APC* gene encodes a large protein that contains β-catenin binding sites that allow linkage to the cytoskeleton and E-cadherin. In this manner, APC probably plays a role in linking the extracellular matrix to intracellular signaling pathways, and it may play a role in apoptosis. Germline mutations in *APC* cause the development of multiple benign colonic polyps. Most mutations result in truncation of the protein and, because of the size of the gene, mutations can be screened using a protein truncation test. Tumorigenesis caused by *APC* mutations follows the two-hit model that charaterizes classic tumor suppressor genes. In FAP, neoplasia is initiated on inactivation of the remaining normal allele. *APC* mutations are also very common in sporadic colon cancers, which occasionally demonstrate inactivation of both *APC* alleles.

CELL-CYCLE CONTROL PROTEINS Not unexpectedly, a number of tumor suppressor genes play a role in control of the cell cycle. *Rb* was the first of these to be recognized. As shown in Fig. 7-2, Rb acts primarily at the restriction point in G_1 of the cell cycle. Early in G_1, Rb is hypophosphorylated and binds transcription factors E2F 1–3. E2Fs dimerize with a family of DP proteins (DP 1–3). The E2F/DP complexes bind to a consensus sequence, TTTCGCGC, which is present in the promoters of many genes, including *thymidine kinase*, *dihydrofolate reductase*, c-*myc*, and *E2F* itself. When Rb is bound to E2F/DP complexes, it can function as a repressor. On the other hand, dissociated E2Fs are transcriptional activators. Overexpression of E2F appears to be sufficient to push cells through the restriction point in G1. Phosphorylation of Rb by cyclin D/cdk4,6 complexes results in dissociation of E2Fs from Rb. Several pathways can act to prevent Rb phosphorylation and inhibit E2F dissociation from Rb. In the setting of cell damage, p53 levels are increased, and induce the cdk inhibitor, p21, which inhibits the actions of cyclin E/cdk2, another activator of Rb. p16 can also inhibit cyclin D1/cdk4.

In addition to *Rb* mutations in retinoblastoma, somatic mutations in *Rb* are relatively common in small cell lung cancer, sarcomas, and bladder cancer (*see* Chapters 40 and 105). Deletion of *p16* has been observed in small cell lung cancers in which the *Rb* gene is expressed. The absence of p16 would be expected to diminish inhibition of Rb-mediated progression through G_1. Expression of the papilloma virus E7 protein in cervical cancers functionally inactivates Rb. Overexpression of cyclin D1 occurs by amplification in some breast, esophageal, and squamous cell carcinomas. In addition, cyclin D1 is ectopically expressed as a result of translocations in some parathyroid tumors (PTH-cyclin D1) (*see* Chapter 51) and B-cell lymphomas (IgH-cyclin D1).

Mutations of *p53* and LOH at 17p occurs commonly in colorectal, lung, breast, and bladder cancers. Germline mutations of *p53* are found in Li-Fraumeni syndrome, which is characterized by a greatly increased risk for multiple tumors including breast cancer, soft-tissue sarcomas, osteosarcomas, brain tumors, and leukemias. Although *p53* is one of the most prevalent mutations in advanced stages of tumorigenesis, its cellular functions are only partly understood. p53 is capable of acting as a transcription factor and induces the expression of inhibitors (e.g., p21) of the G_1/S transition. p53 also appears to govern entry into the apoptosis pathway (by stimulating *bax*) in response to genotoxic damage. Thus, the absence of p53 not only favors progression through the cell cycle, but it also allows cells with damaged DNA to avoid undergoing apoptosis.

TRANSCRIPTION FACTORS The Wilms' tumor (*WT-1*) suppressor gene causes renal tumors in children (*see* Chapter 71). The *WT-1* locus on chromosome 11p13 was identified based on a contiguous gene syndrome, WAGR (Wilm's, aniridia, genitourinary disorders, retardation). The *WT-1* gene encodes a transcription factor that contains zinc finger domains and is expressed in the urogenital ridge and in the developing kidney. WT-1 appears to suppress gene expression, including the *IGF-II* gene, which is also overexpressed in Beckwith-Wiedeman syndrome (*see* Chapter 116). Mutations in *WT-1* are found in only a minority of cases of Wilm's tumor, suggesting that other loci are also involved in the pathogenesis of this tumor.

Von Hippel-Lindau (VHL) syndrome includes retinal angiomas, predisposition to renal cancer, pheochromocytomas, hemangioblastomas of the central nervous system, and cysts in several tissues. The *VHL* gene was identified on chromosome 3p based on linkage. Tumors in patients with germline mutations of *VHL* show mutations or loss of the remaining normal *VHL* gene. Somatic mutations in both alleles of *VHL* are also found in the majority of clear cell renal cancers (*see* Chapter 71). *VHL* encodes a protein that binds to elongin and is involved in transcriptional elongation. The normal function of VHL appears to be inhibition of elongin activity.

The *BRCA 1* (breast cancer predisposition) and *BRCA 2* genes are located on chromosomes 17q21 and 13q, respectively (*see* Chapter 63). The proteins are weakly homologous and likely function as transcription factors. Germline mutations predispose to early breast and ovarian cancers (especially *BRCA 1*). Although the *BRCA 1* and *2* genes were identified in large pedigrees with early breast cancer, these genes appear to account for a relatively small fraction of increased breast cancer risk, even when there is an affected first-degree relative. Their functional roles and their importance for genetic testing and counseling remain to be determined.

DNA REPAIR PROTEINS The role of DNA repair processes is most clearly illustrated in hereditary nonpolyposis colorectal cancer (HNPCC). Based primarily on studies by Lynch and colleagues, this form of hereditary colon cancer was strongly suspected to be caused by predisposing "cancer genes." HNPCC is now known to be caused mutations in one of several different DNA repair enzymes (*hMSH2*, *hMLH1*, *hPMS2*). Initially, linkage analyses indicated association with chromosomes 2p16 or 3p21. However, unlike the situation with *Rb*, *MEN-1*, and other heritable tumor suppressor genes, tumor samples did not always exhibit loss of heterozygosity in the putative normal allele at these loci. Rather, new microsatellites (highly polymorphic repeat sequences, *see* Chapters 4 and 5) were detected, and these aberrations were present throughout the patient's genome, suggesting microsatellite instability. This type of genomic instability is similar to that found in microorganisms with mutations in mismatch repair (proofreading) enzymes (e.g., mutS, mutL), spurring a search for human homologs of these genes. Germline mutations have now been identified in the human mismatch repair enzyme genes (*hMSH2*, *hMLH1*, *hPMS2*) in kindreds with HNPCC. Of these, mutations in *hMSH2* and *hMLH1* appear to account for the majority of HNPCC cases. Although HNPCC is relatively uncommon (2–4% of colorectal cancer), sporadic mutations in DNA repair enzymes may result in genomic instability in as many as 15% of colorectal cancers. The TGF-β receptor, which mediates apoptosis of colon cells, has been hypothesized as a target of inactivation by microsatellite instability.

The *mutated in ataxia telangiectasia (ATM)* gene represents another example of a DNA repair enzyme defect. Heterozygotes who carry this gene appear to be at increased risk for breast cancer. The defective *ATM* gene product appears to cause impaired p53 responses to DNA damage. Thus, ATM may play an important role in cell cycle checkpoints for DNA damage. Xeroderma pigmentosa represents another example of defects in DNA repair. In this case, a mutation in one of several different genes involved in nucleotide excision and repair leads to a high incidence of skin tumors, particularly in response to UV radiation (*see* Chapter 81).

APOPTOSIS-RELATED PROTEINS Although cancer is frequently conceptualized in terms of cell proliferation, the role of abnormalities in cell death, or apoptosis, is now becoming more fully appreciated. Most malignancies demonstrate abnormalites in programmed cell death. In addition to contributing to the immortality of the replicating cell, alterations in the apoptotic pathway also favor the accumulation of additional genetic alterations that would normally induce cell death. Responses of tumors to certain types of chemotherapy or irradiation also appear to correlate with the ability of tumors to undergo apoptosis.

Bcl-2 was initially discovered based on its translocation in follicular lymphomas. In this case, the recombination of the immunoglobulin locus on chromosome 14 with the *Bcl-2* gene on chromosome 18 causes persistent overexpression of *Bcl-2* in lymphoid cells. It was shown that the clonal expansion of lymphoid cells reflected increased survival rather than enhanced proliferation. *Bcl-2* is a member of a family of proteins that regulate the apoptotic pathway. While Bcl-2 protects against cell death, others such as Bax, favor cell death. Bcl-2 and Bax can form homodimers or heterodimers, and the balance of *Bcl-2* and *Bax* expression regulates the predisposition to cell death.

As noted above, p53 also plays an important role in apoptosis. Since *p53* mutations are found in up to 50% of human cancers, its role in cell-cycle checkpoints and in apoptosis may represent one of the most common lesions in neoplastic cells. The exact function of p53 in the apoptotic pathway has not been fully defined. Thymocytes from mice deficient in p53 fail to undergo apoptosis in response to DNA damage. However, glucocorticoids can still induce apoptosis in the absence of p53. Thus, p53 is not absolutely required for all pathways of cell death. It has been suggested that p53 may induce apoptosis primarily in the presence of DNA damage or when survival factors are limiting. It is notable that p53 can increase *Bax* expression, providing one mechanism for shifting the cell into an apoptotic pathway.

INHERITED CANCER SYNDROMES

Several inherited cancer syndromes have already been described as examples of the functional roles of oncogenes *(MEN-2)*, tumor suppressor genes *(Rb)*, or DNA repair enzymes (HNPCC). Although many of these syndromes cause relatively rare disorders, they have been enormously important for the identification of cancer-related genes and for establishing principles of cellular abnormalities in neoplasia. In addition, many of the genes that cause inherited forms of cancer are frequent targets for somatic mutations in sporadic tumors. Thus, these syndromes often identify candidate oncogenes or tumor-suppressor genes.

Some of the inherited cancer syndromes are listed in Table 7-3. Most of these disorders are discussed in greater detail in specific specialty sections of the book. In general, inherited forms of cancer are caused by a limited number of mechanisms. The classical two-hit model for neoplasia, in which one copy of the mutant gene is inherited and the second normal copy is subsequently lost (*see* Fig. 7-3), is illustrated by disorders such as retinoblastoma *(Rb)*, Li-Fraumeni *(p53)*, MEN-1 *(MENEN)*, and Wilm's tumor *(WT-1)*. MEN-2 (*Ret*), and some of the signaling pathway disorders such as neurofibromatosis type 1 likely involve inherited stimulation of cell growth followed by the accumulation of additional mutations that lead to malignancy. Another group of disorders involve abnormalities in DNA repair, predisposing to a high frequency of genetic alterations at numerous loci. This group includes genes that cause HNPCC, xeroderma pigmentosa, Bloom's syndrome, and ataxia-telangiectasia.

Table 7-3
Inherited Cancer Syndromes

Syndrome/cancer	*Oncogene*	*Function*
Retinoblastoma	Rb	Cell cycle control
Li-Fraumeni	p53	Cell cycle; apoptosis
Familial adenomatous polyposis	APC	Cell-cell interactions
Lynch's syndrome (HNPCC)	MSH2, MLH1, PMS1,2	DNA repair
Von Hippel-Lindau	VHL	Transcriptional elongation
Von Recklinghausen's	NF-1	GAP-like
Neurofibromatosis type 2	NF-2	Ezrin-like
Wilms' tumor	WT-1	Transcriptional repression
Ataxia-telangiectasia	ATM	DNA repair
Nevoid basal cell cancer syndrome	Patched	Transmembrane protein
Multiple endocrine neoplasa type I	MENIN	Tumor suppressor
Multiple endocrine neoplasa type II	Ret	Tyrosine kinase
Xeroderma pigmentosa	XP A-G	DNA repair
Bloom's syndrome	BLM	DNA helicase
Breast cancer	BRCA1, BRCA2	Tumor suppressors

MULTISTEP THEORY OF NEOPLASIA

Pathologists have long recognized a spectrum of histologic abnormalities that correlate with different degrees of tumorigenic ity. These observations have led to various grades of malignancy based on the degree of abnormal cellular morphology or to stages of invasiveness such as dysplasia, carcinoma *in situ*, locally invasive tumors, or metastatic lesions that have spread beyond their original site of growth. There is now strong evidence that these morphological and clinical characteristics of tumors can be explained in molecular terms.

The process of "multistep carcinogenesis" has been studied in many different models. It is sometimes divided into stages of initiation, promotion, and progression. These categories are undoubtedly oversimplistic, and it is likely that different tumor types involve distinct pathways for progression. In addition to developing altered pathways for proliferation and escape from apoptosis, tumors require angiogenesis and escape from immune surveillance in order to continue clonal expansion. Early models for cellular transformation demonstrated cooperation among different classes of oncogenes such as *ras* and *myc*. However, analogous events do not hold true for all malignancies. Many hematologic malignancies harbor distinct translocations that are not found in other tumor types. In some of these cases, however, it remains true that progression to more aggressive tumors involves the acquisition of additional genetic abnormalities. In fact, surveys of most

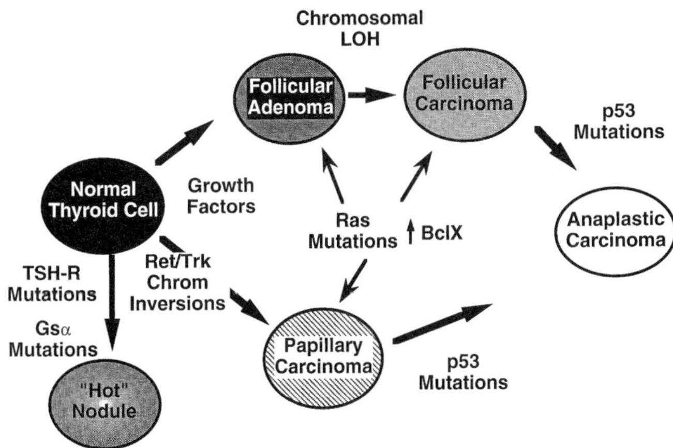

Figure 7-7 Example of multistep carcinogenesis involving thyroid carcinoma. There is evidence for multistep carcinogenesis for most cancers. In the case of thyroid cancer, various mutations affect the differentiated phenotype of the cancer as well as the degree of invasiveness. The normal thyroid follicular cell can be converted to an autonomously functioning "hot" nodule by two different types of mutations. Mutations in the TSH-receptor can activate Gsα and the cAMP signaling pathway, which is mitogenic in the thyroid. Gsα is a guanine nucleotide-binding protein that is structurally related to Ras. Gsα mutations that inhibit GTP hydrolysis also cause constitutive activation of the cAMP pathway. Follicular adenomas exhibit *ras* mutations (~30%) and, in the progression to follicular cancers, there is an increasing prevalence of loss of heterozygosity (LOH) at several distinct loci. Papillary cancers have a high frequency (20–40%) of a unique mutation caused by an inversion on chromosome 10 that brings the ret tyrosine kinase receptor under the control of several different genes. *Ras* mutations are found in papillary cancer with similar prevalence to follicular neoplasms. Mutations in *p53* are relatively common in anaplastic cancer, most of which are thought to arise from follicular cancers. Adapted with permission. (Jameson JL. Applications of molecular biology in endocrinology. In: Degroot LJ, ed. Endocrinology, 3rd ed. Philadelphia, PA: WB Saunders, pp. 119-147.)

hematologic malignancies for genetic alterations reveal numerous examples of gene amplification or loss of heterozygosity.

The concept of multistep carcinogenesis has been particularly well-studied for colon cancer by Vogelstein and colleagues. In colon cancer, it appears that seven or more genetic events (*APC*, *ras*, *DCC*, mismatch repair, *TGF-b-R*, *p53*, and others) may be required before an invasive carcinoma or metastases develop. Based on this list of genetic alterations, it is apparent that colon cancers can contain nearly every type of oncogene, tumor-suppressor gene, and DNA repair defect. Patients with germline *APC* mutations may first develop a second hit in this gene and subsequently develop additional growth promoting mutations such as mutations in *ras* or *p53*. However, the order in which these mutations occurs is variable in different patients.

Another example of multistep carcinogenesis is depicted for thyroid cancer in Fig. 7-7. Thyroid cancer is appealing as a model because several mutations give rise to distinct tumor phenotypes and because some of the growth promoting factors have been well-characterized. Proliferation of the thyroid follicular cell is largely dependent on thyroid-stimulating hormone (TSH) and IGF-1 (*see* Chapter 50). TSH stimulates growth through a Gsα-coupled receptor that acts via the cAMP pathway, whereas IGF stimulates a tyrosine kinase receptor that activates IRS-1, PI-3 kinase, and the Ras pathway. These pathways function synergistically to induce cellular proliferation. Activating mutations in the TSH-R, or in Gsα, cause constitutive activation of the cAMP pathway. These mutations cause clonal proliferation of a highly differentiated (benign) nodule that functions autonomously and secretes excess thyroid hormone. Although these mutations cause cellular proliferation, this mutation pathway is rarely observed in malignant thyroid cancers, which are not well-differentiated and rarely produce excess hormone. A group of inversions on chromosome 10 bring the *ret* oncogene under the control of various promoters. These fusion genes were initially termed papillary thyroid cancer (PTC) because they are essentially unique to this histologic variant. Approximately 20–30% of papillary thyroid cancers contain PTC rearrangements. *Ras* mutations (*K-ras*, *N-ras*, *H-ras*) have been found in all types of thyroid neoplasms, including benign macrofollicular adenomas, papillary cancers, and follicular cancers. As in most other cancers, the more malignant thyroid tumors show numerous examples of loss of heterozygosity, presumably involving tumor-suppressor gene loci. LOH is particularly common in follicular thyroid cancer, which has a greater tendency to metastasize. Anaplastic thyroid cancers have a very poor prognosis and show a marked increase in *p53* mutations. Although it is unclear whether tumors show a gradual progression from *ras* mutations to loss of tumor suppressor loci, to *p53* mutations, this seems likely, as anaplastic lesions are often noted to develop within a pre-existing follicular cancer. The loss of *p53* may represent a pivotal step in which there is a defect in normal apoptosis pathways and a more rapid accumulation of additional genetic abnormalities. Superimposed on these genetic abnormalities, it is well-established that thyroid cancers respond to normal growth factors such as TSH, leading clinicians to suppress TSH with thyroid hormone as one means of therapy. This feature of the thyroid tumors emphasizes the overlap between normal and abnormal influences on cell growth. Thus, in the model of thyroid cancer, there are examples of mutations that are associated with specific tumor phenotypes (e.g., *TSH-R*, *PTC*), but other mutations are less specific (e.g., *ras*) for distinct tumor types.

IMPLICATIONS FOR DIAGNOSIS AND TREATMENT

Ideally, one would hope to "genotype" a tumor to establish a specific diagnosis and to aid in prognosis. In some cases, such as hematologic malignancies, specific translocations can be used for diagnostic purposes. Characteristic genetic changes can also be used to detect minimal residual disease using PCR or other sensitive techniques. However, for most malignancies, the array of genetic alterations is too large and the pattern of mutations is too variable to provide a diagnostic or prognostic code. It is possible in the future that the growing body of correlations between clinical course and genetic alterations will allow such analyses, at least for some tumors.

In the short term, the greatest advances are likely to involve assessment of genetic risk based on inheritance of predisposing cancer genes. Thus, in kindreds with autosomal dominant MEN-2, it is now possible to determine early in life whether or not an individual carries the mutant *ret* gene. In conjunction with genetic counseling and clinical assessment, this has allowed careful monitoring for characteristic tumors (medullary thyroid cancer, pheochromocytoma, parathyroid adenomas) and, in some cases, prophylactic thyroidectomy to prevent thyroid cancer. In addition, unaffected family members can be spared the anxiety associated with repeated testing for possible malignancy. By analogy, earlier and more careful screening procedures can be anticipated in affected individuals with inherited cancer syndromes such as FAP and HNPCC. In addition to issues of medical intervention, the assessment and detection of genetic risk carries an obligation for genetic counseling and raises numerous ethical issues involving health insurance, effects on the individual's sense of self, and interpersonal relationships.

For many disorders, there is an opportunity for prevention as well as enhanced surveillance. In patients with increased risk of colon cancer, changes in diet to reduce red meat and to increase fiber content are reasonable, and nonsteroidal anti-inflammatory agents may be protective. Patients with xeroderma pigmentosa have increased sensitivity to UV light and need to avoid or block UV exposure.

In the long term, it is hoped that an improved understanding of the molecular basis of neoplasia will provide new avenues for therapy. The field is still very new and, given the usual timeline for drug discovery, it is not surprising that there are relatively few successes at this stage. The recognition that *ras* and *p53* are commonly involved in many types of tumors has led to aggressive efforts to find agents that can alter their functions. In the case of Ras, it has been possible to inhibit farnesylation, which is required for the protein to function. Efforts are underway to search for drugs that might mimic some of the actions of p53. The recognition that the retinoic acid receptor was involved in a translocation in promyelocytic leukemia led to trials of its ligand, all *trans*-retinoic acid, which has proven to differentiate the tumor cells. Glucocorticoids induce apoptosis in many lymphoid malignancies, and antagonists of estrogens have been useful in hormonally responsive breast cancers. Further studies of the mechanisms of oncogene action and apoptosis may provide additional therapeutic strategies.

Finally, gene therapy holds some promise for cancers. Because of the large number of abnormalities in most cancer cells and because of rapid clonal selection, it is unlikely to be practical to replace or to correct mutant genes. However, strategies to target toxic genes to malignant cells hold some promise. The primary challenge (as with many chemotherapeutic approaches) is to achieve specificity for the tumor and to target a very high fraction of the tumor cells. Several strategies are underway to augment immunologic responses (using cytokines) or to alter the drug sensitivity of tumors. Attempts are also being made to genetically modify (e.g., with multidrug resistance genes) normal bone marrow constituents to make them more resistant to chemotherapy.

SELECTED REFERENCES

Bale AE, Li FP. Principles of cancer management: cancer genetics. In: DeVita VT, Hillman S, Rosenberg SA, eds. Cancer: Principles and Practice of Oncology, 5th ed. Philadelphia, PA: Lippincott-Raven, 1997; pp. 285–294.

Baserga R. Oncogenes and the strategy of growth factors. Cell 1994; 79:927–930.

Cooper GM. Oncogenes, 2nd ed. Boston, MA: Jones and Bartlett, Boston, 1995.

Fearon ER, Vogelstein B. Tumor suppressor and DNA repair gene defects in human cancer. In: Holland J, Frei E, eds. Cancer Medicine, 4th ed. Baltimore, MD: Williams and Wilkins, 1997; pp. 97–118.

Haber D, Harlow E. Tumor-suppressor genes: evolving definitions in the genomic age. Nat Genet 1997;16:320–322.

Hunter T. Oncoprotein networks. Cell 1997;88:333–346.

Kastan MB. Molecular biology of cancer: the cell cycle. In: DeVita VT, Hillman S, Rosenberg SA, eds. Cancer: Principles and Practice of Oncology, 5th ed. Philadelphia, PA: Lippincott-Raven, 1997; pp. 121–134.

Kinzler KW, Vogelstein B. Lessons from hereditary colorectal cancer. Cell 1996;87:159–170.

Korsmeyer SJ. Regulators of cell death. Trends Genet 1995;11: 101–105.

Levine AJ. p53, the cellular gatekeeper for growth and division. Cell 1997;88:323–331.

Oltvai ZN, Korsmeyer SJ. Checkpoints of dueling dimers foil death wishes. Cell 1994;79:189–192.

Perkins AS, Stern DF. Molecular biology of cancer: oncogenes. In: DeVita VT, Hillman S, Rosenberg SA, eds. Cancer: Principles and Practice of Oncology, 5th ed. Philadelphia, PA: Lippincott-Raven, 1997; pp. 79–102.

Rabbitts TH. Chromosomal translocations in human cancer. Nature 1994;372:143–149.

Roth JA, Cristiano RJ. Gene therapy for cancer: what have we done and where are we going? J Natl Cancer Inst 1997;89:21–39.

Schichman SA, Croce CH. Oncogenes. In: Holland J, Frei E, eds. Cancer Medicine, 4th ed. Baltimore, MD: Williams and Wilkins, 1997; pp. 85–96.

Sherr CJ. Cancer cell cycles. Science 1996;274:1672–1677.

Weinberg RA. E2F and cell proliferation: a world turned upside down. Cell 1996;85:457–459.

8 Molecular Diagnostic Testing

C. Sue Richards and Patricia A. Ward

BACKGROUND

Molecular diagnostic testing is a rapidly evolving field that currently includes analysis for single-gene disorders, multifactorial disorders, some forms of cancer, infectious disease, microbial epidemiology, and personal identification. The era of molecular medicine began in the late 1970s with the cloning of the β-globin gene and identification of the point mutation responsible for sickle-cell anemia. At the same time, population-based carrier testing, using other technologies, for common genetic diseases such as Tay-Sachs and sickle-cell disease and prenatal diagnosis for chromosomal abnormalities were becoming widely available. The diagnostic capability of molecular technology has expanded tremendously, and there are now tests available for more than 300 genetic diseases being performed in greater than 200 diagnostic laboratories, academic and commercial, throughout the country (information provided by *Helix*; Seattle, Washington). The completion of the Human Genome Project will facilitate the identification of all disease genes, making a greater number of molecular diagnostic tests possible. While improved technological tools are essential for molecular diagnostics to move forward, the basic strategies for designing and implementing testing, which we describe in this chapter, will be long-lasting. To illustrate these principles, we will focus on the application of molecular diagnostic testing for single-gene disorders using DNA technology.

METHODS AND MUTATIONS

DNA testing becomes feasible when the disease gene responsible is mapped or identified. If the gene has been mapped but not identified or if the mutations in a particular gene have not been characterized, then linkage analysis may be possible. If the gene has been cloned and mutations characterized, then it may be possible to perform direct mutation analysis. Direct mutation analysis is the method of choice, since it is more accurate and offers confirmation of diagnosis, in addition to precise carrier and fetal risk prediction. In contrast, linkage analysis cannot be used to confirm a diagnosis and provides a less accurate statistical prediction of carrier or fetal risk based on analysis of DNA markers surrounding a gene.

DIRECT MUTATION DETECTION

Both the technology and the strategy used for mutation detection is determined by the nature of the specific mutation. The availability of gene sequence information and probes specific for the gene are essential for technology transfer from research to diagnostic laboratory. For the purpose of this limited discussion we will present examples of well-characterized mutation types represented in several common genetic diseases.

DELETION AND DUPLICATION MUTATIONS IN DUCHENNE MUSCULAR DYSTROPHY

Duchenne muscular dystrophy (DMD) is an X-linked recessive neuromuscular disorder affecting approximately 1 in 3500 males with one-third of isolated cases resulting from a new mutation in the *dystrophin* gene. The *dystrophin* gene, located on Xp2l, is the largest gene identified to date, having greater than two megabases encompassing 79 exons. Two-thirds of patients have structural mutations with approximately 60% having intragenic deletion mutations and 6% duplication mutations. In addition, these mutations occur more frequently in certain regions of the gene reported as "hot spots for recombination." This knowledge, gene sequence information, and the full-length cDNA *dystrophin* probe provide the tools needed to design a comprehensive and efficient strategy for molecular analysis of DMD.

MULTIPLEX PCR DNA from affected males can be analyzed for the presence or absence of specified exons in the *dystrophin* gene, utilizing multiplex PCR reactions. Our laboratory examines 32 of the 79 *dystrophin* exons in three multiplex amplification reactions. These exons have been shown to account for over 98% of detectable deletions in the *dystrophin* gene. In addition, careful design of multiplexing strategy allows for establishment of deletion endpoints, which may be useful for phenotype–genotype correlations. Results from the multiplex reactions are analyzed for the presence or absence of specified exons, using agarose gel electrophoresis and ethidium bromide detection of DNA fragments (Fig. 8-1A). A positive result—i.e., the absence of a single PCR product or several gene contiguous PCR products from this multiplex—is virtually diagnostic of Duchenne or Becker muscular dystrophy. In contrast, a negative result—i.e., the presence of all exonic PCR products—neither confirms nor refutes the diagnosis. *Dystrophin* gene duplications can be problematic to detect by PCR analysis as band intensity can be modified by PCR conditions. Various approaches to overcome this technical challenge have included fluorescence-labeled primers and automated gene analyzer equipment to visualize fragment intensities compared to normal male and female control DNAs.

From: *Principles of Molecular Medicine* (J. L. Jameson, ed.), ©1998 Humana Press Inc., Totowa, NJ.

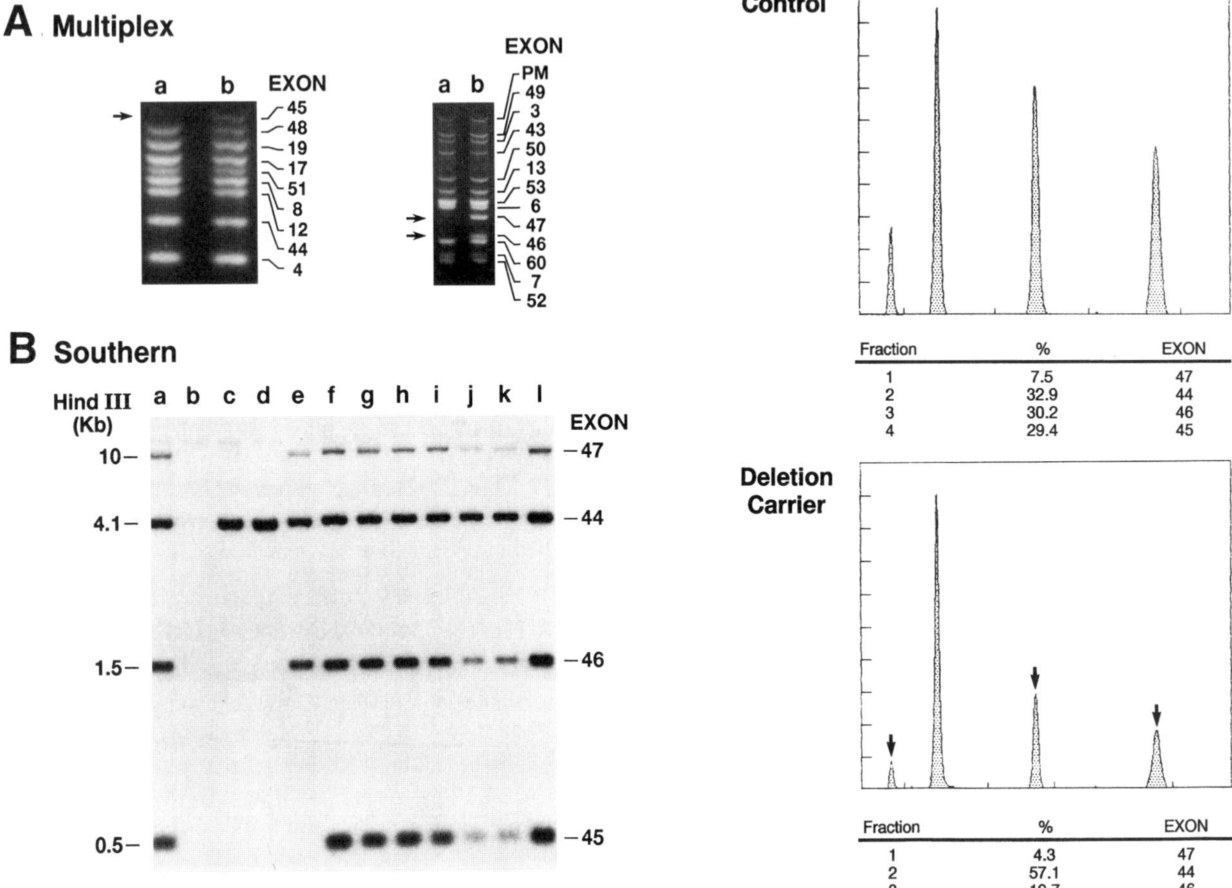

Figure 8-1 *Dystrophin* DNA analysis for deletion and duplication mutations. **(A)** Multiplex PCR analysis. For the two multiplex PCR panels shown, lanes represent: (a) a patient deleted in exons 46 through 48, and (b) a normal male control. Arrows point to deleted exons. **(B)** Southern analysis of *Hin*dIII fragments using cDNA probe 47-4B. Patient samples are in lanes b–k; male control (a), male patients (b–f); female patients (g–k); female control (l). Patient b is deleted for exons 44–47; patients c and d, deleted for exons 45–47; patient e, deleted for exon 45 only; patient f, no deletion detected. Carrier analysis of female relatives (lanes j and k) of affected male in lane c identifies the familial deletion (*see* Fig. 8-2).

Figure 8-2 *Dystrophin* gene dosage analysis by scanning densitometry. Scans of Southern *dystrophin* analysis in Fig. 8-1B, control female (lane 1), and deletion carrier female (lane k). Arrows indicate deleted exons at approximately half gene dosage as compared to the normal female control.

SOUTHERN DELETION ANALYSIS For male probands with a negative result by multiplex PCR or in the absence of endpoint resolution, Southern analysis should be done to examine the entire *dystrophin* gene for deletions and duplications. In our laboratory we use eight cDNA probes that cover the entire *dystrophin* gene to probe *Hin*dIII-digested patient DNAs to examine for the presence or absence of *Hin*dIII-fragments and their intensity as compared to a known male control DNA (Fig. 8-1B). Carrier detection in females can also be performed using Southern and dosage analysis for deletions and duplications (Fig. 8-2). Dosage analysis is also used for identification of duplication mutations in male probands. Ideally, a male proband is analyzed first to determine whether an identifiable mutation is present. If a mutation is identified in the affected male, then females at risk are examined for the presence or absence of the specific mutation using scanning densitometry to determine gene dosage as compared to a known female control DNA. Whereas two copies of each *dystrophin* exon are normal for females, one copy indicates a gene deletion in a female, and three copies indicate a duplication. In the event that an affected male is unavailable for DNA analysis, females can undergo DNA testing for carrier determination. However, in the absence of a male proband, female mutation analysis using DNA dosage analysis is less reliable. Recently, deletion and duplication analysis by fluorescence *in situ* hybridization (FISH) has proven useful for diagnosis of female carriers of DMD when the familial deletion or duplication has been previously identified by DNA analysis.

In the family shown in Fig. 8-3, the proband II-1 with a suspected diagnosis of DMD is analyzed by multiplex PCR and found to have a deletion of exons 45 through 50, confirming the diagnosis. Thus, molecular analysis of a blood specimen has avoided the invasive and costly procedure of muscle biopsy to confirm the diagnosis. The mother, I-2, who prior to DNA analysis has a 66% carrier risk, is analyzed by Southern deletion analysis and densitometry and found to carry the same deletion in one of her *dystrophin* genes. Similar analysis of the daughter, II-2, who has a prior carrier risk of 33%, does not identify this deletion mutation in either *dystrophin* gene. Thus her carrier risk is the same as a female from the general population, less than 1 in 2000. The male fetus, II-3, has a prior risk of 33% to be affected with DMD and is analyzed using multiplex PCR and does not have the familial

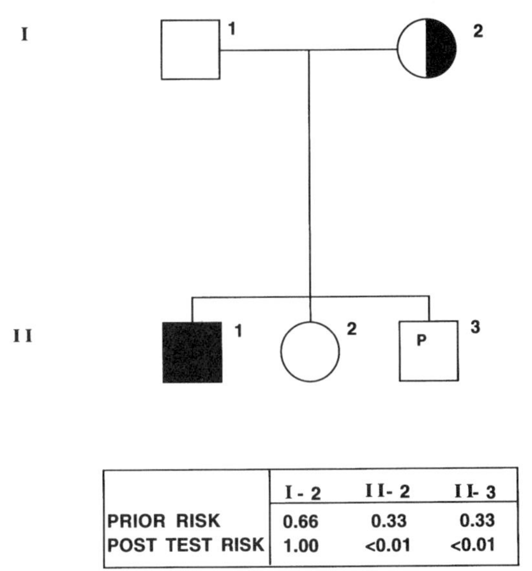

	I-2	II-2	II-3
PRIOR RISK	0.66	0.33	0.33
POST TEST RISK	1.00	<0.01	<0.01

Figure 8-3 DMD risk modification following direct mutation detection.

deletion mutation. Additional comparative studies using highly polymorphic DNA markers are performed on the maternal and fetal samples in order to rule out maternal cell contamination and demonstrate inheritance of one maternal allele. These results indicate that this fetus is unaffected with DMD. Accurate prenatal diagnosis is available for future pregnancies of I-2 and for her other female relatives at risk.

POINT MUTATION ANALYSIS IN CYSTIC FIBROSIS

Cystic fibrosis (CF) is a common autosomal recessive disorder that, in US Caucasians of Northern European background, has an incidence of approximately 1 in 2000 and a carrier frequency of 1 in 25. With the cloning of the *cystic fibrosis transmembrane regulator gene (CFTR)* in 1989 and the subsequent identification of a number of common mutations, a DNA-based laboratory test was quickly put in place to provide more precise carrier detection and prenatal diagnosis for CF families. In addition, molecular analysis is helpful to confirm a CF diagnosis for some patients and is indicated for abnormal fetal ultrasound suggesting echogenic bowel. Recent guidelines recommend that potential gamete donors also have CF carrier screening performed, as appropriate to the donor's ethnic background. Although debate in the genetics community has inhibited general population screening protocols, the general trend has been for progressive genetics centers to offer such testing. While hundreds of mutations have been identified, a detection rate of approximately 90% in US Caucasians can be achieved with the analysis of only 20–30 mutations. Carrier frequency and detection rate will vary, depending on ethnicity and geographical location of a specific population.

Although various mutation detection methods exist, we will present the method used in our laboratory, allele-specific oligonucleotide (ASO) hybridization. This test uses multiplex PCR to analyze 10 exons and one intron in the *CFTR* gene for the presence or absence of 30 CF mutations. A partial test result illustrating the most common CF mutation, ΔF508, is shown in Fig. 8-4. This

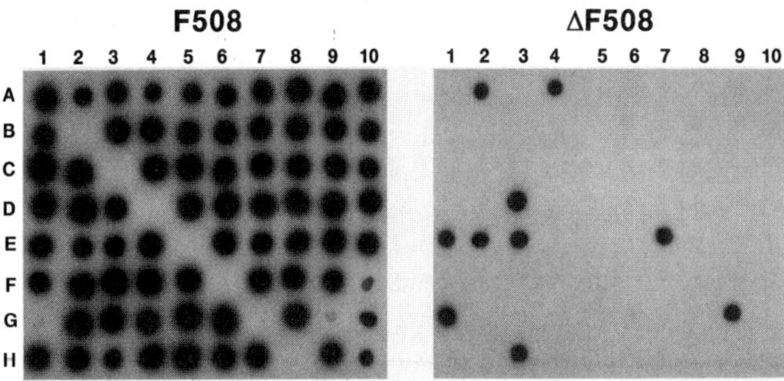

Figure 8-4 CF mutation analysis for ΔF508. Autoradiogram from exon 10 PCR products from appropriate controls and patient DNAs spotted on membranes and hybridized to the normal (F508) and mutant (ΔF508) radiolabeled ASOs. For example, patient specimens in positions GI, E1, and E2 represent an affected child and both parents, respectively. Homozygote G1 shows hybridization only to ΔF508, while heterozygotes E1 and E2 hybridize to both F508 and ΔF508.

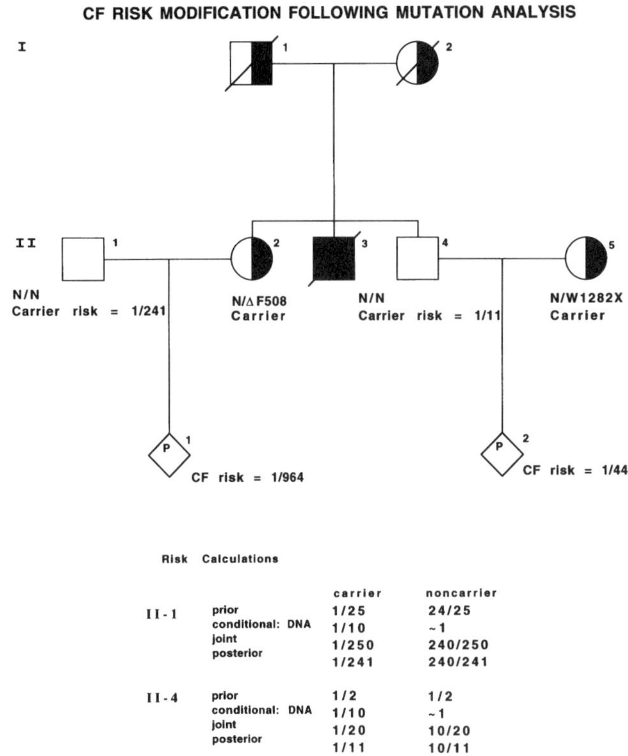

		carrier	noncarrier
II-1	prior	1/25	24/25
	conditional: DNA	1/10	~1
	joint	1/250	240/250
	posterior	1/241	240/241
II-4	prior	1/2	1/2
	conditional: DNA	1/10	~1
	joint	1/20	10/20
	posterior	1/11	10/11

Figure 8-5 CF modification following mutation analysis.

analysis can be partially automated using robotics, multiplexing, and pooling strategies. In addition, this strategy is applied in our laboratory to other genetic diseases, including Tay-Sachs, Gaucher, Canavan, Fanconi anemia, achondroplasia, sickle-cell and hemoglobin SC disease, and α-1-antitrypsin deficiency.

The case shown in Fig. 8-5 illustrates the impact of molecular analysis on CF risk modification. All individuals are of Northern European Caucasian descent. Individuals II-2 and II-4 had a brother affected with CF who died prior to CF testing and the two carrier parents, I-1 and I-2, are also deceased. Thus, the prior carrier risk for II-2 and II-4 is two-thirds and their fetuses are both at 1 in 150 risk to be affected. CF testing reveals that II-2 is a CF carrier with one copy of a ΔF508 mutation. Individual II-1, the spouse of individual II-2, has a negative family history for CF; thus his prior carrier risk is 1 in 25. His CF mutation analysis is negative. His modified carrier risk is 1 in 241. Thus, the modified CF risk for fetus III-1 is now 1 in 964 and prenatal diagnosis is not recommended. In contrast, individual II-4 does not have a ΔF508 or any of the other 29 CF mutations tested. The carrier risk for II-4 can be modified using Bayesian analysis. Based on detection of a ΔF508 mutation in II-2, the prior risk for II-4 is 1 in 2, since only one parental mutation has been identified. Based on a ~90% detection rate using this panel of 30 CF mutations, the prior risk of 50% can be conditionally modified using a 10% chance that a mutation will not be detected. Thus, II-4s modified carrier risk is 1 in 11. The reproductive partner, individual II-5, who has a negative family history of CF and a prior carrier risk of 1 in 25, is found by molecular analysis to carry a W1282X mutation, and thus, is a definite CF carrier. As a result, fetus III-2 is at a 1-in-44 risk to be affected with CF. This presents a complex prenatal diagnosis situation. If prenatal diagnosis is performed and the results are negative for W1282X, the fetus is unaffected with CF, but carrier risk is ambiguous at a 1-in-22. However, if the fetus inherits the W1282X mutation, then the fetus is a definite carrier and at 1 in 22 risk to be affected with CF.

TRINUCLEOTIDE REPEAT MUTATION AND METHYLATION ANALYSIS IN FRAGILE X MENTAL RETARDATION SYNDROME

Fragile X syndrome was the first disorder in which the molecular basis was explained by the expansion of a trinucleotide repeat. Fragile X is the most common cause of inherited mental retardation, occurring in approximately 1 in 1500 males and 1 in 2500 females in all ethnic groups studied. Prior to the cloning of the *FMR-1* gene, cytogenetic analysis was used for diagnostic confirmation. However, cytogenetic analysis proved unreliable, particularly for carrier detection and prenatal diagnosis. With the cloning of the *FMR-1* gene and identification of a trinucleotide repeat expansion, the phenomenon of anticipation and reduced penetrance in fragile X families, the Sherman Paradox, was explained, and molecular analysis became the method of choice for fragile X testing. A CGG repeat occurs within the 5' untranslated region of the *FMR-1* gene, which in normal individuals varies in size up to approximately 40 repeats and is inherited stably over generations. However, in affected individuals this CGG repeat region expands to greater than 200 repeats and becomes hypermethylated. In unaffected carriers, an intermediate size repeat region, termed as premutation, is seen ranging from approximately 60 to 200 repeats, but hypermethylation is not present. Premutation alleles are unstable during female meiosis and, depending on size (>70 repeats), have a significant likelihood of expanding to a full mutation in the next generation. However, unstable premutation alleles found in normal transmitting males generally do not expand to a full mutation in transmission to their carrier daughters. An indeterminate range between 40 and 60 repeats presents a challenge in counseling families regarding the potential risk of fragile X occurring in their future generations. Alleles in this range can be either normal stable alleles or unstable premutations, but have never been shown to be transmitted as full mutations. Fragile X testing is indicated for individuals with mental retardation or developmental delay of unknown cause, or individuals with a positive family history of fragile X. While general population carrier screening for fragile X carrier detection has been done primarily on an investigational basis, this application may become more widely accepted in the future.

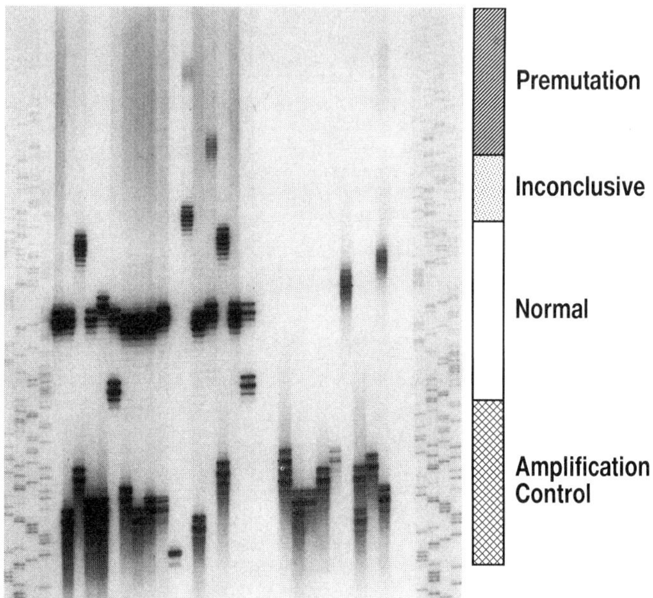

Figure 8-6 Fragile X PCR analysis. Radiolabeled PCR products from patient DNA generated from primers flanking CGG repeat are separated by electrophoresis and analyzed by comparison to a standardized sizing ladder to determine allele size. An amplification control is included to rule out test failure in males with large expansions that fail to amplify by PCR. Normal alleles range up to 42 repeats; inconclusive, 43–59 repeats; premutation, 60 to approximately 200 repeats.

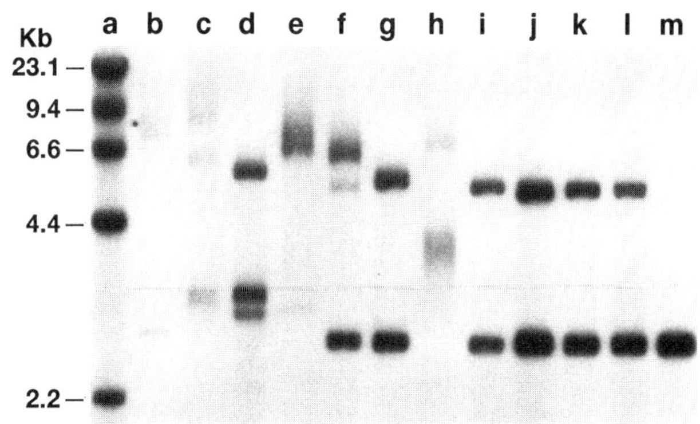

Figure 8-7 Fragile X Southern analysis. *Eco*RI- and *BSS*HII-restricted DNAs from patients (b–k) and normal control (female, l and male, m) hybridized to radiolabeled pE5.1 probe isolated from the CGG repeat region of FMR-1. The normal *Eco*RI fragment size detected by this probe is 5.2 kb. In normal males additional digestion using the methylation-sensitive enzyme, *BSS*HII, results in a 2.8-kb fragment only, representing an active X chromosome. Normal females have one 5.2-kb fragment, due to normal X inactivation, and one 2.8-kb fragment. Lanes b and e show affected males with full hypermethylated mutations; lane c and h, mosaic males having a full mutation and a premutation, respectively; lane d, a female with two premutations, the mother of affected male in lane e; lane f, a female with a full mutation; lane g, a female with a small premutation (68 repeats); lanes i, j, k, females having no detectable expansion.

Fragile X analysis is performed in our diagnostic laboratory using simultaneous PCR analysis to determine the size of normal and small premutation alleles (Fig. 8-6), and Southern analysis to examine methylation status and to estimate the size of large premutation and full mutation alleles (Fig. 8-7).

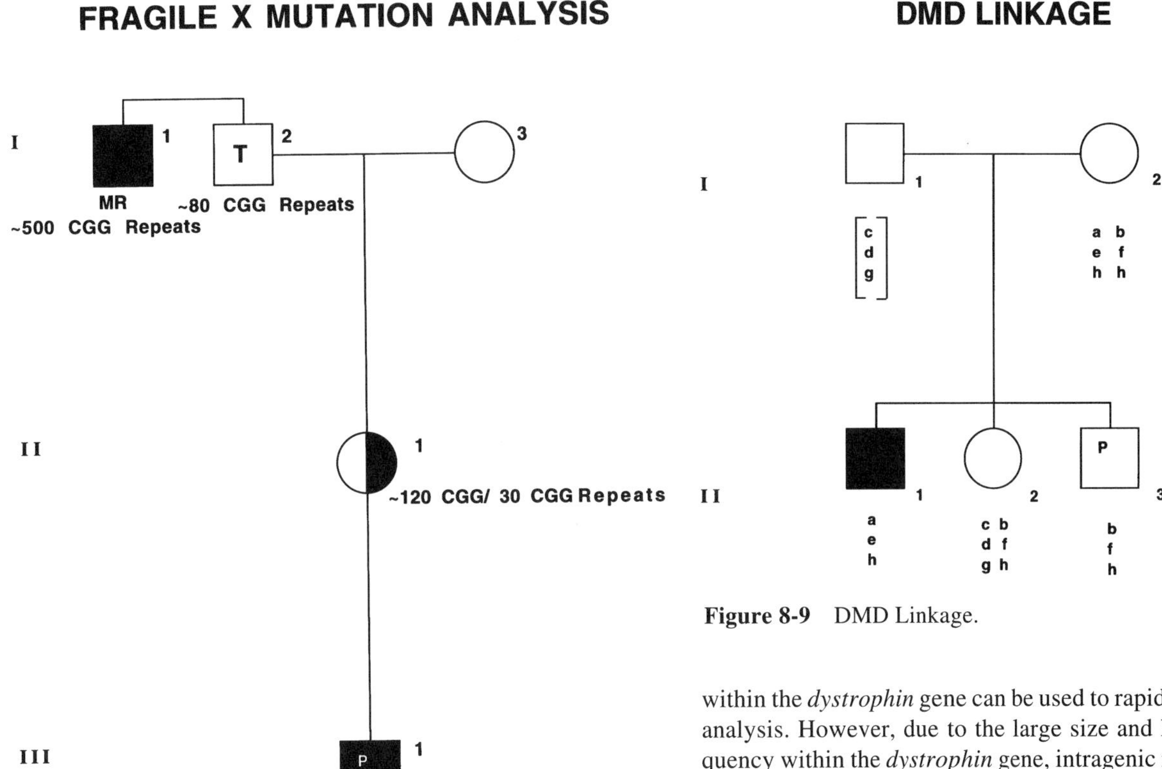

Figure 8-8 Fragile X mutation analysis.

Figure 8-9 DMD Linkage.

The family shown in Fig. 8-8 illustrates the impact of direct mutation detection for fragile X for diagnostic clarification as well as carrier and fetal risk prediction. Individual II-1 reports to her obstetrician that she has a paternal uncle with mental retardation of unknown cause. DNA analysis of the uncle, I-1, reveals an expansion of approximately 500 CGG repeats, thus confirming his diagnosis as fragile X. Subsequent PCR analysis of her father, I-2, who is of normal intelligence, identifies a premutation allele of 80 repeats, thus indicating that he is a normal transmitting male. His daughter, II-1, is found to have one normal allele of 30 repeats and one premutation allele of 150 repeats, confirming her carrier status. Thus, her male fetus, III-1, is at a 1-in-2 risk to be affected with fragile X. PCR analysis of fetal DNA indicates a null allele, i.e., failure of amplification across the CGG region, suggesting the presence of a full mutation. Southern analysis of this fetus reveals a CGG expansion of >700 repeats with hypermethylation, thus predicting that this fetus is affected with fragile X mental retardation syndrome.

LINKAGE ANALYSIS

When direct mutation detection is not possible, either because the gene has not been cloned or a particular family does not have an identifiable mutation, then linkage analysis may be possible, provided that key family members are available and willing to be studied and that the necessary molecular tools are available for the analysis. For example, in the Duchenne muscular dystrophy case depicted in Fig. 8-3, if molecular analysis did not detect a mutation in the affected male, then linkage analysis in this family would be possible and could provide risk modification for the sister and the fetus. PCR analysis of highly polymorphic intronic DNA markers within the *dystrophin* gene can be used to rapidly accomplish this analysis. However, due to the large size and high mutation frequency within the *dystrophin* gene, intragenic recombinations do occur and must be accounted for in the risk analysis. We analyze DNA markers at the 5', central, and 3' regions of the *dystrophin* gene. Those females whose two-*dystrophin* marker patterns (haplotypes) can be distinguished are termed "informative." If all markers are informative, a 1% chance of unrecognized recombination remains. If 5' and central, 3' and central, or only central markers are informative, a 5% chance for unrecognized recombination exists. If only 5' or 3' markers are informative, a 10% chance of recombination is used in the risk calculation.

In this example shown in Fig. 8-9, the affected male, II-1, does not have an identified deletion or duplication mutation. Linkage analysis of the mother is informative at the 5' and central sites, but not at the 3' site. The sister of the affected and the male fetus has inherited the opposite maternal haplotype. The paternal haplotype of II-2 can be deduced from the data without the analysis of her father's DNA. Based on the new mutation rate in DMD, I-2's carrier risk is 67% and linkage analysis does not modify her risk. The carrier risk for individual II-2 based on family history is 33%; but, using linkage data and taking into account two possible recombination events with a 5% recombination frequency for each event, this risk can be modified to 6.4%. Similarly, the risk that the male fetus, II-3, is affected can also be modified from 33 to 6.4%, based on linkage analysis.

FUTURE DIRECTIONS

With the expansion of molecular diagnostics will come improved health care. To date, the major impact of molecular analysis has been reproductive decision making regarding single gene disorders, which occur in a small percentage of the population. Future trends in genetic testing will include more predictive tests for susceptibility to common diseases, including cancer, cardiovascular disease, diabetes, and psychiatric disorders. When offering genetic testing, particularly for those disorders with adult onset, the molecular laboratory must be aware of the legal and ethical implications. Comprehensive protocols attentive to national guidelines must be implemented that should include genetic counseling, medical and (in some instances), psychological evaluations, and informed consent. Predictive testing is currently being performed for several adult onset diseases having trinucleotide repeat expansion mutations, including Kennedy disease, myotonic dystrophy, Huntington's disease, spinocerebellar ataxia type 1, dentatorubral-pallidoluysian atrophy, and Machado Joseph/spinocerebellar ataxia type 3. In addition, cancer susceptibility genes, including those responsible for some inherited breast and ovarian cancer and colorectal cancer, have been identified, and tests have been developed for individuals at risk. While susceptibility testing is currently performed under research protocols, it is likely that testing will become more widely available. Predictive testing, while having positive implications for the individual and family, has the potential risk of insurance or employment discrimination and other negative implications. Such legal, social, and ethical issues specific to genetic testing are currently being debated and addressed at a national level. A key component to the future success of this discipline is the evolution of technology development to address volume and cost issues. Laboratory testing, which is now routinely done in highly specialized genetic testing laboratories in both academic and industrial settings, may eventually be done in hospital chemistry laboratories and physician offices. Gene and technology patenting issues further complicate and potentially limit the widespread application of genetic testing. However, the major challenge to ensure widespread access to genetic testing is education of health care professionals, consumers, and insurance carriers.

SELECTED REFERENCES

Broholm J, Cassiman JJ, Craufurd D, et al. Guidelines for the molecular genetics predictive test in Huntington's disease. Neurology 1994; 44:1533–1536.

Chamberlain JS, Gibbs RA, Ranier JE, et al. Deletion screening of the Duchenne muscular dystrophy locus via multiplex DNA amplification. Nucleic Acid Res 1988;16:11,141–11,156.

Clemens PR, Fenwick RG, Chamberlain JS, et al. Carrier detection and prenatal diagnosis in Duchenne and Becker muscular dystrophy families, using dinucleotide repeat polymorphisms. Am J Hum Genet 1991;49:951–960.

DeMarchi JM, Caskey CT, Richards CS. Population-specific screening by mutation analysis for diseases frequent in Ashkenazi Jews. Hum Mut 1996;8:116–125.

DeMarchi JM, Richards CS, Fenwick RG, Pace R, Beaudet AL. A robotics-assisted procedure for large scale cystic fibrosis mutation analysis. Hum Mut 1994;4:281–290.

Fu YH, Kuhl DPA, Pizzuti A, et al. Variation of the CGG repeat at the fragile X site results in genetic instability: Resolution of the Sherman Paradox. Cell 1991;67:1047–1058.

Fu YH, Pizzuti A, Fenwick RG, et al. An unstable triplet repeat in a gene related to myotonic muscular dystrophy. Science 1992;255: 1256–1258.

Grompe M. The rapid detection of unknown mutations in nucleic acids. Nat Genet 1993;5:111–117.

Hejtmancik JF, Ward P, Tantravahi U et al. Genetic analysis: a practical approach to linkage, pedigrees, and Bayesian risk. In: Rowland LP, Wood DS, Schon EA, DiMauso S, eds. Molecular Genetics of Brain, Nerve and Muscle. New York: Oxford University Press, 1989; pp. 191–207.

Kan YW, Dozy AM. Antenatal diagnosis of sickle-cell anemia by D.N.A. analysis of amniotic-fluid cells. Lancet October 28, 1978:910,911.

Kawaguchi Y, Okamoto T, Taniwaki M, et al. CAG expansions in a novel gene for Machado-Joseph disease at chromosome 14q32.1. Nat Genet 1994;8:221–228.

Kerem B, Rommens JM, Buchanan JA, et al. Identification of the cystic fibrosis gene: Genetic analysis. Science 1989;245:1073–1080.

Koenig M, Hoffman EP, Bertelson CJ, et al. Complete cloning of the Duchenne muscular dystrophy (DMD) cDNA and preliminary genomic organization of the DMD gene in normal and affected individuals. Cell 1987;50:509–517.

Korf B. Molecular Medicine Molecular Diagnosis (first of two parts). New Engl J Med 1995;332:1218–1220.

Korf B. Molecular Medicine Molecular Diagnosis (second of two parts). New Engl J Med 1995;332:1499–1502.

MacDonald ME, Ambrose CM, Duyao MP et al. A novel gene containing a trinucleotide repeat that is expanded and unstable on Huntington's disease chromosomes. Cell 1993;72:971–983.

Miki Y, Swensen J, Shattuck-Eidens D, et al. A strong candidate for the 17q-linked breast and ovarian cancer susceptibility gene BRCA1. Science 1994;266:66–71.

Orr HT, Chung MY, Banfi S, et al. Expansion of an unstable trinucleotide CAG repeat in spinocerebellar ataxia type 1. Nat Genet 1993;4:221–226.

Shiang R, Thompson LM, Zhu YZ, et al. Mutations in the transmembrane domain of FGFR3 cause the most common genetic form of dwarfism, Achondroplasia. Cell 1994;78:335–342.

Tsui LC. Mutations and sequence variations detected in the cystic fibrosis transmembrane conductance regulator (CFTR) gene: a report from the Cystic Fibrosis Genetic Analysis Consortium. Hum Mut 1992;1:197–203.

Verkerk AJMH, Pieretti M, Sutcliffe JS, et al. Identification of a gene (FMR-1) containing a CGG repeat coincident with a breakpoint cluster region exhibiting length variation in Fragile X syndrome. Cell 1991;65:905–914.

Warren ST, Nelson DL. Advances in molecular analysis of fragile X syndrome. JAMA 1994;271:536–542.

Zielenski J, Rozmahel R, Bozon D, et al. Genomic DNA sequence of the cystic fibrosis transmembrane conductance regulator (CFTR) gene. Genomics 1991;10:214–228.

9 Genetic Counseling

BETH A. FINE

INTRODUCTION

The practice of genetic counseling has evolved in the last quarter century into a communication process between an appropriately trained health professional and a patient/client, couple, and/or family, regarding the occurrence or risk of occurrence of a genetic condition and relevant implications. In response to advances in molecular genetics and diagnostic technologies, a new health care professional, the master's-level genetic counselor, emerged in the early 1970s to participate in a multidisciplinary team approach to meeting the informational, psychosocial, and medical needs of individuals and families affected with or at risk for genetic conditions.

In this chapter, a historical perspective on the profession and practice of genetic counseling in the United States will be followed by a discussion of the principles and types of service delivery in the settings in which genetic counseling is conducted. Next, the philosophical underpinnings of genetic counseling along with a review of the psychosocial, ethical, religious, and ethnocultural contexts in which patients experience genetic counseling and testing will be reviewed. The chapter will end with a description of genetic-counselor education, training, and credentialing. Since more nongenetics health professionals are participating and will continue to participate in aspects of genetic-counseling activities, the aim of this chapter is to introduce the components of genetic counseling together with the relevant issues faced by professionals and patients and their families as the Human Genome Project progresses. Resources for referrals to genetic counselors are included in Table 9-1.

THE PROFESSIONAL GENETIC COUNSELOR

Genetic counselors are health professionals with specialized graduate degrees and experience in medical genetics and counseling, often with undergraduate education in biology, genetics, psychology, public health, social work, or nursing. Approximately 1500 genetic counselors are members of the National Society of Genetic Counselors (NSGC); most practice in university or community hospitals.

Genetic counselors work as members of a health-care team, providing information and support to individuals and families who have members with birth defects or genetic disorders, and to families who may be at risk for a variety of inherited conditions. They identify individuals and families at risk for genetic conditions, birth defects, or disease-susceptibility, and investigate the problem in the family. Genetic counselors analyze inheritance patterns and risk of occurrence/recurrence, interpret and communicate information about the disorder, and explore and discuss available options with the family.

Genetic counselors aim to communicate complex genetic and medical information to individuals and families in a manner that makes sense within the context of the patients' lives. A patient's educational level, culture, religion and psychosocial issues inform the way that genetic counselors frame risks and discuss the implications of genetic risk with families. Therefore, the information must be presented in a culturally sensitive manner in order to facilitate informed decision-making. Genetic counselors often work with patients and families in crisis, at the time of a diagnosis, or during loss of a pregnancy or family member. They provide supportive counseling to families, serve as patient advocates, and refer individuals and families to community resources/services.

Some genetic counselors also serve as educators and consultants for other health-care professionals and for the general public. Genetic counselors work in the public-health setting, in academic and commercial laboratories as liaisons to clinicians, and are involved in clinical research and public policy.

THE GENETIC-COUNSELING PROCESS

In 1974, an *ad hoc* committee of the American Society of Human Genetics defined genetic counseling as a communication process that deals with the human problems associated with the occurrence or risk of occurrence of a genetic disorder in a family. This process involves an attempt by one or more appropriately trained persons to help the individual or family to:

1. Comprehend the medical facts, including the diagnosis, probable course of the disorder, and the available management.
2. Appreciate the way heredity contributes to the disorder and the risk of recurrence in specified relatives.
3. Understand the options for dealing with the risk of recurrence.
4. Choose the course of action that seems appropriate to them in view of their risk and the family goals and act in accordance with that decision.
5. Make the best possible adjustment to the disorder in an affected family member and/or to the risk of recurrence of that disorder (Fraser, 1974).

Historically, the practice of genetic counseling, defined as providing information about recurrence risks for particular conditions within a family, began in the early part of this century. Genetic

From: *Principles of Molecular Medicine* (J. L. Jameson, ed.), ©1998 Humana Press Inc., Totowa, NJ.

Table 9-1
Resources for Referrals to Genetic Counselors

Clinical Genetics Web Sites
http://www.faseb.org/genetics
http://www.kumc.edu/gec/geneinfo.htm
http://members.aol.com/nsgcweb/nsgchome/htm

National Cancer Institute Familial Cancer Risk Counseling and Genetic Counseling Information Genetic Counselor Directory
http://cancer net.nci.nih.gov/www.prot/genetic/genesrch.shtml

Genetic Counseling Resources
National Society of Genetic Counselors
233 Canterbury Drive
Wallingford PA 19086-6617
610-872-7608
E-mail: nsgc@aol.com

American Board of Genetic Counseling
9650 Rockville Pike
Bethesda MD 20814-3998
301-571-1825

American College of Medical Genetics
9650 Rockville Pike
Bethesda MD 20814-3998
301-530-7127

American Society of Human Genetics
9650 Rockville Pike
Bethesda MD 20814-3998
301-571-1825

Alliance of Genetic Support Groups
35 Wisconsin Circle, Suite 440
Chevy Chase MD 20815-7015
1-800-336-GENE

counseling was conducted by biologists with research interests in particular conditions. The goal of providing risk information in the absence of diagnostic or preventive measures reflected the eugenic philosophy of the time. In fact, the first genetic-counseling clinic, the Eugenics Records Office, was established in the early 1900s in Cold Spring Harbor, NY. The only options available to these families were to "take their chances" and initiate a pregnancy or to refrain from having biological children.

In the 1940s, heredity clinics staffed by physicians who were interested in genetic diseases were established. Genetic counseling at that time was conducted by physicians and PhD geneticists. They primarily used a medical/preventive model that involved providing "facts"—risk figures, natural history, and treatment information—so that couples and families could make informed reproductive decisions. Geneticists assumed that these decisions were based on the patients' perception of the risk, while studies revealed the importance of the perception of the burden of the disease. In essence, the genetic counseling was primarily an education process.

With the advent of carrier testing and prenatal diagnosis in the late 1960s and early 1970s, families' range of choices broadened. Geneticists recognized that information alone regarding genetic conditions and testing procedures was not enough to facilitate decision making and to truly serve the patients and families. Dr. Melissa Richter, a visionary, initiated the development of a master's degree program in genetic counseling at Sarah Lawrence College to prepare a new professional to address the needs of families at genetic risk. These new professionals would also serve as "physician-extenders," providing the genetic information in a psychosocial context using skills the physicians did not possess. Thus, the team approach to genetics services began.

As genetic counseling and related services moved from a more preventive focus to a more client-centered approach, some practitioners adhered to the decision-making model in which information is presented within the psychological and cultural context, so that patients can come to an appropriate decision regarding genetic testing and reproductive options. Genetic counselors came to espouse a nondirective approach to genetic counseling about reproductive issues to demonstrate respect for the patients' autonomy and to move away from the eugenic underpinnings of earlier genetic counseling.

Today, it is recognized that many psychosocial and medical factors influence the genetic-counseling process. The information communicated in most genetic-counseling sessions is emotion-laden, often leading to a crisis. Therefore, many contemporary genetic counselors adhere to the psychotherapeutic genetic counseling model that involves psychosocial assessment, provision of information, psychological support and counseling, and referrals to other mental-health professionals as needed. It is often true that the genetic counselor functions as a liaison to the other specialists dealing with a patient and the family, providing a forum for sharing feelings, having them validated, and for processing information and resources. Genetic counselors work in pediatric or obstetric settings as well as in a wide array of specialty clinics, focusing on a particular disorder or group of disorders. While the contexts may differ, the process remains the same.

Genetic counseling involves developing a relationship and rapport with a patient or family, usually in a short time period. In many instances, there is only one encounter between a patient and a genetic counselor, although many individuals affected with genetic conditions are followed on a long-term basis. The goal of genetic counseling is to make genetic and medical information relevant to the patient or family accessible and useful so that they can optimize their health care and lifestyle decisions. The genetic counselor begins each session by asking the patient what his or her goals are for the session and the relationship, e.g., their questions about diagnosis, testing, options for dealing with risks, therapeutic modalities, support, access to resources. The genetic counselor then places the patient's expectations in context for what is possible within the limitations of scientific knowledge and available technology. Whether the genetic-counseling process occurs in one clinic visit or on a periodic basis over many years, the following components are necessary for the goals that the patient and professional wish to meet.

INFORMATION GATHERING Geneticists and genetic counselors have been compared to detectives with regard to their work in making a diagnosis or discovering an underlying etiology for a condition that runs in a family. The sleuth work begins with gathering a great deal of information from the patient, his or her physician, and other family members. Whereas an accurate diagnosis is the most important component of quality genetic counseling, several types of histories must be obtained to arrive at that diagnosis.

First, the genetic counselor will elicit a detailed ***family history***, constructing a pedigree or a family tree. The purpose of the pedigree is to create a graphic record of the family history for use in the medical record. The pedigree may lead to an accurate diagnosis and precise risk assessment for a particular condition in family members. Approaches to testing or treatment may be determined at least partially by information gathered for a pedigree.

There are standard symbols used for pedigree notation that have been approved by the National Society of Genetic Counselors and the American Society of Human Genetics (Bennett et al., 1996). The pedigree should include at least three generations, including the proband (the affected person about whom the consultation is sought) or consultand (an unaffected individual seeking risk information), their children, siblings, parents, grandparents and aunts, uncles and cousins. Since most patients do not have complete medical information on all family members, it is important to encourage them to inquire about health histories from their relatives. They should inquire about symptoms or traits that run in families, as they can provide clues to a diagnosis. For example, if several relatives in more than one generation experienced sudden death from aortic dissection, one might consider the diagnosis of Marfan syndrome.

The genetic counselor will pose questions about any medical, developmental, or physical abnormalities that may run in the family. In addition, questions will be asked about pregnancy losses, stillbirths, environmental exposures during pregnancy, birthdates or ages of individuals, ages and causes of death, and about ethnicity and possible consanguinity. When necessary, medical records may be requested to confirm diagnoses. This type of questioning also helps build a rapport with the patient, so that difficult or emotional issues can be addressed more easily. Genetic conditions are considered taboo or shameful in some families, so that the patient must feel safe and comfortable in discussing such matters.

The questioning may be focused on features of specific conditions when the patient seeks genetic counseling for a particular disorder. For preconceptual counseling or prenatal diagnosis because a woman is over 35 years of age, the family history should be more general. However, if a family history of a particular condition is discovered, genetic counseling can address the risks for that condition if the patient is interested.

The pedigree is useful as a communication tool in genetic counseling. When the patient or family is involved in constructing the diagram, it often jars their memory about other family members. It can be used to illustrate modes of inheritance and how risk figures are calculated.

Finally, when genetic testing in a family is conducted, the pedigree is useful in determining which family members need to be tested and in interpreting their test results. In general, the pedigree is the genetic counselor's primary tool for conducting risk assessment and counseling.

Second, if there is an affected individual in the family, the genetic counselor must gather information about the ***medical history***. This should include symptoms prior to diagnosis, age at diagnosis, confirmatory tests, course of the disorder, and current treatment. Confirmation of a diagnosis is necessary for accurate genetic counseling.

Third, a ***developmental history*** is important, particularly in pediatric genetic counseling, since a large proportion of children with inherited conditions have developmental disabilities. Knowledge of specific disabilities is essential for accurate diagnosis in some cases. In other situations, a geneticist may make recommendations for special education or other therapies based on the specific condition or constellation of problems.

Finally, the genetic counselor gathers information about ***patient*** and/or ***family concerns***, fears and questions regarding the genetic counseling process, the condition, or possible testing or treatment. It is also important to understand the ***family dynamics*** and ***support systems*** that often influence the care for the affected individual. In addition, the genetic counselor must assess the ***level of baseline knowledge*** and understanding of genetics, the genetic disorder, and the medical components of the condition. This information will guide the genetic counselor in presenting the information being offered to the patient and family.

DIAGNOSIS An accurate diagnosis is central to providing appropriate and effective genetic services. A genetic diagnosis can be made in a variety of ways, depending on the age of the patient and the nature of the symptoms or characteristics leading to the referral to a genetics center.

The physical examination provides a great deal of information, particularly in the case of dysmorphic features. The identification of physical findings, which include a constellation of characteristics and symptoms that represent a known syndrome, is important in providing answers about prognosis, natural history, and possible therapies or management strategies. In addition, a genetic diagnosis may lead to prevention of adverse symptoms or amelioration of a particular condition. For example, a healthy baby born with macrosomia, macroglossia, characteristic facies, and creases in the earlobes may carry the diagnosis of Beckwith-Wiedemann syndrome. While the features described here are not medical problems, infants with this syndrome are at increased risk for hypoglycemia, which, if left untreated, can lead to mental retardation. In addition, these children are at increased risk for Wilms' tumor. Thus, by making the diagnosis, mental retardation can be prevented by monitoring blood sugar levels, and screening for early diagnosis of the kidney malignancy is possible.

Many genetic diagnoses are made in the laboratory. Cytogenetic analysis performed on a blood sample from a child or adult, or on amniocytes or chorionic villi obtained by prenatal diagnosis leads to the preparation of a karyotype that reveals aneuploidy or chromosomal rearrangements. Chromosome analysis is the most frequently ordered genetic test, since the majority of women who have prenatal diagnosis are age 35 or older and are therefore at increased risk for chromosomal abnormalities such as Down syndrome.

Biochemical assays are available to diagnose many inborn errors of metabolism in individuals and in fetuses. These conditions are primarily autosomal recessive conditions in which the gene product has been identified. For example, an assay to measure the level of α-iduronidase in a child with coarse facial features, hepatosplenomegaly, and developmental delay may lead to the diagnosis of Hurler syndrome. Biochemical assays are also used for carrier detection for rare recessive disorders. In most cases, carrier testing is offered for individuals with a specific ethnic origin who are at increased risk for carrying a gene for a specific condition. For example, carrier testing for Tay Sachs disease among Ashkenazi Jews involves measurement of the level of hexosaminidase A in a blood sample. The accuracy, specificity, and sensitivity of such tests vary; genetic counselors remain current on the standard procedures of this type of testing.

Increasing numbers of genes for inherited conditions have been mapped and sequenced over the last several years. With the completion of the Human Genome Project, the genes for all genetic conditions will be mapped and sequenced. While the goal of the

Human Genome Project is to understand how genes work under normal circumstances, many of these discoveries have resulted in the availability of DNA-based genetic tests. The large number and varied frequencies of mutations in each disease gene result in a range of accuracy for each test. The complexity of the interpretation of DNA test results necessitates genetic counseling that involves an informed consent process and psychosocial counseling before, during, and after testing. Again, as technology changes rapidly, genetic counselors are obligated to remain current on standard clinical tests and to identify appropriate research studies for their patients and families.

Imaging techniques, such as ultrasonography, particularly in prenatal diagnosis, and X-rays for diagnosis of skeletal dysplasias and other syndromes, are often useful in diagnosing specific conditions. The use of ultrasonography in pregnancy to identify fetuses at increased risk for chromosomal abnormality or syndromes that involve structural abnormalities is increasing. Again, genetic counseling to explain the benefits and limitations of ultrasound diagnosis and issues surrounding uncertainty and loss is important to maximize patients' ability to cope successfully.

RISK ASSESSMENT Many patients seek genetic counseling with the explicit question, "What is the chance that this condition will occur in one of our family members?" or "What is the chance that this will happen again?" Geneticists use a variety of sources to attempt to answer one or both of these questions. While many patients and clinicians believe that arriving at a specific, accurate number to quantify the risk is the information desired, studies have shown that reproductive decisions are more likely to be based on a patient's perception of the burden of the disease, rather than the magnitude of the risk of occurrence or recurrence. Also, the risk must be considered within the context of the patients' lives, including an understanding of how the individual processes numerical values such as percents or ratios. Risk assessment followed by communication is a prerequisite to any type of decision making regarding reproduction or taking genetic tests.

Recurrence or occurrence risks may be calculated by pedigree analysis in which a known mode of inheritance is identified. If two parents are found to be carriers of a recessive gene, then the risk for each future offspring is 25%. This information will affect different couples' reproductive decisions in different ways. Empiric risks are often used when disorders are not caused by single genes, but are polygenic or multifactorial in nature. Empiric risks are derived from studying disease frequencies in a given population. If the data is gathered in an unbiased manner, using appropriate study design, the risk figures provide a sound basis for counseling. However, one must critically evaluate whether such studies are applicable to an individual patient because of differences in ethnic groups, factors that modify gene expression, and whether new developments led to reclassification of disorders that were once thought of as multifactorial.

Calculations based on genetic testing results can also lead to risk assessment that is specific to a particular family. For example, a woman, with a brother affected with cystic fibrosis (CF), and her husband, who has no family history of CF, asked about their risk of having a child with CF. This risk, prior to any testing, is 1/120. The affected brother is found to have two copies of the common dF508 mutation; DNA analysis for the woman revealed that she carries this mutation. Her husband, of Northern European descent, tested negative for 30 common mutations. Since this test detects about 90% of all mutations, his risk of being a carrier is about 1/240. Thus, after testing, their risk to have an affected child is 1/1920, much lower than the *a priori* risk. Again, changes in the detection rates for many DNA tests occur often; genetic counselors must remain aware of new standards in testing and counseling.

PROVISION OF INFORMATION Genetic counseilng is truly a communication process, designed to answer the concerns of patients and their health care providers about diagnosis, prognosis, and treatment/management options. Genetic counseling can be thought of as a conversation between genetic counselor and the patient and his or her family members. In meeting the needs of patients, genetic counselors often discuss the risk of recurrence or occurrence of a disorder in the patient and/or other relatives. The genetic counselor assesses the patient's emotional and cognitive status so as to present the information in an appropriate manner.

A significant component of genetic counseling involves a discussion of genetic testing as an option for patients. While not all genetic-counseling sessions involve a discussion of genetic testing, genetic counseling should be part of any genetic testing process. Obtaining informed consent for testing includes reviewing the risks, benefits, limitations, costs, ramifications, and accuracy of any genetic test. The genetic counselor must then facilitate the decision-making process regarding testing, based on the patient's response to the informed consent process. If a patient elects to undergo genetic testing, either in the form of prenatal diagnosis of chromosomal disorders by amniocentesis, or in the form of a blood test on an individual, plans are made for the disclosure of results either by telephone or in person.

Once a patient consents to testing, the genetic counselor must disclose test results when they become available. Usually, a genetic counselor will review the possible results and the patient's reaction to each outcome prior to testing. A plan for communicating results either by telephone, mail, or in person is arranged. Finally, the genetic counselor facilitates an exploration of possible options following particular results. Communication, exploration of options, and support for the patient's decision follow the provision of results. Genetic counselors can continue to be resources to the family and referring professionals in such circumstances.

It is standard practice to provide written documentation of the session(s) to the patient and referring physician. This letter or report may also include diagrams or figures that illustrate the information shared with the family. Written communication serves as a record the patient and physician can refer to at a later time; it can also be used to assist in explaining the information with other family members.

PSYCHOLOGICAL ASSESSMENT AND COUNSELING Since most genetic-counseling relationships are short-term, the genetic counselor must assess the psychological state of the patient and family rather quickly and tailor the plan for counseling and testing to meet the patient's needs. A new diagnosis or possible diagnosis often presents a crisis to the patient; the genetic counselor must determine how to intervene in the time of crisis, providing the proper amount and type of information, or planning for a more comprehensive approach at a later date. After establishing a rapport with the patient and family, the genetic counselor elicits the patient's perceptions about the genetic condition, testing, and the genetic-counseling process. The genetic counselor identifies the anxieties, fears, concerns, and hopes of the patient, accomplishing this by assessing verbal and nonverbal cues, and speaking with the patient, family members, and, occasionally, the referring physician.

The diagnosis of a genetic condition, or the realization that a health problem exists, leads to many emotions and reactions for the patient. By providing anticipatory guidance for the possible outcomes of genetic counseling and testing, the genetic counselor assists the patient by exploring issues of loss, grief, and survivor guilt. The genetic counselor can also assist the patient in examining the meaning of the diagnosis or possible outcomes of testing in the context of religious, spiritual, ethical, and cultural beliefs. When a patient faces difficulty in coping with the diagnosis and its implications, genetic counselors will make appropriate referrals to mental-health professionals or to any type of resource that will provide support financially, medically, or emotionally.

SUPPORT FOR DECISION-MAKING AND ONGOING PATIENT SUPPORT In many genetic-counseling relationships, one goal of the session or sessions is to assist a patient in informed decision making regarding reproductive options, pursuing genetic testing, or acting on a test result. The genetic counselor aims to facilitate decision-making by providing a forum for discussion of the patient's reactions to any and all possible outcomes for each choice. A supportive environment in which a patient or family does not feel judged by the genetic counselor for any option they choose is essential to successful genetic counseling. Once a decision is made, the genetic counselor will facilitate arrangements for the patient to act on the choice. For example, if an asymptomatic son of a man who died of hereditary nonpolyposis colon cancer elects to have predictive testing, the genetic counselor will make arrangements with an appropriate laboratory and arrange for follow-up counseling either in person or on the telephone. In many cases, the genetic counselor can help meet the support needs of patients by making referrals to peer-support volunteers or support groups on a local or national level. Often, patients who learn they have a family history of a genetic condition feel alone, not knowing anyone else with the disorder. While professionals can be supportive, many patients seek the true empathy that only an individual in the same situation can provide. The Alliance of Genetic Support Groups is an excellent resource for providing contacts for this type of support (*see* Table 9-1).

Genetic counselors refer patients to a variety of medical specialists who can provide long-term care or treatment for patients with genetic conditions affecting a variety of systems. Ideally, a multidisciplinary continuity clinic can provide integrated, comprehensive care for such patients. Genetic counselors often serve on these clinic teams; others are aware of such clinics on a local, regional, and national basis. For example, a patient diagnosed with Marfan syndrome would benefit from attending a clinic staffed by specialists in cardiology, genetics, ophthalmology, and medicine. Many institutions have a Craniofacial Clinic at which children are followed and treated by otolaryngologists, orthodontists, plastic surgeons, speech pathologists, and audiologists. When patients are eligible for research protocols for diagnosis, treatment, and management, genetic counselors are excellent resources for referral to such programs.

The experience of loss and related grief occurs with the diagnosis of many genetic conditions, whether or not the disorder leads to the death of an individual or a pregnancy loss. Parents of newborns diagnosed with a genetic condition often grieve the loss of the expected healthy child they had planned for and dreamed about. A woman who learns she has the Huntington disease gene grieves the loss of a healthy future. Genetic counselors maintain relationships by contacting patients by telephone or mail at the time of the anniversary of a diagnosis or at the time a birth would have occurred if a pregnancy loss had not taken place. Plans for follow-up visits are also often made. In some cases, the genetic counselor provides support when seeing a patient or family when there are subsequent pregnancies or when new information on a disorder or test becomes available.

GENETIC TRIAGE: THE GENETIC COUNSELOR/ PRIMARY CARE PROVIDER PARTNERSHIP

Since increasing numbers and types of disorders are being identified as genetic conditions, primary care providers are being faced with questions from patients regarding etiology, risk assessment, and management of genetic conditions. Most practicing physicians, physician assistants, and nurses have had little genetics education during their training or in postgraduate courses and therefore are unable to provide comprehensive genetic services. An important role for primary care providers is to identify patients at risk for genetic conditions and to make appropriate referrals to a genetics center. After eliciting a genetic family history, the primary care provider can consult with a genetics professional for risk assessment and identification of patients who may benefit from genetic counseling and/or testing. The primary care provider can prepare patients for the genetic-counseling process by providing anticipatory guidance, explaining what to expect from the genetics consultation. Genetic counselors maintain ongoing communication with the referring health professional and the patient, informing them of new developments when appropriate. Genetics professionals and the primary care provider will establish a cooperative plan for follow-up, medical management, and support for the patient as needed. For example, a 57-year-old, Ashkenazi Jewish woman, who was diagnosed with breast cancer at age 41, came for genetic-susceptibility testing, learning that she has the common BRCA1 mutation, 185delAG. Her unaffected daughter, age 32, came for risk assessment, genetic counseling, and testing. She was found to have the same mutation, indicating that she has an increased lifetime risk of developing breast cancer. The genetic counselor referred the young woman to her internist with recommendations for surveillance by mammography and clinical breast exam as determined by her physician. The team approach is one used by geneticists and genetic counselors since the beginning of the profession. Genetics professionals usually function as consultants to those who provide ongoing care to the patient.

PROFESSIONAL VALUES OF GENETIC COUNSELORS

The practice of genetic counseling grew out of the medical model, whereby information was provided to patients, followed by advice from the clinician about reproductive choices. This prescriptive advice reflected the clinician's perception of the genetic condition and the burden the disorder placed on an individual and his family. This view has been associated eugenic policies and practices of the early part of this century. However, the eugenic Nazi atrocities led clinical genetics in America away from directive, prescriptive practice. The birth of the genetic-counseling profession was concomitant with the women's movement, the self-help movement, and the reproductive-rights movement. Thus, genetic counselors developed a technique of nondirectiveness with regard to reproductive decision making and prenatal-diagnosis counseling that reflects a respect for patient autonomy. It became obvious that in a situation that involved reproductive decisions, such as deciding whether or not to continue a pregnancy after a fetal diagnosis of Down syndrome, there was no one right choice for all couples. Therefore, genetic counselors strive to provide information, support, and counseling in a context that is unique for each family. By demonstrating empathy, respect, and unconditional positive regard for their patients, genetic counselors can guide patients and families in understanding their own values, in making decisions that are appropriate for them, and in helping them cope with their grief. Nondirectiveness does not imply that genetic counselors give information, refuse to answer the question posed by many patients, "What would you do in this situation?" and remove themselves from the relationship when difficult decisions need to be made. The role of the genetic counselor is to elicit beliefs, values, and feelings from patients so that they can understand for themselves which decision is best for them. When there is clearly a better option for a couple, genetic counselors are often faced with a dilemma: a conflict of the bioethical principles of respect for autonomy and beneficence. These types of dilemmas are difficult, if not impossible, to resolve since the principles are not assigned varying levels of importance.

Thus, when the National Society of Genetic Counselors (NSGC) considered the format for its Code of Ethics, it elected to draft the Code as an "ethic of care," since this approach emphasizes the interdependence of individuals and best reflects the values, principles, and beliefs of genetic counselors. The relationships are: genetic counselors themselves; genetic counselors and their clients; genetic counselors and their colleagues, and genetic counselors and society. The NSGC Code of Ethics provides guidance and a framework for approaching dilemmas that genetic counselors face in practice. It includes the value of respect for client autonomy as an important focus. Genetic counselors, therefore, function within the health care system as patient advocates who aim to empower patients and families to find solutions to problems and ways of coping that are optimal for them.

GENETIC-COUNSELOR EDUCATION AND TRAINING

In response to the development of amniocentesis for prenatal diagnosis and carrier screening for several recessive conditions, the first master's-level program in genetic counseling was established at Sarah Lawrence College in 1969. By 1977, there were six programs that collectively graduated about 50 genetic counselors per year. These programs had unique curricula designed by faculty at each university. In 1979 a conference was convened to explore the training, role, and function of the genetic counselor. This was the first organized effort to standardize curriculum and training. The recommendations from this meeting have provided the backbone of education for genetic counselors. Some curricular modifications have resulted from the development of new diagnostic technologies in the laboratory, in the clinic, and from genetic counseling research. As the role of the genetic counselor expanded into specialty areas, the curricula changed to address the educational and practice needs of the students. For example, as questions from health professionals and pregnant women regarding the risks of exposures in pregnancy to the fetus arose with increasing frequency, genetic counselors (with their knowledge of birth defects, embryology, epidemiological literature, and methods for presenting risks in a meaningful way) led the way in developing and staffing Teratogen Information Services. Similarly, as academic clinical molecular genetics laboratories and commercial biotechnology companies developed, their directors recognized the need to have a "customer service representative" for referring physicians and patients. Again, genetic counselors have filled many of these positions because of their skill in bridging the gap between the laboratory and the clinic.

Throughout the 1980s, leaders in the field recommended course topics and approaches to clinical training, yet there were no requirements or guidelines for programs to adhere to. Today, 23 master's-degree-granting programs are accredited by the American Board of Genetic Counseling (ABGC). Approximately 130 new graduates enter the field each year. Graduates of accredited programs must demonstrate proficiency in a wide range of appropriately supervised cases in the form of a log book and letters of recommendation to be eligible to take the ABGC certification examination.*

Each program comprises didactic courses, clinical rotations, academic departmental activities such as case conferences, journal clubs, rounds, and clinical research (optional). Within this framework, each program is unique and reflects the approaches of the faculty and the nature and culture of the patient populations. Each program can guide students in developing these skills in any way it chooses: in the classroom, the clinic, or both. Instructional curricular content must include the following topics:

1. Principles and applications of human genetics and related sciences.
2. Principles and practice of clinical/medical genetics.
3. Methods of genetic testing.
4. Theory and application of interviewing and counseling.
5. Social, ethical, and legal issues.
6. Health care delivery systems/public health.
7. Teaching skills.
8. Research methods.

Curricula and program accreditation are based on each program's ability to support the development of 27 practice-based competencies in genetic counseling drafted by a consensus development team comprised of program directors and the ABGC Board of Directors. These competencies define what an entry-level genetic counselor should be able to do upon graduation from an accredited program. The 27 competencies fall into four skill categories: communication, critical thinking, interpersonal counseling and psychosocial assessment, and professional ethics and values. The competencies are published in the September 1996 issue of the *Journal of Genetic Counseling*.

Graduate programs undergo an accreditation process every 6 years. A written self-study document is reviewed by the ABGC Accreditation Committee and recommendations are made regarding areas to explore during the 2-day site visit. Administrative/institutional support, curricular content and design, clinical training, and student supports are several areas that are explored as part of the accreditation process. Programs are required to submit an annual report to document that the program is remaining in compliance with ABGC requirements.

*The 2-part national certification examination includes a general genetics examination taken by all geneticists (doctoral and masters level) and a separate specialty examination in genetic counseling.

The interdisciplinary academic training of genetic counselors is essential if patients' needs are to be met successfully. The integration of course work in genetics, psychology, communication, ethics, and medicine, with supervised clinical experience, is essential for effective practice in the clinic and in society.

SELECTED REFERENCES

Alliance of Genetic Support Groups. Directory of National Genetic Voluntary Organizations and Related Resources. Chevy Chase, MD, 1995.

Andrews LB, Fullarton JE, Holtzman NA, Motulsky AG. Issues in genetic counseling. In: Assessing Genetic Risks: Implications for Health and Social Policy. National Academy Press, Washington, DC: National Academy, 1995; pp. 146–184.

Bartels DM, LeRoy BS, Caplan AL. Prescribing Our Future: Ethical Challenges in Genetic Counseling, Hawthorne, NY: Aldine de Gruyter, 1993.

Benkendorf JL, Callanan NI, Grobstein R, Schmerler S, FitzGerald KT. An explication of the National Society of Genetic Counselors Code of Ethics. J Genet Counseling 1992;1:31–40.

Bennett RL, Steinhaus KA, Uhrich SB, et al. Recommendations for standardized human pedigree nomenclature. J Genet Counseling 1995;4: 267–280.

Fine BA, Baker DL, Fiddler MB, et al. Practice-based competencies for accreditation of and training in graduate programs in genetic counseling. J Genet Counseling 1996;5:113–122.

Fraser FC. Genetic counseling. Am J Hum Genet 1974;26:636–659.

Harper PS. Practical Genetic Counseling, 4th ed. Oxford, UK: Butterworth Heinemann, 1993.

Kelly PT. Dealing with Dilemma: A Manual For Genetic Counselors. New York: Springer-Verlag, 1977.

Kessler S. Genetic Counseling: Psychological Dimensons. New York: Academic, 1979.

National Society of Genetic Counselors. National Society of Genetic Counselors Code of Ethics. J Genet Counseling 1992;1:41–44.

Robinson A, Linden MG. Clinical Genetics Handbook, Cambridge, UK: Blackwell Scientific, 1993.

Thompson MW, McInnes RR, Willard HF. Thompson & Thompson Genetics in Medicine, 5th ed. Philadelphia, PA: WB Saunders, 1991.

Walker AP. Genetic counseling. In: Rimoin DL, Connor JM, Pyeritz RE, eds. Emery and Rimoin's Principles and Practice of Medical Genetics, 3rd ed. New York: Churchill Livingstone, 1997; pp. 595–618.

Walker AP, Scott JA, Biesecker BB, Conover B, Blake W, Djurdijinovic L. Report of the 1989 Asilomar meeting on education in genetic counseling. Am J Hum Genet 1990;46:1223–1230.

10 Transgenic Mice as Models of Disease

T. RAJENDRA KUMAR AND MARTIN M. MATZUK

BACKGROUND

Efforts to manipulate the genome have been the constant pursuit of geneticists since the end of the 19th century. Methods to improve the quality of the species have been practiced and perfected by plant breeders. Induction of random mutations by UV-radiation and consequent screening for interesting phenotypes in bacteriophage or fruit flies have set forth a trend to identify the genetic basis of structural and functional malformations in these organisms. The advent of chromosomal mapping and gene cloning techniques and the availability of breeding data in many animal species have made it possible to selectively manipulate the genomes of species such as mice, rats, pigs, and cattle. This technology, called "transgenic animal" technology, has already revolutionized our current understanding of how organisms develop and how several physiological processes are regulated. In addition, transgenic models have increased our understanding of the genetic basis for many human diseases, including cancer. Although gene manipulation is theoretically possible in many species, the mouse has become the obvious choice for several reasons. Mice are relatively inexpensive to maintain and easy to breed, and an exhaustive store of information is already available on chromosomal mapping and linkage analysis of many genes in the mouse. In addition, micromanipulation of mouse embryos is technically easier and more feasible compared to that of other species.

The manner in which transgenic technology has been used until today and will be used in the future has implications for basic and clinical research. Using essentially the same principles, but with specific modifications in the approach, it is now possible to create mice with precise targeted genetic lesions or generate mice that express any gene product at a designated time and place. As a result, numerous strains of mice have been created to address diverse issues such as early development, organogenesis, growth and differentiation, and the molecular basis of many diseases. In the following sections, we will briefly discuss the principles of transgenic technology and illustrate the efficacy and power of this novel approach by drawing some important examples in several physiological systems.

PRINCIPLES OF TRANSGENIC TECHNOLOGY

Foreign DNA can be introduced into the chromosomal DNA of mice essentially in three ways. The first method, originally developed years ago, involves the infection of mouse embryos at different developing stages by retroviruses. Because of many technical constraints, this method presents problems for the routine production of transgenic mice. The second method, which has been the most widely used procedure, involves the direct microinjection of foreign DNA into the pronuclei of one-cell fertilized mouse embryos (Fig. 10-1). This results in the chromosomal integration of one or more copies of the injected foreign DNA ("transgene") at a random site, and all cells of the embryo including the extraembryonic tissues will carry the injected DNA, since the injected transgenes usually integrate into the genome prior to embryo cleavage. The injected embryos are then transferred back to foster pseudopregnant mothers, and the offspring eventually are screened for the introduced transgene by standard protocols involving either Southern blot or polymerase chain reaction. The offspring generated are termed founder mice, and lines are eventually generated from these founder mice and maintained for successive generations by breeding to determine the transmission of the stably integrated transgene to the progeny. Because a wealth of information is available on different promoter or regulatory sequences of many genes, it is possible to over- or underexpress a given gene in a cell- or tissue-specific manner. Specific promoters or regulatory sequences can be used to selectively express reporter genes, toxin genes, oncogenes, or antisense constructs, as well as wild-type and mutant genes, in transgenic mice. Promoters can be constitutive, inducible, or even conditionally regulated, depending on the situation. In instances in which cell transfection studies are not possible, transgenic mouse technology can be exploited as a powerful expression system. Promoters containing hormone-responsive elements, enhancers, silencers, and locus-controlling regions can be finely mapped and functionally dissected. By targeting coding sequences of commercially and pharmacologically important proteins using mammary gland-specific promoters, bulk purification of these products is also possible.

The third method for generating transgenic mice is based on a gene-targeting approach in embryonic stem (ES) cells (Fig. 10-2). ES cells are derived from the cells of the inner cell mass of the blastocyst. The ES cells are pluripotent and can contribute to all tissues of the embryo. ES cells can be genetically manipulated in vitro and so-called "gene-targeting" vectors can be used to manipulate DNA at specific loci. The locus to be manipulated can be deleted, and this deletion can span a region as small as a base pair to as large as several megabases. Different types of vectors (insertional or replacement) can be designed, depending on the

From: *Principles of Molecular Medicine* (J. L. Jameson, ed.), ©1998 Humana Press Inc., Totowa, NJ.

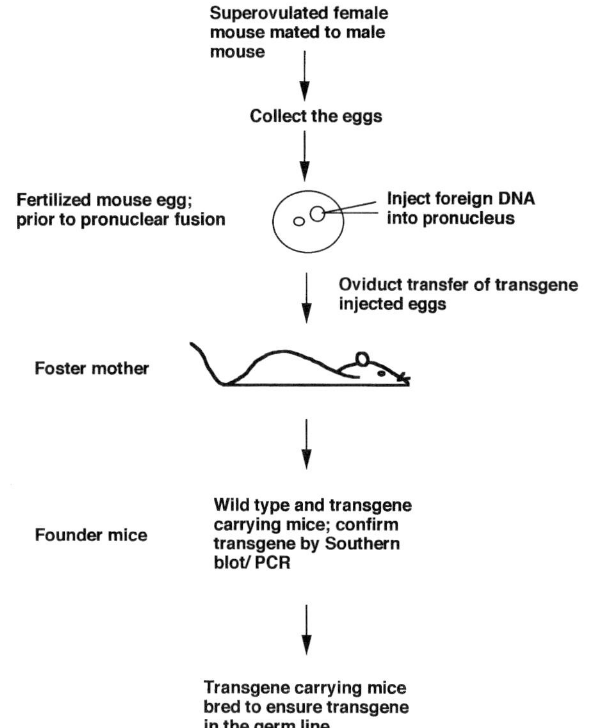

Figure 10-1 Production of transgenic mice.

situation. Typically, replacement vectors are used that have positive and negative selectable markers, and sequences homologous to the target gene flank the positive selectable marker. The targeting vector DNA is then introduced into ES cells in culture, and a simultaneous double-selection procedure is used to enrich for the correct homologous recombination event. The negative selection eliminates many of the cells with random integrations. Cell clones that survive the double selection are expanded, and the DNA from these clones is analyzed by the polymerase chain reaction or Southern blot analysis to identify clones that contain the correctly targeted recombinant allele. ES cells carrying the desired mutation are microinjected into 3.5-day-old blastocysts and implanted back into uteri of the foster mice. Most ES cell lines are derived from mice that have an agouti coat color, and the blastocysts are usually collected from mice that have either a white or black coat color. Therefore, when the genetically manipulated ES cells mix with the inner cell mass cells of the injected blastocysts, the offspring are chimeric because of the patchy appearance of these distinct coat colors. The chimeric mice are subsequently mated to wild-type mice to obtain germline transmission of the mutant allele. The heterozygous mice (i.e., mice carrying one copy of the mutant allele) are bred, if viable and fertile, to obtain homozygous null mice (i.e., mice with two mutant alleles). If the mutation is not lethal in embryos, then theoretically 25% of the offspring will be homozygous for the mutation, following a typical Mendelian inheritance pattern.

Recently, it has also been possible to generate "tissue-specific" knockout mice. The mutation in the gene of interest is achieved as described above in ES cells but with insertion of phage sequences called lox sites that flank (f) the region to be deleted. These "flox-mice" are then mated to another line of transgenic mice that harbor a transgene containing the phage Cre protein coding sequences, driven by a cell/tissue-specific promoter. The Cre protein can excise the gene sequences between the lox sites and thus result in a tissue-specific gene deletion. This method has many advantages in situations where the regular mutation is embryonic lethal or the mice eventually develop multiple defects in several tissues. In this manner, the specific function of a gene product in a given cell type can be studied by loss of function in that cell without affecting its expression in other cell types of the mouse. Alternatively, it is also possible to "knock-in" or replace a different new gene into a locus and disrupt the actual gene at that locus. In the following sections, we will describe the successful application of transgenic technology to study whole-animal biology and the development of mouse models for many human diseases. We will illustrate the functional analysis of each physiological system with a few examples.

APPLICATIONS OF TRANSGENIC TECHNOLOGY

CELL-CYCLE CONTROL The process of cell multiplication involves a complex series of regulatory steps. Each of these steps is either activated, inhibited, or blocked by several protein kinases, phosphatases, cyclin proteins, growth factors, proto-oncogenes, or tumor suppressor proteins. Gain of function and/or loss of function mutations in the genes encoding these regulatory proteins often will lead to important insights into the origin and/or development of many tumors.

p53 is an important tumor-suppressor protein. It is ubiquitously expressed in mouse and human tissues. Under normal physiological situations, p53 is phosphorylated by cdc2 kinase in a cell-cycle–dependent manner. Thus, activation leads to the binding to and inhibition of a yet unidentified cell-replication protein and prevents the cells from entering the S phase. Mutations and allelic loss of the *p53* gene have been associated with many human tumors. These genetic lesions are frequently observed in spontaneous human cancers. Mutations in p53 are associated with the inherited cancer-susceptibility Li-Fraumeni syndrome in humans. To study the function of p53 in an animal model, mice carrying mutations in one or both copies of the *p53* gene have been generated.

Surprisingly, p53-deficient mice develop normally. Therefore, p53 does not play an essential role in cell-cycle control during embryonic development. However, these mutant mice develop tumors at a very early age with 100% penetrance. The tumors are often derived from multiple cell lineages, suggesting that the loss of growth control is not cell-type-restricted. Mice heterozygous for the mutant *p53* allele also develop tumors, although it usually takes more time to develop these tumors. The analysis of tumors from the heterozygous mice demonstrates that the tumor cells usually lose the remaining wild-type *p53* allele. Heterozygous *p53* mutant mice are more susceptible to tumors when challenged with carcinogens, which supports a role of p53 in DNA damage-response pathways. Because p53-deficient mice are highly susceptible to a wide spectrum of tumors as diverse as sarcomas, lymphomas, choriocarcinomas, and gonadoblastomas, these mice are invaluable for testing suspected carcinogens and cancer therapeutic agents.

Several proteins are known to interact with p53 under different conditions in a given cell. One of the proto-oncogene products called Mdm2 (named after a gene located on a mouse double-minute chromosome present in 3T3 fibroblast cells) forms a complex with the p53 protein and inhibits the p53-mediated transregulation of gene expression. The human *Mdm2* gene is amplified in 30–40% of sarcomas and is overexpressed in many

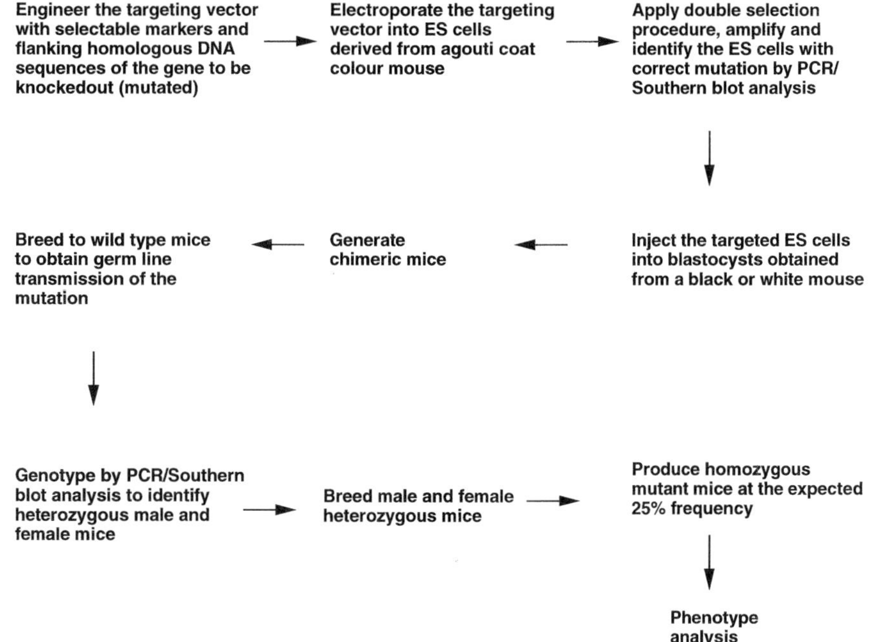

Figure 10-2 Production of knockout mice.

leukemic cells. To understand the biological role of Mdm2 during development, null mice have been created. This mutation leads to lethality of the mice between embryonic day 4.5–7.5. In normal mice, both p53 and Mdm2 are ubiquitously expressed on embryonic days 6.0–6.5, and at this point in normal mouse development, there is a sudden increase in cell-cycle rate. To further resolve the issue of whether the embryonic lethality in Mdm2-deficient mice is a result of alterations in Mdm2-mediated gene expression or a loss in the ability of Mdm2 to downregulate p53 activity, double-homozygous mutants for both *Mdm2* and *p53* are generated by intercrossing the corresponding compound heterozygotes. Interestingly, absence of p53 rescues the embryonic lethality in Mdm2-deficient mice. These results indicate that Mdm2 functions normally in development primarily as a downregulator of p53 activity. *Mdm2/p53* double-mutant mice develop normally, are fertile, and they appear phenotypically similar to mice deficient in only p53.

The retinoblastoma susceptibility gene *(Rb)* is another tumor suppressor gene associated with a wide variety of tumor types, including retinoblastomas, sarcomas, and breast, prostate, and lung carcinomas. The inheritance of a mutant form of the *Rb* gene by an individual is associated with a 90% incidence of multifocal, bilateral retinoblastomas. Loss of heterozygosity has been observed at the *Rb* locus in these tumors, confirming that both copies of the *Rb* gene must be mutated for the development of retinoblastoma. Rb protein has been implicated to play key role(s) in cell-cycle control, and the gene is ubiquitously expressed in different cell types. However, homozygous mice with mutations in both *Rb* genes develop to mid-gestation but exhibit defects in the hematopoietic system and central and peripheral nervous systems leading to embryonic lethality. In contrast, heterozygous mice, like humans, exhibit a dramatic predisposition to tumor development with 100% penetrance by 18 months of age. However, the mice do not develop retinoblastoma, indicating that there are species differences in the susceptibility of differentiated cell types to loss of function mutations in *Rb*. Instead, these heterozygous mice develop multifocal tumors of the intermediate lobe of the pituitary gland and demonstrate elevated serum levels of α-melanocyte-stimulating hormone.

It is now feasible to consider using mice with specific genetic mutations as an assay system for the identification of tumor-suppressor genes because the effects of such targeted mutations in either known or unknown genes can be directly tested in vivo. For example, using this principle, inhibin has been shown to be the first secreted tumor-suppressor protein with specificity restricted only to the gonads and adrenals. Inhibins are heterodimers (α:β), which belong to the transforming growth factor (TGF)-β superfamily. They share the β-subunits (βA- or βB-subunits) with activins. Inhibins were originally discovered as Sertoli and granulosa cell products that had FSH-suppressing activity. These peptides are also expressed in other tissues outside the reproductive tract. Mice deficient in the α-subunit of inhibin are viable, indicating that inhibin is not essential for embryonic development. However, between 5 and 20 weeks, both male and female mice deficient in inhibin develop hemorrhagic and bilateral gonadal sex cord-stromal tumors with nearly 100% penetrance. As the tumors progress, they secrete high levels of activin, leading to a human-cancer cachexia-like wasting syndrome in the mice with hepatocellular necrosis and weight loss leading to eventual death. In contrast, gonadectomized, inhibin-deficient mice survive beyond 20 weeks but develop adrenal cortical tumors and also die of a similar wasting syndrome. These knockout mouse studies have provided an excellent opportunity to examine similar human gonadal tumors for mutations in the inhibin α-subunit gene, which was not previously envisioned.

DEVELOPMENTAL BIOLOGY Highly programmed molecular events triggered by the process of fertilization between the mammalian sperm and egg lead to distinct layers of cells and pattern formation in the embryo. The changing topography of the body axis during normal development eventually results in organogenesis. Mutations affecting critical events associated with early embryogenesis may result in severe deformities of the developing embryo at distinct steps or even embryonic lethality. Several human mutations affecting the fetus have been described, and many interesting lines of mutant mice have been generated with the aim of dissecting the critical molecular events during early embryogenesis. Numerous genetic manipulation studies on fruit flies, zebrafish, and *C. elegans* have paved the way to identify homeobox genes and other related pattern-regulating genes. Many of these genes encode transcription factors involved in organogenesis, body axis determination, and distinct layer formation. The corresponding mouse homologs have been identified, and mice with mutations in these genes have been created and characterized. In some cases, these critical factors have been ectopically expressed to follow the cell fate and consequences of this aberrant expression.

Cleft palate is a commonly occurring craniofacial developmental disorder in humans. It has been possible to identify some of the critical factors during craniofacial development by generating different strains of mutant mice. For example, the majority of the mice that are deficient in activin βA, a member of TGF-β family, develop cleft palate, tooth defects, and lack of whiskers. Some of the mice that do not have cleft secondary palate exhibit either incomplete or complete failure of hard-palate formation. As a result, these mice cannot nurse and die perinatally. Similarly, mice deficient in follistatin, an activin-binding protein, also exhibit cleft palate and have hard-palate defects. In addition, mice that are deficient in a transcription factor MSX-1 display similar phenotypic characteristics. Thus, using transgenic mice, one can verify the in vitro observations in an in vivo context and also draw conclusions on the involvement of several factors in a common pathway controlling a physiological process.

Several lines of transgenic mice have also been created to study embryonic formation of limbs, notochord, different brain regions, musculoskeletal structures, and body-axis. Mice with mutations in the presumptive "mesoderm-inducers" have also been generated. It has been possible to dissect out the early developmental events in the formation of virtually every organ system using transgenic mice. A few examples are given below.

The *Wnt*-1 (*int*-1) proto-oncogene, which encodes a putative signaling molecule, is expressed exclusively in the developing central nervous system (CNS) and adult testes. To test the presumptive function of Wnt-1 in mammalian neural-tube organization and patterning role in CNS development, Wnt-1 null mice have been generated. These mice develop to term but die within 24 h after birth as a result of abnormal brain development. Most of the neural tube and nonneural tissues appear normal. However, as early as embryonic day 14.5, a substantial portion of the midbrain fails to develop. This includes a large contiguous domain, comprising approximately the caudal two-thirds of the midbrain, the normal midbrain-metencephalic junction, and rostral metencephalon. Thus, for the first time, using an in vivo approach, it has been established that Wnt-1 acts as a determinant for the development of a specific region of the CNS.

Defining and understanding the nature of vertebrate organizers in molecular terms have been among the fundamental issues in embryology. Toward this end, several putative DNA transcription factors that are expressed in the organizer region have been identified in *Xenopus*, chick, and mouse. The Lim 1 transcription factor is the mouse homolog of xlim-1 in *Xenopus*, which is expressed in the node, the developing kidney, and portions of the CNS. Lim-1-deficient mice lack head structures anterior to the optic vesicle but develop the remaining body axis normally. The mutant embryos lack forebrain and midbrain because of the absence of an organized node, head process, and prechordal mesoderm by embryonic day 7.5. Some mutant embryos develop a partial anterior secondary axis as a result of a disrupted early organizing region. By embryonic day 10.5, most of the embryos die but a few "headless" pups (4/1000) are delivered stillborn. These mutant mice also lack kidneys and gonads. Thus, using knockout mouse technology, the requirement of Lim-1 in head-organizer formation has been clearly confirmed.

Combinatorial interactions between products of clusters of Hox genes direct regional development in the embryo. Hox genes encode transcriptional regulators that contain sequence-specific DNA binding motifs called homeodomains. Mutations in most of these genes often result in homeotic transformations. In the mouse, four clusters of Hox genes exist that are homologous to the *Drosophila* homeotic complex. Both gain-of-function and loss-of-function mutations in these genes have been created in transgenic mice. These experiments have demonstrated that Hox genes act as key selector genes and have led to the "Hox code"-hypothesis, in which several Hox genes control the specification of regional identity (i.e., they control the formation of the anteroposterior body axis and secondary axis of the limb). By either overexpression or deletion of a particular set(s) of Hox genes, it has been possible to specify and demarcate the boundaries of expression of each gene during development and determine the consequences of such a perturbation.

One of the models developed to establish the specific role of a *Hox* gene in a specific cluster has been to introduce *Hoxb-4* mutations into the mouse germline. Hox genes are organized in tightly linked clusters with poorly understood and complex mechanisms of transcriptional regulation. Because the conventional "replacement" gene-targeting strategy introduces exogenous sequences that may affect transcription of the *Hox* gene cluster and disrupt normal regulation at several important genetic loci, genetic subtle mutations have been engineered into the *Hoxb-4* locus. Hoxb-4 is a member of the Hoxb cluster on mouse chromosome 11. Hoxb-4 is first expressed at embryonic day 8.5 from the posterior end of the prospective spinal cord and eventually the anterior limit at the boundary between rhombomeres 6 and 7 in the hindbrain. In addition, Hoxb-4 is widely expressed in tissues including spinal ganglia, the nodose ganglion of cranial nerve X, prevertebrae up to the second cervical vertebra or axis (C2), and in mesodermal components of lung, kidney, and gut. Mutant mice that harbor a disrupted first exon of *Hoxb-4* show two obvious skeletal changes—a partial homeotic transformation of C2 from axis to atlas and a defective morphogenesis of the sternum. These phenotypes are variable in penetrance and expressivity depending on the genetic background. Mice generated from ES cells that are engineered to have a premature stop codon in the second exon, by an insertion of a oligonucleotide using the "hit-and-run" method, also show partial homeotic transformation of axis to atlas; these mice, however, do not show abnormalities in sternum. Whereas only a portion of the first-category mice survive to adulthood, mice that carry the second type of mutation are viable, healthy, and fertile. These experiments illustrate that ES cell technology can be effectively used to introduce subtle mutations into the mouse genome, and this can be used as an assay system to study their effects on functions of complex clusters of *Hox* genes. Selected genetic crosses between individual mutant mice belonging to individual clusters give important clues to the combinatorial interactions that operate among these key regulatory molecules.

MUSCLE BIOLOGY A distinct set of transcription factors called myogenic basic helix-loop-helix (HLH) factors have been implicated in the regulation of skeletal-muscle differentiation. These include MyoD, Myogenin, Myf-5, and Myf-6/MRF-4. Each of these factors, when ectopically expressed in nonmuscle cells, can activate the skeletal-muscle differentiation program. Each factor can induce other factors, including a number of skeletal muscle-specific genes. Null mutations in each of these factors have been introduced into the germline of mice. Further, mice with multiple genetic lesions in these factors have also been obtained by breeding. It has been possible to formulate a hierarchical network of interactions involved in the program of muscle differentiation based on the functional analyses on these mutant mice.

Mice deficient in MyoD are viable and show no skeletal-muscle abnormalities. The inactivation of this gene causes a twofold increase in *Myf5* mRNA expression, whereas *myogenin* and *MRF4* levels are not altered. Myf-5-deficient mice also develop normal skeletal muscle, but die at birth because of the absence of the distal parts of the ribs, which leads to breathing problems. Double-mutant mice that lack both MyoD and Myf5 produce no detectable skeletal-muscle-specific markers (skeletal-actin, troponin T, and so on) and appear to lack skeletal myoblasts, suggesting that both of these factors function similarly in myoblast formation. Mice lacking myogenin have normal numbers of skeletal myoblasts at birth, but show a severe reduction of skeletal-muscle fibers. Both MyoD and Myf5 are expressed in undifferentiated myogenic cells, suggesting that they act earlier in development than myogenin. MRF4-deficient mice show only a slight reduction in a subset of muscle-specific genes. Consistent with the in vitro observations that MRF4 downregulates the expression of myogenin, myogenin levels are elevated in adult skeletal muscle from MRF4-deficient mice. Surprisingly, MRF4-null mice exhibit multiple rib abnormalities, possibly through an indirect mechanism affecting the rib primordia.

Duchenne muscular dystrophy (DMD) is an X-linked recessive disease in humans caused by defective expression of dystrophin. Progressive skeletal-muscle weakness and wheelchair confinement are the most obvious symptoms of DMD. Most patients die of respiratory failure resulting from progressive atrophy of the diaphragm. There is a naturally occurring mutant mouse strain called the *mdx* mouse that has been identified. This mouse has a point mutation that eliminates the expression of the 427-kDa muscle and brain isoforms of dystrophin. These *mdx* mice do not display muscle weakness or impaired movement, but the diaphragm muscles show progressive myofibre degeneration and fibrosis similar to the human condition. Transgenic mouse technology has demonstrated the feasibility of gene therapy for DMD. High-level and tissue-specific expression of a full-length murine dystrophin was achieved in transgenic mice by using the regulatory regions of the mouse muscle creatinine kinase gene, and the transgene was introduced into the *mdx* genetic background by crossbreeding. The transgene positive *mdx* mice show complete correction of the dystrophic pathology in skeletal muscles and the diaphragm as assessed by both functional and immunohistochemical tests. It is now feasible to generate viral vectors that encode the full-length human dystrophin to treat and/or cure human patients with DMD.

HEMATOLOGY/IMMUNOLOGY The most thoroughly studied aspects of mammalian physiology using transgenic technology are perhaps the immune and hematopoietic systems. Both by conventional microinjection techniques and using ES cell technology, mutant mice have been generated that either overexpress or lack cell-specific transcription factors, immune cell-specific light chains, the recombination-associated proteins, receptors for antibodies, MHC antigens, and immune cell-specific growth factors (lymphokines/ cytokines). Because many human disorders involve aberrations in hematopoietic/immune systems, these mice serve as excellent models to understand and treat these human disorders. Mice that lack an important component of these systems often are more prone to many microbial diseases and are often sensitive to immediate and/or delayed hypersensitivity reactions. These transgenic mice can be effectively used to screen for the efficacy of various anti-inflammatory drugs and other chemotherapeutic products and are also useful models in transplantation biology.

β2-microglobulin is a 12-kDa polypeptide and is associated with the heavy chain of the polymorphic MHC class I proteins encoded by the H2-K, H2-L/D, and Qa/Tla loci. One of the first mouse models generated using ES cell technology involved the targeted disruption of the β2-microglobulin gene. Mice deficient in β2-*M* microglobulin were generated to precisely understand its biological function. These mice are normal and fertile but have no mature $CD4^{-}CD8^{+}$ T cells in either the thymus or peripheral lymphoid organs and are defective in $CD4^{-}CD8^{+}$ T-cell-mediated cytotoxicity. Although it was widely believed that γδ T cells interact with class-I molecules, this subset of cells develops normally in these mutant mice.

TGF-βs are homodimeric peptides that control a wide variety of cellular processes such as cell proliferation, differentiation, embryonic development, extracellular matrix formation, bone development, wound healing and hematopoiesis, and immune and inflammatory cell response. Three distinct TGF-β genes (*TGF-b1*, *-b2*, and *-b3*) have been identified in mammals. The three mammalian TGF-βs are structurally highly similar (75% identity at the amino acid level) and are often coexpressed and colocalized in a spatiotemporal manner. Many additional functions are also attributed to TGF-βs based on in vitro observations. Obviously, to delineate the individual functions of these peptides, gene-targeting approaches have begun to be employed. Approximately 50% of TGF-β1 null mice show no gross developmental abnormalities. By 3–4 weeks of age, however, these viable mutant mice succumb to a wasting syndrome and die. All mutant mice exhibit a marked but variable degree of mixed inflammatory cell infiltration and tissue necrosis in multiple organs. Many of these lesions resemble those found in human autoimmune disorders, graft vs host diseases, and some viral diseases, and suggest that the TGF-β1–deficient mice are an important model to study these diseases.

Gene-targeting approaches have also recently helped to understand the molecular basis of human inflammatory bowel disease (IBD). These studies have led to the unexpected discovery that mice with deletions in genes encoding specific cytokines and T-cell receptor subunits develop chronic intestinal inflammation. In humans, IBD manifests as a chronic, noninfectious, inflammation limited to the large bowel, known as ulcerative colitis, or as a granulomatous inflammation anywhere along the gastrointestinal tract, known as Crohn's disease. Several lines of evidence suggest that human patients with IBD are hyperresponsive to normal gut constituents. Mutant mice that are deficient in T-cell receptor (TCR)-α, TCR-β, both TCR-β/δ, or class II major histocompatibility complex all develop chronic intestinal inflammation. This intestinal disorder resembles ulcerative colitis but without ulceration or bleeding. These mice have normal number of B cells but lack class II-MHC-restricted CD4+ αβ T cells. It was hypothesized that, in the absence of a tolerance to dietary or microbial antigens, an autoimmune attack on the intestinal epithelium results in the inflammatory response. This suggests that the αβ T-cell-mediated suppression of B cells does not occur in these mice.

Interleukins are cytokines of the immune system. Interleukin-2 (IL-2) is produced by activated T cells. It is a key regulator of immune and inflammatory responses. T-cell proliferation in vitro, differentiation of B cells, activation of macrophages, and NK cells are all dependent on IL-2 signaling. IL-2–deficient mice at 4 weeks of age develop normal thymus glands, with unaltered thymocyte and peripheral T-cell subset composition. The in vitro responses to T-cell mitogens on isolated T cells from these mice are reduced. The differentiation of B cells is affected in these mice, with a drastic increase of serum levels of immunoglobulin (Ig) G1 and IgE. IL-2–deficient mice beyond 6 weeks of age develop an IBD similar to ulcerative colitis in humans. These mice develop ulcerations and bloody diarrhea, and the mucosa and submucosal tissue of the large bowel shows pronounced thickening. Crypt abscesses are found, and the epithelial layer shows loss of goblet cells. Similar to IL-2–deficient mice, mice with a gene deletion in *IL-10* also develop mucosal inflammation. However, the inflammation in these mice is restricted to the villi. The crypt is associated with pseudopolyps and villous atrophy. These mice show elevated levels of interferon-γ. The intestinal disease in these mice may result from the absence of a suppressive effect of IL-10 on macrophage production of inflammatory cytokines. However, these knockout mouse models are not identical to patients with IBD, because IBD patients have T cells and produce IL-2 and IL-10. However, the mouse models elucidate that T-cell abnormalities could be the cause of many forms of intestinal inflammation. These mice may also prove useful in testing the involvement of other genetic and nongenetic factors in the etiology of human IBD.

PULMONARY BIOLOGY Transgenic mouse technology has successfully been used in four major aspects of pulmonary biology research. First, the molecular mechanisms controlling epithelial-cell gene expression have been determined. Second, the cellular interactions that contribute to lung morphogenesis and maturation have been elucidated. Third, models that may be clinically relevant for developing new strategies for therapy have been developed. Fourth, functional analysis of genes by targeted expression or mutation and their consequences in lung growth and development has been undertaken.

The respiratory-cell epithelium produces distinct gene products, including surfactant proteins A, B, and C (SP-A, B, C), clara cell secretory protein (CCSP) or uteroglobulin. The most exhaustively studied genes are *SP-C* and *CCSP*. Expression studies using transgenic mice have identified that a 3.7-kb human SP-C promoter contained the necessary elements to drive a chloramiphenicol acetyltransferase reporter gene correctly to bronchiolar and alveolar respiratory epithelial cells. The same promoter has been used to express diphtheria toxin-A chain in transgenic mice. These mice die immediately after birth as a result of cytotoxic lesions of the respiratory epithelium induced by the diphtheria toxin expression. Similarly, to study lung epithelial-mesenchymal interactions in vivo, transgenic mice have been created that express human TGF-α under the control of the 3.7-kb *SP-C* promoter sequences. These mice develop marked pulmonary fibrosis, exhibit increased collagen deposition, and demonstrate disruption of elastin fibers. Two other mutant strains of mice have been created with lung-specific promoter sequences. In one case, a dominant negative FGF-receptor mutant is expressed in transgenic mice, and in the second case, SV40 large T-antigen expression is directed from the 5' flanking sequences of the uteroglobin gene. While the mice expressing the former transgene die of respiratory failure similar to the 3.7-kb SP-C diphtheria toxin-A-bearing mice, the latter mice die because of the development of pulmonary adenocarcinoma. These models are highly useful for the study of molecular pathogenesis and therapy for adenocarcinoma of the lung in humans.

Transgenic mice have also been created to study the human disease cystic fibrosis. Cystic fibrosis is the most common fatal autosomal-recessive disorder, affecting about 1 in 2500 newborns. The disease is characterized by defective chloride transport in epithelial cells leading to excess mucus secretion. Meconium ileus, or intestinal blockage, is also a diagnostic feature of the disease. Associated defects include pancreatic insufficiency, malabsorption in the gut, chronic opportunistic lung infections, and reproductive tract defects. To develop mouse models, both insertional mutagenesis, which disrupts exon 10 of the *CF* gene, and a replacement-type vector to delete the same exon, have been employed. The cystic fibrosis transmembrane regulator *(CFTR)* mutant mice demonstrate many similarities in their pathology to human patients. The majority of mutant mice die from intestinal perforation and peritonitis following intestinal blockage. This is primarily caused by dehydrated secretions in the crypts of the intestine. The pancreatic effects seen in humans are not recapitulated in mice, however. Pathological changes in the respiratory tract of mutant mice mimic those in humans-goblet cell number increases, gland ducts in the nasal and proximal trachea dilate, and destructive changes in the upper-airway epithelia occur. Interestingly, there are no reproductive defects in male mice that survive to the adult stage, but female mice show infertility.

Mice deficient in N-*myc* proto oncogene exhibit markedly slow growth rates in embryonic lungs, resulting in hypoplastic lungs at birth. Targeted disruption of a novel homeobox gene, *Gsh*-4, similarly results in neonatal respiratory failure in the mutant mice. The expression of *Gsh*-4 mRNA is confined only to the CNS, suggesting that the mice die as a result of a respiratory-center failure in the brain at birth. Both of these mouse models have provided previously unanticipated results demonstrating the power and the advantage of transgenic mouse technology to establish novel functions of known gene products.

CARDIOVASCULAR BIOLOGY Hypertension and atherosclerosis are the most common human disorders. Many transgenic animal models have been developed to study cardiovascular function. Cardiovascular function is dependent on a multitude of hormones, regulatory peptides, and cell-signaling pathways, in addition to the genetic background. Only a few candidate genes have been identified thus far, and many quantitative trait analyses are being performed to identify loci that control cholesterol levels in mice.

Antidiuretic hormone (ADH) is a nona-peptide synthesized in the hypothalamus as a precursor and later transported to and stored in the posterior pituitary. The major endocrine function of ADH is to increase reabsorption of water in collecting ducts of the kidney. ADH also increases blood pressure by constricting the arterioles.

Absence of ADH results in diabetic insipidus, a common human disease with problems of water retention. Surprisingly, transgenic mice that chronically express a preproarginine vasopression, by using a metallothionein promoter, have a mild nephrogenic diabetes insipidus.

Atrial natriuretic peptide (ANP) is released from the heart in response to cardiac atrial stretch. This peptide is also involved in sodium balance. It is highly concentrated in the preoptic and median eminence areas within the CNS. A 10-fold overexpression of ANP by using a *transthyretin* promoter in transgenic mice resulted in lowered blood pressure without affecting the electrolyte balance. ANP has been implicated to mediate its natriuretic and vasorelaxant effects through the guanylyl cyclase-A (GC-A) receptor. Approximately half of all humans with essential hypertension are resistant to salt. However, a gene defect for this phenotype has not been described. Recently, GC-A gene knockout mice have been generated. As a result of this mutation, these mice have chronic elevations in blood pressure when placed on a normal diet, and even in response to either minimal or high-salt diets, the blood pressure remains elevated and unchanged. Aldosterone and ANP concentrations are not affected in these mice. Therefore, mice with GC-A mutations can be useful models to study some salt-resistant forms of essential hypertension in humans.

The renin-angiotensin system is a major regulator of blood pressure and sodium and volume homeostasis. Transgenic mice that overexpress the rat or human renin or angiotensin genes develop high blood-pressure levels. Recently, knockout mice have been generated to systematically address the issues of hypertension in relation to the angiotensin system. Mice carrying one, two, three, or four functional copies of the murine *angiotensinogen* gene at its normal chromosomal location have been created by gene targeting. These mice demonstrate plasma angiotensinogen levels corresponding to the number of gene copies they carry (i.e., mice with four copies show 145% elevated levels compared to one-copy animals). Accordingly, the blood pressures also show significant and linear increases in each of these mice. These elegant experiments have established a direct causal relationship between angiotensinogen genotypes and blood pressure.

Atherosclerosis and other lipid-associated disorders are very common in humans. There are four major types of plasma lipoproteins—chylomicrons, very low-density lipoproteins (VLDL), intermediate density, and low-density lipoproteins (IDL and LDL), and high-density lipoproteins (HDL). These are synthesized either in liver or intestine. The lipid-free protein components of plasma lipoproteins are termed apolipoproteins. These are represented by five major types (A, B, C, D, and E), and some of them also can be categorized further into subtypes, for example, A-I, II, IV and C-I, II, III. The coordinated network of interactions between these complexes and the corresponding receptors regulates cholesterol homeostasis in blood.

To mimic human atherosclerosis in mice, several candidate genes have been either overexpressed or knocked-out in transgenic mice. Apolipoproteins A-I (apo A-I) is the major protein associated with HDL. It is synthesized in the liver and small intestine. Apo A-I serves as a cofactor for the enzyme lecithin-cholesterol acetyltransferase that catalyzes cholesterol ester formation. Human individuals deficient in apo A-I because of various types of mutations are more prone to developing atherosclerosis. The human *apo AI* transgene has been genetically transferred into the atherosclerosis-susceptible inbred mouse strain C57BL/6. This results in elevated levels of apo A-1 and HDL and correction of atherosclerosis. Mice that are deficient in apo A-1 have low levels of HDL cholesterol, but interestingly, do not develop atherosclerosis when supplemented with an atherogenic diet. This suggests that low levels of HDL may only predispose, but low HDL does not by itself, accelerate atherosclerosis. Transgenic mice that overexpress apo E do not show atherosclerotic plaques, even when fed a high-fat diet. In contrast, apo E-deficient mice accumulate VLDL and remnant particles in plasma. Young mice lacking apo E that are fed a low-fat diet develop atherosclerosis similar to that seen in humans. Transgenic mice that overexpress dominant apo E mutants have also been generated. These types of mutations are associated with a dominant form of type III hyperlipoproteinemia in humans. Mice overexpressing these mutant forms of apo E develop hypertriglyceridemia and hypercholesterolemia. Finally, the "familial hypercholesterolemic mouse" has been developed by knocking-out the LDL-receptor gene. These mice have elevated cholesterol levels and demonstrate delayed plasma clearance of VLDL and LDL. When placed on an atherogenic diet for prolonged time, the mice develop extensive fibroproliferative atherosclerosis and thus are a useful model to study human disease. In contrast, high levels of LDL-receptor expression in transgenic mice results in eight times faster clearance of blood LDL than normal. This has exciting possibilities of genetically correcting some human familial hypercholesterolemia syndromes caused by LDL-receptor defects.

Mutant mice with gene deletions in the endothelial receptor tyrosine kinase *tek* die in utero. These mice have defects in the integrity of endothelium and show abnormalities in heart development. These in vivo studies have identified that the tek signaling pathway plays a critical role in the differentiation, proliferation, and survival of endothelial cells in the mouse embryo. Vascular-system defects are the major phenotypic characteristics in mutant mice that lack ras GTPase-activating protein. The ras family consists of small guanine-nucleotide-binding proteins that are known to participate in normal- and oncogenic-signaling pathways. Four GTPase-activating proteins (GAPs) specific for ras proteins have been identified. These function as negative modulators of ras activity. One of the proteins, p120-ras GAP, interacts with various proteins, including tyrosine kinases, through its src-homology 2 (SH2)-binding domains. Mutant mice that lack this important biological signaling protein die by embryonic day 10.5. These embryos have a reduced number of somites and show a failure in reorganization of endothelial cells into a vascular network. The mutant embryos also exhibit a thinning of the dorsal aorta and aberrant ventral branches. In later stage mutants, local ruptures in the embryonic vasculature result in leakage of blood into the body cavity. At this stage, the pericardium is distended. These mutant mice have provided important insights into the understanding of the molecular mechanisms involving the interactions between SH signaling proteins and downstream targets of tyrosine kinases.

RENAL BIOLOGY Kidney development requires the coordinated differentiation of two distinct tissues, the ductal epithelium and the nephrogenic mesenchyme. Both of these tissues are derivatives of the early embryonic-intermediate mesoderm. The ductal epithelium gives rise to the genital tracts, ureters, and collecting duct system. The mesenchymal components undergo epithelial transformation to form nephrons, the functional unit of the kidney. The nephron consists of the renal corpuscle and proximal and distal tubules, which are derived from the metanephric blastema.

Mutations in genes expressed during kidney development have been created using transgenic mice technology. The phenotypes of these mutant mice, in many cases, resemble many of the well-known human renal disorders. The most striking phenotype of the Wilms' tumor *(WT)*-1 gene knockout mouse is the absence of kidneys. WT-1 encodes a protein with a proline/glutamine rich N-terminal domain and with four Cys-His zinc fingers at the C-terminal domain. Germline mutations in *WT-1* gene are associated with human urogenital malformations and a childhood kidney tumor called Wilms' tumor. Mutant mice that are deficient in WT-1 protein die at embryonic day 11.5. At this stage, the metanephric blastema cells undergo cell death, and the embryos show a failure in ureteric bud growth and an absence of the inductive events, which lead to the formation of a definitive kidney. Whereas human individuals with the WAGR (Wilms' tumor, aniridia, genitourinary, and mental retardation) syndrome, with retention of one functional copy of the *WT-1* gene, are predisposed to develop kidney tumors, *WT-1* heterozygous mutant mice are normal. This situation is reminiscent of the absence of retinoblastomas in *Rb*-heterozygous mice as described above.

Abnormal kidney development is also seen in mutant mice that lack either the ligand, platelet-derived growth factor (PDGF) B or its cognate receptor PDGFβ-R. In both cases, the kidney glomerular tufts do not form because of the absence of mesangial cells, and there are also cardiovascular defects. Failure of kidney mesenchymal-epithelial interactions is also obvious in bone morphogenetic protein-7 (BMP-7) mutant mice. BMP-7 is a member of the TGF-β superfamily. BMP-7 is expressed in the kidney at the time of the earliest inductive event. BMP-7–deficient mice die within 48 h of birth as a result of small dysgenic kidneys with hydroureters. The kidneys show a severe reduction in the number of glomeruli, lack identifiable metanephric mesenchyme, and do not show any evidence of glomerular formation in the cortical region. At embryonic day 14.5, all mesenchymal derivatives are absent in the mutant embryos. The expression of the early markers in kidney development, for example, WT-1 and Pax-2, are either reduced or completely absent in BMP-7–deficient embryos. These studies have thus identified BMP-7 as an early glomerular inducer. The BMP-7 mutant mice may also be a useful animal model to dissect the genetic pathway for several human genetic diseases accompanied by impairment of glomerular formation.

Recently, a prostaglandin synthase-2 gene knockout mouse model has been created that accurately mimics the human congenital renal disease called oligomeganephronia. This condition is characterized by small kidneys with reduced number of nephrons. The glomeruli and tubules are hypertrophied, and the kidneys eventually develop focal segmental glomerular sclerosis. These mice will be important models for studying human oligomeganephronia.

Transgenic mice have been generated using glomeruli-specific promoters driving the expression of SV40 T antigen. These mice develop tumors of the glomeruli, and cell lines derived from these tumors are useful for studying renal-cell biology in vitro. Transgenic mice that express a constitutively activated allele of the human c-erbB2 growth factor receptor gene under the regulatory control of a MMTV-LTR promoter develop hyperplastic lesions in kidney, in addition to defects in other organs. In the kidney, multifocal, severe hyperplasia of renal tubules appear that may lead to microcyst formation. Within the tubules, the epithelial cells show atypical proliferation into the intraluminal compartment. The morphology of these cells also shows dramatic changes, with increased cell volume and enlarged nuclei.

Renal cysts also appear in transgenic mice that chronically overexpress TGF-α under the control of a metallotheionein (MT) promoter. TGF-α is a member of the epidermal growth factor (EGF) family of proteins. Like EGF, TGF-α binds to the EGF receptor and elicits its cellular function. In human autosomal-dominant polycystic kidney disease, EGF and its stimulation have been implicated to cause this renal pathology, and thus the MT–TGF-α transgenic mice may be mimicking the human pathology.

NEUROBIOLOGY One of the challenging areas of research in present-day modern biology is to understand the development of the mammalian nervous system. Many naturally occurring mutant mice provide excellent models to study human disorders associated with this complex system. The identification of many neuronal cell-specific genes that encode receptors, neurotransmitters, growth factors, surface antigens, and structural proteins has resulted in generation of a vast array of transgenic and knockout mice strains. These aid in understanding many neurological diseases like Prion disease, Alzheimer's disease, poliomyelitis, many myelination disorders, leukodystrophy, Amylotropic lateral sclerosis, peripheral neuropathy, Down's syndrome, Parkinsonism, and many others. Transgenic mice that express viral oncogenes in specific neural-cell types are excellent sources of generating immortalized cell lines. In addition, the development of mouse models has made it possible to probe into the early developmental aspects of the nervous system. Generation of transgenic and knockout mice for neurotrophins and their receptors has helped to obtain a clearer picture of the factors necessary for survival of many types of neurons. Transgenic and mutant mice are also currently being extensively used to explore the genetic basis of complex behavioral patterns and cognitive functions such as learning and memory. Numerous mouse models are already available for understanding the development and function of special sense organs; for example, the eye, ear, and skin. Transgenic-mouse models that mimic many human neurodegenerative disorders have been developed. We will give examples of mouse models for neurodegenerative disorders in the following section.

Amyotrophic lateral sclerosis (ALS) in humans is a degenerative disease of motor neurons. It is characterized by accumulation of neurofilaments in the perikarya and proximal axons. Neurofilaments (NF) belong to the intermediate filament family, are approximately 10 nm in diameter, and show polymorphism depending on the cell type. Transgenic mice that overexpress the human NF-heavy-subunit gene *(NF-H)* show neuropathological symptoms close to those seen in human patients. These include neuronal and axonal swellings of α motoneurons and dorsal root ganglion cells, distal axonopathy, and secondary muscular atrophy. The L5 ventral roots from NF-H transgenic mice at old age reveal massive degeneration of large axons derived from spinal motor neurons. Metabolic labeling experiments and ultrastructural analyses on these mice have provided valuable insights into the mechanism of neurodegeneration resulting from disorganized neurofilaments. Most importantly, there are dramatic defects in axonal transport of neurofilaments, tubulin, and actin. Ultrastructural analysis on these mice indicate significant reduction of mitochondria in the degenerating axons. Because this affects the energy metabolism, neuropathy may result in these mice. Similar phenotypic characteristics are also apparent in some human familial ALS cases induced by mutations in the superoxide dismutase gene *SOD-1* and in transgenic mice that express a mutant form of human *SOD-1*. The NF-H transgenic-mouse model, therefore, provides an important assay system to test drugs that are capable of downregulating neurofilament expression and consequently help to devise therapeutic approaches to treat human ALS.

Huntington's disease (HD) is a dominant neurodegenerative disorder. Typical symptoms of the disease include chorea, psychiatric alterations, and intellectual decline. The disease results from the presence of an expanded stretch of CAG trinucleotides (37–40 U) in one copy of the gene encoding huntingtin. It is a ~350-kDa cytoplasmic protein with unknown biological function, found in fetal and adult peripheral tissues and nervous system. Because the CAG repeat, when translated, elongates the N-terminus of huntingtin protein by a polyglutamine segment, it may reduce the normal activity of the protein. However, humans with one copy of the normal gene inactivated because of translocations do not develop HD. Similarly, a loss of function or a gain of function mutation in huntingtin *(Hdh)* leading to HD may also exist. To assess these possibilities, the mouse *Hdh* gene has been inactivated by gene targeting. Heterozygous mice are viable, fertile, and display no phenotypic abnormalities, similar to individuals with translocations. The homozygous *Hdh* mouse embryos implant normally, exhibit abnormal gastrulation at embryonic day 7.5, and resorb by day 8.5. These results suggest that Hdh is critical for embryonic development in mice, before the emergence of neural tube, presumably between embryonic days 8.0 and 8.5. Because the Hdh inactivation does not lead to the development of Hd neuropathology, this suggests that the human disease involves a gain of function. These experiments now open up the possibility of generating an accurate model of HD by producing transgenic mice that carry the Hdh with an expanded polyglutamine segment. A similar strategy has recently been adopted by generating a mouse model for another neurodegenerative disorder, called spinocerebellar ataxia-1 (SCA-1). SCA-1 is an autosomal-dominant inherited adult-onset human neurologic disorder characterized by loss of Purkinje cells in the cerebellar cortex and neurodegeneration within the brain stem and spinocerebellar tracts. Both the human and mouse *SCA1* genes have been isolated and genetically mapped. Whereas the human gene normally has 6–40 CAG repeat units, the mouse homolog has only two CAGs. The human gene encodes a protein called ataxin-1 with 792–826 amino acids, depending on the number of glutamine residues. It is expressed in a variety of both neuronal and nonneuronal cell types and can be localized to nucleus and cytoplasm, respectively. In contrast, in cerebellar Purkinje cells, ataxin-1 has both nuclear and cytoplasmic localization. To study the intergenerational stability of trinucleotide repeats in mice, the human *SCA-1* gene with normal or an expanded CAG tract containing 30 or 82 repeats, respectively, has been introduced into the mouse germline under the regulatory control of Purkinje cell-specific gene *Pcp2* sequences. Several lines of heterozygous mice carrying the human transgene have been obtained. Some lines are bred to homozygosity. Transgenic mice that carry the normal human *SCA1* allele are neurologically normal even after 1 year of age, indicating intact Purkinje cell function. In contrast, as early as 8–10 weeks of age, transgenic mice that carry the expanded repeats show slightly reduced cage activity, a gentle swaying of the head while walking, and early signs of general incoordination. By 16–30 weeks, these mice become clearly ataxic when walking. The onset of the neurological abnormalities and ataxia phenotype vary in independent 82-repeat-transgenic lines, without any correlation to the mRNA levels of the transgene. Those lines of mice that show earliest onset of ataxia tend to have the most severe neuropathologic disease. Typical phenotypic characteristics include significant loss of Purkinje cell population, with Bergmann glial proliferation, and shrinkage and gliosis of the molecular layer. These mice also show numerous ectopic Purkinje cells in the molecular layer, sometimes in the granular layer, and abnormal dendritic arrays. Heterozygous 82-repeat-transgenic mice do not show ataxia symptoms but display only mild cerebellar pathology. These mice do not show loss of Purkinje cells or gliosis, but exhibit only occasional Purkinje cells in both the molecular and granular layers. In humans, CAG repeats in the expanded range are subject to intergenerational instability, but those in the unexpanded range are stable. Eighty-two CAG repeat-containing *SCA-1* transgenic mice show no variation in repeat length with parent-to-offspring transmission. These results suggest that the mechanisms of DNA repair, replication, and the higher order structure of chromatin may be important factors in determining the CAG repeat instability in humans. Irrespective of the molecular mechanisms that control CAG repeat instability, this in vivo transgenic approach has successfully resulted in the generation of a mouse model that phenocopies the human SCA-1 disorder. These mice may also be amenable for further manipulation to devise therapeutic strategies and for targeting SCA-1 transgene expression to different tissues within the CNS. In addition, loss of function mutations can be engineered into the murine SCA-1 locus to explore its biological function during normal development of the mouse.

Po is a cell-adhesion protein that belongs to the immunoglobulin (Ig) superfamily of recognition molecules. It contains only one variable-like Ig-related extracellular domain. Members of this family have been implicated in cell migration, axon outgrowth, fasciculation, and myelination. The other mammalian members of this neural-cell-adhesion molecule superfamily include neural-cell-adhesion molecule (N-CAM) proteins, L1, and MAG. Each of these molecules can exhibit both homophilic or heterophilic interactions, and their signal transduction pathway includes regulation of cytoskeletal and second-messenger systems. Po is uniquely expressed by myelinating Schwann cells of the peripheral nervous system during the first 3 weeks after birth and accounts for almost 60% of the protein in the peripheral myelin sheath. These characteristic features have been taken into consideration in generating the Po-deficient mouse model. The mutant mice exhibit lack of normal motor coordination, tremors, and occasional convulsions. The peripheral nerve axons show severe hypomyelination and degeneration. Many of the molecules involved in myelination are abnormally regulated in Schwann cells of the mutant mice. These results suggest that Po is essential for the normal spiraling, compaction, and maintenance of the peripheral myelin sheath and for the continued integrity of associated axons. In addition, these Po mutant mice may help to decipher the molecular mechanisms of genetically transmitted peripheral neuropathies in humans.

Although the above-mentioned mouse models mimic human neurodegenerative disorders, the initial efforts to develop a useful transgenic mouse model for the fatal Alzheimer's disease have not been successful. However, several attempts have been made to develop such a mouse model. Alzheimer's disease (AD) is an irreversible neurodegenerative disorder that affects the human CNS. The disease is characterized by massive deposition of fibrillary aggregates, intracellularly as neurofibrillary tangles, extracellularly as amyloid plaques. Patients with Down's syndrome also show similar pathological symptoms. Principally, the plaques are deposited in parenchyma of amygdala, hippocampus, and neocortex. The human β-amyloid protein (Aβ) is derived from the amyloid precursor protein (APP), encoded by at least 18 exons located on chromosome 21. Four distinct transcripts of APP pre-mRNAs are generated by alternate splicing. The rationale for developing an APP overexpressing mouse model is based on the fact that AD may be initiated or accelerated by high levels of APP. In addition, high levels of APP have been observed in Down's syndrome patients. Unfortunately, most of the transgenic mice that harbor several copies of human APP cDNA do not show any pathological symptoms of AD. Only in one case, in which the expression of a human APP cDNA is driven by a mouse metallothionein promoter, have behavioral changes been noticed.

Because in many instances, the introduction of foreign cDNA does not result in high levels of transgene expression, a different strategy has been used to derive APP transgenic mice. A yeast artificial chromosome (YAC) containing 400-kb human APP gene and approximately 250 kb of flanking sequences has been transfected into mouse ES cells. These cells have been used to generate transgenic mice that retain the APP-YAC transgene with stable integration and transmission. These mice show high levels of human APP mRNA and protein in brain and peripheral tissues. In particular, human APP is expressed in cell bodies of neurons in the hippocampus, neocortex, and cerebellum in a 3-month-old APP YAC transgenic mouse. Surprisingly, this mouse also does not show any AD-type pathology.

While transgenic mice that express human APP cDNAs or gene (through YAC) do not show any AD symptoms, recently two other mouse models have been generated to understand the AD pathology and to explore the normal function of APP in mouse. The first model is a transgenic-mouse model in which the mouse Aβ expression is restricted to only neuronal cells by using 1.8 kb of 5' flanking sequences from the mouse neurofilament-light (NF-L) gene. This promoter is transcriptionally active throughout adult life. Several independent lines overexpressing this NF-L–transgene have been generated. Although transgene expression is also seen in peripheral tissues, only brains from these mice show pathological changes. Similarly, in humans, even though Aβ deposits are seen in skin and intestine without much clinical consequence, the CNS is the main target of the APP toxicity. At least three independent lines of transgenic mice show extensive neuronal degeneration. *In situ* hybridization analysis suggests that apoptosis is the predominant cause for this degeneration. These mice also show reactive gliosis. Over 50% of the transgenic mice die by 12 months of age. However, the mice do not show neurofibrillary tangles and senile plaques characteristic of human AD. It may be possible that factors required for plaque formation in humans may be absent in mice. Nevertheless, this model is important in understanding the APP toxicity and the mechanisms of apoptosis that lead to neuronal-cell death and degeneration.

Lastly, to understand the physiological function of APP, the mouse *APP* gene was disrupted by insertion of a premature stop codon in exon 2 in ES cells, and mutant mice have been generated from these ES cells. Homozygous mutant mice continue to express the *APP* mRNA in brain and other tissues, although at 5- to 10-fold lower levels than wild-type mice. This could possibly result from skipping of the disrupted exon during splicing. A shortened β-APP–specific protein has also been detected in low levels in different regions of brain. These mutant mice show severe impairment of spatial learning and exploratory behavior. Most strikingly, these mice show an increased incidence of agenesis of the corpus callosum. Although the original goal of generating a true APP null mouse has not been produced here, this model does help to understand the normal physiological function of APP during mouse development.

ENDOCRINOLOGY Mouse models for human hypothalamic-pituitary disorders, thyroid disorders, pancreas disorders, and adrenal disorders have, in general, been useful for analysis of the endocrine function in mammals. Transgenic mice that overexpress either growth hormone (GH) or growth hormone-releasing hormone (GHRH) are excellent models for both acromegaly and hyperprolactinemia, common endocrine disorders in humans. MT-GH transgenic mice are historically one of the earliest mouse models developed and were used to correct a genetic defect in the dwarf *little* mouse. The little mouse, a naturally occurring mouse strain, shows a deficiency of GH, which causes its short stature. Several MT-GH fusion genes have been injected to generate transgenic mice that overexpress growth-hormone mRNA in several tissues and consequently elevated serum-GH levels. These mice show accelerated growth rates. When the transgene is introduced into the "little" background, the phenotype is rescued, and fertility is also restored.

Using cell ablation techniques in transgenic mice, the development of somatotropes, lactotropes, and thyrotropes can be suppressed. These experiments have clarified the lineage relationships and identification of common progenitor cells for these types of anterior pituitary cells. A similar strategy has also been helpful to study proopiomelanocortin (POMC) producing corticotropes and melanotropes. Transgenic mice that express the SV-40 T antigen oncogene, driven by a human α-glycoprotein hormone or a rat POMC promoter sequences, develop anterior and intermediate lobe of pituitary tumors, respectively, and have provided novel cell lines to study the function of these cell types.

Transgenic mouse models for analyzing the etiology of human type-I diabetes have been useful in the validation of the current hypothesis on the human disorder. Essentially different types of transgenes have been targeted to β cells of the pancreas to selectively destroy these cells. Transgenic mice in which the autoimmune response is evoked in pancreatic β cells by induction of MHC antigens develop diabetes accompanied by a selective loss of these cells. To mimic the typical autoimmune response in β cells, transgenic mice have been created that express a viral protein in pancreatic islet cells. Because the virus shares some antigenic epitopes common to mouse proteins, the immune response generated against the viral proteins also destroys the β cells. As a result, these mice develop diabetes. Although this model is useful in understanding the pathogenesis of human type-I diabetes, it differs from the human disease in two aspects. First, the presence of virus is required to elicit the response in mice, whereas in humans, the autoimmunity is maintained by endogenous β-cell-specific proteins. Second, the β cells are destroyed at a rapid rate in the mouse model unlike in the human situation, where the disease process is rather prolonged. Finally, transgenic mice that express a rat-insulin promoter-SV40 oncogene sequences develop heritable pancreatic β-cell tumors. They have β-cell hyperplasia and elevated serum insulin levels. The α and δ cells of the islets of Langerhans are disordered, and their number is drastically reduced in the pancreatic tumor tissue. These mice develop highly vascularized solid pancreatic tumors that cause premature death of the mice around 9–12 weeks of age. This animal model has become invaluable in studying the biogenesis of islet cells, cell–cell interactions within the endocrine pancreas, and understanding of the pathobiology of human insulinomas.

The three pituitary glycoprotein hormones—namely, luteinizing hormone (LH), follicle stimulating hormone (FSH), and thyroid stimulating hormone (TSH)—are heterodimeric proteins. They share a common α-subunit that is noncovalently linked to a hormone-specific β-subunit. Whereas LH and FSH control gonadal functions, TSH regulates thyroid function. Mice deficient in the glycoprotein hormone α-subunit (α-GSU) have been generated by gene targeting in ES cells. These mice are viable, but exhibit growth insufficiency and are hypothyroid and hypogonadal. The thyroids are hypoplastic and contain small disorganized follicles. The animals are infertile and show lack of some secondary sexual characteristics, although the sex organs differentiate normally. Within the pituitary, the thyrotropes exhibit hypertrophy and intensely stain for TSH-β subunit antibody. The gonadotrope cell population is normal, whereas both somatotropes (GH expressing cells) and lactotropes (prolactin-expressing cells) are reduced and absent, respectively. Absence of α-GSU does not affect the distribution and appearance of gonadotropin-releasing-hormone (GnRH) neurons that migrate to different regions of the hypothalamus. Experiments with these mice have thus established the physiological functions of these important trophic hormones in mammalian growth and differentiation.

REPRODUCTIVE BIOLOGY The hypothalamic-pituitary-gonadal axis, commonly known as the reproductive axis, is regulated by a complex network of interactions between neuropeptides, trophic hormones, gonadal steroids, and peptides and growth factors. Distinct genes encoding several critical factors are activated during the establishment of the primitive reproductive axis, functional maturation of the gonads, and maintenance of their differentiated function. Disruption of any key step may lead to aberrant reproductive function and may even cause sterility as demonstrated in the analysis of several transgenic and knockout mice. Still, many mouse models are currently being generated to understand human infertility and associated disorders to test and design novel strategies for contraception. These many transgenic models have been extensively summarized elsewhere, and we will only discuss a few models related to sex determination.

Mammalian sex differentiation is dependent on interactions between several factors. The early molecular events that dictate the choice between the pathways of male and female sex-organ development in mammalian early embryo are poorly understood, including those in humans. Several genetic lesions have been characterized in humans that affect this complex pathway. Successful application of the transgenic-mouse technology in recent years has given important clues toward identifying functions of regulatory molecules that control the sexual-differentiation process. Most important among these are transcription factors including WT-1 (described in an earlier section) and steroidogenic factor-1 (SF-1), SRY, and Mullerian inhibiting substance (MIS), a member of the TGF-β superfamily. Gene deletions of WT-1 or SF-1 by homologous recombination in ES cells and generation of knockout mice show drastic phenotypes. Absence of either WT-1 or SF-1 results in failure of development of the gonads. Transgenic mice that express SRY, a testis-determining gene, demonstrate testis formation in XX females. The function of MIS in mammalian reproductive development has been elucidated both by gain-of-function transgenic mice that chronically overexpress MIS and by an MIS knockout mouse model. Absence of MIS in males prevents regression of the Mullerian duct, and therefore male mice develop uteri and testicular Leydig cell hyperplasia.

METABOLIC DISORDERS Metabolic defects most often result from an accumulation of a substrate because of absence or reduced activity of an enzyme, often causing formation of a toxic side product or absence of an important product for a subsequent enzyme reaction. Such defects can cause life-threatening problems during childhood or adulthood. There are many transgenic-mouse models available to investigate the pathogenesis and to evaluate therapeutic approaches for such human diseases. Some of the transgenic mice that are useful models in understanding these human metabolic disorders are discussed below.

The Lesch-Nyhan syndrome in human males is a rare neurological and behavioral disorder. The disorder is caused by an inherited deficiency in the level of activity of the X-chromosome–linked purine salvage enzyme hypoxanthine-guanosine phosphoribosyl transferase (HPRT). Hemizygous mutant male mice have been generated that carry a mutation in the HPRT gene. Interestingly, these mice are viable and normal. No gross neurological symptoms have been apparent in male mice. Even though these mutant mice do not show any metabolic, neurological, or behavioral symptoms characteristic of the human syndrome, the basic principles of gene-targeting technique were originally developed during the creation of this animal model.

Urate oxidase, or uricase, is a purine metabolic enzyme. The enzyme catalyzes the conversion of uric acid to allantoin in most mammals. In humans and other primates during evolution, deleterious mutations in the urate oxidase gene resulted in the loss of this enzyme. Therefore, the sparingly soluble uric acid is the end product of purine metabolism in humans, instead of a more soluble allantoin. Because humans lack urate oxidase, they are predisposed to metabolic disorders, such as gouty arthritis and renal stone formation, as a result of elevated uric acid levels. To understand the biological function of urate oxidase in lower mammals and to develop an animal model for human hyperuricemia, knockout mice have been created by gene-targeting techniques. Approximately 65% of mice deficient in urate oxidase die at 3–4 weeks of age. Both serum and urinary uric acid levels are elevated 10- and 5-fold higher, respectively, in mutant mice compared to wild-type control mice. Consistent with the biochemical action of the enzyme, mutant mice show a decrease in urinary allantoin content. Urate oxidase-deficient mice show small cortical cysts and white yellow deposits of uric acid in both kidney cortex and medulla as early as 6 days after birth. With the progression of the deposition, the mice show kidney tubular degeneration leading to severe hydronephrosis at 5 weeks. This eventually results in glomerular atrophy and occurrence of chronic inflammation within the kidney interstitium, similar to acute hyperuricemia nephropathy in humans. Similar to human patients, urate oxidase-deficient mice, when treated with allopurinol, an inhibitor of xanthine oxidase, show dose-dependent reduction in serum uric acid levels. Although urate oxidase is absent in humans, most humans do not develop hyperuricemia at a young age and do not show increased mortality, unless in conjunction with other environmental and genetic factors. However, generation and analysis of urate oxidase knockout mice resolved the long-standing debate on the biological function of urate oxidase in mice and other lower mammals that retain it.

DERMATOPATHOLOGY The application of transgenic technology to skin research has resulted in many advances in our understanding of skin development and function. The skin is a complex organ system. It consists of two different layers, epidermis and dermis, derived from ectoderm and mesoderm, respectively. Cells of the outermost layer of the epidermis, called periderm, continually undergo keratinization and are replenished by cells arising from the basal layer that lies beneath. The fully developed epidermis consists of five distinct layers—stratum corneum, stratum lucidum, stratum granulosum, stratum spinosum, and stratum germinativum. The epithelial cells of the epidermis are called keratinocytes. They produce important proteins that regulate the epidermal–dermal interactions.

The epidermis has been the major target for several gene-manipulation studies. The epidermis exerts its protective function through an extensive cytoskeletal network. The major structural components of this network are called keratins. Keratins are members of the intermediate filament (IF) superfamily. They are α-helical proteins that can assemble into 10-nm filaments. Based on amino acid sequence, keratins can be subdivided into two groups—the acidic, type I, keratins and the basic, type II, keratins. Type I keratins include K9–K20 and are in the molecular-weight range of 64–40 kDa, whereas type II keratins include K1–K8 and weigh 67–53 kDa. Heteropolymeric combinations of type I and type II can result in the formation of 10-nm filaments. Proliferating basal cells express K5 and K14 mRNAs, and they differentiate in the first suprabasal layer, inducing the expression of K1 and K10. During the wound-healing process and in cultured epidermal cells, K6 and K16 are induced. Many of the human and mouse keratin genes and other epidermal-specific genes have been isolated and characterized in detail. This structural analysis has led to the design of many transgenic and knockout mice to understand cutaneous development and functions including hair development and skin cancer.

Epidermolytic hyperkeratosis (EHK) in humans is a dominantly inherited disorder of keratin, characterized by hyperplasia of the stratum corneum. Mutations in highly conserved regions of K1 and K10 genes have been identified in patients with EHK. Transgenic mice expressing a mutant form of K1 have been generated. Most of the homozygous mice with two copies of the mutant transgene die within 24–36 h after birth resulting from progression of skin erosions. Similar to EHK patients, the spinous layer shows many clear cells that have clumping of keratin filaments around the nucleus. Mice that survive to the juvenile and adult stage do not show suprabasal epidermal splitting (blistering) in their back skin, but their footpad epithelium, which lacks hair follicles, show cell lysis and splitting in the spinous layer, similar to human EHK disorder. Hyperkeratosis is also seen in mice deficient in follistatin, an activin-binding protein. Both granular and stratum corneum layers show increased thickness in these follistatin-mutant mice.

Psoriasis is a hyperproliferative inflammatory skin disorder in humans. Approximately 2% of the world's population is affected by this skin disorder. Transgenic mice that express either human integrin β1-subunit or heterodimers of β1- and α2- or β1- and α5-subunits in the suprabasal layers of epidermis exhibit a phenotype that resembles the human disorder. Integrins are extracellular matrix receptor proteins; three types are expressed by epidermal keratinocytes. They share a common β-subunit. The α2β1 complex is a collagen receptor, and the α3β1 is a laminin receptor; both of these are expressed in normal epidermis. The α5β1 is the keratinocyte fibronectin receptor and is upregulated during wound-healing, in psoriasis, and in cultured keratinocytes. Normally, integrin expression is confined to the keratinocytes in the basal layer of the epidermis. Since their expression is often seen in suprabasal layers during wound-healing and in psoriasis, integrin subunits are targeted to this layer in transgenic mice, using a suprabasal layer cell specific promoter called involucrin. Several lines of mice have been obtained that express each of the integrin subunits, α2, α5, and β1, separately. Subsequently, β1 transgene-bearing mice have been mated to α2 or α5 mice to generate mice that express the heterodimers. A majority of the α5, β1, and α5β1 transgenic mice have defects in eyelid closure, hair, and whisker development. The eyelids noticeably fail to fuse prior to birth, and often an inflammatory exudate in the cornea and eyelid is apparent. The hair of the coat does not display a uniform orientation, with disorganized follicles, and the whiskers are short and curly. These phenotypic features are characteristic of those seen in many other mutant mice in which the growth factor signaling is disrupted. For example, activin/inhibin βB knockout mice display eyelid-closure defects. Similarly, TGF-α and EGF receptor-deficient mice and BMP-2, BMP-4 overexpression transgenic mice exhibit abnormal skin development. In mice deficient in activin βA-subunit, the whisker follicles differentiate in a delayed manner, with abnormal hair papilla and irregularly positioned cells at the base of the hair bulb. These observations are all consistent with the fact that growth factors regulate integrin levels in keratinocytes and may explain the consequences of perturbances in integrin expression during embryonic development. The β1 alone or β1α2 or β1α5 integrin–transgenic mice also show the typical features of psoriasis (i.e., increased keratinocyte proliferation, abnormal differentiation, increased dermal mitoses, capillary dilation, and an influx of $CD4^+$ and $CD8^+$ T-lymphocytes). The abnormal keratinocyte development and inflammation in these mice result in flaking of the epidermis on the chin, behind the ears, reddening of skin and paws, and pustule formation on dorsal-skin surface. Consistent with the belief that psoriasis in humans is influenced by several genetic and environmental factors, all transgenic mice that express the integrin subunits do not show the symptoms. Thus, the transgenic technology has provided important answers to the understanding of the etiology of psoriasis. These mice have a potential as important models in the treatment of psoriasis using immunosuppressive agents.

Recently, gene-targeting approaches have been used to create knockout mice to mimic the human disease xeroderma pigmentosum (XP). XP is a rare autosomal disease in humans, resulting from a defective nucleotide excision repair process. It is characterized by hypersensitivity of the skin to sunlight and a very high risk of skin-cancer incidence in body parts exposed to sunlight. There are eight complementation groups in XP (A–G and a variant form). Mice deficient in XPC are viable and fertile and do not exhibit an increased susceptibility to spontaneous tumor generation. However, following 10 d of UV exposure, the ears of the mutant mice exhibit marked atrophy. By 20 weeks of exposure, they develop skin cancers of different types. Most of these belong to the squamous-cell carcinoma category. These mice also show epidermal hyperplasia with focal areas of hyperkeratosis and varying degrees of dysplasia, acantholysis, and/or dyskeratosis. The UV treatment of the mutant mice also results in keratitis and corneal ulceration of the eye. The spectrum of these phenotypic features are characteristic of human XPC. Similar to XPC-deficient mice, mice deficient in XPA also are viable and fertile and are highly susceptible to chemical and UV-induced skin carcinogenesis. These mice also develop squamous-cell carcinoma and eye defects. These knockout mouse models are useful in two ways. First, they can be used to understand XP disorders, and cells from these mice can be used to study the molecular mechanisms of nucleotide excision. Second, sensitive short-term in vivo carcinogenicity of genotoxic agents can be tested using these excision repair enzyme-deficient mice.

CONCLUSIONS AND FUTURE DIRECTIONS

Transgenic animal technology has become highly popular in recent years. The primary reasons are because this is an in vivo manipulative approach, and the specificity with which a target gene can be expressed makes it an extremely powerful approach. Virtually every physiological system has been and will continue to be investigated from a developmental and functional perspective (i.e., both physiological and pathological). In many instances, the clinical data and the naturally occurring mutant strains of mice complement the efforts on gene-manipulation research.

What can we envision in future with this technology? Animal species such as goat and cattle can routinely be used as bioreactors to produce pharmacological products in high quantities. The functional redundancies or specificities between close members of a superfamily can be resolved by breeding and generating mice with combinations of mutations in distinct or unrelated pathways. Large-scale deletions that mimick many human chromosomal haploidy situations can be created in mice, and thus sets of genes on a specific chromosome can be identified structurally and functionally. The "cre-lox" system will be used in many cases to generate tissue-specific knockout mice. Many mouse models will be generated to address the genetic basis for the complex issues of behavior, learning, and memory. The potential possibilities of generating ES cells from species other than mouse and rat can be anticipated. The rapid pace with which the genome-mapping data are being accumulated in parallel will set a continued pace to identify and define the biological functions of many newly discovered genes. The final goal is to generate cheap, convenient, and easily manipulative animal models that exactly reflect many human-disease conditions. Both human health and health-care management will thus benefit richly from this fascinating technology.

SELECTED REFERENCES

Aguzzi A, Brandner S, Sure U, Ruedi D, Isenmann S. Transgenic and knockout mice: Models of neurological disease. Brain Path 1994;4:3–20.

Bradley A, Hasty P, Davis A, Ramirez-Solis R. Modifying the mouse: design and desire. Bio/Technology 1992;10:534–539.

Burright EN, Clark HB, Servadio A, et al. SCA1 transgenic mice: a model for neurodegeneration caused by an expanded CAG trinucleotide repeat. Cell 1995;82:937–948.

Capecchi MR. Targeted gene replacement. Sci Amer 1994;270:52–59.

Cox GA, Cole NM, Matsumura K, et al. Overexpression of dystrophin in transgenic mice eliminates dystrophic symptoms without toxicity. Nature 1993;364:725–729.

Giese KP, Martini R, Lemke G, Soriano P, Schachner M. Mouse Po gene disruption leads to hypomyelination, abnormal expression of recognition molecules, and degeneration of myelin and axons. Cell 1992;71: 565–576.

Gilbert SF. Developmental Biology. Sunderland, MA: Sinauer Associates, 1994.

Glasser SW, Korfhagen TR, Wert SE, Whitsett JA. Transgenic models for study of pulmonary development and disease. Am J Physiol 1994;267: L489–L497.

Grandaliano G, Choudhury G G, Abboud HE. Transgenic animal models as a tool in the diagnosis of kidney diseases. Semin Nephrol 1995;15:43–49.

Greenhalgh DA, Roop DR. Dissecting molecular carcinogenesis: development of transgenic mouse models by epidermal gene targeting. Adv Cancer Res 1994;64:247–296.

Gu H, Marth JD, Orban PC, Mossmann H, Rajewsky K. Deletion of a DNA polymerase beta gene segment in T cells using cell type-specific gene targeting. Science 1994;103–106.

Hammer RE, Palmiter RD, Brinster RL. Partial correction of murine hereditary growth disorder by germ-line incorporation of a new gene. Nature 1984;311:65–67.

Hanahan D. Heritable formation of pancreatic β-cell tumours in transgenic mice expressing recombinant insulin/simian virus 40 oncogenes. Nature 1985;315:115–122.

Henkemeyer M, Rossi DJ, Holmyrad DP, et al. Vascular system defects and neuronal apoptosis in mice lacking Ras GTPase-activating protein. Nature 1995;377:695–701.

Jones SN, Roe AE, Donehower LA, Bradley A. Rescue of embryonic lethality in Mdm2-deficient mice by absence of p53. Nature 1995; 378:206–208.

Kendall SK, Samuelson LC, Saunders TL, Wood RI, Camper SA. Targeted disruption of the pituitary glycoprotein hormone alpha-subunit produces hypogonadal and hypothyroid mice. Gen Devel 1995; 9:2007–2019.

Kreidberg JA, Sariola H, Loring JM, et al. WT-1 is required for early kidney development. Cell 1993;74:679–691.

Kuehn MR, Bradley A, Robertson EJ, Evans MJ. A potential animal model for Lesch-Nyhan syndrome through introduction of HPRT mutations into mice. Nature 1987;326:295–298.

Kumar TR, Donehower LA, Bradley A, Matzuk MM. Transgenic mouse models for tumor-suppressor genes. J Int Med 1995;238: 233–238.

Lamb BT. Making models for Alzheimer's disease. Nat Genet 1995;9:4–6.

Luo G, Hofman C, Bronckers ALJJ, Sohocki M, Bradley A, Karsenty G. BMP-7 is an inducer of nephrogenesis, and is also required for eye development and skeletal patterning. Gen & Devel 1995;9: 2808–2820.

Luo X, Ikeda Y, Parker KL. A cell-specific nuclear receptor is essential for adrenal and gonadal development and sexual differentiation. Cell 1994;77:481–490.

Matzuk MM, Finegold MJ, Su J-GJ, Hseuh AJW, Bradley A. α-Inhibin is a tumor-suppressor gene with gonadal specificity in mice. Nature 1992;360:313–319.

Matzuk MM. Functional analysis of mammalian members of the transforming growth factor-β superfamily. Trends Endocrinol Metab 1995;6:120–127.

Matzuk MM, Kumar TR, Vassalli A, Bickenbach JR, Roop DR, Bradley A. Functional analysis of activins during mammalian development. Nature 1995;374:354–356.

McMahon AP, Bradley A. The Wnt-1 (int-1) proto-oncogene is required for development of a large region of the mouse brain. Cell 1990;62: 1073–1085.

Molkentin JD, Black BL, Martin JF, Olson EN. Cooperative activation of muscle gene expression by MEF 2 and myogenic bHLH proteins. Cell 1995;83:1125–1136.

Morham SG, Langenbach R, Loftin CD, et al. Prostaglandin synthase 2 gene disruption causes severe renal pathology in the mouse. Cell 1995;83:473–482.

Nishimori K, Matzuk MM. Transgenic mice in the analysis of reproductive development and function. Reviews of Reproduction, 1996;1:203–212.

Paigen B, Plump AS, Rubin EM. The mouse as a model for human cardiovascular disease and hyperlipidemia. Curr Opin Lipidol 1994;5: 258–264.

Palmiter RD, Brinster RL. Germ-line transmission of mice. Annu Rev Genet 1986;20:465–499.

Ramirez-Solis R, Liu P, Bradley A. Chromosome engineering in mice. Nature 1995;378:720–724.

Ramirez-Solis R, Zheng H, Whiting J, Krumlauf R, Bradley A. Hoxb-4 (Hox-2.6) mutant mice show homeotic transformation of a cervical vertebra and defects in the closure of the sternal rudiments. Cell 1993;73:279–294.

Sands AT, Abuin A, Sanchez A, Conti CJ, Bradley A. High susceptibility to ultraviolet-induced carcinogenesis in mice lacking XPC. Nature 1995;377:162–165.

Shawlot W, Behringer RR. Requirement for Lim-1 in head-organizer function. Nature 1995;374:425–430.

Smithies O, Kim H-S. Targeted gene duplication and disruption for analyzing quantitative genetic traits in mice. Proc Natl Acad Sci USA 1994;91:3612–3615.

Snouwaert JN, Brigman KK, Latour AM, et al. An animal model for cystic fibrosis made by gene targeting. Science 1992;257:1083–1088.

Stewart TA. Models of human endocrine disorders in transgenic rodents. Nature 1993;4:136–141.

Strober W, Ehrhardt RO. Chronic intestinal inflammation: an unexpected outcome in cytokine or T cell receptor mutant mice. Cell 1993;75:203–205.

Taverne J. Transgenic mice in the study of cytokine function. Int J Exp Path 1993;74:525–546.

Wagner J, Thiele F, Ganten D. Transgenic animals as models for human disease. Clin Exp Hyperten 1995;17:593–605.

Wu X, Wakamiya M, Vaishnav S, et al. Hyperuricemia and urate nephropathy in urate oxidase-deficient mice. Proc Natl Acad Sci USA 1994;91:742–746.

Zijlstra M, Bix M, Simister NE, Loring JM, Raulet DH, Jaenisch R. Beta 2-microglobulin deficient mice lack $CD4^{-}8^{+}$ cytotoxic T cells. Nature 1990;344:742–746.

CARDIOLOGY II

SECTION EDITOR:
ANTHONY ROSENZWEIG

11 Molecular Cardiology

An Overview

ANTHONY ROSENZWEIG

Not too long ago a textbook section entitled "Molecular Cardiology" would have seemed curiously paradoxical and impractical. Molecular biology appeared to have little to do with either clinical cardiology or even its scientific foundations. Classical large animal physiology experiments provided insights that were readily extrapolated from the laboratory to the bedside. In contrast, the clinical relevance of molecular biology seemed remote. This perception is changing because of the substantial progress made in applying the tools of molecular biology to cardiovascular biology and medicine.

An imperfect measure of these changes is reflected in the number of papers published in these fields over the past 30 years. Acknowledging that the number of papers published in all fields has burgeoned, some insight may be gained from comparing the relative changes in publications related to cardiology, molecular biology, or the intersection of these disciplines (Fig. 11-1). As one might expect, the number of publications in molecular biology has increased over 30-fold during this period, which has witnessed the genesis of many important technologies under this general umbrella. The number of papers in cardiology has also increased over this period by approximately fivefold. However, the number of papers over the past 30 years within what might be termed "molecular cardiology" has increased nearly 75-fold, perhaps reflecting the growing realization of valuable connections between these two fields.

Molecular biology provides a set of powerful tools that can be brought to bear on clinical and scientific problems. These tools are rapidly elucidating the molecular basis of many clinical phenomena. One example highlighted by Dr. Michel in Chapter 15 is the identification and molecular cloning of the enzymes responsible for production of endothelium-dependent relaxing factor (EDRF), now recognized as nitric oxide (NO). Absence or dysfunction of endothelial cells results in less NO production. This is recognized in the catheterization laboratory as a paradoxical vasoconstrictive response to acetylcholine that dilates normal vessels through an endothelium-dependent mechanism. Such an abnormality is seen both in atherosclerotic vessels and patients with risk factors for atherosclerosis even in the absence of angiographically demonstrable lesions. Identification of the nitric oxide synthase (NOS) genes responsible for NO production has permitted a demonstration of their role in vascular tone homeostasis. Such studies form the essential foundation for future analysis of the role of NOS and other regulators of vascular tone in a variety of cardiovascular conditions, including hypertension and atherosclerosis.

Molecular technologies that are particularly relevant to the clinical arena include molecular genetics, generation of genetic animal models, and somatic gene transfer. The exponential increase in available genetic markers has dramatically hastened analysis of monogenic disorders. Genetic analysis of such disorders is of immediate interest to clinicians because of its the potential to provide both diagnostic and prognostic insights. These themes are echoed repeatedly throughout this section in chapters on congenital heart disease, cardiomyopathies, arrhythmia, and hypertension. In Chapter 12, Dr. Chin reviews the growing list of genetic defects linked to congenital heart disease. Furthermore, he illustrates the importance of animal models for understanding the molecular basis of cardiac development, especially in relationship to congenital heart disease. Although standard genetic models are limited for congenital heart disease, there is great potential in the study of mutant zebrafish. Clinicians are occasionally skeptical of such studies both because the animals studied seem so far from clinical experience and because even human monogenic conditions represent only a small subset of a broad clinical spectrum of sporadic and polygenic disorders. However, both genetic animal models and mendelian conditions provide a rare window of opportunity for observations that can have much broader relevance. In addition, identification of disease-causing mutations can illuminate unanticipated molecular functions or interactions. Admittedly most of the cardiovascular diseases encountered routinely by clinicians result in fact from a complex interaction between multiple genetic loci and superimposed environmental influences. Using hypertension as an example, Drs. Koike and Jacob (Chapter 16) illustrate evolving approaches to understanding the genetic bases of polygenic disorders. Surprisingly, little is known about the genetic basis of most coronary artery disease, despite the prevalence of the phenotype. It is likely that approaches similar to those described by Drs. Koike and Jacob will shed light on the genetic bases of this problem as well.

Somatic gene transfer is of interest not only as a potential experimental tool for the development of local overexpression models, but also as a vehicle for somatic gene therapy. Gene therapy within the cardiovascular system has been broadly defined to include not only replacement of a defective gene but also overexpression of a beneficial gene product. This approach to gene therapy within the cardiovascular system differs from gene

From: *Principles of Molecular Medicine* (J. L. Jameson, ed.), ©1998 Humana Press Inc., Totowa, NJ.

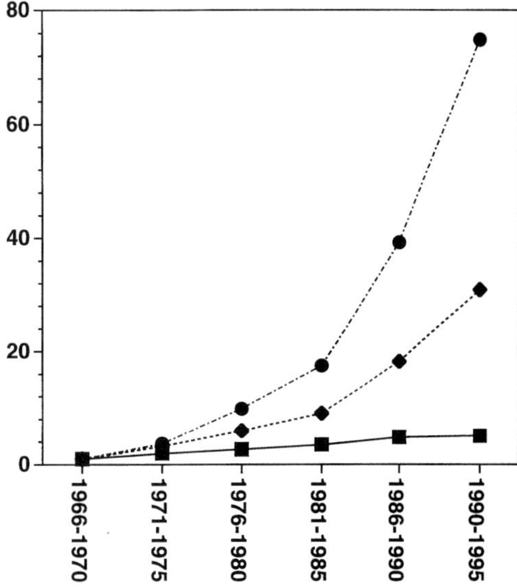

Figure 11-1 Relative number of papers published 1966–1995. The MEDLINE database was searched using BRS Colleague to identify papers published between January 1966 and December 1995. Papers were identified as relating broadly to cardiology (contain the word "heart" or the root "cardi-"), molecular biology (contain the word-root "gene-" or "molecul-"), or molecular cardiology (falling into both categories). For each group, the number of papers was normalized to the initial reference period (1966–1970), which is arbitrarily assigned the value 1. The number of papers in subsequent 5-year periods is displayed relative to this initial reference period. ■, cardiology; ◆, molecular, ●, molecular cardiology.

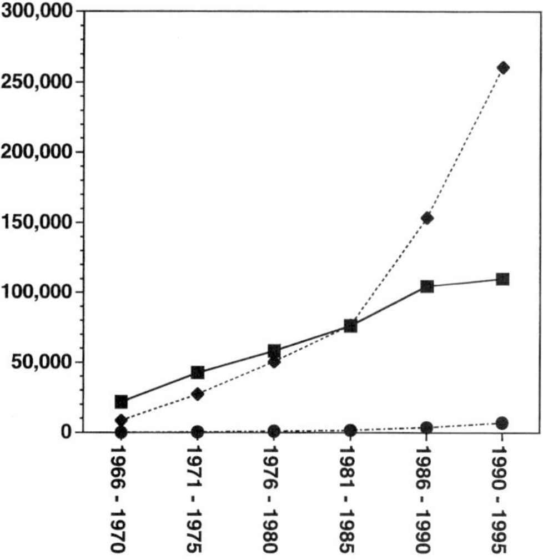

Figure 11-2 Absolute number of papers published 1966–1995. The MEDLINE database was searched as described for Fig. 11-1. Here the absolute number of papers published in each 5-year period is shown graphically for each of the three categories as defined previously. ■, cardiology; ◆, molecular; ●, molecular cardiology.

replacement therapy in other disciplines in several important ways. Access to the target tissue is often more difficult than in other systems, and may require specific catheter delivery systems. In addition, the target cells for gene transfer within the cardiovascular system (endothelial cells, vascular smooth muscle cells, or cardiomyocytes) replicate either slowly or not at all and are notoriously resistant to gene transfer techniques. These limitations have sparked interest in viral vectors to achieve acceptable efficiencies in vivo. On the positive side, gene therapy for several potential cardiovascular applications (such as restenosis) has the advantage that transient expression of beneficial gene products may be sufficient to mediate significant clinical benefit. Drs. Vassalli and Dichek discusses the status of cardiovascular gene therapy in Chapter 18.

The potential power of molecular approaches to clinical cardiology is perhaps best illustrated in the evolving story of hypertrophic cardiomyopathy, recounted by Dr. Seidman et al. in Chapter 13. This clinically important, often familial condition has been recognized for approximately 30 years. However, the fundamental etiologies remained obscure. The Seidman laboratory first established genetic linkage for this condition in several large affected families. They then went on to identify disease-causing mutations in multiple genes, including cardiac myosin, troponin T, and tropomyosin. This work has had important implications for our understanding of hypertrophic cardiomyopathy and basic muscle biology. The clinical prognosis of patients with this condition is dramatically affected by the specific mutation they carry. As one might expect, more conservative mutations, in general, carry a better prognosis than more radical alterations. In addition, these genes all participate in forming the sarcomere, and elucidating the genetic abnormalities responsible for the clinical phenotype will likely continue to provide insights into their molecular functions and interactions.

The genetic analysis of the long QT syndrome (LQTS) discussed by Dr. London in Chapter 17 is a similar evolving success story, which also illustrates the potential synergism between basic and clinically focused research. The LQTS is an uncommon but life-threatening condition. Afflicted individuals suffer high rates of syncope and sudden cardiac death. The condition is clinically and genetically heterogeneous. Genetic pedigree analysis has implicated three ion channel genes in the condition. Simultaneously, basic investigation has substantially advanced our understanding of the contribution of these channels to the cardiac action potential. We are just beginning to realize the substantial promise of synergism between these fields. For example, one recent report suggests it may become feasible to tailor pharmacological therapy to the individual LQTS genotype. Specifically, patients in whom LQTS is due to delayed inactivation of the sodium channel benefit from mexiletene, which decreases inward sodium current. In contrast, in patients in whom LQTS is due to reduced function of a potassium channel, no benefit is seen with mexiletene. It should be noted that this particular potassium channel was initially cloned as a homolog of a mutant drosophila gene not then known to be relevant to cardiovascular disease. Further evidence that the dividends of basic research are far-reaching and difficult to predict.

The ability to manipulate putative disease-causing genes in the germline of mice allows such genetic analysis to be brought full-circle, and provides an invaluable animal model for analysis of pathophysiology and potential therapeutic interventions. Altering cardiac expression of ion channels in mice through germline manipulation has improved our understanding of the molecular basis of the cardiac action potential and offers promise of animal models of arrhythmia in general as well as LQTS in particular.

This may well become the paradigm for future investigation in molecular medicine: genetic analysis of human conditions providing the basis for development of genetically manipulated animal models. Those models, in turn, provide a unique opportunity to return to the fundamental physiologic focus with which cardiovascular investigation began. The dog lab of the past may be supervened by the mouse lab of the future to allow analysis of physiology and pathophysiology with full advantage of the power of modern genetics. Moreover, such models will likely become the optimum testing ground for pharmacological or genetic therapies.

It is clear that clinical cardiology has only begun to feel the impact of these advances in molecular biology. Although, as pointed out earlier, there has been a dramatic increase in the relative number of papers published in "molecular cardiology," these papers still constitute an exceedingly small minority of the absolute number of papers published in either cardiology or molecular biology as a whole (Fig. 11-2). The transformation has only begun. It is likely that the most dramatic changes lie ahead. The chapters in this section provide a glimpse of a revolution very much in progress, but whose repercussions have yet to fully impact clinical cardiology.

12 Congenital Heart Disease

ALVIN J. CHIN

BACKGROUND

Sufficient progress has occurred in identifying, characterizing, and surgically repairing physiologically important congenital cardiac defects (which occur at the rate of 20,000/yr in the United States) that 85% of these infants can now expect to survive to adulthood. Since only the most severe structural malformations thwart current management schemes, prevention and early *in utero* detection are the remaining strategies to further reduce the impact of heart malformation on the health of infants and children; however, any prevention approach would depend largely on knowing the percentage of congenital heart defects that are genetic. For example, if the vast majority of congenital heart anomalies are due to intrauterine insults (infectious agents, toxins, mechanical stress, and so on) to the embryo during the first 30 days of gestation, then a prevention strategy would be ineffective; since most pregnancies are already monitored by ultrasound at least once for accurate dating, perhaps adding a "cardiac surveillance" portion to the imaging protocol would suffice to increase the chance of prenatal identification. However, evidence has begun to accumulate for the hypothesis that the majority of congenital heart malformations are due to gene alterations. Therefore, the scientific challenge of the next several decades will be to unravel the sequence of molecular decisions that result in the construction of the heart and blood vessels from the first embryonic tissue layers. Although more than 50 genes have already been reported to be involved in cardiovascular morphogenesis (Table 12-1), the way they function to form the heart and great vessels correctly (in space and time) remains obscure. Both forward and reverse genetic approaches are being tried, and a variety of organisms are being scrutinized since the underlying mechanisms of patterning appear to be widely shared among vertebrates. Murine cardiac development is difficult to study in vivo without new imaging techniques because of the relatively inaccessible embryo. Furthermore, a systematic screen of the mouse genome for embryonic lethal mutations affecting organogenesis is impractical. Other vertebrates such as the chick *Gallus gallus* and the African clawed frog *Xenopus laevis* have long generation times. The teleost fish *Danio* (formerly *Brachydanio*) *rerio* (zebrafish) has emerged as a model system because of its prolific egg production, rapid (90-d) generation time, optically transparent embryo, and extremely rapid heart development (48 h). Despite the advantages of the zebrafish system for mutational analysis, there are some aspects of cardiovascular construction, namely septation and pulmonary artery formation, that must be studied in higher vertebrates.

This overview will discuss the anatomical malformations that make up the vast majority of cases of human congenital heart disease but will specifically exclude heritable cardiomyopathies (Chapter 13), long QT syndrome (Chapter 17), and Marfan syndrome, and will only briefly mention diGeorge syndrome, since this is also covered in Chapter 120.

CLINICAL FEATURES

The majority of human newborns with hemodynamically significant heart defects present in the first 2 weeks of life with one of four physiological arrangements: obstruction to pulmonary arterial circulation, obstruction to systemic arterial circulation, inadequate mixing between pulmonary and systemic circulations, or pulmonary venous obstruction. Because of the two-connected-pumps-working-in-parallel construction of fetal cardiac circulation (Fig. 12-1), these four types of hemodynamic aberration are well-tolerated for a 40-week gestation. An obstruction to either the pulmonary or aortic flow is reliably compensated for by blood flow shifting to the contralateral side of the heart. Transposition of the great arteries with intact ventricular septum does not have antenatal hemodynamic consequences since it merely constitutes a different variety of two-connected-pumps-working-in-parallel configuration. Finally, anomalous pulmonary venous connection with pulmonary venous obstruction does not substantially alter prenatal hemodynamics because very little blood flow is normally allowed into the lungs *in utero*.

The four physiological derangements are unmasked when the circulation is acutely changed at birth to a two-unconnected pumps-working-in-series arrangement, with lungs but without placenta (Fig. 12-1). The rapidity of presentation is critically dependent on the time course of foramen ovale closure or ductal closure or both. Obstruction to pulmonary arterial circulation (Fig. 12-2A,B) manifests as cyanosis. Obstruction to systemic arterial circulation manifests as "low output syndrome." Inadequate mixing between the pulmonary and systemic circulations also appears as cyanosis. Pulmonary venous obstruction (Fig. 12-2C) initially manifests as tachypnea out of proportion to arterial desaturation.

Although these four hemodynamic subsets account for virtually all cases of heart defect appearing early, severe cases of the rare malformation "absent pulmonary valve syndrome," whose cardinal feature is ventilatory failure due to airway impingement by adjacent markedly dilated pulmonary arteries, may also show up on the first day of life.

From: *Principles of Molecular Medicine* (J. L. Jameson, ed.), ©1998 Humana Press Inc., Totowa, NJ.

Table 12-1
Genes Involved in Cardiovascular Morphogenesis

Gene family	Temporal and spatial expression of mRNA/phenotype of knockout homozygote/overexpression (mRNA injection) data		
	Drosophila	*Xenopus*	*Mus*
Transcription factors			
NK		*XNkx2.3* in pharyngeal endoderm and cardiac mesoderm @ stage 16	
	tinman: no heart or gut muscle precursors	*XNkx2.5*(similar to *XNkx2.3*)	*Nkx2.5* in myocardial progenitors@7.5 d, in myocardium@8.5 d, also in sinus venosus @9.0 d, venosus@9.0 d, but not in aorta; *Nkx2.5* knockout@8.5 d shows no looping, cushions, trabeculae carnae
Hox			a-2 in aorta @ 9.75 d, in vasculature @11.5 d; knockout does not have heart phenotype
			a-3 in atrium and aortic trunk@12.5 d; a-3 knockout has defective aortic and pulmonary valves, thin aortic wall, atrial and left ventricular hypertrophy, dilatation of systemic veins
Sox			Sox-4 knockout die @ 14 d from dysplasia of both semilunar valves; there is also a defect in septation of the outflow of the heart
GATA			*GATA-4* in caudal end of heart tube @8.0 d, in endocardium and myocardium (stopping at distal outflow tract) @ 9.0 d, in endocardial cushions and myocardium @10 d; knockout dies by 9.5 d, showing cardia bifida and absence of the pericardial coelom, defects rescuable by wild-type endoderm
		XGATA-5 in ventral cardiac mesoderm @stage 18, by stage 34, only in endocardium	*GATA-5* in precardiac mesoderm @7.0 d, in atrium and ventricle @ 9.5 d, in only atrial endocardium @ 12.5 d
MADS	*Dmef2* in all cardial cells @ 5.5 h; lies directly downstream of *tinman*		*GATA-6* in precardiac mesoderm and primitive streak @ 7.0 d, in atrium and ventricle @ 9.5 d, throughout atrial and ventricular endocardium and myocardium @ 12.5 d
			Mef2a in heart @ 8.5 d
			Mef2c in heart primordia@7.5 d, in sinus venosus @8.0 d, in atrium and ventricle @ 8.5 d; knockout dies by 10.5 d
			Mef2d in heart @ 8.5 d
			No looping occurs; the right ventricle and sinus venosus fail to form
bHLH			*dHAND*; knockout dies @ 10.5 d, showing hypoplastic right ventricle and outflow tract but a dilated aortic sac
			eHAND in outflow tract and left ventricle @ 8.0 d
	twist activates *tinman*	*Xtwist* in cephalic neural crest @ stage 16	*M-twist* in first branchial arch @ 8.0 d, in atrioventricular canal endocardial cushion @ 10.0 d; knockout does not have heart phenotype
HLH			Id in ventral, aortae, aortic arch, and dorsal aortae @9.0 d; in atrioventricular cushions and outflow tract ridges @ 10.0 d
Myc			1/3 of c-*myc* knockouts show enlarged heart and pericardial effusion; die by 10.5 d
			N-*Myc* in heart @ 9.5 d in only compact layer of ventricular myocardium @10.5 d; knockout shows reduction in compact layer of ventricular myocardium
MFH-1			Knockout shows type B interruption of left aortic arch in 10/12 and perinatal death
Pax			Homozygous splotch^{2H} show truncus arteriosus @ 13.5 d approximately 50% of the time

Table 12-1 *(continued)*

Gene family	*Drosophila*	*Xenopus*	*Mus*
Transcription factors			
Zfh-1	In dorsal vessel cardioblasts @ stages 11–15; mutant manifests breaks in anterior region of heart and kink in heart shape		
Evi			In truncal and conal ridges and valves @12.5 d
Secreted proteins			
TGF-β			β1 in yolk-sac blood islands and heart mesoderm @ 7.0 d, in endocardium @8.0 d, only in endocardial cushions (both atrioventricular canal and outflow tract) @9.5 d. Knockout does not have heart phenotype (due to transplacental passage of maternal TGF-β1) unless mother is TGF-β1 null. In the latter case, knockout shows poorly formed ventricular lumina and disorganized valves and ventricular myocardium; half die @ 10.5 d due to defective yolk sac vasculogenesis, endothelial differentiation, and hematopoiesis. β2 in sinus venosus @ 8.0 d, in outflow tract and aortic sac @ 8.5 d, in atrioventricular canal and proximal outflow tract myocardium @ 9.5 d β3 in pericardium @ 9.0 d
Vg-1		Injection of mRNA into right-dorsal blastomere randomizes heart looping	
DVR	*dpp* required for activation of dorsal mesoderm genes	*Xbmp4* overexpression ventralizes mesoderm; inhibition dorsalizes mesoderm	*bmp2* in atrial myocardium @9.5 d (low levels in truncus and dorsal aortae), in myocardium of atrioventricular canal (not truncus) @10.5 d *bmp4* in myocardium @8.5 d, more localized to atrioventricular canal region @ 9.0 d, more localized to truncus (aorta) @10.5 d; knockout: heart phenotype varies, depending on genetic background, dies between 7.5 and 10.5 d
Wnt	*wg*^{ts} shifted to nonpermissive temperature @3–5h: ↓#pericardial and cardial cells		
VEGF			In myocardium @ 8.5 d; heterozygotes die @ 11.0 d showing no blood vessels
Neuregulin			In endocardium @ 10.5 d; knockout shows absent ventricular trabeculae and distorted endocardial cushions
Nodal		Xnr-1 in left lateral plate mesoderm @ stage 19	Mouse nodal is in left side of node @ 4-somite stage and in left lateral plate mesoderm @ 5-somite stage
Extracellular proteins			
Tenascin	*odd Oz* in cardioblasts @9.5 h; encodes tenascin like protein		Tenascin-X is in epicardial layer of sinus venosus and atrium @ 12.0 d
Fibronectin			In mesoderm during primitive streak stage, in endocardium @ 5-somite stage; knockout may not develop a heart, depending on genetic background (heart primordia not fused @ 8.5 d)
Laminin	Heart is "broken" (dissociation of pericardial cells)		Knockout does not have heart phenotype
Receptors			
Receptor for PDGF			In dorsal aortae @9.5 d; in ventricular trabeculae, cushions, and pericardium @ 11.5 d; in valves @ 15 d; *Patch* mutation (deletion for PDGFRα) homozygotes show truncus arteriosus, and >50% die by 9.5 d

(continued)

Table 12-1 *(continued)*
Genes Involved in Cardiovascular Morphogenesis

Gene family	*Temporal and spatial expression of mRNA/phenotype of knockout homozygote/overexpression (mRNA injection) data*		
	Drosophila	*Xenopus*	*Mus*
Receptors for neuregulin			*ErbB4* knockout dies @ 10.5 d and shows absent ventricular trabeculae. *ErbB2* knockout dies @ 10.5 d and shows absent ventricular trabeculae
Receptors for TGF-β–like ligands		Injection of truncated activin receptor type IIB mRNA into left-dorsal blastomere (16-cell stage) randomizes heart looping	Activin receptor type II B knockout dies perinatally, showing randomized heart position (and double-outlet right ventricle, right atrial appendage isomerism, and other anolmalies)
VEGF receptors			*flk-1* in heart mesoderm @ 7.0 d, in yolk-sac blood islands @ 8.0 d, in vasculature and endocardium @ 8.5 d; knockout shows no yolk sac blood islands, endocardium, or blood vessels; dies by 9.5 d *flt-1* knockout forms endothelial cells but cannot assemble blood vessels, shows disorganized endocardium, and dies by 9.0 d *tie-1* in vasculature and endocardium @ 8.5 d; knockout shows edema (followed by hemorrhage) due to leaky blood vessels; dies @ birth *tie-2* (also called *tek*) in yolk sac blood islands @ 8.0 d, in vasculature and endocardium @ 8.5 d; knockout shows malformation of vascular network including coronary vessels; dies by 10.5 d showing disorganized dorsal aorta and heart trabeculae
Integrins			α1 α4 knockout shows no epicardium or coronary vessels and dies @ <15.5 d α5 knockout does develop a heart; dies by 11 d (abnormal blood vessel formation) α6 in myocardium@8.5 d; in endothelial cells of atrioventricular canal @ 11.5 d av in heart @ 8.5 d
Ig superfamily			
N-CAM			
PECAM-1			In endothelium of dorsal aorta, endocardium of conotruncus and ventricle@8.5 d
VCAM-1			Knockout has no epicardium and shows reduction in compact layer of ventricular myocardium and ventricular septum, and dies @12.5 d
Retinoic acid receptors			
RXR			α-/-: shows reduction in compact layer of ventricular myocardium and ventricular septum and dies @9.5 d RXRα-/-/RARα-/-: shows reduction in compact layer of ventricular myocardium, truncus arteriosus; aberrant right subclavian artery RXRα-/-/RARγ-/-: shows reduction in compact layer of ventricular myocardium, truncus arteriosus; proximal aorticopulmonary window; isol rpa
RAR			α1β2: TOF, right arch, aberrant left subclavian artery; truncus arteriosus αβ2+/–: truncus arteriosus, right arch; double arch, isol rpa and lpa αβ2: truncus arteriosus, right arch, absent lpa; left arch, aberrant right subclavian artery; right cervical arch, aberrant left subclavian artery; left cervical arch, aberrant right subclavian artery α1γα2+/–:TOF, aberrant right subclavian artery; double-outlet right ventricle αγ: truncus arteriosus, right arch, isolated lpa

Table 12-1 *(continued)*

Gene family	*Drosophila*	*Xenopus*	*Mus*
Channels			
connexin 43			*cx43* in ventricle @ 9.5 d; knockout shows cyanosis, dies shortly after birth, with severe subpulmonary stenosis
Other			
NF-1			Knockout dies @ 13.5 d, shows double-outlet right ventricle with obstruction of both outflow tracts
ET-1			Knockout shows ventricular septal defect in approximately 50%
l-r dynein			*iv* homozygote shows heterotaxy

bHLH, basic helix-loop-helix; *bmp*, bone morphogenetic protein; *cx*, connexin; *dpp*, *decapentaplegic*; DVR, *decapentaplegic*-Vg1-related; Evi, ecotropic viral integration site-1; *flk*, fetal liver kinase; *flt,fms*-like tyrosine kinase; Hox, homeobox; Id, inhibitor of differentiation; Ig, immunoglobulin; isol, isolation of the; lpa, left pulmonary artery; MADS, MCM1, Agamous, Deficiens, Serum Response Factor; Mef, Myocyte enhancer factor; N-CAM, neural cell adhesion molecule; PDGF, platelet-derived growth factor; PDGFR, platelet-derived growth factor receptor; PECAM, platelet endothelial cell adhesion molecule; rpa, right pulmonary artery; TGF-β, transforming growth factor-β; TOF, tetralogy of Fallot; ts, temperature-sensitive; VCAM, vascular cell adhesion molecule; VEGF, vascular endothelial growth factor; *wg*, *wingless*.

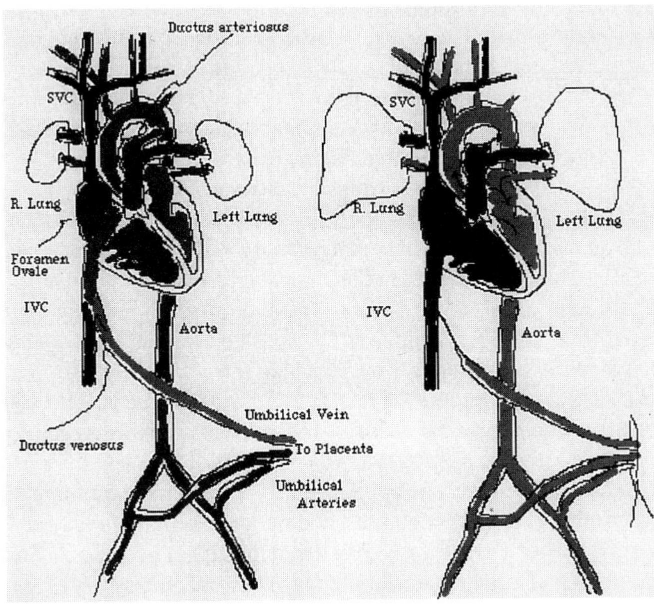

Figure 12-1 (Left) Fetal circulation in the human. Oxygenated blood travels from the placenta to the fetus via the umbilical vein and then the ductus venosus. After combining with deoxygenated inferior vena caval blood, it preferentially streams across the foramen ovale into the left heart and eventually supplies the ascending aorta. Deoxygenated superior vena caval blood preferentially fills the right heart and supplies the descending aorta via the ductus arteriosus. Since they do not function as the gas exchange site, the lungs are not inflated *in utero* and receive very little blood flow. The two sides of the heart function as parallel pumps, communicating at the level of the atria (foramen ovale) and the great arteries (ductus arteriosus). (Right) Neonatal circulation in the human. The lungs inflate, assume their gas exchange function, and begin to receive more blood flow. Ductus venosus and ductus arteriosus constrict in the first few days. The two sides of the heart function as pumps-in-series now; any blood passing through the right heart must eventually also pass through the left heart. (*See* color insert following p. 684.)

A few types of malformation show up after 2 weeks of age. Isolated large septation defects resulting in left-to-right shunt physiology typically do not present in the first 2 weeks of age because the magnitude of the left-to-right shunt depends mostly on the pulmonary vascular resistance, the latter parameter falling to its adult value gradually over the first 6 months. The uncommon condition of anomalous origin of the left coronary artery from the pulmonary artery, which results in gradual-onset myocardial ischemia, also manifests after the neonatal period since the reduction in perfusion of the left ventricle is closely linked to the fall in pulmonary vascular resistance.

DIAGNOSIS

Although the screening protocol includes physical examination, arterial blood gas, electrocardiogram, and chest roentgenogram, currently the principal tool for detailed characterization of both morphology and hemodynamics in the human newborn is ultrasound imaging. With progressive refinement over the last 15 years, its accuracy in assessing anatomy and circulatory physiology in the newborn and young infant now approaches that of cardiac catheterization.

Taking a detailed family history and surveying the patient for even subtle extracardiac anomalies is an increasingly important part of the initial workup. For the detection of deletions, translocations, or duplications, fluorescence *in situ* hybridization (FISH) will become standard as more probes become widely available.

GENETIC BASIS OF DISEASE

Until recently, the prevailing view of the etiology of congenital heart disease was that 8% of defects were single-gene defects, 2% due to teratogens, and 90% were "multifactorial." Three recent classes of observation argue that this view is incorrect. First, as the number of adult survivors of congenital heart disease in the US exceeds 600,000, surveys of the F1 generation reveal a much higher incidence of congenital heart malformation than previously reported. Second, an increasing number of genes responsible for syndromes involving the heart are being identified by positional cloning, a technique based on identifying a DNA marker with which a phenotype cosegregates (Table 12-2). Third, mutations producing phenotypes similar to human congenital heart disease are being identified in several lower vertebrates. In mice, the technique of targeted gene disruption has uncovered models for diGeorge syndrome (*Hox a-3* knockout) and subpulmonary stenosis (*connexin 43* knockout). Spontaneous mutations in the *iv* and

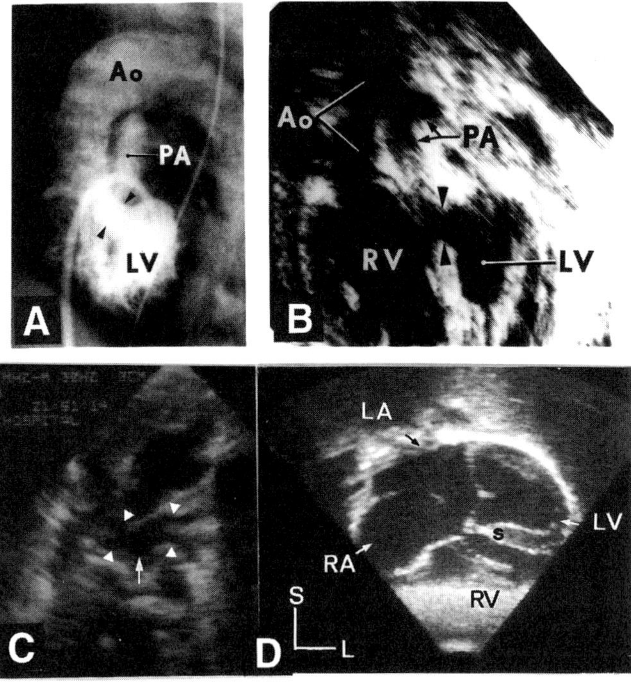

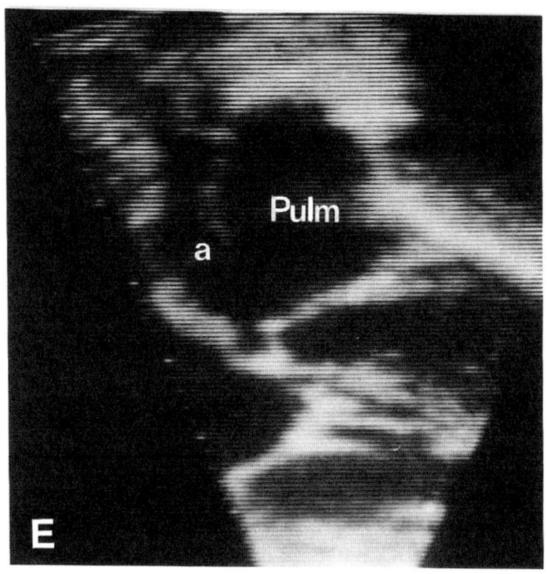

Figure 12-2 **(A,B)** Double-outlet right ventricle with severe subpulmonary stenosis, angiographic and echocardiographic sagittal views, respectively. The ductus arteriosus has already closed. **(C)** Suprasternal frontal echocardiogram showing the pulmonary venous confluence (arrow) in an infant with obstructed total anomalous pulmonary venous connection. The arrowheads point to the individual pulmonary veins. **(D)** Subcostal 4-chamber view of complete common atrioventricular canal. s = muscular ventricular septum. **(E)** Subcostal frontal view of an infant with truncus arteriosus as well as interrupted aortic arch. Note how the truncal root has been separated unequally such that the ascending aortic (a) component is very small compared to the pulmonary arterial (Pulm) component. Other abbreviations: Ao, aorta; L, left; LA, left atrium; LV, left ventricle; PA, pulmonary root; RA, right atrium; RV, right ventricle; S, superior.

pax-3 genes produce models for heterotaxy and truncus arteriosus, respectively. In zebrafish, saturation mutagenesis screens carried out in two laboratories (C. Nüsslein-Volhard at the Max-Planck-Institut, Tübingen, Germany and W. Driever at Massachusetts General Hospital, Boston, MA) have revealed mutants lacking endocardium or valves, manifesting tachyarrhythmias, and demonstrating underdevelopment of particular chambers.

Reverse genetics in the human has been very successful in the last decade as exemplified by the mapping of several familiar disorders to specific chromosomal regions.

Familial supravalvar aortic stenosis (SVAS), an autosomal dominant disorder affecting many large arteries (particularly the pulmonary arteries and the ascending aorta), was found to be coinherited with a DNA polymorphism at 7q11.23. Analysis of a SVAS family in which a balanced translocation involving chromosome 7 cosegregated with the phenotype showed that the elastin gene was disrupted. Another SVAS family manifested a large deletion in the elastin gene. In addition, SVAS also occurs as part of Williams syndrome (supravalvar aortic or pulmonary stenosis, stenoses of other systemic arteries, elfin facies, precocious verbal ability, hypersensitivity to sounds, poor visual-motor integration). Hemizygosity at the elastin locus is present in both sporadic and familial Williams syndrome. Finally, Williams syndrome patients have a very large deletion extending beyond the elastin gene, raising the possibility of a contiguous gene syndrome. This concept has been proposed for diGeorge and Shprintzen (velocardiofacial) syndromes, part of the CATCH 22 (Cardiac defects, Abnormal facies, Thymic hypoplasia, Cleft palate, and Hypocalcemia from chromosome 22 deletions) spectrum (*see* Chapter 120).

Approximately 85% of complete atrioventricular canal patients exhibit Down syndrome. In the complete form of common atrioventricular canal, the atria and ventricles are incompletely septated (Fig. 12-2D); in addition, the atria drain into the ventricles via a single (common) atrioventricular valve with typically five leaflets. Through studies of families with various partial 21 trisomies, a critical region of 9 Mb for atrioventricular canal defects has been identified (21q22.2-21q22.3).

Holt-Oram syndrome (an autosomal dominant condition with forelimb anomalies, ostium secundum atrial septal defects, and atrioventricular block), which mapped to 12q2 in two large families, results from mutations in the human Tbx5 gene.

Although the association of both IAA type B and truncus arteriosus (Fig. 12-2E) with diGeorge syndrome has long been known, the finding that chromosome 22 deletions occurred in many diGeorge patients suggested the hypothesis that a specific gene defect could control arch formation and/or outflow tract development. Chapter 120 discusses the hunt for the diGeorge syndrome gene(s) in much greater detail; although the cloning of a balanced translocation between chromosomes 2 and 22 in a patient with "partial" diGeorge syndrome suggests that the section of DNA disrupted by the translocation breakpoint is responsible for much of the diGeorge phenotype, it may not be responsible for the heart disease (the affected individual had only aortic coarctation and no intracardiac malformation).

The further discovery that many nonsyndromic patients with interrupted aortic arch, truncus arteriosus, and tetralogy of Fallot have chromosome 22 microdeletions has instigated an effort to reclassify our patient populations genetically or developmentally. Because of its noninvasive nature, ultrasound imaging will emerge as the dominant postnatal screening method to construct the large pedigrees that form the substrate for investigation.

Table 12-2
Developmental Classification Scheme

Phenotype in H. sapiens	*Gene product*	*Chromosomal locus in H. sapiens*
Heart malposition		
Ectopia cordis		
Heterotaxy syndrome		(Familial variant—Xq24-q27.1)
Isolated dextrocardia		
Looping		
L-loop		
Supero-infero ventricles		
Ascending aorta/aortic arch/pulmonary artery (obstruction, interruption, dilatation, arch sidedness)		
Peripheral pulmonic stenosis (Alagille syndrome)	Jagged1	20p12
Coarctation (Turner syndrome)		Monosomy X
Familial supravalvar aortic stenosis and Williams syndrome	Elastin	7q11.23 deletion
Aortic dilation (Marfan syndrome)	Fibrillin-1	15q21.1
Aortic dilation (Ehler-Danlos syndrome, type IV)	Type III collagen	2q31
Arch interruption, right arch, anomalous origin of arch vessels (diGeorge syndrome)		
Conotruncus (outflow valve development, alignment, septation)		
Truncus arteriosus, TOF (malalignment VSD with subpulmonary stenosis), TOF with pulmonary atresia, TOF with isol rpa or lpa, double-outlet RV, malalignment VSD with subaortic stenosis (diGeorge syndrome)		22q11.2 deletion
Double-outlet RV, TOF	Trisomy 18	
Transposition of the great arteries		
Double-outlet left ventricle		
Anatomically corrected malposition of the great arteries		
Valvar aortic stenosis		
Valvar pulmonary stenosis (Noonan syndrome)		
Atrioventricular canal (valve development, septation)		
Complete AV canal, partial AV canal (Down syndrome)		Trisomy 21q22
Mitral and tricuspid prolapse (Marfan syndrome)	Fibrillin-1	15q21.1
Mitral and tricuspid dysplasia		Trisomy 18
Single ventricle		
Ventricles (septation, dysplasia, hypoplasia)		
Tricuspid atresia		
Ebstein's anomaly (RV dysplasia)		
Spongy myocardium		
Muscular VSDs		
Atria, systemic veins, pulmonary veins (septation, alignment)		
Sinus venosus type "ASDs"		
Ostium secundum ASDs (Holt-Oram syndrome)	Tbx5	12q2
Anomalous systemic venous connection		
Anomalous pulmonary venous connection		
Hypoplastic left heart syndrome		

ASD, atrial septal defect; isol, isolation of the; lpa, left pulmonary artery; rpa, right pulmonary artery; RV, right ventricle; TOF, tetralogy of Fallot; VSD, ventricular septal defect.

MOLECULAR PATHOPHYSIOLOGY OF DISEASE

Although the physiologically based schema mentioned in the Clinical Features section works quite well for the clinician, a developmentally oriented classification of defects (taking advantage of the fact that all vertebrate hearts appear to go through a straight heart tube stage) may be more appropriate for the molecular biologist (Table 12-2): heart malposition (i.e., abnormal positioning of the heart vis-à-vis the ventral-dorsal, rostral-caudal, and left-right body axes), looping, ascending aorta/aortic arch/pulmonary artery, conotruncus, atrioventricular canal, ventricles, and atria/systemic veins/pulmonary veins. Notice that situs inversus totalis is not listed since these rare individuals are a left-right mirror-image of normal and do not necessarily have any heart disease.

Since few gene products have yet been identified, the way gene alterations contribute to pathology is still obscure. For example, how a reduced level of elastin results in the gradual development of supravalvar aortic stenosis is unclear. One hypothesis is that recurring damage to the endothelium of relatively inelastic arteries provokes intimal proliferation followed by fibrosis. Consistent with this hypothesis is the clinical observation that pulmonary arterial stenoses tend not to progress (the normal pulmonary vascular resistance decline results in gradual lowering of right ventricular pressure after birth, presumably lowering the shear forces on the main pulmonary branches).

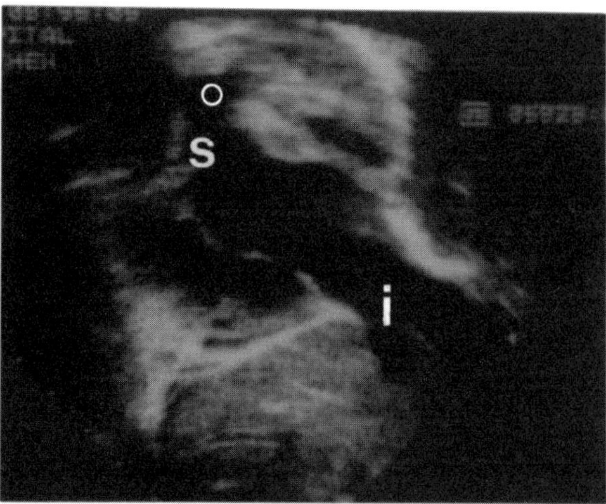

Figure 12-3 Sagittal echocardiographic view of a modified Fontan repair. The superior (s) and inferior vena caval (i) flows have been rerouted directly into the proximal right pulmonary artery (open circle).

The anomalies in the CATCH 22 phenotype are in structures to which migrating neural crest cells contribute, so it is understandable that much attention is being focused on genes known to be important in cell–cell signaling and cell movement. However, other work centering on transcription factors that may function as master controls is also important. Vertebrate homologs to the *Drosophila* homeodomain-containing gene *tinman* (without which the fly does not form a heart) have been cloned recently, showing that control of cardiac formation is likely to have been conserved over 600 million years.

MANAGEMENT/TREATMENT

The vast majority of congenital heart malformations have now become rather straightforward to correct surgically. Even the varieties with hypoplasia of one or the other ventricle can be palliated well with a modified Fontan operation, in which the systemic venous circulation is rerouted directly into the pulmonary arteries (Fig. 12-3); the remaining questions for cardiologists and cardiovascular surgeons center around the prevention of arrhythmic and effusive complications and the search for ways of manipulating neonatal pulmonary vascular impedance so that the Fontan operation would not need to be staged as it is now.

Assessment of the quality of the surgical repair is no longer done 6 or 12 months postoperatively but rather in the operating room or shortly before hospital discharge. Long-term follow-up is typically done using noninvasive techniques such as ultrasound, magnetic resonance scanning, and exercise testing.

The only ways of further lowering the morbidity of congenital heart defects are prevention (by genotyping and counseling), termination *in utero* upon phenotype recognition, and better prenatal or postnatal screening. While the second may be practiced in some countries, for religious and ethical reasons it is doubtful whether it will ever be widely implemented in the US. The third way has so far not proved cost-effective. Hence, efforts will likely be concentrated on the first approach. As a prerequisite, more work needs to be done to understand the construction of the heart and vessels at the molecular level.

FUTURE DIRECTIONS

Some of the questions that biologists hope to answer are:

1. How do the myocardial, endocardial, and vascular endothelial lineages become specified?
2. How is the heart tube "patterned" and situated? (Do the same families of molecules responsible for body axis patterning get reused in the patterning of organs?)
3. How are the cardiac valves formed?
4. How is the conduction system formed? Humans with abnormal lateralization or looping have anomalous conduction systems.
5. Given that in mammalian hearts two atria and two ventricles function in parallel and develop in tandem *in utero*, how is growth of the left heart exquisitely matched to that of the right heart throughout gestation?
6. How are mechanisms constructed during embryonic development that allow heart rate and contractility to be modulated by both the nervous system and circulating hormones?
7. How are myocardial cells maintained in a state of terminal differentiation?

A variety of organisms will yield answers to these questions.

Although laboratories studying the mouse system will continue to create knockouts including double and triple knockouts, mice carrying specific mutations rather than null mutants may be more illuminating. Furthermore, tissue-specific mutations will also become feasible. Zebrafish labs will continue to analyze more than 100 recessive mutations affecting cardiovascular development that have been isolated in the Tübingen and Boston saturation mutagenesis screens. Cloning the genes affected in these mutants will be facilitated by the completion of a genetic map. Finally, positional cloning will continue to be utilized for large human families with single-gene disorders.

SELECTED REFERENCES

Budarf M, Collins J, Gong W, et al. Cloning a balanced translocation associated with diGeorge syndrome and identification of a disrupted candidate gene. Nat Genet 1995;10:269–277.

Chen J-N, Haffter P, Odenthal J, et al. Mutations affecting the cardiovascular system and other internal organs in zebrafish. Development 1996;123:293–302.

Goldmuntz E, Emanuel BS. Genetic disorders of cardiac morphogenesis. The DiGeorge and Velocardiofacial syndromes. Circ Res 1997; 80:437–443.

Harvey RP. NK-2 homeobox genes and heart development. Dev Biol 1996;178:203–216.

Keating M. Elastin and vascular disease. Trends Cardiovasc Med 1994;4:165–169.

Kimmel CB. Genetics and early development of zebrafish. Trends in Genetics 1989;5:283–288.

Kuo CT, Morrisey EE, Anandappa R, et al. GATA 4 transcription factor is required for ventral morphogenesis and heart tube formation. Genes Dev 1997;11:1048–1060.

Lee RY, Luo J, Evans RM, Giguere V, Surov HM. Compartment-selective sensitivity of cardiovascular morphogenetics to combinations of retinoic acid receptor gene mutations. Circ Res 1997; 80:757–764.

Lin Q, Schwarz J, Bucana C, Olson EN. Control of mouse cardiac morphogenesis and myogenesis by transcription factor MEF2C. Science 1997;276:1404–1407.

Molkentin JD, Lin Q, Duncan SA, Olson EN. Requirement of the transcription factor GATA4 for heart tube formation and ventral morphogenesis. Genes Dev 1997;11:1061–1072.

Reaume AG, deSousa PA, Kulkarni S, et al. Cardiac malformation in neonatal mice lacking connexin 43. Science 1995;267:1831–1834.

Srivastava D, Thomas T, Lin Q, Kirby ML, Brown D, Olson EN. Regulation of cardiac mesodermal and neural crest development by the bHLH transcription factor dHAND. Nat Genet 1997;16:154–160.

Stainier DYS, Fouquet B, Chen J-N, et al. Mutations affecting the formation and function of the cardiovascular system in the zebrafish embryo. Development 1996;123:285–292.

Supp DM, Witte DP, Potter SS, Brueckner M. Mutation of an axonemal dynein affects left-right asymmetry in inversus viscerum mice. Nature 1997;389:963–966.

Tonissen KF, Drysdale TA, Lints TJ, Harvey RP, Krieg PA. *XNkx*-2.5, a *Xenopus* gene related to *Nkx-2.5* and *tinman*: evidence for a conserved role in cardiac development. Dev Biol 1994;162: 325–328.

Weinstein B, Stemple DL, Driever W, Fishman MC. *Gridlock*, a localized heritable vascular patterning defect in the zebrafish. Nature Medicine 1995;1:1143–1147.

Wu X, Golden K, Bodmer R. Heart development in *Drosophila* requires the segment polarity gene *wingless*. Dev Biol 1995; 169:619–628.

Yang JT, Rayburn H, Hynes RO. Cell adhesion events mediated by α4 integrins are essential in placental and cardiac development. Development 1995;121:529–560.

13 Inherited Cardiomyopathies

CHRISTINE E. SEIDMAN, CALUM MACRAE, AND J. G. SEIDMAN

INTRODUCTION

The cardiomyopathies are primary disorders of the myocardium that traditionally are classified as hypertrophic, dilated, or restrictive. Although these descriptors reflect a common anatomy and/or the pathophysiology exhibited by affected individuals, the natural history of these disorders often encompasses more than one subclassification. That is, some individuals with hypertrophic cardiomyopathy exhibit little myocardial hypertrophy; others develop increased cardiac chamber size with clinical manifestations that typify idiopathic dilated cardiomyopathy. Similarly, myocyte hypertrophy is a common histopathologic manifestation of dilated cardiomyopathy. To understand the molecular signals that cause cardiac remodeling, researchers have sought to elucidate the genetic bases for hypertrophic, dilated, and restrictive cardiomyopathies. These studies may help to define pathways of cardiac remodeling that also occur in response to common cardiovascular pathologies.

Application of molecular genetic approaches to the study of inherited cardiomyopathies has yielded much progress. This approach requires the identification of affected families with multiple affected individuals. As a first step, linkage studies are performed to identify the chromosome location (or loci) of the disease gene. Subsequent analyses of candidate genes that map to the defined region and/or positional cloning of novel genes enables identification of mutations that cause the pathology. Molecular genetic studies have been particularly productive in elucidating many gene defects that cause hypertrophic cardiomyopathy. Although disease genes have yet to be identified that cause dilated cardiomyopathies inherited as a dominant trait, an ever-increasing number of loci responsible for these disorders have been mapped in the genome. Further, the molecular etiologies of several X-linked dilated cardiomyopathies have been elucidated. Unfortunately, application of molecular genetics to the restrictive cardiomyopathies remains limited, probably because these disorders occur infrequently and familial cases are extremely rare. Because neither the disease genes nor loci that cause restrictive cardiomyopathies are known, this disorder will not be reviewed further.

Elucidation of the genetic basis of inherited cardiomyopathies has refined classification of hypertrophic and dilated cardiomyopathies into distinct gene (or locus) defects. While compilation of the complete spectrum of genetic etiologies that cause these cardiomyopathies remains an ongoing effort, the data reviewed in this chapter and future progress will have significant relevance to patient diagnosis and management. Identification of cardiomyopathy genes allows characterization of a preclinical stage in these disorders. This provides a new perspective on the natural history of the cardiomyopathies that may ultimately foster early intervention. More immediately, individuals at risk for inherited cardiomyopathies can be recognized, and appropriate longitudinal evaluation can be initiated. Genetic studies have also clarified the relationship of sporadic and familial disease in some cardiomyopathies. Because sporadic disease can be due to *de novo* mutations in genes that cause familial disease, assessment of risk and genetic counseling of individuals with sporadic disease can be guided by the experiences of individuals with known familial disease. Perhaps most importantly, these studies have demonstrated substantial genetic heterogeneity in the cardiomyopathies; distinct genetic etiologies appear to account in part for the variable clinical phenotypes of dilated and hypertrophic cardiomyopathies. In dominant hypertrophic cardiomyopathy, genotype has been shown to influence clinical outcome. When the genetic basis for cardiomyopathies is more fully solved, our understanding of the complex relationship between genotype and phenotype will undoubtedly improve management of these disorders.

HYPERTROPHIC CARDIOMYOPATHY: A DISEASE OF THE SARCOMERE

CLINICAL STUDIES Hypertrophic cardiomyopathy is a disorder characterized by an increase in cardiac mass accompanied by myocyte and myofibrillar disarray. Outmoded clinical terms such as asymmetric septal hypertrophy (ASH), idiopathic subaortic hypertrophic stenosis (IHSS), and hypertrophic obstructive cardiomyopathy described the marked increase in myocardial septal mass found in some patients. However the widespread use of two-dimensional echocardiograms, family studies, and recent genetic research have demonstrated considerable variation in the location, symmetry, and extent of hypertrophy in affected individuals. Clinical diagnosis is generally based on finding unexplained left ventricular wall thickness greater than 13 mm at any location. Hypertrophic cardiomyopathy can occur without symptoms, but most individuals experience dypsnea, angina, and palpitations. Presyncopal symptoms are of particular concern because of the increased risk for sudden death in some affected individuals. Arrhythmias, embolic events, and congestive heart failure contribute to the premature morbidity and mortality of this disorder.

From: *Principles of Molecular Medicine* (J. L. Jameson, ed.), ©1998 Humana Press Inc., Totowa, NJ.

Table 13-1
Features of Familial Hypertrophic Cardiomyopathy Loci

Locus	*Gene*	*Penetrance*	*Prognosis*
1q32	Cardiac troponin T	Incomplete	Poor
7q3	Unknown	Variable for WPW	Unknown
11q1	Cardiac myosin binding protein C	Incomplete	Limited data; generally good
14q1	β Cardiac myosin heavy chain	Usually complete	Variable; Mutation-dependent
15q2	α Tropomyosin	Usually complete	Limited data

Family studies have demonstrated hypertrophic cardiomyopathy to be a heritable disorder that is transmitted as autosomal dominant trait or as a sporadic disease. Hypertrophic cardiomyopathy is not a rare condition; a recent report of more than 7000 two-dimensional echocardiograms of young individuals in the United States (obtained to screen for coronary artery disease) demonstrated the disorder in 0.2% of this population. No racial nor ethnic groups are predisposed to the condition.

GENETIC STUDIES Molecular genetic analyses of familial hypertrophic cardiomyopathy (FHC) have identified disease loci (Table 13-1) on five chromosomes. To date, four disease genes have been identified: cardiac troponin T (chromosome 1), cardiac myosin binding protein C (chromosome 11), β cardiac myosin heavy chain (chromosome 14), and α tropomyosin. Collectively these genes account for approximately 60–70% of all FHC, thus indicating that other disease genes are yet to be identified. Only one other FHC locus has been mapped to chromosome 7; in one family, a mutation in this locus causes both FHC and Wolff-Parkinson-White syndrome (WPW).

More than 30 different mutations in the β cardiac myosin heavy-chain gene have been demonstrated to cause FHC. All are point mutations that alter one amino acid residue in the globular head or head-rod junction of the myosin heavy chain. In some instances, affected members from unrelated families have identical mutations. However, genetic (haplotype) analyses indicate that most mutations arose as an independent event; there is little evidence for a mutation founder effect in FHC. In addition to causing familial disease, *de novo* mutations in the β cardiac myosin heavy-chain gene have been demonstrated to cause sporadic hypertrophic cardiomyopathy.

While there is clinical variation in the phenotype associated with β cardiac myosin heavy-chain gene mutations, these defects are usually quite penetrant by adulthood. That is, although children may not exhibit signs or symptoms of disease, demonstrable hypertrophy (detected by two-dimensional echocardiograms) is typically evident in gene carriers by age 20. Figure 13-1 shows the parasternal long axis view of a two-dimensional echocardiogram from an 18-year-old with FHC caused by a missense (Arg453Cys) mutation in exon 14; there is significant interventricular septal and posterior ventricular wall hypertrophy. Marked myocardial hypertrophy characterizes many β cardiac myosin heavy-chain mutations; analyses of affected individuals from six families with different myosin mutations found a mean maximal left ventricular wall thickness = 23.7 ± 7.7 mm. Despite nearly complete disease penetrance and significant hypertrophy that is associated with β cardiac myosin heavy-chain gene mutations, survival varies considerably and is, in part, mutation-specific. That is, individuals with the Arg403Gln mutation have markedly shortened life expectancies (average age of death = 45 years), whereas survival is near normal in individuals carrying the Val606Met mutation. The change (or absence) of amino acid charge appears to influence outcome in FHC. In general, conservative mutations are associated with a better prognosis than nonconservative mutations. A mouse model of FHC has been created using the Arg403Gln mutation. Homozygous mice die soon after birth, but cardiac histopathology and dysfunction in heterozygotes resemble human FHC. This model may be useful to help define the natural history and pathophysiology of FHC. Although more data is required to provide a complete profile of the phenotypes associated with each myosin mutation, preliminary data clearly indicate that genotype may assist in risk stratification of premature death in FHC.

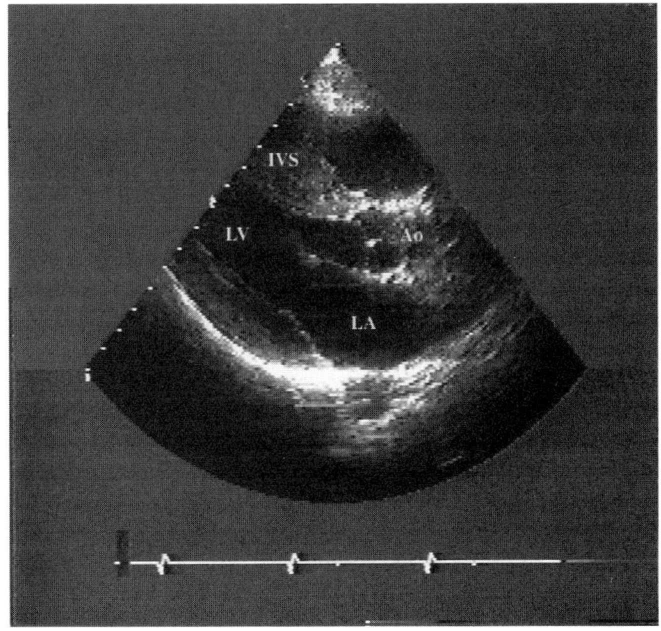

Figure 13-1 The echocardiographic findings of hypertrophic cardiomyopathy. Parasternal long axis view of the heart shows significant hypertrophy of the interventricular septum (IVS) and posterior ventricular wall. Cavity size of the left ventricle (LV) is normal, but the left atrium (LA) is enlarged. The aorta (Ao) is indicated.

β Cardiac myosin heavy chains are abundantly expressed in the adult ventricle and at much lower levels in slow twitch skeletal muscles. Expression of this isoform outside of the heart has prompted evaluation of skeletal muscle structure and function in FHC patients. Intriguingly, there is histologic evidence of central core disease (*see* Chapter 104) in some patients with β cardiac myosin heavy-chain gene mutations, although a clinically significant skeletal myopathy has not been observed.

Mutations in cardiac troponin T account for approximately 15% of all FHC. Unlike FHC mutations in myosin, these gene defects include small deletions and mutations in splice signals, in addition to missense mutations. The FHC phenotype produced by each of these mutations is, however, strikingly similar. Affected individuals have substantially less cardiac hypertrophy than that observed with myosin mutations; mean maximal left ventricular wall thickness =16.7 ± 5.5 mm for cardiac troponin T mutations ($p < 0.001$; [5]). The hypertrophy found in some adult individuals with cardiac troponin T mutations is less than standard criteria for diagnosis. Despite this reduced penetrance, all reported cardiac troponin T mutations are associated with markedly reduced survival.

α Tropomyosin gene mutations are a rare cause of FHC; less than 5% of cases are caused by these gene defects. Because of their infrequent occurrence, less information is available regarding the correlation between genotype and phenotype. However these mutations are biologically interesting, because unlike all other FHC genes, α tropomyosin is widely expressed outside of the heart. The mechanism by which a cardiac-specific phenotype is produced by these mutations is unknown. Because some FHC mutations in α tropomyosin occur in regions that interact with troponin T, the tissue-specific isoform cardiac troponin T may restrict dysfunction to the myocardium. Alternatively, FHC mutations in α tropomyosin may perturb a function that is unique and/or critical to cardiac myocytes.

Recent studies have demonstrated that cardiac myosin binding protein-C mutations cause FHC. This polypeptide participates in thick filament assembly by binding myosin heavy chain and titin. In addition, the protein appears to modulate myosin ATPase activity and participates in adrenergic regulation of cardiac contraction. Three FHC mutations have been reported in cardiac myosin binding protein-C: two of these alter splice signals; the third mutation is a six amino acid insertion. The location of these mutations predict that each will perturb the ability of the peptide to bind myosin. Despite the limited number of known FHC mutations in cardiac myosin binding protein-C, linkage studies suggest that this locus contributes 10–15% of all FHC cases. Available clinical data suggests that cardiac myosin binding protein-C mutations are associated with reduced disease penetrance and better prognosis than that observed with cardiac troponin T and some myosin mutations.

SIGNIFICANCE OF GENETIC STUDIES Molecular genetic analyses of FHC have demonstrated mutations in β cardiac myosin heavy chain, α tropomyosin, cardiac troponin T, and cardiac myosin binding protein-C, thus defining this as a disease of the sarcomere. This result has implications for further basic research and clinical studies of cardiac hypertrophy. First, because four disease genes encode sarcomere proteins, it is likely that FHC genes yet to be identified will similarly encode proteins involved in cardiac contraction. Second, because most mutations are missense or alter splice signals, they are likely to encode stable proteins that are incorporated into the multimeric components of the sarcomere. These dysfunctional components presumably produce a dominant negative effect on the myocardial sarcomere. Third, the dysfunctional sarcomere must trigger intracellular signals that result in the clinical features of FHC.

There are several clinical ramifications of these data. First, based on genotype, a preclinical phenotype has been identified in children at risk. Although two-dimensional echocardiograms of young children with an FHC mutation are typically normal, their electrocardiograms usually demonstrate minor abnormalities. Second, disease penetrance appears to be dependent on both age and mutation type. Cardiac hypertrophy in affected adults is quite variable and can be subtle. Despite its name, FHC can occur with little hypertrophy. Third, genotype can provide prognostic information in FHC.

Definition of the precise mutation that causes FHC in an affected individual remains a difficult task. The FHC genes currently identified appear to encompass only 70% of cases. Further, because most mutations appear to be family-specific, there is considerable cost and complexity in mutation identification. While this remains a research tool at present, the rapid advances in DNA technologies are likely to make genotyping of FHC patients a useful clinical test in the near future.

HYPERTROPHIC CARDIOMYOPATHIES OF CHILDHOOD

CLINICAL STUDIES Recent clinical studies estimate that 30% of cardiomyopathy in children may be familial. The clinical presentations of these pediatric disorders differs significantly from the hypertrophic cardiomyopathies discussed in prior sections. That is, FHC that is caused by sarcomere gene mutations generally does not present until after childhood. Accurate clinical diagnosis of FHC in children at risk can actually be quite difficult until after the growth spurt of puberty. Similarly, many familial dilated cardiomyopathies are rare in childhood, and the age of onset of those associated with conduction system disease is generally after the third decade. In addition to syndromic disorders that are not discussed, molecular genetic studies of pediatric cardiomyopathies have identified defects of mitochondrial genes (*see* Chapter 103), and mutations in nuclear genes involved in fatty acid β-oxidation. Recent progress in understanding autosomal cardiomyopathies caused by mutations encoding proteins involved in fatty acid β-oxidation is reviewed here.

Patterns of inheritance, age of onset, and natural history of infantile cardiomyopathies have demonstrated significant differences from clinically related adult disorders. The clinical genetics of these pediatric disorders demonstrates autosomal recessive transmission. Affected children have two mutated alleles of genes encoding proteins involved in cardiac energy metabolism. Their heterozygous parents, with one normal and one mutated allele, are clinically well. The cardiomyopathies produced by these mutations are often hypertrophic, but cardiac dilation also occurs. The hemodynamic consequences of infantile hypertrophic cardiomyopathy are different from that of FHC. Infantile hypertrophic cardiomyopathies typically cause impaired systolic function, which usually occurs late in the natural history of FHC. In contrast, the dilated phenotype is not dissimilar from that of affected adults. Endomyocardial biopsy is useful in diagnosing infantile cardiomyopathies: lipid-laden cytoplasmic inclusion bodies help to define those disorders due to defects in energy metabolism.

The natural history of these cardiomyopathies can include heart failure, pulmonary edema, arrhythmias, and sudden death. As in FHC, sudden death may be the presenting manifestation of the disorder. However, symptoms and episodic cardiac dysfunction are generally precipitated by fasting states, such as childhood illnesses. Although these recessive cardiomyopathies can be severe and progressive, careful management of these children enables them to become clinically well and less susceptible to cardiac episodes. The biochemical basis for the age-dependent improved outcome is unknown.

GENETIC STUDIES Molecular genetic analyses of infantile cardiomyopathies have identified several defects in transport proteins or enzymes involved in fatty acid β-oxidation, the major source of energy in the myocardium during periods of hypoglycemia. Carnitine is a required cofactor for entry of long-chain fatty acids into mitochondria and carnitine deficiency blocks metabolism of these fatty acids and ketones. Carnitine deficiency results from mutations in several genes including a transporter for intracellular uptake, carnitine-acylcarnitine shuttling (for translocation of carnitine into mitochondria [12]), and carnitine palmitoyltransferase II, which catalyzes carnitine derivatives into acyl-CoA (chromosome 1p32). Although limited numbers of mutations have been identified in each of these genes, recognition of these defects enables therapy. In some instances, pharmacologic doses of carnitine may provide clinical improvement.

The cardiac substrates for mitochondrial β-oxidation are fatty acids of variable chain lengths. Four acyl-CoA dehydrogenases (CAD) selectively act on very-long-chain, long-chain, medium-chain, and short-chain fatty acids. Mutations in the genes encoding very-long-chain, long-chain (chromosome 7), and medium-chain acyl-CoA (chromosome 1p) dehydrogenases result in cardiomyopathies. Estimates of the incidence of these mutations in the general population range from 1 in 10,000 to 1 in 15,000.

Several different types of mutations have been identified in each dehydrogenase, including splice signal, insertion, and missense mutations. Mutations in the medium chain acyl-CoA dehydrogenase are most common at nucleotide residue 985. An A-to-G transition at this site accounts for approximately 90% of individuals with medium chain acyl-CoA dehydrogenase deficiency. Haplotype analyses provide data strongly suggesting a founder effect.

SIGNIFICANCE OF GENETIC STUDIES Molecular genetic studies have demonstrated that childhood hypertrophic cardiomyopathy results from energy deprivation. This hypothesis is furthered by analyses of mitochondrial respiratory gene mutations; these similarly cause cardiomyopathies. The mechanisms by which defects in energy result in cardiac hypertrophy is unknown. However, these studies clearly demonstrate that energy deprivation causes cardiac remodeling and dysfunction. It is particularly intriguing that these mutations can produce both the hypertrophic and dilated phenotype; there may be common signals in these different cardiac remodeling pathways. Understanding the biochemical consequences of these metabolic defects may help to elucidate important mechanisms in other non heritable forms of cardiac remodeling.

Genetic studies of fatty acid β-oxidation mutations have improved clinical management of patients with these defects. First, definition of the molecular bases for these disorders has enabled presymptomatic diagnosis of children at risk. This is particularly important because of the impact that dietary therapy can have on survival. Further, these studies define a novel basis for cardiac arrhythmias. Defects in these pathways have been shown to increase intracellular long-chain fatty acylcarnitines, which are toxic to mitochondria and may induce ventricular arrhythmias that contribute to sudden death. In addition to usual therapeutics to manage life-threatening arrhythmias, understanding the biochemical defect has provided effective approaches to restore energy supplies to the heart, thereby reducing sudden cardiac death in affected children.

DILATED CARDIOMYOPATHIES

CLINICAL STUDIES Dilated cardiomyopathy is characterized by cardiac chamber dilatation and contractile dysfunction. A large number of acquired and inherited disorders can cause this phenotype, and estimated prevalence of dilated cardiomyopathy approximates 37 per 100,000 individuals. In most cases the cause is unknown. Dilated cardiomyopathy is the most common indication of heart transplantation in the United States and accounts for up to one-third of severe heart failure in individuals 25–65 years old.

Although there has been significant progress in identifying the cellular changes that may contribute to the cardiac dysfunction of dilated cardiomyopathy, these studies have not provided a unifying pathophysiologic mechanism nor suggested a molecular mechanism. Findings include impaired sarcoplasmic reticulum calcium handling, atypical myocyte potassium currents and autoantibodies to myosin, adrenergic receptors, and other antigens. Animal models of dilated cardiomyopathy have also been studied including a natural occurring recessive hamster cardiomyopathy and murine models generated by autoimmunization with myosin or infection with cardiotropic enteroviruses. The relationship, if any, of these models to human disease is unknown.

Recent systematic screening of probands' families has suggested a genetic component to dilated cardiomyopathy. Over 25% of probands had first-degree relatives with evidence of dilated cardiomyopathy. In addition, up to 20% of first-degree relatives had evidence of ventricular enlargement without contractile dysfunction. Figure 13-2 shows the parasternal long axis view of a two-dimensional echocardiogram from a 14-year-old with family history of dilated cardiomyopathy; her study exhibited significant left atrial and ventricular chamber dilation. The precise relationship between this phenomenon and clinically significant dilated cardiomyopathy is currently unknown. These studies are supportive of two primary modes of inheritance in familial dilated cardiomyopathy: X-linked and autosomal-dominant.

Family studies of probands with dilated cardiomyopathy have demonstrated cardiac abnormalities in family members. Findings include atrial cardiomyopathy, atrioventricular block, hypertrophic cardiomyopathy, and ventricular tachycardia. This clinical diversity has implied that familial dilated cardiomyopathy is a genetically heterogeneous disorder. To elucidate the molecular bases for the many phenotypes observed in conjunction with cardiac dilatation, large families have been clinically evaluated and DNA isolated for linkage analysis. Unfortunately the majority of study families are small, in part due to the significant premature mortality associated with these disorders. The limited numbers of families appropriate for genetic studies has also hindered progress of gene identification. Autosomal-dominant dilated cardiomyopathy loci are often defined by analyses of a single family, which often has insufficient power to move from a genomic location to disease gene. Hence our knowledge of the genetic bases for dilated cardiomyopathies is currently limited to identification of disease loci.

GENETIC STUDIES Three X-linked syndromes with associated dilated cardiomyopathies have been mapped and disease-causing mutations identified. Cardiomyopathy can be found in patients with Duchenne/Becker muscular dystrophy and in some patients represents the dominant clinical phenotype. Deletions in the 5' muscle promoter of the dystrophin gene are associated with an "isolated" cardiac phenotype. Although muscle biopsies can demonstrate classical features of these dystrophies, these are often subclinical. A recently described mutation causing a premature stop codon has also been found in a family with no clinical skeletal myopathy. However, genetic analyses of the dystrophin promoter in patients with isolated idiopathic cardiomyopathy failed to detect any mutations, thereby suggesting that this is a rare cause of sporadic, adult onset dilated cardiomyopathy.

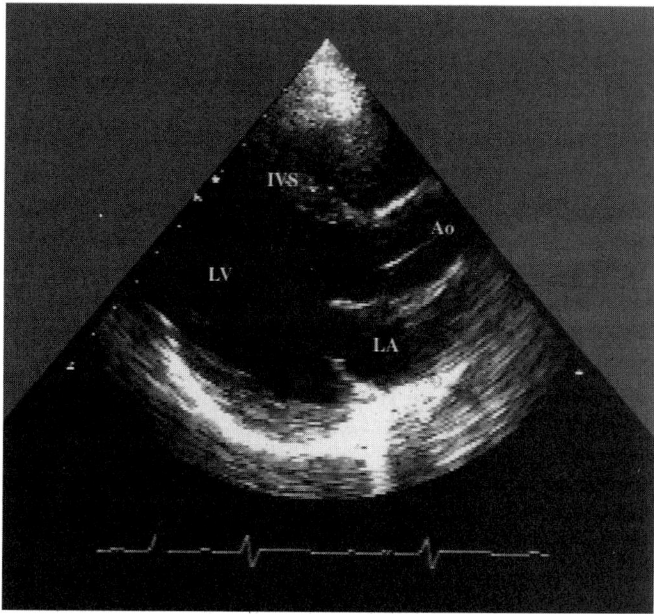

Figure 13-2 The echocardiographic findings of familial dilated cardiomyopathy. Parasternal long axis view of the heart shows normal wall thickness (compare interventricular septum [IVS] with hypertrophic septum in Fig. 13-1), but left ventricular (LV) chamber dilation. The left atrium (LA) is normal; the aorta (Ao) is indicated.

Table 13-2
Clinical Features of Dilated Cardiomyopathy Loci

Locus	*Gene*	*Inheritance*	*Associated Phenotypes*
1p1-1q1	Unknown	Dominant	Conduction system disease
1q24	Unknown	Dominant	None
3p2	Unknown	Dominant	Conduction system disease; CVA
9q13	Unknown	Dominant	None
Xp21	Dystrophin	X-linked	Variable involvement of skeletal muscles
Xq2	Tafazzin	X-linked	Short stature; neutropenia
Xq28	Emerin	X-linked	Skeletal muscle and conduction system disease

Emery-Driefuss muscular dystrophy causes progressive skeletal muscle dysfunction, contractures, and cardiomyopathy, typically associated with atrioventricular conduction abnormalities (*see* Chapter 94). Atrial paralysis, atrial fibrillation, and atrial flutter are common; symptoms often result from infra nodal conduction with slow junctional rhythms and atrioventricular block. The disorder has been mapped to the distal end of the X chromosome, and is therefore genetically (and clinically) distinct from the Duchenne/Becker muscular dystrophy locus. The genetic cause of this disorder has recently been identified (Emerin) through genetic mapping strategies. Although the function of the novel protein Emerin, remains unknown, it is localized to the nuclear membrane of muscle cells.

Barth's syndrome is a rare X-linked infantile disorder that is often lethal in childhood. Affected individuals exhibit a dilated cardiomyopathy, short stature, and neutropenia. Genetic mapping studies defined a locus that overlaps the Emery-Driefuss muscular dystrophy critical region. However, recent positional cloning have demonstrated these disorders to be due to different gene defects. Barth's syndrome is caused by mutations in a novel gene called tafazzin. Alternative splicing of this gene produces multiple transcripts that are expressed in a variety of tissues. Whether distinct mutations in tafazzins will correlate with clinical findings of this disease is unknown.

Dilated cardiomyopathies that are transmitted as an autosomal-dominant trait also provide evidence for clinical and genetic heterogeneity. The relationship of these to the X-linked disorders remains unknown, because at present no autosomal disease genes have been defined.

The first autosomal-dominant kindreds to be mapped were classified as conduction disease with dilated cardiomyopathy (Table 13-2). In one large kindred, affected individuals over the age of 30 years developed progressive conduction system disease characterized by atrial arrythmias, atrial fibrillation, atrioventricular block. In conjunction with the conduction system disease, myocardial disease was evident and culminated in ventricular chamber dilation and congestive heart failure. Longitudinal studies have demonstrated some improvement with pacemaker implantation, but in other affected individuals disease progression continued. Genetic linkage studies mapped this disorder to the centromeric region of chromosome 1. A second family with autosomal-dominant conduction disease and dilated cardiomyopathy has been studied. Sinoatrial node dysfunction progressed to supraventricular tachyarrhythmias, and His-Purkinje system conduction delay and was accompanied by chamber dilation. Despite similarities to the clinical phenotype produced by the disease locus on chromosome 1, molecular genetic studies mapped the cardiomyopathy in this family to a distinct locus, on chromosome 3p25-p22.

Several kindreds with isolated dilated cardiomyopathy, unaccompanied by conduction system disease, have also been studied. Adult onset, dominant transmission of chamber dilation, and systolic dysfunction has been mapped to chromosome 9q13 in one family; dilated cardiomyopathy in two other unrelated families also appears to map here. A clinically similar disorder has been identified in anther family, but genetic mapping studies have defined linkage to chromosome 1q42.

SIGNIFICANCE OF GENETIC STUDIES Although the clinical impact of these studies remains limited at present, they provide evidence of the power of genetic approaches to the study of inherited cardiovascular disease. Undoubtedly the disease genes at each of these dilated cardiomyopathy loci will be identified. These findings promise to provide substantive new insights into the complex relationship of the excitation, contraction coupling, and the mechanisms of cardiac failure. As with hypertrophic cardiomyopathy, identification of genes that cause inherited dilated cardiomyopathies can be expected to improve classification based on genetic subtypes, define the relationship of inherited dilated cardiomyopathies to isolated (idiopathic) cases, and improve risk stratification in affected individuals.

ACKNOWLEDGMENTS

We are grateful for the generous assistance of Mr. Mark Adams in formatting echocardiograms for reproduction. This work was supported in part by grants from the Howard Hughes Medical Institutes and National Institutes of Health to JGS and CES.

SELECTED REFERENCES

Bione S, D'Adamo P, Maestrini E, Gedeon AK, Bolhuis PA, Toniolo D. The novel X-linked gene G4.5 is responsible for Barth syndrome. Nat Genet 1996;12:385–389.

Bonne G, Carrier L, Bercovici J, et al. Cardiac myosin binding protein-C gene spice acceptor site mutation is associated with familial hypertrophic cardiomyopathy. Nat Gene 1995;11:438–440.

Cuda G, Fananapazir L, Shu W-S, Sellers JR, Epstein ND. Skeletal muscle expression and abnormal function of β-myosin heavy chain gene mutations in hypertrophic cardiomyopathy. J Clin Invest 1993;91:2861–2865.

Dracopoli NC, Haines JL, Korf BR, Moir DT, Morton CC, Seidman CE, Seidman JG, Smith DR, eds. Current Protocols in Human Genetics. New York: Wiley, 1994; pp. 1:1–1.7.

Dec GW, Fuster V. Idiopathic dilated cardiomyopathy. N Engl Med 1994;331:1564–1575.

Durand JB, Bachinski LL, Bieling LC, et al. Localization of a gene responsible for familial dilated cardiomyopathy to chromosome 1q32. Circ 1995;15:92:3387–3389.

Franz WM, Herrmann R, Cremer M, et al. Molecular pathogenesis of X-linked dilated cardiomyopathy by stop mutation and alternative splicing of the dystrophin exon 29. Circ 1995;92:1–184.

Geisterfer-Lowrance AA, Christe M, Conner DA, Ingwall JS, Schoen FJ, Seidman CE, Seidman JG. A mouse model of familial hypertrophic cardiomyopathy. Science 1996;272:731–734.

Kass S, MacRae C, Graber HL, et al. A gene defect that causes conduction system disease and dilated cardiomyopathy maps to chromosome 1p1-1q1. Nature Genet 1994;7:546–552.

Kelly DP, Strauss AW. Inherited Cardiomyopathies. N Engl J Med 1994;330:913–919.

Krajinovic M, Pinamonti B, Sinagra G, et al. Linkage of familial dilated cardiomyopathy to chromosome 9. Am J Hum Genet 1995;57:846–852.

Maron BJ, Gardom JM, Flack MN, Gidding SS, Kurosakiu TT, Bild DE. Prevalence of Hypertrophic Cardiomyopathy in a General Population of Young Adults. Circ 1995;92:785–789.

Michels V, Moll PP, Miller FA, et al. The frequency of familial dilated cardiomyopathy in a series of patients with idiopathic dilated cardiomyopathy. N Engl J Med 1992;326:77–82.

Michels VV, Pastores GM, Moll PP, et al. Dystrophin analysis in idiopathic dilated cardiomyopathy. J Med Genet 1993;30:955–957.

Muntoni F, Cau M, Banau A, et al. Deletion of the dystrophin muscle-promoter region associated with X-linked dilated cardiomyopathy. N Engl J Med 1993;329:921–925.

Mutoni F, Wilson L, Marrosu G, et al. A mutation in the dystrophin gene selectively affecting dystrophin expression in the heart. J Clin Invest 1995;96:693–699.

Nagano A, Koga R, Ogawa M, Kurano Y, Kawada J, Okada R, Hayashi YK, Tsukahara T, Arahata K. Emerin deficiency at the nuclear membrane in patients with Emery-Dreifuss muscular dystrophy. Nat Genet 1996;12:254–259.

Olson TM, Keating MT. Mapping a cardiomyopathy locus to chromosome 3p22-p25. J Clin Invest 1996;97:528–532.

Pyeritz RE, Genetics and Cardiovascular Disease. In: Braunwald E, ed. Heart Disease. Philadelphia: WB Saunders, 1992; pp. 1622–1655.

Rosenzweig A, Watkins H, Hwang D-S, et al. Preclinical diagnosis of familial hypertrophic cardiomyopathy by genetic analysis of blood lymphocytes. N Engl J Med 1991;325:1753–1760.

Siciliano G, Fanin M, Angelini C, et al. Identification of a novel X-linked gene responsible for Emery-Dreifuss muscular dystrophy. Nat Genet 1994;8:323–327.

Small K, Iber J, Warren ST. Emerin deletion reveals a common X-chromosome inversion mediated by inverted repeats. Nat Genet 1997;16: 96–99.

Stanley CA, Hale DE, Berry GT, Deleeuw S, Boxer J, Bonnefont J-P. A deficiency of carnitine-acylcarnitine translocase in the inner mitochondrial membrane. N Engl J Med 1992;327:19–23.

Strauss AW, Powell CK, Hale DE et al. Molecular basis of human mitochondrial very-long-chain acyl-CoA dehydrogenase deficiency causing cardiomyopathy and sudden death in childhood. Proc Natl Acad Sci USA 1995;92:10,496–10,500.

Taroni F, Verderio E, Fiorucci S, et al. Molecular characterization of inherited carnitine palmitoyltransferase II deficiency. Proc Natl Acad Sci USA 1992;89:8429–8433.

Tein I, De Vivo DC, Bierman F, et al. Impaired skin fibroblast carnitine uptake in primary systemic carnitine deficiency manifested by childhood carnitine-responsive cardiomyopathy. Pediatr Res 1990;28: 247–255.

Watkins H, Conner D, Thierfelder L, et al. Mutations in the cardiac myosin binding protein-C gene on chromosome 11 cause familial hypertrophic cardiomyopathy. Nat Genet 1995;11:434–437.

Watkins H, McKenna W, Thierfelder L, et al. The role of cardiac troponin T and a-tropomyosin mutations in hypertrophic cardiomyopathy. N Engl J Med 1995;332:1058–1064.

Watkins H, Seidman JG, Seidman CE. Familial hypertrophic cardiomyopathy: a genetic model of cardiac hypertrophy. Hum Molec Genet 1995;4:1721–1727.

Yokota I, Indo Y, Coates PM, Tanaka K. Molecular basis of medium chain acyl-coenzyme A dehydrogenase deficiency: an A to G transition at position 985 that causes a lysine-304 to glutamate substitution in the mature protein is the single prevalent mutation. J Clin Invest 1990;86:1000–1003.

14 Coronary Atherosclerosis

ROBERT E. GERSZTEN AND ANTHONY ROSENZWEIG

BACKGROUND

Atherosclerotic coronary artery disease is a complex biological process resulting in the narrowing of arterial vessels supplying blood to the heart. This process can clinically remain silent, but it commonly gives rise to clinical signs and symptoms when the narrowing becomes sufficiently severe that blood flow is unable to meet the metabolic needs of the heart muscle. If this condition is transient without permanent myocardial cell damage, it is termed myocardial ischemia. If the condition is sufficient in severity and duration to cause irreversible, clinically detectable myocardial cell damage, it is termed myocardial infarction. The clinical symptoms associated with myocardial ischemia are termed angina pectoris. In myocardial ischemia, the blood flow is insufficient relative to the requirements of the myocardium. Therefore, ischemia can be influenced by both alterations in the coronary blood flow (supply) and changes in the metabolic state of the myocardium (demand). Many patients with coronary disease experience exertional symptoms in a consistent and predictable pattern termed chronic stable angina. A marked acceleration in the frequency, severity, or duration of angina, or a significant decrease in the level of exertion inducing angina, constitutes unstable angina and carries a substantial risk of progression to myocardial infarction. Together, unstable angina and myocardial infarction comprise the acute or unstable coronary syndromes. The biological basis for the transition from either no clinical symptoms or chronic stable angina to an unstable coronary syndrome is the subject of intense investigation and has important clinical implications.

First, we will review the clinical features of these two general presentations of patients with atherosclerotic coronary disease: the acute coronary syndromes and stable angina. Salient features of the history, physical exam, and diagnosis of each will be discussed. We then turn to the molecular pathophysiology of atherosclerosis and examine the putative role(s) of multiple constituents of the blood vessel wall in the development, progression, and stability of atherosclerotic plaques.

CLINICAL FEATURES

Atherosclerotic cardiovascular diseases constitute a major cause of morbidity and mortality among both men and women in the United States, accounting for 500,000 deaths each year, approximately half of which are sudden. Atherosclerosis is a chronic and complicated process in humans and develops over many years. Large epidemiological studies and interventional trials have identified a number of contributory elements to the development of these lesions, including genetic predisposition, elevated lipid levels, diabetes, tobacco smoking, and hypertension. This has led to a significant decline in age-adjusted mortality rates for patients with cardiovascular disease over the past several decades. Over the past 25 years, important advances have been made in the treatment of severe coronary stenoses, including bypass surgery and subsequently percutaneous transluminal coronary catheter-based interventions. Since the mid 1980s, thrombolytic therapy has become a mainstay in our treatment of acute myocardial infarction. From this wealth of clinical experience, our theories about the pathogenesis of the atherosclerotic plaque and the propensity towards acute coronary syndromes (i.e., myocardial infarction and unstable angina) have also evolved.

Surprisingly, serial angiographic studies have demonstrated that it is often not the most angiographically severe lesions that become unstable clinically. This data suggest that nonobstructive lesions may progress rapidly to obstruction through plaque rupture and/or thrombosis. Furthermore, the angiographic appearance of a lesion is a poor predictor of its clinical behavior. Lessons learned from recent clinical trials with lipid lowering agents have been equally intriguing. While lipid reduction only modestly improves the angiographic severity of high grade atherosclerotic lesions, it substantially improves the risk of acute coronary events, such as unstable angina or myocardial infarction. Our clinical experience has therefore served as the impetus to better understand the fundamental mechanisms of lesion biology.

DIAGNOSIS OF UNSTABLE CORONARY SYNDROMES

HISTORY The hallmark of the unstable coronary syndromes is rapidly progressing exertional substernal chest pressure, often radiating to the jaw or left arm. However, the initial presentation may be symptoms at rest. The discomfort of acute myocardial infarction is qualitatively similar, although it is often more severe and prolonged. It is acute in onset and often associated with diaphoresis, dyspnea, and a sense of impending doom. Elderly and diabetic patients often have less typical symptoms. One must also consider underlying illnesses such as anemia or infection that may precipitate the presentation of coronary disease. Acute infarction is present in a minority of patients presenting with chest pain of presumed cardiac origin. Chest discomfort described as "pressure" or "burning" is most associated with acute infarction. Positional or pleuritic pain should prompt consideration of other

From: *Principles of Molecular Medicine* (J. L. Jameson, ed.), ©1998 Humana Press Inc., Totowa, NJ.

etiologies. It should be noted that approx 25% of myocardial infarctions are silent and associated with either no symptoms, or only mild and atypical symptoms. The prognosis of such silent infarctions appears similar to that of more classical presentations.

PHYSICAL EXAMINATION Physical examination neither establishes nor excludes the diagnosis of acute myocardial infarction or unstable angina. It does, however, provide critical clinical information of practical importance in patient management. Evaluation of the vital signs is particularly important in patients with chest pain. The heart rate is usually normal or slightly elevated, though infarctions involving the diaphragmatic portion of the heart are often accompanied by bradycardia and nausea. An irregular rhythm should raise the suspicion of ventricular ectopy or atrial fibrillation. Hypotension in the setting of chest pain may be secondary to pump failure and is a particularly ominous finding. Mild hypertension is more commonly found with acute onset of symptoms. Tachypnea may be secondary to evolving congestive heart failure.

The jugular venous pulsation is usually normal. An elevated measurement may denote chronically elevated right-sided filling pressures but should raise the possibility of right ventricular involvement. The diagnosis of right ventricular infarction may also be suggested by a paradoxical rise in venous pressure with inspiration, known as the Kussmaul's sign.

Evaluation of the arterial pulse amplitude and duration provides important clues to possible valvular disease or associated, noncoronary arterial disease. The pulse contour also reflects the patient's cardiac output. This evaluation may be confounded in elderly patients by noncompliant arteries in that the pulse amplitude may appear normal despite a significantly reduced cardiac output. The status of peripheral arteries, as well as the quality of the lower extremity veins, should be carefully assessed prior to consideration of interventions such as cardiac catheterization, angioplasty, intra-aortic balloon counterpulsation, or bypass surgery.

The possible auscultatory findings in atherosclerotic heart disease are protean. An S4 heart sound is common, often a reflection of long-standing diastolic dysfunction secondary to hypertension. On the other hand, a third heart sound reflects significant systolic impairment. Cardiac murmurs may be fixed or transient, emphasizing the importance of serial examinations. Both stable and unstable symptoms may be precipitated or exacerbated by underlying valvular heart disease such as aortic stenosis. The murmur of papillary muscle dysfunction is often transient while mechanical complications such as ventricular septal defect may not occur until days into the hospital stay. A pericardial friction rub often occurs several days after infarction. Evaluation of the lungs centers on the presence of rales consistent with congestive heart failure. In the acute coronary syndromes, the presence of pulmonary rales consistent with congestive heart failure, coupled with an S3 gallop, is a poor prognostic sign.

LABORATORY EVALUATION The classic electrocardiographic pattern of acute myocardial infarction includes ST-segment elevation in multiple leads reflecting a coronary distribution, followed by evolution of T-wave inversion and significant Q waves in these same leads, reflecting a Q-wave myocardial infarction. However, patients with infarction can also present with ST-segment depression or T-wave inversion alone without evolution of Q waves, termed non–Q-wave myocardial infarction. The correlation of these electrocardiographic findings with pathologic findings of transmural or subendocardial infarction is sufficiently imprecise to favor exclusive use of the electrocardiographic descriptors in clinical practice.

Serologic markers of myocardial necrosis remain the cornerstone in establishing the diagnosis of myocardial infarction. The serum creatine kinase (CK) and its myocardial-specific isozyme, CK-MB, are the most widely used tests. The degree of elevation in these markers correlates approximately with the amount of myocardium damaged but is influenced by many other factors. Elevated levels of serum transaminase and lactate dehydrogenase (LDH) with isoform reversal occurs later after infarction. Measurement of these levels generally adds little to clinical management and should not be routinely employed in evaluation of acute chest pain. Recent work has emphasized the utility of CK-subforms and myocardial-specific isoforms of troponin T and I, noting advantages in sensitivity in early diagnosis.

In evaluating acute coronary syndromes, studies by Dr. Lee Goldman and colleagues have been particularly instructive. His group integrated historical features to assess pretest probability, along with electrocardiographic findings, in a computer algorithm to predict myocardial infarction, and used this tool to prospectively analyze almost 5000 emergency room patients with chest pain. Of note, the incidence of acute myocardial infarction in the setting of a normal or near-normal electrocardiogram is approx 10%, but these patients are at lower risk for the life-threatening complications of infarction.

DIAGNOSIS OF STABLE ANGINA

HISTORY Angina is classically described as a substernal chest pressure brought on by exertion and relieved by rest. Radiation of this discomfort (to the arm or jaw) and associated symptoms such as dyspnea or diaphoresis are common. Other precipitants include emotional stress, cold weather, or even large meals in some patients. Comorbid diseases such as anemia, thyrotoxicosis, or infection should be considered as possible contributors. Angina is most frequently the result of epicardial coronary stenoses that impair the coronary flow reserve. As the coronary flow reserve is decreased, the stress-induced myocardial ischemia typically results in anginal chest discomfort. Classical studies have shown that angina often correlates with coronary stenoses of 70% of the luminal cross section. Rest angina may develop with coronary stenoses of 90% or greater. Many patients with coronary artery disease have documented episodes of ischemia in the absence of anginal symptoms. The full implications and management of this silent ischemia remain controversial.

PHYSICAL EXAMINATION As described above for acute myocardial infarction, the physical exam provides important insights into the status of the patient's cardiovascular system and general health. In particular, evidence of valvular heart disease, systolic and diastolic ventricular dysfunction, and peripheral vascular disease should be sought.

LABORATORY EVALUATION Two goals form the rationale for further evaluation of patients with suspected coronary artery disease: the first is to establish (or refute) the diagnosis; the second is to acquire prognostic information in patients with coronary disease. This information can be extremely useful by identifying not only candidates for more aggressive management, but also those who do not need it.

As with all clinical testing, a positive or negative result must be interpreted in the context of the prior probability that a diagnosis such as ischemic heart disease exists in the patient or population under study. Further testing is most useful when clinical evaluation places the prior probability of coronary disease in an intermediate level. If the prior probability of disease is extremely low, a positive test is most likely to be a false-positive and may precipitate a cascade of expensive and otherwise unnecessary further tests. If the prior probability is extremely high, a negative test is likely false-negative, and a positive test contributes little to the diagnosis. However, testing can be extremely useful even in patients with known coronary disease as a functional assessment and a prognostic rather than a diagnostic tool.

Evocative testing is necessary because, as previously indicated, ischemia connotes a relative deficiency of blood flow. Therefore, clinical or electrocardiographic evaluation of a well-compensated patient at rest is often unrevealing, even in the presence of significant coronary artery disease. Several objective methods of inducing and measuring myocardial ischemia are useful. Exercise testing while monitoring the patient's blood pressure and 12-lead ECG remains the most widely used approach. The patient must be able to exercise adequately, and the baseline ECG must be normal to rely on this test alone. Furthermore, drugs that alter the repolarization phase, such as digoxin, are a significant source of false-positive ECG changes. This incremental study is usually symptom limited, and the test is discontinued if there is evidence of chest discomfort, profound shortness of breath, a fall in systemic blood pressure of more than 15–20 mmHg, marked ECG changes, or ventricular arrhythmia. The total duration of exercise, the time to the onset of ischemic ST-segment change and chest discomfort, the total work performed (calculated by the heart rate-blood pressure product), the depth of the ST-segment depression, and the time needed for recovery to baseline all have important prognostic implications. When exercise is not possible, pharmacologic manipulations such as intravenous adenosine or dipyridamole can be useful but do not provide the same functional information as exercise testing. These compounds produce a dose-dependent myocardial hyperemia secondary to dilation of the coronary microvasculature. Coronary pressure distal to an epicardial stenosis declines in response to pharmacologic vasodilation, and this results in an impaired microvascular perfusion pressure. Therefore, in the setting of severe epicardial stenoses, these drugs cause an intramyocardial "steal" such that endocardial blood flow acutely declines while epicardial blood flow is either unchanged or increased. If no stenoses are present, both endocardial and epicardial blood flow will increase. Relative differences in blood flow can then be detected by radionuclide imaging. Of note, patients with bronchospastic pulmonary disease may not tolerate this form of pharmacologic testing. Dobutamine, a selective β-adrenergic agonist that produces a positive inotropic and chronotropic effect on the heart, has also been used to provide a pharmacologic stress.

Noninvasive assessment of myocardial perfusion is most commonly accomplished with radionuclide scintigraphy following the intravenous administration of a radioisotope such as thallium-201. Such radionuclide scintigraphy improves both the sensitivity and specificity of evocative testing. In addition, these techniques often allow differentiation between ischemic and infarcted zones. In the former, isotope uptake is initially reduced but normalizes over time. In the latter, uptake is persistently decreased. Newer agents using Technetium -99m have the advantage of higher energy and shorter half-life. The increased radionuclide dose improves image quality and is less subject to artifacts of soft-tissue attenuation. An indirect indication of coronary flow is provided by examination of systolic wall movement and thickening by echocardiography. Therefore, dobutamine-induced ischemia can be detected as transient left-ventricular dysfunction by 2D-echocardiography. The sensitivity and specificity of stress echocardiography are similar to that of thallium stress testing.

GENETIC BASIS OF DISEASE

Atherosclerosis is a complex phenotype that most commonly appears modulated by interactions between environmental factors and multiple genetic loci, only some of which have been identified. Genetic dyslipoproteinemias can substantially accelerate disease progression. Assessment of serum lipid levels should be included in the evaluation of all patients with coronary disease and therefore provides an initial screen for genetic dyslipoproteinemias as well. Similarly, understanding the genetic bases for other recognized clinical risk factors such as diabetes mellitus or hypertension will have an important impact on the development and progression of coronary disease. Some studies have suggested an association between the deletional allele of the angiotensin converting enzyme (ACE) gene and the risk of myocardial infarction. However, this was not confirmed in a prospective study of a large cohort of US physicians. Elevated serum levels of homocysteine can result from genetic defects in certain metabolic enzymes and is independently associated with ischemic heart disease. The epidemiological relationship of coronary artery disease and markers of thrombosis such as fibrinogen levels are also currently being investigated. However, the genetic basis of most ischemic heart disease remains elusive.

MOLECULAR PATHOPHYSIOLOGY Hypotheses concerning the molecular pathogenesis of ischemic heart disease seek to explain two related but distinct phenomena: the gradual development of obstructive atherosclerotic lesions responsible for stable angina and the rapid progression of these lesions to the acute coronary syndromes. Dr. Russell Ross and colleagues first proposed that atherosclerotic lesions develop as a "response to injury" of the vascular endothelium, and much of our current view of atherogenesis arises from these concepts. The work of Dr. Michael A. Gimbrone, Jr., Dr. Myron Cybulsky, and colleagues has suggested that atherogenesis may begin with endothelial activation or dysfunction rather than actual injury. This endothelial dysfunction may represent a common response to a wide variety of factors (Fig. 14-1). This work has also emphasized the dynamic role of the endothelium as the interface between circulating leukocytes and subintimal constituents of the vessel wall (Fig. 14-2). Activation of vascular endothelium may initiate a cascade of events leading to mononuclear leukocyte recruitment into the vessel wall with subsequent release of cytokines and growth factors contributing to smooth muscle cell migration and proliferation, as well as abnormalities of extracellular matrix formation. The precise molecular mechanisms involved in vivo are not completely understood.

Abrupt clinical change from stable angina (or no symptoms at all) to the unstable coronary syndromes appears to have its basis in acute plaque rupture. Exposure of the atherosclerotic fatty gruel to the blood serves as a substrate for the propagation of clot. Pathological studies have emphasized the importance of a central lipid core in the process of plaque fissuring and confirmed the role of thrombosis in unstable angina and myocardial infarction.

ROLE OF LIPIDS Autopsy studies have shown that fatty streaks frequently exist in the coronary arteries and aortae of chil-

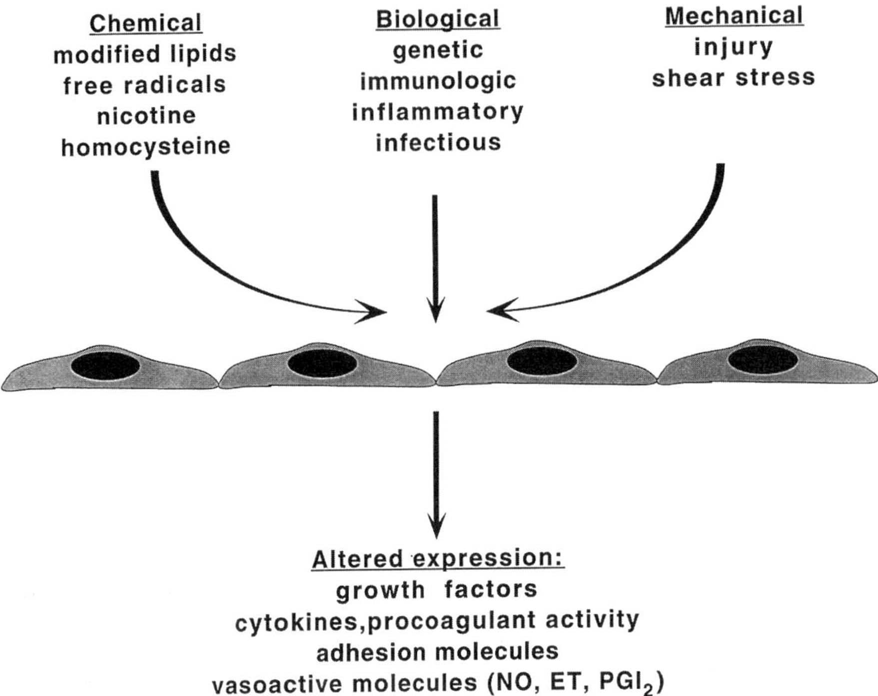

Figure 14-1 The central role of vascular endothelium. Many different stimuli may induce a similar repertoire of dysfunctional endothelial responses that ultimately contribute to clinical atherosclerosis. The endothelium provides a potential pathophysiologic link between well-established clinical risks factors such as hypercholesterolemia, cigaret smoking, hypertension, and atherogenesis. The role of the endothelial effects of other agents such as homocysteine or viral infection, as well as inflammatory cascades, remains more controversial.

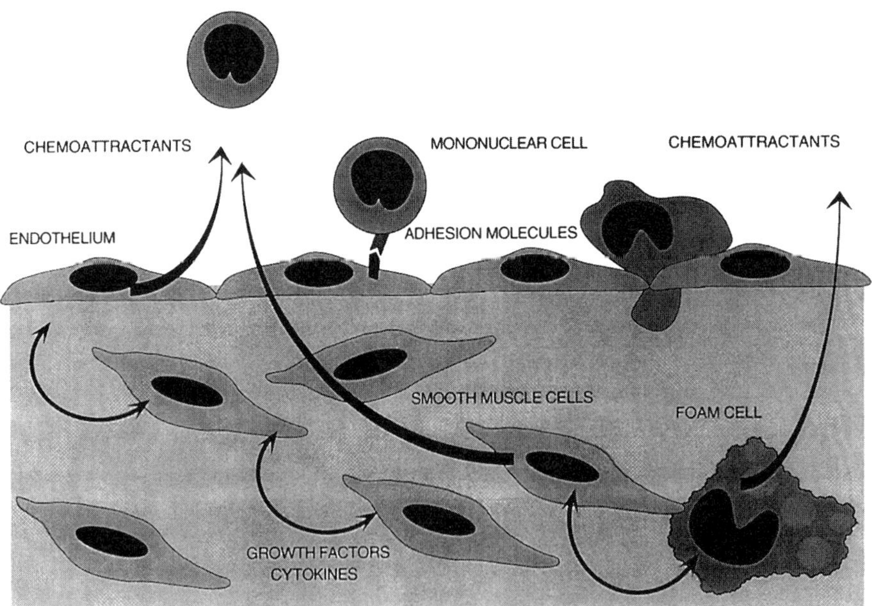

Figure 14-2 Leukocyte interactions with the vessel wall. An activated or dysfunctional endothelium may initiate a cascade of events that augment atherogenesis. These events include the recruitment of leukocytes through endothelial expression of cytokines and adhesion molecules, as well as alterations in smooth muscle cell function mediated by growth factors, cytokines, and vasoactive substances (indicated by arrows). Mononuclear cells and the foam cells they give rise to, as well as vascular smooth muscle cells, can also release growth factors and cytokines, further perpetuating this cycle.

dren in their teens. These lesions may constitute the earliest recognizable precursor of atherosclerotic plaques. The major lipid component of these lesions is oxidized LDL. In vitro experiments have shown that oxidized LDL stimulates the adherence of monocytes to vascular endothelium most likely through increased expression of endothelial adhesion molecules. Oxidized LDL also stimulates transcription and secretion of monocyte chemotactic protein-1 (MCP-1) by human aortic and smooth muscle cells in vitro. MCP-1

Table 14-1
Please Provide Table Title

Factor	*Source*	*Target*
Growth Factors		
PDGF	EC, WBC	SMC
bFGF	EC, SMC, WBC	EC, SMC
M-CSF	EC	WBC
VEGF	SMC	
Cytokines		
IL-1	EC, SMC, WBC	EC, WBC, SMC
TNF-α	EC, SMC, WBC	EC, WBC, SMC
IFN-γ	WBC	EC, WBC, SMC
Chemokines (MCP-1)	EC, SMC, WBC	WBC
Vasoactive substances		
Nitric oxide	EC	SMC, WBC
Endothelin	EC	SMC
Prostaglandin	EC	SMC

is a powerful chemoattractant for monocytes and memory T cells in vitro, which are the predominant leukocytes populations present in atherosclerotic lesions. Lysophosphatidylcholine, which constitutes a significant fraction of oxidized LDL, is itself a chemoattractant for monocytes and also induces expression of the endothelial adhesion molecules vascular cell adhesion molecule-1 (VCAM-1) and intercellular adhesion molecule-1 (ICAM-1). In addition, oxidized LDL can stimulate platelet aggregation and promote procoagulant activity on the surface of macrophages by an increase in tissue thromboplastin activity and by stimulating the expression and secretion of tissue factor by monocytes or aortic endothelial cells. Finally, oxidized LDL may also contribute to the vasomotor dysfunction that can promote or exacerbate the atherosclerotic lesion. Therefore, in many patients with atherosclerosis, lipids (particularly oxidized lipids) likely constitute an early and persistent precipitant of endothelial activation and dysfunction.

CELLULAR COMPONENTS: SMOOTH MUSCLE CELLS

Abnormal growth of vascular smooth muscle cells (SMCs) is prominent in atherosclerosis. At least two phenotypes have been described of the smooth muscle cells that make up the vascular wall. This is based on examination of myosin filaments and details of the secretory protein apparatus. When cells are in a contractile phenotype, they respond to elements that promote vasoconstriction or vasodilation such as endothelin, angiotensin II, prostaglandin I_2, or nitric oxide. A second synthetic phenotype has also been identified. In this state, SMCs synthesize numerous growth factors and their receptors—cytokines, as well as matrix proteins. Multiple factors may be able to stimulate smooth muscle cell proliferation and migration from the vessel media through the internal elastic membrane. These activated smooth muscle cells, in turn, release substances that act in complex paracrine and autocrine manners, involving vascular endothelial and smooth muscle cells, as well as blood borne elements such as white cells and platelets (Table 14-1 and Fig. 14-2). A particularly dramatic example of this process occurs after mechanical injury of the vessel during angioplasty, but a similar process may contribute to atherogenesis. A central issue in the investigation of atherogenesis is to define the source(s) of the critical factors that initiate and perpetuate the shift in smooth muscle cell phenotype. Peripheral leukocytes have been postulated to play a role in this process.

LEUKOCYTES Because of their early and consistent association with atherosclerotic lesions, mononuclear cells appear to be central to atherogenesis. The mononuclear cells in atherosclerotic lesions are predominantly monocytes and lymphocytes of the memory T-cell phenotype (CD45 RO^+). Monocyte-derived foam cells are a major component of atheroma, comprising as much as 60% of cells found in the necrotic lipid core and 10–20% of cells in the fibrous cap. Mononuclear cells serve as both as the progenitors of foam cells and as a potential source of growth factors and cytokines (Fig. 14-2). In turn, these chemical signals may mediate both intimal and smooth muscle hyperplasia and amplify recruitment of more leukocytes to the vessel wall. Even as atherosclerotic plaques increase in size, mononuclear leukocyte recruitment may continue to play an important role, particularly in the plaque borders. Furthermore, mononuclear cells may contribute to the plaque rupture underlying acute coronary syndromes, as suggested by correlative clinical studies of atherectomy specimens and autopsy series. When blood flow is restored after acute coronary occlusion, infiltrating leukocytes (particularly granulocytes) appear to be key mediators of reperfusion injury. Although considerable circumstantial evidence suggests a role of mononuclear cells in atherogenesis, their contribution remains unproven in vivo.

MOLECULAR SIGNALS

ADHESION MOLECULES Nevertheless, much work has focused on the molecular signals responsible for recruitment mononuclear leukocytes into the vessel wall. Recent findings have indeed pointed to a multistep sequence of events that guides the emigratory behavior of leukocytes in the vasculature. Leukocyte-endothelial interaction often begins with a relatively weak adhesive interaction manifested as leukocyte rolling, followed by firm adhesion to the vessel wall, and finally diapedesis. Local expression of adhesion molecules and cytokines by vascular cells appears to be an important determinant of this interaction.

Vascular cell adhesion molecule-1 (VCAM-1; CD106) is an intriguing candidate for a role in mononuclear cell recruitment in atherogenesis (Fig. 14-3). VCAM-1 was identified and cloned in rabbits by Dr. Myron Cybulsky and colleagues using an expression-cloning strategy designed to identify adhesion molecules potentially involved in the development of atherosclerotic lesions, so-called athero-ELAMs. VCAM-1 is an inducible 110-kDa member of the immunoglobulin superfamily (previously termed INCAM-110), which supports monocyte adhesion and is expressed by vascular endothelium and smooth muscle cells early in atherogenesis in the hypercholesterolemic rabbit model. VCAM-1 expression has been documented adjacent to infiltrating leukocytes in advanced human coronary atheroma. Expression of other adhesion molecules such as intercellular adhesion molecule-1 (ICAM-1) has also been observed in association with atheroma in rabbit models and human plaques. However, this expression appears less specific and often extends into noninvolved endothelium. In addition, VCAM-1 (but not ICAM-1) could explain, at least in part, the specificity of mononuclear leukocyte recruitment since its counter-ligand, VLA-4, is expressed exclusively on these leukocytes. Furthermore, VCAM-1 (again in contrast to ICAM-1) has recently been demonstrated to support attachment of mononuclear leukocytes under flow without prior participation of selectin-mediated interactions.

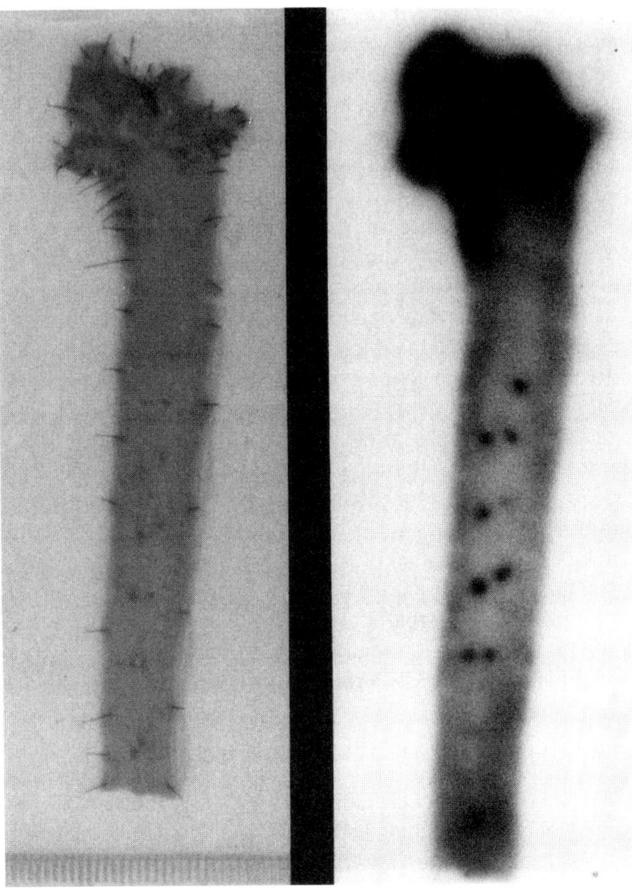

Figure 14-3 Expression of VCAM-1 at sites of atherogenesis. In the left panel, the aorta of a hypercholesterolemic rabbit has been stained with Oil-Red-O to reveal characteristic sites of fat deposition and atherogenesis (darker red) involving areas of disturbed flow including the aortic arch and intercostal branch points. In the right panel, an autoradiograph of the same aorta using radiolabeled antibody to rabbit vascular cell adhesion molecule-1 (VCAM-1) demonstrates that these areas of fat deposition and atherogenesis correlate well with surface VCAM-1 expression. (Courtesy of Dr. Myron Cybulsky, Brigham and Women's Hospital, Boston, MA.) (*See* color insert following p. 684.)

Multiple clinically recognized modulators of atherogenesis also modulate expression of VCAM-1 in the appropriate direction. As noted above, VCAM-1 expression is inducible in vitro and in vivo by atherogenic lipids. Decreased nitric oxide activity increases VCAM-1 expression. VCAM-1 transcriptional induction is repressed by antioxidants, and this could explain the beneficial effects of these agents on atherogenesis in animal studies. The laboratory of Dr. Tucker Collins has demonstrated that the VCAM-1 promoter contains functional NF-κB binding sequences, which may represent a common pathway for activation of genes involved in the development of atherosclerosis. Intriguingly, aspirin, shown in many circumstances to have beneficial effects on the progression of ischemic vascular disease, inhibits VCAM-1 expression through an NF-κB pathway. Obviously, each of these manipulations produces multiple effects, and a causal role for VCAM-1 in atherogenesis remains speculative. Moreover, since VCAM-1 supports adhesion of both lymphocytes and monocytes, it alone cannot explain the predominance of monocytes in atherosclerotic plaque. One would predict an important contribution of other molecules modulating either leukocyte recruitment or retention to fully explain the specificity of the populations observed.

CHEMOATTRACTANT CYTOKINES In addition to cell surface expressed adhesion molecules such as VCAM-1, smaller secreted proteins may also play important roles in atherogenesis. The chemoattractant cytokines, also known as "chemokines," are proinflammatory cytokines that have been postulated to contribute to the recruitment of specific mononuclear leukocyte subpopulations into atherosclerotic plaques. Monocyte chemoattractant protein-1 (MCP-1) is a chemokine that acts specifically on monocytes and memory T cells, the two leukocyte populations most prevalent in atheroma. As noted above, expression of MCP-1 by vascular smooth muscle cells is induced in vitro by oxidized lipids. Furthermore, *in situ* studies have documented increased MCP-1 mRNA in vascular smooth muscle cells, mesenchymal intimal cells, and macrophages in atherosclerotic lesions, as compared to normal vessels. This chemokine may therefore play an important role in the local specific recruitment of monocytes and subsequent lesion formation. Chemokines are likely to augment leukocyte recruitment both by supplying a local chemoattractant signal and by enhancing the avidity of leukocyte counterligand binding to locally expressed adhesion molecules.

HEMODYNAMIC FORCES It has long been clinically recognized that certain sites within the vasculature are more prone to development of atherosclerosis. These are often sites of disturbed flow, such as vessel branch points. Hemodynamic forces induce various functional changes in vascular endothelium, including morphological changes and alterations in the production of important product such as coagulation factors, fibrinolytic factors, growth factors and cytokines. However, only recently has a precise connection between hemodynamic forces and control of endothelial gene expression been elucidated. Work by Drs. Nitzan Resnick and Michael A. Gimbrone, Jr, has identified a *cis*-acting shear stress response element (SSRE) in the promoters of several genes, including PDGF-A and ICAM-1, which appears to mediate increased expression of ICAM-1 in cultured human endothelial cells subjected to a physiological range of laminar shear stress. The SSRE is a functional NF-κB binding site in vascular endothelial cells under these conditions. This SSRE may represent a common pathway by which mechanical forces influence gene expression. Other adhesion molecules such as VCAM-1 or E-selectin, whose promoters lack this motif, are not upregulated under these conditions. Identification of the molecular basis of upregulation of expression of VCAM-1 under more complex hemodynamic conditions may provide insights into the differential regulation of these genes and their role in atherogenesis.

MANAGEMENT/TREATMENT

In approaching an individual patient, several goals must be considered simultaneously. These include prevention of disease progression, control of symptoms, and optimization of prognosis. The tools available to achieve these goals include patient education, risk-factor modification, pharmacologic therapy, and mechanical interventions including surgical- and catheter-based approaches. All these considerations must be integrated into a coherent clinical approach, which, in practice, is often influenced dramatically by the acuity of the patient's clinical presentation.

Patient education and behavior modification form the cornerstone of primary and secondary prevention. Recent clinical trials have demonstrated that aggressive risk factor modification, particularly reduction in serum lipids, can have a dramatic clinical impact, even over a few years in populations with documented atherosclerotic coronary disease. Randomized trials have documented angiographic regression of plaques, establishing for the first time that regression is possible, in principle. However, even more intriguing is the observation that while the degree of regression has been modest, the improvement in clinical endpoints has been more dramatic. Reduction in serum lipids appears to have clinical benefits that are only imperfectly reflected in the angiographic appearance of lesions. These clinical benefits can be realized during a relatively brief (2–3 year) period of treatment, which underscores the importance of secondary prevention efforts. Although lifestyle modifications are emphasized as the first step in this process, it is often necessary to move to pharmacologic lipid-lowering therapies. The particular agent(s) employed is determined by the specifics of the patient's lipid profile.

Other therapies of proven clinical benefit in patients who have a prior history of myocardial infarction include aspirin, β-blockade, and angiotensin-converting enzyme inhibitors in patients with a reduced left-ventricular ejection fraction. These agents reduce the incidence of clinical cardiovascular events and mortality. For this reason, they should be considered in all patients after myocardial infarction, even if they are asymptomatic. Medications that may be useful in the chronic treatment of coronary patients but that have not been demonstrated to improve prognosis include calcium channel blockers and nitrates. In fact, in the setting of non–Q-wave infarction, the calcium channel blocker diltiazem had a deleterious effect on one year survival in patients manifesting congestive heart failure during the initial hospitalization. On the other hand, these medications may help control anginal symptoms, hypertension, or arrhythmias, but should not be routinely prescribed independent of a specific indication because of the lack of proven benefit in outcome.

Therapy for chronic stable angina includes both pharmacologic and mechanical interventions. The three classes of pharmacologic agents primarily employed are β-blockers, calcium channel blockers, and nitrates. As noted above, only the first has documented survival benefit in postinfarction patients, but all three have been demonstrated to improve exercise tolerance and can reduce ischemic symptoms—a valid goal in and of itself. Mechanical interventions encompass a variety of catheter-based approaches, such as percutaneous translumenal angioplasty (PTCA) and coronary artery bypass surgery (CABG). Early randomized trials established that CABG provides a survival benefit over medical therapy alone in patients with significant left main coronary disease or severe three-vessel coronary disease (particularly in the setting of compromised left ventricular function). In patients with one or two vessel coronary disease and mild symptoms, CABG does not confer a survival benefit. However, surgery eliminates or reduces anginal symptoms more effectively than medical therapy alone. Catheter-based interventions are also highly effective at reducing ischemic symptoms but are all plagued by a significant rate of restenosis. In addition, no survival benefit has been demonstrated for clinically stable patients using catheter-based interventions. Nevertheless, the number of these procedures performed each year continues to grow rapidly. Randomized comparisons of surgery and PTCA are currently underway.

In acute myocardial infarction, the immediate goal is restoration of adequate coronary flow as quickly as possible to minimize or avoid irreversible myocardial damage. Two general approaches are widely employed to achieve this goal: primary angioplasty and thrombolytic therapy. Several randomized trials have demonstrated additional clinical benefit to primary angioplasty, if it can be accomplished quickly by experienced interventionalists. However, in most communities this is not practical, and immediate administration of thrombolytic agents becomes preferable. The two most widely used are streptokinase (SK) and tissue plasminogen activator (tPA), both of which have been documented to improve survival and left ventricular function after infarction. The large GUSTO trial demonstrated a modest survival benefit of the substantially more expensive tPA as compared with SK. Whether this modest clinical benefit justifies the additional expense remains controversial. Interestingly, thrombolytic agents have not been beneficial in the treatment of unstable angina. However, therapy with heparin and aspirin—alone and in combination—reduces the rate of progression to frank infarction. Patients with unstable symptoms which cannot be controlled by heparin/aspirin and maximal anti-ischemic therapy should undergo early catheterization to define possible options for immediate mechanical intervention.

While heparin and aspirin remain the mainstay of antithrombotic therapy for unstable angina and non–Q-wave myocardial infarction, newer agents are currently being evaluated. Recently, basic investigation has pointed to the key role of the platelet glycoprotein IIb/IIIa receptor as the pivotal mediator of platelet aggregation. Platelet adhesion, the first step in the process of hemostasis, can be triggered endothelial dysfunction or injury and subsequent interaction of platelets with the subendothelial matrix. Adhesion molecules of the vessel wall, along with clotting proteins such as fibrinogen, interact with platelet-membrane glycoproteins—of which integrins such as IIb/IIIa play a key role. Currently, clinical trials are evaluating monoclonal antibodies directed at the IIb/IIIa receptor in the unstable coronary syndromes. Furthermore, lessons gleaned from the molecular biology of the thrombin receptor have spurred interest in the role of the naturally occurring leach anticoagulant hirudin in the clinical arena. Evaluation of the clinical role of hirudin, which binds thrombin with remarkable avidity, is currently underway. Molecular analysis of the human thrombin receptor has elucidated the role of a "hirudin-like" domain close to the site where thrombin cleaves its receptor. Future pharmaceuticals may include the creation of monoclonal antibodies or smaller synthetic molecules directed at this thrombin receptor domain, thus producing a direct receptor antagonist.

FUTURE DIRECTIONS

Several areas of investigation appear particularly fertile over the coming decade. Further genetic analysis of atherosclerosis as a complex trait will be imperative. Such studies should provide substantial insight into the significant proportion of clinical coronary risk that currently remains unattributable. Improved assessment of genetic risk for atherosclerosis would focus and facilitate efforts at primary prevention and intervention. Ultimately, the identification of the relative contribution of specific genes will also improve our understanding of the fundamental biology of atherogenesis.

Our understanding of atherogenesis may benefit more immediately from the ongoing development of genetically altered animal models. Germline manipulation of mice has already produced lines prone to atherosclerosis. These will continue to help define events in atherogenesis and to elucidate the modulating effects of other genes through crossbreeding experiments. Somatic gene transfer will also help define the role of local vascular expression of individual molecules in disease pathogenesis, as well as the potential for therapeutic local gene delivery.

Finally, translation of these advances to the clinical arena will be vitally important. As described above, the tools available for assessing atherosclerosis in individual patients and for predicting the clinical behavior of individual lesions remain quite poor. One hopes that an improved understanding of genetic risks and lesion biology should enable us to develop better clinical markers. The ability to discriminate between biologically stable and unstable lesions would have far-reaching clinical implications. Two aspects of this problem are equally important: the identification of reliable markers of lesion behavior and the development of technologies for the practical detection of these markers in the clinical setting.

SELECTED REFERENCES

Berliner JA, Navab M, Fogelman AM, et al. Atherosclerosis: basic mechanisms. Oxidation, inflammation, and genetics. Circulation 1995; 91:2488–2496.

Breslow JL. Transgenic mouse models of lipoprotein metabolism and atherosclerosis. Proc Natl Acad Sci USA 1993;90:8314–8318.

Collins T. Endothelial nuclear factor-kappa B and the initiation of the atherosclerotic lesion. Lab Invest 1993;68:499–508.

Cybulsky MI, Gimbrone MA. Endothelial expression of a mononuclear leukocyte adhesion molecule during atherogenesis. Science 1991; 251:788–791.

Davies MJ, Gordon JL, Gearing AJ, et al. The expression of the adhesion molecules ICAM-1, VCAM-1, PECAM, and E-selectin in human atherosclerosis. J Pathol 1993;171:223–229.

Davies MJ, Richardson, PD, Woolf N, Katz DR, Mann J. Risk of thrombosis in human atherosclerotic plaques: role of extracellular lipid, macrophage, and smooth muscle cell content. Br Heart J 1993;69: 377–381.

Dzau VJ, Gibbons GH, Kobilka BK, Lawn RM, Pratt RE. Genetic models of human vascular disease. Circulation 1995;91:521–531.

Fuster V. Lewis A. Conner Memorial Lecture. Mechanisms leading to myocardial infarction: insights from studies of vascular biology [published erratum appears in Circulation 1995;91(1):256]. Circulation 1994;90:2126–2146.

Gimbrone MA. Vascular endothelium: an integrator of pathophysiologic stimuli in atherosclerosis. Am J Card 1995;75:67B–70B.

Jang Y, Lincoff AM, Plow EF, Topol EJ. Cell adhesion molecules in coronary artery disease. J Am Coll Card 1994;24:1591–1601.

Khachigian LM, Resnick N, Gimbrone MA Jr, Collins T. Nuclear factor-kappa B interacts functionally with the platelet-derived growth factor B-chain shear-stress response element in vascular endothelial cells exposed to fluid shear stress. J Clin Invest 1995;96:1169–1175.

Khan BV, Harrison DG, Olbrych MT, Alexander RW, Medford RM. Nitric oxide regulates cell adhesion molecule 1 gene expression and redox-sensitive transcriptional events in human vascular endothelialalles. Proc Natl Acad Sci USA 1996;93:9114–9119.

Lee TH, Cook EF, Weisberg M, Sargent RK, Wilson C, Goldman L. Acute chest pain in the emergency room—identification and examination of low risk patients. Arch Intern Med 1985;145:65–69.

Resnick N, Collins T, Atkinson W, Bonthron DT, Dewey CF Jr, Gimbrone MA Jr. Platelet-derived growth factor B chain promoter contains a cis-acting fluid shear-stress-responsive element. Proc Natl Acad Sci USA 1993;90:4591–4595.

Ross R. The pathogenesis of atherosclerosis: a perspective for the 1990s. Nature 1993;362:801–809.

Scandinavian Simvastatin Study Group. Randomized trial of cholesterol lowering in 4444 patients with coronary heart disease: the Scandinavian Simvastatin Survival Study (4S). Lancet 1994;344:1383–1389.

Springer TA. Traffic signals for lymphocyte recirculation and leukocyte emigration: the multistep paradigm. Cell 1994;76:301–314.

15 Endothelium-Derived Nitric Oxide and Control of Vascular Tone

SANTIAGO LAMAS AND THOMAS MICHEL

PHARMACOLOGIC AND ENDOGENOUS SOURCES OF NITRIC OXIDE

Endothelium-derived nitric oxide is a key determinant of vascular tone. Nitric oxide (NO) is a free radical gas, highly lipophilic and chemically reactive, and can be formed either by endogenous synthesis catalyzed by a family of nitric oxide synthase enzymes or consequent to the metabolism of organic nitrate vasodilator drugs. These drugs—which include such important cardiovascular agents as nitroglycerin, isosorbide dinitrate, and sodium nitroprusside—are metabolized to form NO by poorly understood enzymatic and nonenzymatic pathways.

NO has had an important role in cardiovascular therapeutics for more than a century: nitroglycerin and other organic nitrate compounds were first used in the treatment of angina pectoris in the late 19th century. Pharmacologists discovered in the 1950s that nitroglycerin and related organic nitrate drugs relax smooth muscle cells from diverse tissues, including the vasculature, gut, and lung. By the 1970s, nitroglycerin and the other organic nitrate vasodilators were discovered to be prodrugs that are metabolized in the body to form their biologically active metabolite, NO.

The NO formed from organic nitrate vasodilators leads to characteristic pharmacologic effects in diverse target tissues. An important molecular target of NO is the soluble isoform of guanylate cyclase, which is expressed in many tissues, including vascular smooth muscle cells, blood platelets, and cardiac myocytes. In vascular as well as nonvascular smooth muscle cells, guanylate cyclase activation, and the consequent rise in intracellular cyclic GMP (cGMP), leads to muscle relaxation. In blood platelets, elevated cGMP levels lead to an inhibition of platelet aggregation; guanylate cyclase activation in cardiac myocytes may attenuate myocardial contractility. The presence in these numerous tissues of molecular targets responding to NO metabolized from exogenously administered drugs suggested that endogenous pathways might exist that are modulated by NO-dependent signaling. Only in the past decade was the endogenous synthesis of NO documented in mammalian cells.

The discovery of the endogenous synthesis of NO represents the convergence of independent lines of investigation pursued variously by vascular pharmacologists, neuroscientists, and chemically inclined immunologists. In 1980, Furchgott and Zawadzki discovered that the vascular endothelium produces a labile molecule that relaxes smooth muscle, and termed this substance "endothelium-derived relaxing factor," or EDRF. In 1986, several groups discovered that EDRF is NO. In entirely independent studies in the mid-1980s, researchers investigating nitrate metabolism in inflammatory cells discovered that immunoactivated macrophages synthesize NO. High concentrations of macrophage-derived NO were shown to be toxic to cells, including tumor cells and bacteria, and it was proposed that NO synthesis by inflammatory cells represents a primitive immune response. A third line of investigations in the late 1980s led to the discovery that NO is synthesized by specific neuronal populations in the brain, and a role for NO in neurotransmission was proposed. In 1991 and 1992 several laboratories isolated a family of enzymes that make NO, termed NO synthases; during the past several years, three distinct nitric oxide synthases (NOS) were purified, cloned, and characterized at the molecular level. More than a century passed between the clinical use of NO in the form of organic nitrate vasodilators and the discovery of an endogenous pathway for NO synthesis in humans.

From: *Principles of Molecular Medicine* (J. L. Jameson, ed.), ©1998 Humana Press Inc., Totowa, NJ.

THE NITRIC OXIDE SYNTHASE GENE FAMILY

The different mammalian NOS were originally isolated from neuronal, immunocyte, and endothelial cell sources. One nomenclature for the three NO synthases, still in wide use, identifies the isoforms based on the cell types from which they were originally characterized (nNOS, iNOS, and ecNOS). However, it has since become clear that the different isoforms have a much wider tissue distribution than was originally appreciated; this has led to a numerical designation for the three isoforms, in order of their discovery (NOS1, NOS2, and NOS3, respectively). There are important differences in the physiologic roles subserved by the distinct NOS isoforms, as well as important differences for the same isoform as expressed in various tissues. The activity of the ecNOS isoform present in the vascular endothelium represents a key determinant of vascular tone under physiologic conditions.

The different NOS isoforms share a common overall catalytic scheme, as shown in Fig. 15-1. In ecNOS catalysis, as well as for the other enzyme isoforms, the amino acid L-arginine is oxidized to form NO plus L-citrulline in a complex reaction requiring molecular oxygen, as well as numerous redox cofactors.

Binding of the calcium-binding regulatory protein calmodulin is required for full NOS activation. The multitude of cofactors

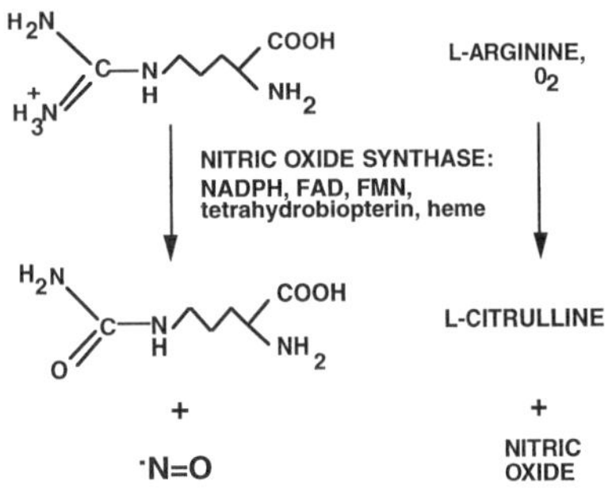

L-ARGININE, O_2

NITRIC OXIDE SYNTHASE: NADPH, FAD, FMN, tetrahydrobiopterin, heme

L-CITRULLINE + NITRIC OXIDE

Figure 15-1 NOS catalysis.

involved in NO formation provide for numerous potential points of regulation of the enzyme. Other forms of regulation occur at the level of the NOS genes themselves or the proteins once they have been synthesized. The different NOS isoforms can all be regulated by control of their genes (transcriptional regulation) or by alterations in the mRNA encoded by the gene (posttranscriptional regulation). A modification unique to ecNOS is *N*-myristoylation, in which the fatty acid myristic acid is added onto one end of the protein while it is being synthesized; ecNOS undergoes a second importantly regulated fatty acid modification termed palmitoylation. The fatty acid modifications of ecNOS are important determinants of the enzyme's targeting to specialized regions of the endothelial plasma membrane termed caveolae. All three NOS isoforms appear to be subject to regulation by reversible phosphorylation.

Other regulatory pathways influence NOS signaling, and may involve modulation of substrate availability or the metabolism of enzyme cofactors. For example, experiments in animal models and in humans have shown that dietary supplementation with the amino acid L-arginine, the NOS substrate, can influence atherogenesis. Another NOS substrate, molecular oxygen, may also play a role in regulation of NO-dependent relaxation: hypoxia may influence enzyme abundance and activity as well as NO metabolism. NO produced by the NOS enzymes themselves, as well as NO formed from pharmacologic sources, may also influence NOS activity and may relate to the mechanisms of pharmacologic tolerance to organic nitrate vasodilator drugs. The fate of NO once it is made may also be controlled by intracellular as well as extracellular pathways that importantly influence its biologic activity. These metabolic fates of NO may include binding to hemoglobin or other proteins, as well as interactions with reactive oxygen species, which may lead either to the degradation or stabilization of NO.

VASOACTIVE SUBSTANCES PRODUCED BY THE VASCULAR ENDOTHELIUM

The vascular endothelium is a specialized monolayer of cells that subserves numerous dynamically regulated functions in its role as the interface between blood components and the vascular wall. The endothelium is involved in the coordinated regulation of processes as diverse as thrombosis, smooth muscle mitogenesis, cell adhesion, and vascular tone. Furchgott and Zawadzki observed in 1980 that the vasodilatory effect exerted by acetylcholine was dependent on the presence of endothelial tissue, and deduced the existence of an EDRF, later shown to be NO. These and subsequent studies established the concept of the vascular endothelium as a major regulator of blood pressure homeostasis, and showed that NO represents the quantitatively most important endothelium-derived substance controlling vascular tone. Other endothelium-derived vasoactive mediators have been characterized, but appear to contribute less importantly to the dynamic regulation of vascular tone than does NO. Two extensively studied vasoactive endothelial products include prostacyclin and endothelin.

Prostacyclin was characterized in aortic strips as a substance capable of inhibiting platelet aggregation and promoting the relaxation of vascular smooth muscle. Prostacyclin, a dienoic bicyclic eicosanoid derived from arachidonic acid, is produced not only in endothelial cells, but is also synthesized within vascular smooth muscle cells and platelets, in which it contributes to the regulation of vascular tone and platelet aggregation. Prostacyclin synthesis from arachidonic acid is catalyzed by cyclooxygenase(s); after binding to its cognate G-protein–coupled cell-surface receptors, at least some of the physiologic effects of prostacyclin are mediated through activation of adenylate cyclase and the consequent increase in intracellular levels of cyclic AMP. Though prostacyclin may indeed play an important role in the regulation of platelet aggregation, this substance does not seem to be a major determinant of blood pressure under physiologic circumstances.

Endothelin is a peptide with powerful vasoconstrictor properties that was isolated and characterized as a novel product synthesized and secreted by cultured endothelial cells. Numerous lines of investigation have studied the synthesis, metabolism, and genetic regulation of endothelin. The role of endothelin in vascular homeostasis is less clearly established. Indeed, mice in which the endothelin-1 gene has been disrupted demonstrate a rather surprising phenotype. Inactivation of the gene encoding this vasoconstrictor peptide leads to significant developmental abnormalities and an unexpected vascular phenotype in which the endothelin-deficient mice are actually hypertensive. Despite numerous studies of the effects of endothelin in vitro, this substance has yet be definitively established as a major regulator of vascular tone in vivo.

By contrast, a variety of experimental approaches have shown that NO is a major determinant of vascular tone. Administration of arginine analogs that serve as competitive NOS inhibitors (e.g., N^G-monomethyl L-arginine) leads to an increase in blood pressure in experimental animals as well as human subjects. This observation suggests that tonic synthesis of NO plays an important role in vascular homeostasis. Proof for this hypothesis came from the analysis of mice in which the ecNOS gene had been genetically inactivated (by targeted gene disruption using homologous recombination in mouse embryo-derived stem cells). These ecNOS-deficient mice are fully viable but are hypertensive relative to their wild-type littermates, suggesting that compensatory mechanisms are unable to overcome the absence of endothelium-derived NO. Therefore, the ongoing synthesis of NO establishes a tonic state of vasodilation vital for vascular homeostasis.

The important role of ecNOS in blood pressure homeostasis has led to numerous investigations into the possible association of genetic defects in this enzyme with human hypertension. One report failed to find any convincing genetic linkage between the ecNOS gene and hypertension in a large population-based study. The genetic relationship between NOS and hypertension is likely to be complex. In other studies, the iNOS gene was discovered to map to a region in the rat genome linked to hypertension in SHR rats, but disease association or the relevance of this finding to human disease has yet to be established. A recent study found an association between polymorphisms in noncoding regions of the human ecNOS gene and atherosclerosis in cigaret smokers; the

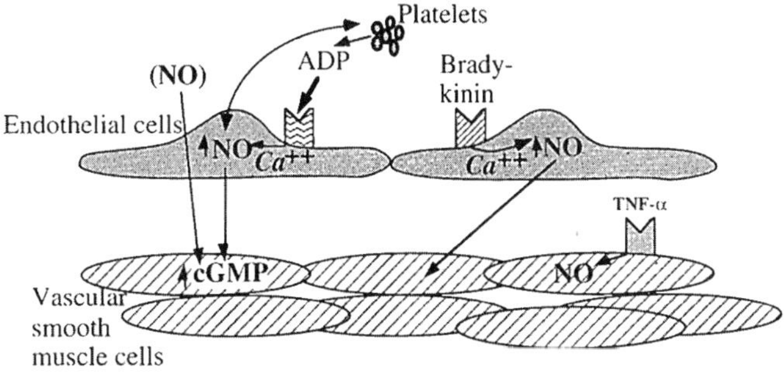

Figure 15-2 NO signaling in vascular cells.

significance of this association remains to be established. A polymorphism in the ecNOS complementary DNA (cDNA) sequence, predictive of a conservative amino acid change, was found with higher frequency in a cohort of patients with vasospastic angina than in control patients, but the functional consequences of this genetic polymorphism have yet to be clarified.

REGULATION OF ECNOS IN THE VASCULAR WALL

The nitric oxide synthase in vascular endothelial cells (ecNOS) is activated by specific receptors and by increases in blood flow, and NO diffuses from the endothelium to inhibit platelet aggregation and to relax vascular smooth muscle (Fig. 15-2). Both cell surface receptors and increases in blood flow transiently activate ecNOS by increasing intracellular calcium. Perhaps the most important autacoid agonist for ecNOS activation is bradykinin. Bradykinin, a potent vasodilator peptide, is synthesized by cells in the vascular wall, and is degraded by angiotensin-converting enzyme, an enzyme that is expressed on the surface of endothelial cells. The clinically important angiotensin converting enzyme inhibitors (e.g., captopril, enalapril, lisinopril) exert at least some of their therapeutic effects by inhibiting the breakdown of bradykinin, which in turn promotes ecNOS activation leading to vasodilation. As a consequence of ecNOS activation, NO synthesized by ecNOS diffuses out of the endothelial cells, and relaxes smooth muscle and inhibits platelet aggregation by activating guanylate cyclase, thereby causing a rise in cGMP in these target cells.

The NO-dependent signaling scheme outlined in Fig. 15-2 appears to be affected in a variety of diseases. The ability of vascular endothelial cells to promote vasorelaxation is impaired ("endothelial dysfunction") in several important disease states, including hypertension, diabetes mellitus, atherosclerosis, hypercholesterolemia, and heart failure. Endothelial dysfunction may be an early marker of atherosclerosis and can be detected in patients before the onset of clinically apparent disease. Treatment of hypercholesterolemia by lipid-lowering drugs or diet appears to reverse endothelial dysfunction. Restoration of endothelium-dependent relaxation may also be seen after the oral administration of L-arginine, the amino acid substrate for NOS, to hypercholesterolemic rabbits or humans. The abundance of the endothelial NO synthase enzyme does not appear to be decreased in these disease states, and may even be increased. It seems likely that abnormalities in the activation of ecNOS or in the metabolism of NO are likely concomitants of endothelial dysfunction, but the molecular details remain obscure.

In addition to its acute effects on vascular tone, endothelium-derived NO may also serve to modulate the growth of vascular smooth muscle cells. For example, a recent report studied in vivo gene transfer of ecNOS to rat carotid arteries in which an intimal lesion was created by intravascular balloon injury. Gene therapy with ecNOS restored vascular NO activity in the injured vessel, and was associated with a marked attenuation of neointima formation, suggesting that NO is an endogenous inhibitor of neointimal proliferation.

NITRIC OXIDE AND PULMONARY HYPERTENSION

Structurally abnormal pulmonary endothelial cells have been documented in the lung vessels of patients with pulmonary hypertension. In these abnormal tissues, the expression of ecNOS appears to be markedly decreased; this was observed in patients with either primary or secondary pulmonary hypertension. It is not clear whether the abnormality in ecNOS is causal for these disorders, or whether reduced expression of ecNOS in pulmonary hypertension reflects a more general endothelial abnormality. Because NO is a gas, and its half-life in the systemic circulation is short, it was hypothesized that NO administered as an inhaled gas might selectively promote pulmonary vasodilation, with potential benefit to patients exhibiting pulmonary hypertension from a number of causes. Inhaled NO has been used to treat patients with the adult respiratory distress syndrome, as well as neonates with primary pulmonary hypertension of the newborn. Beneficial hemodynamic effects are observed in many such patients with pulmonary hypertension, in whom the inhaled NO indeed does selectively dilate the pulmonary vasculature, and because NO is rapidly inactivated in the bloodstream, there is little systemic hypotension. The efficacy and toxicity of longer-term therapy with inhaled NO is being studied in several ongoing clinical trials.

NO PRODUCTION AND SEPTIC SHOCK

A wide variety of cells possess the capacity to synthesize NO in response to immune activators. NO production by immunoactivated cells appears to have a beneficial function in host defense; however, the cellular synthesis of NO needs to be carefully regulated because of the potentially harmful cytotoxic and hypotensive effects of NO. Because NO is a reactive free radical molecule, high concentrations of NO can cause cytotoxic effects. The mechanisms underlying NO's cytotoxicity are multifactorial and include the inhibition of enzymes involved in DNA synthesis in addition to metabolic enzymes, as well as direct effects on cell lipids and DNA. In immunoactivated cells, the iNOS gene is induced, and the NO formed by these cells may play an important role in host defense against bacterial, viral, and protozoan infection. In contrast with cells that constitutively synthesize low levels of NO (such as vascular endothelial cells), immunoactivated cells are generally characterized by much higher levels of NO production. This reflects both the higher level of iNOS protein expression in many immunoactivated cells, as well as the fact that the iNOS protein remains persistently activated, whereas ecNOS (and nNOS) is only transiently activated in response to the short-lived increases in intracellular calcium consequent to receptor activation. The resulting NO production may produce profound hypotension and, not uncommonly, may lead to a fatal outcome. In addition to direct effects of NO on the vasculature to produce vasorelaxation, NO (generated by iNOS induced within the myocytes) may have a direct effect on myocardial contractility. Thus, inappropriate or unregulated NO synthesis may have deleterious effects, either because of direct cytotoxic effects or as a result of NO-induced hypotension.

The delicate balance of NO production in host defense is exemplified in studies of mice in which the iNOS gene has been genetically inactivated. These iNOS-deficient mice show a lower mortality from sepsis-induced hypotension, but are less able to resist infection compared with wild-type mice.

In pathologic states, such as sepsis, smooth muscle cells themselves may activate the iNOS gene in response to cytokines such as TNF-α (tumor necrosis factor-α, generated by immunoactivated cells) or in response to bacterial endotoxin. This leads to excessive NO formation in the smooth muscle cells, and the consequent vasorelaxation can lead to hypotension or even shock, as discussed below. In addition to vascular smooth muscle cells, a wide variety of other cells and tissues express the iNOS gene after immunostimulation by cytokines or bacterial endotoxins. The acute mortality from septic shock derives in part from NO-induced hypotension, and several studies have tried to inhibit sepsis-induced NO production in both experimental and clinical settings. Administration of glucocorticoids does attenuate the genetic induction of iNOS; but, likely because of their pleiotropic effects, steroids do not appear to reduce mortality from sepsis and may in fact be deleterious. Recent experimental studies have administered different growth factors and cytokines in an effort to more selectively block iNOS induction. The greatest amount of clinical experience is in the use of agents that directly block NOS enzyme activity.

NOS inhibitors have been studied in case reports describing treatment of septic shock and are being investigated in ongoing clinical trials. The iNOS inhibitors that have been most widely investigated are analogs of arginine, the substrate for all three NOS isoforms. Infusion of these arginine analogs increases systemic blood pressure in normal humans, and there are anecdotal reports in which administration of arginine analogs stabilized blood pressure in profoundly hypotensive patients in septic shock. Unfortunately, the therapeutic window for the administration of arginine analogs appears to be rather narrow. Complete NOS blockade may result in unopposed vasoconstriction, ultimately leading to tissue ischemia and death. It would be ideal to inhibit just the iNOS because concomitant inhibition of ecNOS could lead to unopposed vasoconstriction and tissue ischemia. Numerous academic investigators and pharmaceutical companies are trying to develop NOS inhibitors that selectively block the iNOS isoform.

The past decade has witnessed the confluence of multiple lines of investigation that together establish the central homeostatic role of NO in control of vascular tone. Ongoing investigations into the structure of NOS isoforms, as well as studies of their cellular regulation, will likely lead to therapeutic advances in the treatment of hypertension and septic shock.

SELECTED REFERENCES

Cuevas P, Garcia-Calvo M, Carceller F, et al. Correction of hypertension by normalization of endothelial levels of fibroblast growth factor and nitric oxide synthase in spontaneously hypertensive rats. Proc Natl Acad Sci USA 1996;93:11,996–12,001.

Furchgott RF, Zawadzki JV. The obligatory role of endothelial cells in the relaxation of arterial smooth muscle by acetylcholine. Nature 1980;288:373–376.

Giaid A, Saleh D. Reduced expression of endothelial nitric oxide synthase in the lungs of patients with pulmonary hypertension. N Engl J Med 1995;333:214–221.

Harrison DG, Armstrong ML, Freiman PC, Heistad DD. Restoration of endothelium-dependent relaxation by dietary treatment of atherosclerosis. J Clin Invest 1987;80:1808–1811.

Hirata Y. Endothelin peptides. Curr Opin Nephrol Hypertens. 1996;5:12–15.

Huang PL, Huang Z, Mashimo H, et al. Hypertension in mice lacking the gene for endothelial nitric oxide synthase. Nature 1995;377:239–242.

Ignarro LJ. Biosynthesis and metabolism of endothelium-derived nitric oxide. Annu Rev Pharmacol Toxicol 1990;30:535–560.

Khan BV, Harrison DG, Olbrych MT, Alexander RW, Medford RM. Nitric oxide regulates vascular cell adhesion molecule 1 gene expression and redox-sensitive transcriptional events in human vascular endothelial cells. Proc Natl Acad Sci USA 1996;93:9114–9119.

Lamas S, Michel T. Molecular biological features of nitric oxide synthase isoforms. In: Zapol W, Bloch KD, eds. Nitric Oxide and the Lung. New York: Marcel Dekker, 1996; pp. 59–73.

Lamas S, Marsden PA, Li GK, Tempst P, Michel T. Endothelial nitric oxide synthase: molecular cloning and characterization of a distinct constitutive enzyme isoform. Proc Natl Acad Sci USA 1992;89:6348–6352.

MacMicking JD, Nathan C, Hom G, et al. Altered responses to bacterial infection and endotoxic shock in mice lacking inducible nitric oxide synthase. Cell 1995;81:641–650.

Marletta MA. Nitric oxide synthase: aspects concerning structure and catalysis. Cell 1994;78:927–930.

Moncada S, Gryglewski R, Bunting S, Vane JR. An enzyme isolated from arteries transforms prostaglandin endoperoxides to an unstable substance that inhibits platelet aggregation. Nature 1976;262:663–665.

Myers PR, Minor RL Jr, Guerra R Jr, Bates JN, Harrison DG. Vasorelaxant properties of the endothelium-derived relaxing factor more closely resemble S-nitrosocysteine than nitric oxide. Nature 1990;345:161–163.

Nathan C, Xie Q-w. Regulation of biosynthesis of nitric oxide. J Biol Chem 1994;269:13,725–13,728.

Palmer RMJ, Ferrige AG, Moncada S. Nitric oxide release accounts for the biological activity of endothelium-derived relaxing factor. Nature 1987;327:524–526.

Shesely EG, Maeda N, Kim HS, et al. Elevated blood pressures in mice lacking endothelial nitric oxide synthase. Proc Natl Acad Sci USA 1996;93:13,176–13,181.

Simonson MS. Endothelins: multifunctional renal peptides. Physiol Rev 1993;73:375–411.

Stamler JS, Simon DI, Osborne JA, et al. S-nitrosylation of proteins with nitric oxide: synthesis and characterization of biologically active compounds. Proc Natl Acad Sci USA 1992;89:444–448.

Von der Leyen HE, Gibbons GH, et al. Gene therapy inhibiting neointimal vascular lesion: in vivo transfer of endothelial cell nitric oxide synthase gene. Proc Natl Acad Sci USA 1995;92:1137–1141.

Wei XQ, Charles IG, Smith A, et al. Altered immune responses in mice lacking inducible nitric oxide synthase. Nature 1995;375:408–411.

Yanagisawa M, Kurihara H, Kimura S, Tomobe Y, Kobayashi M. Endothelin, a vasoconstrictor peptide produced by vascular endothelial cells. Nature 1988;332:411–415.

16 Hypertension

George Koike and Howard J. Jacob

INTRODUCTION

The explosion of genetic markers and analytical techniques in the field of molecular genetics makes the dissection of the genes conveying risk for multifactorial (multiple genes and gene–environment interaction) disorders, such as essential hypertension, possible. This chapter will discuss the application of molecular genetic techniques to the genetic dissection of hypertension. It is important to note that, although the topic discussed in this chapter is hypertension, the approaches and techniques described are applicable to other multifactorial disorders, such as diabetes mellitus, renal failure, and myocardial infarction.

Essential hypertension, defined by an increased blood pressure that exceeds an epidemiologically significant threshold, is a major risk factor for cardiovascular disease as well as a major cause of heart failure, renal failure, and stroke. Although hypertension is a qualitative trait (either a patient has it or not), blood pressure is a continuous trait that exhibits a normal distribution or a quantitative trait in the population. As illustrated in Fig. 16-1 from the Hypertension Detection and Follow-Up Program (HDFP), the threshold level has continued to decrease as the epidemiological significance of a new threshold becomes apparent. If the threshold is inaccurate, its use may reduce statistical power and may introduce bias.

In recent years, there have been several genetic studies using a variety of study designs, most typically association studies (case control studies). These studies have focused on a limited number of candidate genes. The majority of the results from these studies are conflicting (Table 16-1). This may be owing to the difference of study method, phenotyping method (what kind of criteria is used to define hypertensives, what kind of protocol is used to measure blood pressure), number of subjects, gender, and genetic background. These issues are very important and must be considered when designing a genetic study properly. Clinicians/scientists have to be careful to evaluate each study. Currently, there is only one gene, angiotensinogen, that has met relatively stringent criteria, including replication in independent studies by more than one group. However, not all studies with angiotensinogen have been confirmatory, and the causal mutation of this gene has not been identified, leaving open the possibility that this is not the causal gene, but rather near the causal gene or linked to the causal gene.

From: *Principles of Molecular Medicine* (J. L. Jameson, ed.), ©1998 Humana Press Inc., Totowa, NJ.

The goal of this chapter is:

1. To outline how molecular genetic techniques can be brought to bear on hypertension.
2. To illustrate how study design and phenotyping play an essential role in discovering genetic underpinnings of human hypertension.
3. To extend results from studies of experimental animal models.

GENETIC STUDIES FOR HYPERTENSION IN HUMANS

EVIDENCE FOR A GENETIC BASIS Epidemiological studies for many years have revealed that hypertension clusters in families, which could be the result of sharing genes, sharing the same environment, or both. Segregation analyses (which tests for a genetic transmission pattern of disease within a pedigree) suggest that there is a fairly strong genetic component to this disease. The best studies for estimating heritability of a disease are those involving monozygotic and dizygotic twins. Since twins of both classifications share the same womb, there is a control for maternal environment. However, dizygotic twins share 50% of their genomes (same as any other sibling), whereas monozygotic twins are genetically identical. If the monozygotic rate of disease is significantly higher than the dizygotic one, there is a strong genetic component. In monozygotic twins, the chance of a twin developing hypertension if his or her sibling has hypertension is 58%, whereas in dizygotic twins, the risk of developing hypertension if his or her sibling has hypertension is 19%. These data are interpreted as follows: Since the risk to a monozygotic twin is three times higher than for the dizygotic twin, there is a strong genetic component. Interestingly, it is remarkable that even in monozygotic twins, hypertension and other diseases are not fully penetrant (a subject has the genetic predisposition, but does not develop the disease). The reasons for the diseases not being fully penetrant are still unknown, but the most common explanation is that environmental interaction may be required for disease expression. However, it is not hard to see how incomplete penetrance further increases the difficulty in determining the genetic cause of hypertension.

Although genetic and epidemiological studies demonstrated that hypertension has a genetic component, a problem with determining the genetic basis of hypertension is that it results from multiple genes (polygenic nature) and is very common, ranging from a prevalence of 20–40% in humans. The combination of multiple genes and a very common disease translates to most humans carrying at least one hypertensive gene, which means nor-

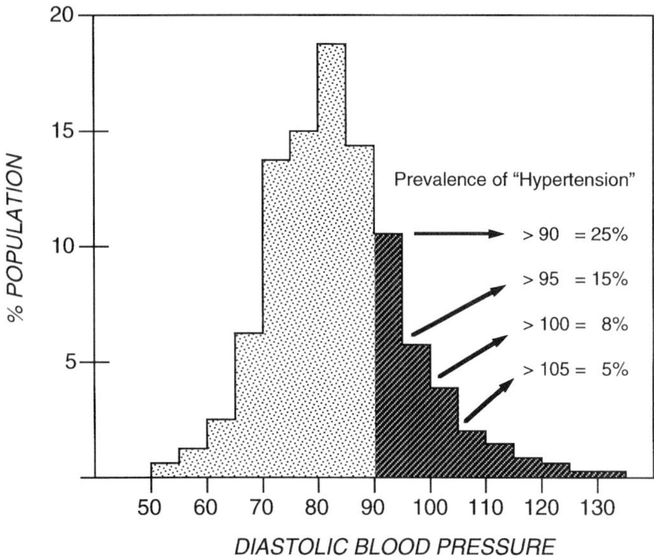

Figure 16-1 Frequency distribution of diastolic blood pressure at home screen of 158,906 persons, 30–69 years of age, HDFP (1974). H. D. a. F.-U. P. C. Group Circ Res 1997.

Table 16-1
Genetic Studies of "Hypertensive loci" in Humans

Candidate genes	*Study design*	*Segregation with High blood pressure*
Renin	Case control	No
ACE	Case control	Yes
	Affected sib-pairs	No
	Four corners	No
Angiotensinogen	Affected sib-pairs	Yes
	Case control	No
S_A	Case control	Yes
	Case control	No

motensive family members will carry hypertensive genes that are shared with hypertensive family members. This problem is further exacerbated by the relatively late age of onset. Will the normotensive subject always be normotensive?

BLOOD PRESSURE AS A PROTOTYPICAL QUANTITATIVE TRAIT Hypertension is a clinically and epidemiologically defined disease. However, as shown in Fig. 16-1, blood pressure shows a normal distribution. There are two key words for the basic principals of the trait (phenotype), "qualitative" and "quantitative." The qualitative trait is a discontinuous variation. For example, Mendel's peas were either green or yellow: the coats of the peas were either smooth or wrinkled. The qualitative trait could be easily followed from one generation to the next with a defined mode of inheritance (additive, dominant, or recessive). In contrast, the quantitative trait is a continuous variation, in which the difference of the phenotype slowly integrates. The quantitative trait is usually described from one extreme to the other. Height and weight are typical examples of a quantitative trait. As described in Fig. 16-1, the distribution of the blood pressure shows from low (normotensive) to high (hypertensive) continuously, and blood pressure is a prototypical quantitative trait. This concept of quantitative genetics has been applied to the agriculturally important crops and experimental models, and several trait-causing genes have been mapped. In a last decade, this has also been applied to several complex traits in humans. Genetic studies for hypertension have used clinical thresholds to defined hypertension as a qualitative trait. To study hypertension as a quantitative trait, it is essential to collect "natural" blood pressure. However, in most cases, patients have been on medication for hypertension, preventing the use of blood pressure as a quantitative trait. Even if medication is removed, there is no guarantee that blood pressure measured is identical to what would have been found if the patients had not been treated. One solution to overcome this conflict is to study hypertension as a qualitative trait. This strategy worked for the human insulin-dependent diabetes mellitus (IDDM) study and human non–insulin-dependent diabetes mellitus (NIDDM) study (*see* Chapter 47). However, if the threshold to defining disease that has quantitative trait is inaccurate, its use may reduce statistical power and may introduce bias.

DETERMINING THE GENETIC BASIS OF HYPERTENSION Prior to 1980, genetic dissection of hypertension or any other diseases in human was practically impossible owing to a paucity of genetic markers. In 1980, Botstein and colleagues demonstrated that sequence variation can be used as a genetic marker. Recent progress of the human genome project has provided several tools, such as genetic markers, genetic linkage maps, expressed sequence tag sites (ESTs), large insert libraries (yeast artificial chromosome [YAC], and bacterial artificial chromosome [BAC]), and radiation hybrids, enabling investigators to carry out gene hunting for genetic disorders. Using these tools, causal genes for many genetic disorders, such as familial hypertrophic cardiomyopathy (*see* Chapter 13), Huntington's disease (*see* Chapter 97), and Liddle's syndrome, have been identified. However, all these diseases have been caused by one gene exhibiting simple Mendelian genetics. To date multifactorial diseases, such as hypertension, have remained elusive.

With the tools required for genetic dissection largely in place, genetic studies into the etiology of hypertension have become quite common. In general, these studies can be broken into two different study designs, as well as by how the subjects were ascertained. It is essential that the clinician/scientist interested in these studies understand the study designs used for dissecting the genetic basis of hypertension.

The study designs can be divided into two different ways: candidate gene approach and total genome scan.

Candidate Gene Approach This strategy focuses on a single gene of interest and has been the most widely applied to the study of human hypertension, as well as other disorders. Generally, to perform candidate gene approach, targeted genes have been picked because they have been known to play a role in blood pressure regulation. For example, since the renin-angiotensin system has been known to play an important role in blood pressure regulation, renin and angiotensin-converting enzyme (ACE) have been favorite targets for studying human hypertension. Furthermore, this study design has frequently been combined with the easiest population ascertainment scheme, association study. (Please *see* Association Study *below* for details.) The concept of this strategy is to find an association between the sequence (allele) difference of a candidate gene and phenotype of interest, in this case, blood pressure. This strategy works well for simple Mendelian diseases. However, since hypertension is a polygenic (polygeneity: simultaneous abnormalities of multiple genes cause one phenotype [hypertension] and genetically heterogeneous [genetic heterogeneity]:

Table 16-2
Comparison of Genetic Studies

Linkage analysis (pedigree analysis)
- Advantages
  - Suitable for total genome scan
  - Suitable for simple Mendelian traits
  - No need to collect a control population
  - May be useful for multifactorial disorders when isolated population is studied
- Disadvantages
  - Difficult to collect large informative pedigrees
  - Difficult to obtain enough statistical power for complex traits

Allele-sharing method
- Advantages
  - Suitable for total genome scan
  - Suitable for multifactorial traits
  - No need to collect a control population if the information of allele frequency in general population is available
- Disadvantages
  - Difficult to collect population

Affected sib-pairs study
- Advantage
  - More statistical power with parent's information (IBD information)
- Disadvantage
  - Same as above

Affected pedigree member study
- Advantage
  - More statistical power with the more information of IBS to infer IBD
- Disadvantage
  - Difficult to collect relatives in addition to sib-ships

Discordant sib-pairs study
- Advantages
  - To save genotyping effort (requires fewer genotypes and fewer patients to be ascertained)
  - To use same population for several different traits of interest
- Disadvantage
  - Need to collect a large number of sib-ships, affected and unaffected; especially difficult to collect unaffected sib-ships
  - Discordant unaffected sibs need to be defined based on the distribution within the population

Association study (case control study)
- Advantages
  - Suitable for candidate gene approaches
  - Easiest for subjects ascertainment
- Disadvantages
  - Need a large number of population
  - Need a control population
  - Difficult to obtain enough statistical power
  - High probability of false linkage without the correct control population

abnormalities in any one of several genes cause one identical phenotype [hypertension]) disease and a lot of genes have been considered as candidates, with current technology it is not an efficient way to study hypertension owing to hundreds of combinations of candidate genes within the population.

Total Genome Scan Strategy This strategy, reported in 1986 by Lander and Botstein, has become more favored as the number of genetic markers have increased. The concept of this strategy is that once a complete genetic linkage map is available, the total genome could be scanned simultaneously to find genetic markers that cosegregate (is genetically linked) with phenotypes that have a genetic basis; in this case, blood pressure. This approach is more systematic compared to the candidate gene approach. Therefore, this strategy is suitable to studying a polygenic and genetically heterogeneous disease, such as hypertension. Using this strategy, the region or genetic locus containing a gene responsible for a disease could be mapped without any *a priori* knowledge, having a great potential to identify novel genes.

Study designs and the methods to collect study population (patient ascertainment) available for genetic dissection of multifactorial traits in humans, such as hypertension, can be broken down roughly into three methods:

1. Linkage analysis (pedigree analysis).
2. Allele-sharing method (affected sib-pairs study, discordant sib-pairs study, affected pedigree member study).
3. Association study (case control study).

A brief comparison of these studies is summarized below and in Table 16-2. For more detailed information, several reviews are available.

Linkage Analysis Linkage analysis involves proposing a model to explain the inheritance pattern of phenotypes and genotypes observed in a pedigree. For simple Mendelian traits, this model is straightforward and powerful. Among hypertension-related diseases, identification of the genes for Liddle's syndrome and glucocorticoid-remediable aldosteronism provides typical examples. On the other hand, for multifactorial traits, such as essential hypertension, this model could become more complicated and less powerful owing to the difficulty of phenotyping (difficult to define disease state, especially with late-onset traits among generations) and the loss of transmission of the linkage among generations. Since hypertension is polygenic and common, unaffected pedigree members will carry some of the genes, but not express the disease. This situation is the biggest limitation to studying hypertension with this strategy. One solution would be to divide hypertension patients into multiple subgroups based on phenotype. Unfortunately, we do not have any agreed upon clinical end points to accomplish this. It may be possible to apply this strategy to an isolated population, such as Chicoutimi-Saguenay-Lac St. Jean French-Canadian population. Isolated populations frequently exhibit a founder effect, meaning that only a few disease genes are segregating in the population. Therefore, the disease has less heterogeneity, improving the likelihood that hypertension is a single disease. For this strategy, multiple consecutive generations (generally at least three) in a pedigree are required to specify the correct model to obtain a enough statistical power. Without the information of multiple consecutive generations, linkage analysis could not be carried out. However, it is highly likely that a model for a pedigree assumed with this limited information could be wrong, resulting in missing true linkage and sometimes accepting false linkage.

Allele-Sharing Method The allele-sharing method can obviate many of these restrictions in the dissection of polygenic traits. Affected sib-pairs, affected pedigree member (APM), and discordant sib-pairs studies are included in this method. Prior information regarding the mode of inheritance, penetrance of the disease, or other assumptions is not required. Analysis is based on significant sharing of alleles between affected relatives at the disease loci. Both the candidate gene approach and the total genome scan strategy can be applied with this method. Affected sib-pairs study compares the number of alleles shared between sib-ships. On average (with fully informative markers), sib-ships are expected to share an allele 50% of the time. However, if a disease-causing gene resides near a genetic marker, then affected sib-pairs will exhibit allele sharing significantly different from 50%. In practice, if parental genotypes are not known, shared alleles are identical-by-state (IBS), because one does not know if the parents shared the same allele. If parental genotypes are known, the allele sharing is identical-by-descent (IBD) (with a fully informative marker). Consequently, multiplex families provide more genetic power than simply looking at affected sib-pairs. In contrast, APM study requires affected relatives (uncles, aunts, cousins, and so forth) and in some cases is more informative than the affected sib-pairs study. Recently, discordant sib-pairs study design has been described and is based on most of the linkage information being derived from both extremes of the traits of population. For this strategy, affected sibs and unaffected sibs are collected to reflect the extremes of the general population in contrast to the other studies. Therefore, fewer patients need to be ascertained and genotyped. Unfortunately, ascertainment is based on the unaffected individuals being at the extreme of the population. Consequently, this study design requires population data and selective ascertainment.

Two examples of using allele-sharing method in human are the identification of the region of the human genome linked to NIDDM by Hanis et al. and of several regions linked to IDDM by Davies et al. (*see* Chapter 47).

Association Study Association study is the most common strategy used to carry out genetic study for hypertension, and does not require familial inheritance patterns of diseases at all. This study design is based on a comparison of unrelated affected and unaffected individuals from a given population, and to test whether a particular allele is observed at higher frequency among affected than unaffected individuals. Therefore, criteria to collect individuals are less stringent (subjects could be collected randomly) than other studies discussed above. An essential component is the selection of the unaffecteds (controls) and to study a large number of subjects followed by ascertaining a second population set for confirmation. Otherwise, the chance of a false linkage is high. This approach has widely been applied. For example, association studies for ACE insertion/deletion (I/D) polymorphism, and several diseases, such as myocardial infarction, hypertrophic cardiomyopathy, left ventricular hypertrophy, and hypertension have been carried out. However, replications of these findings have been limited and may be owing to the following reasons:

1. The criteria to collect human subjects (affecteds and unaffecteds) may differ among studies.
2. The number of subjects is relatively small.
3. The two-allele system (D allele and I allele) for ACE does not provide enough information, since it is highly possible that these alleles may be commonly observed among subjects.
4. It is extremely unlikely that this sequence variance represents a biologically relevant mutation.
5. Most of the studies are the retrospective that potentially introduces biased data set. For example, in the first paper demonstrating an association of myocardial infarction (MI) and ACE polymorphism, the subjects studied were the survivors from the initial MI. This study did not include the subjects who died at the initial MI.

Each one of these decreases the statistical power to analyze the data set. If these criteria are well-covered, this approach is a powerful method to perform genetic dissection of multifactorial disease, such as the association between apolipoprotein E and Alzheimer's disease. This study involved the use of the multiple-allele system and relatively large population, and has been replicated numerous times.

How then does one design a study that has enough power to detect genes responsible for hypertension against a backdrop of multiple genes, moderate penetrance, environmental interaction, and when many of the causal genes are frequent in the general population? Despite the recent advances in molecular genetics (because of the success of the international human genome project), only one locus, the angiotensinogen gene locus, has been shown to segregate with essential hypertension in several studies and several study designs (although not all studies find a positive association). Major limitations in human studies are as follows:

1. To collect the large number of samples in a well-controlled study with accurate phenotyping remains a daunting challenge.
2. Genetic heterogeneity (several genes or gene combinations are able to cause the same phenotype).
3. Polygeneity (multiple genes are necessary to express the phenotype).

4. Environmental factors (for example, it is well-known that stress and salt in some people are able to increase blood pressure).
5. Statistical concerns and challenges in evaluating collected data, particularly with respect to studying hypertension as a quantitative trait.

These limitations have restricted the genetic dissection of hypertension in humans to the candidate gene approach instead of scanning the total genome, although they are now under way in several laboratories around the world. One solution that we have taken is to attack the genetic basis of hypertension using two approaches, allele-sharing methods and studies of experimental animal models.

As described *above*, we are still facing several difficulties that have to be overcome. Therefore, the points that we have to be careful to evaluate in genetic studies, especially in human, are as follows: (1) Is positive result real or not? (2) Negative result does simply not mean there is no linkage. If the study is carried out with enough genetic power, there may potentially be a linkage identified, or the gene may play a role in another population or ethnic group.

GENETIC STUDIES FOR HYPERTENSION IN EXPERIMENTAL ANIMAL MODELS

Another approach to carrying out the genetic study for hypertension is the genetic analysis of large crosses in experimental animal models, particularly in rat. Experimental animal models offer several advantages for genetic research:

1. They are inbred (maternal and paternal chromosomes are identical), thereby solving the problem of heterogeneity.
2. Mating can be controlled and optimized.
3. Large numbers of progeny can be generated.
4. Invasive phenotyping protocol can be used.

These attributes of inbred animals are allowing dissection of various genes affecting multifactorial traits, such as hypertension. The coding region of the rat genome is more than 90% similar to the human genome. Therefore, once disease genes are identified in animal models, these genes can then be studied in the regions of conserved gene order between human and model genomes. Not all genes discovered in this manner are expected to play a role in the human disease; however, historically, more complete understanding of the physiology in model animals has aided understanding of human biology. Of course, genetic dissection of human hypertension has made progress recently, and the physiology and pathophysiology of the experimental animal models are not identical with human. For example, in the case of humans and rat (experimental animal model for hypertension), cardiovascular parameters, such as blood pressure and heart rate, and onset age of hypertension are different. However, recent progress in the human cannot account for the etiology of hypertension completely. Therefore, the complementary investigations in both humans and experimental animal models should continue toward our complete understanding of genetic causes for hypertension and other multifactorial diseases (e.g., diabetes and renal failure). In the last 30 years, several experimental animal models of hypertension have been used to study the etiology of hypertension and the blood pressure regulation. Among several experimental animal models, the rat has been extensively characterized in physiology. Most importantly, several hypertensive and normotensive rat strains are available as inbred strains. Table 16-3 lists major hypertensive and normotensive inbred rat strains. As described in this table, each hypertensive strains has a unique character(s).

Table 16-3
Major Hypertensive and Normotensive Inbred Rat Strains

Hypertensive rat
Dahl salt-susceptible rat (SS/Jr): Model for salt-sensitive hypertension
Fawn-Hooded hypertensive rat (FHH): Model for hypertension and renal failure
Genetically hypertensive rat (GH): Model for hypertension and cardiac hypertrophy
Lyon hypertensive rat (LH): Model for hypertension
Milan hypertensive rat (MHS): Model for mild hypertension
Sabra hypertensive rat (SBH): Model for DOCA salt-sensitive hypertension
Spontaneously hypertensive rat (SHR): Model for hypertension
Stroke-prone spontaneously hypertensive rat (SHRSP): Model for hypertension, stroke and cardiovascular diseases
Normotensive rat
AxC irish rat (ACI)
Brown Norway rat (BN)
Dahl salt-resistant rat (SR/Jr)
Donryu rat (DRY)
Fischer rat (F344)
Lewis rat (LEW)
Lyon normotensive rat (LN)
Milan normotensive rat (MNS)
Wistar-Kyoto rat (WKY)

Based on genetic infrastructure, the mouse is the best-characterized experimental model. However, there is only one mouse strain that develops severe hypertension, and the physiology of the mouse cardiovascular system is very rudimentary. Even though the rat genetic infrastructure is less developed than the mouse, a tremendous effort has been made to understand the physiology of hypertension using this species. For example, there have been more than 2000 reports that have used the spontaneously hypertensive rat (SHR), a genetically hypertensive rat, with most of these reporting differences between the SHR and a normotensive control, typically the Wistar-Kyoto rat (WKY). Similar studies have been carried out using various genetically hypertensive rats. However, these studies focused on simple differences in physiological characteristics between the strains without genetics.

Clearly experimental animal models have some physiological and pathophysiological differences with human, so how useful will these models be? The issue of relevancy to the human pathobiology is frequently associated with there being a 100% correlation between human and experimental animal models. It would be extremely unlikely that the rat strains developed by simply selecting for animals with the highest blood pressure would be identical to human hypertension. It would be equally unlikely that any human pedigree or small set of affected sib-pairs would represent all patients with hypertension. In fact, the very definition of hypertension remains limited to the clinical presentation and various attributes found in some patients with hypertension. In practice, however, it is very likely that some genes found in animal models will be concordant with human disease, but in all cases, the information learned is important in understanding the etiology of hypertension. For example, Cicila et al. reported that 11-β hydroxylase is responsible for mineralocorticoid hypertension in the SS/Jr. These data appear to confirm the study by Lifton et al. (1992), which found that an unequal crossover between 11-β hydroxylase and aldosynthase resulted in glucocorticoid-remediable aldosteronism. A recent genome-wide scan of humans for IDDM located two quantitative trait loci (QTLs) in homologous regions with the NOD mouse, confirming that total genome search in animal models may provide insight. We believe that using the rat QTLs as genetic pointers to highlight the regions of the human genome to genotype with markers at 1-cM intervals will increase our chances of locating novel and important regions involved in hypertension.

Our laboratory has been building the infrastructure, genetic markers, and genetic map for the rat. We and others have used this infrastructure to carry out genetic dissection of multifactorial traits, such as hypertension, renal failure, type I and II diabetes mellitus, and cardiac hypertrophy using the rat as an animal model. In this chapter, we would like to focus on how these data can be used to study hypertension in human.

RECENT PROGRESS IN RAT Over the last few years, investigators have begun to use molecular genetic techniques to find genes responsible for hypertension using rats. Initial studies began with "candidate gene" studies hypothesizing that the gene is a cause of hypertension. Previously, Dr. John Rapp set four criteria to define a causal gene:

1. A biochemical and/or physiological difference between two strains (people) must be established.
2. The locus or loci must segregate in a Mendelian fashion.
3. The locus or loci identified must account for a significant portion of the blood pressure.
4. There must be some logical link between the locus or loci and its control of blood pressure.

More recently, the definition of a candidate gene has expanded to include an unknown gene within an interval that cosegregates with hypertension, and these genes are "positional candidate genes."

Complete genome scans in the rat models of hypertension have become more popular as the number of markers available for the rat genome have increased. These studies involve genotyping a large number of genetic markers and observing if any of these markers cosegregate with any of the recorded phenotypes, offering the possibility of locating previously unknown genes responsible for hypertension. A glance at Table 16-4, listing the loci found in several studies, shows that many of the genetic regions that cosegregate with high blood pressure contain a candidate gene. Several key points are evident from Table 16-4. First, there appears to be a "hypertension-causing" gene on practically every rat chromosome. One might conclude that genetic dissection does not appear to be simplifying the process of determining the causal genes for high blood pressure. However, the blood pressure regulatory pathway is very complex and contains a large number of potential sites, which, if disrupted, could result in high blood pressure. It is quite likely that this list will expand as the genetic map of the rat improves and the number of crosses studied increases. Second, when studying this table, it is apparent that different crosses utilizing one or both of the same strains may or may not have the same QTL(s) cosegregating with blood pressure. A limitation of all genetic dissection is that it can only identify differences between strains or people. It cannot identify genes in common between two strains, even if those genes are also critical to the development of hypertension.

This table also details, quite surprisingly, that very few studies (except for those in the recombinant inbred strains) have identified QTLs associated with baseline blood pressure, despite a spread of more than 2 SD between the blood pressure of the two parental strains. Why so few QTLs have been identified for baseline blood pressures remains to be determined. A logical hypothesis is that the critically important system of blood pressure regulation involves a large number of genes, some involved in increasing low blood pressure and others involved in reducing blood pressure. If this hypothesis is correct, there may be several genes involved in hypertension in any one cross, each one contributing only a few mmHg to the overall blood pressure. In this case, a very large number of animals will be required before "linkage" can be determined. Therefore, it may be necessary to induce various stresses to the cardiovascular system in order to uncover which regulatory mechanism of the blood pressure system cannot respond. This may also explain why most of the studies have identified linkage to a particular QTL after inducing a salt-load stress.

In sum, the initial studies utilizing a genetic dissection approach have located several regions in the rat genome that play a role in hypertension; however, several points need to be emphasized. Many of the initial studies have not utilized a complete genetic linkage map and may have missed additional QTLs. Also many of the crosses studied are quite small (<200 animals) and lack enough power to identify additional QTLs.

Newly identified QTLs have become synonymous with candidate genes in or near the QTL. This association with any candidate is likely to be premature and may cause future research to focus on the candidate, rather than identifying previously unknown genes in the region that may also be involved with blood pressure regulation. If the initial candidate does not prove to be causative in additional studies, the initial finding may be discounted based on studying the wrong candidate. For example, renin is a candidate gene because it is important in blood pressure regulation, and it also has been shown to cosegregate with high blood pressure. However, there is no direct evidence that the renin gene is a causal gene for hypertension in the original cross.

Based on previous rat studies in Table 16-4, another aspect that we have to pay attention to is genetic background. The influence of genetic background on the expression of hypertension has been largely ignored. Studies using the same hypertensive strain crossed with different normotensive strains showed different results (each study identified different loci), suggesting that the gene(s) derived from normotensive strain may play a role in the development of hypertension. This may also be a result of differences in phenotypes. Presently, the only method to control for these effects is to use a 2 × 2 study design, where two different hypertensive strains are crossed with the same normotensive strain, which has not been reported.

The effect of gender on blood pressure also has been largely overlooked, since most cross-structures reported have used a single-cross approach (typically the male hypertensive animal crossed with a female normotensive animal) and most studies have only focused on males. The use of single cross and/or the use of male animal prevents determining if a phenotypic difference between the male and female animals is the result of a sex-linked (gene carried on the sex chromosomes X or Y) gene or genes, or the sex-specific (the result of hormonal differences or other factors that distinguish the two sexes).

LESSONS FROM RAT STUDIES In addition to identifying loci responsible for blood pressure regulation, results from our rat studies revealed significantly important aspects regarding gender

Table 16-4
Summary of Hypertensive Loci Identified by Genetic Mapping of Rat[a]

Cross	*Hypertensive loci*	*Phenotype*
SHRSP	Chr. 10 (ACE), Chr. 18 (?)	SBP after salt
	Chr. 10 (ACE), X Chr.(?)	SBP after salt
	Chr. 1 (SA)	SBP after salt
	Chr. 10 (?)	basal SBP
	Chr. 10 (ACE)	SBP after salt
		DBP after salt
SHRSP/Izu × WKY/Izu	Chr. 10 (ACE)	SBP after salt
SHR × WKY	Chr. 1 (SA)	SBP, DBP
	Chr. 1 (MT1PA)	SBP
SHR × WKY	Chr. 4 (NPY, SPR)	SBP, DBP, MAP
SHR × WKY	Y-Chr.(?)	SBP
SHR × WKY	Chr. 13 (Renin)	SBP, DBP
SHR × BN	Chr. 2 (GCA, MT1PB)	SBP after salt
	Chr. 4 (NPY), Chr 8 (?), Chr. 16 (?)	
SHR × DRY	Chr. 10 (NGF)	MAP
SHR × LEW	Chr. 13 (Renin)	MAP
RI (SHR × BN)[b]	Chr. 20 (HSP70)	SBP
RI (SHR × BN)[b]	Chr. 12 (HSP27)	SBP
RI (SHR × BN)[b]	Chr. 13 (Renin)	SBP
RI (SHR × BN)[b]	Chr. 1 (Kallikrien)	SBP
RI (SHR x BN)[b]	Chr. 19 (?)	SBP
	Chr. 2 (?)	DBP
	Chr. 4 (IL6)	MAP
SS/Jr/Hsd/Mcw × BN	Chr. 3 (ADRFLP, AVP)	SBP after salt
SS/Jr × SR/Jr	Chr. 13 (Renin)	SBP after salt
SS/Jr × SR/Jr	Chr. 3 (ET3)	SBP after salt
SS/Jr × MNS	Chr. 2 (GCA), Chr. 10 (ACE)	SBP after salt
	Chr. 2 (NaKα1-CAMK)	SBP after salt
	Chr. 10 (iNOS)	SBP after Salt
SS/Jr × WKY	Chr. 2 (GCA)	SBP after salt
	Chr. 2 (NaKα1-CAMK)	SBP after salt
SS/Jr × LEW	Chr. 5 (ET2), Chr.17 (HITH)	SBP after salt
SS/Jr × LEW	Chr. 1 (SA)	SBP after salt
	Chr. 1 (P450)	SBP after salt
GH × BN	Chr. 2 (GCA), Chr10 (ACE)	SBP
LH × LN	Chr.2 (?)	PP
	Chr.13 (Renin)	DBP

[a]Candidate genes: α2b adrenergic receptor (ADRFLP); angiotensin-converting enzyme locus (ACE); arginine vasopressin (AVP); calmodulin-dependent protein kinase II-Δ locus (CAMK); cytochrome P450 (P450); endothelin-2 locus (ET2); endothelin-3 locus (ET3); guanylyl cyclase A/atrial natriuretic peptide receptor locus (GCA); heat-shock protein locus (HSP); inducible nitric oxide synthase locus (iNOS); metallothionein-1 pseudogene-A (MT1PA); metallothionein-1 (MT1PB); $Na^{+}K^{+}$ATPase α locus (NaKα1); nerve growth factor locus (NGF); neuropeptide Y locus (NPY); substance P receptor locus (SPR); the testis-specific histon locus (HITH); no known candidate gene reported (?).

Phenotypes: blood pressure (BP); diastolic blood pressure (DBP); mean arterial pressure (MAP); pulse pressure (PP); systolic blood pressure (SBP).

Strains of rats: donryu (DRY); genetically hypertensive (GH); Lyon hypertensive (LH); Lyon normotensive (LN); Milan normotensive strain (MNS); spontaneously hypertensive rat (SHR); stroke prone SHR (SHRSP); Dahl salt-susceptible rat (SS/Jr); Dahl salt-resistant rat (SR/Jr).

[b]RI, recombinant inbred strains. This methodology, although not as powerful as a cross-study, does offer some insight. A problem with this approach is that the same phenotyping information is "scanned" repeatedly, increasing the chance of false linkage, and the segregation of genes is fixed in only 28 strains.

differences and phenotyping that may also be critical for human genetic studies. In this section, we discuss how these issues potentially relate to genetic studies of human hypertension.

Gender Effect The difference in blood pressure levels between males and females and the putative regulatory mechanisms involved have been extensively addressed in the literature. Even though the sex effects have been reported by several investigators, controversy over the existence of sex-linked (the result of gene[s] on the X or Y chromosome) and/or sex-specific (differences because of sex: the result of hormonal differences or other factors that distinguish the two sexes) effects remains. Previously, Tanase et al. used several estimates of heritability to carry out genetic analysis of hypertension in three crosses (Table 16-5). The progenies of these crosses were phenotyped over many weeks. Several interesting points arise from this study. One of them is that an estimate of the number of loci is different between male and

Table 16-5
Number of Genetic Loci Estimated to be Responsible for Blood Pressure at Different Sexes and Ages[a]

					Week						
Cross	*5*	*7*	*9*	*11*	*13*	*15*	*17*	*19*	*20*	*25*	*30*
SHR × WI											
Male	0.2	1.6	3.1	4.0	4.2	5.7	6.3	5.4			
Female	0.2	1.2	3.9	3.4	4.8	4.9	4.0	4.0			
SHR × WKY											
Male						2.5			2.6	2.2	2.8
Female						4.1			3.2	4.3	4.0
SHR × WM											
Male						1.6			1.4	2.5	2.4
Female						2.7			3.1		

[a]WI, Wistar/Imamichi; WKY, Wistar/Kyoto; WM, Wistar/Mishima.

female in the same cross at the same time-point, indicating the gender difference responsible for hypertension. Recently, differences between sexes also observed in the SHRSP/Hei X WKY/Hei and the GH X BN cross suggest that there maybe sex-specific (not sex-linked) QTLs influencing blood pressure. An example for sex-linked effect is the Y chromosome effect on blood pressure. In 1990, Ely and Turner reported a Y chromosome effect that accounted for a significant proportion of the genetic variance in blood pressure. The notion of a hypertensive gene on the Y chromosome is consistent with producing all hypertensive progeny in the fourth generation after initiating the selection for hypertension when deriving the original SHR. They have generated a set of congenic animals where a Y chromosome from the WKY was placed on an SHR background (SHR-Y^{WKY}) and a Y chromosome from the SHR was placed on a WKY background (WKY-Y^{SHR}). These congenic rats' blood pressures were measured and compared to the parental strains. The SHR-Y^{WKY} has a lower pressure than the SHR, and the WKY-Y^{SHR} has a higher blood pressure than the WKY.

To address the gender effect, a study design, reciprocal cross-setup, allows one to investigate if there are any sex-linked genes, sex-specific genes, or epigenetic factors (imprinting, mitochondrial genes) in a cross. Reciprocal crossdesign is to setup two different grandparents combination; hypertensive male × normotensive female, and normotensive male × hypertensive female, resulting in maximum power to carry the genetic study to elucidate gender effect and potentially reveal any epigenetic effects (mitochondrial or imprinting). However, the majority of previous rat studies used only single grandparent setup (generally hypertensive male × normotensive female), not able to see sex-linked genes or epigenetics. Our study addressing these effects is being analyzed, but this stage is too early to show our conclusion. Nevertheless, we are confident that our studies will be very useful in understanding sex-linked, gender, and epigenetic effects on blood pressure regulation and provide us with clues for searching for genes in affected sib-pairs and case control studies.

Phenotyping Window Effects It is important to realize that rat genetic studies described in this chapter can distinguish differences between the only two strains studied. (This is an advantage to use animal models instead of human.) Because the selection of strains determines the number of genes segregating within the cross, it is meaningless to talk about the number of genes responsible for hypertension without specifying the strains studied. The number of genes responsible for phenotype can theoretically be estimated. For example, again using the study of Tanase et al. described in Table 16-5, another interesting point is that the estimated number of loci are changing at the different time-points and are different between male and female in the same cross at the same time-point. Recently, we identified two genes, *Rf-1* and *Rf-2*, responsible for renal failure using the FHH × ACI cross. In this study, we only used male population, because females did not develop renal failure at the age of 6–9 months, but males do develop renal failure. However, when we let the females live to 2 years of age, they developed renal failure, and we could identify *Rf-1* with the female population. In this case, age of onset for renal failure is completely different. These two studies imply the following question: Are phenotypes collected at a correct time-point? Especially when a gender-mixed population is studied, investigators have to be careful to set a phenotyping time-point.

In humans, women generally develop hypertension later than men (in early adulthood until late middle age, the rise in men's blood pressure is bigger than women's), indicating that phenotyping time-point should be different between males and females. Therefore, this "phenotyping window effect" has to be considered, leading one to ask; "Are gender-matched, age-matched study designs appropriate?" Otherwise, human genetic studies with gender-mixed populations and age-matched controls may not be appropriate because of this "phenotyping window effect."

Phenotyping Is Critical There are a variety of methods to measure blood pressure of the rat, such as direct catheter measurement, tail-cuff method, and telemetry method. One of our studies using F_2 intercross of GH X BN measured blood pressure by two different methods, direct catheter measurement and tail-cuff method. Even if we could measure blood pressure under the same conditions by different methods, the same QTLs should be detected if the methodology has no effect. However, we could detect QTLs on chromosome 2, 6 and 18 by tail-cuff method, and only on chromosome 6 by the direct catheter method, suggesting these two phenotypes represented different blood pressure phenotypes. It is obvious that these two methods are totally different. The tail-cuff method is a stressful method for the rat (stress induces blood pressure increase) because of the use of anesthesia, heating, and tail-cuff itself in contrast to the direct catheter method, which is less stressful. This could explain why several studies identified different QTLs with the use of the same rat strains. Consequently, determination of blood pressure in human is not as easy as it

Table 16-6
Cosegregation of Hypertensive Loci in the Human and Rat Genome

Hypertensive loci	*Species*	*Cosegregation with high blood pressure*	
Renin	Rat	Yes:	SS/Jr × SR/Jr
			SHR × WKY
		No:	SHRSP/Hei × WKY/Hei
			SHR × BN
	Human No:		
ACE	Rat	Yes:	SHRSP/Hei × WKY/Hei
			SIIRSP/Izu × WKY/Izu
	Human Yes:		
		No:	
Angiotensinogen	Rat	No:	SHRSP/Hei × WKY/Hei
	Human Yes:		
		No:	
S_A	Rat	Yes:	SHRSP/Hei × WKY/Hei
			SHR × WKY
			SS/Jr × LEW
			FHH × ACI
		No:	SHR × BN
	Human Yes:		
		No:	

appears, since the following factors are likely to influence the level of blood pressure:

1. Type of method.
2. When.
3. How many times.
4. Which position, and so forth.

CLINICAL IMPLICATIONS OF THE RAT STUDIES In Table 16-6, a comparison of the recent studies between human and rat is summarized. Of course, we are not simply able to compare human and rat studies because of the difference in the experimental design. Table 16-6 can be interpreted several ways. Optimistically, we could say that the ACE locus and the S_A locus, found to be important in the rat for the increase in blood pressure after a salt-load, play a role in human hypertension. However, we could say just the opposite, which the majority of investigators would support based on the strength of each study's design. We take these data at face value to mean that the genetic dissection of hypertension in the rat and human will at times lead to conflicting results. These differences come from several sources. For human study, etiological heterogeneity and study designs are the major reasons for the conflicts, as Lander and Schork recently observed. For the rat studies (Table 16-4), genetic background effects are a major problem that should prevent investigators from making sweeping conclusions, but do not. Even when using the rat, the number of the rats in some studies is relatively small and may not have enough power to identify QTLs, which control a small portion of the variance.

Given these difficulties in the rat studies and the successes of molecular genetics in dissection hypertension in humans, many investigators may ask next the following simple questions: Is there still a role for experimental animal models? Will the genes important in determining hypertension in animal models also be important in humans? Data outlined in Table 16-6 suggest that the rat genes may not be important for human hypertension. Furthermore, a study by Hübner et al. reported that angiotensinogen, thc only known gene responsible for hypertension in humans, does not cosegregate with hypertension in the SHRSP/Hei x WKY/Hei. However, we must consider several points. First, as discussed earlier, the data connecting the QTL with any candidate genes are largely circumstantial. Additionally, most of the genetic "hypertensive" loci have not yet been tested as candidate regions in affected sib-pair studies or in various ethnic groups. Second, the negative study with angiotensinogen in a single cross has very little meaning, since genetic studies can only distinguish differences between the two strains studied, and a negative finding can have several causes and is not definitive for the candidate gene in a more general context.

After finding a gene responsible for hypertension in either human or experimental animal models, the next step in the research would be to investigate its molecular mechanism and physiology. Because of the difficulty of carrying out a physiological study in humans, experimental animal models have been studied instead. These studies have been providing us with the detailed physiology for the understanding of the pathogenesis of hypertension. Even a novel gene responsible for hypertension is found based on human genetic study, experimental animal models will remain one of the best ways to understand the detailed physiology and gene functions.

SUMMARY

Despite the recent progress of molecular genetics, there are several challenges to dissect the genetic basis of human essential hypertension using human subjects. Although there is an argument regarding whether the experimental animal models could represent humans, there is no question that this is one of the powerful approaches to performing genetic study. Genetic analysis using experimental animal models (rat for hypertension) provides: (1) understanding of the multifactorial basis of hypertension (e.g., genetic basis, environmental factors, and gene–gene interaction) and (2) the direction of the regions of the human genome to be studied before the genes are identified, thereby revealing clues about the genetic basis of human hypertension. The detailed physiology known about the animal models (this is also another advantage for the animal models) combined with this new genetic information is likely to provide more complete understanding of the pathogenesis of hypertension. Taking this advantage, clinical diagnosis of essential hypertension will be divided into more detailed subcategories (no longer essential hypertension with unknown etiology), resulting in increasing the efficiency of drug therapy and potentially in future gene therapy.

SELECTED REFERENCES

Aitman TJ, Gotoda T, Evans AL, et al. Quantitative trait loci for cellular defects in glucose and fatty acid metabolism in hypertensive rats. Nat Genet 1997;16:197–201.

Anastos K, Charney P, Charon RA, et al. Hypertension in women: what is really known? Ann of Intern Med 1991;115:287–293.

Botstein D, White RL, Skolnick M, Davis RW. Construction of a genetic linkage map in man using RFLP's. Am J Hum Genet 1980;32:314.

Brown DM, Provoost AP, Daly MJ, Lander ES, Jacob HJ. Renal disease susceptibility and hypertension are under independent genetic control in the fawn-hooded rat. Nat Genet 1996;12:44–51.

Cambien F, Poirier O, Lecerf L, et al. Deletion polymorphism in the gene for angiotensin-converting enzyme is a potent risk factor for myocardial infarction. Nature 1992;359:641–644.

Caulfield M, Lavender P, Farrall M, et al. Linkage of the angiotensinogen gene to essential hypertension. N Engl J Med 1994;330:1629–1633.

Cicila GT, Rapp JP, Wang JM, Lezin E, Ng SC, Kurtz TW. Linkage of 11β-hydroxylase mutations with altered steroid biosynthesis and blood pressure in Dahl rat. Nat Genet 1993;3:346–353.

Cicila GT, Rapp JP, Bloch KD, et al. Cosegregation of the endothelin-3 locus with blood pressure and relative heart weight in inbred Dahl rats. J. Hypertens 1994;12:643–651.

Corder EH, Saunders AM, Risch NJ, et al. Protective effect of apolipoprotein E type 2 allele for late onset Alzheimer disease. Nat Genet 1994;7:180–184.

Davies J, Kawaguchi Y, Bennett S, et al. A genome-wide search for human type1 diabetes susceptibility genes. Nature 1994;371:130–136.

Deng AY, Rapp JP. Locus for the inducible, but not a constitutive, nitric oxide synthase cosegregates with blood pressure in the Dahl salt-sensitive rat. J Clin Invest 1995;95:2170–2177.

Deng AY, Dene H, Rapp JP. Mapping of a quantitative trait locus for blood pressure on rat chromosome 2. J Clin Invest 1994a;94:431–436.

Deng AY, Dene H, Pravenec M, Rapp JP. Genetic mapping of two new blood pressure quantitative trait loci in the rat by genotyping endothelin system genes. J Clin Invest 1994b;93:2701–2709.

Deng Y, Rapp JP. Cosegregation of blood pressure with angiotensin converting enzyme and atrial natriuretic peptide receptor genes using Dahl salt-sensitive rats. Nat Genet 1992;1:267–272.

Dubay C, Vinent M, Samani NJ, et al. Genetic determinants of diastolic and pulse pressure map to different loci in Lyon hypertensive rats. Nat Genet 1993;3:354–357.

Dzau V. Circulating vs. local renin-angiotensin system in cardiovascular homeostasis. Circ 1988;77:I4–I13.

Ely DL, Turner ME. Hypertension in the spontaneously hypertensive rats is linked to the Y-chromosome. Hypertension 1990;16:282–289.

Ely DL, Daneshvar H, Turner ME, Johnson ML, Salisbury RL. The hypertensive Y Chromosome elevates blood pressure in F_{11} Normotensive rats. Hypertension 1993;21:1071–1075.

Feinleib M, Garrison R, Borhani N, Rosenman R, Christian J. Studies of hypertension in twins. In: Paul O, ed. Epidemiology and Control of Hypertension. Miami: Symposia Specialists, 1975; pp. 3–20.

Galli J, Li L-S, Glaser A, et al. Genetic analysis of non-insulin dependent diabetes mellitus in the GK rat. Nat Genet 1996;12:31–37.

Gu L, Dene H, Deng AY, et al. Genetic mapping of two blood pressure quantitative trait loci on rat chromosome 1. J Clin Invest 1996;97: 777–788.

Hamet P, Kong D, Pravenec M, et al. Restriction fragment length polymorphism of hsp70 gene, localized in the RT1 complex, is associated with hypertension in spontaneously hypertensive rats. Hypertension 1992;19:611–614.

Hanis CL, Boerwinkle E, Chakraborty R, et al. A genome-wide search for human non-insulin-dependent (type 2) diabetes genes reveals a major susceptibility locus on chromosome 2. Nat Genet 1996;13:161–166.

Hansson JH, Nelson-Williams C, Suzuki H, et al. Hypertension caused by a truncated epithelial sodium channel γ subunit: genetic heterogeneity of Liddle syndrome. Nat Genet 1995;11:76–82.

Harrap S, Davidson R, Connor J, et al. The angiotensin I-converting enzyme gene and predisposition to high blood pressure in man. Hypertension 1993;21:455–460.

Harris EL, Dene H, Rapp JP. A gene and blood pressure cosegregation using Dahl salt-sensitive rats. Am J Hypertens 1993;6:330–334.

Harris EL, Phelan EL, Thompson CM, Millarm A, Grigor MR. Heart mass and blood pressure have separate genetic determinants in the New Zealand genetically hypertensive (GH) rat. J Hypertens 1995; 13:397–404.

H. D. a. F.-U. P. C. Group. The hypertension detection and follow-up program: a progress report. Circ Res 1977;40:I-106–I-109.

Hilbert P, Lindpaintner K, Beckmann JS, et al. Chromosomal mapping of two genetic loci associated with blood pressure regulations in hereditary hypertensive rats. Nature 1991;353:521.

Hübner N, Kreutz R, Takahashi S, Ganten D, Lindpaintner K. Unlike human hypertension, blood pressure in a hereditary hypertensive rat strain shows no linkage to the angiotensinogen locus. Hypertension 1994;23:797–801.

Iwai N, Ohmichi N, Hanai K, Nakamura Y, Kinoshita M. Human SA gene locus as a candidate locus for essential hypertension. Hypertension 1994;23:375–380.

Jacob HJ, Lindpaintner K, Lincoln SE, et al. Genetic mapping of a gene causing hypertension in the stroke-prone spontaneously hypertensive rat. Cell 1991;67:213–224.

Jacob HJ, Pettersson A, Wilson D, Mao Y, Lernmark A, Lander ES. Genetic dissection of autoimmune type I diabetes in the BB rat. Nat Genet 1992;2:56–60.

Jeunemaitre X, Lifton RP, Hunt SC, Williams RR, Lalouel JM. Absence of linkage between the angiotensin converting enzyme locus and human essential hypertension. Nat Genet 1992a;1:72–75.

Jeunemaitre X, Soubrier F, Kotelevtsev YV, et al. Molecular basis of human hypertension: role of angiotensinogen. Cell 1992b;71:169–180.

Kapuscinski M, Charchar F, Mitchell G, Harrap S. The nerve growth factor gene and blood pressure in the spontaneously hypertenive rat. (abstract) J Hypertens 1994;12:S191.

Katsuya T, Higaki J, Zhao Y, et al. A neuropeptide Y locus on chromosome 4 cosegregates with blood pressure in the spontaneously hypertensive rat. Biochem Biophys Res Commun 1993;192:261–267.

Kureutz R, Hübner N, James MR, et al. Dissection of a quantitative trait locus for genetic hypertension on rat chromosome 10. Proc Natl Acad Sci USA 1995;92:8778–8782.

Kurtz TW, Simonet L, Kabra PM, Wolfe S, Chan L, Hjelle BL. Cosegregation of the renin allele of the spontaneously hypertensive rat with an increase in blood pressure. J Clin Invest 1990;85:1328–1332.

Lander ES, Botstein D. Strategies for studying heterogenous genetic traits in humans by using a linkage map of RFLP. Proc Natl Acad Sci USA 1986;83:7353.

Lander ES, Botstein D. Mapping Mendelian factors underlying quantitative traits using RFLP linkage maps. Genetics 1989;121:185–199.

Lander ES, Schork NJ. Genetic Dissection of Complex Traits. Science 1994;265:2037–2048.

Lifton RP. Genetic determinants of human hypertension. Proc Natl Acad Sci USA 1995;92:8545–8551.

Lifton RP. Molecular genetics of human blood pressure variation. Science 1996;272:676–680.

Lifton RP, Dluhy RG, Powers M, et al. A chimeric 11-beta-hydroxylase/aldosterone synthase gene causes glucocorticoid-remediable aldosteronism and human hypertension. Nature 1992;355:262–265.

Lindpaintner K, Hilbert P, Ganten D, Nadal-Ginard B, Inagami T, Iwai N. Molecular genetics of the SA-gene: cosegregation with hypertension and mapping to rat chromosome 1. J Hypertens 1993;11:19–23.

Lindpaintner K, Pfeffer MA, Kreutz R, et al. A prospective evaluation of an angiotensin-converting-enzyme gene polymorphism and the risk of ischemic heart disease. N Engl J Med 1995;332:706–711.

Marian AJ, Yu QT, Workman R, Greve G, Roberts R. Angiotensin-converting enzyme polymorphism in hypertrophic cardiomyopathy and sudden cardiac death. Lancet 1993;342:1085,1086.

Meilahn EN. Hemostatic factors and risk of cardiovascular disease in women. Arch Pathol Lab Med 1992;116:1313–1317.

Nabika T, Bonnardeaux A, James M, et al. Evaluation of the SA locus in human hypertension. Hypertension 1995;25:6–13.

Nara Y, Nabika T, Ikeda K, Sawamura M, Endo J, Yamori Y. Blood pressure cosegregates with a microsatellite of angiotensin converting enzyme (ACE) in F2 generation from a cross between original normotensive Wistar-Kyoto rat (WKY) and stroke-prone spontaneously hypertensive rat (SHRSP). Biochem Biophys Res Commun 1991;181: 941–946.

Nishimura S, Kario K, Kayaba K, et al. Effect of the angiotensinogen gene Met^{235}-Thr variant on blood pressure and other cardiovascular risk factors in two Japanese population. J Hypertens 1995;13:717–722.

Os I, Kjeldsen SE, Nordby G, et al. Sex differences in essential hypertension. J Int Med 1993;233:13–19.

Pravenec M, Kren V, Kunes J, et al. Cosegregation of blood pressure with a kallikrein gene family polymorphism. Hypertension 1991a;17: 242–246.

Pravenec M, Simonet L, Kren V, et al. The rat renin gene: assignment to chromosome 13 and linkage to the regulation of blood pressure. Genomics 1991b;9:466–472.

Pravenec M, Gauguier D, Schott J-J, et al. Mapping of quantitative trait loci for blood pressure and cardiac mass in the rat by genome scanning of recombinant inbred strains. J Clin Invest 1995;96:1973–1978.

Rapp JP, Wang SM, Dene H. A genetic polymorphism in the renin gene of Dahl rats cosegregates with blood pressure. Science 1989;243: 542–544.

Risch N, Zhang H. Extreme discordant sib pairs for mapping quantitative trait loci in humans. Science 1995;268:1584–1589.

Rubattu S, Volpe M, Kreutz R, Ganten U, Ganten D, Lindpaintner K. Chromosomal mapping of quantitative trait loci contributing to stroke in a rat model of complex human disease. Nat Genet 1996;13: 429–434.

Samani N, Lodwick D, Vincent M, et al. A gene differentially expressed in the kidney of the spontaneously hypertensive rat cosegregates with increased blood pressure. J Clin Invest 1993;92:1099–2005.

Schork NJ, Chakravarti A. A nonmathematical overview of modern gene mapping techniques applied to human diseases. In: Mockrin SC, ed. Molecular Genetics and Gene Therapy of Cardiovascular Disease. New York: Marcel Dekker, 1996; pp. 79–109.

Schork NJ, Krieger JE, Trolliet MR, et al. A biometrical genome search in rats reveals the multigenic basis of blood pressure variation. Genome Res 1995;5:164–172.

Schunkert H, Hense HW, Holmer SR, et al. Association between a deletion polymorphism of the angiotensin-converting enzyme gene and left ventricular hypertrophy. N Engl J Med 1994;330:1634–1638.

Schuster H, Wienker TE, Bahring S, et al. Severe autosomal dominant hypertension and brachydactyly in a unique Turkish kindred maps to human chromosome 12. Nat Genet 1996;13:98–100.

Seidman CE, Seidman JG. Molecular Genetic Studies of Inherited Cardiomyopathies. In: Mockrin SC, ed. Molecular Genetics and Gene Therapy of Cardiovascular Disease. New York: Marcel Dekker, 1996; pp. 153–172.

Shimkets RA, Warnock DG, Bositis CM, et al. Liddle's syndrome: heritable human hypertension caused by mutations in the B subunit of the epithelial sodium channel. Cell 1994;79:407–414.

Soubrier F, Jeunemaitre X, Rigat B, Houot A, Cambien F, Corvol P. Similar frequencies of renin gene RFLPs in hypertensives and normotensives. Hypertension 1990;16:712–717.

Sun L, McArdle S, Chun M, Wolff DW, Pettinger WA. Cosegregation of the renin gene with an increase in mean arterial blood pressure in the F2 rats of SHR-WKY cross. Clin Exp Hypertens 1993;15:797–805.

Tanase H, Suzuki Y, Ooshima A, Yamori Y, Okamoto K. Genetic analysis of blood pressure in spontaneously hypertensive rats. Jpn Circ J 1970;34:1197–1212.

T. H. S. D. C. R. Group. A novel gene containing a trinucleotide repeat that is expanded and unstable on huntington's disease chromosomes. Cell 1993;72:971–983.

Vincent M, Kaiser MA, Orea V, Lodwick D, Samani NJ. Hypertension in the Spontaneously Hypertensive Rat and the sex chromosomes. Hypertension 1994;23:161–166.

Ward R. Familial aggregation and genetic epidemiology of blood pressure. In: Laragh JH, Brenner BM, eds. Hypertension: Pathophysiology, Diagnosis and Management. New York: Raven, 1990; pp. 81–100.

Wright S. Evolution and the Genetics of Populations, vol. IV. Chicago and London: The University of Chicago Press, 1978.

Zee R, Lou Y-K, Griffiths L, Morris B. Association of a polymorphism of the angiotensin I-converting enzyme gene with essential hypertension. Biochem Biophys Res Commun 1992;184:9–15.

17 Cardiac Arrhythmias

BARRY LONDON

BACKGROUND

Modern experimental electrophysiology began earlier this century with the explanation of the basis of the action potential by Hodgkin and Huxley in the squid giant axon, and clinical cardiac electrophysiology with the development of the electrocardiogram by Einthoven. The fields continued to diverge in two rather independent directions. The development of intracellular electrodes, the voltage clamp, and the single-channel patch clamp revealed the subcellular events that underlie cardiac excitability and automaticity. Meanwhile, arrhythmia mapping, devices, and clinical trials have defined the mechanisms of the more common human arrhythmias and assessed the efficacy of therapeutic interventions. The advent of molecular biology has been invaluable to the understanding of channel biophysics during the last decade; the relation of single-channel properties to clinically relevant electrophysiology has lagged behind. The promise of molecular electrophysiology as a unifying element in the field is only now becoming apparent.

The genetic basis of one condition, the autosomal dominant long QT syndrome, has recently been revealed through positional cloning. I will discuss the molecular genetics, pathophysiology, and implications of these findings in considerable detail. It is important to realize, however, that arrhythmias remain a major cause of cardiovascular morbidity and mortality, and that the vast majority of arrhythmias result not from Mendelian genetic defects but from more common ischemic or cardiomyopathic disorders. Molecular mechanisms undoubtedly predispose these more common disorders to cardiac arrhythmias; they are unlikely to yield their secrets as rapidly as the genetic disorders. I will highlight some of the avenues of future research that are most likely to yield results.

THE LONG QT SYNDROME

CLINICAL SYNDROME Romano and Ward described the autosomal dominant form of the long QT syndrome in the early 1960s. The condition is rare, and while the exact gene frequency is not known, it is one of the more common causes of sudden cardiac death among otherwise healthy adolescents and young adults (along with hypertrophic cardiomyopathy and myocarditis). It is characterized by recurrent presyncope and syncope, unexplained seizures, and sudden death. Symptoms often begin near adolescence and are preceded by emotional events such as surprise and fear. The electrocardiographic manifestation of the disease is a prolonged QT interval and an abnormal T-wave morphology on the surface EKG, although the QT interval has considerable variability and some symptomatic affected individuals have QT intervals within the normal range. The most common arrhythmia is *torsade de pointes*, or polymorphic ventricular tachycardia with a rotating axis (Fig. 17-1). The symptoms often respond to treatment with β blockers, although some patients are refractory and require sympathectomy.

An autosomal recessive long QT syndrome was reported by Jervell and Lange-Nielsen and is associated with congenital deafness. Other conditions also prolong the QT interval and lead to similar arrhythmias. Causes of these "acquired long QT syndromes" include medications (particularly Type IA antiarrhythmics but also certain antibiotics and antihistamines), ischemia, metabolic disorders, and neurologic disorders.

MOLECULAR BASIS OF THE DISEASE Ion-channel defects were considered likely candidates for this disease, whose hallmark is a prolonged QT interval. A sodium or calcium channel that fails to inactivate properly could delay repolarization by producing an inward leak current. This would explain the dominant nature of the disease. A defective potassium channel could also cause the syndrome by interfering with the outward currents, which repolarize heart cells following each action potential (Fig. 17-2). The dominant nature of the syndrome might be explained by insufficient outward repolarizing current owing to the presence of only one functional copy of the gene; the large number of potassium channel subunits expressed in the heart makes this seem somewhat unlikely. Alternately, the syndrome's dominant nature could be explained by taking into account that four potassium channel α-subunits (with or without assorted β-subunits) are required to form functional channels. A single defective gene product could homomultimerize or heteromultimerize with normal subunits (translated from the normal copy of that gene or from related genes) and produce a large number of the nonfunctional potassium channels through a dominant negative mechanism (Fig. 17-3).

Dr. Mark Keating mapped the gene of one large family to the H-ras locus on chromosome 11p15.5. His group and others quickly mapped additional families to that locus and to unrelated loci on other chromosomes; mutations of at least four genes cause the long QT syndrome. In 1995, Dr. Keating's laboratory identified three of these genes. Multiple mutations of two potassium channels (HERG and KVLQT1) and one sodium channel (SCNA5) cause the long QT syndrome. HERG and SCNA5 were identified by a candidate gene approach; KVLQT1 was identified by exon trapping of potassium channel-like elements from cloned genomic

From: *Principles of Molecular Medicine* (J. L. Jameson, ed.), ©1998 Humana Press Inc., Totowa, NJ.

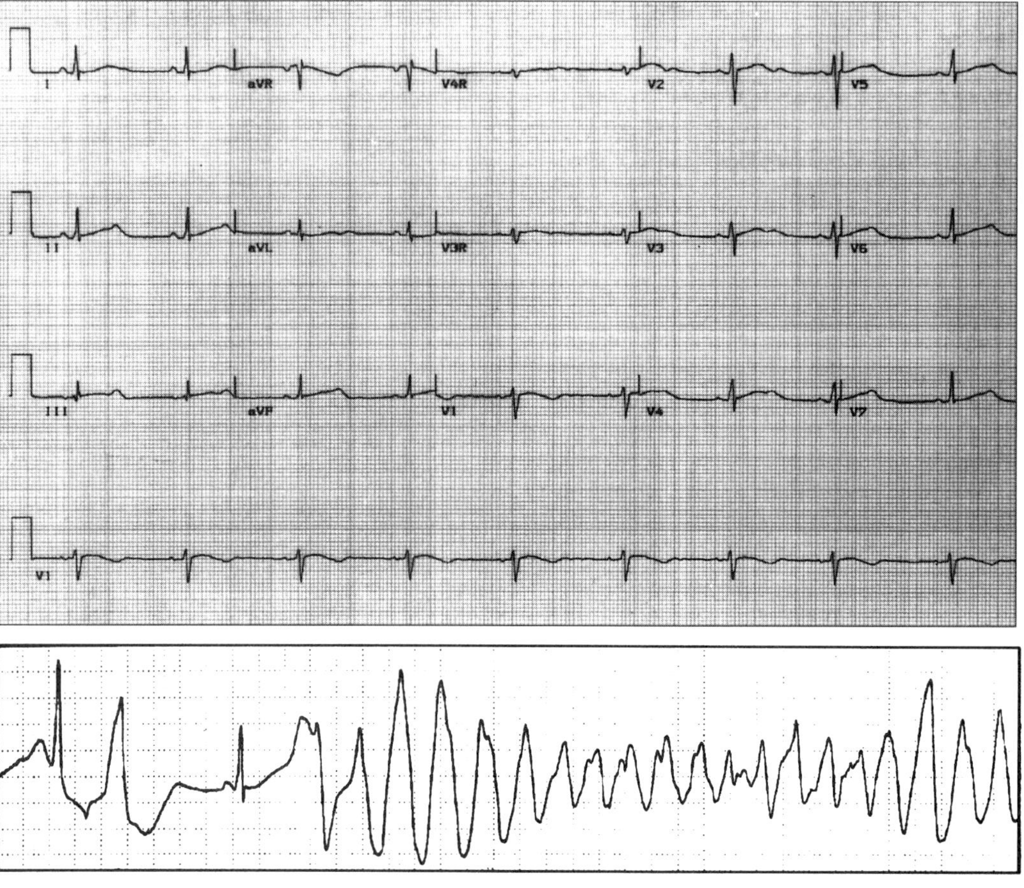

Figure 17-1 Electrocardiographic manifestations of the long QT syndrome. (Top) EKG of a child with the Romano-Ward autosomal dominant long QT syndrome. (Bottom) Lead II rhythm strip demonstrating *torsade de pointes*. (Figure courtesy of Carol A. Satler, Children's Hospital, Boston, MA.)

DNA. In vitro studies of SCNA5 mutants confirm a disruption of inactivation, and in vitro studies of HERG suggest that mutations affect the inwardly rectifying potassium current I_{Kr} in the heart. This inward rectification arises from a voltage-dependent inactivation process that reduces conductance at positive voltages. The inactivation resembles C-type or the slow inactivation mechanism of other K^+ channels. The exact mechanism by which potassium channel mutations cause disease is currently a subject of intense investigation.

Of interest, neither HERG nor KVLQT1 was known to be important to the function of the heart prior to their identification as causes of the long QT syndrome by positional cloning. This is the case despite the prior cloning of more than 30 potassium channel genes, of which at least 10 are expressed in the heart. In addition, the fact that markedly different underlying channel disorders produce indistinguishable phenotypes underscores the importance of the balance between depolarizing and repolarizing forces in the heart.

MANAGEMENT AND TREATMENT The mapping of the long QT syndrome and the identification of the responsible genes allow prenatal and presymptomatic testing for many families with this disorder. In addition, knowledge of the underlying channel pathology will allow testing of channel-specific therapies: sodium channel blockers such as mexilitine for patients with the SCNA5 defect, and manipulation of serum potassium levels for patients with potassium channel defects. Preliminary studies by Dr. Peter Schwartz and colleagues have shown QT-interval shortening in response to mexilitine in patients with SCNA5 sodium channel mutations but not in patients with HERG potassium channel mutations.

The long QT syndrome story remains incomplete. Other genes remain to be cloned. The molecular causes of the acquired forms are unknown; it is possible that defects of other channels may prolong the QT interval only in the presence of certain drugs. The exact mechanisms by which mutations lead to disease are not entirely understood. The efficacy of gene-specific treatments on symptoms and survival remains to be shown. The work of the last several years is a major advance, however, in the understanding not only of the cause of this rare syndrome but also of the relationships in vivo between ion channels, currents, and clinical cardiac electrophysiology.

OTHER ARRHYTHMIAS

CLINICAL SYNDROMES Certain arrhythmias are poorly understood but effectively treated. Bypass tract-mediated (Wolf-Parkinson-White syndrome) and AV node re-entrant tachycardias usually respond well to either radiofrequency ablation or medication. Bradyarrhythmias most commonly result from idiopathic deterioration of the conduction system; electronic pacemakers are usually safe and effective.

Most cardiac arrhythmias, however, occur in adults and in the presence of other heart disease. Atrial tachyarrhythmias such as atrial fibrillation and flutter usually result from conditions that

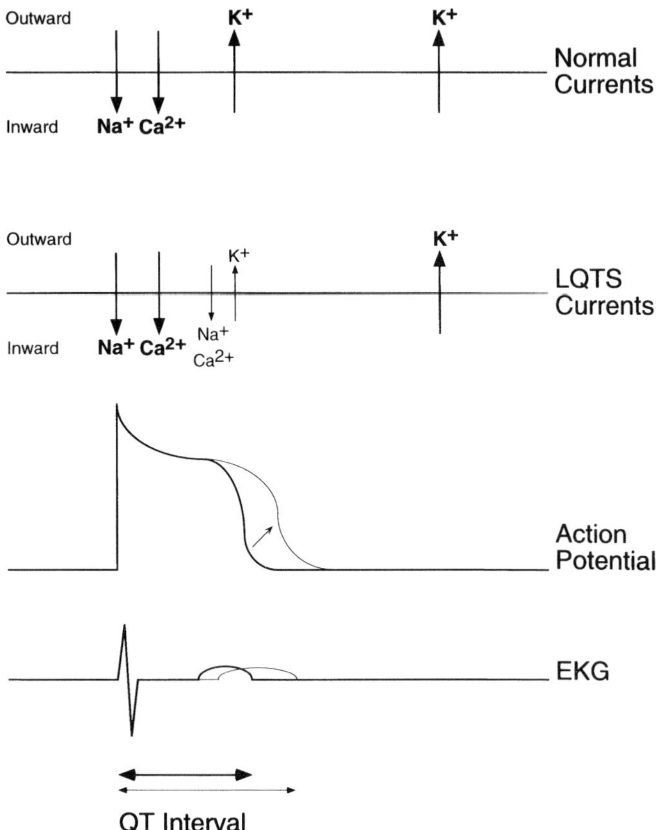

Figure 17-2 Ionic basis of the long QT syndrome. Schematic representation of transmembrane ionic currents (top), intracellular potential (middle), and surface electrocardiogram (bottom) of a normal individual contrasted with one having the long QT syndrome (LQTS). A prolonged inward sodium (Na^+) current, a prolonged inward calcium (Ca^{2+}) current, or insufficient repolarizing potassium (K^+) current can prolong the cellular action potential (arrow) and the QT interval.

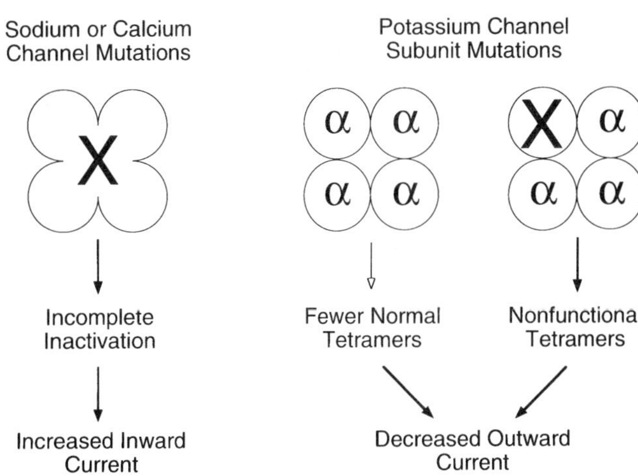

Figure 17-3 Molecular basis of the long QT syndrome. Schematic representation of the mechanisms by which channel mutations (designated by X) can cause increased inward currents (left) or decreased outward currents (right). Note that sodium and calcium channels have a single α-subunit with four homologous domains, whereas potassium channels have four α-subunits, all of which multimerize to form tetramers. Mutations of one sodium or calcium channel gene could produce dysfunctional channels to allow increased inward current and cause the disease. Mutations of a single potassium channel gene could decrease the number of functional channel tetramers and cause disease either by decreasing the pool of normal α-subunits or by multimerizing with normal subunits to form nonfunctional channels.

mechanically stretch the atria, including hypertension and valvular heart disease. Ventricular tachyarrhythmias accompany acute myocardial ischemia and infarction, occur postinfarction in the scarred ventricle, and are also common in myocarditis and idiopathic dilated cardiomyopathies. Re-entry through intraventricular electrical circuits is often documented by electrophysiological (EP) studies. Treatment for these conditions remains limited, as sudden death can be the presenting symptom, the long-term efficacy of drug therapy is often poor, and devices carry the problems of high cost and limitation of lifestyle.

MOLECULAR BASIS OF THE DISEASES Atrial and ventricular arrhythmias accompany a vast array of diseases. Most are considered "structural," and little is known about them at the molecular level. In human cardiomyopathies, for example, the action potential is prolonged and a decrease of outward potassium currents has been noted. It is likely that molecular changes in ion channel and/or ion pump expression accompany and predispose to these diseases.

Molecular changes may predispose to disease in ways other than mutated channel proteins (the mechanism responsible for the long QT syndrome). Gene polymorphisms could contribute to familial inheritance in some of these cardiac disorders. Ion-channel gene promoters contain binding sites for regulatory molecules including glucocorticoids and cyclic AMP; these mediators are altered in disease and are proven to modify channel expression in vitro. In addition, electrical coupling of adjacent myocytes through gap junctions is tightly regulated and clearly plays a major role in the genesis and maintenance of arrhythmias.

FUTURE DIRECTIONS

ANIMAL MODELS One promising direction involves the use of animals to study the function of channel genes in vivo and to design interventions on arrhythmias. As one example, recombinant adenoviral vectors have been used to express potassium channels and shorten the action potential in heart cells of rats and dogs. Clearly gene therapy for arrhythmias remains far away, and much progress would need to be made both technically (e.g., obtaining sufficiently uniform gene transfer to prevent electrical inhomogeneities) and in understanding the complex interactions among the many cell systems tied to ion fluxes (*see* Chapter 18). The usefulness of this technique to dissect those elements important for normal cardiac function and for arrhythmias is more immediately apparent.

The recent ability to manipulate the mouse genome using transgenic and knockout techniques also provides a novel avenue for research. Our laboratory and others have used gene targeting to disrupt ion channels thought to be important in the heart. These methods should allow the engineering of a mouse model of human genetic diseases such as the long QT syndrome. Of equal importance, however, will be the information obtained regarding the relationship of individual gene products to the function of the heart as an electrical entity.

FROM ION CHANNEL TO ARRHYTHMIA A great many ion channels, pumps, and exchangers have been cloned during the past decade and studied in vitro using isolated membranes, vesicles, *Xenopus* oocytes, and cultured cells. These proteins form the basis of the currents that depolarize and repolarize the heart. A complete catalog of their identity, a model of their structure, and an understanding of the biophysical mechanisms by which they open, close, inactivate, interact, and distinguish between different ions are rapidly becoming reality. The regulation of gene expression, the role of posttranslational modifications, and the relationship of individual genes to the cardiac currents, to the action potential, to the EKG, and to arrhythmias will not be solved in the near future. Establishing the link between these basic and clinical parameters is essential, however, if the molecular analysis of cardiac electrophysiology is to have maximal impact in the understanding and treatment of arrhythmias. Future possibilities include (but are not limited to) rational drug design, arrhythmia prediction, arrhythmia prevention, and gene-directed therapies. The recent advances related to the long QT syndrome highlight the possibilities.

SELECTED REFERENCES

Bennett PB, Yazawa K, Makita N, George AL, Jr. Molecular mechanism for an inherited cardiac arrhythmia. Nature 1995;376:683–685.

Braunwald E. Heart Disease: A Textbook of Cardiovascular Medicine, 5th ed. Philadelphia: WB Saunders, 1996; pp. 548–741.

The Cardiac arrhythmia suppression trial (CAST) investigators. Preliminary report: effect of encainide and flecainide on mortality in a randomized trial of arrhythmia suppression after myocardial infarction. N Engl J Med 1989;321:406–412.

Curran ME, Splawski I, Timothy KW, Vincent GM, Green ED, Keating MT. A molecular basis for cardiac arrhythmias: HERG mutations cause long QT syndrome. Cell 1995;80:795–803.

Grace AA, Chien KR. Congenital long QT syndromes. Toward molecular dissection of arrhythmia substrates. Circulation 1995;92:2786–2789.

Hille B. Ion Channels in Excitable Membranes, 2nd ed. Sakmann B, Neher E, eds. Sunderland MA: Sinauer Associates, 1992.

Jiang C, Atkinson D, Towbon JA, et al. Two long QT syndrome loci map to chromosomes 3 and 7 with evidence for further heterogeneity. Nat Genet 1994;8:141–147.

Johns DC, Nuss HB, Chiamvimonvat N, Ramza BM, Marban E, Lawrence JH. Adenovirus-mediated expression of a voltage-gated potassium channel in vitro (rat cardiac myocytes) and in vivo (rat liver). J Clin Invest 1995;96:1152–1158.

Keating MT, Sanguinetti MC. Molecular genetic insights into cardiovascular disease. Science 1996;272:681–685.

Pongs O. Molecular biology of voltage-dependent potassium channels. Physiol Rev 1992;72:S69–88.

Romano C. Congenital cardiac arrhythmia. Lancet 1965;1:658,659.

Sanguinette MC, Jiang C, Curran ME, Keating MT. A mechanistic link between an inherited and an acquired cardiac arrhythmia: HERG encodes the I_{Kr} potassium channel. Cell 1995;81:299–307.

Schwartz PJ, Locati EH, Napolitano C, Priori SG. The long QT syndrome. In: Zipes DP, Jalife J, eds. Cardiac Electrophysiology: From Cell to Bedside, 2nd ed. Philadelphia: WB Saunders, 1995; pp. 788–811.

Schwartz PJ, Priori SG, Locati EH, et al. Long QT syndrome patients with mutations of the SCN5A and HERG genes have differential responses to Na^+ channel blockade and to increases in heart rate. Implications for gene-specific therapy. Circulation 1995;92:3381–3386.

Sanguinetti MC, Curran ME, Spector PS, Keating MT. Spectrum of HERG K+-channel dysfunction in an inherited cardiac arrhythmia. Proc Natl Acad Sci USA 1996;93:2208–2212.

Smith PL, Baukrowitz T, Yellen G. The inward rectification mechanism of the HERG cardiac potassium channel. Nature 1996;379:833–836.

Tomaselli GF, Beuckelmann DJ, Calkins HG, et al. Sudden cardiac death in heart failure: the role of abnormal repolarization. Circulation 1994;90:2534–2539.

Wang Q, Curran ME, Splawski E, et al. Positional cloning of a novel potassium channel gene: KVLQT1 mutations cause cardiac arrhythmias. Nat Genet 1996;12:17–23.

Ward OC. A new familial cardiac syndrome in children. J Irish Med Assoc 1964;54:103–106.

18 Cardiovascular Gene Therapy

GIUSEPPE VASSALLI AND DAVID A. DICHEK

INTRODUCTION

Recombinant DNA technology has provided invaluable tools for understanding the molecular basis of cardiovascular diseases. Elucidation of the underlying molecular genetic mechanisms of cardiovascular disease has led to the emergence of gene therapy as an appealing therapeutic approach. Gene therapy involves the introduction and expression of recombinant DNA in order to ameliorate or cure a disease condition. Despite the extensive publicity devoted to gene therapy, it must be emphasized that this field is still very much in its infancy, and fundamental questions regarding efficacy, safety, and clinical benefit remain unanswered. Initial clinical trials in cardiovascular gene therapy are at an early stage, and the place of gene therapy within the armamentarium of cardiovascular therapeutics remains uncertain. This chapter is devoted principally to a review of the theoretical basis for cardiovascular gene therapy, as established by in vitro and preclinical animal experiments. In addition, the two currently approved human cardiovascular gene-therapy trials (familial hypercholesterolemia [FH; MIM # 14389] and peripheral arterial disease) are discussed, and the likely future directions of the field are summarized.

CARDIOVASCULAR DISEASES POTENTIALLY AMENABLE TO GENE THERAPY

MONOGENIC DISEASES Cardiovascular diseases potentially amenable to gene therapy are summarized in Table 18-1. The potential of gene therapy is most obvious in those rare cases of cardiovascular disease due to a defect in a single gene. Specific examples of monogenic cardiovascular disease include the cardiomyopathy associated with Duchenne muscular dystrophy (DMD; MIM # 31020), an X-linked genetic disease caused by a defect in the gene that encodes dystrophin (*see* Chapter 94) and atherosclerotic disease resulting from homozygous FH, an autosomal dominant disease with a gene dosage effect, caused by low-density lipoprotein (LDL) receptor deficiency. Both DMD and homozygous FH are caused by the absence of normal alleles (i.e., lack of one normal allele for DMD and lack of two normal alleles for the homozygous form of FH). If heterozygotes are either asymptomatic (as in DMD) or have a less severe form of the disease (as in FH), then homozygotes might be treated by introduction of a normal allele. However, not all cardiovascular diseases arising from monogenic defects are clearly treatable by introduction of a normal allele. Hypertrophic cardiomyopathy (HCM), caused frequently by dominant mutations in the gene encoding the β-myosin heavy chain (*see* Chapter 13), cannot be treated with current gene therapy technology because the heterozygotes may have a severe disease phenotype despite the presence of a normal allele. Gene therapy for this type of dominant mutation would require replacement of the mutated allele, not simply addition of a normal allele. The technology for widespread gene replacement in vivo does not yet exist.

POLYGENIC DISEASES Complex cardiovascular disease processes such as atherosclerosis (*see* Chapter 14), thrombosis, and hypertension (*see* Chapter 16) have a polygenic basis and are also subject to significant modulation by environmental factors. Nevertheless, several gene therapy approaches to polygenic cardiovascular diseases have been described, each of which is based on delivery of a normal allele of a single gene (Fig. 18-1). In each of these gene therapy strategies, delivery and expression of the chosen therapeutic gene are intended to drive specific metabolic pathways for which the therapeutic gene product is rate-limiting. The metabolic pathways that are driven by the introduced gene act to reverse the pathophysiology of the targeted disease. Thus, delivery of a single gene may be an effective therapy for complex disease processes. This approach to gene therapy is strikingly similar to traditional pharmacotherapy, in which a therapeutic drug (e.g., a diuretic for essential hypertension or coumadin for atrial thrombosis) is given to counteract a disease process rather than to correct the underlying cause.

Specific single-gene therapies for the polygenic diseases of atherosclerosis, thrombosis, and hypertension have each been tested in animal models. Gene therapy for primary atherosclerosis has focused primarily on manipulation of lipid metabolism. For example, transfer of the gene that encodes 7α-hydroxylase (which catalyzes the rate-limiting step in bile acid synthesis) into the livers of hamsters reduced plasma LDL to nearly undetectable levels. Transfer of the genes that encode either tissue-type or urokinase plasminogen activator into baboon endothelial cells decreased thrombus deposition in ex vivo arteriovenous shunts. Finally, transfer of the gene that expresses human tissue kallikrein reduced blood pressure in spontaneously hypertensive rats. In each of these studies, the overexpression of a single normal allele in animals not known to have a specific genetic defect produced a potentially therapeutic effect.

From: *Principles of Molecular Medicine* (J. L. Jameson, ed.), ©1998 Humana Press Inc., Totowa, NJ.

Table 18-1
Cardiovascular Diseases Potentially Amenable to Gene Therapy

Disease	*Therapeutic gene(s)*	*Anticipated mechanism*[a]	*Results*
Familial hypercholesterolemia (LDL receptor defective or absent)	LDL receptor	LDL clearance	Ex vivo gene transfer in humans: 6–23% decrease in LDL cholesterol in three of five patients
Hyperlipidemia with no specific genetic defect	LDL receptor	LDL clearance	In vivo gene transfer into normal mice: decrease in LDL cholesterol
	7α-Hydroxylase	Biliary elimination of cholesterol	In vivo gene transfer into hamsters: reduction in LDL cholesterol
	Apolipoprotein A-I	Increase in HDL	In vivo gene transfer of human apolipoprotein A-I into mice: 35% increase in HDL
Hypertension	Tissue kallikrein	Vasodilation	Prolonged (6 weeks) blood pressure reduction in spontaneously hypertensive rats
Peripheral artery disease	VEGF	Angiogenesis	Gene transfer into patients with stage IV peripheral artery disease (in progress)
Occlusive arterial disease	Constitutively active retinoblastoma gene, hirudin, thymidine kinase, NO synthase	Cytostatic, cytotoxic, inhibition of smooth muscle cell proliferation	In vivo gene transfer into injured rat carotid or pig femoral arteries: 35–70% reduction in neointima formation
Thrombosis	Prostaglandin H synthase	Prostacyclin production	In vivo gene transfer into pig carotid arteries: decreased thrombosis
	t-PA and glycosyl-phosphatidylinositol-anchored urokinase	Fibrinolysis	Ex vivo gene transfer into endothelial cells seeded onto vascular grafts in baboons: reduction in platelet deposition and fibrin accumulation
Hypertrophic cardiomyopathy	Gene replacement of mutated with normal allele of myosin heavy chain	Normalized function of cardiac myosin	None; currently technically unfeasible

[a]The anticipated mechanism has not always been experimentally verified in individual studies.

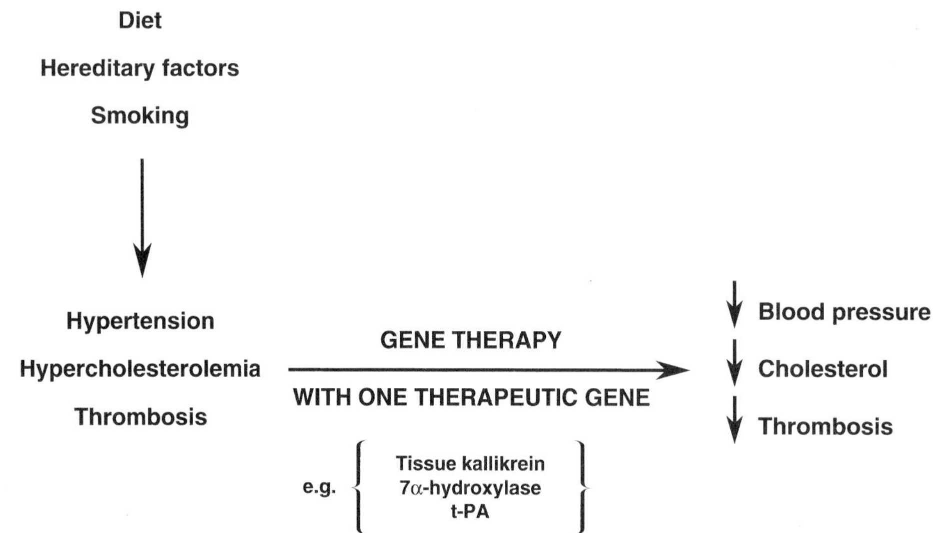

Figure 18-1 Gene therapy approaches to polygenic cardiovascular diseases. Environmental and hereditary factors are involved in the development of polygenic diseases such as hypertension, hypercholesterolemia, and thrombosis. These diseases can be potentially corrected by transfer of one therapeutic gene.

METHODS OF CARDIOVASCULAR GENE TRANSFER

To achieve delivery of a recombinant gene product in vivo, the following steps must occur:

1. Recombinant DNA sequences must be introduced into the nucleus.
2. The DNA must be transcribed into RNA.
3. The RNA must be translated into a functional protein.

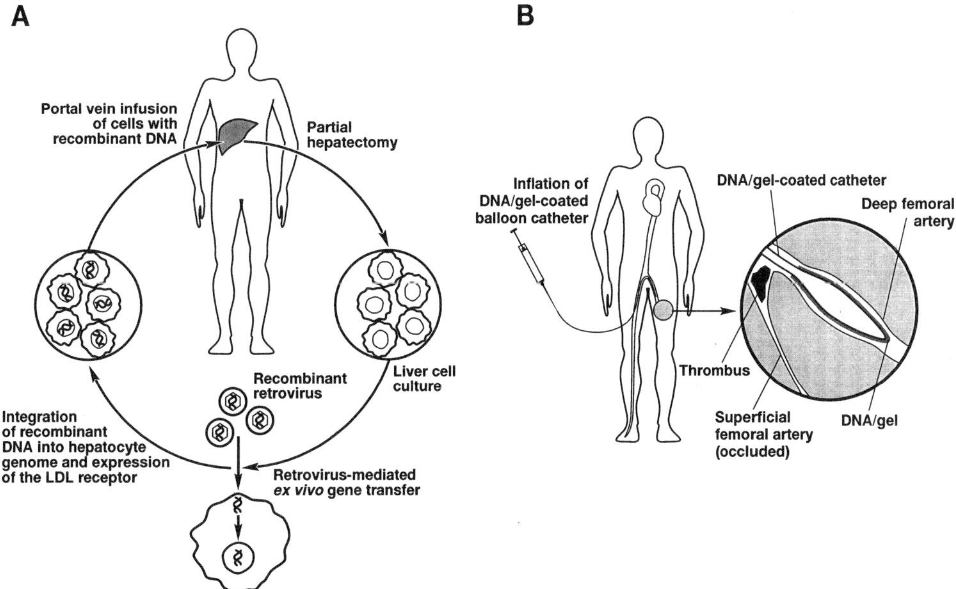

Figure 18-2 Methods in gene therapy. **(A)** Ex vivo gene transfer. This approach has been used to deliver the gene that encodes the LDL receptor to the liver in patients with familial hypercholesterolemia. Following partial hepatectomy, hepatocytes are transduced in vitro using a retrovirus vector, and recombinant DNA is integrated into the hepatocyte genome. Finally, transduced hepatocytes are reinfused into the portal vein and target the liver. **(B)** In vivo gene transfer. This approach has been used to deliver the gene that encodes vascular endothelial growth factor (VEGF) to peripheral arteries.

Steps 2 and 3 must occur in vivo; however, step 1, gene delivery, may be accomplished either in vivo or ex vivo. Stated differently, therapeutic genes may be delivered to cells within an intact animal (or human) tissue or, alternatively, cells may be removed from the targeted tissue, subjected to gene transfer ex vivo, and then reimplanted within the tissue from which they were derived. These two strategies are referred to as "in vivo" and "ex vivo" gene therapy, respectively, and have each been used in cardiovascular gene therapy studies (Fig. 18-2). Each strategy possesses advantages and disadvantages, which we will discuss herein.

EX VIVO GENE THERAPY In ex vivo gene therapy, cells are removed from an animal, maintained in culture, targeted with a therapeutic gene, and then reintroduced into the donor animal. The role of the reintroduced cells is uniquely to deliver a recombinant gene product. The cells are not required to reconstitute a particular organ or tissue; therefore, the excised cells may be reimplanted in a location different from their site of excision. For example, hepatocytes harvested from one liver lobe and genetically modified ex vivo may be reinfused throughout the donor liver. Endothelial cells harvested from a donor vein may be reimplanted in the arterial circulation.

The primary advantages of ex vivo gene therapy are:

1. Gene delivery is performed under controlled, optimized conditions in which the efficiency of gene transfer into the targeted cells may be very high.
2. Gene delivery may be restricted to one specific cell type in which expression is optimized by careful design of a cell-type-specific transgene construct.
3. The potential for an immune response to the gene transfer vector is minimized by performing gene delivery in a setting remote from the host immune system (i.e., a tissue culture dish).

The disadvantages of ex vivo gene transfer derive primarily from technical considerations:

1. Except in rare cases of monozygotic siblings, the requirements of histocompatibility mandate that the excised cells be reintroduced only into the donor individual. Thus, every animal (or human) receiving ex vivo gene therapy must undergo two invasive procedures: cell harvest and cell reintroduction.
2. Cell culture and ex vivo gene transfer must be performed under strict aseptic conditions to avoid the introduction of pathogenic microorganisms at the time of cell reimplantation.
3. The requirement that cells be removed and reinfused in ex vivo gene therapy imposes limitations on the type and number of cells that can be used.

The cells must be nonessential, and their removal and reimplantation must be practical. Thus, ex vivo cardiovascular gene therapy may be attempted with hepatocytes derived from partial hepatectomy and with endothelial and smooth muscle cells derived from excised, nonessential vessels. However, the ex vivo approach is not feasible with other cell types (e.g., cardiac myocytes).

IN VIVO GENE THERAPY The advantages and disadvantages of in vivo gene therapy are the reverse of those of ex vivo gene delivery. Advantages of in vivo gene therapy include:

1. Only one invasive procedure is required (i.e., injection of the gene vector).
2. Laborious and technically demanding steps of cell harvesting and reimplantation are eliminated.
3. Any cell within an intact tissue or organ is theoretically a target for in vivo gene therapy.

Table 18-2
Major Advantages and Disadvantages of Currently Available In Vivo Gene-Transfer Techniques

Method	*Advantages*	*Disadvantages*
Naked DNA	Not a known pathogen No integration into host genome[a] Permits large DNA inserts Easy to manipulate	Low efficiency
Liposomes	Not a known pathogen Wide range of target cells Permits large DNA inserts Commercially available	Low efficiency
Adenovirus	High efficiency Transduces nonreplicating cells No integration into host genome[a]	Derived from potential pathogen DNA insert size limited (≤8 kb) Direct toxicity Short duration of expression Inflammatory response Complex construction
Retrovirus	Stable, long-term gene expression To date, safe in human use	Low efficiency Potential reversion to replication competence Transduces replicating cells only Integration into host genome[a]

[a]Integration into host genome might be favorable with respect to the duration of transgene expression; however, there is a theoretical risk of insertional mutagenesis.

The disadvantages of in vivo gene therapy are:

1. Gene delivery to remote, technically difficult locations may be required; for example within the myocardium or in the presence of flowing blood in a narrow end artery supplying an ischemic territory. In clinical settings such as these, the gene transfer vector may be washed away or undesirable clinical consequences (ischemia, infarction) may intervene prior to successful gene delivery.
2. Systemic release of the vector is unavoidable; therefore, the target cells for in vivo gene delivery are likely to be a heterogeneous population in which optimization of expression is difficult.
3. There is an obligatory exposure of the gene delivery vector to the immune system. This exposure may produce an immune response that causes rejection of the transduced cells or abrogation of gene delivery if the recipient organism is already immune to the gene transfer vector.

Despite these disadvantages, the practical advantages of in vivo versus ex vivo gene transfer are overwhelming. If cardiovascular gene therapy is ever to become practical as well as economically feasible, it will likely be with in vivo gene transfer technology.

VECTORS FOR CARDIOVASCULAR GENE THERAPY

In general, the uptake of foreign genetic material (naked DNA or RNA) by mammalian cells is an inefficient process. This inefficiency makes sense teleologically, as there is little advantage for a cell to allow its highly regulated and evolved genetic program to be altered at random by pieces of DNA or RNA that land on its membrane. While there are notable exceptions, in order to introduce genetic material into mammalian cells with reasonable efficiency, it has generally been necessary for investigators to associate the genetic material with a "vector" that can mediate entry, nuclear transport and, in some cases, chromosomal integration. Vectors for mammalian gene therapy belong to two general categories: nonviral vectors, which mediate gene transfer largely by physical means; and viral vectors, which make use of viral proteins and nucleic acids to mediate efficient gene transfer (Table 18-2).

NAKED DNA AND NONVIRAL VECTORS Nonviral means of gene transfer include naked DNA, liposomes, protein-polylysine complexes, and microparticle bombardment. The principal theoretical advantage of nonviral gene transfer is that the components can be prepared as standardized pharmaceutical reagents. This standardization might maximize reproducibility and minimize toxicity. Individual investigators have reported both promising animal data and plans for clinical trials in humans using naked DNA for cardiovascular gene therapy. However, the efficiency of gene transfer with nonviral vectors is low when compared to that obtainable with viral vectors, and in no case have nonviral gene transfer approaches achieved long-term, stable expression in the cardiovascular system.

VIRAL VECTORS Both retroviral and adenoviral vectors are currently in use for cardiovascular gene therapy in animal models. Retroviral vectors are able to mediate integration of recombinant DNA into the target cell chromosome, permitting long-term expression of transgenes and ensuring transmission of inserted DNA to the progeny of transduced cells. Use of retroviral vectors in cardiovascular gene therapy has been limited, however, by their inability to achieve reasonable levels of gene transfer in vivo. The estimated efficiency of in vivo retrovirus-mediated arterial gene transfer is 0.01% or less. In contrast, adenovirus vectors are capable of high efficiency in vivo gene transfer: About 35% of smooth muscle cells in a local segment of injured artery and about 90% of hepatocytes express recombinant genes following in vivo gene transfer in animal models. The clinical use of adenovirus vectors is limited, however, by their toxicity and immunogenicity. Despite the promise demonstrated by adenovirus vectors in animal models of cardiovascular disease, it is likely that significant improvements in adenovirus vector design will be required prior to their widespread use in humans.

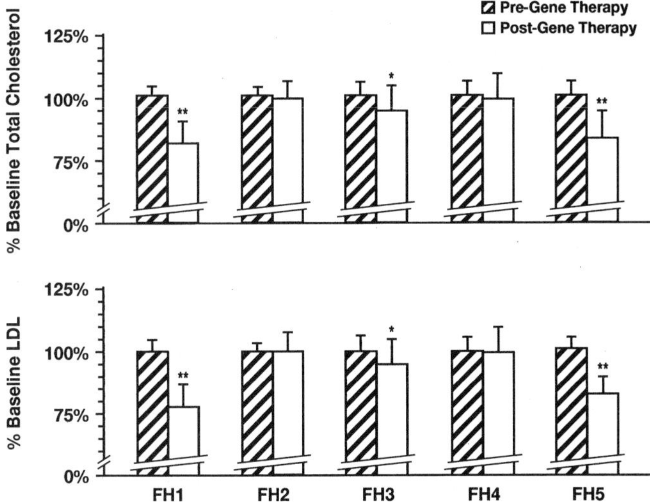

Figure 18-3 Cholesterol and LDL levels before (hatched box) and after (white box) retrovirus-mediated ex vivo transfer of the LDL receptor gene in five patients with familial hypercholesterolemia (FH). A significant decrease in these two parameters was observed in three out of five patients (*p = 0.05, **p < 0.01 vs before gene therapy). (Reproduced with permission from Grossman et al.)

CARDIOVASCULAR GENE THERAPY: CURRENT STATUS AND FUTURE DIRECTIONS

ATHEROSCLEROSIS RESULTING FROM HYPERLIPIDEMIA Because plasma LDL cholesterol is a genetically determined, major modifiable risk factor for the development and progression of atherosclerotic cardiovascular disease, it is logical that gene therapy approaches have focused on lowering plasma LDL cholesterol. An extensive set of in vitro data with cultured hepatocytes and preclinical experiments with both rabbits and primates led Grossman et al. to develop and implement an ex vivo clinical gene therapy protocol for homozygous FH (Fig. 18-3). Treatment of five FH patients revealed that introduction of a normal LDL receptor allele was capable of increasing LDL catabolism and lowering LDL cholesterol in individual patients; however, in no case was LDL lowered to such an extent that any of the patients' cardiovascular disease risk was appreciably diminished. Moreover, the response of the patients was heterogeneous, with two of five showing no change in plasma LDL levels following gene therapy. The authors acknowledged that their inability to reconstitute more than a small fraction of the liver with genetically modified cells placed a severe limitation on this approach, forcing them to forego further clinical trials and refocus their attention on the more basic issue of effecting higher levels of hepatic gene transfer.

Additional approaches to gene therapy of hyperlipidemia include adenovirus-vector-mediated overexpression of apolipoprotein A-I to raise plasma high-density lipoprotein (HDL) levels (which are negatively correlated with the development of cardiovascular disease) and hepatic overexpression of 7α-hydroxylase, to expedite hepatocyte catabolism of cholesterol to bile acid with subsequent elimination via the gastrointestinal tract. While both of these approaches have appeared powerful and feasible in animal studies, the key questions of efficiency and safety that have been raised in human studies with retrovirus vectors and in animal studies with adenovirus vectors will require resolution, prior to the commencement of clinical studies with these potentially therapeutic genes.

RESTENOSIS FOLLOWING ANGIOPLASTY The initial success of percutaneous transluminal coronary angioplasty in enlarging the lumen of stenotic coronary arteries is reversed by recurrent stenosis ("restenosis") in 30–50% of patients. Demonstration of successful in vivo gene transfer into injured mammalian arteries with both viral and nonviral gene transfer systems, along with the availability of animal models of local arterial injury, have stimulated several groups to propose gene therapy approaches to prevent restenosis. Transfer of cytotoxic genes, such as herpesvirus thymidine kinase, or cytostatic genes, such as a mutant retinoblastoma protein, into injured arteries results in decreased neointima formation in animal models. Alternatively, transfer of "protective" genes, such as nitric oxide synthase or hirudin, at the time of arterial injury results in a similar reduction in neointima formation. None of these animal studies, however, has demonstrated a decrease in arterial stenosis following gene delivery.

The success of gene transfer in limiting neointima formation in animal models has suggested to some that a gene therapy trial for restenosis in humans is imminent. Indeed, restenosis appears to be a reasonable candidate for gene therapy in that it is a focal disease for which there is currently no accepted therapy. There are, nevertheless, important caveats that should be considered prior to the initiation of human trials:

1. The pathophysiology of human restenosis is almost certainly different from that found in animal models of arterial injury; cell proliferation (the target of several gene therapy approaches) may not play a significant role in human restenosis.
2. Local gene delivery in the human coronary circulation is far more challenging than in an isolated peripheral animal artery. In contrast to the animal experiments with isolated peripheral arteries, it is currently unfeasible to isolate a human coronary artery lumen (with both proximal and distal occlusion as well as prevention of leakage via side branches) and maintain an elevated infusion pressure during 20 min of gene delivery. Thus, without significant technical improvements, gene transfer efficiency in human coronaries will almost certainly be lower, and systemic gene delivery will be far higher, than in animal models (Fig. 18-4).
3. Direct vascular toxicity and proinflammatory effects of adenovirus may counteract any salutary effects of expressed transgenes. As 50–70% of angioplasty patients are cured of their disease without gene therapy, it would appear that careful consideration of pros and cons as well as resolution of the above major clinical issues should precede human trials.

PERIPHERAL ARTERY DISEASE The identification and cloning of genes that control the development and growth of blood vessels has inspired several investigators to propose gene therapy for deficient peripheral circulation. According to this paradigm, delivery of a gene to the wall of an artery supplying an ischemic territory will result in the release of angiogenic peptides into the distal circulation. These peptides will, in turn, stimulate the growth of blood vessels that relieve the peripheral ischemia. A human clinical trial has been initiated to treat severe peripheral arterial disease by delivery of the gene encoding vascular endothelial

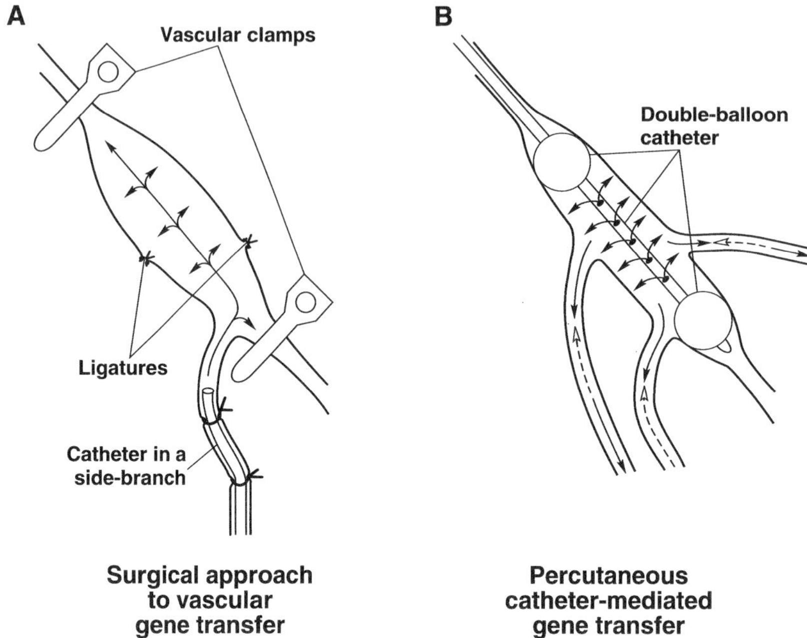

Figure 18-4 In vivo arterial gene transfer. (**A**) Surgical approach. Side branches are ligated, and the target segment vessel is clamped proximally and distally. Infusion is performed under direct vision, and the vessel wall is maintained in a distended state by the infusion pressure. Systemic spread of the recombinant gene is limited. (**B**) Potential percutaneous approach. The recombinant gene is delivered through a double-balloon catheter. Systemic leakage via the side branches cannot be avoided, and distension cannot be maintained. In addition, collateral flow (dotted arrows) may enter the occluded artery and dilute the vector solution. Gene delivery will likely be decreased and systemic exposure increased compared to the surgical approach. The use of double-balloon catheters for arterial gene delivery has, to date, largely been accomplished via a surgical approach using direct vision and ligation of branch vessels, as in (A).

growth factor (VEGF) to the iliofemoral artery wall. If effective in engendering the growth of physiologically significant collateral vessels, it is anticipated that this protocol will result in the salvage of severely ischemic limbs. Furthermore, any success encountered in the peripheral circulation will certainly inspire efforts to direct gene therapy toward the enhancement of coronary collaterals to relieve myocardial ischemia.

HYPERTENSION A recent animal study demonstrated the feasibility of gene therapy for hypertension. Intravenous injection of a naked DNA construct expressing human tissue kallikrein reduced systolic blood pressure for 6 weeks in spontaneously hypertensive rats (Fig. 18-5). The authors did not present any results obtained by using a gene transfer vector, such as retrovirus, that may have provided longer-lasting gene expression. Thus, it remains possible that, with a more stable gene transfer system, the hypotensive effect would have persisted even longer. These findings therefore raise the exciting possibility that human hypertension, a lifelong disease treated with a lifetime of expensive and inconvenient medication, might someday be treated by the transfer and stable expression of a single gene. The promise and attraction of gene therapy lie precisely herein: the potential that the delivery of a single gene could reprogram and correct systemic physiology for the lifetime of a patient. Just as the inheritance of a single dominant disease allele can produce a lifetime of disease, a single dominant therapeutic allele might prevent a lifetime of disease. The power of gene therapy and the potential that it might someday revolutionize medical care is perhaps most evident in the context of such common diseases as hypertension.

Prior to the initiation of therapeutic trials of gene therapy for hypertension in humans, it will be important to address several issues:

1. The applicability of studies in specific animal models to the pathophysiology of hypertension in humans.
2. The requirement for long-term stable expression in a significant number of cells.
3. The need to develop practical means for the adjustment or reversal of antihypertensive gene therapy, should the effect of the inserted gene prove detrimental over time.

THROMBOSIS Gene therapy for thrombosis has focused on the thrombotic problems of intravascular prosthetic devices such as grafts and stents. Because these devices are acellular and cannot be targeted by in vivo gene transfer, an ex vivo, cell-based gene therapy strategy is obligatory. According to this strategy, endothelial cells may be harvested from a superficial vein and transduced with genes that express either tissue plasminogen activator (t-PA) or urokinase. These fibrinolytically "enhanced" cells would then be seeded onto the surface of prosthetic devices prior to device implantation. When these cells are implanted in vivo, increased expression of t-PA or urokinase might prevent device thrombosis. With this approach, overexpression of plasminogen activators from seeded endothelial cells decreased thrombus deposition onto a synthetic baboon arteriovenous shunt (Fig. 18-6). The antithrombotic effect was unaccompanied by evidence of systemic fibrinolysis, proving the concept that genetic manipulation of endothelial cells can decrease local thrombosis without creating a systemic fibrino(geno)lytic state. While theoretically promising, these data are derived from very short-term experiments (1 h), whereas the clinical problem they address (device thrombosis) may extend over years. The clinical applicability of the seeding of vascular devices with genetically "enhanced" cells will depend on the generation of data that demonstrate that these cells or their

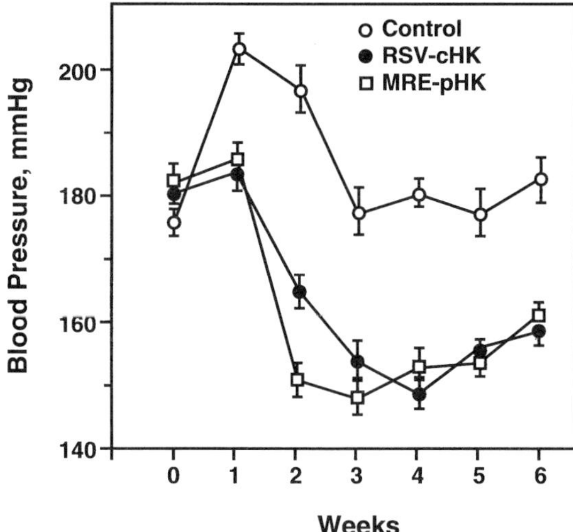

Figure 18-5 Systolic blood pressure of spontaneously hypertensive rats after intravenous injection of plasmid DNA. Rats received injections of control plasmid DNA (open circles), plasmid DNA expressing a human tissue kallikrein cDNA under the control of the Rous sarcoma virus 3'-long terminal repeat promoter (RSV-cHK; solid circles), or plasmid DNA expressing a human tissue kallikrein cDNA under the control of a metal response element-containing (MRE) promoter (MRE-pHK; open squares). Blood pressure values are expressed as mean ± SEM ($n = 6$). Bars represent standard deviation. $*p < 0.05$ vs control. Blood pressure differences were no longer significant at 7 weeks (not shown). (Reproduced with permission from Wang et al.)

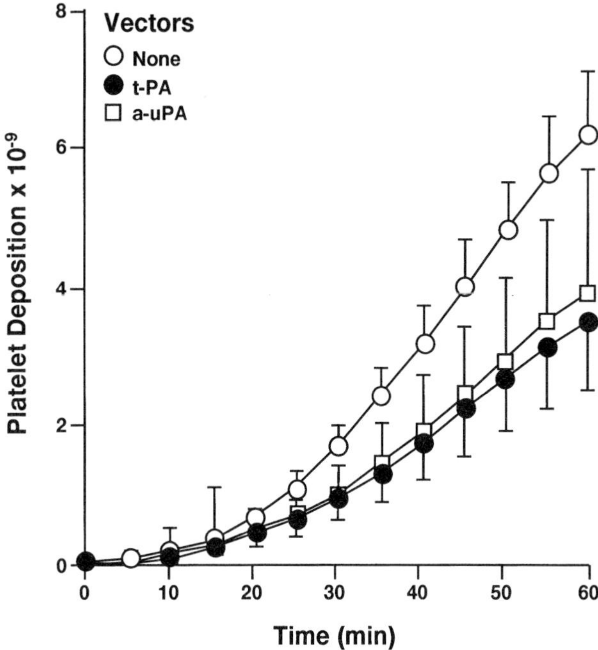

Figure 18-6 Deposition of In-labeled platelets on thrombus tails propagated downstream from grafts seeded at equivalent densities with either untransduced or transduced endothelial cells and exposed to flowing blood in a baboon ex vivo arteriovenous shunt. Platelet deposition is shown in real time for untransduced endothelial cells (open circles; $n = 13$), endothelial cells transduced with a retroviral vector expressing human tissue plasminogen activator (t-PA; closed circles; $n = 8$), and a retroviral vector expressing glycosylphosphatidylinositol (GPI)-anchored human urokinase plasminogen activator (a-uPA; closed squares; $n = 5$). Bars represent SEM. (Reproduced with permission from Dichek et al.)

progeny survive for prolonged periods of time following introduction in vivo. Such data have not yet been forthcoming, despite substantial experimental efforts in animal models. Furthermore, the logistical issues mentioned above surrounding ex vivo manipulation of autologous cells are particularly daunting in this clinical setting, given the extreme importance of avoiding microbial contamination of a prosthetic device.

CONCLUSIONS

A variety of mono- and polygenic cardiovascular diseases are potentially treatable with gene therapy. Initial animal studies have confirmed that genes with potentially therapeutic effects within the cardiovascular system may be introduced in vivo. Nevertheless, practical concerns relating to the achievement of safe, efficient, and long-lasting gene therapy continue to dominate the field. To become useful therapeutic approaches, gene transfer techniques must, in general, achieve high efficiency, prolonged gene expression, and tissue-specific targeting, without the induction of systemic immunity. Each of these goals represents a substantial technical challenge. In addition, as we progress beyond the initial excitement associated with overcoming these technical hurdles, gene therapy must ultimately prove its safety as well as its efficacy in relation to more traditional therapeutic interventions. Only then will gene therapy gain acceptance as a treatment for cardiovascular disease.

SELECTED REFERENCES

Chang MW, Barr E, Seltzer J, et al. Cytostatic gene therapy for vascular proliferative disorders using a constitutively active form of RB. Science 1995;267:518–522.

Clowes MM, Lynch CM, Miller AD, Miller DG, Osborne WR, Clowes AW. Long-term biological response of injured rat carotid artery seeded with smooth muscle cells expressing retrovirally introduced human genes. J Clin Invest 1994;93:644–651.

Dichek DA, Anderson J, Kelly AB, Hanson SR, Harker LA. Enhanced in vivo antithrombotic effects of endothelial cells expressing recombinant plasminogen activators transduced with retroviral vectors. Circulation 1996;93:301–309.

Dzau VJ, Mann MJ, Morishita R, Kaneda Y. Fusigenic viral liposome for gene therapy in cardiovascular diseases. Proc Natl Acad Sci USA 1996;93:11,421–11,425.

Flugelman MY, Jaklitsch MT, Newman KD, et al. Low level in vivo gene transfer into the arterial wall through a perforated balloon-catheter. Circulation 1992;85:1110–1117.

Grossman M, Rader DJ, Muller DWM, et al. A pilot study of ex vivo gene therapy for homozygous familial hypercholesterolaemia. Nat Med 1995;1:1148–1154.

Herz J, Gerard RD. Adenovirus-mediated transfer of low density lipoprotein receptor gene acutely accelerates cholesterol clearance in normal mice. Proc Natl Acad Sci USA 1993;90:2812–2816.

Isner JM, Walsh K, Symes J, et al. Arterial gene therapy for therapeutic angiogenesis in patients with peripheral artery disease. Circulation 1995;91:2687–2692.

Kopfler WP, Willard M, Betz T, Willard JE, Gerard JE, Meidell RS. Adenovirus-mediated transfer of a gene encoding human apolipoprotein A-I into normal mice increases circulating high-density lipoprotein cholesterol. Circulation 1994;90:1319–1327.

Ledley FD. Nonviral gene therapy: the promise of genes as pharmaceutical products. Hum Gene Ther 1995;1129–1144.

Lee SW, Trapnell BC, Rade JJ, Virmani R, Dichek DA. In vivo adenoviral vector-mediated gene transfer into balloon-injured rat carotid arteries. Circ Res 1993;73:797–807.

Nabel EG, Plautz G, Nabel GJ. Site-specific gene-expression in vivo by direct gene transfer into the arterial wall. Science 1990;249:1285–1288.

Nabel E. Gene therapy for cardiovascular disease. Circulation 1995;91: 541–547.

Newman KD, Dunn PF, Owens JW, et al. Adenovirus-mediated gene transfer into normal rabbit arteries results in prolonged vascular cell activation, inflammation, and neointimal hyperplasia. J Clin Invest 1995;96:2955–2965.

O'Brien ER, Schwartz SM. Update on the biology and clinical study of restenosis. Trends Cardiovasc Med 1994;4:169–178.

Ohno T, Gordon D, San H, et al. Gene therapy for vascular smooth muscle cell proliferation after arterial injury. Science 1994;265:781–784.

Rade JJ, Schulick AH, Virmani R, Dichek DA. Local adenoviral-mediated expression of recombinant hirudin reduces neointima formation after arterial injury. Nat Med 1996;2:293–298.

Schulick AH, Newman KD, Virmani R, Dichek DA. In vivo gene transfer into injured carotid arteries. Optimization and evaluation of acute toxicity. Circulation 1995;91:2407–2414.

Spady DK, Cuthbert JA, Willard MN, Meidell RS. Adenovirus-mediated transfer of a gene encoding cholesterol 7α-hydroxylase into hamsters increases hepatic enzyme activity and reduces plasma total and low density lipoprotein cholesterol. J Clin Invest 1995; 96:700–709.

von der Leyen HE, Gibbons GH, Morishita R, et al. Gene therapy inhibiting neointimal vascular lesion: In vivo transfer of endothelial cell nitric oxide synthase gene. Proc Natl Acad Sci USA 1995;92: 1137–1141.

Wang C, Chao L, Chao J. Direct gene delivery of human tissue kallikrein reduces blood pressure in spontaneously hypertensive rats. J Clin Invest 1995;95:1710–1716.

Yang Y, Li Q, Ertl HCJ, Wilson JM. Cellular and humoral immune responses to viral antigens create barriers to lung-directed gene therapy with recombinant adenoviruses. J Virol 1995;69:2004–2115.

Zoldhelyi P, McNatt J, Xu X-M, et al. Prevention of arterial thrombosis by adenovirus-mediated gene transfer of cyclooxygenase gene. Circulation 1996;93:10–17.

HEMATOLOGY III

SECTION EDITOR:
SWEE LAY THEIN

19 Hematopoiesis

Growth Factors and Mechanisms of Regulation

Andrew Haynes and Nigel Russell

INTRODUCTION

The bone marrow of a normal individual represents 5% of the total body weight. Hematopoietic cells first appear in the yolk sac, and migrate first to the liver and finally to the marrow, so that, by 5 months *in utero*, the marrow is the major source of hematopoietic cells. At birth, all bones contain hematopoietic marrow, but in adults, fatty replacement restricts active hematopoiesis to the axial skeleton, upper humeri, and femora. To sustain a healthy peripheral circulation, the bone marrow turns over a trillion cells every day, producing 70 billion neutrophils and 200 billion red cells. The marrow contains a spectrum of cells within each lineage, ranging from immature precursors to mature cells. The latter represent storage compartments released at times of increased demand; 10 times the circulating number of neutrophils are stored in the marrow, whereas the stored and circulating numbers of reticulocytes for red cells are equal. As a consequence in normal marrow, some 50–60% of cells are dedicated to myelopoiesis.

STRUCTURAL ORGANIZATION OF THE BONE MARROW

Bone marrow occupies the intertrabecular spaces inside the marrow cavity of trabecular bone. A framework of reticular cells and collagen supports hematopoietic tissue and vascular channels. Stromal cells, adipocytes, and macrophages provide the necessary microenvironment for hematopoietic cells. Thin-walled vascular sinuses drain blood from the periphery to the center of the marrow cavity. Hematopoietic elements are organized in a perivascular distribution. Discrete islands of erythropoietic cells often with a central macrophage are located near vascular sinuses. The macrophages present growth factors and phagocytose extruded nuclei. Megakaryocytes that produce platelets are also located adjacent to vascular sinuses. In contrast, immature white cell precursors are found next to the bony trabeculae, but as cells differentiate, they become motile; mature cells migrate to the vascular sinuses.

STEM CELLS Hematopoietic activity is sustained by the presence of pleuripotent stem cells which are capable of differentiation to form all of the mature elements of the blood (Fig. 19-1). The existence of such cells was postulated after the demonstration that bone marrow infusion could rescue lethally irradiated mice. The spleens of such animals contained colonies of hematopoietic cells, and the seminal work of Till and McCulloch provided evidence for the existence of self-renewing pleuripotent cells that are capable of sustaining long-term stable hematopoiesis. Single-cell cultures of murine fetal liver stem cells give rise to colonies containing mature lymphoid and myeloid cells, supporting the presence of a pleuripotent stem cell. The pleuripotent stem cells give rise to more differentiated lineage-committed stem cells that, in turn, differentiate into mature end-stage cells. The stem-cell content of human bone marrow can be inferred from the in vitro growth of colonies that produce mature cells in semi-solid media. These colonies arise from lineage-restricted committed stem cells, and those forming myeloid cells (CFU-GM), erythroid cells (CFU-E and BFU-E), and megakaryocytes (CFU-Meg) have been described. It is estimated that 0.1–0.3% of the cells in human marrow are committed stem cells.

PLEURIPOTENT STEM CELLS These most primitive stem cells have been isolated from the lymphocyte fraction of marrow, and at any given time, less than 5% are in active cell cycle. Stable long-term hematopoiesis therefore requires a balance between expansion and differentiation of the pleuripotent stem cell pool. It is estimated that 1 in 10^6 marrow cells are pleuripotent stem cells; hence, the total population of $1–2 \times 10^6$ such cells produces greater than 10^{11} cells each day. Assays for human primitive stem cells have been developed, such as the long-term culture initiating cell (LTCIC) assay. Plastic adherence can also be used to separate long-term culture repopulating cells from more committed stem cells. Civin et al. described the expression of a specific antigen—now designated CD34—on the surface of 1–3% of bone marrow mononuclear cells. This fraction of marrow cells contains committed stem cells but is also capable of stable long-term reconstitution of hematopoiesis in humans after myeloablative doses of chemoradiotherapy. Furthermore, marking by transfection of the Neomycin resistance gene has confirmed its ability to cause long-term production of all lineages, hence the presence of pleuripotent stem cells within the CD34-positive fraction. Expression of the CD34 antigen is stage-specific and lost upon maturation. Further characterization of CD34-positive cells can be made by studying their expression of surface antigens. Cells expressing high levels of CD34 ($CD34^{bright}$) are the most primitive. Analysis of the expression of CD38, Thy-1, CD45 isoforms and the uptake of the dye Rhodamine 123 has identified a subpopulation of CD34 cells that are $CD34^{bright}$, Thy-1^+, $CD38^-$, $CD45RO^+$, and Rhodamine 123^{dull}. These cells can establish LTCIC capable of self-renewal in

From: *Principles of Molecular Medicine* (J. L. Jameson, ed.), ©1998 Humana Press Inc., Totowa, NJ.

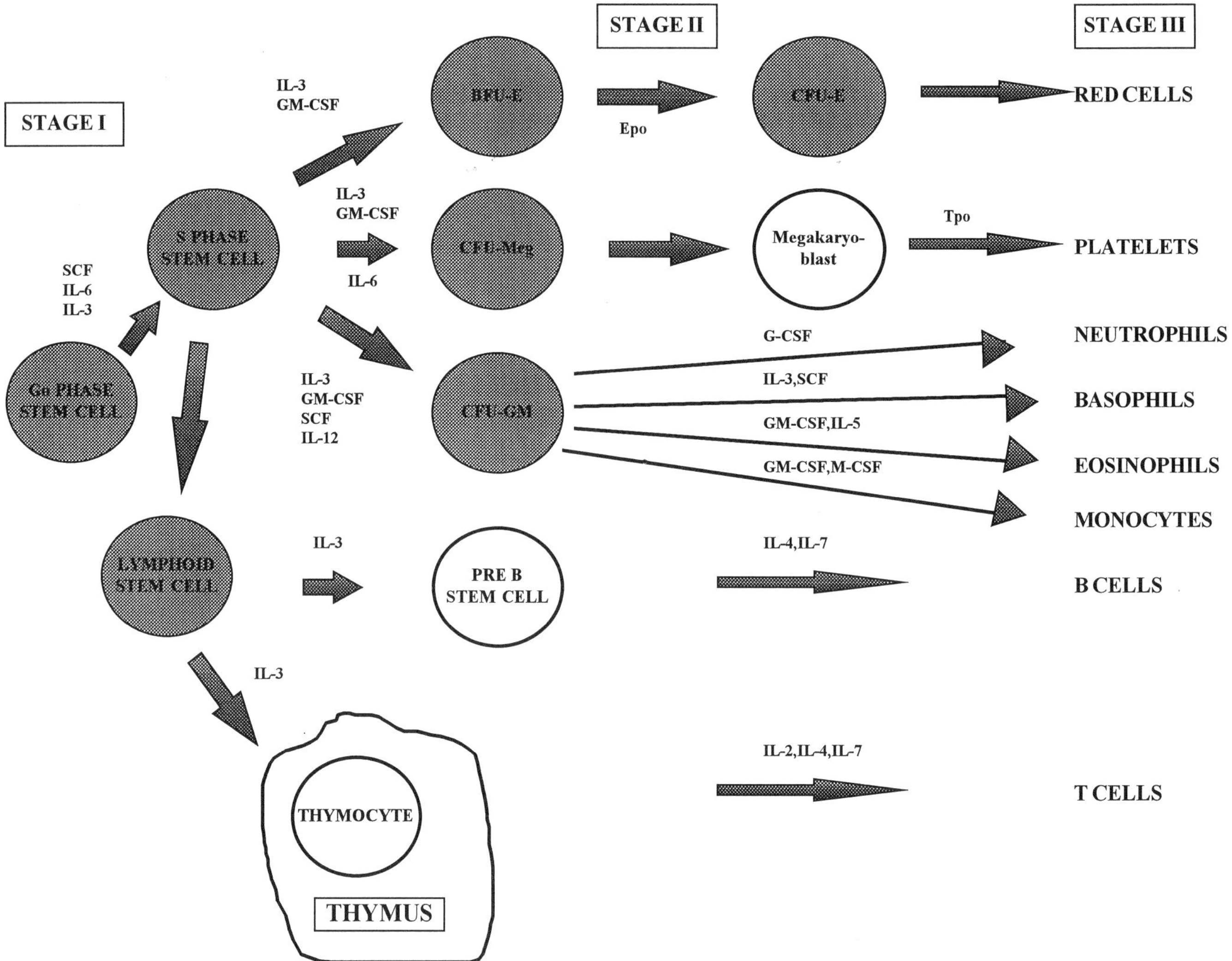

Figure 19-1 Hierarchy of stem-cell development. At stage I, the pleuripotent stem cell is capable of differentiation to form all of the mature elements in the blood under the influence of appropriate growth factors. At stage II, stem cells become lineage-committed and differentiate only to form particular mature elements (stage III). Shaded cells express CD34 antigen; expression is lost at stage II of differentiation. SCF, stem-cell factor; IL, interleukin; GMCSF, granulocyte macrophage colony-stimulating factor; G-CSF, granulocyte colony-stimulating factor; M-CSF, macrophage colony-stimulating factor; Epo, erythropoietin; Tpo, thrombopoietin.

vitro and represent less than 10% of the CD34-positive cell fraction. The gene for the CD34 antigen is present on chromosome 1 at 1q32 and encodes for a 110-kDa glycoprotein. The function of CD34 remains unknown; it may play a role in cell adhesion, with its expression upregulated after intracellular phosphorylation by protein kinase C.

GROWTH FACTORS

The survival, proliferation, and differentiation of normal progenitor cells in vitro is dependent on the presence of growth factors or colony-stimulating factors. A growing family of such factors is emerging with their evolutionary significance underlined by interspecies homology, homology between different factors in the same species, and the common use of certain receptors and signaling mechanisms by different factors. Growth factors prevent apoptosis in stem cells, and their crucial role in normal hematopoiesis is highlighted by genetic studies in mice. Murine production of stem-cell factor (SCF) and its receptor, c-kit, occur at the *Steel* (Sl) and *W* loci, respectively. Homozygous deletion of these loci results in animals with diminished erythropoiesis and mast cell production. In the O*p* mouse, a stop codon in the macrophage colony-stimulating factor (M-CSF) gene results in osteopetrosis and decreased macrophage production.

It is beyond the scope of this chapter to give a detailed account of all of the growth factors contributing to hematopoiesis. An overview of stem-cell hierarchy and the important growth factors is presented in Fig. 19-1. We intend to focus on a number of growth factors that illustrate common mechanisms and that have achieved a place in the management of clinical problems (Table 19-1).

Some factors play a crucial role in the basal production of specific lineages; for example, antibodies against Epo or G-CSF produce anemia and neutropenia, respectively, when injected into animals. Other factors, such as GM-CSF and IL-3, exert actions on a variety of lineages. More than one growth factor appears to exert actions on a particular lineage, and the reasons for this apparent redundancy may be several:

Table 19-1
Human Growth Factors

	Human chromosome location	Product, kDa	Origin	Receptor	Action
G-CSF	17q21–q22	19–25	Monocytes Macrophages	Low-affinity monomer (130 kDa) High-affinity oligomer	Proliferation and differentiation of neutrophils upregulates activity of mature neutrophils
Epo	7q	18–32	Kidney Fetal liver	507-Amino acid polypeptide	Proliferation and differentiation of intermediate stage erythroid progenitors
Tpo	3q26–q27	76	Liver Kidney Spleen Marrow	Product of the c-mp1 proto-oncogene	Proliferation and differentiation of megakaryocyte precursors
GM-CSF	5q23–q31	22	Macrophages Endothelium T cells Fibroblasts Mast cells	Low affinity α-subunit (85 kDa) β-subunit (120 kDa) common to IL-3/5 receptors	Growth and differentiation of granulocyte and macrophage committed stem cells upregulates macrophage, neutrophil, eosinophil, and endothelial cell function
IL-3	5q23–q31	28	T cells Mast cells	Low affinity α-subunit (70 kDa) β-subunit (120 kDa) common to IL-3/5 receptors	Proliferation and differentiation of early precursors in multiple lineages
SCF	12q22–q24	20–35	Marrow stroma Fibroblasts	145-kDa Transmembrane protein	Proliferation and differentiation of multiple lineages

G-CSF, granulocyte colony-stimulating factor; Epo, erythropoietin; Tpo, thrombopoietin; GM-CSF, granulocyte macrophage colony-stimulating factor; IL-3, interleukin-3; SCF, stem-cell factor.

1. Sequential action: Regulators may act at specific phases in the differentiation sequence of specific lineages. For example, Epo acts on more mature erythroid precursors, whereas IL-3 and SCF act on early progenitors.
2. Recruitment: Purified stem cells require a combination of two or more growth factors for proliferation, for example, SCF plus IL-3 or IL-6. Stem-cell factor alone maintains the survival of stem cells but induces little division, unless a second regulator is present. This need for simultaneous signaling by two receptors is an example of recruitment.
3. Synergy: Enhancement of proliferation by combinations of growth factors such as SCF plus G/GM-CSF results, not in an increased number of colonies formed, but a 10- to 20-fold increase in the number of cells per colony, compared to either growth factor alone.

These processes of sequential action, recruitment and synergy overlap in normal development. The injection of G-CSF not only increases circulating neutrophil numbers, but it also increases the levels of progenitor cells of all lineages in the peripheral blood. The failure to produce mature cells in other lineages results from the absence of the relevant factors, emphasizing the need for synergy and sequential action. If G-CSF is injected into mice bearing the *Steel* or *W* loci mutations that abrogate responses to SCF, a much smaller rise in circulating neutrophils and progenitors is observed, emphasizing the need for recruitment.

REGULATION OF GROWTH FACTOR PRODUCTION

Regulation of expression of growth factors lie predominantly at the posttranscriptional level that involves mRNA stabilization. The genes encoding growth factors belong to the family of early response genes (ERGs) which are characterized by a rapid and transient activation of transcription. ERG mRNAs are usually short-lived with half-lives of 10–30 min, compared to those of most mammalian mRNAs, which typically survive for hours or days. ERG mRNAs are characterized by the presence of multiple copies of the sequence motif AUUUA in the 3' untranslated region (UTRs); this sequence appears to function as a potent mRNA destabilizing determinant.

For instance, the mRNA encoding G-CSF has a half-life of less than 15 min owing to rapid degradation of the mRNA by cytoplasmic RNase. In contrast, although the mRNAs of other cytokines (such as GM-CSF, IL-1, and IL-6) also contain poly-AUUUA sequence, these mRNAs are stabilized by IL-1 and thus allowed to accumulate. In normal cells, G-CSF gene expression is transient, with levels diminishing after 8–12 h, even in the face of continued simulation. In solid tumors, aberrant production of G-CSF in association with abnormal mRNA accumulation, may be responsible for a "leukemoid reaction" with marked increase in circulating neutrophils.

At the transcriptional level, two upstream regulatory elements important in transcription have been identified: an octamer sequence (ATTTGCAT) 110 bp upstream of the TATA box, a decanucleotide sequence (GAGATTCCCC) 180 bp upstream of the transcription start-site, which is conserved between species. Similar sequences are present in the GM-CSF and IL-3 genes.

GROWTH FACTOR RECEPTORS

Growth factors exert their actions via interaction with receptors; different receptor families specific to groups of growth factors have been recognized on the basis of their molecular structure (Fig. 19-2).

Receptors with intrinsic tyrosine kinase activity stimulated by ligand binding, are distinguished by a single membrane spanning

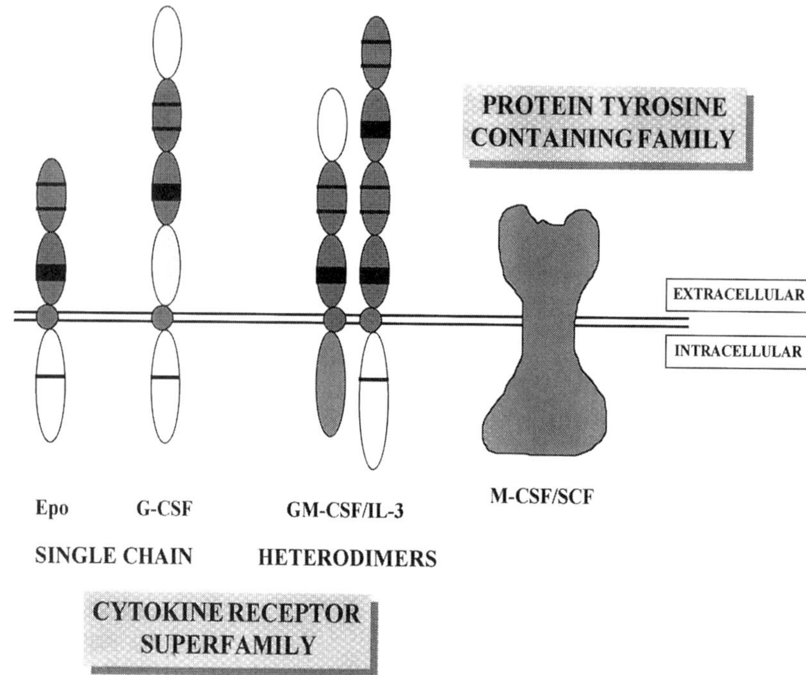

Figure 19-2 Molecular structure of human growth factor receptors. Two families are recognized: those with intrinsic tyrosine kinase activity and those without, which are members of the cytokine receptor superfamily. Trp-Ser-X-Trp-Ser motif, thick black bar; conserved cysteine residues, double thin black bar; conserved box 1/2 domains, single thin black bar.

domain and five immunoglobulin-like extracellular domains that identify them as part of the immunoglobulin superfamily. Examples include the SCF and M-CSF receptors.

Receptors with common motifs in their extracellular domains identify them as part of the cytokine receptor superfamily. Examples include Il-2/3/4/5/6/7, G-CSF, GM-CSF, Epo, and Tpo receptors. The extracellular motifs include four conserved cysteine residues and a conserved five amino acid sequence of Trp-Ser-X-Trp-Ser where X can be any amino acid. The latter domain is present in complement proteins, thrombospondin and properdin, where it mediates protein–protein interaction. These receptors have some sequence homology in their cytoplasmic membrane proximal regions termed the box 1 and 2 domains that are important for signaling.

In the cytokine receptor superfamily, some members are single chain such as the Epo or G-CSF receptors whereas others have two or more subunits such as the GM-CSF or IL-3 receptors (Fig. 19-2). A better understanding of the structure of these receptors has helped to explain some of the observed effects of and the cellular events triggered by growth factors.

ERYTHROPOIETIN RECEPTOR The gene for the human Epo receptor is on chromosome 19p and encodes a 507-amino acid, 68-kDa, single polypeptide chain protein with a single transmembrane domain. The cytokine superfamily motifs divide the extracellular portion of the receptor into two subdomains linked by disulfide bonds; the regions of this structure crucial for particular functions have been studied in vitro by site-directed mutagenesis.

1. Mutations affecting the Trp-Ser-X-Trp-Ser motif result in sequestration of the protein in the endoplasmic reticulum and failure of expression.
2. The cytoplasmic portion of the receptor consists of 236 amino acids with the two regions, box 1 and box 2, which share sequence homology with other cytokine receptors. Mutations truncating the carboxyl terminus and removing the box 1 and 2 domains abolish growth-signaling, establishing the importance of the membrane proximal domains in this process.
3. A mutation changing Arg^{129} to cysteine in the extracellular domain results in receptor dimerization and constitutive signaling not dependent on the presence of Epo. This indicates a requirement for the normal receptor to oligomerize to permit growth signaling.
4. A mutation truncating 70 amino acids at the carboxy terminal of the cytoplasmic domain results in abnormal signaling and produces familial erythrocytosis in humans. This area is important for limiting signaling after stimulation.

GRANULOCYTE COLONY-STIMULATING FACTOR RECEPTOR This is a 100- to 120-kDa single polypeptide chain protein that is a member of the cytokine receptor superfamily. The monomeric protein has low affinity for G-CSF but forms a high affinity receptor after oligomerization. In addition to the cytokine family motifs, the extracellular domain also has three fibronectin-like repeats. The first 57 amino acids of the cytoplasmic domain contain the box 1 and 2 sequences that are required for growth signaling. A murine knockout of the transcription factor, CAAT enhancer-binding protein (C/EBP) α, causes loss of G-CSF receptor expression and a block in neutrophil development.

GRANULOCYTE–MACROPHAGE COLONY STIMULATING FACTOR AND IL-3 Both of these growth factors have actions on a wide range of hematopoietic cells. Binding of GM-CSF to its receptor is completed by IL-3 and vice versa; this cross-competition is explained by the molecular structure of their receptors. Ligand binding occurs with low affinity to a specific α-chain, which for GM-CSF and IL-3 are encoded by genes in the pseudoautosomal regions of the X and Y chromosomes. Both receptors share a common 120-kDa β chain encoded by a gene on chromosome 22q12-13 that is necessary for signaling. The αβ chain heterodimer displays high affinity specific binding. Transfection of the cell line NIH-3T3 with GM-CSF α, IL-3 α, and common β-subunits has confirmed that the basis for cross-competition is competition among specific α-subunits for the common β-subunit. The extracellular domains of both chains carry the motifs associated with the cytokine receptor superfamily. The membrane proximal portion of the β-subunit has box 1 and 2 domains, and truncated mutations that retain the 60 amino acids containing these domains still induce growth signals. The cytoplasmic domains of the α chains are also required for signaling, indicating that an intact αβ heterodimer is required for this process.

STEM-CELL FACTOR RECEPTOR This 145-kDa product of the c-*kit* proto-oncogene is a transmembrane glycoprotein. Receptor–ligand interaction is associated with oligomerization and activation of endogenous tyrosine kinase activity that is essential for signaling.

The response of a given hematopoietic precursor will thus depend on the nature of the receptor units expressed by that cell and their relative numbers. This may explain some of the pleiotropic actions of human growth factors.

RECEPTOR SIGNALING MECHANISMS

TYROSINE PHOSPHORYLATION The intrinsic protein tyrosine kinase activity of the SCF and M-CSF receptors is essential for signal transduction. Similarly, a number of common proteins are tyrosine phosphorylated after stimulation by IL-3, GM-CSF, and Epo. In the Epo receptor, deletion of 20 amino acids (numbers 280–301) in the conserved region of the cytoplasmic domain inactivates growth promotion, tyrosine phosphorylation, and early gene induction. Finally, tyrosine kinase inhibitors prevent the action of growth factors. These lines of evidence suggest that although members of the cytokine receptor superfamily do not have intrinsic tyrosine kinase activity, an associated activity is essential for receptor signaling. Tyrosine kinase activity is rapidly induced after stimulation of these receptors at 4°C, suggesting that the kinase activity must be closely associated to the receptor, if not an integral part of its structure.

A family of cytoplasmic tyrosine kinases, the Janus or Jak kinases, are associated with activated growth factor receptors (Table 19-2). The four members of this family contain two kinase domains, the carboxy-terminal one being a protein tyrosine kinase. The region of the box 1 and 2 domains in the cytoplasmic tail of cytokine receptor superfamily members is required for receptor association with Jaks. This association may be constitutive e.g., Epo receptor or occurs only after ligand binding, e.g., IL-3 receptor. Oligomerization of the receptors brings the associated Jak kinases into sufficient proximity to allow crossphosphorylation and activation of their protein tyrosine kinase domains. A single chain may associate with a single Jak, e.g., Epo receptor and Jak 2 or with multiple Jaks, e.g., G-CSF receptor and Jaks 1 and 2. These observations explain many of the structural requirements of growth factor receptors necessary for signaling to occur.

PATHWAYS ACTIVATED BY TYROSINE PHOSPHORYLATION Receptor autophosphorylation by Jaks creates crucial docking sites for a number of important proteins that propagate the growth signal (Fig. 19-3).

Table 19-2
The Janus Kinase Family and Hematopoietic Growth Factor Receptors

	Size	*Chromosome*	*Receptors linked to*
JAK-1	135	1p31.3	IL-2, -3, -4, -5, -6, -7, -11 G-CSF GM-CSF IFN-α/β/γ
JAK-2	130	10p23–24	IL-2, -3, -4, -5, -6, -7, -11, -12 Epo G-CSF GM-CSF
Tyk-2	140	19p13.2	IL–6, -11, -12 IFN-α/β/γ

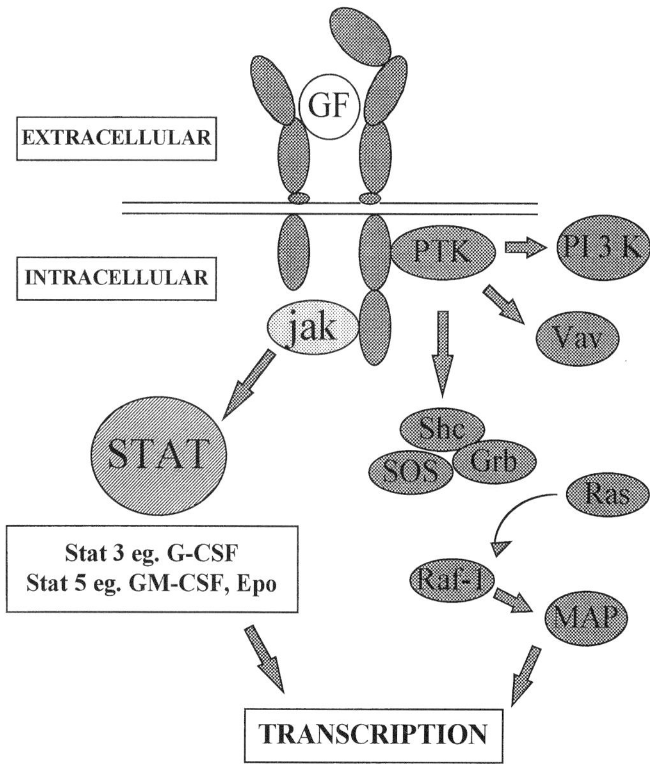

Figure 19-3 Signal transduction mechanisms used by growth factor receptors. The PTK activity intrinsic to or associated with the growth factor receptor activates a series of phosphorylation cascades. PI-3-kinase phosphorylates inositol phosphates, whereas activation of the Ras pathway stimulates the intrinsic GTPase activity of this GTP-binding protein. The latter induces a further phosphorylation cascade that culminates in early gene induction. The Jak kinases have tyrosine phosphorylation activity and rapidly associate with activated growth factor receptors. These molecules phosphorylate a second family of molecules, termed Stats, which then acquire DNA binding properties. PTK, protein tyrosine kinase; Jak, Janus kinase; STAT, signal transducer and activator of transcription; GF, growth factor.

Ras Pathway Activation Receptor associated Jaks activate the protein SHC that, in turn, associates with the adaptor protein Grb 2. The latter associates with SOS, a GDP-GTP exchange factor that controls the intrinsic GTPase activity of a small molecular-weight membrane associated GTP-binding protein termed Ras.

Phosphorylated Ras activates a phosphorylation cascade that activates Raf-1 and MAP kinase, which in turn leads to early gene induction.

Phosphatidyl Inositol 3 Kinase (PI-3 Kinase) Activation The box 1 and 2 domains of the cytoplasmic tail of receptors can bind the p85 subunit of PI-3 kinase, increasing its activity. This kinase phosphorylates inositol phosphates that are known to play a role in signal transduction for non–growth factor receptors.

Vav Activation The vav gene is only expressed in hematopoietic cells and is tyrosine phosphorylated by a number of growth factors. Expression of antisense vav in hematological malignancies reduces CFU-GM colony formation and BFU-E activity. However, function of this gene remains incompletely understood.

Signal Transducer and Activator of Transcription (Stat) Activation This novel family of proteins acquire DNA-binding properties after tyrosine phosphorylation and oligomerization. These proteins were identified as important links in mediating signal transduction between interferon receptors and interferon responsive genes. Stats share sequence homology and coprecipitate with Jaks after growth factor stimulation. A growing family of Stats has been identified that appear to be important in initiating altered gene transcription after growth factor signaling (Fig. 19-3).

Hematopoietic Cell Phosphatase (HCP) Activation This protein contains a carboxy-terminal tyrosine phosphatase domain that binds to the tyrosine phosphorylated carboxy-terminal domains of the Epo, SCF, and IL-3 receptors. Its expression is restricted to hematopoietic cells. The importance of this factor for limiting the action of growth factors has been confirmed by study of "motheaten" mice. These animals have a mutation that deletes HCP and is rapidly lethal in the homozygous state owing to accumulation of activated macrophages in the lung. It is associated with increased sensitivity to Epo. Similarly, the familial erythrocytosis seen with mutations that remove 70 amino acids at the carboxy-terminal of the human Epo receptor is a result of loss of the phosphorylation residue recognized by HCP and continued signaling after receptor stimulation.

Gene Transcription Growth factor tyrosine phosphorylation is associated with upregulation of c-*myc*, which, in turn, upregulates expression of the enzyme ornithine decarboxylase (ODC). Inhibition of this enzyme blocks growth factor stimulation.

Other genes upregulated by growth factors include c-*fos*, c-*jun*, and *pim*-1. The latter is expressed only in hematopoietic cells and produces a serine-threonine kinase that may influence cell-cycle control.

CLINICAL APPLICATION OF GROWTH FACTORS Our expanding knowledge of the mechanism of action of human hematopoietic growth factors is shedding light on the pathophysiology of a number of disease states. Furthermore, in the decade since the cDNAs for G and GM-CSF were identified, recombinant human growth factors have become established in therapeutic use. In the next section, we will outline some of the clinical consequences arising from our understanding of the basic science of hematopoietic growth factors.

GRANULOCYTE COLONY-STIMULATING FACTOR (G-CSF) Recombinant human G-CSF expressed from bacterial or yeast cells is available for clinical use. After subcutaneous or intravenous injection of 2.5–10 µg/kg of these products, up to a 10-fold rise in the peripheral neutrophil count, beginning with the first dose and sustained for the duration of therapy, is seen. In concert with this, up to a 100-fold increase in circulating progenitors of all lineages is seen during treatment. These observations have led to a number of clinical applications.

Minimizing Chemotherapy-Induced Neutropenia The use of myelosuppressive chemotherapy to treat hematological malignancies and solid tumors is associated with a period of neutropenia. Septicemia from endogenous organisms colonizing the gut is a cause of patient morbidity and mortality during periods of neutropenia. The risk of such sepsis is directly related to the duration and degree of neutropenia. By administering G-CSF after the chemotherapy, the depth and duration of neutropenia can be reduced. Trials have shown that for a number of diseases, including lymphoma and acute leukemia, as well as solid tumors, G-CSF support during chemotherapy reduces the number of infections, hence patient morbidity. These trials have not demonstrated definitive benefits for treatment outcome. Other growth factors, such as GM-CSF or IL-3, have no superior efficacy to G-CSF but are associated with more side effects.

Maximizing Dose Intensity of Chemotherapy By minimizing the duration of neutropenia induced by chemotherapy, the interval between courses of treatment can be shortened with an increase in the delivered dose intensity. Using G-CSF, it has been possible to reduce the duration between courses, but thrombocytopenia remains a limitation. Only modest increases in dose intensity can be achieved by this approach, and major clinical benefit has not resulted. With the isolation of Tpo, new approaches to prevent dose-limiting thrombocytopenia may be feasible. Animal studies have demonstrated the ability of Tpo to decrease the depth and duration of thrombocytopenia and its safe combination with G-CSF.

High-Dose Therapy and Transplantation Independent observers have documented the "mobilization" of stem cells from the bone marrow into the peripheral blood after G-CSF treatment or upon recovery from myelosuppressive chemotherapy. The combination of both treatments is synergistic for this effect. Stem cells can be harvested from the peripheral blood mononuclear fraction by leukapheresis. Such collections contain CD34-positive stem cells and can be used for bone marrow rescue after high-dose therapy (Fig. 19-4). The aim of such treatment is to give maximum dose intensity to eliminate the disease and use peripheral blood stem cells (PBSC) to rescue the patient from the resultant myeloablation. The PBSC may be collected from the patient and used for a later autologous procedure or from a sibling donor in an allogeneic transplant. Gene-marking studies have documented the ability of PBSC to restore long-term stable hematopoiesis in this setting, hence the presence of pleuripotent stem cells in these collections. The stem-cell content of PBSC can be inferred from the numbers of CD34-positive cells collected. Patients receiving greater than 2.5×10^6 CD34-positive cells per kilogram body weight engraft rapidly after autologous PBSC transplants. This engraftment is more rapid than that seen with bone marrow rescue as the source of stem cells and is accounted for by the number of CD34 positive cells, which is up to 10-fold higher in PBSC collections. The number of natural killer (NK) cells is up to 20-fold greater in PBSC and the distribution of lymphocyte subsets differs. For these reasons, the use of PBSC for allogeneic transplantation may offer enhanced immunological reactions against malignant cells, the so-called "graft vs leukemia" effect and speedier immune reconstitution with a reduction in the risk of infection. For hematological diseases that affect the bone marrow, PBSC may provide

A AUTOLOGOUS TRANSPLANT

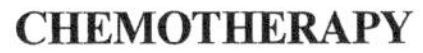

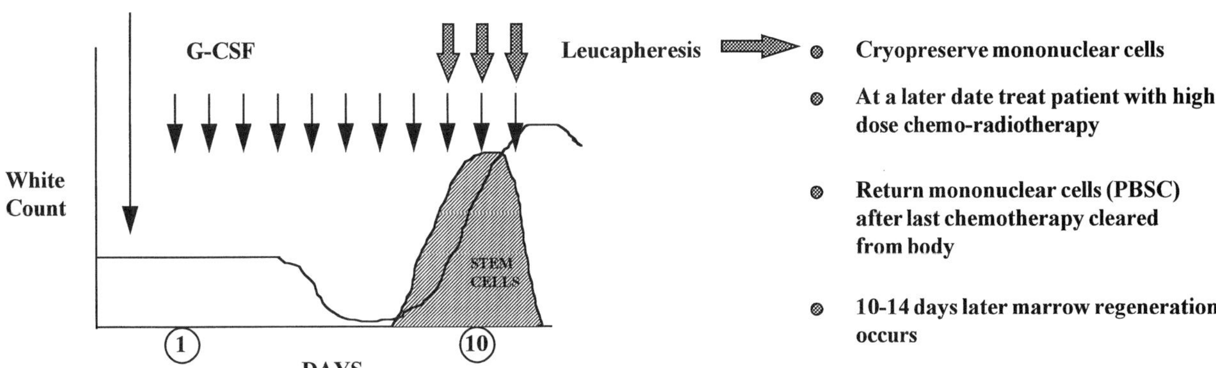

B ALLOGENEIC TRANSPLANT

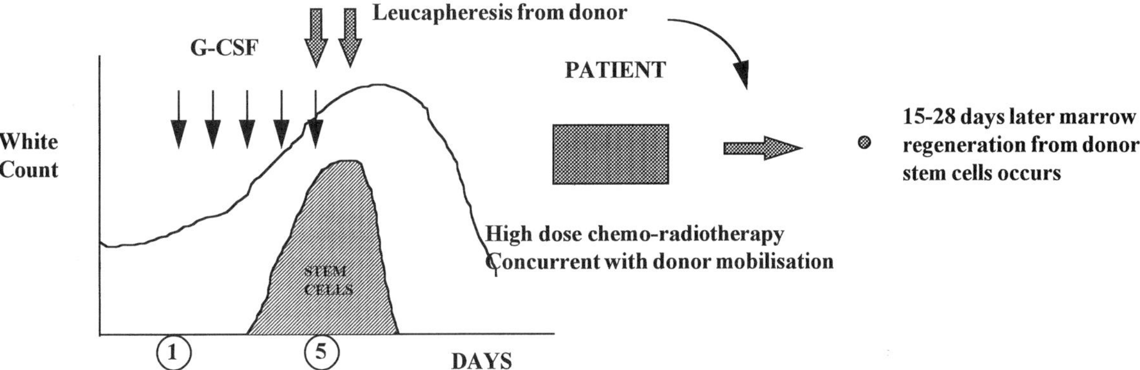

Figure 19-4 Use of G-CSF to obtain stem cells for **(A)** autologous and **(B)** allogeneic transplantation.

a source of autologous rescue that is less contaminated with tumor cells than bone marrow. In practice, however, tumor-cell contamination has been documented and may relate to the degree of marrow contamination at the time of mobilization.

The use of PBSC has now virtually replaced marrow in autologous rescue after high-dose therapy, and we expect their use for allogeneic transplantation to expand. These procedures are still associated with a period of absolute neutropenia and thrombocytopenia; the use of growth factors to further reduce these remains to be explored. Combinations of other growth factors such as SCF or IL-3 with G-CSF are being explored for synergy in mobilizing CD34 positive stem cells for collection.

Congenital Neutropenia Congenital neutropenias are a spectrum of disorders with various etiologies. Kostmann's syndrome is one example in which severe neutropenia at birth is associated with maturation arrest at the promyelocyte/myelocyte stage of development in the marrow. Inheritance may be autosomal dominant or recessive. These babies experience severe pyogenic infection and historically have a median survival of approximately 3 years. Circulating levels of G-CSF are raised in Kostmann's syndrome, with normal expression and affinity of G-CSF receptors. Studies on G-CSF receptor structure have largely been normal, but abnormal protein phosphorylation has been described raising the possibility of a downstream signal transduction block. The majority of these patients respond to G-CSF therapy with a rise in their neutrophil counts, a reduction in infections, and improvements in survival. Prior to the use of G-CSF, some of these patients developed myelodysplasia and acute myeloid leukemia. Many patients have now been treated with G-CSF for several years, and an increased incidence of this progression to acute leukemia has been documented in such patients. This is probably a result of increased survival highlighting this feature of the natural history of Kostmann's syndrome. Patients developing leukemia usually have an antecedent monosomy 7 cytogenetic abnormality, and one report detailed the presence of mutations in the G-CSF receptor in this group. The latter may also account for the rare cases that are refractory to G-CSF therapy.

Neonatal Sepsis Newborn babies have immature host defense systems that predispose them to increased mortality during bacterial sepsis. Depletion of storage pool neutrophils associated with neutropenia during neonatal sepsis is associated with a poor prognosis that can be improved by granulocyte transfusions. Studies have documented decreased production by effector cells of a number of growth factors in neonates, including G-CSF, GM-CSF, IL-3, and IL-6. Other studies have documented the safety of administration of G- and GM-CSF in this setting, with increases in peripheral neutrophil counts. Trials are pending to show the clinical benefits of such treatment.

ERYTHROPOIETIN **Renal Failure** Erythropoietin was the first human growth factor to be available for clinical use. The first patient group targeted for therapy were patients with renal failure. Since Epo is made by peritubular cells in the kidney, nephron loss is associated with decreased Epo production. Patients with renal failure thus have a hypoproliferative anemia with low Epo levels for the degree of anemia. The anemia is responsible for much of the morbidity of renal failure with poor exercise tolerance and exacerbation of the symptoms of ischemic heart disease, which is not uncommon in this patient group. Greater than 95% of renal patients treated with recombinant Epo will improve their hemoglobin and derive clinical benefit. Other benefits include improvement in cardiovascular parameters, such as reduction in left ventricular hypertrophy and normalization of the bleeding time. The increased blood viscosity may exacerbate hypertension, and an increased incidence of shunt thrombosis has been reported. Iron stores must be adequate prior to starting Epo, and supplementation may be necessary.

Chronic Disease Some, but not all, patients with chronic disease such as malignancy or rheumatoid arthritis have a hypoproliferative anemia associated with Epo levels that are reduced for the degree of anemia. These patients have been documented to respond to pharmacological doses of Epo with an increase in hemoglobin and improvement in morbidity.

Premature Neonates Some premature neonates experience a hypoproliferative anemia 2–12 weeks postnatally. Erythropoietin levels are detectable in cord blood of babies born from 25 weeks gestation but show an increase after 32 weeks. Levels of SCF and IL-6 had no relationship to gestation, and those of GM-CSF and IL-3 were undetectable. In a randomized study, recombinant Epo reversed the anemia of prematurity in about 30% of premature infants, suggesting low levels of Epo may be a contributory factor.

Diamond Blackfan Anemia This is a rare congenital pure red cell aplasia, presenting with macrocytic anemia in infancy. The disease behaves heterogeneously with regard to associated dysmorphic features, inheritance, and clinical course. These patients have appropriate Epo levels, and no clinical response to treatment with recombinant Epo has been demonstrated. Over 70% of patients respond to steroid therapy, and the majority are steroid dependent. Some become refractory to treatment, and, ultimately, some 40% will be transfusion dependent. Levels of stem-cell factor and the expression of c-*kit*, the SCF receptor, are normal. In vitro erythroid colony formation is reduced but shows some response to IL-3. Clinically, IL-3 has produced responses in approximately 10% of patients, some achieving steroid independence for several years. All of the responders had at some point been steroid responsive. At least a third of patients had side effects, including fever, fluid retention, and local reactions at injection sites. Further studies to better define the molecular lesions in these patients are pending.

CONCLUSION

Our understanding of the molecular factors that stimulate and regulate hematopoiesis is a good example of the impact basic scientific knowledge can have on the practice of clinical medicine. New factors, both stimulatory and inhibitory, continue to be defined, offering insights into the pathogenesis of inherited and acquired disease and the potential for novel therapeutic strategies.

SELECTED REFERENCES

Bearpark AD, Gordon MY. Adhesive properties distinguishing subpopulations of hemopoietic stem cells with different spleen colony forming and marrow repopulating capacities. Bone Marrow Transplantation 1989;4:625–628.

Cairo MS. Therapeutic implications of dysregulated colony stimulating factor expression in neonates. Blood 1993;82:2269–2272.

Civin CI, Strauss LC, Brovall C, Fackler MJ, Schwarz JF, Shaper JH. Antigeneic analysis of hematopoiesis III. A hematopoietic progenitor cell surface antigen defined by a monoclonal antibody raised against KG-1a cells. J Immunol 1984;133:157–165.

Cumano A, Paige CJ, Iscove NN, Brady G. Bipotential precursors of B cells and macrophages in murine fetal liver. Nature 1992;356:612–615.

Cytokines and growth factors. Balliere's Clinical Hematology. Brenner M, ed. London: Balliere Tindall, 1994.

Dunbar CE, Cottler Fox M, O'Shaughnessey JA, Doren S, Carter C, Berenson R et al. Retrovirally marked CD34 enriched peripheral blood and bone marrow cells contribute to long term engraftment after autologous transplantation. Blood 1995;85:3048–3057.

Ford CE, Hamerton JL, Barnes DWH, Loutit JF. Cytological identification of radiation chimeras. Nature 1956;177:452–454.

Goldman J. Peripheral blood stem cells for allografting. Blood 1995; 85:157–165.

Haynes AP, Russell NH. Clinical use of hemopoietic growth factors. In: Hoffbrand AV, ed. Recent Advances In Hematology, vol 8. London: Churchill Livingstone, 1996.

Haynes AP, Russell NH. Blood stem cell allografting. Current Opinion in Hematology 1995;2:431–435.

Holyoake TL, Alcorn MJ. CD34 positive hemopoietic cells: Biology and clinical applications. Blood Rev 1994;8:113–124.

Ihle JN, Kerr IM. Jaks and Stats in signalling by the cytokine receptor superfamily. Trends in Genetics 1995;11:69–74.

Kaushansky K. Thrombopoietin: The primary regulator of platelet production. Blood 1995;86:419–431.

Lathja LG. Stem cell concepts. Differentiation 1979;14:23–29.

Luger SM, Ratajczak J, Ratajczak MZ, et al. A functional analysis of protooncogene Vav's role in adult human hematopoiesis. Blood 1996;87:1326–1334.

Pike BL, Robinson WA. Human bone marrow colony growth in agar gel. J Cell Physiology 1976;76:77–84.

Taswell C. Limiting dilution assays for the determination of immunocompetent cell frequencies. J Immunol 1981;126:1614–1619.

Teppermann AD, Curtis JE, McCulloch EA. Erythropoietic colonies in cultures of human marrow. Blood 1974;44:659–669.

Till JE, McCulloch EA, Siminovitch L. A stochastic model of stem cell proliferation based on the growth of spleen colony forming cells. Proc Natl Acad Sci 1964;51:24–36.

Vainchenker W, Bouguet J, Guichard J, Breton-Gorius J. Megakaryocyte colony formation from human bone marrow precursors. Blood 1979;54:940–945.

Wu H, Klingmuller U, Acurio A, Hsiao JG, Lodish HF. Functional interaction of erythropoietin and stem cell factor receptors is essential for erythroid colony formation. Proc Natl Acad Sci USA 1997;94:1806–1810.

Zhang DE, Zhang P, Wang ND, Hetherington CJ, Darlington GJ, Tenen DG. Absence of granulocyte colony-stimulating factor signaling and neutrophil development in CCAAT enhancer binding protein alpha-deficient mice. Proc Natl Acad Sci USA 1997;94:569–574.

20 Disorders of Hemoglobin Structure and Synthesis

SWEE LAY THEIN AND JACQUES ROCHETTE

INTRODUCTION

All human hemoglobins have a tetrameric structure, consisting of two identical α-like (α or ζ) and two β-like (ε, γ, δ, or β) globin chains, each linked to a heme group.

Human hemoglobin production is characterized by two "switches," production of embryonic hemoglobin switches after the first 2 months of gestation to the production of fetal hemoglobin and then just before birth to adult hemoglobin (Fig. 20-1). These different types of hemoglobin have been adapted to the changes in physiological requirements that occur during development. Fetal hemoglobin (Hb F) exhibits a higher oxygen affinity than the adult hemoglobins in vivo; the higher oxygen affinity of Hb F relative to adult hemoglobin facilitates the transfer of oxygen across the placenta from the maternal circulation to the fetal circulation.

The α- and β-like globin chains are encoded by genetically distinct loci on the tip of chromosome 16p and chromosome 11p15.5, respectively (Fig. 20-1). In both clusters, the genes are arranged 5'→3' in the order in which they are expressed during development. While the α-like genes undergo a single developmental switch (embryonic → fetal/adult), the β-like genes undergo two switches (embryonic → fetal → adult).

Expression of the individual genes within each cluster is controlled by complex interactions between regulatory sequences within each gene, and regulatory elements upstream of the cluster. In the β cluster, the upstream element is referred to as the β locus control region (β-LCR) and a corresponding element in the α cluster is referred to as HS-40 (Fig. 20-1). The products of the two gene clusters are expressed in equal amounts, maintaining a balance in globin chain production throughout development.

Much interest has focused on the mechanisms by which the globin genes are expressed in a tissue- and developmental-stage–specific manner. Tissue-specific expression may be explained by the presence of the binding sites for two proteins, GATA-1 and NF-E2, in the upstream regulatory elements and the local promoter of the globin genes. GATA-1 and NF-E2 are specifically expressed in erythroid cells, and it seems likely that these two *trans*-acting factors form part of a network of factors that commit hemopoietic stem cells to erythroid differentiation. The mechanisms by which developmental regulation is controlled are less clear; autonomous control of the embryonic ε and ζ genes and the γ genes implicates negatively acting factors, referred to as silencers. So far, the best-defined example of a developmental–stage-specific regulatory factor is the erythroid Krüppel-like factor (EKLF) that appears to be essential for the final steps of definitive erythropoiesis, at least in mice.

The vast majority of hemoglobin disorders are inherited and can be classified into those that are characterized by a quantitative deficiency of one or more of the globin chains of hemoglobin (thalassemias); those in which there is a structural change in a globin chain (hemoglobin variants) and the thalassemic hemoglobinopathies in which a structurally abnormal hemoglobin produces the phenotype of thalassemia. The acquired abnormalities can also be classified into those characterized by a reduced synthesis of the globin chains (e.g., acquired Hb H disease) and those that alter the structure and function of hemoglobin so that oxygen transport is affected (e.g., carboxyhemoglobinemia, methemoglobinemia).

THE THALASSEMIAS

BACKGROUND Thalassemia was first recognized by Cooley and Lee in 1925 as a form of severe anemia that is associated with splenomegaly and bone changes in children. The term thalassemia is derived from the Greek θαλασσα (the sea), because many of the early cases came from the Mediterranean region. However, it is now clear that the disorder is not only limited to the Mediterranean region, but it occurs also throughout the world, prevalent in the tropical and subtropical regions including the Middle East, parts of Africa, the Indian subcontinent, and Southeast Asia. It appears that heterozygotes for thalassemia are protected from the severe effects of *falciparum* malaria, and natural selection has increased and maintained their gene frequencies in these malarious regions.

The thalassemias can be classified according to the type of globin chain(s) that is produced in reduced amounts (i.e., α-, β-, δβ-, γδβ-, δ-, γ-, and εγδβ-thalassemias). The two major categories are the α- and β-thalassemias, whereas the rare forms include the γ-, δ-, and εγδβ-thalassemias. Hereditary persistence of fetal hemoglobin (HPFH) syndromes refer to the group of disorders in which the switch from fetal to adult hemoglobin production is incomplete, and the fetal hemoglobin levels are elevated in otherwise normal individuals. Because of their concomitant increased Hb F levels, the δβ- and γδβ-thalassemias are often

From: *Principles of Molecular Medicine* (J. L. Jameson, ed.), ©1998 Humana Press Inc., Totowa, NJ.

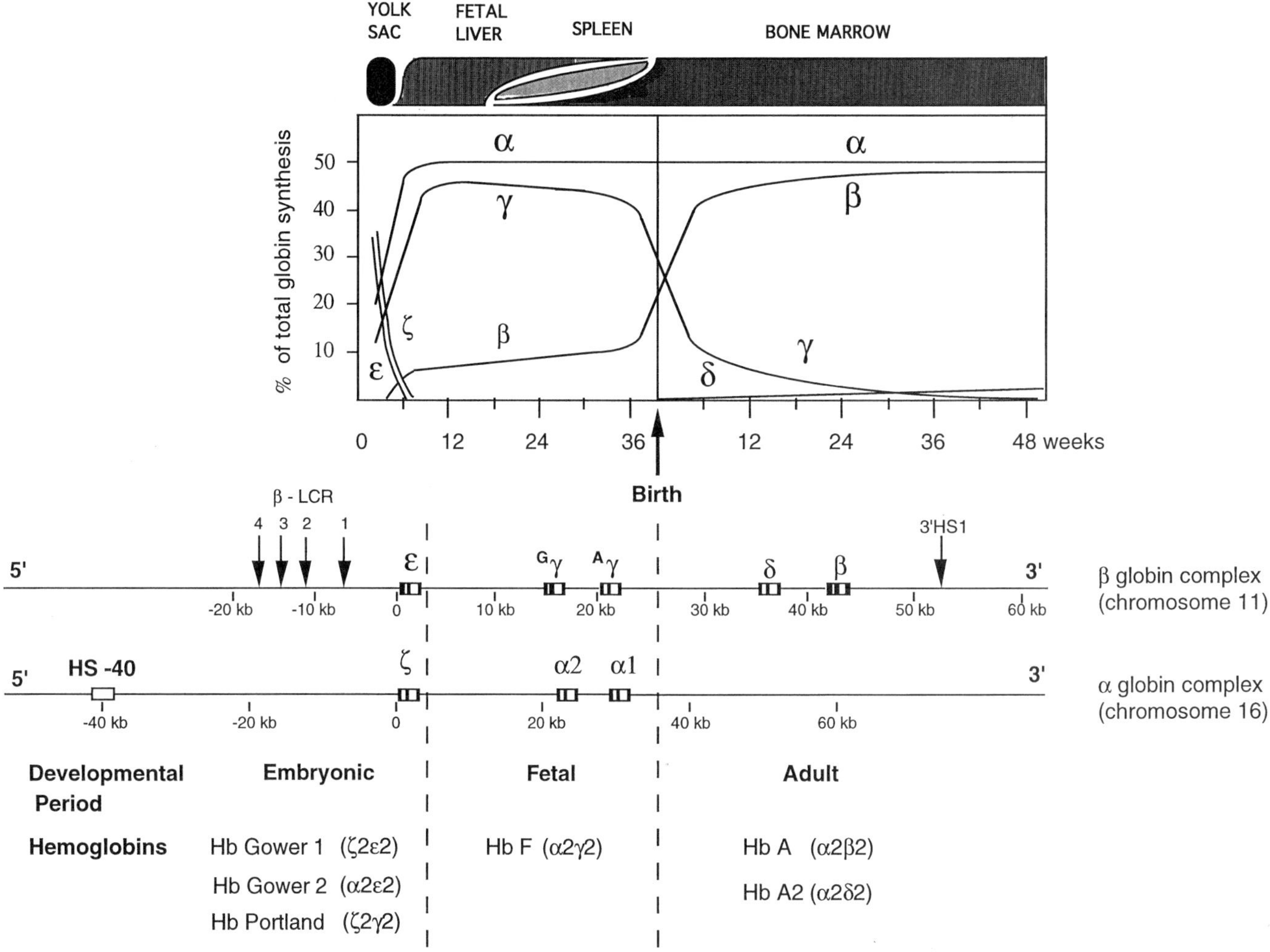

Figure 20-1 Sequence of human hemoglobin synthesis *(above)* and the organization of the globin gene clusters on chromosome 11p and 16p *(below)* with the types of hemoglobin synthesized during the different developmental periods. Solid arrows represent the erythroid-specific deoxyribonuclease I hypersensitive sites (HSs) in the β cluster. HSs 1–4 upstream of the β cluster form the β-LCR; the 3'HS1 site is a downstream enhancer. HS –40 form the equivalent of the β-LCR in the α-globin complex.

considered with the HPFH syndromes. In many populations, the α- and β-thalassemias coexist with a variety of different structural hemoglobin variants. In these populations, it is quite common to inherit a combination of genes; these complex interactions give rise to an extremely wide spectrum of clinical phenotypes that together constitute the thalassemia syndromes. It has been estimated that about 300,000 individuals severely affected with thalassemia are born each year, posing a heavy burden on health services. Mass migration of populations from high prevalence areas has resulted in the hemoglobin disorders being increasingly observed in parts of the world where they were not previously recognized.

THE β-THALASSEMIAS Clinical Features The clinical features of β-thalassemia range from the major forms to a completely silent carrier state.

Infants affected with β-thalassemia major are well at birth. Anemia usually develops during the first few months of life, when adult hemoglobin synthesis becomes established. There are no specific clinical signs, and further clinical manifestations of the disease depend on whether the child is maintained on an adequate transfusion regime.

The inadequately transfused child develops the typical features of Cooley's anemia. They show marked retardation of growth and development with progressive hepatosplenomegaly. A typical "thalassemia" facies develops with frontal bossing, prominent cheek bones, and protruding upper jaw as a result of extension of the marrow in the skull and facial bones. Radiography of the skull shows the typical "hair-on-end" appearance. The long bones and phalanges become rarefied from marrow expansion and show a lacy trabecular pattern on radiography. These changes may be associated with repeated pathological fractures. Occasionally, the expanding marrow extends from the rib or vertebrae and forms large paraspinal extramedullary masses. The massive marrow expansion causes a hypermetabolic state that is accompanied by intermittent fevers and weight loss. Gall stones and leg ulcers are common complications. Without any transfusion, death occurs within the first 2 years. "Palliative" transfusion allows the child to live somewhat longer, but the bony deformities remain unchanged; the child normally succumbs to an overwhelming infection. If these children survive to puberty, they develop complications of iron overload. Iron accumulation results from an increased rate of gastrointestinal absorption, as well as that derived from the blood transfusions.

When transfused adequately to maintain a hemoglobin level of >11 g/dL, these children grow and develop normally until early puberty, when they begin to show signs of progressive hepatic, cardiac, and endocrine disturbances, including liver failure, diabetes, hypoparathyroidism, and delayed or absent secondary sexual development. These changes are owing largely to tissue siderosis from the progressive accumulation of iron derived from transfusions. Unless iron overload is controlled by regular chelation therapy, death results in the second or third decade, from acute or intractable congestive cardiac failure.

Individuals with β-thalassemia minor are typically asymptomatic. Splenomegaly is rare.

Diagnosis Untransfused hemoglobin levels in β-thalassemia major can be as low as 2–3 g/dL. The red cells show severe hypochromia, marked anisopoikilocytosis, target cell formation, and basophilic stippling. Poorly hemoglobinized nucleated red cells are frequently found in the peripheral blood and may reach very high levels after splenectomy. Despite the severe anemia, the reticulocyte count is usually not very high because of the massive destruction of erythroid precursor cells in the bone marrow (i.e., ineffective erythropoiesis). The bone marrow shows marked erythroid hyperplasia, characterized by poorly hemoglobinized normoblasts. Ragged inclusions (α-chain aggregates) in the normoblasts are revealed under phase microscopy or after supravital staining (e.g., methyl violet). Increased iron deposition is also seen in the bone marrow; the majority of the iron granules are randomly distributed. Biochemical evidence of hemolysis and progressive iron loading are observed. Other biochemical changes may include evidence of diabetes and endocrine dysfunction, such as parathyroid insufficiency.

The findings on Hb electrophoresis vary with the β-thalassemia genotype and is informative only in the previously untransfused patient. In homozygous β^o-thalassemia, Hb A is completely absent, and the hemoglobin consists of F and A_2 only. In β^+-thalassemia (homozygous or compound heterozygous), a variable amount of Hb A is present. The Hb F is usually elevated and vary from 10 to 90% of the total hemoglobin. The Hb A_2 level is of no diagnostic value. In vitro globin chain biosynthesis of peripheral blood reticulocytes or bone marrow shows globin chain imbalance with a marked excess of α- over β- and γ-chain production. In β^o-thalassemia, there is a complete absence of β-chain synthesis.

The heterozygous state for β-thalassemia (β^o or β^+) is remarkably uniform hematologically. If present, anemia is mild, and the diagnosis is based on a low MCV and MCH, accompanied by an increased proportion of Hb A_2, from 3.5 to 5.5%, with the exception of a subgroup that has a normal level of Hb A_2. Globin chain biosynthesis shows α chains in excess of about twofold.

Normal A_2 heterozygous β-thalassemia may be difficult to distinguish hematologically from heterozygous α-thalassemia, since both cases are characterized by hypochromic microcytic red cells and a normal Hb A_2 level. The distinction is made by globin chain biosynthesis and DNA analysis. Type I normal A_2 β-thalassemia is "silent," in that the red cell indices are almost normal, and the phenotype is caused by very mild mutations that cause only a minimal deficit in β-chain production (e.g., C-T mutation in position −101 of the β gene). Other cases (type 2 normal Hb A_2 β-thalassemia) are a result of the coinheritance of δ-thalassemia *in cis* or *in trans* to the β-thalassemia gene.

DNA analysis frequently shows the β-globin cluster to be intact and point mutations within the β gene or its immediate flanking regions.

Genetic Basis of Disease The β-thalassemias are considered to be autosomal recessive disorders, because individuals who have inherited one abnormal β gene (carrier) are asymptomatic and the inheritance of two abnormal β-globin genes is required to produce a clinically detectable phenotype. Molecular analysis of the β-thalassemia genes has demonstrated a striking heterogeneity. Although >150 β-thalassemia alleles have been characterized, population studies indicate that probably only 20 β-thalassemia alleles account for >80% of the β-thalassemia mutations in the whole world. This is because in each of the high-frequency areas, only a few (four to six) mutations are common, with a varying number of rare ones; each of these populations has its own unique group of mutations. This is particularly relevant to prenatal diagnosis, because direct detection of these mutations by DNA analysis becomes feasible.

The vast majority of β-thalassemia mutations are single-base substitutions, small insertions or deletions of one to two bases involving the critical sequences that control the various stages of gene expression (Fig. 20-2A). Approximately half of these mutations completely inactivate the β gene and cause a phenotype of β^o-thalassemia. Mutations that allow the production of some β globin lead to the phenotype of β^+-thalassemia. Mutations affecting the conserved sequences in the 5' promoter (i.e., TATA box, proximal CACCC and distal CACCC box), typically cause a 70–80% reduction in promoter activity and are often very mild. Mutations affecting the polyadenylation signal (AATAAA) at the 3' end also generally result in a mild β^+-thalassemia phenotype.

Studies show that the different inphase termination mutants exhibit a "positional" effect. Frameshifts and nonsense mutations that result in premature termination early in the sequence (in exon 1 and 2) are associated with minimal amounts of mutant β mRNA. In such cases, no β chain is produced from the mutant allele, and only half the normal β globin is present, resulting in a phenotype of typical heterozygous β-thalassemia. In contrast, mutations that produce inphase terminations later in the β sequence—in exon 3—are associated with substantial amounts of mutant β-mRNA. Such mutations, even when present in a single copy, result in a moderately severe anemia and are said to be "dominantly inherited." Small amounts of truncated β-variant chains have been isolated in one case (heterozygous β codon 121). However, these truncated β chains are nonfunctional and not able to form viable tetramers, resulting in ineffective erythropoiesis and clinical disease, even in the heterozygous state.

β-thalassemia is rarely caused by deletions (Fig. 20-2B). Of these, only the 619-bp deletion at the 3' end of the β gene is common, but even that is restricted to the Sind populations of India and Pakistan, where it constitutes approximately 30% of the β-thalassemia alleles. The other deletions, although extremely rare, are of particular phenotypic interest, because they are associated with an unusually high level of Hb A_2 in heterozygotes. The mechanism underlying the markedly elevated levels of Hb A_2 and the variable increases in Hb F in heterozygotes for these deletions is related to the removal of the 5' promoter region of the β-globin gene that removes competition for the upstream β-LCR, leading to an increased interaction of the LCR with the γ and δ genes *in cis*, thus enhancing their expression. Even more rare are three upstream deletions that remove all or part of the β-LCR, but leave the β gene itself intact, yet cause β-thalassemia. Because of the vast number of different β-thalassemia mutations, many patients with thalassemia major are compound heterozygotes for two different molecular lesions.

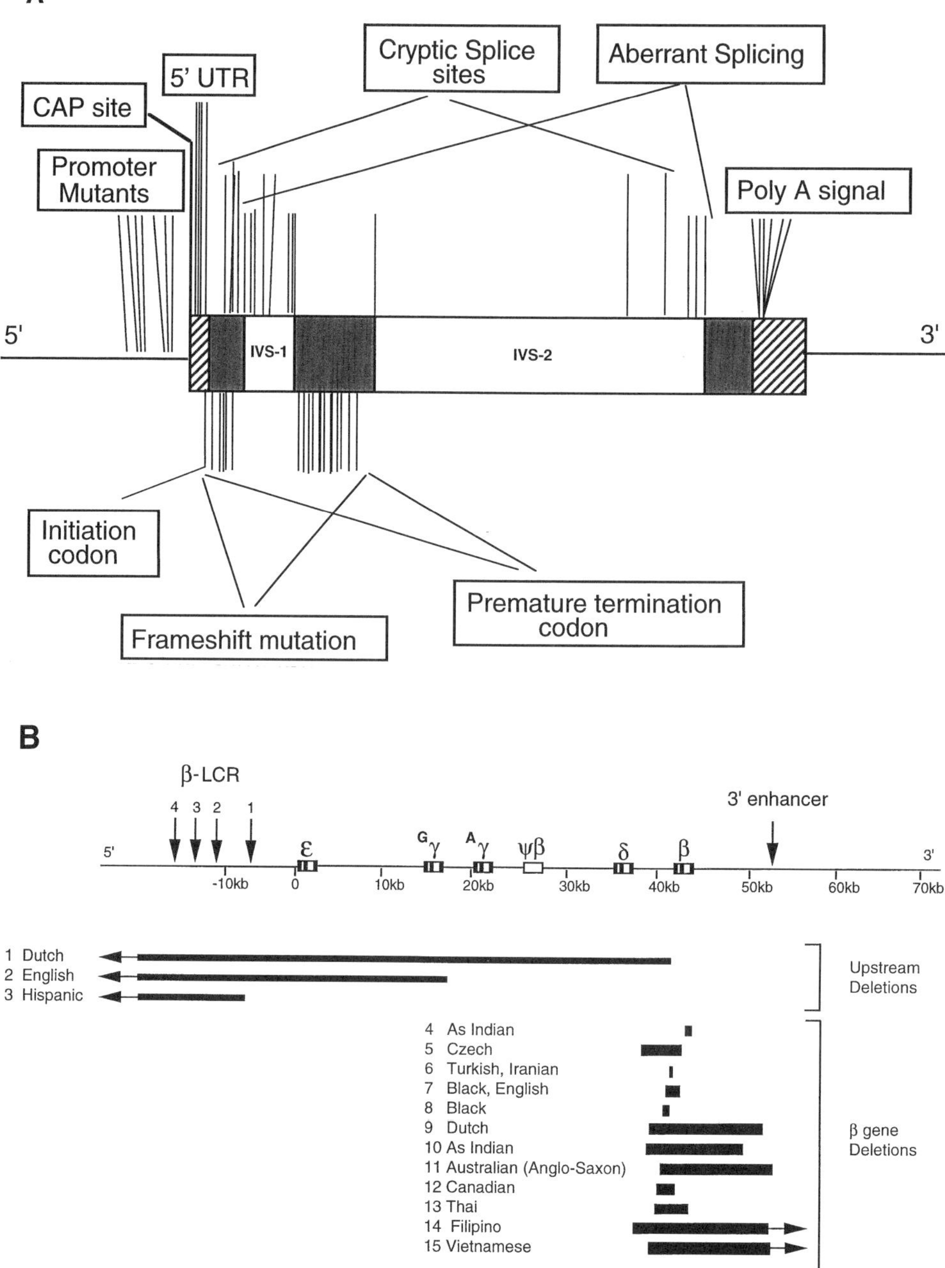

Figure 20-2 **(A)** Point mutations causing β-thalassemia. The β-globin gene is represented by 3 exons (gray) interrupted by 2 introns with the 5' and 3' untranslated regions (UTRs, striped boxes). The vertical lines represent the sites of the different mutations that can be found in the UTRs, exons and introns. **(B)** Deletions causing β-thalassemia. Two groups of deletions are shown: (1) group of upstream deletions which remove extensive regions (30–100 kb) of the 5' end of the β cluster but leave the β gene intact; (2) deletions that remove part or all of the β gene. These range from 290 bp to >45 kb in size. The 619-bp deletion (number 4) removes the 3' end of the β gene but leaves the 5' end intact, whereas the other deletions remove, in common, the 5' promoter region of the β gene, including sequences from positions –125 to +78 (relative to the β mRNA cap site).

Pathophysiology The molecular defects in β-thalassemias result in absent or reduced β-chain production, whereas α-chain synthesis proceeds at a normal rate. This imbalance in globin synthesis in β-thalassemia gives rise to excess α chains (Fig. 20-3A), which are extremely unstable and precipitate in the red cell precursors, forming inclusion bodies. These inclusions interfere with the red cell maturation and are responsible for the intramedullary destruction of the erythroid precursors, hence, the ineffective erythropoiesis that characterizes all β-thalassemias. The anemia of β-thalassemia results from a combination of underproduction of hemoglobin and ineffective erythropoiesis and is ultimately related to the degree of imbalance between the α- and non–α-globin chains.

HB E/β-THALASSEMIA Throughout Southeast Asia and the Indian subcontinent, it is not uncommon to encounter individuals who are compound heterozygotes for Hb E and β-thalassemia. Because Hb E is also insufficiently synthesized, the compound heterozygous state results in a clinical picture closely resembling homozygous β-thalassemia, ranging from severe anemia and transfusion dependency to thalassemia intermedia. The diagnosis of Hb E/β-thalassemia is confirmed by finding Hb E and F on hemoglo-

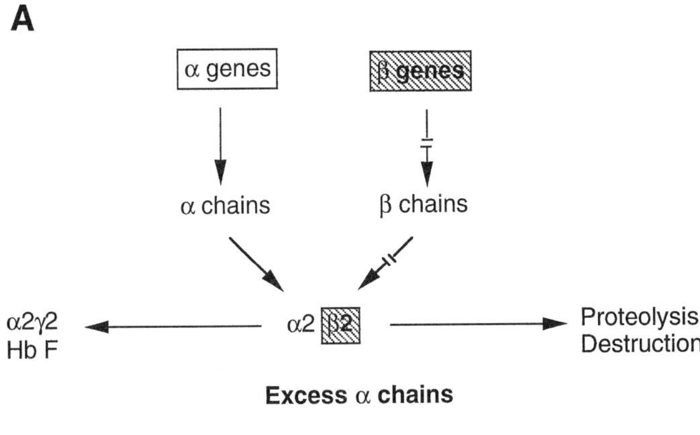

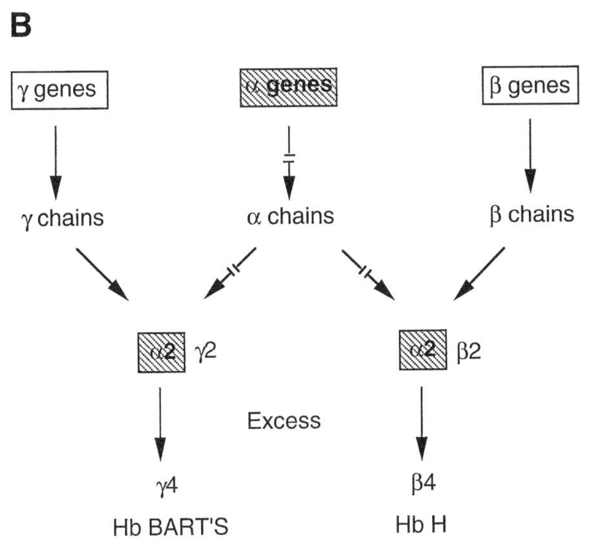

Figure 20-3 Diagrammatic representation of the pathophysiology of **(A)** β-thalassemia; **(B)** α-thalassemia.

bin electrophoresis and by demonstrating Hb E trait in one parent and β-thalassemia trait in the other.

THE δβ-, γδβ-THALASSEMIAS AND HPFH SYNDROMES This group of disorders is characterized by a reduced synthesis of β- and δ-globin chains and a variable increase in γ-chain production. They are remarkably heterogeneous at the molecular level. In some cases, they result from extensive deletions of the β-gene cluster, removing the β- and δ- or β-, δ- and γ-globin genes, whereas in others, they result from point mutations in the γ-globin promoters (HPFH). Occasionally, δβ-thalassemia results from unequal crossing over between the δ- and β-genes producing a δβ-fusion gene. The δβ-fusion chains combine with α chains to form Hb Lepore ($\alpha_2(\delta\beta)_2$). In a subgroup of HPFH, heterocellular HPFH, the β cluster—including the γ-globin genes—is intact. The distinction between HPFH and δβ-thalassemia is subtle and made on both clinical and hematological grounds.

HPFH is characterized in heterozygotes by levels of Hb F of up to 30% with normal red cell indices and near normal hematocrit levels, whereas heterozygotes for δβ-thalassemia tend to have elevated levels of Hb F that are lower (up to 20%) with mild anemia and hypochromic microcytic red cells. The importance of this group of conditions lie in their interaction with β-thalassemia. Compound heterozygotes for HPFH and β-thalassemia tend to have a mild disease compared to β-thalassemia homozygotes, whereas compound heterozygotes for δβ- and β-thalassemia exhibit a wide spectrum in disease severity, ranging from mild anemia to thalassemia major.

INTERMEDIATE FORMS OF β-THALASSEMIA Thalassemia intermedia is an ill-defined clinical term used to describe patients with phenotypes that are more severe than the asymptomatic thalassemia trait but milder than the transfusion-dependent thalassemia major. The criteria on which the diagnosis is based is that patients present later in life relative to thalassemia major and that they are capable of maintaining a reasonable level of hemoglobin (≥ 6 g/dL) without transfusion. At the severe end of the spectrum, patients present between the ages of 2 and 6 years; although they are just capable of surviving without blood transfusion, it is clear that growth and development are retarded. Many will show the skeletal and facial changes and progressive splenomegaly, as seen in untreated thalassemia major. As they become older, they develop iron-overload because of increased gastrointestinal absorption of iron. At the other end of the spectrum, patients are completely asymptomatic until adulthood and are transfusion-independent with hemoglobin levels of 10–12 g/dL. Such patients are diagnosed either during episodes of infection, when they become anemic, or by a chance hematological examination. There is usually some degree of splenomegaly. Table 20-1 lists some of the molecular interactions associated with the phenotype of thalassemia intermedia.

Because of the extreme variability of these disorders, these patients should be regularly followed from early childhood and the growth charts and iron accumulation carefully monitored.

THE α-THALASSEMIAS The geographical distribution of α-thalassemia is very similar to that of β-thalassemia. Although the α-thalassemias are more common, they pose less of a public health problem because the severe homozygous states cause death *in utero*, and the milder forms that survive into adulthood do not cause a major disability.

Clinical Features The clinical disorders resulting from α-thalassemia range from death *in utero* (Hemoglobin Bart's hydrops syndrome) to a completely silent carrier state.

Hb Bart's hydrops is a frequent cause of stillbirths in Southeast Asia. Affected infants are usually stillborn with gross pallor, generalized edema, and massive hepatosplenomegaly. The placenta is enlarged and friable, frequently causing obstetric difficulties. The intermediate form of α-thalassemia is Hb H disease, commonly seen in the Mediterranean, Middle East, and Southeast Asia. A spectrum of disease severity is also encountered in Hb H disease. Generally, these individuals have a moderately severe anemia and splenomegaly but are usually transfusion-independent, except during episodes of hemolysis associated with infection. The skeletal deformities and growth retardation characteristic of β-thalassemia are not common.

Diagnosis Diagnosis is based on the hemoglobin level, red cell indices, examination of the peripheral blood smear, and hemoglobin analysis. Infants with Hb Bart's hydrops are severely ane-

Table 20-1
Molecular Basis of β-Thalassemia Intermedia

1. Homozygous or compound heterozygous state for β-thalassemia.
   a. Inheritance of mild β^+-thalassemia alleles.
      - e.g., βIVS1-6 T-C, β promoter mutations.
   b. Coinheritance of α-thalassemia.
      - Effect more evident in β^+ thalassemia.
   c. β Thalassemia with elevated γ-chain production.
      - Polymorphism at position –158 Gγ gene. (Xmn I-Gγ site).
      - γ Promoter mutations.
      - Heterocellular HPFH. X-linked, 6q-linked.
2. Compound heterozygotes for β-thalassemia and deletion forms of HPFH or δβ-thalassemia.
3. Compound heterozygotes for β-thalassemia and β-chain variants (e.g., Hb E/β-thalassemia).
4. Heterozygotes for β-thalassemia.
   a. Coinheritance of extra α-globin genes. (ααα/αα or ααα/ααα)
   b. Dominantly inherited forms of β-thalassemia (including some thalassemic hemoglobinopathies).

mic with hemoglobin levels of 6–8 g/dL. The blood film shows severe thalassemic changes with numerous hypochromic nucleated red cells. There is no Hb A or F, the hemoglobin consists mainly of Hb Bart's (γ_4 tetramers), with small amounts of embryonic hemoglobin and Hb H (β_4 tetramers). Biosynthetic studies confirm the complete absence of α chains. Patients with Hb H disease run an hemoglobin level of 7–10 g/dL, with moderate reticulocytosis. Again, typical thalassemic changes are seen in the blood film. On incubation of the red cells with brilliant cresyl blue, numerous inclusion bodies are generated by precipitation of the Hb H, forming typical "golf balls." Hemoglobin analysis shows 5–40% Hb H, with the major component being Hb A and a normal or reduced level of Hb A_2. Sometimes, there is also a small amount of Hb Bart's. Carriers for α-thalassemia may be slightly anemic with hypochromic microcytic red cells or "silent," with minimal hematologic changes. The Hb electrophoretic pattern is normal, and globin biosynthetic studies show a deficit of α-chain production.

Diagnosis of α-thalassemia is confirmed by DNA analysis, which commonly reveals deletions of the α-gene cluster, removing one or both α genes. Less commonly, the α genes are present and DNA sequence analysis reveals point changes within the α2 gene or its immediate flanking regions.

Genetic Basis of Disease Normal individuals (αα/αα) have two α-globin genes, α2 and α1, on each chromosome 16. The α-thalassemia syndromes result from underproduction of α chains and are frequently caused by deletions that remove one of the linked α genes ($-\alpha^{3.7}$/αα or $-\alpha^{4.2}$/αα). Extensive deletions that remove both the linked α2 and α1 genes tend to be geographically isolated, and so are often referred to by their geographical origin for example, $—^{SEA}$/αα. More rarely, upstream deletions that remove the HS –40 region but leave the α genes themselves intact can also cause α-thalassemia.

Loss of one functioning α gene (αα/–α) is almost completely silent with normal or only slightly hypochromic red cells. Loss of two α genes (—/αα or –α/–α) produces a mild hypochromic microcytic anemia. Individuals who have inherited only one α gene (—/–α) have Hb H disease, whereas inheritance of no α genes (—/—) gives rise to a lethal, intrauterine hemolytic anemia termed the Hb Barts hydrops fetalis syndrome. Deficiency of α chains gives rise to an excess of γ chains (in fetal life) or β chains (in adult life) that form γ_4-tetramers (Hb Barts) and β_4-tetramers (Hb H). The presence of Hb Barts or Hb H is thus diagnostic of α-thalassemia. Anemia results from a combination of the underproduction of hemoglobin and hemolysis owing to the intracellular precipitation of Hb Barts and Hb H, and is ultimately directly related to the degree of α-chain deficiency.

Less commonly, α-thalassemia results from point mutations involving the critical sequences that control the various stages of gene expression, as encountered in β-thalassemia. With the exception of one phenotypically mild α thalassemia mutant, all of these mutations affect the dominant α_2-globin gene. In general, the nondeletion α-thalassemia variants ($\alpha^T\alpha/\alpha\alpha$) give rise to a more severe reduction in α-chain synthesis than the single α-gene deletions (–α/αα), the homozygous state ($\alpha^T\alpha/\alpha^T\alpha$) for such variants often result in Hb H disease. A common nondeletion α-thalassemia variant in Southeast Asia is Hb Constant Spring (Hb CS), which is caused by a single base substitution (TAA → CAA) in the α2 globin termination codon. This results in read through of the 3' untranslated sequence until another inphase termination codon is encountered 31 codons later. Homozygotes ($\alpha^{CS}\alpha/\alpha^{CS}\alpha$) or compound heterozygotes ($\alpha^{CS}\alpha$/—) for Hb CS have a less severe form of Hb H disease. Very low levels of this elongated α globin chain (5–8% of the total hemoglobin in homozygotes) are found; the defective α^{CS} chain production is a consequence of the instability of the α^{CS} mRNA. Three other variants (Hb Icaria, Hb Seal Rock, and Hb Koya Dora) involving different base substitutions in the α2 termination codon have been identified.

Pathophysiology There is a fundamental difference in the pathophysiology of the α- and β-thalassemias (Fig. 20-3). Because γ_4 and β_4 tetramers are soluble, they do not precipitate to a significant degree in the bone marrow (i.e., erythropoiesis is more effective than in β-thalassemia). However, these β_4 tetramers do precipitate as the red cells age, forming inclusion bodies. Hemolysis occurs because of the red cell membrane damage and obstruction in the spleen.

α-THALASSEMIA WITH MENTAL RETARDATION (ATR) SYNDROMES There are two distinct syndromes of α-thalassemia and mental retardation. One group, ATR-16, results from

Table 20-2
Clinical Disorders Caused by Structural Hemoglobin Variants

1. Sickle syndromes causing hemolysis and tissue damage.
   Hb S and interaction of Hb S with other Hb variants.
   (Hbs S/C, S/O-Arab, and S/D-Punjab) and β-thalassemia (S/β-thal).
2. Chronic hemolysis—unstable hemoglobin variants (congenital Heinz body anemia, CHBA).
   e.g., Hb Köln, Hb Bristol.
3. Congenital polycythemia—high oxygen affinity Hb variants.
4. Congenital cyanosis—Low oxygen affinity Hb variants.
   M hemoglobins.
5. Hypochromic microcytic anemia (thalassemic hemoglobinopathy).
   e.g., Hb E—β structural variant.
   Hb Constant Spring—α structural variant.
   Hyperunstable hemoglobin variants.
6. Drug-induced hemolysis (e.g., Hb Zurich).

extensive deletions of 1–2 Mb of the tip of chromosome 16, which remove the α-globin gene cluster. The mental retardation is associated with variable dysmorphic features and is thought to result from loss of a variable number of genes at the tip of chromosome 16p. ATR-X is characterized by more severe mental retardation, characteristic dysmorphic facies, and genital abnormalities. In these cases, the α-globin gene cluster is intact; the underlying mutation is a *trans*-acting abnormality encoded in the *XH2* gene on the X chromosome.

ACQUIRED HB H DISEASE Hb H disease is occasionally seen in individuals with a variety of hematological disorders within the myelodysplastic syndromes. These individuals are predominantly elderly males and hematologically normal before the onset of the disease. The α-globin gene cluster is intact, and the acquired α-thalassemia is likely to be caused by reduced α-gene transcription, but the nature of the specific defect remains completely unknown.

MANAGEMENT The thalassemias are a major health problem in many populations; because there is no definitive treatment, major efforts are concentrated on prevention.

Preventive programs in the past were based on education, population screening, heterozygote detection, and genetic counseling, but they were not entirely effective. Most countries now combine this approach with screening programs at antenatal clinics. When heterozygous mothers are detected, their partners are tested; if their partners are also carriers, the couples are offered prenatal diagnosis and selective termination of pregnancy.

Regular transfusion and iron chelation remain the cornerstones of treatment for severe β-thalassemia and are primarily palliative. Currently, the most useful chelating agent is desferrioxamine (Desferal). Unfortunately, Desferal is not only expensive, but it also has to be administered parenterally via an infusion pump. It is not surprising that noncompliance becomes a problem, particularly during adolescence. Considerable effort is directed towards the development of a safe and effective oral iron chelator. The most promising of these is deferiprone (L1); results of recent clinical trials suggest that although deferiprone is initially effective, there is a loss of efficacy in the long term. Another alternative that is currently being developed is a new formulation of depot desferrioxamine which can be given as a single bolus dose subcutaneously once a week. The development of hypersplenism as shown by the falling platelet and white-cell counts, and increasing blood transfusion requirements is an indication for splenectomy.

Bone marrow transplantation is the only form of treatment that can cure the severe forms of β-thalassemia, but it is dependent on the availability of an HLA-compatible related donor. Young well-chelated patients without evidence of liver disease are the best candidates, having 80% chance of cure.

With increasing knowledge of cell and molecular biology, a long-term aim would be the replacement of the defective β gene with its normal counterpart. Although, significant progress has been made in addressing the problems of gene transfer and expression, major biological problems remain. It has long been known that the severity of disease in β-thalassemia can be ameliorated by coinheritance of genetic factors that increase Hb F production. Thus, activation of the normal γ genes in patients with β-thalassemia represent a potentially important approach of therapy for this disorder. Several compounds, including 5-azacytidine, hydroxyurea, butyrate and butyrate analogs, have been tried, but, to date, none could achieve the therapeutic levels of Hb F needed without inducing significant toxic side effects.

STRUCTURAL HEMOGLOBIN VARIANTS

More than 600 structurally different hemoglobin variants have been described. Many of them are harmless and have been discovered in population surveys using electrophoretic analyses of human hemoglobin. Because only variants that alter the charge of the hemoglobin molecule are detectable in routine electrophoresis, this number is probably an underestimate. Diseases resulting from structural abnormalities of hemoglobin are shown in Table 20-2. In this section, only those abnormal hemoglobins of clinical importance are described.

SICKLE-CELL DISEASE

Background Sickle-cell anemia was first described by Herrick from Chicago in 1910, in a West Indian student. Peculiar elongated and sickle-shaped red blood cells were observed in the peripheral blood films and suggested the term sickle cell anemia. In 1949, Pauling et al. demonstrated that this sickling phenomenon was related to an abnormal hemoglobin present in all patients with sickle-cell anemia; this hemoglobin had an abnormally slow electrophoretic migration. Subsequently, in 1956, the sickle hemoglobin was chemically characterized by Ingram and was shown to differ from normal adult hemoglobin (Hb A, $\alpha_2\beta_2$) by the single substitution of glutamic acid to valine at position six in the β-

Table 20-3
The Major Sickling Disorders

	β Genotype	*α Genotype*	*Hb Electrophoresis*
Sickle-cell trait	β^A/β^S	αα/αα	Hb S approx 40%; Hb A 60%
Sickle-cell trait	β^A/β^S	α–/αα or α–/α–	Hb S 20–35%; Hb A 65–80
Sickle-cell Anemia	β^S/β^S	αα/αα	Hb S 80–100%; Hb F 0–20%
SC disease	β^S/β^C	αα/αα	Hb S 50%; Hb C 50%
SO-Arab disease	β^S/β^{OArab}	αα/αα	Hb S, HbO Arab[a]
SD-Punjab disease	$\beta^S/\beta^{D\text{-}Punjab}$	αα/αα	Hb S 50%; Hb D Punjab 50%[b]
$S\beta^+$ thal	β^S/β^{Th}	αα/αα	Hb S 50–80%; Hb F 0–20% Hb A 10–30%; Hb A_2 3–6%
$S\beta^o$ thal	β^S/β^{Th}	αα/αα	Hb S 75–100%; Hb F 0–20% Hb A_2 3–6%
S HPFH	β^S/β^c	αα/αα	Hb S 70–80%; Hb F 20–30%; Hb A_2 decreased

[a]HbC, HbO-Arab, and HbE are not separated on routine alkaline electrophoresis.
[b]Quantitation based on agar gel electrophoresis.
[c]Deletion of β-globin cluster.

subunit. Since then, molecular characterization has shown that, apart from the homozygous state for the β^s gene, the syndrome of sickle-cell disease can also arise from the compound heterozygous state for HbS and other structural variants such as Hbs C and D and β-thalassemia (Table 20-3).

The sickling disorders occur predominantly in black African populations, but they are also prevalent throughout the Mediterranean, Middle East and parts of India. It appears that heterozygotes for the β^s gene are protected from the severe effects of *Plasmodium falciparum*, thus explaining the high gene frequencies in those malarious regions. The β^s gene in these diverse population groups is caused by the same molecular defect (β codon 6 GAG to GTG).

Recent investigations using β haplotypes constructed from the linked-groupings of DNA sequence polymorphisms in the β globin cluster have provided some insights into the origins and migration of the β^s gene. The β^s gene occurs on four different β haplotypes in Africa, known as the Senegal, Benin, Central African Republic (or Bantu), and the Cameroon types. In addition, it is associated with a different β haplotype in Saudi Arabian and Asian Indian sickle patients. The evidence suggests multiple independent origins of the β^s mutation, although gene conversion on regionally specific β haplotypes cannot be excluded.

Clinical Features Sickle-cell trait is a benign condition and generally does not cause any clinical disability. However, under certain extreme conditions such as severe pneumonia, flying in unpressurized aircraft, and exercise at high altitude, vaso-occlusive episodes can occur.

The clinical manifestations of sickle cell disease range from a chronic hemolytic anemia interspersed with painful crises to a completely asymptomatic state, detected only by chance on routine hematological examination. Most patients fall between these two extremes and are relatively asymptomatic, except for the occasional clinical crisis.

Sickle-cell anemia normally presents in infancy with attacks of painful dactylitis, the so-called "hand-foot syndrome," with swelling of the fingers and feet. At this stage, the infant is usually anemic with mild jaundice and the spleen palpable. Splenomegaly usually resolves owing to repeated infarctions of the spleen, the "autosplenectomy" manifested by typical postsplenectomy changes in the peripheral blood film. It is unusual to feel the spleen after the first decade of life. Typically, these children have a chronic hemolytic anemia. The hemoglobin level varies between 6 and 8 g/dL, with a reticulocyte count of 10–20%, slight elevation of the serum bilirubin level, and increased urinary urobilinogen. Examination of the peripheral blood smear shows polychromasia and poikilocytosis, with a variable number of sickled erythrocytes.

The chronic hemolysis of sickle-cell anemia is punctuated by acute exacerbations of the illness termed sickling crises traditionally classified as vaso-occlusive, sequestration, aplastic, or hemolytic.

The most common are the vaso-occlusive crises, characterized by acute painful episodes caused by blockage of small vessels with sickled erythrocytes and tissue infarction. Commonly, the patient experiences a rapid onset of deep throbbing bone pain in the lumbosacral spine and limb bones, usually without physical findings but sometimes accompanied by local tenderness, warmth, and swelling. Marrow aspirated from areas of bone tenderness have revealed infarction of the marrow tissue. Occasionally, abdominal pain is the major symptom and can pose a difficult problem in differential diagnosis. The abdominal crisis is accompanied by distension and rigidity with loss of bowel sounds—findings typical of an acute surgical abdomen.

Vaso-occlusion in the lung, acute chest syndrome, is characterized by acute dyspnea and pleuritic pain and often accompanied by a significant fall in the hemocrit that may reflect sequestration of the sickled cells in the pulmonary vessels. The distinction from pulmonary infection is often very difficult, particularly as infection and infarction usually coexist. Acute chest syndrome is the most common cause of death after 2 years of age; the patient with acute chest syndrome is extremely vulnerable because hypoxia has a profound effect on sickling. Acute vaso-occlusion in the central nervous system (CNS) usually presents in childhood, either as fits, transient neurological symptoms resembling ischemia attacks, or with a fully developed stroke. Recurrent attacks are common, 70% of patients experience a recurrence within 3 years, and many are left with permanent motor and intellectual disabilities. Priapism is a distressing problem resulting from vaso-occlusion of the outflow vessels from the corpora cavernosa by sickled erythrocytes. This complication may present as multiple short-lived episodes ("stuttering" priapism) that may progress to "severe prolonged" priapism, lasting several days and leading to permanent sexual dysfunction.

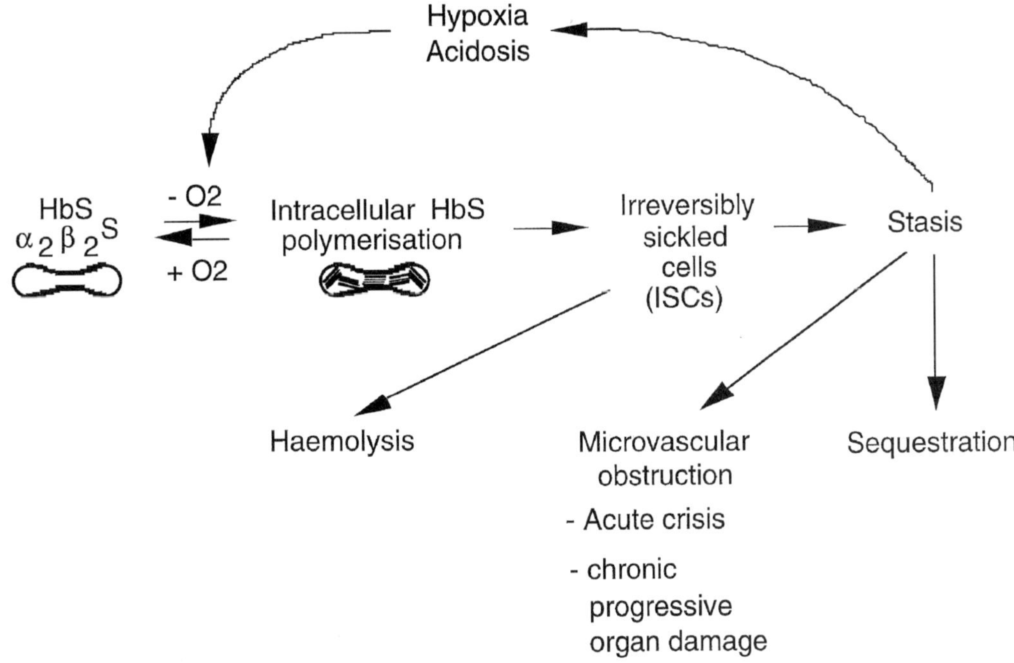

Figure 20-4 Pathophysiology of sickle-cell disease. Initially, intracellular polymerization is reversible, but repeated cycles of polymerization-depolymerization in the circulating red cell results in membrane damage, and the cell becomes irreversibly sickled. This results in two main effects; first, sickled erythrocytes are mechanically fragile with a short intravascular life-span resulting in a chronic hemolytic anemia. Second, sickled erythrocytes are not so flexible, particularly in the microvasculature; they adhere abnormally to the vascular endothelium and form aggregates leading to vascular stasis, local hypoxia, and further sickling, complete vaso-occlusion and tissue infarction.

Temporary marrow aplasia can have a profound effect with reticulocytopenia and a very sudden drop in hematocrit. These aplastic crises appear to result from intercurrent infections, particularly owing to parvovirus B19 and often occur in epidemics, frequently involving more than one sibling in the same family.

Sequestration crises are the most serious of the acute crises and commonly involve the spleen in the first 2 years of life. Acute splenic sequestration is characterized by sudden rapid massive enlargement of the spleen that becomes engorged with sickled erythrocytes. As the crisis progresses, a large proportion of the circulating red cell mass may be trapped in the spleen, leading to profound anemia and death. Splenic sequestration shows a tendency to recur in the same individual. A similar type of sequestration may occur in the liver in adult life, causing a dramatic fall in the hematocrit.

Patients with sickle-cell disease are particularly susceptible to infection because of Streptococcus pneumonia, Salmonella, *Escherichia coli*, and Hemophilus influenza. Osteomyelitis is common and results from infection of bone infarcts. Pneumococcal pneumonia and overwhelming septicemia are particularly important causes of death in infancy and childhood because of hyposplenism.

Repeated vaso-occlusive events ultimately result in end-organ damage and almost any organ can be affected. The vertebral bodies and femoral heads are particularly prone to infarction. A vascular necrosis of the femoral head may lead to total disability, frequently requiring a total hip prosthesis. Virtually every patient with sickle-cell anemia has some form of renal impairment. Sickling of the erythrocytes is enhanced in the hypertonic, hypoxic, and acidotic environment of the renal medulla, leading to progressive infarction of the medullary papillae. There is progressive inability to concentrate urine, polyuria, nocturia, and enuresis, which is common in children. Eventually, the glomerular damage causes chronic renal failure, particularly in patients over 40 years of age. Because of chronic hemolysis, gallstones are very common and are seen in one-third of SS patients by 10 years of age. However, it is difficult to assess its clinical significance, because only a minority develop clear-cut cholecystitis. Recurrent chronic leg ulceration is common and can be a major handicap. The lesions normally occur just above the medial malleoli and seem to be more common in those patients with severe anemia. Proliferative retinopathy leading to progressive visual loss is an important ocular complication, although this is more common in Hb SC disease.

Diagnosis Diagnosis is established by the combination of several tests: hemoglobin electrophoresis on cellulose acetate (pH 8.6) and agar (pH 6.2) and positive sickling or solubility tests. Diagnostic difficulties can often be resolved by family studies.

Genetic Basis and Molecular Pathophysiology of Disease Sickle hemoglobin (Hb S, $\alpha_2\beta_2^S$) is produced by a single base substitution (G<u>A</u>G→G<u>T</u>G resulting in Glu to Val) in codon 6 of the β-subunit of hemoglobin. Fundamental to the sickle-cell pathophysiology is the insolubility of deoxy-Hb S in the red cells (Fig. 20-4). This leads to intracellular polymerization, which alters successively the cytoplasmic viscosity, the topography, and microrheology of the membranes, the ion fluxes, and the cell–cell interactions in their adherence to the vascular endothelium. The rate of polymerization varies exponentially with the intracellular hemoglobin concentration and composition (percentage of Hb S and non-S hemoglobin), as well as oxygen saturation. Oxygen binding to HbS has a dramatic effect on polymerization.

Sickling is influenced by a wide variety of inherited and acquired factors, both intracellular and extracellular. Abnormal endothelial adherence of the sickled erythrocytes is also influenced by cellular constituents such as von Willebrand factor, cytokines, and vascular tone.

Management Currently, there is no specific treatment that is useful in sickle cell disease. Management consists of continuous general medical care and treatment of complications as they arise. In high-risk populations, neonatal screening programs should be established to identify babies with sickle-cell anemia as soon as possible. These babies should be given prophylactic penicillin, followed by polyvalent pneumococcal vaccine between the ages of 6 and 12 months.

Folate supplements should be given during pregnancy and in patients with severe anemia. Transfusions are not usually required except in special circumstances. Episodes of infection should be treated early and sudden exposure to cold and high altitudes avoided.

All but the mildest of crises should be managed in hospital. The patient should be examined for any underlying infection, kept warm and adequately hydrated, either orally or intravenously, and given appropriate antibiotics. Prompt and adequate relief of pain is of prime importance. In selected patients, exchange transfusion may be effective in preventing recurrent painful crises.

Most patients with sickle-cell anemia tolerate the relatively low levels of hemoglobin quite well, and blood transfusion is usually not required. However, a blood transfusion is indicated when there is a sharp fall in the hemoglobin because bone marrow failure (aplastic crisis) or increased hemolysis. A sequestration crisis requires very close surveillance, and urgent transfusion is usually indicated because of the prompt development of profound anemia. "Acute chest syndrome" and the "brain syndrome" should be treated by partial exchange transfusion to maintain a level of sickle hemoglobin of <30% of the total Hb.

Proliferative retinopathy may require photocoagulation or diathermy to reduce the risk of vitreous hemorrhage. Chronic leg ulcers may respond to conservative treatment, such as rest and elevation of the affected limb and zinc sulfate dressings. Occasionally, a regime of regular blood transfusions is helpful. Priapism occurs in approximately 40% of SS male patients. Preliminary data suggest that stilboesterol (5 mg daily) may be effective in preventing a major episode in patients with "stuttering" priapism. Initial management should be conservative and include sedation, adequate hydration and analgesia, and partial exchange transfu sion to maintain the level of Hb S at <30%. Failure to respond after 24 hours requires immediate surgical intervention, rather than waiting in hope of resolution. Patients who develop a long-standing impotence may benefit from a penile prosthesis.

There is no special treatment during pregnancy except for close supervision and folate supplementation. Blood transfusions are not normally indicated, except for when there is a significant drop in hemoglobin level or recurrent crises. In such cases, a regular transfusion regime should be started to maintain the Hb S level below 30% throughout pregnancy and delivery. Although there is no evidence that oral contraceptives increase the risk of veno-occlusive episodes, it may be prudent to use a low estrogen preparation. Any surgical procedure should be undertaken with caution, and scrupulous care taken to avoid factors known to precipitate crisis, including hypoxia, dehydration, cold, acidosis, and circulatory stasis. Major surgical procedures may be best carried out after exchange transfusions.

Prenatal Diagnosis Despite the advances in prenatal diagnosis, there has been little uptake of these services with little impact on the prevention of SS disease. The situation may be a reflection of the extreme clinical variability of disease and ineffective genetic counseling.

Anti-Sickling Therapy Currently, treatment to prevent sickling follows three approaches; chemical inhibition of Hb S polymerization itself, reduction of mean cell hemoglobin concentration (MCHC), and pharmacological induction of fetal hemoglobin.

Numerous chemical antisickling agents have been promoted, but none can be regarded as safe and effective. The rationale of reducing MCHC by inducing hyponatremia thereby causing an osmotic swelling of red cells is sound, but it is too cumbersome and risky. Induction of Hb F as a form of therapy was initially based on clinical and epidemiological observations that showed that even slight elevations of fetal Hb have an ameliorating effect on the clinical severity. These observations were subsequently supported by biophysical studies. An increase in intracellular Hb F effectively reduces the concentration of Hb S and mixed hybrids of Hb S and Hb F ($\alpha_2\gamma\beta^s$) do not form polymers. Pharmacological agents used include 5-azacytidine, a potent inhibitor of DNA methylation, arabinosylcytosine (Ara-C), hydroxyurea, erythropoietin, and the butyrate analogs. Hydroxyurea is currently the agent of choice. It is relatively nontoxic, its myelosuppressive effects are reversible, and it is not known to induce secondary malignancies. A recent trial in the United States suggests that SS patients given daily hydroxyurea increase their Hb F levels and have fewer crises. Hydroxyurea has also been shown to be highly effective in a group of Greek sickle/β-thalassemia patients.

Bone Marrow Transplant Bone marrow transplant may have a role in certain cases of sickle-cell disease. Until more is known about the natural history of the disease and the ability to predict the disease severity, bone marrow transplant as a form of curative treatment for all cases is not recommended.

OTHER SICKLING DISORDERS These include mainly the compound heterozygous states for HbS, together with Hbs C, O-Arab, and D-Punjab, as well as the inheritance of the β^s gene with the different forms of thalassemia (Table 20-3).

Sickle/β-thalassemia is the most common sickling disorder in individuals of Mediterranean origin. The severity of disease ranges from a completely asymptomatic state to one similar to that seen in sickle-cell anemia. Much of this heterogeneity depends on the type of β-thalassemia mutation and the amount of Hb A produced. Because the majority of the β-thalassemia alleles in Africans causes a minimal deficit in β-chain production, sickle/β-thalassemia in Africans is generally milder than in the Mediterranean populations. The presence of β-thalassemia is indicated by the presence of hypochromic microcytic red cells, more than 50% of Hb S on electrophoresis and an elevated level of Hb A_2. Family studies are often crucial in distinguishing between the two disorders. Globin chain biosynthetic studies are also useful; in S/β-thalassemia, the β^S/α ratio is 0.5, whereas in SS disease, it is close to one.

OTHER HEMOGLOBIN VARIANTS The other hemoglobin variants that are encountered commonly are Hbs C, E, and D (Table 20-4). Hb C is the second most common variant among individuals of African ancestry. Hb C is less soluble than Hb A and tends to crystallize within the red cells leading to their reduced deformability. The important interactions of Hb C are with Hb S (to produce Hb SC disease) and β-thalassemia. Individuals with Hb C/β^o-thalassemia have a mild to moderate hemolytic anemia.

Hb E (β26 Glu—Lys) is the second most common hemoglobin variant in the world, occurring in a region extending from

Table 20-4
Common Hemoglobin Variants (Other than HbS)

Variant	*Phenotype*	*Genotype*	*Diagnosis*
HbC ($\alpha 2\beta 2^{6\ Glu\rightarrow Lys}$)[a]	Trait (asymptomatic)	β^A/β^C	Hbs A, C, target cells,
	HbC Disease (mild to moderate hemolytic anemia)	β^C/β^C	Hb C 100% target cells 100%
HbE ($\alpha 2\beta 2^{26\ Glu\rightarrow Lys}$)[a]	Trait (asymptomatic)	β^A/β^E	Very mild hypochromic microcytosis, Hbs A, and E
	HbE disease (asymptomatic mild anemia)	β^E/β^E	Hypochromic microcytosis Hb E 100%
HbD-Punjab[b] ($\alpha 2\beta 2^{121\ Glu\rightarrow Gln}$)	Trait, asymptomatic	$\beta^A/\beta^{D\text{-}Punjab}$	Hbs A and D
	HbD disease (asymptomatic, very mild anemia)	β^D/β^D	Hb D approx 100%

[a]Hbs C and E are not separated from Hb A_2 on routine alkaline electrophoresis.
[b]HbD^{Punjab} has the same electrophoretic mobility as HbS at alkaline pH.

Bangladesh through to China, including Southeast Asia. Gene frequencies of 50–70% have been recorded in parts of Thailand, Laos, and Kampuchea. The pathophysiology of Hb E is thought to result from a combination of inefficient synthesis of Hb E owing to activation of a cryptic site in exon 1 of the β-globin gene and reduced stability of Hb E itself. The overall reduction in splicing is the molecular basis for the mild β^+-thalassemia phenotype of Hb E. The importance of Hb E lies in the interaction with β-thalassemia (see Hb E/β-thalassemia).

THE UNSTABLE HEMOGLOBIN DISORDERS Structural changes in the globin subunits can lead to instability of the hemoglobin molecule, causing it to precipitate intracellularly, forming Heinz bodies and a chronic hemolytic anemia. This group of unstable hemoglobin disorders are generally referred to congenital Heinz body hemolytic anemia (CHBA); the true incidence of CHBA is not known. The majority follows an autosomal dominant pattern of inheritance; affected individuals are almost exclusively heterozygotes. In many families, only the proband is affected, suggesting that the mutation has arisen by a *de novo* mutation. Instability of the hemoglobin can be demonstrated by the presence of flocculent precipitates on heating a dilute hemoglobin solution at 50°C for 15 min or by the addition of isopropanol.

Most patients with CHBA do not require treatment. General supportive measures include folic acid supplements, prompt treatment of infection, and reduction of fever. Oxidant drugs should be avoided. Transfusions are indicated only rarely, such as during an aplastic crisis.

HEMOGLOBIN VARIANTS WITH ABNORMAL OXYGEN BINDING The hemoglobin tetramer exists in equilibrium between two quaternary conformations: R and T. When fully deoxygenated, hemoglobin assumes the "T" or "tense" state, in which it has a relatively low affinity for oxygen and relatively high affinity for allosteric effectors such as Bohr protons and 2,3-DPG. On the other hand, oxyhemoglobin exists in the "R" or "relaxed" state, in which it has a high affinity for oxygen and a low affinity for effectors. The transition between these two conformations requires "heme–heme interaction" which involves a series of structural changes. Thus, mutations that result in a structural alteration that affects the equilibrium between the R and T states would have a marked effect on hemoglobin binding of oxygen. Both high and low oxygen affinity variants have been described.

Individuals with high oxygen affinity hemoglobin variants have an increased red cell mass, as shown by the unusually high hemoglobin level or hematocrit. Diagnosis is made by excluding other causes for erythrocytosis and by demonstrating a left-shifted oxygen dissociation curve with a reduced p50 value and a normal 2,3-diphosphoglycerate (2,3'-DPG) value. High-affinity variants follow an autosomal dominant inheritance pattern; all affected individuals are heterozygotes. A positive family history is helpful, but occasionally, the variants rise from *de novo* mutations.

Far fewer hemoglobin variants with low oxygen affinity have been described, but they should always be considered in any patient with unexplained congenital cyanosis—the differential diagnosis being methemoglobinemia.

HEMOGLOBINS M A group of seven hemoglobin variants known as Hbs M is characterized by the presence of ferric atoms in either α or β chains, owing to amino acid substitutions in the heme pocket. The most common substitutions are tyrosine for the proximal (F8) or the distal (E7) histidine in either the β or α chain. As a result of these substitutions, these Hbs M are resistant to the reduction by methemoglobin reductase. These variants do not combine fully with oxygen.

The predominant clinical feature associated with Hbs M is a change in the coloration of skin and mucous membranes that can vary from brownish to slate gray. Cyanosis is a result of an excess of deoxyhemoglobin. Hbs M have a dominant form of inheritance; affected individuals are heterozygous and present early in life with cyanosis. Furthermore, if the cyanosis is present from birth, it is normally because of an α-chain variant, whereas β-chain Hb M produces cyanosis after the first few months of life, when adult hemoglobin synthesis becomes established.

The most reliable diagnostic test is based on examination of the hemolysate by recording spectrophotometry. The underlying molecular lesion is identified by DNA analysis of the globin genes.

THE THALASSEMIC HEMOGLOBINOPATHIES

This group of hemoglobin disorders includes structural hemoglobin mutants, presenting with a clinical phenotype that ranges from the mild forms of heterozygous thalassemia to that resembling thalassemia intermedia. Despite the extensive clinical heterogeneity, these patients have in common a typical hematological phenotype, including the thalassemic red cell morphology with hypochromic microcytic anemia and basophilic stippling; in some cases, chronic severe hemolytic anemia with splenomegaly is a feature. The molecular abnormalities are remarkably heterogeneous and include single amino acid mutations, amino acid dele-

Table 20-5
Molecular Abnormalities Observed in Thalassemic Hemoglobinopathies

Unstable variants	e.g., Hb Suan Dok ($\alpha2^{109\ Leu\rightarrow Arg}$)
Hyperunstable variants	e.g., Hb Quong Sze ($\alpha2^{125\ Leu\rightarrow Pro}$) Hb Showa Yakushiji ($\beta^{110\ Leu\rightarrow Pro}$)
Variants that cause abnormal splicing	e.g., Hb E (β26Glu→Lys) Hb Knossos ($\beta^{27\ Ala\rightarrow Ser}$)
Variants with mutations in the termination codon	e.g., Hb Constant Spring ($\alpha2^{142\ Term\rightarrow Gln}$)[a]
δ/β fusion globin subunits	e.g., Hb Lepore

[a]Hb Constant Spring is a particularly common form of nondeletion α-thalassemia in Thailand.

tions, elongated or truncated globin chains, and fusion globins (Table 20-5). In contrast to β-thalassemia, thalassemic hemoglobinopathies are often inherited as autosomal dominants.

SELECTED REFERENCES

Beutler E. Hemoglobinopathies associated with unstable hemoglobin. In: Beutler E, Lichtman MA, Coller BS, Kipps TJ, eds. Williams Hematology, 5th ed. New York: McGraw-Hill, 1995.

Bianco I, Cappabianca MP, Foglietta E, et al. Silent thalassemias: genotypes and phenotypes. Haematologica 1997;82:269–280.

Bunn HF, Forget BG. Hemoglobin: Molecular, Genetic and Clinical Aspects. Philadelphia: WB Saunders, 1986.

Charache S, Terrin ML, Moore RD, et al. Effect of hydroxyurea on the frequency of painful crises in sickle cell anemia. N Engl J Med 1995;332:1317–1322.

Craig JE, Rochette J, Fisher CA, et al. Dissecting the loci controlling fetal haemoglobin production on chromosomes 11p and 6q by the regressive approach. Nat Genet 1996;12:58–64.

Crossley M, Orkin SH. Regulation of the β-globin locus. Curr Opin Genet Dev 1993;3:232–237.

Dover GJ, Smith KD, Chang YC, et al. Fetal hemoglobin levels in sickle cell disease and normal individuals are partially controlled by an X-linked gene located at Xp22.2. Blood 1992;80:816–824.

Embury SH, Hebbel RP, Mohandas N, Steinberg MH. Sickle Cell Disease: Basic Principles and Clinical Practice. New York: Raven, 1994.

Gibbons RJ, Picketts DJ, Villard L, Higgs DR. X-linked mental retardation associated with α thalassaemia (ATR-X syndrome) results from mutations in a putative global transcriptional regulator. Cell 1995;80: 837–845.

Grosveld F, van Assendelft GB, Breaves DR, Kollias G. Position-independent, high-level expression of the human γ-globin gene in transgenic mice. Cell 1987;51:975–985.

Higgs DR, Weatherall DJ. Baillière's Clinical Haematology. International Practice and Research: The Haemoglobinopathies. London:Baillière Tindall, 1993.

Ho PJ, Hall GW, Luo LY, Weatherall DJ, Thein SL. Beta thalassemia intermedia: is it possible to consistently predict phenotype from genotype? Br J Haemat 1998;100:70–78.

Lau YL, Chan LC, Chan YY, et al. Prevalence and genotypes of alpha- and beta-thalassemia carriers in Hong Kong—implications for population screening. N Engl J Med 1997;336:1298–1301.

Miyoshi K, Kaneto Y, Kawai H, et al. X-linked dominant control of F-cells in normal adult life: characterization of the Swiss type as hereditary persistence of fetal hemoglobin regulated dominantly by gene(s) on X chromosome. Blood 1988;72:1854–1860.

Olivieri NF, Brittenham GM. Iron-chelating therapy and the treatment of thalassemia. Blood 1997; 89:739–761.

Olivieri NF, Brittenham GM, Matsui D, et al. Iron-chelation therapy with oral deferiprone in patients with thalassemia major. N Engl J Med 1995;332:918–922.

Orkin SH. Transcription factors and hematopoietic development. J Biol Chem 1995;270:4955–4958.

Pászty C. Transgenic and gene knock-out mouse models of sickle cell anemia and the thalassemias. Curr Opin Hematol 1997;4:88–93.

Pászty C, Brion CM, Manci E, Witkowska HE, Stevens ME, Mohandas N, Rubin EM. Transgenic knockout mice with exclusively human sickle hemoglobin and sickle cell disease. Science 1997;278: 876–878.

Perkins AC, Gaensler KM, Orkin SH. Silencing of human fetal globin expression is impaired in the absence of the adult beta-globin gene activator protein EKLF. Proc Natl Acad Sci USA 1996;93:12,267–12,271.

Rochette J, Craig JE, Thein SL. Fetal hemoglobin levels in adults. Blood Reviews 1994;8:213–224.

Rodgers GP, Rachmilewitz EA. Novel treatment options in the severe β-globin disorders. Br J Haematol 1995;91:263–268.

Ryan TM, Ciavatta DJ, Townes TM. Knockout-transgenic mouse model of sickle cell disease. Science 1997;278:873–876.

Serjeant GR. Sickle Cell Disease, 2nd ed. Oxford: Oxford University Press, 1992.

Stamatoyannopoulos G, Nienhuis AW, Majerus PW, Varmus HE. The Molecular Basis of Blood Diseases, 2nd ed. Philadelphia: WB Saunders, 1994.

Stamatoyannopoulos JA, Nienhuis AW. Therapeutic approaches to hemoglobin switching in treatment of hemoglobinopathies. Annu Rev Med 1993;43:497–521.

Stasiak A, West SC, Egelman EH. Sickle cell anemia research and a recombinant DNA technique. Science 1997;277:460–462.

Steinberg MH, Lu Z-H, Barton FB, Terrin ML, Charache S, Dover GJ. Multicenter Study of Hydroxyurea: fetal hemoglobin in sickle cell anemia: determinants of response to hydroxyurea. Blood 1997;89:1078–1088.

Thein SL. Dominant β thalassaemia: molecular basis and pathophysiology. Br J Haematol 1992;80:273–277.

Weatherall DJ, Clegg JB. The Thalassaemia Syndromes. Oxford: Blackwell Scientific, 1981.

Wilkie AOM, Buckle VJ, Harris PC, et al. Clinical features and molecular analysis of the a thalassemia/mental retardation syndromes. I. Cases due to deletions involving chromosome band 16p13.3. Am J Hum Genet 1990;46:1112–1126.

Yang B, Kirby S, Lewis J, Detloff PJ, Maeda N, Smithies O. A mouse model for beta 0-thalassemia. Proc Natl Acad Sci USA 1995;92: 11,608–11,612.

21 Disorders of the Red Cell Membrane

JEAN DELAUNAY

BACKGROUND

The red cell membrane is composed of a lipid bilayer, studded with transmembrane proteins, and the membrane skeleton, also termed the erythrocyte skeleton. The latter is a bidimensional network that laminates the inner surface of the bilayer. Skeleton proteins are connected to transmembrane proteins through anchoring proteins (Fig. 21-1). The main features of the proteins of interest and their genes are enumerated in Table 21-1. A number of hereditary hemolytic anemias, usually associated with red cell shape abnormalities, stem from mutations affecting a variety of genes that encode membrane, skeletal, or anchoring proteins. We will focus on hereditary spherocytosis (HS), hereditary elliptocytosis (HE), and its aggravated form, hereditary pyropoikilocytosis (HPP).

CLINICAL FEATURES

The conditions mentioned above share in common icterus, anemia, and splenomegaly. Their severity can range from the absence of symptoms to death *in utero* (hydrops fetalis). Complications may occur, including gallstones and parvovirus infections (HS). HE/HPP is encountered in one out of 5000 Caucasian kindreds, and up to 1 out of 100 families in some black populations. The prevalence of HE/HPP coincides with some malarious regions. In comparison to HE/HPP, HS is relatively more common (with a frequency of approximately 1 in 2000 kindreds); it is uniformly distributed throughout all ethnic groups, although studies show that it seems to be absent among black people.

DIAGNOSIS

Routine laboratory data are based on the red cell indices, the levels of bilirubin, and haptoglobin, the reading of blood smears and the study of the osmotic fragility (its increase is a key sign in HS). More sophisticated techniques, such as ektacytometry or electron microscopy, may be used. Electrophoresis of membrane proteins on polyacrylamide gel in the presence of SDS (SDS-PAGE) (Fig. 21-2) and, if necessary, spectrin partial digests, often provides clues to the primarily altered proteins. Because the genes encoding these proteins have been cloned and sequenced and polymorphic sequences, including variable number of dinucleotide repeats (VNDRs) and variable number of tandem repeats (VNTRs) identified, it is possible to track these genes by linkage to these polymorphic sites using polymerase chain reaction (PCR). For further analysis, exons or portions of cDNA are PCR-amplified in view of finding single strand conformational polymorphisms (SSCPs). Polymorphic fragments are then cloned and submitted to nucleotide sequencing.

From: *Principles of Molecular Medicine* (J. L. Jameson, ed.), ©1998 Humana Press Inc., Totowa, NJ.

GENETIC BASIS

HEREDITARY SPHEROCYTOSIS Based on genomic lesions, it is possible to divide HS into 6 subsets.

HS Associated with ANK1 Gene Mutations In 75% of the HS Caucasian kindreds, the disease stems from a mutation in the ANK1 gene, encoding erythroid ankyrin. The ankyrin gene contains 42 exons that are distributed over about 160 kb. Dominantly inherited HS cases are often owing to nonsense or frameshift mutations (heterozygous state). Upon SDS-PAGE, the lacking haploid set is mainly manifested by a reduction of ankyrin isoform "band 2.1." An elevated reticulocyte count is likely to mask this decrease because the reticulocyte part of band 2.1 has not yet been proteolyzed into components of lower molecular weights, a process applying to normal and pathological red cells (Fig. 21-2A). Mutations indifferently involve the three domains of ankyrin: domain "89 kDa" (carrying the binding site for band 3), domain "63 kDa" (binding site for β-spectrin), and domain "55 kDa" (regulatory domain). The reduction of ankyrin is accompanied by a nearly constant reduction in protein 4.2 although no direct contact between ankyrin and protein 4.2 has been demonstrated so far, and a less constant decrease of spectrin (Fig. 21-2A). When occurring near the 3' end of ANK1 gene, a truncated ankyrin molecule may be generated (Fig. 21-2B). Recessively transmitted HS cases imply the occurrence of two mutations *in trans* to one another (homozygous or compound heterozygous states). Ankyrin (band 2.1) is also reduced, but, again, a high reticulocyte count may mask this decrease. Only in a very few instances have the two changes been elucidated unambiguously, and some described changes possibly represent functionally neutral polymorphisms.

HS Associated with EPB3 Gene Mutations and Band 3 Deficiency In 15–20% of HS families, the condition stems from mutations (heterozygous state), affecting the EPB3 gene that encodes band 3—that is, the erythroid anion exchanger 1 (AE1). Nonsense or frameshift mutations may occur in the cytoplasmic domain (positions 1–403), or the transmembrane (TM) domain of the molecule (positions 404–881) comprising 14 membrane-spanning segments. They result in the absence of one haploid set of band 3 (Fig. 21-3). SDS-PAGE shows a 20–40% decrease of band 3 and, in a secondary fashion, of protein 4.2, which binds to the cytoplasmic domain of band 3 (Figs. 21-2C and 21-3). The mode of inheritance is dominant; blood smears disclose occasional

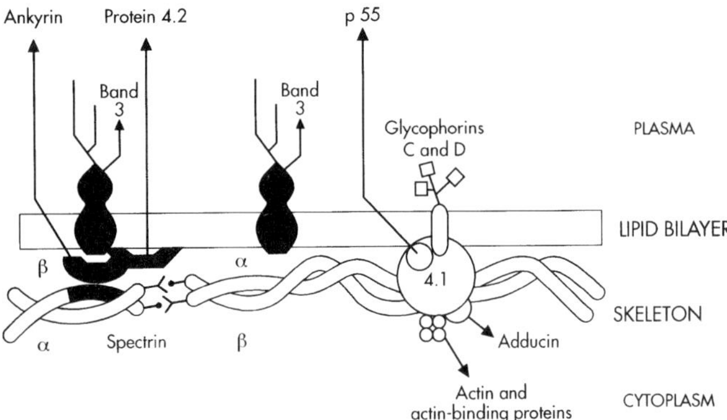

Figure 21-1 Section of the erythrocyte membrane and skeleton. Only relevant proteins and some other major proteins are shown. Band 3, anion exchanger; GPC and GPD, glycophorins C and D, respectively; horizontal interactions, spectrin αβ dimers self-associate head-to-head to form an $\alpha_2\beta_2$ heterotetramer—each of the extremities of the tetramer interacts with actin and protein 4.1 (junctional complex). Vertical interactions: β-spectrin interacts with ankyrin that, in turn, interacts with the cytoplasmic domain of band 3; protein 4.2 also interacts with the latter. Protein 4.1, p55 and GPC (GPD) form another vertical (ternary) complex.

"pincered" red cells, the shape of which evokes mushrooms. Single amino acid substitutions at highly conserved positions in membrane spanning segments result in an identical picture, presumably because they impede band 3 incorporation into the membrane. The only known homozygous case of mutations of this category was lethal *in utero* (Alloisio et al., unpublished results); however, no generalization can be made at this time. Red blood cells from mice with targeted disruption of the band 3 gene spontaneously shed membrane vesicles and tubules, leading to severe spherocytosis. However, the synthesis of spectrin and skeletal architecture were nearly normal, suggesting that band 3 does not regulate membrane skeleton assembly, but it is necessary for membrane stability.

HS Associated with EPB3 Gene Mutations and the Absence of Protein 4.2 Quite rarely, homozygous state mutations lying in the cytoplasmic domain of band 3 leave the amount of band 3 virtually unchanged but yield a total, or at least a substantial lack of protein 4.2; only Western blots may reveal traces of this protein and some lower compounds that could be degradation products (Figs. 21-2D and 21-3). The inheritance pattern is strictly recessive; the mutations are thought to disrupt the binding site of band 3 cytoplasmic domain for protein 4.2.

HS Associated with ELP42 Gene Mutations and the Absence of Protein 4.2 Also rarely, homozygous or compound heterozygous state mutations affecting the ELP42 gene, encoding protein 4.2, result in the complete—or nearly complete—absence of protein 4.2 (Fig. 21-2E). Again, these conditions are recessively transmitted. The picture is that of an atypical form of HS: spherocytes are rare, and the osmotic fragility is little increased. Apart from one case—allele ELP42 Lisboa, carrying a frameshift mutation—single amino acid substitutions come into play and must disrupt the binding site for the cytoplasmic domain of band 3 or disturb the overall stability of protein 4.2.

HS Associated with SPTB Gene Mutations Several mutations responsible for dominantly transmitted HS have been found in the SPTB gene, encoding erythroid β-spectrin. Usually, nonsense or frameshift mutations, scattered over the β chain except for homologous segment β17 (in this case, the mutations would engender HE or HPP; *see below*, abolish the synthesis of one haploid set of β chain. Because the β-chain synthesis, though in excess, is limiting with respect to that of α chain, the lack of one haploid set of β-spectrin causes a deficit in spectrin $\alpha_2\beta_2$ tetramer. One mutation that defines spectrin Kissimmee carries a simple amino acid substitution and alters the binding capacity of β-spectrin for protein 4.1 and F-actin.

HS Associated with SPTA1 Gene Mutations So far, mutations responsible for recessively transmitted HS have been encountered in the SPTA1 gene, encoding erythroid α-spectrin. They are frameshift mutations and occur *in trans* to one another. Because of the large excess of spectrin α-chain synthesis, heterozygosity is nonexpressed.

HEREDITARY ELLIPTOCYTOSIS AND HEREDITARY PYROPOIKILOCYTOSIS HS/HPP Associated with SPTA1 and SPTB Gene Mutations Numerous mutations responsible for HE/HPP have been found in SPTA1 and SPTP genes. Both spectrin chains are comprised of approximately 106 amino acid homologous or repeating segments: 22 in the α chain and 17 in the β chain. Each homologous segment contains three α-helical stretches—h3, h1, and h2—and is folded into conformational units with a shift of 26 amino acids. As a result, a conformational unit harbors helices 1 and 2 of a homologous segment and helix 3 of the following segment (Fig. 21-4). The HE/HPP mutations stand in or near α-spectrin, the self-association region—that is, the region at which two spectrin αβ dimers interact head-to-head through complementary binding sites to form an $\alpha_2\beta_2$ tetramer (Fig. 21-4). As a consequence, the self-association process is weakened. Most of the α mutations lie in helices 3 of homologous segment α1–α8. No mutations have been found in segment 6; however, it must be a matter of chance. Mutations in helices 2 are rare. The insertion of a leucine at position 154—helix 3, homologous segment α2—is endemic in West Central Africa. It followed population migrations to the Indies and North America and to both banks of the Mediterranean Basin. Mutation Saint Louis—helix 2, segment α2)—which is less frequent, may have had a similar history.

Many mutations of the β17 homologous segment (helix 2) yield a truncation of the β chain in one way or another and disclose a dominant inheritance pattern (Fig. 21-2F). Others are single amino acid substitutions, a cluster of which exists in helix 1 of segment β17. Silent in the heterozygous state, they produce a severe phenotype in the homozygous state.

Allele α^{LELY} A salient feature concerns alleles of the SPTA1 gene (α^{HE} alleles). For a given mutation, some members disclose a mild HE phenotype or are symptomless, whereas other members are severely affected, often exhibiting HPP. It has long been assumed that this situation reflected the presence of a low expression allele *in trans* to the α^{HE} allele. That allele had to be widespread, for it manifested itself in nearly all families already carrying an α^{HE} allele. The key to the problem was the discovery of allele α^{LELY} (LELY: Low Expression LYon). Allele α^{LELY} appears to be uniformly distributed at a polymorphic frequency of 0.2–0.3 of all α alleles among all ethnic groups (Caucasians, blacks, Japanese, Chinese). It is invariably characterized by mutations at position 1817 (exon 40), at positions - 12 of introns 45 and 46 (however, the latter mutation is nonspecific). The mutation in intron 45 is associated with a partial skipping (50%) of exon 46 (18 nt) on α-spectrin transcript processing. Lack of exon 46 is thought to disrupt the binding site of the α-chain site (C-

Table 21-1
Main Features of the Considered Proteins and Their Genes

	Amino acids (actual mol wt)	*Monomers per cell*	*Gene symbol and chromosomal location*	*Gene size (kb) and exon number*	*Size of mRNA, kb*	*Disease*	*Inheritance pattern[b] (autosomal)*
Spectrin α chain	2429 (281)	242,000	SPTA 1; 1q22–q23	80; 52	8	HE	Dominant
						HS	Recessive
Spectrin β chain	2137 (246)	242,000	SPTB; 14q23–q24.2	> 100; 36	7.5	HE	Dominant or recessive
						HS	Dominant
Ankyrin	1880 (206)	124,000	ANK1; 8p11.2	> 120; 42	6.8–7.2	HS	Dominant or recessive
Band 3	911 (102)	1,200,000	EPB3; 17q12–q21	17; 20	4.7	HS	Dominant or recessive
Protein 4.1	588 (66)	~ 200,000	EL1; 1p33–p34.2	> 250; > 23	5.6	HE	Dominant
Protein 4.2	691 (77)	~ 200,000	ELP42; 15q15–q21	20; 13	2.4	HS[a]	Recessive

[a]Atypical form of HS.
[b]The inheritance pattern depends on complex factors in addition to the mere nature of the mutations.

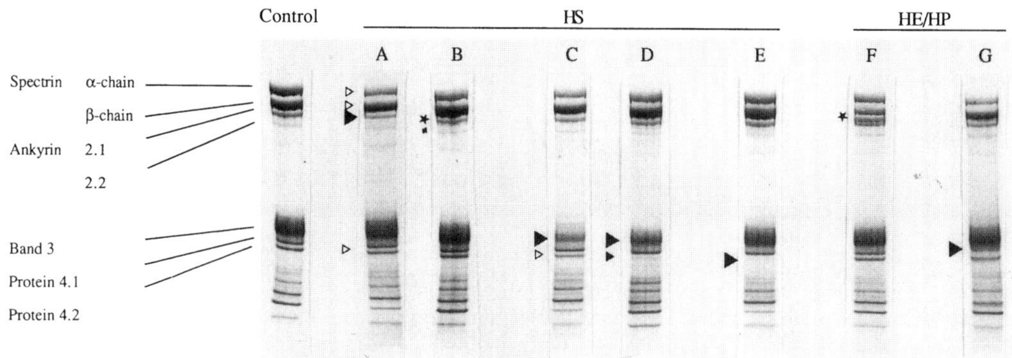

Figure 21-2 A series of changes in the SDS-PAGE profile in HS and HE/HPP. (▶), primary decrease or absence; (▷), secondary decrease; (*), duplication (+ decrease). A and B: HS associated with ANK1 gene mutations. A: one allele (heterozygosity) carries an early frameshift mutation. It abolishes one haploid set of ankyrin and leads to the secondary reduction of spectrin and protein 4.2 (Morlé et al., unpublished results). B: one allele (heterozygosity) carries a nonsense mutation near the 3' end of the gene. It yields a truncated ankyrin molecule (Hayette et al., unpublished results). C and D: HS associated with EPB3 gene mutations. C: compound heterozygosity for two abnormal alleles generates a sharp reduction of band 3 and, secondarily, a noticeable decrease of protein 4.2 (Alloisio et al., unpublished results). D: compound heterozygosity for two other abnormal alleles yields a total absence of protein 4.2; one allele is of the same type as in C (abolishing one haploid set of band 3) and the other allele disrupts the binding site of band 3 cytoplasmic domain for protein 4.2 (Kanzaki et al., unpublished results). E: HS associated with a frameshift mutation in the ELP42 gene (homozygosity). F: HE associated with an exon skipping near the 3' end of SPTB transcript (heterozygosity), yielding a truncated β-spectrin molecule. G: HE associated with the abolition of the downstream initiation codon (homozygosity) of the EL1 gene. (Electrophoreses done by Ms. M.-A. Schreiner.)

terminal region) for a complementary site in the β chain (N-terminal region). As a consequence, the nucleation process, i.e., the onset of dimerization, becomes impossible, and all exon 46-lacking spectrin α chains are discarded. However, this remains innocuous, even in the homozygous state, because a large excess of α chains is normally synthesized. Half of the α^{LELY} products—those bearing exon 46—are sufficient to meet the needs of the erythrocyte. On the contrary, in the $\alpha^{HE}/\alpha^{LELY}$ situation, there is a twofold excess of α^{HE} chains compared to α^{LELY} chain having retained exon 46. An increased proportion of $\alpha^{HE}\beta$ dimers are assembled. Subsequently, those dimers prove unable to self-associate, hence the aggravation of the disease. Of course, some α^{HE} alleles, coined $\alpha^{HE\text{-}LELY}$ alleles, carry the LELY mutations in *cis* of a HE mutation. As one would anticipate, the expression of HE is attenuated.

4.1(-) Hereditary Elliptocytosis Among Caucasians, approximately 30% of HE results from defects involving protein 4.1, usually in the heterozygous state and rarely in the homozygous state (Fig. 21-2G). Protein 4.1 is a key element of the junctional complex (Fig. 21-1). Heterozygous 4.1(–) HE is symptomless and discloses numerous, smooth and well-elongated elliptocytes. Homozygous 4.1(–)HE achieves a picture of HPP. Owing to the size of EL1 gene (>250 kb) and of its introns, and also because of the extraordinary complexity of the alternative splicing characterizing protein 4.1 transcript, only two mutations have been elucidated at the gene level so far. One of them cancels the downstream initiation codon for translation—the only initiation codon used in the erythroid cells—whereas the other disrupts the binding site of protein 4.1 for spectrin and actin.

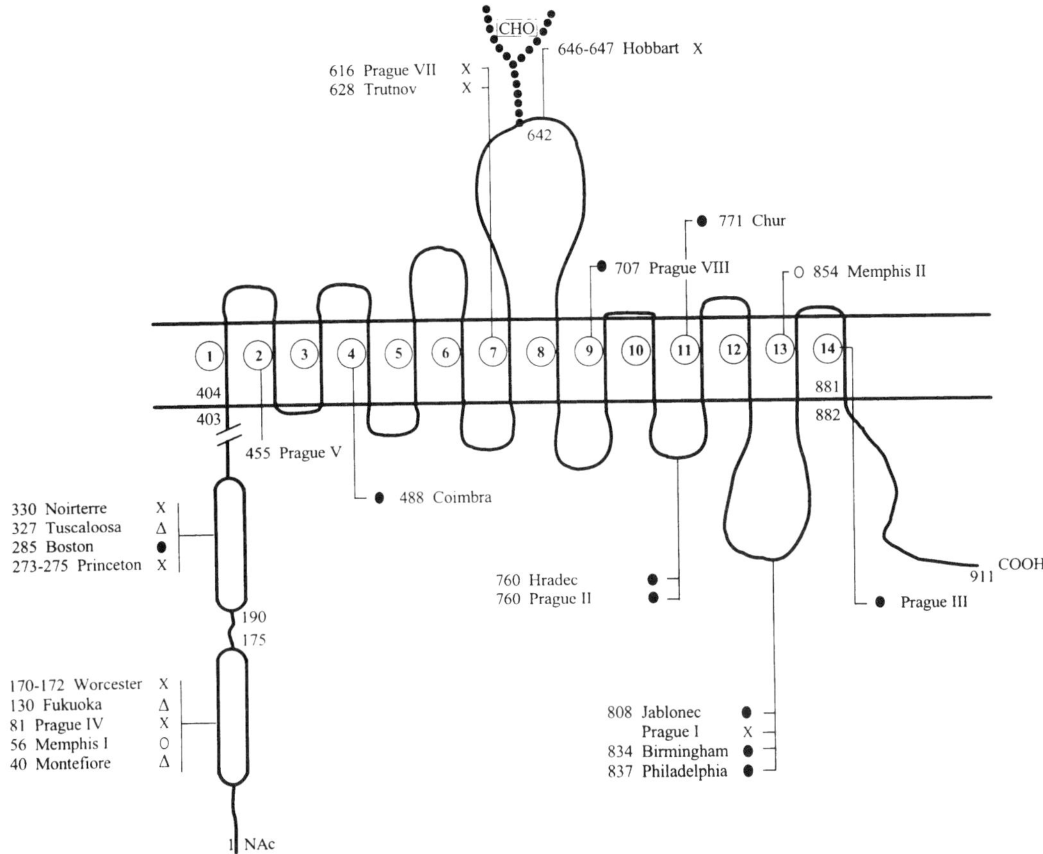

Figure 21-3 Location of mutations in band 3 (cDNA level) (recorded 8/31/95). The cytoplasmic domain (positions 1 to 403) and the membrane domain (404–881) with its transmembrane segments (circled numbers) are individualized. ●, single base mutations; ○, polymorphisms; x, frameshift or nonsense mutations; △, mutations abolishing the binding of protein 4.2.

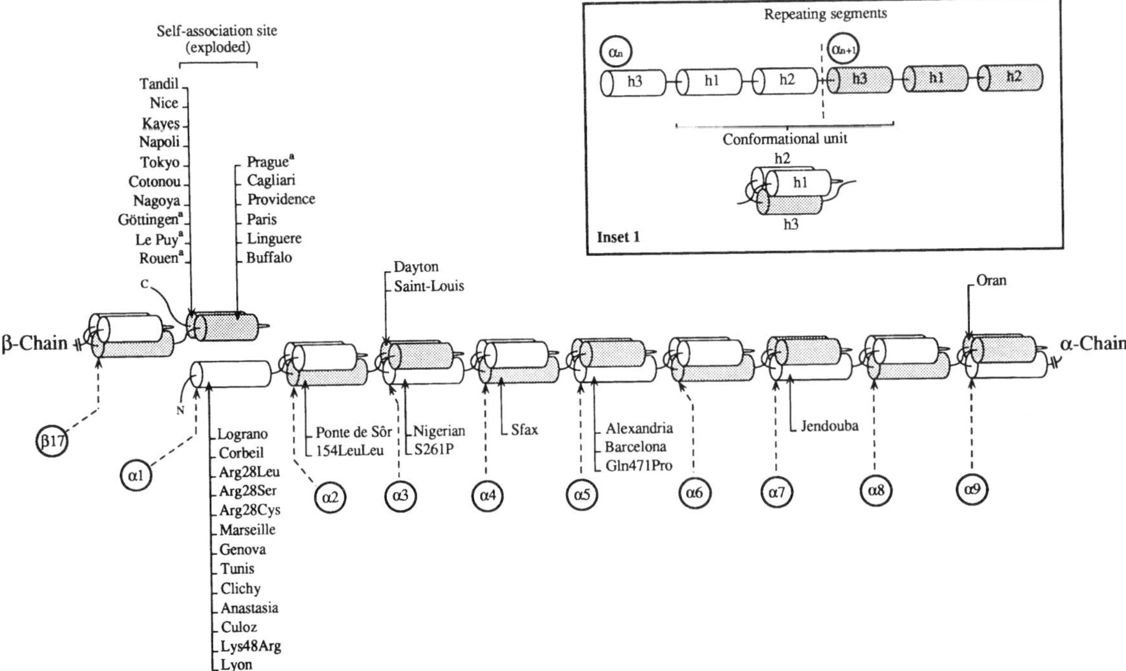

Figure 21-4 Clustering of mutations responsible for HE/HPP at/or in the vicinity of the self-association region (recorded 8/31/95). Circled numbers designate the homologous segments at the point where they begin. [a]: intronic mutations that yield skipping of SPTB gene exons 30 or 31. Inset: correspondence between the homologous (or repeating) segments (linear) and the conformation units (three-dimensional). Each conformational unit contains one helix with a color, h3, belonging to a homologous segment, and two white helices, h1 and h2, belonging to the preceding homologous segment. (Courtesy of Dr. P. Maillet.)

In homozygous 4.1(–)HE, the total absence of protein 4.1 causes a sharp reduction of transmembrane glycophorin C and the total absence of a third protein, called p55 (not shown). This reflects a triangular interaction between these proteins (a vertical interaction; *see* Fig. 21-1). On the other hand, the Leach phenotype, a rare blood group resulting from the primary absence of glycophorin C, is associated with elliptocytosis. Protein 4.1 is slightly diminished (hence the elliptocytosis) and p55 is, again, entirely missing.

MOLECULAR PATHOPHYSIOLOGY

Few studies have tried to bridge the abnormalities at the molecular and cellular levels. In a simple fashion, spherocytes stem from discocytes by "spleen conditioning," i.e., the removal of microvesicles (50–80 nm) that yield a reduction of the membrane surface area. It is intriguing that mutations in at least five distinct proteins result in the same cellular phenotype. Elliptocytes do not recover the discocyte shape following shear stress in large vessels. This lack of elastic deformability generates increased mechanical fragility. In severe cases, the cells shatter against the walls of major arteries, achieving pyropoikilocytosis. Again, it is remarkable that mutations in spectrin and protein 4.1 have a similar cellular phenotype.

TREATMENT

Molecular genetics has allowed reclassification HS and HE/HPP and provide a rational basis of diagnosis. Treatment is based on occasional or regular blood transfusions. Splenectomy is beneficial; it is nearly curative in HS. Identification of the causative mutation at the DNA level allows prenatal diagnosis when a mutation, that is severe or lethal in the homozygous state, occurs in consanguineous couples (Alloisio et al., unpublished data). The efficiency of prenatal and postnatal managements do not justify gene therapy.

FUTURE PROSPECTS

Beside the practical interest in describing mutations, many of the latter offer precious natural models. They allow far-reaching studies on gene expression and structure–function relationships within proteins.

SELECTED REFERENCES

Alloisio N, Morlé L, Maréchal J, et al. SpαV/41: a common spectrin polymorphism at the αIV-αV domain junction. Relevance to the expression level of hereditary elliptocytosis due to α-spectrin variants located in *trans*. J Clin Invest 1991;87:2169–2177.

Alloisio N, Texier P, Vallier A, et al. Modulation of clinical expression and band 3 deficiency in hereditary spherocytosis. Blood 1997;90:414–420.

Amin KM, Scarpa AL, Winkelmann JC, Curtis PJ, Forget BG. The exon-intron organization of the human erythroid β-spectrin gene. Genomics 1993;18:118–125.

Conboy JG. Structure, function, and molecular genetics of erythroid membrane skeletal protein 4.1 in normal and abnormal red blood cells. Semin Hematol 1993;30:58–73.

Dalla Venezia N, Gilsanz F, Alloisio N, Ducluzeau MT, Benz EJ Jr, Delaunay J. Homozygous 4.1(-) hereditary elliptocytosis associated with a point mutation in the downstream initiation codon of protein 4.1 gene. J Clin Invest 1992;90:1713–1717.

Delaunay J, Dhermy D. Mutations involving the spectrin heterodimer contact site: clinical expression and alterations in specific functions. Semin Hematol 1993;30:21–33.

Eber SW, Gonzalez JM, Lux ML, et al. Ankyrin-1 mutations are a major cause of dominant and recessive hereditary spherocytosis. 1996;13:214–218.

Gallagher PG, Ferriera JD. Molecular basis of erythrocyte membrane disorders. Curr Opin Hematol 1997;4:128–135.

Gallagher PG, Kotula L, Wang Y, et al. Molecular basis and haplotyping of the alphaII domain polymorphisms of spectrin: application to the study of hereditary elliptocytosis and pyropoikilocytosis. Am J Hum Genet 1996;59:351–359.

Gallagher PG, Tse WT, Scarpa AL, Lux SE, Forget BG. Structure and organization of the human ankyrin-1 gene. Basis for complexity of pre-mRNA processing. J Biol Chem 1997;272:19,220–19,228.

Hassoun H, Vassiliadis JN, Murray J, et al. Characterization of the underlying molecular defect in hereditary spherocytosis associated with spectrin deficiency. Blood 1997;90:398–406.

Hayette S, Dhermy D, dos Santos ME, et al. A deletional frameshift mutation in protein 4.2 gene (allele 4.2 Lisboa) associated with hereditary hemolytic anemia. Blood 1995;85:250–256.

Jarolim P, Murray JL, Rubin HL, et al. Characterization of 13 novel band 3 gene defects in hereditary spherocytosis with band 3 deficiency. Blood 1996;88:4366–4374.

Jenkins PB, Abou-Alfa GK, Dhermy D, et al. A nonsense mutation in the erythrocyte band 3 gene associated with decreased mRNA accumulation in a kindred with dominant hereditary spherocytosis. J Clin Invest 1996;97:373–380.

Kotula L, Laury-Kleintrop LD, Showe L, et al. The exon-intron organization of the human erythrocyte α-spectrin gene. Genomics 1991;9: 131–140.

Lorenzo F, Dalla Venezia N, Morlé L, et al. Protein 4.1 deficiency associated with an altered binding to the spectrin-actin complex of the red cell membrane skeleton. J Clin Invest 1994;94:1651–1656.

Lux SE, Palek J. Disorders of the red cell membrane. In: Handin RI, Lux SE, Stossel TP, eds. Blood, Principles and Practice of Hematology. Philadelphia: JB Lippincott, 1995; pp. 1701–1818.

Peters LL, Lux SE. Ankyrins: structure and function in normal cells and hereditary spherocytes. Semin Hematol 1993;30:85–118.

Peters LL, Shivdasani RA, Liu SC, et al. Anion exchanger 1 (band 3) is required to prevent erythrocyte membrane surface loss but not to form the membrane skeleton. Cell 1996;86:917–927.

Randon J, Miraglia del Giudice E, Bozon M, et al. Frequent de novo mutations of the ANK1 gene mimic a recessive mode of transmission in hereditary spherocytosis: three new ANK1 variants: ankyrins Bari, Napoli II and Anzio. Br J Haematol 1997;96:500–506.

Sahr KE, Laurila P, Kotula L, et al. The complete cDNA and polypeptide sequences of human erythroid α-spectrin. J Biol Chem 1990;265: 4434–4443.

Sahr KE, Taylor WT, Daniels BP, Lubin HL, Jarolim P. The structure and organization of the human erythroid anion exchanger (AE1) gene. Genomics 1994;24:491–501.

Schofield AE, Martin PG, Spillett D, Tanner MJA. The structure of the human red blood cell anion exchanger (EPB3, AE1, Band 3) gene. Blood 1994;84:2000–2012.

Tanner MJA. Molecular and cellular biology of the erythrocyte anion exchanger (AE1). Semin Hematol 1993;30:34–57.

Tanner MJ. Physiology: The acid test for band 3. Nature 1996;382: 209,210.

Wilmotte R, Maréchal J, Morlé L, et al. Low expression allele α^{LELY} of red cell spectrin is associated with mutations in exon 40 ($\alpha^{V/41}$ polymorphism) and intron 45 and with partial skipping of exon 46. J Clin Invest 1993;91:2091–2096.

Winkelmann JC, Chang JG, Tse WT, Scarpa AL, Marchesi VT, Forget BG. Full-length sequence of the cDNA for human erythroid β-spectrin. J Biol Chem 1990;265:11,827–11,832.

Winkelmann JC, Forget BG. Erythroid and nonerythroid spectrins. Blood 1993;81:3173–3185.

Yawata Y. Red cell membrane protein band 4.2: phenotypic, genetic, and electron microscopic aspects. Biochim Biophys Acta 1994;1204: 131–148.

22 Red Cell Enzymopathies

Lucio Luzzatto and Rosario Notaro

INTRODUCTION

The mature red cell is the product of a developmental pathway that brings the phenomenon of differentiation to an extreme. An orderly sequence of events produces synchronous changes, whereby the gradual accumulation of a huge amount of hemoglobin in the cytoplasm (to a final level of 340 g/L, i.e., about 5 m*M*) goes hand in hand with the gradual loss of cellular organelles and of biosynthetic abilities. In the end, the erythroid cell undergoes a process that has features of apoptosis, including nuclear pycnosis and actual loss of the nucleus. However, the final result is more altruistic than suicidal; the cytoplasmic body, instead of disintegrating, is now able to provide oxygen to all cells in the human organism for some remaining 120 days of the red cell life-span.

This unique behavior has important consequences, not only with respect to the physiology of red cells (which cannot be covered here), but also with respect to their pathophysiology. Specifically, the chemical machinery of intermediary metabolism is drastically curtailed in mature red cells (Fig. 22-1); for instance, because cytochrome-mediated oxidative phosphorylation has been lost with the loss of mitochondria, there is no backup to anaerobic glycolysis for the production of adenosine triphosphate (ATP). Also, because the capacity of making protein has been lost with the loss of ribosomes, the existing metabolic machinery is always at risk: if any component deteriorates, it cannot be replaced, as in most other cells. Another consequence of the relative simplicity of red cells is that they have a very limited range of ways to manifest distress under conditions of hardship: in essence, any sort of metabolic failure will eventually lead either to membrane damage or to failure of the cation pump. In the former, the cell will suffer direct mechanical breakdown; in the latter, it will undergo osmotic lysis. In either case, the life-span of the red cell is reduced, which is the definition of a hemolytic disorder. If the rate of red cell destruction exceeds the capacity of the bone marrow to produce more red cells, the hemolytic disorder will manifest as hemolytic anemia.

Inherited abnormalities of red cell enzymes (enzymopathies for short) are a distinct set of genetic disorders. Most of the enzymes involved are housekeeping enzymes that, by definition, are present in all cells. Therefore, it is of interest first of all to consider the possible consequences of the deficiency of any of them. On one hand, we might expect that a severe reduction in the activity of any housekeeping enzyme would have generalized clinical manifestations, because in principle, all organs would be affected. On the other hand, in many cells there might be "metabolic redundancy," whereby other enzymes provide the missing function in a surrogate capacity; or, if the deficiency is not total, an increase in the synthesis of the enzyme involved might provide the minimum of activity compatible with cell viability. Because both of these compensatory mechanisms are not available to red cells, they would be more severely affected than other cells. In practice, we observe a clinical picture somewhere within this spectrum for each individual enzymopathy. In the majority of cases the main problem is hemolytic anemia; in some cases, hemolytic anemia is associated with other clinical manifestations; and in others the latter—particularly neurological damage—may dominate the clinical picture.

In this chapter, we shall concentrate on those enzymopathies affecting red cell metabolism of which the molecular basis has been elucidated. We will not cover conditions in which an enzyme abnormality is expressed also in red cells, but the main clinical manifestations are elsewhere (e.g., the porphyrias, acatalasemia, galactosemia, the Lesch-Nyhan syndrome). For the sake of brevity, some enzymopathies will be discussed as a group, with details of individual enzymes given in additional notes and within the illustrative material.

From: *Principles of Molecular Medicine* (J. L. Jameson, ed.), ©1998 Humana Press Inc., Totowa, NJ.

ENZYMOPATHIES OF GLYCOLYSIS

PREVALENCE All of these defects are rare to very rare (Table 22-1, pp. 200–201).

CLINICAL FEATURES All of these defects cause hemolytic anemia with varying degrees of severity (the detailed description of the clinical features and of the pathophysiology of hemolytic anemia is not within the scope of this book). If the anemia is severe, it will usually present very early in life, sometimes with severe neonatal jaundice that may require exchange transfusion; if the anemia is less severe, it may present later in life, or it may even remain asymptomatic and be detected incidentally when a blood count is done for unrelated reasons. The spleen is often enlarged. When other systemic manifestations occur, they involve either the neuromuscular system, or the central nervous system (CNS)—sometimes entailing severe mental retardation—or both.

DIAGNOSIS The diagnosis of hemolytic anemia is usually not difficult, based on the triad of normo-macrocytic anemia, reticulocytosis, and hyperbilirubinemia. Enzymopathies should be considered in the differential diagnosis of any chronic Coombs-negative hemolytic anemia. Once hemoglobinopathies have been ruled out, the field is narrowed down to membrane abnormalities and enzymopathies. Red cell morphology is usually conspicuously

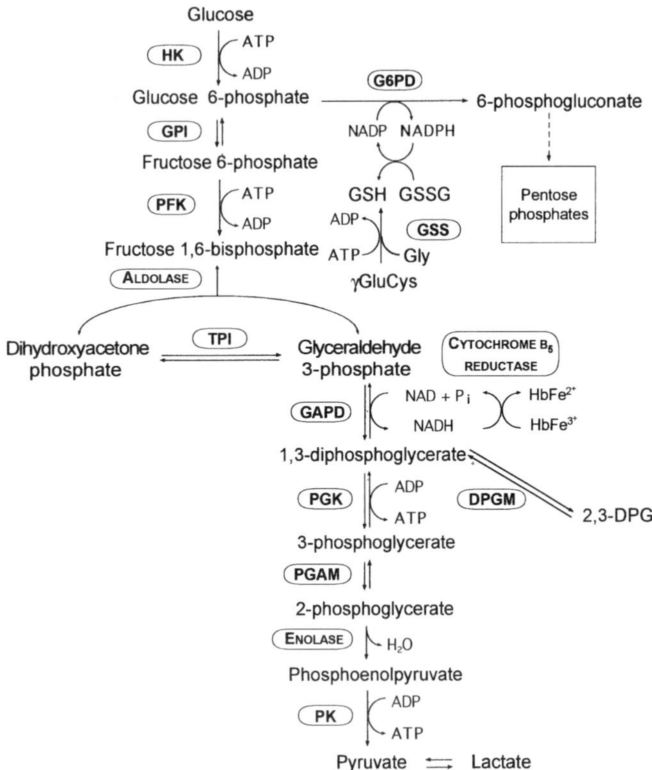

Figure 22-1 Intermediary metabolism in red cells. The diagram shows the glycolytic pathway and related reactions (not the complete metabolic machinery of the red cells). Enzymes are enclosed in rounded boxes. Abbreviations are as in Table 1. Additional abbreviations: DPG, diphosphoglycerate; GSH, reduced Glutathione; GSSG, Glutathione; $HbFe^{2+}$, hemoglobin; $HbFe^{3+}$, methemoglobin; γGluCys, γ-Glutamylcysteine.

abnormal in membrane disorders, but conspicuously normal in glycolytic enzymopathies. A useful test is the so-called autohemolysis test, in which red cells are simply incubated at 37°C under defined conditions, and the percent lysis measured after 48 hours. With membrane abnormalities, an abnormal hemolysis takes place, but this can be limited or abolished by the addition of sufficient concentrations of glucose; with glycolytic enzyme abnormalities, this "glucose correction" is only partially or totally lacking. This test has been criticized because it is unspecific: however, in our hands, it can be used as a reliable screening for enzymopathies. If the test is abnormal, the final diagnosis must be done by assaying individual glycolytic enzymes by the appropriate spectrophotometric method. For the sake of economy, it makes sense to carry out these rather laborious tests in order of frequency of the various enzymopathies (i.e., first PK, then GPI, and so on; Table 22-1). If a particular molecular abnormality is already known in the family, of course one can test for that directly on the patient's DNA, bypassing the need for enzyme assays.

GENETIC BASIS Because these conditions are all recessive, there are usually no affected members in the previous generations. However, inquiries for consanguinity should always be made, and there may be of course an affected sibling.

MOLECULAR PATHOPHYSIOLOGY At the biochemical level, all glycolytic enzymopathies have something in common, because their main consequence is to reduce the capacity of the red cell to produce chemical energy in the form of ATP. As seen in Table 22-1, the majority of mutations so far identified in the genes encoding glycolytic enzymes are of the missense type, causing single amino acid replacements. This is important, because in all these cases, the activity of the respective enzyme is reduced, but it is not completely lost. Thus, the residual activity can still support a decreased but nonzero flow through the glycolytic pathway: this explains how red cells survive in circulation, even though their life-span is reduced. As for the molecular basis for the reduction in enzyme activity, we must consider two basic mechanisms:

1. In the majority of cases, loss of activity is probably owing to a decreased stability of the protein. In such cases, we would predict that other cells might be much less affected than red cells, because the former can compensate for decreased stability through increased synthesis of the enzyme.
2. In some cases, the amino acid replacement may affect the active center of the enzyme. This, in turn, may affect either substrate binding (K_m) or the catalytic rate of the enzyme (k_{cat}), or both: in this case, other cells in which the rate of glycolysis is critical will be affected, as well as red cells.

MANAGEMENT Currently, there is no specific treatment for these conditions. Patients with moderate anemia may require occasional blood transfusion when they experience exacerbations of the anemia because of increased rate of hemolysis, or because of decreased red cell production secondary to infection (the most extreme example being "aplastic crisis" from parvovirus infection). Very rarely, chronic anemia may be sufficiently severe to require regular blood transfusion treatment with associated iron chelation. In some patients, splenectomy has been beneficial. In severe cases, bone marrow transplantation would be a rational form of treatment for patients who have a suitable donor, provided there are no systemic manifestations other than hemolytic anemia, and provided it is carried out before there is organ damage (e.g., from iron overload).

ADDITIONAL NOTES ON INDIVIDUAL GLYCOLYTIC ENZYMOPATHIES

HEXOKINASE (HK) Several isoenzymes of HK are known. The main isoenzyme in normal red cells is type 1. In the very rare cases of HK deficiency, this defect is only expressed in red cells, presumably because the other isoenzymes contribute sufficient HK activity in other cells. It is possible that even in red cells HK2 (normally present as a minor species) might help in damage limitation.

GLUCOSE 6-PHOSPHATE ISOMERASE (GPI) Most mutations entail single amino acid replacements, compatible with some residual enzyme activity (Fig. 22-2, p. 202). The splicing defects near exon 16 and the stop codon mutation in exon 18 might still result in the production of some enzymatically active protein. The nonsense mutation in exon 4 might be lethal in the homozygous state, but it has been found, together with a missense mutation, in two brothers with HA who were genetic compounds for these GPI mutations.

PHOSPHOFRUCTOKINASE (PFK) In many metabolic pathways, the first reaction is the one most exquisitely regulated (Fig. 22-3, p. 202). In the case of glycolysis in red cells it appears that PFK, the second kinase of the pathway, is more subject to regulation, particularly by ATP and adenosine monophosphate (AMP), which affect both k_{cat} and K_m^{F6P}. An interesting point of potential physiological significance is that this step is downstream of the pentose phosphate shunt; thus, the two pathways can be regulated independently. Five isoenzymes encoded by two genes are present in red cells. In PFK deficiency, all the mutations have been in the M subunit (Table 22-1), which explains the basis for the myopathy (glycogenosis type VII). In all these cases, we presume that the contribution of the L_4 species of PFK will be unaffected, and hybrid tetramers may be partially active. This may explain why the HA associated with PFK deficiency is rather mild. Conversely, it is possible that L subunit mutations may exist, but they may not cause HA as long as the M subunit is normal.

ALDOLASE Aldolase A, present in red cells, is a different enzyme from that which, when deficient in liver, causes fructose intolerance. Very few families with this red cell enzymopathy have been reported, and in only two was the molecular defect identified. In one family it was a missense mutation, causing an amino acid replacement of glycine for aspartic acid at position 128, a change that was shown to cause marked instability of the enzyme. Two members of the family were homozygous for this mutation and had enzyme levels of about 5% of normal, showing convincingly that aldolase deficiency can cause HA.

TRIOSEPHOSPHATE ISOMERASE (TPI) This is a very rare but one of the most serious red cell enzymopathies, because HA is usually associated with severe involvement of the CNS (Fig. 22-4, p. 203). One might reasonably surmise that this is owing to the fact that a low level of TPI compromises some crucial metabolic step in the CNS; however, there is a single report in the literature of two brothers with TPI deficiency, one of whom died with severe mental retardation, whereas the other lives at the age of 22 with only hemolytic anemia. This intriguing observation would be consistent with the CNS manifestations requiring the coexistence of a mutation in some other unlinked gene. Another extraordinary finding has been that of the same missense mutations (105 Glu→Asp) in 17 unrelated families from distant parts of the world. In addition, this mutation is in strong linkage disequilibrium with several polymorphic sites.

DIPHOSPHOGLYCERATE MUTASE (DPGM) DPGM is the only enzyme in the table that is not housekeeping; on the contrary, it is probably erythroid-specific. It is important in controlling the level of DPG, which is a regulator of the hemoglobin–oxygen dissociation curve. With DPGM deficiency, the DPG level is reduced, with consequent decreased delivery of oxygen to tissues, functional hypoxia, and polycythemia.

PHOSPHOGLYCERATE KINASE (PGK) Like most other enzymes in the table, the X-linked gene encoding PGK is expressed in virtually all cells: a notable exception are sperm cells, in which a closely related autosomal PGK gene is expressed (Fig. 22-5, p. 203). Apart from HA, patients with PGK deficiency often have either CNS involvement, a myopathy, or both. Attempts have been made to correlate various combinations of clinical manifestations with the extent of enzyme instability produced in red cells and in muscle cells by individual mutations. However, the correlation does not always hold.

PYRUVATE KINASE (PK) PK deficiency is by far the most common glycolytic enzymopathy (Fig. 22-6, p. 204), and it is also that for which the largest number of mutant alleles has been reported (Table 22-1). In a recent survey of 30 patients (60 alleles), 19 different mutations were observed. A single mutant, 1529A (corresponding to 510 Arg→Gln in Fig. 22-6), accounted for 42% of the total. This mutation had been already found in several families, and it is in strong linkage disequilibrium with a polymorphic site elsewhere in the gene, consistent with a single ancient origin. Although this might be an example of founder effect, it is also compatible with some selective advantage of this allele in heterozygotes, possibly related to a slightly increased DPG level in these subjects. Homozygotes are at a disadvantage because of HA, but this is often characteristically well-tolerated, as a markedly increased DPG favors oxygen supply to the tissues. One patient with PK deficiency is known to have successfully completed a marathon run (EC Gordon-Smith, personal communication). PK deficiency is also the only glycolytic enzymopathy for which a significant proportion of mutant alleles are of the "null" variety, by virtue of having nonsense or frameshift mutations. In most cases, residual activity can be provided by the other allele in genetic compounds. However, several patients have been identified who were homozygous for the frameshift mutation called Gipsy. In these patients, some residual activity may be contributed by the M isoenzyme, present at low abundance in red cells. A mouse model of PK deficiency has been described that exhibits splenomegaly and nonspherocytic hemolytic anemia. This strain may be useful as an experimental model of PK deficiency.

GLUCOSE 6-PHOSPHATE DEHYDROGENASE (G6PD) DEFICIENCY

EPIDEMIOLOGY G6PD deficiency is distributed worldwide. Areas of high prevalence are found in Africa, Southern Europe, the Middle East, South East Asia, and Oceania. In the Americas and in parts of Northern Europe, G6PD deficiency is also quite prevalent as a result of migrations that have taken place in relatively recent historical times. The overall geographic distribution of G6PD deficiency and its heterogeneity, together with clinical field studies and in vitro culture experiments, strongly support the view that this common genetic trait has been selected by *Plasmodium falciparum* malaria, by virtue of the fact that it confers a relative resistance against this highly lethal infection.

CLINICAL FEATURES Three types of clinical presentations are well characterized: acute hemolytic anemia, neonatal jaundice, and chronic nonspherocytic hemolytic anemia.

1. The vast majority of G6PD deficient people are asymptomatic most of the time, but they are at risk of developing acute hemolytic anemia (AHA), which may be triggered by drugs, infections, or fava beans. During a hemolytic attack, the hemoglobin may fall very little, or it may plummet to values as low as 40 g/L or less; however, even if severe, the anemia is usually self-limited and tends to resolve spontaneously. Depending on the proportion of red cells that have been destroyed (reflected in the severity of the anemia), the hemoglobin level may be back to normal in 3–6 weeks.
2. The risk of developing neonatal jaundice (NNJ) is much greater in G6PD deficient than in G6PD normal newborns. NNJ related to G6PD deficiency—unlike "classical" Rhesus-related NNJ—is very rarely present at birth; the clinical onset is usually between day 2 and day 3. The severity varies enormously from being subclinical, to overlapping with "physiological jaundice," to imposing the threat of kernicterus, if not treated. Prematurity, infection, and environmental factors (e.g., the use of naphthalene—camphor balls—used in baby bedding and clothing) are known aggravating factors.

Table 22-1
Synopsis of Red Cell Enzymopathies[a]

Enzyme	Isoenzyme[b] characteristic of red cells	Prevalence of enzyme deficiency	Main clinical features associated with enzyme deficiency[c]	Benefit from splenectomy[d]	Chromosomal localization	Number of exons
Hexokinase (HK)	1	Very rare	HA	Partial	10q22 (q11?)	18
Glucose 6-phosphate isomerase (GPI)		Rare	HA, NM, CNS	Partial	19q13.1	18
Phosphofructokinase (PFK)[h]	M	Very rare	HA, myopathy		1cen-q32	24
	L				21q22.3	22
Aldolase	A	Very rare	HA, myopathy		16q22–24	12
Triosephosphate isomerase (TPI)		Very rare	HA, CNS, NM,	None	12p13	7
Glyceraldehyde 3-phosphate dehydrogenase (GAPD)[k]		Very rare	HA		12p13.31–p13.1	9
Diphosphoglycerate mutase (DPGM)		Very rare	Polycythemia		7q31-q34	3
Phosphoglycerate kinase (PGK)	1	Very rare	HA, CNS, NM	Partial	Xq13	11
Monophosphoglycerate mutase (PGAM-B)	B				10q25.3	
Enolase[k]	1 (α)	Very rare	HA		1pter-p36.13	
Pyruvate kinase (PK)	R[m]	Rare	HA	Partial	1q21	12
Glucose 6-phosphate dehydrogenase (G6PD)	B	Common	HA	None	Xq28	13
Cytochrome-b_5 reductase		Rare	pseudocyanosis, CNS		22q13.31–qter	9
Adenylate kinase (AK)	1	Very rare	HA, CNS	Partial	9q34.1	7
γ-Glutamylcysteine synthetase (GLCLC)[k,q]		Very rare	HA		6p12	
Glutathione synthetase (GSS)		Very rare	HA, CNS		20q11.2	12
Glutathione peroxidase (GSH-Px)		Very rare[r]	?[r]		3q11–q12	

		Number of known mutations[f]						
					Deletion–insertion			
Enzyme	Number of amino acids[e]	5′UTR[j]	Missense	Nonsense	In frame	With frameshift	Affecting splicing	Total
Hexokinase (HK)	917		1		3–0			4[g]
Glucose 6-phosphate isomerase (GPI)	558		19	2			2	23
Phosphofructokinase (PFK)[h]	780		7	1		1–0	6	15
	784							
Aldolase	364		2					2[i]
Triosephosphate isomerase (TPI)	249	1	9	2		1–0		13
Glyceraldehyde 3-phosphate dehydrogenase (GAPD)[k]	335							
Diphosphoglycerate mutase (DPGM)	259		1		1–0			2[l]
Phosphoglycerate kinase (PGK)	417		8		1–0		2	11
Monophosphoglycerate mutase (PGAM-B)	254							
Enolase[k]	434							
Pyruvate kinase (PK)	574[m]	1	65	7	2–2	7–3	9	96
Glucose 6-phosphate dehydrogenase (G6PD)	515		115[n]	1	6–0		1	123
Cytochrome-b_5 reductase	276[o]		7	2	2–0		2	13
Adenylate kinase (AK)	194		2	1				3[p]
γ-Glutamylcysteine synthetase (GLCLC)[k,q]	637							
Glutathione synthetase (GSS)	474		13		1–0	1–0	1	16
Glutathione peroxidase (GSH-Px)	201							

[a]We have listed all enzymes in the intermediary metabolism of red cells for which—to the best of our knowledge—the corresponding cDNA/gene has been cloned. There are other enzymes the deficiency of which may be associated with HA, but for which no molecular information is yet available: for instance pyrimidine 5'-nucleotidase.

[b]No entry in this column means that there are no known isoenzymes; therefore, it is assumed that the same enzyme type is present in all tissues.

[c]The following abbreviations have been used. CNS, central nervous system involvement; HA, hemolytic anemia; NM, neuromuscular manifestations.

[d]Data available only on some patients.

[e]Including N-terminal methionine, which is cleaved off in most or all cases.

[f]Each individual molecular change, if observed in more than one patient, has been counted only once.

[g]Two HK mutations were found in the same patient: 529 Leu→Ser and Δ162-193. Two large deletions were found in another patient: △ exons 3–14, Δ exons 5–8.

[h]PFK in normal red cells consists of a mixture of the five tetrameric species that can be formed from random association of the M (muscle) and L (liver) highly homologous subunits (i.e., M_4, M_3L, M_2L_2, ML_3, L_4).

[i]The only known aldolase mutations are 128 Asp→Gly and 206 Glu→Lys.

[j]5'UTR, 5' Untranslated region.

[k]Since no mutations have yet reported, there is no formal proof that HA associated with this enzyme deficiency is due to mutation of the corresponding gene.

[l]The only two DPGM mutations known were found in the same patient. They were: 89 Arg→Cys and Δ C205 (or 206). The deletion causes a frameshift resulting in an abnormal protein of 46 amino acids in which only the first 19 N-terminal amino acids are correct.

[m]The red cell form of PK called R is produced by the gene encoding the L (liver) subunit. Because a different promoter is used (*see* Fig. 22-5) the size of liver PK is 543 amino acids.

[n]The 115 missense mutations include two variants with normal activity, A and São Borja. Seven variants have 2 missense mutations each: these include G6PD Santamaria, G6PD Mount Sinai and the three variants that are called G6PD A—both of which have the mutation of G6PD A plus another mutation; G6PD Honiara and G6PD Bangkok. G6PD Vancouver variant has 3 different missense mutations (*see* Fig. 22-6).

[o]The cytoplasmic form of this enzyme, present in red cells, differs from the microsomal form present in other cells because, as a result of an alternative splicing pathway, it lacks the first 25 N-terminal amino acids. Therefore, in other cells, the size of the enzyme is 301 amino acids.

[p]The known AK mutations are: 128 Arg→Trp, 164 Tyr→Lys, and 107 Arg→Stop.

[q]γ-glutamylcysteine synthetase consist of two subunits, a catalytic subunit and a regulatory subunit; the data concerning the catalytic subunit are shown here.

[r]There is no clear evidence that inherited deficiency of glutathione peroxidase exists.

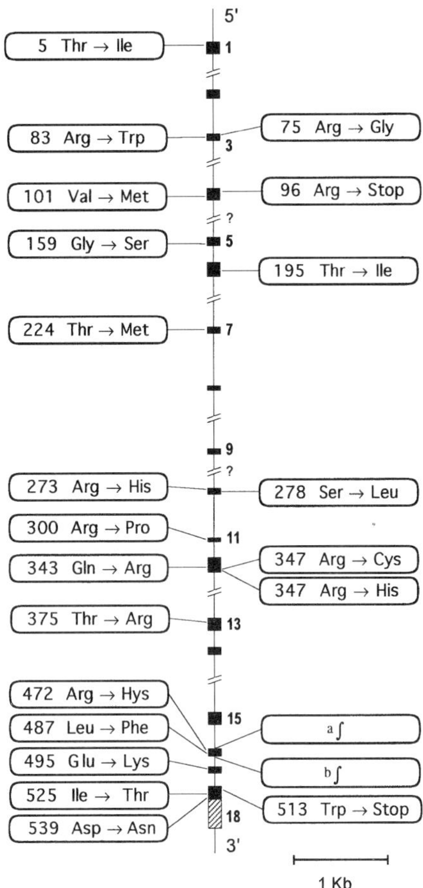

Figure 22-2 Diagram of mutations in the *GPI* gene. In this and in the following figures, the central vertical line represents the genomic structure, with exons shown as thick blocks and introns as thin lines. Exons are numbered. Long introns are signalled by a diagonal double line. Additional symbols are as follows: ■, translated exon region; ▨, untranslated exon region; △, deletion; Ins, insertion; ∫, splicing error. The *GPI* genomic gene spans approximately 40 kb. A question mark (?) next to a diagonal double line indicates that the exact length of the intron is unknown. [a]This variant has a mutation in the acceptor site that causes an aberrant splicing of exon 16. [b]This variant has a deletion of the last 2 nucleotides of exon 16 and of the first 2 nucleotides of intron 16, with possible abnormal splicing.

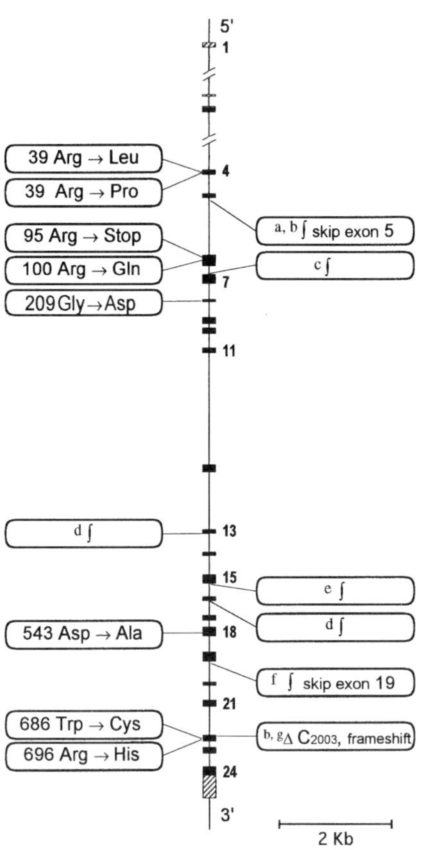

Figure 22-3 Diagram of known mutations in the *PFK-M* gene. The *PFK-M* genomic gene spans approximately 30 kb. [a]This mutation at the donor site of intron 5 causes exon 5 to be skipped (in frame) and thus a protein lacking 26 amino acids is produced. [b]Each one of these two *PFK* mutations has been found recurrently in several Ashkenazi families. [c]This mutation at the acceptor site of intron 6 causes the production (thanks to the presence of two cryptic splice sites in exon 7) of two abnormal mRNA species, one lacking 5-bp and the other lacking 12-bp: the latter is more abundant and in frame, thus producing a protein lacking 4 amino acids. [d]The mutation in the donor site causes splicing to a cryptic site in the intron, resulting in the retention of some intronic sequence and a premature stop. [e]The mutation at the donor site of intron 15 causes splicing to a cryptic splicing site in exon 15 (in frame) and thus a protein lacking 25 amino acids is produced. [f]This mutation at the donor site of intron 19 causes exon 19 to be skipped (in frame), thus, a protein lacking 55 amino acids is produced. [g]This single basepair deletion causes a frameshift with a stop codon 47 nucleotides downstream and a truncated protein of 683 amino acids, with the last 16 C-terminal amino acids being incorrect. (For other symbols, *see* legend to Fig. 22-2.)

3. Chronic nonspherocytic hemolytic anemia (CNSHA). In contrast to the large majority of G6PD deficient subjects who have minimal and subclinical hemolysis in the steady state, a small minority of G6PD deficient individuals have chronic anemia of variable severity. This rare condition is rather similar to CNSHA associated with glycolytic enzymopathies *(see above)* and, again, it is of variable severity. However, it is characteristically exacerbated by the same agents that can cause acute hemolytic anemia in people with the ordinary type of G6PD deficiency.

DIAGNOSIS When there is anemia, it is usually normocytic and normochromic, and it may be from moderate to extremely severe. In AHA, the anemia results from intravascular hemolysis; and hence, it is associated with hemoglobinemia, hemoglobinuria, and low or absent plasma haptoglobin. The blood film shows anisocytosis, polychromasia, and other features associated with acute hemolysis, including spherocytes. In severe cases, the poikilocytosis is very marked, with presence of bizarre forms, numerous red cells that appear to have an uneven distribution of hemoglobin within them (hemighosts), and red cells that appear to have had parts of them bitten away ("bite cells," or "blister cells"). Supravital staining with methyl violet, if done promptly, reveals the presence of Heinz bodies, consisting of precipitates of denatured hemoglobin. In CNSHA, the morphology is less characteristic. The final diagnosis must rely on the direct demonstration of decreased activity of G6PD in red cells. In most cases, one of the commercially available "spot tests" is adequate, but the gold standard is, as for all other enzymes, a spectrophotometric assay.

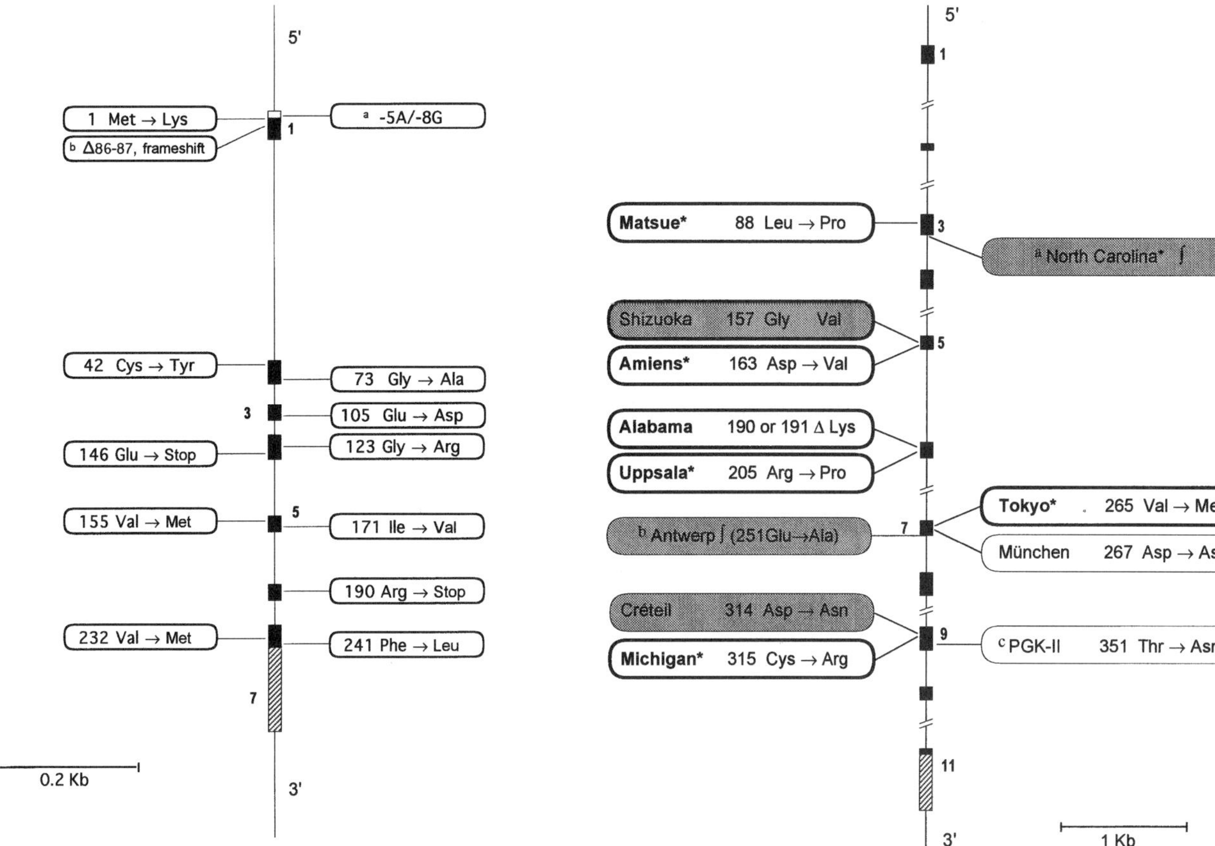

Figure 22-4 Diagram of mutations in the *TPI* gene. The *TPI* genomic gene spans 3.2 kb. [a]Sequencing of this variant reveals of two single base change in the 5' untranslated region. It is not clear whether and how this causes enzyme deficiency. [b]The deletion of these two nucleotides causes a frameshift. (For other symbols, *see* legend to Fig. 22-2.)

Figure 22-5 Diagram of known mutations in the *PGK* gene. The *PGK* genomic gene spans approximately 23 kb. The methionine initiator is counted as residue zero. ⬭, hemolytic anemia; ⬬, myopathy; *, CNS involvement. [a]This mutation in the donor site of intron 3 causes splicing to a cryptic site within intron 3 with the consequent insertion of 10 extra amino acids in the protein. [b]This mutation in exon 7 causes either a missense mutation and the alteration of the consensus donor splice sequence site with alternative splicing to a cryptic site in intron 7 and a premature stop. [c]The variant PGK-II, found at a polymorphic frequency in New Guinea, has normal activity. (For other symbols, *see* legend to Fig. 22-2.)

GENETIC BASIS G6PD is a homodimeric molecule, and its single subunit is encoded by an X-linked gene (Table 22-1). Therefore, in areas with high prevalence of G6PD deficiency, male hemizygotes and female heterozygotes are common, but female homozygotes are rare. As a result of the phenomenon of X-chromosome inactivation in somatic cells, female heterozygotes are genetic mosaics, in whom approximately one-half of the red cells are normal and approximately one-half are G6PD deficient; however, sometimes the ratio is greatly imbalanced. Clinical manifestations in heterozygotes are milder than in hemizygotes and in homozygotes, roughly in proportion to the fraction of red cells that are G6PD deficient.

MOLECULAR PATHOPHYSIOLOGY AHA associated with G6PD deficiency results from the action of an exogenous factor on intrinsically abnormal red cells. Although the sequence of events ending in hemolysis is not completely understood, it is clear that the exogenous agent taxes the capacity of the red cell to detoxify oxygen radicals, which is impaired by the short supply of NADPH in G6PD deficient red cells. Hence, the notion of oxidative hemolysis. AHA is seen with variants of G6PD that retain some 10% of the normal enzyme activity, or even less, if the kinetic parameters are favorable. By contrast, with some other variants the steady-state level of G6PD is so low that, even in the absence of any oxidant challenge, it becomes limiting for red cell survival. This is the case in the patients with CNSHA, who may have a red cell life-span of between 10 and 50 days. Very numerous point mutations in the *G6PD* gene causing CNSHA have been identified (*see* Fig. 22-7). Although we cannot explain the reason for a severe clinical phenotype in every case, a cluster of mutations causing CNSHA in exons 10 and 11 corresponds closely to the region of the molecule where the two subunits interface. It is not surprising that amino acid replacements in this region will interfere with dimer formation or will cause marked instability of the dimer.

MANAGEMENT The most common manifestations of G6PD deficiency, NNJ and AHA, are largely preventable or controllable by screening, surveillance, and avoidance of triggering factors, particularly fava beans, by G6PD deficient subjects. When a patient presents with AHA, and once the cause is diagnosed, no specific treatment may be needed if the episode is mild. However, at the other end of the spectrum—especially in children—AHA may be a medical emergency requiring an immediate blood transfusion. The management of NNJ does not differ from that of NNJ owing to causes other than G6PD deficiency. To prevent neurological damage, it may have to include phototherapy and/or exchange blood transfusion. The management of CNSHA is simi-

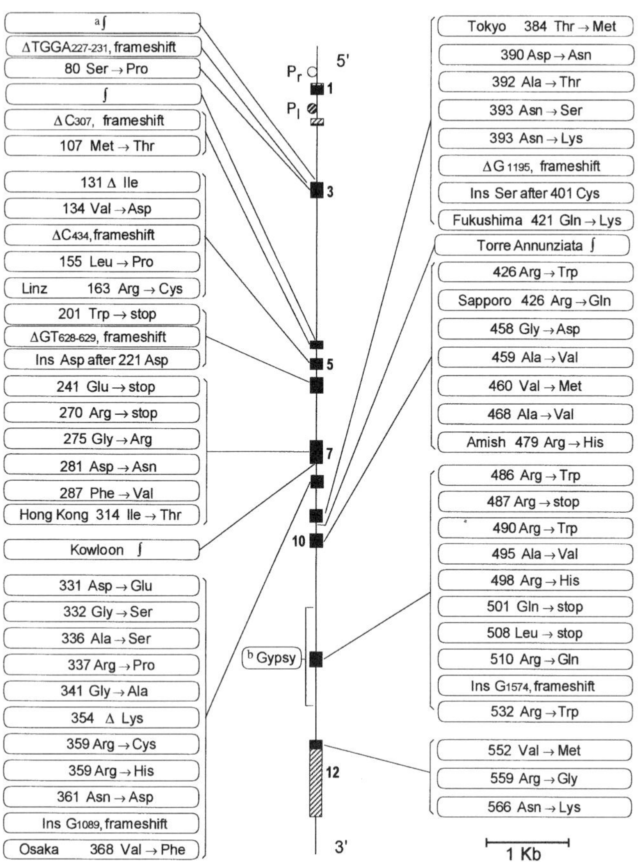

Figure 22-6 Diagram of mutations in the *PK* gene. The *PK* genomic gene spans 8.6 kb. The same gene encodes the R (red cell) and L (liver) form of PK. In the erythroid cell transcription starts from the upstream promoter (P_r ○); in the liver transcription starts from the downstream promoter (P_l ⊘). Thus, exon I of erythroid *PK* mRNA is missing in liver *PK* mRNA. [a]The consequences of this mutation at the acceptor site of intron 2 on RNA processing are not known. [b]This deletion removes the entire exon 11 and parts of intron 10 and intron 11 (total 1149 bp); it also causes a frameshift. (For other symbols, *see* legend to Fig. 22-2.) For reasons of space not all mutations can be shown.

lar to that of CNSHA caused by glycolytic enzymopathies, but, in addition, it is important to avoid exposure to potentially hemolytic drugs. Again, although there is no evidence of selective red cell destruction in the spleen (e.g., as seen instead in hereditary spherocytosis), splenectomy has proven beneficial in severe cases.

GLUTATHIONE SYNTHETASE DEFICIENCY

Glutathione (GSH) is a ubiquitous tripeptide with a range of important biological functions. In red cells, the main function of GSH is protection against oxidative damage. GSH is produced from glutamic acid, cysteine, and glycine through the action first of γ-glutamylcysteine synthetase and then glutathione synthetase (GSS) (*see* Fig. 22-1). GSS deficiency is a rare autosomal recessive disorder resulting in very low levels of GSH in red cells. Clinically, GSS deficiency may present in two different clinical forms: a mild form that causes only a compensated hemolytic anemia, and a severe form that causes also 5-oxyprolinuria and neurological manifestations. Twelve unrelated patients with GSS deficiency have been studied for mutations in the *GSS* gene and 16 different mutations have been identified: three patients were homozygotes, six were compound heterozygotes, and in three only a missense mutation was found in heterozygosity (Fig. 22-8).

CYTOCHROME B$_5$ REDUCTASE DEFICIENCY

A small amount of methemoglobin is formed in red cells continuously as a by-product of the cyclic oxygenation and deoxygenation of hemoglobin. It is estimated that methemoglobin would accumulate in blood at the rate of about 2% per day, unless it was continuously reduced. Red cells have both a NADPH-dependent and a NADH-dependent mechanism for the reduction of methemoglobin, but several lines of evidence indicate that the latter is by far more important physiologically. Cytochrome-b$_5$ reductase (formerly called diaphorase) is the currently accepted name for the enzyme that reduces methemoglobin using NADH as the electron donor. Patients with cytochrome-b$_5$ reductase deficiency can be also described as having methemoglobinemia. However, because this is caused by an enzyme defect rather than to a hemoglobin abnormality (Hb M), the former term is preferable.

PREVALENCE Cytochrome-b$_5$ reductase deficiency is relatively common in Alaskan Eskimos, but it is a rare condition elsewhere.

CLINICAL FEATURES The main finding is cyanosis, because since this is a result of the presence of methemoglobin rather than deoxyhemoglobin, it is sometimes referred to as pseudocyanosis, but with the naked eye, the two are not easily distinguished. There may be also a mild erythrocytosis, resulting from the erythropoietin-drive associated with the reduced oxygenation of tissues. A subset of patients with cytochrome-b$_5$ reductase deficiency (i.e., designated as having type II disease) may have also mental retardation, which can be severe, and other neurological signs including microcephaly, opisthotonus, and athetoids movements.

DIAGNOSIS Usually a patient presenting with cyanosis is suspected to have congenital heart disease or acquired cardiac or pulmonary disease; the suspicion may be reinforced by the coexistence of erythrocytosis. When the appropriate investigations are negative, a test for methemoglobin will explain the (pseudo)-cyanosis. The differentiation of methemoglobinemia caused by cytochrome-b$_5$ reductase deficiency from that caused by Hb M is based on electrophoretic and spectral studies of hemoglobin. An enzyme assay or a therapeutic trial of methylene blue will clinch the diagnosis.

GENETIC BASIS Clinically affected individuals are homozygotes or genetic compounds; therefore, methemoglobinemia secondary to cytochrome-b$_5$ reductase deficiency exhibits an autosomal recessive pattern of inheritance. This is in contrast to methemoglobinemia associated with Hb M, in which the pattern of inheritance is autosomal dominant.

MOLECULAR PATHOPHYSIOLOGY Several point mutations have been identified in the cytochrome-b$_5$ reductase gene in patients with congenital methemoglobinemia (Fig. 22-9). Not surprisingly, patients with type II disease have mutations that are different from those found in patients with type I disease: indeed, they include amino acid deletions and splicing mutations. Presumably, the resulting abnormal molecules are more unstable, or compromised in catalytic efficiency; therefore, the level of enzyme activity becomes severely reduced, not only in red cells, but also in nerve cells. In the latter, the enzyme is thought to be involved in lipid synthesis.

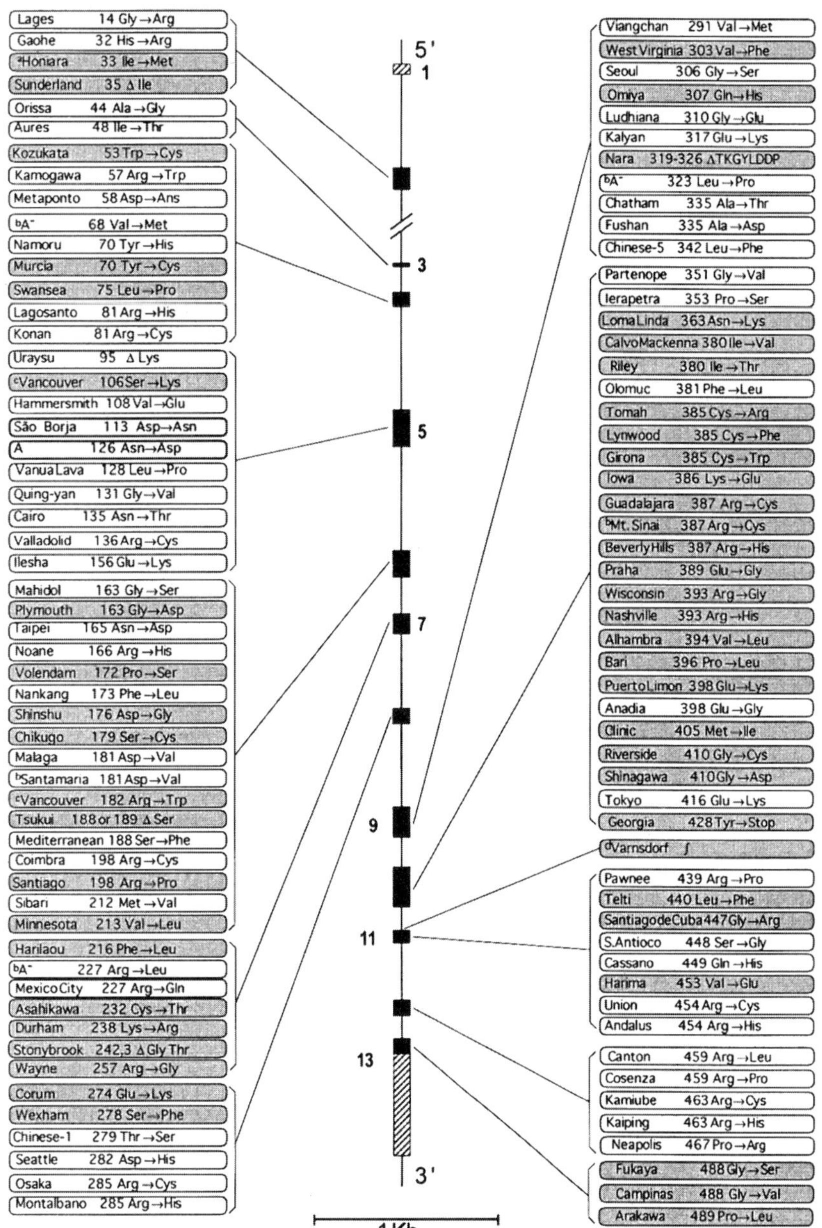

Figure 22-7 Diagram of mutations in the *G6PD* gene. The *G6PD* genomic gene spans approximately 18 kb. ⬭, variant with normal enzymatic activity; ⬭, variant that cause acute hemolytic anemia; ⬬, variant that cause chronic nonspherocytic hemolytic anemia (CNSHA). [a]This variant has, in addition to the mutation shown, also the mutation (454 Arg→Cys) of G6PD Andalus. [b]These variants have, in addition to the mutation shown, also the mutation (126 Asn→Asp) of G6PD A. [c]This variant has been reported to have three different mutations; two are unique (106 Ser→Lys and 182 Arg→Trp), whereas one is the mutation (198 Arg→Cys) of G6PD Coimbra. [d]The deletion of the last two nucleotides of intron 10 destroys the acceptor site with unknown effect on the processing of the transcript. (For other symbols, *see* legend to Fig. 22-2.) For reasons of space not all mutations can be shown.

MANAGEMENT Most patients with type I disease suffer little disability. However, if they are fair-skinned, their discoloration may create a cosmetic problem: this responds very well to the administration of methylene blue or ascorbic acid. The former activates the NADPH-dependent pathway of methemoglobin reduction; therefore, it is not effective if the patient happens to be also G6PD deficient. Unfortunately, no treatment is known for the neurological manifestations of type II disease. Knowledge of the molecular lesion makes it possible to offer prenatal diagnosis to a couples at risk for type II disease.

FUTURE DIRECTIONS

Red cells have been for decades a model system in the study of intermediary metabolism, and red cell enzymes have been a classical tool of biochemical genetics and of population genetics. With the cloning of most of the genes encoding red cell enzymes, it has been possible to validate many of the items predicted in earlier times: for instance, the prediction that most of the individuals affected with rare autosomal enzymopathies—barring inbreeding—would be genetic compounds rather than true homozygotes. From the point of view of genotype–phenotype correlations, the

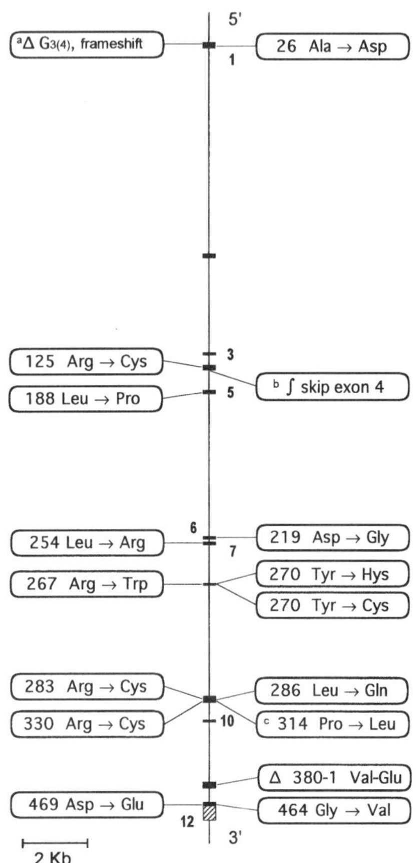

Figure 22-8 Diagram of mutations in the *GSS* gene. The *GSS* genomic gene spans approximately 23 kb. [a]This single base deletion causes a frameshift. [b]The mutation in the donor site results in aberrant splicing, whereby exon 4 is skipped. [c]This varient has normal activity. (For other symbols, *see* legend to Fig. 22-2.)

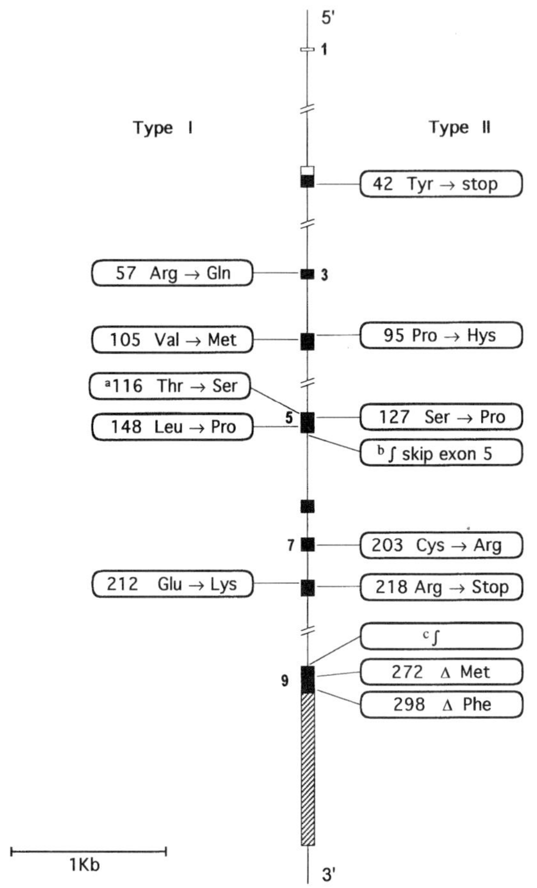

Figure 22-9 Diagram of known mutations in the *cytochrome b5 reductase* gene. The genomic gene spans approximately 31 kb. ▒, region of exon 1 and 2 encoding for transmembrane domain (25 aa), missing in the erythrocyte cytoplasmic form of the enzyme. The methionine initiator is counted as residue zero. There are two types of cytochrome-b_5 reductase deficiency. In type I, the enzyme deficiency is limited to the red cell cytoplasmic form, and its main clinical manifestation is pseudocyanosis. In type II, the enzyme deficiency involves both the cytoplasmic and the microsomal forms of the enzyme, and all tissues are affected. In addition to pseudocyanosis, there is mental retardation and other neurological signs. It is likely that type I mutations affect mainly the stability of the enzyme, whereas type II mutations either produce no viable protein or compromise drastically its catalytic activity. [a]This variant, found at a polymorphic frequency in African American, has normal activity. [b]The mutation at the donor site of intron 5 causes the skipping of exon 5 and produces in red cells a truncated protein of 102 amino acids. [c]The consequences of this mutation at the acceptor site of intron 8 on the RNA are not exactly known, but the protein product is undetectable by immunological analysis. (For other symbols, *see* legend to Fig. 22-2.)

analysis of at what point mutations cause what degree of change in stability or in catalytic properties of each enzyme has only just begun. The universe of patients with enzymopathies constitutes a living spontaneous mutagenesis laboratory in which structure–function relationships are, so to speak, displayed in vivo. From the practical point of view, the molecular analysis has not yet had any impact on management, which is still unsatisfactory, but it does provide the option of prenatal diagnosis in cases where previous family history has led to identifying a specific enzymopathy. Because chronic hemolytic anemia is the main clinical problem associated with these enzymopathies (in the majority of cases), they are an ideal target for correction by gene transfer into hematopoietic stem cells. Indeed, since the deficiency of most of these enzymes is likely to be a disadvantage even before erythroid cell differentiation reaches the end point of the mature red cell, it is conceivable that phenotypic correction might be self-selecting, thus abrogating the need for bone marrow ablation in future gene therapy protocols.

ACKNOWLEDGMENTS

We thank our colleagues F Alfinito, L Baronciani, S Miwa, L Pastore, A Rovira, JL Vives-Corrons, TJ Vulliamy, and A Zanella, for kindly communicating information on mutations not yet published. We are also very grateful to Professor A Afolayan and Professor B Rotoli for their support and critical reading of the manuscript.

SELECTED REFERENCES

Baronciani L, Bianchi P, Zanella A. Hematologically important mutations: Red cell pyruvate kinase. Blood Cells Mol Dis 1996;22:259–264.

Baronciani L, Beutler E. Molecular study of pyruvate kinase deficient patients with hereditary nonspherocytic hemolytic anemia. J Clin Invest 1995;95:1702–1709.

Beutler E. Hemolytic anemia in disorders of red cell metabolism. New York, Plenum Medical Book Company, 1978.

Beutler E, West C, Britton HA, et al. Glucosephosphate Isomerase (GPI) Deficiency Mutations Associated with Hereditary Nonspherocytic Hemolytic Anemia (HNSHA). Blood Cells Mol Dis 1997;23:402–409.

Bianchi M, Magnani M. Hexokinase mutations that produce nonspherocytic hemolytic anemia. Blood Cells, Mol Dis 1995;21:2–8.

Cappellini MD, Martinez di Montemuros F, De Bellis G, Debernardi S, Dotti C, Fiorelli G. Multiple G6PD mutations are associated with a clinical and biochemical phenotype similar to that of G6PD Mediterranean. Blood 1996;87:3953–3958.

Cohen-Solal M, Valentin C, Plassa F, et al. Identification of new mutations in two phosphoglycerate kinase (PGK) variants expressing different clinical syndromes: PGK Creteil and PGK Amiens. Blood 1994;84:898–903.

Dacie JV. Haemolytic anaemias. In: The Hereditary Haemolytic Anaemias, vol I, 3rd ed. London: Churchill Livingstone, 1985.

Dacie JV, Lewis SM. Practical Haematology, 8th ed. London: Churchill Livingstone, 1995.

Dahl N, Pigg M, Ristoff E, et al. Missense mutations in the human glutathione synthetase gene result in severe metabolic acidosis, 5-oxoprolinuria, hemolytic anemia and neurological dysfunction. Hum Mol Genet 1997;6:1147–1152.

Harris RW. The red cell—production, metabolism, destruction: normal and abnormal. Cambridge: Harvard University Press, 1963.

Hollan S, Fujii H, Hirono A, et al. Hereditary triosephosphate isomerase (TPI) deficiency: two severely affected brothers, one with and one without neurological symptoms. Hum Genet 1993;92:486–490.

Kanno H, Fujii H, Wei DC, et al. Frame shift mutation, exon skipping, and a two-codon deletion caused by splice site mutations account for pyruvate kinase deficiency. Blood 1997;89:4213–4218.

Kishi H, Mukai T, Hirono A, Fujii H, Miwa S, Hori K. Human aldolase A deficiency associated with a hemolytic anemia: thermolabile aldolase due to a single base mutation. Proc Natl Acad Sci USA 1987;84: 8623–8627.

Kreuder J, Borkhardt A, Repp R, et al. Inherited metabolic myopathy and hemolysis due to a mutation in aldolase A. N Engl J Med 1996;334:1100–1104.

Lemarchandel V, Joulin V, Valentin C, et al. Compound heterozygosity in a complete erythrocyte bisphosphoglycerate mutase deficiency. Blood 1992;10:2643–2649.

Lukens JN. Hereditary hemolytic anemias associated with abnormalities of erythrocyte anaerobic glycolysis and nucleotide metabolism. In: Lee GR, Bittell TC, Foerster J, Athens JW, Lukens JN, eds. Wintrobe's Clinical Hematology, 9th ed. Philadelphia: Lea & Febiger, 1993; pp. 990–1005.

Luzzatto L, Mehta A. Glucose 6-phosphate dehydrogenase deficiency. In: Scriver CR, Beaudet AL, Sly WS, Valle D, eds. The Metabolic and Molecular Bases of Inherited Disease, 7th ed. New York: McGraw-Hill, 1995; pp. 3367–3398.

Manabe J, Arya R, Sumimoto H, et al. Two novel mutations in the reduced nicotinamide adenine dinucleotide (NADH)-cytochrome b_5 reductase gene of a patient with generalized type, hereditary methemoglobinemia. Blood 1996;88:3208–3215.

Matsuura S, Igarashi M, Tanizawa Y, et al. Human adenylate kinase deficiency associated with hemolytic anemia: a single base substitution affecting solubility and catalytic activity of the cytosolic adenylate kinase. J Biol Chem 1989;264:10,148–10,155.

McCaneu JR, Thomas K. Human testis-specific PGK gene lacks introns and possesses characteristics of a processed gene. Nature 1987;326:501–504.

Miwa S, Fujii H. Molecular basis of erythroenzymopathies associated with hereditary hemolytic anemia: tabulation of mutant enzymes. Am J Hematol 1996;51:122–132.

Naylor CE, Rowland P, Basak AK, et al. Glucose 6-phosphate dehydrogenase mutations causing enzyme deficiency in a model of the tertiary structure of the human enzyme. Blood 1996;87:2974–2982.

Qualtieri A, Pedace V, Bisconte G, et al. Severe erythrocyte adenilate kinase deficiency due to homozygous A→C substitution at codon 164 of human AK1 gene associated with chronic haemolytic anaemia. Br J Haematol 1997;99:770–776.

Raben N, Sherman JB. Mutations in muscle phosphofructokinase gene. Hum Mutat 1995;6:1–6.

Schneider A, Cohen-Solal M. Hematologically important mutations: Triosephosphate isomerase. Blood Cells Mol Dis 1996;22:82–84.

Schneider A, Westwood B, Yim C, et al. The 1591C mutation in triosephosphate isomerase deficiency, tightly linked polymorphism and a common haplotype in all known families. Blood Cells Mol Dis 1996;22:115–125.

Sierra-Rivera E, Summar ML, Dasouki M, Krishnamani MRS, Phillips JA, Freeman ML. Assignment of the gene (GLCLC) that encodes the heavy subunit of gamma-glutamylcysteine synthetase to human chromosome 6. Cytogenetics and Cell Genetics 1995; 70: 278–279.

Vieira LM, Kaplan JC, Kanh A, Laroux A. Four new mutations in the NADH-cytochrome b5 reductase gene from patients with recessive congenital methemoglobinemia type II. Blood 1995;85: 2254–2262.

Vulliamy T, Luzzatto L, Hirono A, Beutler, E. Hematologically important mutations: glucose-6-phosphate dehydrogenase. Blood Cells Mol Dis 1997;23:302–313.

Yoshida A. Molecular Abnormalities of phosphoglycerate kinase. Blood Cells Mol Dis 1996;22:265–267.

23 Coagulation Disorders

MARTINA DALY, ANNE GOODEVE, PETER WINSHIP, AND IAN PEAKE

INTRODUCTION

Inherited disorders of the coagulation system have been recognized for many years, and their study formed the basis of laboratory experiments from which grew the concept of clotting factors and the coagulation cascade with its subsequent refinements. The genes encoding these factors have now also been identified and cloned (Table 23-1), and, in most cases, a series of causative mutations have been detected. The gene for von Willebrand factor (VWF) has also been identified and cloned. Although not a procoagulant factor, VWF plays an integral part in the primary hemostatic process, and its deficiency results in von Willebrands disease (VWD), the most common bleeding disorder. This chapter will concentrate on the genetic basis of the three most common disorders, hemophilia A (factor VIII deficiency), hemophilia B (factor IX deficiency), and VWD. Reference to rarer defects in other factors will also be made.

THE GENETIC BASIS OF HEMOPHILIA A

Hemophilia A is a recessively inherited X-linked disorder of coagulation factor VIII (FVIII) with an incidence of 1 in 5000 in the male population. The gene for FVIII was identified and cloned in 1984 and is found on the long arm of the X chromosome at Xq28.

Human FVIII is synthesized primarily in hepatocytes as an approximately 300-kDa single-chain polypeptide, having a repeated domain structure A1-A2-B-A3-C1-C2. Activation of FVIII occurs by thrombin cleavage at sites within the B-domain, giving rise to a heterodimer comprised of a constant sized light chain (A3-C1-C2) and a heavy chain (A1-A2). FVIII circulates in complex with VWF, an association that protects it from proteolytic degradation. Thrombin activation releases FVIII from VWF and allows it to function as a cofactor for FIXa in the conversion of FX to its activated form (FXa).

FACTOR VIII GENE STRUCTURE The factor VIII gene is 186 kb in length and contains 26 exons. The FVIII mRNA is approximately 9 kb long and contains 7053 nucleotides of coding sequence. The mature factor VIII protein contains 2332 amino acids (Fig. 23-1).

Of particular interest is intron 22 of the gene that contains a CpG island from which two adjacent genes, F8A and F8B are encoded in opposite orientations. This was the first example in humans of genes being found wholly contained within another gene. The F8A gene is in the opposite orientation to the FVIII gene, is intronless, and produces a mRNA transcript of 1.8 kb found in many tissues. F8B is transcribed in the same direction as FVIII. Its first exon, encoding eight amino acids, is within intron 22 and, in the mRNA, is spliced to exons 23–26 of the FVIII gene. The function of the F8A and F8B genes and their predicted protein products are not known. F8A lies within a 9.5-kb region of DNA (int22h) repeated two additional times approximately 400 kb telomeric to FVIII. The three homologous regions (int22h 1, 2 and 3) are identical in over 99.9% of their sequence, and each of the three F8A genes is transcribed.

DEFECTS IN THE FACTOR VIII GENE Following the cloning of the FVIII gene in 1984, it became possible to begin analysis for mutations resulting in hemophilia A. Southern blotting analysis initially revealed a few patients with total or partial deletions or point mutations at specific restriction enzyme sites (e.g., C to T transitions at CpG sites identified by TaqI digestion—*see below*). The more sensitive techniques now applied to mutation detection are all based on amplification of DNA by the polymerase chain reaction (PCR), followed by mismatch detection methods (e.g., SSCP, DGGE, and so on) and DNA sequencing to characterize the mutations found. These techniques can be applied to genomic DNA or cDNA, produced by reverse transcription and PCR amplification (RT-PCR) from FVIII mRNA. The current hemophilia A database demonstrates the variety of mutations responsible for FVIII defects and is summarized in Table 23-2. The mutations reported have not been located by a systematic search/analysis of the gene and thus cannot be taken as a true representation of the relative incidence of the different mutations within the hemophilia A population. The table demonstrates that mutations can occur throughout the entire coding region of the FVIII gene, although no promoter or polyadenylation signal mutations have been identified to date. Twenty-five percent of single basepair substitutions occur at CpG dinucleotides; multiple mutations at these sites are frequent in the database and reinforce its "mutation hotspot" nature. Despite this, most of these mutations are "private," and are found in only one or a few unrelated families.

In contrast to the above, a novel type of mutation is now known to occur in the FVIII gene and accounts for nearly 50% of cases of severe hemophilia A. This DNA inversion is mediated by the three copies of int22h one located in intron 22 of FVIII, the other two 400 kb 5' and telomeric to the gene (Fig. 23-1). Homologous recombination appears to occur between the intron 22 copy (int22h-1) and either the distal (telomeric, int22h-3) or more proximal (int22h-2) copy, and this process occurs most readily at male meiosis when the X chromosome is largely unpaired. Recombina-

From: *Principles of Molecular Medicine* (J. L. Jameson, ed.), ©1998 Humana Press Inc., Totowa, NJ.

Table 23-1
Blood Coagulation Factor Genes

Clotting factor	*Gene, kb*	*Location*	*mRNA, kb*	*Inheritance pattern*
Fibrinogen (I)	α5.4		α2.2	Autosomal dominant or recessive
	β8.2	4q23–q23	β~2.5	
	γ8.4		γ~2.5	
Prothrombin (II)	20.2	11p	2	Autosomal recessive
Factor V	~80	1q21–q25	7	Autosomal recessive
Factor VII	13	13q34	~2.5	Autosomal recessive
Factor VIII	186	Xq28	8.8	X-linked recessive
Factor IX	34	Xq27.1	1.8	X-linked recessive
Factor X	25	13q34–qter	1.5	Autosomal recessive
Factor XI	23	4q32–q35	2	Autosomal recessive
Factor XII	12	5q33–qter	2-4	Autosomal recessive
Factor XIII	A160	A 6p24–25	A4	Autosomal recessive
	B28	B 1q31–32;1	B > 2	
von Willebrand Factor (VWF)	178	12p12–pter	9	Autosomal dominant or recessive

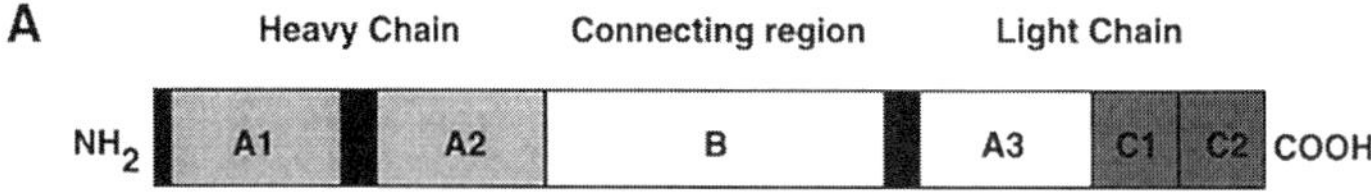

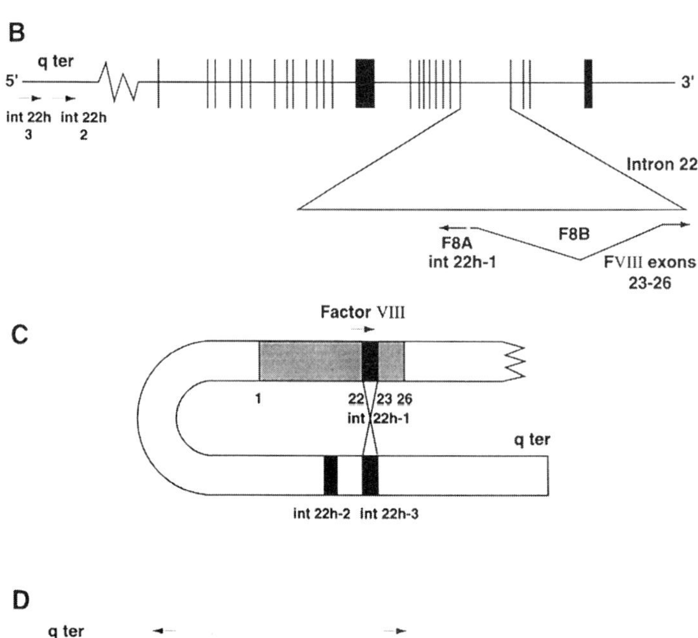

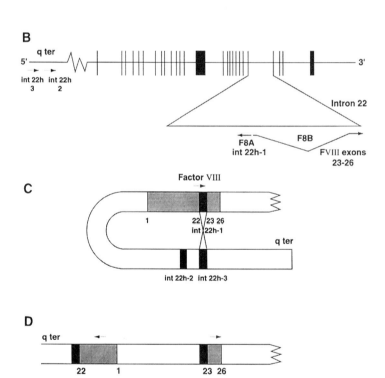

Figure 23-1 The factor VIII gene. (**A**) Structural domains of factor VIII. Triplicated A domains of 330 amino acids, the unique B domain of 980 amino acids and duplicated C domain of 150 amino acids, are shown. (**B**) Exon (vertical bar) and intron (horizontal line) structure of factor VIII gene. Intron 22 is shown expanded, the locations of F8A and F8B transcripts are shown and the three homologous regions int22h-1 within factor VIII, and -2 and -3 400 kb 5' and telomeric to factor VIII are indicated. (**C**) An intrachromosomal crossover event, mediated by homologous recombination between int22h-1 and -3 is shown. This results in the common distal form of factor VIII gene inversion shown in (**D**). (D) Following an inversion event, introns 1–22 of the factor VIII gene now lie 400 kb 5' and telomeric to exons 23–26 of the gene, in the opposite transcriptional orientation.

tion results in FVIII exons 1–22, in addition to adjacent DNA becoming inverted and relocated some 400 kb from its normal position, with exons 23–26 remaining in their original location. Therefore, intact FVIII transcript and protein cannot be produced. Crossover with the most distal int22h sequence results in a type 1 inversion. This is the most common inversional event, accounting for 82% of all inversions and 35% of all patients with severe disease. Crossover involving the proximal int22h results in a type 2

Table 23-2
Summary of 1998 Database for Mutations in the FVIII and FIX Genes in Patients with Hemophilia A and B[a]

	Hemophilia A[a,b]	*Hemophilia B[c]*
Patient entries	536	1713
Unique molecular events	304	652
Short deletions or insertions	48	132
Large deletions	80	29[d]
Different amino acid substitutions	155	389
STOP mutations	27	55
Percentage involving CpG transitions	48	58

[a]From Kemball-Cook et al. Nucleic Acids Res 1998;26:216–219. http://europium.mrc.rpms.ac.uk
[b]Does not include the FVIII gene inversion responsible for up to 50% of all severe hemophilia A.
[c]From Giannelli et al. Nucleic Acids Res 1998;26:265–268. http://www.umds.ac.uk/molgen/haemBdatabase.htm.
[d]Not included in Giannelli et al. (1998) database.

Table 23-3
Useful DNA Polymorphisms Within or Flanking the Human Factor VIII, Factor IX and von Willebrand Factor Genes

Gene	*Type of polymorphism*	*Restriction enzyme*	*Location*	*Detection method[d]*	*Heterozygosity (Caucasian)[a]*
F VIII	RFLP	*Taq*I	5'	Probe	0.40
	(G/A)	—	Int7	PCR	0.33
	VNTR CA repeat	—	Int13	PCR	0.80 (10 alleles)
	RFLP	*Bcl*I	Int18	PCR	0.39
	RFLP	*Hind*III	Int19	PCR	0.38
	RFLP	*Msp*I	Int22	Probe	0.01[b]
	RFLP	*Xba*I	Int22	PCR	0.49
	VNTR CA repeat	—	Int22	PCR	0.55 (6 alleles)
	RFLP	*Bgl*I	3'	Probe	0.25
	RFLP	*Msp*I	3'	Probe	0.43
F IX	RFLP	*Mse*I	5'	PCR	0.44
	RFLP	*Bam*HI	5'	PCR	0.04
	DEL/INS[e]	—	Int1	PCR	0.36
	RFLP	*Bam*HI	Int3	PCR	0.11
	RFLP	*Xmn*I	Int3	PCR	0.41
	RFLP	*Taq*I	Int4	PCR	0.45
	RFLP	*Msp*I	Int4	PCR	0.32
	RFLP	*Mnl*I	Codon 148	PCR	0.44
	(A/G)	—	Codon 192	PCR	0.01[c]
	RFLP	*Hha*I	3'	PCR	0.48
VWF RFLP: Over 30 have been reported.					
VNTR (AGAT repeats): two regions in intron 40. Multiallelic.					

[a]Heterozygosity rates can vary in different ethnic groups.
[b]0.13 in Asians.
[c]0.11 in Asians.
[d]Probe (Southern blot) method when PCR-based technique has not been reported.
[e]Dimorphic with two major forms differing by 50 bp.

inversion and occurs less frequently (15%). The number of copies of int22h outside the FVIII gene appears to be polymorphic, with some individuals having extra complete or partial copies that can result in rarer types of inversion (3A, 3B, or other variants). Inversions can be readily detected by Southern blotting following DNA digestion with BclI and using a probe for part of the int22h sequence. Overall, this inversion is the causative mutation in 43% of patients with severe disease and accounts for 20% of all cases of hemophilia A.

GENETIC SCREENING FOR HEMOPHILIA A In families affected by hemophilia A, female relatives of patients wish to know their carrier status. This can be achieved either by tracking the defective FVIII gene through the family by using polymorphic genetic markers or by detection of the causative mutation. The latter procedure is the most technically demanding and expensive, unless the inversion mutation is present, but is the ideal approach.

Since mutation detection is not available in many laboratories, the approach most frequently adopted for noninversion families is that of gene tracking, using DNA polymorphism analysis. A number of intragenic restriction fragment length polymorphisms (RFLP) in the FVIII gene have been described. However, the CA dinucleotide repeat polymorphisms located in introns 13 and 22 are the most useful (*see* Table 23-3). Heterozygosity rates in females from different ethnic backgrounds vary from 30 to 90%.

The suggested strategy for hemophilia A analysis is thus to first determine whether the FVIII gene inversion is present. If not, then dinucleotide repeats should be examined; if these are not informative, try RFLPs. Approximately 85% of families examined will be informative by using one of these intragenic polymorphisms. The probability of error caused by crossover at meiosis between a factor VIII gene mutation, and the intragenic polymorphism used to track its inheritance is <1%. For the families remaining uninformative, two extragenic markers at loci St14 and DX13 can be used with caution, since an approximate 5% crossover rate at meiosis has been reported between these loci and the FVIII gene locus. Overall, about 5% of families are uninformative for the FVIII gene inversion and the intragenic and extragenic polymorphisms outlined *above*. For these kindred, direct mutation analysis is the only option. Approximately, one-third of all cases of hemophilia have no prior family history of the disorder (sporadic hemophilia A). Prior to recognition of the FVIII gene inversion, 85% of mothers of these isolated cases were estimated to be true carriers of hemophilia, based on phenotypic analysis or by retrospective diagnosis following the birth of a second affected male child. A further proportion were thought to be mosaics for the mutation (i.e., it was present in only a proportion of their tissues). Since the recognition of the FVIII gene inversion and its ready detection, 96% of mothers of sporadic cases of hemophilia A caused by the inversion have been shown to carry the mutation. It should be noted that in families without the FVIII gene inversion and with no prior history of hemophilia, carrier diagnosis by linkage analysis is only able to exclude carrier status.

Prenatal diagnosis of hemophilia A is generally achieved by chorionic villus sampling (CVS) at 10–13 weeks' gestation. Karyotype analysis is performed to determine fetal sex and eliminate any chromosomal abnormalities. Fetal sex can also be determined by PCR. Chorionic villus DNA can be used for the detection of a previously identified familial mutation, or of a polymorphic allele in phase with hemophilia A in that particular family.

MOLECULAR PATHOPHYSIOLOGY OF HEMOPHILIA A Patients with hemophilia A can either have levels of FVIII activity and protein reduced in parallel (crossreacting material negative [CRM$^-$]) or have dysfunctional protein present at normal (CRM positive [CRM$^+$]) or reduced (CRM reduced) level. The mutations found in CRM$^+$ and CRM-reduced patients are important in understanding the functional significance of particular amino acids. Only the small proportion of mutations that result in FVIII protein production in vivo and in vitro enable the effect of the mutation on the protein to be elucidated. Thus, mutations at Arg 372 and Ser 373 that abolish thrombin cleavage in the heavy chain and at Arg 1689 that abolishes thrombin cleavage in the light chain result in CRM$^+$ hemophilia A where FVIII cannot be activated.

VWF binds to FVIII in a region between Lys 1673 and Glu 1684. There are two sulfated tyrosines in this region—Tyr 1664 and Tyr 1680. Several unrelated instances of Tyr 1680 Phe have been reported that result in moderate CRM-reduced hemophilia A. Replacement of tyrosine by phenylalanine results in loss of high-affinity binding to VWF. Other mutations appear to create new glycosylation sites

Approximately one-third of all hemophilia A patients will develop inhibitors (antibodies) directed against FVIII, following replacement therapy with FVIII. A small number of these inhibitors are persistent, of high titer, and cause considerable problems in the management of bleeds. Inhibitor development appears to be related to some extent to the severity of the causative mutation, with, for example, patients having major gene deletions being more likely to develop an inhibitor than those with a missense mutation. However, this is not the sole influence, and it is now clear that the patient's genetic background (HLA type) and the FVIII concentrate with which they are treated can also contribute to inhibitor development.

THE GENETIC BASIS OF HEMOPHILIA B

Hemophilia B (Christmas Disease), a sex-linked recessive blood coagulation disorder occurring at a frequency of approximately 1 in 30,000 males, is caused by reduced levels of biologically active coagulation factor IX in the plasma and is clinically indistinguishable from hemophilia A. The biochemical distinction between classical hemophilia and Christmas disease first became apparent in 1952, with the realization that one of two different components of the plasma could be reduced or absent in patients with "hemophilia." Laboratory clotting tests have subsequently been developed to permit the differential diagnosis of these two conditions. The clinical similarities between the two conditions can be rationalized, once it is appreciated that both factor VIII and factor IX participate at the same step in the middle phase of the blood coagulation cascade. Indeed, factor VIII acts as a cofactor in the enzymatic cleavage of coagulation factor X by the activated form of factor IX. Christmas disease patients can be broadly classified into one of two categories on the basis of biochemical tests for factor IX antigen (FIXAg) and factor IX clotting (FIXc) levels. Sixty percent of patients are termed CRM$^-$ and show characteristically low circulating levels of biologically active factor IX. The remaining 40% of patients have lowered or near normal levels of circulating factor IX with a low biological activity and are therefore referred to as CRM$^+$. Approximately 1% of patients have absolutely no detectable plasma factor IX and raise antibodies to the exogenous factor IX administered during replacement therapy.

FIX GENE STRUCTURE FIX cDNA clones were isolated from both bovine and human cDNA libraries in the early 1980s and showed the full-length human cDNA to be 2.8 kb, including a 296p 5' noncoding and a 1.39-kb 3' noncoding region (Fig. 23-2). These clones were then used as hybridization probes to screen human genomic libraries, and the entire 34-kb factor IX gene was isolated as a series of clones. The human FIX gene has been assigned to Xq27.1. The gene has been shown to comprise eight exons, separated by seven intervening regions of variable length, and the entire 34-kb region of DNA has been sequenced.

DEFECTS IN THE FACTOR IX GENE Recent advances in DNA technology and mutation detection methods combined with the relatively small size and low complexity of the factor IX locus mean that defining the causative mutation in each individual patient has become a possibility. An international database has been established, and the most recent data is summarized in Table 23-2. As with hemophilia A and the FVIII gene, a large number of different mutations have been found within the FIX gene in individuals with hemophilia B. Indeed, ongoing research programs directed towards establishing national databases listing the precise molecular defect in each individual with hemophilia B are being established in the United Kingdom, Sweden, and New Zealand. Once established, these will serve as a valuable resource, enabling precise mutation information to be made available in these countries to all families with a history of the disease *(see below)*.

GENETIC SCREENING FOR HEMOPHILIA B As with hemophilia A, the X-linked nature of hemophilia B inheritance and the resulting silent transmission of the condition through

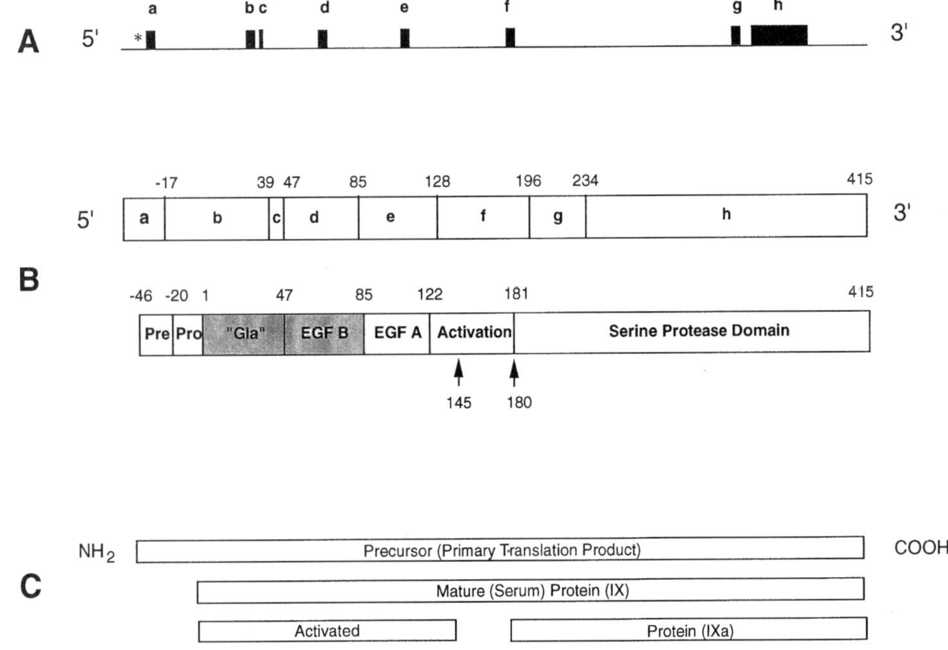

Figure 23-2 Organization of the factor IX gene and protein. **(A)** Line diagram of the 34 kb factor IX gene locus showing the location of the 8 exons, a–h. *Promoter region of the gene. **(B)** Factor IX mRNA and protein domain structure *(below)* showing the close correspondence between the 8 exons and 7 protein domains are numbered relative to the 1st residue of the mature serum protein. The peptide bonds cleaved to produce the two chain activated form of factor IX (IXa) are shown by arrows. **(C)** Sequential processing of the precursor molecule to the mature serum protein is achieved by excision of the pre- and proleader sequences. The cysteine-bridged two-chain activated protein (IXa) is produced by removal of the activation peptide (amino acid residues 145–180) from the mature serum protein.

the female line to male offspring means that screening for female "carriers" and prenatal screening of potentially affected male fetuses forms the major focus of any genetic screening program.

Original carrier screening methods based on a combination of measured circulating factor IX protein levels and estimating prior risk by pedigree analysis were at best only 80% accurate. Accordingly, as with hemophilia A, this procedure has been largely superceded by the more reliable methods of linkage analysis with intragenic RFLP markers or direct detection of the genetic defect itself in a particular kindred.

Useful RFLPs have been characterized either within the factor IX structural gene itself or in the immediate 5' and 3' flanking sequences. (Table 23-3). The use of any of these polymorphic markers to "tag" the defective gene and follow it through the affected pedigree will, where diagnosis is possible, allow carrier status (or prenatal diagnosis) to be made with 99.9% certainty. Varying levels of overall heterozygosity for the polymorphisms are observed in different ethnic groups and range from approximately 95% in Caucasians to less than 50% in Chinese. However, approximately one third of hemophilia B cases arise in pedigrees with no prior history of the condition. As with hemophilia A and the FVIII gene, whether these represent genuine cases of *de novo* mutation in either the patient or his mother, or simply the silent transmission of an existing mutation through the female line for a number of generations, cannot be deduced without first knowing the exact nature of the molecular defect. Fortunately, the identification of causative mutations within the FIX gene in patients with hemophilia B is becoming increasingly possible *(see above)* and, in several laboratories, polymorphism-based family studies have been replaced by direct mutation analysis.

MOLECULAR PATHOPHYSIOLOGY OF HEMOPHILIA B

The eight exons, a–h, of the factor IX gene each encode, at least in part, distinct protein domains of the mature protein (Fig. 23-2). Hence, the first exon, a, contains the 5' noncoding region of the mRNA and also encodes the hydrophobic signal domain of the primary translation product (precursor molecule). Exon b encodes the hydrophilic pro sequence of the precursor molecule. The prepro 46-amino acid leader sequence must be cleaved to allow release of the blood-borne 415-amino acid single-chain mature glycoprotein from its site of synthesis in the liver. The bulk of exon b encodes the first domain of the mature factor IX molecule. The posttranslational γ-carboxylation of 12 glutamic acid residues in this domain is instrumental in the formation of calcium bridges between this protein domain of the molecule and the phospholipid surface at its site of action on the vascular endothelium. The third exon, c, encodes a hydrophobic stack domain that is essential for the interaction of factor IX with its cofactor factor VIII. Two domains with homology to epidermal growth factor (EGF) are encoded by exons d and e; the EGF-B domain (encoded by exon d) containing a high-affinity calcium binding site required for the expression of full biological activity. Cleavage of the activation domain (encoded by exon f) during the coagulation process yields the two chain-activated forms of the mature protein molecule. Finally, the seventh and eighth exons, g and h, encode the catalytic activity domain seen in all members of the vitamin K dependent serine protease family, of which factor IX is one example.

Inspection of the current 1998 worldwide database of 1713 hemophilia B mutations (summarized in Table 23-2) indicates that just over one-third (652) are unique molecular events and confirms the extreme genetic diversity of the condition alluded to in

Table 23-4
Diagnosis and Molecular Basis of von Willebrand's Disease

Type	*Diagnostic criteria*	*Inheritance*	*Location of mutations*
Type 1	Quantitative deficiency of VWF	Autosomal dominant or recessive	Generally unknown, no specific region
Type 2A	Qualitative defect of VWF Reduced platelet binding Lack of HMW VWF multimers	Autosomal dominant	A2 domain
Type 2B	Qualitative defect of VWF Decreased platelet binding	Autosomal dominant	A1 domain Cys509–Cys695 loop region
Type 2N	Qualitative defect of VWF Reduced FVIII binding	Autosomal recessive	FVIII binding domain D1-D3
Type 2M	Qualitative defect of VWF Reduced platelet binding Normal VWF multimer profile	Autosomal dominant	A1 domain
Type 3	Severe quantitative deficiency of VWF	Autosomal recessive	Throughout VWF gene Deletion, termination codon, and so on

an earlier section. As with many genetic disorders, any repeat mutations at specific residues in apparently unrelated patients are explicable on the basis of CpG dinucleotides acting as mutational "hot spots." Other commonly occurring mutations are accounted for by founder effects.

The study of naturally occurring mutations has helped define and confirm the proposed importance and functions of the domains described in the previous section. Hence, mutations at 9 of the 12 γ-carboxylated residues in the Gla domain and the CRM^+ phenotype of these patients confirms the functional importance of these residues and this domain (Fig. 23-2). Similarly, the identification of CRM^+ patients with mutations at critical residues in the high-affinity calcium binding EGF-B domain serve to highlight its functional significance (Fig. 23-2).

One of the most interesting insights into gene/protein structure function relationships to emerge from these studies is the identification of the Leyden subgroup of hemophilia B patients. These patients are characterized by classic symptoms of hemophilia B in early life but have only very mild—if any—symptoms in later years. This clinical recovery, apparently triggered by the onset of puberty in the affected individual, is accompanied by a corresponding rise in circulating plasma levels of FIXc and FIXAg. This subtype of hemophilia B has generated considerable interest and has led to the identification of a complex array of transcription factors responsible for the regulation of factor IX expression. A picture is emerging of a series of liver-specific transcription factor binding sites directing the tissue restricted mode of expression of factor IX. To date, all patients with the Leyden subtype have a mutation at one of these sites in the factor IX promoter region (Fig. 23-2). Although controversial, it has been postulated that the clinical recovery of these patients is partly triggered by a compensatory mechanism, whereby the increased levels of testosterone present following puberty interact with and activate an androgen response element in the FIX gene promoter.

THE DIAGNOSIS AND GENETIC BASIS OF VWD

VWD is the most common human inherited bleeding disorder, occurring in a mild form in up to 1% of some populations. It occurs as a result of quantitative and/or qualitative deficiency of VWF, a multifunctional plasma glycoprotein synthesized in vascular endothelial cells and megakaryocytes and found in plasma, platelets, and in the subendothelial cell vascular matrix. VWF exists in plasma and platelets as a series of high-molecular-weight multimers, ranging from 5×10^5 to 2×10^7 Dalton. The two major functions of VWF are to form a link between exposed subendothelium and platelets and to bind to and protect coagulation factor VIII from premature proteolytic inactivation in plasma. The former function is multimer dependent with the largest multimers an essential requirement. VWD diagnosis is made by quantitative analysis of plasma VWF as VWF antigen (VWFAg), or qualitative analysis of VWF multimeric profile (i.e., its ability to bind to platelet glycoprotein GPIb/IX [measured as VWF Ristocetin Cofactor Activity], to collagen and to factor VIII).

The clinical and genetic heterogeneity of VWD is reflected in its recently revised classification (Table 23-4). Types 1 and 3 VWD refer to partial quantitative and virtually complete quantitative deficiency of VWF respectively. Type 2 VWD refers to qualitative VWF deficiency and is subdivided into four further categories, depending on the physicochemical properties exhibited by the VWF: Types 2A and 2M VWD refer to variants having decreased platelet-binding function associated with the presence (type 2M) or absence (type 2A) of high mol wt VWF multimers. Type 2B VWD refers to those qualitative variants having increased affinity for the platelet VWF receptor, GpIb/IX, and type 2N VWD refers to variants with reduced binding affinity for factor VIII.

Considerable variability in the severity of clinical symptoms and penetrance has been documented in VWD families and combined dominant and recessive inheritance within the same kindred has been described. The latter most likely reflects the multimeric structure of VWF and the possibility for mutated subunits to interact with normal subunits in a "dominant-negative" manner. Type 1 disease is usually dominantly inherited, whereas the most severe type 3 disease is often a recessive disorder. Some type 2 variants (e.g., type 2B) show dominant inheritance, and others (e.g., type 2N) are characterized by recessive inheritance. Molecular genetic analysis has revealed that compound heterozygosity, particularly coinheritance of types 1 and 2N VWD (indicated type 1/2N) is a relatively common event with important consequences for diagnosis and genetic counseling.

VWF GENE STRUCTURE The VWF gene is located on chromosome 12 at p12-pter and comprises 52 exons spanning some 178 kb of genomic DNA. The gene is transcribed to yield an approximately 9-kb mRNA encoding the preproVWF signal peptide (22 aa), propeptide (741 aa), and mature subunit (2050 aa)

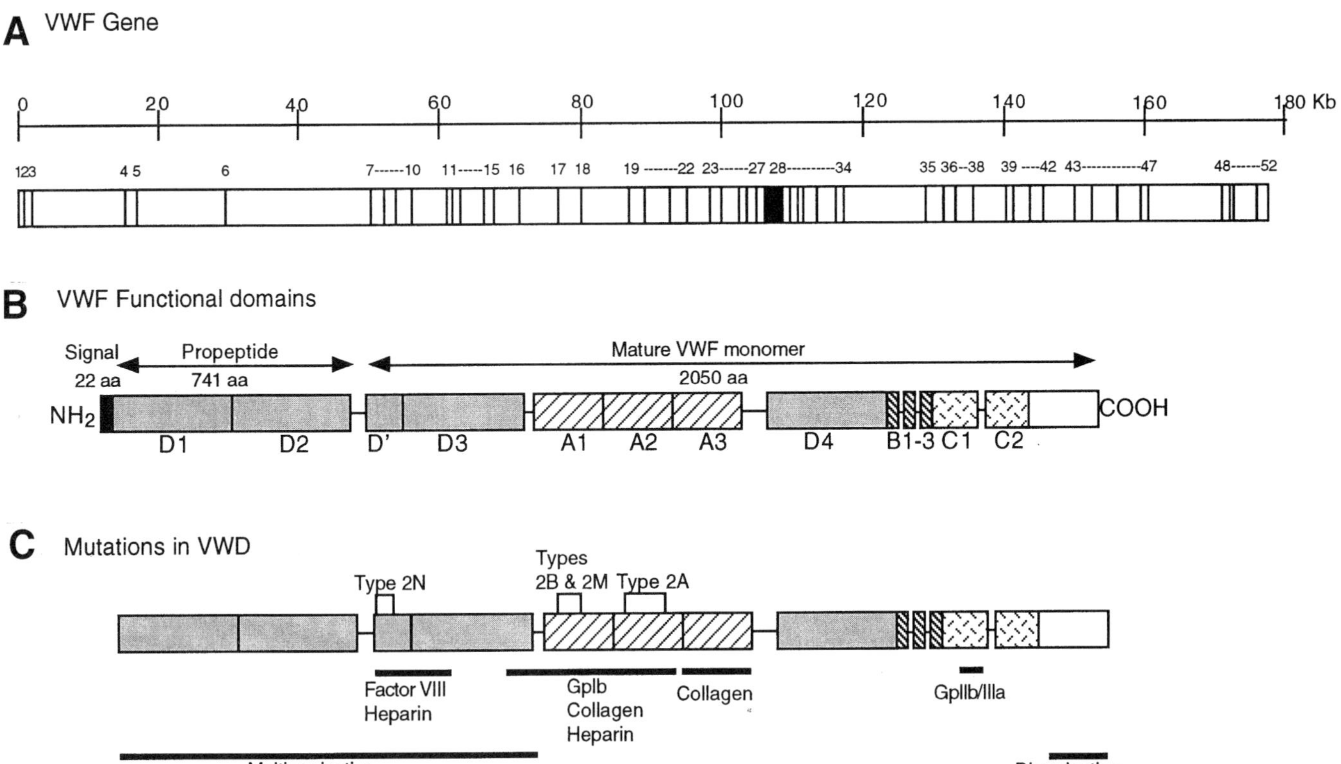

Figure 23-3 Schematic representation of the VWF gene encoding the prepro-VWF subunit. VWF gene exons (not drawn to scale) are represented by vertical lines in part A. The repeated domain structure of the prepro-VWF and sites of signal and propeptide cleavage are indicated in part B. The approximate location of regions involved in VWF structure and function are indicated by thick bars below the figure in part C. The locations of clusters of mutations in the D', A1, and A2 domains identified in patients with type 2 VWD are indicated in part C.

(Fig. 23-3). VWF contains four types of homologous regions (A,B,C, and D), which, in the complete translated nonprocessed peptide, are present in the order of D1-D2-D'-D3-A1-A2-A3-D4-B1-B2-B3-C1-C2. During processing, the D1-D2 domains (the signal and propeptide regions) are cleaved to yield the mature subunit, which, as a dimer, forms the basis of the multimeric structure of VWF. Also present on chromosome 22 (q11.22–q11.23), is a partial highly homologous pseudogene corresponding to exons 23–34 of the VWF gene and showing only 3% divergence in sequence. The presence of the pseudogene, along with the size and complexity of the VWF gene have, until recently, hampered molecular genetic analysis in VWD kindred. However, sequencing of the pseudogene has allowed sequence differences between it and the VWF gene to be exploited in selective PCR-based analyses of those regions of the VWF gene encoding specific functional domains. This has led to an acceleration in understanding the molecular basis of VWD and the characterization of almost 100 specific VWF gene mutations correlating with distinct VWD subtypes. Numerous polymorphisms within the VWF gene have also been reported. Of particular importance in family studies are the multiallelic polymorphic tetranucleotide repeat regions found within intron 40 (Table 23-3).

MOLECULAR PATHOLOGY OF VWD Recent progress made in understanding the molecular basis of different phenotypic variants of VWD will be summarized here. For more detailed descriptions of the mutations giving rise to VWD, the reader is referred to the database of point mutations, insertions and deletions giving rise to VWD, first published in 1993 and now maintained and updated on the Internet.

Type 2 VWD By stabilizing circulating FVIII and mediating platelet adhesion to sites of injury, VWF has two major roles in hemostasis. Structure–function studies using proteolytic fragments of VWF, synthetic peptides, and monoclonal antibodies have localized FVIII binding moieties in the N-terminal 272 amino acids of the mature VWF subunit (D'-D3 region). Although the GpIb binding domain has not been fully characterized, several peptide sequences in the A1 domain are involved. Normal platelet adhesion also requires the assembly of high-molecular-weight VWF multimers. Expression studies using deletion mutants of VWF have indicated that the C-terminal 151 amino acids are required for dimerization to take place, whereas, in addition to the propeptide, both the D' and D3 domains are required for multimer assembly. Therefore, investigation of the molecular basis of qualitative VWF deficiency has concentrated on the regions of the VWF gene encoding specific functional domains.

Type 2A VWD Type 2A VWD is dominantly inherited and is characterized by lack of high mol wt VWF multimers and reduced binding to GPIb/IX on platelets. The increased concentration of a 176-kDa proteolytic fragment derived from the C-terminus of VWF in plasma from affected individuals suggested that the phenotype may well have been caused by a mutation causing increased susceptibility to proteolysis and focused attention on the corresponding region of the VWF gene (exon 28). This has led to the identification of a number of mutations in type 2A VWD, the majority of which are clustered within the A2 domain. Expression of mutated type 2A alleles in mammalian cells has revealed two possible mechanisms for the lack of high-molecular-weight multimers in plasma. Certain mutations can lead to a defect in intracellular transport with the retention of large multimers in the endoplasmic reticulum, whereas others appear to cause increased sensitivity of the largest multimers to proteolysis after their appearance in plasma.

Type 2B VWD VWF in plasma from patients with type 2B VWD shows an increased affinity for platelet GpIb/IX. This results in a preferential loss of high-molecular-weight VWF multimers from plasma. At least 13 different mutations have been identified in type 2B disease, the majority causing amino acid substitutions within the A1 domain loop, which is formed by disulfide bonding between cysteine residues 509 and 695. The integrity of this loop appears to be important in VWF binding to GpIb/IX. Expression of recombinant type 2B variants has established the causative nature of the mutations, since the expressed material has increased affinity for platelet GpIb/IX.

Type 2N VWD VWF from individuals with type 2N VWD has reduced affinity for FVIII in the absence of other qualitative or quantitative abnormalities. The most immediate consequence of this is the reduction in plasma FVIII levels, which contributes to the bleeding episodes that are experienced by affected patients and sometimes results in misclassification as mild hemophilia A. However, unlike hemophilia A, type 2N VWD shows autosomal recessive inheritance. At least six type 2N mutations have been characterized, and all cause substitutions of specific amino acids located in the N-terminal region of VWF implicated in FVIII binding *(see above)*. Interestingly, one of these mutations—Arg91Gln—has an allele frequency of approximately 1% in the Dutch population.

Type 2M VWD The sequence of events leading to initial platelet adhesion to the vascular subendothelium is believed to involve binding of VWF to subendothelial components, followed by a conformational change, which causes binding of VWF to platelet GpIb/IX. Type 2M mutations presumably prevent VWF from undergoing this conformational change, resulting in decreased platelet-dependent function; at the same time, this does not have any effect on multimer structure. The number of such type 2M variants is small, and two missense mutations causing amino acid substitutions in the A1 domain have been described.

Type 3 VWD VWF gene analysis by Southern blotting in patients with recessively inherited type 3 VWD—virtually complete quantitative VWF deficiency—has revealed complete or partial deletions of the VWF gene in a few families. Several individuals in these families have developed alloantibody inhibitors to VWF following replacement therapy.

In addition to gene deletions, direct sequencing of the entire VWF gene from members of kindred with type 3 VWD has identified several frameshift, splice-site, and nonsense mutations, often leading to introduction of early termination codons and a lack of expression from defective alleles either at the mRNA or protein levels. Of particular interest is the frameshift mutation, caused by the deletion of a single cytosine from exon 18 and the subsequent introduction of an early termination codon. This was shown to be inherited in either homozygous or compound heterozygous form in 15/24 Swedish type 3 families, probably as a result of a founder effect within the population.

Type 1 VWD Although type 1 VWD—partial quantitative VWF deficiency—accounts for approximately 70% of all VWD, its genetic basis is poorly understood. Considerable variability in the clinical and laboratory features of type 1 VWD can occur, even within the same family. Molecular genetic analysis of the VWF gene in a number of type 1 families showing heterogeneity of clinical symptoms and VWF profiles has revealed that clinically relevant VWD is often associated with compound heterozygosity for a null allele and a mutated allele. This causes a qualitative defect and indicates that inheritance is actually recessive rather than dominant with the severity of disease depending on the particular combination of mutations inherited. In addition, although heterozygous relatives of type 3 patients who have a quantitative null allele sometimes meet the criteria for type 1 VWD, they are generally asymptomatic, and perhaps they should not be classified as having type 1 VWD. Therefore, quantitative defects caused by the presence of a null allele appear to result in heterozygous carriers of type 3 VWD, rather than type 1 VWD.

Dominant inheritance of type 1 VWD, the molecular mechanism of which is still unknown, is the most common form. However, it is believed that type 1 patients may have functional VWF defects that interfere with the products of the normal allele, the so-called "dominant-negative" effect. The products of both normal and mutated alleles may therefore form dimers, but only normal homodimers form normal multimers that may then be secreted.

RARE COAGULATION DISORDERS

Inherited defects of fibrinogen, prothrombin, and factors V, VII, X, XI, XII, or XIII are rare and are invariably inherited in an autosomal recessive manner. Most give rise to mild to moderate bleeding disorders, although some abnormal fibrinogens can predispose the individual to thrombotic problems. The incidence of these defects is often 1 per 10^6 or more of the population, although factor XI deficiency is relatively common with 5–10% of the Ashkenazi Jewish population being heterozygous for a defective FXI gene and having reduced FXI levels. Four mutations have been described, and two mutations account for 98% of cases (a nonsense mutation; GAA to TAA in exon 5, or Phe 283 Leu). The relatively high frequency of these mutations in this population is undoubtedly because of founder effects, as is the high incidence of FX Fruili (Pro 344 Ser) found in the area of the same name in Northern Italy. This factor X defect results in decreased clotting activity in both the extrinsic and intrinsic systems, since it impairs the interaction of FX with other coagulation factors.

FV deficiency is rare, even though the structure and function of FV are similar to those of factor VIII. The higher frequency of FVIII deficiency may be because of the X-chromosome location of the factor VIII gene, or because true homozygous FV deficiency is lethal in utero. Indeed this has been recently confirmed in mice in which both FV genes have been "knocked out." The same may apply to other severe clotting-factor deficiencies, accounting for their low incidence in the general population.

MANAGEMENT AND TREATMENT OF COAGULATION FACTOR DEFICIENCIES

Specific factor replacement therapy is the goal of treatment for clotting-factor deficiencies, and an industry has grown up to provide optimum treatment for hemophilia A, B, and VWD, in particular. Factors purified from large pools of human blood have been the mainstay of treatment since the early 1970s, and high purity material extracted from plasma and purified by affinity chromatography (i.e., ion exchange or monoclonal antibody-based) is now available in most parts of the developed world for treatment of hemophilia. It should be remembered, however, that hemophilia is either treated ineffectively or not at all in 80% of the world. Less purified plasma products that contain VWF can be used to treat VWD.

The use of material prepared from large donor pools (often over 20,000 donors) has led to the infection of large numbers of patients with blood-borne viruses, in particular HIV, hepatitis B and hepatitis C. Virus inactivation has been achieved but the possibility of "new" resistant viruses in the blood supply is always a concern. The cloning and expression of factor VIII and IX (and VWF) in mammalian cells has led not only to the production of recombinant products but also to the possibility of gene therapy. Recombinant factor VIII, free of all human protein apart from albumin added as a stabilizer, is now available for treatment, and recombinant factor IX and VWF have also been produced.

Gene therapy studies using viral (i.e., retrovirus, adenovirus) and nonviral vectors have been reported for several years, in particular using the factor IX gene as a model system. It has been amply shown that normal factor IX will be produced by many cell types when transfected with a suitable vector containing the necessary promoter sequences and the FIX cDNA. In vitro studies have been followed by ex vivo experiments in which transduced cells have been transplanted into a recipient and have continued to produce factor IX that can be detected in the blood. Adeno-associated virus (AAV) has been used to deliver persistent therapeutic levels of factor IX in mice. In vivo studies, particularly in the hemophilia B dog model, have also shown promise. By targeting the liver (injection of factor IX cDNA-containing vectors into the hepatic portal vein) Mark Kay and colleagues in Chapel Hill, NC, were able to show prolonged low level factor IX production using retroviral-based vectors and transient high-level production using adenoviral-based vectors. These experiments confirmed the essential properties of these two-vector systems, and also showed that antibodies produced in the dogs to adenoviral antigens after the first adenoviral vector administration prevented subsequent successful therapy.

Nonviral-based systems targeting specific receptors have several advantages over viral vectors. The insert size constraints associated with viral systems which mean, for example, that the complete factor VIII cDNA cannot be used in these systems are not a problem. Also, there are continuing concerns about the use of viruses, although modified and inactivated, originate from oncogenic or highly infective and destructive pathogens.

Gene therapy for hemophilia will no doubt be available in some form in the future. Before this happens, however, improvements in the level of expression, intracellular stability, and cell specificity of the vectors will be essential.

SELECTED REFERENCES

Antonarakis SE, Rossiter JP, Young M, Horst J and a consortium of 65 other authors. Factor VIII gene inversions in severe haemophilia A. Results of an International Consortium Study. Blood 1995;86:2206–2212.

Cahill MR, Colvin BT. Haemophilia. Postgrad Med J 1997;73:201–206.

Crossley M, Ludwig M, Stowell KM, de Vos P, Olek K and Brownlee GG. Recovery from haemophilia B Leyden; an androgen-responsive element in the factor IX promoter. Science 1992;257:377–379.

Eikenboom JC, Matsushita T, Reitsma PH, et al. Dominant type 1 von Willebrand disease caused by mutated cysteine residues in the D3 domain of von Willebrand factor. Blood 1996;88:2433–2441.

Furie B, Furie BC. The molecular basis of blood coagulation. Cell 1988;53:505–518.

Giannelli F, Green PM. The molecular basis of haemophilia A and B. Baillieres Clin Haematol 1996;9:211–228.

Giannelli F, Green PM, Sommer SS, et al. Haemophilia B: database of point mutations and short additions and deletions—8th ed. Nucleic Acids Res 1998;26:265–268.

Ginsburg D, Sadler JE. von Willebrand Disease: a database of point mutations, insertions and deletions. Thromb Haemost 1993;69:177–184.

Ginsburg D, Walter Bowie EJ. Molecular genetics of von Willebrand disease. Blood 1992;79:2507–2519.

Girma JP, Ribba AS, Meyer D. Structure-function relationship of the A1 domain of von Willebrand factor. Thromb Haemost 1995;74:156–160.

High KA, Roberts HR. In: The Molecular Basis of Thrombosis and Haemostasis. New York: Marcel Dekker, 1995.

Kemball-Cook G, Toddenham EGD, Wacy AI. The factor VIII structure and mutation resource site: Hamsters version A. Nucleic Acids Res 1998;26:216–219.

Lakich D, Kazazian H, Antonarakis SE, Gitschier J. Inversions displaying the FVIII gene as a common cause of haemophilia A. Nat Genet 1993;5:236–241.

Mazurier C, Meyer D. Molecular basis of von Willebrand disease. Baillieres Clin Haematol 1996;9:229–241.

Nichols WC, Ginsburg D. von Willebrand disease. Medicine (Baltimore) 1997;76:1–20.

Peake IR. Molecular genetics and counselling in haemophilia. Thromb Haemost 1995;74:40–44.

Peake IR, Lillicrap DP, Boulyjenkov V, et al. Report of a joint WHO/WFH meeting on the control of haemophilia: carrier detection and prenatal diagnosis. Blood Coag Fibrinol 1993;4:313–314.

Naylor JA, Brinke A, Hassock S, Green PM, Giannelli F. Characteristic mRNA abnormality found in half the patients with severe haemophilia A is due to large DNA inversion. Hum Mol Genet 1993;2:1773–1778.

Sadler JE. A revised classification of von Willebrand disease. Thromb Haemost 1994;71:520–525.

Sadler JE, Matsushita T, Dong Z, Tuley EA, Westfield LA. Molecular mechanism and classification of von Willebrand disease. Thromb Haemost 1995;73:161–166.

Snyder RO, Miao CH, Patijn GA, et al. Persistent and therapeutic concentrations of human factor IX in mice after hepatic gene transfer of recombinant AAV vectors. Nat Genet 1997;16:270–276.

Thompson AR. Progress towards gene therapy for the haemophilias. Thromb Haemost 1995;74:45–51.

Tuddenham EGD, Schwaab R, Seehafer J, et al. Haemophilia A: database of nucleotide substitutions, deletions, insertions and rearrangements of the factor VIII gene. 2nd Ed. Nucl Acids Res 1994;22:3511–3533.

24 Thrombotic Disorders

ROBIN J. OLDS, DAVID A. LANE, AND SWEE LAY THEIN

BACKGROUND

Normal intravascular fluidity is maintained by a balance between the procoagulant and the anticoagulant mechanisms. Small amounts of activated coagulation factors, like factors Xa and Va, are generated continuously, producing small amounts of thrombin. Therefore, natural anticoagulant mechanisms are required to counteract this procoagulant effect. The importance of the coagulation inhibitors was demonstrated in 1965, when Egeberg described a family with familial venous thrombotic disease that was associated with an inherited reduction in antithrombin (AT) activity in the plasma. There followed a systematic search for other proteins that participate in regulation of coagulation and in which inherited deficiency might predispose to thrombosis. Identification of deficiencies of protein C and protein S resulted. However, before 1993, specific inherited inhibitor deficiencies could be identified in only approximately 5% of patients presenting with an unexplained thrombosis. In 1994, resistance to activated protein C (aPC) was described; in the vast majority of cases, this is caused by a single defect (506 Arg to Gln) in the factor V (FV) gene. The FV 506 Arg→Gln mutation can be identified in up to 50% of patients with thrombophilia. An important conceptual development is the recognition that mutations of single inhibitor genes on their own predispose towards—but do not cause—thrombosis. Clinical thrombotic manifestations of disease require either interaction of two or more genes, or interaction of acquired and genetic factors. This chapter will concentrate on the two principal endogenous anticoagulant pathways—AT/heparin and the protein C/protein S/thrombomodulin, the inhibitor protein deficiencies involved with and the nature of genetic mutations responsible for these deficiencies.

CLINICAL FEATURES AND DIAGNOSIS

EPIDEMIOLOGY The prevalence of venous thrombosis in the population is not well documented and, in part, the notorious unreliability of diagnosis based solely on clinical findings has contributed to this. An approximate prevalence is 1 in 1000 of the general population. The frequency with which individuals with confirmed venous thrombosis have family histories of thrombosis is about 25%. Venous thromboembolism appears to be uncommon in certain populations, such as Asians and Africans. The incidence of specific deficiencies in patients with objectively confirmed episodes of venous thrombosis and in the general population is shown in Table 24-1.

From: *Principles of Molecular Medicine* (J. L. Jameson, ed.), ©1998 Humana Press Inc., Totowa, NJ.

PRESENTATION OF VENOUS THROMBOSIS Venous thrombosis is the most common mode of clinical presentation in individuals deficient for the various inhibitor protein deficiencies. The usual sites of thrombosis are the superficial or deep veins of the leg, including the iliac and femoral veins. Individuals may also present with pulmonary embolism. Less commonly, venous occlusion may occur at other sites, including pelvic, renal, cerebral, retinal, hepatic, portal, axillary, and mesenteric vessels and the inferior vena cava. While presentation with arterial thrombosis is much rarer than with venous thrombosis, there is emerging evidence that inhibitor deficiency may constitute a low but significant risk for myocardial infarction.

Most clinically affected individuals are heterozygous for the abnormal gene. Homozygous protein C and protein S deficiencies typically present shortly after birth with purpura fulminans, the result of widespread microvascular thrombosis, leading to extensive skin necrosis and severe disseminated intravascular coagulation. Homozygous AT deficiency is very rare, and the few reported individuals usually have deficiency caused by mutations altering heparin binding and suffer arterial events or severe and recurrent venous thromboembolic disease. Homozygous factor V gene mutation has been identified much more frequently, and the clinical consequences seem less severe than with the other homozygous deficiencies.

In all heterozygous deficiencies, the incidence of thrombosis is age related. It is unusual for an episode to occur before teenage years. Although events such as immobilization, hospitalization, or pregnancy may trigger a thrombosis, in approximately 50% of cases, no predisposing event can be identified. Incidence rates of thrombosis in affected individuals are difficult to ascertain from the literature, but for aPC resistance, about 25% of aPC resistant relatives of probands presenting with venous thrombosis will also suffer a thrombotic episode before the age of 50. The risk for homozygously affected individuals is higher, with about 40% suffering an event by the time they are in their thirties. In heterozygotes for aPC resistance, the risk of thrombosis is increased sevenfold, compared to the unaffected population, with a 30-fold increased risk in the subgroup of affected females taking oral contraceptives. The risk of thrombosis caused by a genetic defect in PS has recently been estimated as ~10-fold. A general impression, not yet adequately supported by quantitative population-based data, is that the risk of thrombosis for heterozygotes increases in the order FV 506 Arg to Gln/protein C/protein S/antithrombin deficiency.

Table 24-1
Incidence of Defects Associated with Venous Thrombosis

	Normal population	*Patients with DVT, %*
AT Deficiency	1:5000 to 1:350	2–5
PC Deficiency	1:16000 to 1:250–300	2–4
PS Deficiency	1:15000	~ 5
aPC resistance	1–5%	30–60
Fibrinogen defects	?	<1

LABORATORY ASSESSMENT Standard laboratory assays—both functional and immunological—are used to measure AT, protein C, and protein S in those presenting with thrombosis. For protein S deficiency, both total and free protein S antigen are assayed, the free protein S being that fraction that is unbound to C4b binding protein. At present, there is an awareness that functional assays for protein S are far from satisfactory. Resistance to aPC is identified in the laboratory by using clotting assays from commercially available kits and followed up by DNA analysis for the factor V 506 Arg to Gln mutation. This defect can be identified by *Mnl*I restriction analysis of a specifically amplified FV gene sequence.

There is no consensus as to precisely which patients should be screened biochemically for defects predisposing to thrombosis. Guidelines suggested by the British Society for Hematology includes those suffering from venous thromboembolism before age 40–45 years, recurrent venous thrombosis or thrombophlebitis, thrombosis in an unusual site (e.g., mesenteric vein, cerebral vein) unexplained neonatal thrombosis, arterial thrombosis before age 30, patients with a clear family history of thrombosis, and patients with recurrent fetal loss.

GENETIC BASIS OF DISEASE AND MOLECULAR PATHOPHYSIOLOGY

PRINCIPLE ENDOGENOUS ANTICOAGULANT PATHWAYS Figure 24-1 depicts the site of action of the major anticoagulant pathways that have been identified; AT/heparan sulfate, protein C/protein S/thrombomodulin and tissue factor pathway inhibitor (TFPI), and the fibrinolytic system. Additionally, several other proteins have minor anticoagulant activities, as indicated. The generation of the activated serine proteinase thrombin, factor IIa, is the crucial event in the coagulation pathway in that it promotes the formation of the fibrin clot. The anticoagulant proteins act at various strategic points to downregulate the coagulation cascade. Antithrombin directly inactivates the coagulation proteinases—reactions that can be accelerated by heparin-like molecules, such as heparan sulfate. Another anticoagulant mechanism involves thrombin as the trigger. Thrombin, when complexed to an endothelial cell surface protein, thrombomodulin, is able to activate protein C. aPC, in association with protein S as a cofactor, downregulates the coagulation cascade by inactivation of activated coagulation factors Va and VIIIa. Tissue factor pathway inhibitor also has anticoagulant activity, inhibiting tissue factor/factor VIIa/factor Xa. As yet, no clear association between TFPI deficiency and thrombosis has been recognized. This chapter will only consider the first two major pathways.

AT/HEPARAN SULFATE PATHWAY

Normal Structure and Function of AT Plasma AT is a 58-kDa single-chain glycoprotein, primarily synthesized in the hepatocytes, where a 32 amino acid signal peptide is removed prior to export of the 432 residue mature protein. Six cysteines form three intramolecular disulfide bonds, 8 Cys—128 Cys, 21 Cys—95 Cys, and 247 Cys—430 Cys, and there are four glycosylation sites at Asn residues 96, 135, 155, and 192 (Fig. 24-2). AT shares sequence and structural homology with other members of a family of serine proteinase inhibitors (collectively referred to as the serpins), which include members such as α_1-antitrypsin and ovalbumin. AT structure conforms to the helical/β-sheet model with 30% helices (nine helices, denoted A–I) and 40% β-sheet (five sheets). The reactive site bond of AT is located towards the C-terminus of the protein between residues Arg393 and Ser394 (designated P_1-P_1') in a protruding reactive center loop that is exposed to attack by the proteinases.

The other important functional domain is the glycosaminoglycan binding region, which is involved in the interaction with heparin and endothelial cell surface heparan sulfate proteoglycans. This domain is remote from the reactive center and includes the amino-terminal end and helix D, a region that contains a relatively high density of positively charged amino acids. The two functional domains—reactive center and heparin binding site—are conformationally linked, so that induced perturbations of one may influence the function of the other. AT inhibits the activated serine proteinases by acting as a pseudosubstrate. The proteinases attack and attempt to cleave the reactive site bond, P_1-P_1' (393 Arg-394 Ser) of AT, which subsequently undergoes a major conformational change. This involves partial insertion of one end of the reactive site loop into the β-sheet as an extra strand (strand 4), trapping the proteinase in an irreversible 1:1 complex. The inactive AT-proteinase complex is subsequently rapidly removed from the circulation. The rate at which AT and thrombin interact is accelerated in the presence of heparin, or in vivo, by (heparin-like) heparan sulfate proteoglycans that are located on the surface of endothelial cells. Heparin is a heterogeneous mixture of oligosaccharides of varying chain length. A minimum of five specific saccharide units is required to enhance anticoagulant activity of AT against factor Xa, whereas at least 18 monosaccharides (including the specific pentasaccharide sequence) are required for effective enhancement of AT inhibition of thrombin. Endothelial surface heparan sulfate is structurally much more heterogeneous than heparin, but it is known to contain elements that enable binding of AT and facilitate enhanced proteinase inhibition.

AT Gene Structure The *AT* gene is located on chromosome 1q23–q25 and is 13.8 kb in length with seven exons, encoding a signal peptide of 32 aa and a mature protein of 432 aa (Fig. 24-2). The complete nucleotide sequence of the AT has now been determined; of particular interest is the presence of nine full-length and one partial-length Alu repeat elements located within the introns of the AT gene. These repeats comprise 25% of the intron sequence, which is considerably higher than the estimated 5% of the human genome accounted for by Alu repeats. Two of the Alu repeats, Alu 5 and Alu 8 within intron 4, have tails composed of trinucleotide (ATT) repeats that are polymorphic in copy number.

Commonly identified control regions such as the TATA box, the CCAAT box, or GC elements are not found in the 5'-untranslated region of the gene. Two regions have been identified in the 5' end of the gene, which appear to act as regulatory elements

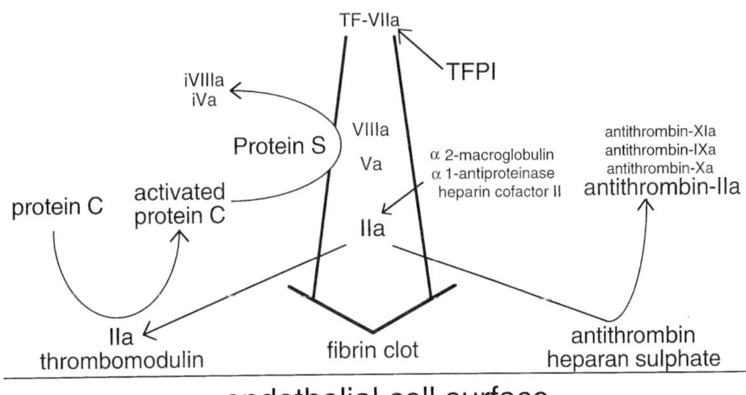

Figure 24-1 Plasma anticoagulant pathways. The events of coagulation are summarized by the large arrow, with initiation by tissue factor (TF)-factor VIIa. The three major anticoagulant pathways, involving AT, protein C-protein S-thrombomodulin, and tissue factor pathway inhibitor (TFPI), and their targets are indicated, as well as other proteins which have some antithrombin activity.

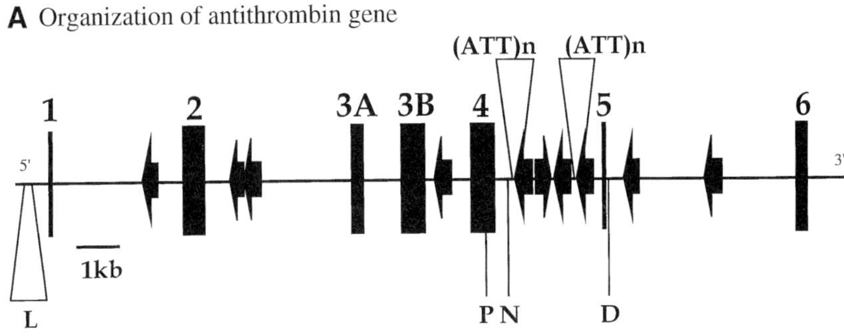

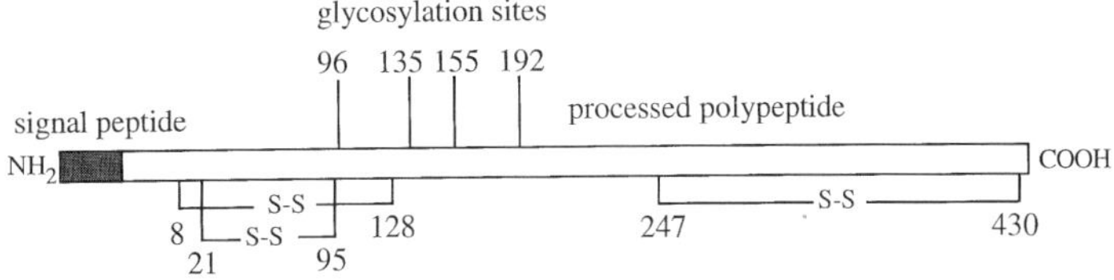

Figure 24-2 Structure of the AT gene and protein. (**A**) Genomic organization with the exons numbered according to convention. Arrows indicate the positions of 10 Alu repeat sequences within the introns. Sequence polymorphisms are marked: L, length dimorphism; P, *Pst*I site; N, *Nhe*I site; D, *Dde*I site; (ATT)n trinucleotide repeat length polymorphisms in the tails of Alu 5 and Alu 8. (**B**) AT protein (not to scale), showing residues involved in disulfide bonds and Asn-linked glycosylation sites.

and that apparently confers some tissue-specific control of expression. A single transcription start site is localized 72 bp 5' of the ATG initiation codon, whereas the 3' end of the gene contains the polyA sequence, AATAAA, located 49 bp 3' to the termination codon. The cleavage/polyadenylation site is located 24 bp downstream from the AATAAA sequence. In addition to the polymorphic tails of the Alu repeats in intron 4, the AT gene contains a number of sequence polymorphisms that include a 76 bp length polymorphism at the 5' end of the gene and four single base variations, three of which involve restriction enzyme cleavage sites (*see* Fig. 24-2). These polymorphisms have proven to be extremely useful in the construction of *AT* gene haplotypes for tracking particular *AT* alleles within families and for tracing the origin of repeated *AT* mutations.

AT Deficiency AT deficiency may be inherited or acquired. This short article will concentrate on the hereditary AT deficiencies.

The incidence of hereditary AT deficiency has been estimated at between 1 in 2000 and 1 in 5000 in the normal population. However, according to a recent survey of Scottish blood donors, the incidence may be much higher—1 in 350—with most of these individuals being clinically asymptomatic.

Inherited AT deficiency is associated with a venous thrombotic tendency that increases with increasing age, although there is still uncertainty regarding the prevalence of thromboembolism in affected individuals. The risk of thromboembolism varies with the type of molecular defects *(see below)*. Defects causing AT deficiency are distributed mainly in the coding regions of the gene. In the most recently published AT mutation database, a total of 256 mutations were reported, 143 of which were unique molecular events. AT deficiency is classified as two main types: type I and type II. Type I deficiency is characterized by a quantitative reduction of AT at both the antigen and functional level to approximately 50% of normal, whereas in type II deficiency the antigen level is near normal, but functional activity is reduced, indicating the presence of a dysfunctional variant.

Type I AT Deficiency The database of mutations lists 113 cases, 92 of which are unique molecular events. The majority of cases are caused by single nucleotide changes and short insertions or deletions; most of these mutations result in premature translation termination codons. Mutations that potentially affect mRNA splicing have also been identified but, unlike protein C, only a small number of type I deficiencies are associated with missense mutations. Large deletions of the AT gene are detected in less than 10% of cases of type I deficiency; only 12 cases are listed in the database. In one of these that has been fully characterized, exon 5 and flanking intron sequences were deleted, the deletion having arisen by homologous recombination between Alu repeat elements located in introns 4 and 5 of the AT gene.

Type II AT Deficiency Type II deficiency can be subdivided according to the properties of the variant AT into those with abnormalities primarily affecting heparin binding, those with impaired reactive site function and those with pleiotropic or multiple abnormalities that demonstrate disturbance of both heparin-binding and proteinase inhibition. Additionally, many of the latter variants are present at reduced concentration in the plasma.

Analysis of variants with reduced heparin affinity has contributed to the delineation of the heparin-binding site of the normal AT protein. Substitution of two classes of residue produce reduced heparin affinity: residues making direct contact with the heparin chains and residues that control access to or overall conformation of the heparin-binding surface. Substitutions affecting positively charged Arg residues at positions 24, 47 (in exon 2 of the AT gene) and 129 (in exon 3 of the AT gene) probably alter contact sites with the chains of negatively charged heparin oligosaccharides. Modeling of normal AT shows that these residues are clustered to form a positively charged surface, involving the A and D helices of the protein. Other substitutions affecting 41Pro, 99Leu, 116Ser, and 118Gln probably affect heparin affinity by altering conformation of the heparin-contact domain.

AT variants in which primary abnormality is defective reactive site function have mutations confined to two distinct regions of the protein, near the C terminus. The residues 393 Arg-394 Ser form the reactive site bond, P_1-P_1', of AT protein. Substitutions affecting 392Gly, 393Arg, and 394Ser all result in reduced inhibition of serine proteinases. Another group of reactive site variants have mutations affecting the P_{12} and P_{10} residues, 382Ala and 384Ala; in addition to being functionally inactive, these variants act as substrates for thrombin and are cleaved at their reactive sites by thrombin. An explanation for the substrate behavior can be derived by considering the structures of cleaved and uncleaved serpins. Following cleavage of the reactive site loop the P_1 and P_1' residues move to opposite poles of the protein, and the P_4-P_{14} residues of the reactive site α-helix insert as strand 4 into a now six-stranded β-sheet. Partial insertion of the reactive site loop into the β-sheet appears essential to stabilization of the serpin–proteinase complex. It is likely that insertion is inhibited by the bulkier side chains of the substituted P_{10}–P_{12} amino acids that are situated in the hinge region, and failure or delay of strand insertion results in substrate rather than inhibitor activity.

AT variants with pleiotropic abnormalities have substitutions in residues 402–407 and 429, in or adjacent to strand 1C at the C terminal end of the protein. These variants demonstrate reduced heparin affinity, as well as impaired proteinase inhibition. The combination of these properties may be explained by a conformational disturbance transmitted to both the reactive site and the heparin-binding domains.

There is clinical benefit in defining the type of AT deficiency, as individuals with heterozygous type II deficiency resulting from AT variants with reduced heparin affinity alone have a substantially reduced risk of thrombosis when compared to other AT deficient individuals.

PROTEIN C/PROTEIN S/THROMBOMODULIN SYSTEM

Normal Structure and Function of Protein C and Protein S Protein C (mol wt 62,000) is synthesized in the hepatocytes and is found in plasma principally as a two-chain molecule, generated by proteolysis at the 156Lys–157Arg bond (Fig. 24-3). The N-terminal end of the mature protein contains six residues that undergo posttranslational vitamin K-dependent modification to γ-carboxyglutamic acid (the Gla domain). This region is involved in the interaction of protein C with Ca^{2+} and phospholipid surfaces and is crucial for the anticoagulant activity of the inhibitor. Other structural motifs include two epidermal growth factor (EGF)-like domains, the activation domain and the catalytic domain. Thrombomodulin-bound thrombin activates protein C by cleavage of the 169Arg–170Lys bond, resulting in the release of a 12 amino acid activation peptide from the N-terminal end of the heavy chain. The catalytic domain shows considerable sequence similarity with other serine proteinases, containing the characteristic catalytic site formed by 211His, 257Asp, and 360Ser.

Protein S (mol wt 70,000) is synthesized as a precursor of 676 amino acids, with a leader sequence of 41 residues, by hepatocytes, endothelial cells, and megakaryocytes. Like protein C, protein S has a number of recognizable structural motifs, including a Gla domain, a thrombin-sensitive region, four EGF-like domains, and a large C-terminal region that has homology to sex hormone binding globulin (Fig. 24-4). Approximately 60% of protein S in the plasma is bound to C4b-binding protein, the complexed fraction not demonstrating anticoagulant cofactor activity; the noncomplexed fraction is known as free protein S. Precisely how protein S functions as an anticoagulant cofactor is unknown and is subject of ongoing investigation.

Protein C Deficiency The structure of the protein C gene is shown in Fig. 24-3. The gene spans 12 kb and has been mapped to chromosome 2q13–q14. Protein C deficiency can also be classified into type I and II subtypes, with a similar definition as that for AT. In the recently reported mutation database, 315 cases are listed, with 334 mutations, comprising 160 unique molecular events. Most deficiencies are associated with point changes or short insertions or deletions affecting the coding region of the gene, mRNA splicing or the promoter region. Included in the database are 18 homozygotes and 17 compound heterozygotes. By far, the greatest number of cases, 243 total with 107 unique mutations, to have missense mutations, causing mainly type I deficiency. Why so many amino acid substitutions should give rise to type I (quantitative) deficiency is not clear, but it suggests that the primary amino acid sequence is crucial to the correct ternary structure and stability of the protein. Substitutions within the Gla domain, at the

should be begun slowly and under full heparin cover. The degree of anticoagulation induced by warfarin is monitored by the International Normalized Ratio (INR); for a first episode of thrombosis or following pregnancy, the INR should be maintained within the 2.0–3.0 range, whereas the higher range of 3.0–4.0 is required for treatment of recurrent disease. The duration that treatment is required is not established, although a minimum of 3–6 months is reasonable, and many consider that two distinct clinical events merits lifelong prophylaxis. Protein C concentrates are used to treat the severe complications of homozygous deficiency, in addition to anticoagulation, and maintenance therapy with blood product may be required. AT concentrates are also available and may be used in the management of venous thromboembolism or at parturition in heterozygous deficient patients but are probably best reserved for those cases not responding to standard treatment, as no definitive clinical trials have been performed.

PREGNANCY Pregnancy represents an extremely high-risk situation, and its management is both difficult and complex. Individuals with previous history of thrombosis should be treated and the treatment may include oral warfarin or heparin. Warfarin may be teratogenic during the first trimester and is associated with an increased risk of fetal hemorrhage. Accordingly, care should be taken to change from oral anticoagulants to heparin as soon as pregnancy is confirmed, or preferably, when a pregnancy is planned. Heparin can be self-administered and continued until the second or early third trimesters. At this time, oral anticoagulants can be given until just before term. At the time of delivery, anticoagulants should be discontinued. It has been recommended that heparin plus oral anticoagulants be resumed 48–72 h after delivery and continued for 3 months postpartum. The reference list contains articles detailing therapeutic options in greater detail.

ASYMPTOMATIC INDIVIDUALS The management of asymptomatic individuals with an anticoagulant deficiency is problematic. Most would agree that the patient should be counseled as to the additional risk factors that may predispose to a thrombotic episode and that following diagnosis, family members should be investigated to identify affected—but asymptomatic—individuals. A retrospective survey of individuals with hereditary AT deficiency carried out in the Netherlands found no excess in the mortality rate, the authors concluding that anticoagulant prophylaxis for asymptomatic affected individuals was not indicated. This view must be tempered by clinical judgment, however, because of the marked variability of clinical presentation observed between different kindreds. Lifelong prophylaxis with anticoagulants is not justified in asymptomatic individuals, but prophylactic anticoagulation should be offered to deficient individuals in situations presenting a recognized risk of thrombosis, such as pregnancy and surgery. In view of its remarkably high incidence and ease of detection, it is being debated whether individuals in high-risk situations (e.g., before major surgery, pregnancy, and before starting oral contraception) should be routinely screened for aPC resistance.

FUTURE DIRECTIONS

Many individuals with deficiency of the naturally occurring anticoagulant mechanisms remain asymptomatic for much of their lives. In a proportion of individuals suffering thrombosis, no predisposing abnormality can be identified, suggesting that other genetic factors remain to be discovered. In addition to defects resulting in recognizable deficiency of the anticoagulant pathways, it seems likely that genetic effects on "normal" levels of anticoagulant activity may also be important. This has been shown for protein C, where sequence differences in the promoter region of normal protein C genes significantly influence the plasma levels of the protein. It is clear that the phenotype of venous thrombosis develops from multiple interacting genetic and environmental factors; it may be that analysis of interacting genetic factors will improve the risk prediction for thrombotic events in affected families. Until recently, inhibitor deficiencies were of too low prevalence to enable properly controlled clinical trials of prophylaxis and treatment to be undertaken. The high prevalence of the factor V 506 Arg to Gln mutation has transformed the prospects for progress in this area. The challenge remains to identify additional genetic risk factors that predispose to thrombosis and that interact with known acquired/genetic factors. Recently, the 20210 G-to-A mutation in the prothrombin gene found in 1% of the population was shown to be a significant but weak risk factor for venous thrombosis and a significant risk factor for myocardial infarction in young women. Hyperhomocysteinemia has been shown to be associated with venous thrombosis, and some, but not all studies have implicated a mutation in the methylenetetrahydrofolate reductase gene (C to T at 677). Finally, thrombomodulin gene mutations are increasingly being found in association with venous and arterial thrombosis.

SELECTED REFERENCES

Aiach M, Borgel D, Gaussem P, Emmerich J, Alhenc-Gelas M, Gandrille S. Protein C and protein S deficiencies. Semin Hematol 1997;34:205–216.

Bayston TA, Lane DA. Antithrombin; molecular basis of deficiency. Thromb Haemost 1997;78:339–343.

Bertina RM, Koeleman BPC, Koster T, et al. Mutation in blood coagulation factor V associated with resistance to activated protein C. Nature 1994;369:64–67.

Borgel D, Gandrille S, Aiach M. Protein S deficiency. Thromb Haemost 1997;78:351–356.

British Committee for Standards in Haematology. Guidelines on the investigation and management of thrombophilia. J Clin Pathol 1990;43:703–709.

Carrell RW, Stein PE, Fermi G, Wardell MR. Biological implications of a 3Å structure of dimeric antithrombin. Structure 1994;2:257–270.

Cattaneou M, Tsai MY, Bucciarelli P, Taioli E. Zighetti ML, Bignell M, Mannucci PM. A common mutation in the methylenetetrahydrofolate reductase gene (C677T) increase the risk for deep vein thrombosis in patients with mutant factor V (factor V:Q506). Arterioscler Thromb Vasc Biol 1997;17:1662–1666.

Dahlback B. Inherited thrombophilia: resistance to activated protein C as a pathogenic factor of venous thromboembolism. Blood 1995;85:607–614.

Dahlback B, Carlsson M, Svensson PJ. Familial thrombophilia due to a previously unrecognised mechanism characterized by poor anticoagulant response to activated protein C: prediction of a cofactor to activated protein C. Proc Natl Acad Sci USA 1993;90:1004–1008.

Dahlback B, Stenflo J. A natural anticoagulant pathway: proteins C, S C4b-binding protein and thrombomodulin. In: Bloom AL, Forbes CD, Thomas DP, Tuddenham EGD, eds. Haemostasis and Thrombosis, vol. 1, 3rd ed. Edinburgh: Churchill Livingstone, 1994; pp. 671–698.

Fernandez-Rachubinski FA, Weiner JH, Blajchman MA. Regions flanking exon I regulate constitutative expression ot the antithrombin gene. J Biol Chem 1996;271:29,502–29,512.

Gandrille S, Borgel D. Ireland H, Lane DA, Simmonds R, Reitsma PH, Mannhalter C, Pabinger I, Saito H, Suzuki K, Formstone C, Cooper DN, Espinosa Y, Sala N, Bernardi F, Aiach M. Protein S deficiency: a database of mutations. Thromb Haemost 1997;77: 1201–1214.

Koeleman BP, Reitsma PH, Bertina RM. Familial thrombophilia: a complex genetic disorder. Semin Hematol 1997;34:256–264.

Koster T, Rosendaal FR, de Ronde H, Briet E, Vandenbroucke JP, Bertina RM. Venous thrombosis due to poor anticoagulant response to activated protein C: Leiden thrombophilia study. Lancet 1993;342: 1503–1506.

Lane DA, Bayston T, Olds RJ, Fitches AC, Cooper DN, Millar DS, Jochmans K, Perry DJ, Okajima K, Emmerich J. Antithrombin mutation database: 2nd (1997) update. Thromb and Haemost 1997;77:197–211.

Lane DA, Olds RJ, Boisclair M, et al. Antithrombin III mutation database: first update. Thromb Haemostas 1993;70:361–369.

Lane DA, Olds RJ, Conard J, et al. Pleiotropic effects of antithrombin strand 1C substitution mutations. J Clin Invest 1992;90: 2422–2433.

Lane DA, Mannucci PM, Bauer KA, Bertina RM, Bochkov NP, Boulyjenkov V, Chandy M, Dahlback B, Ginter EK, Miletich JP, Rosendaal FR, Seligsohn U. Inherited thrombophilia: Part 1. Thromb Haemost 1996;76:651–662.

Lane DA, Mannucci PM, Bauer KA, Bertina RM, Bochkov NP, Boulyjenkov V, Chandy M, Dahlback B, Ginter EK, Miletich JP, Rosendaal FR, Seligsohn U. Inherited thrombophilia: Part 2. Thromb Haemost 1996;76:824–834.

Ohlin AK, Norlund L, Marlar RA. Thrombomodulin gene variations and thromboembolic disease. Thromb Haemost 1997;78:396–400.

Olds RJ, Lane DA, Thein SL. The molecular genetics of antithrombin deficiency. Brit J Haematol 1994;87:221–226.

Poort SR, Rosendaal FR, Reitsma PH, Bertina RM. A common genetic variation in the 3'-untranslated region of the prothrombin gene is associated with elevated plasma prothrombin levels and an increase in venous thrombosis. Blood 1996;88:3698–3703.

Prins MH, Turpie AGG. Diagnosis and treatment of venous thromboembolism. In: Bloom AL, Forbes CD, Thomas DP, Tuddenham EGD, eds. Haemostasis and Thrombosis, vol. 2, 3rd ed. Edinburgh: Churchill Livingstone, 1994; pp. 1381–1414.

Reitsma PH. Protein C deficiency: from gene defects to disease. Thromb Haemost 1997;78:344–350.Reitsma PH, Bernadi F, Doig RG, Gandrille S, Greengard JS, Ireland H, Krawczak M, Lind B, Long GL, Poort SR, Saito H, Sala N. Witt I, Cooper D. Protein C deficiency: a database of mutations, 1995 update. Thromb Haemost 1995;73:876–889.

Simmonds RE, Ireland H, Lane DA, Zoller B, Garcia de Frutos P, Dahlback B. Clarification of the risk for venous thrombosis associated with hereditary protein S deficiency. Annals of Internal Medicine 1998;128:8 14.

Simmonds RE, Zöller B, Ireland H, Thompson E, de Frutos PG, Dahlbäck B, Lane DA. Genetic and phenotypic analysis of a large (122 member) protein S-deficient kindred provides an explanation for the familial coexistence of type I and type III plasma phenotypes. Blood 1997;89:4364–4370.

Spek CA, Koster T, Rosendaal FR, Bertina R, Reitsma PH. Genotypic variation in the promoter region of the protein C gene is associated with plasma protein C levels and thrombotic risk. Thromb Vasc Biol 1995;15:214–218.

van Boven HH, Lane DA. Antithrombin and its inherited deficiency states. Semin Hematol 1997;34:188–204.

Vandenbroucke JP, Koster T, Briët E, Reitsma PH, Bertina RM, Rosendaal FR. Increased risk of venous thrombosis in oral contraceptive users who are carriers of factor V Leiden mutation. Lancet 1994;344:1453–1457.

van't Veer C, Kalafatis M, Bertina RM, Simioni P, Mann KG. Increased tissue factor-initiated prothrombin activation as a result of the Arg506→ Gln mutation in factor VLEIDEN. J Biol Chem 1997;272:20,721–20,729.

25 Paroxysmal Nocturnal Hemoglobinuria

BRUNO ROTOLI AND KHEDOUDJA NAFA

INTRODUCTION

Paroxysmal nocturnal hemoglobinuria (PNH) is a complex hematological disorder probably first described three centuries ago, and regarded as a mystery until the 1980s, when most of its pathophysiology was elucidated, followed by the 1990s, when the underlying molecular defect was finally unraveled. The original denomination, PNH, stresses only one component of the disease (i.e., a hyperhemolytic state). A more complete contemporary definition could read as follows: an acquired blood disorder characterized by the expansion of one or a few hematopoietic cell clones that are unable to produce the glycosyl-phosphatidyl inositol (GPI) anchor, against the background of a reduced bone marrow activity. Some landmarks in the history of understanding this disorder are listed in Table 25-1. Because of its complex pathophysiology, this disorder has been variously classified among hemolytic anemias, myelodysplasia, myeloproliferative disorders, or bone marrow failure syndromes; indeed, PNH has some features of each of these. Here we will briefly summarize clinical, diagnostic, and therapeutic features, and we will then review in some detail recent progress on the genetic and pathophysiological aspects of PNH.

CLINICAL FEATURES The disease is rare (prevalence about 1–2 per million), but it occurs throughout the world, with increased prevalence in parts of Asia (i.e., Thailand, China), where an unexplained higher incidence of aplastic anemia is also observed. PNH is characterized by chronic hemolytic anemia with erratic exacerbations, frequent leukopenia and thrombocytopenia, tendency to thrombosis and, to a lesser extent, tendency to infection. The clinical picture can be anything from mild to severe, severity being dictated by extreme pancytopenia (the PNH/aplastic anemia syndrome), hyperhemolysis, or recurrent thrombosis (hemolytic type). Although the disease is not malignant (progression to acute leukemia is very rare, and the frequency may have been overestimated), with a median survival of 10 years in large series, the course may be stormy and the quality of life poor.

DIAGNOSIS A mild jaundice without splenic enlargement, anemia with moderate reticulocytosis, raised serum LDH, episodes of dark urine, and hemosiderinuria are clues to the diagnosis. Until the late 1980s, the only confirmatory test was the Ham test (lysis of a portion of red cells in acidified serum); simpler but less specific tests are the sucrose and the sugar-water tests (red cell lysis in serum with reduced ionic strength). At present, flow cytometry studies on blood cells *(see below)* are more sensitive and more specific than hemolytic tests. More recently, with the discovery of the causative gene, molecular studies on DNA or mRNA from nucleated blood cells have become valuable diagnostic tools.

GENETIC BASIS

Although this disease has a well-recognized genetic cause, it is neither inherited nor transmitted to the progeny. Indeed, it is a clonal disorder arising from a somatic mutation in the phosphatidyl inositol glycan class A *(PIG-A)* gene of an early hematopoietic progenitor.

THE *PIG-A* GENE AND THE GPI-ANCHOR *PIG-A* is a housekeeping gene located on the short arm of the X chromosome (Xp22.1), the cDNA of which was first isolated by Kinoshita's group in 1993 through expression cloning and complementation of GPI-deficient cell lines. The organization of the genomic gene was established by Bessler in 1994 (Fig. 25-1). *PIG-A* is a conserved gene that encodes for a protein involved in the synthesis of the glycosyl-phosphatidyl inositol (GPI) anchor. This molecule is used by cells to bind a number of proteins without a transmembrane portion on the outer surface. The functional implications of the GPI-anchoring of proteins are not completely understood; they include ease of assemblage and of shedding, lateral mobility, capping, involvement in endo-, exo-, and potocytosis (a clathrin-independent form of endocytosis and recycling). There are examples of proteins existing in both a transmembrane and a GPI-linked configuration. The adhesion molecule LFA-3 (CD58) is encoded by a gene that may undergo alternative splicing, producing the two different configurations; FcγR-III (CD16) is encoded by two different genes, one of which provides the site for GPI-anchor attachment. The strongest evidence that this type of membrane anchorage is important in cell biology is its high conservation among eukaryotic cells (e.g., it is found in yeast and in trypanosomes). The protein encoded by *PIG-A*, in combination with at least two other proteins, is essential in the very first step of the complex GPI-anchor biosynthesis pathway (i.e., in the transfer of *N*-acetyl glucosamine to phosphatidyl inositol [Fig. 25-2]). By experimental mutagenesis, GPI-deficient cell lines showing defects in any of the various metabolic steps have been produced. However, the study of PNH has shown, perhaps surprisingly, that the same early step is impaired in all patients, and all patients have a mutation in the *PIG-A* gene. The favored explanation for this finding is that among the various genes involved in GPI-anchor synthesis, *PIG-A* may be the only one that is X-linked. As a result, a single mutation in that gene will produce an abnormal cell in either sex: males have

From: *Principles of Molecular Medicine* (J. L. Jameson, ed.), ©1998 Humana Press Inc., Totowa, NJ.

Table 25-1
Landmarks in the History of PNH

Author	*Report*
Schmidt (1678)	First clinical report
Strübing (1882)	First detailed description
Marchiafava (1911)	Recognition as a disease entity
Ham (1937); Dacie (1938)	Specific diagnostic test
De Sandre (1956)	PNH erythrocytes are AchE deficient
Lewis and Dacie (1965)	PNH granulocytes are NAP-deficient
Rosse and Dacie (1966)	Two types of PNH erythrocytes
Lewis and Dacie (1967)	Relation with aplastic anemia
Oni and Luzzatto (1970)	Evidence of clonal origin
Nicholson-Weller (1983)	PNH cells are DAF-deficient
Rotoli and Luzzatto (1984)	In vitro evidence of clonal origin
Medof (1986)	Relation to GPI-anchoring system
Rotoli and Luzzatto (1989)	The "relative advantage" hypothesis
Ueda (1992); Hillmen (1993)	PNH lymphoblastoid cell lines
Kinoshita (1993)	Cloning of the *PIG-A* gene
Bessler and Luzzatto (1994)	*PIG-A* gene organization and mutations

AchE, acetylcholinesterase; NAP, neutrophil alkaline phosphatase; AF, decay accelerating factor (CD55).

only one allele and females have only one functional allele (as a result of X-chromosome inactivation). Although females have two *PIG-A* alleles, only one half of the mutations will occur in the functional X; thus, the risk of having the disease is the same in both genders. Since a defect causing a metabolic block is generally recessive, it is very unlikely (although not impossible) that a double mutation targeting both alleles of an autosomal gene in the same cell may occur in vivo.

***PIG-A* MUTATIONS IN PNH** Practically all types of mutations have been found in the *PIG-A* gene of PNH cells: small deletions or insertions with frameshift, nucleotide substitutions resulting in a stop codon, missense mutations causing amino acid substitution or new sites for alternative splicing, and large deletions. Most of the mutations occur in exon 2, which is the largest; however, no particular clustering of mutations has emerged, and almost all mutations are unique to each patient (*see* Fig. 25-1).

If we compare the type of mutations found in PNH with those found in another—this time inherited—X-linked disorder of a housekeeping gene (i.e., G-6PD deficiency) a clear discrepancy is apparent. In PNH, the vast majority of mutations lead to truncated proteins, whereas missense mutations are rare; in G-6PD deficiency almost all mutations are missense. Two considerations may be relevant to this discrepancy.

1. In hereditary disorders, a complete lack of a housekeeping gene product is probably lethal; thus, we only see mutations with residual activity. By contrast, if a mutation is somatically acquired, it will not affect organ development and, once occurred, it will affect the genetic make-up of only a small fraction of somatic cells.
2. If missense mutations in PNH are rare, this means that for a clonal expansion to take place, the gene damage must be serious.

Indeed, several of the missense mutations found in PNH patients are associated with a complete absence of GPI-linked proteins, indicating that they affected seriously either mRNA stability, protein function, or both.

MOLECULAR PATHOPHYSIOLOGY

The *PIG-A* mutation responsible for PNH arises in a multipotent hematopoietic stem cell, which is then capable of differentiating along several lineages: erythroid, myeloid, and megakaryocytic differentiation capabilities are almost always preserved, whereas lymphoid differentiation (along B- and/or T-lineages) is observed in only a minority of patients. As a consequence of the damage of the GPI-anchor synthesis pathway, all the affected cells in any state of maturation are deficient in all the GPI-linked molecules, and deficiency is often complete. Up to now, at least 19 different proteins sharing the GPI-anchoring system have been described on the surface of human blood cells (Fig. 25-3). Our understanding of their functional significance is rather limited; in some cases, the very study of PNH patients or cells has been an important source of information. CD59/MIRL and CD55/DAF are the most typical examples: we now know that they are two complement-regulatory proteins, the absence of which renders PNH erythrocytes extremely sensitive to complement activation, and this is translated in vivo into a hemolytic state and in vitro into a positive Ham or sucrose test. A low level of complement activation is probably a constant physiological phenomenon, which is greatly amplified during inflammatory or infectious diseases; thus, PNH erythrocytes are chronically lysed with paroxysmal exacerbations. It is still unclear why exacerbation occurs mainly during the night. In a functional hierarchy, CD59 plays the major role. This was discovered by studying rare inherited conditions in which a single molecule is lacking: a CD59-deficient patient had a PNH-like picture, whereas subjects deficient in CD55 on red cell membrane (those carrying the rare Inab blood group phenotype) are almost normal. Although CD59 and CD55 are deficient also on leukocytes, there is no evidence of reduced leukocyte lifespan in PNH patients, probably because nucleated cells have an additional transmembrane (i.e., non–GPI-linked) molecule (CD46) that protects them from complement activation. Sensitivity to complement is the best known, but not the only defect, of PNH cells. Table 25-2 lists other molecules that are deficient with the specific function of each of them, if known. The surface abnormalities of PNH cells can be

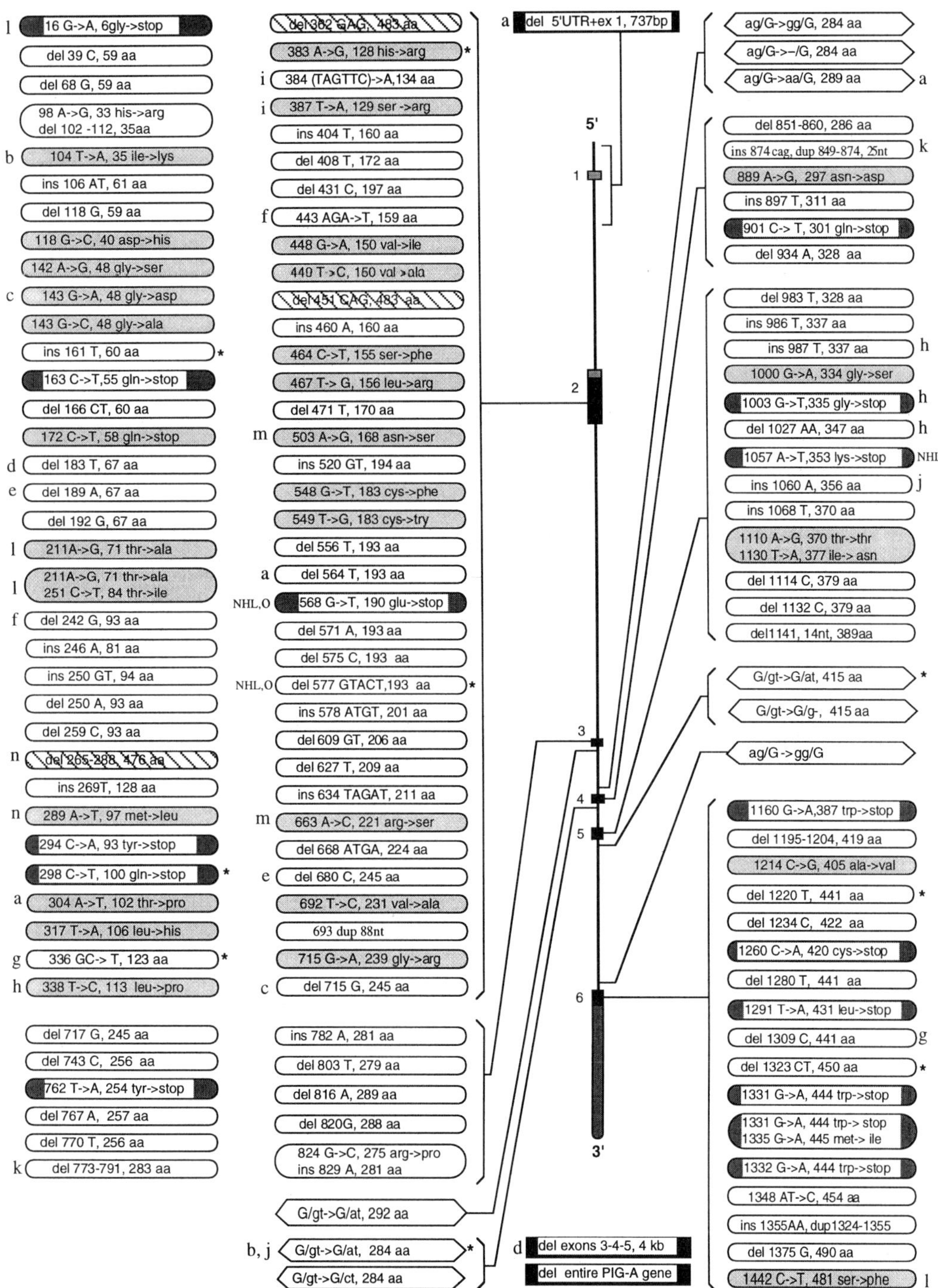

Figure 25-1 *PIG-A* gene structure and mutations. The genomic gene spans approximately 17 kb. Exons (thick blocks, numbered) and introns (thin lines) are represented in the central bar; untranslated exon regions are in gray. Three mRNA transcripts arising from alternative splicing were found by Bessler et al., who also described an unproductive pseudogene mapped to 12q21. All the mutations found so far are displayed. (rounded box), small deletion or insertion, with frameshift and truncated protein; (dark-ended box), nonsense mutation; (pointed box), mutation causing altered splicing; (black box), vast deletion; (hatched box), deletion, in frame; (gray box), missense mutation. *Mutations found in more than one patient. A small letter outside the box identifies multiple mutations found in a single patient. Only one polymorphism has been described so far (55C→T, 19 art→trp).

also used for diagnostic purposes. Flow cytometry using fluoresceinated antibodies against GPI-linked molecules (Fig. 25-4) is a very sensitive contemporary diagnostic tool, by which a PNH abnormality can be identified even at a very early stage. In addition, it makes it possible to pinpoint which cell lineages are involved and to what extent.

CLONAL DOES NOT NECESSARILY MEAN MONOCLONAL The presence of more than one abnormal cell population in a single PNH patient was first inferred by functional studies. In 1966, Rosse and Dacie found in a single patient a proportion of red cells that were three- to fivefold more sensitive to complement (which they called PNH II cells) and a proportion that were 15- to

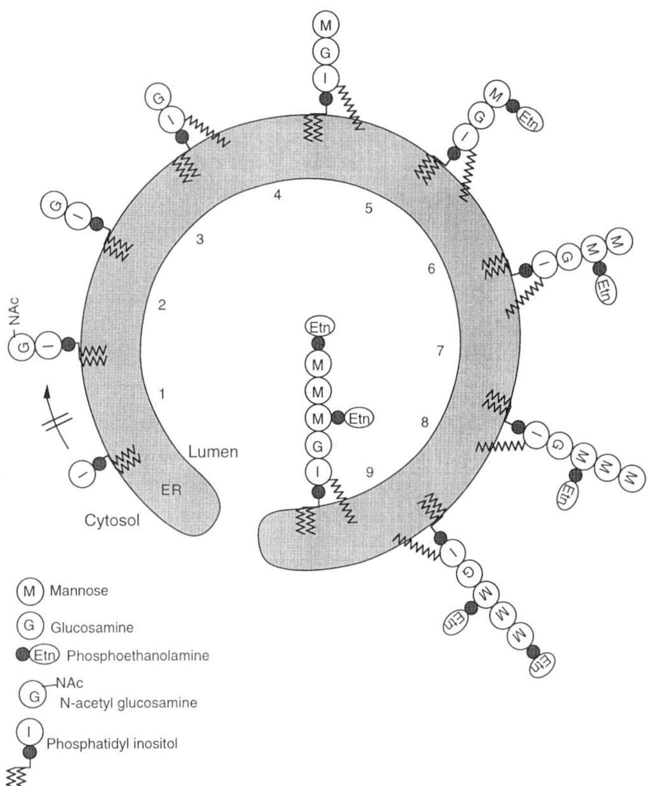

Figure 25-2 GPI-anchor biosynthesis. The anchor synthesis is a multistep (1–9) process that occurs in the endoplasmic reticulum (ER), starting in the cytoplasmic side, then flipping into the luminal side. It is then transferred *en bloc* on the C-terminal of the protein, which is cleaved of a short sequence of 20–30 amino acids led by a signal sequence called ω. While GPI-deficient cell lines obtained by experimental mutagenesis have shown defects in any step of the synthesis, all PNH patients studied so far are defective in the first step (↛).

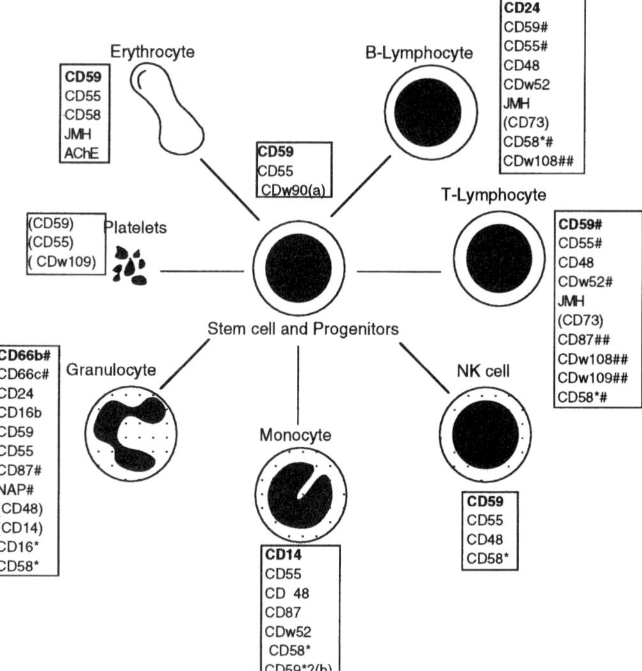

Figure 25-3 GPI-linked molecules on blood cell surface. For each cell type, molecules are listed in order of sensitivity for detecting deficient cells (in bold: highest sensitivity). (. . .), weak expression; *, also transmembrane; #, increased upon cell activation; ##, expressed only upon cell activation. (a) About 25% of early hematopoietic progenitors express CDw90, which is an analog of the murine Thy-1. (b) In our hands, CD59 was always present on PNH monocytes. We have omitted a few other molecules that may need better characterization (HRF, NB1, Group 8, Mo3, p50 8). (Reprinted with permission from B. Rotoli et al., Blood Reviews, 1993;7:78.)

25-fold more sensitive (PNH III) as compared to normal red cells. In the early 1990s, the establishment of lymphoblastoid cell lines has confirmed this finding: in a number of cases, two cell lines differing in their cytofluorometric pattern were obtained. Finally, DNA analysis has shown two different *PIG-A* mutations in several patients (Fig. 25-1).

A mechanism that may explain the expansion of more than one clone carrying the same functional defect, but arising from different mutations, is positive selection. A theory based on this mechanism was developed for PNH in 1989 and termed the "relative advantage" or the "escape" hypothesis; it is supported by several pieces of circumstantial evidence and still requires a direct confirmation. According to the relative advantage theory, a mutation in the *PIG-A* gene might be a fairly common phenomenon, which has no biological consequences, because the mutated cell has no chance of expanding or even of survival. However, if normal hematopoiesis is inhibited by a primary cause, and if the inhibition mechanism is mediated by one or more proteins that are GPI-linked on the surface of progenitor cells, *PIG-A* mutated cells acquire a relative advantage and may undergo clonal expansion. Because only cells severely GPI-deficient may escape, this explains why serious molecular lesions (i.e., frameshift, stop codon, deletion) prevail over single amino acid substitutions. A recent observation from Germany indirectly supports this hypothesis: in a few patients with B-cell non-Hodgkin lymphoma experimentally treated with Campath-1H (a monoclonal antibody that kills T lymphocytes using the GPI-linked protein CDw52) severely GPI deficient T cells appeared; they were cloned and showed mutations in the *PIG-A* gene. On Campath-1H discontinuation, the GPI-deficient T cells gradually disappeared. In order to explore experimentally the growth of PNH hematopoietic stem cells, the mouse *PIG-A* gene was inactivated in embryonic stem (ES) cells using the conventional knockout gene targeting technique. In vitro preliminary studies demonstrated that *PIG-A* deficient ES cells were able to differentiate into mature cells of various hematopoietic lineages. However, when tested in vivo, in the few surviving chimeras the proportion of GPI-deficient blood cells was low at birth and decreased with aging, thus proving that there is no absolute growth advantage for PNH cells as compared to normal cells coexisting in the same organism. If the escape theory is confirmed, several implications must be borne in mind:

1. PNH patients always have two concomitant defects: (a) one (or a few) early hematopoietic progenitor cells carrying a *PIG-A* mutation; and (b) a bone marrow failure syndrome, the mechanism of which is permissive for the expansion of GPI-deficient cells. This would explain the frequent association of PNH with aplastic anemia (AA) and the increased incidence of PNH in countries where AA is more frequent.

Table 25-2
Functions of GPI-Linked Proteins on Blood Cells

Antigen	*Alternative denomination*	*Function*
CD14	LPS-LPB-r	Monocyte adhesion and activation
CD16b	FcγR-IIIb	Low affinity receptor for IgG
CD24		Ca^{2+} flux, triggers H_2O_2 production by PMN
CD48	BLAST-1	Counter-receptor for CD2
CD55	DAF	Accelerates C3 and C5 convertase decay
CD58	LFA-3	Counter-receptor for CD2
CD59	MIRL	Binds C8/C9, thus inhibiting MAC assembly
CD66b	CGM6 (CEA family member)	Granulocyte adhesion/activation
CD66c	NCA	Granulocyte adhesion/activation
CD73	5'-NT	Purine/pyrimidine ribo/deoxyribonucleoside phosphorilation
CD87	uPAR	Urokinase receptor
CDw52	Campath-1	Unknown
CDw90	Thy-1	Adhesion
CDw108		Unknown
CDw109	Platelet Gove/b alloantigen	Unknown
ACHE		Enzyme, unknown substrate on RBC
NAP		Enzyme, granulocyte function
JMH		Unknown

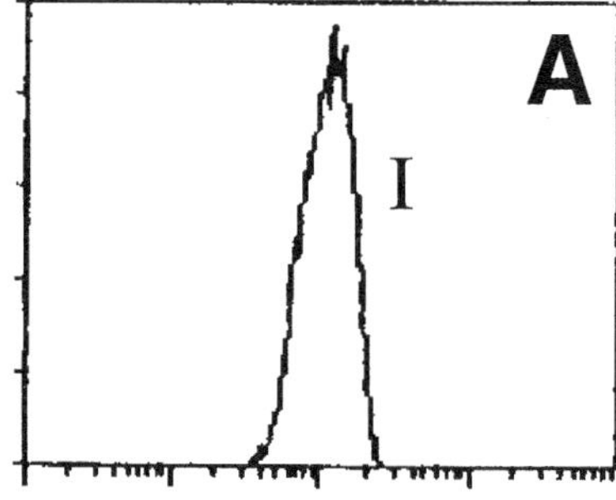

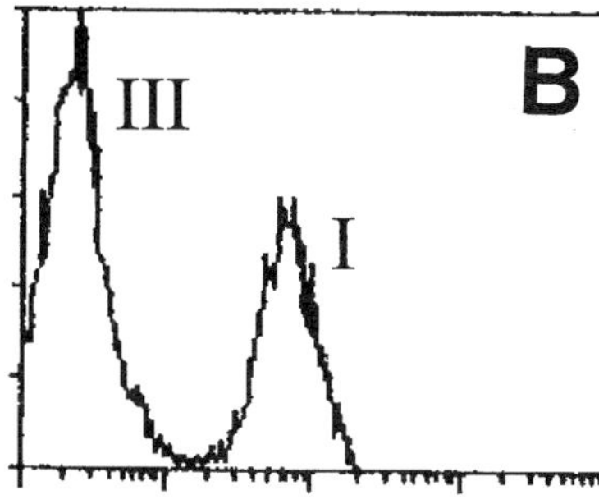

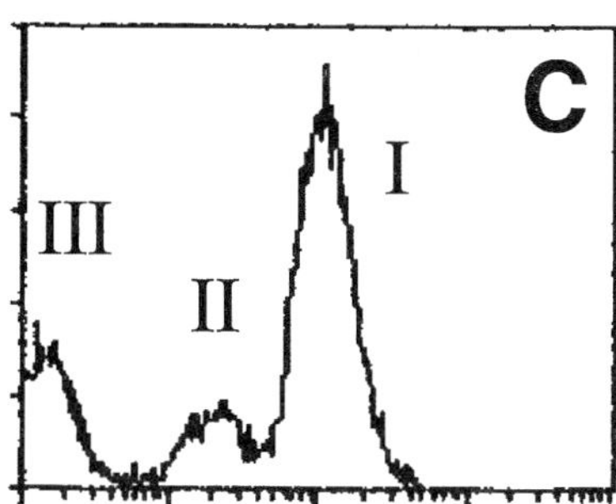

Figure 25-4 Red blood cell flow cytometry analysis of CD59-defined antigen expression in a normal subject and two representative PNH patients. *x*-axis: log green fluorescence; *y*-axis; relative cell counts. (**A**) The unimodal distribution of $CD59^+$ cells in the normal subject. (**B**) Two cell populations are present in this patient, one normally expressing and the other completely lacking CD59. (**C**) Three cell populations are distinguishable in this patient (normal, dim, and negative). (Reprinted with permission from P. Hillman et al. BrJ Haematol 1992;80:402.)

2. The PNH clones, although responsible for a number of clinical consequences, are not invasive; rather, they should be considered "salvage" clones, which positively mitigate the consequences of bone marrow failure.
3. The aim of treatment should be to recover normal hematopoiesis rather than to destroy or to repair the PNH clone(s).

TREATMENT

At present, the treatment of PNH patients is essentially supportive. Prevention and early treatment of concurrent infectious or inflammatory diseases may help in reducing the frequency and severity of paroxysmal exacerbations. Folate supplement and red cell transfusion are the basis for ameliorating anemia. Iron supplements—to balance the persistent urinary loss of iron in the form of hemosiderinuria—or iron chelation, if iron overload develops due to frequent transfusions, may be needed in selected patients. Anticoagulants are used to treat or to prevent thrombosis.

Bone marrow transplant is a curative approach for PNH patients with severe bone marrow failure, less than 45 years of age, and having a related HLA-identical donor. If the escape theory is correct, there is little room for futuristic approaches with cell therapy (insertion of molecules on the outer surface of blood cells) or with gene therapy (insertion of a functioning *PIG-A* gene in early hematopoietic progenitors) in PNH, since a repair of the damaged cell may result in cell destruction; in fact, in most PNH patients, a residual population of normal hematopoietic progenitors already exists, but it is unable to repopulate the bone marrow. Immunosuppression using antilymphocyte globulin and/or cyclosporin could be a valid alternative, aiming to treat the underlying bone marrow failure syndrome; it has been used in a few patients in recent years, with promising results.

FUTURE DIRECTIONS

Although so many pathophysiological aspects of PNH have been unraveled, several important items still require clarification, such as:

1. The functional properties of the GPI-anchoring system in human cells.
2. The structure and the function of the protein encoded by *PIG-A*.
3. The exact role of each GPI-linked molecule on blood cell development and function.
4. The amount of transfer of GPI-linked molecules (if any) that takes place in vivo from one cell to another.
5. The hierarchy by which the various molecules are preferred in the cell for anchor attachment, when a reduced amount of anchor is produced.
6. The reason for the nocturnal exacerbation of hemolysis.

Also, a formal proof of the escape theory is needed. If it is confirmed, PNH could be regarded as a special type of nonneoplastic clonal disease, in which the expansion of the mutated cell is due to a survival advantage rather than to a growth advantage.

ACKNOWLEDGMENTS

The experimental work on PNH carried out by the authors was performed in Prof. Lucio Luzzatto's laboratories in several countries; we also thank Prof. Luzzatto for reviewing the manuscript. We thank Dr. Luigi Del Vecchio for useful discussion and updated information on surface antigens and flow cytometry data.

SELECTED REFERENCES

Bessler M, Hillmen P, Longo L, Luzzatto L, Mason PJ. Genomic organization of the X-linked gene *(PIG-A)* that is mutated in paroxysmal nocturnal haemoglobinuria and of a related autosomal pseudogene mapped to 12q21. Hum Mol Gen 1994;3:751–757.

Bessler M, Mason P, Hillmen P, Luzzatto L. Somatic mutations and cellular selection in paroxysmal nocturnal hemoglobinuria. Lancet 1994;343:951–953.

Hertenstein B, Wagner B, Bunjes D, et al. Emergence of CD52-, phosphatidyl inositol glycan-anchor-deficient T lymphocytes after in vivo application of Campath -1H for refractory B-cell non-Hodgkin lymphoma. Blood 1995;86:1487–1492.

Hillmen P, Lewis SM, Bessler M, Luzzatto L, Dacie JV. Natural history of paroxysmal nocturnal hemoglobinuria. New Engl J Med 1995;333: 1253–1258.

Kawagoe K, Kitamura D, Okabe M, et al. Glycosylphosphatidylinositol-anchor-deficient mice: implications for clonal dominance of mutant cells in paroxysmal nocturnal hemoglobinuria. Blood 1996;87: 3600–3606.

Kinoshita T, Inoue N, Takeda J. Defective glycosyl phosphatidylinositol (GPI)-anchor synthesis and paroxysmal nocturnal hemoglobinuria. Adv Immunol 1995;60:57–103.

Luzzatto L, Bessler M. The dual pathogenesis of paroxysmal nocturnal hemoglobinuria. Curr Opin Hematol 1996;3:101–110.

Luzzatto L, Bessler M, Rotoli B. Somatic mutations in paroxysmal nocturnal hemoglobinuria: a blessing in disguise? Cell 1997;88:1–4.

Miyata T, Takeda J, Lida Y, et al. The cloning of *PIG-A*, a component in the early step of GPI-anchor biosynthesis. Science 1993;259: 1318–1320.

Nafa K, Mason PJ, Hillmen P, Luzzatto L, Bessler M. Mutations in the *PIG-A* gene causing paroxysmal nocturnal hemoglobinuria are mainly of the frameshift type. Blood 1995;86:4650–4655.

Oni SB, Osunkoya BO, Luzzatto L. Paroxysmal nocturnal hemoglobinuria: evidence for monoclonal origin of abnormal red cells. Blood 1970;36:145–152.

Plesner T, Hansen NE, Carlsen K. Estimation of PI-bound proteins on blood cells from PNH patients by quantitative flow cytometry. Br J Haematol 1990;75:585–590.

Rosse WF. Paroxysmal nocturnal hemoglobinuria as a molecular disease. Medicine (Baltimore) 1997;76:63–93.

Rosse WF, Dacie JV. Immune lysis of normal and paroxysmal nocturnal hemoglobinuria (PNH) red blood cells. I. The sensitivity of PNH red cells to lysis by complement and specific antibody. J Clin Invest 1966;45:736–748.

Rosse WF, Ware RE. The molecular basis of paroxysmal nocturnal hemoglobinuria. Blood 1995;86:3277–3286.

Rotoli B, Robledo R, Scarpato N, Luzzatto L. Two populations of erythroid cell progenitors in paroxysmal nocturnal hemoglobinuria. Blood 1984;64:847–851.

Rosti V, Tremml G, Soarez V, Pandolfi PP, Luzzatto L, Bessler M. Murine embryonic stem cells without *PIG-A* gene activity are competent for PNH-like hematopoiesis but not for clonal expansion. J Clin Invest 1997;100:1028–1036.

Rotoli B, Luzzatto L. Paroxysmal nocturnal haemoglobinuria. Baillière's Clinical Haematology 1989;2:113–138.

Schlossman SF, Boumsell L, Gilks W, et al. Leucocyte typing V. White cell differentiation antigens. In: Proceedings of the Fifth International Workshop and Conference. Boston: Oxford University Press, 1995.

Takeda J, Miyata T, Kawagoe K, et al. Deficiency of the GPI anchor caused by a somatic mutation of the *PIG-A* gene in paroxysmal nocturnal hemoglobinuria. Cell 1993;73:703–711.

Telen MJ, Hall SE, Green AM, Moulds JJ, Rosse WF. Identification of human erythrocyte blood group antigens on decay-accelerating factor (DAF) and an erythrocyte phenotype negative for DAF. J Exp Med 1988;167:1993–1998.

Yamashina M, Ueda E, Kinoshita T, et al. Inherited complete deficiency of 20-kilodalton homologous restriction factor (CD59) as a cause of paroxysmal nocturnal hemoglobinuria. N Engl J Med 1990;323: 1184–1189.

Yomtovian R, Prince GM, Medof ME. The molecular basis for paroxysmal nocturnal hemoglobinuria. Transfusion 1993;33:852–873.

26 Leukemias

JEFFREY E. RUBNITZ AND CHING-HON PUI

INTRODUCTION

The acute and chronic leukemias arise from the uncontrolled clonal expansion of hematopoietic progenitor cells blocked in differentiation. The different types of leukemia represent distinct clinicopathologic entities that have characteristic biological and clinical properties and respond to specific therapies. The identification of specific molecular lesions helps us to understand the molecular mechanisms that contribute to leukemogenesis. Here we review the epidemiology, clinical features, and molecular genetics of acute lymphoblastic leukemia (ALL), acute myeloid leukemia (AML), chronic myelogenous leukemia (CML), and chronic lymphocytic leukemia (CLL).

EPIDEMIOLOGY

Acute leukemia is the most common malignancy in children, accounting for approximately one-third of all childhood cancers. ALL predominates during childhood, with 2000 new cases diagnosed in the United States each year, compared to 500 new cases of AML. CML accounts for less than 100 cases of pediatric leukemia each year, whereas CLL is extremely rare in children. The 4:1 ratio of ALL:AML is reversed in adults, with AML being more common and occurring in approximately 5000 adults each year. Chronic leukemias are also common in adults, with approximately 6000 cases of CML and 12,000 cases of CLL diagnosed each year in the United States.

Environmental and genetic factors are linked to an increase in the risk of leukemia. Exposure to ionizing radiation, toxic chemicals (e.g., benzene), and specific chemotherapeutic agents are all associated with a higher risk of acute leukemia. In particular, alkylating agents used to treat a primary malignancy can induce secondary AML that is characterized by a prior myelodysplastic syndrome and abnormalities of chromosomes 5 and 7. Also, exposure to topoisomerase II inhibitors, especially the epipodophyllotoxins teniposide and etoposide, can lead to the rapid development of secondary AML with rearrangements of the *MLL* gene.

Genetic diseases associated with chromosomal instability, such as Bloom's syndrome, Fanconi's anemia, and ataxia–telangiectasia, are also characterized by an increased risk of acute leukemia. Similarly, children with congenital immunodeficiencies, such as Wiskott-Aldrich syndrome, are predisposed to develop leukemia. The 10- to 20-fold increased risk of acute leukemia in patients with trisomy 21 is further evidence for a role of genetic factors in the development of leukemia. However, the vast majority of leukemia cases—especially in children—have no clear etiology.

From: *Principles of Molecular Medicine* (J. L. Jameson, ed.), ©1998 Humana Press Inc., Totowa, NJ.

CLASSIFICATION

Leukemias are classified according to morphological, immunological, biochemical, and cytogenetic characteristics. The French-American-British (FAB) system of morphological classification distinguishes three types of ALL (L1 through L3, Table 26-1), but has not proven to be clinically useful. ALLs are further classified by their expression of normal lymphoid-associated surface markers (Table 26-1). Eight types of AML (M0–M7, Table 26-2) are defined morphologically and show correlations with clinical features, cytogenetics, and outcome. Immunophenotyping is also performed in AML but is used primarily to distinguish undifferentiated cases of AML from ALL.

Leukemias can also be classified according to specific chromosomal abnormalities, which can be identified in over 90% of ALL, AML, and CML cases. Difficulties in obtaining sufficient metaphases have hampered cytogenetic analysis in CLL, but approximately two-thirds of CLL patients have clonal chromosomal abnormalities. Recurring chromosomal abnormalities, including changes in both chromosome structure and number, are associated with specific biological and clinical features. For example, hyperdiploidy with a chromosome number greater than 50 is identified in approximately one-fourth of childhood ALL cases and is associated with favorable prognostic factors, such as lower leukocyte count and a better treatment outcome, even with antimetabolite-based therapy. Several structural chromosomal abnormalities also have prognostic and therapeutic implications; the t(9;22)(q34;q11) or t(4;11)(q21;q23) confers a particularly poor prognosis in ALL, whereas the dic(9;12)(p11-12;p12) is associated with a favorable prognosis. In AML, cases with t(8;21)(q22;q22) or inv(16)(p13q22) respond well to chemotherapy regimens that contain high-dose cytarabine, whereas leukemic cells containing the t(15;17)(q21;q21) differentiate in response to all-*trans*-retinoic acid. In contrast, cases of AML with monosomy 7 have a particularly poor outcome and require allogeneic bone marrow transplantation for cure.

MOLECULAR ANALYSIS OF LEUKEMIA

Cytogenetic analysis has been the standard method of identifying translocations, but it is technically difficult and dependent on an adequate diagnostic specimen. The molecular characterization of translocation breakpoints has led to alternative approaches,

Table 26-1
Classification of Acute Leukemias

		Frequency, %	
		Adult[a]	*Childhood*[b]
Acute lymphoblastic leukemia			
Morphologic classification			
L1	Small, homogeneous cells with scanty cytoplasm	30	80
L2	Larger, heterogeneous cells with irregular nuclei and at least one large nucleolus	60–70	17
L3	Large, homogeneous cells with deep basophilic cytoplasm and prominent cytoplasmic vacuoles	5	3
Immunophenotype			
Early pre-B	CD19+, CD22+, cIg–, sIg–	50–60	57
Pre-B	cIg+	15–25	25
Transitional pre-B	cIg+, sIg+, sIgκ–, sIgλ	Unknown	1
B cell	sIg+	5	2
T cell	CD3+, CD7+, and CD5+ or CD2+	20–25	15
Ploidy			
Hypodiploid (<45 chromosomes)		5–10	7
Diploid (normal 46 chromosomes)		25–35	8
Pseudodiploid (46 chromosomes with structural abnormalities)		50–60	42
Hyperdiploid (47–50 chromosomes)		5–10	15
Hyperdiploid (>50 chromosomes)		5–10	27
Triploid or tetraploid (>65 chromosomes)		1	1
Acute myeloid leukemia			
M0	Minimal differentiation	2–3	2
M1	Poorly differentiated myeloblasts	10–20	13
M2	Differentiated myeloblasts	30–35	28
M3	Promyelocytic	10–15	6
M4	Myelomonoblastic	15–25	19
M5	Monoblastic	10–15	21
M6	Erythroleukemia	1–4	1
M7	Megakaryoblastic	1	10

[a]Based on literature review.
[b]Based on 600 consecutive cases of newly diagnosed ALL and 180 cases of AML in children less than 18 years of age studied at St. Jude Children's Research Hospital from 1984–1992 (N Engl J Med 1995;332:1618).

including fluorescence *in situ* hybridization (FISH), Southern blot analysis, and reverse transcriptase-polymerase chain reaction (RT-PCR). These techniques can be performed on samples inadequate for cytogenetic analysis and are quicker, more sensitive, and more specific than cytogenetics. For example, molecular rearrangements of *MLL* (located at 11q23) are seen in approximately 80% of infants with ALL, whereas only about 60% of these cases have 11q23 alterations by cytogenetics.

Molecular approaches can also detect important submicroscopic genetic abnormalities not visible by cytogenetics. The *TEL-AML1* gene fusion, which results from the t(12;21)(p12-13;q22), occurs in greater than one-fourth of B-lineage childhood ALL cases, few of which have cytogenetic evidence of the t(12;21). Likewise, *TAL1* gene rearrangements (Table 26-1), the most common abnormality in T-cell ALL, are generally detectable only at the molecular level. Finally, the tumor suppressor gene *p16*, located at 9p21, is homozygously deleted in about one-fourth of ALL cases, including many that have cytogenetically normal chromosome 9p.

Moreover, some lesions can appear identical by cytogenetics, yet they differ when analyzed at the molecular level. RT-PCR assays have detected *E2A-PBX1* fusions in patients with normal or unsuccessful cytogenetic studies and have identified patients who have the t(1;19) but lack the fusion gene. The distinction is clinically important, because patients with *E2A-PBX1* fusions fare poorly on nonintensive therapies, whereas patients with t(1;19) who lack *E2A-PBX1* do quite well on standard antimetabolite-based protocols.

MOLECULAR ABNORMALITIES IN LEUKEMIA

Chromosomal rearrangements can cause leukemogenesis by two mechanisms: the activation of dominant cellular proto-oncogenes, and the inactivation of tumor suppressor genes (Fig. 26-1). Proto-oncogenes are activated by at least four pathways. First, in T- and B-cell leukemias, cellular oncogenes may be activated by transcriptional deregulation, following their juxtaposition with T-cell receptor (TCR) or immunoglobulin (Ig) genes (Fig. 26-1A, Table 26-2). Second, in B-precursor ALL and in AML, translocations frequently create chimeric fusion genes that encode novel oncogenic proteins (Fig. 26-1B, Table 26-2). Third, gene amplification can lead to oncogene overexpression, an event that is less common in leukemias than in certain solid tumors. Fourth, point mutations of the *ras* gene, reported in up to 50% of AML cases, are likely key events in leukemogenesis.

Many of the genes at the breakpoints of leukemia-specific translocations are oncogenic transcription factors involved in cellular proliferation and differentiation. Oncogenic transcription factors are classified by their structural motifs, including basic helix-loop-helix (bHLH), leucine-zipper, and LIM domains (Table 26-2) (*see also* Chapter 3). Other oncogenes identified in this manner include protein kinases, growth factors, and proteins involved in signal transduction (*see* Chapter 7).

Table 26-2
Translocations in Leukemia

Translocation	Genes involved	Protein products	Frequency (%)[a]	
			Adult	Childhood
B-lineage ALL				
t(9;22)(q34;q11)	*BCR-ABL*	Tyrosine kinase	15–25	3–5
t(1;19)(q23;p13.3)	*E2A-PBX1*	Homeodomain protein (PBX1)	3–5	5–6
t(17;19)(q22;p13.3)	*E2A-HLF*	Basic leucine-zipper (HLF)	<1	<1
t(5;14)(q31;q32)	*IL3 (IgH)*	Cytokine	<1	<1
t(4;11)(q21;q23)	*MLL-AF4*	DNA-binding trans. factor	5	2
t(12;21)(p13;q22)	*TEL-AML1*	Transcription factors	1–3	25[b]
B-cell ALL				
t(8;14)(q24;q32)	*MYC (IgH)*	Basic helix-loop-helix-zipper	5–8	1–2
t(2;8)(q12;q24)	*MYC (IGκ)*	Basic helix-loop-helix-zipper	1	<1
t(8;22)(q24;q11)	*MYC (IGλ)*	Basic helix-loop-helix-zipper	1	<1
T-cell ALL				
t(8;14)(q24;q11)	*MYC (TCRδ)*	Basic helix-loop-helix-zipper	<1	<1
t(10;14)(q24;q11)	*HOX11 (TCRδ)*	Homeodomain	3	<1
t(7;10)(q35;q24)	*HOX11 (TCRβ)*	Homeodomain	<1	<1
t(11;14)(p15;q11)	*TTG1 (TCRδ)*	Cysteine-rich (LIM)	<1	<1
t(7;11)(q35;p13)	*TTG2 (TCRβ)*	Cysteine-rich (LIM)	<1	<1
t(11;14)(p13;q11)	*TTG2 (TCRδ)*	Cysteine-rich (LIM)	1	1
t(1;7)(p32;q35)	*TAL1 (TCRβ)*	Basic helix-loop-helix (bHLH)	<1	<1
t(1;14)(p32;q11)	*TAL1 (TCRδ)*	bHLH	1	<1
t(7;9)(q34;q32)	*TAL2 (TCRβ)*	bHLH	<1	<1
t(7;19)(q34;p13)	*LYL1 (TCRβ)*	bHLH	<1	<1
t(1;7)(p34;q34)	*LCK (TCRβ)*	Tyrosine kinase	<1	<1
t(7;9)(q34;q34)	*TAN1 (TCRβ)*	Transmembrane protein	<1	<1
AML				
t(3;21)(q26;q22)	*AML1-EAP*	Runt homology (AML1)	<1	<1
t(8;21)(q22;q22)	*AML1-ETO*	Runt homology (AML1)	6–12	8–10
t(6;9)(p23;q34)	*DEK-CAN*	Probable transcription factors	1	<1
t(9;22)(q34;q11)	*BCR-ABL*	Tyrosine kinase	3	<1
t(15;17)(q21;q21)	*PML-RARα*	Transcription factor	5–15	6–10
t(11;17)(q23;q21)	*PLZF-RARα*	Transcription factor	<1	<1
t(11;16)(q23;p13.3)	*MLL-CBP*	Transcription factor	<1	<1
inv(16)(p13q22)	*CBFβ-MYH11*	Transcription factor	3	8–10
inv(3)q21q26)	*EVI1*	Transcription factor	1	<1
t(9;11)(p21-22;q23)	*MLL-AF9*	Transcription factor	1–2	7–9
t(1;22)(p13;q13)	Unknown	Unknown	<1	2–3
CML				
t(9;22)(q34;q11)	*BCR-ABL*	Tyrosine kinase	95	95

[a]Based on literature review.
[b]Based on molecular analysis.

COMMON TRANSLOCATIONS IN ALL

t(9;22)(q34;q11)

The balanced translocation t(9;22)(q34;q11), also referred to as the Philadelphia chromosome (Ph), occurs in about 95% of all CML cases, 25% of adult ALL cases, 3–5% of pediatric ALL cases, and less than 1% of AML cases. In both CML and ALL, the t(9;22) results in the translocation of the *ABL* proto-oncogene from the distal long arm of chromosome 9 into the *BCR* gene on chromosome 22, forming a *BCR-ABL* fusion gene (Fig. 26-2). In the majority of CML cases, and in about one-half of adult Ph+ ALL cases, the *BCR* breakpoints are located in the major breakpoint cluster region (M-bcr), producing chimeric mRNAs that encode a fusion protein of approximately 210 kDa (p210). p210 has enhanced tyrosine kinase activity, compared to ABL, a cytoplasmic intracellular location, and the ability to transform hematopoietic precursors in experimental systems. Most cases of childhood Ph+ ALL and the other half of adult Ph+ ALL cases are characterized by *BCR-ABL* fusions in which the breakpoints in the *BCR* gene are distributed in a second breakpoint cluster region (m-bcr). The resulting fusion gene encodes a 190-kDa protein (p190) in which tyrosine kinase activity and transforming potential are enhanced compared to those of p210.

t(1;19)(q23;p13.3) The t(1;19)(q23;p13.3) is present in 1% of early pre-B ALLs and 25% of cases with a pre-B (cytoplasmic Ig positive) immunophenotype. The t(1;19) breakpoint on chromosome 19 involves the *E2A* gene, which encodes the Ig enhancer binding proteins E12 and E47. E12 and E47 both contain N-terminal transactivation domains and C-terminal helix-loop-helix DNA-binding and dimerization motifs. In pre-B ALL, the t(1;19) disrupts *E2A* and fuses the N-terminal transactivation domain of E12/E47 to the DNA binding domain of PBX1, a homeodomain protein (Fig. 26-3). Transformation by E2A-PBX1 presumably results

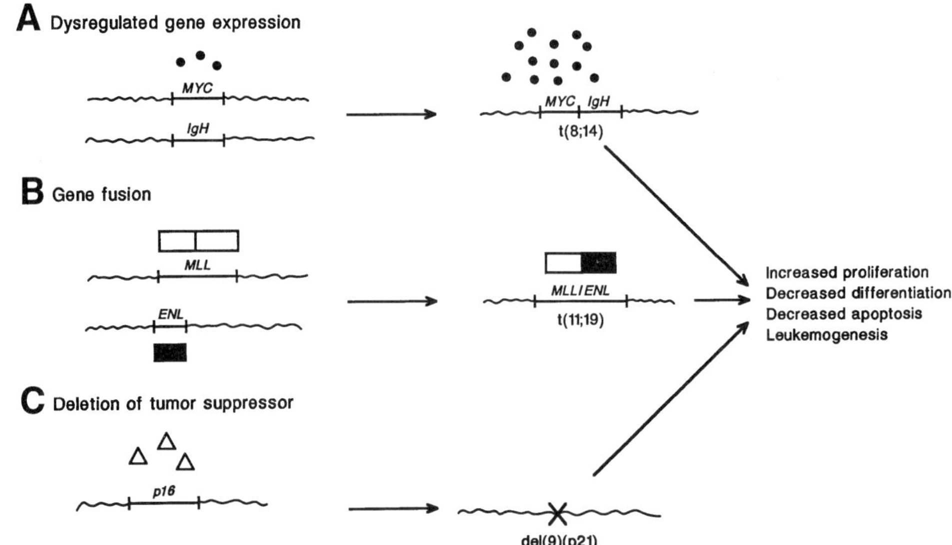

Figure 26-1 Mechanisms of leukemogenesis. **(A)** Cellular proto-oncogenes, such as *MYC*, may become deregulated, following their juxtaposition with transcriptionally active genes, such as the immunoglobulin heavy-chain gene *(IgH)*. **(B)** Gene fusion activates cellular oncogenes. The t(11;19) fuses the N-terminal portion of the *MLL* gene with the *ENL* gene to create the chimera *MLL/ENL*. **(C)** The tumor suppressor gene *p16* is inactivated by deletion of the 9p21 region.

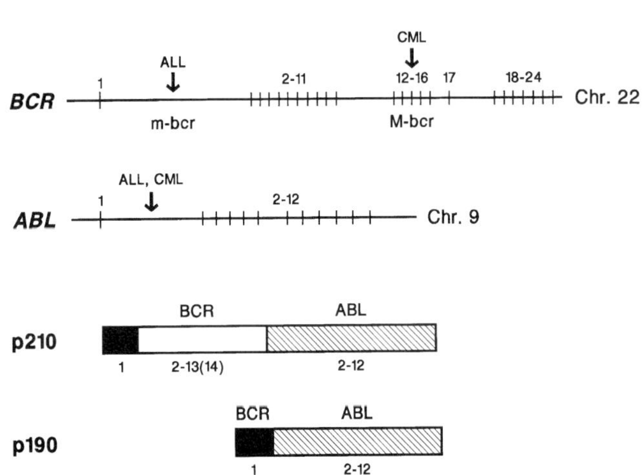

Figure 26-2 BCR-ABL fusion as a result of the t(9;22). *BCR* is a schematic representation of the *BCR* gene, which lies on chromosome 22 and contains 24 exons (depicted as vertical bars). ALL (m-bcr) and CML (M-bcr) breakpoints are indicated by arrows. *ABL* shows the genomic structure of the *ABL* gene on chromosome 9, with ALL and CML breakpoints indicated between exons 1 and 2. p210 and p190 represent BCR-ABL fusion proteins created as a result of CML (p210) or ALL (p190) breaks. p210 is encoded by exons 1 through 13 or 14 of *BCR* fused to exon 2 of *ABL*, whereas p190 is encoded by exon 1 of *BCR* fused to exon 2 of *ABL*.

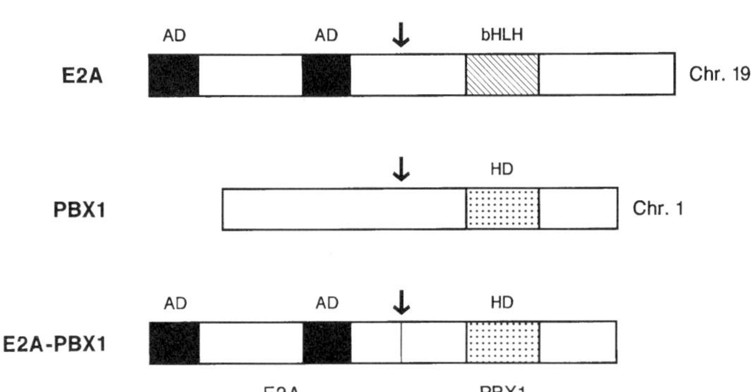

Figure 26-3 E2A-PBX1 fusion created by t(1;19). E2A contains two activation domains (AD) and a basic helix-loop-helix domain (bHLH), whereas PBX1 contains a homeodomain (HD). The t(1;19) results in the fusion of the N-terminal portion of E2A to the C-terminal portion of PBX1. Arrows indicate breakpoints.

from the inappropriate expression of PBX1 in lymphoid cells, allowing PBX1 to bind specific DNA sequences and transactivate unknown target genes. As predicted by this model, E2A-PBX1 is a transactivator in vitro, transforms NIH-3T3 fibroblasts, and induces lymphomas in transgenic mice. In contrast to pre-B ALL, cytogenetically indistinguishable early pre-B (cytoplasmic Ig negative) ALL cases containing the t(1;19) do not involve either *E2A* or *PBX1*.

11q23 Rearrangements Structural lesions involving chromosome 11, band q23, occur in approximately 80% of infant ALL cases and in 85% of secondary leukemias (generally AML) that arise in patients treated with topoisomerse II inhibitors. Over 40 reciprocal chromosomal loci participate in 11q23 translocations, the most common being 4q21, 9p22, and 19p13. The gene on chromosome 11 that is disrupted by these translocations is designated *MLL* (mixed lineage leukemia), but is also referred to as *HRX*, *ALL-1*, and *HTRX1*. *MLL* rearrangement in ALL identifies a high-risk subgroup of patients who are unlikely to be cured with conventional chemotherapy. In contrast, cases that have 11q23 abnormalities but lack *MLL* rearrangements have an intermediate prognosis.

MLL is a 431-kDa protein with two central zinc finger domains, a C-terminal region that shows high homology to the *Drosophila* trithorax protein, a region with homology to DNA methyltransferases, and an N-terminus that contains three AT hooks (Fig. 26-4). 11q23 translocations cluster in an 8.5–kb region of *MLL* and fuse

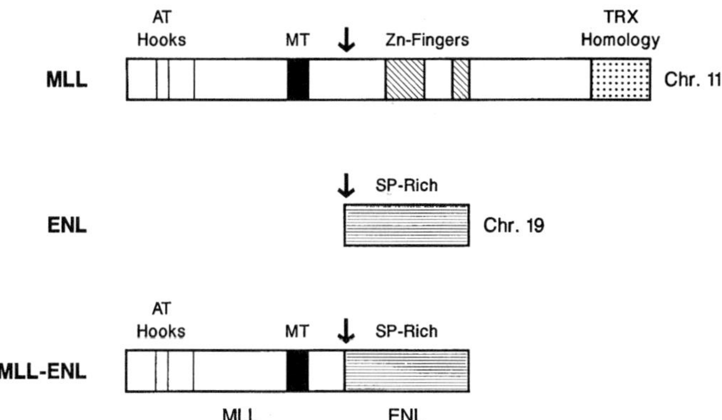

Figure 26-4 The *MLL* gene, located at 11q23, encodes a protein (MLL) with 3 AT-hooks near the N-terminus, a methyltransferase domain (MT), two zinc fingers (Zn-fingers), and a region of homology to the Drosophila trithorax protein (TRX homology). The t(11;19) involves the *ENL* gene at 19p13, which encodes a small serine/proline-rich (SP-rich) protein. The MLL-ENL fusion protein includes the N-terminal portion of MLL fused to nearly all of ENL. Breakpoints are indicated by arrows.

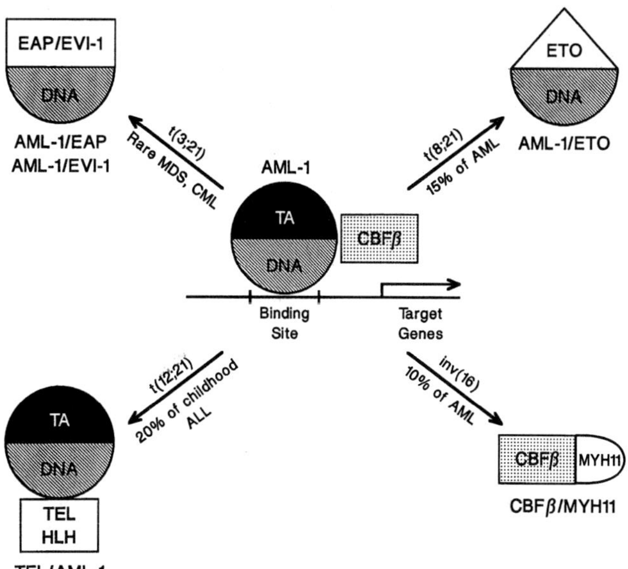

Figure 26-5 The transcription factor complex AML-1/CBFβ (center) is the target of a variety of translocations. TA and DNA represent the transactivation and DNA-binding domains of AML-1. The t(3;21) (upper left) fuses the DNA binding domain of AML-1 to either EAP or EVI1 in rare cases of myelodysplastic syndrome (MDS) or CML. In ALL, the t(12;21) (lower left) creates a chimeric protein consisting of AML-1 fused to the helix-loop-helix (HLH) portion of TEL. In AML, CBFβ is fused to MYH11 as a result of inv(16) (lower right), and in the t(8;21) the DNA-binding portion of AML-1 fuses to ETO (upper right).

the N-terminal portion of MLL—containing the AT hooks and methyltransferase domains—to a variety of proteins. In ALL with the t(11;19), for example, MLL is fused to a small serine/proline-rich protein (ENL) that has in vitro transactivation activity (Fig. 26-4). Accordingly, MLL fusion proteins are thought to function as chimeric transcription factors in early hematopoietic progenitor cells.

t(12;21)(p13;q22) The *TEL* gene, located at 12p13 and encoding a novel ETS-like transcription factor, is fused to the DNA-binding and transactivation domains of *AML1* as a result of a cryptic t(12;21)(p13;q22) in ALL. *AML1* encodes the DNA-binding component of the AML1/CBFβ transcription factor complex, which is also targeted by the myeloid-associated translocations t(8;21), t(3;21), and inv(16) (Fig. 26-5). Although the t(12;21) is detected by standard cytogenetic techniques in less than 1 in 1000 cases, molecular analyses have demonstrated that *TEL-AML1* is actually the most common genetic lesion in pediatric ALL, occurring in approximately one-fourth of B-lineage cases. In addition, this fusion gene is associated with an excellent prognosis. Because the relationship of *TEL-AML1* expression to a favorable prognosis is independent of recognized prognostic features in B-precursor leukemia, including age and leukocyte count, *TEL-AML1* identifies a large subset of children with favorable-prognosis B-precursor leukemia who cannot be identified by clinical features. These patients may be candidates for less intensive therapy, designed to reduce both early and late adverse effects.

Translocations in B-Cell ALL B-cell ALL is characterized by the presence of surface immunoglobulin, FAB L3 morphology, frequent extramedullary disease, and translocations involving the *MYC* gene on chromosome 8, band q24 (Table 26-2). Approximately 80% of B-cell cases contain the t(8;14)(q24;q32), in which *MYC* is translocated to the immunoglobulin heavy chain gene locus. Nearly all of the remaining cases contain the t(2;8)(p12;q24) or the t(8;22)(q24;q11), in which either the κ (located at 2p12) or λ (located at 22q11) light chain gene is translocated to chromosome 8 adjacent to *MYC*. All three translocations result *MYC* dysregulation and ultimately lead to transformation.

Translocations in T-Cell ALL Recurring translocations in T-cell ALL often involve the TCR β locus (7q34) or the TCR α/δ locus (14q11) (Table 2). For example, the t(1;14)(p32;q11) results in abnormal *TAL1* expression, following translocation of *TAL1* into the TCR α/δ locus. *TAL1* encodes a bHLH transcription factor that is also involved in the t(1;7) (Table 26-2). *TAL2* and *LYL1* encode related members of the bHLH family that are translocated to TCR sites in cases of T-cell ALL. Other proteins involved in T-cell leukemias include MYC, the cysteine-rich proteins TTG1 and TTG2, the homeodomain transcription factor HOX11, the tyrosine kinase LCK, and the transmembrane protein TAN-1 (Table 26-2).

COMMON TRANSLOCATIONS IN AML

t(8;21)(q22;q22)

Approximately 15% of AML cases carry the t(8;21)(q22;q22), which is associated with a tendency to form tumor masses (granulocytic sarcomas) in extramedullary sites and a favorable response to therapy. The t(8;21) disrupts *AML1* (located at 21q22), which encodes a transcription factor that contains a transactivation domain near its C-terminus and a DNA-binding region of homology with the *Drosophila runt* gene near its N-terminus. *AML1* shares homology with the alpha subunit of core-binding factor (CBFα), which binds conserved sites in the enhancers of murine leukemia viruses, the T-cell receptor gene, and several myeloid-specific genes. In the t(8;21), the runt domain of *AML1* is translocated to the derivative 8 chromosome and joined to *ETO* (Fig. 26-5). In vitro, AML1-ETO binds AML1 sites and represses transcription of reporter genes. Thus, the t(8;21) may lead to transformation by creating a protein that competes in vivo with AML1 and inhibits AML1-mediated expression of myeloid-specific genes.

inv(16)(p13q22)and t(16;16)(p13;q22) Approximately 10% of AML cases carry pericentric inversions or translocations of chromosome 16. These cases are associated with myelomonocytic differentiation, the presence of abnormal bone marrow eosinophils (commonly FAB subtype M4Eo), a propensity for central nervous system (CNS) involvement, and a favorable prognosis. In the inv(16) and t(16;16), sequences from the β-subunit of core binding factor *(CBFb)* at 16q22 are joined to the smooth muscle myosin heavy chain gene *(MYH11)* at 16p13. CBFβ interacts with and increases the DNA-binding affinity of AML1. Thus, disruption of the AML1/CBFβ transcription complex by inv(16), t(8;21), t(3;21), or t(12;21) may lead to leukemia (Fig. 26-5).

t(15;17)(q21;q21) Acute promyelocytic leukemia (APL, AML-M3), characterized by coagulopathy and severe bleeding diathesis, is frequently associated with a balanced translocation that involves the retinoic acid receptor-alpha *(RARa)* gene (17q21) and the *PML* gene (15q21). RARα, a transcription factor, binds various retinoids, including all-*trans*-retinoic acid, and interacts directly with DNA. PML contains a putative DNA-binding domain, a potential dimerization domain, a serine/proline-rich region, and a phosphorylation site. The PML-RARα fusion protein formed by the t(15;17) contains the PML dimerization and DNA-binding domains fused to the DNA-binding and retinoid-binding portion of RARα. The PML-RARα fusion retains the ligand binding and dimerization properties of RARα, but displays altered transactivation activities.

SECONDARY AML Therapy-induced secondary AML, involving 11q23 translocations, is typically seen in patients treated with topoisomerase II inhibitors, particularly the epipodophyllotoxins etoposide and teniposide. Unlike the secondary leukemias that occur after treatment with alkylating agents, secondary AMLs containing 11q23 abnormalities have a short latent period, lack a prior myelodysplastic phase, and generally have features of monocytic differentiation (M4 and M5 subtypes). Molecular analyses have shown that the majority of patients with topoisomerase-induced secondary AML have *MLL* rearrangements analogous to those seen in ALL.

TRANSLOCATIONS IN CML Greater than 95% of CML patients have cytogenetic evidence of the t(9;22)(q34;q11). As stated earlier, this translocation creates a *BCR-ABL* fusion gene that encodes a 210-kDa protein with altered kinase activity. Detection of *BCR-ABL* has important implications for diagnosis and the detection of minimal residual disease. In general, the persistence or increase in the level of minimal residual disease detectable by RT-PCR after allogeneic bone marrow transplantation is closely correlated with subsequent relapse.

TRANSLOCATIONS IN CLL Clonal abnormalities occur in approximately two-thirds of CLL patients, of which about one-third has trisomy 12. Although the biological significance of trisomy 12 is unknown, patients with this abnormality have a worse prognosis than patients with other single abnormalities. The most common structural cytogenetic abnormality in CLL is partial deletion of the long arm of chromosome 13, including band q14, the site of the retinoblastoma type 1 gene *(RB1)*. Homozygous deletion of a region telomeric to *RB1* suggests that a new tumor suppressor gene might be involved in CLL.

TUMOR SUPPRESSOR GENES Tumor suppressor genes, in which loss of function may cause transformation, include *RB1*, the Wilms' tumor gene, and *p53*. Although *p53* is mutated or deleted in a variety of human malignancies, it does not play a significant role in the development of pediatric leukemia. Mutations in *p53* occur in only 1–2% of B-precursor and T-cell ALLs at diagnosis but are present in about 25% of relapsed T-cell leukemia cases. Among the relapsed T-cell cases, patients with *p53* mutations have a shorter second remission than those patients without *p53* mutations. Therefore, *p53* mutations may be important in the development of drug-resistant disease.

Recently, two candidate tumor suppressor genes, designated *p16 (MTS1, INK4a)* and *p15 (MTS2, INK4b)*, were localized to 9p21, a site of nonrandom chromosomal abnormalities in gliomas, melanomas, esophageal carcinomas, lung carcinomas, and leukemias. p16 and p15 are highly homologous and function as specific cell cycle inhibitors by targeting activated cyclin D-cdk4/6 complexes. Deletions of *p16* have been detected in 46% of cell lines and 10–20% of primary tumor samples. In ALL, homozygous deletions of *p16* and *p15* have been detected in 20–30% of B-precursor ALLs and 70–80% of T-cell ALLs. In other leukemias, however, *p16/p15* deletions are quite rare, being reported in less than 10% of AML, CLL, and CML cases.

CLINICAL APPLICATIONS OF MOLECULAR ANALYSIS

Molecular analyses have improved our abilities to diagnose and risk-stratify patients, monitor response to therapy, and detect minimal residual disease. In ALL, the presence of *BCR-ABL* or *MLL-AF4* is associated with poor prognostic indicators, such as hyperleukocytosis, organomegaly, and CNS leukemia. Furthermore, despite overall improvements in outcome for ALL, patients with these genetic abnormalities still have a dismal prognosis and are candidates for innovative therapies or allogeneic bone marrow transplantation in first remission. Because cytogenetic studies fail to detect these abnormalities in some patients, molecular detection methods become even more valuable. Similarly, molecular techniques are essential to identify patients with *E2A-PBX1* fusions, because these patients fare poorly on standard moderately intense therapies, but they do quite well when treated more aggressively. This observation was first made at St. Jude Childrens Research Hospital, where patients with *E2A-PBX1* fusions had a 4-year EFS of about 50% on Total Therapy Study X, but a 4-year EFS of 79% on the more intensified Study XI.

Molecular detection of *PML-RARa*, *AML1-ETO*, and *CBFb-MYH11* also has significant therapeutic implications. Approximately 95% of patients with acute promyelocytic leukemia and *PML-RARa* achieve complete remission when treated with all-*trans*-retinoic acid. Treatment with all-*trans*-retinoic acid is associated with leukemic promyelocyte differentiation, onset of normal hematopoiesis without bone marrow aplasia, and correction of the associated coagulopathy that was formerly a leading cause of death during induction therapy. The combination of all-*trans*-retinoic acid with anthracycline-based chemotherapy has greatly improved the overall outcome of these patients. Detection of *AML1-ETO* or *CBFb-MYH11* is associated with a high rate of long-term remission following treatment with high-dose cytarabine chemotherapy.

Finally, early detection of minimal residual disease by use of molecular techniques can potentially improve cure rates for patients with leukemia. Adoptive immunotherapy with donor leukocytes forestalls clinical relapse in patients who have CML and molecular evidence of minimal residual disease after allogeneic bone marrow transplantation. Therefore, molecular techniques can be used to monitor the minimal residual disease level and potential for relapse in these patients.

FUTURE DIRECTIONS

Molecular characterization of translocation breakpoints has identified new oncogenes and tumor suppressors, and it has led to the development of molecular diagnostic assays that have improved therapeutic management and detection of residual disease. To further elucidate the pathways leading to malignant transformation, research will focus on oncogenic transcription factors and their downstream targets. These proteins may represent molecules to which novel tumor-specific therapies can be directed. In addition, gene replacement therapy of inactivated tumor suppressor genes could play a role in the future treatment of leukemia. Finally, attempts to induce leukemic cells to undergo normal differentiation and apoptosis will be the basis of important future research.

SELECTED REFERENCES

Bash RO, Hall S, Timmons CF, et al. Does activation of the TAL1 gene occur in a majority of patients with T-cell acute lymphoblastic leukemia? A Pediatric Oncology Group study. Blood 1995;86:666–676.

Berger R. Acute lymphoblastic leukemia and chromosome 21. Cancer Genet Cytogenet 1997;94:8–12.

Cleary ML. Oncogenic conversion of transcription factors by chromosomal translocations. Cell 1991;66:1–3.

Crist WM, Carroll AJ, Shuster JJ, et al. Philadelphia chromosome positive childhood acute lymphoblastic leukemia: clinical and cytogenetic characteristics and treatment outcome. A Pediatric Oncology Group Study. Blood 1990;76:489–495.

Guerrasio A, Serra A, Gottardi E, et al. Molecular events in chronic myeloid leukemia progression. Leukemia 1997;11 Suppl 3:519–521.

Hirama T, Koeffler HP. Role of the cyclin-dependent kinase inhibitors in the development of cancer. Blood 1995;86:841–854.

Mackinnon S, Papadopoulos EB, Carabasi MH, et al. Adoptive immunotherapy evaluating escalating doses of donor leukocytes for relapse of chronic myeloid leukemia after bone marrow transplantation: separation of graft-versus-leukemia responses from graft-versus-host disease. Blood 1995;86:1261–1268.

Nucifora G, Rowley JD. AML1 and the 8;21 and 3;21 translocations in acute and chronic myeloid leukemia. Blood 1995;86:1–14.

Pui C-H. Childhood leukemias. N Engl J Med 1995;332:1618–1630.

Pui C-H, Crist WM. Cytogenetic abnormalities in childhood acute lymphoblastic leukemia correlates with clinical features and treatment outcome. Leuk Lymphoma 1992;7:259–274.

Pui C-H, Crist WM, Look AT. Biology and clinical significance of cytogenetic abnormalities in childhood acute lymphoblastic leukemia. Blood 1990;76:1449–1463.

Pui C-H, Ribeiro RC, Hancock ML, et al. Acute myeloid leukemia in children treated with epipodophyllotoxins for acute lymphoblastic leukemia. N Engl J Med 1991;325:1682–1687.

Rabbitts TH. Chromosomal translocations in human cancer. Nature 1994;372:143–149.

Raimondi SC, Behm FG, Roberson PK, et al. Cytogenetics of pre-B-cell acute lymphoblastic leukemia with emphasis on prognostic implications of the t(1;19). J Clin Oncol 1990;8:1380–1388.

Rowley JD, Reshmi S, Sobulo O, et al. All patients with the T(11;16)(q23;p13.3) that involves MLL and CBP have treatment-related hematologic disorders. Blood 1997;90:535–541.

Rubnitz JE, Behm FG, Downing JR. 11q23 rearrangements in acute leukemia. Leukemia 1996;10:74–82.

Rubnitz JE, Downing JR, Pui C-H, et al. *TEL* gene rearrangement in acute lymphoblastic leukemia: A new genetic marker with prognostic significance. J Clin Oncol 1997;1150–1157.

Shurtleff SA, Bujis A, Behm FG, et al. TEL/AML1 is the most common genetic lesion in ALL and is associated with an excellent prognosis. Leukemia 1995;9:1985–1989.

Trueworthy R, Shuster J, Look T, et al. Ploidy of lymphoblasts is the strongest predictor of treatment outcome in B-progenitor cell acute lymphoblastic leukemia of childhood: a Pediatric Oncology Group study. J Clin Oncol 1992;10:606–613.

Warrell RP Jr, de The H, Wang Z-Y, Degos L. Acute promyelocytic leukemia. N Engl J Med 1993;329:177–189.

27 Lymphomas

FINBARR E. COTTER

INTRODUCTION

Molecular analysis of chromosomal translocations in human lymphoma cells has led to the identification of new cellular proto-oncogenes that contribute to lymphoma formation. Genes encoding for the B-cell immunoglobulin heavy chain *(IgH)* and T-cell antigen receptors *(TCR)* are frequent targets for such rearrangements. Many of these rearrangements are detectable by Southern blot analysis, hybridizing with the immunoglobulin *(Ig)*, *TCR*, or appropriate DNA probes for other genes involved at the point of translocation.

An increased incidence of lymphoma has followed the era of organ transplantation and more recently, acquired immunodeficiency syndrome (AIDS). The development of lymphoma in human immunodeficiency, congenital and acquired, is approximately 100 times greater than expected and is predominantly associated with Epstein-Barr virus (EBV) genome within tumor cell DNA. The lymphomas are B cell in origin and may often be associated with specific oncogene deregulation.

The process of lymphoma formation probably represents a multistep process that requires a number of mutations leading to the development of clinically malignant disease, the described translocations being an essential step. However, further progression may occur following additional mutations involving the p53 or tumor suppressor genes such as the retinoblastoma gene (*see* Chapter 7). Ultimately, defining the mechanism of oncogenesis at a molecular level may increase the therapeutic options and include those based on the biological action of the lymphoma. The molecular alterations and their role in the pathogenesis of lymphoma is presented in this chapter.

EPIDEMIOLOGY OF LYMPHOMAS Lymphomas are a heterogeneous group of disease with varying incidence, geographical distribution, etiology, and response to therapy. The incidence of lymphoma in the Western world has been steadily increasing over the last few decades. The cause for this is unclear, although the increased occurrence of organ transplantation, human T-cell lymphotrophic virus human (HTLV1), and human immunodeficiency virus (HIV) may in part be contributory factors. Interestingly an association between *Helicobacter pylori* and stomach lymphomas of mucosa-associated lymphoid tissue (MALT) is observed and responds to antibacterial treatment, suggesting a role for infective organisms in the etiology of some lymphomas. In America and Europe, 85% of lymphomas are B cell in origin. B-cell lymphomas, however, have a considerably lower incidence in the Far East; T-cell lymphomas account for half the number of lymphomas in Japan, although this is mainly owing to the prevalence of HTLV1 in that country. In general, there is a slightly increased incidence in males and with rising age. Follicular and large cell diffuse lymphomas account for 23 and 20%, respectively, of all lymphomas and make up the largest subgroups by far.

CLASSIFICATION The classification of lymphoma has been a consistent cause for debate with divided views predominantly between the two sides of the Atlantic. During the 1980s, attempts at a unification were made with the working formulation that basically divided the lymphomas into three groups—low, intermediate, and high grade—according to the morphological appearance (low equating to small mature-looking lymphoid cells and high to large immature cells). However, with the advent of cytogenetic and molecular analysis of lymphoma, it became increasingly clear that these alterations could be of considerable importance indicating prognosis and treatment and that the classifications based solely on morphology were inadequate. Over the last 3 years, significant attempts have been made in reclassification, taking into account specific morphological, clinical, and molecular cytogenetic features. This unifying classification termed, the Revised European American Lymphoma (REAL) Classification, is far from perfect, but it is practical and applicable for the pathologist, clinician, and molecular hematologist (Fig. 27-1).

MOLECULAR PATHOLOGY OF B-CELL LYMPHOMA

The first molecular alteration involved the *C-MYC* proto-oncogene associated with Burkitt's lymphoma (BL). The t(11;14)(q13;q21) translocation involving the *IgH* locus and the B-cell lymphoma/leukemia-1 *(BCL-1)* region was next described almost exclusively in Mantle cell lymphoma and indicating a poor prognosis. Soon after this, the t(14;18)(q32;q21) seen in follicular lymphomas (FL) and some high grade B-cell lymphomas was cloned owing to its involvement of a J_H segment of the *IgH* locus. The translocation partner gene is *BCL-2* proto-oncogene which has subsequently been found to play a vital role in preventing programmed cell death—also termed apoptosis (after the Greek word referring to the falling of leaves from at tree or petals from a flower, being descriptive for the morphological appearances). Subsequently, the t(10;14)(q24;q32) found in 7% of low grade and occasional high grade B-cell lymphomas was cloned and found to involve the *LYT-10* transcriptional factor on chromosome 10, which becomes juxtaposed to the *IgH* gene. Most recently the *BCL-6* and *BCL-7* genes have been cloned on chromosomes 3 and

From: *Principles of Molecular Medicine* (J. L. Jameson, ed.), ©1998 Humana Press Inc., Totowa, NJ.

Neoplasm	Phenotype	Genetic changes	Comments
Entities seen mainly in lymph node biopsies			
Small lymphocytic lymphoma/leukaemia	Usually B, less commonly T	No common abnormalities	Includes chronic, lymphocytic, prolymphocytic, and large granular T lymphocyte leukaemias
Lymphoplasmacytoid lymphoma	B cell	No common abnormalities	Also known as immunocytoma
Mantle cell lymphoma	B cell	t(11;14), *bcl-1* rearrangement and *PRAD1/cyclin D1* overexpression in many cases	'Centrocytic' lymphoma in the Kiel scheme
Follicular lymphoma	B cell	t(14;18). *bcl-2* rearrangement	'Centroblastic/centrocytic' lymphoma in the Kiel scheme; the official title is 'follicle centre lymphoma, follicular'
Burkitt's lymphoma	B cell	t(2;8), t(8;14) or t(8;22); *c-myc* rearrangement	
Diffuse large B-cell lymphoma	B cell	t(14;18) in some cases	Combines 'immunoblastic' and 'centroblastic' lymphomas
Lymphoblastic leukaemia/lymphoma	B cell, less commonly T	t(1;19), in a few B lineage cases; *Tal-1/SCL* rearrangement in some T cell cases	Official title; 'precursor B-(or T-) lymphoblastic leukaemia/lymphoma'
Peripheral T-cell lymphomas, unspecified	T cell	No common abnormalities	'Unspecified' reflects the strong conviction that this is a heterogenous category
Adult T-cell leukaemia/lymphoma	T cell	No common abnormalities; integrated HTLV1 genome	
Angiommunoblastic T-cell lymphoma (AILD)	T cell	No common abnormalities	
Anaplastic large cell lymphoma	T cell, B cell or null	t(2;5) in some cases	Sometimes known as 'Ki-1 lymphoma'
Entities seen mainly at extranodal sites			
Hairy cell leukaemia	B cell	No common abnormalities	Localized to spleen and bone marrow
Plasmacytoma/myeloma	B cell	t(11;14) in a few cases	Seen in bone marrow
MALT lymphoma	B cell	Trisomy 3 in some cases	Arises in gut and other epithelial sites
Intestinal T-cell lymphoma	T cell	No common abnormalities	Seen in gut, with or without associated enteropathy
Angiocentric lymphoma	T cell	No common abnormalities	Arises in nose and other extranodal sites; includes mid-line granuloma; also known as 'nasal T-cell lymphoma'
Mycosis fungoids/Sezary syndrome	T cell	No common abnormalities	Seen in skin

Figure 27-1 REAL Classification for lymphoma.

12, respectively, because of their involvement of the *IgH* locus as the reciprocal partner gene on chromosome 14. Little is known at present about *BCL-7*. All these translocations are thought to occur as a mistake during the process of variable-diversity-joining (V-D-J), joining under the influence of recombinase enzyme responsible for normal V-D-J rearrangement, which is an essential mechanism for B-cell development (Fig. 27-2). Other chromosomal alterations have been observed; however, their significance is not always clear. For example, MALT lymphoma is commonly associated with chromosome 3 alterations. Although this may be helpful diagnostically, the role in the disease process remains unclear. Some of the more common translocations are described in the following section.

B-CELL LYMPHOMAS INVOLVING PROTO-ONCOGENE DEREGULATION

The majority of lymphomas are of B-cell lineage in origin. Translocations involving the q32 region of chromosome 14, the site of *IgH*, are most often observed (Figs. 27-2, 27-3). Rearrangement of one of the two alleles of this *IgH* gene is essential for development of the pre–B cell into a functional B cell and takes place normally under the influence of a DNA recombinase enzyme system. B-cell lymphomas predominantly involve the deregulation of proto-oncogenes following their juxtaposition to Ig genes. Their occurrence in part must be a result of their obligate DNA breaks and rearrangement within the Ig loci and probably involves a mistake mediated by the recombinase enzyme system responsible for normal Ig rearrangement.

MYC GENE DEREGULATION IN LYMPHOMA t(8;14) *C-MYC* plays an important role in the regulation of cell growth and differentiation mediated by a transcriptional role. Characteristically, *C-MYC* rearrangement in malignant lymphoma is associated with a t(8;14) translocation (90%), or more rarely, a t(2;8) or t(8;22) translocations of Burkitt's lymphoma. The breakpoint regions for the t(8;14) translocation, on both chromosomes differ between African (endemic) BL and non-African (sporadic) BL,

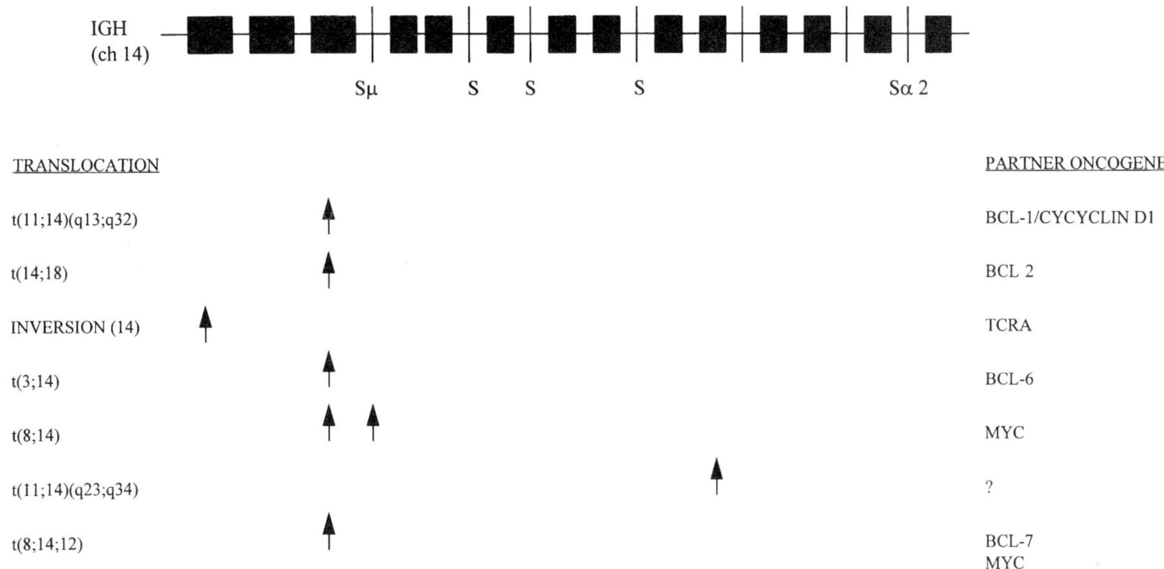

Figure 27-2 Schematic representation of the Immunoglobulin heavy chain *(IgH)* gene on chromosome 14. The arrows indicate the sites of common breakage within the *IgH* gene in reciprocal chromosome translocations, indicated on the left. The partner gene involved in the translocation is indicated on the right.

suggesting differing translocation mechanisms (Fig. 27-4). In sporadic BL, there is a loss of promoter sequences in exon 1 of the *C-MYC* gene and can be detected with exon 2 or 3 probes, whereas the break on chromosome 14 occurs within the switch region for the *IgH* μ constant region with loss of the enhancer sequence between the *IgH* joining and switch regions. Endemic BL predominantly has a breakpoint on chromosome 8 upstream of the *C-MYC* gene, too far for detection by exon 2 or 3 probes. The breakpoint on chromosome 14 differs, breaking within the *IgH* joining region. HIV-associated t(8;14) translocation predominantly has a breakpoint pattern similar to the endemic form of BL. Endemic BL t(8;14) associated translocation is thought to involve an error brought about by the recombinase enzyme system at the time of V-D-J rearrangement of the *IgH* locus on chromosome 14 and is supported by the introduction of point mutations into the *C-MYC* promoter region in exon 1 or either of the two coding exons 2 and 3 on chromosome 8, during or following the translocation. This is less common in sporadic BL, for which the translocation mechanism remains unclear; however, the suggestion is that the translocation takes place at an earlier stage in B-cell development.

Translocation involving the *C-MYC* gene in both varieties of BL leads to deregulation of the gene and excessive C-MYC mRNA and C-MYC protein production in the BL cell. This leads to excessive production of *C-MYC* in B-lineage cells with continuous growth and division. However, the quantitative changes may be less important than the inability of the rearranged gene to respond to regulatory factors, owing to loss of promoter or enhancer sequences or point mutations. The *C-MYC* gene may be deregulated as a result both of transcriptional enhancement by the proximity to the IgH locus and of point mutations in the structure of the *C-MYC* gene.

An oncogenic potential for the deregulated *C-MYC* gene is suggested by study of transgenic mice, in which lymphomas frequently develop when *C-MYC* is linked to an Ig enhancer. Excessive production of C-MYC in B-lineage cells appears to leads to immortalization by preventing the B-cell from leaving the cycling pool leading to oncogenesis. Downregulation of *C-MYC* expression results in a return to normal B-cell development. Additional steps such as *p53* mutations may be important with a 37% frequency in BL.

THE ROLE OF *BCL-2* IN LYMPHOMAS t(14;18)(q32;q21) The t(14;18) translocation is the most common alteration seen in lymphomas (Fig. 27-5). It is found in 85% of FL and 25% diffuse lymphomas. It involves the B-cell lymphoma/leukemia-2 *BCL-2* gene on chromosome 18. FL starts usually as a low-grade disease, consisting mainly of small mature-looking lymphoid cells; however, progression to a high-grade aggressive histology, with diffuse large cells frequently occurs and is associated with the accumulation of additional cytogenetic defects. The presence of the t(14;18) translocation persists and confers a poor prognosis. The breakpoint was first cloned in 1984 and led to the discovery of the *BCL-2* gene, consisting of three exons. The human *BCL-2* gene transcripts generate two proteins, p26 α and p22 β. These two proteins have in common the first 196 amino acids at the NH_2-terminus and two highly conserved (from *Candida elegans* through to the human) dimerization motifs, BH1 and BH2. These motifs are found in a range of "survival" and "death" molecules, including BAX, $BCLX_l$, and $BCLX_s$. Dimerization to form homo- and heterodimers affects the ability of the cell to avoid or induce programmed cell death (apoptosis). An excess of *BCL-2* protects against apoptosis even in the presence of apoptosis inducing chemotherapeutic agents.

The t(14;18) translocation breakpoint occurs within two very short breakpoint regions on chromosome 18. The first contains 60% of the breakpoints, is approximately 150 bases long at the downstream (3' or telomeric) untranslated region of the BCL-2 on exon III and is known as the major breakpoint region *(mbr)*. The second is known as the minor cluster region *(mcr)*, approximately 20 kb downstream of the gene where an additional 25% of breakpoints are found. The coding regions of the *BCL-2* gene are left intact, so that a *BCL-2/IgH* fusion gene is created and leads to

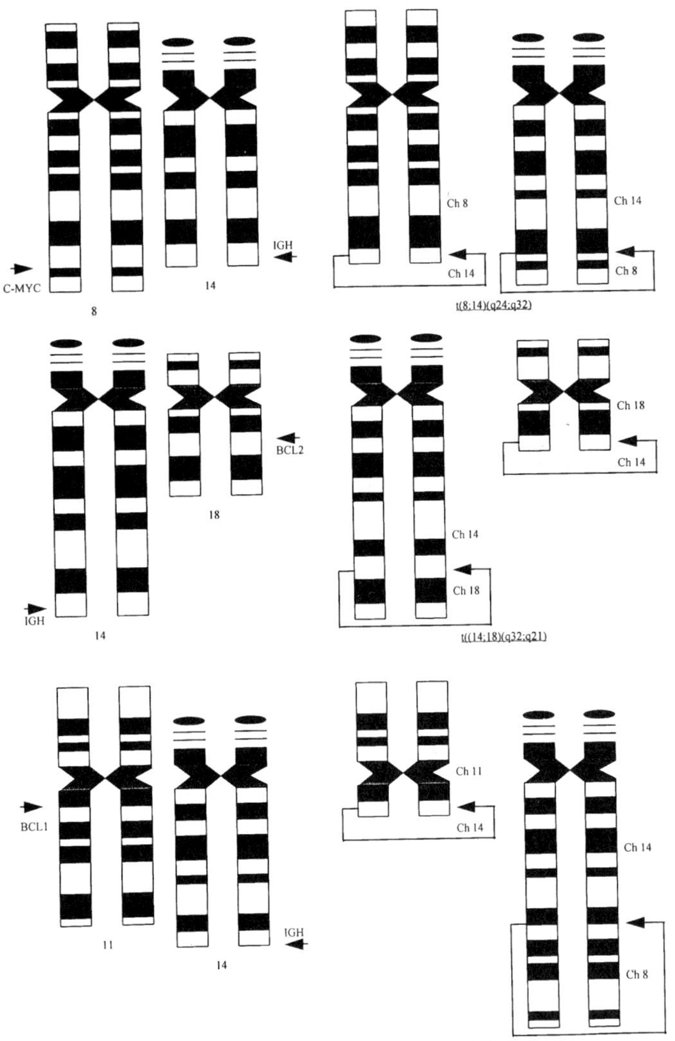

Figure 27-3 Schematic representation of three common B-cell lymphomas associated translocations involving the IgH gene. The normal chromosomes, with arrows indicating the breakpoint positions, and the genes involved are on the left. The derivative chromosomes formed following the translocations are indicated on the right.

marked deregulation both in transcription and efficiency of RNA processing with ensuing elevation of BCL-2-IG chimeric RNA as well as normal-sized 25-kDa protein. The excess of BCL-2 protein effectively "immortalizes" the lymphoma cell by preventing apoptosis and protects against chemotherapy induced cell death. This may in part explain the lack of "curability" associated with the t(14;18) translocation in B-cell lymphoma. The breakpoint on chromosome 14 occurs within the joining region of the *IgH* gene predominantly involving the J5 and J6 segments placing the IgH enhancer μ alongside the *BCL-2* gene. An error mediated by the recombinase enzyme system, normally responsible IgH rearrangement, has again been implicated in the mechanism of this translocation supported by the presence of N regions between the breakpoints and somatic point mutations within the translocated joining regions. Although the physiological role of BCL-2 appears to be the generation and maintenance of long-term B-cell memory, its role as an oncogene is suggested by the development of lymphoma in mice with the *BCL-2/IgH* fusion gene placed into the germline. Interestingly, involvement of the *C-MYC* is often seen

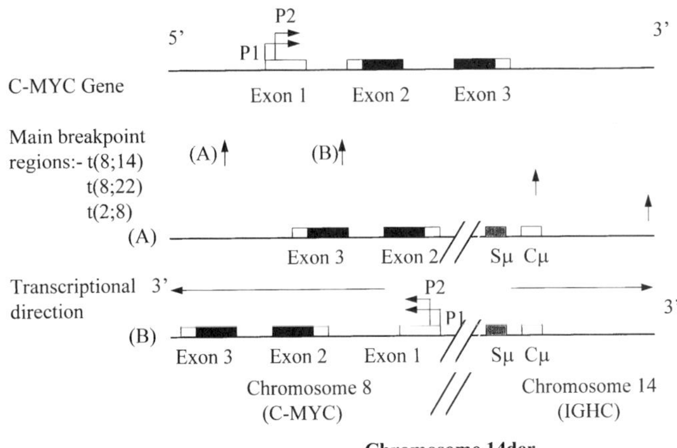

Figure 27-4 Schematic diagram of the *C-MYC* gene orientated 5' ("upstream"/cetromeric) to 3' ("downstream"/telomeric) and two possible derivative 14q+ chromosomes (A) and (B) from translocation t(8;14) in Burkitt lymphoma (BL). P1 and P2 indicate the sites of the two promotors for *C-MYC* gene transcription, and the arrows indicate the direction of transcription. The filled boxes indicate the C-MYC protein coding segments. The major breakpoint regions in BL and their associated translocations are indicated below the *C-MYC* gene by arrows. //, translocation junction between chromosomes 8 and 14; Sμ, μ switch; Cμ, μ constant Region of the immunoglobulin heavy chain constant region (IgHC). In (A), the derivative 14 chromosome has lost exon 1 and the promotor sequences unlike (B). Both (A) and (B) derivative 14 chromosomes have reversed their *C-MYC* orientation with a loss of Cμ enhancer sequence.

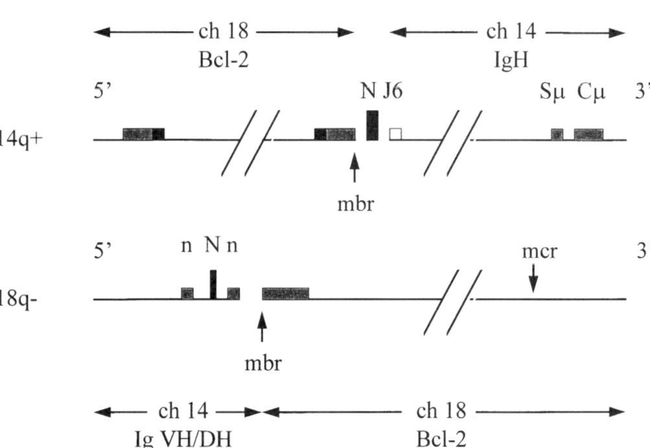

Figure 27-5 Schematic diagram of the derivative 14q+ and 18q– chromosomes resulting from the t(14;18) translocation in lymphoma, at the major breakpoint region *(mbr)*. V_H, D_H, J_H, represent the *IgH* gene variable, diversity, and joining regions respectively. N, "N" segment (insertions of random nucleotides found between the two breakpoints, reminiscent of "N insertions" normally observed between recombining segments following *IgH* rearrangement and mediated by the recombinase enzyme system); Sμ, μ switch region; Cμ, μ constant region; *mcr*, minor cluster region. It is of note that the BCL-2 protein encoding region remains intact on the 14q+ derivative chromosome and that a portion of the J_H segment is deleted on the 18q- derivative chromosome.

in these lymphomas and complements prolonged survival by promoting proliferation. It is also of note that the majority of t(14;18) bearing lymphomas overexpress *C-MYC*. Retroviral introduction of human *BCL-2* complementary DNA into human B-lineage cells constitutionally expressing C-MYC gene promotes proliferation of B-cell precursors, some of which become tumorigenic. Finally, downregulation of *BCL-2* with antisense oligonucleotides overcomes the malignant phenotype of lymphoma cells showing the essential role *BCL-2* plays in the lymphoma process. These experimental findings suggest *BCL-2* protein contributes to neoplasia and suggest a multistep progression to tumorigenesis.

***BCL-1* IN MANTLE CELL LYMPHOMA t(11;14)(q13;q32)** The *BCL-1* gene was first described in association with the t(11;14) translocation of mantle cell lymphoma (MCL). It was subsequently realized that the gene involved in this translocation was the *Cyclin D1* gene, also known as *PRAD1* (at chromosome 11 band q13); however, it was not directly disrupted. BCL-1 now describes a breakpoint region of 120 kb upstream of the *Cyclin D1* gene and following the characteristic t(11;14) translocation high expression of the 4.5-kb Cyclin D1 transcript occurs. Although low levels of this gene are seen in many lymphoproliferative disorders, overexpression of the gene is restricted to MCL and some hairy cell leukemias. It maybe a reliable marker for the classification of MCL being detectable by both immunocytochemistry and immunoblotting. *Cyclin D1* is a cell cycle control gene that is localized predominantly to nuclei, with a striking variation of protein levels among the exponentially growing cells, reflecting the maximum levels reached in mid/late G1 and the lowest levels in S-phase. This cell cycle dependent oscillation is owing to the requirement of Cyclin D1 protein for G1 phase progression (*see* Chapter 6). In MCL, the excess of *Cyclin D1* overcomes the G1 phase control essentially driving the cell into continual proliferation. In normal cell cycle, as the cell progresses through G1, the dephosphorylated (active form) of retinoblastoma combines with *Cyclin D1*, which in turn dimerizes with the cdk4 and cdk6 protein kinases in order to deactivate retinoblastoma by phosphorylating the molecule (Fig. 27-6). In the active form, retinoblastoma inhibits cell cycle by preventing DNA synthesis. This is carried out by inhibiting E2F, a transcription factor that normally initiates the DNA synthesis required for the cell to progress from G1 to the S phase of cell cycle. As the retinoblastoma gene is progressively deactivated by phosphorylation in G1 (mediated by Cyclin D1), so E2F loses its inhibition and activates DNA synthesis, thus permitting the cell-cycle to progress into S phase (Fig. 27-7). In mantle cell lymphoma, the excess of Cyclin D1 and loss of normal homeostasis loops controlling cell cycle causes excessive deactivation of retinoblastoma, greatly increased E2F activity, and consequent increased cycling of the lymphoma cells. Interestingly, a protein called p16 is an inhibitor of cdk4 and cdk6, which, in the presence of excess Cyclin D1, may slow down cell cycling by decreasing the necessary protein kinases (e.g., cdk4 and 6). However, as the mantle cell lymphoma progresses, becoming more resistant to treatment, mutations in p16 (inactivating the protein) have been detected. Mutation of p16 removes an antitumor control by removing a mechanism of controlling the rate of cell cycle (Fig. 27-7). From this, it can be seen how stepwise progression can occur as malignancy progresses and how retinoblastoma and p16 genes are essential suppressors of tumor in which loss of function permits malignancy. Comprehension of these pathways makes them attractive targets for therapeutic intervention in mantle cell lymphoma.

***BCL-6* IN DIFFUSE LARGE CELL LYMPHOMA (DLCL) t(3;R)(q27;R)** The *BCL-6* gene (also known as *LAZ3*) was identified by its rearrangement in 3q27 translocations associated with 45% of DLCL, 10% of diffuse mixed cell lymphomas and 6% of follicular lymphomas. In addition, an association with immunodeficiency state lymphomas has been observed: all are of B-cell type. The reciprocal partner chromosomes are considerable, including chromosomes 14q32 (site of IgH gene) (Fig. 27-2) and 22q11, as well as 1p32, 1p34, 3p14, 6q23, 12p13,14q11, and 16p13. The breakpoints on chromosome 3 cluster within the 5' regulatory region of *BCL-6* spanning its first noncoding exon and results in deregulated expression of a normal BCL-6 protein, analogous to BCL-2 following the t(14;18) translocation. *BCL-6* is predicted to be a transcriptional factor and has a punctuated nuclear localization in most germinal center B cells and a small number of marginal zone B cells, suggesting that *BCL-6* is important in the maturation of immune responses and may play some physiological role in germinal center B cells. In vivo homodimerization of the protein is observed. The exact role of *BCL-6* in oncogenesis has yet to be determined; however, deregulated expression may contribute to malignancy by preventing postgerminal center differentiation.

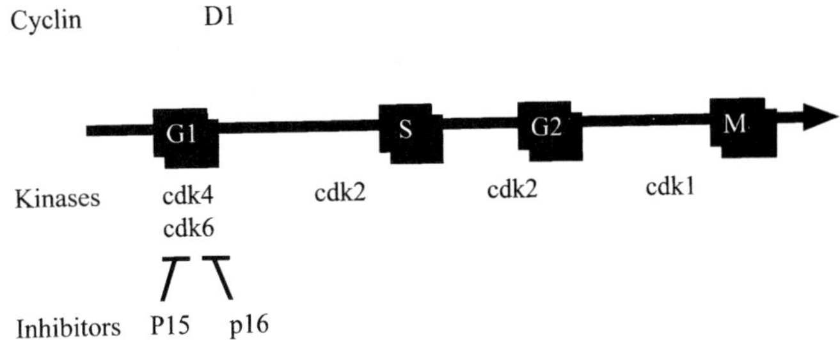

Figure 27-6 Normal cyclin D1, cell cycle kinases, inhibitors, and their association with different stages of the cell cycle as indicated.

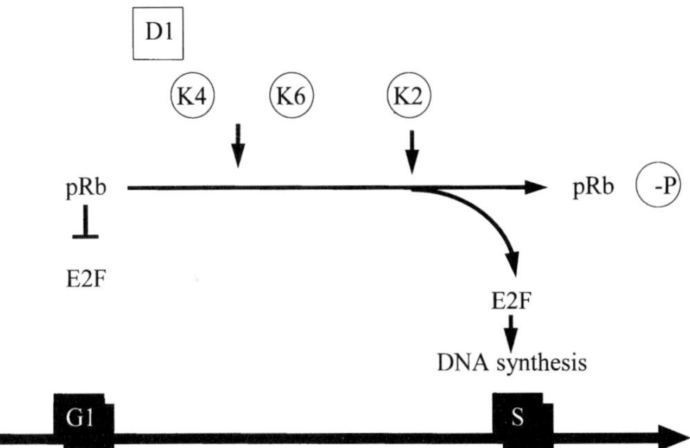

Figure 27-7 The association of protein kinases (K4, K6, and K2), Cyclin D1 (D1), retinoblastoma protein (pRb) and E2F with DNA synthesis, and cell cycle. (pRb-P) represents the phosphorylated form of retinoblastoma. The lower dark arrow and boxes represent the G1 and S phases of cell cycle. pRb inhibits E2F and thus DNA synthesis and cell cycle. Inactivation of pRb by phosphorylation to pRb-P by the Cyclin D1 and K2 protein kinase permits E2F to initiate DNA synthesis and subsequent cell cycle progression.

MOLECULAR PATHOLOGY OF T-CELL LYMPHOMA

T-cell lymphomas are rare compared to B-cell tumors. The prognosis is considerably worse, with the majority dying of their disease similar to T-cell leukemias. Much of the identification of genes involved in T-cell malignancy oncogenesis has been through their consistent involvement of TCR genes. As with B-cell lymphomas, it is postulated that this involves a mistake within the recombinase enzyme mechanism during antigen receptor rearrangement. Consistent translocations involving the TCR genes predominantly affect the 14q11-12 regions where the *TCR* α and δ loci are situated. Less frequently, the *TCR* γ or β loci on the long arm and short arm respectively of chromosome 7 are involved in T-cell lymphoma associated translocations. Frequently, genes encoding transcriptional factors are involved as the reciprocal partner in the translocation. The first two recurrent abnormalities defined were the t(8;14)(q24;q11) and inversion 14 [inv(14)(q11q32)] (the latter also described in ataxia-telangiectasia). The inversion 14 is heterogeneous at a molecular level, involving a variable region of the IgH locus and a TCR J_α segment leading to transcription of a hybrid IgH–TCR mRNA. The function of the hybrid fusion product is unknown, although suspicion is high that it has a role in oncogenesis, particularly as the inversion 14 has additionally been described in B-cell lymphoma. Interestingly, there is another recurring translocation in T-cell lymphomas involving the V_H region of the IgH locus and the region containing the TCR beta chain gene on chromosome 7, the t(7;14)(q35-q36;q32). It is not clear as yet if the same sequences are involved. Other reciprocal translocations in T-cell malignancies include t(11;14)(p15;q11) involving the TCR delta locus with the TTG-1 (or Rhombotin) on chromosome 11 and the t(10;14)(q24;q11), where a putative protooncogene called *TCL3* (T-cell leukemia/lymphoma 3) has now been characterized as a new homeobox gene, *HOX11*, on chromosome 10, which is redirected into the δ TCR locus. The t(10;14) is particularly associated with T-ALL and high grade T-cell lymphomas. The significance of translocations involving TCR genes is less clear than for those involving Ig genes; however, their recur rent involvement leads to speculative implication in the development of malignant transformation. Some of the more common translocations are described *below*.

T-CELL TRANSLOCATIONS AND TRANSCRIPTIONAL FACTORS

Much of the understanding of T-cell neoplasia is based on studies of T-cell leukemias and have been shown to involve both T-cell antigen receptors and transcriptional factor genes in reciprocal translocations (*see* Chapter 3). Those implicated in lymphomas relate to one of four specific transcriptional families, namely, helix-loop-helix (e.g., *C-MYC*), Homeobox (e.g., *TCL3/HOX11*), LIM motif (e.g., *TTG-1/rhombotin-1*), and REL (e.g., *LYT-10*). Altered transcription factor expression appears to be the consequence of translocations, involving them in lymphomas. The mechanism of oncogenesis can be divided into three broad categories (deregulation ectopic expression, and formation of a chimeric gene) examples of which are given *below*.

Deregulation The first involves deregulation, illustrated by the t(8;14)(q24;q11) involving *C-MYC*, as seen in T-cell high grade lymphomas and ALL. The mechanism of oncogenesis is similar to that of Burkitt's Lymphoma.

Ectopic Expression The second involves ectopic expression in a cell type that normally has none or low levels. For example, *HOX11* is not normally detectable in T-cells. Following the t(10;14)(q24;q11) in T-cell neoplasia, high ectopic expression occurs. Possibly aberrant expression of *HOX11* is initiated by transcriptional factors acting on the *TCR* loci δ and the *HOX11* is exposed to other transcriptional factors in the T cell with which it interacts. As it would not normally be exposed to the T-cell specific transcriptional factors, this interaction would not normally take place. The alteration within the T cell may lead to a growth advantage, and additional steps are required for a frankly malignant cell to arise. *TTG-1/rhombotin-1* acts in the same manner.

Formation of a Chimeric Gene The third mechanism is the formation of a chimeric gene, following a reciprocal chromosomal translocation leading to a fusion protein with altered transcriptional properties. This is illustrated by the t(10;14)(q24;q32) translocation of B-cell lymphomas. The *LYT-10* protein normally contains an amino-terminal DNA-binding (REL-like) domain and a carboxy-terminal domain homologous to ankyrin and mediates protein–protein interaction. Following the translocation, the ankyrin domain is deleted in the fusion protein and replaced by IgH C α sequences. This produces a fusion protein with greatly increased DNA-binding properties, deregulated transcription, and the potential for oncogenesis.

t(2;5)(p23;q35) Translocation This translocation is a consistent finding in many cases of anaplastic large-cell lymphoma (ALCL) that express the Ki-1 (CD30) antigen, a cytokine receptor for a ligand related to a tumor necrosis factor family. The result of the translocation is the chimeric Nucleophosmin-anaplastic lymphoma kinase (*NPM-ALK*) gene. *NPM* is a nucleolar phosphoprotein gene on chromosome 5, whereas ALK is a member of the insulin receptor subfamily. As a result of the t(2;5) translocation, transcription of the portion of the *ALK* gene encoding its kinase domain is driven by the strong *NPM* gene promoter, leading to its inappropriate expression in lymphoid cells, where it is normally not expressed. The fusion genes oncogenic potential is demonstrated by its ability to transform fibroblast cell lines. ALCL is frequently misdiagnosed as other conditions, such as Hodgkin's disease, malignant histiocytosis, and mycosis fungoides. Detection of the translocation is beneficial in making the correct diagnosis that in turn leads to appropriate therapy.

LYMPHOMA IN THE IMMUNOCOMPROMISED PATIENT

Immunodeficiency, both congenital and acquired, predisposes to lymphoma. The majority are high grade and are often associated with EBV genome within the tumor. It is possible that a failure of immune surveillance may play a role. In the setting of organ transplantation, much of the immunosuppression is aimed at reducing T-cell function; this seems to greatly increase the risk of lymphoma, suggesting a pivotal role for T cells in preventing lymphoproliferation and malignancy. Therefore, it is not surprising that patients with HIV infection have a greatly increased risk of developing lymphoma.

HIV AND LYMPHOMA HIV-associated lymphomas are predicted to account for up to 27% of all cases of lymphoma in the United States. The HIV does not appear to directly induce lymphoma, but it may participate in the process indirectly by inducing cytokine release, such as IL-6 from monocytes/macrophages. IL-6 is a differentiating factor for B-lymphocytes and has been demonstrated as an autocrine growth factor in non-HIV and non-EBV lymphomas. It has also been shown that IL-10, which may have a role in B-cell growth and immortalization, is expressed in large amounts in HIV-related BL. HIV stimulates a cascade of cytokine release that subsequently stimulates B-cell proliferation and development. This, accompanied by DNA rearrangement and the increased possibility of developing mutations and chromosomal translocations involving the *IgH* and *IgL* genes, will lead to the increased development of lymphoma. This hypothesis is supported by the high incidence of Burkitt's type translocations and subsequent *C-MYC* deregulation and, more recently, the recognition of *BCL-6* rearrangements (including involvement of the IgH gene) in HIV-associated lymphomas.

Present evidence indicates that in HIV lymphomas, EBV integration occurs before clonal B-cell expansion and suggests EBV may play a significant role in the development of lymphoma. However, not all HIV-associated lymphomas contain EBV, and many of these contain *BCL-6* rearrangements. The etiology of lymphoma in these patients must be diverse with HIV, EBV, or both, creating the environment for mutations within oncogenes or tumor suppressor genes and translocations leading to *C-MYC* or *BCL-6* activation, clonal selection, and development of monoclonal B-cell lymphoma.

POST TRANSPLANT LYMPHOPROLIFERATIVE DISORDERS (PTLD) PTLDs are a well-known complication of iatrogenic immune deficiency and almost certainly result from EBV-infected lymphocytes, as described for HIV above. Many will progress to frank lymphoma, usually of high-grade type, if immunosuppression continues. Similar to HIV lymphomas, an association with BCL-6 translocations has been detected.

HTLV1 AND LYMPHOMA HTLV-I is the etiological agent in some cases of T-cell lymphoma and leukemia. There appears to be a multistep process following HTLV-I infection of T-cells, with an initial polyclonal proliferation and immortalization progressing to a monoclonal tumor. HTLV-I carries a unique region located at the 3' end called pX, and this confers the immortalizing function, as well as playing an important role in regulating the virus life cycle. The pX region encodes for three proteins, one of which is the 40-kb transcriptional transactivator protein—*Tax*—a transactivator of viral transcription acting through a 21-bp enhancer element in the long terminal repeats in HTLV-I. *Tax* also stimulates the expression of selected cellular genes in the infected T-cell, leading to their immortilization. These genes are predominantly early mitogen response genes and play a role in the initiation and maintenance of cellular proliferation in T-cells. This is in a similar manner to HIV, creating an environment for further DNA alterations and the induction of a malignant clonal T-cell proliferation.

CLINICAL APPLICATION OF MOLECULAR ABNORMALITIES

Detection of the defect within a lymphoma cell owing to the molecular alterations described above may provide pathological information for the diagnosis, prognosis, and management of the disease. Presence of specific molecular alterations such as the t(11;14) of mantle cell lymphoma and t(8;14) of Burkitt's lymphoma can assist with the diagnosis, and it can additionally act as prognostic markers, suggesting a poor outcome with a need for more aggressive therapy, such as autologous or even allogeneic bone marrow transplantation. Such DNA-related analysis is primarily the role of molecular pathology and should be performed alongside conventional histopathology and immunophenotyping. Methods to detect these alterations are being refined and are evolving from the research to the diagnostic laboratory. Southern analysis was one of the earliest molecular techniques, but it is essentially limited to diagnosis or frank relapse because of its relative insensitivity (maximum sensitivity of 1%, although in real terms, this is nearer 5%). One of the single most powerful techniques in this new branch of pathology has been the polymerase chain reaction (PCR), which has greatly increased the sensitivity of detection. An added bonus of the PCR is that it is highly robust; the technique can enzymatically amplify specific sequences from high-quality template DNA prepared from fresh frozen tissue as well as degraded DNA extracted from paraffin-embedded tissue.

The t(14;18) translocation detected by PCR has been extensively investigated. Detection of this translocation prognostically suggests that lymphoma that will not be cured by conventional chemotherapy. Detection of minimal disease using t(14;18) PCR has a useful role. The disappearance of the marker in the bone marrow setting may suggest effective therapy, whereas persistence or return of the marker may suggest that a clinical return of the disease will occur. However, the time course can be very variable from weeks to years. With quantitative techniques, it may become easier to determine rising or falling levels of disease in a more predictive manner. The t(8;14) translocation of Burkitt's lymphoma and the t(2;5) translocation of Ki 1 positive lymphoma are also amenable to PCR, although their clinical application is less well investigated. Disappearance of the disease marker suggests a good response to therapy.

Other markers, such as the t(11;14) of mantle cell lymphoma are not readily detected by PCR or Southern blot analysis owing to the relatively large area of chromosome breakage on chromosome 11. This has been overcome recently in part by the use of a number of less sensitive but as powerful techniques, including fluorescence *in situ* hybridization (FISH). This uses a large DNA probe that covers the whole breakage region and has the advantage of being applicable on interphase as well as metaphase chromosomes.

Molecular therapy, such as antisense oligonucleotides, are now entering the clinical setting, using the basic understanding of the molecular basis of disease to obtain an antilymphoma effect. For example, high *BCL-2* expression in follicular lymphoma leads to a failure of apoptosis and chemoresistance. Treatment with *BCL-2* antisense has been shown to lower *BCL-2* expression and permit improved lymphoma cell kill. In order to determine the most useful therapy option, it will become essential to determine the molecular alteration. In turn, the molecular marker will allow monitoring of the disease response and predict potential "cure" at an earlier stage

SUMMARY

Chromosomal translocations in both B- and T-cell lymphomas appear to be the prime initiating step in the development of malignancy. They predominantly involve proto-oncogenes and transcriptional factors that are juxtaposed to the *Ig* or *TCR* genes, leading to the deregulation of the oncogenes expression. Selective protection against apoptosis is achieved by the lymphoma cell permitting a clone to persist until other oncogenes are activated in a multistep progression to tumorigenesis. The occurrence of these translocations is assisted by obligatory DNA breaks and rearrangements of *Ig* and *TCR* that have to occur in order for B and T cells to mature and function. The molecular alterations specific to lymphomas provide a potential for detection of disease, indicate prognosis, permit monitoring of therapy, and in the future may suggest specific target for molecular therapy.

SELECTED REFERENCES

Cotter F. Molecular pathology of lymphomas. Cancer Surveys 1993;16: 157–174.

Cotter F, Johnson P, Hall P, et al. Antisense oligonucleotides suppress B-cell lymphoma growth in a SCID-hu mouse model. Oncogene 1994;9:3049–3055.

de Boer CJ, van Krieken JH, Schuuring E, Kluin PM. Bcl-1/cyclin D1 in malignant lymphoma. Ann Oncol 1997;8 Suppl 2:109–117.

Korsmeyer SJ. Bcl-2: an antidote to programmed cell death. Cancer Surveys 1992;15:105–118.

Mason DY, Gatter KC. Annotation. Not another lymphoma classification! Br J Haematol 1992;90:493–497.

Monni O, Joensuu H, Franssila K, Klefstrom J, Alitalo K, Knuutila S. BCL2 overexpression associated with chromosomal amplification in diffuse large B-cell lymphoma. Blood 1997;90:1168–1174.

Rabbitts TH. Translocations, master genes and differences between the origins of acute and chronic leukemia. Cell 1991;67:641–644.

Rabbitts TH. Chromosomal translocations in human cancer. Nature 1994;372:143–149.

Tycko B, Sklar J. Chromosomal translocations in lymphoid neoplasia: a reappraisal of the recombinase model. Cancer Cells 1990;2:1–8.

Ye BH, Chaganti S, Chang CC, et al. Chromosomal translocations cause deregulated BCL6 expression by promotor substitution in B cell lymphoma. EMBO J 1995;14:6209–6217.

IMMUNOLOGY IV

SECTION EDITOR:

RALPH C. WILLIAMS, JR.

28 Regulation of Humoral Immunity

RALPH C. WILLIAMS, JR.

BACKGROUND

Any discussion of mechanisms involved in the regulation of humoral immunity must address what we think we know in terms of factors that influence antibody production and the vast spectrum of human disorders that may be directly or indirectly related to B-cell function and production of a humoral immune antibody response. Many human diseases cannot get a foothold in the susceptible host if the host already has manifest humoral immunity—e.g., specific protective antibodies to the prospective pathogen. Thus, prior vaccination with a mixture of 23 pneumococcal polysaccharides from the current most prevalent pathogenic pneumococcal serotypes will often protect an individual who otherwise might develop a serious bacterial infection with the pneumococcal organisms. Similarly, childhood and subsequent youthful booster immunizations with tetanus toxoid can also protect from otherwise nearly certain fatal tetanus infection. However, humoral antibody alone cannot itself provide fail-safe protection or successful defense against many human diseases. This is readily illustrated by the still unsolved problem of human immunodeficiency virus (HIV) infection (acquired immunodeficiency syndrome, or AIDS) as well as the ongoing long-term difficulty that has faced research scientists in producing a successful, fully protective malaria vaccine. Thus, naturally occurring humoral antibodies alone do not appear to afford sufficient protection to arrest the inevitable progression of HIV. Similarly, although initial reports looked extremely promising, the falciparum malaria vaccine designed around the unique repeat motifs of Asn-Ala-Asn-Pro in the malarial pathogen currently does not appear to be the whole solution.

In a similar fashion a number of other human disorders of unknown primary cause—often called autoimmune diseases—clearly are associated with the presence of important autoantibodies. Perhaps one of the first autoimmune diseases felt to be directly associated with an autoantibody response was idiopathic thrombocytopenia, or ITP, in which production of antiplatelet antibody was invariably linked to initiation of the disease. Several other common human diseases—also felt to be produced by immune mechanisms, including systemic lupus erythematosus (SLE), rheumatoid arthritis (RA), and insulin-dependent diabetes mellitus (IDDM)—have been strongly associated with autoantibodies such as anti-DNA antibody (SLE), rheumatoid factor (RA), or anti–islet cell antibody (IDDM). Although such antibodies are undoubtedly an important aspect of each of these human disease states, there are also other important key features of cell-mediated immune responses that represent critical features of these same diseases. This section will cover several key elements of the humoral immune response including B-cell activation, the molecular mechanisms that have been identified as contributing to autoantibody production, and what is known concerning the specificity of various autoantibodies including anti-DNA and other antinuclear antibodies in SLE, rheumatoid factors in RA, antineutrophil cytoplasmic antibodies (anti-cANCA) in Wegener's granulomatosis and polyarteritis, and islet cell antibodies in IDDM.

Much of the new information concerning humoral antibody responses in many human diseases derives from our recent insight into precise molecular mechanisms that constitute the genomic basis for antibody production and the eventual pathways involved in antibody affinity maturation and binding specificity. Antibody molecules achieve their specificity by forming a combining site that expresses exquisite binding capacity for three-dimensional structures representing the primary antigenic determinants actually involved in reaction with the receptor structures of the antibody. Despite intensive focus on the specifics involved in making up antigenic determinants, surprisingly little solid evidence has yet emerged as to exactly what constitutes antigenic determinants. Much of the recent conceptualization of precise antigenic components or conformations, crucial for antigenic determinants, has come from computer-assisted modeling of three-dimensional simulations of critical interactive molecules. Within the immune system, examples of available crystal structures include the HLA class I or class II structures and the few monoclonal antibodies or myeloma proteins that have now been studied to provide general shape–function relationships. With respect to antibodies, molecular identification of general families of variable region (V-region) genes making up crucial antibody-combining site structures recently has at last begun to make some sense out of basic biologic mechanisms leading to antibody specificity.

In this chapter we will explore several molecular mechanisms that have now been identified to generate both humoral antibody and specificity. Another important aspect of humoral immunity is control of antibody production and the basic mechanisms involved in regulation of the humoral immune response.

From: *Principles of Molecular Medicine* (J. L. Jameson, ed.), ©1998 Humana Press Inc., Totowa, NJ.

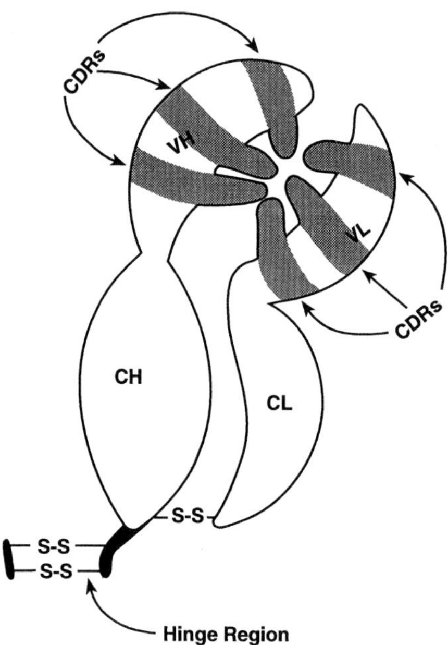

Figure 28-1 Diagram of one-half of the IgG molecule showing three hypervariable regions located within the V_H and V_L segments. These regions, designated CDRs for complementarity-determining regions, are most directly involved in forming the actual antibody-combining site.

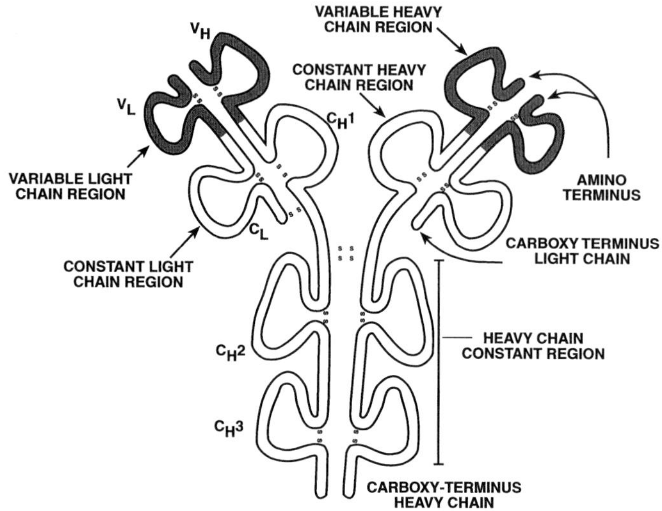

Figure 28-2 Diagram of an IgG molecule indicting constant and variable regions of both heavy and light chains. Both heavy and light chains have domains consisting of intrachain disulfide-linked loops. The variable regions of heavy (V_H) and light chains (V_L) are involved in forming the actual antibody combining sites.

MOLECULAR BASIS FOR ANTIBODY SPECIFICITY

Antibody molecules derive their specific combining activity by way of their variable or V-region segments. These portions of all antibody molecules are made up of the variable regions of immunoglobulin Ig heavy and light chains. The V-regions of both Ig heavy and light chains each contain three loops that participate in forming the antibody-combining site. These loops are referred to as complementarity-determining regions, or CDRs, which contribute to the three dimensional structure of the antibody-combining site itself (Fig. 28-1). The remarkable diversity of the antibody repertoire is derived from the combinatorial rearrangement of a relatively small number of gene segments composed of variable (V_H) diversity (D), and joining (J_H) segments for the heavy chain V region and variable (V_L) and joining (J_L) segments for the light chain V region. During the gene rearrangement process, the J_H and J_L segments are spliced to the constant region genes coding for the (C_H) and (C_L) segments of the heavy and light chains (Fig. 28-2 and 28-3). The V_H segment itself encodes a hydrophobic leader peptide and between 96 and 101 amino acids of the V_H domain, which includes two antigen-binding loops (H1 and H2). The third antigen-binding loop (H3) is a part of the region produced by the joining together of V_H, D, and J_H gene segments. This third H3 antigen-binding loop is considered to represent the most critical region contributing to the antibody-combining site because it is actually situated exactly within the center of the site. Additional diversity for each individual antibody produced by the rearrangement process is generated by the association of the variable regions of the heavy chain with the variable portions of the light chain that encode three additional antigen-binding loops (L1, L2, and L3) and represents itself the product of a similar combining rearrangement of V_L and J_L gene segments.

Human V_H segments have been classified into seven families, which have been designated as V_H1–V_H7, with different members of each family being at least 80% homologous within the nucle-

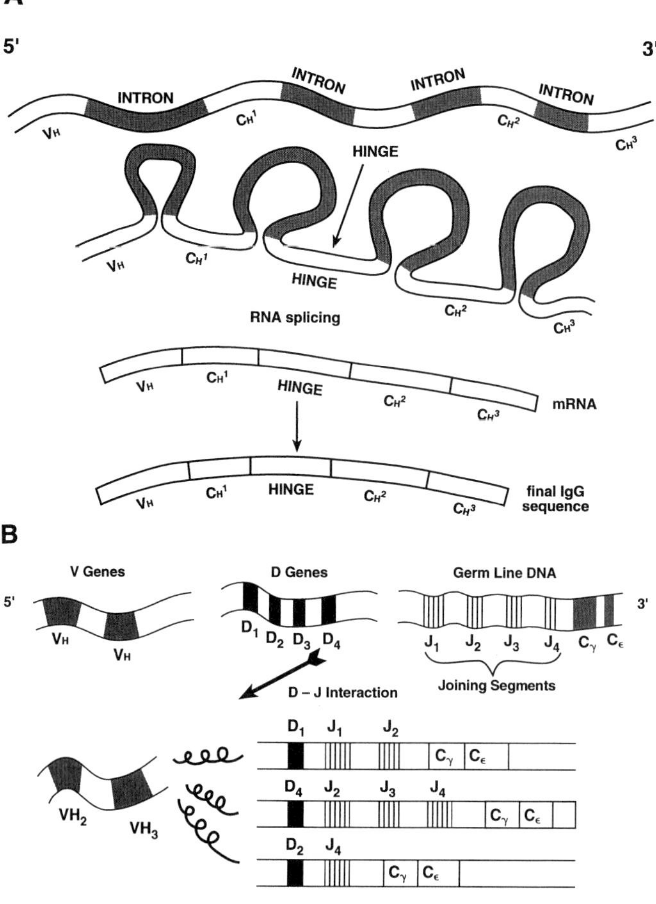

Figure 28-3 (**A**) Sequential process of splicing out of introns whereby widely separated exons coding for variable and constant region domains, and hinge region of IgG are brought close together and rearranged to make the final mRNA and hence the final IgG heavy-chain sequence. (**B**) Gene groups for κ chains and λ light chains are located on chromosomes 2 and 22, respectively. The gene families making up variable (V), diversity (D), joining (J), and constant (C) regions of heavy chains are located on chromosome 1.

otide sequence level. Southern blot hybridization using different V_H-family-specific probes has been employed to provide estimates of the approximate number of V_H segments within the human genome, as well as the dimensions of the V_H locus. These estimates have varied from 60 to 200 V_H segments ranging over a region of 1000–3000 kb on chromosome 14. Unfortunately this strategy has the disadvantage of the fact that different V_H gene segments or restriction fragments of the same length will comigrate on a gel, thereby leading to underestimates of total numbers of separate gene segments. Also, hybridization studies actually produce no direct information about the sequences of the gene segments or more importantly whether the gene segments represent functional genes or only pseudogenes. Based on a number of recent improvements in genomic analysis, a much more direct examination of the germline human V_H repertoire has become possible, as follows.

GERMLINE V_H REPERTOIRE ANALYSIS

Because members of a particular V_H family show considerable conservation of germline nucleotide sequence, sets of oligonucleotide primers for analysis have been designed with the polymerase chain reaction (PCR). Such primers anneal to the leader V-intron region and to the recombination signal sequence (RSS), which is situated just downstream of the coding region. Because the RSS is deleted by the rearrangement process and V_H-D joining, these primers only amplify germline V_H segments. Using this approach recently, 74 germline sequences were obtained from a single normal donor, and an additional 14 segments subsequently identified.

PHYSICAL MAPPING OF THE V_H LOCUS ON CHROMOSOME 14q32.3

The V_H locus is 1100 kb in length and includes approximately 95 V_H gene segments. Actually, the exact dimensions and numbers of V_H segments vary with the individual haplotype. Different members of the seven different V_H families are interspersed throughout the locus unlike the organization of the murine V_H locus in which V_H family constituents are clustered together.

In humans, the heavy chain V gene repertoire is assembled from a comparatively small number of basic genomic segments: there are 51 V_H segments, approximately 30 D segments, and six J_H segments (Fig. 28-4). The relatively small size within the germline repertoire underlines the importance of both junctional diversity and the cojoining with different variable regions on light chains to provide a broad final diversity of antibody molecule products. In addition to gene segment rearrangement, additional antibody diversity is also generated by somatic mutations within antibody V-regions. Very little is currently understood about mechanisms stimulating such mutation.

POSSIBLE V-REGION RESTRICTION IN AUTOIMMUNE DISEASE

Considerable present experimental evidence suggests that, in some autoimmune diseases, both the B- and T-cell repertoires may be restricted. Such a view suggests the possibility that V-region restriction might allow a single antigenic epitope derived from a single antigen (possibly an infectious agent or part of a self-antigen) to produce expansion of a small number of immunologically committed cells, which then become critical for disease pathogenesis. It follows that characterization of such a population of restricted lymphoid cells might then lead to identification of the

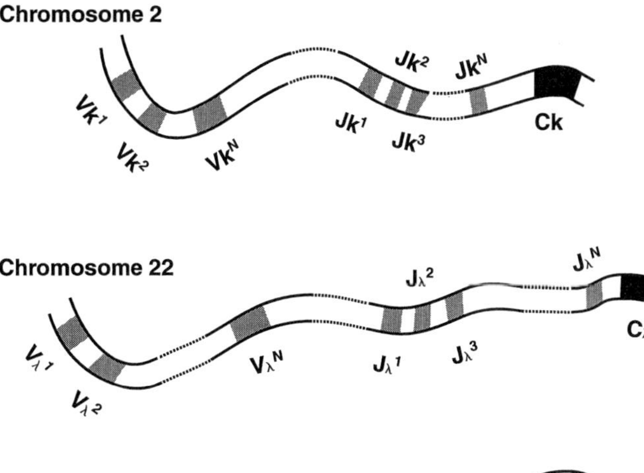

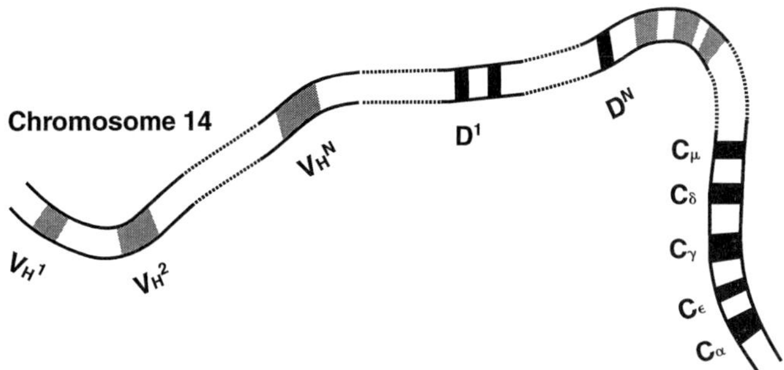

Figure 28-4 The interposition of D segments provides for additional variability within antibody genes. D segments connected to J segments are capable of combining with any variable region gene sequence.

original target antigen. Such an approach could conceivably provide important insights into etiology of many autoimmune diseases.

V-GENE RESTRICTION

Considering the fact that there are several hundred V, D, and J gene segments in the germline—and adding to that the combinatorial, junction, N segment, and somatic mutation in B-cells thus contribute to antibody diversity—clearly no focused immune response would use the entire genomic repertoire. Restricted V-gene use usually indicates dramatic overuse of a few V-gene segments. Thus, if more than 75% of a given B-cell response is limited to a maximum of three gene segments, it would be labeled restricted for V-gene usage. V-gene restriction, on the other hand, does not imply clonality.

From a theoretical point of view, the notion of V-gene restriction implies possible uniformity or focusing of both the immunizing antigen as well as the genetic profiles of individuals who are responding. However, all of the important genetic elements involved in the immune response are polymorphic. Besides the remarkable polymorphism of HLA class I and class II genes, T-cell receptor genes of the α, β, γ, and σ complex contribute polymorphism, as do the immunoglobulin genes of the heavy, κ, and λ loci. In addition, the degree of polymorphism at each of these loci results in every individual being heterozygous at most of the loci contributing to immune responses, which further complicates the notion of V-gene restriction.

Following on the initial studies of idiotypes in various human diseases, it was demonstrated that many autoantibodies obtained from different unrelated patients contain crossreactive idiotypes. Moreover, most idiotypes have been localized to specific V-gene segments and often represent the products of single germline genes. Patients with the same disease (SLE, RA, or scleroderma [PSS]) often express these idiotypes in their signal autoantibody populations.

Direct sequencing of heavy and light polypeptide chains of a large number of human autoantibodies from a broad variety of autoimmune disorders has shown almost no restriction of V-gene segments, with the exception of the clear-cut restriction of the V_H 4–21 gene segment in cold agglutinin disease. Thus, sequencing of more than 20 V_H and V_L gene segments from specific rheumatoid factors from patients with RA has not revealed restriction of one particular set of genes for this particular autoantibody. Instead, the data suggest that almost any combination of V_H and V_L gene segments can be selected to make a rheumatoid factor. Similar results have been found when individual V_H and V_L gene segments have been examined in other autoantibodies, such as anti–acetylcholine receptor antibodies, anti–striational antibodies or antibodies to thyroglobulin. These findings, therefore, do not support the concept of a conventional superantigen (SAg) being responsible for these various autoimmune diseases. Rather, the heterogeneous V-gene repertoire recorded in the large variety of autoantibodies from autoimmune diseases thus far examined suggests that they are the products of an antigen-driven process.

B-CELL SUPERANTIGENS—A POSSIBLE ALTERNATIVE PATHWAY FOR B-CELL ANTIBODY PRODUCTION

For a number of decades, B-cell interactions involving membrane-anchored immunoglobulin (mIg) triggered by direct reaction with antigen were felt to represent the only way in which B-cells could be activated to produce antibody and subsequently to induce clonal activation and further antibody secretion. This conventional clonal activation mechanism involved mIg antibody-combining sites produced through the hypervariable regions of mIg molecules. Recently an additional mode of interaction has been recognized in which various molecules termed B-cell superantigens can bind to human B cells bearing immunoglobulin receptors of a given variable V-gene family. Such a mechanism involves interaction from antibody regions outside the conventional hypervariable V-region CDR loops and appears to be able to initiate a B-cell response of considerably increased magnitude. Studies of the expressed repertoires of certain V_H-gene families have shown that these particular subsets interact in a specific way with a newly recognized group of antigens, called B-cell superantigens (SAgs).

SAgs were initially recognized for T cells and, in contradistinction to conventional antigens, do not appear to require presentation by allelic and isotypic forms of major histocompatibility complex (MHC) molecules. Instead of the conventional or usual way of binding, the T-cell SAgs bind directly with a site on the Vβ segment of the T-cell receptor (TCR) heterodimer that is different from the region for binding of self-MHC and foreign antigenic peptides. It has recently been recognized that this Vβ specificity of T-cell SAgs has a parallel analogy in the humoral B-cell response. Thus, protein A of the *Staphylococcus aureus* (SPA) may actually represent a B-cell SAg because 40% of human polyclonal IgM binds to protein A. Moreover, the binding of human IgM, IgA, and IgG to SPA is highly restricted to the V_H3 gene family. Additional observations now indicate that 60% of Ig Fab fragments from V_H3, derived from at least 15 different germline V_H-gene segments, also showed SPA-binding activity. In addition, there appears to be a hierarchy within the binding affinities of V_H3 genes that seems to reflect V-gene usage. Additional B-cell SAgs may also be present in viral components, such as the gp120 major envelope protein of HIV-1. Thus, HIV-1 gp120 has been found to bind to V_H3^+ B cells and to serum V_H3^+ IgG from normal individuals independent of the L-chain isotype. In addition, staphylococcal enterotoxin D (SED) appears to target preferentially a subset of B cells by way of a V_H-specific mechanism without any restricted distribution of J_H and D_H elements.

ATTEMPTS TO DELINEATE IG DOMAINS INTERACTING WITH B-CELL SAgS

Several experimental approaches have attempted to delineate the structural basis for V_H3 SAg binding. Initially it was suggested that the SAg-binding area included the amino acid residues both in the framework 1 (FR1) or FR3 regions or both. These particular immunoglobulin domains are known to be highly conserved among V_H3 gene products. Experiments in which residue 57 within the hypervariable region CDR2 was mutated from glutamic acid to lysine altered a V_H3-family member from a non-SPA binder to one which bound SPA, suggesting that CDR2 may be directly involved in the actual SPA contact binding site. Other studies, however, have shown that an epitope encompassing the amino acid residues of FR1, the 3' end of CDR2, and even FR3 may be involved in direct nonconventional IgG-SPA binding. This work suggests that some motif or Ig-binding region for SPA may be present between residues 75 and 84—entirely outside the conventional paratope or antibody combining sites of the three hypervariable CDR loops making up conventional antibody molecules. A theoretical model of how staphylococcal SAgs bind to V_H3 or Ig molecules is shown in Fig. 28-5. Despite the experimental evidence cited above, the precise linear or three-dimensional immunoglobulin sites binding to SAgs have still not been definitively identified. Indeed, several other portions of immunoglobulin structure besides the conventional combining site CDRs may be involved.

IN VITRO STIMULATION OF B CELLS BY SAgS

The precise mechanism of how B cells may be activated by SAgs remains unclear. SPA has repeatedly been demonstrated to be a highly effective stimulator for human peripheral blood B cells. Moreover, SPA activation of such B cells selects for V_H3-associated idiotypes. Subsequent experimental data also indicate that SPA can selectively activate V_H3^+ IgM-positive B cells and, in addition, such a stimulus can activate their differentiation and immunoglobulin secretion. Furthermore, the HIV gp120 interaction with V_H3-gene segment products appears selectively to induce Ig secretion by V_H3^+ B cells. Finally, another SAg encoded by the *Mycoplasma arthritidis* (MAM) can also activate resting human B cells and induce a polyclonal Ig response through MAM-stimulated B cells.

There also seem to be other alternative mechanisms of B-cell SAg activation that must be considered—such as the *Peptostreptococcus magnus* protein L, which specifically binds to VK1, VK3, and VK4 chains without blocking the parallel antibody combining sites of IgG molecules. This same protein L is also capable of activating mast cells and basophiles by binding to IgE.

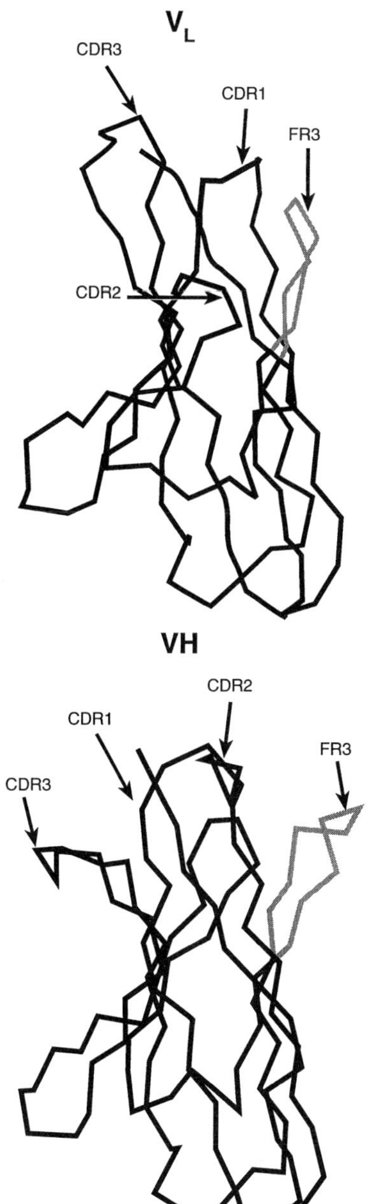

Figure 28-5 Alpha carbon representations of the V_L and V_H domains of an antibody molecule from approximately equal orientations. The view above shows the hypervariable regions (CDR1, CDR2, and CDR3) merging together to form the combining site. In the other view, in which the boundaries of framework 3 (FR3) are shown, it can be noted that FR3 of V_L is folded toward the CDRs. In contrast, because the folding occurs in FR3 of V_H toward the solvent, it is less favorably situated for antigen contact, but has a protruding region (lighter gray) that can interact with superantigens (SAg).

It has been hypothesized that there may also exist B-cell SAgs of endogenous origin, such as autologous protein Fv, which is synthesized in the human liver and released in the digestive tract and which can bind secretory IgA. A single protein Fv molecule is able to bind six $F(ab)'_2$ fragments by way of the V_H domains of all Ig isotypes. The majority of V_H3 and V_H6 IgM molecules bind protein Fv. An additional self-protein, human CD4, can bind to 78% of human myeloma proteins by way of the Fab region representing the portion of the IgG molecules containing the antibody-combining sites.

WHAT HAPPENS TO B CELLS AFTER ACTIVATION?

After interaction with antigen, B-cell activation is dependent on the stage of B-cell maturation, the actual antigen-binding affinity, and crosslinking of the B-cell antigen receptors. This can lead to a spectrum of results, including clonal expansion, differentiation, anergy, clonal deletion, or a newly recognized homeostatic mechanism that has been called receptor editing. Because B-cell-activating SAgs appear to differ from ordinary antigens in that they trigger much greater numbers of B cells than ordinary antigens, and also differ by their ability to react with different sites on B-cell receptors, the ultimate fate or result of such SAg–B-cell interaction is still unclear.

For HIV, recent data appear to indicate that gp120 can be within the B-cell repertoire. Thus, in patients with progressive disease, HIV-specific B-cell activation decreases while polyclonal B-cell activation increases. Understanding the mechanisms involved in gp120 as a B-cell SAg could lead to the design of new therapeutic strategies for this disease.

B-CELL ACTIVATION AND SIGNALING

Considerable basic investigation into both B-cell and parallel T-cell activation indicates that in each cell type, transmembrane signaling and activation are linked to similar enzymatic and phosphorylation mechanisms. In B cells, membrane IgM (mIgM) is the first isotype expressed with mIgD appearing later on in maturing cells.

The B-cell receptor complex appears to be a substrate for receptor-triggered tyrosine kinases and phosphatases. Currently it has been proposed that Ig-associated proteins interacting with other components within or close to the B-cell membrane actually provide biochemical transducers at early stages of a strictly tyrosine or serine kinase activity and also are linked to phosphatidyl inositol pathways as well. Anti-Ig or B-cell mIg interacting with antigen triggers a complex cascade of events in which kinase and phosphatase activities are sequentially released. Tyrosine kinases (and phosphatases) have repeatedly been demonstrated to act as key elements in signal transduction within B cells. Tyrosine kinase activation is followed by phosphorylative changes generated through Ig crosslinking.

Two highly conserved hydrophobic sequences have been identified within transmembrane regions of mIgM. Mutagenesis experiments indicate that the TAST sequence in humans is critical for transport from endoplasmic reticulum to the cell membrane but itself is not crucial for either signal transduction or antigen presentation. A second amino acid motif YSTTVT, which is closer to the cytoplasmic boundaries appears to be involved in antigen presentation and Ca^{2+} mobilization.

SIGNALING PATHWAYS

A picture has now emerged that suggests that the C_H4 Ig domain and the amino terminus proximal transmembrane sequence TAST represent the key elements for membrane transport. The carboxyl proximal sequence (YSTTVT), the cytoplasmic tail, and also possibly the α and β associated proteins contribute to transduction of signals by providing sites for one or more nonreceptor kinases. Crosslinking of IgM or IgD activates the enzymatic activity of such Ig receptor-bound enzymes. A tyrosine kinase is probably the first active component to be released. Later activation pathways almost certainly lead to G-protein-dependent phospholipase C

(PLC) activation, Ca^{2+} fluxes, and activation of protein kinase C (PKC) and Ca^{2+}–calmodulin-dependent kinase. These interactions are shown schematically in Fig. 28-6. Recently B-cell activation has also been linked to CD22, a membrane immunoglobulin (mIg)-associated B-cell protein that is tyrosine-phosphorylated after mIg is ligated.

DELINEATION OF ANTIGENIC DETERMINANTS OR STRUCTURES IN AUTOIMMUNE DISEASE

For some time there has been a simplistic attempt to define what really constitutes precise antigenic moieties generating an immune response—particularly with respect to autoimmune disorders such as RA, SLE, Wegener's granulomatosis, or scleroderma. Not surprisingly, antigenic structures have been sought within the various molecules or tissue components that our sometimes fumbling laboratory tests have demonstrated actually react with the presumed autoantibodies being studied. The most familiar example of such a broad line of investigation can be illustrated in the case of rheumatoid factors (RFs). RFs were first recognized as probable autoantibodies to γ-globulins based on the primary observations of Waaler more than five decades ago. The finding that these anti-γ-globulin antibodies were often present in very high titer of serum dilutions from patients with a common chronic crippling disorder, rheumatoid arthritis, produced the name rheumatoid factors. These strange autoantibodies have now been exhaustively studied literally by thousands of investigators. Their primary specificity—felt to be structures on the Cγ3 and Cγ2 domains of IgG or the Fc portion—has been presumed principally based on the laboratory test procedures used to measure RFs, e.g., hemagglutination or sensitized particle agglutination, later succeeded by turbidity measurements of the 19S RF interacting with 7S IgG autologous γ-globulin molecules. Levels of serum RFs in patients with RA have repeatedly been correlated with vasculitis, neurovascular disease complications, severe rheumatoid nodulosis or parenchymal organ involvement, and unrelenting progressive disease. The major specificity of RF has always been presumed to be epitopes on the Fc portion of autologous IgG—principally because we can demonstrate that RFs agglutinate particles coated with this same autologous IgG. In this way as in most other presumed autoantibodies associated with various autoimmune or connective tissue diseases, the positive results obtained in the original type of antibody detection assay later strongly influenced how the clinicians would subsequently regard this particular autoantibody.

Recently we have been interested in attempts to precisely map or delineate the real antigenic determinants on autologous proteins or other well-defined self components. This approach has often employed overlapping heptamers of primary amino acid sequence or the presumed antigenic regions of the protein previously established to be the principal antigenic molecule reacting with the autoantibodies in question. Thus, overlapping heptamers of Cγ3 and Cγ2 of IgG can be demonstrated to have strong enzyme-linked immunosorbent assay (ELISA) reactivity with several selected regions of the Ig domain primary sequences. In like manner these same RFs can be shown to react with similar, but not exactly the same, linear heptamer peptides from other immunoglobulin supergene related molecules, such as β_2-microglobulin or HLA class I MHC molecules. Perhaps if β_2-microglobulin or HLA class I MHC molecules had been the first sort of test substrate employed, RFs would go by another name and have entirely different connotations.

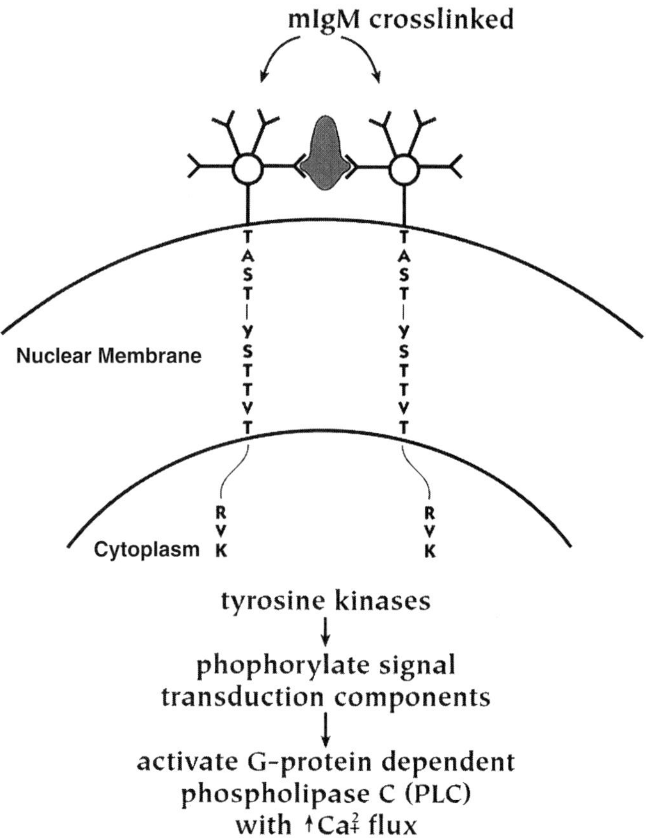

Figure 28-6 When IgM membrane Ig is crosslinked by antigen or anti-IgM antibody, a series of events is initiated, including eventual tyrosine kinase activation, phosphorylation of transduction components, and eventual activation of G-protein-dependent phospholipase C (PLC). The highly conserved hydrophobic transmembrane sequence TAST is crucial for export from endoplasmic reticulum to the cell membrane. The second region YSTTVT is involved in antigen presentation and Ca^{2+} mobilization. The short RVK sequence within the cytoplasmic tail is required for signal transduction and antigen presentation.

In a similar fashion we have recently tried to map antigenic epitopes on proteinase-3 or PR-3, the major cytoplasmic neutrophil antigen that reacts with anti-cANCA, the autoantibody closely associated with Wegener's granulomatosis or occasionally polyarteritis nodosa. In the case of anti-cANCA antibodies, again a number of well-defined linear heptamers derived from the primary amino acid sequence of PR-3 were found to represent reactive antigenic epitopes.

DEFINITION OF ACTUAL ANTIGENS

When a complex structure such as the Cγ3 and Cγ2 of IgG or the entire PR-3 is analyzed for regions that apparently represent antigenic determinants, the reactive linear regions cannot be assumed to constitute all of the reactive antigenic moieties involved because the reactive antigenic determinants must be composed of noncontiguous loops or folds of the primary structure that also make up important antigenic determinants. Nevertheless, the use of similar or parallel strategies of molecular modeling and epitope analysis has recently provided an additional potent tool to examine what make up antigenic sites on a number of molecules or autoantigens of interest.

REGULATION OF THE IMMUNE RESPONSE

Despite an immense amount of investigative effort and much focus on the question of immune system regulatory control, there is still very little clear insight into what features in a particular disease actually play the key roles in immune regulation. Some years ago there were strong proponents of a probably much oversimplified yin-yang theory that both humoral and cell-mediated immune responses were largely controlled by an appropriate balance between helper and suppressor cells that either upmodulated or downregulated various immune reactions. This still may be true in a limited way; however, the entire subject of immune regulatory response and balanced control of immune responsiveness has now become considerably more complex—particularly with the virtual explosion of knowledge in the area of active immunocyte-produced cytokines. This area will be discussed in a separate chapter within this section.

IDIOTYPES (Id) AND ANTI-Id REGULATION

Jerne and coworkers first proposed the concept of idiotypic control of the immune system based on the idea that both antibodies and T-cell receptors must have some sort of mechanism that was individually specific and could provide ultimate stable modulation. Currently there is considerable evidence that the Id–anti-Id feedback loops do indeed influence and to some extent control both normal immune reactivity as well as abnormal disease states, such as myasthenia gravis or SLE. The concept of individual antibody responses stimulating a self-modulating counter influence is based on the model originally proposed by Jerne of Ab1, Ab2, and Ab3 and is derived from the idea that the body or immune system sees internal images of antibody-combining sites or T-cell receptors and reacts to them in such a way as to gently downregulate their magnitude and overall effect.

Presently clinical medical problems in which Id–anti-Id mechanisms may actively be involved have not been defined to an extent that exquisite specific turning on or off of an anti-Id response is possible either through drugs given or other strategies under the control of the treating primary physician. It has been postulated, however, that the use of intravenous γ-globulins (IVGG), as in dermatomyositis, juvenile rheumatoid arthritis, or some patients with intractable ITP, may actually involve administration of generic polyclonal anti-idiotypic antibody capable of downregulating pathogenic autoantibodies associated with a patient's primary disease. Hopefully, as our understanding of Id–anti-idiotype regulation increases, our ability to incorporate such an approach into common therapeutic protocols will progressively improve and become a rational method of treatment.

SELECTED REFERENCES

Amador R, Moreno A, Valero V, et al. The first field trials of the chemically synthesized malaria vaccine: SPf66: safety, immunogenicity and protectivity. Vaccine 1992;10:179–184.

Bensimon C, Chastagner P, Zouali M. Human lupus anti-DNA autoantibodies undergo essentially Vk gene rearrangements. EMBO J 1994;13:2951–2962.

Berberian L, Goodglick L, Kipps TJ, Braun J. Immunoglobulin VH3 gene products: natural ligands for HIV gp 120. Science 1993;261:1588–1591.

Cook GP, Tomlinson IM. The human immunoglobulin VH repertoire. Immunol Today 1995;16:237–242.

Doody GM, Justement, LB, Delibrias CC, et al. A role in B cell activation for CD22 and the protein tyrosinase phosphatase SHP. Science 1995;269:242–244.

Forsgren A, Svedjelund A, Wigzell H. Lymphocyte stimulation by protein A of staphylococcus. Eur J Immunol 1976;6:207–213.

Greally JM. Short analytical review, the physiology of anti-idiotypic interactions: from clonal to paratopic selection. Clin Immunol Immunopathol 1991;60:1–112.

Hillson JL, Karr NS, Oppliger IR, Mannik M, Sasso EH. The structural basis of germline-encoded VH3 immunoglobulin binding to staphylococcal protein A. J Exp Med 1993;178:331–336.

Hunter T, Cooper JA. Protein-tyrosine kinases. Annu Rev Biochem 1985;54:897–930.

Jerne NK. Towards a network theory of the immune system. Ann Immunol (Paris) 1974;125C:373–377.

Jerne NK, Roland J, Cazenove P-A. Recurrent idiotopes and internal images. EMBO J 1982;1: 243–247.

Karpatkin S, Lackner HL. Association of anti-platelet antibody with functional platelet disorders autoimmune thrombocytopenic purpura, systemic lupus erythematosus and thrombopathia. Am J Med 1975;59:599–604.

Kelton JG, Gibbons S. Autoimmune thrombocytopenia. Sem Thromb Hemost 1982;8:83–104.

Levy JA. Pathogenesis of human immunodeficiency virus infection. Microbiol Rev 1993;57:183–289.

Maizels N. Somatic hypermutation: how many mechanisms diversify V region sequences? Cell 1995;83:9–12.

Nilson BHK, Solomon A, Björck L, Akerström B. Protein L from peptostreptococcus magnus binds to the κ light chain variable domain. J Biol Chem 1992;267:2234–2239.

Parlevliet KJ, Henzen-Logmanns SC, Oe PL, et al. Antibodies to components of neutrophil cytoplasm; a new diagnostic tool in patients with Wegener's granulomatosis and systemic vasculitis. QJM 1988;249:55–63.

Pascual V, Capra JD. Human immunoglobulin heavy chain variable region genes: organization, polymorphism, and expression. Adv Immunol 1991;49:1–74.

Pascual V, Randen I, Thompson, et al. The complete nucleotide sequences of the heavy chain variable regions of six monospecific rheumatoid factors derived from Epstein-Barr virus-transformed B cells isolated from the synovial tissue of patients with rheumatoid arthritis: further evidence that some autoantibodies are unmutated copies of germ line genes. J Clin Invest 1990;86:1320–1328.

Pascual V, Wictor K, Lelsz D, et al. Nucleotide sequence analysis of the variable regions of two IgM cold agglutinins: evidence that the VH4-21 gene segment is responsible for the major cross-reactive idiotype. J Immunol 1991;146:4385–4391.

Peterson C, Malone CC, Williams RC Jr. Rheumatoid-factor-reactive sites on CH3 established by overlapping 7-mer peptide epitope analyses. Mol Immunol 1995;32:57–75.

Sasano M, Burton DR, Silverman GJ. Molecular selection of human antibodies with an unconventional bacterial B cell antigen. J Immunol 1993;151:5822–5839.

Sasso EH, Silverman GJ, Mannik M. Human IgA and IgG F(ab)2 that bind to staphylococcal protein A belong to the VHIII subgroup. J Immunol 1991;147:1877–1883.

Schultz PG, Lerner RA. From molecular diversity to catalysis: lessons from the immune system. Science 1995;269:1835–1842.

Shaw AC, Mitchell RN, Weaver YK, et al. Mutations of immunoglobulin transmembrane and cytoplasmic domains: effects on intracellular signaling and antigen presentation. Cell 1990;63:381–392.

Shokri F, Mageed RA, Maziak BR, Jefferis R. Expression of VHIII-associated cross-reactive idiotype on human B lymphocytes. Association with staphylococcal protein A binding and *Staphylococcus aureus* Cowan I stimulation. J Immunol 1991;146:936–940.

Tomlinson IM, Walter G, Marks JD, Llewelyn MB, Winter G. The repertoire of human germline VH sequences reveals about fifty groups of VH segments with different hypervariable loops. J Mol Biol 1992;227:776–798.

Tonegawa S. Somatic generation of antibody diversity. Nature 1983;302:575–581.

Tumang JR, Posnett DN, Cole BC, Crow MK, Fridman SM. Helper T cell-dependent human B cell differentiation mediated by a mycoplasmal superantigen bridge. J Exp Med 1990;171:2153–2158.

Valero MV, Amador LR, Galindo C, et al. Vaccination with SPf66, a chemically synthesized vaccine, against *Plasmodium falciparum* malaria in Columbia. Lancet 1993;1:705–710.

Waaler E. On the occurrence of a factor in human serum activating the specific agglutination of sheep blood corpuscles. Acta Pathol Microbiol Immunol Scand 1940;17:172–188.

Walter MA, Surti U, Hofker MH, Cox DW. The physical organization of the human immunoglobulin heavy chain gene complex. EMBO J 1990;9:3303–3313.

White J, Herman A, Pullen AM, Kubo R, Kappler JW, Marrack P. The Vb-specific superantigen staphylococcal Enterotoxin B: stimulation of matrix T cells and clonal deletion in neonatal mice. Cell 1990;56:27–35.

Williams GT, Venkitaraman AR, Gilmore DJ, Neuberger MS. The sequence of the m transmembrane segment determines the tissue specificity of the transport of immunoglobulin M to the cell surface. J Exp Med 1990;171:947–952.

Williams RC Jr, Kunkel HG, Capra JD. Antigenic specificities related to the cold agglutinin activity of IgM globulins. Science 1968; 161:379–381.

Williams RC Jr, Malone CC. Rheumatoid-factor-reactive sites on CH2 established by analysis of overlapping peptides of primary sequence. Scand J Immunol 1994;40:443–456.

Williams RC Jr, Malone CC, Harley JB. Rheumatoid factors from patients with rheumatoid arthritis react with tryptophan 60 and 95, lysine 58 and arginine 97 on human beta 2-microglobulin. Arthritis Rheum 1993;36:916–926.

Williams RC Jr, CC Malone. Human IgM rheumatoid factors react with class I HLA molecules. Arthritis Rheum 1993;36:D202, S265.

Williams RC Jr, Staud R, Malone CC, et al. Epitopes on proteinase-3 recognized by antibodies from patients with Wegener's granulomatosis. J Immunol 1994;152:4722–4737.

Zouali M. B-cell superantigens: implications for selection of the human antibody repertoire. Immunol Today 1995;16:399–405.

29 Molecular Regulation of Cellular Immunity

ERIC SOBEL

INTRODUCTION

The task of the immune system is a formidable one. Out of the enormous array of antigens encountered daily, it must respond to eliminate the harmful (i.e., foreign and self altered by malignancy and infection) and ignore the useful (i.e., normal self). The response must be rapid, sensitive, and specific. Moreover, the immune system must be extremely adaptable, because it must provide a defense for all possible invaders, including novel ones. All of these demands are finely balanced. If the immune response is deficient, the individual risks recurrent and life-threatening infections or malignancy. If the response is too vigorous or not restricted to unique aspects of the pathogen, autoimmunity ensues.

Impressive strides in the understanding of how the immune system accomplishes these tasks have been made in the past 10–15 years. Although the normal immune response has classically been divided into humoral and cell-mediated arms, in reality, the generation of a response is governed by a complex interplay of cellular interactions and the elaboration of a number of soluble factors (cytokines). Antibody- and cytokine-mediated regulation will be discussed in more detail in separate chapters (28 and 30, respectively). Advances in our understanding of the molecular basis of autoimmunity (Chapter 34) and immunodeficiency (Chapter 33) will also be presented elsewhere, as will the role of the major histocompatibility complex (Chapter 31). This chapter will focus on a general understanding of the molecular basis for the regulation of the immune response, with an emphasis on a few key advances in antigen presentation, coactivation, and programmed cell death (apoptosis).

MOLECULAR BASIS FOR ANTIGEN RECOGNITION

It has long been recognized that antibodies, produced by cells of B-lymphocyte lineage, are the effector molecules of the humoral arm of the immune system and that these molecules bind directly to antigen. The nature of the antigenic determinant recognized is unrestricted, and numerous examples of antibodies specific for determinants on protein, polysaccharide, lipids, nucleoprotein complexes, nucleic acid, and simple chemicals have been described. In some cases, antibodies recognize linear epitopes on protein, but in many other cases, the determinants are conformational and require that the macromolecule be in its native state. In contrast, the molecular basis for antigen recognition by T cells is a relatively recent discovery, dating back to the identification and cloning of the T-cell receptor in 1983 and X-ray crystallographic resolution of the structure of major histocompatibility complex (MHC) molecules in 1989. Since then, progress has been rapid. T cells recognize peptide fragments of protein antigens only when bound to and "presented" by MHC molecules (Chapter 31). Thus, MHC molecules act as restriction factors, and the interaction between T cells and target is said to be "MHC-restricted."

There are two major types of MHC molecules. Class I molecules are ubiquitously expressed on virtually every nucleated cell. The class I antigen is a heterodimer consisting of β2 microglobulin (not encoded in the MHC) noncovalently linked to a 300-amino acid protein. This heterodimer forms a β-sheeted floor with two opposing α helical "walls" (Fig. 29-1). Within the groove separating the helixes lies the peptide antigen. Residues from both the peptide and the MHC molecule act as contact points for the T-cell receptor. Class II molecules are very similar in structure to class I (Fig. 29-2), but differ in three fundamental ways. First, class II molecules are expressed by a more limited population of hematopoietically derived "professional antigen-presenting cells." The major cell types expressing class II are B cells, monocytes or macrophages, and dendritic cells. In humans, but not mice, activated T cells also express class II, the role of which is unclear. Second, class II molecules are composed of αβ heterodimers. Third, bound peptides have less stringent size requirements and can be significantly larger than the 9 to 11-amino acid-length peptides found in class I molecules. This is because the groove in which the peptide sits has closed ends in class I molecules. Class I and class II molecules differ in one other crucial respect: class I molecules preferentially interact with T cells having the CD8 coreceptor whereas class II molecules interact with the CD4 coreceptor.

Numerous studies have been conducted on identification of motifs of peptides that bind to specific MHC molecules. In general, residues near the amino and carboxy terminal ends determine binding to the MHC class I molecule and are called anchor residues. The interior peptides are more variable and are more likely to determine whether a given T-cell receptor will bind. Frequently, the interior residues can kink and protrude from the groove. Binding to class II has fewer restrictions, not only in size but in sequence, so that anchor residues are not as readily recognized. This is presumably because the open ends of the class II molecule allow more flexibility in the alignment of the peptide within the groove. Peptides up to 30 amino acid residues in length have been described. Compared with class I, peptides in class II molecules tend to be in an extended conformation.

From: *Principles of Molecular Medicine* (J. L. Jameson, ed.), ©1998 Humana Press Inc., Totowa, NJ.

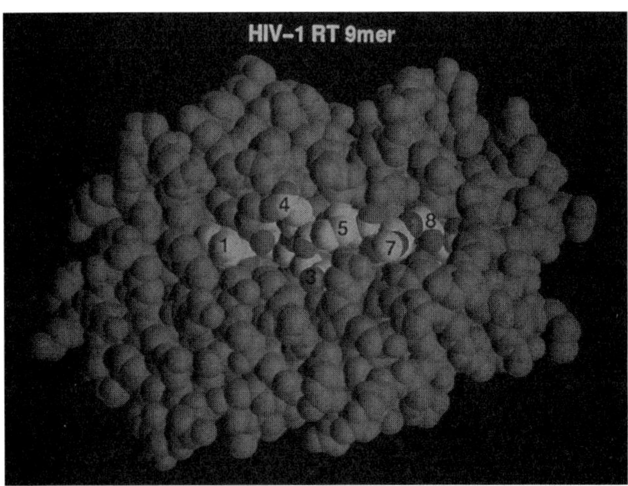

Figure 29-1 Peptide-binding constraints differ between class I and class II molecules. Size of peptide constrained to 8–10 amino acids in length by "closed ends" of class I molecule.

THE T-CELL RECEPTOR

STRUCTURE OF THE T-CELL RECEPTOR One of the major puzzles of immunology was how the immune system could encode for the staggering number of immunoglobulin and T-cell receptors found. It is now known that diversity in both classes of molecules is generated during maturation of the cell by a unique process of somatic genomic rearrangements. This is done in a clonal fashion such that an individual B or T cell expresses a single immunoglobulin or T-cell receptor. Although a detailed description of the structure and development of the T-cell receptor is beyond the scope of this chapter, it is important to appreciate in a general sense how receptor diversity is generated.

T-cell receptors are covalently linked heterodimers. The majority are composed of α and β polypeptide chains, each containing a variable and constant region. A significant minority of T cells express instead a γδ heterodimer, the function of which is still incompletely understood but may recognize nonpeptide antigens. The variable region itself is encoded by the combination of different gene segments. In the case of the α and γ chain, the variable region is produced by combining a variable (V) and a joining (J) gene segment by gene rearrangement (Fig. 29-3). There are approximately 50–75 different V and 70 different J gene segments available for the α chain. The β (and γ) chain has an additional diversity (D) gene segment inserted between the V and J segments. The constant region, as the name implies, is much less diverse. There are two gene segments available for recombination in the case of the β chain and one for the α.

GENERATION OF THE T-CELL REPERTOIRE Recombination proceeds in an orderly fashion, mediated by the products of the RAG-1 and RAG-2 genes. As of this writing, it is still unclear whether these genes are physically part of the recombinase machinery or are regulatory proteins. The β-chain locus on one allele is the first to attempt to rearrange, with first a DJ joining, followed by joining of the V segment. Functional rearrangement of the β chain triggers the rearrangement of the α gene in a similar fashion, except that, lacking the D region, it is a direct VJ joining. Additional junctional diversity is introduced through the random addition of nucleotides at the VD, DJ, and VJ regions, mediated by the enzyme terminal deoxyribonucleotidyl transferase (TdT). If an attempted rearrangement is nonproductive (through frameshift mutations or other problems), the rearrangement of the alternate allele is activated. With successful rearrangement, further rearrangement activity ceases. Thus, a given T cell expresses only one α chain and one β chain, a phenomenon known as allelic exclusion. If all attempts at productive rearrangement fail, the developing T cell will die, a very common event. It is the huge number of combinatorial possibilities arising from random rearrangements that generates the diversity of the T-cell repertoire.

ANTIGEN PROCESSING

In the past 5–6 years, there have been major advances in our understanding of the pathway by which protein antigens are degraded and displayed bound to MHC. It has been appreciated for some time that antigenic peptides bound to class II are predominantly extracellular, whereas peptides of endogenous origin are presented by class I. It has also been known that fixed cells could present protein as antigen only if the protein had been cleaved into peptide fragments. This clearly demonstrated the need for an active process.

THE CLASS II PATHWAY The difference in source of antigens between class I and class II is reflected in the difference in antigen processing pathways (Figs. 29-4 and 29-5). Exogenous antigens destined for class II presentation are taken up by different antigen-processing cells (APC) by different mechanisms. The nature of the antigen may dictate which type of APC is dominant and affect the outcome. Macrophages internalize antigen primarily by phagocytosis, whereas dendritic cells use endocytosis or pinocytosis. Unlike the nonspecific binding of most APCs, B cells can bind antigens with high selectivity through immunoglobulin receptors. Once bound, the antigens become localized to intracellular membrane-bound vesicles called endosomes. It is in these acidic vesicles that protein is degraded by proteases and the resulting peptides associate with the class II molecules. The class II molecules themselves have been synthesized and assembled with the invariant chain (Ii) in the endoplasmic reticulum and transported to the endosomes in vesicles derived from the Golgi apparatus. The invariant chain serves to assist in assembly of class II molecules and to prevent endogenous antigen from binding prematurely. Furthermore, evidence suggests that the invariant chain contains endosomic targeting signals for the class II molecule. In the acidic environment of the vesicles and in the presence of peptides, the invariant chain dissociates and allows binding of processed peptide. From here, the class II molecule with peptide is transported to the cell surface. Interestingly, a number of peptides from class II molecules have been sequenced, and many of them have been found to be cell surface molecules derived from self.

THE CLASS I PATHWAY Endogenously synthesized cytosolic antigens follow a different pathway. Proteins targeted for proteolysis are bound covalently by a small molecule (ubiquinin). Such bound proteins are degraded by a large cytoplasmic organelle called a proteasome, which is composed of as many as 24 protein subunits. Interestingly, two of these subunits map to the class II region of the MHC and, although not absolutely required, seem to enhance processing. In addition to the proteasome subunits, two "transporter in antigen processing" (TAP) genes have also been mapped to the class II region. The products of these two genes form an endoplasmic reticulum membrane-bound heterodimer that serves to transport proteasome-produced peptides into the endoplasmic reticulum. Here the peptides bind to and stabilize the

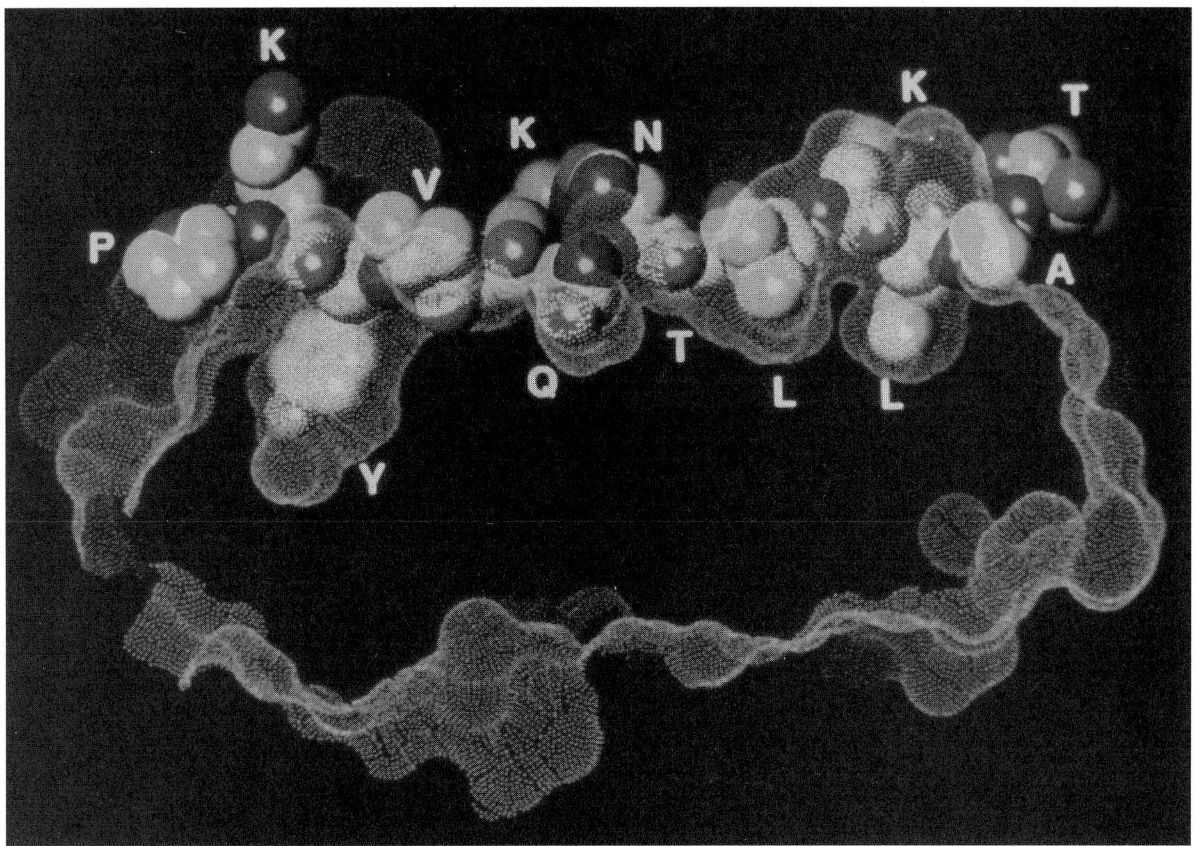

Figure 29-2 The "open ends" of class II molecule permit larger peptides and overhanging residues. (*See* color insert following p. 684.)

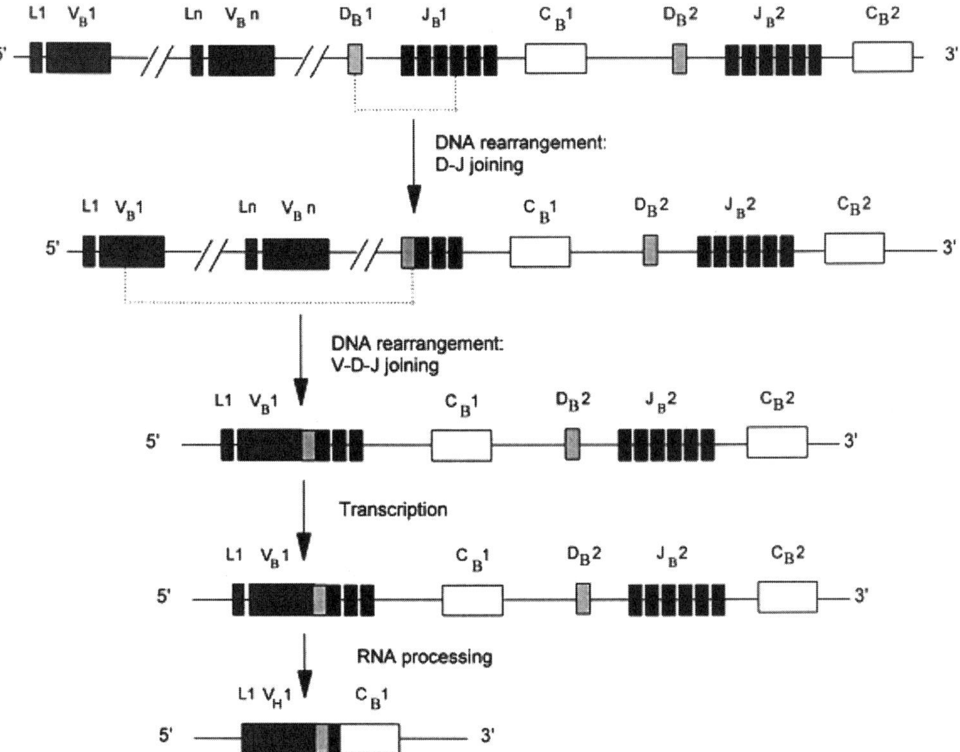

Figure 29-3 DNA gene rearrangement, also seen in immunoglobulins, is responsible for the enormous diversity of T-cell receptors. Individual T cells undergo somatic and random rearrangement of germline DNA. There are approximately 75 V_β segments available. The α chain follows a similar process except that no D regions exist and subsequently, the first step is V-J rearrangement. With the addition of N-region diversity at the D-J and V-D junctions, total available diversity has been estimated to be greater than 10^{15}.

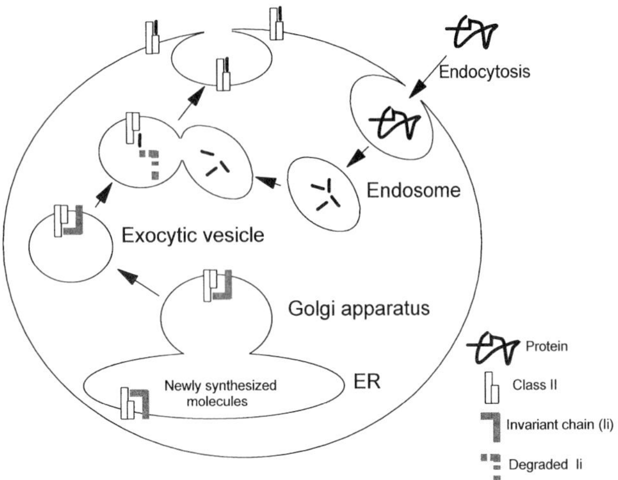

Figure 29-4 Antigen-processing pathways differ for class I and class II molecules. Presentation by class II is limited to "professional" antigen-presenting cells and is tailored to present preferentially peptide derived from exogenous sources. This is accomplished by the invariant chain (Ii), which prevents binding of peptide within the class II cleft until the Golgi-derived exocytic vesicle has fused with the endosome.

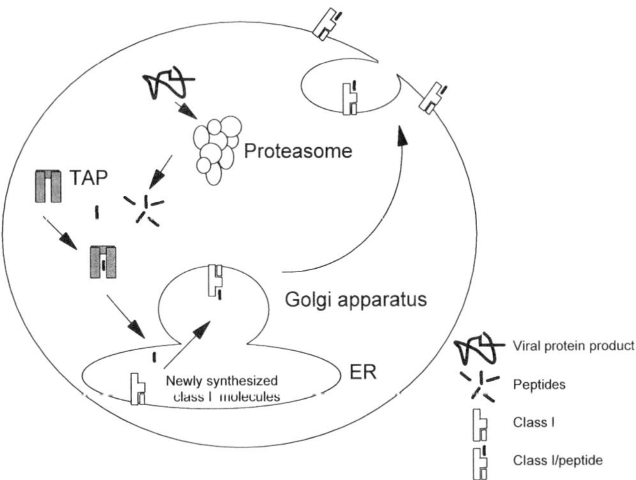

Figure 29-5 Presentation by class I molecules is performed by virtually all nucleated cells. Peptides, derived from cytosolic proteins, are targeted for degradation by proteasomes and transported to the endoplasmic reticulum (ER) by specific transporter (TAP) proteins.

formation of nascent class I molecules. Thus, the class I pathway is well-suited to present neoantigens derived from malignant or viral transformation. Compared with the restricted expression of class II, the wide expression of class I allows the immune system to survey most nucleated cells.

T- AND B-CELL MATURATION AND THE DEVELOPMENT OF TOLERANCE

CENTRAL T-CELL TOLERANCE Tolerance mechanisms have been classified as either central (thymic) or peripheral. Intrathymic tolerance involves clonal deletion whereas peripheral tolerance can occur either through deletion or anergy. Cells committed to the T-cell lineage migrate to the cortex of the thymus from the bone marrow, probably homing there through as yet uncharacterized receptors. As immature thymocytes, their T-cell receptors (TCR) are in the germline configuration, and none of the mature T-cell markers, such as CD4 or CD8, is expressed. Within the cortex, the thymocytes begin the process of random somatic rearrangement of their TCR genes. Once a thymocyte has successfully rearranged and expressed its TCR (at low levels), it can coexpress CD4 and CD8 and migrate from the cortex to the medulla. It is at this point that positive and negative selection occur. For positive selection, some threshold affinity of TCR for MHC molecule is required. However, those maturing T cells having a TCR that engages a self-MHC molecule too avidly are deleted from the repertoire through negative selection. An understanding of the selection process has been greatly enhanced by the discovery of endogenous superantigens and the development of transgenic and targeted deletion technology. Negative selection by clonal deletion was first conclusively demonstrated for superantigens, which are molecules that activate a much larger subset of T cells than conventional antigen. It has now been shown that this occurs because superantigens can bind to certain V_β genes regardless of which D_β, J_β, or even α chains are used. Moreover, these superantigens have binding sites that can engage certain class II molecules by binding to nonpolymorphic regions outside the peptide-binding cleft. In mice, some superantigens are encoded by endogenous retroviruses and are thus considered self. For example, one well-studied superantigen present in certain strains of mice engages Vβ17a in the presence of the class II molecule I-E. In these mice, Vβ17a$^+$ CD4$^+$CD8$^+$ thymocytes were found. However, mature Vβ17a$^+$ cells were not found in the periphery. Further analysis showed that these cells were deleted at the CD4$^+$CD8$^+$ stage within the thymus, because no CD4$^+$ or CD8$^+$ thymocytes expressing high levels of TCR could be detected.

Positive selection was demonstrated in a similar way by the use of TCR transgenic mice. One of the best-studied introduced a TCR that, in the context of the class I molecule H-2D^b, was specific for a peptide derived from the male-associated antigen H-Y. Transgenic female mice expressing H-2D^b had T cells expressing the transgene, whereas male mice of the same haplotype did not. To demonstrate that the female mice expressed this transgene through positive selection and not through the absence of negative selection, the transgene was bred onto another MHC background. In the presence of only irrelevant class I molecules, T cells from female mice did not express the transgene.

Those cells that survive this selection process emerge as CD4$^+$ or CD8$^+$ cells bearing high levels of TCR. For TCRs that engage class II, CD8 expression is downregulated and the converse is true for TCRs engaging class I. The exact mechanism for this downregulation is still unclear, but an individual T cell probably commits to the CD4 or CD8 lineage before selection. Cells that are negatively selected or have TCR that do not engage MHC die from apoptosis, a series of regulated steps characteristically resulting in endonuclease activation, DNA fragmentation, cell fragmentation, and blebbing. In contrast to necrosis, death by apoptosis causes little inflammation.

The cells within the thymus responsible for positive and negative selection arise from different populations. Positive selection is mediated by non–bone marrow-derived thymic epithelial cells, whereas negative selection can apparently be mediated by more than one cell type. This has been shown most convincingly in some recent bone marrow cell transfer experiments using a mouse strain with a mutation induced in its class II molecule. Such mice, lacking expression of class II, failed to express $CD4^+$ T cells in the periphery, owing to a lack of positive selection on class II. When these mice were lethally irradiated and reconstituted with bone marrow from normal mice, few $CD4^+$ T cells were found in the periphery, indicating that bone marrow-derived cells expressing class II could not mediate positive selection. Conversely, infusion of class II-negative bone marrow into normal mice resulted in normal expression of $CD4^+$ T cells. In both cases, the mice were tolerant to donor and host cells.

B-CELL TOLERANCE A similar process of tolerance occurs in the bone marrow for developing B cells. As for T cells, through random rearrangements, a vast repertoire of immunoglobulin receptors develops. Again, transgenic technology has been vital in demonstrating negative selection. In a particularly elegant set of experiments, mice transgenic for an antibody to hen egg lysozyme (HEL) were generated. The construct was such that expression of both IgM and IgD through alternative splicing was possible, and easily detectable anti-HEL antibody was found in the serum. Two other transgenic strains, one expressing HEL on the cell membrane and the other expressing HEL in secreted form, were also created. When the anti-HEL transgenic was crossed with the strain expressing membrane-bound HEL, essentially no B cells expressing anti-HEL were found in the periphery and no anti-HEL was found in the serum of the F_1 offspring. In contrast, when the anti-HEL mice were crossed with the strain expressing only secreted HEL, the B cells in the offspring were not deleted but had downregulated their IgM (but not IgD) expression on the cell surface. Again, no anti-HEL was found in the serum. Moreover, these mice could not be induced to produce anti-HEL with immunization. Thus, in the case of the cross with membrane-bound HEL, B-cell tolerance through clonal deletion was induced, whereas in the case of soluble HEL, B-cell tolerance by clonal anergy was induced.

PERIPHERAL T-CELL TOLERANCE This pathway of intrathymic (central) negative selection goes a long way in explaining T-cell tolerance to self-antigens that are secreted or common to all cells. However, it does little to explain organ-specific tolerance, as it is hard to see how all such antigens could be efficiently transported to the thymus. Other hypotheses, such as the presence of thymus-specific peptides inducing tolerance, have been proposed but have found little experimental support. Clonal anergy in B cells could be understood as a result of stimulation in the absence of T-cell help. However, T-cell tolerance by clonal anergy was more difficult to explain. In the last few years, the discovery of coactivation molecules and the two-signal hypothesis for T-cell activation has provided a molecular framework for the concept of clonal anergy (*see below*).

REGULATION OF CELLULAR INTERACTIONS IN THE DEVELOPMENT OF AN ANTIBODY RESPONSE

It is now possible to outline, in some detail, the specific steps leading to a T-cell-dependent antibody response. Classic experiments in the 1970s, using the hapten-carrier system, demonstrated that, for effective T-B collaboration, both T and B cells must recognize the same antigen. The actual epitope need not be the same, but they must be physically linked. Early experiments also showed that soluble factors were important. However, for optimal help, physical contact (i.e., cognate interactions) between T and B cells must be established. It is now apparent that effective activation of T and B cells requires at least two signals, one acting through the TCR or immunoglobulin receptor, respectively, and the other a costimulatory signal generated by recently described molecules. The following section will outline the current understanding of these interactions.

THE ROLE OF COSTIMULATORY MOLECULES The first costimulatory pair to be identified was CD28-B7, important in the activation of T cells. B7 has now been shown to be a family composed of at least three members: B7-1 (CD80), B7-2 (CD86), and B7-3. B7-1 is a 55- to 60-kDa glycoprotein not normally expressed on resting B cells, but which can be induced by a variety of stimuli, including polysaccharides and crosslinking of cell surface IgM or class II. B7-1 expression can also be induced on monocytes by interferon-γ (IFN-γ). Expression after induction is slow in onset, with peak expression occurring 2–3 days after exposure. In contrast, expression of B7-2, a 70-kDa glycoprotein can be induced on B cells much more rapidly with the same stimuli. B7-2 is also constitutively expressed on monocytes at a low level and on dendritic cells at a higher level. Less is known about B7-3. Its expression is slow in onset, similar to B7-1. The first receptor to be discovered for B7 was CD28. This is an 88-kDa, disulfide-linked homodimer constitutively expressed on T cells but subject to further upregulation in vitro with phorbol ester or anti-CD3 stimulation. It is expressed by $CD4^+CD8^+$ thymocytes, but its role in intrathymic selection is unclear inasmuch as thymocyte development appears normal in CD28-deficient mice. CTLA-4, a second receptor for B7, is found only on activated T cells. Both B7 and CD28 are members of the immunoglobulin supergene family.

In contrast to the CD28–B7 receptor–ligand interactions, the CD40L–CD40 system is important in B-cell activation. CD40L, a 39-kDa glycoprotein also called gp39, is expressed on activated T cells. CD40, a member of the tumor necrosis receptor family, is a 45 to 50-kDa glycoprotein expressed constitutively on B cells and dendritic cells. Crosslinking of CD40 on B cells induces class switching and stimulates proliferation. The importance of this system has been dramatically illustrated by the discovery that the hyper-IgM syndrome, characterized by poor germinal center formation in response to foreign antigen and deficient class switching, is caused by a defect in CD40L. The reciprocal interactions between B7–CD28 and CD40L–CD40 are crucial to the development of the immune response. Engaging CD28 on activated T cells causes an increased expression of CD40L. Conversely, engagement of CD40 on B cells causes an increased expression of B7-1 and B7-2.

TRACING A T-CELL-DEPENDENT B-CELL RESPONSE IN VIVO With this as background, the sequence of events leading to a T-cell-dependent antibody response can be outlined. When foreign antigen enters the organism, it is taken up into the cortex of draining lymph nodes. Into these same areas, naive T cells migrate by passing through venules specialized for diapedesis, called high endothelial venules. Here, they encounter the processed antigen presented, in the context of class II, on "professional" antigen-presenting cells, primarily thought to be the bone marrow-derived dendritic cells. These cells express high levels of class II and B7-2. If the APC can interact with the naive T cell through engagement of the TCR while simultaneously crosslinking CD28 through B7, the T cell becomes an activated effector cell. One of the end results of activation is expression of CD40L on the T cell.

The activated T cell is now capable of interacting with naive B cells, which also circulate through this area of the lymph node.

B cells that express surface immunoglobulin that can bind the foreign antigen will preferentially display peptides derived from this antigen and will be efficient APCs for the activated T cells. When such an encounter occurs, the B cells are stimulated to upregulate B7 expression through engagement of constitutively expressed CD40 by the activated CD40L$^+$ T cells, and the B cells are themselves activated. These activated B cells begin secreting antibody and migrate to nearby primary lymphoid follicles, where they interact with follicular dendritic cells. The follicular dendritic cells are epithelial-derived cells that bear no relationship to the dendritic cells of bone marrow origin mentioned earlier. Furthermore, they have the unique and critical property of binding and trapping antibody–antigen complexes for interaction with the germinal center B cells. B cells under this stimulation are driven to somatically hypermutate and, through additional T-cell signals delivered by cytokines (Chapter 30), to begin undergoing class switching. As the immune response develops, competition for binding to the follicular dendritic cells ensues such that those B cells expressing the highest affinity immunoglobulin receptors are preferentially selected, while those that have mutated to a lower affinity antibody die through apoptosis. This results in the phenomenon of affinity maturation that marks an adaptive immune response. With an ongoing immune response, the selected cells undergo rapid clonal expansion, and some of these cells begin migrating into the circulation. With additional help from activated T cells, some of these cells will be triggered to develop into long-lived memory B cells. The remainder will become short-lived plasma cells designed to secrete enormous amounts of antibody.

Although the CD28–B7 and CD40–CD40L costimulation signals are crucial to development of the immune response, other molecules are also clearly important. The best-studied of these are lymphocyte function-associated antigen-1 (LFA-1) and CD2 present on T lymphocytes. The counterreceptors for LFA-1, present on antigen-presenting cells, are the intercellular adhesion molecules ICAM-1, ICAM-2, and ICAM-3, whereas the counterreceptor for CD2 is LFA-3. Although antibodies to CD2 or LFA-1 can block activation of T cells, activation can occur normally in induced mutants deficient in either of these molecules, suggesting a redundancy of function. The exact function of these and other activation molecules, such as CD43, CD73, and CD7, for which counterreceptors have not yet been identified, is still uncertain. However, it is thought that these nonspecific interactions provide for a multivalent low-affinity system between T cell and APC, thus allowing prolonged contact and the opportunity for the T cell to sample numerous MHC molecules with peptide. When signaling occurs through the TCR, a conformational change is induced in LFA-1 causing an increased affinity for the ICAMs. ICAM-2 is also constitutively expressed on vascular endothelial cells, and ICAM-1 is inducibly expressed in the presence of inflammatory mediators. Thus, these molecules also subserve the important function of lymphocyte migration into the areas of active inflammation and may have an important role in the pathogenesis of vasculitis. The potential clinical importance of these interactions has also been illustrated by recent studies in primates, which showed that attachment and subsequent infection by rhinoviruses could be blocked by soluble analogs of ICAM.

REGULATION OF CELL-MEDIATED IMMUNITY

The pathway outlined above for a specific antibody response to antigen results in the development of Th2 CD4 effector cells. These cells produce interleukin-4 (IL-4), IL-5, IL-6, IL-9, and IL-10, all important in the regulation of antibody production (Chapter 32). CD4$^+$ cells are also capable of becoming Th1 effector cells, characterized by the elaboration of IL-2 and IFN-γ, crucial to the activation of macrophages for elimination of intracellular pathogens such as *Listeria* species. The specific mechanisms in vivo leading to activation of a polarized Th1 or Th2 response is unclear but probably reflects the microenvironment in which the T cells were activated. For example, in vitro studies have shown that addition of IL-4 during T-cell stimulation with antigen resulted in a Th2 response. Conversely, addition of IFN-γ stimulated a Th1 pattern. The costimulatory molecules may also play a role. In experimental allergic encephalomyelitis, an animal model of multiple sclerosis, specific blockage of B7-2 by antibody treatment caused an increased Th1 response, whereas blockage of B7-1 led to a Th2-predominant response and less disease. Finally, there is evidence to suggest that undetermined genetic factors are involved.

REGULATION OF CELL-MEDIATED CYTOTOXICITY

The molecular basis for the interactions leading to a specific immune response by CD8$^+$ T cells is less well-understood than for CD4$^+$ responses but basically follows the same paradigm. The importance of B7 as a costimulator has been illustrated by a number of studies in which B7 has been transfected into tumor cells and transferred to a naive host. Under these conditions, the tumor is cleared much more readily. Conversely, blockage of the B7–CD28 pathway can lead to reduced rejection. In infections or malignancies involving cells that cannot express B7, CD4$^+$ Th1 cells stimulating CD8$^+$ cells are important, and the role of B7 as the direct costimulator of CD8$^+$ T cells is less clear. The CD4$^+$ cells themselves are presumably activated through professional APCs as outlined above and are therefore stimulated to secrete IL-2. It has been shown that engagement of the TCR on CD8$^+$ cells in the presence of sufficient IL-2 can circumvent the need for costimulation. Inasmuch as CD8$^+$ cells are responding to peptide plus class I, whereas CD4$^+$ cells are responding to peptide with class II, it is not yet clear whether CD4$^+$ T cells are stimulating CD8$^+$ T cells through a common APC or by bystander effects.

Only two different effector mechanisms appear to account for cell-mediated cytotoxicity. In the first mechanism, death is caused by a secretory pathway mediated by perforin and granzymes. Perforin, structurally related to the terminal component of complement C9, performs a similar function by creating large pores in the membrane of the target cell. Serine proteases (granzymes) are cosecreted, resulting in target lysis. The perforin and granzymes are stored in specialized vesicles and are released by a Ca^{2+}-dependent mechanism that spares the effector cell from self-lysis. In the second mechanism, target cells are induced to undergo programmed cell death (apoptosis) by crosslinking of a specific receptor called Fas (CD95). The regulation of apoptosis is an area of intense investigation. Although the exact pathway leading to apoptosis remains to be elucidated, recent evidence points to ceramide, a product of sphingomyelin hydrolysis, as a second messenger.

Although the intramolecular signals leading to apoptosis are still being delineated, more is understood about the cell surface molecules involved. Fas, the receptor signaling apoptosis, is a 48-kDa glycoprotein and member of the tumor necrosis factor (TNF) receptor family. It is expressed on activated T and B lymphocytes. Mutations of Fas have arisen spontaneously, the best known of which is called *lpr*. Mice homozygous for the *lpr* mutation develop a systemic autoimmune disease characterized by the accumulation of a massive number of peripheral T cells that bear neither CD4 nor CD8 and express decreased levels of TCR. Furthermore, these mice develop high titers of autoantibodies. The *gld* mutation, which causes disease phenotypically identical to *lpr*, has been shown to be a point mutation of the ligand binding Fas, rendering it nonfunctional. Fas ligand (FasL), a 40-kDa glycoprotein expressed on cytotoxic T cells, is without an intracellular signal sequence, suggesting it functions purely as a ligand. The physiologic roles of Fas and FasL are still under investigation. Despite the expression of Fas on $CD4^+CD8^+$ thymocytes, central tolerance appears to be intact, pointing to a role in peripheral tolerance by clonal deletion.

T-CELL SIGNALING PATHWAYS

Complementing the great progress in understanding the cell surface interactions leading to immune responses has been the elucidation of the intracellular signaling pathways involved. This is a complicated field, and, although a great number of detailed steps are known, full integration of all of the events leading to activation is still incomplete. Therefore, a broad overview will be provided, mentioning some of the steps that have been shown to be potentially clinically relevant.

The T-cell receptor itself has little in the way of a cytoplasmic component and therefore does not itself transduce the intracytoplasmic signals. Instead, the TCR has associated with it a number of additional invariant proteins, collectively called CD3. CD3 consists of three proteins (CD3γ, CD3δ, and CD3ε), which have homology to immunoglobulins, and two additional proteins, η and ζ, which do not. The ζ chain is an alternatively spliced variant of the η chain and, in the TCR complex, exists as either ζ-ζ or ζ-η disulfide-linked dimers. The CD3ε chain is present in two copies per TCR complex; ε, γ, and δ all have large extracellular domains, whereas ζ and η do not. All five proteins associate with the TCR through noncovalent bonds and can associate with cytosolic tyrosine kinases.

PHOSPHORYLATION With crosslinking of the TCR complex, a set of four interdependent events occurs: (1) tyrosine phosphorylation of membrane and cytosolic proteins; (2) hydrolysis of membrane inositol phospholipids; (3) intracellular calcium fluxes; and (4) increased protein kinase C activity. All members of the CD3 complex have intracytoplasmic tyrosine residues that become phosphorylated with activation. In addition, three major phosphotyrosine kinases have been described: lck, fyn, and ZAP (ζ-associated protein) kinase. Lck is physically associated with the intracytoplasmic domains of CD4 and CD8. It is a crucial protein, as shown by the lack of T-cell development in lck-deficient mice created by homologous recombination. Fyn is weakly associated with the ζ chain of the TCR. In contrast to lck, however, deletion of fyn has shown no effect on development and relatively little effect on T-cell activation. ZAP 70, the third protein, becomes tightly associated with the ζ chain after activation. Interestingly, a form of immunodeficiency characterized by deficient T-cell signaling and an absence of CD8 cells has been described in patients lacking ZAP 70 (*see* Chapter 32). The specific substrates for each of these phosphotyrosine kinases are still being defined. Also regulating phosphorylation is the cell surface molecule CD45, also called leukocyte common antigen, which has intrinsic intracytoplasmic phosphatase activity. One of the functions of CD45 is to remove phosphate from carboxy terminal tyrosine residues on lck and fyn, thereby increasing their activity. Mice deficient in CD45 have deficient B-cell responses and undergo defective intrathymic positive selection.

TRANSCRIPTION After these early events, a number of transcription factors are expressed, now thought to number greater than 70. These factors are divided into three broad groups: immediate, which require no *de novo* protein synthesis; early factors, which require synthesis but appear before mitosis; and late factors, which occur only after mitosis. Some of the most important immediate factors are in the Jun/Fos family of proto-oncogenes. They are activated by phosphorylation by JNK kinase and bind to the transcription factor called nuclear factor of activated T cells (NF-AT). This complex binds to the DNA regulatory sites of many cytokine genes. Other important regulatory proteins include the NF-κB complex, which, when activated, translocates to the nucleus and is a regulatory factor for IL-2. Other factors, such as calcineurin, a calcium-dependent phosphatase, are important in regulation of the activity of these transcription factors. Dephosphorylation causes activation and translocation to the nucleus. The potent immunosuppressant cyclosporin A, which binds to calcineurin, prevents the association of calcineurin with NF-AT, thus blocking transcription of IL-2 (*see* Chapter 30).

THE TWO-SIGNAL HYPOTHESIS AND REGULATION OF ACTIVATION The requirement for costimulatory molecules would predict that, on a molecular level, engagement of TCR alone vs TCR plus CD28 would lead to differences in phosphorylation and gene transcription. Originally, in fact, the two-signal hypothesis arose out of observations that engagement of TCR alone in some $CD4^+$ clones resulted in lack of IL-2 production and a poor proliferative response. The defect appears selective; IL-4 gene expression can be induced in an anergic cell having little IL-2 production. In previously anergized cells, the anergy can again be overcome in vitro by stimulation in the presence of IL-2 but not by B7. Conversely, use of altered peptides designed to bind within the MHC cleft but not engage TCR effectively results in secretion of IL-4 but little proliferation. A current hypothesis for the molecular role of costimulators is that engagement of CD28 causes its phosphorylation and a cascade of events that ultimately converges with the TCR pathway to increase levels of Jun. Without maximal activation of Jun provided by both pathways, there is no transcription of IL-2, a cytokine critical for the development of an armed effector cell. Costimulation provides the means for autocrine production, a requirement that can be overcome in vitro by an exogenous source. However, the hyporesponsiveness of anergic T cells has been shown to be an active response, as it is blocked by protein synthesis inhibitors in vitro. Thus, suboptimal production of a kinase alone seems unlikely to explain all aspects of tolerance. The complete elucidation of stimulatory and costimulatory pathways affords the possibility of developing novel therapies to enhance specific anergy, particularly in transplantation.

DOWNREGULATION OF THE IMMUNE RESPONSE

In the past, it had been assumed that the downregulation of the immune response was a passive process, the natural result of decreased stimulation resulting as antigen was cleared. It has become increasingly clear in recent years that there is also an active component to this regulation, and that apoptosis is an important mechanism by which this operates. Again, it appears that the Fas-FasL system is important. In vitro experiments have shown that activated T cells express Fas but become susceptible to anti-Fas antibodies after only a few days of stimulation. Cells derived from *lpr* mice, deficient in Fas, failed to undergo activation-induced apoptosis. Fas-mediated apoptosis, then, may be a means by which chronic inflammatory reactions are limited. In vivo and in vitro studies have suggested that, at least for T cells, Fas can be crosslinked by FasL present either on its own cell surface or on a neighboring cell. The relative importance of these two pathways in normal circumstances remains to be determined. In addition, there is evidence that the second receptor for B7, CTLA-4, may act to downregulate activation. As an area of research for the treatment of autoimmunity, the activation-induced apoptosis pathway holds promise, because its manipulation may allow downregulation of an ongoing immune response.

SELECTED REFERENCES

Berke G. The CTL's kiss of death. Cell 1995;81:9–12.

Bevan MJ, Hogquist KA, Jameson SC. Selecting the T cell receptor repertoire. Science 1994;264:796,797.

Clark EA, Ledbetter JA. How B and T cells talk to each other. Nature 1994;367:425–428.

Davis MM, Bjorkman PJ. T-cell antigen receptor genes and T-cell recognition. Nature 1994;334:395–402.

Davis MM, Chien Y. Issues concerning the nature of antigen recognition by $\alpha\beta$ and δ T-cell receptors. Immunol Today 1995;16:316–318.

Foy TM, Laman JD, Ledbetter JA, Aruffo A, Claassen E, Noelle RJ. gp39-CD40 interactions are essential for germinal center formation and the development of B cell memory. J Exp Med 1994;180: 157–163.

Germain RN, Margulies DH. The biochemistry and cell biology of antigen processing and presentation. Annu Rev Immunol 1993;11:403–450.

Goodnow CC. Transgenic mice and analysis of B-cell tolerance. Annu Rev Immunol 1992;10:489–518.

Kuchroo VK, Das MP, Brown JA, et al. B7-1 and B7-2 costimulatory molecules activate differentially the Th1/Th2 developmental pathways: application to autoimmune disease therapy. Cell 1995;80: 707–718.

Liblau RS, Singer SM, McDevitt HO. Th1 and Th2 CD4(+) T cells in the pathogenesis of organ-specific autoimmune diseases. Immunol Today 1995;16:34–38.

Linsley PS. Distinct roles for CD28 and cytotoxic T lymphocyte- associated molecule-4 receptors during T cell activation? J Exp Med 1995;182:289–292.

Markowitz JS, Auchincloss H Jr., Grusby MJ, Glimcher LH. Class II-positive hematopoietic cells cannot mediate positive selection of $CD4^+$ T lymphocytes in class II-deficient mice. Proc Natl Acad Sci U SA 1993;90:2779–2783.

Marrack P, Ignatowicz L, Kappler JW, Boymel J, Freed JH. Comparison of peptides bound to spleen and thymus class II. J Exp Med 1993; 178:2173–2183.

Miller JFAP, Flavell RA. T-cell tolerance and autoimmunity in transgenic models of central and peripheral tolerance. Curr Opin Immunol 1994;6:892–899.

Mondino A, Jenkins MK. Surface proteins involved in T cell costimulation. J Leukoc Biol 1994;55:805–815.

Nagata S, Suda T. Fas and Fas ligand: lpr and gld mutations. Immunol Today 1995;16:39–43.

Pieters J, Bakke O, Dobberstein B. The MHC class II-associated invariant chain contains two endosomal targeting signals within its cytoplasmic tail. J Cell Sci 1993;106:831–846.

Pushkareva M, Obeid LM, Hannun YA. Ceramide: an endogenous regulator of apoptosis and growth suppression. Immunol Today 1995; 16:294–297.

Robey E, Allison JP. T cell activation: integration of signals from the antigen receptor and costimulatory molecules. Immunol Today 1995;16:306–310.

Rotzschke O, Falk K. Origin, structure and motifs of naturally processed MHC class II ligands. Curr Opin Immunol 1994;6:45–51.

Steinman RM, Swanson J. The endocytic activity of dendritic cells. J Exp Med 1995;182:283–288.

Stern LJ, Brown JH, Jardetzky TS, et al. Crystal structure of the human class II MHC protein HLA-DR1 complexed with an influenza virus peptide. Nature 1994;368:215–221.

30 Cytokines

WILLIAM L. LOWE, JR., AND BARBARA A. DA SILVA

BACKGROUND

Cytokines encompass diverse groups of multifunctional proteins that play key roles in a variety of biological processes, including cell growth and activation, inflammation, immunity, hematopoiesis, tumorigenesis, tissue repair, fibrosis, and morphogenesis. Chemotaxis is stimulated by a recently defined group of cytokines, the chemokines. Consistent with their relatively diverse functions, cytokines are synthesized in a variety of cell types, including cells of the mononuclear phagocyte system, lymphocytes, epithelial cells, fibroblasts, endothelial cells, and chondrocytes. These peptides interact with receptors on a wide variety of cell types to initiate intracellular signaling cascades that are responsible for mediating their effects. Interactions of the cytokines with these receptors can occur locally in an autocrine fashion on the cells that produced the cytokine or in a paracrine fashion on cells adjacent to the site of production. Finally, cytokines can function at distant sites in an endocrine fashion. This chapter will provide an overview of the major cytokines and their actions, their receptors and intracellular signaling cascades, and the role of cytokines and their receptors in specific disease processes.

CLASSES AND ACTIONS OF CYTOKINES AND CHEMOKINES

Given the diverse nature of cytokines, their pleiotropic effects, and, in some cases, their functional redundancy, it has proven difficult to categorize them into families based on structure or function. Families of cytokines that are important for immune function and inflammation include the interferons, interleukins, tumor necrosis factors, and colony-stimulating factors. Details about their sites of production and action are reviewed in Table 30-1. In addition to those cytokines, a variety of others also have been characterized, including: (1) hormones such as growth hormone, prolactin, and leptin; (2) hematopoietic factors such as erythropoietin and thrombopoietin, which are required for erythrocyte and megakaryocyte maturation and differentiation, respectively; (3) the neurotrophins, including brain-derived neurotrophin factor, nerve growth factor, neurotrophin-3, neurotrophin-6, and glial-derived neurotrophic factor, which are important for growth and differentiation of neurons; (4) neuropoietic factors such as ciliary neurotrophic factor (CNTF), oncostatin M, and leukemia inhibitory factor (LIF), which modulate neuronal differentiation; and (5) the transforming growth factor-β (TGF-β) family, which includes the TGF-βs, bone morphogenic proteins, activins, and inhibins, whose members have diverse effects on cell growth and differentiation in various organ systems.

Chemokines are chemotactic cytokines that attract leukocytes to sites of inflammation and are generally 8- to 10-kDa proteins that can be divided into four different subfamilies based on structural characteristics. The CXC or α-chemokines contain four cysteines, the first two of which are separated by a single amino acid. Some members of this family contain the sequence glutamic acid-leucine-arginine near the N-terminus and are chemotactic for neutrophils, whereas those members of the subfamily that do not contain that sequence are chemotactic for lymphocytes. A second subfamily is the CC or β-chemokines, which, like the α-chemokines, contain four cysteines, but the first two cysteines are adjacent to each other. These chemokines are chemotactic for eosinophils, basophils, and lymphocytes but not, in general, for neutrophils. The sole member of the third subfamily is fractalkine. In fractalkine, the first two cysteines are separated by 3 amino acids, and it is chemotactic for natural killer cells, monocytes, and activated T cells. The last subfamily of chemokines also contains a single member, lymphotactin. Lymphotactin contains only two cysteines and is chemotactic for T cells. Over 40 different chemokines have been identified, and almost all cell types are able to produce them. The different inflammatory infiltrates that are characteristic of different disease processes are controlled, in part, by the chemokines that are expressed locally at the site of disease. Stimuli for chemokine production include several pro-inflammatory cytokines (e.g., IL-1 and TNF-α), T cell products like IL-4 and IFN-γ, bacterial products (e.g., lipopolysaccharide), and viral infection.

MECHANISM OF CYTOKINE-MEDIATED SIGNAL TRANSDUCTION

CYTOKINE RECEPTORS The effects of cytokines are mediated by specific receptors that initiate signal transduction pathways with subsequent activation of gene transcription (*see* Chapter 46). Cytokine receptors contain extracellular, transmembrane, and cytoplasmic domains and are grouped into five classes based on unique amino acid motifs (Table 30-2).

1. Class 1 receptors: These receptors contain conserved amino-terminal cysteine pairs and an extracellular tryptophan-serine-X-tryptophan-serine (WSXWS) motif proximal to the transmembrane domain. The class 1 cytokine receptors can be further subdivided into the IL-2R, IL-3R, and IL-6R subgroups based on use of one of

From: *Principles of Molecular Medicine* (J. L. Jameson, ed.), ©1998 Humana Press Inc., Totowa, NJ.

Table 30-1
Features of the Major Cytokines

Cytokine	Major sites of production	Principal targets	Major effects
IFN-α/β	leukocytes, epithelial cells, fibroblasts, produced by most cell types in culture	lymphocytes, receptors present on most cell types	stimulates natural killer cells; MHC class I induction; antiviral effect
IFN-γ	T lymphocytes, natural killer cells	lymphocytes, monocytes, multiple other cell types	activates monocytes; MHC class I and II induction; enhances lymphocyte adherence to endothelial cells via increased expression of adhesion molecules
IL-1α,β	major source is macrophages but made in other cell types (e.g., B cells, fibroblasts, endothelial cells)	essentially all cell types have receptors for and can respond to IL-1	stimulates T and B cells; proinflammatory mediator; pyrogen; increases ACTH release from pituitary gland; induces production of acute phase proteins
IL-2	T cells	T cells, B cells, monocytes	T cell proliferation and differentiation; activation of cytotoxic lymphocytes and macrophages
IL-3	T cells, mast cells	stem cells, basophils	multi-lineage colony stimulating factor; chemotactic for basophils
IL-4	T cells	B cells, T cells	growth and differentiation factor for B cells leading in particular to IgG1 and IgE production; T cell growth and activation factor
IL-5	TH2 lymphocytes, macrophages	eosinophils, lymphocytes	Growth and differentiation factor for eosinophils; activates lymphocytes
IL-6	most cell types with greatest production by T cells, macrophages, B cells, fibroblasts, and endothelial cells	acts on most cells types	B cell differentiation; activates B cells; induces production of acute phase proteins; proinflammatory mediator; growth factor for multiple myeloma
IL-7	Bone marrow and thymic stroma	pre-B and T cells	Growth factor for pre-B and -T cells; activates T cells
IL-9	Activated T cells	hematopoietic stem cells, mast cells	Mast cell growth and differentiation; growth factor for hematopoietic stem cells
IL-10	TH2 and TH1 lymphocytes, other cell types	B lymphocytes, TH1 lymphocytes, macrophages	inhibits IFN-γ and IL-3 production by TH1 lymphocytes; inhibits macrophage production of multiple cytokines, including IL-1, IL-6, and TNF-α; activates B cells
IL-11	mesenchymal cells	hematopoietic stem cells, receptor present in wide variety of tissues	stimulates production and maturation of megakaryocytes
IL-12	monocytes, B cells	TH1 lymphocytes, natural killer cells	stimulates natural killer cells; stimulates activation and proliferation of TH1 lymphocytes; induces IFN-γ secretion by resting and activated T and natural killer cells
IL-13	activated T lymphocytes	B lymphocytes, monocytes	IL-4-like effects; anti-inflammatory via effects on monocytes; stimulates immunoglobulin synthesis
IL-14	T lymphocytes	B lymphocytes	growth factor for B lymphocytes
IL-15	monocytes, multiple tissues including skeletal muscle and placenta	T and B lymphocytes, NK cells	T and NK cell growth factor; chemoattractant for T cells; B cell proliferation and differentiation
IL-16	T lymphocytes	T lymphocytes, eosinophils, monocytes	competence factor for growth of T cells; induces cytokine synthesis by T cells; chemoattractant for T cells; chemotactic factor for eosinophils and monocytes
IL-17	T lymphocytes	receptor is ubiquitously expressed	limited information suggests that it functions as a pro-inflammatory cytokine
TNF-α	neutrophils, lymphocytes, macrophages, NK cells, neutrophils and many nonlymphoid cells including endothelial cells, adipocytes, and smooth muscle cells	macrophages, neutrophils, lymphocytes, fibroblasts, endothelial cells and multiple other non-lymphoid cell types	activation of macrophages, leukocytes, and cytotoxic cells; pro-inflammatory cytokine; increases leukocyte adhesion to endothelial cells; induces acute phase response; induces cachecia; pyrogen; stimulates angiogenesis; enhances MHC class I production
TNF-β	T lymphocytes	same as above	same as above
M-CSF	monocytes, fibroblasts, endothelial cells, epithelial cells	macrophage precursors	proliferation of macrophage precursors; chemotactic factor for monocytes
GM-CSF	T and B lymphocytes, monocytes, fibroblasts, and endothelial cells	stem cells; monocytes	induces proliferation and differentiation of bone marrow precursors (macrophages, neutrophils, and eosinophils); enhances monocyte migration into inflamed tissue
G-CSF	monocytes, macrophages, endothelial cells, fibroblasts	stem cells	stimulates division and differentiation to promote differentiation of neutrophils

IFN, interferon; IL, interleukin; TNF, tumor necrosis factor; CSF, colony stimulating factor.

Table 30-2
Cytokine Receptors

Cytokine receptor class	Subgroup	Cytokine receptors
Class 1	IL-2R - share γc	IL-2R, IL-4R, IL-7R, IL-9R, IL-13R (does not use γc but may dimerize with ligand binding subunit of IL-4R), IL-15R
	IL-3R - share βc	IL-3R, IL-5R, GM-CSF receptor
	IL-6R - share gp130	IL-6R, IL-11R, cardiotrophin-1 receptor, CNTF receptor, LIF receptor, oncostatin M receptor, leptin receptor (no evidence demonstrating association with gp130), IL-12R (uses a subunit related to but distinct from gp130)
	Others	growth hormone receptor, erythropoietin receptor, prolactin receptor
Class 2		IFN-α/β-R, IFN-γ-R, IL-10R
Immunoglobulin		type I and II IL-1R
TNF receptors		p55 TNF-α-R, p75 TNF-α-R, Fas receptor, lymphotoxin-β receptor, CD-40 ligand receptor
Chemokine receptors		four receptors for CXC chemokines (CXCR1-4), eight receptors for CC chemokines (CCR1-8), and one receptor for fractalkine (CX_3CR1)

three common subunits, which are required for ligand-mediated signal transduction: γc for the IL-2R subgroup, βc for the IL-3R subgroup, and γp-130 for the IL-6R subgroup (Table 30-2). The ligand-binding and signal transduction subunits each contain a single transmembrane domain and heterodimerize upon ligand binding.

2. Class 2 receptors: These receptors contain conserved amino- and carboxy-terminal cysteines without a WSXWS motif. The receptors in this class include the IFN-α/β, IFN-γ, and IL-10 receptors. Interferon-α and -β bind to the type I interferon receptor, whereas interferon-γ binds to the type II interferon receptor.
3. Ig class receptors: This class of receptors contains three immunoglobulin motifs in the extracellular domain. These immunoglobulin motifs have a specific tertiary structure that may be involved in ligand binding. The type 1 and type 2 IL-1 receptors, both of which bind to IL-1α and IL-1β, are members of this class of receptors. It is thought that the type 2 receptor does not have a role in signaling, but may be more important in modulating signal transduction by preventing ligand binding to the type 1 receptor.
4. TNF receptor class: These receptors contain conserved cysteine rich repeats in the extracellular domain. There are several members of this receptor class, including the two receptors for TNF-α, p55 and p75.
5. Chemokine receptors: These receptors are members of the family of seven transmembrane domain receptors that are coupled to G proteins. To date, four receptors for the CXC chemokines, eight receptors for the CC chemokines, and one receptor for fractalkine have been identified. Activation of these receptors results in stimulation of signaling pathways characteristic of G-protein-coupled receptors (*see* Chapter 46), including activation of phospholipases and protein kinase C and release of intracellular calcium. In addition to expression on hematopoietic cells, chemokine receptors also have been found on nonhematopoietic cells, including neurons, astrocytes, epithelial cells, and endothelial cells, suggesting that they have other, as yet, unknown functions.

With the exception of the chemokine receptors, many of the cytokine receptors also exist as soluble forms, generated by either alternative splicing or proteolytic cleavage of the extracellular domain. The function of these soluble receptors is incompletely understood, but they may block cytokine action, stabilize the cytokine by acting as a carrier protein in the circulation, and/or contribute to receptor activation (which has been observed for IL-6). In some cases, circulating levels of the soluble receptors may be a marker for activation of a cytokine network and disease activity. For example, increased levels of the soluble receptors for TNF-α are present in patients with sepsis and rheumatoid arthritis.

INTRACELLULAR SIGNALING PATHWAYS ACTIVATED BY CYTOKINE RECEPTORS Cytokine binding to the class 1 and 2 receptors activates one or more members of a family of cytoplasmic tyrosine kinases, the Janus kinases (Jaks). Cytokine receptors do not possess intrinsic kinase activity, so they depend on the Jaks for this function. The Jaks are a family of four tyrosine kinases (Jak1, Jak2, Jak3, and Tyk1) that associate with specific cytokine receptors and catalyze phosphorylation of tyrosine residues in the cytoplasmic domain of the cytokine receptor. These phosphorylated residues then serve as docking sites for proteins with phosphotyrosine binding (PTB) or Src homology 2 (SH2)-binding domains. Binding of these proteins is important for ligand-mediated signal transduction and helps to confer specificity to the intracellular effects of the different cytokines.

Among the proteins with an SH2 domain that bind to these phosphorylated tyrosine residues are the signal transducers and activators of transcription (STATs). The STATs are a family of transcription factors with at least seven members: STAT1, STAT2, STAT3, STAT4, STAT5a, STAT5b, and STAT6. The SH2 domain of the STATs is important for binding to the phosphorylated receptor, and, like the Jaks, specific STATs interact with specific cytokine receptors. Once the STAT protein binds to the receptor, it is phosphorylated on tyrosine residues by Jak, which allows it to form either homo- or heterodimers with other phosphorylated STAT proteins. These activated STAT complexes translocate to the nucleus, where they can interact with specific DNA sequences to induce gene transcription. In addition to the STATs, other signal transduction pathways, e.g., the Ras/Raf/ERK and phosphatidylinositol 3-kinase pathways, can be activated in response to cytokine binding (*see* Chapter 46). The mechanisms for the termination of signal transduction via activated cytokine receptors are currently less clear, but may involve phosphotyrosine phosphatases and/or degradation of the STAT proteins.

ROLE OF CYTOKINES IN PATHOLOGIC AND PHYSIOLOGIC PROCESSES

The cytokines are intimately involved in a wide variety of physiologic and pathologic processes, a complete description of which is beyond the scope of this chapter. Rather, a description of the role of cytokines in the pathophysiology of rheumatoid arthritis and sepsis and the physiology of weight regulation will be provided as examples of the pleiotropic effects of cytokines, their potentially synergistic interactions, as well as their potentially opposing and antagonizing effects.

RHEUMATOID ARTHRITIS Rheumatoid arthritis is a chronic polyarthritis characterized by an inflammatory synovitis that involves the peripheral joints, typically in a symmetrical fashion. The disease is characterized by additional systemic symptoms, including fatigue, anorexia, weight loss, and a low-grade fever. The etiology of rheumatoid arthritis is not fully understood and is likely secondary to both genetic and environmental factors.

Table 30-3
Effects of the Cytokines that Contribute to the Pathogenesis of Rheumatoid Arthritis

Cytokine	Manifestations of rheumatoid arthritis
IL-1	Contributes to fever and constitutional symptoms; stimulates the acute phase response; contributes to tissue destruction by increasing matrix metalloprotease and PGE_2 production; increases fibroblast proliferation via increased PDGF production; T cell activation and proliferation; activates endothelial cells; stimulates production of itself, IL-6, IL-8, LIF, and GM-CSF
TNFα	Synergizes with IL-1 to increase PGE2 and matrix metalloprotease production; stimulates fibroblast proliferation; activates endothelial cells; increases production of IL-1, IL-6, IL-8, LIF, TGF-β, and MCP-1; contributes to constitutional symptoms; stimulates acute phase response
IL-6	Stimulates antibody production; participates in T cell activation; stimulates the acute phase response; stimulates production of TNF-α and Fc receptors
GM-CSF	Increases expression of HLA class II antigens; increases macrophage number by helping to maintain macrophage viability; participates in the induction of IL-1 and TNF-α production
LIF	Induces expression of IL-1, IL-6, IL-8, and itself; activates monocytes, proinflammatory effects similar to IL-6
M-CSF	Stimulates TNF-α production; promotes macrophage survival
IL-2	T cell proliferation
IFN-γ	Endothelial cell activation; stimulates antibody production

PG, prostaglandin; PDGF, platelet-derived growth factor; LIF, leukemia inhibitory factor; MCP, monocyte chemoattractant protein

The synovitis is characterized by hyperplasia and hypertrophy of synovial lining cells, perivascular infiltration by mononuclear cells, microvascular injury, and neovascularization. The synovial fluid also demonstrates acute inflammatory changes, with large numbers of polymorphonuclear leukocytes and limited numbers of mononuclear cells being present.

Cytokines play a critical role in the maintenance of active synovitis, tissue destruction, and systemic symptoms characteristic of rheumatoid arthritis (Table 30-3), although the role of cytokines in the initiation of the synovitis is unclear. IL-1 and TNF-α are the two proinflammatory cytokines that make major contributions to the pathogenesis of rheumatoid arthritis. In addition to mediating many of the inflammatory and constitutional symptoms, cytokines also establish positive feedback loops to help sustain the inflammatory process. For example, IL-1 regulates not only its own production but that of TNF-α, whereas TNF-α is capable of increasing IL-1 production. Moreover, both IL-1 and TNF-α stimulate the production of a variety of other cytokines, including IL-6, IL-8, and LIF, that are important for the inflammatory process. Finally, IL-1 and TNF-α act synergistically to stimulate a variety of other inflammatory effects, e.g., matrix metalloprotease and prostaglandin production, fibroblast proliferation, and endothelial cell activation.

Interestingly, not only inflammatory cytokines, but a variety of anti-inflammatory cytokines are present in synovial fluid and/or tissue. For example, increased levels of a naturally occurring antagonist of IL-1, IL-1ra, are present in synovial tissue from patients with rheumatoid arthritis. IL-1ra is a member of the IL-1 gene family that is a competitive inhibitor of IL-1 and, as such, binds to, but does not activate, the IL-1 receptor. It is produced by monocytes, neutrophils, and other cell types in response to a variety of cytokines, including IL-1, IL-4, and IL-10. High levels of TGF-β1 and -β2 are also present in synovial fluid. Both of these cytokines have anti-inflammatory effects that include inhibition of T cell, B cell, and fibroblast proliferation and antibody production. Moreover, they are able to deactivate macrophages, decrease production of TNF-α and IL-1 by macrophages, and stimulate production of extracellular matrix. A third inhibitory cytokine present in inflammatory synovial fluid is IL-10. IL-10 inhibits expression of IL-1, IL-6, IL-8, GM-CSF, and TNF-α by monocytes, which may help to inhibit synovitis. It is unclear whether exacerbations and remissions of the disease may be related to shifts in the balance between production of the proinflammatory and inhibitory cytokines.

Chemokines also contribute to the pathogenesis of rheumatoid arthritis. The C-C chemokines monocyte chemoattractant protein-1 (MCP-1), macrophage inflammatory protein-1α (MIP-1α), and RANTES (regulated upon activation normal T-cell expressed and secreted) are produced by fibroblasts and macrophages in response to IL-1 and TNF-α. These peptides are chemotactic for monocytes and T cells. In addition to the above, the C-X-C chemokines IL-8, gro, and epithelial cell-derived neutrophil-activating peptide 78 (ENA-78) are produced by macrophages and chondrocytes in response to TNF-α and IL-1. These peptides are chemotactic for neutrophils and, in the case of IL-8, also for lymphocytes. Thus, chemokines contribute to the inflammatory process by attracting inflammatory cells into the synovium and synovial fluid.

Given the critical role of cytokines in the pathogenesis of rheumatoid arthritis, they have served as targets for novel therapies for the disease. Since IL-1ra is a competitive antagonist for binding to the IL-1 receptor, it has been tried as a therapeutic agent. In humans, early phase I and now phase II trials of IL-1ra administered subcutaneously have resulted in improvement of several clinical measures of disease, including the number of painful and swollen joints. Other clinical trials have examined the efficacy of monoclonal antibodies directed against specific cytokines in patients with rheumatoid arthritis. Antibodies to both IL-6 and TNF-α have demonstrated potential efficacy in early trials. Cytokines may represent, therefore, an important target for novel therapeutic strategies for rheumatoid arthritis.

SEPSIS Cytokines are also important in septic shock, which occurs secondary to the systemic inflammatory response to an overwhelming infection. It is characterized by fever, hypotension, and tissue hypoperfusion with resulting organ dysfunction and lactic acidosis. Sepsis, in addition to trauma, burn injuries, and meningitis, is one of the conditions in which large amounts of TNF-α are released into the circulation. Cytokine production, and specifically release of TNF-α, is induced by bacteria themselves or soluble bacterial products, including lipopolysaccharide (LPS), exotoxins, and cell-wall glycopeptides. A primary role for TNF-α in the host response to sepsis is suggested by several findings. For one, infusion of TNF-α into humans results in fever, myalgias, headaches, hypotension, a vascular leakage syndrome, and increased protein degradation, all of which are characteristic of the response to sepsis. TNF-α–induced hypotension is secondary to decreased cardiac contractility and decreased vascular resistance mediated by increased nitric oxide release. A second piece of evidence supporting a primary role for TNF-α in septic shock is the observation that mice with a null mutation of the TNF-α gene are protected from the lethal effects of LPS.

Although TNF-α is a primary mediator of the manifestations of septic shock, a cascade of cytokines is released during sepsis, many in response to TNF-α. One of the other primary cytokines that contributes to septic shock and acts synergistically with TNF-α is IL-1. Similar to TNF-α, IL-1 infusion in humans induces fever, sleepiness, anorexia, generalized myalgias, arthralgias, headache, and, in high doses, hypotension. Hypotension occurs secondary to the release of nitric oxide, prostaglandins, and platelet-activating factor. Two other effects of IL-1 contribute to the body's response to stress. For one, IL-1 increases production of adrenocorticotropic hormone (ACTH) by the pituitary gland, which stimulates glucocorticoid production by the adrenal gland. Interestingly, glucocorticoids decrease IL-1 and TNF-α production and may serve to modulate the inflammatory response. Second, IL-1 stimulates IL-6 production and, together, these cytokines mediate the hepatic acute phase response, which helps to maintain systemic homeostasis. The hepatic acute phase response is characterized by fever, leukocytosis, and increased hepatic production of C-reactive protein, α_1-acid glycoprotein, serum amyloid A, fibrinogen, factor B, haptoglobin, complement C3, α_1-proteinase inhibitor, α_1-chymotrypsin, ceruloplasmin, and C1 esterase inhibitor and decreased production of albumin, transferrin, and lipoprotein lipase. Finally, additional cytokines are released either directly or indirectly in response to TNF-α, including IL-2, IL-4, IL-6, IL-10, IL-12, IFN-γ, and TGF-β.

Like rheumatoid arthritis, cytokines have been the target of therapeutic interventions in sepsis. Both IL-1ra and monoclonal antibodies directed against TNF-α have been used. Results with both agents have been similar in that early mortality was reduced and a trend toward reduced 28-day mortality was apparent, although statistically significant reductions in 28-day mortality have not, as yet, been demonstrated. These cytokines likely represent important therapeutic targets, and additional studies to address this issue are underway.

BODY-WEIGHT REGULATION Apart from their known immunologic, proinflammatory, and growth and differentiation functions, cytokines are involved in body-weight regulation and metabolic perturbations such as insulin resistance. At least three cytokines are important for these metabolic effects. Leptin, an adipose-derived factor, is secreted in proportion to body fat mass and is transported across the blood–CSF and blood–brain barriers via a saturable transporter, which is likely an isoform of the leptin receptor. It then exerts at least some of its effects, including regulation of food intake and energy expenditure, by binding to leptin receptors in hypothalamic nuclei. Second, TNF-α is secreted by adipose cells and increases leptin output from adipose cells. TNF-α also interferes with the insulin signaling pathway and, thus, contributes to obesity-related insulin resistance. Finally, neural-derived ciliary neurotropic factor (CNTF) has been implicated in body-weight regulation because of its effects on hypothalamic neuropeptide Y (NPY). NPY production by the hypothalamus increases food intake and decreases thermogenesis. CNTF interferes with NPY production and/or secretion, which results in anorexia and weight loss. The ability of leptin to inhibit food intake also is mediated, in part, by decreasing NPY production in the hypothalamus.

ROLE OF CYTOKINE RECEPTORS IN DISEASE

Alterations in cytokine receptors and associated signal transduction molecules are now being recognized as important in the etiology of specific disease processes. A dramatic example of this is the severe combined immunodeficiencies (SCIDs). SCID occurs in ~1 in 100,000 live births, with 50% of cases having X-linked SCID (XSCID). Males with XSCID exhibit a profoundly decreased number of T cells with normal to increased B cells. The B cells, however, are nonfunctional, and the patients exhibit hypogammaglobulinemia. These children present with failure to thrive, severe and recurrent infections, and premature death in the absence of a curative bone marrow transplant. Insight into the etiology of XSCID came with the recognition that the gene encoding the γ-subunit of the IL-2R was localized to a region of the X-chromosome, Xq13, known to contain the XSCID locus. A variety of mutations, including premature stop codons, truncations, insertions, deletions, frame shifts, and single amino acid changes, in the

Table 30-4
Disorders Associated with Cytokine Receptor Mutations

Cytokine Receptor	Type of Mutation/Inheritance	Effect of mutation/disorder associated with mutation
Growth hormone receptor	Inactivating mutation; autosomal recessive	Laron Dwarfism (growth hormone resistant dwarfism)
IL-2 receptor α chain	Inactivating mutation; autosomal recessive	Immunodeficiency characterized by decreased peripheral T cells which proliferate abnormally, normal B cell development, and lymphocytic infiltration of multiple tissues accompanied by tissue atrophy and inflammation
γc subunit	Inactivating mutation, X-linked recessive	X-linked severe combined immunodeficiency
Interferon-γ receptor 1	Inactivating mutation; autosomal recessive	Immunodeficiency characterized by altered IFN-γ-induced TNF-α production, defective antigen processing and presentation, and susceptibility to mycobacteria infections
Erythropoietin receptor	Activating mutation; autosomal dominant	Familial erythrocytosis
IL-4 receptor α chain	Activating mutation; autosomal dominant with incomplete penetrance	Hyper-IgE syndrome, severe atopic dermatitis, atopy
Receptor common β chain (βc)	Decreased expression of βc (mechanism unclear - missense mutation present in one subject)	Probable molecular defect in some cases of childhood-onset pulmonary alveolar proteinosis

γ-subunit now have been demonstrated in these patients. All of these mutations abrogate ligand-activated function of the γ-subunit. Initially, the γ-subunit was known to be associated with only the IL-2 receptor, but with the recognition that the phenotype of patients with XSCID was more severe than that of patients with IL-2 deficiency, it was subsequently demonstrated that the γ-subunit, which was renamed γc (for common), was associated with the receptors for several cytokines, including IL-4, IL-7, IL-9, and IL-15. Comparison of the phenotype of patients with γc mutations to that of patients with IL-2 deficiency or mutations of the IL-2 receptor α chain *(see below)*, demonstrates that all or some subset of these cytokines are required for normal development of the immune system. A subset of patients with an autosomal recessive form of SCID have now been shown to have mutations in Jak3. This was predicted, since Jak3 associates with γc. Recognition of the molecular defects responsible for XSCID and some cases of autosomal recessive SCID likely will facilitate development of new and more targeted therapies for treatment of these patients, especially those for whom a bone marrow transplant is not available.

As the number of cytokine receptors continues to grow, an increasing number of disease processes have been ascribed to mutations in cytokine receptors (Table 30-4). Although many of these mutations are associated with rare syndromes, the activating mutation in the IL-4R α chain appears to be a relatively common mutation that underlies, in part, the genetic predisposition to allergic diseases. This mutation was initially identified by screening a small group of patients with the hyper-IgE syndrome and severe atopic dermatitis for IL-4R mutations. Six of the ten patients were found to be heterozygous for a missense mutation (substitution of arginine for glutamine at position 576) in the IL-4R α chain gene. Subsequent screening of the general population demonstrated that the frequency of the mutant allele was 35% in those with a history of atopy and only 10% in those without a history of atopy, thus demonstrating a strong association of the mutation with atopy. Additional studies demonstrated a probable molecular basis for this increased susceptibility. IL-4 is important for production of IgE by B cells, and enhanced signaling of the mutant compared to the wild-type receptor was demonstrated. This recent elucidation of the contribution of an IL-4 receptor mutation to a common problem like atopy will be important for future attempts to identify susceptible individuals and, possibly, for developing and/or targeting the use of new therapeutic modalities.

REFERENCES

Bazzoni F, Beutler B. The tumor necrosis factor ligand and receptor families. N Engl J Med 1996;334:1717–1725.

Bray GA, York DA. Clinical review 90: leptin and clinical medicine: a new piece in the puzzle of obesity. J Clin Endocrinol Metab 1997;82:2771–2776.

Darnell Jr JE. STATs and gene regulation. Science 1997;277:1630–1636.

Dinarello CA. Proinflammatory and anti-inflammatory cytokines as mediators in the pathogenesis of septic shock. Chest 1997;112:321S–329S.

Dirksen U, Nishinakamura R, Groneck P, Hattenhorst U, Nogee L, Murray R, Burdach S. Human pulmonary alveolar proteinosis associated with a defect in GM-CSF/IL-3/IL-5 receptor common β chain expression. J Clin Invest 1997;100:2211–2217.

Ebadi M, Bashir RM, Heidrick ML, Hamada FM, Refaey HE, Hamed A, Helal G, Baxi MD, Cerutis DR, Lassi NK. Neurotrophins and their receptors in nerve and injury repair. Neurochem Int 1997;30:347–374.

Gregg XT, Prchal JT. Erythropoietin receptor mutations and human disease. Semin Hematol 1997;34:70–76.

Khurana Hershey GK, Friedrich MF, Esswein LA, Thomas ML, Chatila TA. The association of atopy with a gain-of-function mutation in the a subunit of the interleukin-4 receptor. N Engl J Med 1997;337:1720–1725.

Ihle JN. Cytokine receptor signaling. Nature 1995;377:591–594.

Ivashkiv LB. Cytokine expression and cell activation in inflammatory arthritis. Adv Immunol 1996;63:337–376.

Leonard WJ. Dysfunctional cytokine receptor signaling in severe combined immunodeficiency. J Invest Med 1996;44:304–311.

Luster AD. Chemokines—chemotactic cytokines that mediate inflammation. N Engl J Med 1998;338:436–445.

Newport MJ, Huxley CM, Huston S, Hawrylowicz CM, Oostra BA, Williamson R, Levin M. A mutation in the interferon-γ-receptor gene and susceptibility to mycobacterial infections. N Engl J Med 1996;335:1941–1949.

O'Shea JJ, Notarangelo LD, Johnston JA, Candotti F. Advances in the understanding of cytokine signal transduction: the role of Jaks and STATs in immunoregulation and the pathogenesis of immunodeficiency. J Clin Immunol 1997;17:431–447.

Sharfe N, Dadi JK, Shahar M, Roifman CM. Human immune disorder arising from mutation of the a chain of the interleukin-2 receptor. Proc Natl Acad Sci USA 1997;94:3168–3171.

Taga T. gp130 and the interleukin-6 family of cytokines. Annu Rev Immunol 1997;15:797–819.

Woodcock JM, Bagley CJ, Lopez AF. Receptors of the cytokine superfamily: mechanism of activation and involvement in disease. Ballieres Clin Haematol 1997;10:507–524.

31 The HLA Complex

ROBERT W. KARR

INTRODUCTION

The human major histocompatibility complex (MHC), or HLA (for human leukocyte antigen), is located on chromosome 6 and contains multiple genes that encode proteins which play central roles in the generation of immune responses. The HLA complex can be divided into three regions, each of which contains genes that encode molecules of similar structures: the class I and II genes encode the HLA class I and II molecules, respectively, and the class III genes encode the C4, C2, and Bf components of the complement system. The HLA class I and II molecules are intimately involved in the process of discriminating self from nonself, and these molecules share the characteristic of being highly polymorphic in the population.

STRUCTURE OF CLASS I AND II MOLECULES

The HLA class I molecules, HLA-A, -B, and -C, are heterodimers composed of a polymorphic, HLA-encoded, 44-kDa transmembrane glycoprotein, referred to as the heavy or α chain, and β-2-microglobulin (β2m), a nonpolymorphic, 12-kDa protein encoded outside the MHC that noncovalently associates with the extracellular portion of the heavy chain (Table 31-1). HLA class I molecules are expressed on virtually all cells, and these molecules restrict recognition of antigenic peptides by $CD8^+$ T cells. Based on analysis of the linear sequences of the genes and proteins, it was shown that HLA class I molecules belong to the immunoglobulin supergene family, that the extracellular region of the α chain can be divided into three domains (α1, α2, and α3), each containing approximately 90 amino acids, and that the polymorphism in the α chain is localized to hypervariable regions in the α1 and α2 domains.

A seminal contribution to our understanding of the structure and function of class I molecules was the solution of the three-dimensional structure of the HLA-A2 molecule by X-ray crystallography by Bjorkman et al. in 1987. These data demonstrated that the membrane-proximal α3 and β2m domains are associated with each other and are folded into structures resembling immunoglobulin constant regions (Fig. 31-1). The membrane-distal α1 and α2 domains form a platform composed of a single eight-stranded β-pleated sheet topped by two α-helices with a long groove between the helices. Importantly, this groove was shown to be the binding site for antigenic peptides. The α1 and α2 domains each contribute half of the platform or floor and one of the α-helices. The previously identified polymorphic residues in the α1 and α2 domains are located in the floor of the peptide-binding site or on the α-helices where they are likely to influence function through effects on peptide binding or T-cell receptor (TCR) recognition. Additional key concepts about class I molecules emerged from subsequent determination of the three-dimensional structures of HLA-A68 and -B27 molecules. Polymorphic differences between class I molecules create unique subsites or pockets within the peptide-binding groove that determine the physical characteristics of peptides that may be bound by each molecule. In general, the grooves of class I molecules contain about three peptide-binding pockets.

Considerable progress has been made in understanding the nature of the peptides bound by HLA class I molecules. Although there is some variation in length, most peptides bound by class I molecules are 9 amino acids and bind in an N-to-C orientation with the C-terminus to the right end of the groove and the N-terminus to the left end of the groove (Fig. 31-1B). Peptides bound to class I molecules usually have an arched conformation with a kink in the middle. The termini of the peptides are anchored by hydrogen bonds with conserved class I residues located in relatively deep pockets at the ends of the peptide-binding site, and a polymorphic peptide-binding pocket in the central portion of the groove determines allele-specific peptide binding. The physical characteristics of peptides that bind to a specific class I molecule are referred to as the peptide motif for that molecule. For example, HLA-B27 molecules bind nonamers, almost all of which have an arginine at the P2 position of the peptide that fits into the B pocket of the B27 groove.

The HLA class II molecules, HLA-DR, -DQ, and -DP, are heterodimers in which both chains, an α chain of ~32 kDa and a β chain of ~28 kDa, are MHC-encoded, transmembrane glycoproteins (Table 31-1). DRβ, DQα and β, and DPα and β chains are polymorphic, whereas the DRα chain is nonpolymorphic. HLA class II α and β chains are also members of the immunoglobulin supergene family, and α and β chains each contain two extracellular protein domains, referred to as α1 and α2, and β1 and β2, respectively. Whereas β2 domains have minimal sequence variability, β1 domains are highly polymorphic, and like class I heavy chains, the polymorphisms are localized to specific regions of the linear sequences, called hypervariable regions. For example, in DRβ chains, three such regions have been identified: the first hypervariable region encompasses amino acids 9–13, the second, amino acids 26–37, and the third, amino acids 67–74.

From: *Principles of Molecular Medicine* (J. L. Jameson, ed.), ©1998 Humana Press Inc., Totowa, NJ.

Table 31-1
Comparison of HLA Class I and Class II Molecules

	Class I	*Class II*
Name	HLA-A, -B, and -C	HLA-DR, -DQ, and -DP
Structure	Heterodimer ~44 kDa heavy chain ~12 kDa β2m	Heterodimer ~32 kDa α chain ~28 kDa β chain
Distribution	Virtually all cells	B cells, macrophages, and activated T cells
Function	Bind and present antigenic peptides to CD8+ T cells	Bind and present antigenic peptides to CD4+ T cells
Peptide length	8–10 residues	10–25 residues

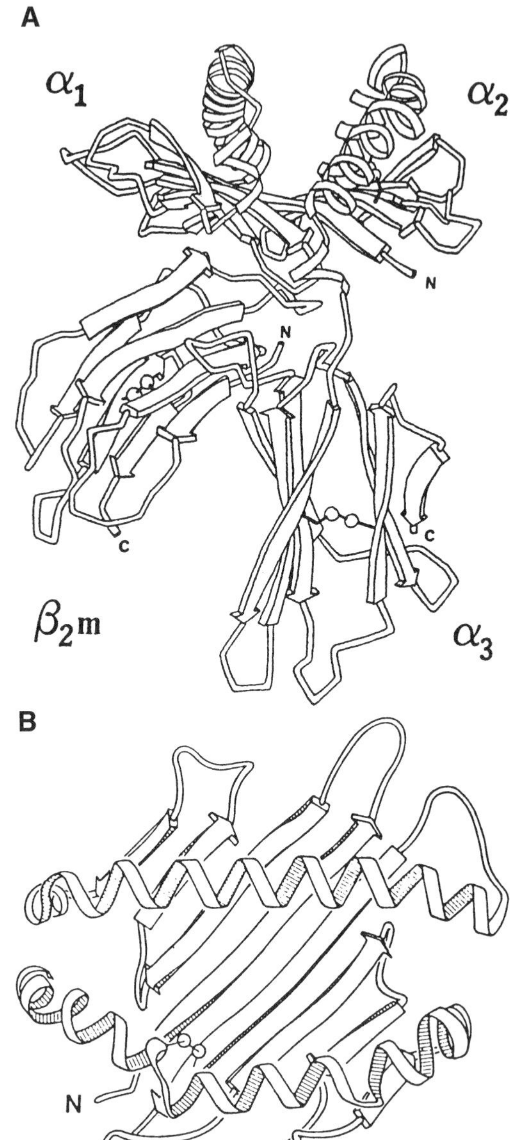

Figure 31-1 The three-dimensional structure of a class I molecule, HLA-A2. **(A)** Schematic representation of the A2 molecule shown in the side view, with the α1, α2, and α3 domains of the HLA heavy chain and β2m labeled. The peptide binding groove is formed by two α-helices rising above the floor of β-pleated sheets. **(B)** Top view of the molecule showing the peptide-binding groove. (Reprinted with permission from Nature 1987;329:506–512. Copyright 1987 Macmillan Magazines Limited.)

The three-dimensional structures of the HLA-DR1 molecule with a mixture of peptides or a single peptide bound were reported in 1993 and 1994. As predicted in an earlier hypothetical model of a class II molecule based on the class I HLA-A2 structure, the general organization of the DR1 molecule is similar to class I molecules. In the DR1 structures (Fig. 31-2), the α1 and β1 domains form a membrane-distal peptide-binding groove composed of two α-helices that rise above a floor of β strands. The α1 and β1 domains each contribute half of the floor and one of the α-helices. As with class I molecules, the polymorphisms previously noted in the linear sequences are located in regions where they seem very likely to determine function. The DRβ chain first and second hypervariable regions are located in the floor of the peptide-binding groove, where the polymorphic residues may influence peptide binding or conformation, and the third hypervariable region is located on the α-helix. The side-chain orientations of these third hypervariable region residues suggest that some may influence peptide conformation, whereas others may directly contact the TCR. DR1 molecules also contain peptide-binding pockets, although the number of pockets is larger than that found in class I molecules. For example, pocket 1, formed by residues β85, β86, β89, β90, α24, α31, α32, and α43, is deep and plays a key role in anchoring the bound peptide. The side chains of DRβ residues 13, 70, 71, 74, and 78, as well as α9, form a shallow pocket, referred to as pocket 4, that exerts a major and disproportionate influence on the outcome of T-cell recognition. The recently reported structure of the HLA-DR3 molecule with a bound peptide is similar to the DR1 structures.

Although class I and class II molecules have very similar structures overall, class II molecules bind peptides differently than class I molecules. Class II molecules bind peptides of variable lengths, ranging from 12 to 25 amino acids. In contrast to class I molecules, which use conserved residues at each end of the groove to make hydrogen bonds near the ends of the peptide, class II molecules use multiple, mostly conserved, residues throughout the groove to make hydrogen bonds with the main chain of the peptide. For example, in the DR1 structure with a single peptide bound, there are hydrogen bonds between 12 nonpolymorphic and 3 polymorphic DR1 residues and main-chain atoms of the peptide. Peptides bind to class II molecules in an N-to-C orientation and in a fully extended or straight conformation. The combination of polymorphic residues in the class II peptide-binding pockets determine the characteristics or motif of the peptides that may be bound by each class II molecule. The motif of peptides that bind to DR1 is best characterized based on the three-dimensional structure, peptide-binding studies, and sequencing of naturally occurring peptides eluted from the DR1 molecules. These motifs usually include four anchor residues, for example P1, P4, P6, and P9, that are known or thought to interact with pockets 1, 4, 6, and 9, respectively, in the class II binding groove. It is important to note that these motifs are usu-

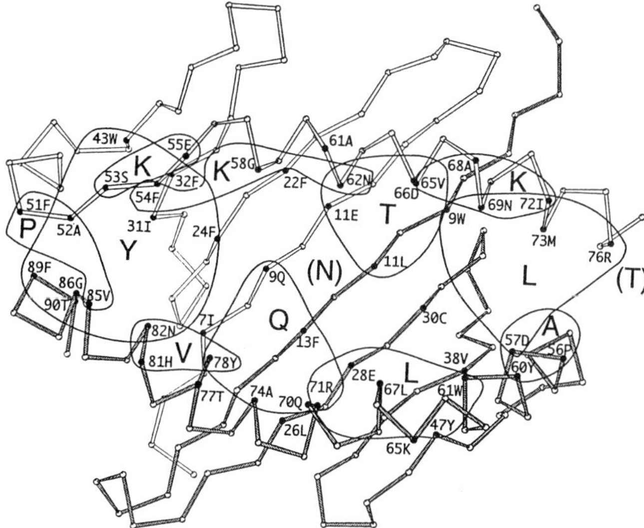

Figure 31-2 Schematic representation of the structure of HLA-DR1 and DR1–peptide contacts. DR1 was cocrystallized with the influenza hemagglutinin peptide, PKYVKQNTLKLAT. The top view of DR1 is shown in the Cα trace with the peptide binding groove formed by the α chain α-helix at top, the β chain α-helix at bottom, and the floor of the groove. Lines enclose all DR1 residues in contact with each peptide side chain (large letters). The DR residues in contact with the same peptide residue define the peptide-binding pockets. For example, the residues in pocket 1 (residues β85, β86, β89, β90, α24, α31, α32, and α43) contact the P1 residue (Y), and pocket 4 (DRβ residues 13, 70, 71, 74, and 78, as well as α9) contacts Q, the P4 residue. (Reprinted with permission from Nature 1994;368:215–221. Copyright 1994 Macmillan Magazines Limited.)

ally located in the central portions of the 12–25 residue peptides, suggesting that the N- and C-termini of bound peptides extend out the ends of the peptide-binding groove. The first residue in the DR1 peptide motif, P1, which fits into pocket 1, is hydrophobic, with a strong preference for aromatic residues, whereas the P4 residue is often aliphatic, but is polar in some DR1-binding peptides. DR1 molecules have a strong preference for peptides with alanine or glycine at P6. In contrast, P9 is said to be degenerate, because there is no preference for the residue at this position. The sum of the restricted or degenerate requirements at each peptide position results in an allele-specific peptide-binding motif that is determined by the unique combination of polymorphic residues in the peptide-binding groove of that class II molecule.

The tissue distribution of class II molecules is more restricted than class I molecules; class II molecules are expressed primarily on immunocompetent cells, including macrophages, monocytes, dendritic cells, B cells, and activated T cells (Table 31-1). Class II expression may also be induced on other cell types, such as endothelial cells, by cytokines, such as interferon-γ. HLA class II molecules restrict the recognition of antigenic peptides by $CD4^+$ T cells, in contradistinction to class I molecules that restrict the recognition by $CD8^+$ T cells. Although the details of the interactions are not yet known, the TCR is thought to simultaneously contact portions of the α-helices of the class II molecule and the bound peptide. In addition, the CD4 molecule on the same T cell interacts with specific conserved residues in the membrane-proximal β2 domain of the class II molecule.

GENETIC ORGANIZATION, POLYMORPHISM, AND NOMENCLATURE OF THE HLA SYSTEM

More than 100 genes have been mapped in the 4000 kb of DNA that comprise the HLA complex on the short arm of chromosome 6 (Fig. 31-3). The class II region, which contains the genes encoding HLA class II molecules, as well as other genes, is located most centromeric in the HLA complex. The class III region, which contains complement and other genes, is located between the class II region and the most telomeric region, the class I region, which contains the genes encoding HLA class I heavy chains. The class I region contains the genes that encode the classic HLA-A, -B, and -C heavy chains of class I molecules, as well as other genes that encode the more recently described nonclassic HLA-E, -F, and -G heavy chains. The class II region is organized into three subregions, DR, DQ, and DP, each of which contains the corresponding α and β chain genes. In addition, the class II region contains the LMP and TAP genes, which encode molecules involved in class I antigen processing and transport, as well as the gene that encodes HLA-DM, a molecule recently shown to be involved in class II peptide loading. The class III region contains genes encoding a variety of proteins, including the complement components C4, C2, and properdin factor B, tumor necrosis factor-α and -β, 21-hydroxylase, and heat shock protein 70.

A notable hallmark of HLA-A, -B, -C, -DR, -DQ, and -DP genes and molecules is their extensive polymorphism or sequence variability in the population. As of 1995, these numbers of alleles had been identified at the various loci based on DNA sequencing: HLA-A, 59; HLA-B, 118; HLA-C, 36; HLA-DRB1, 128; HLA-DQA1, 16; HLA-DQB1, 25; HLA-DPA1, 8; and HLA-DPB1, 62. During the evolution of the current understanding of the HLA system, a variety of nomenclature schemes, often resulting in a seemingly self-defeating alphabet soup of names, have been used. In recent years, a standard nomenclature has evolved for HLA class I and II genes and molecules. Alleles at each locus are named by this convention: the locus name is followed by an asterisk and four or five digits to denote the specific allele. When possible, the first two digits of the allele designation correspond to the historical serologic specificity associated with a family of alleles. For example, 2 of the 10 HLA-B locus alleles related to the B27 serologic specificity are named B*2701 and B*2704. Likewise, DRB1 alleles related to the DR4 serologic specificity are named DRB1*0401 through DRB1*0422. Class II A and B genes, such as DRA1*0101 and DRB1*0401, encode α and β chains, respectively. Although each chromosome 6 contains an HLA-A, -B, -C, -DRA, -DRB1, -DQA1, -DQB1, -DPA1, and -DPB1 gene that encodes an expressed protein, haplotypes containing different DRB1 alleles may also contain and express one of three other DRB genes, DRB3, DRB4, or DRB5. Haplotypes with DRB1*15 or 16 alleles also express β chains encoded by a DRB5 allele; haplotypes with DRB1*03, 11, 12, 13, or 14 alleles also express a DRB3 allele, and haplotypes with DRB1*04, 07, or 09 alleles also express DRB4. DRB1*01 and 08 haplotypes do not express a second DRβ chain. Because the two copies of chromosome 6 usually contain different alleles at each of the HLA loci, most individuals express six class I molecules (two each of HLA-A, -B, and -C) and eight class II molecules (two each of HLA-DRβ1, -DQ, and -DP and two of DRβ3, 4, or 5).

HLA-typing methods have evolved over time with changes in the understanding of the HLA genes and molecules and improved technology. Historically, HLA typing was done by complement-

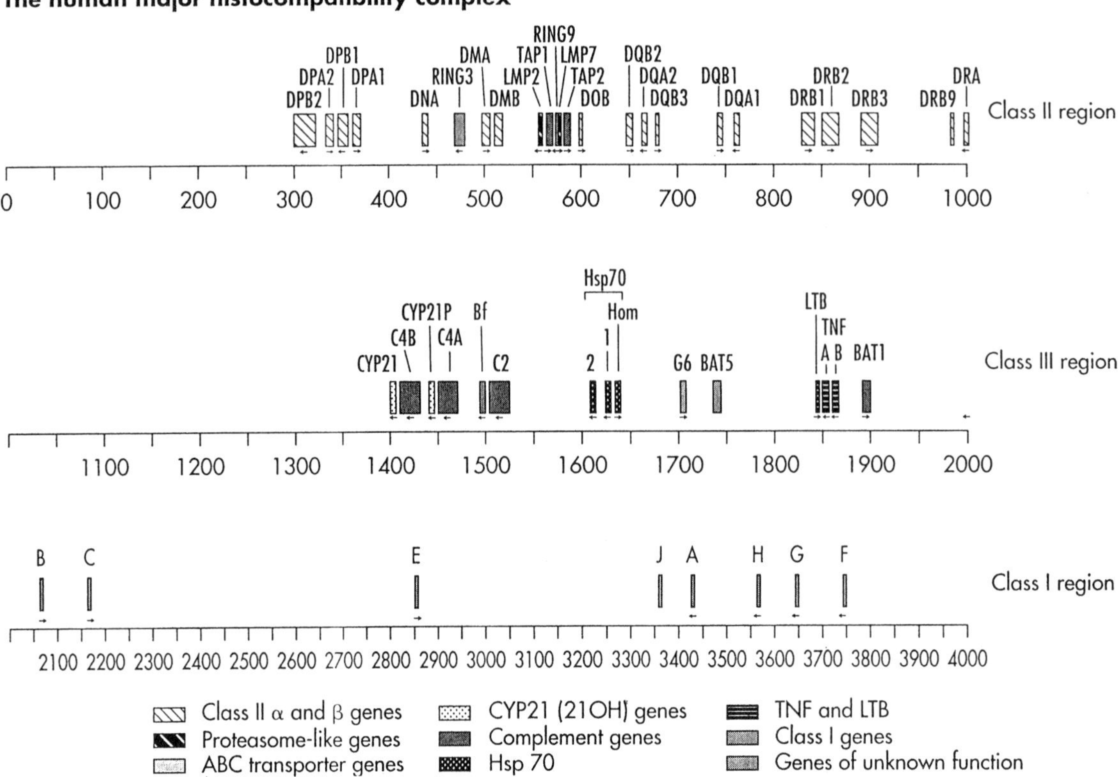

Figure 31-3 Map of the HLA complex. The three regions of the HLA complex, class II, class III, and class I, were named for the class of genes first mapped to each region. The numbers below the line denote kilobases of DNA within the 4000-kb HLA complex. This material was originally published in Immunology Today 1993;14:349–352. (Copyright Elsevier Science Ltd, from whom permission has been obtained. This adaptation of the figure is reproduced by permission from Rich RR, editor in chief. Clinical Immunology: Principles and Practice. St. Louis: Mosby, 1995.)

mediated cytotoxicity using alloantisera from multiparous women. Panels of sera were accumulated that detected many of the HLA-A, -B, -C, -DR, and -DQ polymorphisms subsequently characterized at the nucleotide and amino acid sequence levels. Other class II polymorphisms, including HLA-DP and those on DR molecules referred to as HLA-D, are detected by T cells in primary or secondary mixed lymphocyte reactions and are termed T cell-defined specificities. With the wide availability of molecular genetic methods, DNA typing for HLA alleles has been applied recently, especially for class II. Analysis of DNA using restriction fragment length polymorphism (RFLP) or, more recently, sequence-specific oligonucleotides permits identification of the specific alleles that an individual possesses at the locus of interest.

HLA-DISEASE ASSOCIATIONS

With the availability of serologic testing for HLA class I specificities in the early 1970s, investigators began to search for associations between specific HLA antigens and diseases. HLA-disease associations have been described for more than 100 diseases. The experimental approach in HLA-disease association studies is to compare the frequencies of HLA antigens (serologic or cellular typing) or alleles (DNA typing) in persons with the disease of interest and a control population without the disease. Because the frequencies of HLA antigens and alleles normally vary in different ethnic and racial groups, it is important that the disease and control groups be composed of individuals of the same ethnic and racial background. The relative risk or incidence is used to quantify the strength of the HLA-disease association or how many times more frequent the disease is in individuals positive for the HLA antigen than in individuals negative for the antigen. After determining the percentages of patients and controls with (P^+ and C^+, respectively) and without (P^- and C^-) the antigen or allele, the relative risk is calculated by the formula $(P^+ \times C^-) / (P^- \times C^+)$. The greater the relative risk above 1, the stronger the association between the HLA antigen or allele and the disease.

The first HLA-disease association described, that of B27 and ankylosing spondylitis (AS), remains the prototypical example because of the high relative risk (Table 31-2). B27 was present in 88% of American white patients with AS and in 8% of controls, resulting in a relative risk of 81. Among African-Americans, B27 occurred in 50% of AS patients and 2% of controls, with a relative risk of 49. B27 is also associated with Reiter's syndrome and reactive arthritis, other spondyloarthropathies.

Multiple diseases are associated with HLA class II antigens. The HLA class II associations with insulin-dependent diabetes mellitus (IDDM), multiple sclerosis, and pemphigus vulgaris will be briefly summarized (Table 31-2), and the association with rheumatoid arthritis will be reviewed in detail, as an example of how these data might begin to influence clinical practice. HLA-DR3 and 4 are individually associated with IDDM, and DR3, 4 heterozygotes have a relative risk (RR), 20, that is much higher than the sum of the relative risks for DR3 and 4 alone. The HLA allele most highly associated with IDDM is DQB1*0302 (also referred to as DQ3.2 in earlier literature), which is found in linkage with

Table 31-2
HLA-Disease Associations

Disease	*Associated HLA antigen*	*Patients, %*	*Controls, %*	*Relative risk*
Ankylosing spondylitis				
Whites	B27	88	8	81
African-Americans	B27	50	2	49
Insulin-dependent diabetes mellitus	DR3	69	27	6.1
	DR4	66	20	7.8
	DQB1*0302	59	12	11
Pemphigus vulgaris				
Ashkenazi Jews	DR4	97	30	25
Multiple sclerosis	DRB1*1501	63	30	3.9

HLA-DR4–positive haplotypes and appears to account for the DR4 association. Examination of the amino acid sequences of DQβ chains positively or negatively associated with IDDM led to the observation that negatively associated chains often have aspartic acid at position 57, whereas chains associated with IDDM, such as DQβ1*0302, have an amino acid other than aspartic acid (usually serine or alanine) at this position. Based on these data, it was proposed that DQβ aspartic acid 57 was protective for IDDM. However, others have argued that this hypothesis is not correct, because the DQB genes most highly associated with IDDM in some ethnic groups encode aspartic acid 57. Pemphigus vulgaris is strongly associated with DR4 in Ashkenazi Jews; DRB1*0402 was subsequently shown to account for the DR4 association. Multiple sclerosis is associated with the DRB1*1501-DQA1*0102-DQB1*0602 haplotype.

HLA ASSOCIATIONS WITH RHEUMATOID ARTHRITIS

In retrospect, the first evidence for an HLA association with rheumatoid arthritis (RA) was presented in 1969 by Astorga and Williams, who found that lymphocytes from 64% of RA patients did not activate each other in a mixed lymphocyte culture. However, it was not until 1976 that a definite HLA association with RA was established; 68% of white RA patients, but only 12% of controls (RR, 15.6), typed for the class II antigen, HLA-Dw4. As serologic reagents became available to detect HLA class II antigens, Stastny reported in 1978 that HLA-DRw4 (later referred to as DR4) was present in 70% of white RA patients, compared with 28% of controls (RR, 6.0).

By 1987, the list of HLA-D antigens associated with RA had expanded to include the DR4-associated T-cell-defined specificities Dw14 and Dw15, and DR1, in addition to DR4, Dw4. Notably, no association between RA and two other DR4-associated specificities, Dw10 or Dw13, was reported. In the mid-1980s, important progress was made in the understanding of the molecules that bear the DR4-associated class II antigens and in the isolation of cDNAs and genes encoding these molecules. The latter studies established that the β chains of the five DR4-associated HLA-D specificities defined at that time (Dw4, 10, 13, 14, and 15) were largely identical except for differences of 2–4 amino acids at positions 57, 67, 70, 71, 74, and 86 (Table 31-3). In the current nomenclature, these chains are referred to as DRβ1*0401, 0402, 0403, 0404, and 0405, respectively. Based on the amino acid sequences of the DRβ1 chains that are or are not associated with RA, Gregersen et al. proposed the shared epitope hypothesis in 1987 to explain how different class II molecules might predispose to the same disease. They proposed that amino acids at DRβ1 positions 67–74 in the different RA-associated chains form a group of related epitopes that confer the risk to RA. The DRβ1*1402 and 1001 chains, which were subsequently found to be associated with RA in some populations, also have similar sequences in this region. Although the shared epitope was originally discussed in terms of residues 67–74, in more recent times, most authors have focused their discussions on residues 70–74. This segment of sequence has subsequently been referred to by multiple names, including rheumatoid or RA epitope. The sequences of amino acids 70–74 of the RA epitope differ slightly at positions 70 or 71 in different molecules: QKRAA in DRβ1*0401; QRRAA in DRβ1*0404, 0405, 0101, and 1402; and RRRAA in DRB1*1001.

Table 31-3
RA-Associated and -Non-Associated DRβ1 Chains

DRβ1 chain	*Serologic specificity*	*T-cell-defined specificity*	*Amino acids*					*RA association*
			70	*71*	*72*	*73*	*74*	
0401	DR4	Dw4	Q	K	R	A	A	+
0404	DR4	Dw14	Q	R	R	A	A	+
0405	DR4	Dw15	Q	R	R	A	A	+
0101	DR1	Dw1	Q	R	R	A	A	+
1402	DR14	Dw16	Q	R	R	A	A	+
1001	DR10	—	R	R	R	A	A	+
0402	DR4	Dw10	D	E	R	A	A	–
0403	DR4	Dw13	Q	R	R	A	E	–

In general, the association of DRβ1 molecules bearing the rheumatoid epitope with RA has been found in most ethnic and racial groups analyzed (Table 31-4). HLA-DR4 is associated with RA in most white populations studied as a result of increased frequencies of DRB1*0401 and 0404 in patients. Notably, two other DR4-associated alleles, DRB1*0402 and 0403, are not associated with RA in any population studied. Four other alleles that encode the rheumatoid epitope, DRB1*0101, 1402, 1001, and 0405, another DR4-associated allele, are associated with RA in other ethnic and racial groups. The DRB1*0101 association was found in Basque, Israeli Jew, and Indian RA patients, whereas DRB1*1001 is associated with RA in Greeks, Spanish, Israeli Jews, and Basques. The DR4 association in Japanese, Chinese, New Zealand Polynesians, and Spanish is caused by increased frequencies of DRB1*0405, in contrast to the increased frequencies of DRB1*0401 and 0404 noted above. Among Yakima Indians in the United States, DRB1*1402 is the RA-associated allele. Arabs in Kuwait are

Table 31-4
HLA Associations with Rheumatoid Arthritis in Different Ethnic and Racial Groups

Ethnic/racial group	*Associated HLA antigen or allele*	*Patients, %*	*Controls, %*	*Relative risk*
British whites	DR4	68	17	10.4
Shared epitope		83	46	7.2
Norwegians	DR4	80	34	7.9
White Americans				
Nashville/Dallas	DR4	63	33	3.5
Seattle	DR4	63	32	3.7
Italians				
Genoa	DR4	44	10	6.9
Bologna	DR4	29	15	2.4
Black South Africans				
Sotho origin	DR4	56	9	12.4
Zulu origin	DR4	82	7	59.0
Western Cape	DR4	38	13	3.9
Durban	DR4	44	10	7.4
African-Americans				
St. Louis	DR4	46	14	5.1
Washington, DC	DR4	58	18	6.3
Israeli Jews	Shared epitope	56	13	8.6
Greeks	DR4	23	12	2.1
	DR10	7	0	12.7
Japanese	DR4	67	40	3.0
	DRB1*0405	38	16	3.2
Chinese	DR4	42	18	3.3
	DRB1*0405	25	9	3.4
Spanish	DR4	41	23	2.4
	DR10	13	4	3.8
New Zealand Polynesians	DR4	67	26	5.8
	DRB1*0405	37	5	11.0
Yakima Indians	DRB1*1402	83	60	3.3
Arabs (Kuwait)	DR3	34	2	23.6

notable for the absence of an association with the shared epitope; DR3 is associated with RA in this population.

Based on a provocative series of studies of white RA patients examined at the Mayo Clinic in Rochester, Minnesota, Weyand, et al. have called attention to the role of DRB1 alleles in determining disease severity, in addition to disease susceptibility. In their initial study, 81 patients with seropositive, erosive rheumatoid arthritis were stratified into three groups based on disease manifestations: those without or with rheumatoid nodules and those with extraarticular manifestations in addition to nodules. DR4 and the RA epitope were found at high frequencies in the three groups: nonnodular (78 and 93%), nodular (100 and 100%), and extra-articular (95 and 100%). They also noted a strong correlation of the HLA-DRB1 alleles possessed by the patients with their clinical manifestations. Half of the patients with extraarticular manifestations in addition to nodules (vasculitis, Felty's syndrome, rheumatoid lung disease, and neuropathy) were homozygous for DRB1*0401, suggesting that a double dose of this disease-associated allele may predispose to more severe disease. In contrast, in the patients with nodules but no major organ involvement, homozygosity for DRB1*0401 occurred in only 1 of the 36 patients. However, 56% of the latter group had two DRB1 alleles with the RA epitope, but only 11% of the nonnodular patients were homozygous for the RA epitope. These data suggested a hierarchy among RA-associated DRB1 alleles, with 0401 and 0404 being associated with more severe disease.

In another study from the Mayo Clinic of 102 patients with seropositive, erosive RA, 89% were positive for the RA-associated alleles DRB1*0401, 0404, or 0408, 96% possessed alleles with the RA epitope, and 46% were homozygous for the disease-associated epitope. One hundred percent of patients with two disease-associated DRB1*04 alleles had nodular disease, and 61% had additional extra-articular disease. In contrast, patients heterozygous for DRB1*04 and the RA epitope-containing DRB1*0101 or 1402 alleles and those heterozygous for a DRB1*04 allele and a non-RA-associated B1 allele had comparable frequencies of nodular disease (58 vs 59%) and little or no extraarticular disease (in addition to nodules). Based on these data, the authors suggested that genotyping for both DRB1 alleles may provide prognostic information that could be used to select patients for early aggressive therapy.

This approach has recently been extended to compare DRB1 alleles in white seropositive and seronegative RA patients. Seropositive patients were more likely to have DRB1*04 alleles and seronegative patients were more likely to have DRB1*0101. DRB1*04 alleles were present in 22% of controls, 91% of seropositive patients, and 42% of seronegative patients, whereas DRB1*01 alleles occurred in 27, 23, and 42%, and the RA epitope occurred in 41, 97, and 68%, respectively. Among the seronegative patients, DRB1*04 alleles were enriched in patients with early erosive disease and those requiring aggressive therapy, whereas patients without an RA-associated DRB1 allele had milder dis-

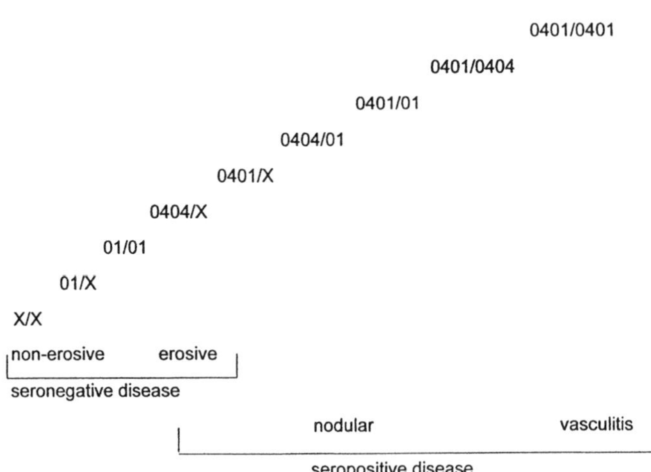

Figure 31-4 Proposed hierarchy of HLA-DRB1 alleles in determining disease severity in seronegative and seropositive RA. DRB1*0404 in this sheme represents the group of alleles including DRB1*0404, 0405, and 0408. (Reproduced by permission from The Journal of Clinical Investigation 1995;95:2120–2126 by copyright permission of The American Society for Clinical Investigation.)

ease, as judged by the frequent use of nonaggressive therapy and the presence of nonerosive or late erosive disease. The frequencies of the DRβ1 amino acid 70–74 sequence QKRAA encoded by DRB1*0401 and 0409 and the QRRAA sequence encoded by DRB1*0404, 0405, 0408, 0410, 0101, and 0102 were also compared. QKRAA occurred much more frequently in seropositive (65%) than seronegative (35%) patients, and 35% of the seropositives, but none of the seronegatives, expressed both QK and QR alleles. QRRAA alleles occurred at similar frequencies (57 vs 58%) in the two groups. Based on this series of studies, a hierarchy of DRB1 alleles and allelic combinations for determining disease severity in RA has been proposed (Fig. 31-4). In this scheme, DRB1*0401, which encodes lysine at position 71, has the strongest effect and is associated with the most severe disease, especially when present in the homozygous combination. DR4-associated alleles that encode arginine 71 (DRB1*0404 and 0405) have less potent effects, and DRB1*0101, which encodes the rheumatoid epitope in the context of a different sequence in the floor of the peptide-binding groove, is less potent than DRB1*0404 and 0405. Finally, the presence of two non-RA-associated alleles correlates with the mildest disease.

The possibility, based on studies in whites, that determining DRB1 alleles in patients with early RA may permit prediction of eventual disease severity and selection of patients for early aggressive therapy has stimulated a reassessment of the role of DRB1 alleles and the shared epitope in African-Americans with RA. Analysis of 86 African-American patients with RA from Alabama and southeast Texas found that most patients do not have the rheumatoid epitope; only 32% of the seropositive patients and 40% of the seronegative patients have the rheumatoid epitope. In addition, disease severity did not correlate with the presence of the RA epitope in these patients. The frequencies of DRB1 alleles were similar in the patients and controls, except for a modest increase of DRB1*04 alleles in seropositive (27%; RR, 2.5) and seronegative patients (25%; RR, 2.2), compared with 13% of controls. These investigators concluded that determination of DRB1 alleles in African-American RA patients cannot be used to predict disease severity, and they suggested that the products of other undefined non-HLA genes that may interact with RA-associated DRβ1 chains in whites may not be present in African-Americans. However, the absence of a significant DRB1 association in this study differs somewhat from other studies of black RA patients in the United States and Africa (Table 31-4). In earlier studies from St. Louis and Washington, DC, DR4 was present by serologic typing in 46 and 58%, respectively, of patients and 14 and 18% of controls. In studies of other black populations, DRB1*04 (29 vs 4%) and DRB1*1001 (19 vs 2%) were significantly increased in Shona patients with RA from Zimbabwe compared with controls. DRB1*04 was also associated with RA in black South Africans of Sotho and Zulu origin and patients in Durban and the Western Cape region.

Although the influence of DRB1 alleles on RA disease severity is clearly demonstrated in the studies of white Americans examined at the Mayo Clinic, the results have been variable in other studies. The presence of DR4 was associated with seropositivity and more severe radiographic changes, in a study of whites from Nashville. Among British patients with erosive, seropositive RA being treated with disease-modifying drugs, the frequency of DRB1*04 homozygotes was increased significantly. The relative risks for the DRB1*0401/0401, 0404/0404, and 0401/0404 allelic combinations were 15, 20, and 49, respectively. On the other hand, disease severity did not correlate with the presence of the RA epitope in other studies. In agreement with the study of African-Americans from Alabama and Texas, there was not an association between the presence of the RA epitope and disease severity among African-American RA patients in Atlanta.

POSSIBLE MECHANISMS UNDERLYING HLA-DISEASE ASSOCIATIONS

Although many HLA-disease associations have been described, the molecular basis for these associations remains undefined. Several hypotheses have been proposed to explain HLA-disease associations. The first hypothesis proposes that the disease-associated HLA molecule is a receptor for the etiologic agent, such as a virus or bacteria. In the second hypothesis, the peptide-binding groove of the disease-associated HLA molecule uniquely binds a peptide that is the cause of the disease. The third hypothesis suggests that a specific T-cell receptor, which corecognizes the complex of HLA molecule and peptide, is ultimately responsible for the disease. The fourth hypothesis proposes that the disease-associated HLA molecule is structurally similar to a microbial antigen and that the HLA antigen becomes a target for T cells in the course of the normal immune response to the microbe. This possible scenario has been termed the molecular mimicry hypothesis. The fifth hypothesis postulates that a gene in the HLA complex that encodes a protein involved in antigen processing, such as a TAP gene, is defective, resulting in lower expression levels of class I molecules or more molecules on the cell surface without peptides bound in their grooves (empty molecules). An alternative version of this hypothesis is that a normal TAP allele preferentially transports a disease causing peptide.

Recent studies strongly support the hypothesis that selective binding of peptides is the major mechanism underlying some HLA-disease associations. Hammer et al. have established that peptides with different characteristics bind to DR molecules containing the RA-associated DRβ1*0401 and 0404 chains and the nonassociated DRβ1*0402 chains. As noted in Table 31-3, within the shared

Table 31-5
Disease-Associated DRβ and DQβ Polymorphisms Determine Selective Binding of Self Peptides

Disease	*Disease-associated polymorphism*	*Self-peptide characteristics*
Rheumatoid arthritis	DRβ1*0401 71 Lys	P4 Asp or Glu
	DRβ1*0404 71 Arg	P4 Asp or Glu
Pemphigus vulgaris	DRβ1*0402 71 Glu	P4 Lys or Arg
	DQβ1*05032 57 Asp	P9 Lys or Arg
IDDM	DQβ1*0302 57 Ala	P9 Asp or Glu

epitope, DRβ1*0401 and 0404 chains both have glutamine at position 70 and a highly conservative lysine to arginine difference at position 71, whereas non-RA-associated DRβ1*0402 chains have aspartic acid at 70 and glutamic acid at 71. Using designer peptides in which positions P3 to P7 of the peptide were individually substituted with all natural amino acids (except cysteine), significant differences between DRβ1*0402 molecules and the two RA-associated molecules were observed in the effect of charged peptide residues on peptide binding. The most striking difference is that peptides with positively charged residues, lysine or arginine, at P4 or P6 bind 100 to 1000-fold better to DRβ1*0402 molecules than to DRβ1*0401 or 0404 molecules. Conversely, peptides with negative charges, aspartic acid or glutamic acid, at P4 or P5 bind 100 to 500-fold less well to DRβ1*0402 molecules than to DRβ1*0401, and ~50-fold less well to DRβ1*0404 molecules. A site-directed mutant molecule in which DRβ1*0401 lysine 71 was changed to glutamic acid exhibited a binding specificity similar to that of DRβ1*0402 molecules. Thus, the position 71 lysine to glutamic acid difference in DRβ1*0401 and DRβ1*0402 chains seems to account for most of the difference in peptide binding specificity between these RA-associated and nonassociated molecules. In other experiments, the position 71 lysine to arginine acid difference in DRβ1*0401 and DRβ1*0404 chains was also shown to account for minor differences in peptide binding between these molecules. In summary, residue 71 of the RA-associated DRβ1*0401 or 0404 chains determines that these molecules bind peptides in which P4 has a negative, but not a positive, charge (Table 31-5).

Based on these data on selective binding of peptides to RA-associated DR molecules and other related studies, a model has been proposed in which charge–charge interactions between specific disease-associated HLA polymorphic residues and specific residues of self peptides result in selective binding of self peptides by disease-associated molecules, the HLA-self peptide complexes become the targets of autoreactive T cells, and autoimmune disease develops. In addition to the data with RA-associated polymorphisms cited above, these authors have cited other examples in which DR or DQβ polymorphisms linked to pemphigus vulgaris (PV) or IDDM may determine selective binding of disease-associated self peptides (Table 31-5). In some ethnic groups, PV is associated with DRβ1*0402. The prediction is that the disease-associated DRβ1*0402 molecules, with a negatively charged glutamic acid at DRβ71, bind peptides with a positive charge at P4. Within the target antigen of PV, desmoglein 3 (an epithelial adhesion molecule), seven peptides were identified with the common anchor residues at P1 and P6 and lysine or arginine at P4. According to the model, one or more of these peptides may be involved in the autoimmune process in PV. In other ethnic groups, PV is associated with DQβ1*05032, which has aspartic acid at position 57 and is modeled to be located in pocket 9 of DQ molecules. In IDDM, many disease-associated DQβ chains, such as DQβ1*0302, do not have aspartic acid at position 57. Therefore, the model predicts that P9 of a pemphigus-associated peptide that binds to DQβ1*05032 molecules will have a positive charge. According to the model, the non-IDDM-associated DQ molecules with Asp 57 should bind peptides with a positively charged residue at P9. However, because many IDDM-associated DQβ chains have serine or alanine, residues that are not strongly charged, at position 57, it is more difficult to predict the characteristics of the P9 residue, but it may be negatively charged.

SELECTED REFERENCES

Astorga GP, Williams RC. Altered reactivity in mixed lymphocyte culture of lymphocytes from patients with rheumatoid arthritis. Arthritis Rheum 1969;12:547–554.

Bjorkman PJ, Parham, P. Structure, function, and diversity of class I major histocompatibility complex molecules. Annu Rev Biochem 1990;59:253–288.

Bjorkman PJ, Saper MA, Samraoui B, Bennett WS, Strominger JL, Wiley DC. Structure of the human class I histocompatibility antigen, HLA-A2. Nature 1987;32:506–512.

Bjorkman PJ, Saper MA, Samraoui B, Bennett WS, Strominger JL, Wiley DC. The foreign antigen binding site and T cell recognition regions of class I histocompatibility antigens. Nature 1987; 329:512–518.

Bodmer JG, Marsh GE, Albert ED, Bodmer WF, et al. Nomenclature for factors of the HLA system, 1995. Hum Immunol 1995;43: 149–164.

Bodmer JG, Marsh SGE, Albert ED, et al. Nomenclature for factors of the HLA system, 1991. Hum Immunol 1992;34:4–18.

Brown JH, Jardetzky TS, Gorga JC, et al. Three-dimensional structure of the human class II histocompatibility antigen HLA-DR1. Nature 1993;364:33–39.

Caillat-Zucman S, Garchon H-J, Timsit J, et al. Age-dependent HLA Genetic Heterogeneity of Type 1 insulin-dependent diabetes mellitus. J Clin Invest 1992;90:2242–2250.

Campbell RD, Trowsdale J. Map of the human MHC. Immunol Today 1993;14:349–352.

Fu X-T, Bono CP, Woulfe SL, et al. Pocket 4 of the HLA-DR(α,β1*0401) molecule is a major determinant of T cell recognition of peptide. J Exp Med 1995;181:915–926.

Garrett TPJ, Saper MA, Bjorkman PJ, Strominger JL, Wiley DC. Specificity pockets for the side chains of peptide antigens in HLA-Aw68. Nature 1989;342:692–696.

Ghosh P, Amaya M, Mellins E, Wiley DC. The structure of an intermediate in class II maturation: CLIP bound to HLA-DR3. Nature 1995;378:457–462.

Gregersen PK, Silver J, Winchester RJ. The shared epitope hypothesis. An approach to understanding the molecular genetics of susceptibility to rheumatoid arthritis. Arthritis Rheum 1987; 30:1205–1213.

Hammer J, Gallazzi F, Bono E, et al. Peptide binding specificity of HLA-DR4 molecules: Correlation with rheumatoid arthritis association. J Exp Med 1995;181:1847–1855.

Jardetzky T. Not just another Fab: the crystal structure of a TcR-MHC-peptide complex. Structure 1997;5:159–163.

Jonas BL, Gonzalez EB, Callahan L et al. The shared epitope is not associated with disease severity in an African-American population with rheumatoid arthritis. Arthritis Rheum 1995;38:S193.

Madden DR, Gorga JC, Strominger JL, Wiley DC. The structure of HLA-B27 reveals nonamer self-peptides bound in an extended conformation. Nature 1991;353:321–325.

McDaniel DO, Alarcon GS, Pratt PW, Reveille JD. Most African-American patients with rheumatoid arthritis do not have the rheumatoid antigenic determinant (epitope). Ann Intern Med 1995;123:181–187.

Nepom GT. Immunogenetics and IDDM. Diabetes Rev 1993;1:93–103.

Olsen NJ, Callahan LF, Brooks RM et al. Associations of HLA-DR4 with rheumatoid factor and radiographic severity in rheumatoid arthritis. Am J Med 1988;84:257–264.

Rammensee H-G, Friede T, Stevanovic S. MHC ligands and peptide motifs: first listing. Immunogenetics 1995;41:178–228.

Schlosstein L, Terasaki PI, Bluestone R, Pearson CM. High association of an HL-A antigen, W27, with ankylosing spondylitis. N Engl J Med 1973;288:704–706.

Schwartz BD. Infectious agents, immunity, and rheumatic diseases. Arthritis Rheum 1990;33:457–465.

Stastny P. Mixed lymphocyte cultures in rheumatoid arthritis. J Clin Invest 1976;57:1148–1157.

Stastny P. Association of the B-cell alloantigen DRw4 with rheumatoid arthritis. N Engl J Med 1978;298:869–871.

Stern LJ, Brown JH, Jardetzky TS, et al. Crystal structure of the human class II MHC protein HLA-DR1 complexed with an influenza virus peptide. Nature 1994;368:215–221.

Tiwara JL, Terasaki PI. HLA and Disease Associations. New York: Springer-Verlag;1985.

Todd JA, Bell JI, McDevitt HO. HLA-DQβ gene contributes to susceptibility and resistance to insulin-dependent diabetes mellitus. Nature 1987;329:599–604.

Weyand CM, Hicok KC, Conn DL, Goronzy JJ. The influence of HLA-DRB1 genes on disease severity in rheumatoid arthritis. Ann Intern Med 1992;117:801–806.

Weyand CM, McCarthy TG, Goronzy JJ. Correlation between disease phenotype and genetic heterogeneity in rheumatoid arthritis. J Clin Invest 1995;95:2120–2126.

Weyand CM, Xie C, Goronzy JJ. Homozygosity for the HLA-DRB1 allele selects for extraarticular manifestations in rheumatoid arthritis. J Clin Invest 1992;89:2033–2039.

Wordsworth P, Pile KD, Buckely JD, et al. HLA heterozygosity contributes to susceptibility to rheumatoid arthritis. Am J Hum Genet 1992;51:585–591.

Wucherpfenning KW, Strominger JL. Selective binding of self peptides to disease-associated major histocompatibility complex (MHC) molecules: a mechanism for MHC-linked susceptibility to human autoimmune diseases. J Exp Med 1995;181:1597–1601.

32 Inherited Immune Deficiency

Richard Hong

INTRODUCTION

The immune system provides protection from infectious agents, using two major lymphocyte subsets, known as T cells and B cells. The immune system can respond specifically to millions of different stimuli (epitopes) by virtue of the vast clonal repertoire created by the processes described in other chapters of this volume (Chapters 28 and 29). Because the numerous complicated and varied steps that lead to a competent immune system provide many sites that can be affected by genetic disease, the potential causes of primary immunodeficiency are legion. Granulocytes, although an important member of the host defense system, are not components of the immune system. Therefore, granulocyte disorders are considered elsewhere, in the section on Molecular Hematology.

To place the many events into a framework that highlights the unique developmental aspects of the host defense system, I will divide the processes of an immune response into three phases. First, multipotential stem cells, which give rise to hematopoietic cells as well as lymphocytes, generate cells destined to become mature T and B lymphocytes. Second, an immense repertoire is created through a complex set of differentiation steps. Finally, antigen engagement initiates effector functions (e.g., recruitment of other cells and secretion of molecules) that result in containment or death of infectious agents. Tables 32-1 and 32-2 summarize, respectively, events in T- or B-cell biology necessary to yield a competent immune response. Because of space considerations, only diseases for which the biochemical basis is known are described in this chapter and are tabulated in Tables 32-3 (T cell) and 32-4 (B cell). For further discussion of immune deficiency in general, the reader should refer to other standard texts. Secondary immunodeficiency states, i.e., those secondary to another disorder such as cancer, will not be included, except for acquired immunodeficiency syndrome (AIDS), secondary to infection with human immunodeficiency syndrome (HIV), which is considered in Chapter 33.

SYMPTOMS OF IMMUNE DEFICIENCY

Regardless of the specific cause of the defect, the clinical presentations are similar for the various diseases. The manifestations depend upon the degree of incompetence of the T cells or B cells, or whether combined T- and B-cell disorders coexist. Unique symptoms, associated with specific diseases, will be described in the relevant sections.

The major symptoms of immune deficiency are increased susceptibility to infection. Because the T and B cells are effective against different groups of agents, defects in either system produce different patterns of susceptibility. Antibodies protect against infections from extracellular pyogenic bacteria, whereas T cells prevent viral, fungal, tuberculous, and opportunistic infections, such as *Pneumocystis carinii* pneumonia.

Patients with immune deficiency are susceptible to agents that are nonpathogenic for those with intact host defense systems, and also will experience unusually severe and sometimes fatal manifestations of infections caused by ordinarily benign bacteria or viruses. Thus, in immunodeficiency states, cytomegalovirus causes retinitis and severe pneumonia, atypical mycobacteria or parasites can cause severe protracted diarrhea, and measles is a fatal disease. Overwhelming pneumonia is a particularly virulent and often fatal complication of varicella, rubeola, or parainfluenza.

LABORATORY ASSESSMENT

QUANTITATIVE TESTS Tests of the immune status can be either quantitative or qualitative. If an element of the immune system, e.g., lymphocyte subset or immunoglobulin (Ig) level, is completely absent, obviously no immune function is possible, but this degree of deficiency is usually not seen. An absolute lymphocyte count of less than 1200/mm^3 is abnormal. T and B cells are enumerated most conveniently by the technique of flow cytometry, using a panel of antibodies that identify surface markers characteristic of each of the lymphocyte subsets (Table 32-5). In addition, the absence of certain markers are diagnostic of some diseases, e.g., CD43 in Wiskott-Aldrich syndrome. Serum immunoglobulin levels provide a quantitative measure of B-cell secretion. However, immunoglobulin levels should be compared with age-adjusted normal ranges because serum values increase with age. The Ig levels in patients with clinically significant B-cell disease hardly ever overlap with normal ranges. Therefore, 95% confidence limits are not useful in differentiating between deficient and normal immunoglobulin values. In the presence of low levels of lymphocytes or Igs, a functional or qualitative test is the only reliable assessment to decide whether the patient is at risk.

QUALITATIVE (FUNCTIONAL) TESTS T-cell function can be assessed by measuring in vitro proliferative responses to various stimuli. Three types of stimuli are used: mitogens, allogeneic cells, and antigens. Mitogen-induced proliferation implies the

From: *Principles of Molecular Medicine* (J. L. Jameson, ed.), ©1998 Humana Press Inc., Totowa, NJ.

Table 32-1
Events in T-Cell Immune Response

Stem-cell generation	*Repertoire generation*	*Effector function*
Lineage commitment	Lineage commitment Gene rearrangement Thymic differentiation Thymic selection (+ or –) Extrathymic differentiation Signal transduction Cytokine secretion and response	MHC-presented antigen recognized by T-cell receptor Homing Signal transduction Cytokine secretion and response Target lysis Macrophage recruitment

Table 32-2
Events in B-Cell Immune Response

Stem-cell generation	*Repertoire generation*	*Effector function*
Lineage commitment	Gene rearrangement Isotype switching Signal transduction Cytokine secretion and response	Antigen recognition Immunoglobulin secretion Complement activation Signal transduction Cytokine secretion and response

Table 32-3
T-Cell and Combined T- and B-Cell Disorders

Process at fault	*Defect*	*Disease [OMIM]*[a]
Generation of stem cell	Recombinase failure to date seen only in mice	Severe combined immunodeficiency (SCID);
Development of thymus gland	Faulty facial neural crest tissue development; related to chromosome 22 deletion	DiGeorge anomaly [*188400]
Cytokine or cytokine response	γ Chain of IL-2 receptor mutated	SCID (X-linked)[*312863]
	Defects in multiple cytokines; IL-2 synthesis and response, IL-1	Various forms of SCID[*147680]
MHC antigen expression	Faulty transactivators, promoters, DNA-binding stabilizers, transporters	Barc lymphocyte syndrome [#209920,*600006,*1720261]
Expression of surface protein CD43	Defect in WASP (Wiskott-Aldrich syndrome protein)	Wiskott-Aldrich syndrome [*30100]
Expression of T-cell receptor complex	CD3 ζ chain defect	SCID caused by TCR defect [*186780]
Maintenance of adequate numbers of lymphocytes	Mutation of ADA gene	Adenosine deaminase deficiency [*102700]
	Mutation of PNP gene	Nucleoside phosphorylase deficiency [*164050]
Defective signal transduction	ZAP-70	SCID caused by ZAP-70 defect [#600802,*176947]
	Jak3	Autosomal form of SCID [#600802,*600173]
	Mutation of ATM gene; product homologous to PI–3 kinases	Ataxia–telangiectasia [*208900]

[a]OMIM from Online Mendelian Inheritance in Man, OMIM (TM). Center for Medical Genetics, Johns Hopkins University, Baltimore, MD, and National Center for Biological Information, National Library of Medicine, Bethesda, MD, 1995.

Table 32-4
B-Cell Disorders

Process at fault	*Defect*	*Disease [OMIM]*[a]
Development of B-cell lineage	Bruton tyrosine kinase	X-linked agammaglobulinemia (Bruton's disease) [*300300,*186973]
Isotype switching	CD40 ligand	X-linked hyper-IgM [*308230]
Isotype switching	CD40 transduction	X-linked hyper-IgM

[a]OMIM from Online Mendelian Inheritance in Man, OMIM (TM). Center for Medical Genetics, Johns Hopkins University, Baltimore, MD, and National Center for Biological Information, National Library of Medicine, Bethesda, MD, 1995.

Table 32-5
Surface Markers

Marker	*Comment*
T-cell series	
CD 1a, b, c	Cortical thymocytes
CD2	T cells, natural killer (NK) cells, LFA–3 receptor
CD3	Part of the T-cell receptor complex; a pan-T-cell marker
CD4	T cells reactive with class II HLA-presented antigen (helper T cell)
CD5	Pan-T-cell marker; present on a B-cell subset
CD8	T cell reactive with class I HLA-presented antigen (killer T cell)
CD28	T-cell subset, activated B cell, thymocytes, site of second signal stimulus
CD43	Leukocytes except B cells (leukosialin); deficient in Wiskott-Aldrich syndrome
CD45RA	Naive T cell (has not reacted with antigen); recent emigrant from thymus
CD45RO	Memory T cell
CD56	Natural killer cell
B-cell series	
CD10	Common acute lymphatic leukemia antigen (CALLA)
CD19	Pan-B-cell marker
CD20	Pan-B-cell marker
CD21	Epstein-Barr virus receptor
CD23	Activated B cells, macrophages, eosinophils, platelets; the low affinity $Fc_{\varepsilon}RII$
Myeloid series	
CD14	Monocytes, granulocytes, Langerhans' cells, macrophages
CD16	NK cells, granulocytes, macrophages; the $Fc_{\gamma}RIIIA$, $Fc_{\gamma}RIIIB$ receptor
CD34	Hematopoietic precursor cells, endothelial cells
CD35	Granulocytes, monocytes, NK, B cells; the CR1/C3b receptor
Other	
CD 11a, b, c	LFA–1 integrin chains; adhesion molecule on leukocytes
CD62E, L, P	Selectin adhesion molecules on endothelial cells, leukocytes, platelets
CD69	Early activation marker of T cells

presence of T cells with surface receptors characteristic of T cells; allogeneic cells stimulate on the basis of transplantation-antigen differences. Of the three stimuli, antigens are the most informative, and a positive response provides the best correlate of the ability of the patient to resist infection. However, antigen response occurs only after sufficient exposure to the agent and, therefore, may not be elicited in young children during the first year of life. A delayed hypersensitivity skin test in which the antigen is injected intradermally and localized swelling of the puncture site measured 48 h later is a classic test of T-cell responses; it can be considered an in vivo correlate of the in vitro antigen-induced proliferation response. Other tests of T-cell capability involve the release of cytokines and the lysis of target cells (T-killer-cell assay). The functional capability of B cells is tested by measuring the specific antibody response to ubiquitous or vaccine antigens.

CARRIER STATE AND PRENATAL DIAGNOSIS Once the gene has been cloned, the availability of specific molecular DNA probes allows definition of the specific cause of the deficiency and also can be used for prenatal diagnoses. When the molecular basis has not been defined at the gene level, a diagnosis of the carrier or disease state can be made if an informative probe (i.e., near the chromosome lesion) is available and used in conjunction with restriction fragment length polymorphism (RFLP) analysis (*see* Chapter 4). When the restriction fragments are electrophoresed, then probed, two bands will be seen, one corresponding to each parentally inherited chromosome. In an X-linked disease, an identical size fragment will be found in the heterozygote mother and her affected male child, because both carry the disease-associated chromosome. Family analysis may reveal that the carrier mother inherited the disease-associated chromosome from her mother. Healthy boys will show the chromosome band of the healthy maternal allele. RFLP analysis has been most informative for X-linked diseases because of the larger numbers of probes available and the greater knowledge of the approximate gene location as compared with autosomal chromosomes.

A carrier status can be defined in females, based upon nonrandom inactivation of the X chromosome by carriers in cell lines affected by the disease. If one prepares DNA from carrier lymphocytes and granulocytes (or fibroblasts), it will be seen that T or B lymphocytes will show only one restriction digest band, whereas nonlymphocyte populations will show two bands. If the disease affects both T and B cells, all lymphocytes will show only the pattern of the healthy allele; if the disease is restricted to B cells, e.g., hypogammaglobulinemia, T lymphocytes will show two bands and B lymphocytes will show the single pattern of the healthy allele. Apparently, cell lines using the disease-carrying X chromosome in healthy heterozygotes suffer a growth disadvantage and, with time, the population is converted entirely or nearly so, to lymphocytes that use the healthy X chromosome. Thus, RFLP analysis of cell lines of a putative obligate heterozygote will confirm the carrier state and the X-linked inheritance pattern, and define the cell lines affected by the disorder. Carrier detection studies have shown that in lethal X-linked diseases, a third to a half of the patients are affected by a new mutation, thus giving a negative family history. At the present time, informative probes are available for investigation of Wiskott-Aldrich syndrome, X-linked severe combined immunodeficiency disease, X-linked proliferative syndrome, and X-linked agammaglobulinemia.

As will be described later, the genes for Wiskott-Aldrich syndrome, ataxia telangiectasia, X-linked hyperimmunoglobulin M, X-linked agammaglobulinemia, and autosomal and X-linked severe combined immunodeficiency have been cloned. Thus, these disorders may be analyzed precisely at the DNA level.

Prenatal diagnosis is accomplished by biochemical testing of cultured amniotic fibroblasts (enzyme deficiency) or molecular analysis of chorionic villus biopsies.

THERAPY

INTRAVENOUS GAMMA-GLOBULIN For isolated B-cell deficiency, γ-globulin, prepared from Cohn Fraction II, provides excellent replacement therapy. Intramuscular preparations, used extensively in the past, have now been replaced by intravenous products, which provide much higher body stores and serum levels. Intravenous γ-globulin (IVIG) will not provide significant amounts of IgA or IgM. Paradoxically, it may contain a sufficient amount of IgA to sensitize patients with isolated IgA deficiency, endangering them for anaphylaxis as a result of anti-IgA antibodies in the future. Therefore, IVIG therapy for selective IgA deficiency is not recommended.

Some preparations of IVIG have been associated with transmission of hepatitis C. Patients on IVIG therapy should be monitored for occult liver disease by periodic transaminase studies. Transmission of HIV has not been reported and seems unlikely because the virus is being eliminated by the methods of preparation of the product.

BONE MARROW TRANSPLANTATION Because the defects of immune deficiency disorders are caused by faulty cell lines, replacement by means of bone marrow transplants will cure the disease. Transplantation in patients with sufficiently profound T-cell disease will not require ablation, so the morbidity associated with radiation or chemotherapy can be avoided. Also, for reasons not entirely clear, patients with immune deficiency (with the notable exception of Wiskott-Aldrich syndrome) tend to have little or no graft-vs-host disease. In general, if the recipient is in reasonable health and does not have a serious infection at the time of transplant, his clinical course is much less complicated than that seen in the usual bone marrow transplant recipient suffering from hematologic malignancy.

The donor may be a matched sibling, a haploidentical family member (usually a parent), or a matched unrelated individual. Results are in general better with a matched sibling donor, but nearly equal results are seen with alternative donors.

It is not necessary to know the defect precisely because the transplanted cells will replace all of the cell lines in patients receiving ablation therapy or, when ablation is not used, the transplanted healthy cell lines will manifest a growth advantage over the diseased lines of the recipient. Overall, success rates with permanent cure of the disease range from 25 to 75% when the recipient is in good health at the time of transplant for both matched and mismatched transplants.

GENE THERAPY Because bone marrow transplantation is essentially stem cell replacement therapy, immunodeficiency patients are ideal candidates for gene therapy. The outcome depends on successful transfection of the stem cells with the appropriate gene, resulting in normalized stem cells that then mature into competent T and B lymphocytes. At present, a major stumbling block is the technology for transfection, which is quite inefficient. This, combined with the low frequency of stem cells in the bone marrow, makes the total number of successfully transduced cells quite small. Other problems depend on the level of gene expression obtained and the complexity of the gene product, i.e., single versus multiple polypeptide chain structures.

Adenosine deaminase deficiency, a major cause of autosomally transmitted combined immunodeficiency, is ideally suited for gene therapy. The enzyme is a single polypeptide chain that is constitutively produced, and close regulation of cell levels is not required. An injectable form of adensosine deaminase can be used to support the patient while undergoing gene correction. An encouraging response has been obtained recently. The details are described more fully later.

COMBINED T- AND B-CELL DISEASES

X-LINKED SEVERE COMBINED IMMUNODEFICIENCY The term combined immunodeficiency refers to involvement of both T and B lymphocytes; severe was used in the original descriptions because most children had a severe clinical disease with death occurring within the first 2 years of life. However, with more sensitive diagnostic tests and with improved treatment, the arbitrary 2-year limit on lifespan in untreated patients is no longer valid. The term "severe" is of little descriptive value today.

The genetic fault in X-linked severe combined immunodeficiency (SCID) involves the γ_c chain of the interleukin-2 (IL-2) receptor. IL-2 is a cytokine that is necessary for the antigen-induced proliferative response. Impairment of the IL-2 response would cripple the immune system, but does not readily explain the magnitude of the immune system deficit seen in this disease. Indeed, mice lacking the IL-2 gene show only mild disease and no infectious susceptibility at all. The explanation for the global effects of IL-2R γ_c chain deficiency was shown by Kondo et al., Noguchi et al., Russell et al. The receptors for IL-4, IL-7, IL-9, and IL-2 all share the same γ_c chain, and thus, deficiency involving multiple cytokines is present. These cytokines affect T- and B-cell development and differentiation as well as mast cell enhancement (IL-9), thus accounting for the multicellular nature of the defect. The transduction of these receptor signals involves the tyrosine phosphorylation of multiple cellular substrates, including the Janus family kinases Jak1 and Jak3; the γ_c chain associates with Jak3. Hence, it is not surprising that mutations in Jak3 have now been shown to result in an autosomally transmitted SCID phenotype.

Most patients present during the first year of life with a history of excessive numbers of severe, often life-threatening infections, cutaneous or oral candidiasis not responding to local therapy, or opportunistic infections. Bone marrow transplantation is curative.

BARE LYMPHOCYTE SYNDROME Transplantation antigens, which determine the acceptance or rejection of tissue transplants between individuals, are controlled by genes on chromosome 6 that form the major histocompatibility complex (MHC). In actuality, this highly polymorphic system is related to transplantation only because humans transplant tissues or organs.

The actual biologic role of the MHC products is to present antigen to T cells. The class I MHC antigens, expressed on virtually all nucleated cells and denoted human leukocyte antigens (HLA) -A, -B, and -C, present antigens digested in the cytosol to CD^{8+} cytolytic T cells, forming an important mechanism of viral control. The Class II MHC antigens (HLA-DP, -DQ, and -DR), are expressed constitutively by phagocytes and B cells; cytokines such as interferon-γ (IFN-γ) may induce class II MHC expression on other cells. Antigens that are phagocytosed or organisms that multiply in intracellular vesicles are protected from cytosolic degradation, but digested by the acidic lysosomal enzymes and incorporated into class II molecules for antigen presentation to CD^{4+} helper T cells. Patients may manifest deficiency of class I MHC products only, class II MHC products only, or both classes.

Of the two types, the MHC class II deficiencies have been the most extensively studied and are caused by a heterogeneous array of abnormalities in autosomal recessive genes that regulate MHC expression. Complementation studies suggested four complementation groups; however, most defects described to date are of two varieties. *Trans*-acting genes, not linked to the MHC, control the transcription of MHC class II structural genes. A class II transactivator splicing mutant has been found. Other genes initiate gene transcription by means of proteins that bind to *cis*-active promoter elements (X and Y boxes). Reith et al. found a defect in one such DNA-binding protein, RF-X; defects in accessory proteins that stabilize or enhance DNA binding have been described. Class I MHC deficiency can be caused by a defect of a transporter protein (TAP) necessary for peptide incorporation into the MHC cleft. Without an associated peptide, the MHC molecules are not expressed on the cell surface. The lack of MHC antigen expression is usually complete, but a few patients may express low levels, which in some cases can be upregulated by cytokines, such as interferon, or Epstein-Barr virus infection.

The lack of MHC antigens results in the inability to present peptide to T cells, thus subverting an immune response. In addition, thymic selection, which is controlled in large part by MHC expression, is affected, so that the bare lymphocyte syndrome is also manifested by inappropriate thymopoiesis with mature T-cell subset deficiencies. For example, in class II MHC deficiency, there is often a lack of CD^{4+} T cells.

Symptoms of excessive and overwhelming infections usually begin in the first year of life, and without therapy, death is the usual outcome by 4 years of age. Bone marrow transplantation is curative. Because the patients cannot be typed for transplantation by the usual methods, newer techniques of MHC typing by DNA are required for matching.

WISKOTT-ALDRICH SYNDROME Wiskott-Aldrich syndrome (WAS) is characterized by thrombocytopenia with small platelets, frequent infections, eczema, and a high incidence of malignancy. It is inherited as an X-linked defect. Characteristic immunologic abnormalities include inability to respond to polysaccharides and a characteristic immunoglobulin pattern of low IgM and high IgA. Lymphocyte counts and functional analysis may be fairly normal at first, but diminish with time.

The first abnormality noted in WAS lymphocytes was a defective expression of CD43 (sialophorin). However, the X-linked inheritance pattern could not be reconciled with the location of the CD43 gene on chromosome 16. Recently, the WAS gene was cloned, and the product, the Wiskott-Aldrich syndrome protein (WASP) was shown to be a 501-amino acid proline-rich structure. How it is related to CD43 is as yet unknown, but WASP may play a central role in formation of cell surface microvilli, which play an important role in antigen responses evoked by large inflexible molecules such as polysaccharides. Characteristically, patients with WAS do not make polysaccharide antibodies.

The bleeding manifestations caused by the thrombocytopenia are usually the first clinical symptoms. The onset of infections may be delayed for some years. The patients are unusually susceptible to herpetic infections. Malignancy may occur in as many as 15% of the untreated patients.

Bone marrow transplantation is curative. Use of T-cell depleted marrows when a matched sibling donor is unavailable has met with variable results, often with less success than other immunodeficiency diseases treated by other than HLA matched donors. The less than salutary results are because of the high incidence of B-cell lymphomas and severe graft versus host disease. B-cell lymphomas may respond to monoclonal antibodies or cellular infusions, however.

PURINE ENZYME (ADENOSINE DEAMINASE, PURINE NUCLEOSIDE PHOSPHORYLASE) DEFICIENCY Two enzymes of purine metabolism, adenosine deaminase (ADA, located on chromosome 2) and purine nucleoside phosphorylase (PNP, located on chromosome 14), are associated with immune deficiency. ADA deficiency accounts for 40% of autosomal recessively inherited combined immunodeficiency. PNP deficiency is much rarer (4%) and usually involves only the T-cell system, with relative sparing of the B cells.

Adenosine deaminase and purine nucleoside phosphorylase are enzymes of the purine salvage pathway, which recycle purines resulting from cell breakdown for re-use in synthesis of new DNA required for cell proliferation. ADA deaminates adenosine to yield inosine, which is then converted to hypoxanthine by PNP. In the absence of either enzyme, toxic metabolites accumulate. ADA absence leads to high levels of deoxyadenosine, which, in the presence of the high levels of deoxycytidine kinase in lymphocytes, becomes phosphorylated to deoxyadenosine triphosphate. The excessive amounts of deoxyATP interfere with ribonucleotide reductase, an enzyme essential for synthesis of DNA precursors. In PNP deficiency, deoxyguanosine triphosphate accumulates with similar consequences. The reason for sparing of the B cells in PNP deficiency is at present unknown. In addition to the accumulation of deoxyATP and deoxyGTP, inactivation of *S*-adenosyl homocysteine hydrolase occurs, leading to inhibition of methylation, which has further toxic effects. Although ADA and PNP are present in all cells, clinically evident pathology involves only a few tissues, probably because of differing susceptibility of various tissues to the toxic metabolites. In addition to the lymphocytes, lesions involving the growing ends of bones and neurologic disturbances are apparent clinically. However, at autopsy, renal and adrenal lesions have also been found.

In symptomatic patients, the defect in ADA must be nearly complete because only 1–5% of normal amounts is necessary for competent immunity. Patients with ADA deficiency have been divided into four groups, in order of increasing serum levels of ADA. Group 1 (ADA-SCID) shows the usual symptomatology of early life-threatening infections and severe lymphopenia. Groups 2 and 3 show delayed onset, and autoimmune diseases are a prominent feature. Group 4, designated partial ADA deficiency, has normal immunity and the defect is discovered only incidentally. Asymptomatic PNP-deficient patients have not been described as yet. A high incidence of neurologic disorders are found, including mental retardation and developmental delay. Autoimmune disease is common.

Most mutations of ADA are missense; only two PNP mutants have been studied. One was a missense and the other a frameshift mutant.

A number of treatments are available for ADA deficiency. Bone marrow transplantation is curative. In milder deficiency states, benefit from a polyethylene glycol-modified preparation of bovine ADA, PEG-ADA, has been observed.

Patients with ADA deficiency are ideal candidates for gene therapy. ADA has a single polypeptide chain and overexpression should not present a problem. At first, two children were treated with their own T cells that had been transfected with the ADA gene. After seven monthly infusions, totaling 7×10^{10} cells, the first patient showed persistent ADA activity in her peripheral T cells to levels 25% of normal. Improvement in many immune function tests and clinical well-being have persisted for at least 6 months after the last infusion. Results in the second patient are less dramatic, but both children participate fully in school and social activities and tolerated the infusions without incident.

These encouraging results led to the treatment, by insertion of the ADA gene in the cord blood stem cells, of three neonates in whom the diagnosis of ADA deficiency had been made prenatally. Transfected umbilical cord stem cells were reinfused into the infants without cytoablation and have persisted for 18 months. PEG-ADA, given at first to support the patients while the transfected cells were engrafting, has been dropped to 50% of normal treatment doses. With the decrease in PEG-ADA, although the total numbers of lymphocytes has decreased, the numbers of vector-containing lymphocytes has increased, demonstrating that transduced ADA-producing cells can expand in response to the demand for more immunocompetent cells.

ATAXIA-TELANGIECTASIA Ataxia-telangiectasia (AT) is an autosomal recessively inherited immunodeficiency disorder with an extremely diverse clinical phenotype characterized by ataxia, conjunctival telangiectasia, combined immunodeficiency, predisposition to lymphoreticular malignancies, and sensitivity to ionizing radiation. Studies at the cellular level suggest checkpoint defects at the G1 and G2 phases of the cell cycle, reduced life-span, and higher growth factor requirements.

The cloning of the AT gene provides insight into a number of biochemical mysteries and helps to explain the multitude of clinical manifestations of AT. The gene, located on the long arm of chromosome 11 (region q22–23) has been named ATM (AT, mutated) and bears strong homology to phosphatidylinositol-3' (PI-3) kinases, enzymes important in signal transduction, meiotic recombination, and cell cycle control. The demonstration of a PI-3 kinase role in maintaining brain growth factors may explain the Purkinge cell loss in the cerebellum, a hallmark of AT. Similar pivotal roles of PI-3 kinases probably account for defective cellular responses to insulin and immunologic deficiency.

A role for ATM in DNA damage repair has particularly profound implications. Not only does it explain the sensitivity of AT patients' cells to radiation, but it may define a group of women who possess a single copy of the mutant and are at increased risk for breast cancer, as suggested by previous epidemiologic studies. In such patients routine diagnostic X-rays and mammograms may be contraindicated.

T-CELL DISEASES

DIGEORGE ANOMALY The DiGeorge anomaly (DGA) is characterized by facial abnormalities (hypognathia, hypertelorism, downward slope of the lateral aspects of the eyes, defective ear pinnae), hypoparathyroidism, conotruncal heart abnormalities, and T-cell deficiency. Other organ involvement, namely brain, gastrointestinal, thyroid, eye, and renal have been described.

The pathogenesis of DGA is understood in developmental terms, but the mechanistic correlation with the observed chromosome 22 defect has not been elucidated. A failure of incorporation of the facial neural crest tissue into branchial arch derivatives is at the heart of the symptom complex, and explains the symmetrical character of the lesions. Facial neural crest tissue is injured by the multitude of causations that have been incriminated in DGA. These include first-trimester infections, alcohol exposure, retinoic acid, and maternal diabetes.

Usually, the DiGeorge anomaly occurs sporadically. However, familial cases have been described with various modes of transmission. Parents may have asymptomatic mild versions of the anomaly and only on careful questioning or examination will the subtle manifestations be revealed. A deletion of chromosome 22q11 was found in 33 of 35 DGA patients when sufficiently sensitive methodology was employed and, thus, most likely represents the genetic basis for the disorder.

Diagnosis should be considered in all cases of neonatal hypocalcemia or conotruncal heart defects. The facies, particularly hypognathia and defective ear pinnae formation are other highly suggestive signs. T-cell lymphopenia is common, but immunodeficiency requiring therapy is necessary only in about 25% of the cases; in the remainder, spontaneous correction is seen. Phytohemagglutinin responses less than 10% of the lowest acceptable normal value or CD^{4+} lymphocytes less than 300/mm^3 define patients in whom spontaneous remission of immune deficiency is extremely unlikely; they should be considered for transplantation. Hypoparathyroidism is associated with parathormone deficiency. This problem may spontaneously improve with time or disappear completely. The chromosome 22 deletion is readily demonstrated by fluorescence *in situ* hybridization.

Symptoms of T-cell deficiency occur, but the clinical course is mostly punctuated by the serious heart disease and hypocalcemia.

Thymus transplantation is curative. Bone marrow transplantation from a matched sibling donor has been successfully accomplished twice. T-cell-depleted haploidentical transplants from the parents will not succeed because the T-cell defect is caused by absence of the thymus and bone marrow stem cells cannot be differentiated. The hypoparathyroidism is controlled by vitamin D and calcium. The heart defects usually require corrective surgery that are well-tolerated despite the defects in the immune system.

ZAP-70 DEFICIENCY Most instances of T-cell deficiency are associated with lymphopenia involving both major subsets, CD^{4+} and CD^{8+} T cells. In an unusual variety marked by a normal to slightly elevated lymphocyte count, CD^{8+} T cells are virtually absent. The CD^{4+} T cells will respond to stimuli that bypass the T-cell receptor (TCR), e.g., phorbol ester plus calcium ionophore, but not to crosslinking of CD3, phytohemagglutinin, or allogeneic cell stimuli. A protein tyrosine kinase (PTK), ZAP-70, is lacking in such patients.

Other PTKs involved in TCR signal transduction, Lck, Fyn, and Syk, are normal in these patients, but cannot compensate for the defect. Further, ZAP-70 appears to be unnecessary for CD^{4+} T-cell thymic maturation, selection, and export to the periphery, whereas CD8+ thymopoiesis is ZAP-70-dependent. This defect is inherited as an autosomal recessive trait.

T-CELL RECEPTOR (TCR) DEFECT The T-cell receptor is a heterodimer of α and β or γ and δ chains. The $\alpha\beta$ TCR is the most common variety and accounts for essentially all of the routine protection from infectious agents. The $\gamma\delta$ TCR may represent a more primitive structure capable of reacting without the restraints required for usual T-cell activation (e.g., MHC antigen presentation) and may respond to nonpeptidic epitopes, such as those found in lipids, mycobacteria, and heat shock proteins. Immunodeficiency involving $\gamma\delta$ TCRs has not been described. Surface expression of the $\alpha\beta$ TCR requires complexing with proteins of the CD3 complex, a mixture of γ, δ, ε, ζ, and η subunits. The TCR α and β chains lack cytoplasmic tails and, therefore, would not transduce activation signals effectively. The CD3 complex provides the necessary cytoplasmic extensions that allow TCR stimulation to initiate the intracellular events necessary for a competent T-cell antigen response. Mutations of chains of the CD3 complex, most commonly the γ or ε chains, have been described and are associated with abnormal or diminished expression of the TCR. The γ chain defect results in a more clinically severe disease.

TRANSDUCTION DEFECTS A number of primary signal transduction defects have been described, characterized by failure to proliferate after ligation of TCR-CD3, CD2, or CD3 surface molecules. If membrane activation is bypassed, using phorbol ester plus calcium ionophore or G-protein activators, the T cells will respond, thus placing the lesions early in the activation pathway.

In another variety, a structural defect in the nuclear factor of activated T cells (NF-AT) was found. Thus, lesions from the beginning to the end of the signal transduction pathway have been described.

B-CELL DISEASES

X-LINKED AGAMMAGLOBULINEMIA (XLA) The first immunodeficiency disease was described by Ogden Bruton in 1952. The patient was a 4-year-old boy with a history of repeated septic episodes. Using the new technique of serum protein electrophoresis, Bruton showed that gamma globulin was lacking. Following treatment with intramuscular gamma globulin injections, the patient remained infection free. Subsequently, autosomal recessive forms of agammaglobulinemia and late onset ("acquired") varieties were described. To date, the molecular bases for those variants have not been delineated.

The development of mature immunoglobulin-secreting B cells involves, first, the differentiation from pre-B cells into progressively more mature stages, next, switching to isotype commitment, and ultimately, antigen-driven terminal differentiation with synthesis and secretion of Ig. The first step, from pre-B to B cell, is blocked in X-linked agammaglobulinemia as a result of a fault in the Bruton tyrosine kinase (*Btk*) gene, located in the midportion of the long arm of the X chromosome, at Xq22. Several varieties of mutations have been described, resulting in inactivity or deficient expression of *Btk*. *Btk* is related to the *src* family of cytoplasmic protein tyrosine kinases and is vital to supporting the clonal expansion of pre-B cells.

Recently, a point mutation in the SH2 domain, which was associated with a milder form of disease, was found in a family with three affected males. In two of the brothers, the levels of IgG were higher than usually seen (470 and 590 mg/dL). In all three, the peripheral blood B cells numbered from 0.3 to 2% in contrast to the mean value of 0.1% for XLA patients. The clinical disease was much milder in all three; in fact, one patient had no serious infections even though he complied poorly with therapy.

Recurrent infections with extracellular pyogenic pathogens resulting in meningitis, pneumonia and septicemia characterize hypogammaglobulinemia.

The disease is usually well-controlled by replacement gamma globulin. Intramuscular injections can be used in small infants in whom access is difficult, but intravenous preparations have largely supplanted this route and are necessary to achieve appropriate therapeutic levels in older children and adults. A critical factor in the ultimate prognosis in these patients is the degree of pulmonary involvement by chronic infection leading to bronchiectasis and pulmonary fibrosis. Therefore, close monitoring of the pulmonary status by regular function studies is important.

HYPER-IgM (HIM) The initial response of the cell system to antigen stimulates IgM clones. With continued stimulation or with a booster injection, the antibody response is shifted to IgG, IgA, or IgE clones that have developed by T-cell-dependent isotype switching of the IgM precursors. Isotype switching is dependent on the interaction of CD40, a B-cell surface growth factor receptor, with CD40 ligand (CD40L or gp39) expressed primarily on CD^{4+}T cells shortly after activation. HIM shows X-linked, autosomal recessive, and autosomal dominant forms of inheritance. Most patients with X-linked hyper-IgM (X-HIM) lack CD40L and, as a result, show increased levels of IgM, with virtually no IgG, IgA, or IgE. Four of 17 male patients with suspected X-linked HIM, however, were shown to have normal CD40L but defective CD40-mediated signal transduction. It is not certain that the $CD40L^+$ variety is also X-linked; one of the patients had affected male relatives, whereas the others did not.

HIM patients have two problems not seen in agammaglobulinemia because of B cell defects, infections with opportunistic infections and neutropenia. These complications are more common in the $CD40L^-$ type of HIM. The clinical course is otherwise similar to panhypogammaglobulinemia.

In contrast to carriers of most immunodeficiency disorders studied to date, phenotypically normal mothers of X-HIM patients may show a significant number of cells of the affected (T-cell) line that express the diseased maternally derived chromosome; in some cases as many as 68% are CD40L negative. Thus, normal levels of immunoglobulins and freedom from infectious susceptibility can be attained with levels of only 30% $CD40L^+$ cells. These observations also suggest that CD40-CD40L interactions are not critical for intrathymic T-cell selection and export to the periphery.

Most patients with HIM respond to intravenous immunoglobulin therapy. When the clinical history warrants, bone marrow transplant can be performed.

SUBCLASS DEFICIENCY The immunoglobulins are divided into subclasses, based on minor amino acid sequence differences in the constant region. IgG has four subclasses, denoted IgG1 through IgG4. The subclasses have slightly different biologic activity. Most importantly, the major carbohydrate antibody response shifts from IgG1 in children to IgG2 in adults. It can be argued that a deficiency of the IgG2 subclass could impair the antibody response to many bacteria. Furthermore, if a subclass is missing or low, total IgG determinations will usually not reflect this deficiency. Other subclasses are normal or elevated to mask this defect. However, whether IgG subclass deficiency is a clinically significant defect is a debatable issue. The major disclaimer is the fact that individuals completely lacking in IgG2, IgA1, IgG4, and IgE because of a structural gene defect have been described who have no increased susceptibility to infectious disease whatever. It is postulated that subclass deficiency as a result of gene deletion is an asymptomatic condition with compensatory antibody formation by other subclasses, whereas subclass deficiency because of immune dysregulation is symptomatic because antibody formation is impaired. The distinction can be made by measuring specific antibody responses.

SELECTED REFERENCES

GENERAL

Abbas AK, Lichtman AH, Pober JS. Cellular and Molecular Immunology. Philadelphia:WB Saunders, 1994.

Conley ME. Molecular approaches to analysis of X-linked immunodeficiencies. Annu Rev Immunol 1992;322:1063–1066.

Janeway CA Jr., Travers P. Immunobiology. The Immune System in Health and Disease. New York:Garland, 1994.

Stiehm ER. Human gamma globulins as therapeutic agents. Adv Pediatr 1988;35:1–72.

Stiehm ER. Immunologic Disorders in Infants and Children. ed. Philadelphia: WB Saunders, 1989.

THERAPY

Anderson WF. Human gene therapy. Science 1992;256:808–813.

Filipovitch AH, Shapiro RS, Ramsay NKC, et al. Unrelated donor bone marrow transplantation for correction of lethal congenital immunodeficiencies. Blood 1992;80:270–276.

Fischer A, Griscelli C, Friedrich W, et al. Bone marrow transplantation for immunodeficiencies and osteopetrosis: European survey 1968–1985. Lancet 1986;2:1080–1084.

Moen RC, Horowitz SD, Sondel PM, et al. Immune reconstitution after haploidentical bone marrow transplantation for immune deficiency disease: treatment of bone marrow cells with monoclonal antibody CT-2 and complement. Blood 1987;70:664–669.

O'Reilly RJ, Keever CA, Small TN, Brochstein J. The use of HLA-non-identical T-cell-depleted marrow transplants for correction of severe combined immunodeficiency disease. Immunodefic Rev 1989;1: 273–309.

SEVERE COMBINED IMMUNODEFICIENCY

Kondo M, Takeshita T, Ishii N, et al. Sharing of the interleukin-2 (IL-2) receptor γ chain between receptors for IL-2 and IL-4. Science 1993;262:1874–1877.

Macchi P, Villa A, Giliani S, et al. Mutations of Jak–3 gene in patients with autosomal severe combined immune deficiency (SCID). Nature 1995;377:65–68.

Noguchi M, Nakamura Y, Russell SM, et al. Interleukin-2 receptor γ chain: a functional component of the interleukin-7 receptor. Science 1993;262:1877–1880.

Noguchi M, Yi H, Rosenblatt HM, et al. Interleukin-2 receptor gamma chain mutation results in X-linked severe combined immunodeficiency in humans. Cell 1993;73:147–157.

Puck JM, Deschenes SM, Porter JC, et al. The interleukin-2 receptor symbol γ chain maps to Xq13.1 and is mutated in X-linked severe combined immunodeficiency. Hum Molec Genet 1993;2:1099–1104.

Russell SM, Johnston JA, Noguchi M, et al. Interaction of IL-2Rβ and γ_c chains with Jak1 and Jak3: implications for XSCID and XCID. Science 1994;266:1042–1045.

Russell SM, Keegan AD, Harada N, et al. Interleukin-2 receptor γ chain: a functional component of the interleukin-4 receptor. Science 1993;262:1880–1883.

BARE LYMPHOCYTE SYNDROME

Benichou B, Strominger JL. Class II-antigen-negative patient and mutant B cell lines represent at least three and probably four distinct genetic defects defined by complementation analysis. Proc Natl Acad Sci USA 1991;88:4285–4288.

de Preval C, Lisowska-Grospierre B, Loche M, Griscelli C, Mach B. A trans-acting class II regulatory gene unlinked to the MHC controls expression of HLA class II genes. Nature 1985;318:291–293.

Kara CJ, Glimcher LH. Promoter accessibility within the environment of the MHC is affected in class II-deficient combined immunodeficiency. EMBO J 1993;12:187–193.

Reith W, Satola S, Herrero-Sanchez C, et al. Congenital immunodeficiency with a regulatory defect in MHC class II gene expression lacks a specific HLA-DR promoter binding protein RF-X. Cell 1988;53:897–906.

Salter RD, Alexander J, Levine F, Pious D, Cresswell P. Evidence for two trans-acting genes regulating HLA class II antigen expression. J Immunol 1985;135:4235–4238.

Stimac E, Urieli-Shoval S, Kempkin S, Pious D. Defective HLA DRA X box binding in the class II transactive transcription factor mutant 6.1.6 and in cell lines from class II immunodeficient patients. J Immunol 1991;146:4398–4405.

WISKOTT-ALDRICH SYNDROME

Brochstein JA, Gillio AP, Ruggiero M et al. Marrow transplantation from human leukocyte antigen-identical or haploidentical donors for correction of Wiskott-Aldrich syndrome. J Pediatr 1991; 119:907–912.

Derry JMJ, Ochs HD, Francke U. Isolation of a novel gene mutated in Wiskott–Aldrich syndrome. Cell 1994;78:635–644.

Fischer A, Blanche S, Le Bidois J, et al. Anti-B cell monoclonal antibodies in the treatment of severe B-cell lymphoproliferative syndrome following bone marrow and organ transplantation. N Engl J Med 1991;324:1451–1456.

Klein C, Lisowska-Grospierre B, LeDeist F, Fischer A, Griscelli C. Major histocompatibility complex class II deficiency: Clinical manifestations immunologic features and outcome. J Pediatr 1993;123:921–928.

Molina IJ, Kenney DM, Rosen FS, Remold-O'Donnell E. T cell lines characterize events in the pathogenesis of the Wiskott-Aldrich syndrome. J Exp Med 1992;176:867–874.

Rooney CM, Smith CA, Ng CY et al. Use of gene–modified virus-specific T lymphocytes to control Epstein-Barr-virus-related lymphoproliferation. Lancet 1995;345:9–13.

Rumelhart SL, Trigg ME, Horowitz SD, Hong R. Monoclonal antibody T-cell-depleted HLA-haploidentical bone marrow transplantation for Wiskott-Aldrich syndrome. Blood 1990;75:1031–1035.

ADENOSINE DEAMINASE AND NUCLEOSIDE PHOSPHORLYASE DEFICIENCY

Blaese RM. Development of gene therapy for immunodeficiency: adenosine deaminase deficiency. Pediatr Res 1993;33(Suppl): S49–S55.

Hirschhorn R. Overview of biochemical abnormalities and molecular genetics of adenosine deaminase deficiency. Pediatr Res 1993; 33(Suppl):S35–S41.

Kohn DB, Weinberg KI, Nolta JA, et al. Engraftment of gene-modified umbilical cord blood cells in neonates with adenosine deaminase deficiency. Nat Med 1995;1:1017–1023.

Markert ML. Purine nucleoside phosphorylase deficiency. Immunodef Rev 1991;3:45–81.

Santisteban I, Arrendondo-Vega FX, Kelly S, et al. Novel splicing missense and deletion mutations in seven adenosine deaminase-deficient patients with late/delayed onset of combined immunodeficiency disease. J Clin Invest 1993;92:2291–2302.

ATAXIA-TELANGIECTASIA

Nowak R. Discovery of AT gene sparks biomedical research bonanza. Science 1995;268:1700,1701.

Savitsky K, Bar-Shira A, Gilad S, et al. A single ataxia telangiectasia gene with a product similar to PI-3 kinase. Science 1995;268: 1749–1753.

DIGEORGE ANOMALY

Conley ME, Beckwith JB, Mancer JFK, Tenckhoff L. The spectrum of the DiGeorge syndrome. J Pediatr 1979;94:883-890.

Hong R. The DiGeorge anomaly. Immunodef Rev 1991;3:1–14.

ZAP-70 DEFICIENCY

Arpaia E, Shahar M, Dadi H, Cohen A, Roifman CM. Defective T cell receptor signaling and CD8+ thymic selection in humans lacking zap-70 kinase. Cell 1994;76:947–958.

Chan AC, Kadlecek TA, Elder ME, et al. ZAP–70 deficiency in an autosomal recessive form of severe combined immunodeficiency. Science 1994;264:1599–1601.

Elder ME, Lin D, Clever J, et al. Human severe combined immunodeficiency due to a defect in ZAP-70, a T cell tyrosine kinase. Science 1994;264:1596–1599.

T-CELL RECEPTOR DEFECTS

Alarcon B, Regueiro JR, Arnaiz-Villena A, Terhorst C. Familial defect in the surface expression of the T-cell receptor-CD3 complex. N Engl J Med 1988;319:1203–1208.

Arnaiz-Villena A, Timon M, Corell A, Perez-Aciego P, Martin-Villa JM, Regueiro JR. Brief report: primary immunodeficiency caused by mutations in the gene encoding the CD3-gamma subunit of the T-lymphocyte receptor. N Engl J Med 1992;326:529–533.

Arnaiz-Villena A, Timon M, Rodriguez-Gallego C, et al. Human T-cell activation deficiencies. Immunol Today 1992;13:259–265.

Born WK, O'Brien R, Modlin RL. Antigen specificity of γδ T lymphocytes. FASEB J 1991;5:2699–2705.

Constant P, Davodeau F, Peyrat M-A, et al. Stimulation of human γδ T cells by nonpeptidic mycobacterial ligands. Science 1994; 264:267–270.

Raulet DH. The structure, function, and molecular genetics of the γ/δ T cell receptor. Annu Rev Immunol 1989;7:175–207.

Thoenes G, Soudais C, Le Deist F, et al. Structural analysis of low TcR-CD3 complex expression in T cells of an immunodeficient patient. J Biol Chem 1992;267:487–493.

TRANSDUCTION DEFECT

Chatila T, Wong R, Young M, Miller R, Terhorst C, Geha RF. An immunodeficiency characterized by defective signal transduction in T lymphocytes. N Engl J Med 1989;320:696–702.

X–LINKED AGAMMAGLOBULINEMIA

Bruton OC. Agammaglobulinemia. Pediatrics 1952;9:722–728.

Kinnon C, Hinshelwood S, Levinsky RJ, Lovering RC. X-linked agammaglobulinemia—gene cloning and future prospects. Immunol Today 1993;14:554–558.

Saffran DC, Parolini O, Fitch-Hilgenberg ME, et al. Brief report: a point mutation in the SH2 domain of Bruton's tyrosine kinase in atypical X-linked agammaglobulinemia. N Engl J Med 1994; 330:1488–1491.

Tsukada S, Saffran DC, Rawlings DJ et al. Deficient expression of a B cell cytoplasmic tyrosine kinase in human X-linked agammaglobulinemia. Cell 1993;72:279–290.

Vetrie D, Vorechovsky I, Sideras P, et al. The gene involved in X-linked agammaglobulinaemia is a member of the src family of protein-tyrosine kinases. Nature 1993;361:226–233.

HYPER–IGM SYNDROME

Aruffo A, Farrington M, Hollenbaugh D, et al. The CD40 ligand gp39 is defective in activated T cells from patients with X-linked hyper-IgM syndrome. Cell 1993;72:291–300.

Callard RE, Armitage J, Fanslow WC, Spriggs MK. CD40 ligand and its role in X-linked hyper-IgM syndrome. Immunol Today 1993;14:559–564.

Conley ME, Larche M, Bonagura VR et al. Hyper IgM syndrome associated with defective CD40-mediated B cell activation. J Clin Invest 1994;94:1404–1409.

Hollenbaugh D, Wu LH, Ochs HD, et al. The random inactivation of the X chromosome carrying the defective gene responsible for X-linked hyper IgM syndrome (X-HIM) in female carriers of HIGM1. J Clin Invest 1994;94:616–622.

Thomas C, de Saint Basile G, LeDiest F et al. Brief report: correction of X-linked hyper-IgM syndrome by allogeneic bone marrow transplantation. N Engl J Med 1995;333:426–429.

IGG SUBCLASS DEFICIENCY

Lefranc MP, Lefranc G, Rabbits TH. Inherited deletion of immunoglobulin heavy chain constant regions in normal human individuals. Nature 1982;1982:760–762.

Plebani A, Ugazio AG, Meini A, et al. Extensive deletion of immunoglobulin heavy chain constant region genes in the absence of recurrent infections: When is IgG subclass deficiency clinically relevant? Clin Immunol Immunopathol 1993:68:46–50.

33 Human Immunodeficiency Virus and Acquired Immune Deficiency Syndrome (AIDS)

John W. Sleasman and Maureen M. Goodenow

AIDS AND HUMAN RETROVIRUSES

Acquired immunodeficiency syndrome (AIDS) is a result of infection with human immunodeficiency virus type 1 (HIV-1), a human retrovirus. Retroviruses cause a variety of diseases ranging from immunodeficiency to malignancy. Human retroviruses are divided into two major families. Oncornaviruses, including human T-cell lymphotropic viruses (HTLV-1 and HTLV-2), have the capacity to cause tumors. Lentiviruses, which include HIV, are a second family of retroviruses that have the capacity to be cytopathic and cause cell death, usually after a long period of incubation. There are two recognized subtypes of HIV: HIV-1, which causes AIDS and related complexes worldwide; and HIV-2, which may be less pathogenic and is more geographically restricted than HIV-1. HIV-2 is genetically more closely related to simian immunodeficiency virus than to HIV-1.

AIDS was initially described in 1981 as an immunodeficiency syndrome restricted epidemiologically to gay males living in the United States. The disease was quickly recognized to affect men, women, and children living throughout the world. By 1983 the causal relationship between HIV-1 infection and the development of AIDS was realized. Today AIDS has become a major worldwide cause of death in both adults and children. The World Health Organization estimates that there are more than 20 million infected individuals worldwide. In the United States, AIDS is the leading cause of death of men between the ages of 25 and 45 and the fifth leading cause of death of women of reproductive age. HIV-1 is transmitted primarily through sexual contact, intravenous (iv) exposure to contaminated blood or blood products, and vertical transmission from mother to child. The clinical manifestations of AIDS result from a profound deficiency in cell-mediated immunity, and to a lesser extent, humoral immunity. The clinical manifestations of HIV-1 infection, as categorized by the Centers for Disease Control and Prevention, are summarized in Table 33-1.

NATURAL HISTORY OF HIV-1 INFECTION

The pathogenesis from initial HIV-1 infection to the development of AIDS results from a dynamic interaction between the virus and the host immune system. The principal mechanism leading to immunodeficiency is the progressive loss of $CD4^+$ lymphocyte number and function. Immunologic abnormalities can be demonstrated soon after initial infection before the loss of $CD4^+$ T lymphocytes, indicating that attrition of $CD4^+$ T lymphocytes alone does not explain completely all of the clinical and immunologic manifestations seen in HIV-infected individuals.

The clinical history of HIV-1 infection generally follows three stages: an acute "flulike" illness, a relatively asymptomatic "latent" period, and the reappearance of symptoms and immunodeficiency ultimately resulting in AIDS (Fig. 33-1). Primary symptomatic HIV-1 infection is generally characterized by an acute febrile illness, lymphadenopathy, and malaise, which occur 3–4 weeks after exposure. However, not all HIV-1-infected individuals exhibit symptoms during this acute stage of viral infection. This acute phase is associated with high levels of HIV-1 replication and plasma viremia. Laboratory evaluation reveals evidence of T-cell activation, transient inverted CD4 to CD8 T-lymphocyte ratio, and mild hypergammaglobulinemia. During this stage of acute infection, individuals are HIV-1-antibody negative yet potentially infectious. Seroconversion and the production of antibody to core and envelope proteins occurs 4–6 weeks after viral exposure. The emergence of immunologic suppression of HIV, as measured by the production of antibodies to viral proteins, results in a decline in plasma viremia and clinical symptoms. At this point the patient enters a period of clinical latency. However, viral replication continues in the lymphoid system often at subclinical levels.

In adults, the diagnosis of HIV-1 infection is based on the detection of serum antibodies to HIV proteins using enzyme-linked immunosorbent assay (ELISA) and is confirmed by Western blot analysis. In newborn infants, antibody-based assays of detection of HIV infection are not helpful because of the presence of passively acquired maternal antibody. Because only about a third of infants born to HIV-infected mothers are infected, a direct means of detecting the virus is required to differentiate infected from uninfected infants. The most sensitive means for identifying infected infants is the use of the polymerase chain reaction to amplify HIV proviral DNA within infected $CD4^+$ T lymphocytes.

Although a small percentage of infected infants will develop a rapid progression to the AIDS, the majority of infected adults and

From: *Principles of Molecular Medicine* (J. L. Jameson, ed.), ©1998 Humana Press Inc., Totowa, NJ.

Table 33-1
1993 CDC Clinical Categories for Adolescents and Adults[a]

Category A
Asymptomatic HIV infection
Persistent generalized lymphadenopathy
Acute (primary) HIV infection with accompanying illness or history of acute HIV infection
Category B
Bacillary angiomatosis
Candidiasis, oropharyngeal (thrush)
Candidiasis, vulvovaginal; persistent, frequent, or poorly responsive to therapy
Cervical dysplasia (moderate or severe) and cervical carcinoma *in situ*
Constitutional symptoms, such as fever (38.5°C) or diarrhea lasting >1 month
Hairy leukoplakia, oral
Herpes zoster (shingles), involving at least two distinct episodes or more than one dermatome
Idiopathic thrombocytopenic purpura
Listeriosis
Pelvic inflammatory disease, particularly if complicated by tubo-ovarian abscess
Peripheral neuropathy
Category C
$CD4^+$ T-lymphocyte count <200 cells/μL or $CD4^+$ percentage <14%
Candidiasis of bronchi, trachea, or lungs
Candidiasis, esophageal
Cervical cancer, invasive
Coccidioidomycosis, disseminated or extrapulmonary
Cryptococcosis, extrapulmonary
Cryptosporidiosis, chronic intestinal (>1 month's duration)
Cytomegalovirus disease (other than liver, spleen, or nodes)
Cytomegalovirus retinitis (with loss of vision)
Encephalopathy, HIV-related
Herpes simplex: chronic ulcer(s) (>1 month's duration); or bronchitis, pneumonitis, or esophagitis Histoplasmosis, disseminated or extrapulmonary
Isosporiasis, chronic intestinal (>1 month's duration)
Kaposi's sarcoma
Lymphoma, Burkitt's (or equivalent term)
Lymphoma, immunoblastic (or equivalent term)
Lymphoma, primary, of brain
Mycobacterium avium complex or *Mycobacterium kansasii*, disseminated or extrapulmonary
Mycobacterium tuberculosis, any site (pulmonary or extrapulmonary)
Mycobacterium, other species or unidentified species, disseminated or extrapulmonary
Pneumocystis carinii pneumonia
Pneumonia, recurrent
Progressive multifocal leukoencephalopathy
Salmonella septicemia, recurrent
Toxoplasmosis of brain
Wasting syndrome due to HIV

[a]The revised CDC classification system for HIV-infected adolescents and adults categories persons on the basis of clinical conditions associated with HIV infection and $CD4^+$ T-lymphocyte counts.

children will enter an asymptomatic latent period after acute infection that may last from months to 10 years or more. Factors that may play a role in the length of latency include viral virulence, the magnitude of the immune response, infection with other pathogens, age of the patient, and the use of antiretroviral drugs. The events that trigger the onset of clinical symptoms and mark the end of latency are poorly understood. During the end of latency, blood $CD4^+$ T-lymphocyte numbers decline and plasma viremia levels increase. Although $CD4^+$ T lymphocytes are the principal reservoir of HIV-1 in peripheral blood, less than 10% of blood $CD4^+$ T cells harbor HIV-1. HIV-1 infection of other cell types plays an important role in the progression to AIDS. Expression of the CD4 peptide is not limited to helper T lymphocytes. Cells of macrophage lineage, including dendritic cells, Langerhans cells, and microglia, also express CD4, which renders them susceptible to HIV-1 infection. HIV-1 has been detected in macrophages from blood, lung, and brain of infected individuals. Viral particles are localized primarily in the cytoplasm of infected macrophages and are not particularly cytopathic. HIV-1 isolates obtained from individuals soon after infection display a greater ability to replicate in monocytes and macrophages and are not as cytopathic as viral isolates obtained at late-stage disease. HIV-infected macrophages may play a critical role in many of the organ-specific manifestations of AIDS, particularly in the brain where infection leads to a chronic inflammatory process that ultimately results in HIV-1 encephalopathy.

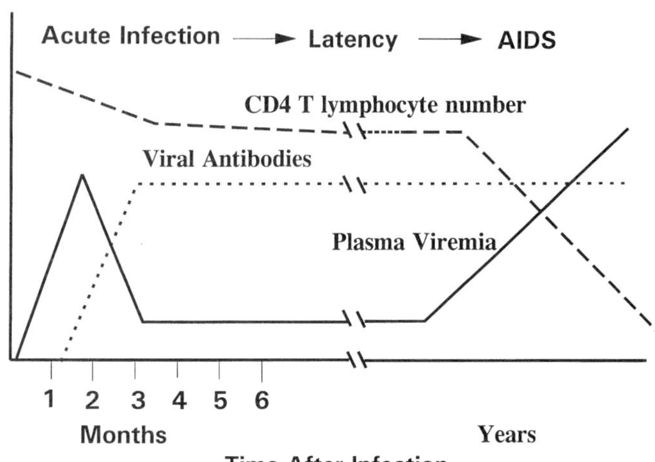

Figure 33-1 Natural history of HIV infection. After initial infection there is an acute phase of plasma viremia, as represented by the solid line. Acute viremia peaks 2–6 weeks after exposure but falls soon after the appearance of antibodies to HIV viral proteins, as represented by the dotted/dashed line. HIV antibodies develop within 4–8 weeks after exposure and remain detectable throughout infection. During the acute phase of infection there is evidence of T-cell activation, inverted CD4 to CD8 T-cell ratios, and a suppression of $CD4^+$ T-lymphocyte number, as indicated by the dashed line. During latency $CD4^+$ lymphocyte number is mildly depressed and viremia is low. Latency may last months to years. As $CD4^+$ T-lymphocyte counts fall plasma viremia reappears. Continued attrition of $CD4^+$ T-cell number finally results in depletion of cell-mediated immunity and the development of AIDS.

HIV-1 MOLECULAR ORGANIZATION AND VIRAL LIFE CYCLE

The basic structure of HIV-1 is similar to that of other retroviruses. The virus particle is surrounded by a lipid envelope containing the envelope glycoproteins protruding from the surface. Within the virus particle, core proteins surround the HIV-1 genome, which is composed of ribonucleic acid (RNA). The inner core also contains enzymes required for HIV-1 replication.

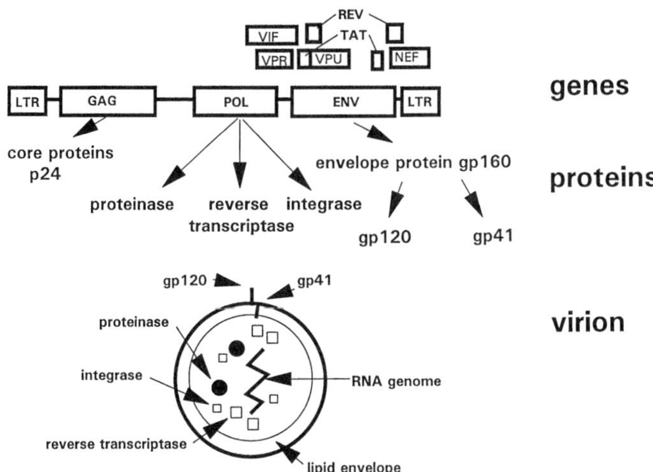

Figure 33-2 HIV-1 genetic organization, proteins, and viral structure. The principal HIV-1 structural genes, *gag*, *pol*, and *env*, a flanked by the long terminal repeats (LTRs). The regulatory genes, *vif*, *vpr*, *vpu*, *tat*, *rev*, and *nef*, overlap *pol*, *env*, or the 3' LTR. *Gag* encodes the core proteins including p24. *Pol* encodes the HIV proteinase, reverse transcriptase, and intergrase. *Env* encodes gp160, which is cleaved by a cellular proteinase into gp120 and gp4l. Viral enzymes and genomic RNA are wrapped within the core proteins and packaged into a complete virion. The lipid envelope contains gp120, which is anchored to gp4l.

Proteins and enzymes involved in the structure and replication of HIV-1 are encoded by the linear viral genome, which is organized into three major genes; *gag*, *pol*, and *env* (Fig. 33-2). These genes are transcribed into RNA and ultimately translated into the viral proteins that are generally identified by their molecular size. For example, p24 refers to a 24-kDa core protein, whereas gpl20 is a 120-kDa glycoprotein located in the envelope. *Gag* is a major gene encoding the HIV-1 core proteins. *Pol* encodes at least three enzymatic activities: proteinase, an enzyme involved in cleavage of *gag*- and *pol*- encoded protein precursors; reverse transcriptase, essential for transcribing the RNA genome into DNA; and integrase, required for the covalent linkage between the viral DNA and the host cell chromosomal DNA. *Env* encodes gpl60, a glycoprotein that is processed into gp4l and gpl20. The smaller gp4l spans the lipid envelope membrane and serves as an anchor for gpl20, which interacts with receptors on the surface of target cells. In addition to *gag*, *pol*, and *env*, the HIV-1 genome contains a set of regulatory genes that are involved in positive and negative modulation of virus replication. The regulatory genes include *Tat*, a potent transactivator of HIV gene expression that facilitates the initiation of RNA transcription; *Rev*, which facilitates the transport of unspliced mRNA from the nucleus to the cytoplasm; and less well-understood regulatory and accessory genes, which include *Nef*, *Vpr*, *Vpu*, and *Vif*. The regulatory genes, which overlap *pol* and *env*, and are expressed by complex splicing mechanisms, are unique to the lentiviruses and do not appear in the genomes of the oncogenic retroviruses. Flanking the coding regions of the HIV-1 genome are long terminal repeats (LTRs) composed of sequences that regulate virtually every aspect of the virus life cycle, including replication, integration, and viral gene expression. Some of the proteins encoded by the regulatory genes of HIV-1 act directly or indirectly on target elements in the LTRs.

HIV-1 LIFE CYCLE Knowledge of the viral life cycle is essential to understanding the natural history of HIV-1 infection and is vital to the development of medical strategies to attenuate the disease (Fig. 33-3A). The first step in HIV-1 infection is attachment of the virus to its receptor. The HIV-1 envelope glycoprotein gpl20 binds directly to a molecule called CD4, a protein found on the surface of T helper cells and macrophages. This second step is viral penetration. CD4 is necessary, but not sufficient, for HIV-1 entry into target cells. Interactions between gp120 and CD4 increases the affinity of gp120 for a second class of cell surface molecules, the chemokine receptors, which contribute to virus entry. Chemokine receptors are seven-transmembrane, G-protein-coupled proteins that normally function in cell trafficking and response to inflammation. CCR5 and CXCR4 are two

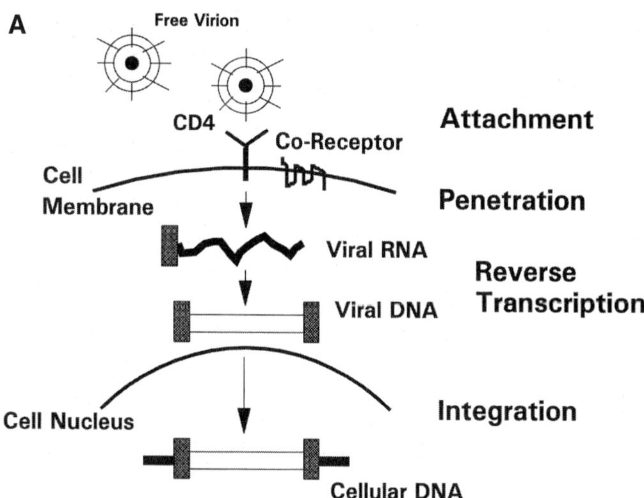

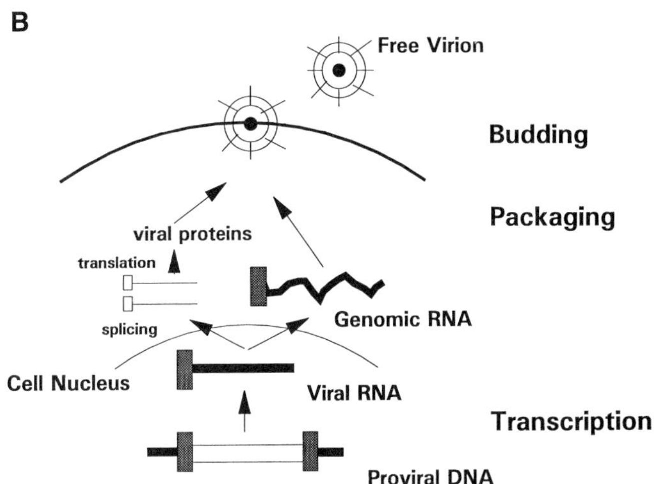

Figure 33-3 HIV life cycle **(A)** Phase of viral replication. Free virus attaches to CD4+ T cells by the binding of gpl20 to the CD4 molecule. The virus penetrates the cell, and viral RNA is reverse transcribed into double-stranded DNA. This process is initiated at the 5' LTR, indicated by the shaded box. Proviral DNA is transported to the nucleus where it integrates into host cellular DNA. **(B)** Phase of viral expression. Viral transcription is initiated at the LTR and depends on cellular proteins and host cell activation. Viral RNA is spliced into genomic RNA or mRNA, which are ultimately translated into viral proteins. Viral proteins are further cleaved by the HIV proteinase for packaging and budding into new virions.

chemokine receptors that function as major coreceptors for HIV-1. CCR5 and CXCR4 are differentially expressed on distinct subsets of CD4-positive cells and are critical in determining viral tropism for primary T lymphocytes, macrophages, or transformed T-cell lines. Viruses that use CCR5, which is expressed by macrophages and lymphocytes, are macrophage-tropic and most commonly found during acute and early infection. Viruses that use CXCR4, which is expressed by lymphocytes and transformed T-cell lines, can evolve during disease progression. The lipid envelope membrane of the virus containing gpl20 and gp4l fuses with the cell membrane of the target cell, allowing viral entry and uncoating of the core proteins, enzymes, and genomic RNA in the cytoplasm of the target cell. Within the cytoplasm viral RNA is transcribed into double-stranded DNA by the unique retrovirus enzyme, reverse transcriptase. The viral DNA is transported into the nucleus of the cell and is poised for the next step in the viral life cycle, integration.

The viral-encoded integrase enzyme enables integration of viral DNA by a covalent linkage to the chromosomal DNA of the host cell, resulting in the HIV-1 DNA becoming an actual component of the host cell genome. Viral DNA is replicated along with host DNA as the infected cell divides. The integrated DNA form of HIV-1 is termed the provirus. HIV-1 provirus DNA can remain hidden in the host cell DNA and evade immunologic recognition. Viral latency describes the state of the provirus in which it is integrated within the host DNA but the virus proteins are not expressed and viral replication is dormant.

Proviral expression results in transcription of viral DNA into viral RNA (Fig. 33-3B), which is dependent on host cell activation and host cell enzymes. Lymphokines that activate T cells also activate provirus expression through target sequences in the LTR. The full-length RNA transcripts are spliced and transported to the cytoplasm, where HIV-1 RNA is then translated into viral proteins by normal cellular mechanisms. The regulatory gene products for *Tat* and *Rev* are thought to play a key role during this phase of the viral life cycle. Viral proteins are processed, assembled into new viral particles, and bud from the surface of the HIV-1-infected cell. Because replication of HIV-1 does not always result in cell death, persistence of HIV-1 can result from the chronic production of low levels of virus in infected individuals.

It is now obvious that the factors leading to $CD4^+$ T-cell depletion involve more than the cytopathic effects of HIV-1 replication. One hypothesis is that the slow attrition of $CD4^+$ T cells that leads to AIDS is an HIV-induced apoptosis of $CD4^+$ T lymphocytes. $CD4^+$ T cells are destroyed by a two-step process. First, HIV-1 gpl20 crosslinks CD4 on the target T cells. Second, antigen stimulation through the T-cell receptor results in an aberrant signal transduction pathway to the nucleus leading to cell death. HIV-1 infection results in the loss of $CD4^+$ T-cell capacity for regeneration and self-renewal. Over time the total $CD4^+$ T-cell number falls and a profound defect in cell-mediated immunity occurs. This ultimately leads to the clinical manifestations of opportunistic infections and malignancy that characterize AIDS, the final stage of HIV-1 infection.

IMPLICATIONS OF HIV-1 GENETIC VARIABILITY IN THE TREATMENT AND PREVENTION OF AIDS

Lentiviruses in general, and HIV-1 in particular, demonstrate extensive variability among virus genomes. Errors introduced by HIV-1 reverse transcriptase occur as frequently as 1 in 10,000 nucleotides, the approximate size of the HIV-1 genome. This error rate can produce one genetic change during each replication cycle of the virus. In addition to nucleotide substitutions, nucleic acid deletions, insertions, and duplications can occur in the process of reverse transcription of HIV-1. Genetic variability is modulated by selective pressures for virus viability and host interactions. The result of genetic variability is that every HIV-1 genome is unique. The HIV-1 genome evolves into a collection of genetically different viruses, or a quasi-species. Genetic variability in HIV-1 manifests itself not only among different infected individuals, but within each infected individual as well. The virus population within an individual changes over time. The extent of genetic variability among strains of HIV-1 has important implications for tracking the epidemiology of HIV-1 as it is transmitted from one person to another.

Although nucleotide changes can occur anywhere within the viral genome, the extent of genetic variability is not uniform within the various gene segments. Regions in *gag* and *pol* display less variability than *env* presumably because the function of proteins encoded by *gag* and *pol* are easily disrupted by amino acid changes. In contrast, the most variable regions of the virus genome are centered in five hypervariable regions, Vl through V5, in *env* gpl20. Within these regions there is a high ratio of nonsynonymous to synonymous substitutions, an indication that changes in the nucteotide sequences are likely to result in amino acid changes of the gpl20 protein. This finding suggests that this region of HIV-1 is driven by positive selection, perhaps as a result of the influence of the host immune response, thereby providing the virus with an escape mechanism from immune surveillance. There is a highly conserved region of gpl20, localized between V4 and V5, which is part of the CD4-binding site.

HIV VACCINES HIV-1 genetic diversity has profound implications in the management and treatment of disease progression. Although a vigorous antibody and cellular immune response is generated by infected individuals against HIV-1, the life cycle pattern of infection, latency, and replication, in combination with genetic changes, particularly within gp120, results in evasion of the immune response and ultimately disease progression. Furthermore, the intimate relationship between HIV-1 infection and the immune response creates several potential pitfalls to the development of an effective vaccine. There is evidence that vaccination with gpl20-subunit vaccines results in the production of neutralizing antibody against the vaccine strain of HIV-1 but not for infecting viral strains. Alternatively, cytotoxic $CD8^+$ T cells directed against HIV-1 epitopes expressed on infected $CD4^+$ T cells may contribute to $CD4^+$ T-cell attrition and accelerate the development of AIDS. These and other factors may render traditional vaccine development difficult as a strategy in preventing infection.

ANTIRETROVIRAL THERAPY The current therapeutic strategies to slow disease progression in infected individuals uses antiretroviral agents that act at distinct stages of the viral life cycle. Dideoxynucleoside reverse transcriptase inhibitors, such as zidovudine (also known as AZT), act only on the infection phase of the viral life cycle by competing with endogenous deoxynucleotides for incorporation into proviral DNA during reverse transcription from viral RNA. Once the drug is incorporated into proviral DNA further elongation of the DNA chain is terminated. In addition to zidovudine and related analogs, there are several other nondeoxynucleoside analogs that inhibit the infective phase of the viral life cycle but have no activity against the phase of viral replication.

A new class of antiretroviral agents targeted against the HIV aspartyl protease have been approved for clinical use. The HIV protease is a unique enzyme that is responsible for the cleavage of the large *gag* and *pol* polyprotein gene products, an essential requirement for the production of infectious virus. Protease inhibitors compete with the substrate for binding to the enzymatic active site. This results in incomplete processing of the polyprotein precursors into viral structural proteins and enzymes, and ultimately in the production of immature noninfectious virions.

Compared with genes that display a high degree of genetic variability, such as *env*, the sequences of *gag* and *pol* that encode the HIV reverse transcriptase of protease and its cleavage sites, exhibit only a small degree of genetic drift because of the essential role of these enzymes in infection and replication. However, emergence of drug-resistant variants occurs in a short period of time because the genes are placed under selective pressure by potent inhibitors of reverse transcriptase or protease. The future direction of HIV-1 therapy will be the use of combinations of antiviral agents that act at different stages of the viral life cycle. The goal of therapy will be to reduce viral load, thereby prolonging latency and perhaps reducing the risk of transmission from an infected individual. This therapeutic strategy has been greatly enhanced by the development of sensitive diagnostic techniques, such as quantitative competitive PCR amplification of viral RNA and branched chain DNA, which can quantify the precise number of viral particles in a patient's blood. These methods are currently being used to monitor response to therapy. The recent advances in drug therapy and monitoring of disease progression have been demonstrated to prolong survival and improve the quality of life of HIV-infected individuals.

SELECTED REFERENCES

1993 Revised classification system for HIV infection and expanded surveillance case definition for AIDS among adolescents and adults. MMWR Morb Mortal Wkly Rep 41 1992;(RR-17):1–19.

Barre SF, Chermann JC, Rey F, et al. Isolation of a T-lymphotropic retrovirus from a patient at risk for acquired immune deficiency syndrome (AIDS). Science 1983;220:868–871.

Bates P. Chemokine receptors and HIV-1: an attractive pair? Cell 1996;86:1–3.

Bonhoeffer S, Coffin JM, Nowak MA. Human immunodeficiency virus drug therapy and virus load. J Virol 1997;71:3275–3278.

Broder CC, Collman RG. Chemokine receptors and HIV J Leukocyte Biol 1997;20–29.

Capon DJ, Ward RHR. The CD4-gpl20 interaction and AIDS pathogenesis. Annu Rev Immunol 1991;9:649–678.

Cavert W, Notermans DW, Staskus K. Kinetics of response in lymphoid tissues to antiretroviral therapy of HIV-1 infection. Science 1997; 276:960–964.

Clark S, Saag MS, Decker D, et al. High titers of cytopathic virus in plasma of patients with symptomatic primary HIV-1 infection. N Engl J Med 1991;324:954–960.

Coffin, JM. HIV population dynamics in vivo: Implications for genetic variation pathogenesis, and therapy. Science 1995;267:483–489.

Deng H, Liu R, Ellmeier W. Identification of a major co-receptor for primary isolates of HIV-1. Nature 1996;381:661–666.

Deng HK, Unutmaz D, KewalRamani VN, Littman DR. Expression cloning of new receptors used by simian and human immunodeficiency viruses. Nature 1997;388:296–300.

Goodenow M, Huet T, Saurin W, Kwok S, Sninsky J, Wain-Hobson S. HIV-1 isolates are rapidly evolving quasispecies: evidence for viral mixtures and preferred nucleotide substitutions. J Acquir Immune Defic Syndr 1989;2:352.

Gottlieb MS, Schroff R, Schanker HM, et al. *Pneumocystis carinii* pneumonia and mucosal candidiasis in previously healthy homosexual men: evidence of a new acquired cellular immunodeficiency. N Engl J Med 1981;305:1425–1431.

Groux H, Torpier G, Monte D, Mouton Y, Capron A, Ameisen, JC. Activation-induced death by apoptosis in CD4+, T cells from human immunodeficiency, virus-infected asymptomatic individuals. J Exp Med 1992;175:331–340.

Klotman ME, Wong-Stall F. Human immunodeficiency virus (HIV) gene structure and genetic diversity. In: The Human Retroviruses. Gallo RC, Jay G, eds. San Diego: Academic, 1991; pp. 35–68.

Lamers S, Sleasman JW, Barrie K, Pomeroy S, Barrett DJ, Goodenow MM. Persistence of multiple maternal genotypes of human immunodeficiency virus type 1 in infants infected by perinatal transmission. J Clin Invest 1994;93:380–390.

Liu R, Paxton WA, Choe S. Homozygous defect in HIV-1 coreceptor accounts for resistance of some multiply-exposed individuals to HIV-1 infection. Cell 1996;86:367–377.

McCune JM. HIV-1: the infective process in vivo. Cell 1991;64:351–363.

McCune JM. Viral latency in HIV disease. Cell 1995;82:183–188.

Meltzer M, Skillman DR, Gomatos PJ, Kalter DC, Gendelman HE. Role of mononuclear phagocytes in the pathogenesis of human immunodeficiency virus infection. Annu Rev Immunol 1990;8:169–194.

Miedema F, Tersmette M, van Lier RAW. HIV and the immune system, AIDS pathogenesis: a dynamic interaction between HIV and the immune system. Immunol Today 1990;11:293–297.

Pantaleo G, Graziosi C, Demarest JF, et al. HIV infection is active and progressive in lymphoid tissue during the clinically latent stage of disease. Nature 1993;362:355–362.

Paul WE. Can the immune response control HIV infection? Cell 1995;82:177–182.

Pleskoff O, Treboute C, Brelot A, Heveker N, Seman M, Alizon M. Identification of a chemokine receptor encoded by human cytomegalovirus as a cofactor for HIV-1 entry. Science 1997;276:1874–1878.

Schnittman SM, Fauci AS. Human immunodeficiency virus and acquired immunodeficiency syndrome: an update. Adv Intern Med 1994; 39:305–355.

Schwartz, DH. Potential pitfalls on the road to an effective HIV vaccine. Immunol Today 1994;15:54–56.

Shearer WT, Quinn TC, LaRussa P. Viral load and disease progression in infants infected with human immunodeficiency virus type 1. Women and Infants Transmission Study Group. N Engl J Med 1997;336: 1337–1342.

Trono D. HIV accessory proteins: leading roles for the supporting cast. Cell 1995; 82:189-192.

Varmus H. Retroviruses. Science 1988;240:1427–1435.

Wei X, Ghosh SK, Taylor ME, et al. Viral dynamics in human immunodeficiency virus type1 infection. Nature 1995;373:117–122.

World Health Organization. World AIDS Day 1995: shared rights, shared responsibilities. Press Release, WHO/17, 3, Geneva, Switzerland, March 1995.

Zhu T, Mo H, Wang N, et al. Selection for specific sequences in the external envelope protein of human immunodeficiency virus type 1 upon primary infection. J Virol 1993;67:3345–3356.

34 Autoimmune Diseases

N. Lawrence Edwards

BACKGROUND

Our current understanding of the immune system and the diseases associated with its aberration has evolved from the work of countless investigators over the past century. Initially conceived of as a mechanism to simply discriminate "infectious nonself" from "noninfectious self," the immune system is now recognized as a tightly regulated process by which the antibody response to both foreign and endogenous antigens requires the interaction of B cells, T cells, and specialized antigen-presenting cells (usually macrophages). In the early 1900s, the concept that the immune system might not be able to distinguish self from nonself lead to Erhlich's projection of a "horror autotoxicus," in which the individual's immune system would attempt to destroy itself. Burnett and other investigators in the mid-1900s postulated that diseases in which antibodies or immune competent cells reacted against normal body tissue were caused by the release of "forbidden clones" of immunologic cells and such rare occurrences were the result of faulty immune mechanisms.

Autoimmunity as we now understand it bears little resemblance to Erhlich's "horror autotoxicus," but rather is a common phenomenon that is often under normal immune regulation. In some circumstances this "self-attack" is beneficial, as in the natural clearing of exhausted red blood cells or in the response to cancer cells. These housekeeping and surveillance functions of the immune system are mediated by natural autoantibodies. The failure to distinguish these from pathogenic autoantibodies has lead to great confusion and slowed the progress in our understanding of autoimmune diseases.

Autoimmune diseases are conventionally grouped under the headings of organ-specific diseases and non-organ-specific (systemic) diseases (Table 34-1). In organ-specific autoimmunity, antigens peculiar to one cell type or tissue are the targets of an aggressive immune reaction. Examples of this type of targeting include the insulin-producing cells of the pancreas in type I diabetes mellitus, the acetylcholine receptors of muscle endplates in myasthenia gravis, and thyroid tissue in Hashimoto's disease. The non–organ-specific disorders include the rheumatic or connective tissue diseases. Because of their systemic manifestations, this group was the first to be associated with autoimmune mechanisms and they will be the subject of this chapter. The connective tissue diseases are frequently lumped together because of shared clinical and pathologic features (Table 34-2). However, the molecular mechanisms that initiate and maintain each of these conditions vary greatly.

From: *Principles of Molecular Medicine* (J. L. Jameson, ed.), ©1998 Humana Press Inc., Totowa, NJ.

In this chapter I will discuss the common clinical features of the connective tissue diseases and discuss the criteria used to diagnose and distinguish these conditions. These diseases of systemic autoimmunity are generally considered to be antigen-driven processes that occur in genetically predisposed individuals (Fig. 34-1). In the final sections of this chapter, I will discuss the genetic basis for susceptibility and the molecular mechanisms that foster and perpetuate antigenic stimulation. Finally, I will attempt to describe how new molecular understanding of immunity and autoimmunity may improve our ability to treat these conditions.

CLINICAL FEATURES

RHEUMATOID ARTHRITIS (RA) Rheumatoid arthritis is a systemic autoimmune disease in which initial and primary manifestations involve the joints and soft tissue structures of the musculoskeletal system. The hallmark of the disease is the chronic, symmetric polyarthritis with proliferative and destructive changes that progress over years to decades. The most universal feature of active RA is morning stiffness in the joints that lasts in excess of 1 h and may be present for most of the day. There are marked undulations in the clinical symptoms over time with periods of severe and debilitating inflammation followed by spontaneous partial abatement of symptoms. Virtually any joint in the body can be involved with RA although the distal interphalangeal joints of the hand and the thoracic and lumbar spine are usually spared. Associated extra-articular manifestations of RA include subcutaneous nodules and inflammatory changes in the lungs, pericardium, and eye. These manifestations may be severe and life-threatening and are correlated with the presence of rheumatoid factor in the serum and the MHC class II DR B1 allele, 0401. Other nonarticular manifestations, such as fatigue and malaise, are common to all individuals with RA.

Rheumatoid arthritis is the most common of the inflammatory arthritides, affecting between 1 and 2% of the world's adult population. Although it can be found worldwide, the prevalence of RA does vary among races with whites living in temperate climates being primarily affected. This may be related to MHC class II differences between blacks, Asians, and whites. Like most of the systemic autoimmune diseases, RA is predominantly a disease of women, with an overall female to male ratio of 2.5:1. There has been an apparently subtle shift in the epidemiology of RA during the past few decades with a tendency for later onset of disease activity. However, women of the child-bearing ages of 20–45 years remain the group at greatest risk for this disease.

Table 34-1
Disorders of Autoimmunity

Organ-specific disorders	*Non–organ-specific disorders*
Hashimoto's thyroiditis	Rheumatoid arthritis
Grave's disease	Systemic lupus erythematosus
Type I diabetes mellitus	Systemic sclerosis
Pemphigus vulgaris	Polymyositis and dermatomyositis
Thrombocytopenic purpura	Sjögren's syndrome
Myasthenia gravis	Various vasculitic syndromes
Multiple sclerosis	
Primary biliary sclerosis	
Pernicious anemia	

Table 34-2
Common Features of Connective Tissue Diseases

Predilection for symptoms in joints, muscles, and skin
Polyclonal hypergammaglobulinemia
Demonstrable circulating autoantibodies
Deposition of autoantibodies in multiple tissues and organs
Clinical improvement with corticosteroids or immunosuppressive drugs

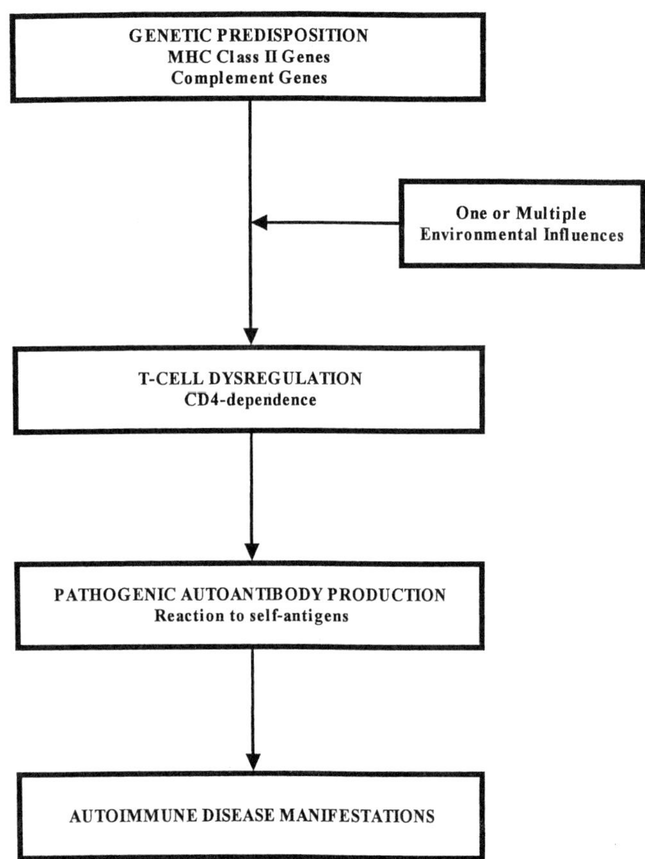

Figure 34-1 Immunologic and genetic basis of autoimmune disease.

SYSTEMIC LUPUS ERYTHEMATOSUS (SLE) Because of the high level of antibody expression in SLE, this disease is considered by many to be the prototypic autoimmune disorder. It is truly a multiorgan disease with marked variability in clinical manifestations as well as in morbidity and mortality. The organ systems most frequently involved include the skin, joints, kidneys, lungs, and brain. The gastrointestinal and cardiac systems may also be affected by the immune complex-mediated tissue injury associated with SLE.

The clinical spectrum of SLE ranges from patients having only mild "nuisance" symptoms of rash and arthritis to acute, life-threatening involvement of the central nervous system or kidneys. Although most patients with SLE require close clinical supervision, only a small fraction will develop potentially catastrophic illnesses. SLE is considered a rare disorder with a prevalence in the general population of 0.05%. This is primarily a disease of young women with a peak age of onset between 15 and 40 years. The overall female-to-male ratio is 5:1. The prevalence in young and middle-age women is 0.14%. For black and Hispanic women in this same age group, the prevalence is even higher at 0.4%. Although the exact genetics of SLE are not understood, it has been shown clinically to cluster in first-degree relatives of patients. SLE is concordant in 25–50% of monozygotic twins and 5% of dizygotic twins. Despite these high percentages, most cases of SLE are considered to be sporadic.

SYSTEMIC SCLEROSIS (PSS) Systemic sclerosis is a rare connective tissue disease that also goes by the names progressive systemic sclerosis and scleroderma ("hard skin"). Although the edematosis and indurative and atrophic changes in the skin are the most common and recognizable manifestations of PSS, most of the morbidity associated with the disease is because of vascular involvement of the gastrointestinal tract, lungs, kidneys, and heart. Underlying the pathogenesis of PSS is an increased fibrosis in skin and internal organs associated with marked increased production and deposition of collagens in the extracellular matrix leading to small vessel occlusive disease.

Cold and stress-induced vasospasm causing blanching or cyanosis of the digits (Raynaud's phenomenon) is the most common presenting manifestation of PSS and will eventually be present in 75–100% of these patients. The skin manifestations occur in stages, with the early diffuse edematous changes leading to the characteristic "hidebound skin." This leathery tightening of the skin can cause contractures in the extremities and limited facial mobility. In time, this "hard skin" gives way to some atrophy and softening. Disuse atrophy of muscles is a common feature, as is pulmonary fibrosis. Renal involvement is rare but may be life-threatening and is frequently associated with poorly controlled hypertension. Esophageal and other gastrointestinal hypomotility are common clinical problems that may affect the nutritional and health status of these patients.

PSS is probably best viewed as a spectrum of fibrosing disorders. On the milder end of the spectrum is a condition called the CREST syndrome. CREST is an acronym for the clinical manifestations of calcinosis of the skin, Raynaud's phenomenon, esophageal dysmotility, sclerodactyly (thickened skin over the digits) and telangiectasias appearing on the fingers, face, or mucosal surface.

The exact prevalence of PSS is difficult to assess because of the lack of a specific diagnostic test. However, recent estimates of the prevalence in this country range from 20 to 70 cases per 100,000 population (0.0004–0.001%). Women are more commonly affected than men with a female-to-male ratio similar to that of SLE. Peak incidence of onset is in the third and fourth decades of life. Most PSS appears to be idiopathic, but some sclerodermalike syndromes have been associated with environmental exposures (silica and vinyl chloride), certain drugs (bleomycin and methysergide), or adulterated food products (rapeseed oil in Spain and *L*-tryptophan in the United States).

POLYMYOSITIS AND DERMATOMYOSITIS (PM AND DM) PM and DM are inflammatory diseases of skeletal muscle that may present as distinct connective tissue diseases or as "overlap syndromes" with SLE, PSS, or RA. The dominant feature of these conditions is symmetric muscle weakness involving the proximal muscles of the upper or lower extremities. The muscle weakness may begin acutely, but more characteristically has an insidious onset. Patients will describe difficulty climbing stairs, getting out of chairs, or combing their own hair. If the disease goes unrecognized or untreated the patient can become bedridden and occasionally even require assisted ventilation.

DM and PM differ only in the appearance of skin lesions with DM. The skin manifestations may precede, follow, or appear concomitantly with the muscle symptoms. The only pathognomonic skin changes in DM are Gottron's papules. These are flat-topped, red-to-purple papules that occur over the interphalangeal joints of the hand. Another characteristic rash of DM is the heliotrope (lavender-colored) rash of the eyelids. The eyelids are usually edematous.

Malignant neoplasms are found in a higher than expected percentage of patients with PM and DM. The highest incidence of coincidental muscle disease and malignancy is with DM and is approximately 15%. This association is found only in adult populations and the most frequently associated cancers are adenocarcinomas of the lungs, ovaries, breasts, and stomach.

Inflammatory muscle diseases can occur at any age but have their peak onset in the fifth decade. Women are twice as likely as men to get either PM or DM. These conditions are rare with an annual incidence of 5–10 cases per million population.

SJÖGREN'S SYNDROME (SS) Sjögren's syndrome is a chronic autoimmune exocrinopathy primarily involving the lacrimal and salivary glands. Chronic inflammation of these glands results in dry eyes (xerophthalmia), dry mouth (xerostomia), and recurrent salivary gland pain and swelling. The persistent lack of good tear production results in destruction of corneal and bulbar conjunctival epithelium (keratoconjunctivitis sicca). This accounts for the ocular burning and itching and light sensitivity experienced by patients with SS. Sjögren's syndrome may occur as a primary connective tissue disease or as a secondary condition when associated with any of the organ-specific or non–organ-specific autoimmune diseases listed in Table 34-1. In the first 5–10 years of their disease, 50% of patients with primary Sjögren's syndrome will develop organ involvement in extraglandular sites, such as lungs, kidney, or the blood vessels of the central or peripheral nervous systems.

SS is the second most common systemic autoimmune disease, behind RA. Ninety percent of SS patients are women with a peak age of onset in the fourth and fifth decades of life. SS can affect all age groups and patients as young as 3 years old have been identified.

DIAGNOSIS

RHEUMATOID ARTHRITIS (RA) In 1987, the American Rheumatism Association introduced revised criteria for the diagnosis of RA. A person is said to have RA if they fulfill at least four of the seven criteria listed in Table 34-3. A requirement for the first four criteria is that these symptoms be present for at least 6 weeks.

Table 34-3
Classification Criteria for Rheumatoid Arthritis

Morning stiffness
Arthritis of three or more joint areas
Arthritis of hand joints
Symmetric arthritis
Rheumatoid nodules
Serum rheumatoid factor
Typical radiographic changes

Table 34-4
Classification Criteria for Systemic Lupus Erythematosus

Malar rash
Discoid rash
Photosensitivity
Oral ulcers
Arthritis
Serositis
Renal disorder
Neurologic disorder
Hematologic disorder
Antinuclear antibody
Other immunologic disorder

This provision helps to differentiate RA from various acute viral arthritides that may mimic RA in its earliest stage. As mentioned above, morning stiffness of at least 1 hour is present in most all patients with active RA. Prolonged stiffness after periods of rest is also common in other systemic autoimmune disorders. The 14 possible "joint areas" referred to in criterion 2 (Table 34-3) are the right and left proximal interphalangeal (PIP), metacarpal phalangeal (MCP), wrist, elbow, knee, ankle, and metatarsal phalangeal (MTP) joints. Further criteria are fulfilled if the same joints are involved on both the right and left side of the body and if the PIP, MCP, or wrist joints are affected.

Rheumatoid nodules are hard, rubbery subcutaneous masses measuring several millimeters to several centimeters in size and are present in 25–50% of individuals with RA. These nodules occur around joints or over bony prominences or extensor surfaces. Rheumatoid nodules occur almost exclusively in patients with a positive serum rheumatoid factor. Rheumatoid factors are the prototypic autoantibodies, although their role in the etiopathogenesis of RA remains unclear. They are present in 85% of patients with RA, as well as in approximately 3% of healthy persons. The prevalence of rheumatoid factor positively increases with age in the general population. The rheumatoid factors measured in clinical laboratories are IgM molecules that react with the Fc portion of IgG molecules. Rheumatoid factors may play an important "housekeeping" role in normal immune defense by promoting clearance of small antigen–antibody complexes (immune complexes) from the circulation or by enhancing removal of micro-organisms.

The final criterion in the diagnosis of RA is the presence of "typical" bony changes on radiographs of the hands and wrists. These bony changes include marked decalcification localized to areas around involved joints or actual erosions of the bony cortex adjacent to the joint.

SYSTEMIC LUPUS ERYTHEMATOSUS (SLE) A person is said to have SLE if they fulfill 4 of the 11 criteria listed in Table 34-4. These criteria may be present serially or simulta-

Table 34-5
Criteria for Classification of Systemic Sclerosis

Major criterion
Proximal scleroderma
Minor criteria
Sclerodactyly
Pitting scars at tips of fingers or loss of digital pad tissue
Bibasilar pulmonary fibrosis

neously over the course of observation. The first six criteria represent the distinguishing clinical manifestations of the disease whereas the remaining five are the laboratory parameters used to define SLE. The three cutaneous criteria of (1) a fixed erythematous rash over the bridge of the nose and cheeks; (2) the raised discoid lesions with atrophic scarring; and (3) the unusual sensitivity to sunlight are but a few of the dermal eruptions associated with SLE, but these three are the most specific for lupus. The oral and nasal mucosal ulcers are usually painless. The arthritis generally involves the same joints as RA but, unlike RA, the arthropathy of SLE tends to be nonerosive and nondestructive. Inflammation of the serosal surfaces of the pleura or pericardium are common manifestations of SLE.

Renal involvement with SLE is evidenced by either persistent proteinuria of greater than 0.5/d or the presence of cellular casts in the urine. Neurologic abnormalities are extremely common in SLE and vary from persistent headaches to coma and stroke. For the purpose of classifying SLE, however, only the symptoms of seizure and nonmetabolic psychosis are considered. The reduction of red blood cells, granulocytes, lymphocytes, or platelets by immune mechanisms is considered a criterion for diagnosing lupus.

The immunologic features of SLE include a positive antinuclear antibody test (ANA), a false-positive serologic test for syphilis, and the more specific serologies of antibodies against native (double-stranded) DNA or the Smith (Sm) nuclear antigen. The detection of ANAs by indirect immunofluorescence is highly sensitive for SLE (>98%) but not very specific because most other forms of systemic autoimmune diseases have circulating antinuclear antibodies. A negative ANA test is strong evidence against a diagnosis of lupus although a few patients with photosensitivity, arthritis, and Raynaud's phenomenon will occasionally fall into a diagnosis of seronegative SLE. Most of these individuals will demonstrate laboratory autoimmunity to other cellular (nonnuclear) components.

SYSTEMIC SCLEROSIS (PSS) The diagnosis of advanced PSS is quite obvious with the typical features outlined above. The clinical criteria used to classify this disease are listed in Table 34-5 and a person is said to have systemic sclerosis if the one major or at least two of the minor criteria are present. For these criteria to be meaningful, the localized form of cutaneous sclerosis, such as linear scleroderma, morphea, and eosinophilia fasciitis, need to be excluded. Proximal scleroderma refers to thickened, hidebound skin proximal to the metacarpophalangeal (MCP) joints, whereas sclerodactyly is similar skin tightening over the fingers.

Virtually all individuals with PSS have serum antinuclear antibodies. The specificity of several of the autoantibodies found in PSS is quite remarkable. Antibodies to the nuclear centromere are found almost exclusively in PSS and the CREST syndrome. Anti-topoisomerase I autoantibodies (also called SCL-70) are selective for PSS and tend to occur in subjects with diffuse cutaneous involvement. In addition to these two specific autoantibodies, PSS may be associated with numerous other nonspecific antibodies such as anti-ribonucleoprotein (anti-RNP), and SS-A (anti-Ro) and SS-B (anti-La).

POLYMYOSITIS AND DERMATOMYOSITIS (PM AND DM) The diagnosis of PM and DM is made in patients with proximal muscle weakness who also have at least two of the three laboratory abnormalities associated with these autoimmune muscle diseases. These laboratory findings are, (1) elevated serum levels of various muscle-associated enzymes; (2) myopathic changes on electromyography (EMG) and nerve conduction velocity (NCV); and (3) typical pathologic changes of inflammatory myositis on muscle biopsy.

Serum creatine kinase or aldolase is elevated in virtually all patients with PM and DM. In rare cases in which these serum muscle enzymes are not elevated, the other two diagnostic parameters should be abnormal. Even without treatment, muscle enzyme levels will fall in patients after they have lost substantial muscle mass.

The characteristic findings of autoimmune muscle disease on EMG or NCV are (1) small-amplitude, short-duration, polyphasic motor-unit potentials; (2) spontaneous fibrillations, positive spike waves at rest, and increased irritability; (3) bizarre, high-frequency complex discharges; and (4) absence of neuropathic changes. The muscle biopsy is the single most accurate parameter for establishing the diagnosis of PM and DM. However, the site of biopsy must be carefully chosen to select a muscle that is actively inflamed and weak although not having undergone clinical evidence of atrophy. Also sites of needle probes for EMG or NCV should be avoided. The characteristic pathologic changes are those of focal or diffuse inflammatory infiltrates of lymphocytes and macrophages surrounding muscle fibers and small blood vessels. The myocytes themselves show features of both degeneration and regeneration, such as size variation, fiber necrosis, and centralization of nuclei.

Antinuclear antibodies are detected in one-third to one-half of individuals with PM and DM. A speckled ANA pattern is usually associated with antibodies to ribonucleoprotein or antihistidyl-transfer RNA (t RNA) synthetase (Jo 1). Anti Jo 1 occurs primarily in patients with PM and significant pulmonary involvement. A nucleolar ANA pattern is usually associated with anti-PM and Scl and occurs in patients with the overlap disease of polymyositis and systemic sclerosis.

SJÖGREN'S SYNDROME (SS) The combination of dry eyes and dry mouth are quite common in elderly patients and persons taking various medications. The diagnosis of SS requires not only documenting significant dryness in the eyes and mouth but also evidence of autoimmunity on laboratory evaluation. Decreased lacrimal gland function is documented by an abnormal Schirmer's test. This test uses a strip of filter paper placed in the lower palpebral fissure. After 5 min, if 5 mm or less of wetting occurs, the test is abnormal. Oral dryness is usually documented by the patient's history of difficulty swallowing or chronic thirst and the absence of saliva pools in the mouth on physical examination.

Biopsy of the minor (lip) or major (parotid) salivary glands should reveal clusters of lymphocytic infiltrates with acinar atrophy. Other evidence of autoimmunity in SS is the frequent occurrence of autoantibodies. Rheumatoid factors are present in 70% patients with primary and secondary Sjögren's syndrome. Antinuclear antibodies are present in about 90% of patients. Antibodies to SS-A (anti-Ro) are detected in 55% of SS patients and may be associated with vasculitis. Antibodies to SS-B (anti-La) are more likely to be found in patients with secondary Sjögren's syndrome.

GENETIC BASIS OF AUTOIMMUNITY

The current theories of autoimmune susceptibility generally support a multifactorial paradigm with contributions from both genetic and environmental influences (Fig. 34-1). The relative importance of each of these factors may vary greatly among the different autoimmune diseases and may, in fact, differ substantially between individuals presenting with the same autoimmune disease. Familial clustering of single autoimmune diseases has been reported, but it is even more common to find kindreds in which multiple family members are affected with different autoimmune diseases. In monozygotic twin studies, the concordance rates for any autoimmune disease is less than 50% and in general the genetic contribution to autoimmune susceptibility is thought to be about 30%. This low level of penetrance for genetic risk factors in autoimmunity may be explained by the fact that otherwise genetically identical individuals have dissimilar immune systems as a result of unpredictable rearrangement of gene segments in the immunoglobulin and T-cell receptor genes. In addition, immunoglobulin genes undergo somatic mutation throughout life.

The major and minor genetic factors that regulate normal immune function also play key roles in permitting and perpetuating autoimmunity. These genes include those encoding the histocompatibility antigens, T-cell receptors, immunoglobulins, the complement molecules, and the genes affecting antigen processing and presentation. In addition to these genetically controlled systems, the sex-linked genes are also important in the pathogenesis of autoimmunity. The marked female predominance of most systemic autoimmune disorders offers circumstantiated evidence of an important endocrine-immune regulatory mechanism that is corroborated by in vitro and animal studies.

The major histocompatibility complex (MHC) genes are some of the most polymorphic in the immune system and impart a great deal of the individuality of responses to endogenous and foreign antigens. The MHC molecules have been divided into two classes: class I and class II. Class I molecules are present on the surface of most nucleated cells and bind short peptides arising from the cytoplasm of the cell. The MHC class I molecule "charged" with its peptide antigen alerts CD8 (cytotoxic) T cells to the presence of virus infection or an alteration of normal cells and thus provides important immune surveillance. Class II molecules are sometimes designated "DR" and are normally found on monocytes, B cells, and other antigen-presenting cells. MHC class II molecules bind larger peptides derived from extracellular proteins and interact with T-cell receptors on $CD4^+$ lymphocytes that regulate delayed hypersensitivity and immunoglobulin production. Most autoimmune diseases have been associated with genes in the class II region of the MHC. Hypotheses of how a particular MHC class II molecule could predispose to autoimmunity include altered binding of a "self" peptide increasing its autoantigenicity; altering the T-cell repertoire by generating peptides within the thymus; or the intrathymic deletion of T-cell populations that help control infection.

The T-cell receptor (TCR) complex is another extremely polymorphic immune system. The TCR complex is a heterodimer composed of polypeptide chains with variable and constant domains. There are two types of receptors: the abundant α-β heterodimers and the minor component of γ-δ heterodimers. The TCRs encoded by the γ and δ genes may play a role in the inflammatory response that characterizes autoimmunity. Some γ-δ T cells react with autologous antigens on stressed cells. Certain γ-δ T cells also recognize bacterial heat shock proteins without the usual requirement of an MHC molecule to present this antigen.

Table 34-6
MHC Gene Association with Autoimmune Diseases

Autoimmune disease	*MHC antigen*
Rheumatoid arthritis	DR4
	Dw4
	Dw14
	Dw15
Systemic lupus erythematosus	DR2
	DR3
	DQ1/DQ2
	C1q
	C1r-C1s
	C4 total
	C4A
Systemic sclerosis	DR5 (PSS)
	DR3 (PSS/PM)
Polymyositis and dermatomyositis	DR3
Sjögren's syndrome	DR3

Immunoglobulins are the products of differentiated, activated B cells and may be secreted from the cell as antibodies or may adhere to the surface of the B cell and function as receptors. The importance of immunoglobulins in helping to define autoimmunity is obvious because circulating autoantibodies are hallmarks of this group of diseases. However, the mere presence of autoantibodies does not necessarily imply a causative role in the etiopathogenesis of disease. Rheumatoid factors are unique autoantibodies whereas immunoglobulins serve both as antibody and antigen. Despite a high frequency of occurrence in autoimmune disease (especially rheumatoid arthritis), no pathogenic role for these autoantibodies has been proved.

In human fetal B cells certain light- and heavy-chain variable region genes are expressed in cell surface immunoglobulins much more frequently than would be anticipated from their representation in the genome. In fact, a single human κ light-chain variable region gene (Humkv 325) accounts for 10–20% of all κ rearrangements even though there are over 50 variable region genes in the κ locus. This particular κ variable gene is used to encode several important autoantibodies including rheumatoid factors and anti-DNA autoantibodies.

Genetic deficiencies of the early complement components may also predispose to autoimmunity. These complement proteins are important for rapid removal of immune complexes from the circulation and their deficiencies greatly enhance the damaging effects of immune complexes on vascular endothelium. The complement genes are inherited in an autosomal codominant fashion with null alleles encoding for nonsynthesis of the particular protein. The inheritance of a single null allele results in half normal levels whereas the inheritance of two null alleles for the same complement factor will result in a complete deficiency. Complete deficiencies of the complement proteins, C1, C2, and C4 are associated with autoimmune syndromes, including SLE, vasculitis, inflammatory myositis, and glomerulonephritis.

RHEUMATOID ARTHRITIS A clear association between an MHC haplotype and the development of clinical disease is difficult to establish. In 1978, Peter Stastny demonstrated a genetic risk for developing rheumatoid arthritis in individuals expressing the HLA-DR4 and -Dw4 class II proteins. Since the initial observations, multiple subtypes of DR4 have been recognized with some conferring susceptibility (Dw4, Dw14, and Dw15), while others (Dw10 and Dw13) do not (Table 34-6). The distinguishing region of the class II molecule that appears to impart susceptibility resides in the α-helical rims of the peptide-binding cleft. Specifically the RA-associated alleles of DR4 share an amino acid sequence of QK/RRAA at position 70–74 of the DR β chain. It should be stated that most people who carry this DR4 "RA epitope" will not develop any autoimmune disease and at least 10% of whites with RA do not express the QK/RRAA sequence. It remains unclear whether these DR4 subtypes actually enhance susceptibility to the initiation of synovitis or are responsible for imparting a more severe clinical expression in people who have the disease. The latter hypothesis appears to be gaining acceptance and other MHC and non-MHC genetic factors are probably responsible for actual disease initiation.

SYSTEMIC LUPUS ERYTHEMATOSUS (SLE) The first recognized genetic marker for SLE was the MHC class I allele B8. However, subsequent correlations have been stronger with the MHC class II DR2 and DR3 alleles. The DR3 allele was later proved to be in linkage disequilibrium with HLA-B8. These class II associations are strongest for whites of western European ancestry, but in other racial and ethnic groups no MHC associations have been detected. The class II DQ alleles, DQ1 and DQ2, exist in linkage disequilibriums with DR2 and DR3, respectively. Correlation with these markers are primarily for the SS-A (anti-Ro) and SS-B (anti-La) autoantibodies, which may be present in either SLE or Sjögren's syndrome. Patients with homozygous deficiencies of the complement proteins, C1q, C1r-C1s, C4, C3, or C2 have a high frequency of SLE or a lupuslike illness. In general, homozygous complement deficiencies are rare although the homozygous deficiency of C4 is more common. The C4A and C4B genes are located in the MHC region of human chromosome 6. The null allele of C4A exists in linkage disequilibrium with DR3. Interestingly, the homozygous and heterozygous deficiencies of the C4A complement protein are strongly associated with SLE even in ethnic populations in which no association between DR3 and SLE exists.

SYSTEMIC SCLEROSIS Although no clear MHC association has been observed for disease susceptibility in systemic sclerosis (PSS), there are several scleroderma-specific autoantibodies that do have class II associations. The anti-topoisomerase I (Scl-70) autoantibody is associated with DR5 and the polymyositis and scleroderma overlap marker, anti-PMScl, is associated with DR3.

NON-MHC GENETIC ASSOCIATIONS WITH AUTOIMMUNITY Dr. Betty Diamond and her colleagues have had a special interest in the origin and pathogenicity of anti-DNA antibodies in patients with SLE. These investigators generated monoclonal antibodies to the specific antigen-binding areas, or idiotypes, of anti-DNA antibodies from a patient with SLE. One of these anti-idiotypes, designated 3I, recognizes a specific determinant on the κ light chain of anti-DNA antibodies. The anti-DNA antibodies from 85% of 200 unrelated patients with SLE exhibited strong reactivity with 3I. These patients with SLE also had antibodies that reacted with 3I but were not directed against DNA. Healthy individuals use the 3I κ chain segments only rarely, and none are directed against DNA. In one study, a cluster of patients with familial SLE were examined for 3I reactivity in their immunoglobulins. High percentages of patients with SLE (6 of 8) and family members (15 of 19) had strong 3I reactivity. The 3I reactivity in family members without SLE was with antibodies that did not bind DNA. These data suggested that the preferential use of the immunoglobulin variable region gene, 3I, in the normal immune response may contribute to the genetic predisposition to SLE.

These same investigators have also examined the role of somatic mutation in autoimmunity. A mouse myeloma cell line, S107, produces an antibody against the pneumococcal cell wall antigen, phosphorylcholine (PC). A point mutation in the gene controlling the hypervariable region of the heavy chain of this antibody results in a single amino acid substitution. This mutation greatly alters the antigenic specificity of the antibody to that of low affinity for PC but with a newly acquired high affinity for DNA. This study demonstrates that a somatic mutation of immunoglobulin genes can convert antibacterial antibodies (protective immune response) to anti-DNA antibodies (pathologic response). Thus, part of the genetic predisposition to SLE may result from the preferential use in the normal immune response of specific variable region genes that require only a few mutations to acquire pathogenic autoreactivity.

MOLECULAR PATHOPHYSIOLOGY

If the entire genetic basis for each of the autoimmune diseases was known—including the preferential expressions or deletions of specific MHC and non-MHC genes—we would still be a long way from unraveling the critical events leading to the induction of autoimmunity. Most investigators now believe that autoimmunity results from a failure of immune tolerance for specific self-antigens and that this failure of tolerance is driven by repeated exposures to autoantigens. This premise leads to two important questions: What is the initiating antigen? And why does immune tolerance fail? While the answers to these questions remain unknown, many theories have been promoted.

Several lines of investigation now support the notion that tolerance at the T-cell level is critical to the prevention of autoimmunity. Three models have been promoted to explain how T-cell tolerance for self-antigens develops. Any one or all of these proposed schemes may be important in the normal regulation of the immune system. And any one or all of these schemes may be defective in autoimmune diseases.

The first model of tolerance for self-antigens states that T cells with self-reactivities undergo clonal deletion in the thymus. Direct evidence for this model has been presented by Kappler and colleagues in mouse thymus. Immature T cells from the bone marrow migrate to the thymus and develop an unselected repertoire of T-cell receptors on their surface because of unrestricted T-cell receptor gene rearrangements. This unselected T-cell repertoire comes in contact with thymic epithelial cells, which express histocompatibility complexes on their surface and function as antigen-presenting cells. The antigens being presented are ubiquitous self-antigens contained in the thymus. Any immature T cell with high affinity for the self-peptide/self-MHC on the thymic epithelium is passed on to thymic macrophages or dendritic cells for elimination. In this way, the T-cell repertoire that is allowed to

Table 34-7
Management of Rheumatoid Arthritis

General	Rest Physical therapy Occupational therapy
Symptomatic therapy	Aspirin or other NSAIDs Corticosteroids (systemic or intra-articular)
Second line agents	Antimalarials Sulfasalazine Intramuscular gold Methotrexate Azathioprine Cyclophosphamide Cyclosporine
Corrective surgery	Synovectomy Arthroplasty Arthrodesis

mature and leave the thymus has been selected for low T-cell reactiveness to self peptides. One problem with this scheme is that certain organ-sequestered self-antigens (e.g., from the brain, uveal tract, or testes) may never be in the thymus, and, therefore, T cells with high-affinity receptors for these peptides may exist in the peripheral lymphocyte population.

The second model of T-cell tolerance for self peptides theorizes that certain suppressor T cells are capable of controlling the reactiveness of T cells with self-recognizing receptors. This suppressor activity may be directed against specific antigen-combining sites in the T-cell receptor or may be directed against entire families of receptors that share similar variable regions (idiotypes). This model has been criticized because it is not clear which immune cell might exert this postthymic suppression.

The final model of self tolerance may be important for preventing certain organ-specific forms of autoimmunity. In immunologically privileged sites (such as the islet cells of the pancreas, central nervous system, and uveal tract) a natural deficiency of MHC class II antigen-presenting cells may be the primary defense against self-reactivities. If infection or other nonspecific inflammation was to attract class II-bearing cells to these sites, then autoimmunity may occur.

Immunologic tolerance is strongly influenced by both antigen availability and antigen presentation. An increased availability of self-antigens or an altered mode of self-antigen presentation may lead to autoimmunity. The availability of autoantigens may be increased by specific deficiencies in complement components or natural autoantibodies that would normally be involved in removal of cellular debris and immune complexes. Repeated exposure to certain environmental antigens may cause tissue destruction with increased release of self-antigens, or the environmental antigen may mimic certain host antigens leading to autoimmunity. Molecular mimicry is a much more common phenomenon in nature than previously thought. A microbe that mimics part of its host structure at the molecular level is at an advantage because it may avoid immunologic detection by the host. Alternatively, if an antibody response is generated against the microbe then these same antibodies may interact with host peptides, making them more antigenic and promoting autoimmunity. The most convincing example of molecular mimicry resulting in a disease is the role of β-hemolytic group A streptococci in causing acute rheumatic fever (ARF). All the relevant organs that are involved in clinical manifestations of ARF share crossreacting determinants with various components of the streptococcus cell wall. For instance, antibodies against the cell wall M protein will crossreact with synovial structures leading to arthritis. Similarly, antibodies to the specific streptococcus group A carbohydrate will crossreact with heart valves leading to tissue damage.

An experimental model of autoimmunity that involves molecular mimicry is the adjuvant arthritis induced in rats when they are injected with heat-killed mycobacteria suspended in mineral oil. The rats develop an arthritis 2–3 weeks after the injection that is histologically similar to human rheumatoid arthritis. The microbial antigen participating in this mimicry is a 9-amino acid epitope on a mycobacterium heat-shock protein (hsp65). The crossreactive host epitope appears to be in the proteoglycan component of the joint cartilage. The overall importance of molecular mimicry in the etiopathogenesis of human autoimmune diseases remains to be established.

MANAGEMENT AND TREATMENT

RHEUMATOID ARTHRITIS (RA) The ideal management of RA involves not only a complex selection of pharmacotherapeutics but additional input from physical and occupational therapists and orthopedic surgeons. Until recent years the early stages of mild to moderate RA were treated with rest, nonsteroidal anti-inflammatory drugs (NSAIDs), and occasionally intra-articular steroids. The "second-line" drugs were reserved for patients with severe disease or deformities (Table 34-7). A new therapeutic trend is to use these second-line or disease-modifying drugs sooner in the course of disease with the hope that suppressing the inflammatory process earlier will improve the long-term outcome for people with this disease. Antimalarials (hydroxychloroquine, 200–400 mg/d) and sulfasalazine (1500–4000 mg/d) are good adjunctive therapies but by themselves are usually not adequate to suppress active disease. Intramuscular gold salt injection has been a mainstay of treatment for RA for many decades. Despite the potential toxicity to the lungs, kidneys, and bone marrow, gold salt injections continue to be used because of their effectiveness. Over the past 10 years, low-dose weekly methotrexate has become the most widely used second-line agent in the treatment of RA. Oral dosing with 7.5–20 mg/wk yields excellent benefits in the majority of patients. Methotrexate toxicity in the liver and lungs needs to be monitored carefully.

Several products of recent molecular advances have already been used in trials as immunotherapies for RA. Various antilymphocytic monoclonal antibodies (MAb) are undergoing clinical trials to determine their efficacy in RA. CAMPATH-1H is a lymphocyte-depleting IgG humanized MAb directed against the surface antigen CD52, which is present on all lymphocytes and some monocytes. Patients with refractory RA developed immediate, profound, and sustained reduction in peripheral lymphocyte count after the intravenous infusion of CAMPATH-1H. Although side effects were frequent, 65% of the study patients did develop a clinical response. Surprisingly, there was no correlation between the level of lymphocyte depletion and the clinical response. Immunotherapy with a chimeric anti-CD4 MAb (cM-T412) significantly decreased the number of circulating CD4 cells, which are believed to be important in the initiation and perpetuation of autoimmunity. The reduction of $CD4^+$ T cells was associated with decreased synovial inflammation histologically and reduced expression of adhesion molecules in the synovium. However, clinical effectiveness has not been demonstrated with this form of therapy. The experiences with both CAMPATH-1H and anti-CD4 MAb suggest that a treatment strategy directed at depleting circulating lymphocytes may have insufficient effects in the target tissue to result in clinical improvement of the disease process.

SYSTEMIC LUPUS ERYTHEMATOSUS (SLE) The improvements in medical management of SLE during the past 30 years has greatly reduced morbidity and mortality, so that now the 15-year survival rate is at least 90%. Part of this improvement can certainly be attributed to the more effective and judicious use of corticosteroids and cytotoxic agents. Advances in general medical support of patients with severe renal, pulmonary, and hematologic problems have also been key factors in our improved management of SLE.

For patients with photosensitivity, avoidance of sun exposure is essential. Other more chronic rashes may respond to topical corticosteroids or hydroxychloroquine. Non-life-threatening manifestations of SLE, such as low-grade fever, myalgia, arthritis, or pleuritis, are most commonly treated with nonsteroidal anti-inflammatory drugs or low-dose prednisone (less than 10 mg/d or less than 20 mg on an alternate day dosage). High dose corticosteroids (1–2 $mg \cdot kg^{-1} \cdot d$ oral prednisone or 1 g/d of iv methylprednisolone daily for 3 days) are usually reserved for acute fulminant nephritis, CNS disease, hemolytic anemia or thrombocytopenia. Occasionally, intravenous cyclophosphamide (0.75–1.0 g/m^2 body surface) is given monthly for severe and unresponsive cases. Other cytotoxic agents, such as azathioprine and chlorambucil, are sometimes used instead of cyclophosphamide, although their effectiveness remains controversial.

SYSTEMIC SCLEROSIS (PSS) Scleroderma or PSS is certainly one of the most difficult management problems in all of the connective tissue diseases. Unlike most other forms of autoimmunity, PSS does not generally respond well to corticosteroid therapy and in fact prednisone may be deleterious because of its enhancing effects on blood pressure. Raynaud's phenomenon can be effectively treated with hand warming, stress reduction, and calcium channel blockade (nifedipine). Esophageal dysmotility can be improved with metoclopramide and octreotide acetate. The sclerodermatous skin changes can be debilitating, but little therapeutically can be done other than preventing dryness. The only treatment measure that has ever been shown to improve survival rates in PSS is an aggressive approach to blood pressure control. Using calcium channel blockers or angiotensin converting enzyme (ACE) inhibitors, even borderline or mildly elevated blood pressures should be treated. Target diastolic pressures of 70 mmHg or less and systolic pressures of 125 mmHg or less may prevent the hypertensive renal crisis that is almost universally fatal in this disease.

POLYMYOSITIS AND DERMATOMYOSITIS (PM AND DM) Corticosteroids are the mainstay of therapy for PM and DM. When the disease is newly diagnosed and active, prednisone is begun in doses of 60–100 mg/d in divided doses. When a therapeutic response has been obtained and creatine phosphokinase (CK) levels have returned to normal, the prednisone is consolidated into a single morning-time dose and the steroid is gradually tapered. If the disease proves to be recalcitrant (requiring high-dose prednisone for greater than 3 months) or if the patient is showing evidence of early steroid toxicity, another immunosuppressive or cytotoxic agent may be used for the steroid-sparing effect. Methotrexate in initial doses of 7.5–10.0 mg/wk orally or azathioprine (2–3 mg/kg body weight) can be given to allow a more rapid steroid taper. It is important to remember that corticosteroids may actually cause muscle weakness and atrophy. In the setting of high-dose prednisone and worsening muscle symptoms, a steroid myopathy should be considered. Even with optimal medical care the patient's strength will lag far behind other evidence of disease improvement such as normalization of serum muscle enzyme levels. A muscle-strengthening program should be started after muscle inflammation has been controlled with medication.

SJÖGREN'S SYNDROME (SS) In most patients with primary SS, therapy is directed at relief of "sicca symptoms," i.e., dry eyes and dry mouth. Artificial tears should be used every 2–3 hours throughout the day to prevent keratoconjunctivitis sicca. The treatment of dry mouth is more problematic and patients are seldom seen without a glass of water in their hands. Sugar-free lemon drops can help stimulate whatever salivary gland function remains. Systemic corticosteroids and cytotoxic drugs are generally reserved for patients with life-threatening extraglandular involvement of the brain, lungs, or kidneys. Through the course of therapy, patients should be evaluated for the development of lymphoma or Waldenstrom's macroglobulinemia. These malignant complications of SS may occur years to decades after the initial diagnosis of Sjögren's syndrome.

FUTURE DIRECTIONS

Molecular technologies and genetic-based therapies will soon have an impact on the treatment of the autoimmune diseases. I described in the preceding section how monoclonal antibodies are currently being used to selectively delete lymphocyte subsets. Other forms of immune manipulation that are currently being developed include cytokines, cytokine antagonists, and recombinant proteins that block adhesion or migration of immune cells. Several drugs that interfere with genetically mediated T-cell activation are already undergoing clinical trials for various autoimmune diseases. These include cyclosporine and FK506, which inhibit T-cell differentiation and replication. The efficacy of these drugs in early trials is encouraging but their toxicities and lack of specificity of immune suppression make it clear that we are still a long way from the breakthrough remedies we are seeking for autoimmune disease.

The therapeutic dilemma in autoimmunity is that as long as the autoantigens and autoreactive lymphocytes persist, the autoimmune disease will be self-perpetuating. All of the new therapies mentioned so far in this section may effectively interfere with the inflammatory process created by the interaction of autoantigens, class II MHC molecules, and T-cell receptors. However, these therapies would have to be given for the patient's lifetime or the autoimmunity would rekindle. The truly futuristic approaches to therapy will include ways of eliminating the source of autoantigens and selectively eliminating the pathogenic population of autoreactive lymphocytes.

Another therapeutic approach for the future would require a much more complete identification of the susceptibility genes responsible for each of the autoimmune diseases. Monitoring genetically susceptible individuals for preclinical serologic evidence of autoimmunity may permit treatment options that would not be possible or appropriate once target tissue damage has occurred. Advances in gene therapy may allow for selective DNA-based therapeutics, such as antisense drugs, that could combine with the susceptibility genes and downregulate their expression.

SELECTED REFERENCES

Carson DA. Genetic factors in the etiology and pathogenesis of autoimmunity. FASEB J 1992;6:2800–2805.

Chervonsky AV, Wang Y, Wong FS, et al. The role of Fas in autoimmune diabetes. Cell 1997;89:17–24.

Condemi JJ. The autoimmune diseases. JAMA 1992;268:2882–2892.

Davidson A, Shefner R, Livneh A, Diamond B. The role of somatic mutation of immunoglobulin genes in autoimmunity. Annu Rev Immunol 1987;5:85–108.

Ehrlich E; Boldman C, trans. Collected Studies on Immunity. New York: John Wiley and Sons, 1906;586.

Hall R. Molecular mimicry. Adv Parasitol 1994;34:81–132.

Hohlfeld R, Meinl E, Weber F, et al. The role of autoimmune T lymphocytes in the pathogenesis of multiple sclerosis. Neurology 1995; 45:S33–S38.

Kappler JW, Roehm N, Marrrack P. T cell tolerance by clonal elimination in the thymus. Cell 1987;49:273–282.

Kretz-Rommel A, Duncan SR, Rubin RL. Autoimmunity caused by disruption of central T cell tolerance. A murine model of drug-induced lupus. J Clin Invest 1997;99:1888–1896.

Krieg AM, Steinberg AD. Retroviruses and autoimmunity. J Autoimmun 1990;3:137–166.

LaCava A, Nelson JL, Ollier WER, et al. Genetic bias in immune responses to a cassette shared by different microorganisms in patients with rheumatoid arthritis. J Clin Invest 1997;100:658–663.

Lippman SM, Arnett FC, Conley CL, Ness PM, Meyers DA, Bias WB. Genetic factors predisposing the autoimmune diseases. Am J Med 1982;73:827–840.

Masi AT, Rodnan GP, Medsger TA Jr, et al. Preliminary criteria for the classification of systemic sclerosis (scleroderma). Arthritis Rheum 1980;23:581–590.

Nepom GT, Ehrlich H. MHC class II molecules and autoimmunity. Annu Rev Immunol 1991;9:493–525.

Odeh M. New insights into the pathogenesis and treatment of rheumatoid arthritis. Clin Immunol Immunopathol 1997;83:103–116.

Pascual V, Capra JD. Human immunoglobulin heavy chain variable region genes: organization, polymorphic, and expression. Adv Immunol 1991;49:1–74.

Rassenti LZ, Pratt LF, Chen PP, Carson DA, Kipps TJ. Autoantibody encoding kappa L chain genes frequently rearranged in lambda L chain expressing chronic lymphocytic leukemia. J Immunol 1991; 147:1060–1066.

Rose LM, Latchman DS, Isenberg DA. BCL-2 and Fas, molecules which influence apoptosis, a possible role in systemic lupus erythematosus. Autoimmunity 1994;17:271–278.

Schwartz BD. Infectious agents, immunity and rheumatic diseases. Arthritis Rheumat 1990;33:457–465.

Stastny P. Association of the B-cell alloantigen DRw4 with rheumatoid arthritis. N Engl J Med 1978;298:869–874.

Tan EM, Cohen AS, Fries JF, et al. The 1982 revised criteria for the classification of systemic lupus erythematosus (SLE). Arthritis Rheum 1982;25:1271–1277.

Vyse TJ, Kotzin BL. Genetic basis of sytemic lupus erythematosus. Curr Opin Immunol 1996;8:843–851.

Webb SR, Hutchinson J, Sprent J. Mls antigens: immunity and tolerance. In: Biological Significance of Superantigens. Fleischer B, ed. Chem Immunol, Basel: Karger, 1992;55:87–144.

35 Allergic Diseases

Asthma as a Model

SUSAN M. MACDONALD

BACKGROUND

Allergic disease and asthma affect approximately 12 million people in the United States and account for 1% of total health care costs. Between 1965 and 1983, hospitalizations of adults with asthma increased 50%, whereas hospitalizations of children increased 200% (*see* Chapter 36). Additionally, both the lay press and scientific publications report that, from 1985 to 1991, mortality from asthma has increased. The prevalence, the tremendous cost, the increased mortality, as well as the time lost from work or school, mandate investigations to curtail or prevent these diseases.

Previously, asthma was viewed as a respiratory disease of acute airway obstruction related to bronchospasm. The mast cell and its products, histamine, sulfidopeptide leukotrienes, and prostaglandins, became the primary focus for pharmacologic interventions. More recently, asthma has been defined (by the Expert Panel Report 2, *Guidelines for Diagnosis and Management of Asthma*, NIH publication) as a disease of the airways characterized by "airway inflammation, airway hyperresponsiveness, and reversible airway obstruction." Antigen exposure in an allergic asthmatic individual results in an acute reaction resulting in a decrease in forced expiratory volume in 1 second (FEV_1). This acute reaction subsides, but if the initial antigenic stimulus is sufficiently high, there is a recrudescence of symptoms termed the late-phase reaction (LPR) some 6–24 hours later. With its bronchial inflammation and enhanced bronchial responsiveness, the LPR is a useful tool to explore the pathogenesis of asthma.

The LPR is characterized by edema and erythema in the skin, and increased resistance to air flow in the nose and lungs. There are several reasons why the LPR may be a more appropriate model of allergic inflammation than is the acute response to antigen. The duration, susceptibility to oral steroids, and characteristic infiltration by eosinophils, neutrophils, and basophils resembles that of chronic allergic inflammation. The role of specific cell types in the LPR has not been proven, but several lines of evidence suggest that the basophil, and not the mast cell, plays a significant role in the LPR. First, the mast cell mediators that are found associated with the symptoms of the acute reaction, i.e., histamine, prostaglandin D_2 (PGD_2), tryptase, and leukotriene C_4 (LTC_4) are clearly different than those found in the late reaction, i.e., histamine and LTC4 but no PGD_2 or tryptase. Basophils do not contain tryptase or PGD_2. Second, by morphologic and flow-cytometric evidence, basophils clearly appear during antigen-induced LPR in skin chambers and in the nose. Furthermore, the IgE-bearing cells in late-phase nasal lavages express CD18, an adhesion molecule found primarily on basophils and other leukocytes, but not on the mast cell. Additionally, basophils have been identified as the histamine-containing cells in bronchoalveolar lavage fluids obtained during the late response. Of the alcian blue-positive cells that increased 15-fold in the antigen versus the saline site in late-phase bronchoalveolar lavage fluids, 96% were morphologically and functionally defined as basophils. Finally, basophils have been shown to increase dramatically in the airways of those subjects experiencing asthmatic episodes and in biopsies of patients dying of asthma. These data would suggest that the infiltration of proinflammatory cells, including basophils, is of critical importance in the LPR of allergic asthmatic diseases.

The pathogenesis of the late reaction is complex and not well-understood. An initial event in the human response to antigen might well be mast cell degranulation and release of mediators that, in turn, attract inflammatory cells and upregulate adhesion molecules on endothelium and leukocytes. The basophils and eosinophils that infiltrate are known to be activated or primed to be hyperresponsive to stimuli. Elevated levels of histamine and neutrophil chemotactic factor have been found in the blood hours after antigen bronchoprovocation. Using an in vivo model of intranasal antigen challenge, mediators such as histamine have been shown to be elevated in nasal washes coincident with symptoms in those individuals experiencing an LPR. In both the skin and nasal models, this late mediator release is not caused by continued antigenic stimulation. Furthermore, cytokines known to potentiate mediator release, such as interleukin-1 (IL-1), IL-3, and granulocyte-macrophage colony-stimulating factor (GM-CSF), have been found to be released locally during the cutaneous allergic LPR. Thus, mediator release clearly occurs in vivo during the late response to antigen, and there can be selective recruitment of cells that seem to be important in this late response. However, the actual stimulus for activation remains unknown.

Although mediators and cells have been identified in the LPR, two key questions remain: (1) what is the stimulus for basophil activation during the late response? and (2) why do only some people have this response? These questions prompted our initial investigation of a histamine-releasing factor (HRF). HRF was first reported as a factor that was present in late-phase skin blister fluid that caused basophil histamine release. This factor was not present in early blister fluids when antigen was present. Subsequently,

From: *Principles of Molecular Medicine* (J. L. Jameson, ed.), ©1998 Humana Press Inc., Totowa, NJ.

such a factor was found to exist in nasal lavages obtained during the LPR and that these HRFs have functional and physicochemical characteristics similar to those of HRF from macrophages and from the macrophagelike cell line, U937. One working hypothesis is that these factors are related and that this family of molecules is responsible for stimulation of basophils during the IgE-mediated LPR in an allergic asthmatic individual.

Much of what is known concerning the pathogenesis, epidemiology, diagnosis, and management of asthma has been reviewed previously. The purpose of this chapter is to update the reader with regard to new molecular discoveries that might impact on the thinking and eventual treatment of this disease. The emphasis of these new discoveries will relate to the LPR as mentioned above. As previously stated, this LPR clearly mimics the inflammation of chronic allergic asthma. Additional topics will address the genetics of asthma (although no current gene therapy is available), the relatively new concept of heterogeneity of the IgE molecule, and clinical trials of new therapies for asthma. All of this will be discussed in the context of the traditional management of asthma.

CLINICAL FEATURES

For comprehensive reviews of the clinical features and diagnosis of asthma, the reader is referred to references listed at the end of this chapter. It is now well-established that there are several epidemiologic parameters that demonstrate asthma is an increasing problem. The prevalence is high, approximately 5% in adults and 10% in children. The incidence, morbidity, and mortality of asthma have been increasing. The actual reasons for these increases are not defined. Several factors, such as decreased access to medical care for those of lower socioeconomic status, increased indoor allergens, in modern central air-conditioned homes, such as house dust mite, the increased incidence of smoking mothers, and the exposure to viral infections at day care centers and in the preschool environment are several potential factors that contribute to the apparent rise in morbidity and mortality of this disease.

Asthma is classically divided into two types: extrinsic, synonymous with allergic asthma, intrinsic, not associated with atopy. There is an interesting correlation among bronchial reactivity, the diagnosis of asthma, and the total serum level of immunoglobulin E (IgE). In fact, the presence of allergic disease associated with asthma ranges from 50 to 90%, with the highest association existing in children. The existence of a history of allergies and the exposure to an environmental allergen that is associated with exacerbation of the symptoms of asthma point to allergies as having an important role in the pathogenesis of asthma.

The symptoms of asthma—wheezing, dyspnea, cough, and chest tightness—can be explained by airway obstruction. This airway obstruction is caused by edema, mucous production, epithelial cell sloughing, smooth muscle constriction, and mucosal inflammation. The inflammatory changes that are seen in asthma include cellular infiltrates, including basophils, eosinophils, mast cells, and mononuclear cells; epithelial cell damage and cellular mediators, including histamine, sulfidopeptide leukotrienes, tryptase, prostaglandins, kinins, eosinophil-derived proteins, and several cytokines, such as IL-4, IL-5, and GM-CSF. This inflammatory process can lead to enhanced vascular permeability, mucous production, smooth muscle contraction, and reflex bronchospasm.

DIAGNOSIS

Asthma is episodic in nature, with asymptomatic periods intermingled with symptomatic exacerbations. Table 35-1 has a list of causes of asthma and conditions that exacerbate it. A careful history should be taken to detect any of these factors. In the majority of patients, a thorough history by the physician will lead to the diagnosis of asthma. Table 35-2 illustrates other considerations that are important for the differential diagnosis of asthma. Because asthma is characterized by reversible bronchial obstruction and airway hyperresponsiveness, it is very useful to document the presence of these hallmarks. Formal pulmonary function tests showing a decrease in the forced expiratory volume in 1 s (FEV_1) and a decrease in the forced vital capacity (FVC) can be used to document obstruction. This decrease in FVC can be attributed to air trapping in the asthmatic lung. As a general rule, the ratio of FEV_1 to FVC is less than 0.80. Normally, the decrease in these two parameters is readily reversible with the inhalation of a β_2-adrenergic bronchodilator. The major drawback of formal pulmonary function testing is the cost. This can be overcome to some degree with the use of an inexpensive hand-held peak flow meter that measures the peak expiratory flow rate, which correlates with FEV_1. The other advantage of this device is the ability of the patient to use it at home to monitor exacerbations of asthma and effectiveness of therapy. In some patients it may be necessary to demonstrate airway hyperresponsivesness with the use of a standardized methacholine or histamine inhalation challenge. A detailed list of all the laboratory tests useful in diagnosing asthma is beyond the scope of this chapter but is summarized in Table 35-3.

GENETIC BASIS OF DISEASE

The ability to identify the genes responsible for human diseases has markedly expanded during the last several years. Indeed, as illustrated in other chapters, genes associated with cystic fibrosis, myotonic dystrophy, neurofibromatosis, Duchenne's muscular dystrophy, and Huntington's disease have been identified. Atopic allergies and asthma are complex diseases and it is unlikely that a single gene will be responsible for allergic diseases or asthma. Instead, the interaction of different classes of genes combined with environmental factors are more likely to be responsible. For a comprehensive review of the potential genes that are likely to be associated with allergic asthma, the reader is referred to the references.

There are three major categories of genes that appear to be associated with asthma. The first are genes that are disease-specific, and that may be responsible for increasing the inflammatory response leading to hyperreactive airways. The second type of genes determine the ability of an individual to synthesize total IgE antibody. As previously mentioned, several epidemiologic studies have shown that the risk of asthma is related to the total serum IgE level. Furthermore, in patients with very low IgE levels, no asthma was found. Finally, a third group of genes, the immune response (*Ir*) genes, determines the ability of patients to make specific immune responses, such as IgE antibody to specific inhaled allergens. Classical *Ir* genes map to the major histocompatibility complex. It is this group of genes that is influenced by environmental factors, such as the level of exposure to indoor allergens and seasonal allergens.

APPROACH TO GENE MAPPING Molecular genetic analysis of human diseases involves two approaches, forward and reverse genetics. The forward approach examines candidate genes.

Table 35-1
Causes of Asthma and Exacerbating Conditions

Causes	*Exacerbating conditions*
Allergy	Infections
Allergic asthma	Bronchiolitis
Allergic bronchopulmonary aspergillosis	Upper respiratory tract infections
Industrial-occupational or environmental exposure	caused by viruses (influenza, rhinovirus, respiratory syncytial virus)
Chemicals (e.g., toluene diisocyanate, TDI)	Bronchitis
Allergens (e.g., plicate acid)	Sinusitis
Vasculitis (Churg-Strauss allergic angiitis and granulomatosis)	Gastroesophageal reflux
Idiopathic (intrinsic)	Pregnancy
Aspirin or other nonsteroidal anti-inflammatory agents (associated with nasal polyps, Samter's triad)	Hyperthyroidism
Sulfiting agents	Psychological stress
β-adrenergic antagonists	
Exercise	

Modified from Kaliner M, Lemanske R, Rhinitis and asthma. JAMA 1992;268:2807–2829. Copyright 1992, American Medical Association.

Table 35-2
Differential Diagnosis of Asthma

More common	*Less common*	*Rare*
Aspiration (gastroesophageal reflux)	Cystic fibrosis	α1-Antitrypsin deficiency
Bronchiectasis	Laryngeal edema	Allergic bronchopulmonary aspergillosis
Cardiac failure ("cardiac asthma")	Laryngeal or tracheal obstruction	Carcinoid syndrome
Chronic bronchitis and emphysema	Pulmonary embolism	Foreign bodies
Factitious wheezing		Hyperventilation syndrome
Sarcoidosis		Löffler's syndrome
Tumors in the central airways		Tropical eosinophilia

Modified from Kaliner M, Lemanske R, Rhinitis and asthma. JAMA 1992;268:2807–2829. Copyright 1992, American Medical Association.

Before discussing the forward approach it is necessary to describe the likely candidate genes associated with asthma. The reverse genetic approach, also called positional cloning, tries to establish linkage between a disease and anonymous DNA markers. Both of these approaches use the polymerase chain reaction (PCR) to amplify DNA markers.

An example of the latter approach is the Cookson and Hopkin hypothesis. Their initial family studies suggested an autosomal dominant mode of inheritance of atopy. In genetic linkage studies the putative atopy gene was linked to the DNA marker, D11S97, which is located on chromosome band 11q13. Their data showed that the β-subunit of the high-affinity IgE receptor on chromosome 11 is maternally linked to atopy. Furthermore, a common polymorphism of this receptor subunit, Leu 181–Leu 183, was identified in 4.5% of the population in a rural town of Australia. The children who inherited this variant from their mothers were atopic and had an increased risk of positive skin-prick test to house dust mite and grass pollen, antigen-specific IgE antibody levels, and bronchial hyperresponsiveness. Thus, this is one particular chromosomal localization of a gene associated with atopy.

To discuss the forward approach to gene mapping, the candidate genes associated with allergies and in particular allergic asthma must be discussed. To accomplish this, it is necessary to summarize the T helper cell, Th1 versus Th2 dichotomy. Th1 cells are associated with cell-mediated immunity, including delayed-type hypersensitivity, whereas Th2 cells facilitate the humoral immune response, including IgE antibody production. The cytokine production profiles of these T helper cell subsets are very different. Th1 cells produce IL-2 and interferon-γ (IFN-γ), whereas Th2 cells secrete IL-4, IL-5, and IL-13.

In humans, IL-4 or IL-13 is absolutely required for the immunoglobulin heavy-chain isotype switching that produces ε germline transcripts. Interestingly, basophils, which are an important cell type in the allergic LPR, also produce IL-4 and IL-13. IFN-γ downregulates IgE production. IL-5 is important for eosinophil activation and recruitment, and the eosinophil is another cell found in large numbers in allergic LPR. It is noteworthy that the genes encoding IL-13, IL-4, IL-5, and interferon regulatory factor 1 map to a cluster of a few million basepairs on chromosome 5. Because of the pivotal role that IL-4 and IL-13 play in IgE production,

Table 35-3
Utility of Various Tests in the Evaluation of Patients Suspected of Having Asthma

Test	*Diagnostic utility*
Pulmonary function testing	
Peak flow monitoring ± bronchodilators	Document pulmonary function, its variability, and response to therapy
FEV_1/FVC ± bronchodilators	Distinguish reversible vs fixed obstruction or restriction
Residual volume, total lung capacity	Distinguish obstruction vs restriction
Diffusion capacity (DL_{co})	Document impaired gas exchange in COPD and interstitial lung disease
Flow volume loops	Distinguish extra- vs intrathoracic obstruction
Histamine/methacholine challenge	Document airway hyperreactivity
Exercise testing	Document oxygen desaturation, exercise-induced asthma
X-rays	
Chest X-ray	Document hyperinflation, infiltrates, hilar lymphadenopathy, tumors, heart failure
Esophagram	Document reflux
Sinus X-rays	Document acute sinusitis
Sinus CT	Document chronic sinusitis, polyposis
Blood testing	
Total IgE	Allergic bronchopulmonary aspergillosis
Total eosinophil count	Often elevated in asthma
Aspergillus precipitants	Allergic bronchopulmonary aspergillosis
α1-Antitrypsin levels	Emphysema
Angiotensin converting enzyme	Sarcoidosis
Arterial blood gases (oximetry)	Document degree of hemoglobin desaturation, oxygenation
Other tests	
Skin testing (RAST)	Evaluate allergic status
Esophageal pH monitoring	Document gastroesophageal reflux
ECG	Document arrhythmia, ischemia, cor pulmonale, left ventricular hypertrophy
Sputum culture/Gram stain/cytology	Document infection, eosinophilia
Sweat chloride test	Assess for cystic fibrosis
Serum immunoglobulin levels	Assess for humoral immunodeficiency

Reproduced with permission from Bochner BS, Togias A, Lichenstein M. The outpatient management of asthma, in Wilson JD, Braunwald E, Isselbacher KJ, Martin JB, Fauci AS, Kasper DL, eds., Harrison's Principles of Internal Medicine. New York: McGraw-Hill;1993; pp. 1–15.

COPD, chronic obstructive pulmonary disease; CT, computed tomography; ECG, electrocardiogram; FEV_1, forced expiratory volume in 1; FVC, forced vital capacity.

likely candidate genes for atopy would be in this IL-4 gene cluster on chromosome 5, in particular 5q31.1.

As previously mentioned, there is a striking correlation between the total serum IgE level and the prevalence of asthma. Using the candidate gene approach, Marsh and coworkers measured concentrations of total serum IgE and analyzed 349 sib pairs. These data demonstrated linkage between total serum IgE concentrations and a marker in the IL-4 gene cluster located in chromosome 5q31.1. Markers mapping outside 5q31.1 showed no evidence of linkage. These findings are supported by other groups who showed evidence for linkage of various markers in the 5q31 and q33 region with total IgE level and an association between the total serum IgE level and a polymorphism in the IL-4 gene.

In conclusion, although the genetics of asthma are complex, there is evidence to suggest a link between asthma and genes in the IL-4 gene cluster. Work is ongoing to investigate other candidate genes for atopy.

MOLECULAR PATHOPHYSIOLOGY OF DISEASE

As mentioned in the Background section of this chapter, the LPR mimics the chronic inflammation that is the hallmark of asthma. Many laboratories have been working to decipher the etiology of this LPR. As previously noted, basophils and eosinophils are increased in the LPR, and the stimuli that cause mediator release from these cells have been under intense investigation.

During the last decade, there has been an explosion of interest in cytokines that either augment basophil histamine release or are direct agonists (Table 35-4). One type of HRF was shown to interact with the IgE molecule, and that only a subpopulation of atopic donors basophils are responsive to this HRF. Work by MacDonald et al. designated the

Table 35-4
Histamine Releasing Factors

Direct agonists
IgE-dependent HRF
IL-3
MCP-1
MCP-3
MIP-1α
RANTES
CTAP III
NAP-2
IL-8
Augment histamine release
IL-1α and ß
IL-3
IL-5
IL-6
IL-7
c-kit ligand

NAP-2, neurotrophil-activating peptide 2; CTAP-III, connective tissue activating peptide III; MCP, monocyte chemotactic protein; RANTES, regulated on activation, T cell expressed and secreted; MIP-1α, macrophage inflammatory protein-1 alpha.

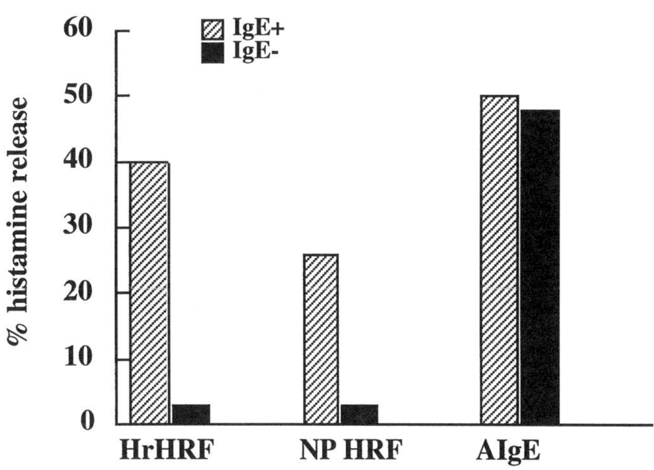

Figure 35-1 Representation of the histamine release produced by various stimuli: human recombinant histamine-releasing factor (HrHRF), native, nasal pool HRF (NP HRF) and polyclonal anti-IgE antibody (AIgE) on lactic acid-treated basophils passively sensitized with IgE$^+$ (hatched bars) or IgE$^-$ (closed bars).

IgE that interacts with this HRF, IgE$^+$, and therefore, by definition, the remaining IgE molecules that do not interact with HRF are IgE$^-$.

In the context of purifying this IgE-dependent HRF, and with the availability of recombinant cytokines, it became imperative to investigate whether our HRF was a known, stimulatory cytokine. Of the interleukins that caused direct histamine release from basophils, namely IL-3 and IL-8, it was evident that the kinetics of release and the lack of crossdesensitization of basophils differentiated these interleukins from our HRF, and, indeed, their mechanism of release is IgE-independent. The possibility also developed that the chemokines, a family of low molecular weight (8–11 kDa) molecules, might be involved in the LPR. The chemokines are divided into two groups, C-X-C or α chemokines, found on chromosome 4, including PF-4, IL-8, NAP-2, and CTAP-III, and the C-C chemokines or β chemokines, found on chromosome 17, including MCP-1, MCP-3, RANTES, and MIP-1α. It is clear from recent reports that MCP-3 is a potent histamine secretagog, as is MCP-1. RANTES is an eosinophil chemokine attractant, and to a lesser degree, a histamine-releasing agent. However, again, the kinetics of histamine release caused by these stimuli are very rapid and do not mimic that induced by the IgE-dependent HRF.

PURIFICATION OF THE IgE-DEPENDENT HRF The IgE-dependent HRF was purified from 50 L of supernatant from the human U937 monocyte-macrophage cell line and subcloned. It was found to have a 94% homology to p21, a protein from mouse tumor cells, as well as identity to p23, the human homolog. Both molecules were cloned on the basis of their abundant expression in tumor cells, and no function could be ascribed to either molecule. The cDNA for rp21 was kindly supplied by Drs. Margaret Koots and George Brawerman of Tufts University, Boston, MA. Primers were designed and the PCR product was expressed in *Escherichia coli* as protein fused to glutathione-*S*-transferase (GST). The fusion protein was purified by affinity chromatography using immobilized glutathione. The same primers were used to generate the human rp23 from the U937 cell line, which was also expressed as a GST fusion protein and affinity purified.

Both recombinant fusion proteins, and their cleaved products, caused IgE-dependent histamine release from IgE$^+$ donors' basophils. Figure 35-1 shows a comparison of IgE-dependent histamine release using three stimuli: human recombinant HRF (HrHRF), native, nasal lavage-derived HRF (NP HRF), and anti-IgE antibody (AIgE). Cell surface IgE was removed using lactic acid, and the cells were then passively sensitized using sera containing either 200 ng of known IgE$^+$, or IgE$^-$. On washing and stimulation, the IgE-sensitized basophils did not support release to HrHRF or to NP HRF, whereas histamine release occurred to both stimuli only when IgE$^+$ was placed on the basophils. As expected, release induced by anti-IgE did not discriminate between IgE$^+$ and IgE$^-$.

In a separate series of Western blot experiments, a polyclonal rabbit antibody generated against cleaved human recombinant p23 recognized mouse recombinant p21, human recombinant p23, native HRF from the U937 cell line, and native HRF from supernatants of peripheral blood mononuclear cell cultures. Thus the recombinant HRF produced in *E. coli* was identical to the native material found in vivo.

As previously mentioned, basophils infiltrate tissues and are thought to play an important role in the pathogenesis of chronic allergic diseases. This concept is supported by recent studies showing that basophils generate and secrete high levels of IL-4, a proinflammatory cytokine having immunoregulatory properties that affect many different cell types that interact during allergic inflammation. The secretion of IL-4 protein from basophils, however, unlike that described for histamine release, seems more dependent on IgE-dependent stimulation, with little evidence thus far that other, non-IgE-dependent physiologic stimuli can induce secretion of this cytokine. Because the recombinant protein caused IgE-dependent basophil histamine release, MacDonald et al. asked whether this HRF could also cause IL-4 protein production. In basophil cell cultures challenged for 4 h with recombinant HRF, the secretion of IL-4 correlated with histamine release in 14 donors ($r = 0.9$, $p = 0.001$). Figure 35-2 shows histamine release and IL-4 production in three IgE$^-$ donors and three IgE$^+$ donors. As is evident, none of IgE$^-$ donors' cells released histamine or IL-4 protein when stimulated with recombinant HRF. In contrast, his-

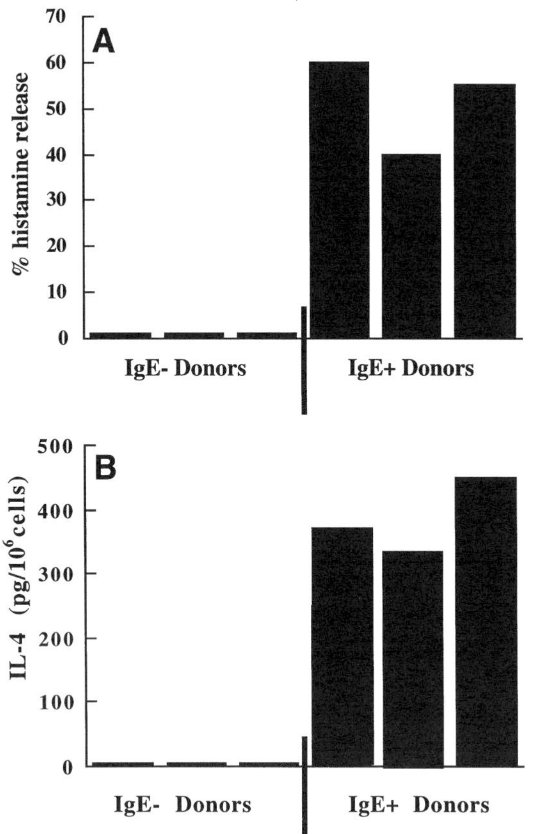

Figure 35-2 The % histamine release **(A)** and the IL-4 protein production **(B)** in basophils stimulated with 4×10^{-7} *M* HrHRF from 3 IgE^- and 3 IgE^+ donors is shown.

tamine release and IL-4 production occurred with the IgE^+ donors' basophils stimulated with HRF. These data strongly support the concept that the IgE-dependent HRF has the potential to play a key role in the pathogenesis of human allergic disease.

CLINICAL RELEVANCE Chemokines with IgE-independent histamine-releasing activity have been found in vivo; MCP-1 levels were increased, and IL-8 levels decreased, in resting nasal lavages of symptomatic patients during the appropriate pollen season, and bronchoalveolar lavage fluids of asthmatic subjects have higher levels of RANTES and MIP-1α than do those of normals. Furthermore, MCP-1 expression has been shown by immunohistochemical techniques to be increased in bronchial tissue from asthmatic patients. The IgE-dependent HRF also has been detected in human respiratory secretions, late-phase skin blister fluids, and nasal lavages. Knowing that the IgE-dependent HRF caused basophil histamine release in approximately 50% of allergic donors and that it is found in vivo in late-phase blister fluids and nasal lavages, it was questioned whether responsiveness to HRF was associated with disease severity. In a previous study of 55 ragweed-sensitive hay fever patients, a significant correlation ($p < 0.02$) was found between the intensity of symptoms in the LPR and basophil histamine release to the IgE-dependent HRF. Also, when an IgE-dependent, platelet-derived HRF was investigated, basophils from allergic asthmatics, and not from nonallergic asthmatics, responded to this stimulus. Of those allergic subjects who responded in vitro, methacholine sensitivity and symptoms of asthma were highly correlated ($r = 0.87$, $p < 0.005$).

Sampson et al. showed that production of HRF also is associated with the clinical status of food allergy and atopic dermatitis. Using blood from food-allergic children with atopic dermatitis, they found that the children's basophils have a high spontaneous release of histamine and their mononuclear cells spontaneously produce an IgE-dependent HRF in culture. When these children are placed on an avoidance diet that eliminates the offending food allergen, they improve clinically, their basophils no longer spontaneously secrete histamine, and their mononuclear cells no longer spontaneously produce HRF.

With the availability of recombinant material, MacDonald et al. examined the lymphocytes of allergic and nonallergic patients for the generation of HRF mRNA and protein. Twelve patients (four allergic IgE^+, four allergic IgE^-, and four nonallergic) were recruited. Peripheral bood mononuclear cells (PBMCs) were cultured for HRF protein production and processed for mRNA extraction and subsequent reverse transcription PCR (RT-PCR) for HRF message. The quantity of mRNA for HRF, when compared with β-actin, did not appear different among the groups. However, the bioactivity of the IgE-dependent HRF protein produced by mononuclear cells from IgE^+ donors, when tested on lactic acid-treated cells passively sensitized with IgE^+ serum was greater than in the allergic IgE^- patients and the nonallergic subjects. Thus it appears that all individuals make mRNA for HRF but atopics are more effective at translating it to protein.

CONCLUSION The gene for the IgE-dependent HRF has been subcloned. The recombinant protein has biologic activity and shows a band of identity with the native material from nasal lavage and peripheral blood mononuclear cell supernatants by Western blots. The availability of recombinant material will enable us to determine its exact relationship to the severity of allergic disease and to determine the nature of IgE heterogeneity. Currently, several hypotheses that could explain the heterogeneity of the IgE molecule (i.e., IgE^+ vs IgE^-) include a genetic polymorphism, differential glycosylation, or alternatively spliced forms of IgE found in atopic sera. Investigations are in progress to determine whether HRF binds IgE^+ directly or alternatively interacts with its own receptor.

MANAGEMENT AND TREATMENT

For more details, the reader is referred to the Selected References. Additionally, specific strategies for treatment are outlined in Guidelines for the diagnosis and Management of Asthma. The first line of treatment is patient education. The patient must understand that asthma is episodic in nature and that certain situations, such as exposure to an allergen or an upper respiratory infection, can exacerbate the disease. Patient recognition of a change in symptoms can lead to early therapy that can control the inflammation of asthma. Because asthma has triggers specific to the individual, avoidance of the particular allergen is recommended. Pets should be removed from the home if the family is in agreement. In the case of dust mite sensitivity, mattresses and pillows should be encased in plastic and, if possible, carpets removed. The following nonspecific irritants should be avoided: cigaret smoke, cold air, air pollution, and, in some patients, perfumes. Because viral infections are a frequent cause of asthma exacerbations, influenza vaccination is recommended.

Pharmacologic treatment of asthma has changed in the last 10 years. It is now appreciated that bronchodilators that provide immediate symptomatic relief do not alleviate the inflammatory process involved in asthma. For this reason, the treatment of the

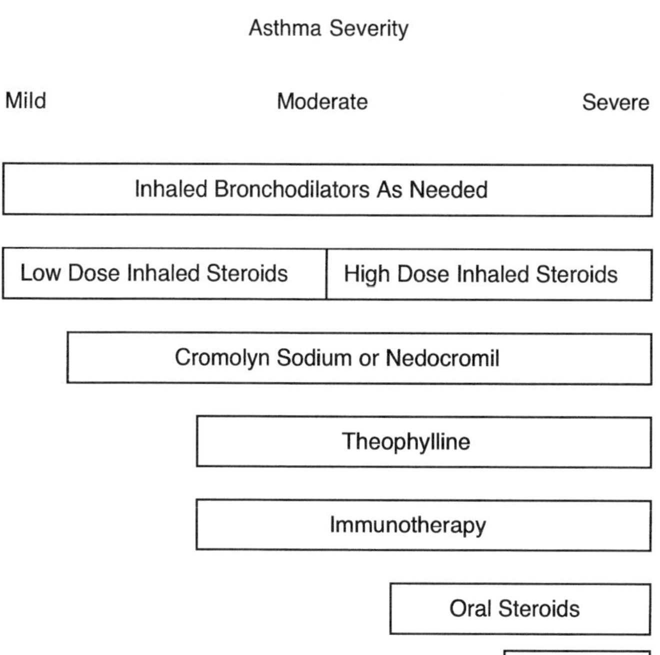

Figure 35-3 Pharmacologic management of asthma. Treatment choices are used in a stepwise fashion based on asthma severity. (Reproduced with permission from Bochner B, et al. The outpatient management of asthma. In: Harrison's Textbook of Internal Medicine, 1993.)

asthmatic patient needs to be individualized according to the severity of disease. Figure 35-3 outlines the current approach. The use of inhaled bronchodilators alone is for patients with mild disease with symptoms occurring less than once or twice a week. This therapy is made more effective by use of a metered dose inhaler with a spacer that increases the amount of inhaled medication reaching the lower airways by reducing particle size and can reduce side effects such as candidiasis. The available selective β_2 agonists in the United States are albuterol, metaproterenol, terbutaline, bitolterol, pirbuterol, and isoetharine. Their duration of action is 6 h. Salmeterol, a longer acting β2 agonist, has recently become available. For mild disease, these agents are used "as needed." If the patient uses the inhaler more than three times per day, then addition of an anti-inflammatory medication is necessary to control the disease. Corticosteroids are the most potent anti-inflammatory treatment. The newer inhaled corticosteroids, such as fluticasone have much less systemic side effects than oral corticosteroids. As a general rule, oral short-acting steroids, such as prednisone, are used only in patients whose disease is not controlled. Cromolyn sodium is another locally acting treatment with apparent anti-inflammatory activity. If it is used, one must wait 6–10 weeks before a full effect is seen. Often cromolyn sodium is tried in children before to initiating corticosteroids. It has been proven to be efficacious for exercise-induced asthma. Nedocromil sodium, another anti-inflammatory medication, has the same indications for use as does cromolyn. Theophylline, a methylxanthine with bronchodilating effects, and a previous mainstay in the treatment of asthma for a century and a half, is now used as a third-line agent for patients who have not responded to inhaled bronchodilator or anti-inflammatory agents. An obvious inconvenience with the use of this medicine is the necessity to monitor blood levels, which should be in the range of 5–15 μg/mL. Also the side effect profile necessitates setting levels for individual patients.

FUTURE DIRECTIONS

The management and therapy of asthma is likely to change in the future. Several investigational treatments are in place. Cytokines such as IL-4 and IL-13 are important in immunoglobulin switching to IgE, and trials in severe combined immunodeficient mice (SCID) transplanted with human fetal thymus and bone have demonstrated suppression of ongoing IgE synthesis when treated with IL-4 and IL-13 receptor antagonists. It is logical to assume that these successful trials in an animal model will progress to clinical trials in man.

Several pharmaceutical companies have ongoing clinical trials with pharmacologic agents that block leukotrienes. These compounds are aimed at directly antagonizing the actions of these mediators or inhibiting the enzyme, 5-lipoxygenase, that is responsible for the production of leukotrienes. These treatments appear promising and might lead to additional medications that could be used in conjunction with known drug therapy.

Classic immunotherapy has been used with varied efficacy in some patients with allergic asthma. This treatment, which was first reported almost a century ago, is hampered by the availability of purified allergen extracts. A new approach in this field is the use of purified peptide epitopes of the known allergen. In mice, administration of these peptides results in T-cell tolerance such that T cells no longer proliferate to the allergen, and no longer secrete the cytokines responsible for the maintenance of allergic inflammation. These peptides do not react with specific IgE antibody and therefore do not produce allergic symptoms. The advantage of this treatment is the ability to administer much larger quantities of the peptides vs the intact allergen. These studies are already in phase 2 clinical trials and may provide an exciting new form of therapy.

Finally, the use of an anti-IgE antibody is in clinical trials. At first glance, the concept of using an anti-IgE antibody to treat allergic asthma might seem contradictory. Two groups have produced monoclonal antibodies that recognize epitopes on the IgE antibody molecule when it is bound to B cells but not when it is bound to the high-affinity IgE receptor, FχεR1. Thus these monoclonal antibodies would recognize IgE bound to B cells and IgE in the circulation, but not IgE bound to mast cells or basophils. The hypothesis is that treatment with this type of antibody will clear IgE from the circulation and downregulate IgE synthesis from B cells. In clinical trials these anti-IgE antibodies have been shown to reduce IgE without producing symptoms of allergic disease. Currently ongoing clinical trials are designed to test the efficacy of this treatment in the early stages and LPR of allergic disease. The future of treatment of allergic asthma might be drastically altered by any of the above-mentioned therapies.

SELECTED REFERENCES

Alam R, York J, Boyars M, et al. Detection and quantitation of RANTES and MIP-1 alpha in bronchoalveolar lavage (BAL) fluid and their mRNA in lavage cells. J Allergy Clin Immunol 1994;93:183.

Bochner BS, Togias A, Lichtenstein LM. The outpatient management of asthma. In: Harrison's Principles of Internal Medicine. Wilson JD, Braunwald E, Isselbacher KJ, Martin JB, Fauci AS, Kasper DL, eds. McGraw-Hill, 1993; pp. 12–15.

Carballido JM, Schols D, Namikawa R, et al. IL-4 induces human B cell maturation and IgE synthesis in SCID-hu mice. J Immunol 1995; 155:4162–4170.

Chang RW, Davis FM, Sun N-C, Sun CRY, MacGlashan J DW, Hamilton RG. Monoclonal antibodies specific for human IgE-producing B cells: a potential therapeutic for IgE-mediated allergic diseases. Biotechnology 1990;8:122–126.

Dahinden CA, Geiser T, Brunner T, et al. Monocyte chemotactic protein 3 is a most effective basophil- and eosinophil-activating chemokine. J Exp Med 1994;179:751–756.

Holgate ST. Asthma genetics: waiting to exhale. Nat Genet 1997;15: 227–229.

Diaz-Sanchez D, Zhang K, Nutman TB, Saxon A. Differential regulation of alternative 3' splicing of ε messenger RNA variants. J Immunol 1995;155:1930–1941.

Kaliner M, Lemanske R. Rhinitis and asthma. JAMA 1992;268:2807.

Koshino T, Arai Y, Miyamoto Y, et al. Mast cell and basophil number in the airway correlate with the bronchial responsiveness of asthmatics. Int Arch Allergy Immunol 1995;107:378,379.

Kuna P, Lazarovitch M, Kaplan AP. Studies of MCAF/MCP-1, RANTES, MIP-1 alpha, IL-8, histamine, ECP and tryptase in allergic rhinitis sufferers and asymptomatic subjects. J Allergy Clin Immunol 1994;93:321.

Langdon J, Anders K, Lichtenstein LM, MacDonald SM. Atopics translate mRNA for the IgE-dependent histamine releasing factor (HRF) more effectively than normals. J Allergy Clin Immunol 1995;95:336.

MacDonald SM. Histamine releasing factors and IgE heterogeneity. In: Allergy: Principles and Practice. Middleton E, Reed CE, Ellis EF, Adkinson NF, Yunginger JW, Busse WW, eds. St. Louis, MO: Mosby Yearbook:1993; pp. 1–11.

MacDonald SM, Lichtenstein LM, et al. Studies of IgE-dependent histamine releasing factors: heterogeneity of IgE. J Immunol 1987; 139:506–512.

MacDonald SM, Rafnar T, Langdon J, Lawrence LM. Molecular identification of an IgE-dependent histamine-releasing factor. Science 1995;269:688–690.

Marsh DG. Genetics of atopy and IgE. In: Frank MM, Austen KF, Claman HN, Unanue ER, eds. Samter's Immunologic Diseases. Boston, MA: Little, Brown, and Co. 1995; pp. 1257–1272.

Marsh DG. Molecular genetic studies of atopic allergy. In: Eibl, Huber, Peter, Wahn, eds. Symposium in Immunology IV. Berlin:Springer-Verlag, 1995; pp. 65–74.

Marsh DG, Neely JD, Breazeale DR, et al. Linkage analysis of IL4 and other chromosome 5q31.1 markers and total serum immunoglobulin E concentrations. Science 1994;264:1152–1156.

Postma DS, Bleecker ER, Amelung PJ, et al. Genetic susceptibility to asthma—bronchial hyperresponsiveness coinherited with a major gene for atopy. N Engl J Med 1995;333:894–900.

Ruffilli A, Bonini S. Susceptibility genes for allergy and asthma. Allergy 1997;52:256–273.

Saban R, Haak-Frendscho M, Zine M, et al. Human FcERI-IgG and humanized anti-IgE monoclonal antibody MaE11 block passive sensitization of human and rhesus monkey lung. J Allergy Clin Immunol 1994;94:836–843.

Schroeder JT, MacGlashan DW, Kagey-Sobotka A, White JM, Lichtenstein LM. IgE-dependent IL-4 secretion by human basophils. The relationship between cytokine production and histamine release in mixed leukocyte cultures. J Immunol 1994;153: 1808–1817.

Schroeder JT, Lichtenstein LM, Langdon J, Kagey-Sobotka A, MacDonald SM. An IgE-dependent recombinant histamine releasing factor induces IL-4 secretion from human basophils. J Exp Med 1996;183:1265–1270.

Sheffer AL, et al. Guidelines for the diagnosis and management of asthma. Bethesda, MD: National Institutes of Health; 1991, US Department of Health and Human Services, publication 91–3042.

Sousa AR, Lane SJ, Nakhosteen JA, Yoshimura T, Lee TH, Poston RN. Increased expression of the monocyte chemoattractant protein-1 in bronchial tissue from asthmatic subjects. Am J Respir Cell Mol Biol 1994;10:142–147.

Warner JA, Pienkowski MM, Plaut M, Norman PS, Lichtenstein LM. Identification of histamine releasing factor(s) in the late phase of cutaneous IgE-mediated reactions. J Immunol 1986;136:2583–2587.

Wilkinson J, Holgate ST. Candidate gene loci in asthmatic and allergic inflammation. Thorax 1996;51:3–8.

PULMONOLOGY V

SECTION EDITOR:

MICHAEL J. HOLTZMAN

36 Asthma

MICHAEL J. HOLTZMAN, DWIGHT C. LOOK, MICHAEL F. IADEMARCO, DOUGLAS C. DEAN, DEEPAK SAMPATH, AND MARIO CASTRO

INTRODUCTION

Asthma is often defined as a lung disease with three characteristics: reversible airway obstruction, increased airway responsiveness (hyperreactivity) to inhaled stimuli, and airway inflammation. The disease is generally a chronic condition, and it affects between 7 and 20 million Americans, 2 to 5 million of whom are children. The impact of asthma on any individual is highly dependent on the control of the disease that can be achieved by elimination of precipitating factors and the effective use of medical therapy. Despite improved understanding of these factors and the availability of more effective drugs for treatment of the condition, the prevalence of asthma, the numbers of hospitalizations for asthma, and deaths attributed to the disease have all been increasing, especially among minority and inner-city populations. At least some of the increases in mortality and morbidity are based on poor use of medication and, in particular, inadequate long-term treatment with anti-inflammatory drugs. Nonetheless, the marked increases in frequency and severity of asthma during the past decade serve to underscore the need for a better understanding of the molecular basis for the disease.

Perhaps the single most important conceptual "advance" in defining molecular mechanisms of asthma has been the recognition that it is an inflammatory disease. Evidence that inflammation is an important component of asthma was evident even in early descriptions of the cytopathology and histopathology of the disease. For example, analysis of sputum samples and airway tissue indicated that epithelial desquamation and airway eosinophilia were invariably present during acute attacks. However, the critical role of inflammation as a cause of the abnormal physiology was only firmly established in two important ways: first, in experimental models of the disease induced by nonallergic and allergic stimuli, asthmatic pathophysiology was closely linked to the development of an inflammatory response; second, in studies of asthmatic subjects under baseline conditions and during spontaneous or provoked flares of the disease, evidence of abnormal airway function was again closely correlated with the presence of inflammatory cells and mediators. Both types of studies were strongly influenced by the development of bronchoscopic techniques for obtaining airway tissue and histochemical techniques for analyzing the types of inflammatory cells and mediators in the tissue. In the context of the three characteristics of asthma (airway obstruction, hyperreactivity, and inflammation), morphologic studies of asthma now appear to indicate that an overexuberant inflammatory response is what causes the hyperreactivity of airway end-organs (e.g., increases in airway smooth muscle contraction and mucous gland secretion), and this hyperreactivity may in turn be responsible for the characteristic asthmatic attacks of airway obstruction.

From: *Principles of Molecular Medicine* (J. L. Jameson, ed.), ©1998 Humana Press Inc., Totowa, NJ.

Accordingly, the challenge that now confronts researchers and clinicians is twofold: first, defining the biochemical mechanisms responsible for asthmatic airway inflammation, and then determining the pharmacologic means to more effectively inhibit inflammatory pathways or potentiate anti-inflammatory ones. Thus, this chapter is aimed mainly at reviewing prominent biochemical pathways responsible for airway immunity and inflammation. Defining these pathways has provided initial clues to the identity of genes activated in the course of asthmatic disease. Consequently, we also review initial studies aimed at linking the loci for these immune-response genes to the asthmatic phenotype.

MECHANISMS OF AIRWAY INFLAMMATION

The concept that inflammation leads to airway hyperreactivity and narrowing has led to a widening search for the types of inflammatory cells and mediators responsible for the cascade of events linking the initial stimulus to the final abnormality in airway function. Cell types implicated in the development of airway inflammation include immune cells (including basophils, eosinophils, mast cells, lymphocytes, neutrophils, and macrophages) as well as sentinel parenchymal cells (including airway epithelial cells, vascular endothelial cells, and airway smooth muscle cells). Cell–cell interactions are attributed to classes of mediators that include lipids, proteases, peptides, cytokines, and chemokines. It is not yet possible to integrate all of this information into a single model for the development of airway inflammation; however, a useful framework for this system may be based on the classification of T-cell responses to allergic and nonallergic stimuli that are inhaled into the airway.

Using a scheme that was developed in murine models of the immune response, T-cell-dependent responses may be classified into T-helper-1 (Th1) or Th2 types. Th1 cells characteristically mediate delayed-type hypersensitivity reactions and selectively produce interleukin (IL)-2 and interferon (IFN)-γ, whereas Th2 cells promote B-cell–dependent humoral immunity and selectively

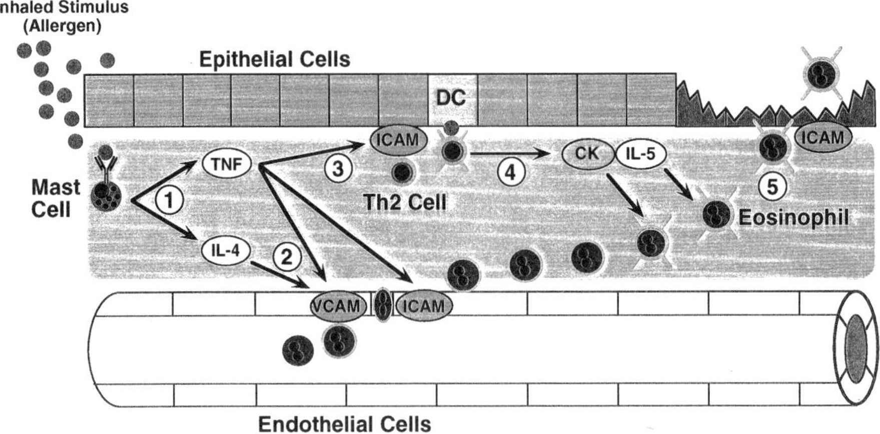

Figure 36-1 Cell–cell interaction cascade for a Th2-type response in the airway. Proposed steps include: (1) inhaled allergen stimulates mast cells (by crosslinking surface IgE) and Th2 cells (via antigen-presenting dendritic cells, DC) to cause release of IL-4 and TNF-α; (2) IL-4 and TNF-α synergistically induce VCAM-1 expression on the endothelium causing VLA-4-dependent eosinophil adhesion; (3) TNF-α also induces ICAM-1 expression on the endothelium for Mac-1- or LFA-1-dependent transendothelial migration; (4) activated T cells also release chemokines (CK) and IL-5 that in combination with IL-4 and TNF-α promote recruitment, survival, and activation of eosinophils; and (5) activated eosinophils release additional IL-4, IL-5, and TNF-α that autoamplifies eosinophil influx and local production of eosinophil-derived arachidonate products, matrix metalloproteinases, toxic peptides, and other mediators contributing to epithelial damage.

produce IL-4 and IL-5. In the simplest case, a Th2-type reaction may underlie the bronchial hyperreactivity and inflammation characteristic of the delayed response to allergen inhalation and (by extension) the allergen-dependent inflammatory response in patients with extrinsic asthma. Alternatively, a Th1-type reaction may be responsible for the hyperreactivity and inflammation that results from exposure to nonallergic stimuli (such as respiratory viruses). However, this dichotomous concept may not be completely accurate for several reasons. First, the separation between these two types of immune responses is less distinct in humans than in mice, and some evidence suggests that both responses may be triggered by allergic and nonallergic stimuli. In addition, there is cross regulation of the two types of responses, so that a Th2-derived mediator (e.g., IL 10) may serve to downregulate Th1-type responses, and a Th1-derived mediator (e.g., IFN-γ) may downregulate Th2-type responses. Nonetheless, the classification still forms a useful basis for beginning to organize a molecular scheme of airway inflammation.

TH2-TYPE T-CELL RESPONSE The percentage of asthma that is caused by an abnormal sensitivity to inhaled allergen is uncertain, but there is little question that allergen is a primary stimulus of airway inflammation and asthma in at least some subjects. Thus, it is natural to propose that a Th2-type allergic response, already incriminated in other types of antibody-dependent allergic responses, may also be invoked in the IgE-driven response to inhaled antigens that is characteristic of atopic individuals with asthma. This possibility is supported by evidence of increased numbers of activated T cells exhibiting a Th2 phenotype in airway tissue from atopic asthmatic subjects.

A scheme for the cascade of cell–cell interactions during a Th2-type response in the airway is depicted in Fig. 36-1. In this scheme, inhaled allergen provides the trigger for the first step in the cascade, and allergen triggering may occur in two ways: (1) allergen is bound to the surface of IgE-bearing mast cells for antibody (Ab) crosslinking and subsequent production or release of mast cell mediators; or (2) allergen is taken up by an antigen-presenting cell (e.g., a dendritic cell recruited to the mucosal epithelium) followed by antigen presentation to the T-cell receptor (TCR) and TCR-dependent cytokine production. In the context of a scheme for airway inflammation calling for recruitment of immune cells, it would appear that some of the most critical mediators are derived from the cytokine class (e.g., IL-4, IL-5, and tumor necrosis factor-α [TNF-α]). In this regard, studies of asthmatic airway tissue indicate that: (1) mast cells and Th2 cells generate IL-4, IL-5, and TNF-α; (2) the level of cellular production is increased relative to nonasthmatic subjects; and (3) the levels can be further increased by inhalation challenge with antigen.

IL-4 Generation By comparison with other cytokines (especially IL-2), little is known concerning the regulation of IL-4 production. In other cases, the control of cytokine levels may depend on the status of cytokine gene activation and the consequent rate of transcription, and in turn, the level of transcription depends on specific DNA–protein interactions within the gene promoter region. In the case of IL-4, only preliminary information has been obtained incriminating the involvement of specific transcription factors that bind to the promoter region and trigger IL-4 gene activation. Initial work indicated that a nuclear factor of activated T cells (NFAT) may exert some control over the T-cell specificity of IL-4 production, but this factor does not yet explain the capacity of T cells to regulate IL-4 production during inflammation. As described in more detail below, a member of a new family of transcription factors designated the STAT family (for *s*ignal *t*ransduction and *a*ctivation of *t*ranscription) may serve to regulate IL-4 production. The newest member of this family (designated Stat6) binds to the IL-4 gene promoter region (suggesting it may regulate transcription of IL-4) and appears to mediate the capacity of IL-4 to activate its target genes (e.g., those controlling IgE production). Thus, Stat6 may serve to create an autoamplifying loop whereby its activation leads to further IL-4 production and consequently further Stat6 activation. Such a positive feedback loop is consistent with observations that IL-4 is a product of Th2 cells and, once produced, IL-4 also promotes further Th2-type T-cell differentiation.

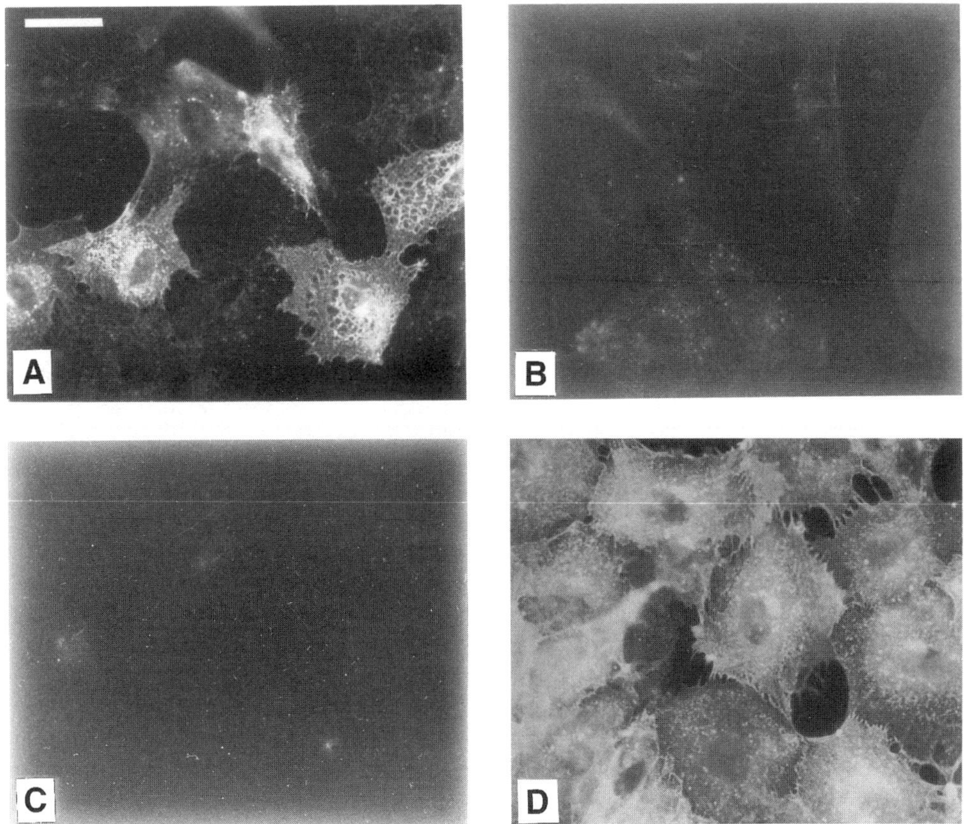

Figure 36-2 IL-4 and TNF-α synergistically induce expression of VCAM-1 on vascular endothelial cells. Human umbilical vein endothelial cell (HUVEC) monolayers were stimulated with 10 ng/mL TNF-α (**A**), 0.2 ng/mL TNF-α (**B**), 100 U/mL IL-4 (**C**), or both 0.2 ng/mL TNF-α and 100 U/mL IL-4, and then fixed in methanol, pretreated with 2% fish gelatin to block nonspecific Ig binding, and incubated with Abs against VCAM-1. Primary antibody binding was detected with FITC-conjugated goat antimouse IgG. Bar = 40 μm.

IL-4–Dependent Recruitment of Immune Cells IL-4 has a number of actions that influence the development of airway inflammation. As noted above, it is critical for the gene activation underlying differentiation of B cells into Ab-forming cells and consequent production of IgE and IgG isotypes. In the context of the scheme for Th2-type immune cell recruitment to the airway, IL-4 may also exert a separate but critical influence. In particular, IL-4-driven expression of a cell adhesion molecule (VCAM-1) on the endothelial cell surface may serve in the recruitment of inflammatory cells (especially T cells and eosinophils bearing the $\alpha_4\beta_1$- and $\alpha_4\beta_7$-integrins) from the circulation. This possibility is supported by evidence of increased levels of immune cell IL-4 and endothelial cell VCAM-1 in tissue from asthmatic subjects as well as inhibition of allergen-induced airway inflammation in animals lacking the IL-4 gene or treated with anti–VCAM-1 antibodies. The precise mechanism for how IL-4 exerts its effect on VCAM-1 expression is uncertain, but it appears that it is not dependent on Stat6-driven gene activation. Instead, IL-4 acts in concert with other cytokines (TNF-α and IL-1). These cytokines are responsible for transcriptional activation of the VCAM-1 gene through two adjacent NF-κB sites in the promoter region, whereas IL-4 stabilizes the resulting mRNA. This cytokine synergy results in exaggeration and prolongation of VCAM-1 levels on the endothelial cell surface (Fig. 36-2). As depicted in Fig. 36-1, this cytokine synergy may also reflect an important cell–cell interaction in which TNF-α (and in some cases IL-1) derived from mast cells and eosinophils acts in concert with IL-4 (and in some cases IL-13) derived from mast cells, eosinophils, Th2 cells, and possibly basophils to promote immune cell recruitment to the airway.

Other Mechanisms for Recruitment of Immune Cells In addition to IL-4 and TNF-α effects on VCAM-1, other events in endothelial cells and immune cells are also critical for full development of the Th2-type inflammatory response. For example, at least two other cell adhesion systems appear to be activated during allergen-triggered airway inflammation: (1) selectin binding to mucin-like molecules; (2) other cell adhesion molecules of the Ig supergene family that bind to integrin receptors. In the case of endothelial cells, allergen may trigger endothelial-leukocyte adhesion molecule-1 (E-selectin) expression, which enables binding to a corresponding leukocyte sialyl-Lewis X carbohydrate ligand; and intercellular adhesion molecule-1 (ICAM-1) expression, which allows for binding to the leukocyte β_2-integrins LFA-1 ($\alpha_L\beta_2$) and Mac-1 ($\alpha_M\beta_2$). In addition to these cell adhesion systems for direct cell–cell contact, endothelial cells and immune cells also appear capable of generating a series of *chemo*attractant cyto*kines* (or chemokines) that may act over a greater distance to direct immune cell movement and activation in airway tissue. These three systems—selectin binding to mucinlike molecules, cell adhesion molecules binding to integrins, and chemokine binding to G-protein–coupled receptors—may act in a specific combination to dictate the type of immune cells that enter or get retained in the airway tissue (Fig. 36-3). These same systems also serve to control the activation status of immune cells acting at least in some cases through distinct signal transduction pathways.

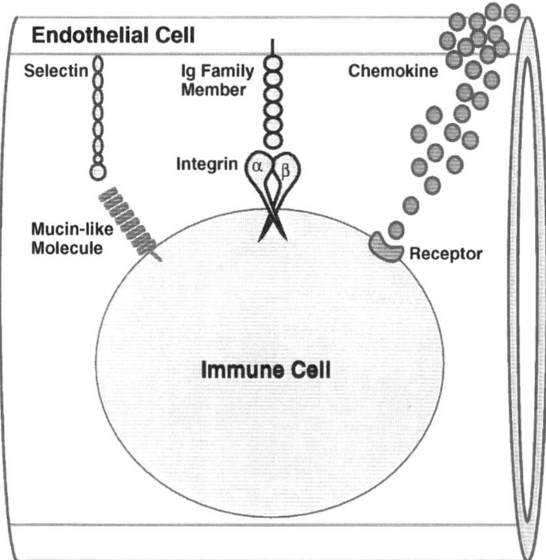

Figure 36-3 Endothelial cell-dependent recruitment of immune cells from the circulation during inflammation. Proposed steps include: (1) selectin interaction with its carbohydrate ligand (e.g., E-selectin interaction with sialyl Lewis X); (2) Ig family member interaction with the corresponding integrin receptor (e.g., VCAM-1 and ICAM-1 interaction with VLA-4 and Mac-1 or LFA-1, respectively); and (3) α- or β-chemokine interaction with a corresponding chemokine receptor (e.g., RANTES interaction with the serpentine superfamily of G protein-coupled receptors). These three steps may occur sequentially in some but not all cases. For example, VCAM-1–VLA-4-integrin interaction may by itself initiate immune cell rolling as well as subsequent adhesion to endothelium.

Once inflammatory cells are recruited from the circulation, they are often directed toward the epithelial surface. It appears that epithelial cells (along with other parenchymal cells and resident immune cells) also possess at least two important mechanisms for influencing the movement of inflammatory cells after they arrive in the airway tissue: (1) concomitant activation of cell adhesion molecules on the epithelial cell surface that may interact with corresponding integrin receptors on the immune cell surface; (2) release of chemotactic factors that bind to specific receptors on the immune cell. In the case of airway epithelial cells (as noted *below*), these systems appear to be more responsive to Th1-type cytokines, but there is evidence that they are also influenced by the level of TNF-α. Thus, even in the absence of a Th1-type response, epithelial levels of cell adhesion molecules (especially ICAM-1) and certain chemokines (from the α- and β-chemokine families) are capable of supporting transepithelial migration and activation of immune cells.

Interestingly, there is no evidence of selectin or VCAM-1 expression on airway epithelial cells (or fibroblasts and smooth muscle cells); thus, it is likely that these cell types present fewer ligands than do endothelial cells for directing leukocyte movement. The biologic basis for this difference is not certain, but it makes sense: endothelial cells must be armed with ligands that slow down passing leukocytes (to allow tethering and triggering) and then select a specific leukocyte subset (to allow adhesion and transmigration) from the diverse circulating pool. This requires multiple specific molecular interactions. By contrast, parenchymal cells (epithelial cells, fibroblasts, and smooth muscle cells) come into contact with immune cells after selection and some degree of activation, so that they are required only to facilitate further leukocyte migration and retention. ICAM-1 is well-suited to mediate this process because nearly all immune cells constitutively express the β_2-integrins LFA-1 or Mac-1. In the case of T-cell traffic, the endothelial cells (and likely epithelial cells) also express a series of receptors (designated homing receptors or addressins) that serve to direct distinct subsets of lymphocytes to appropriate locations of lymphoid tissue. This type of cell adhesion (exemplified by some of the β_7-integrin interactions) is probably most important in maintaining a resident population of immune cells, but whether this system is also regulated during airway inflammation remains uncertain.

Eosinophil-Derived Mediators Causing Inflammation Several lines of evidence indicate that eosinophils, once recruited to the airway, are a source of substances that mediate epithelial damage and endorgan dysfunction in asthma. As noted above, eosinophils may contribute to the local concentrations of IL-4, IL-5, and TNF-α that augment immune cell recruitment and activation. In addition, they contain a series of inflammatory mediators capable of causing dysfunction of airway smooth muscle, nerves, and glands, as well as damage to epithelial tissue. For example, eosinophils represent an active source of mediators derived from phospholipid arachidonic acid metabolism. This metabolic pathway leads to the production of bioactive compounds (including prostaglandins, leukotrienes, and platelet-activating factor) at higher than normal levels in asthmatic airways. Enzymes (including prostaglandin synthases, lipoxygenases, and phospholipases) and cell surface receptors for this pathway have been structurally characterized, and, in some cases, this information has led to the development of specific pharmacologic antagonists. For example, recombinant 5-lipoxygenase and its accompanying docking protein—the 5-lipoxygenase activating protein (designated FLAP) have been expressed and used as targets for drug development. The functional significance of 5-lipoxygenase and its capacity to generate biologically active leukotrienes is underscored by the efficacy of 5-lipoxygenase and leukotriene antagonists to diminish airway responsiveness and improve airway function in asthmatic subjects.

Eosinophils also store and release a variety of substances (including major basic protein, eosinophilic cationic protein, and eosinophil-derived neurotoxin) that are toxic to cells. Because these substances are potent cytotoxins, some have suggested that epithelial detachment is a consequence of cell death. However, denudation of the epithelium may require proteolysis of the extracellular and membrane-associated proteins involved in cell adhesion to the basal lamina. This proteolytic activity may be provided by matrix metalloproteinases. For example, eosinophils are selectively capable of synthesizing and releasing an abundance of a specific matrix metalloproteinase (the 92-kDa gelatinase) with a substrate specificity capable of mediating epithelial detachment. This enzyme, as well as other proteases, may also aid in immune cell movement through tissue. Other matrix metalloproteinases (as well as members of the cysteine and serine protease families) derived from diverse cell types (including mast cells and T cells) may also influence immune cell movement and contribute to epithelial damage and end-organ dysfunction.

Other Mechanisms of Epithelial Damage and End-Organ Dysfunction In addition to lipid mediators and proteases, it is also possible that local production of nitric oxide is a component of airway inflammation in asthma. As noted below, this concept

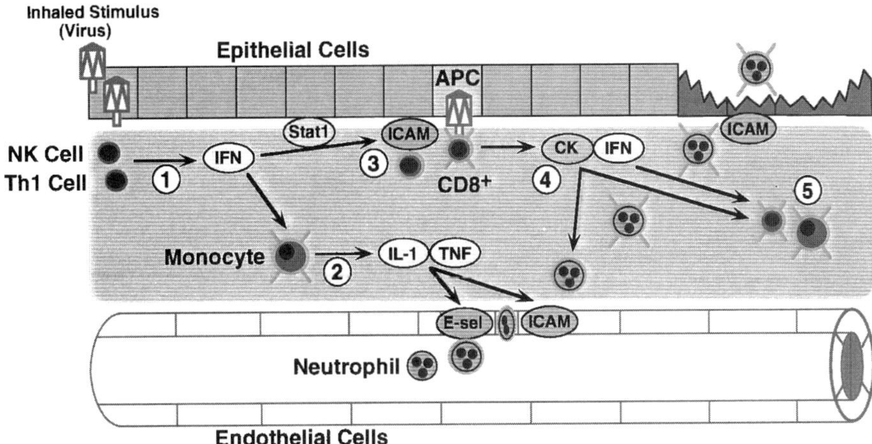

Figure 36-4 Cell–cell interaction cascade for a Th1-type response in the airway. Proposed steps include: (1) respiratory virus (or other nonallergic stimulus) triggers NK cells (as well as Th1 cells and CD8$^+$ T cells) to release IFN-γ; (2) IFN-γ triggers monocyte and macrophage release of IL-1 and TNF-α that in turn induce E-selectin (E-sel) and ICAM-1 expression on the endothelium and Mac-1 or LFA-1-dependent transendothelial migration of neutrophils; (3) IFN-γ also drives Stat1-dependent expression of ICAM-1 on epithelial cells that enables epithelial–T cell interaction and antigen presentation of virus to CD8$^+$ T cells; (4) activated T cells (and epithelial cells) also release α- and β-chemokines (CK) that serve to direct neutrophils and mononuclear cells, respectively, to the airway; and (5) activated neutrophils and later mononuclear cells release additional cytokine and chemokine that autoamplifies immune cell influx and activation and local production of mediators contributing to epithelial damage.

may be more relevant to Th1-type models of host defense against respiratory pathogens, but in either case, it appears that local production of IL-1 can drive expression of an inducible nitric oxide synthase (i-NOS) in airway epithelial cells. Thus, the damaging effects of IL-1 on the epithelium may depend on overproduction of nitric oxide by the respiratory epithelium itself or by adjacent leukocytes. The precise cellular sources of IL-1 and nitric oxide in asthmatic airways, the pathway and specificity of nitric oxide-mediated damage, the effects of IL-1 and nitric oxide on epithelial repair, and the possibilities for therapeutic intervention by inhibiting nitric oxide production are still under study. For example, an i-NOS inhibitor given to asthmatic subjects is capable of reducing nitric oxide levels in the airway, but possible effects on airway inflammation are still uncertain.

TH1-TYPE T-CELL RESPONSE An abnormal sensitivity to inhaled allergen is responsible for asthma in some cases, but in other cases, it appears that patients develop asthma in response to nonallergic stimuli. Thus, just as IL-4-driven, Th2-dependent hypersensitivity to allergen may underlie allergic asthma, it is also natural to propose that an overexuberant or aberrant IFN-γ–driven, Th1-type reaction, incriminated in delayed-type hypersensitivity reactions, may underlie nonallergic airway inflammation and asthma. This possibility is consistent with evidence of increased IL-4– and decreased IFN-γ–producing T cells in airways of allergic asthmatics, as well as selective overexpression of IFN-γ in intrinsic asthmatics. As noted *above*, however, this concept may not be completely correct. Thus, the capacity for IFN-γ production may be increased even in atopic asthma. In addition, there may be concomitant release of IFN-γ (and IL-4) in response to allergen challenge. Thus, a Th1-type response may contribute to allergic as well as nonallergic asthma, but perhaps the clearest circumstance for a predominantly IFN-γ–driven Th1-type response in the airway may occur in response to infection with respiratory viruses. In some individuals, this response may mediate virus-induced airway inflammation and hyperreactivity. A scheme depicting the cell–cell interactions that might occur in this type of Th1-dependent cascade is depicted in Fig. 36-4.

IFN-γ Generation The precise cellular and molecular events leading to generation of IFN-γ are uncertain, but it would seem likely that, in the case of respiratory viruses, an initiating event may be attachment of virus to the (epithelial) cell surface. Some viruses have learned to subvert the immune response by using epithelial cell adhesion molecules (such as ICAM-1) to gain attachment and possibly entry into the host cell. The next step, in which proliferation of intracellular virus may stimulate cytokine (especially IFN-γ) production is incompletely defined. This effect may occur directly, for example by virus-dependent major histocompatibility complex (MHC) class I repression and consequent stimulation of natural killer (NK) cells, or indirectly, by class I-dependent presentation of viral antigens to Th1 cells or antiviral CD8$^+$ cytotoxic T cells. It is also possible that epithelial cells, once infected with virus, are induced to generate cytokines or chemokines that in turn activate immune cells, including IFN-γ–producing T cells. In either case, it appears that IFN-γ production may be controlled at a transcriptional level, but most information on the regulation of the IFN-γ gene promoter rests on cell model systems that use transformed T cells. In some systems, Th1-cell development and consequent IFN-γ production depends on the activity of IL-12. Interestingly, IL-12 may exert its actions through two additional members of the STAT family of transcription factors (Stat3 and Stat4).

IFN-γ–Dependent Recruitment of Immune Cells Once released, IFN-γ exerts a number of actions aimed to enhance antiviral defense. Perhaps most relevant to inflammation, IFN-γ may act to recruit and activate immune cells (especially T cells and macrophages) in the airway by enhanced expression of cell adhesion molecules and chemokines. As depicted in Fig. 36-4, activation of each of these systems at the level of the airway endothelium and epithelium may influence the development of airway inflammation and hyperreactivity. In the case of endothelial-dependent recruitment of inflammatory cells, IFN-γ–dependent activation of

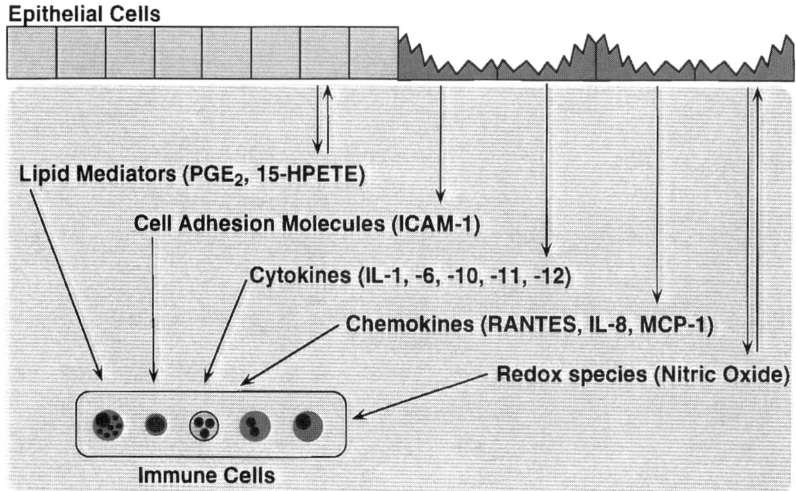

Figure 36-5 Epithelial cell-dependent modulation of immunity and inflammation. Based on studies of airway epithelial cells in vivo and ex vivo, at least five families of mediators have been proposed to act as mediators of inflammation within the epithelium itself and in the underlying tissue: (1) lipid mediators include arachidonic acid metabolites prostaglandin E_2 (PGE_2) and 15-hydroperoxyeicosatetraenoic acid (15-HPETE); (2) cell adhesion molecules include ICAM-1; (3) cytokines include IL-1, IL-6, IL-10, IL-11, and IL-12; (4) chemokines include RANTES, IL-8, and MCP-1; and (5) redox species include nitric oxide (NO). Some of these substances act in autocrine regulation of epithelial cell functions (including ion transport and mucous secretion) whereas others act to regulate immune cell behavior.

tissue macrophages may result in the generation and release of IL-1 and TNF-α. As was the case for allergic inflammation, this mechanism serves to activate endothelial–immune cell adhesion. In particular, IL-1β and TNF-α are potent inducers of endothelial E-selectin and ICAM-1 expression.

As noted above, after inflammatory cells are recruited from the circulation, they are often directed toward the epithelial surface. This observation has led to the specific proposal that epithelial cells are a source of mediators that direct immune cell movement and the general concept that epithelial–immune cell interaction may influence inflammation (Fig. 36-5). In this regard, it appears that airway epithelial–T cell adhesion, transmigration, and activation depend on the cytokine-dependent expression of ICAM-1 on the epithelial cell surface, as well as the concomitant levels of expression and activation of LFA-1 on the T-cell surface. This system appears activated in asthma because there are increased numbers of activated T cells as well as increased ICAM-1 expression in the epithelium of asthmatic subjects. Interestingly, it is often epithelial (and not endothelial) expression of ICAM-1 that is consistently increased in biopsies of asthmatic versus normal airway tissue, and this appears to be the case in both allergic and nonallergic subjects.

Based on studies of isolated airway epithelial cells, it appears that the level of ICAM-1 is regulated by a specific IFN-γ–driven signal transduction pathway that consists of the IFN-γ–receptor, receptor-associated Jak1 and Jak2 tyrosine kinases, additional serine kinase(s), the Stat1 transcription factor, and a specific Stat1–DNA interaction in the ICAM-1 gene promoter region (Fig. 36-6). In this pathway, Stat1 serves to relay the signal from the cytoplasm to the nucleus (Fig. 36-7). Interestingly, Stat1–DNA interaction (as well as Stat1–Sp1 synergy) in the ICAM-1 gene promoter region may also be critical for IFN-γ responsiveness of other epithelial immune-response genes, especially interferon regulatory factor-1 (IRF-1). The IRF-1 gene product is itself a member of a transcription factor family and is responsible for activating the genes for i-NOS and possibly MHC class I molecules. Thus, a cascade of common molecular building blocks enables IFN-γ to efficiently and selectively activate an immune-response subset in the airway epithelial barrier to mediate mucosal immunity and inflammation. Stat1 appears to sit at a critical site in the development of this cascade, but the characteristics of Stat1-dependent gene regulation in airway inflammation in vivo are still poorly defined. Similarly, only alittle has been established for the regulation or expression of chemokines in airway epithelial (or other parenchymal) cells in airway tissue. Initial evidence indicates that members of each chemokine family—α-chemokines (e.g., IL-8) and β-chemokines (e.g., monocyte chemoattractant protein-1 [MCP-1] and regulated upon activation, normal T expressed, and presumably secreted [RANTES])—are expressed in airway epithelial cells ex vivo and *in situ*, and, in some cases, the profile of chemokine activity fits with the pattern of immune cell infiltration (e.g., RANTES acts on T cells and eosinophils).

ASTHMA AS A GENETIC DISEASE

POPULATION AND FAMILY STUDIES Evidence that genetic factors are important in common diseases often comes initially from studies comparing the frequency of disease among genetically related individuals with that in the general population. Accordingly, the evidence for a genetic component to the development of asthma includes: (1) family studies indicating more frequent occurrence of asthma in first-degree relatives of asthmatic subjects; (2) familial aggregation patterns in which the rates of asthma were found to be significantly higher in those families with one or more asthmatic parent; and (3) studies showing that monozygotic twins are significantly more concordant for asthma than dizygotic twins. Reports during the past 50 years have proposed both simple mendelian and multifactorial models to explain the familial clustering of asthma (or allergy). These studies provided the general (not surprising) conclusion that the expression of asthma is likely to be heterogeneic and polygenic and to be the result of an interaction between genetic and environmental factors. Statistical analysis of data was often hampered by the absence

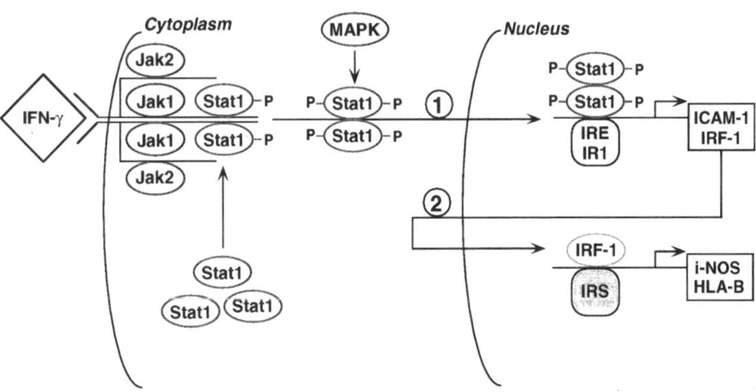

Figure 36-6 IFN-γ–driven signal transduction and gene activation. IFN-γ signal transduction begins when IFN-γ binds to its receptor and triggers activation of α-chain–associated Jak1 and β-chain–associated Jak2 tyrosine kinases and consequent α-chain phosphorylation. This step enables α-chain recruitment of Stat1 via its SH2 domain and subsequent Stat1 phosphorylation and release of the phosphorylated Stat1-homodimer. Additional evidence indicates an additional action of a serine-threonine kinase is needed to convey full activity. Two consequences (labeled 1 and 2) then occur: (1) activated Stat1 homodimer translocates to the nucleus where it binds to an inverted-repeated type motif in the IFN-γ–response element (IRE) or IFN-response 1 (IR1) site and activates (in concert with Sp1) transcription of the corresponding genes (ICAM-1 and IRF-1, respectively); and (2) newly generated IRF-1 mRNA is translated into protein that returns to the nucleus (based on its nuclear localization signal), binds to an IFN-response stimulation (IRS) site, and activates a second wave of transcription (for the i-NOS and HLA-B genes).

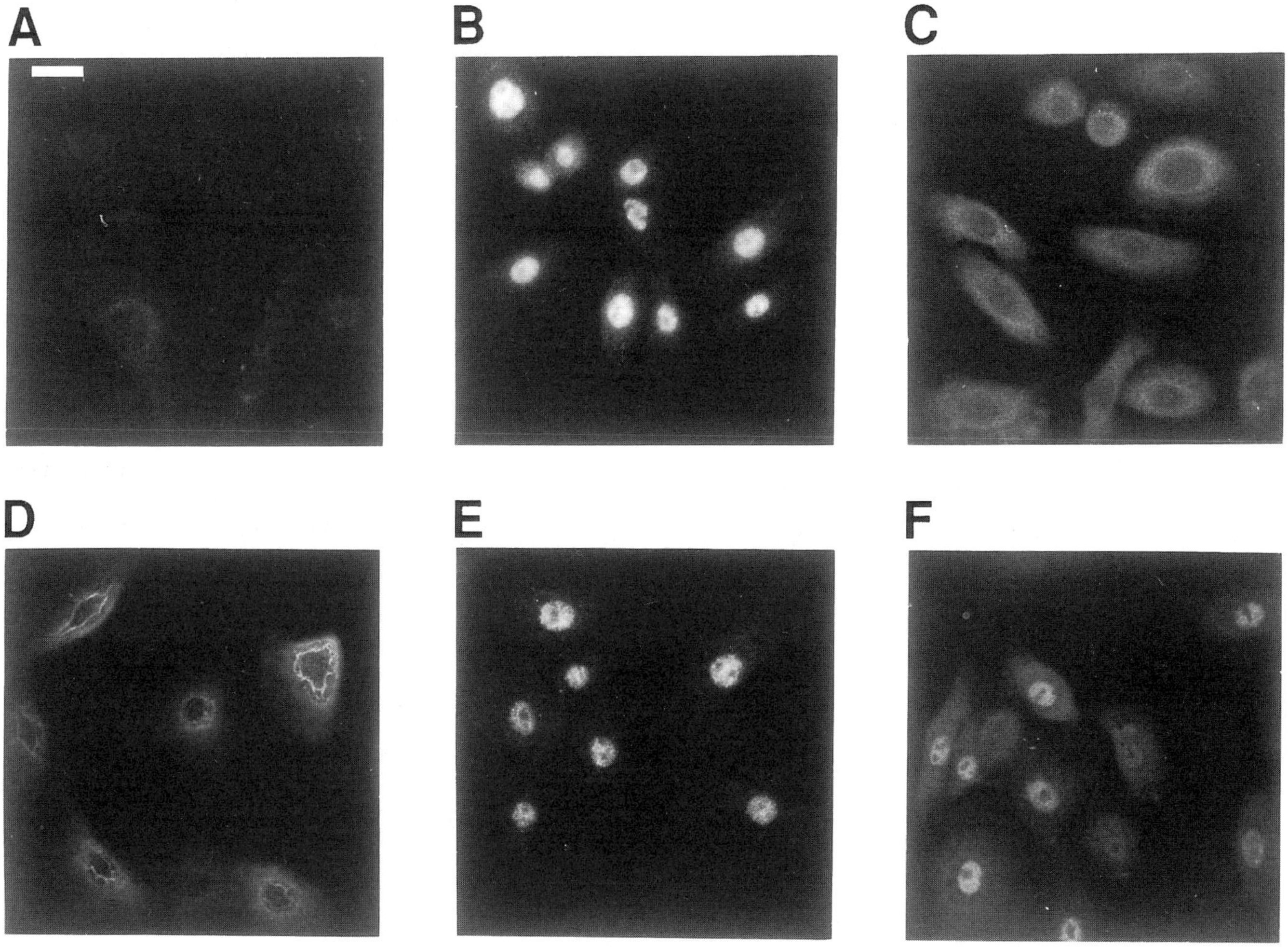

Figure 36-7 IFN-γ activates Stat1 and induces ICAM-1 in airway epithelial cells. Human tracheobronchial epithelial cell (hTBEC) monolayers were unstimulated (top row, A–C) or stimulated (bottom row, D–F) with IFN-γ (100 U/mL), fixed in methanol, pretreated with 2% gelatin to block nonspecific Ig binding, and then incubated with Abs against ICAM-1 (left column; A and D), Sp1 (middle column; B and E), or Stat1 (right column; C and F) in 2% fish gelatin. Primary antibody binding was detected with CY3-conjugated goat anti-mouse IgG. Control nonimmune IgG gave no signal above background. Bar = 40 μm.

of physiologic criteria for a specific asthmatic phenotype, the difficulty in separating inheritance of the atopic predisposition from the inheritance of asthma, or the lack of controls for environmental factors. The development of phenotypic markers for asthma (or subtypes of asthma) has served to facilitate studies of its inheritance.

PHENOTYPIC MARKERS AND INHERITANCE Bronchial hyperreactivity is a common phenotypic marker of asthma, and family studies (and animal models) suggest that hyperreactivity is under genetic influence. In fact, concordance among identical twins is significantly greater for bronchial reactivity than for asthma symptoms. In addition, bronchial hyperreactivity may be found in asymptomatic parents of asthmatic children without evidence of positive allergen skin tests or increased serum IgE, and the hyperreactivity is inherited in an autosomal dominant pattern. Other studies have provided similar results, but some indicate that the trait may not be caused by segregation at a single autosomal locus.

The discovery of IgE and the observation that its levels may increase in association with atopic disease quickly placed IgE (and in particular its level of biosynthesis) as a candidate marker for atopy. Several recent observations indicate that the level of total serum IgE may correlate even better with the development of asthma than for atopy. These results suggested that asthma resulted from IgE-dependent mechanisms even in the absence of identifiable allergen sensitivity. A separate follow-up study confirmed the relationship between asthma and IgE levels and established a similar link between bronchial hyperreactivity and total serum IgE levels. Other investigators have confirmed these results and have added that an increase in circulating eosinophils may also be linked to the asthma phenotype. Genetic models for the inheritance of IgE levels were proposed in a series of population and family studies to support the existence of a relatively common recessive regulatory locus, with recessive homozygotes maintaining persistently high levels of IgE. In addition, a significant multifactorial background was detected.

DNA MARKERS AND MOLECULAR GENETICS By using markers for DNA polymorphisms, at least two genetic loci have been linked to atopy and possibly to asthma. Initial work defined a single dominantly inherited locus located on chromosome 11q13 controlling IgE hyperresponsiveness. The apparent discrepancy in mode of inheritance between results derived from segregation versus linkage analysis may be related to the definition of phenotypes employed by the two types of studies. In the linkage studies, the definition of atopy was expanded to include asymptomatic subjects (identified by abnormal IgE responsiveness). Subsequent work on the 11q13-linked atopy "gene" suggested that it may be genetically linked to the site of the β-subunit of the high-affinity receptor for IgE and that a putative variation within this gene (Ile181Leu) may be associated with atopy. These findings suggest that the IgE receptor (FcεRI-β) is a candidate gene predisposing to atopy. However, at least three other studies failed to reproduce the association of the 11q13 locus with atopy or asthma, perhaps reflecting the variability in clinical expression, a role for environmental effects, or effects of genes at other loci. In further support of the view that there are other genes specific to asthma, additional work has linked markers for chromosome 5q31–33 with atopy (defined by total serum IgE) and bronchial hyperreactivity. The 5q site is near the genes for IL-4, IL-9, and IL-13 (implicated in the control of IgE biosynthesis) as well as additional candidate genes encoding for other cytokines, growth factors, and receptors (including the β_2-adrenergic receptor). Finer mapping of this region is aimed at better definition of candidate genes linked to asthma.

Because antigen-dependent immune and inflammatory mechanisms participate prominently in the expression of the asthmatic phenotype, a number of investigators have also attempted to establish linkage of asthma to loci within the major histocompatibility complex (MHC). The class I (HLA-A, -B, and -C) and class II (HLA-DP, -DQ, and -DR) genes are among the most polymorphic human genes described, with more than 10 alleles defined for each locus. The nature of this polymorphism has been extensively investigated using serologic reagents and more recently using nucleic acid typing probes. In some studies, significant HLA associations with asthma have been found, but in others there is no association between asthma and specific HLA alleles. It is likely that weak or conflicting associations are again realted to the heterogeneity of the phenotype and the possibility that a discrete abnormality may be restricted to a subset of asthmatic subjects. It also appears likely that a particular sequence is a necessary but not sufficient requirement of responsiveness to a particular antigenic epitope and that further genetic and environmental factors are required for the expression of specific immune responsiveness.

SUMMARY

Understanding and treating asthma depends on understanding how inflammatory cells infiltrate the pulmonary airway and how the resulting infiltrate leads to characteristic pathologic changes in airway tissue. In this context, investigators have pursued the regulatory controls over genes encoding for critical components of the immune response to inhaled allergic and nonallergic stimuli. Initial evidence indicates that allergic and nonallergic asthma exhibit separate but overlapping cell–cell interactions orchestrated by immune cells and airway parenchymal cells. In that context, several lines of evidence also point to genetic factors in the development of asthma. Population and family studies indicate that specific biologic abnormalities (increased serum IgE, bronchial hyperreactivity, and blood eosinophilia) may be useful markers of the asthmatic phenotype, and segregation analysis and linkage analysis for the asthmatic phenotype have suggested mendelian and polygenic patterns of inheritance as well as an influence of environmental factors. Taken together, the biochemical and genetic studies offer compatible approaches for further pursuit: (1) biochemical studies will aim to define individual candidate genes and mechanisms for gene regulation under conditions in which confounding environmental and genetic factors are largely eliminated; and (2) genetic studies will aim to link these candidates (forward genetics) and other unknown genes (reverse genetics) to the asthmatic phenotype. Evidence of linkage will in turn lead to finer mapping and perhaps further definition of genes that are abnormally expressed in the airway of asthmatic subjects.

SELECTED REFERENCES

Ben-Baruch A, Michiel DF, Oppenheim JJ. Signals and receptors involved in recruitment of inflammatory cells. J Biol Chem 1995;270:11,703–11,706.

Bentley AM, Durham SR, Robinson DS, et al. Expression of endothelial and leukocyte adhesion molecules intercellular adhesion molecule-1, E-selectin, and vascular cell adhesion molecule-1 in the bronchial mucosa in steady-state and allergen-induced asthma. J Allergy Clin Immunol 1993;92:857–868.

Bleecker ER, Postma DS, Meyers DA. Genetic susceptibility to asthma in a changing environment. Ciba Found Symp 1997;206:90–99.

Bousquet J, Chanez P, Lacoste JY, et al. Eosinophilic inflammation in asthma. N Engl J Med 1990;323:1033–1039.

Bradding P, Roberts JA, Britten KM, et al. Interleukin-4, -5, and -6 and tumor necrosis factor-α in normal and asthmatic airways: evidence for the human mast cell as a source of these cytokines. Am J Respir Cell Mol Biol 1994;10:471–480.

Burrows B, Martinez FD, Halonen M, Barbee RA, Cline MG. Association of asthma with serum IgE levels and skin-test reactivity to allergens. N Engl J Med 1989;320:271–277.

Cippitelli M, Sica A, Viggiano V, et al. Negative transcriptional regulation of the interferon-γ promoter by glucocorticoids and dominant negative mutants of c-Jun. J Biol Chem 1995;270:12,548–12,556.

The Collaborative Study on the Genetics of Asthma (CSGA). A genome-wide search for asthma susceptibility loci in ethnically diverse populations. Nat Genet 1997;15:389–392.

Cookson WOCM, Sharp A, Faux JA, Hopkin JM. Linkage between immunoglobulin E responses underlying asthma and rhinitis and chromosome 11q. Lancet 1989;1:1292–1295.

Dixon RAF, Diehl RE, Opas E, et al. Requirement of a 5-lipoxygenase-activating protein for leukotriene synthesis. Nature 1990;343:282–284.

Hamilos DL, Leung DYM, Wood R, et al. Evidence for distinct cytokine expression in allergic versus nonallergic chronic sinusitis. J Allergy Clin Immunol 1995;96:537–544.

Heiss LN, Lancaster JR Jr, Corbett JA, Goldman WE. Epithelial autotoxicity of nitric oxide: role in the respiratory cytopathology of pertussis. Proc Natl Acad Sci USA 1994;88:3681–3685.

Holgate ST. Asthma Genetics: waiting to exhale. Nat Genet 1997;15: 227–229.

Holtzman MJ. Arachidonic acid metabolism: implications of biological chemistry for lung function and disease. Am Rev Respir Dis 1991; 143:188–203.

Holtzman MJ, Brody SL, Look DC. Does gene therapy call for "STAT" immunity and inflammation at the epithelial barrier? Am J Respir Cell Mol Biol 1995;12:127–129.

Holtzman MJ, Fabbri LM, O'Byrne PM, et al. Importance of airway inflammation for hyperresponsiveness induced by ozone in dogs. Am Rev Respir Dis 1983;127:686–690.

Holtzman MJ, Sampath D, Castro M, Look DC, Jayaraman S. The one-two of T helper cells: does interferon-γ knockout the Th2 hypothesis for asthma? Am J Respir Cell Mol Biol 1996;14:316–318.

Hou J, Schindler U, Henzel WJ, et al. An interleukin-4-induced transcription factor: IL-4 Stat. Science 1994;265:1701–1706.

Huang S-K, Marsh DG. Genetics of allergy. Ann Allergy 1993;70: 347–358.

Iademarco MF, Barks JL, Dean DC. Regulation of vascular cell adhesion molecule-1 expression by IL-4 and TNF-α in cultured endothelial cells. J Clin Invest 1995;95:264–271.

Ihle JN, Witthuhn BA, Quelle FW, Yamamoto K, Silvennoinen O. Signaling through the hematopoietic cytokine receptors. Annu Rev Immunol 1995;13:369–398.

Jacobson NG, Szabo SJ, Weber-Nordt RM, et al. Interleukin 12 signaling in T helper type 1 (Th1) cells involves tyrosine phosphorylation of signal transducer and activator of transcription (STAT)3 and Stat4. J Exp Med 1995;181:1755–1762.

Kamijo R, Harada H, Matsuyama T, et al. Requirement for transcription factor IRF-1 in NO synthase induction in macrophages. Science 1994;263:1612–1615.

Kips JC, Tavernier JH, Joos GF, Peleman RA, Pauwels RA. The potential role of tumour necrosis factor alpha in asthma. Clin Exp Allergy 1993;23:247–250.

Li JT. Mechanism of asthma. Curr Opin Pulm Med 1997;3:10–16.

Lobb RR, Hemler ME. The pathophysiologic role of α4 integrins in vivo. J Clin Invest 1994;94:1722–1728.

Look DC, Pelletier MR, Holtzman MJ. Selective interaction of a subset of interferon-γ response element binding proteins with the intercellular adhesion molecule-1 (ICAM-1) gene promoter controls the pattern of expression on epithelial cells. J Biol Chem 1994;269: 8952–8958.

Marsh DG, Neely JD, Breazeale DR, et al. Linkage analysis of IL4 and other chromosome 5q31.1 markers and total serum immunoglobulin E concentrations. Science 1994;264:1152–1156.

McEver RP, Moore KL, Cummings RD. Leukocyte trafficking mediated by selectin–carbohydrate interactions. J Biol Chem 1995;270:11,025–11,028.

Nakajima S, Look DC, Roswit WT, Bragdon MJ, Holtzman MJ. Selective differences in vascular endothelial- vs. airway epithelial-T cell adhesion mechanisms. Am J Physiol 1994;267:L422–L432.

Nakajima S, Roswit WT, Look DC, Holtzman MJ. A hierarchy for integrin expression and adhesiveness among T cell subsets that is linked to TCR gene usage and emphasizes $V\delta1^+$ $\gamma\delta$ T cell adherence and tissue retention. J Immunol 1995;155:1117–1131.

Postma DS, Bleecker ER, Amelung PJ, et al. Genetic susceptibility to asthma—bronchial hyperresponsiveness coinherited with a major gene for atopy. New Engl J Med 1995;333:894–900.

Raulet DH, Held W. Natural killer cell receptors: the offs and ons of NK cell recognition. Cell 1995;82:697–700.

Robinson DS, Hamid Q, Bentley A, et al. Activation of $CD4^+$ T cells, increased T_{H2}-type cytokine mRNA expression, and eosinophil recruitment in bronchoalveolar lavage after allergen inhalation challenge in patients with atopic asthma. J Allergy Clin Immunol 1993;92:313–324.

Ruffilli A, Bonini S. Susceptibility genes for allergy and asthma. Allergy 1997;52:256–273.

Schindler C, Darnell JEJ. Transcriptional responses to polypeptide ligands: the JAK-STAT pathway. Annu Rev Biochem 1995;64: 621–651.

Sears MR, Burrows B, Flannery EM, et al. Relation between airway responsiveness and serum IgE in children with asthma and in apparently normal children. N Engl J Med 1991;325:1067–1071.

Seminario M-C, Gleich GJ. The role of eosinophils in the pathogenesis of asthma. Curr Opin Immunol 1994;6:860–864.

Shirakawa T, Li A, Dubowitz M, et al. Association between atopy and variants of the β subunit of the high-affinity immunoglobulin E receptor. Nat Genet 1994;7:125–130.

Springer TA. Traffic signals for lymphocyte recirculation and leukocyte emigration: the multistep paradigm. Cell 1994;76:301–314.

Stahle-Backdahl M, Inoue M, Giudice GJ, Parks WC. 92 kDa gelatinase is produced by eosinophils at the site of blister formation in bullous pemphigoid and cleaves the extracellular domain of the 180 kDa bullous pemphigoid autoantigen. J Clin Invest 1994;93:2202–2230.

Ying S, Durham SR, Corrigan CJ, Hamid Q, Kay AB. Phenotype of cells expressing mRNA for TH2-type (interleukin 4 and interleukin 5) and TH1-type (interleukin 2 and interferon γ) cytokines in bronchoalveolar lavage and bronchial biopsies from atopic asthmatic and normal control subjects. Am J Respir Cell Mol Biol 1995;12:477–487.

37 Cystic Fibrosis

DANIEL B. ROSENBLUTH AND STEVEN L. BRODY

INTRODUCTION

Cystic fibrosis (CF) is one of the most common lethal hereditary diseases of monogenic origin. The frequency of the disease is approximately 1 in 2500 births in the white population. CF is characterized by a classic triad that includes an increase in sweat chloride concentration, pancreatic insufficiency, and recurrent pulmonary infections. The onset of symptoms is typically within the first decade of life, often at birth. Lung disease is the most common cause of morbidity and mortality in individuals with CF. More than 90% of all CF deaths are directly related to respiratory disease. Remarkably, survival has increased dramatically during the past 20 years largely because of improved antibiotic therapies, pancreatic enzyme replacement, and nutritional support, so that median survival now exceeds 30 years. The cloning of the "CF gene" in 1989, called the cystic fibrosis transmembrane conductance regulator (CFTR) gene, has led to the identification of one specific mutation in approximately 70% of alleles in individuals with CF and more than 600 other disease-causing mutations. The characterization of CFTR has made possible the development of novel molecular strategies for the treatment of CF-related lung disease and potential cure of CF through gene therapy.

Identification of the CFTR gene has also driven the search for understanding how the genetic defect leads to the disease-causing cellular defect. The CFTR protein has been identified as a cyclic adenosine monophosphate (cAMP)-regulated chloride channel that functions in the apical aspect of epithelial cells. The current concept of pathogenesis of CF-related lung disease is that mutations in the CFTR gene result in inadequate function of the CFTR protein leading to abnormal airway secretions, inflammation, bacterial infection, abnormalities in lung architecture, and decline in lung function. The first major challenge for CF research is to define precisely how the absent or abnormal CFTR protein triggers the cascade of inflammation and infection in the lung, as well as how intestinal and pancreatic dysfunction occur. A second challenge is to use the current information regarding CFTR to further develop therapies that will improve the life of the individual with CF. This chapter will review the current understanding of the CFTR gene and protein function, the pathogenesis of CF, and emerging data from molecular-based therapies, including gene therapy. The major focus of this chapter is CF-related lung disease, the most common cause of morbidity and mortality in CF.

From: *Principles of Molecular Medicine* (J. L. Jameson, ed.), ©1998 Humana Press Inc., Totowa, NJ.

THE CFTR GENE

The CF gene was isolated in 1989 using the technique of positional cloning, based on the relationship of genetic linkage analysis of CF families to known chromosomal markers. Genetic analysis of affected families revealed that the CF gene was inherited in an autosomal recessive pattern and linkage analysis localized the gene to the region of a polymorphic DNA marker on the long arm of chromosome 7 at q31–32. Using other known gene markers, the CF gene was localized to a specific region of the chromosome that could be cloned and sequenced. Final identification of the gene was based on three findings related, in part, to previous observations of CF cell biology. First, on the basis of the predicted chloride or sodium channel functions of the protein, a specific deduced amino acid sequence with conserved features of an ion-transport channel was found. Second, transfection of the putative CFTR cDNA into epithelial cell lines derived from individuals with CF demonstrated an ability to reverse the defect of chloride conductance and to confer cAMP-regulated chloride channel activity. And third, a common 3-bp mutation that resulted in a deletion of a codon for the amino acid phenylalanine at position 508 (ΔF508) was found only in DNA from affected families.

The CFTR gene is located within a 250-kb region of genomic DNA and contains 27 exons. The gene codes for a 6.5-kb mRNA and a deduced protein composed of 1480 amino acid residues. Several alternatively spliced forms of mRNA have been identified. The promoter of the CFTR gene contains a G + C rich region with multiple transcription start sites and does not contain a characteristic TATA transcription complex initiation element. Promoter activity is relatively weak; however, transcription is tightly regulated and transcript abundance varies greatly with cell type. Transcription can be modulated in vitro using cAMP, phorbol esters, and protein kinase C activators. Putative *cis*-acting elements include sites for binding transcriptional activators AP1 and Sp1, factors that may be induced by cAMP and phorbol esters. Analysis of chromatin structure and methylation status of the CFTR promoter region suggests that several other mechanisms may be important for transcriptional regulation.

THE CFTR PROTEIN

Based on the CFTR cDNA sequence, the predicted amino acid sequence was found to contain regions similar to the ABC (ATP-binding cassette) family of transporters. These proteins have highly conserved transmembrane and nucleotide-binding domains and include well-characterized family members, such as the yeast ster-

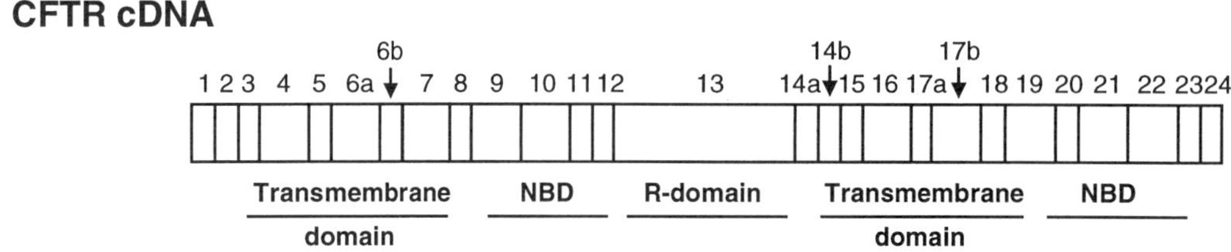

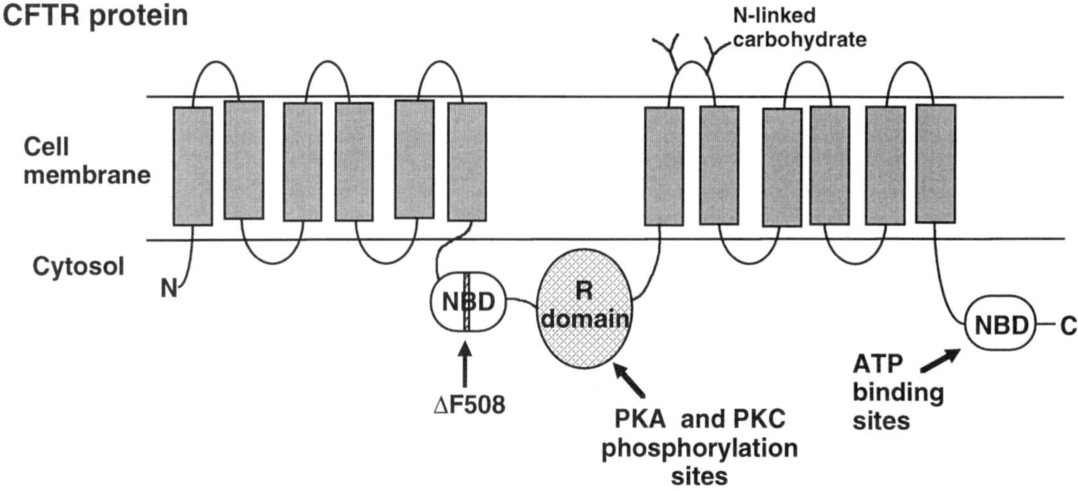

Figure 37-1 Structure of cystic fibrosis transmembrane conductance regulator (CFTR) cDNA and protein. Shown above is a schematic diagram of the structure of the CFTR cDNA with 27 exons indicated by boxes and labeled with the predicted protein domain coded for by the cDNA. A model of the CFTR protein positioned in the apical membrane of the epithelial cell is shown below. The transmembrane domains are flanked by nucleotide-binding domains (NBD) that bind ATP. The regulatory domain (R domain) contains sites for protein kinase A (PKA) and C (PKC) phosphorylation. The location of the ΔF508 mutation is indicated. N is the amino-terminus and C is the carboxy-terminus of the protein. Sites of posttranslational glycosylation by amino (N)-lined carbohydrates are indicated. (Adapted from Zielenski and Tsui with permission from the Ann Rev Gen, 1995; 29; 777–807. © 1995 by Annual Reviews Inc.)

ile 6 protein and the eukaryotic P glycoprotein (the multiple drug-resistance protein). The structure of the CFTR protein consists of two membrane-spanning domains, each containing six transmembrane segments, two nucleotide-binding domains (NBD), and an intracellular hydrophobic regulatory (R) domain (Fig. 37-1). The R domain contains several putative sites for protein kinase A and protein kinase C phosphorylation that play a central role in CFTR regulation. The two NBDs are located intracellularly and flank the membrane-spanning domains. The NBDs represent putative sites for binding and hydrolysis of ATP. The CFTR structure is therefore consistent with a regulated channel molecule. However, unlike other members of the ABC family, CFTR exhibits chloride channel activity.

The function and regulation of the CFTR protein as a chloride channel is based on structural features and is consistent with classic observations in cells obtained from individuals with CF. Before the identification of CFTR, studies in CF cells in the 1980s revealed a defect in cAMP-activated chloride conductance in the epithelial cells of the sweat gland and airway. In the sweat duct, CF cells are unable to normally reabsorb chloride ions, resulting in a high concentration of chloride in the sweat. In the CF airway, epithelial cells are unable to secrete chloride in response to cAMP agonists and sodium reabsorption is markedly increased. Based on alteration in sweat chloride, abnormal chloride conductance across cells, and abnormal sodium reabsorption, it was predicted that the CF gene may be involved with ion transport. Thus, the observation that expression of the normal CFTR cDNA in CF epithelial cell lines corrected the defect in cAMP-regulated chloride permeability was consistent with clinical observations. The specific function of CFTR was more directly verified by demonstrating that purified, reconstituted CFTR fused into lipid bilayers resulted in chloride channel activity with characteristics identical to the CFTR expression in epithelial cell membranes.

The CFTR protein is regulated by phosphorylation of the R domain by cAMP-regulated protein kinase A; however, this alone is not sufficient to activate CFTR chloride channel activity. After phosphorylation, binding and hydrolysis of ATP at the NBD is essential for normal channel gating (opening and closing). Chloride movement through the gate is determined by the electrochemical gradient and does not require further energy. CFTR is proposed to have other functions such as regulating sodium and water channels, transporting other ions, acidification of intracellular vesicles, regulation of endosome fusion, and plasma membrane recycling.

CFTR functions at the apical cell membrane of the epithelial cell to move chloride out of the cell and into the lumen, and also regulates chloride and sodium transport through other channels. In the apical membrane, the alternate chloride channel (Cl_a), the outwardly rectifying chloride channel (ORCC), or other channels also move chloride out of the cell. Recent studies suggest that CFTR directly influences ORCC activity by regulating release of or directly transporting ATP out of cells. The extracellular ATP activates the ORCC in an autocrine fashion, presumably by binding to an apical membrane purinergic receptor, to move additional chloride out of the cell. Intracellular electrical neutrality and sodium and water movement are also regulated at the apical membrane by the epithelial sodium channel (ENaC) and at the basal lateral membrane by sodium–potassium ATPase. In vitro, CFTR has been shown to regulate ENaC by inhibiting sodium reabsorption through ENaC. The absence of CFTR expression results in increased ENaC activity and enhanced sodium reabsorption, likely accounting for the enhanced sodium reabsorption noted in measurements in vitro and in vivo.

LOCALIZATION OF CFTR EXPRESSION Normal CFTR expression exhibits cell specificity and is developmentally regulated. CFTR expression can be detected using RNA blot analysis, *in situ* hybridization, or immunohistochemistry in epithelial cells of the sweat gland, nose, lung, salivary gland, bile ducts, gall bladder, pancreas, small intestine, colon, kidney, epididymis, uterus, and fallopian tube. Unexpectedly, CFTR expression in the airway is at a low level and is difficult to detect, despite a detectable cAMP-regulated chloride transport function. Onset of CFTR expression in the yolk sac, intestine, and lungs of the normal fetus occurs as early as the seventh week of gestation. During lung development, the CFTR gene is expressed in a temporal and spatial pattern within airway epithelial cells. CFTR expression is initially detectable in primitive epithelial cells of the lung bud during the glandular stage (at 5–10 weeks) but at birth is limited to the epithelial cells of the bronchi and small airways, with none detectable in the alveolar sacs. In the normal adult lung, CFTR expression is most marked in epithelial cells of the submucosal glands and is present at lower levels in bronchial and bronchiolar epithelial cells. In general, the expected localization of CFTR appears to be directly related to the sites of pathologic change in CF. However, CFTR can also be detected in some organs not typically affected in individuals with CF, including the salivary glands and kidney, suggesting that CFTR function is not important in these tissues or that nongenetic factors may also play a role in phenotype.

PATHOGENESIS OF CF-RELATED LUNG DISEASE

The relationship between the loss of CFTR function, abnormal chloride and sodium transport, and disease pathology remains a fundamental question. The current paradigm that relates a loss of CFTR function with dysfunction in multiple organ systems is that defective chloride secretion (and sodium reabsorption) results in abnormal, dehydrated secretions within the epithelial cell-lined ducts of the involved organ. The abnormal secretions lead to impaired fluid flow, plugs and obstructions within these ducts, and eventually, end-organ injury and dysfunction. The size and complexity of a duct, the nature of duct secretions, and the flow rate within the duct are all postulated to be important factors that lead to variation in CF phenotype. Many of these pathogenic factors can be appreciated when considering the example of CF-related pathologic changes in the pancreas. The pancreatic ducts become obstructed with inspissated secretions and concretions, and dilated, leading to fatty replacement and fibrosis of the pancreas and pancreatic exocrine insufficiency occurring in greater than 85% of individuals with CF. By similar mechanisms, bile duct obstruction leads to focal biliary cirrhosis. Obstruction of the vas deferens, a long tortuous tube carrying a high glycoprotein load, may account for the obliteration of the vas deferens found in greater than 95% of men with CF. CF-related lung disease may develop by similar mechanisms; however, direct contact with the environment through the airway makes the pathogenesis of lung injury more complex.

As with the pathogenesis of all CF organ injury, the development of the chronic obstructive pulmonary disease typical of CF-related lung injury is incompletely understood. The CF lung at birth appears histologically normal. It is believed that airway epithelial cell defective chloride secretion and excessive sodium absorption contribute to the formation of dehydrated, excessively viscid airway secretions. These secretions are postulated to be ineffectively cleared by the airway mucociliary apparatus because of high viscosity and an inability of the airway epithelial cells to alter the height of the periciliary sol layer for optimal ciliary function. The retained secretions are thought to lead to an increase in airway inflammation and, when infected by bacteria, lead to an ongoing cycle of lung injury. The current concepts of the pathogenesis of lung inflammation, infection, and injury are discussed *below* and are diagrammed in Fig. 37-2.

INITIATION OF AIRWAY INFLAMMATION The initiation of inflammation or infection in the CF lung occurs in the small airways or bronchioles less than 1 mm in diameter. Abnormal mucus results in retained mucous plugs or foreign particles that serve as a nidus for bacterial colonization and infection, and initiate an inflammatory response. Airway inflammation has been demonstrated to begin early in life without evidence of coexisting infection. Analysis of bronchoalveolar lavage fluid obtained from infants with CF, when compared with normal infants, reveals increases in numbers of neutrophils, concentration of neutrophil chemotaxis cytokine interleukin-8 (IL-8), free neutrophil elastase, and elastase–α_1-antitrypsin (α_1-AT) complexes. In these studies, bacterial pathogens could not be isolated in nearly half the infants with CF, indicating that airways inflammation may precede infection. These findings support the hypothesis that airway inflammation may be elicited solely by the accumulation of abnormal secretions. Alternatively, infection may have been present previously but cleared by the inflammatory response, or may have been present below the level of detection. Another interpretation of this data is that there is an obligatory role for CFTR in the regulation of the inflammatory cascade such that the lack of CFTR function results in increased inflammation. Regardless, the lack of proper CFTR expression is clearly associated with the initiation of airway inflammation and infection.

BACTERIAL PATHOGENS SPECIFIC TO THE CF AIRWAY The unique pattern of bacterial infection in the CF lung is a hallmark of the disease. However, the mechanism of bacterial species-specific infection has yet to be elucidated. In infants and children, *Staphylococcus aureus* and *Haemophilus influenzae* are the predominant pathogens. With advancing age, *Pseudomonas aeruginosa* becomes the most common pathogen. Once the CF lung has established colonization with *P. aeruginosa*, the bacteria is rarely eradicated. Several factors may be responsible for *P. aeruginosa* persistence, including virulence factors produced by *P. aeruginosa*, factors related to CFTR function, and host response.

Bacterial factors leading to persistent infection include those elaborated by *Pseudomonas* to enhance bacterial survival. *Pseudomonas aeruginosa* can produce unique ciliotoxins capable of impairing ciliary function and *Pseudomonas*-specific proteases that can cause local lung tissue damage and injure cilia. Persistent colonization is also facilitated by the expression of *Pseudomonas*-specific bacterial genes coding for the production of alginate. Alginate is an exopolysaccharide that causes the mucoid appearance of

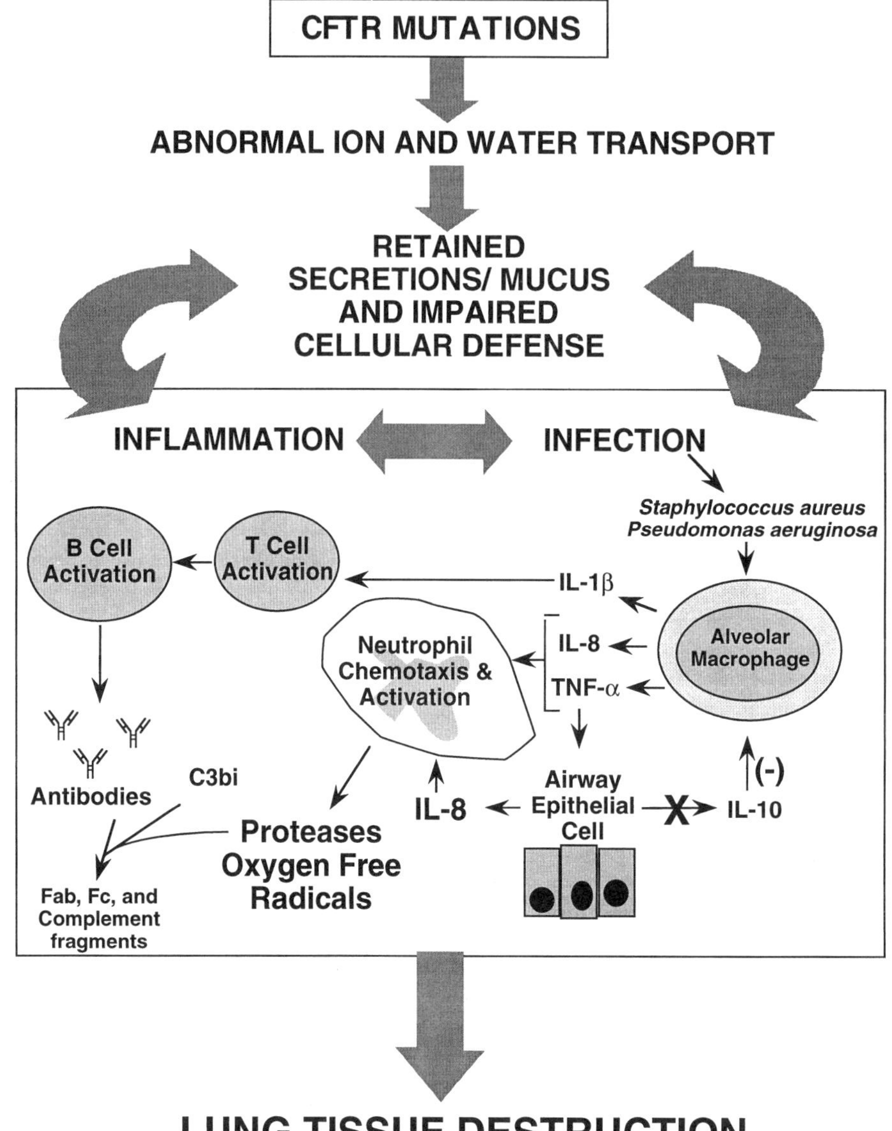

Figure 37-2 Pathogenesis of cystic fibrosis-related lung disease. Proposed mechanism for the development of CF-related lung disease. CFTR mutations lead to abnormal salt and water transport, which in turn result in retained desiccated airway secretions and possibly impaired defensin function. This results in chronic airways infection and inflammation that culminates in lung tissue destruction. The neutrophil is the central component of the inflammatory response being attracted to and activated in the CF airway by IL-8, TNF-α, and components of complement. Proteases and cytokines released by neutrophils attract additional inflammatory cells to CF airways, directly damage the airway, and may even perpetuate infection by cleaving antibodies and complement. (*See text* for further details.)

P. aeruginosa when cultured, and protects the bacterium from host defenses, antibiotics, and phagocytosis by neutrophils.

Loss of CFTR function may specifically allow enhanced epithelial cell infection and impair bacterial clearance. A predisposition for chronic infection of CF airways specifically with *S. aureus* and *P. aeruginosa* is suggested by studies proposing that impaired CFTR function raises the pH within the *trans*-Golgi complex. Alkalinization of the intraorganelle environment decreases sialyltransferase activity and results in the production of undersialylated proteins. Increased numbers of undersialylated proteins and gangliosides have been found in the apical membranes of CF epithelial cells, and in contrast to normally sialylated molecules (in non-CF cells), these asialogangliosides have been shown to specifically bind *S. aureus* and *P. aeruginosa*, but not other bacterial pathogens. Additional studies have shown that a ΔF508 airway epithelial cell line failed to internalize applied *P. aeruginosa*. This effect was specific for *P. aeruginosa*, and growing the cells at 26°C (a process that partially corrects ΔF508 CFTR expression on the cell surface) resulted in epithelial cell *P. aeruginosa* ingestion similar to that of control cells. Last, defensins, antibacterial peptides that possess an ability to specifically kill *S. aureus* and *P. aeruginosa* has been found to be secreted by both normal and CF cells. This bactericidal activity is inhibited by high sodium chloride concentrations, similar to the conditions predicted to be present in the sol layer of CF airway epithelial cells. Transfer of the normal CFTR cDNA to the CF cells results in eradication of the infection. If these conditions can be shown to exist in vivo it may provide a more specific explanation for the relationship between CFTR dysfunction, the chloride impermeability of CF airway epithelial cells, and the development of chronic infection in CF airways.

The antibody-mediated immune response resulting in the clearance of *P. aeruginosa* from the CF lung also appears to be impaired. Anti-*Pseudomonas* IgG titers increase with chronic infection and rising titers correlate with worsening lung disease. The increase in total IgG is primarily caused by an increase in the IgG_2 subclass antibody. The increased IgG_2 impairs *P. aeruginosa* clearance for two reasons. First, IgG_2 has a relatively low affinity for macrophage and lymphocyte Fc and complement receptors, decreasing the efficacy of the normal antibody-mediated antibacterial immune response. Second, IgG_2 is the predominant IgG subclass found in circulating immune complexes that compete with opsonized bacteria for Fc receptors located on phagocytic cells. Thus, the shift in IgG subclass production and consequent inhibition of phagocytosis may contribute to the persistence of *P. aeruginosa* airway colonization and the inflammatory response in the CF lung.

THE CHRONIC INFLAMMATORY RESPONSE The immune response to chronic airways infection is robust, and recruitment and activation of neutrophils is a central feature. Major cytokine mediators of neutrophil chemotaxis that are increased in the CF airway include tumor necrosis factor-α (TNF-α) and IL-8. These cytokines are released from macrophages that are activated by lipopolyscaccharide (LPS), TNF-α, and other mediators of inflammation. TNF-α also may induce airway epithelial cells to express IL-8. Additionally, *P. aeruginosa* directly stimulates respiratory epithelial cells to produce IL-8 via two mechanisms. First, *P. aeruginosa pili* and flagella that mediate *P. aeruginosa* adhesion to epithelial cells can induce IL-8 production by epithelial cells. However, *P. aeruginosa* mutants that do not express either of these adhesins (and which may be present in CF lungs with chronic disease) can stimulate IL-8 production by epithelial cells through a second mechanism. *Pseudomonas aeruginosa* secrete an exoproduct called the *Pseudomonas* autoinducer (PAI). PAI is a homoserine lactone derivative that can stimulate epithelial cell IL-8 production in a dose-dependent manner and this may perpetuate airway inflammation. Neutrophils recruited into the airway also express IL-8 and amplify the inflammatory process.

Inflammation and immune activation is also mediated by interleukin-1β (IL-1β), a cytokine with elevated levels in the bronchoalveolar lavage fluid from individuals with CF. IL-1β is produced by macrophages and activates neutrophils and T cells that, in turn, produce various other cytokines resulting in B-cell differentiation and antibody production. Counterregulatory cytokines capable of decreasing TNF-α and IL-1β levels are inhibited in CF. Interleukin-10 (IL-10) can attenuate inflammation by decreasing LPS-induced macrophage production of TNF-α and IL-1. IL-10 is constitutively produced by normal bronchial epithelial cells but is downregulated in the bronchial epithelial cells of individuals with CF, resulting in unopposed inflammatory cytokine release.

Bacterial products, abnormal mucus, complement activation products (e.g., C5a), and proinflammatory cytokines all contribute to the persistence of a high neutrophil burden in the CF airway. Neutrophils release oxygen free radicals and proteases that result in lung tissue damage, and ultimately can contribute to the development of bronchiectasis that is characteristic of CF. Proteases are released from activated neutrophils during phagocytosis or cell death. Proteases include cathepsin G, proteinase-3, collagenase, and others, but the serine protease neutrophil elastase appears to be most important for several reasons. First, neutrophil elastase can directly damage lung epithelial cells and degrade elastin and other components of lung extracellular matrix. Second, neutrophil elastase is capable of cleaving the Fc portion of intact IgG, and thereby inhibits macrophage-mediated phagocytosis of *P. aeruginosa*. Third, neutrophil elastase also cleaves CR1, which is the neutrophil receptor for C3b (one of the major opsonic components of complement that binds *P. aeruginosa*), and C3bi, which is the other major opsonic component of complement. By inhibiting neutrophil complement-mediated phagocytosis and antibody-mediated phagocytosis, neutrophil elastase likely contributes to the persistence of *P. aeruginosa* infection in the CF airway and ongoing lung destruction. Fourth, neutrophil elastase also stimulates epithelial cells to produce additional amounts of neutrophil chemotactic factor IL-8. Finally, neutrophil elastase induces hyperplasia of goblet cells and mucous-secreting cells of the airway. Mucous hypersecretion and extracellular DNA and actin released from dead neutrophils are added factors that adversely alter the physical properties of the abnormal CF airway secretions and promote the "vicious cycle" of lung inflammation, infection, and injury (Fig. 37-2).

The lung is normally protected from the deleterious effects of neutrophil elastase by the antiprotease α_1-AT and secretory leukoprotease inhibitor (SLPI). Although measured concentrations of α_1-AT and SLPI appear normal in airway epithelial lining fluid obtained from individuals with CF, most of the α_1-AT is complexed with neutrophil elastase or degraded. The persistent increased neutrophil elastase activity found in the airway epithelial fluid of the adult CF lung suggests that the relative level of α_1-AT is inadequate to protect the lung from injury.

CFTR GENOTYPE-PHENOTYPE RELATIONSHIPS

More than 600 disease-causing CFTR mutations have been identified. However, the ΔF508 mutation accounts for 66% of all mutant CFTR alleles identified. The ΔF508 mutation is a three-nucleotide deletion that results in the in-frame deletion of phenylalanine in position 508 of the CFTR protein. The next most common CFTR mutation, G542X, has a frequency of only 2.4%. Although most CFTR mutations are relatively infrequent, mutation frequencies vary considerably between nationalities, ethnic groups, and geographic locations. Some of the most common CFTR mutations are listed in Table 37-1.

TYPES OF MUTATIONS CFTR mutations may be classified by genetic mechanism into categories of missense, nonsense, frameshift, RNA splicing, and amino acid deletions. Mutations can also be separated into five classes based on the biochemical and physiologic consequences of the mutation on CFTR function. Class I mutations are those that result in absent or truncated CFTR protein synthesis because of premature termination of CFTR mRNA translation or the production of unstable mRNA. These mutations are usually caused by nonsense mutations resulting in a premature stop codon, frameshift mutations, or mutations that result in abnormal splicing of the mRNA. Class II mutations result in defective CFTR protein processing. In these mutations, CFTR protein is improperly folded and is degraded in the endoplasmic reticulum. Consequently, CFTR activity at the apical membrane is absent. An important example of this class is the ΔF508 mutation, which results in a partially glycosylated protein that is eventually degraded in the endoplasmic reticulum. It has been observed that,

Table 37-1
Common Cystic Fibrosis Mutations[a]

Mutation	*Frequency (%)[b]*	*Mutation class[c]*	*Phenotypic association*	*Population with increased prevalence[b]*
ΔF508	66	II	Severe disease	
G542X	2.4	I	Severe disease	Spanish
G551D	1.6	III	Severe disease	English
N1303K	1.3	II	Severe disease	Italian
W1282X	1.2	I	Severe disease	Ashkenazi-Jewish
R553X	0.7	I	Severe disease	German
621 + 1G→T	0.7	I	Severe disease	French Canadian
1717-1G→A	0.6	I	Severe disease	Italian
R117H	0.3	IV	Pancreatic sufficiency	
3849+10 kb C→T	0.2	V	Pancreatic sufficiency normal sweat chloride	

[c]Adapted from: Zielenski J, Tsui LC. Cystic fibrosis: genotypic and phenotypic variations. In: Annual Reviews of Genetics. Palo Alto: Annual Reviews, 1995;777–807. Used with permission of Annual Reviews, Inc.

[b]Mutations are designated by the code letter for the normal amino acid, followed by the amino acid position, and the letter of the substituted amino acid or an X, which denotes a nonsense mutation. A Δ indicates deletion of the amino acid whose letter follows it at the noted position. A + or – indicates mutations at various positions within introns relative to the cited position.

[c]Mutation class designated by biochemical or physiologic effect on CFTR protein.

if cells with the ΔF508 mutation are maintained at 26°C, some of the mutant protein becomes fully glycosylated and is transported normally to the apical membrane, where it is functional. Class III mutations result in proper localization of CFTR but in defective CFTR regulation. The degree of dysregulation can be determined by the response to ATP stimulation and may be mild if there is some residual chloride channel function, or severe (e.g., G551D) if the protein is fully dysfunctional. Class IV mutants result in defective chloride channel conductance and are often caused by mutations within regions coding for the transmembrane domains of the CFTR protein. The reduction in chloride channel activity caused by these mutations is variable. Class V mutations are those that result in the reduced synthesis of normal, functional CFTR protein and may be caused by mutations that result in alternative mRNA splicing, altered protein processing, or mutations in promoter sequences.

GENOTYPE-PHENOTYPE CORRELATION Following identification of multiple CFTR mutations, another aim of CF research has been to determine whether specific CFTR mutations and resultant CFTR dysfunction could be correlated with the variability in clinical manifestations of CF. It has been hypothesized that persons with two of the more severe CF mutations (usually from classes I, II, or III), might have different or more severe manifestations of their disease than those with more moderate CF mutations (i.e., class IV or V), in which some residual CFTR function may be expected. Studies have shown that patients who are compound heterozygous for a severe mutation (e.g., ΔF508) and one of a few more moderate mutations (e.g., R117H, A455E, 3849+10kbC→T) are more likely to maintain pancreatic sufficiency than patients with two "severe" mutations. One small study suggests an association between the A455E mutation and mild lung disease. However, in general, good correlation between CF mutations and lung disease has not been demonstrated. Furthermore, no genetically based explanation has been provided to account for differences in clinical manifestations of individuals with identical mutations. These studies may be hindered by the cross-sectional design, mortality bias, and the small number of individuals with various mutations. They also are confounded by environmental, infectious, and other genetic factors that may be important for the development of CF-related problems.

The recognition that chromosomal background affects CF phenotype has been important for understanding some genotype-phenotype correlation. These observations are based on differences in the nucleic acid sequence of the CFTR gene intron 8 splice site acceptor. The normal variant intron 8 splice site acceptor contains a sequence of seven thymidines (7T). Variants containing five thymidines (5T) and nine thymidines (9T) are also found, and these variants affect exon 9 splicing of the CFTR mRNA. In the presence of the 5T allele, the CFTR mRNA lacks exon 9 and codes for a nonfunctional protein. The effect of chromosomal background on phenotype can be observed in the example of the moderate R117H mutation. The R117H mutation can be found on the same allele as a 5T or 7T intron 8 variant. When R117H is found on the 7T background in the compound heterozygous individual, CF is a phenotypically less severe disease than if the mutation is found on the 5T background.

Congenital bilateral absence of the vas deferens (CBAVD) occurs in 95% of individuals with CF (leading to sterility), but may occur in isolation. When individuals with CBAVD who were otherwise asymptomatic were screened for CF mutations and the presence of the 5T variant, it was found that greater than half had either a non-5T variant + CF mutation on each allele, or a non-5T variant + CF mutation on one allele and a 5T variant with a wild-type CFTR on the other allele. These genotypes are correlated with decreases in the level of CFTR function and not necessarily with CF disease. These data, together with other studies, have led to the concept that CFTR-related end-organ dysfunction is based on the amount of active CFTR properly expressed in cells (Fig. 37-3). In this paradigm, the vas deferens is most sensitive to CFTR dysfunction, possibly related to the complex structural and flow aspects of the tubule. Individuals expressing more than 8–12% of normal CFTR mRNA are phenotypically normal, whereas those with only 1–3% of normal CFTR activity have typical pancreatic-insufficient CF with chronic lung disease. Individuals with levels of CFTR activity between these ranges have varying degrees of end-organ involvement, including CBAVD and CBAVD with pancreatic sufficiency and CF-related lung disease.

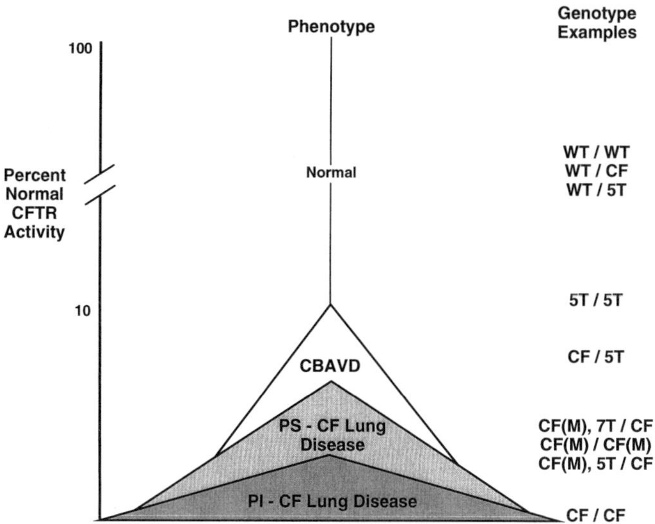

Figure 37-3 The relationship of CFTR activity to CFTR phenotype and genotype. Individuals with greater than approximately 10% normal CFTR activity are unaffected. Levels of normal CFTR activity below 10% are associated with increasingly severe disease ranging from congenital bilateral absence of the vas deferens (CBAVD), to pancreatic-sufficient cystic fibrosis lung disease (PS-CF Lung Disease), to typical pancreatic-insufficient CF lung disease (PI-CF Lung Disease), in a CFTR activity-dependent fashion. Genotype examples are shown on the right, indicating a normal CFTR (WT), an intron 8 polythymidine normal variant (7T) or altered splicing variant (5T), a moderate CFTR mutation [CF(M)], or a mutation associated with typical CF disease (CF). Phenotypes are not strictly correlated with exact thresholds of CFTR activity, therefore the same genotype may express different phenotypes in different individuals. The combination of a CF mutation with a 5T variant on the other allele may be associated with unaffected, CBAVD, or the PS-CF Lung Disease phenotypes. Genotype combinations with one CF(M) may preserve some residual CFTR activity. CF(M) plus one severe CF mutation (CF), or two CF(M) together are associated with CBAVD or PS-CF Lung Disease. The presence of two severe CF mutations is usually associated with typical PI-CF lung disease. (Adapted from Chillón et al. with permission of the publisher.)

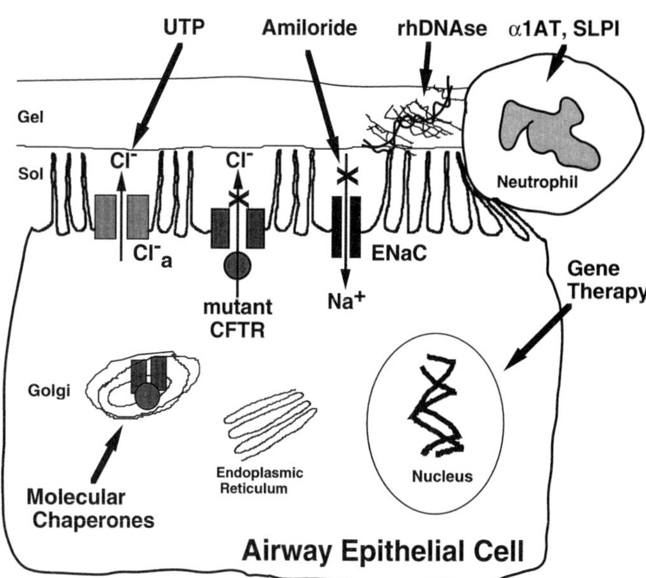

Figure 37-4 Molecular strategies for cystic fibrosis (CF) therapies. Novel molecular-based therapies for CF-related lung disease target several sites within the CF airway epithelial cell. To catalyze the breakdown of viscous secretions present in the CF-lung, recombinant human deoxyribonuclease (rhDNase) is delivered by aerosol. To inhibit neutrophil-mediated proteolytic injury, exogenous protease inhibitors α-1 antitrypsin (α_1-AT) and secretory leukoprotease inhibitor (SLPI) have been administered. To modulate apical membrane ion transport, the alternative chloride channel (Cl-a) can be activated by extracellular nucleotides and their analogs to secrete chloride in compensation for the defective cystic fibrosis transmembrane conductance regulator (CFTR) channel. Also, the hyperabsorption of sodium, mediated by the epithelial sodium channel (ENaC) when CFTR channel function is absent, can be blocked by amiloride and its analogs. Molecular chaperones can correct the abnormal intracellular trafficking of mutant CFTR (e.g., ΔF508) and help deliver mutant CFTR (degraded in the Golgi) to the apical membrane. To complement the mutant CFTR gene, strategies using gene therapy vectors to deliver a normal CFTR cDNA can be used. The gel and sol layers of airway mucus are labeled.

MOLECULAR-BASED THERAPEUTIC STRATEGIES

The increased knowledge of the molecular mechanisms of CFTR structure and function provides opportunities to design innovative therapies aimed at correcting the CF defect at the molecular level. These therapies might include those that attenuate inflammation, normalize CFTR trafficking within the cell, correct the ion transport abnormalities found in CF, deliver normal CFTR to cells within the lung, or deliver the normal CFTR gene to cells (Fig. 37-4). Many of these experimental strategies have been logically directed toward CF-related lung disease. In this regard, the lung is uniquely in communication with the outside environment, allowing novel approaches for aerosolized delivery of therapeutic agents, specifically directing therapy to the affected organ.

DEOXYRIBONUCLEASE I Extracellular DNA released from degraded neutrophils in the CF lung contributes to increased airway mucous viscosity. Deoxyribonuclease I (DNase) is an enzyme that cleaves extracellular DNA in CF airway secretions and is capable of decreasing CF sputum elasticity. When recombinant human DNase is administered via aerosol to the airways of individuals with mild to moderate CF-related lung disease, there is an improvement in lung function and decreased need for administration of intravenous antibiotics. Actin is an additional neutrophil product that increases CF sputum viscosity. Two agents that cleave actin, gelsolin and thymosin β4, are currently under investigation for use in CF-related lung disease.

ANTI-INFLAMMATORY THERAPY Chronic inflammation is present throughout life in the lungs and other organs of individuals with CF and is a major contributor to the structural damage characteristic of CF. It has been hypothesized that modulation of the inflammatory response might favorably alter the progression of CF-related lung disease and improve survival. Systemic nonspecific agents and lung-directed anti-inflammatory therapies have been investigated.

Systemic anti-inflammatory therapy with corticosteroids or nonsteroidal anti-inflammatory agents have been evaluated in clinical trials. Corticosteroids (prednisone, 1 mg/kg) administered orally on alternate days slowed the decline in lung function in individuals with mild to moderate CF-related lung disease compared with the placebo-treated group. This result was attributed to the anti-inflammatory effects of corticosteroids, but after 2 years of therapy, the therapeutic benefit was offset by growth retardation, cataract formation, and a higher incidence of abnormal glucose metabolism in the steroid treated group. The incidence of these adverse effects is decreased by the use of inhaled corticosteroids, although a definite benefit has not been demonstrated. Another anti-inflammatory agent, ibuprofen, in high doses, inhibits migration and aggregation of neutrophils and release of neutrophil lysosomal products. Administration of high-dose ibuprofen to individuals with mild CF-related lung disease was well-tolerated and slowed the decline of lung function in some groups; however, the study size was small.

The benefit of pentoxifylline, a phosphodiesterase inhibitor that blocks TNF-α- and IL-1β-mediated neutrophil chemotaxis and degranulation in vitro, was also evaluated for CF-related lung disease. A small, placebo-controlled trial demonstrated that individuals with CF treated with systemic pentoxifylline for 6 months had no increase in sputum elastase concentrations, whereas elastase concentrations increased significantly in the placebo group. A trend toward improved pulmonary function in the pentoxifylline-treated group was noted and a larger study is underway.

PROTEASE INHIBITORS Endogenous protease inhibitors capable of binding and neutralizing neutrophil elastase have been evaluated in an attempt to blunt neutrophil-mediated lung injury in the CF lung. α_1-Antitrypsin is an endogenous inhibitor of neutrophil elastase produced by the liver that circulates in plasma to all tissues. Secretory leukoprotease inhibitor (SLPI) is an inhibitor of neutrophil elastase produced by the lung airway epithelial cells. Aerosolized inhaled α_1-AT has been shown to increase concentrations of α_1-AT in the respiratory epithelial lining fluid of individuals with CF, inhibit neutrophil elastase activity in the epithelial lining fluid, and restore the ability of neutrophils exposed to CF epithelial lining fluid to kill *P. aeruginosa*. Similarly, aerosolized SLPI decreased neutrophil elastase activity, total neutrophil numbers, and IL-8 levels in CF epithelial lining fluid. These results suggest that the deleterious effects of neutrophil elastase on the CF lung could be mitigated by the exogenous administration of protease inhibitors.

CORRECTION OF CFTR TRAFFICKING Increasingly, strategies to alter abnormalities in CFTR posttranslational processing and protein trafficking are being considered. Most attention has been directed toward ΔF508 CFTR with the prospect of altering the maturation and trafficking of the improperly folded and subsequently degraded protein. Correction of ΔF508 CFTR trafficking will permit some chloride channel function if ΔF508 is expressed in the apical cell membrane. CFTR ΔF508 degradation has been demonstrated to be mediated by the binding of molecular chaperones, including calnexin, to abnormal CFTR protein. These chaperones act as a cellular quality control mechanism, detecting and degrading abnormal or improperly synthesized proteins. It has been proposed that selective inhibition of chaperone function may result in an increase in ΔF508 CFTR at the apical membrane. An alternative strategy is to use a reagent that can function as a chemical chaperone to stabilize immature ΔF508 CFTR and prevent protein degradation. In vitro, glycerol treatment of ΔF508 CFTR stabilizes the abnormal protein and leads to an increase in cellular cAMP-activated chloride conductance, suggesting a gain of CFTR function in the apical membrane.

MODULATION OF ION AND WATER TRANSPORT Correction of electrolyte and water transport abnormalities that result from CFTR deficiency is a promising approach to therapy, especially if used before to the development of structural lung damage. This may potentially be achieved by activating dysfunctional mutant CFTR, inducing higher levels of activity in a smaller number of CFTR channels that are correctly localized in the cell membrane, or by activating or inhibiting alternative cellular electrolyte transport channels.

In vitro, varied classes of compounds have shown an ability to activate CFTR-mediated chloride secretion through different mechanisms. The activity of some of these compounds may be specific for the ΔF508 CFTR mutation. Examples include type III phosphodiesterase inhibitors, amrinone and milrinone, that have been shown to stimulate CFTR-mediated chloride conductance, putatively by affecting cAMP-mediated CFTR regulation. The adenosine$_1$ receptor antagonist CPX activates ΔF508 CFTR in CF cell lines by an unknown mechanism. Another agent, NS004, a substituted benzimidazolone, can activate both wild-type and ΔF508 CFTR. The efficacy of these agents has not been evaluated in vivo.

Activity of alternative ion channels may compensate for deficient CFTR-mediated chloride secretion under certain situations. It is believed that expression of an alternative chloride channel in the lungs and pancreas of CFTR(–/–) mice protect them from the usual lung and pancreatic disease seen in human CF. Nucleotide triphosphates such as ATP and UTP activate chloride secretion in both normal and CF epithelial cells. Their mechanism of action is believed to be activation of the alternative chloride channel by raising intracellular Ca^{2+}. Amiloride, by inhibiting the epithelial sodium channel, may block the hyperabsorption of sodium and water seen in the CF airway. A preliminary clinical study of aerosolized amiloride in CF-related lung disease yielded promising results, but subsequent studies have not conclusively demonstrated a benefit. Further clinical evaluations of amiloride and UTP and some of their longer acting analogs, alone and in combination, are underway.

GENE THERAPY The discovery of the CFTR gene and simultaneous improvements in gene transfer have made possible the consideration of gene therapy for CF. The primary effort for human gene therapy for CF has been directed toward the delivery and expression of a normal CFTR cDNA in bronchial airway epithelial cells, thereby complementing the defective gene. The CF airway epithelial cells represent a difficult challenge for gene transfer for several reasons. First, lung cells cannot be removed, then reimplanted, making in vivo gene transfer necessary. Second, the airway epithelial cells do not rapidly divide, so that vectors such as retroviruses (which only integrate DNA into dividing cells) cannot provide the necessary transfection efficiency. Third, the airway is capable of mounting a marked immunologic response to foreign agents, potentially limiting some viral gene transfer systems. Finally, the presence of abnormal airways, marked inflammation, and increased mucus in the individual with even moderate pulmonary disease may impair efficient gene delivery, particularly to the submucosal glands where normal CFTR expression is more marked. Given these limitations, a variety of vector systems have been evaluated. Currently, adenovirus vectors have been shown experimentally to be advantageous compared with other vectors. However, no single vector is problem-free and liposomes, molecular conjugates of cell receptors, adeno-associated viral vectors, and other viral vectors may also be useful.

Before clinical trials, in vitro and animal gene transfer studies demonstrated that it would be reasonable to attempt gene therapy for CF-related lung disease, even if the gene could be transferred to only 5–10% of the airway epithelial cells. This was based on the observation that in vitro transfer of the CFTR cDNA to 5–7% of CF airway epithelial cells in a monolayer corrected the defect in cAMP-mediated chloride conductance, and that individuals with up to 90% defectively spliced mRNA as a result of the exon 8 splice site acceptor 5T-variant (i.e., producing 90% dysfunctional CFTR) had no lung disease. The CFTR cDNA could be transferred to approximately 5% of airway epithelial cells of experimental animals using adenovirus vectors, and transfer in experimental animals appeared to be safe. Furthermore, the adenovirus vectors carrying the CFTR cDNA can be made to be replication defective and are not known to be oncogenic.

Adenovirus has been investigated as a CFTR cDNA transfer vehicle in several clinical trials for CF therapy. The goal of these trials is to assess the safety of gene transfer vectors and to obtain biologic evidence of gene transfer. Trial design is typically to deliver a replication-defective adenovirus containing the CFTR cDNA in vivo to the nasal or lung epithelium of adults (and some children) with CF. Early evidence suggests that there is minimal expression of the transferred CFTR and that there is no change in chloride channel activity to the normal range. Although no evidence of clinical improvement has been expected in these early trials, there is evidence of immune reaction to the adenovirus. The inflammatory response to the adenovirus vector has been a critical limiting factor for some trials but has been important for driving the development of less immunogenic adenovirus vectors that are also being clinically evaluated. To date, at least 14 CF gene transfer trials (in the United States and Europe) are in progress or have been completed, employing various adenovirus vectors. Also, DNA with liposomes (two trials) and an adeno-associated virus vector (one trial) are being tested. The early studies of gene therapy for CF have been a major stimulus for rapidly developing improvements in gene delivery vectors for many other diseases.

SUMMARY

Information obtained in less than a decade has lead to the burgeoning of the field of basic CF research with important implications for many other diseases found to share common features. A relatively obscure area for investigation until the CF gene was isolated in 1989, it is now known that CF is a genetic disorder that results from mutations in the CFTR gene coding for a cAMP-regulated chloride channel. A rigorous scientific understanding of the pathophysiology of abnormal salt and water movement that leads to the clinical characteristics of CF continues to be a major endeavor in the CF field. Currently, most evidence suggests that a defect in the CFTR protein leads to abnormal salt and water movement in the epithelial cells of the sweat duct, pancreas, lung, and other organs, and the subsequent clinical manifestations of CF. Current observations in CF-related lung disease support the notion that abnormal secretions are linked to an exuberant inflammatory response exacerbated by infection with specific species of bacteria, leading to chronic inflammation and lung injury. Genetic and biochemical studies indicate that if the amount of CFTR functioning in the apical aspect of the epithelial cell is above a specific threshold of about 10% of the normal amount, then salt and water movement is adequate and clinical disease is absent. Based on these and other rapidly acquired data, it is now possible to consider a variety of novel molecular-based therapies for CF.

SELECTED REFERENCES

Anderson MP, Rich DP, Gregory RJ, Smith AE, Welsh MJ. Generation of cAMP-activated chloride currents by expression of CFTR. Science 1991;251:679–682.

Aronoff SC, Quinn FJ, Carpenter LS, Novick WJ. Effects of pentoxifylline on sputum neutrophil elastase and pulmonary function in patients with cystic fibrosis: preliminary observations. J Pediatr 1994;125:992–997.

Birrer P, McElvaney N, Rudegerg A, et al. Protease-antiprotease imbalance in the lungs of children with cystic fibrosis. Am J Respir Crit Care Med 1994;150:207–213.

Biwersi J, Emans N, Verkman AS. Cystic fibrosis transmembrane conductance regulator activation stimulates endosome fusion in vivo. Proc Natl Acad Sci USA 1996;93:12,484–12,489.

Bonfield TL, Konstan MW, Burfeind P, Panuska JR, Hilliard JB, Berger M. Normal bronchial epithelial cells constitutively produce the anti-inflammatory cytokine interleukin-10, which is downregulated in cystic fibrosis. Am J Respir Cell Mol Biol 1995;13:257–261.

Cheng SH, Rich DP, Marshall J, Gregory RJ, Welsh MJ, Smith AE. Phosphorylation of the R domain by cAMP-dependent protein kinase regulates the CFTR chloride channel. Cell 1991;66:1027–1036.

Chillon M, Casals T, Mercier B, et al. Mutations in the cystic fibrosis gene in patients with congenital absence of the vas deferens. N Engl J Med 1995;332:1475–1480.

Crystal RG, McElvaney NG, Rosenfeld MA, et al. Administration of an adenovirus containing the human CFTR cDNA to the respiratory tract of individuals with cystic fibrosis. Nat Genet 1994;8:42–51.

Cystic Fibrosis Foundation. Patient Registry 1996 Annual Data Report, Bethesda, Maryland, August 1997.

The Cystic Fibrosis Genotype-Phenotype Consortium. Correlation between genotype and phenotype in patients with cystic fibrosis. N Engl J Med 1993;329:1308–1313.

Denning GM, Anderson MP, Amara JF, Marshall J, Smith AE, Welsh MJ. Processing of mutant cystic fibrosis transmembrane conductance regulator is temperature-sensitive. Nature 1992;358:761–764.

DiMango E, Zar J, Bryan R, Prince A. Diverse *Pseudomonas aeruginosa* gene products stimulate respiratory epithelial cells to produce interleukin-8. J Clin Invest 1995;96:2204–2210.

Eigen H, Rosenstein BJ, FitzSimmons S, Schidlow DV. A multicenter study of alternate-day prednisone therapy in patients with cystic fibrosis. Cystic Fibrosis Foundation Prednisone Trial Group. J Pediatr 1995;126:515–523.

Engelhardt JF, Zepeda M, Cohn JA, Yankaskas JR, Wilson JM. Expression of the cystic fibrosis gene in adult human lung. J Clin Invest 1994;93:737–749.

Fick R, Naegel G, Squier S, Wood R, Gee J, Reynolds H. Proteins of the cystic fibrosis respiratory tract: fragmented immunoglobulin G opsonic antibody causing defective opsonophagocytosis. J Clin Invest 1984;74:236–248.

Fuchs HJ, Borowitz DS, Christiansen DH, et al. Effect of aerosolized recombinant human DNase on exacerbations of respiratory symptoms and on pulmonary function in patients with cystic fibrosis. The Pulmozyme Study Group. N Engl J Med 1994;331:637–642.

Hart P, Warth JD, Levesque PC, et al. Cystic fibrosis gene encodes a cAMP-dependent chloride channel in heart. Proc Natl Acad Sci USA 1996;93:6343–6348.

Hornick D, Fick R. The immunoglobulin G subclass composition of immune complexes in cystic fibrosis. J Clin Invest 1990;86: 1285–1292.

Imundo L, Barasch J, Prince A, Al-Awqati Q. Cystic fibrosis epithelial cells have a receptor for pathogenic bacteria on their apical surface. Proc Natl Acad Sci USA 1995;92:3019–3023.

Kerem B, Rommens JM, Buchanan JA, et al. Identification of the cystic fibrosis gene: genetic analysis. Science 1989;245:1073–1080.

Kiesewetter S, Macek MJ, Davis C, et al. A mutation in CFTR produces different phenotypes depending on chromosomal background. Nat Genet 1993;5:274–278.

Knowles MR, Clarke LL, Boucher RC. Activation by extracellular nucleotides of chloride secretion in the airway epithelia of patients with cystic fibrosis. N Engl J Med 1991;325:533–538.

Knowles MR, Church NL, Waltner WE, et al. A pilot study of aerosolized amiloride for the treatment of lung disease in cystic fibrosis. N Engl J Med 1990;322:1189–1194.

Knowles MR, Hohneker KW, Zhou Z, et al. A controlled study of adenoviral-vector-mediated gene transfer in the nasal epithelium of patients with cystic fibrosis. N Engl J Med 1995;333:823–831.

Koh J, Sferra TJ, Collins FS. Characterization of the cystic fibrosis transmembrane conductance regulator promoter region. Chromatin context and tissue-specificity. J Biol Chem 1993;268:15912–15921.

Konstan MW, Byard PJ, Hoppel CL, Davis PB. Effect of high-dose ibuprofen in patients with cystic fibrosis. N Engl J Med 1995;332:848–854.

Manson AL, Trezise AE, MacVinish LJ, et al. Complementation of null CF mice with a human CFTR YAC transgene. EMBO J 1997;16:4238–4249.

McElvaney NG, Hubbard RC, Birrer P, et al. Aerosol alpha 1-antitrypsin treatment for cystic fibrosis. Lancet 1991;337:392–394.

Pind S, Riordan JR, Williams DB. Participation of the endoplasmic reticulum chaperone calnexin (p88, IP90) in the biogenesis of the cystic fibrosis transmembrane conductance regulator. J Biol Chem 1994;269:12,784–12,788.

Qu BH, Strickland EH, Thomas PJ. Localization and suppression of a kinetic defect in cystic fibrosis transmembrane conductance regulator folding. J Biol Chem 1997;272:15,739–15,744.

Riordan JR, Rommens JM, Kerem B, et al. Identification of the cystic fibrosis gene: cloning and characterization of complementary DNA. Science 1989;245:1066–1073.

Sato S, Ward CL, Krouse ME, Wine JJ, Kopito RR. Glycerol reverses the misfolding phenotype of the most common cystic fibrosis mutation. J Biol Chem 1996;271:635–638.

Schwiebert EM, Egan ME, Hwang TH, et al. CFTR regulates outwardly rectifying chloride channels through an autocrine mechanism involving ATP. Cell 1995;81:1063–1073.

Smith J, Travis S, Greenberg P, Welsh M. Cystic fibrosis airway epithelia fail to kill bacteria because of abnormal airway surface fluid. Cell 1996;85:229–236.

Stutts MJ, Canessa CM, Olsen JC, et al. CFTR as a cAMP-dependent regulator of sodium channels. Science 1995;269:847–850.

Tizzano EF, Buchwald M. CFTR expression and organ damage in cystic fibrosis. Ann Intern Med 1995;123:305–308.

Tosi M, Zakem H, Berger M. Neutrophil elastase cleaves C3bi on opsonized pseudomonas as well as CR1 on neutrophil to create a functionally important opsonin receptor mismatch. J Clin Invest 1990;86:300–308.

Welsh MJ, Smith AE. Molecular mechanisms of CFTR chloride channel dysfunction in cystic fibrosis. Cell 1993;73:1251–1254.

Xia Y, Haws CM, Wine JJ. Disruption of monolayer integrity enables activation of a cystic fibrosis "bypass" channel in human airway epithelia. Nat Med 1997;3:802–805.

Zielenski J, Tsui LC. Cystic fibrosis: genotypic and phenotypic variations. Ann Rev Genet 1995; 29: pp. 777–807.

38 Pulmonary Emphysema

STEVEN D. SHAPIRO AND ROBERT M. SENIOR

CHRONIC OBSTRUCTIVE PULMONARY DISEASE

EPIDEMIOLOGY Chronic obstructive pulmonary disease (COPD) is defined by the American Thoracic Society as "a disease state characterized by the presence of airflow obstruction due to chronic bronchitis or emphysema; the airflow obstruction is generally progressive, may be accompanied by airflow hyperreactivity, and may be viewed as partially reversible."

COPD occurs worldwide, but it is principally a major health problem in societies in which cigaret smoking is common and the average life-span extends into the sixth decade or beyond. The number of people in the United States afflicted with COPD has been rising sharply in recent decades. Estimates are that about 14 million persons in the United States have COPD, a number that has increased approximately 40% since 1982. The death rate as a result of COPD in the United States has also been increasing in recent decades in contrast to falling death rates from heart and cerebrovascular diseases for the same interval. COPD is now the fourth most common cause of death in the United States, accounting for nearly 4.5% of all deaths, and is a contributory factor in additional 4.3%.

Cigaret smoking is by far the most important risk factor for the development of COPD. Accelerated deterioration of ventilatory function is common among smokers; however, its magnitude is relatively small in most smokers. The relationship between amount of smoking and risk of COPD is quite unpredictable on an individual basis. Many persons with a high number of pack-years of smoking still have a normal or near-normal forced expiratory volume in 1 s (FEV_1), whereas some individuals have a reduced FEV_1 with relatively modest smoking histories. Among smokers who have already sustained reductions in FEV_1, the consequences of continued smoking on ventilatory function are much more impressive than when all smokers are lumped together. The Lung Health Study found that among middle-aged smokers with an FEV_1 between 55 and 90% of predicted, differences of several hundred milliliters of FEV_1 developed within 5 years between those who quit smoking and those who did not quit.

The percentage of smokers in the adult population in the United States has dropped during the past 30 years, particularly among males, from greater than 50% to approximately 25%. However, COPD will continue to be common into the foreseeable future because the United States still has 48 million smokers, and 3000 people, mostly teenagers, take up the habit daily. In fact, smoking is increasing among teenagers. With the large-scale marketing of tobacco products to developing countries that is happening now, an increased prevalence of COPD can be expected throughout the world in the future.

STRUCTURE-FUNCTION In stating that COPD may be caused by either chronic bronchitis or emphysema, it is implied that COPD can result from diseases of either the airways or the lung parenchyma. Although this may be true, COPD is usually a result of pathology and dysfunction of both airways and lung parenchyma.

Cigaret smoking leads to changes in the large airways, small airways, and lung parenchyma (Fig. 38-1). The changes in the large airways, which include mucous gland enlargement and goblet cell hyperplasia, are responsible for chronic bronchitis, defined as cough and sputum on most days for at least 3 months for at least 2 successive years without another explanation. It should be noted that criteria for the diagnosis of chronic bronchitis do not include airflow obstruction and that, in fact, the large airway changes associated with chronic bronchitis do not cause airflow obstruction. Some evidence, however, does implicate chronic bronchitis as a risk factor for chronic airflow obstruction.

Approximately 30 years ago, Hogg and associates found that airways 2 mm or less in diameter were the principal sites of increased airway resistance in COPD. These studies gave rise to the concept that COPD is a "small airway disease," a concept that has stood the test of time. Although from a physiological standpoint the obstruction to airflow in COPD is in the small airways, in most individuals with COPD the relative importance of emphysema vs intrinsic abnormalities of the small airways as the structural basis for the obstruction is complex. It is evident that there is not a single pathologic feature that explains airflow obstruction in every individual with COPD. Emphysema and small airway pathology are both present in most persons with COPD; their relative contributions to obstruction probably vary from one person to another. Emphysema appears to lead to airflow obstruction because the alveolar wall attachments that help maintain the patency of small airways by producing outward traction on their walls are decreased in number and the capacity of the attachments that do remain to develop traction is decreased.

THE PATHOGENESIS OF EMPHYSEMA

Emphysema is defined "as a condition of the lung characterized by abnormal, permanent enlargement of airspaces distal to the terminal bronchiole, accompanied by destruction of their walls, and without obvious fibrosis." Thus, emphysema is a structural

From: *Principles of Molecular Medicine* (J. L. Jameson, ed.), ©1998 Humana Press Inc., Totowa, NJ.

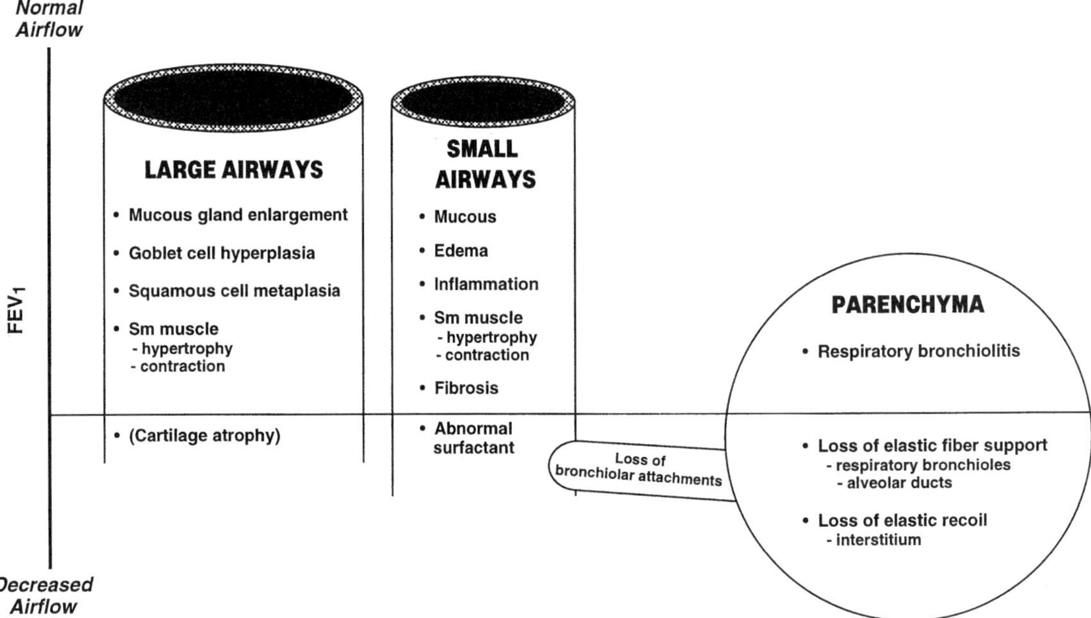

Figure 38-1 Pathologic changes in relation to airflow in chronic obstructive pulmonary disease (COPD). Changes observed in large airways (>2 mm), small airways (<2 mm), and lung parenchyma are depicted. Those abnormalities above the line are associated with normal airflow (normal forced expiratory volume in 1 s [FEV_1]), whereas those below the line are likely to cause decreased airflow (low FEV_1). Note, while controversial, our belief is that most airway changes associated with excess material in the airway do not cause airflow obstruction. A unifying hypothesis for airflow obstruction involves loss of lung elastin resulting in both decreased small airway attachments and decreased parenchymal elastic recoil.

abnormality of the gas-exchanging airspaces, that is, the respiratory bronchioles, alveolar ducts, and alveoli, characterized by obliteration and perforation of airspace walls with coalescence of airspaces into much larger ones than normal.

PROTEINASE–ANTIPROTEINASE HYPOTHESIS In 1963 Laurell and Eriksson reported an association of chronic airflow obstruction and emphysema with deficiency of serum α_1-antitrypsin (α_1-AT); and in 1964 Gross and associates described the first reproducible model of emphysema in experimental animals by injecting papain, a plant-derived proteinase, into the lungs via the trachea. Together these observations indicated that emphysema could be induced by proteolytic injury to the lung extracellular matrix, and eventually they led to the proteinase–antiproteinase hypothesis of emphysema that has been the prevailing concept of the pathogenesis of emphysema ever since. Subsequently, when it was established that α_1-AT is primarily aimed at inhibition of neutrophil elastase and that only proteinases with activity against elastin produce emphysema when given experimentally, emphysema came to be seen as a disease resulting primarily from destruction of lung elastin.

According to the proteinase–antiproteinase hypothesis of emphysema, there is a steady or episodic release of proteolytic enzymes with elastolytic activity into the lung parenchyma (Fig. 38-2). Normally, plasma proteinase inhibitors, especially α_1-AT, permeate lung tissue and prevent proteolytic enzymes from digesting structural proteins of the lungs. Proteinase inhibitors synthesized locally in the lungs also contribute to the antiproteinase shield. Emphysema results from an augmentation of proteinase release in the lungs, a reduction in the antiproteinase defense within the lungs, or a combination of both increased proteinase burden and decreased proteinase inhibitory capacity. Accordingly, emphysema occurs when there is an imbalance between proteinases and antiproteinases in favor of proteinases.

During study of proteinases in emphysema it has become appreciated that events controlling proteolytic injury to the extracellular matrix of the lung do not necessarily operate over the lungs as whole. In fact, important events are tightly controlled and occur at or near the cell membrane of inflammatory cells. Thus, the proteinase–antiproteinase hypothesis has been modified to consider "imbalance" between proteinases and their inhibitors in compartments as small as the microenvironments immediately surrounding inflammatory cells.

Despite the plausibility of the proteinase–antiproteinase hypothesis as the basis for the development of emphysema, many fundamental questions are still unanswered. Inflammatory cells are the presumed source of injurious proteinases, but specifically which inflammatory cells are the culprits? Is it possible that resident cells of the lungs, such as fibroblasts, also contribute to alveolar septal destruction? What are the signals that initiate and perpetuate inflammation in the lungs during the development of emphysema associated with smoking? Which proteolytic enzymes are involved in lung destruction, and how do they make contact with the lung extracellular matrix and maintain their catalytic activity in the presence of an abundance of proteinase inhibitors? Advances in molecular biology will allow investigators to begin to tackle these critical issues.

INFLAMMATION–DESTRUCTION–REPAIR HYPOTHESIS A broader conception of the pathogenesis of emphysema associated with cigaret smoking has been termed the "inflammation–destruction–repair" hypothesis. In this hypothesis, proteolytic enzymes from inflammatory cells and possibly resident lung cells are still central to production of lung injury but, in addition, it is proposed that aberrant repair of the damaged lung also occurs. Abnormal-appearing elastic fibers have been found in human emphysema. Aberrant collagen repair may also contribute to the emphysematous process. Recent studies indicate increased col-

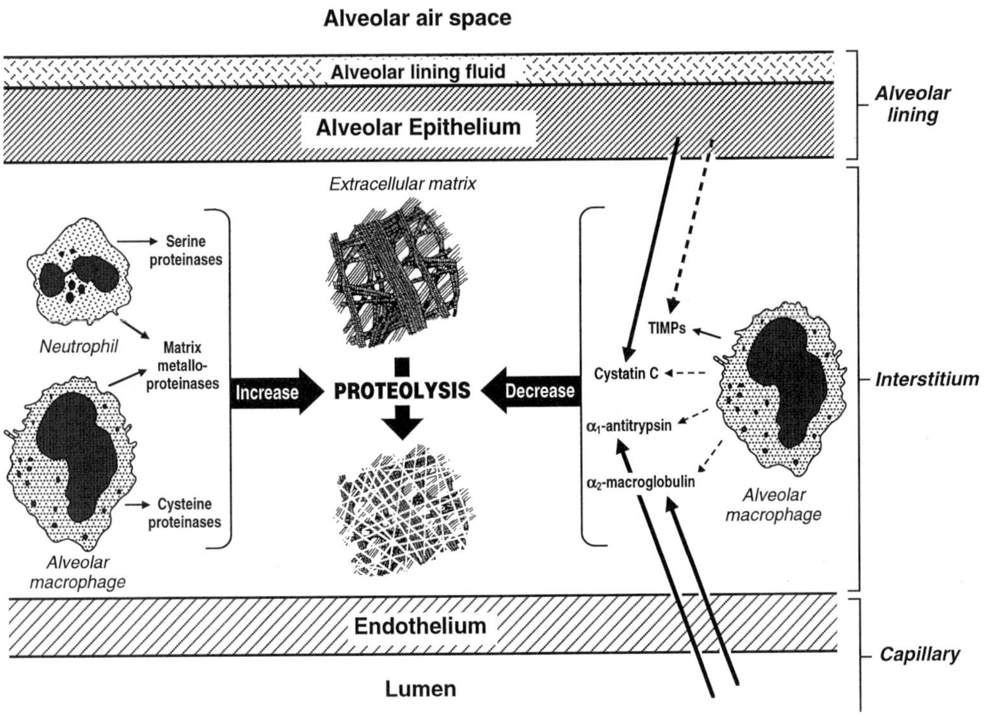

Figure 38-2 Proteinase–antiproteinase balance in the lung parenchyma determines the risk of proteolytic degradation of lung extracellular matrix. Proteinases released by neutrophils, macrophages, and perhaps resident cells have the capacity to degrade lung extracellular matrix components including elastin, thus predisposing to emphysema. Matrix proteolysis is limited by the presence of inhibitors to each class of proteinases. Some inhibitors are locally derived (TIMP, cystatin C), whereas others arrive via the bloodstream (α_1-AT, α_2-macroglobulin). The predominant sources are depicted by solid arrows; lesser sources are indicated by dashed arrows. (Adapted from Evans MD, and Pryor WA. Cigaret smoking, emphysema, and damage to α_1-proteinase inhibitor. Am J Physiol 1994;266:L593–L611.)

lagen per unit volume of airspace wall in emphysematous lungs from smokers and in experimental animals subjected to chronic cigaret smoke inhalation. These findings suggest that the concept of emphysema formation as a purely destructive process may be in error.

INFLAMMATORY CELLS AND THEIR PROTEINASES IN THE LUNGS

Cigaret smoking leads to neutrophil retention in the pulmonary microcirculation circulation and deposition in the lung parenchyma. Cigaret smoking also causes activation and marked accumulation of alveolar (and perhaps interstitial) macrophages. These cells are capable of producing a variety of metallo- and cysteine proteinases that can degrade all components of the extracellular matrix. Other immune and inflammatory cells, such as eosinophils, T lymphocytes, and mast cells, might also contribute to lung destruction; and resident cells within the lung, such as fibroblasts and alveolar type II cells, may be induced to synthesize proteolytic enzymes in response to cigaret smoking.

Defining the cells and proteinases responsible for destruction of lung extracellular matrix associated with cigaret smoking will be critical for development of appropriate proteinase inhibitors for future application in COPD. For example, neutrophils produce predominantly serine proteinases, whereas macrophages synthesize a variety of metallo- and cysteine proteinases as well as some serine proteinases. Neutrophil elastase, a serine proteinase, is almost certainly a critical enzyme in the pathogenesis of the panacinar emphysema associated with marked α_1-AT deficiency, but other elastolytic enzymes that are not serine proteinases, and not necessarily from neutrophils, might be involved in the pathogenesis of emphysema in smokers with normal levels of serum α_1-AT.

Not only do the profiles of proteinases differ between these inflammatory cell types, but regulation of the proteinase expression is quite distinct. Neutrophils are short-lived and package active proteinases into granules ready for quick release, optimal for rapid egress from the vasculature and delivering a lethal blow to microorganisms. Macrophage metalloproteinase expression, on the other hand, is highly regulated by inflammatory cytokines, matrix fragments, and other agents, resulting in much slower release but sustained synthesis. Thus, macrophages appear to monitor and respond to their environment, properties that could allow for tissue remodeling and possibly control of other inflammatory events.

NEUTROPHILS As noted, smoking causes retention of neutrophils in the lungs, apparently by increasing adhesiveness of neutrophils and pulmonary microvascular endothelium, and possibly by increasing neutrophil stiffness so that the cells cannot deform enough to get through pulmonary capillaries normally. Bronchoalveolar lavage (BAL) fluids from smokers contain more neutrophils than lavage fluids from nonsmokers, indicating that smoking leads to recruitment of neutrophils into lung tissue.

Neutrophil Serine Proteinases Serine proteinases are characterized by conserved His, Asp, and Ser residues that form a charge relay system that functions by transfer of electrons from the carboxyl group of Asp to the oxygen of Ser, which then becomes a powerful nucleophile able to attack the carbonyl carbon atom of the peptide bond of the substrate. Serine proteinases are synthesized as preproenzymes in the endoplasmic reticulum that are processed by cleavage of the signal peptide (pre-) and removal of a

Table 38-1
Elastases Present in the Lung Parenchyma

Enzyme class	*Enzyme*	*Molecular mass[a], kDa*	*Cell of origin*	*Matrix substrates other than elastin*	*Relative elastolytic activity, pH 7.5*
Serine	Neutrophil elastase	27–31	Neutrophil (monocyte)[d]	BM components[b]	100%
	Proteinase 3	28–34	Neutrophil (monocyte)	BM components[b]	40%
	Cathepsin G	27–32	Neutrophil (monocyte, mast cell)	BM components[b]	20%
Matrix metalloproteinase	92-kDa gelatinase	92–95	Macrophage, neutrophil, eosinophil	Denatured collagens, types IV, V, and VII collagen	30%
	Metalloelastase	54	Macrophage	BM components[b]	35%
Cysteine	Cathepsin L	29	Macrophage	(Inactive at pH 7.5)	0%[c]
	Cathepsin S	28	Macrophage	(Unknown)	80%[c]

[a]Denotes pre-proenzyme forms.
[b]Basement membrane (BM) components include fibronectin, laminin, entactin, vitronectin, and type IV collagen (nonhelical domains).
[c]These enzymes are significantly more potent than neutrophil elastase at pH 5.5.
[d]Parentheses denote minor cellular sources.

dipeptide (pro-) by cathepsin C, and stored in granules as active packaged proteins. Distinct subsets of serine proteinases are expressed in a lineage-restricted manner in immune and inflammatory cells. Serine proteinases are also expressed in a developmentally specific manner. For example, neutrophil elastase, proteinase 3, and cathepsin G are major components of primary or azurophil granules that are formed at a specific stage during the development of myeloid cells. The fact that neutrophil serine proteinases have a pH optimum of about 7.4 suggests that these enzymes could damage lung tissue if liberated from the neutrophil. Also, the finding that active neutrophil elastase and cathepsin G are concentrated on the outer face of the plasma membrane of activated neutrophils may help explain how these enzymes can function in the extracellular environment despite large excesses of α_1-AT and other inhibitors.

Neutrophil Elastase (HNE) HNE has activity against a broad range of extracellular matrix proteins including elastin (Table 38-1). After the discovery of α_1-AT deficiency and the capacity of HNE to cause emphysema in experimental animals, HNE has been considered to be of primary importance in the pathogenesis of pulmonary emphysema. Further evidence supporting involvement of HNE in this disease process includes (1) the presence of HNE and neutrophils in the lung tissue and BAL of patients with emphysema in some (but not all) studies, (2) the observation that smoking leads to an acute increase in a specific peptide released by HNE action on fibrinogen, and (3) the demonstration that cigaret smoke can oxidize a methionine residue in the reactive center of α_1-AT, inactivating α_1-AT, and thus altering the HNE–α_1-AT balance *(see below)*. Whether oxidative inactivation occurs in vivo is uncertain. Despite these tantalizing pieces of information, however, there are no studies directly linking HNE to the pathogenesis of the common form of emphysema related to cigaret smoking.

Proteinase 3 (PR3) PR3 is roughly 40% as potent as HNE against elastin. PR3 has been shown to cause emphysema in experimental animals. This molecule has been identified as the autoantigen target of cytoplasmic-staining anti–polymorphonuclear neutrophil (PMN) autoantibody in Wegeners granulomatosis.

Cathepsin G (CG) CG is stored in neutrophil primary granules and to a lesser degree in mast cells and a subset of peripheral blood monocytes. CG is chymotryptic, but also has matrix-degrading activity with nearly 20% the elastolytic capacity of HNE. Moreover, CG has been reported to increase elastolytic activity of HNE and may facilitate neutrophil penetration of epithelial and endothelial barriers by increasing their permeability.

Neutrophil Metalloproteinases Neutrophils contain two matrix metalloproteinases (MMPs), the 92-kDa gelatinase (gelatinase B) and neutrophil collagenase. In the neutrophil these MMPs are stored within the specific granules. Neutrophil collagenase can degrade interstitial collagens, but is less active against other extracellular matrix components. Gelatinase B is active against a number of substrates, including denatured collagens (gelatins), basement membrane components, and elastin.

MONOCYTES Monocytes resemble neutrophils in that they contain HNE and CG in peroxidase-positive granules, which are similar to the azurophil granules of neutrophils. These proteinases are synthesized by monocyte precursors in the bone marrow, and can be rapidly released by the circulating cell, perhaps for transvascular migration. Interestingly, expression of both of these serine proteinases is limited to a subset of "proinflammatory" monocytes (~15% of total) that appear to be those capable of tissue penetration. As monocytes differentiate into macrophages in tissues they lose their HNE and CG, but acquire the capacity to synthesize and secrete metalloproteinases.

MACROPHAGES Alveolar macrophages are the most abundant defense cells in the lung under normal conditions and during states of chronic inflammation. Alveolar macrophages are prominent in the respiratory bronchioles of cigaret smokers, where emphysematous changes are first manifest. Because they are capable of producing factors that both promote destruction of extracellular matrix and protect against matrix destruction, macrophages may have a complex role in the pathogenesis of emphysema. Clearly, alveolar macrophages do have the capacity to degrade elastin by means of several different proteolytic enzymes (Table 38-1).

Cysteine (Thiol) Proteinases Cysteine proteinases represent a large, diverse group of plant and animal enzymes with amino acid homology at the active site only. They are inhibited by cystatins, which are produced ubiquitously in local tissue environments (Table 38-2). Human alveolar macrophages produce the lysosomal thiol proteinases, cathepsins B, H, L, and S. These enzymes share similar sizes of 24–32 kDa and high mannose side chains (typical of proteins targeted for lysosomal accumulation).

Table 38-2
Proteinase Inhibitors Present in the Lung Parenchyma

Inhibitor	*Molecular mass, kDa*	*Cell of origin*	*Class of proteinases inhibited*
α_2-Macroglobulin	725	Hepatocyte	Serine
		Lung fibroblast	Metallo
		(Macrophage)[a]	Cysteine
α_1-AT	52	Hepatocyte:	Serine[b]
		(Macrophage)	
SLPI	12	Large airway epithelial cell	Serine[c]
		Type II pneumocyte	
			Serine[c]
Elafin	12	Large airway epithelial cell	Serine
TIMP-1	27.5	Macrophages	Metallo
		Resident lung parenchymal cell	
Cystatin C	13	Bronchial epithelial cell	Cysteine
		(Macrophage)	

[a]Parentheses denote minor cellular sources.
[b]α_1-AT has greater affinity for neutrophil elastase than for proteinase 3 and cathepsin G.
[c]SLPI does not inhibit neutrophil elastase.
α_1-AT, α_1-antitrypsin; TIMP-1, tissue inhibitor of matrix metalloproteinase-1.

Cathepsins B and H have little endopeptidase activity and may function to activate other proteins similar to a distant relative, interleukin converting enzyme. Cathepsins L and S have large active pockets with relatively indiscriminate substrate specificities that include elastin and other matrix components. These enzyme have an acidic pH optimum, but cathepsin S retains ~25% of its elastolytic capacity at neutral pH (making it approximately equal to NE). Thus, these enzymes clearly have the capacity to cause lung destruction if they are targeted to the cell surface or extracellular space (especially if macrophages can acidify their microenvironment). These properties are plausible but remain to be proven. Cathepsin L production is increased in smokers' alveolar macrophages.

Matrix Metalloproteinases (MMPs) MMPs comprise a family of matrix-degrading enzymes believed to be essential for normal development and physiologic tissue remodeling and repair. Abnormal expression of metalloproteinases has been implicated in many destructive processes, including tumor cell invasion and angiogenesis, arthritis, atherosclerosis, arterial aneurysms, and pulmonary emphysema. MMP family members share about 40% identity at the amino acid level, and they possess common structural domains. MMPs are secreted as inactive proenzymes that are activated at the cell membrane surface or within the extracellular space by proteolytic cleavage of the N-terminal domain. Catalytic activity is dependent on coordination of a zinc ion at the active site and is specifically inhibited by members of another gene family, called TIMPs for tissue inhibitors of matrix metalloproteinases (Table 38-2). Optimal activity of MMPs is around pH 7.4. All MMPs except matrilysin have a carboxyl terminal hemopexin-like domain that is important for conferring substrate specificity and for TIMP binding. The 92- and 72-kDa gelatinases have an additional fibronectin-like domain that mediates their high binding affinity to gelatins and elastin.

Individual members of the MMP family can be loosely divided into groups based on their matrix-degrading capacity. As a whole, they are able to cleave all extracellular matrix components. The collagenases have the unique capacity to cleave native triple-helical interstitial collagens but have a restricted substrate specificity, being unable to degrade elastin or basement membrane molecules. There are two gelatinases of 72 kDa (gelatinase A) and 92 kDa (gelatinase B), which differ in their cellular origin and regulation, but share the capacity to degrade gelatins (denatured collagens), type IV collagen, elastin, and other matrix proteins. Stromelysins have a broad spectrum of susceptible substrates, including most basement membrane components. Matrilysin, the smallest MMP (28 kDa as a proenzyme) has the broad substrate specificity of stromelysin plus it has some elastase activity. Macrophage metalloelastase also has a potent broad substrate specificity that includes elastin. The MMP family keeps growing. The newest members are membrane-type metalloproteinases (MT-MMPs). MT-MMP-1 activates the 72-kDa gelatinase; however, the full spectrum of cellular expression of and substrates susceptible to MT-MMPs are currently unknown. MMPs are active against a variety of proteins besides extracellular matrix. They cleave and activate latent tumor necrosis factor-α (TNF-α), thereby regulating inflammation. MMPs degrade and inactivate α_1-AT, thus indirectly enhancing the activity of HNE.

Alveolar macrophages produce several MMPs, including significant amounts of metalloelastase, interstitial collagenase, and 92-kDa gelatinase, and smaller amounts of stromelysin-1 and matrilysin. Expression of these MMPs is highly regulated, and under quiescent conditions, such as in normal mature lung tissue, expression is limited. MMPs are induced and their production and activity are carefully controlled during normal repair and remodeling processes. With chronic inflammation, regulation of MMPs can go awry, and MMPs can be overexpressed and produced at inappropriate sites. There is evidence that expression of metalloelastase and to a lesser degree matrilysin is upregulated in alveolar macrophages of cigaret smokers.

EXPRESSION OF MATRIX METALLOPROTEINASES BY OTHER LUNG CELLS Many cells in the lung have the capacity to produce MMPs. Eosinophils produce significant amounts of the 92-kDa gelatinase. T lymphocytes interacting with endothelial cell vascular cell adhesion molecule-1 (VCAM-1) are induced to express the 72-kDa gelatinase. Various resident lung cells can produce MMPs. Fibroblasts, for example, are a potential promi-

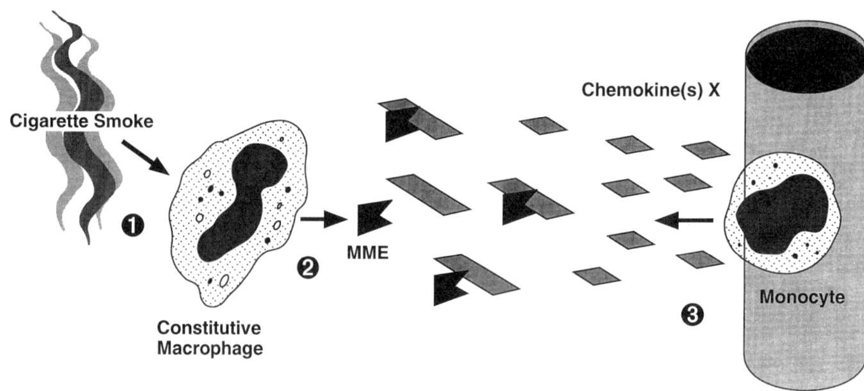

Figure 38-3 Mechanism of metalloelastase-mediated monocyte recruitment in response to cigaret smoke. Inhaled cigaret smoke induces constitutive lung macrophages to produce macrophage metalloelastase (MME). MME proteolytically generates a chemotactic gradient, presumably by cleaving a protein into a chemotactic fragment (chemokine[s] X) that attracts blood monocytes into the lung parenchyma.

nent source of interstitial collagenase, stromelysin, 72-kDa gelatinase, and MT-MMPs. Type II alveolar epithelial cells produce matrilysin and perhaps other MMPs. Considering the variety of lung cells capable of producing MMPs, it seems plausible that MMPs participate in the lung destruction resulting in emphysema.

WHICH ELASTASES ARE INVOLVED IN EMPHYSEMA ASSOCIATED WITH SMOKING?

Efforts to implicate specific elastases in the pathogenesis of emphysema have taken on the form of a criminal trial; attempting to place proteinase X at the scene of the crime (emphysema) with a loaded weapon (elastolytic capacity). Many studies have attempted, with variable success, as noted above, to link neutrophil elastase with emphysema. MMP expression has also been associated recently with emphysema. The chronicity, general absence of smoking late in the disease, and the static nature of these types of studies contribute to the complexity of correlating the presence of elastases with changes in lung architecture.

Based on available literature and our experience with these enzymes, one can rank the relative elastolytic activities of these candidate enzymes (Table 38-1). However, the in vivo situation may defy such simple comparisons. Indeed, even the weakest elastases may contribute to emphysematous changes over many years of cigaret smoking. Other matrix components decorating the elastic fibers must also be degraded. Moreover, the capacity to degrade matrix may be limited to microenvironments of cell matrix interaction that concentrate enzymes and exclude inhibitors.

With the rapidly expanding group of potential candidates capable of causing lung destruction characteristic of pulmonary emphysema, it is imperative to directly determine the relative contribution of these proteinases in smoking-associated emphysema. The most direct methods available to establish protein functions are to perform gain of function and loss of function experiments in complex biologic organisms (mammals). Recently, investigators have taken advantage of transgenic technology to overexpress and delete specific proteinases in mice.

GAIN OF FUNCTION (OVEREXPRESSION) Overexpression of a human collagenase-1 (MMP-1) transgene driven by the haptoglobin reporter unexpectedly resulted in lung-specific expression in several independent founder lines of mice. These mice developed enlarged airspaces characteristic of emphysema. This was the first demonstration that an MMP could directly cause emphysema. Also, because MMP-1 is inactive against mature elastin, this result suggested that collagen degradation was sufficient to cause emphysema. However, it is not certain whether the alveolar pathology in these animals was caused by destruction of collagen in mature lung tissue or whether expression of the transgene during growth and development interfered with normal elastic fiber assembly, perhaps through destruction of the elastic fiber microfibrillar scaffold. Use of cell-specific inducible promoters could circumvent this problem, but none exist at present. Another approach is in vivo transfection of a proteinase to adult animals; however, at present only low levels of non–cell-specific expression are possible.

LOSS OF FUNCTION (UNDEREXPRESSION) Underexpression represents the most direct experimental approach at present. Targeted mutations in genes of embryonic stem cells allow one to generate strains of mice deficient in specific proteins. These mice can be used to directly establish the function(s) of the protein in controlled experiments. Strains of mice deficient in individual candidate elastases can be compared with each other and normal littermates with respect to their capacity to develop emphysema in response to cigaret smoke.

Like humans, wild-type mice chronically exposed to cigaret smoke develop a macrophage predominant inflammatory infiltrate in the lungs, followed by airspace enlargement. In contrast to wild-type littermates, mice deficient in macrophage elastase (MMP-12) failed to recruit macrophages and did not develop pulmonary emphysema in response to cigaret smoke exposure. Whether human emphysema is also dependent on this single MMP is of course uncertain. At the very least, this study demonstrates a critical role of macrophages in the development of emphysema and unmasks a proteinase-dependent mechanism of inflammatory cell recruitment that may have broader biologic implications (Fig. 38-3).

α_1-ANTITRYPSIN (α_1-AT) DEFICIENCY

α_1-AT is a glycoprotein of 52 kDa synthesized primarily by the liver, consisting of a single polypeptide chain of 394 amino acids. Fully processed α_1-AT has three carbohydrate side chains that account for 12% of the molecular mass. The gene for α_1-AT is 12.2 kb located on chromosome 14 near the gene for α_1-antichymotrypsin, the inhibitor for cathepsin G, which like neutrophil elastase is contained in neutrophil azurophil granules. The α_1-AT gene has seven exons and six introns. Exons four through seven code for the mature protein. The first two exons and a 5' segment of exon three are encoded in the transcript expressed in macrophages, but not in hepatocytes. α_1-AT is an acute-phase reactant. Plasma levels of α_1-AT rise with trauma, estrogen therapy, birth control pills, and pregnancy.

Proteolytic inhibition of neutrophil elastase and other serine proteinases by α_1-AT involves cleavage of the "strained" reactive open center of α_1-AT between methionine^{358} and serine^{359}, resulting in an altered, "relaxed" α_1-AT conformation in complex with the proteinase. Formation of the complex renders the proteinase inactive and, because the complex is quite stable, inactivation is essentially permanent. α_1-AT inhibits many serine proteinases and does so on a 1:1 molar basis; however, α_1-AT associates with neutrophil elastase much faster than with trypsin or other serine proteinases suggesting that inhibition of neutrophil elastase is the primary function of α_1-AT. Because α_1-AT inhibits neutrophil elastase and other serine proteinases besides trypsin, some authors prefer the designations α_1-proteinase inhibitor or α_1-antiproteinase, but the name α_1-AT is still commonly used for historic reasons. When α_1-AT is complexed with a proteinase the complex binds to receptors (called serpin-enzyme complex (SEC) receptors) on hepatocytes and monocytes.

α_1-AT is transmitted codominantly. Thus, the gene product from each parent is expressed in the offspring. A large number of α_1-AT alleles are known, but most involve a single amino acid changes that does not alter expression of the protein or its function. The states produced by these different alleles are referred to as follows: normal, in which there is a normal serum concentration of functional α_1-AT; deficient, in which the serum α_1-AT is lower than normal; null, in which there is no measurable serum α_1-AT; and dysfunctional, in which there is a normal serum concentration of α_1-AT, but it does not have the normal antiproteinase activity.

The nomenclature for the α_1-AT polymorphism uses letters to specify the allelic variants. The original letters were chosen to reflect electrophoretic mobility: F for fast; M, medium; S, slow; and Z, ultraslow. The normal phenotype, Pi M, exists in >90% of the population, with the MS and MZ phenotypes the next most common. The MS, MZ, and SS phenotypes, which are associated with modest deficiencies of α_1-AT (about half of the normal serum concentration), do not present an increased risk of emphysema, although there has been an increased frequency of Pi MZ individuals in some COPD populations. Pi MS individuals may have an increased frequency of airway hyperreactivity. Because individuals with Pi SZ, who have an average of 37% of normal α_1-AT serum concentration, rarely develop emphysema, serum levels >35% of normal are thought to be enough to provide protection.

As mentioned above, cigaret smoke can oxidize a methionine residue in the reactive center of α_1-AT, inactivating its capacity as a proteinase inhibitor. The potential consequences of this reaction were demonstrated in a dog model in which animals treated with chloramine-T, an agent that profoundly depresses α_1-AT functional activity, developed pulmonary emphysema. However, the initial studies in smokers that demonstrated oxidatively inactivated α_1-AT in the bronchoalveolar lavage fluid have not been corroborated.

Several α_1-AT phenotypes are associated with very low serum concentrations of α_1-AT. Of these, the Pi Z phenotype is by far the most common, accounting for >95% of such individuals. Pi Z individuals have about 15% of the normal serum concentration of α_1-AT. The prevalence of the Pi Z phenotype in the United States is about one in 3000 people. The Z allele is rare in Asians and African-Americans. The small number of other individuals with marked deficiency of α_1-AT have Pi SZ, Pi null-null, or Pi null-Z phenotypes.

Most Pi Z individuals eventually become symptomatic with COPD as a result of emphysema, but there is considerable variation and some individuals reach advanced age with minimal symptoms. Silverman and colleagues confirmed the wide variability in pulmonary function among Pi Z subjects and found evidence for familial factors that segregated with deterioration in pulmonary function. Smoking has a marked effect on the age at which shortness of breath appears. On the average, Pi Z smokers have symptoms by age 40, about 15 years earlier than Pi Z nonsmokers.

The Pi Z phenotype is caused by a point mutation involving a single nucleotide at codon 342 that results in coding for lysine instead of glutamic acid. This amino acid substitution alters the charge attraction between the amino acids at positions 342 and 290 present in the normal form of α_1-AT and prevents the formation of a fold in the molecule. This change in tertiary structure promotes dimerization of α_1-AT molecules. It is the dimerization that leads to the aggregation of α_1-AT in the endoplasmic reticulum, which impedes secretion of the protein from the cell and results in the low levels of α_1-AT in plasma and other body fluids. The Z form of α_1-AT also has a rate of association with neutrophil elastase that is significantly slower than the association rate of normal α_1-AT with neutrophil elastase. Thus, the Pi Z phenotype leads to both a deficiency of α_1-AT protein and a form of α_1-AT that is less effective than normal α_1-AT as an inhibitor of neutrophil elastase.

The S variant of α_1-AT, which involves a single nucleotide alteration leading to substitution of glutamic acid^{264} with a valine, does not accumulate in the liver. This protein is less stable, presumably because of loss of a salt bridge between the glutamic acid in position 264 and the lysine in position 387. The Pi null phenotype arises because either the α_1-AT gene is missing or there is a mutation in the α_1-AT gene that results in premature termination of the gene's transcription.

REPAIR OF LUNG ELASTIN

The seminal observations about α_1-AT deficiency and production of emphysema in animals with elastolytic enzymes (and only with elastolytic enzymes) led to the concept that destruction of elastin in the lung parenchyma is key to the development of emphysema.

Elastin is the principal component of elastic fibers. Elastic fibers, which possess rubber-like reversible extensibility, come under tension and provide elastic recoil throughout the respiratory cycle. In the lung parenchyma, elastic fibers loop around alveolar ducts, form rings at the mouths of the alveoli, and penetrate as wisps into the alveolar septae, where they are concentrated at bends and junctions.

Elastin is secreted as a soluble protein of 60–70 kDa called tropoelastin (Fig. 38-4). Tropoelastin molecules, encoded by a gene on chromosome 7 in the human, are deposited into the extracellular space and aligned on a "scaffold" of microfibrils that consist of a number of proteins, including fibrillins, microfibril-associated proteins, and latent transforming growth factor-β (TGF-β) binding proteins. In the extracellular space, lysyl oxidase modifies most of the lysine residues in tropoelastin monomers, causing them to crosslink and form elastin, a highly insoluble, rubber-like polymer. The lysine-derived crosslinks in elastin are known as desmosines. Desmosines are unique to elastin, and therefore can be used to quantify elastin in tissues and as markers of elastin degradation in body fluids.

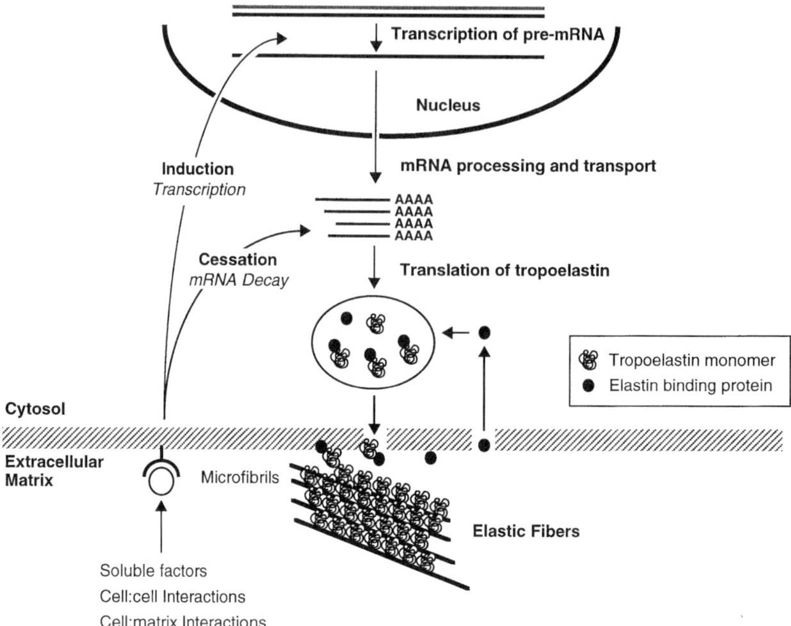

Figure 38-4 The synthesis of tropoelastin and assembly of the elastic fiber. Under the influence of extracellular and intracellular factors, tropoelastin pre-mRNA is transcribed within the nucleus of the elastogenic cell. Differential splicing of tropoelastin pre-mRNA leads to different tropoelastin mRNAs and tropoelastin isoforms. After tropoelastin is secreted from the cell it associates with microfibrils adjacent to the cell surface. Uncertainty exists as to whether there is a carrier protein that facilitates the secretion of tropoelasin. Microfibrils are thought to be a scaffold on which tropoelastin monomers align. On the microfibril, most of the lysines in tropoelastin monomers are modified by lysyl oxidase to form covalent crosslinks (desmosines) between the monomers. The resultant polymer is elastin. (Provided by William C. Parks, PhD).

Elastin is resistant to many proteinases, most notably the collagenases that cleave interstitial collagens, but there are a number of enzymes that may come in contact with the lung that can degrade elastin (Table 38-1). Under normal conditions, elastin synthesis in the lung begins in the late neonatal period, peaks during early postnatal development, continues to a much lesser degree through adolescence paralleling lung growth, and stops in adult life. There is some evidence that the tropoelastin gene always remains transcriptionally active but rapid mRNA degradation prevents expression of the protein. Multiple cell types are responsible for elastin synthesis in the lungs and associated structures. Lung elastin normally lasts a human lifespan, and there is virtually no elastin synthesis in the normal adult lung.

Although destruction of lung elastin appears to be necessary for the development of emphysema caused by smoking, it remains unknown precisely how the breakdown of elastin translates into the deformity recognized as emphysema. Elastin depletion appears to be restricted to the sites of emphysema, rather than being a global deficiency of the lung that contains regions of emphysema. It has also been difficult to determine the capacity of the lung parenchyma to undergo repair after proteolytic injury. It is not known if normal elastic fibers can be properly formed in the lung after the period of growth and development. After an intratracheal injection of human neutrophil elastase into an experimental animal, there is acute depletion of elastin followed by a burst of extracellular matrix synthesis, so that, during the course of a few weeks, the elastin content of the lungs returns to normal, although the lungs develop emphysema. However, the newly synthesized elastic fibers appear disorganized, similar to the elastic fibers in human emphysema. Recent studies of lung growth after pneumonectomy in adult rats indicate that elastin synthesis can be reinitiated in the adult lung and deposited at the sites at which elastin is normally produced during lung development. Nothing is known about the turnover of other extracellular matrix components in human lungs affected by COPD.

CONCLUDING COMMENTS

Intrapulmonary proteolytic activity that degrades lung elastin is generally accepted as the predominant mechanism for emphysema in smokers. Although elastin degradation may be central to emphysema, the biology of emphysema is clearly complex and still poorly understood. Moreover, degradation of extracellular matrix components besides elastin, particularly collagens, may also be essential. To probe the roles of the many factors involved in the development of emphysema and the lung's response to the remodeling called emphysema, researchers are now taking advantage of transgenic mice technology. From these studies, it should be possible to assess more precisely than ever before what is happening in the lung injury that culminates in the development of emphysema.

SELECTED REFERENCES

American Thoracic Society Statement: Standards for the diagnosis and care of patients with chronic obstructive pulmonary disease. Am J Respir Crit Care Med 1995;152:S77–S120.

Bartecchi C, MacKenzie T, Schrier R. The human costs of tobacco use. N Engl J Med 1994;330:907–912; 975–980.

Cantor J. Emphysema, lung disease and retinoic acid. Nat Med 1997;3:817.

Chapman HA Jr, Munger JS, Shi G-P. The role of thiol proteases in tissue injury and remodeling. Am J Respir Crit Care Med 1994;150:S155–S160.

Cox DW. α_1-Antitrypsin deficiency. In: Scriver CR, Beaudet AL, Sly WS, Valle D, eds. The Metabolic and Molecular Bases of Inherited Disease, 7th ed. New York: McGraw-Hill, 1995; pp. 4125–4158.

D'Armiento J, Dalal SS, Okada Y, Berg RA, Chada K. Collagenase expression in the lungs of transgenic mice causes pulmonary emphysema. Cell 1992;71:955–961.

Hautamaki RD, Kobayashi DK, Senior RM, Shapiro SD. Macrophage elastase is required for the development of emphysema induced by cigarette smoke in mice. Science 1997, in press.

Joslin G, Fallon RJ, Bullock J, Adams SP, Perlmutter DH. The SEC receptor recognizes a pentapeptide neodomain of alpha 1-antitrypsin-protease complexes. J Biol Chem 1991;266:11,282–11,288.

Mecham RP, Davis EC. Elastic fiber structure and assembly. In: Yurchenko P, Birk D, Mecham R, eds. Extracellular Matrix Assembly and Structure. San Diego: Academic, 1994; pp. 281–314.

Owen CA, Campbell MA, Sannes PL, Boukedes SS, Campbell EJ. Cell surface-bound cathepsin G on human neutrophils: a novel non-oxidative mechanism by which neutrophils focus and preserve catalytic activity of serine proteinases. J Cell Biol 1995;131:776–789.

Perlmutter DH. Alpha-1-antitrypsin deficiency: biochemistry and clinical manifestations. Ann Med 1996;28:385–394.

Sanford AJ, Weir TD, Pare PD. Genetic risk factors for chronic obstructive pulmonary disease. Eur Respir J 1997;10:1380–1391.

Shapiro SD. The pathogenesis of emphysema: elastase:antielastase hypothesis 30 years later. Proc Assoc Am Physicians 1995;3:346–352.

Shapiro SD, Endicott SK, Province MA, Pierce JA, Campbell EJ. Marked longevity of human parenchymal elastic fibers deduced from prevalence of D-aspartate and nuclear weapons-related radiocarbon. J Clin Invest 1991;87:1828–1834.

Silverman EK, Pierce JA, Province MA, Rao DC, Campbell EJ. Variability of pulmonary function in alpha-1-antitrypsin deficiency: clinical correlates. Ann Intern Med 1989;111:982–991.

Snider GI. Emphysema: the first two centuries—and beyond: a historical overview with suggestions for future research: parts 1 and 2. Am Rev Respir Dis 1992;146:1334–1344; 1615–1622.

Tetley TD. Matrix metalloproteinases: a role in emphysema? Thorax 1997;52:495.

Wright JL. Emphysema: concepts under change—a pathologist's perspective. Mod Pathol 1995;8:873–880.

39 Surfactant Deficiency

Jeffrey A. Whitsett and Timothy E. Weaver

BACKGROUND

Pulmonary surfactant is a complex mixture of phospholipids and associated proteins that reduces surface tension at the air–liquid interface at the alveolar surfaces. In the absence of surfactant, collapsing forces of ~70 dyne/cm^2, generated by unequal intramolecular forces among water molecules at the alveolar surfaces, cause atelectasis, cyanosis, and associated respiratory distress. Pulmonary surfactant is a phospholipid–protein complex produced by type II epithelial cells lining the alveolus of the lung. Surfactant is secreted into the alveolar space, forming an array of macromolecular forms that produce a monolayer or multilayer of phospholipids at the air–liquid interface, reducing collapsing forces and maintaining lung volumes at end-expiration. The critical role of pulmonary surfactant in lung function was first discerned from the studies of respiratory distress syndrome (RDS) in premature infants. Subsequent biochemical, biophysical, and molecular studies have elucidated important features of the pulmonary surfactant system that have led to the widespread application of surfactant replacement therapy for RDS and other clinical abnormalities of surfactant. The present review will discuss the structure, function, and regulation of pulmonary surfactant, focusing attention to the role of surfactant proteins in surfactant function and respiratory distress associated with mutations in the surfactant protein-B gene. Readers are referred to several texts and reviews that are listed in the references.

SURFACTANT DEFICIENCY AND RESPIRATORY DISTRESS

Surfactant deficiency is a life-threatening disorder, the pathophysiology of which is most clearly represented by the respiratory failure associated with infantile respiratory distress (IRDS) that accompanies premature birth. Pulmonary surfactant is composed primarily of phospholipids (PL) that are particularly enriched in dipalmitoylphosphatidylcholine (DPPC). Surfactant phospholipids are packaged in lamellar bodies of type II epithelial cells and secreted into the airspace by exocytotic processes stimulated by stretch, catecholamines, and purinoceptor agonists. After secretion, lamellar bodies form tubular myelin, a highly organized phospholipid–protein mixture that is the most abundant form of extracellular pulmonary surfactant (Fig. 39-1). Surfactant phospholipids move rapidly from tubular myelin to the gas–liquid interface, forming a monolayer in multilayers of phospholipids, thereby creating an interface between alveolar gas and the fluid subphase overlying alveolar cells. The dense packing of phospholipids at this interface is maintained by the parallel packing of the acyl chains of the phospholipids, and further strengthened by interactions of the choline and glycerol head groups of the phospholipid molecules. This dense packing of phospholipids excludes interactions between gas and liquid molecules, reducing surface tension in the alveolus. The reduction of surface tension in the alveolus maintains lung volumes at end-expiration, stabilizing the alveolar spaces from collapse.

Although surfactant proteins represent less than 10% of the mass of pulmonary surfactant, they appear to play a critical role in the routing, storage, secretion, and activity of pulmonary surfactant. Three abundant proteins, surfactant proteins A, B, and C, mediate the packaging of surfactant lipids within the type II cell, contribute to tubular myelin formation, and enhance the spreading and stability of surfactant phospholipids in the alveolar space. Deficiencies in these various components of surfactant contribute to lung dysfunction in a variety of human disorders. Surfactant proteins and lipids are subject to a variety of regulatory stimuli and their expression is precisely controlled during perinatal development, the concentrations of surfactant lipid and protein synthesis increasing markedly with advancing gestational age. In infants, the paucity of surfactant lipids and proteins related to prematurity is associated with a lack of biochemical and morphologic differentiation of the distal respiratory epithelium. Surfactant deficiency is also associated with respiratory failure in adult respiratory distress syndrome (ARDS), a disorder often associated with aspiration, infection, trauma, or shock in older patients. Advances in our understanding of the structure and function of surfactant have recently led to the widespread clinical use of exogenous surfactant replacement for prevention and therapy of IRDS in premature infants. Surfactant replacement is also being studied in the care of infants with other pulmonary disorders, including meconium aspiration, and is under investigation for therapy of ARDS and other lung disorders in older patients.

STRUCTURE AND FUNCTION OF SURFACTANT PROTEINS

The recognition that mixtures of surfactant phospholipids alone do not form a fully active surfactant led to the identification of surfactant proteins A, B, and C and the recognition that each plays a unique role in the organization, function, and catabolism of pulmonary surfactant.

From: *Principles of Molecular Medicine* (J. L. Jameson, ed.), ©1998 Humana Press Inc., Totowa, NJ.

SURFACTANT PROTEIN A (SP-A) Gene: SPA-Structure and Regulation of Expression SP-A belongs to a family of proteins, referred to as calcium-dependent lectins (collectins), encoded by a cluster of genes on the long arm of human chromosome 10. There are two SP-A genes in the human that differ by approximately 1% in the coding region. Although both genes are transcribed, the functional significance of two genes remain unclear, particularly in view of the fact that other species (mouse, rat, and rabbit) contain only a single gene. Transcription from the SP-A locus is regulated both temporally and spatially. SP-A expression is restricted to alveolar type II epithelial cells and nonciliated bronchiolar cells (Clara cells) of the respiratory tree. Synthesis of SP-A mRNA is detectable as early as the second trimester of pregnancy, but secretion of SP-A into the amniotic fluid is not generally detectable until approximately 30 weeks' gestation. Accumulation of SP-A in amniotic fluid during late gestation correlates strongly with surfactant function and lung maturity. The developmental, cell-specific, and basal regulation of SP-A expression is complex. Binding of the nuclear transcription protein TTF-1, thyroid transcription factor-1, to the SP-A promoter is required but is not sufficient to direct appropriate temporospatial SP-A gene transcription. The identification of transcription factors that modulate expression of SP-A independent of or by interacting with TTF-1 is an active area of research that will provide new insight into the regulation of SP-A expression during normal growth and development and in response to lung injury.

Structure and Biosynthesis Translation of the human SP-A mRNA gives rise to a preprotein of 248 amino acids. Cotranslational cleavage of the 20-amino acid signal peptide results in an SP-A monomer comprising four discrete functional domains, including (1) a 7-residue amino-terminal domain involved in association of multiple SP-A subunits, (2) a 72-residue collagenlike domain, (3) a 130-residue C-terminal carbohydrate-recognition domain (lectin-binding domain), and (4) a short neck region that links the lectin-binding and collagenlike domains (Fig. 39-2). The cotranslational addition of asparagine-linked carbohydrate and subsequent processing of the oligosaccharide tree(s), including sialation and sulfation, results in multiple forms of monomeric SP-A ranging in size from 28,000 to 36,000 Dalton. Assembly of mature, oligomeric SP-A is initiated in the endoplasmic reticulum and involves the interaction of the collagenlike domains of three SP-A monomers to form a triple helix; subsequent formation of sulfhydryl bonds between the amino-terminal domains of adjacent trimeric subunits leads to the formation of the mature SP-A molecule comprising 18 monomers. Secretion studies in isolated Type II epithelial cells, fetal lung explants, and rabbit lung in vivo suggest that most of the newly synthesized SP-A is secreted independently of surfactant phospholipids.

Functional Domains SP-A avidly binds to surfactant phospholipids, particularly DPPC, a property thought to be mediated by the C-terminal domain of the protein. The role of SP-A in organizing newly secreted surfactant phospholipids in the airway was deduced from in vitro studies demonstrating that SP-A promotes the calcium-dependent aggregation of lipid vesicles and is also required for the formation of tubular myelin. Binding of SP-A to a receptor on the surface of the type II epithelial cell results in an inhibition of secretagog-stimulated secretion of phospholipid consistent with a role for SP-A in modulation of surfactant secretion. SP-A has also been shown to facilitate the uptake of phospholipid by isolated type II cells. The effect of SP-A on structure, secretion, and uptake of surfactant phospholipid by the type II cell is consistent with the key role for this protein in regulation of surfactant homeostasis. This hypothesis, however, requires careful reassessment in view of the apparently normal lung function in mice lacking SP-A protein (SP-A knockout mice): genetic ablation of the mouse SP-A gene in transgenic mice markedly disrupted the formation of tubular myelin in homozygous SP-A(–/–) mice, but did not alter lung structure, phospholipid content, or function in vivo.

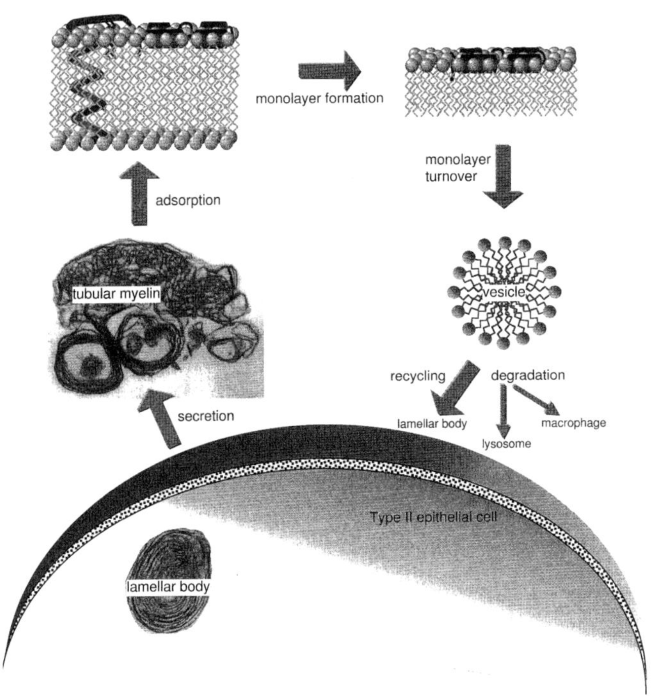

Figure 39-1 Life cycle of surfactant. Newly synthesized surfactant lipids and proteins are stored in the form of lamellar bodies within the type II epithelial cell. Lamellar bodies are secreted into the alveolus and unravel into tubular myelin, a process facilitated by SP-A, SP-B, and calcium. Adsorption of phospholipids to the air–liquid interface and formation of the surface-active monolayer is facilitated by surfactant proteins B and C. Repeated compression and expansion of the monolayer results in the formation of small lipid vesicles, which are taken up by the type II cell and incorporated into lamellar bodies for reuse; a minor proportion of surfactant is degraded in lysosomes of type II cells or macrophages.

Apart from surfactant-related functions, there is growing evidence that SP-A may play an important role in host defense of the airways. SP-A has been shown to stimulate migration of macrophages and to increase production of oxygen radicals involved in the destruction of pathogens internalized by macrophages. SP-A is an opsonin, enhancing phagocytosis of viruses and bacteria, and stimulates phagocytosis of bacteria opsonized by complement or immunoglobulins. Consistent with the broad binding specificity of SP-A, the carbohydrate moieties, the neck region, and the lectin-binding domain have all been implicated in the binding of SP-A to various pathogens. Further insight into the role of SP-A in nonimmune lung defense is certain to come from the study of SP-A knockout mice. Indeed, preliminary evidence with these SP-A(–/–) mice suggests their susceptibility to lung infection.

SURFACTANT PROTEIN B (SP-B) SP-B Gene: Structure and Regulation of Expression SP-B is encoded by a single gene on human chromosome 2. Transcription from the SP-B locus

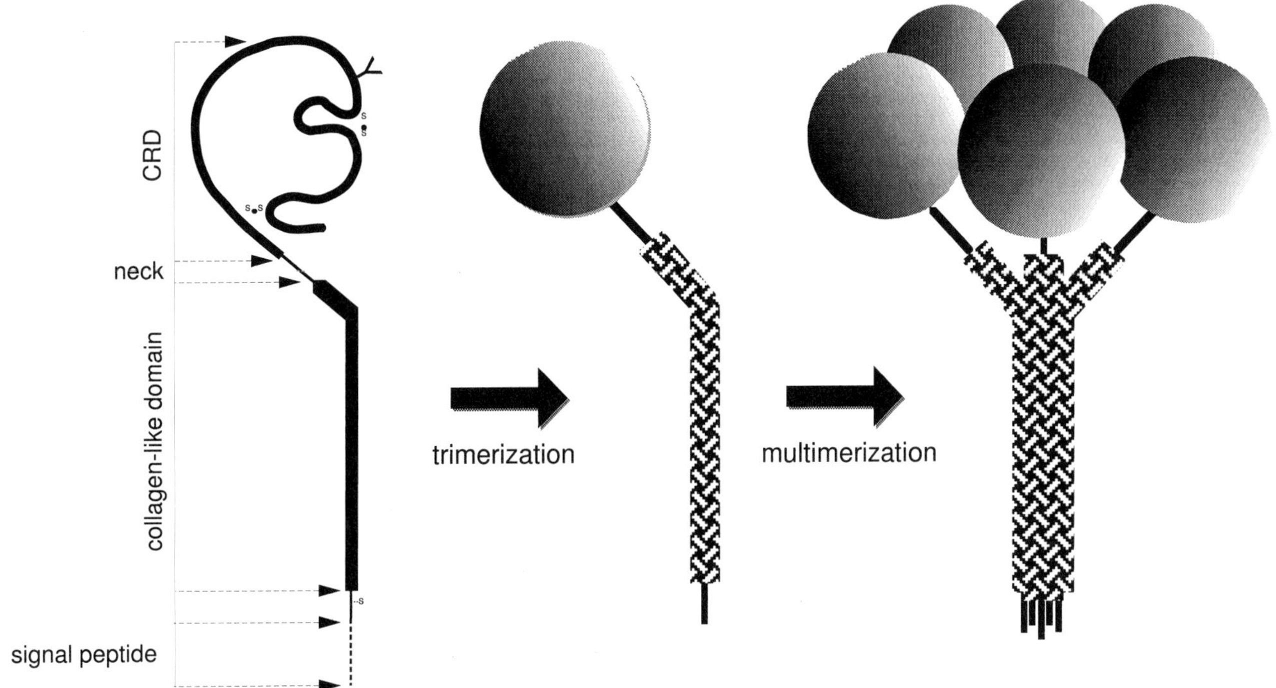

Figure 39-2 Structure of SP-A. SP-A is a 32- to 36-kDa polypeptide that forms trimers, which further assemble into hexamers and larger multimers. The molecules contains a globular lectin domain (C-terminal) and a rigid collagenous domain (N-terminal).

is regulated both developmentally and in a cell-specific manner. As for SP-A, expression of SP-B is restricted to Clara cells and type II cells of the respiratory epithelium. *Cis*-acting elements regulating cell-specific expression have been mapped to the proximal region of the SP-B promoter (–80 to –110) and shown to bind TTF-1 and HNF-3 (hepatocyte nuclear factor-3); in addition, TTF-1 binds at distal sites (–459 to –331) in the promoter resulting in significant enhancement of transcriptional activity. Phosphorylation of TTF-1 by cAMP-dependent protein kinase significantly increases transcription of SP-B consistent with a broad role for cAMP in the regulation of surfactant protein expression. Regulation of developmental expression by binding of specific nuclear proteins to sites within the SP-B promoter has not been systematically evaluated although it is likely that both TTF-1 and HNF-3 are involved in the temporal and spatial determination of SP-B gene expression. SP-B mRNA is detected as early as 12 weeks of gestation but significant amounts of protein are not detected in amniotic fluid before 31 weeks; secretion of SP-B increases significantly to term and is strongly correlated with surfactant function and lung maturity in infants. Overall, the developmental, cell-specific, and basal transcription of the SP-B gene is strongly influenced by TTF-1 and HNF-3; however, the widespread expression of these transcription factors in tissue derived from the embryonic foregut axis indicates that other nuclear proteins may also contribute to the unique pattern of SP-B expression.

Structure and Biosynthesis Human SP-B is synthesized as a preproprotein of 381 amino acids; however, the active peptide associated with surfactant phospholipids is only 79 residues, indicating that extensive proteolytic processing occurs in type II epithelial cells (Fig. 39-3). In the alveolus, SP-B is closely associated with surfactant phospholipids, contributing to tubular myelin formation. Translocation of newly synthesized preproprotein into the endoplasmic reticulum is accompanied by cleavage of a 23-amino acid signal peptide and the addition of asparagine-linked oligosaccharide to the COOH-terminal propeptide. Although glycosylation of the proprotein occurs in all species examined, the functional significance of this modification is not apparent; the mature peptide is not modified by oligosaccharide addition and glycosylation of the proprotein is not required for intracellular trafficking of SP-B. In contrast, the 177-residue NH_2-terminal propeptide is absolutely required for trafficking of SP-B. The propeptide acts as an intramolecular chaperone to prevent nonspecific interactions of the extremely hydrophobic mature peptide with cellular membranes during transport through the secretory pathway; further, the NH_2-terminal propeptide is essential for directing the mature peptide to the lamellar body. Both the NH_2- and COOH-terminal propeptides are proteolytically cleaved before incorporation of the mature peptide into the lamellar body. The function of the COOH-terminal propeptide, the metabolic fate of the cleaved propeptides, and the identity of the endoprotease(s) involved in their cleavage are currently not known.

Functional Domains Mutations in the SP-B gene leading to a complete absence of mature peptide are neonatal lethal in human infants and in SP-B-deficient mice created by gene targeting. Fetal lung development proceeds normally in the absence of SP-B but inflation of the newborn lung is compromised resulting in the rapid onset of respiratory distress. It is likely that many of the histopathologic changes described in SP-B-deficient infants are related to intensive postnatal therapy. Several attempts to rescue SP-B-deficient infants with surfactant preparations containing SP-B have not been successful, suggesting that replacement by the mature peptide alone is insufficient. Consistent with this conclusion, SP-B deficiency is accompanied by aberrant processing of the SP-C proprotein to a diagnostic fragment (M_r = 12,000) detectable in amniotic fluid or alveolar lavage; in addition, mature SP-C peptide is significantly reduced, likely exacerbating RDS in these infants. These findings, coupled with the observation that lamellar body

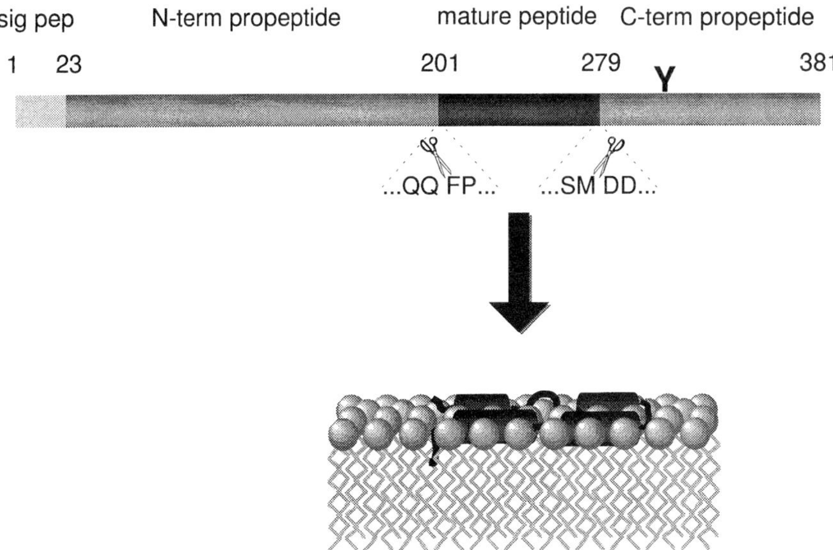

Figure 39-3 Structure of SP-B. Active SP-B, a 79-amino acid polypeptide, is produced by proteolytic processing of a 381-amino acid precursor. SP-B associates with the surfaces of phospholipid membranes, contributing to the adsorption and stability of the phospholipids.

formation is abnormal in SP-B knockout mice, suggest that the SP-B proprotein plays a critical role in assembly of the bioactive pulmonary surfactant complex.

The mature SP-B peptide is very hydrophobic and avidly associates with surfactant phospholipids. There are four regions within the peptide that have the potential to form amphipathic helices, and one or more of these domains may facilitate its interaction with phospholipids. The presence of a large number of cationic residues in SP-B likely accounts for the affinity of this peptide for phosphatidylglycerol, an abundant surfactant phospholipid containing a negatively charged head group. SP-B has been shown to accelerate the transition of newly secreted surfactant to the surface-active film and facilitate respreading of the surface film after dynamic compression and expansion. SP-B has also been shown to stimulate the uptake of phospholipids by type II cells in vitro, suggesting that the peptide may play a role in clearance of surfactant.

SURFACTANT PROTEIN C (SP-C) **SP-C Gene: Structure and Regulation of Expression** SP-C is encoded by a single gene on human chromosome 8. As for surfactant proteins A and B, transcription of the SP-C locus is regulated both developmentally and in a cell-specific manner; however, unlike the other surfactant proteins, expression of SP-C is restricted to type II epithelial cells. Although TTF-1 plays an important role in the regulation of basal and lung-specific transcription of the SP-C gene, other as yet unidentified transcription factor(s) are clearly required to maintain type II cell-specific expression. Elements of the SP-C promoter contained within 3.7 kb of the 5' flanking sequence of the gene have been shown to confer appropriate lung-specific and developmental expression on a reporter gene in transgenic mice. SP-C mRNA is detected at low levels early in the second trimester and increases significantly during the third trimester coincident with mRNAs for SP-A and SP-B. Assessment of SP-C protein levels is complicated by the lack of a monospecific antiserum directed against the active airway peptide; however, immunocytochemical studies with antisera directed against the SP-C proprotein indicate that the time course of SP-C precursor synthesis during lung development approximates that for SP-A and SP-B and therefore parallels overall lung development and functional status.

Structure and Biosynthesis The SP-C gene encodes a proprotein of 197 amino acids (Fig. 39-4); however, differential splicing of the primary mRNA transcript leads to several different SP-C mRNAs, at least one of which results in a reduction in the size of the proprotein to 191 amino acids. It is not known if the multiple SP-C mRNAs are all translated and whether this apparent redundancy is functionally significant. Unlike SP-A and SP-B, the SP-C proprotein is not glycosylated and does not contain an NH_2-terminal signal peptide. The hydrophobic mature peptide (amino acids 24–58) mediates translocation of the NH_2-terminal propeptide into the lumen of the endoplasmic reticulum resulting in a transmembrane protein. As for the SP-B proprotein, the mature 35-amino acid SP-C peptide is generated by proteolytic cleavage of the NH_2- and COOH-terminal propeptides, an event that likely occurs in the multivesicular body of type II cells. The identity of the protease(s) involved in propeptide cleavage and the fate and function of the liberated propeptides are not known. It is also not clear how the mature SP-C peptide, which is presumably oriented within the interior of the vesicle membrane, is assembled with surfactant phospholipids for secretion into the airspace.

Functional Domains Mature SP-C is an extraordinarily hydrophobic peptide consisting of 77% nonpolar amino acids. The most hydrophobic portion of the peptide is the 23-residue, valine-rich C-terminal region that forms a rigid α-helix capable of spanning the membrane bilayer. The relatively hydrophilic NH_2-terminal portion of the peptide contains several positively charged residues that likely anchor SP-C to one side of the membrane by interacting with the negatively charged phospholipid head groups; in addition, the covalent attachment of palmitic acid to cysteines at positions 5 and 6 ensures that the NH_2-terminus of SP-C is firmly anchored to the membrane. Although the function of SP-C is not entirely clear, the membrane-spanning helical region of the peptide is required for rapid adsorption of surfactant phospholipids to the air–liquid interface. The role of SP-C in the surface-active monolayer remains much less clear. Recent studies in vitro suggest that SP-C may play in important role in the clearance of alveolar surfactant lipids by the type II epithelial cell.

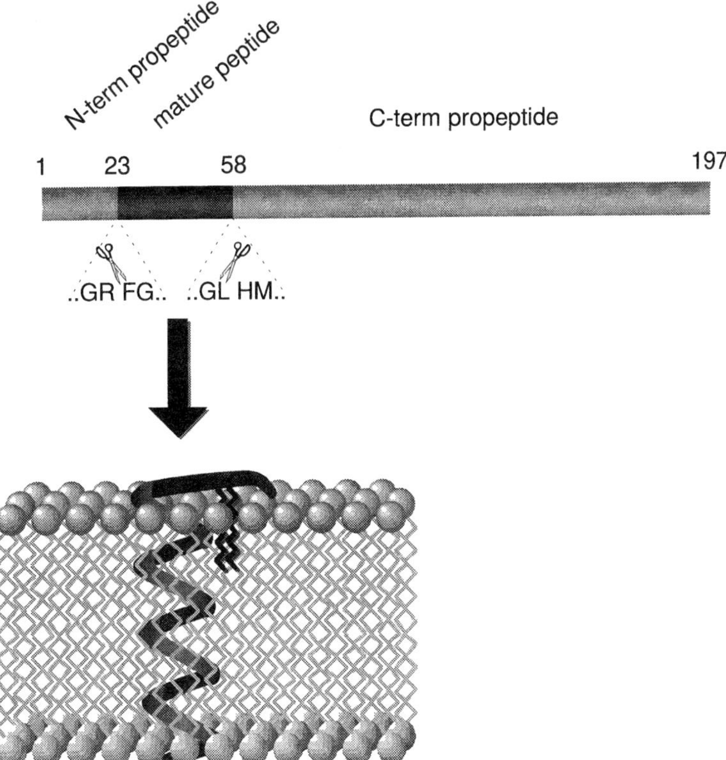

Figure 39-4 Structure of SP-C. SP-C is produced by proteolytic processing of a 197-amino acid precursor. The active SP-C peptide of 33–35 amino acids inserts deeply into lipid monolayers and bilayers, enhancing the surface activity of the phospholipids.

LIFE CYCLE OF PULMONARY SURFACTANT

Pulmonary surfactant phospholipids and proteins are synthesized by type II epithelial cells lining the alveolar surface of the lung. Phospholipids are synthesized *de novo* and are re-used at high rates by the type II epithelial cell in a highly regulated, conservative manner. Phospholipids and proteins are synthesized and trafficked to membranous structures of the endoplasmic reticulum, Golgi, and multivesicular bodies, and ultimately packaged in lamellar bodies, the storage form of phospholipids and proteins in the type II cell. Surfactant, in the form of lamellar bodies, is secreted into the airway by exocytosis. The presence of calcium, SP-A, SP-B, and phospholipids produces tubular myelin, the most abundant form of alveolar surfactant. Monolayers or sheets of monolayers are likely formed by the actions of surfactant proteins B and C and phospholipids. The membranes spread over the alveolar surface, reducing surface tension at the air–liquid interface. The dynamic compression of surfactant during the respiratory cycle generates a variety of structural forms containing surfactant lipids and proteins, and it is likely that some of these forms determine whether the particles are catabolized or taken back up by type II cells for reutilization. Inactive particles, in the form of small, less dense vesicles, that are relatively depleted in surfactant proteins are likely catabolic forms that are taken up by the respiratory epithelium. Surfactant proteins B and A serve to maintain the large aggregates (tubular myelin) that are highly surface active. Differences in the abundance or type of surfactant proteins associated with the various lipid particles may influence the rates of uptake and recycling. Although surfactant proteins and lipids are taken up by the type II epithelial cell and recycled at high rates, a subfraction of surfactant lipids and proteins are taken up and degraded by alveolar macrophages. Although only approximately 15% of phospholipids are catabolized by alveolar macrophages in vivo, this process may be a critical determinant of the steady state concentrations of surfactant, which are maintained at precise levels in the alveolar spaces of the adult animal. Thus, the life cycle of pulmonary surfactant represents a balance between synthesis, secretion, formation of distinct structural forms, reuptake, and catabolism. Each of these processes is influenced at various regulatory levels.

HEREDITARY SURFACTANT PROTEIN B DEFICIENCY

The critical role of surfactant protein B (SP-B) in lung function was emphasized by the finding that full-term infants lacking SP-B develop lethal respiratory distress immediately after birth. Hereditary SP-B deficiency was first recognized in 1993 in a kinship of three full-term infants dying of respiratory failure at birth. Affected infants develop respiratory distress with grunting, retraction, cyanosis, pulmonary hypertension, and radiographic findings consistent with diffuse atelectasis after birth, similar to the findings in premature infants with IRDS. Initial chest radiograms show reticular-granular infiltrates that progress to severe atelectasis. Infants require intubation and intensive care immediately after birth. Therapy with oxygen and positive-pressure ventilation fails in spite of vigorous and continued respiratory management. Although the number of treated infants is not extensive to date, the infants do not have a consistent or prolonged response to exogenous surfactant replacement. Where available, SP-B-deficient infants are often treated with extracorporeal membrane oxygenation (ECMO) before the diagnosis is entertained. Hereditary SP-B deficiency has been consistently fatal and infants usually succumb in the first months of life in spite of continued intensive respiratory support. Several infants with hereditary SP-B deficiency have undergone lung transplantation.

DIAGNOSIS OF HEREDITARY SP-B DEFICIENCY The diagnosis of SP-B deficiency is made on the basis of family history. All infants diagnosed to date have two defective SP-B genes inherited as autosomal recessive genes. The infants develop respiratory distress in the first 24 h and are generally critically ill with increasing respiratory distress in the absence of prematurity, infection, or other underlying causes of respiratory failure. Tracheal aspirates from infants lack the active SP-B peptide and contain a diagnostic fragment of proSP-C (of approximately 12 kDa), which accumulates in the air spaces. Amniotic fluid from these infants contains the 12-kDa proSP-C fragment, a paucity of phospholipids, a decreased lecithin:sphinyomyelin (L:S) ratio, and the absence of the SP-B active peptide and phosphatidylglycerol (PG). Lung biopsy samples generally reveal diffuse lung disease with accumulation of proteinaceous material in the air spaces of affected infants. This material is distinct from that detected in adults with alveolar proteinosis, the former being devoid of the SP-B and enriched in the proSP-C fragment. Electron microscopic examination of lung tissue from SP-B-deficient infants demonstrated the lack of lamellar bodies and tubular myelin, as well as abnormal and injured epithelial cells likely related to prolonged intensive care and oxygen therapy. The definitive diagnosis is made by genetic analysis of the SP-B alleles from the infants and family members.

MOLECULAR DIAGNOSIS OF CONGENITAL SP-B DEFICIENCY The most common genetic defect associated with SP-B deficiency results from a frameshift mutation in exon 4 (121 ins 2), which has been detected in approximately 75% of the affected infants analyzed to date. At present, 38 infants with this disease have been diagnosed since the recognition of the disorder in 1993. Missense and nonsense mutations have also been identified, with the infants generally presenting as compound heterozygotes in concert with the common exon 4 mutation. Definitive diagnosis is made by sequence analysis of the SP-B alleles.

PATHOPHYSIOLOGY OF HEREDITARY SP-B DEFICIENCY IN SP-B GENE-TARGETED MICE The murine SP-B gene was disrupted by homologous recombination in embryonic stem cells used to make SP-B gene-targeted (knockout) mice. Like affected infants, SP-B-deficient mice succumb from respiratory distress postnatally, but are otherwise unaffected. Abnormalities in these mice are confined to the lungs, which are atelectatic but have developed normally. Type II cells of the SP-B(–/–) mice lack lamellar bodies and contain large atypical multivesicular bodies. Tubular myelin is lacking in the air spaces, and there is decreased content of the active SP-C peptide and a complete lack of both proSP-B and SP-B in the gene-targeted mice. Insertional mutagenesis in exon 4 of the mouse gene and the missense mutation in exon 4 of the human gene both result in an unstable messenger RNA and the lack of synthesis of proSP-B. Mutations in other regions of the human gene are associated with expression of abnormal forms of SP-B and proSP-B, which are detected intracellularly and extracellularly. ProSP-C, normally routed through the secretory pathway of the type II epithelial cell in concert with proSP-B, is aberrantly processed, resulting in the secretion and accumulation of proSP-C of $M_r = 12$ kDa in the air spaces of SP-B(–/–) in humans and mice. Thus, in addition to the lack of SP-B, SP-B(–/–) mice and patients are deficient in SP-C active peptide and accumulate high concentrations of proSP-C fragments in the air spaces that likely further impair surfactant function. The aberrant packaging, storage, and organization of surfactant lipids in the SP-B deficiency also are likely to contribute to surfactant dysfunction, leading to respiratory failure in hereditary SP-B deficiency.

HETEROZYGOUS SP-B DEFICIENCY SP-B deficiency is generally inherited as an autosomal recessive gene. Although clinical lung disease has not been associated with heterozygous family members of SP-B-deficient infants, these families have not been intensively studied to date. Heterozygous SP-B gene-targeted mice develop normally for more than a year in the laboratory without apparent abnormalities. However, SP-B mRNA, proSP-B, and the mature SP-B peptide are reduced by approximately 50% in SP-B(+/–) offspring. Careful analysis of lung function in the SP-B-deficient heterozygous mice revealed air trapping and decreased lung compliance, consistent with abnormalities of small airway function. Whether SP-B(+/–) humans have abnormalities of lung function or are susceptible to lung dysfunction is unknown at present. The small airway dysfunction and air trapping seen in the SP-B(+/–) mice suggests that phenotypic alterations in SP-B deficiency might include asthma and other forms of small airway disease.

DISTINCTION OF HEREDITARY SP-B DEFICIENCY FROM PULMONARY ALVEOLAR PROTEINOSIS (PAP) Although associated with the accumulation of surfactant lipids in the air space, the hereditary form of SP-B deficiency is distinct from infants or adults with pulmonary alveolar proteinosis in which both surfactant lipids and proteins accumulate in the alveolar space. Adult forms of alveolar proteinosis are generally idiopathic and are associated with malignancy, immune disorders, and exposure to inhaled particles and are not associated with the acute respiratory failure seen in SP-B-deficient infants. Alveolar proteinosis appears to be caused by disruption in surfactant homeostasis that leads to decreased clearance of surfactant by alveolar macrophages or by the respiratory epithelium. Genetic ablation of granulocyte-macrophage colony-stimulating factor (GM-CSF) or its receptor causes severe alveolar proteinosis in transgenic knockout mice. Unlike hereditary SP-B deficiency, surfactant from these animals or patients with PAP is highly surface-active, contains normally processed surfactant proteins, and lacks the proSP-C fragment, the latter being diagnostic for hereditary SP-B deficiency. The analysis of the GM-CSF of knockout mice has provided novel insight into the role of GM-CSF in lung homeostasis consistent with a critical role for GM-CSF in autocrine-paracrine signaling within the lung. These findings support a role for GM-CSF in the modulation of surfactant homeostasis in the postnatal lung and suggest the potential role of GM-CSF and its receptor subunits in the pathogenesis of alveolar proteinosis in humans.

SECONDARY CAUSES OF SP-B DEFICIENCY Hereditary SP-B deficiency must be distinguished from other causes of surfactant or surfactant protein B deficiency in newborn infants. Secondary causes of SP-B deficiency may be related to infection, prematurity, or to other as yet unknown factors. SP-B content was below the level of detectability in lung lavage fluid from some infants with severe respiratory failure and with no discernible abnormalities in the SP-B genes. SP-B deficiency has also been observed in the lungs of infants dying of congenital lung disease associated with abnormal lung morphogenesis, such as congenital acinar hypoplasia. Lungs from these infants are also deficient in SP-A and SP-C, and the pathogenesis of this disorder may be related to the lack of synthesis of regulatory factors that influence the expression of surfactant proteins in lung epithelial cell differentiation or on pulmonary organogenesis *per se*.

FUTURE DIRECTIONS FOR DIAGNOSIS AND THERAPY OF HEREDITARY SP-B DEFICIENCY Because of the severe disruption of surfactant homeostasis of hereditary SP-B deficiency and the severity of respiratory distress, these infants generally succumb within the first months of life despite extensive ventilatory support and intensive care. SP-B(–/–) infants have not responded to exogenous surfactant replacement even when initiated relatively early in the course of the disease. Genetic testing of the fetus can be used to identify infants with hereditary SP-B deficiency before birth. Both protein and DNA analyses have been used to identify siblings of previously affected kindred with SP-B deficiency. Such information can be useful in genetic counseling of these families. Several infants with SP-B deficiency have received lung transplants for correction of SP-B deficiency and two of these infants have now survived more than a year. Long-term outcome of neonatal lung transplantation is unknown, however, and this procedure should be considered experimental. SP-B mRNA can be transferred to respiratory epithelial cells for the correction of SP-B deficiency in the laboratory, and adenoviral vectors capable of efficiently transferring SP-B mRNA to type II epithelial cells have been used in animal models. However, correction of hereditary SP-B deficiency in infants will require relatively high levels of SP-B gene expression within type II epithelial cells. At present, the inefficiency of gene transfer vectors and immune responses for the use of such vectors provide formidable barriers to successful gene therapy of SP-B deficiency in the lung. Nevertheless, hereditary lung diseases, such as SP-B deficiency, cystic fibrosis, and α_1-antitrypsin deficiency, may someday be amenable to somatic cell gene transfer.

SELECTED REFERENCES

Hohlfeld J, Fabel H, Hamm H. The role of pulmonary surfactant in obstructive airways disease. Eur Respir J 1997;10:482–491.

Johansson J, Curstedt T. Molecular structures and interactions of pulmonary surfactant components. Eur J Biochem 1997;224:675–693.

Khoor A, Stahlman MT, Gray MF, Whitsett JA. Temporal-spatial distribution of SP-B and SP-C proteins and mRNAs in development respiratory epithelium of human lung. J Histochem Cytochem 1994;42:1187–1199.

Kuroki Y, Voelker DR. Pulmonary surfactant proteins. J Biol Chem 1994;269:25,943–25,946.

Nogee LM. Surfactant protein-B deficiency. Chest 1997;111(Suppl): 129S–135S.

Nogee LM, Garnier G, Dietz HC, et al. A mutation in the surfactant protein B gene responsible for fatal neonatal respiratory disease in multiple kindreds. J Clin Invest 1994;93:1860–1863.

Robertson B, Taeusch HW. Surfactant therapy for lung disease. In: L'Enfant C, Lung Biology in Health and Disease. New York: Marcel Dekker, 1995.

Rooney SA, Young SL, Mendelson CR. Molecular and cellular processing of lung surfactant. FASEB J 1994;8:957–967.

van Golde LMJ. Potential role of surfactant proteins A and D in innate lung defense against pathogens. Biol Neonate 1995;67:2–17.

Whitsett JA, Nogee LM, Weaver TE, Horowitz AD. Human surfactant protein B: structure, function, regulation, and genetic disease. Physiol Rev 1995;75:749–757.

40 Lung Cancer

The Role of Tumor Suppressor Genes

STEVEN JAY WEINTRAUB

BACKGROUND

The leading cause of cancer deaths in the United States is carcinoma of the lung. Despite the innumerable advances in the treatment of other types of cancer, lung carcinomas remain nearly uniformly fatal. In the past few years, however, there have been many new findings regarding the series of events that occur on a molecular level during lung carcinogenesis. These findings should prove to be of value not only in understanding the evolution of lung cancer, but also in its diagnosis and treatment.

The different types of lung cancer have been divided into two categories. Small cell lung cancer (SCLC) is thought to be of neuroendocrine origin. Chemotherapy extends survival of patients with this type of lung cancer by several months. Squamous cell carcinoma, adenocarcinoma, and large cell carcinoma are all thought to arise from a bronchoalveolar progenitor cell. This group of carcinomas has been designated non–small cell lung cancer (NSCLC). Current chemotherapeutic regimens have no effect on survival of patients that are afflicted with NSCLC.

Early cytogenetic studies of both SCLC and NSCLC demonstrated that several chromosomal abnormalities occurred consistently in lung cancer tissue and cell lines derived from these tumors, suggesting that a specific set of mutations occurs in each type of lung cancer. Indeed, it is now known that several genes are frequently expressed aberrantly in lung cancer. Of these, the retinoblastoma gene and the p53 gene, both of which are tumor suppressors, are the best studied. Therefore, the function of the retinoblastoma protein (Rb) and p53 protein (p53) in normal cell growth and differentiation and the mechanism by which alteration of their activity promotes lung carcinogenesis will be the focus of this chapter.

THE RETINOBLASTOMA PROTEIN–E2F PATHWAY

Studies of the neoplastic process initially led to the description of oncogenes, which are genes whose expression induces cellular transformation. However, a consistent finding among human retinoblastomas was the deletion of chromosomal band 13q14, suggesting the existence of a gene whose inactivation is necessary for progression to retinoblastoma (*see* Chapters 7 and 105). Thus the existence of antioncogenes or tumor suppressor genes was postulated. Accordingly, a gene, now known as the retinoblastoma gene and found at this locus, is expressed in all normal retinal cells, as well as all normal adult tissue, but is either absent or mutated in all retinoblastomas. Confirmation that Rb is a tumor suppressor was provided by experiments in which wild-type Rb was artificially introduced into retinoblastoma cells. Restoration of Rb in these cells resulted in growth inhibition and loss of tumorigenicity, indicating that inactivation of Rb is necessary for tumorigenesis.

In addition to retinoblastomas, loss of Rb function has been associated with osteosarcomas and bladder, breast, prostate, cervical, and lung cancers. Among patients with bladder cancer, those with Rb(–) carcinomas have more invasive tumors and their prognosis is significantly worse than those with Rb(+) bladder cancers. In cancer of the cervix, disruption of Rb function must be necessary for tumor progression because almost all cervical cancers fall into one of two categories: either they express the human papilloma virus protein E7, a protein that is known to bind to and inactivate Rb, or they produce only a mutant, inactive form of Rb. Similarly, loss of functional Rb appears to be important in lung cancer since it is mutated in over 90% of SCLCs and 20–30% of NSCLCs. Underscoring the role of disruption of Rb function in the pathogenesis of lung cancer is the finding that relatives of retinoblastoma patients who have germline mutations in the Rb gene are at markedly increased risk of developing SCLC.

Rb has two domains that are strongly conserved across species and among two other cellular proteins, p107 and p130, and the region that encompasses these domains has become known as the pocket (Fig. 40-1). Accordingly Rb, p107, and p130 are collectively known as the pocket proteins. The integrity of the pocket is critical for the interaction of these proteins with several other cellular proteins, including the transcription factor E2F *(see below)*. An intriguing early finding was that most mutations of Rb in tumors that express a stable protein involve the pocket, suggesting that a function of the pocket has an essential role in the tumor suppressing activity of Rb (i.e., disruption of an Rb pocket function is important in tumor pathogenesis). Additionally, several DNA tumor virus oncoproteins bind to the Rb pocket and displace cellular pocket-binding proteins. Any mutation in these oncoproteins that interferes with their capacity to bind Rb and displace these proteins disrupts their oncogenicity, suggesting that they are oncogenic because they block the interaction of the Rb pocket with other cellular proteins.

It is now known that Rb plays a role in regulation of progression through the normal cell cycle (*see* Chapter 6). Rb does so at least

From: *Principles of Molecular Medicine* (J. L. Jameson, ed.), ©1998 Humana Press Inc., Totowa, NJ.

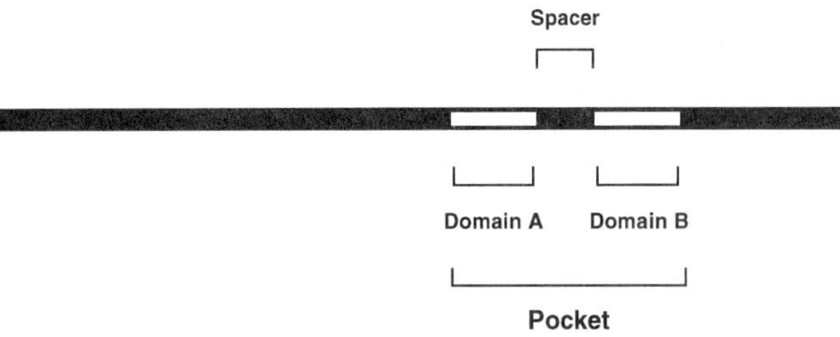

Figure 40-1 Schematic of the pocket proteins. The pockets of Rb, p107, and p130 each consist of two regions, domain A and domain B, that contain amino acid sequences that are conserved both among these three proteins and across species and a nonconserved spacer between these two conserved regions. Most of the cellular functions of the pocket proteins that have been identified to date are dependent on the integrity of the pocket domain. The white areas represent the regions that are conserved between Rb, p107, and p130 and among each of these proteins across different species.

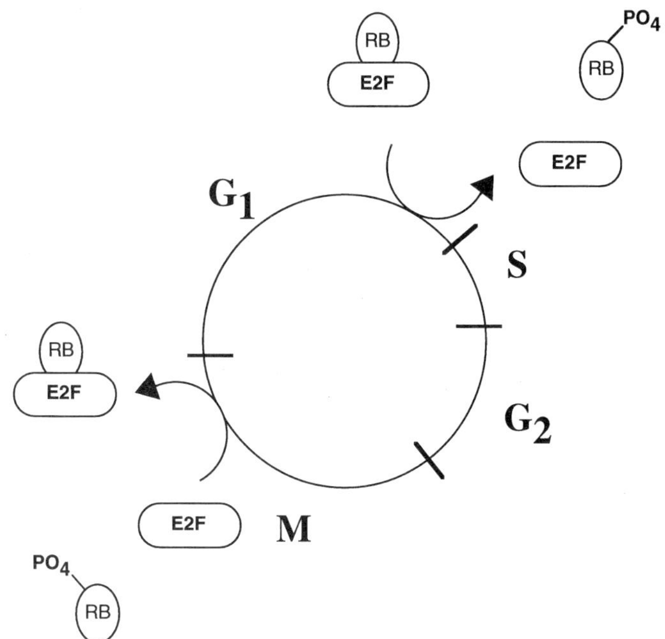

Figure 40-2 Rb is phosphorylated in a cell cycle-dependent fashion and its interaction with E2F is controlled by its phosphorylation state. Rb becomes hyperphosphorylated in late G_1 and remains so until late in mitosis; during anaphase Rb becomes hypophosphorylated. Only the hypophosphorylated form binds E2F. E2F is a family of transcription factors that activate genes whose expression is necessary for progression through the cell cycle. When E2F is complexed with Rb (or one of the other pocket proteins), however, the complex is a transcriptional repressor that inhibits expression of these same genes. Rb is thought to regulate cellular proliferation through its interaction with E2F and the resultant transcriptional repression of these genes.

in part through the interaction of the pocket with a family of transcription factors known collectively as E2F. Binding sites for E2F are found in the promoters of several genes whose expression is necessary for progression through the cell cycle, including thymidylate synthase, dihydrofolate reductase, and DNA polymerase-α. Rb is phosphorylated in a cell cycle-dependent fashion. It is in its "hypophosphorylated" state at the end of mitosis and remains so during most of G_0/G_1, but as the cell enters late G_1 it becomes "hyperphosphorylated." The phosphorylation cycle controls the interaction of Rb with E2F: when it is in its hypophosphorylated form, it binds to E2F; however, when it is hyperphosphorylated in late G_1, it dissociates from E2F leaving free E2F behind on the promoter (Fig. 40-2). Only the hypophosphorylated form of Rb, the form that binds E2F, inhibits growth. The complex of hypophosphorylated Rb and E2F is a transcriptional repressor that inhibits the activity of *trans*-activating factors on the promoter, and the "free" E2F that is left on the promoter upon hyperphosphorylation and dissociation of Rb from E2F is a transcriptional activator. The complex of the Rb-related proteins p107 and E2F are also transcriptional repressors. p107and p130 also bind to E2F in a cell cycle-dependent fashion, but their pattern of binding differs from that of Rb. So it is envisioned that cell cycle progression is regulated by the Rb–E2F pathway as follows: several genes whose expression is necessary for cell cycle progression contain E2F sites and, at specific stages of the cell cycle, free E2F activates these genes; however, when Rb or one of the other pocket proteins bind to E2F, the complex of the pocket protein and E2F inhibits the activity of these same genes. In this fashion Rb and related proteins control the expression of these genes in a cell cycle-specific fashion. If Rb is inactivated through mutation, some of these genes will be constitutively expressed, removing an important constraint on cellular proliferation. It is likely that this is a critical step in the pathogenesis of lung cancer as well as other tumors.

The mechanism by which the Rb–E2F complex represses transcription has recently been elucidated. It was found that the Rb pocket has intrinsic transcriptional repressor activity. This was demonstrated through the use of a chimeric protein in which the pocket was fused to a heterologous DNA binding domain, that of the yeast transcription factor Gal4. The activity of the resultant protein was assessed using an artificial transcriptional reporter construct that contains the Gal4 DNA binding sequence (Fig. 40-3). This facilitated the targeting of Rb to a promoter in an E2F-independent fashion. When the activity of a Gal4-Rb-pocket fusion protein was assessed in this fashion, it was found to be as effective a transcriptional repressor as wild-type Rb when it is tethered to a promoter by E2F. When control proteins or other regions of Rb were fused to Gal4, the resulting chimeric proteins were inactive in this assay. Thus, it is likely that the repressor activity of the Rb–E2F complex is a function of the Rb pocket, and the role of E2F in this complex is to target the repressor activity of Rb to the appropriate promoters. Further, it was shown that this repressor activity is a function of the ability of Rb to disrupt critical interactions of several proteins that activate transcription.

Even though Rb has been shown to interact with several cellular proteins, there is evidence, at least in one cell line, that E2F is the most important mediator of Rb activity. In these cells, overexpression of a form of E2F that lacks Rb, p107, and p130 binding activity, but still encodes a *trans*-activation function will disrupt the growth-inhibitory effect of Rb. When it is overexpressed, this protein will bind to E2F sites and displace cellular proteins that are bound to these sites, such as the Rb–E2F complex, and, like free E2F, it will *trans*-activate promoters that contain E2F sites. Unlike E2F, because it does not bind pocket proteins, it will not mediate transcriptional repression by Rb (or any other effect of the pocket proteins) and it will not affect the interaction of the pocket proteins with other proteins in the cell. The net result of overexpression of this protein then is disruption of the effect of Rb and Rb-related proteins on promoters that contain E2F sites with-

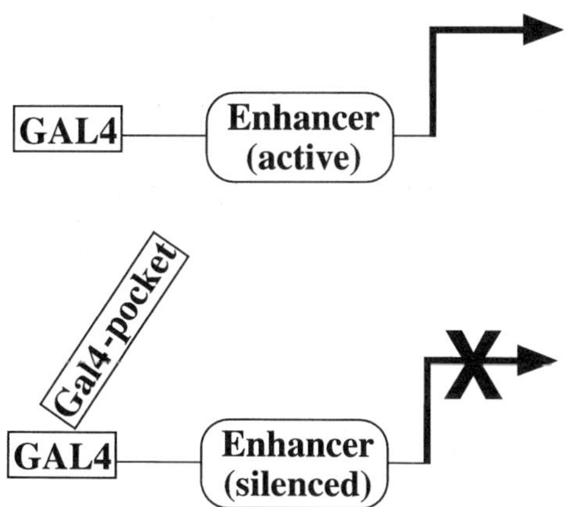

Figure 40-3 The transcriptional repressor activity of Rb is a function of its pocket domain. Chimeric proteins in which the different regions of Rb are fused to the DNA-binding domain of the yeast transcription factor Gal4 are targeted to promoters that contain a Gal4-binding site. This permits an assessment of the activity of the different domains of Rb. When the Rb pocket domain is targeted to a promoter in this fashion it represses the activity of enhancers on the promoter, thereby blocking expression of the gene. The only region of Rb that has repressor activity in this assay is the pocket, suggesting that the repressor activity of Rb is a function of its pocket domain.

out a direct effect on any other function of the Rb family of proteins. The finding that this protein disrupts the growth inhibitory effect of Rb indicates that the interaction of Rb with Rb binding proteins other than E2F is not sufficient for growth suppression. Indeed, it has been suggested that E2F may be the only critical effector of Rb activity.

Although Rb is not inactivated by mutation or deletion in all tumors, it may be functionally inactive in several tumor types that express wild-type Rb. As outlined above, the activity of Rb is controlled by its phosphorylation state, hypophosphorylated Rb being the active growth-inhibitory form and hyperphosphorylated Rb the inactive form. It is becoming apparent that the most important regulators of Rb phosphorylation are the D cyclins and their associated cyclin-dependent kinases (CDKs). The D cyclins activate certain CDKs, which in turn phosphorylate Rb. It has been found that in some NSCLCs that express wild-type Rb, cyclin D_1 is overexpressed. This could lead to constitutive hyperphosphorylation and, therefore, inactivation of the Rb. So even though these cells express wild-type Rb, they are likely to be functionally Rb negative. Additionally, a newly discovered class of proteins has been found that inhibit the activity of cyclin-CDKs. The most relevant one to this discussion appears to be p16. This protein binds to cyclin D–CDK complexes and inhibits phosphorylation of Rb, maintaining Rb in its active growth-suppressive state. Disruption of p16 function would result in inappropriate hyperphosphorylation and, therefore, inactivation of Rb. Accordingly, p16 has been found to be mutated in several different types of cancer and it has been shown that replacement of wild-type p16 into p16(–) cancer cell lines results in inhibition of their growth and suppression of tumorigenicity. It is therefore of note that in a study of 55 SCLC cell lines it was found that whereas the 48 that lacked wild-type Rb expressed p16, 6 of the cell lines expressed wild-type Rb but lacked p16. In the second set of cells, lack of the p16 inhibitor will lead to increased kinase activity of cyclin D–CDK complexes, which in turn should result in increased phosphorylation and functional inactivation of Rb. So although these SCLC cells express wild-type Rb, it is likely to be functionally inactive because of the lack of p16. These findings suggest that inactivation of Rb, whether by mutation or constitutive hyperphosphorylation, is a necessary step in the pathogenesis of lung cancer; in fact, it has recently been postulated that the Rb–E2F pathway may be dysregulated in all human malignancies.

THE p53 CHECKPOINT FOR DNA DAMAGE

p53 plays a critical role in controlling cellular proliferation by either arresting cells in G_1 or by inducing apoptosis under the appropriate conditions (*see* Chapter 7). p53 functions in a pathway that serves as a checkpoint for DNA damage in that various agents that are known to cause mutagenesis of DNA, such as ionizing radiation, will induce either p53-dependent cell cycle arrest or apoptosis. Both of these effects are known to be dependent on p53 activity because mutation of p53 disrupts them and reintroduction of p53 into p53(–) cells restores them. Whether a cell undergoes p53-dependent arrest or apoptosis appears to be cell type-specific.

It is likely that the cell cycle arrest that occurs with DNA damage allows the cell to pause and repair its DNA whereas apoptosis serves to limit proliferation of cells with genomic damage. Evidence for these hypotheses is provided by the finding that cells that lack p53 are one million times more likely to contain abnormally amplified DNA than cells that express p53. Additionally, mice that have homozygous p53 mutations develop normally through birth but invariably develop tumors by 6–9 months. This is probably because of the fact that cells that lack the p53-dependent checkpoint for DNA damage continue to proliferate while accumulating mutations—if the appropriate set of mutations occurs in these cells they will undergo malignant transformation.

The p53 gene is the most frequently mutated gene among cancers of all types. In regard to lung cancer, p53 is mutated in about 90% of SCLCs and 60% of NSCLCs. Additionally, although wild-type p53 is expressed in some lung cancers, it may be inactivated by mechanisms other than mutation. In a recent study, it was found that several NSCLCs that express wild-type p53 overexpress a second protein, mdm2, that binds to and inactivates p53. Overexpression of mdm2 was found to occur only in cells that expressed wild-type p53. These findings suggest that in certain lung tumors the p53 pathway is inactivated by overexpression of mdm2 instead of mutation of p53. This is analogous to the situation with Rb outlined above. Even though Rb is not inactivated by mutation in all SCLCs, it may be functionally inactivated by inappropriate phosphorylation if cyclin D_1 is overexpressed or if CDK inhibitor p16 activity is absent.

After exposure of cells to ionizing radiation there is an increase in cellular p53 levels that is coincident with p53-dependent cell cycle arrest. Like Rb, p53 is a transcription factor, except that p53 is a *trans*-activating protein. Underscoring the role of its *trans*-activating function in cell cycle arrest and, therefore tumor suppression, is the finding that most of the mutant forms of p53 found in tumors have lost this activity. This suggested that wild-type p53 inhibits cellular proliferation by activating the expression of genes that block progression through the cell cycle (Fig. 40-4). It is now known that in nontransformed cells the increase in the cellular level of p53 that occurs with ionizing radiation increases expression of at least two proteins that arrest cellular proliferation, p21 and GADD45. p21, like p16, inhibits the kinase activity of cyclin–CDK complexes. Increased cellular levels of p21 will block phosphorylation of Rb by inhibiting the activity of the Rb-specific cyclin–CDK complexes, thereby maintaining Rb (and possibly

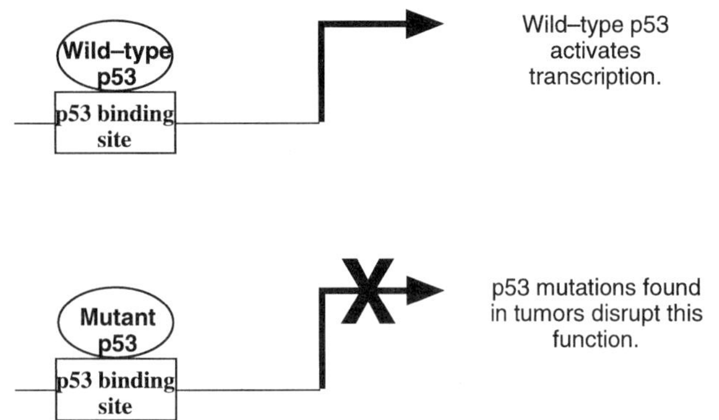

Figure 40-4 The ability of p53 to stimulate transcription is essential for tumor suppression. The critical role that the transcriptional activation function of p53 has in tumor suppression was first suggested by the finding that transforming mutants of p53 do not activate gene expression.

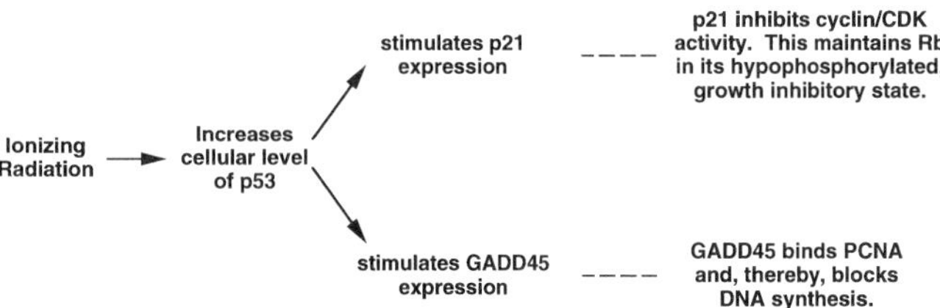

Figure 40-5 Schematic of the mechanism by which p53 mediates ionizing radiation-induced cell cycle arrest. The promoters of the genes for p21 and GADD45 contain binding sites for p53. Ionizing radiation increases p53 in the cell resulting in activation of transcription of the p21 and GADD45 genes. These proteins arrest cell growth.

Rb-related proteins) in its hypophosphorylated growth-suppressive form—resulting in a G_1 cell cycle arrest. GADD45, the other protein whose expression is induced by p53, is thought to arrest cellular proliferation by inhibiting DNA synthesis, probably through an interaction with proliferating cell nuclear antigen (PCNA) (Fig. 40-5).

CONCLUSIONS

A series of mutations resulting in aberrant production of a specific set of proteins culminates in cellular transformation. It is estimated that 10–20 mutations occur during the pathogenesis of lung cancer. Several genes have been identified that are consistently mutated in lung cancers, but the best studied of these are the Rb and p53 genes. Both of these genes encode tumor suppressors. An understanding of the role of these and other tumor suppressors in maintenance of normal cellular physiology and the significance of their inactivation in cancer pathogenesis has advanced significantly during the past decade. The retinoblastoma protein is important for maintaining a controlled progression through the cell cycle by regulating the activity of several growth-promoting genes. p53 limits the transmission of potentially harmful genetic alterations that occur with DNA damage to future generations of cells either by arresting the cell cycle to allow for DNA repair or by inducing apoptosis. Therefore, the inactivation of Rb or p53 disrupts constraints that inhibit the transformation of normal lung tissue to lung carcinoma. The understanding of these processes should allow for more efficient treatment of lung cancer in the future, possibly by the restoration of their function in malignant cells.

SELECTED REFERENCES

Albelda SM. Gene therapy for lung cancer and mesothelioma. Chest 1997;111(Suppl):144S–149S.

Antelman D, Machemer T, Huyghe BG, Shepard HM, Maneval D, Johnson DE. Inhibition of tumor cell proliferation in vitro and in vivo by exogenous p110RB, the retinoblastoma tumor suppressor protein. Oncogene 1995;10:697–704.

Benedict WF. Altered RB expression is a prognostic clinical marker involved in human bladder tumorigenesis. J Cell Biochem 1992; 161(Suppl):69S–71S.

Bookstein R, Lee WH. Molecular genetics of the retinoblastoma suppressor gene. Crit Rev Oncog 1991;2:211–227.

Buchkovich K, Duffy LA, Harlow E. The retinoblastoma protein is phosphorylated during specific phases of the cell cycle. Cell 1989;58:1097–1105.

Cai DW, Mukhopadhyay T, Liu Y, Fujiwara T, Roth JA. Stable expression of the wild-type p53 gene in human lung cancer cells after retrovirus-mediated gene transfer. Hum Gene Ther 1993;4:617–624.

Carbone DP, Minna JD. In vivo gene therapy of human lung cancer using wild-type p53 delivered by retrovirus. J Natl Cancer Inst 1994; 86:1437,1438.

Chen PL, Scully P, Shew JY, Wang JY, Lee WH. Phosphorylation of the retinoblastoma gene product is modulated during the cell cycle and cellular differentiation. Cell 1989;58:1193–1198.

Cordon-Cardo C, Wartinger D, Petrylak D, et al. Altered expression of the retinoblastoma gene product: prognostic indicator in bladder cancer. J Natl Cancer Inst 1992;84:1251–1256.

Donehower LA, Harvey M, Slagle BL, et al. Mice deficient for p53 are developmentally normal but susceptible to spontaneous tumours. Nature 1992;356:215–221.

Dulic V, Kaufmann WK, Wilson SJ, et al. p53-dependent inhibition of cyclin-dependent kinase activities in human fibroblasts during radiation-induced G1 arrest. Cell 1994;76:1013–1023.

el-Deiry WS, Tokino T, Velculescu VE, et al. WAF1, a potential mediator of p53 tumor suppression. Cell 1993;75:817–825.

Ewen ME. The cell cycle and the retinoblastoma protein family. Cancer Metastasis Rev 1994;13:45–66.

Fields S, Jang SK. Presence of a potent transcription activating sequence in the p53 protein. Science 1990;249:1046–1049.

Fujiwara T, Grimm EA, Mukhopadhyay T, Cai DW, Owen-Schaub LB, Roth JA. A retroviral wild-type p53 expression vector penetrates human lung cancer spheroids and inhibits growth by inducing apoptosis. Cancer Res 1993;53:4129–4133.

Harbour JW, Lai SL, Whang-Peng J, Gazdar AF, Minna JD, Kaye FJ. Abnormalities in structure and expression of the human retinoblastoma gene in SCLC. Science 1988;241:353–357.

Harper JW, Adami GR, Wei N, Keyomarsi K, Elledge SJ. The p21 Cdk-interacting protein Cip1 is a potent inhibitor of G1 cyclin-dependent kinases. Cell 1993;75:805–816.

Hu QJ, Dyson N, Harlow E. The regions of the retinoblastoma protein needed for binding to adenovirus E1A or SV40 large T antigen are common sites for mutations. EMBO J 1990;9:1147–1155.

Huang HJ, Yee JK, Shew JY, et al. Suppression of the neoplastic phenotype by replacement of the RB gene in human cancer cells. Science 1988;242:1563–1566.

Kaelin WJ, Pallas DC, DeCaprio JA, Kaye FJ, Livingston DM. Identification of cellular proteins that can interact specifically with the T/E1A-binding region of the retinoblastoma gene product. Cell 1991;64:521–532.

Kastan MB, Canman CE, Leonard CJ. p53, cell cycle control and apoptosis: implications for cancer. Cancer Metastasis Rev 1995;14:3–15.

Kastan MB, Onyekwere O, Sidransky D, Vogelstein B, Craig RW. Participation of p53 protein in the cellular response to DNA damage. Cancer Res 1991;51:6304–6311.

Kastan MB, Zhan Q, el-Deiry WS, et al. A mammalian cell cycle checkpoint pathway utilizing p53 and GADD45 is defective in ataxia-telangiectasia. Cell 1992;71:587–597.

Koh J, Enders GH, Dynlacht BD, Harlow E. Tumour-derived p16 alleles encoding proteins defective in cell-cycle inhibition. Nature 1995;375: 506–510.

Kuerbitz SJ, Plunkett BS, Walsh WV, Kastan MB. Wild-type p53 is a cell cycle checkpoint determinant following irradiation. Proc Natl Acad Sci USA 1992;89:7491–7495.

Livingstone LR, White A, Sprouse J, Livanos E, Jacks T, Tlsty TD. Altered cell cycle arrest and gene amplification potential accompany loss of wild-type p53. Cell 1992;70:923–935.

Marchetti A, Buttitta F, Pellegrini S, et al. Mdm2 gene amplification and overexpression in non–small cell lung carcinomas with accumulation of the p53 protein in the absence of p53 gene mutations. Diagn Mol Pathol 1995;4:93–97.

Minna JD. The molecular biology of lung cancer pathogenesis. Chest 1993;103:449S–456S.

Momand J, Zambetti GP, Olson DC, George D, Levine AJ. The mdm-2 oncogene product forms a complex with the p53 protein and inhibits p53-mediated transactivation. Cell 1992;69:1237–1245.

Nevins JR. E2F: a link between the Rb tumor suppressor protein and viral oncoproteins. Science 1992;258:424–429.

Nevins JR. Transcriptional regulation. A closer look at E2F. Nature 1992;358:375,376.

Otterson GA, Kratzke RA, Coxon A, Kim YW, Kaye FJ. Absence of p16INK4 protein is restricted to the subset of lung cancer lines that retains wildtype RB. Oncogene 1994;9:3375–3378.

Qian Y, Luckey C, Horton L, Esser M, Templeton DJ. Biological function of the retinoblastoma protein requires distinct domains for hyperphosphorylation and transcription factor binding. Mol Cell Biol 1992;12:5363–5372.

Qin XQ, Livingston DM, Ewen M, Sellers WR, Arany Z, Kaelin WG. The transcription factor E2F-1 is a downstream target of RB action. Mol Cell Biol 1995;15:742–755.

Raycroft L, Wu HY, Lozano G. Transcriptional activation by wild-type but not transforming mutants of the p53 anti-oncogene. Science 1990;249:1049–1051.

Roth JA, Nguyen D, Lawrence DD, et al. Retrovirus-mediated wild-type p53 gene transfers to tumors of patients with lung cancer. Nat Med 1996;2:985–991.

Sanders BM, Jay M, Draper GJ, Roberts EM. Non-ocular cancer in relatives of retinoblastoma patients. Br J Cancer 1989;60:358–365.

Schauer IE, Siriwardana S, Langan TA, Sclafani RA. Cyclin D1 overexpression vs. retinoblastoma inactivation: implications for growth control evasion in non–small cell and small cell lung cancer. Proc Natl Acad Sci USA 1994;91:7827–7831.

Scheffner M, Munger K, Byrne JC, Howley PM. The state of the p53 and retinoblastoma genes in human cervical carcinoma cell lines. Proc Natl Acad Sci USA 1991;88:5523–5527.

Serrano M, Hannon GJ, Beach D. A new regulatory motif in cell-cycle control causing specific inhibition of cyclin D/CDK4. Nature 1993;366:704–707.

Shirodkar S, Ewen M, DeCaprio JA, Morgan J, Livingston DM, Chittenden T. The transcription factor E2F interacts with the retinoblastoma product and a p107-cyclin A complex in a cell cycle-regulated manner. Cell 1992;68:157–166.

Slebos RJ, Lee MH, Plunkett BS, et al. p53-dependent G1 arrest involves pRB-related proteins and is disrupted by the human papillomavirus 16 E7 oncoprotein. Proc Natl Acad Sci USA 1994;91:5320–5324.

Smith ML, Chen IT, Zhan Q, et al. Interaction of the p53-regulated protein Gadd45 with proliferating cell nuclear antigen. Science 1994;266: 1376–1380.

Swafford DS, Middleton SK, Palmisano WA, et al. Frequent aberrant methylation of p16INK4a in primary rat lung tumors. Mol Cell Biol 1997;17:1366–1374.

Weinberg RA. The retinoblastoma protein and cell cycle control. Cell 1995;81:323–330.

Weinberg RA. Tumor suppressor genes. Science 1991;254: 1138–1146.

Weintraub SJ, Chow K, Luo RX, Zhang SH, He S, Dean DC. Mechanism of active transcriptional repression by the retinoblastoma protein. Nature 1995;375:812–815.

Weintraub SJ, Prater CA, Dean DC. Retinoblastoma protein switches the E2F site from positive to negative element. Nature 1992;358: 259–261.

Whang PJ, Knutsen T, Gazdar A, et al. Nonrandom structural and numerical chromosome changes in non–small-cell lung cancer. Genes Chromosom Cancer 1991;3:168–188.

Whyte P, Williamson NM, Harlow E. Cellular targets for transformation by the adenovirus E1A proteins. Cell 1989;56:67–75.

Wiest JS, Franklin WA, Otstot JT, et al. Identification of a novel region of homozygous deletion on chromosome 9p in squamous cell carcinoma of the lung: the location of a putative tumor suppressor gene. Cancer Res 1997;57:1–6.

Yin Y, Tainsky MA, Bischoff FZ, Strong LC, Wahl GM. Wild-type p53 restores cell cycle control and inhibits gene amplification in cells with mutant p53 alleles. Cell 1992;70:937–948.

Yonish-Rouach E, Resnitzky D, Lotem J, Sachs L, Kimchi A, Oren M. Wild-type p53 induces apoptosis of myeloid leukemia cells that is inhibited by interleukin-6. Nature 1991;352:345–347.

GASTROENTEROLOGY VI

SECTION EDITOR:
JAMES C. REYNOLDS

41 Hepatology

PIET C. DE GROEN AND NICHOLAS F. LARUSSO

INTRODUCTION

During the past century, hepatology has gradually progressed from a discipline focused on simply describing the signs and symptoms associated with a specific liver disease, via clinical observations, biochemical abnormalities, and organ pathology, to a science that involves describing and understanding abnormal cell function. Rapid progress in the techniques of molecular biology in the last three decades has added an entirely new dimension to the concept of disease; it has led to the development of molecular hepatology as an emerging area of interest that attempts to generate new knowledge of the molecular mechanisms responsible for normal and abnormal liver function.

Recently, several genes responsible for inherited liver diseases have been either localized to a specific part of a chromosome or cloned and characterized. Some of these genes have been found by applying traditional molecular techniques (e.g., the gene was cloned using antibodies to a normal or abnormal protein or cDNA probes were used to screen CDNA libraries [α-1 antitrypsin deficiency]). Other genes have been found using linkage analysis and chromosome jumping or walking (e.g., cystic fibrosis, Wilson's disease, hemochromatosis) or cytogenetic deletions and rearrangements (e.g., Alagille syndrome). Relevant bacterial and viral DNA/RNA compositions have also been identified using a variety of techniques, such as virus purification (Hepatitis B) or cDNA cloning (Hepatitis C and G).

At present, we are beginning to understand why certain genes are expressed only in liver. Hepatocyte-specific promoters have been described and the search for specific transcription factors is ongoing. In vitro as well as in vivo transfection techniques are being developed, and the first human trials of gene therapy in both inherited as well as acquired (e.g., cancer) liver diseases have been started. At least five viruses are now known to preferentially infect the liver, and new therapeutic modalities aimed at selectively interfering with viral metabolism are being developed.

Because of limited space and the fact that substantial components of what might be covered in a chapter on molecular hepatology will be covered in other chapters, our approach will be a very focused one. In this chapter, we briefly describe liver development, bile formation (including the enterohepatic cycle of bile acids), and the molecular mechanisms leading to cirrhosis. Next, we discuss five inherited (i.e., Crigler-Najjar, Gilbert's, Dubin-Johnson, Alagille, and the progressive familial intrahepatic cholestasis [PFIC] syndromes) and two important immune-mediated (i.e., primary biliary cirrhosis [PBC] and primary sclerosing cholangitis [PSC]) cholestatic diseases; finally, we review selected developments in autoimmune hepatitis, polycystic liver disease, amyloidosis, and alcohol- and drug-induced (i.e., acetaminophen, aspirin, and NSAIDS) liver disease.

The classic inherited disorders of the liver are reviewed in Chapter 42 by Ruiz and Wu, who address the molecular basis of Wilson's disease hemochromatosis, α-1-antitrypsin deficiency, cystic fibrosis, the porphyrias, galactosemias, and fructose deficiency. In Chapter 43, Gupta and Shafritz explain in detail the molecular aspects of hepatitis caused by viruses, with particular attention to hepatitis B, C, and D.

MOLECULAR ASPECTS OF LIVER FUNCTION AND BILE FORMATION

During embryogenesis, the liver develops as an extension of cells from the hepatic diverticulum, the caudal portion developing into the gallbladder and cystic duct, and the cranial portion forming the common bile duct and liver bud. The endogenous liver cell population is composed of hepatocytes and intrahepatic bile duct epithelial cells, or cholangiocytes, which are of epithelial cell origin, and a variety of mesenchymal cells, including Kupffer cells, vascular and sinusoidal endothelial cells, fat-storing cells, and pit cells. Within the liver, these cells are organized into histologic and functional units forming the classic hepatic lobules.

The hepatocyte has three important, unique features: first, it is the sole producer of a large number of serum proteins, carbohydrates, and lipids; second, it metabolizes endogenous and foreign substances and excretes the modified products into the biliary system. Third, it synthesizes primary bile acids. All features require hepatocyte-specific promoters and transcription factors for hepatocyte-specific expression of secretary proteins, receptors, or enzymes. Several hepatocyte-specific promoters are now known and include, among others, the albumin, transthyretin, and phosphoenol pyruvate carboxykinase promoters. These specific promoters have been identified by a standard molecular strategy. First, the coding region of the genes was cloned (cDNA) and, subsequently, their genomic structure identified. Next, the upstream untranslated genomic sequence was analyzed for DNA sequences (i.e., *cis*-acting elements) able to drive expression of reporter genes only in hepatocyte-derived cell lines, such as HepG2

From: *Principles of Molecular Medicine* (J. L. Jameson, ed.), ©1998 Humana Press Inc., Totowa, NJ.

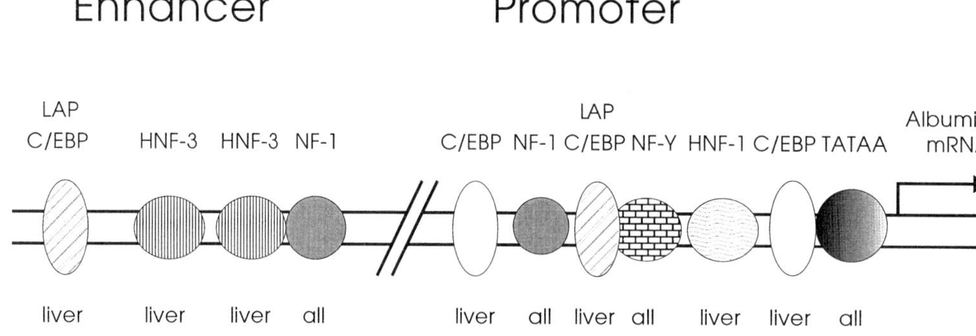

Figure 41-1 Albumin promoter. Transcription factors binding to regulatory elements in the albumin gene are depicted in this schematic, simplified diagram. Parts of the gene (double-stranded DNA) representing the enhancer and promoter regions are shown as a double horizontal line; the distance between the enhancer and the promoter is approximately 10-kb pairs. The arrow to the right of the TATAA box indicates the position and orientation of the transcription start of the albumin mRNA. Transcription factor binding sites are shown as ovals or circles, with the names of several transcription factors that bind to these sites shown above and with the names of representative tissues where these factors have been found shown below. The high degree of tissue specificity of this gene is conferred by the combination of the enhancer as well as promoter regulatory elements. NF-1, nuclear factor 1 or CCAAT transcription factor (CTP); LAP, liver-enriched transcriptional activator protein [also named nuclear factor interleukin-6 (NF-IL6), C/EBPβ, and cysteine-rich protein 2 (CRP2)]; NF-Y, nuclear factor Y. (Adapted from: Zaret KS. Control of hepatocyte differentiation by liver-enriched transcription factors. In: Tavoloni N, Berk PD, eds. Hepatic Transport and Bile Secretion: Physiology and Pathophysiology. New York: Raven, 1993; pp. 135–143.

cells. Finally, the unique DNA sequences able to drive expression were analyzed for binding sites for proteins or transcription factors able to drive hepatocyte-specific transcription. Examples of these factors include CCAAT/enhancer-binding protein (C/EBP) and hepatocyte nuclear factors 1, 3, and 4 (HNF-1,3,4) (Fig. 41-1). Other well-known, unique hepatocyte proteins include the asialoglycoprotein receptor, bile acid formation regulating enzymes, and several transport proteins in the hepatocyte canalicular membrane.

Bile acids are organic acids derived from cholesterol. As natural ionic detergents, they are of vital importance in absorption, transport, and secretion of lipids. The primary bile acids in humans are cholic and chenodeoxycholic acid. Both are excreted predominantly in conjugated form, linked either to glycine or taurine. Dehydroxylation of these bile acids by intestinal bacteria produces the more hydrophobic, secondary bile acids, deoxycholic acid and lithocholic acid. In other mammalian species, alternative hydroxylations can occur. For instance, bears generate ursodeoxycholic acid, the 7β-epimer of chenodeoxycholic acid. After release into the intestine, the majority of bile acids is absorbed and returned to the liver via the portal venous system. This cycling of bile acids between liver and intestine is called the enterohepatic circulation. A small fraction of secondary bile acids is further metabolized in the liver to tertiary, conjugated forms, which are not reabsorbed after excretion. Most enzymes required for cholesterol and bile acid synthesis have been extensively studied, and metabolic defects for several enzymes have been described. For example, deficiency in 26-hydroxylase results in a syndrome of premature arteriosclerosis, cataracts, and dementia, known as cerebrotendinous xanthomatosis. A defect in the final step of the bile acid synthesis pathway, that is, side-chain cleavage in peroxisomes, causes the cerebrohepatorenal syndrome of Zellweger, characterized by severe hypotonia, profound psychomotor retardation, and a characteristic facial appearance. Recently, proteins required for bile acid conjugation and transport have been cloned, either by searching for proteins able to bind to labeled bile acids or by expression cloning for proteins able to transport bile acids. For example, an hepatic sodium/bile acid cotransporter, an ileal bile acid binding protein, an enzyme capable of conjugating bile acids with both glycine and taurine, and the protein responsible for most, if not all, of the sulfation of bile acids in human liver have been cloned.

Secretion of bile acids is coupled to secretion of phosphatidylcholine and cholesterol and thereby provides a major pathway for cholesterol excretion in bile. Deficiency of bile acids results in reduced cholesterol solubility in bile and is thought to contribute to formation of gallstones. On the other hand, expansion of the bile acid pool with ursodeoxycholic acid causes a reduction of biliary cholesterol excretion and has been found to be of therapeutic value in patients with cholesterol gallstones. The exact molecular mechanisms leading to cholesterol gallstone formation are unknown; however, bile with a high cholesterol saturation index strongly predisposes to cholesterol stone formation. Epidemiological studies have shown a familial risk of gallstones and suggest that probably the main cause of this risk is genetic. This concept is supported by the recent description of the lith1 gene associated with development of gallstones in mice.

Until recently, the bile duct epithelial cell, or cholangiocyte, was considered a rather passive cell, that formed a three-dimensional network of interconnecting ducts that served as simple conduits for delivering bile to the intestine. New data show that cholangiocytes actively participate in secretory and absorptive processes. For instance, these cells express the cystic fibrosis transmembrane conductance regulator (CFTR), a regulatory chloride channel, and the chloride/bicarbonate exchanger at their apical domain; the water channel aquaporin 1, or CHIP28, likely at both apical and basolateral domains, and a variety of ion exchangers and ATP-driven pumps at the basolateral domain. Together with cytosolic carbonic anhydrase, these proteins form the basis of a secretory system that is activated, or inhibited by, changes in cytosolic cAMP concentrations. This whole system is finely regulated by peptide hormones. For example, secretin binds to the secretin receptor at the basolateral domain, activates adenyl cyclase, and increases cAMP concentrations, thereby inducing secretion of bicarbonate

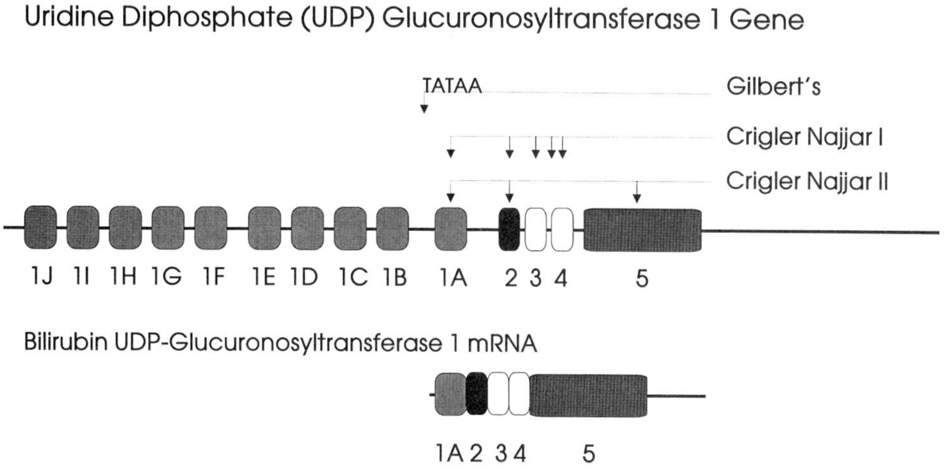

Figure 41-2 The uridine diphosphate (UDP) glucuronosyltransferase 1 gene (UGT1) and bilirubin UDP-glucuronosyltransferase 1 mRNA. The more than 100-kb UGT1 gene is located on chromosome 2. Ten mRNAs are derived from the UGT1 gene, each encoding a different UDP-glucuronosyltransferase. The mRNAs differ only in their most 5' sequence. Each of the 5' exons (exon 1A to 1J) encodes the amino-terminus of one UGT1 isoform. Bilirubin UDP-glucuronosyltransferase 1 mRNA uses exon 1A as is shown. Exon 1A encodes for the substrate binding site, exons 3 and 4 for the uridine diphosphate glucuronic acid binding site and exon 5 for the membrane spanning region and endoplasmatic reticulum retention signal. A (TA) insertion in the TATAA box of the promoter preceding exon 1A has been associated with Gilbert's syndrome; point and splice site mutations, deletions, insertions, and formation of stop codons with Crigler Najjar type I syndrome; and only point mutations with Crigler Najjar type II syndrome. Distances are not to scale. (Adapted from: Janssen PLM, Bosma P. Inherited unconjugated hyperbilirubinemias. AASLD postgraduate course 1995 syllabus, pp. 87–100.)

and water; in contrast, binding of somatostatin to its receptor has the opposite effect.

Kupffer cells are macrophages lining the sinusoidal spaces between rows of hepatocytes. They have a variety of functions, including:

1. Endocytosis of viruses, bacteria, and endotoxins.
2. Antigen processing.
3. Secretion of prostaglandins, interferons, and cytokines.
4. A direct cytotoxicity for parasites and tumor cells.

Pit cells, a population of large granular lymphocytes with natural killer cell activity, are thought to protect the liver from colonization by metastatic tumor cells and viruses. In addition, they may function in the regulation of hepatocyte proliferation. Endothelial cells lining the hepatic sinusoids act as sieves, allowing only free diffusion of particles smaller than 0.2 μm, such as chylomicron remnants, through their fenestrations into the space of Disse. They also are actively engaged in endocytosis and excrete prostaglandins and cytokines in response to various stimuli.

Fat-storing cells, lipocytes, Ito cells, or stellate cells are mesenchymal cells situated in the space of Disse, between endothelial cells and hepatocytes. Under normal conditions, they store large quantities of vitamin A in the form of membrane bound droplets. Recent evidence suggests that fat-storing cells are able to transform into myofibroblast-like cells in response to hepatic injury. The factors involved in activation and transformation of these cells include TNF, TGF-β, PDGF, and, possibly, acetaldehyde. Of these, TGF-β probably is the most important. Secreted by fat-storing cells as well as other nonparenchymal cells in response to injury, it activates fat-storing cells and induces production of collagen and other extracellular matrix proteins. At the same time, synthesis of matrix-degrading proteolytic proteins is inhibited, thereby further disrupting the balance between collagen formation and degradation.

In addition to induction of collagen synthesis, a change in the relative amounts of collagen types occurs. Quiescent cells produce mainly collagen types III and IV, laminin and to a lesser extent collagen type I and fibronectin. Activated myofibroblast-like cells secrete collagens type I, III and IV, fibronectin, laminin and a variety of proteoglycans at a much higher level. In particular, collagen type I, fibronectin and proteoglycans containing chondroitin and dermatan sulfate are expressed at very high levels. Together, these changes result in marked hepatic fibrosis. With continued exposure to agents inducing the abnormal extracellular matrix formation, irreversible fibrosis develops. When this fibrotic process is associated with destruction of the classic hepatic lobule, a histology characteristic of cirrhosis develops: regenerating nodules of hepatocytes separated by dense strands of fibrous tissue.

CHOLESTATIC LIVER DISEASES: INHERITED AND IMMUNE-MEDIATED

A single enzyme, UDP-glucuronosyltransferase 1, is responsible for most of the bilirubin glucuronidating activity in humans. Absence of UDP-glucuronosyltransferase 1 results in a syndrome known as Crigler-Najjar type I, whereas mutations causing severe deficiency of the enzyme result in Crigler-Najjar type II (Fig. 41-2). Both syndromes are inherited in a recessive pattern. Crigler-Najjar type I patients have severe unconjugated hyperbilirubinemia with plasma bilirubin levels fluctuating between 26 and 45 mg/dL. As a result, they develop severe neurologic deficits (kernicterus) and frequently die in their first year of life. Crigler-Najjar type II patients have less severe unconjugated hyperbilirubinemia (usually less than 20 mg/dL) and usually do not develop neurologic symptoms. In contrast to type I, the bile of these patients does contain bilirubin conjugates, and treatment with phenobarbital or glutethimide increases bilirubin metabolism resulting in markedly reduced plasma bilirubin concentrations.

Gilbert's syndrome is characterized by a mild, chronic unconjugated hyperbilirubinemia in the absence of liver disease or overt hemolysis. The mode of inheritance is not clear, as both autosomal dominant as well as recessive patterns of inheritance have been described. The defect is a decreased hepatic glucuronidating activity to approximately 30% of normal, resulting in an increased relative concentration of bilirubin monoglucuronide in bile. The enzyme UDP-glucuronosyltransferase 1 itself is normal (i.e., normal sequence of coding region) in many patients thus far examined, but the 5' promoter region of the gene contains two extra bases (TA) in the TATAA element [A(TA_7)TAA rather than normal A(TA_6)TAA] (Fig. 41-2). The presence of the longer TATAA element results in the reduced expression of a reporter gene, encoding firefly luciferase, in a human hepatoma cell line and therefore appears to be a cause for reduced expression of bilirubin UDP-glucuronosyltransferase 1 in vivo. However, this explanation is not sufficient to explain the complete manifestation of the syndrome.

Dubin-Johnson syndrome is a rare autosomal recessive disorder characterized by chronic conjugated hyperbilirubinemia. Patients have impaired hepatobiliary transport of nonbile salt organic anions. Recently the disease was shown to be caused by a mutation in the canalicular multispecific organic anion transporter, or multidrug-resistance-associated protein 2 (MRP2), on chromosome 10q24. This protein mediates adenosine triphosphate-dependent transport of a broad range of endogenous and xenobiotic compounds across the apical canalicular membrane of the hepatocyte.

Alagille syndrome (also referred to as Alagille-Watson syndrome, syndromic bile duct paucity, or arteriohepatic dysplasia) is an autosomal dominant disorder characterized by abnormal development of liver, heart, skeleton, eye, face, and, less frequently, kidney. Major manifestations of this syndrome are neonatal jaundice and cholestasis in older children; histopathology shows paucity of intrahepatic bile ducts and cholestasis. Analyses of patients with cytogenetic deletions or rearrangements led to the identification of the JAG1 gene on chromosome 20 as the gene mutated or absent in this syndrome. JAG1 encodes a ligand for the Notch transmembrane receptor. This receptor, called Notch for the shape of the malformed wings of fruit flies with only one functional copy, plays a critical role during morphogenesis. The features of Alagille syndrome seem to develop due to the absence of adequate amounts of JAG1 protein during morphogenesis (so-called haploinsufficiency) rather then due to pertubations caused by a mutant protein.

Progressive familial intrahepatic cholestasis (PFIC) is a heterogeneous group of autosomal recessive liver disorders, characterized by early onset of cholestasis that usually progresses to cirrhosis and liver failure before adulthood. Currently, PFIC is divided in three subcategories: PFIC type 1, or Byler disease, is thought to be caused by defective bile salt secretion. Two loci for Byler disease have been found and mapped to chromosome 18q21-q22 and 2q24. The locus on chromosome 18 also maps the gene for benign recurrent intrahepatic cholestasis (BRIC), and it is possible that different mutations in a single gene lead to this variant of Byler disease and BRIC. A second type of PFIC is thought to be caused by defects in bile salt synthesis; multiple genetic loci may be responsible for this phenotype. Patients with this second type and patients with Byler disease have normal serum γ-glutamyltransferase levels. A third type of PFIC can be distinguished from the other two types by high serum γ-glutamyltransferase activity and liver histology showing portal inflammation and ductular proliferation at an early stage. The genetic defect is due to mutations in the multidrug resistance P-glycoprotein MDR3. This protein is responsible for biliary phospholipid excretion at he canalicular membrane of the hepatocyte as was shown by knockout of the mouse homolog MDR2. As patients with MDR3 mutations, the MDR2 knockout mice develop severe liver disease, characterized by inflammation of the portal tracts, proliferation of the bile ducts, and fibrosis.

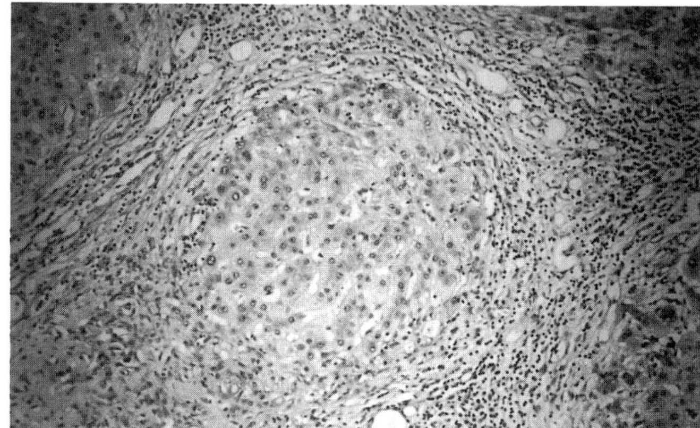

Figure 41-3 Histopathology of primary biliary cirrhosis. This liver specimen, obtained at the time of liver transplantation, shows end stage PBC. A regenerative nodule surrounded by inflammatory tissue and blood vessels can be detected; however, bile ducts and ductules are completely absent. (original magnification ×31.)

Primary Biliary Cirrhosis (PBC) is a liver disease occurring primarily in women and characterized by cholestasis as a result of destruction of septal and interlobular bile ducts (Fig. 41-3) resulting in jaundice and pruritus, hyperlipidemia, fat and fat-soluble vitamin malabsorption, and metabolic bone disease. The liver histology progresses over years to decades from lymphocytic portal infiltrates with bile duct destruction and ductular hyperplasia, to end-stage biliary cirrhosis with complete absence of septal and interlobular bile ducts. At this stage, the usual complications of cirrhosis develop: portal hypertension, variceal hemorrhages, ascites, spontaneous bacterial peritonitis, hepatic encephalopathy, and hepatorenal syndrome.

The molecular defect or abnormality responsible for development of PBC is not known, but an autoimmune basis seems most likely. This presumption is based on the presence of autoantibodies, a possible association with HLA-antigens, known association with other autoimmune diseases, a lymphocytic infiltrate in the early histopathology, and a partial response to a variety of immune-function modifying drugs. The major autoantibodies seen in PBC are directed against the E2 subunit of the mitochondrial pyruvate dehydrogenase enzyme complex and the E2 subunit of the branched chain 2-oxo-acid dehydrogenase complex. It is unclear whether these antibodies are simply a result of the disease process or whether they are actually involved in bile duct destruction. There is an increased frequency of HLA class II antigen DR8 in patients with PBC; how this antigen increases susceptibility to PBC remains unexplained. Exogenous factors also have been implicated; for instance, antibodies as well as T-cell clones derived from patients with PBC crossreact with exogenous antigens such as an *E. coli* pyruvate decarboxylate enzyme complex-E2 peptide.

This suggests that molecular mimicry (i.e., the recognition by the immune system of endogenous proteins with structural similarity to microbial-derived proteins) at the T cell clonal level may be a possible cause of PBC.

Totally effective medical treatment for PBC does not exist. A large number of immune-function modifying and anti-inflammatory drugs have been tried in randomized, controlled, and prospective studies. These drugs included prednisone, azathioprine, chlorambucil, D-penicillamine, cyclosporine, methotrexate, colchicine, and malotilate; none have substantially improved survival, symptoms, or biochemical parameters. However, use of ursodeoxycholic acid has been shown to improve liver tests as well as symptoms, and a recent meta-analysis suggests increased survival or time to liver transplantation; the mechanisms of this apparently beneficial effect are unknown. Finally, liver transplantation clearly has been shown to improve survival, with 1- and 5-year survivals reported as greater than 90 and 80%, respectively.

Unlike PBC, primary sclerosing cholangitis (PSC) is seen predominantly in men. Destruction of bile ducts also forms the basis of this disease, but the inflammatory process is much less pronounced when compared to PBC. Extensive fibrosis of the portal tracts, especially involving the bile ducts (periductal fibrosis), is a histologic hallmark. Unlike PBC, all bile ducts can be affected; that is, the disease can extend from the common bile duct (extrahepatic) to the smallest septal bile ducts (intrahepatic). Involvement of the larger ducts results in a very characteristic radiologic appearance: When the bile ducts are filled with contrast, multiple strictures and localized areas of ectasia are seen (Fig. 41-4). Over years to decades, PSC progresses and end-stage disease is associated with similar complications as discussed for PBC. However, three additional complications are frequently seen. First, stasis of bile in the biliary tree as a result of strictures can lead to intraductal stone formation as well as to development of recurrent infection of the biliary tree (i.e., bacterial cholangitis). Second, in approximately 10% of patients, transformation of bile duct epithelial cells into bile duct cancer occurs. Third, chronic ulcerative colitis, a disease associated with PSC in approximately 70% of cases (*see below*), predisposes to the development of colon cancer.

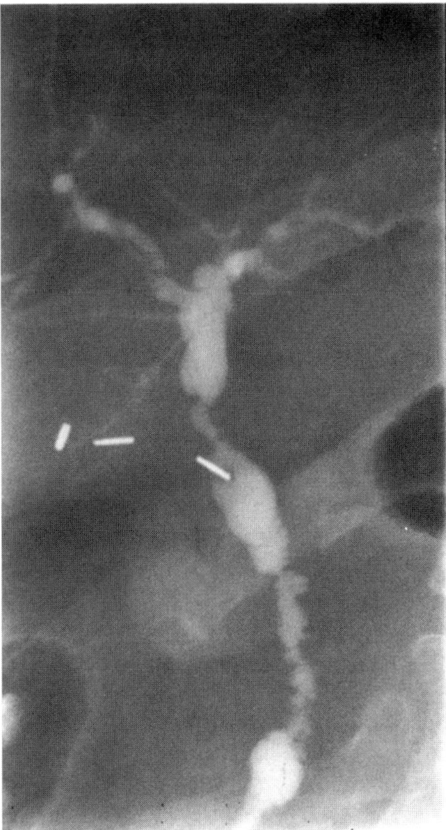

Figure 41-4 Cholangiogram of a patient with primary sclerosing cholangitis. This cholangiogram shows the typical features of primary sclerosing cholangitis: multiple strictures and dilatations throughout the intra- and extrahepatic bile ducts. Three metal clips were placed during cholecystectomy. (Source: LaRusso NF, Wiesner RH, Ludwig J, MacCarty RL. Primary sclerosing cholangitis. N Engl J Med 1984;310:899–903.)

PSC, like PBC, probably is an autoimmune disease. PSC is also associated with other autoimmune diseases, particularly with chronic ulcerative colitis. As mentioned above, this association is seen in approximately 70% of patients and supports the presumed autoimmune basis of the disease. However, antibodies specific for PSC have not been identified, and an obvious, strong association with a particular HLA class I or II phenotype is not seen. Weak associations have been reported for HLA class II DR3, DR8, and DR52 antigens.

All medical regimens tried thus far have been unsuccessful. At present, only liver transplantation offers patients with PSC significant improvement in survival as well as symptoms.

AUTOIMMUNE HEPATITIS

Autoimmune hepatitis can be defined as an idiopathic autoimmune disease in which the hepatocyte is the predominant target of immune-mediated destruction. It can occur at any age but tends to follow a bimodal age distribution (10–30 and above 50 years), most frequently in women. Symptoms and signs are nonspecific and include general malaise, lethargy, and fatigue. The disease is characterized by negative viral serologies, hypergammaglobulinemia, and a number of circulating autoantibodies. Liver histology shows active hepatitis with mononuclear infiltration of portal tracts and surrounding liver lobule (i.e., piecemeal necrosis). Frequently, plasma cells and eosinophils are seen within the infiltrate, in addition to a mixture of helper and suppressor lymphocytes. In general, the disease progresses to cirrhosis. However, treatment with corticosteroids, alone or in combination with azathioprine, markedly delays disease progression and ameliorates symptoms.

As for PBC and PSC, the pathobiology of autoimmune hepatitis is poorly understood. There is a strong linkage with the MHC class II antigens DR3 and DR4 on chromosome 6. In addition, autoimmune hepatitis is also associated with other autoimmune diseases, such as thyroiditis and Sjogren's syndrome. Based on the type of autoantibodies present, several subgroups can be identified. In type I autoimmune hepatitis, autoantibodies are directed against non–organ- and non–species-specific antigens (e.g., antinuclear and antismooth muscle antibodies). These antibodies are unlikely to be involved in the pathogenesis. Type II autoimmune hepatitis is characterized by antibodies against specific cytochrome P450 isoenzymes (anti–liver-kidney microsomal antibodies; putative target cytochrome P450 2D6), which may be expressed on the cell membrane of hepatocytes. Immunogenic cytochrome P450 also can be induced by drug metabolism and haptenation, which indicates that environmental or medicinal xenobiotics may initiate autoimmune liver disease. Finally, a type

III autoimmune hepatitis has been proposed based on the presence of antisoluble liver antigen antibodies.

Treatment goals are to decrease inflammation and prevent progression to cirrhosis. In general, immunosuppressant therapy is only used in symptomatic patients. As mentioned, the therapeutic efficacy of corticosteroids, with or without the addition of azathioprine, is well established. Survival with therapy is excellent. Once cirrhosis and its complications are present, only liver transplantation results in restoration of an acceptable quality of life.

POLYCYSTIC LIVER DISEASE

Simple hepatic cysts are detected in 2–5% of patients undergoing ultrasound examinations of the abdomen. Cysts are seen more frequently in older patients and women. In 60–75%, cysts are solitary and, in general, a maximum of three cysts are detected in patients with multiple lesions. Polycystic liver disease, therefore, should be considered in patients who are found to have four or more hepatic cysts. The most common cause of polycystic liver disease is autosomal dominant polycystic kidney disease (ADPKD). At least three genetic loci are known to predispose to the disease and are located, respectively, on chromosome 16 (ADPKD1), chromosome 4 (ADPKD2), and a still unmapped location (ADPKD3) (*see* Chapter 70). In 1994, the gene from ADPKD1 was cloned and, based on DNA sequence analysis, it codes for a large transmembrane protein called polycystin-1. The function of this protein remains to be determined; a role in cell–cell or cell–matrix interactions is hypothesized. Preliminary evidence suggests that this protein is expressed during fetal development. In normal adults, it is present at very low levels in kidney and biliary epithelial cells; however, its expression is significantly increased in the epithelia lining both kidney and liver cysts of patients with ADPKD1, suggesting that failure to downregulate polycystin expression may be the molecular defect leading to polycystic disease. Recently, the ADPKD2 gene also was cloned; it too seems to encode an integral membrane protein, named polycystin-2, which is ~50% homologous to polycystin-1 at the amino acid level. Polycystin-2 also shows homology to the family of voltage-activated calcium channels. In addition to ADPKD, development of renal as well as hepatic cysts can be a result of other genetic defects, such as autosomal recessive polycystic kidney disease, obstruction of ureter or common bile duct, or a variety of drugs. Finally, multiple families have been described with polycystic liver disease in the absence of significant renal cystic disease; whether these families have a genotype different from all the above-mentioned is unknown.

Liver cysts can range in size from microscopic to several inches in diameter and, therefore, the liver can be normal to massively enlarged (Fig. 41-5). Cysts usually are thin-walled, composed of a single layer of cuboidal epithelial cells, filled with fluid resembling the bile salt independent fraction of bile (i.e., approximate values for sodium, potassium, chloride, and bicarbonate of, respectively, 145, 4, 115, and 25 mEq/L). The cells lining cysts stain positively for biliary epithelial cell markers (i.e., cytokeratin 7 and 19) and secrete ions and water into the cyst in response to secretin, strongly supporting a biliary epithelial origin. Liver cysts are rare in children with ADPKD, but the frequency increases with age to approximately 70% in the seventh decade. Women are likely to have more and larger cysts at an earlier age than men, perhaps related to the use of estrogens and pregnancies. Most patients with polycystic liver disease do not have symptoms. If symptoms occur,

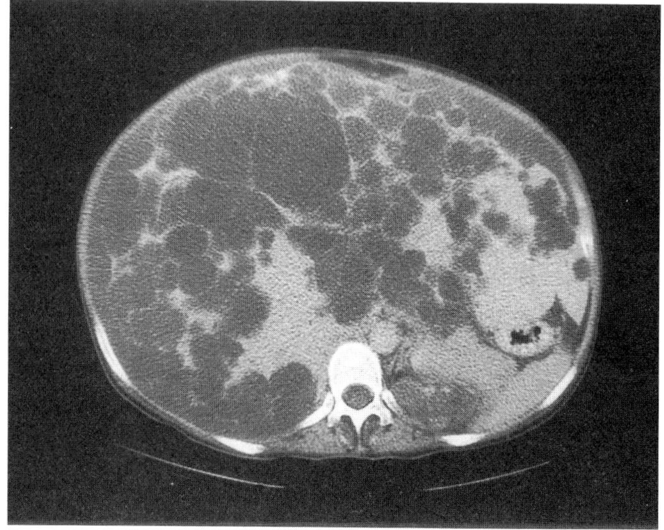

Figure 41-5 CT Scan of a patient with polycystic liver disease. Multiple, large hepatic cysts are present within the liver of this patient with ADPKD.

these reflect abdominal distension due to liver size, venous or biliary obstruction, hemorrhage into cysts, and torsion, rupture, or infection of cysts. Because the volume of the hepatic parenchyma remains normal, overall hepatic function is preserved.

The primary goal of treatment is to reduce the volume of the cysts; this can be established by avoidance of factors associated with cyst development or expansion, such as estrogens and possibly alcohol. Cyst aspiration followed by installation of a sclerosing agent (e.g., 95% alcohol or tetracycline) is used for patients with symptoms a result of one or a few dominant cysts. Finally, surgical fenestration or fenestration combined with cyst resection is performed in patients with advanced disease, whereas liver transplantation is used in the rare patient without liver segments free of cysts.

AMYLOIDOSIS

Amyloidosis is caused by deposition of amyloid substance in the extracellular matrix of various tissues. Frequently the liver is involved, although symptoms and signs because of liver involvement, predominantly hepatomegaly, are nonspecific and relatively infrequent. The amyloid substance is composed of fibrils, which are polymers of low molecular weight proteins in β-pleated sheet conformation. Systemic amyloidoses can be classified into four types as listed in Table 41-1. It is beyond the scope of this chapter to discuss all types in detail; instead, we will discuss the molecular basis of one of the best studied types of hereditary amyloidoses: familial amyloid polyneuropathy caused by point mutations in the transthyretin gene.

Transthyretin is the product of a single copy gene on chromosome 18. This gene has four exons that code for a 127 amino acid mature protein and an 18 amino acid signal peptide. The mature protein functions as a plasma transport protein for both thyroxine and retinol-binding protein. Most of the protein is synthesized in the liver; the remainder is synthesized in the choroid plexuses of the brain and eye. The structure of transthyretin is dominated by eight β strands, which contain approximately 50% of the amino acids and form two four-stranded β sheets. This extensive β-sheet

Table 41-1
Systemic Amyloidoses[a]

Type	*Protein*
Immunoglobulin (AL)/primary	Kappa or lambda light chains
Reactive (AA)/secondary	Serum amyloid A
Hereditary/familial amyloid polyneuropathies	Transthyretin (prealbumin)
	Apolipoprotein A-1
	Gelsolin
β2-microglobulin/dialysis	β2-microglobulin

[a]Source: Reilly MM, King RH. Familial amyloid polyneuropathy. Brain Pathol 1993;3:165–176.

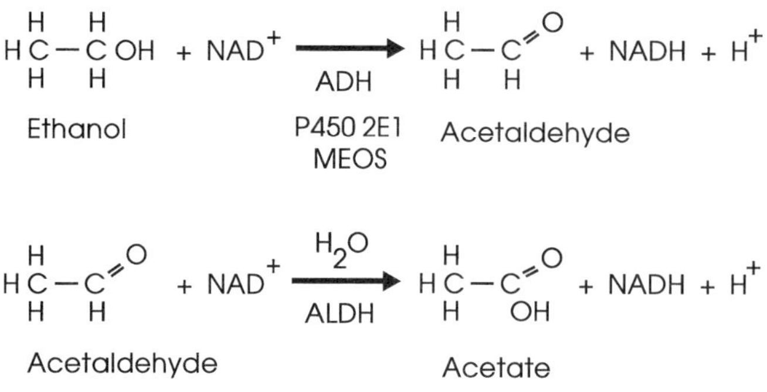

structure makes the transthyretin protein "amyloidogenic." All 30 (approximately) point mutations predisposing to development of neuropathy are located in exons 2, 3, and 4; the most frequent one is a valine to methionine point mutation at amino acid 30. At the genome level, the frequent occurrence of this mutation can be explained by a "CpG hot spot" (i.e., the dinucleotide sequence CpG is more frequently the target sequence of mutations than would be expected on a random basis). Two additional point mutations in exon 2, one mutation in exon 3, and at least three mutations in exon 4 can lead to either hyperthyroxinemia or cardiomyopathy.

Nearly all patients with a transthyretin mutation are heterozygotes; thus, both the normal as well as the mutated protein can be detected in blood. Because the liver is responsible for over 90% of transthyretin production, liver transplantation theoretically should correct the disease. Preliminary results after liver transplantation, performed in patients with familial amyloidosis polyneuropathy as a result of a point mutation converting the valine codon of amino acid 30 into a methionine codon, indeed show dramatic reductions in the abnormal transthyretin serum concentration and, in some cases, associated improvement in autonomic nervous system function.

ALCOHOL-INDUCED LIVER DISEASE

Alcoholic liver disease occurs only in a subset of individuals who consume large amounts of alcohol (10–20%); the precise reason for this is not understood, but a difference in alcohol-metabolizing enzymes caused by genetic differences is suspected to be responsible for the individual variation in the severity of liver disease among heavy drinkers. Alcohol is predominantly metabolized in the liver. Two enzyme systems are of key importance; the first one consists of alcohol dehydrogenase (ADH) and aldehyde dehydrogenase (ALDH) (Fig. 41-6). ADH converts alcohol into acetaidehyde, which in turn is converted to acetate by ALDH. The second enzyme system is the cytochrome P450 2El or microsomal ethanol oxidizing system (MEOS).

Acetaldehyde and increased production of reducing equivalents, such as NADH, are thought to be responsible for most of the hepatotoxicity of alcohol. At least seven different genomic loci are known to encode for over 20 different isoenzymes of ADH. All are expressed in liver and are thought to be derived from a common ancestral gene. They are grouped into five main classes based on the genetic and protein structure. Most are also expressed in other tissues such as the stomach, kidney, and lung. In women, the expression of ADH in the stomach is significantly lower than in men, and this, in part, may explain why women develop alcoholic hepatitis and subsequently progress to cirrhosis sooner, faster, and

$$\underset{\text{Ethanol}}{H_3C-CH_2OH} + NAD^+ \xrightarrow[\text{P450 2E1 / MEOS}]{\text{ADH}} \underset{\text{Acetaldehyde}}{H_3C-CHO} + NADH + H^+$$

$$\underset{\text{Acetaldehyde}}{H_3C-CHO} + NAD^+ \xrightarrow[\text{ALDH}]{H_2O} \underset{\text{Acetate}}{H_3C-COOH} + NADH + H^+$$

Figure 41-6 Metabolic pathway of alcohol. Two enzymes, alcohol dehydrogenase (ADH) and Aldehyde dehydrogenase (ALDH), are responsible for most of the alcohol metabolizing capacity within the liver. Both enzymes require the presence of NAD^+ to convert alcohol via the toxic intermediate product acetaldehyde into the nontoxic product acetate. The cytochrome P450 2El or microsomal ethanol oxidizing system (MEOS) pathway, in general, is not important with infrequent, low-dose alcohol use; however, it is markedly induced during chronic alcohol abuse.

after lower amounts of ethanol consumed than men. Two ALDHs are responsible for more than 90% of acetaldehyde metabolism: ALDH1 and ALDH2. Both are NAD^+-dependent; ALDH1 is cytosolic whereas ALDH2 is mitochondrial.

Many people with an Oriental background develop flushing after moderate alcohol use. This phenomenon is related to a decreased ALDH2 activity that results in relatively high acetaldehyde levels that, in turn, cause the flushing. This side effect of alcohol use may in part explain why alcohol abuse is less common in eastern Asia. Disulfiram is an inhibitor of ALDH; it produces rapid accumulation of acetaldehyde at levels 5–10 times higher than those found during metabolism of the same amount of alcohol alone. The unpleasant effects (flushing, headache, nausea, and vomiting) of high acetaldehyde concentrations caused by disulfiram, even after small amounts of alcohol, are used therapeutically in the treatment of alcoholism; it reminds motivated patients to abstain from alcohol.

Acetaldehyde is known to condense with plasma proteins, forming stable adducts that can be recognized as foreign by the immune system. A prevalence of severe hypersensitivity reactions of 0.54% was found among a large population of non-Oriental individuals. The reactions were severe enough to deter these individuals from consuming all types of alcoholic beverages. Individuals presenting such reactions had significantly elevated levels of circulating anti-acetaldehyde-protein IgE antibodies.

The exact mechanism whereby alcohol induces hepatitis and subsequently cirrhosis is not known. Cytokines and growth factors likely play a major role; interleukin-1, TNF-α, PDGF, EGF, and basic FGF all are known to stimulate Ito cell proliferation or enhance fibrogenesis. Other interleukins, in particular IL-6 and IL-8, also have been implicated in the pathogenesis of alcoholic liver disease. However, more research is needed to explain how alcohol induces production of these growth factors and cytokines.

DRUG-INDUCED LIVER DISEASES

Nearly every drug can cause liver injury, because the liver is the central organ in most drug metabolic pathways. Some drugs cause a predictable, dose-dependent injury, whereas use of others only results in hepatotoxicity in patients with a genetic predisposition.

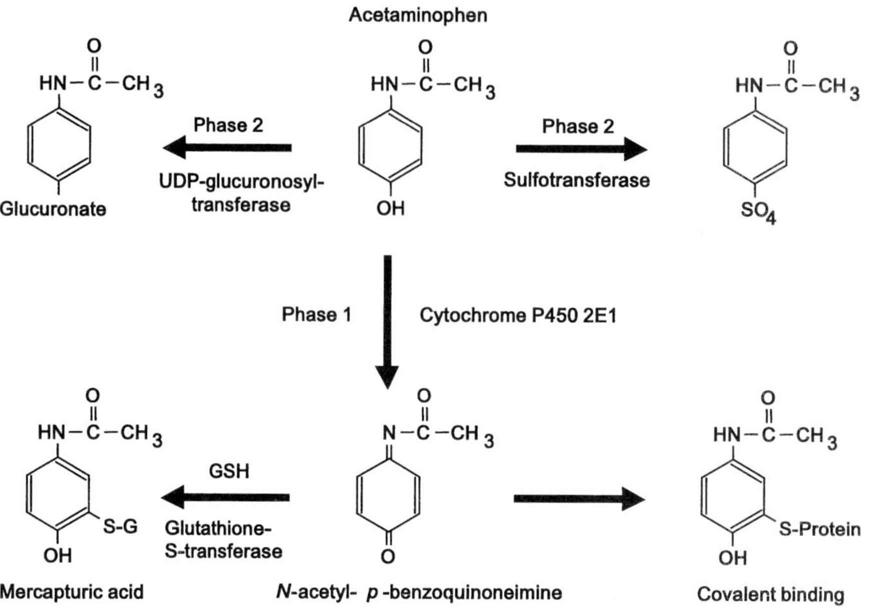

Figure 41-7 Metabolic pathway of acetaminophen. Under physiologic conditions acetaminophen is predominantly metabolized via phase 2 reactions (glucuronidation and sulfation). If the capacity of phase 2 reactions is exceeded, or if the cytochrome P450 complex is induced, increasingly phase 1 biotransformation occurs. In the presence of adequate amounts of reduced glutathione (GSH) the intermediate metabolite *N*-acetyl-*p*-benzoquinoneimine is converted into mercapturic acid; in the absence, covalent binding to cell proteins occurs. UDP, uridine diphosphate. (Adapted from: Lee WM. Drug-induced hepatotoxicity. N Engl J Med 1995;333:1118–1127.)

Two general mechanisms of injury are seen: first, direct disruption of the intracellular function or membrane integrity by the drug or its metabolites; and second, indirect damage from immune-mediated mechanisms.

Most drugs are hydrophobic compounds that require biochemical transformations for excretion, processes that transform the hydrophobic native drug into hydrophilic metabolites that are filtered by the glomerulus or excreted into bile. Biotransformation can be divided into two categories: phase 1 and phase 2 reactions. Phase 1 reactions include oxidation or demethylation and are mediated by the cytochrome P450 enzyme system. For instance, the result of a phase 1 reaction is generation of hydroxyl groups. In phase 2 reactions a large, water-soluble group is attached by glucuronidation or sulfation via ether or ester linkage to the phase 1 intermediate, such as an hydroxylated metabolite, or to the native drug. Enzymes involved in these reactions include the already discussed UDP-glucuronosyltransferases and several species of sulfotransferases. A third metabolic pathway for detoxifying many drugs involves a reduction reaction where an electrophilic compound is inactivated by glutathione-*S*-transferase–mediated glutathione coupling. Some drugs undergo all the processes (e.g., acetaminophen [Fig. 41-7]), others only one or two.

The most common reaction leading to hepatotoxicity is the formation of covalent bonds between a metabolite of the native drug and cell proteins or DNA. Another mechanism likely to lead to cell death is lipid peroxidation. As already mentioned, the toxic effect of a specific drug can directly be related to the dose used (e.g., acetaminophen) or to a genetic variant in the enzymes required for its metabolism (e.g., autosomal recessive deficiency for cytochrome P450 2D6, which is required for metabolism of drugs such as debrisoquin, propranolol, and quinidine). How covalent binding of substrate or lipid peroxidation causes cell death remains unknown.

A commonly used classification of drug reactions is based on three end points: the histologic appearance, the cell type involved, and the clinical picture. Table 41-2 lists examples of toxic reactions and the causative agents. Detailed information regarding individual drugs is readily available and will not be discussed. A few widely used drugs and recently reported drug reactions deserve attention, however.

Acetaminophen has already been mentioned. Its toxicity is enhanced by drugs, inducing the P450 system, such as barbiturates and alcohol, and by depletion of glutathione as seen in starvation and alcohol abuse (Fig. 41-8A). On the other hand, both cimetidine and *N*-acetylcysteine protect against acetaminophen toxicity, the former by inhibition of the P450 2E1 isoenzyme responsible for the conversion of acetaminophen into *N*-acetyl-*p*-benzoquinoneimine, and the latter by replenishing glutathione stores.

Reye's syndrome is defined as acute, noninflammatory encephalopathy in association with liver disease, without a clear explanation for both (Fig. 41-8B). Frequently, it follows a viral illness. Epidemiologic studies have shown a markedly increased risk for development of Reye's syndrome after exposure to aspirin. The molecular mechanisms of aspirin-induced liver injury are poorly understood, but seem to involve inhibition of normal mitochondrial enzyme functions. In patients with hepatitis B, treatment with the nucleoside analog, fialuridine, induced a severe toxic reaction, characterized by hepatic failure, lactic acidosis, pancreatitis, neuropathy, and myopathy. The clinical picture of hepatic failure and the hepatic histology resembled the fulminant hepatic steatosis that occurs with Reye's syndrome. Indeed, this toxic reaction also was a result of widespread mitochondrial damage. Similar toxic reactions may infrequently occur during treatment with other nucleoside analogs.

Finally, recent evidence suggests that bacterial toxins, such as the emetic toxin of Bacillus cereus, also can inhibit hepatic mitochondrial fatty acid oxidation and cause fulminant hepatic failure.

Table 41-2
Types of Toxic Reactions and Examples of Provoking Agents[a]

Type of reaction	*Examples of agents*
Direct reaction	Acetaminophen, carbontetrachloride, mushrooms, phosphorus
Idiosyncratic reaction	Isoniazid, disulfiram, propylthiouracil
Toxic-allergic reaction	Halothane, isoflurane, ticrynafen
Allergic hepatitis	Phenytoin, amoxicillin-clavulonic acid, sulfonamides
Cholestatic reaction	Chlorpromazine, erythromycin estolate, estradiol, captopril, sulfonamides
Granulomatous reaction	Diltiazem, quinidine, phenytoin, procainamide
Chronic hepatitis	Nitrofurantoin, methyldopa, isoniazid, trazodone
Alcoholic hepatitis-like syndrome	Amiodarone, perhexiline maleate, valproic acid
Microvesicular steatosis	Tetracyclines, aspirin, zidovudine, didanosine, fialuridine
Fibrosis or cirrhosis alone	Methotrexate, vitamin A, methyldopa
Veno-occlusive disease	Cyclophosphamide, other chemotherapeutic agents, herbal teas
Ischemic damage	Cocaine, sustained-release nicotinic acid, methylenedioxyamphetamine

[a]Source: WM Lee. Drug-induced hepatotoxicity. N Engl J Med 1995;333:1118–1127.

Nonsteroidal anti-inflammatory drugs (NSAIDS), frequently used anti-inflammatory, and analgesic agents are commonly implicated as causes of liver injury. One of the better studied drugs is diclofenac (Fig. 41-8C). In rare cases, it is associated with the development of fulminant hepatic necrosis. Both direct toxic effects of a diclofenac metabolite and hypersensitivity reactions have been suggested as possible molecular mechanisms of liver injury. In vitro experiments have shown that direct hepatocyte toxicity is increased with inhibition of the glucuronidation pathway and decreased by inhibition of cytochrome P450-dependent oxidative biotransformation. On the other hand, the covalent binding to hepatocellular proteins is greatly reduced when glucuronide formation was selectively blocked. Therefore, diclofenac acyl glucuronide formation is likely associated with covalent binding of a reactive metabolite to hepatocellular proteins, which may be toxicologically relevant for the expression of diclofenac hepatitis.

SUMMARY

We now understand a growing number of the molecular mechanisms responsible for the signs and symptoms, the biochemical abnormalities, and the histopathology of many inherited as well as acquired liver diseases. At present, we are beginning to understand the regulation of gene transcription and translation within the various individual cell types of the liver. Among possible advances, this has resulted in the development of new classes of pharmacological agents and in the possibility of hepatocyte gene transfer. Although much has been learned, even more remains unknown: What are the molecular signals that determine overall liver size and induce the unique phenomenon of liver regeneration to its original size after drug- or virus-induced necrosis or surgical partial hepatectomy? How do different cell types within the liver communicate with each other? Why are genes transfected into

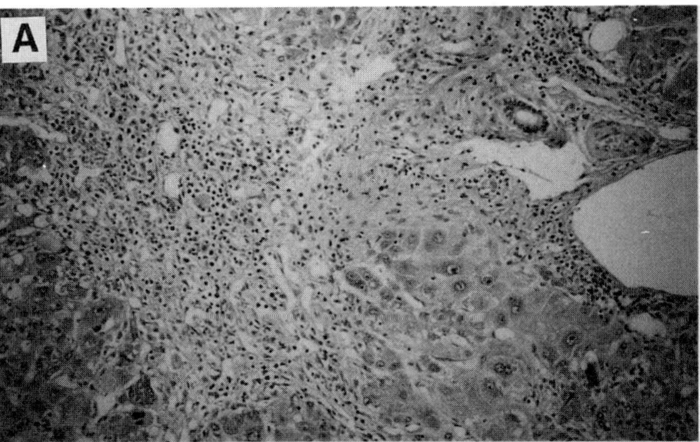

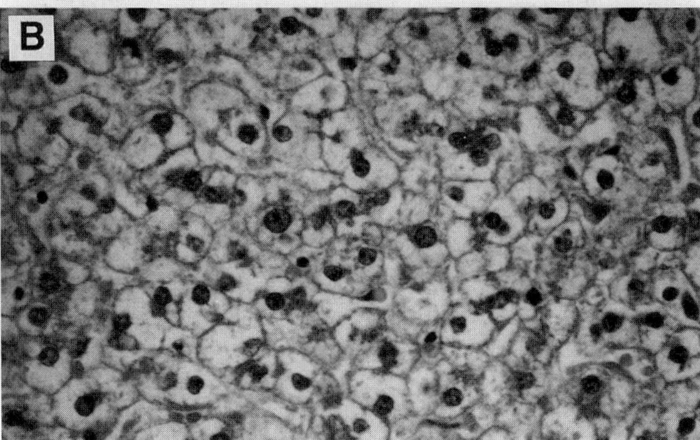

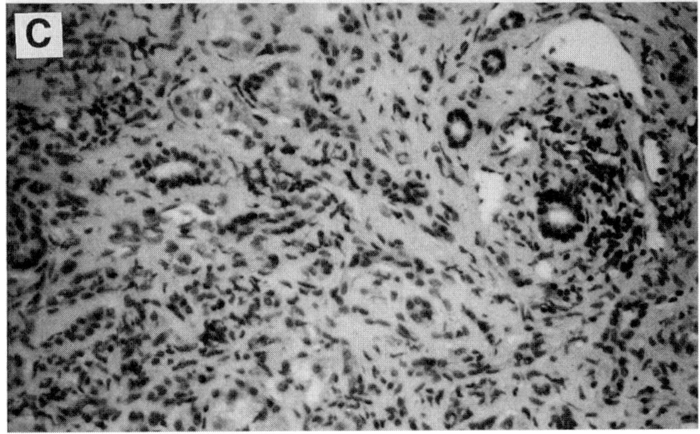

Figure 41-8 Histopathology of drug-induced liver disease. Liver histopathology of acetaminophen-, aspirin-, and diclofenac-hepatotoxicity. **(A)** Shows liver specimen with severe necrosis around the central veins (CV, zone 3 of the hepatic lobule) as the result of an acetaminophen overdose. The hepatic parenchyma around a large portal tract (PT, zone 1 of the hepatic lobule), showing a portal vein branch, an hepatic artery, and a bile duct, is well-preserved. **(B)** Shows the liver parenchyma of a patient with Reye's syndrome after aspirin use. Within the hepatocytes there are abundant fat droplets; the fat has been dissolved and therefore the cells appear white in this illustration. **(C)** The liver specimen is from a patient who had received diclofenac for arthritis. While on the drug, she developed jaundice and therefore diclofenac was discontinued with resolution of symptoms. However, several months later, diclofenac was restarted with recurrence of jaundice. Only a few hepatocytes are seen in the part of the specimen shown in this picture (arrows). The close proximity of several bile ducts and the extensive inflammatory reaction suggest massive destruction of hepatocytes with collapse of the fibrous septa: submassive necrosis. The marked ductular proliferation is evidence of hepatic regeneration. (original magnifications: [A] ×31, [B] ×125, [C] ×62.

hepatocytes only transiently expressed in vivo? Clearly, the answers to many of these important questions will, in part, depend on further molecular studies of the diverse cell types forming the liver.

SELECTED REFERENCES

HEPATOLOGY IN GENERAL

Oxford Textbook of Clinical Hepatology. McIntyre N, Benhamou J-P, Bircher J, Rizzefto M, Rodes J, eds. Oxford: Oxford Medical Publ., 1992.

Sherlock S, Dooley J. Diseases of the Liver and Biliary System. 9th ed. London: Blackwell Scientific Publ., 1993.

Tung BY, Kowdley KV. Inherited liver diseases affecting the adult. Gastroenterologist 1996;4:245–261.

Zakim D, Boyer TD. Hepatology, a Textbook of Liver Disease. 2nd ed. Philadelphia, PA: WB Saunders Company, 1990.

LIVER SPECIFIC GENE EXPRESSION

Lai E, Darnell JE, Jr. Transcriptional control in hepatocytes: a window on development. TIBS 1991;16:427–430.

FIBROSIS AND CIRRHOSIS

Friedman SL. The cellular basis of hepatic fibrosis. Mechanisms and treatment strategies. N Engl J Med 1993;328:1828–1835.

Gressner AM. Activation of proteoglycan synthesis in injured liver—a brief review of molecular and cellular aspects. Eur J Clin Chem Clin Biochem 1994;32:225–237.

CHOLESTATIC LIVER DISEASES

Alpini G, Phillips JO, LaRusso NF. The biology of biliary epithelia. In: Arias IM, Boyer JL, Fausto N, Jakoby WB, Schachter DA, Shafritz DA, eds. The Liver: Biology and Pathobiology, 3rd ed. Eds., New York: Raven, 1994; pp. 623–654.

Bosma PJ, Chowdhury JR, Bakker C, Gantla S, de Boer A, Oostra BA, et al. The genetic basis of the reduced expression of bilirubin UDP-glucuronosyltransferase 1 in Gilbert's syndrome. N Engl J Med 1995;333:1171–1175.

Ciotti M, Obaray R, Martin MG, Owens IS. Genetic defects at the UGT1 locus associated with Crigler-Najjar type I disease, including a prenatal diagnosis. Am J Med Genet 1997;68:173–178.

de Vree JML, Jacquemin E, Sturm E, Cresteil D, Bosma PJ, Aten J, Deleuze J-F, Desrochers M, Burdelski M, Bernard O, Oude Elferink RPJ, Hadchouel M. Mutations in the MDR3 gene cause progressive familial intrahepatic cholestasis. Proc Natl Acad Sci USA 1998; 95:282–287.

Green RM, Gollan JL. Crigler-Najjar disease type I: therapeutic approaches to genetic liver diseases into the next century. Gastroenterology 1997;112:649–651.

Kaplan MM. Toward better treatment of primary sclerosing cholangitis. N Engl J Med 1997;336:719–721.

Lee YM, Kaplan MM. Primary sclerosing cholangitis. N Engl J Med 1995;332:924–933.

Leung PS, Chuang DT, Wynn RM, et al. Autoantibodies to BCOADC-E2 in patients with primary biliary cirrhosis recognize a conformational epitope. Hepatology 1995;22:505–513.

Li L, Krantz ID, Deng Y, Genin A, Banta AB, Collins CC, Qi M, Trask BJ, Kuo WL, Cochran J, Costa T, Pierpont ME, Rand EB, Piccoli DA, Hood L, Spinner NB. Alagille syndrome is caused by mutations in human Jagged1, which encodes a ligand for Notch1. Nature Genetics 1997;16:243–251.

Oda T, Elkahloun AG, Pike BL, Okajima K, Krantz ID, Genin A, Piccoli DA, Meltzer PS, Spinner NB, Collins FS, Chandrasekharappa SC. Mutations in the human Jagged1 gene are responsible for Alagille syndrome. Nature Genetics 1997;16:235–242.

Paulusma CC, Kool M, Bosma PJ, Scheffer GL, ter Borg F, Scheper RJ, Tytgat GN, Borst P, Baas F, Oude Elferink RP. A mutation in the human canalicular multispecific organic anion transporter gene causes the Dubin-Johnson syndrome. Hepatology 1997;25:1539–1542.

Sato H, Adachi Y, Koiwai O. The genetic basis of Gilbert's syndrome. Lancet 1996;347:557–558.

AUTOIMMUNE HEPATITIS

Czaja AJ, Carpenter HA, Santrach PJ, Moore SB. Genetic predispositions for the immunological features of chronic active hepatitis. Hepatology 1993;18:816–822.

AMYLOIDOSIS

Gertz MA, Kyle RA. Amyloidosis: prognosis and treatment. Seminars in Arthritis & Rheumatism 1994;24:124–138.

Reilly MM, King RH. Familial amyloid polyneuropathy. Brain Pathol 1993;3:165–176.

POLYCYSTIC LIVER DISEASE

Torres VE. Polycystic liver disease. In: Watson ML, Torres VE, eds. Polycystic Kidney Disease. Oxford: Oxford University Press, 1996; pp. 498–527.

Mochizuki T, Wu G, Hayashi T, Xenophontos SL, Veldhuisen B, Saris JJ, Reynolds DM, Cai Y, Gabow PA, Pierides A, Kimberling WJ, Breuning MH, Deltas CC, Peters DJ, Somlo S. PKD2, a gene for polycystic kidney disease that encodes an integral membrane protein. Science 1996;272:1339–1342.

ALCOHOL- AND DRUG-INDUCED LIVER DISEASES

Arnon R, Esposti SD, Zern MA. Molecular biological aspects of alcohol-induced liver disease. Alcohol Clin Exp Res 1995;19:247–256.

Lee WM. Drug-induced hepatotoxicity. N Engl J Med 1995;333: 1118–1127.

Lieber CS. Medical disorders of alcoholism. N Engl J Med 1995; 333:1058–1065.

Mahler H, Pasi A, Kramer JM, Schulte P, Scoging AC, Bar W, Krahenbuhl S. Fulminant liver failure in association with the emetic toxin of Bacillus cereus. N Engl J Med 1997;336:1142–1148.

Makin AJ, Wendon J, Williams R. A 7-year experience with severe acetaminophen-induced hepatotoxicity (1987–1993). Gastroenterology 1995;109:1907–1916.

Mehendale HM, Roth RA, Gandolfi AJ, Klaunig JE, Lemasters JJ, Curtis LR. Novel mechanisms in chemically induced hepatotoxicity. FASEB J 1994;8:1285–1295.

McKenzie R, Fried MW, Sallie R, Conjeevaram H, Di Besceglie AM, Park Y et al. Hepatic failure and lactic acidosis due to fialuridine (FIAU), an investigational nucleoside analogue for chronic hepatitis B. N Engl J Med 1995;333:1099–1105.

42 Inherited Liver Disease

JUAN RUIZ AND GEORGE Y. WU

INTRODUCTION

The liver is a major site of metabolism in humans, playing a central role in the metabolism of carbohydrate, protein, lipid, trace elements, and vitamins. In addition, detoxification and biliary excretion of various endogenous and exogenous compounds, especially lipophilic molecules, including most common drugs, and the degradation and elimination of a variety of hormones and hormonal metabolites, are distinct hepatic characteristics. Because of its involvement in so many metabolic pathways, it is not surprising that many inherited diseases of the liver are manifested as inborn errors of metabolism. Disease occurs as a result of lack of the required gene product or accumulation of a toxic metabolite.

Molecular defects responsible for these disorders can be classified as single basepair substitutions, insertions, or deletions, and are exemplified in Fig. 42-1.

ABNORMAL METAL METABOLISM

WILSON DISEASE Wilson disease (hepatolenticular degeneration) was described in 1912 by Kinnear-Wilson. The disease results from a disturbance in hepatic copper metabolism characterized by an inability to secrete copper into bile resulting in hepatic accumulation, progressive liver damage and, after hepatic overflow, accumulation in the brain and other organs. In addition, there is a defect in the incorporation of copper into ceruloplasmin.

Copper is an important metal cofactor present in several enzymes (superoxide dismutase, tyrosinase, lysyl oxidase, dopamine-β-hydroxylase, peptide α-amidating enzyme, cytochrome oxidase, and ceruloplasmin). Although essential, only trace quantities are required and larger amounts are toxic. The normal body content is 70–100 mg and depends on the balance between intestinal absorption and biliary excretion (1–5 mg daily). The liver plays a major role in copper metabolism by the uptake of the recently absorbed metal that is excreted into bile and also incorporated into ceruloplasmin.

Clinical Manifestations (Table 42-1) The disease has a worldwide prevalence of about 1–30,000 (1:200 for the gene) without ethnic preferences. There is a broad organ involvement. Approximately 40% of patients present with hepatic features, followed by neurological (34%) and endocrine, hematological (10%), or neuropsychiatric (12%). Hepatic manifestations tend to appear earlier than those of neurological origin (6–12 years for the hepatic presentation vs 12 years or more for the neurological forms) and will be present always, irrespective of the initial presentation, if adequate treatment is not implemented. There may be a chronic insidious presentation, sometimes punctuated by transient icteric episodes or an acute onset with hemolysis and hepatic or renal failure as a result of an acute release of free nonceruloplasmin bound copper from the liver. Neuropsychiatric symptoms appear later than the hepatic manifestations and are associated with the presence of Kayser-Fleischer rings, which are a manifestation of copper deposition in the Descemet's membrane. There is a strong correlation between the presence of Kayser-Fleischer rings in Wilson disease and copper deposition in the brain. Although the intellect is preserved, there may be a slow deterioration of the personality. Renal changes are related to copper deposition in tubular cells resulting in amino aciduria, glucosuria, uricosuria, hyperphosphaturia, hypercalciuria, renal tubular acidosis, and stone formation.

Diagnosis It is most important to consider Wilson disease in the differential diagnosis of chronic liver disease in children and young adults and whenever liver disease is associated with neurological symptoms.

Important parameters are:

1. Serum ceruloplasmin <20 mg/dL.
2. Hepatic copper concentration >250 μg/g dry weight.
3. Urinary copper excretion >100 μg/d.

Diagnosis can be made by showing either parameter 1 and the presence of Kayser-Fleischer rings or both parameters 1 and 2. However, 50% of patients without neurological symptoms do not have Kayser-Fleischer rings at presentation, and 5–10% of patients have ceruloplasmin levels in the lower normal range. In those patients, the most important determination is liver copper content. If further discrimination is required, orally administered radiocopper (^{67}Cu) incorporation into ceruloplasmin can be used. An absence of an increase in ^{67}Cu serum levels after 24–48 h is diagnostically helpful.

Linkage analysis using specific DNA markers can be applied to siblings. However, because of genetic heterogeneity, it is not useful for screening of potential heterozygotes in the general population. Confirmation in siblings should be sought by measuring serum copper, ceruloplasmin, and urinary copper.

Genetic Basis of the Disease Wilson disease has an autosomal recessive inheritance. The gene (ATP7B), recently identified by positional cloning and the use of the closely related Menke's

From: *Principles of Molecular Medicine* (J. L. Jameson, ed.), ©1998 Humana Press Inc., Totowa, NJ.

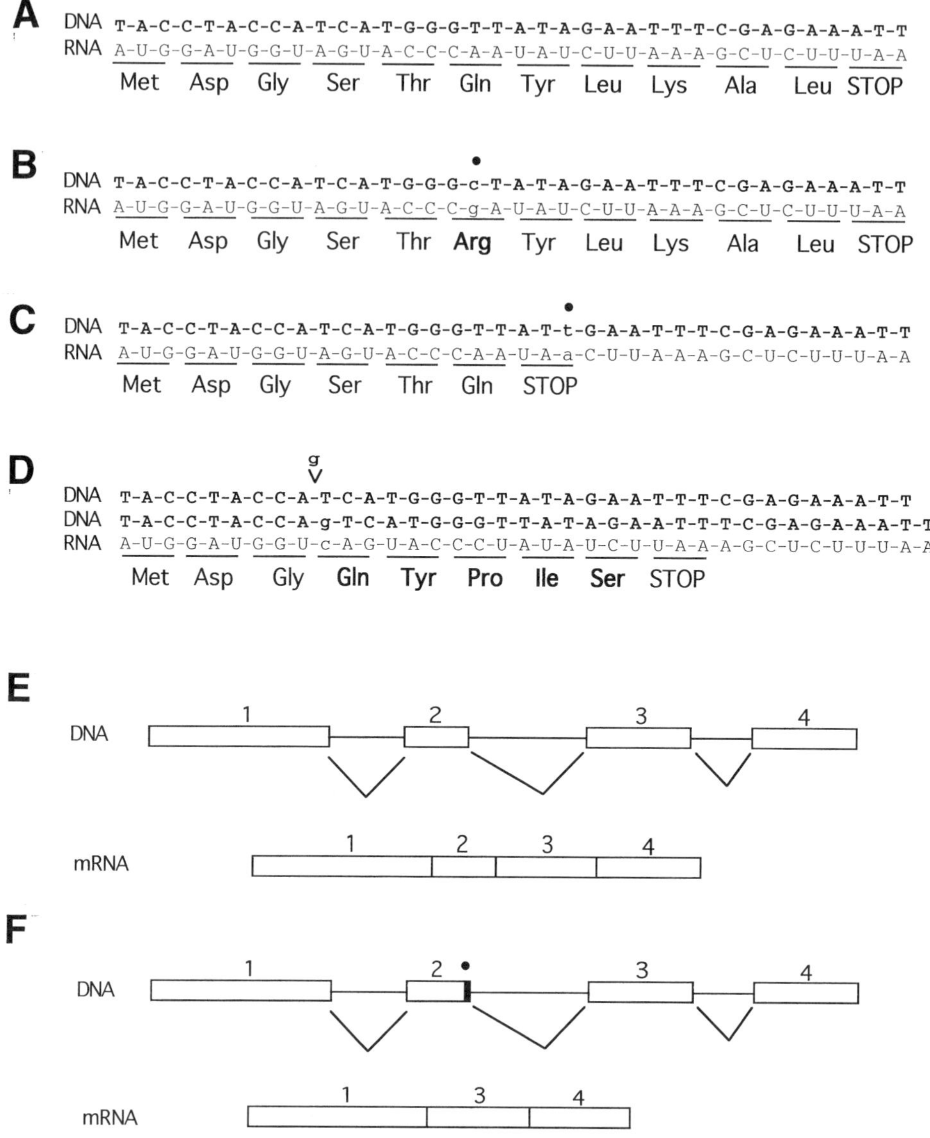

Figure 42-1 Different gene defects and its consequences. **(A)** Normal gene, messenger RNA, and encoded polypeptide. **(B)** Missense mutation leading to a single amino acid substitution: The results can be either a different isoform of the molecule (when the affected amino acid is not functionally essential) or a significant functional alteration of the product. **(C)** Missense mutation resulting in a premature stop codon and termination of the polypeptide: the final product is a truncated protein that has abnormal function or no function at all. **(D)** Insertion of a nucleotide producing a frameshift (modification of the amino acid sequence downstream from the mutation) and a premature stop codon (truncation of the polypeptide): The result is complete abolition of the protein activity (null phenotype). The same effect is produced by nucleotide deletions. **(E)** Scheme of the structure of a gene with the exons (boxes) and introns (lines). After transcription and splicing of the introns, the mRNA is produced. **(F)** Effects of mutations on the splice acceptor or donor sequences: Substitutions in exon/intron splice sites can result in improperly spliced message and abnormal gene product containing intronic sequences or missing exonic elements. In this case, exon 2 is removed from the mature mRNA. The black dot indicates the nucleotide mutation.

disease gene as a probe, is located on chromosome 13. It contains 23 exons and a 4.3-kb region that codes for a membrane-bound cation-transporting P-type adenosine triphosphatase. The family of P-type ATPases also includes the Menke's Disease gene and several related bacterial and yeast genes. There is a 56% identity with the gene for Menke's disease (ATP7A), an X-linked disorder characterized by a defective intestinal absorption of dietary copper. The identity is even higher (75–100%) at the amino acid level of functionally important domains. ATP7B is expressed mainly in the liver, kidney, and placenta. There is alternative splicing for some exons in the liver and the brain. The alternative isoforms may have some functional significance, and the differential splicing may help regulate the amount of functional protein produced.

The genetic defects in Wilson disease are heterogeneous. Using single-strand conformation polymorphism (SSCP) to identify the mutations, followed by sequencing, more than 30 different mutations have been described to date. Genotype analysis has revealed insertions and deletions causing frameshifts, stop codons (nonsense), altered splicing, and missense mutations. In particular, nucleotide substitutions have been described in the phosphorylation consensus sequence and in the hinge region of the ATP-binding site. Unlike Menke's disease, where 20% of patients have

Table 42-1
Clinical Features of Wilson Disease

Hepatic	Acute hepatitis, fulminant hepatitis, chronic hepatitis, liver cirrhosis
Neurological	Akinesia, rigidity, muscle spasms, dystonia, dysarthria, dysphagia, resting and intention tremor, epilepsy, encephalopathy, peripheral neuropathy
Psychiatric	Cognitive impairment, behavioral changes, psychosis, affective disorders
Gastrointestinal	Cholelithiasis, pancreatitis
Ophthalmological	Kayser-Fleischer rings, sunflower cataracts
Hematological	Hemolysis (acute, chronic), coagulopathy, intravascular coagulation, hypersplenism
Renal	Renal tubular dysfunction, nephrolithiasis
Musculoskeletal	Osteoporosis, osteomalacia, osteoarthropathy
Cardiovascular	Cardiomyopathy, arrhythmias
Endocrine	Amenorrhea, miscarriages

large gene deletions, no large deletions have been found. Most patients studied are compound heterozygotes, having two different allelic mutations, a result of the large number of mutations.

Molecular Pathophysiology of Disease It has been shown that copper transport across membranes is an ATP-dependent process. The P-type adenosine triphosphatase involved in Wilson disease contains several domains: six copper binding, nine transmembrane, transduction, channel, phosphorylation, phosphatase, and adenosine triphosphate-binding regions. A decrease in the number of active molecules or a decrease in its activity causes a defect in the secretion of copper into the bile because of a deficiency in the activity of the transporter system. The precise intracellular localization of the transport defect has not yet been elucidated. In addition, a reduction in the incorporation of copper into apo-ceruloplasmin to generate holo-ceruloplasmin, possibly a result of the same genetic defect, causes the accumulation of the metal in the hepatocytes. Damage in tissues where copper has accumulated is probably secondary to membrane lipid peroxidation, glutathione depletion, and polymerization of copper-thionein, resulting in abnormal function of the mitochondria, lysosomes, microtubules, and nuclear DNA.

Wilson disease is an excellent example of a metabolic disease caused by a single gene defect, with a correlation between genotype and phenotype based on the different defects in the mutated protein, e.g., domain modifications or complete absence of gene product. Specific types of mutations may predict the severity of the disease. For example, those mutations that destroy the function of the gene, stop codons truncating the protein or insertions, or deletions causing frameshifts, appear to correlate with an earlier onset of the disease, in one study approximately 7.2 years of age. Interestingly, the same study shows that in those mutations causing modifications in specific domains without affecting the whole molecule (missense mutations), the average age of onset of symptoms is higher, 16.8 years. In fact, some authors suggest than if the genetic defect is so substantial, e.g., large deletions leading to a null phenotype, the result would be a very early onset of the disease that could be misdiagnosed as some cases of Indian Childhood Cirrhosis. Another important phenomenon is that of mutations affecting regions of the gene where a possible alternative splicing can occur. The removal of the mutation in some tissues would mitigate its deleterious effects and lead to a later onset of the disease. As an example, a severely detrimental mutation, 2010del7, located in exon 6, causing a frameshift, results in a later onset, neurological form of Wilson disease by an alternative splicing that removes the deletion.

Ceruloplasmin carries 80% of the copper present in plasma and its function, although not well-understood, can be related to its ferroxidase, amine oxide, and antioxidant properties. The importance of the ferroxidase activity of ceruloplasmin is underlined by the deposition of iron and subsequent damage in the liver, pancreas, retina, and brain in patients with severe ceruloplasmin deficiency. Most patients with Wilson disease show a decrease in serum ceruloplasmin levels that correlate with the clinical manifestations of the disease. However, this decrease is not universal and no pathophysiological correlation has been established. Ceruloplasmin is synthesized in the liver in an inactive form, apo-ceruloplasmin, and is transformed to the active form, holo-ceruloplasmin, by the incorporation of up to six to seven atoms of copper per molecule. Both forms are different antigenically and holo-ceruloplasmin is the form usually detected in plasma in normal subjects. Normal amounts of ceruloplasmin in liver tissue from patients with Wilson Disease, normal ceruloplasmin RNA levels in Long Evans Cinnamon (LEC) rats, an animal model of Wilson Disease, together with the exclusive presence of apo-ceruloplasmin in serum, suggest a posttranslational defect in the incorporation of copper into ceruloplasmin rather than a defect in the ceruloplasmin gene itself.

Management and Treatment Treatment is aimed at reducing the amount of copper in the body and to prevent the toxic effects of free copper in the tissues. *D*-penicillamine (1–2 g/d divided in two doses) is the most common treatment and must be given lifelong. *D*-penicillamine chelates copper, permitting urinary excretion. Additionally, it has detoxifying activity on intracellular copper. In some cases, neurological symptoms may worsen at the beginning of the treatment as copper is released from the liver. In cases of adverse effects to *D*-penicillamine, an alternative agent is trientine, another copper chelator. Other possible agents include tetrathiomolybdate, a chelator that is possibly more effective for neurologic disturbances, and zinc, which decreases intestinal copper absorption and stimulates metallothionein production, which in turn binds copper. Urinary copper determinations are used to monitor the treatment.

Liver transplantation is the treatment of choice for patients with irreversible liver disease or fulminant hepatitis. Its role in cases of neurologic disease without hepatic insufficiency is not clear.

Future Directions LEC rats possess a genetic defect characterized by a deletion of at least 900 bp at the 3' end of the rat-homologous Wilson gene. No mRNA is detected in the liver or other tissues by Northern blots. The same clinical and biochemical features characteristic of Wilson disease have been demonstrated: excessive hepatic copper accumulation, defective holo-ceruloplasmin biosynthesis, and impaired biliary copper excretion. Gene therapy could be a potential option as a curative treatment of Wilson disease in the future and its feasibility can be tested in LEC rats.

HEMOCHROMATOSIS The term hemochromatosis was first used by von Recklinghausen in 1889. The disease is caused by an inappropriately high intestinal absorption of iron that first accumulates in the parenchymal cells of the liver and later in other organs. Unlike most inborn errors of metabolism, the basic defect in hereditary hemochromatosis is not located primarily in the liver. However, its clinical manifestations are largely the result of liver disease and dysfunction.

Iron is absorbed both as heme and nonheme forms (ferrous salt) by the intestinal mucosa. Once inside the enterocyte, it is coupled to transferrin and transported to tissues. Cells having transferrin receptors internalize the protein, and iron is released into the cytoplasm to be incorporated to heme and apoproteins. Because of its high toxicity, excess iron is stored in the body as ferritin or hemosiderin. Iron absorption is a poorly understood but extremely important process, because there is no physiological mechanism for excretion of excess iron. Absorption is responsible for regulation of normal iron balance. Losses because of shedding of mucosal cells along the gastrointestinal and genitourinary tracts and skin desquamation are relatively constant around 1 mg/d, and are compensated by a 10% absorption of the 10–20 mg of iron present in an average diet. Deregulation of the absorption in the presence of fixed losses lead to a constant increase in body iron stores (up to 40 g) with subsequent cell damage.

Clinical Manifestations (Table 42-2) Although all races are affected, hemochromatosis is most common among Caucasoids of Celtic origin, with a prevalence of 1:300–400 and a carrier rate of 1:20. The disease is characterized by a latent period for many years while the iron stores increase in liver. This latent period depends greatly on the dietary iron intake as well as physiologic and pathologic blood loss. This explains the 9-to-1 ratio between affected men and women.

The clinical picture is that of a multisystemic disease. Liver disease has mostly a benign and prolonged course with cirrhosis and liver failure present as late features. However, hepatocellular carcinoma can be the first manifestation of the disease. Hyperpigmentation of the skin is the result of an increase in melanin in the cells of the basal layer. Deposition of iron in the pancreas, heart, pituitary, and joints result in diabetes mellitus, cardiomegaly, arrythmias, heart failure, hypogonadism, hypoparathyroidism, hypothyroidism, chondrocalcinosis, demineralization, and chronic arthropathy.

Diagnosis The introduction of routine serum iron studies for asymptomatic individuals as well as the use of HLA markers in families of affected individuals have improved the rate of early diagnosis and the time of diagnosis before the development of significant disease. This is important because treatment can restore life expectancy to normal if irreversible organ damage, e.g., cirrhosis, has not occurred. Diagnosis is made by serum iron studies, the most important being the transferrin saturation index. An index below 50% excludes the diagnosis, while one above 70% is suggestive of hemochromatosis. Serum ferritin concentration >200 µg/L in asymptomatic homozygotes and >900 µg/L in symptomatic patients is helpful. A high serum iron concentration >30 µmol/L alone is less specific. Confirmation of the diagnosis is made by liver biopsy, the definitive laboratory test, that shows increased iron deposition in hepatocytes (at the periportal areas in early stages) with paucity of iron elsewhere. This is in contrast to secondary iron accumulation in reticuloendothelial cells. Measurement of hepatic iron content allows the quantification of iron in the liver and the calculation of the hepatic iron index (tissue iron in mmol/g liver dry weight/age [years]). The index helps discriminate homozygotes, having indices >1.9, from heterozygotes and individuals with other iron-loading diseases with indices <1.5. Heterozygotes do not develop the disease, even though some may have elevated serum iron and saturations.

All blood relatives of an identified homozygote patient should be investigated. In addition to biochemical studies, HLA haplotyping and other DNA markers, such as microsatellites, have been used until now in order to determine whether any relatives share all four haplotypes of the index patient (homozygotes), half (heterozygotes), or none.

The recent discovery of a candidate gene and the identification of a single mutation present in 83–100% of patients will help in the development of more accurate genetic tests both for diagnosis and population screening.

Genetic Basis of the Disease Hereditary hemochromatosis is an autosomal recessive disease. Numerous studies had previously mapped the hemochromatosis gene to chromosome 6p, closely linked to the HLA-A locus. Recently, a candidate gene responsible for the disease, originally designated HLA-H, has been identified and named HFE. Eighty-three percent of 178 hemochromatotic patients were homozygous for the same missense mutation. Eight out of nine who were heterozygous for this mutation were observed to have a different missense mutation on the other allele. The mutations identified are: (1) a G-to-A transition at nucleotide 845 results in a cysteine-to-tyrosine substitution at amino acid 282 (C282Y). This mutation is homozygous in 83, 91, or 100% of hemochromatosis patients according to different studies. The same mutations are only present in heterozygosity in 5–6% of controls. (2) A second mutation, a C-to G-change that results in a histidine-to-aspartic acid substitution at amino acid 63 (H63D), has also been observed, although at a frequency similar to that of the control population (17–21%).

Before the HFE gene identification, several candidate genes, such as transferrin, transferrin receptor, ferritin or iron-regulating factor, had already been excluded because of their location in chromosomes other than 6p. Tumor necrosis factor-α (TNF-α) gene is located at chromosome 6p, close to the HLA cluster, and had also been implicated because it downregulates iron absorption and its production is decreased in stimulated monocytes of patients with hemochromatosis. However, the TNF-α gene locus does not

Table 42-2
Clinical Features of Hereditary Hemochromatosis

Features	*Percentage*
Weakness and lethargy	100
Hepatomegaly	95
Pigmentation (skin and mucosa)	90
Diabetes mellitus	60
Hypogonadotrophic hypogonadism	50
Splenomegaly	50
Loss body hair, dermal atrophy	50
Anorexia, malaise	45
Confusion, weight loss, vomiting	45
Chronic arthropathy	30
Hepatocellular carcinoma	30
Abdominal pain	30
Cardiomegaly, cardiomyopathy	20
Vertigo, peripheral neuropathy	15
Jaundice	10

coincide with possible sites proposed for the HLA, linked iron-loading gene.

Molecular Pathophysiology of Disease The HFE gene encodes a protein with a strong similarity to MHC class I molecules (HLA-A2) and nonclassical class-I–like molecules (HLA-G and the Fc receptor). The gene comprises seven exons encompassing 12 kb and encodes a 343-amino acid protein. Based on the significant similarity to MHC class I proteins, which are membrane proteins, it was predicted to have three characteristic extracellular domains or loops, a transmembrane domain, and a short cytoplasmic region. The C283Y mutation eliminates a cysteine residue, thus disrupting a disulfide bridge. As a result, the conformation of the α3 domain of the molecule is altered, preventing noncovalent binding to β2-microglobulin. Because the transferrin receptors have also been demonstrated to interact with the β2-microglobulin-HFE protein complex, failure of HFE to bind the complex to the cell surface may prevent normal downregulation of iron transport. Data derived from β2-microglobulin knockout mice support a role for nonclassical class I genes in the control of iron metabolism. β2-Microglobulin-deficient animals develop hepatic iron overload resembling that of hereditary hemochromatosis, and the defect has been related to a failure to limit the transfer of iron from the mucosal cells into the plasma.

Iron can be a very toxic element. Damage in the affected organ is related to:

1. Membrane lipid peroxidation associated with impairment of membrane-dependent functions of mitochondria (oxidative metabolism and calcium sequestration), lysosomes (fluidity, membrane integrity, and pH), microsomes (enzyme activities and calcium sequestration), and cell surface (cellular integrity).
2. Fibrosis resulting from iron-mediated stimulation of collagen synthesis through its action as a cofactor for proline and lysine hydroxylase in collagen synthesis. It appears that Kupffer cells are induced to release cytokines by lipid peroxidation products released from hepatocytes. These cytokines activate stellate cells, resulting in alteration of the extracellular matrix in liver.

Management and Treatment Standard treatment for hereditary hemochromatosis consists of periodic phlebotomies of 500-mL once or twice weekly. One 500-mL unit of blood contains 200–250 mg iron, allowing removal of up to 25 g in a period of 2 years. Gradual decrease in body iron stores is monitored by serum ferritin levels. Plasma transferrin saturation does not change until available iron stores are depleted. Once transferrin saturation is less than 50% and ferritin levels are less than 50 µg/L, phlebotomies can be spaced, usually every 2–4 months. Chelating agents such as desferoxamine are used only when anemia or hypoproteinemia prevents phlebotomy.

Liver transplantation carries a higher mortality in patients with hereditary hemochromatosis, probably because of complications of late pretransplant diagnosis and treatment.

Future Directions Studies on the HLA-H gene and its defects will clarify the complex mechanisms of iron absorption and distribution. Molecular screening tests will be available to identify affected patients and carriers bearing the C282Y mutation. In addition, earlier diagnosis will help prevent the development of the disease.

Table 42-3
Hepatic Manifestations in Alpha-1-antitrypsin Deficiency

Infancy	*Early childhood*	*Adulthood*
Neonatal cholestasis	Hypertransaminasemia	Chronic hepatitis
Prolonged jaundice	Hepatomegaly	Cirrhosis
Hepatomegaly	Cirrhosis	Hepatoma
Splenomegaly		

OTHER RELATIVELY COMMON GENETIC LIVER DISEASES

ALPHA-1-ANTITRYPSIN DEFICIENCY AND LIVER DISEASE

(For a general description of the disease, *see* Chapter 38.) Alpha-1-antitrypsin was isolated in 1955 by Schultze et al. and first associated with liver disease in 1968 by Freier et al. in two brothers with cirrhosis. It is the most important circulating protease inhibitor, and its deficit results in pulmonary emphysema. Liver damage occurs in 10–15% of patients.

Alpha-1-antitrypsin is produced mostly in hepatocytes, but also in other cell types, particularly monocytes and macrophages of the alveoli. Its main function is to neutralize neutrophile elastase. In addition, it represents 90% of the total trypsin inhibitor capacity and inhibits chymotrypsin, plasmin, thrombin, tissue kallikrein, factor Xa, collagenase, renin, and urokinase.

Clinical Manifestations (Table 42-3) Alpha-1-antitrypsin deficiency (PiZZ) affects 1:1600–1800 births in North American and Northern European populations. Development of pulmonary emphysema is the most important clinical manifestation. Neonatal cholestasis is the most frequent hepatic disturbance, present in 10% of PiZZ subjects, and although it usually resolves, it may progress to juvenile cirrhosis, especially in cases of prolonged cholestatic jaundice. Liver disease may also be first diagnosed in late childhood or early adolescence because of the appearance of cirrhosis and its complications. There is an increased risk of cirrhosis and hepatoma in adult life in PiZZ males over the age of 50.

Diagnosis Alpha-1-antitrypsin deficiency should be suspected in patients with emphysema, jaundice in infancy, and chronic liver disease in childhood or adult life. Concentration of alpha-1-antitrypsin in plasma is determined either by functional assays, such as evaluation of trypsin or elastase inhibition, or by immunochemical methods. Although serum concentrations of alpha-1-antitrypsin are decreased to 10–15% of normal values in PiZZ and to a 50% in *PiSS* or *PiMZ*, results can be misleading whenever there is an inflammatory process, because alpha-1-antitrypsin is an acute phase reactant.

Definitive diagnosis is based on alpha-1-antitrypsin phenotype determination of the abnormal protein by isoelectric focusing or agarose electrophoresis at acid pH or by genomic DNA analysis by polymerase chain reaction followed by oligonucleotide probe hybridization.

Liver histology shows periodic acid-Schiff-positive, diastase-resistant globules into hepatocytes, caused by the aggregation of deficient alpha-1-antitrypsin in the rough endoplasmic reticulum. These inclusion bodies may not be present in patients younger than 3 months.

Genetic Basis of the Disease Alpha-1-antitrypsin deficiency has a codominant inheritance pattern. The gene, located in chromosome 14, was identified by linkage studies using markers of the gamma immunoglobulins. It is 12.2 kb in length and contains seven exons. Messenger RNA transcripts from the liver lack the first two exons (1A and 1B) and differ from those of monocytes and macrophages that contain the whole coding sequence (although the first two exons and the 5' region of the third exon remain untranslated in these cell types).

To date, more than 75 different variants of the gene have been identified. They are classified into normal allelic variants, resulting from single mutations that do not modify serum levels or antiprotease activity; deficient variants, representing mutations in important nucleotide-amino acids that lead to decreased serum levels or altered function; and null alleles resulting from insertions or deletions that result in no detectable alpha-1-antitrypsin in serum. Variants were named according to their mobility in acid starch gel electrophoresis: F (fast), M (medium), S (slow), and Z (the most cathodal) and, when more variants with similar mobility were identified, birthplace names were used. PiM is the most common normal allele, present in 89% of the population, and PiZ (Glu 342-Lys) the most frequent deficient variant. Other deficient variants are PiS, PiMMALTON, PiSIIYAMA, or PiMDUARTE. Some variants involve more than one mutation.

Molecular Pathophysiology of Disease Alpha-1-antitrypsin is the most abundant circulating proteinase inhibitor and is the prototypic member of the serine proteinase inhibitor (serpin) superfamily. These proteins have a globular shape and are composed of α-helices and β-pleated A sheets. The reactive centers are situated on a mobile α-helix peptide loop. On interaction with the protease, there is cleavage at the reactive site and a structural rearrangement of the molecule with insertion of the reactive loop into a gap in the β-pleated A sheet molecule. That insertion can also occur with sites on other alpha-1-antitrypsin molecules, leading to polymerization (loop-sheet polymerization). The Z mutation leads to a single amino acid substitution: the negatively charged glutamic acid at position 342 is substituted by a positively charged lysine residue. As a result, the mobility and conformation of the loop changes, leading to a misfolding of the molecule. It also allows the reactive loop to interact spontaneously with the β-sheet of an adjacent molecule. This interaction involves several molecules, leading to the polymerization and aggregation of the molecules within the endoplasmic reticulum of hepatocytes. These aggregates appear as the periodic acid-Schiff-positive, diastase-resistant globules dilating the rough endoplasmic reticulum of hepatocytes in liver biopsies. The polymerization phenomenon is an equilibrium process, and there are some monomeric proteins that are released from the cell, accounting for the 12–15% of Z antitrypsin present in the plasma of patients. Although these monomers retain 85% of the wild-type protein antielastase activity, the number of molecules is not sufficient to protect the lungs against the proteolytic attack by neutrophile elastase that leads to emphysema. However, liver damage is not caused by a deficiency in antiprotease activity, but by accumulation of alpha-1-antitrypsin aggregates in the hepatocytes, resulting in enhanced lysosomal activity within the cell. Supporting this concept are observations in transgenic mice carrying human Z alpha-1-antitrypsin and normal endogenous mouse antiprotease activity. In spite of the presence of normal mouse antiprotease, the mice developed liver injury with PAS-positive globules. Another observation that supports the hypothesis is the fact that patients with a null genotype, who lack the protein altogether, have a more severe pulmonary disease, but do not develop liver disease.

Polymerization and aggregation of alpha-1-antitrypsin have also been observed with other variants like the PiSIIYAMA (Ser 53 to Phe) and the PiMMALTON (Phe 52 deleted). PAS-positive globules and liver disease have been reported in some of these patients.

The aggregation hypothesis for the mechanism of liver injury does not explain why only 10–15% of PIZZ patients develop liver disease. Therefore, it appears that both inherited traits and environmental factors seem to be involved. It has been shown that PiZ homozygous patients that develop liver disease have a delay in the degradation of the accumulated mutant alpha-1-antitrypsin protein in the rough endoplasmic reticulum compared with carriers of the mutation that do not develop liver damage. Other possible explanations include an excessive production of the protein in response to different stimuli or an special sensitivity to the accumulation of the protein. Environmental factors may predispose some individuals to liver disease by upregulating the synthesis of alpha-1-antitrypsin as an acute phase reactant.

An increased prevalence of PiMZ heterozygotes in adult patients with cirrhosis or chronic hepatitis, and the liver disease associated with phenotypes other than PiZZ, has been reported. However, these may represent coincidental findings as other etiologies for the liver disease have been identified.

Management and Treatment There is no specific treatment for liver disease associated with alpha-1-antitrypsin deficiency other than that of the complications of cirrhosis and liver transplantation for the decompensated disease. Plasma-derived or synthetic alpha-1-antitrypsin used for the treatment of lung disease are not effective in preventing liver damage. In fact, they can worsen the evolution of the disease because of the upregulation of alpha-1-antitrypsin synthesis by the interaction of alpha-1-antitrypsin–protease complex and the serpin-enzyme complex (SEC) receptor. Other situations likely to upregulate the synthesis of alpha-1-antitrypsin as an acute phase reactant (infections, inflammatory processes) have to be avoided or promptly corrected. Liver transplantation for end-stage liver disease is the only option.

Future Directions Therapeutics directed toward reducing the retention of the mutant protein in the rough endoplasmic reticulum through the use of synthetic peptides is one of several future therapeutic strategies. These decoy molecules mimic the binding domain of alpha-1-antitrypsin responsible for intracellular retention in the rough endoplasmic reticulum. This strategy could not only prevent the intracellular accumulation of alpha-1-antitrypsin, but also provide the delivery of functionally active protein to extracellular fluid and tissues.

Finally, null phenotypes pose a different challenge because even if alpha-1-antitrypsin could be provided, an immune response against the protein is likely to occur. Transgenic mice carrying the PiZ variant of the alpha-1-antitrypsin deficiency provide a convenient model for testing novel therapeutic agents.

CYSTIC FIBROSIS AND LIVER DISEASE (For a general description of the disease, *see* Chapter 37.) Cystic fibrosis is a common lethal genetic disorder affecting 1 in 2000 live births among Caucasians, with liver and biliary tract disease as frequent complications. The gene for the cystic fibrosis transmembrane conductance regulator (CFTR) encodes a protein that acts as a chloride channel. In addition, it probably has other functions, including the regulation of other channel proteins. There is an intracellular CFTR fraction, on endosomal membranes, that probably participates in the control of the level of intravesicular acidification, an important step in the protein secretory pathway and receptor-mediated endocytosis. The chloride channel is located in

Table 42-4
Hepatobiliary Manifestations of Cystic Fibrosis

Liver	*Biliary tract*
Neonatal cholestasis	Cholelithiasis
Fatty liver	Gallbladder hypoplasia
Hepatosplenomegaly	Common bile duct stenosis
Portal hypertension	Intrahepatic bile duct stenosis
Decompensated cirrhosis	

the liver at the apical membrane of epithelial cells lining the intrahepatic bile ducts. This makes cystic fibrosis the only inherited metabolic disease of the liver in which the primary abnormality is in biliary cells rather than hepatocytes.

Clinical Manifestations (Table 42-4) Liver disease in cystic fibrosis affects 25–30% of patients. It may appear as neonatal cholestasis, fatty change, or progress to biliary cirrhosis when the pulmonary and pancreatic diseases have been present for a long time. Hepatomegaly is the most significant liver feature. Although some authors suggest that liver disease increases with age expectancy, it seems that there is a peak at adolescence and it does not increase after 18 years.

Diagnosis Criteria for diagnosis include any one of the major clinical features (typical pulmonary and/or gastrointestinal manifestations) or history of cystic fibrosis in the immediate family plus a sweat chloride concentration >60 meq/L. Demonstration of pathologic CFTR mutations on both chromosomes is also sufficient to make the diagnosis.

Genetic Basis of the Disease The CFTR gene is assigned to the long arm of chromosome 7, spans 230 kb, and contains at least 27 exons. The mRNA is approximately 6.5 kb long and encodes a protein that contains 12 membrane-spanning domains, two nucleotide (ATP)-binding domains (NBDs), and a regulatory (R) domain that contains consensus sites for phosphorylation by protein kinases. Mutations are well-characterized and a total of more than 300 have been described. The most common (68% of patients) consists of a 3-bp deletion of codon 508 (phenylalanine) in the first NBD (ΔF508). All the other mutations account for less than 5% each, and only 13 different mutations affect more than 1% of the patients. The effect of different mutations includes:

1. Failure to synthesize a full-length protein (splice-site abnormalities, frameshifts, and nonsense mutation-stop codons) leading to a null phenotype.
2. Defective protein processing that leads to improper folding of the molecule and incomplete intracellular transport and glycosylation (fails to traffic to the Golgi). The isolated protein seems to be capable of functioning as a Cl^- channel, but the problem is that it is not present at the apical membrane. This is the mechanism involved in the prevalent ΔF508 mutation and probably most mutations.
3. The protein gets to the membrane, but its function is not regulated (missense mutations).
4. The protein gets to the membrane but its function is slightly altered in the pore size or the opening time. Null mutations and those impairing the intracellular traffic of the protein to the membrane are associated with the more severe phenotypes.

Molecular Pathophysiology of Disease The alteration in the CFTR protein in the liver produces an increase in the bile acid concentration as a result of a decrease in the sodium and water secretion that parallels that of chloride. There is also an impaired mucin secretion that disrupts the protective mucous layer coating the ducts. Finally, the increased fecal loss of taurine-conjugated bile acids increases the proportion of glycoconjugates that, being more hydrophobic than tauroconjugates, are potentially hepatotoxic. The combination of an abnormally concentrated bile containing an excess of hydrophobic bile acids, a lack of mucus protection produces a fibrosing cholangiopathy characterized by multiple constrictions and/or dilatations of the extrahepatic biliary tree. The intrahepatic bile duct lesion causes portal fibrosis and portal hypertension with secondary hepatocyte dysfunction.

It is important to note that liver involvement is not predicted by genotype or severity of lung disease, and only 25% of patients develop liver disease. Possible explanations include individual genetic factors involving other susceptibility genes, HLA A2-B7-DR2-DRw6, the evidence for the latter being the strongest.

Management and Treatment Ursodeoxycholic acid has recently been introduced as a possible therapeutic and preventive agent. The beneficial effects are derived from its choleretic and cytoprotective properties, and it has been shown to improve liver function tests and the hydrophobic/hydrophilic balance of the bile acid pool. Further studies are needed to establish any improvements in histology or prognosis. Liver transplantation has successfully been used for advanced disease without significant respiratory complications.

Future Prospects Introduction of DNases, and novel mucin-clearing agents are undergoing trials. Early gene therapy trials have been disappointing in general. However, much progress in eliminating the immune-mediated disappearance of virally introduced genes is being made.

THE PORPHYRIAS The porphyrias are inherited and acquired disorders caused by enzyme abnormalities in the heme biosynthetic pathway (Fig. 42-2). The liver accounts for 15% of the heme synthesized in the body, utilized for the formation of cytochromes and catalases. The remaining 85% is synthesized in the bone marrow. Partial enzymatic activity of any of the eight enzymes involved in heme synthesis results in excessive accumulation and excretion of porphyrins and their precursors, the porphyrinogens. However, only a small percentage of carriers of the gene defect develop clinical symptoms of the diseases. Thus, additional factors are required to express the phenotype. As a result, the porphyrias represent a complex paradigm for the interaction between genetic and environmental factors that can lead to the clinical manifestation of a disease.

The clinical picture is characterized by a combination of neurological symptoms resulting from toxicity from accumulation of δ-aminolevulinic acid (ALA) and porphobilinogen (PBG), and decreased heme availability; photocutaneous lesions caused by accumulation of porphyrins in the skin that, under UV light stimulation, produce cell damage followed by autolysis and inflammation; or liver damage. Significant liver disease is only present in porphyria cutanea tarda and a subgroup of erythropoietic porphyrias patients. Although classified as erythropoietic, this subgroup can be considered erythrohepatic.

Most porphyrias are inherited in an autosomal dominant pattern, except for δ-aminolevulinic acid dehydratase porphyria, congenital erythropoietic porphyria and some forms of erythropoietic protoporphyria. Patients are heterozygotes for the defect and show a 50% decrease in the activity of the deficient enzymes. The excep-

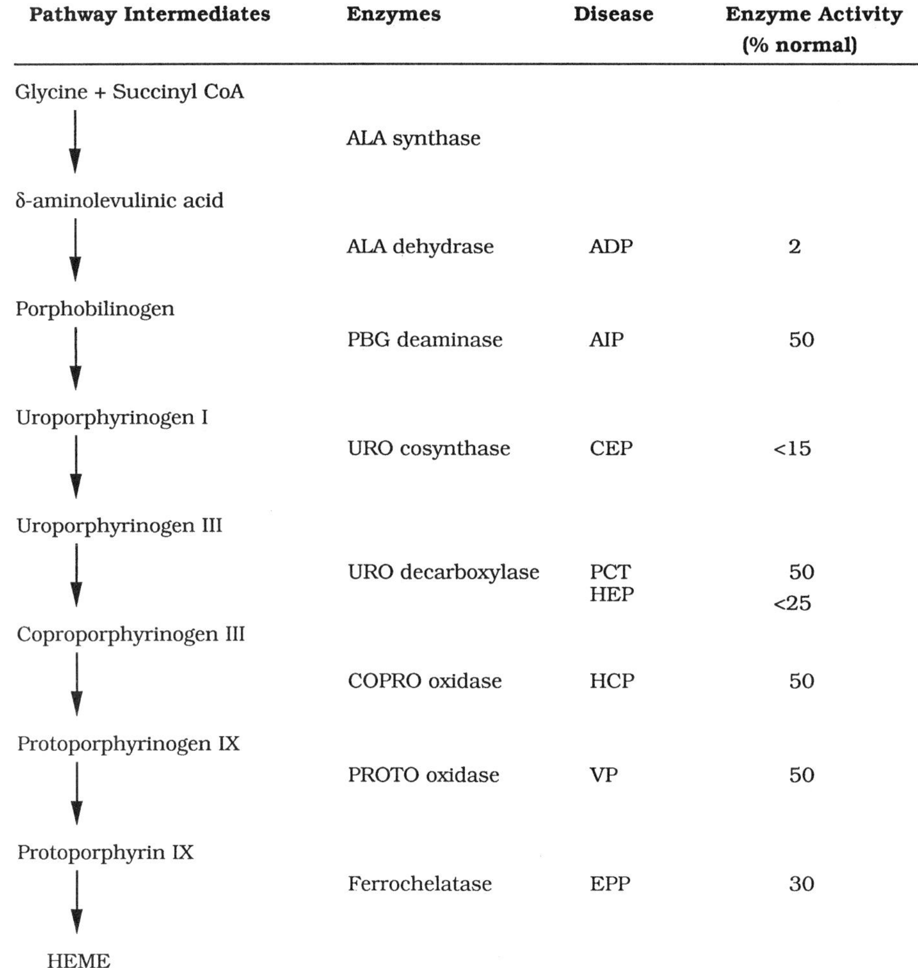

Pathway Intermediates	Enzymes	Disease	Enzyme Activity (% normal)
Glycine + Succinyl CoA			
↓	ALA synthase		
δ-aminolevulinic acid			
↓	ALA dehydrase	ADP	2
Porphobilinogen			
↓	PBG deaminase	AIP	50
Uroporphyrinogen I			
↓	URO cosynthase	CEP	<15
Uroporphyrinogen III			
↓	URO decarboxylase	PCT HEP	50 <25
Coproporphyrinogen III			
↓	COPRO oxidase	HCP	50
Protoporphyrinogen IX			
↓	PROTO oxidase	VP	50
Protoporphyrin IX			
↓	Ferrochelatase	EPP	30
HEME			

Figure 42-2 Enzyme deficiencies of porphyrias ALA, δ-aminolevulinic acid; PBG, porphobilinogen; ADP, ALA dehydratase porphyria; PCT, porphyria cutanea tarda; HEP, hepatoerythropoietic porphyria; EPP, erythropoietic protoporphyria.

tion is hepatoerythropoietic porphyria that is the homozygous form of the defect present in porphyria cutanea tarda (deficit of uroporphyrinogen decarboxylase) and shows a 90–95% reduction in the enzyme activity.

Several environmental factors leading to the clinical manifestation of the disease act through stimulation of the first enzyme in the pathway, the δ-aminolevulinic acid synthase (ALA synthase). This enzyme condenses succinyl CoA and glycine in the mitochondria to form ALA. There are two tissue-specific isozymes encoded by two different genes: the housekeeping ALA synthase gene (ALAS-N or ALAS1, expressed in all tissues, including the liver, assigned to chromosome 3) and the erythroid-specific ALA synthase enzyme (ALAS-E or ALAS2, expressed exclusively in erythroid cells, have been localized to chromosome X). Regulation of the synthesis and activity of the ALAS1 in the liver constitutes the rate-limiting step for the heme synthesis in that organ. The reduction in heme production because of the decrease in activity of any enzyme of the pathway upregulates ALA synthase in an attempt to increase heme synthesis. A new equilibrium is achieved with normal synthesis of heme at the cost of accumulation of more toxic porphyrins and porphyrinogens. In addition, ALAS1 is induced by a large amount of drugs, chemicals, and endogenous compounds, including various steroid metabolites. This step is not rate-limiting in erythroid cells, and ALAS2 is not inducible by compounds that induce the hepatic enzyme. ALAS2 mRNA translation is regulated by iron levels through the interaction of iron-regulatory factor with an iron-responsive element at the 5' untranslated region of the RNA, a characteristic similar to ferritin and transferrin regulation. Patterns of expression of the genes can vary between the liver and the bone marrow, with some of the genes having specific transcripts only present in the erythroid cells. This has led to the classification of porphyrias as hepatic or erythropoietic, according to the principal site of the expression of the enzymatic abnormality.

Acute Intermittent Porphyria (AIP) Hepatic porphyria is caused by a defect of porphobilinogen deaminase that results in increased levels of ALA and PBG in plasma and urine.

Clinical Manifestations Typically, the disease is more frequent in women after puberty and is characterized by acute attacks of abdominal pain, vomiting, constipation, and sometimes psychiatric manifestations, such as anxiety, depression, confusion, or delirium. Motor neuropathy, including muscle weakness or respiratory impairment, is common. There is no cutaneous photosensitivity.

Diagnosis Acute attacks are associated with increased urinary excretion of PBG and, to a lesser extent, ALA. However, levels can be normal in the quiescent phase of the disease. Definite diagnosis includes determination of PBG deaminase activity in erythrocytes and DNA analysis. Gene studies are complicated because of the heterogeneous nature of the genetic defects. Several systems can be used, including denaturing gel electrophoresis when the defect is not known. Relatives to the index case have to be investigated for the defect in order to avoid precipitating factors.

Genetic Basis of the Disease The disease is transmitted as an autosomal dominant trait. The gene responsible for AIP has been mapped to chromosome 11 and contains 15 exons. The use of two separate tissue-specific promoters and alternative splicing produce two different transcripts: nonerythropoietic transcripts contain 52 bp more than the erythropoietic forms, leading to the incorporation of 17 extra amino acids at the amino-terminus of the protein.

Gene defects in AIP are characterized by great heterogeneity, but three groups can be distinguished: the "crossreactive immunological material" negative form (type I) that represents 85% of all patients and is produced by mutations leading to stop codons, frameshifts, or altered splicing whose consequence is a 50% reduction in immunoreactive protein with a parallel 50% decrease in enzyme activity. The type II (<5% patients) is characterized by normal porphobilinogen deaminase activity in the erythroid cells and a 50% reduction in hepatic activity, caused by mutations in exon 1 in the nonerythroid portion of the gene. The "crossreactive immunological material" positive type III (15% patients) is a result of mutations that severely impair the enzyme activity. Only a few mutations related with this phenotype have been described.

Molecular Pathophysiology of Disease The genetic defect itself is not sufficient for the development of the disease, and 90% of the carriers remain asymptomatic throughout life. Factors that increase the synthesis of porphyrins can induce the appearance of clinical symptoms, including hormones, drugs, alcohol, nutritional factors, and so on, that stimulate ALA synthase.

Management and Treatment Treatment is aimed at avoiding precipitating factors. Glucose and hematin infusion are the standard treatments.

Hereditary Coproporphyria (HCP) and Variegate Porphyria (VP) These are also hepatic acute porphyrias, caused by defects in coproporphyrinogen oxidase in hereditary coproporphyria, and protoporphyrinogen oxidase in variegate porphyria. Clinically, they are indistinguishable from acute intermittent porphyria except for the presence of cutaneous photosensitivity in 30% of hereditary coproporphyria and 45–80% of variegate porphyria patients. The gene for coprophyrinogen oxidase has been mapped to chromosome 9 and is now under investigation. The gene responsible for protoporphyrinogen oxidase has not yet been identified. Interestingly, there is a small group of patients in both diseases who are homozygous for the defect. Clinically they are characterized by an early onset of the disease and lifelong photosensitivity.

The diagnosis is similar to AIP but, in addition to PBG and ALA detection in urine, there is increased fecal excretion of coproporphyrin in HCP and protoporphyrin in VP. The most important test is the demonstration of normal PBG erythrocyte activity.

Porphyria Cutanea Tarda (PCT) The most common porphyria, PCT, represents an heterogeneous group of diseases caused by defects in the activity of uroporphyrinogen decarboxylase. These defects can be acquired (sporadic PCT or type I and toxic form) or inherited (familial PCT, types II and III). Inheritance adopts an autosomal dominant pattern.

Clinical Manifestations Clinically, the disease is characterized by bullous cutaneous lesions on the light-exposed areas of the skin. Patients with the familial type of the disease have an early onset compared with sporadic cases. Liver disease is a common feature with the development of cirrhosis and, in some patients, hepatocellular carcinoma. The sporadic PCT (type I) affects more often adults (40–50 years) and is precipitated by alcohol consumption, estrogens, and iron. It has been reported associated with many types of liver disease and, recently, a strong association with hepatitis C infection has been described in Spain and Italy.

Diagnosis The diagnosis is based on the clinical symptoms and confirmed by determination of uroporphyrin and coproporphyrin in plasma, urine, and feces. Uroporphyrin > coproporphyrin in urine is highly indicative of PCT. Gene studies are only useful in type II PCT.

Genetic Basis of the Disease Inheritance occurs in an autosomal dominant pattern. The gene has been assigned to chromosome 1 and contains 10 exons.

No mutations have been found in patients with the sporadic form despite intensive investigation. Several different mutations have been found in patients with familiar PCT. They include missense and splice-site mutations.

Molecular Pathophysiology of Disease Type II familial porphyria cutanea tarda is characterized by a 50% decrease in enzymatic activity and protein immunoreactivity in all tissues, while type III familial porphyria cutanea tarda shows normal enzymatic activity and protein present in all tissues except the liver. The consequence of the mutations, as shown in vitro expression studies, is a significantly shorter half-life of the mutated protein compared with the wild type. In the case of sporadic PCT, the pathogenesis of the disease seems to be a process that specifically inhibits the enzyme without decreasing its concentration. The process could be iron-related.

Management and Treatment Treatment is based on alcohol abstinence and phlebotomies. If phlebotomy is not tolerated, low doses of chloroquine or hydroxychloroquine are used. Treatment of other accompanying diseases may be helpful and, in fact, interferon treatment of HCV infection has been shown to correct the clinical manifestations of PCT in one patient.

Hepatoerythropoietic Porphyria (HEP) This is an extremely rare defect (only 20 patients described) resulting from a homozygous defect in uroporphyrin decarboxylase activity. The mutations described are different from those seen in porphyria cutanea tarda. The activity of the enzyme can be as low as 5% and, as in porphyria cutanea tarda mutations, the cause is a shortened half-life of the molecule.

Erythropoietic Protoporphyria (EPP Protoporphyria) This porphyria belongs to the group of erythroid porphyrias, together with congenital erythropoietic porphyria (CEP), and is caused by a partial deficiency of ferrochelatase, the last enzyme of the heme biosynthetic pathway. The defect results in massive accumulations of protoporphyrin in erythrocytes, plasma, and feces. The inheritance pattern is autosomal-dominant.

Clinical Manifestations Clinically, the most important findings are redness, swelling, burning, and itching of the skin following light exposure. Vesicular lesions (typical of other porphyrias) are uncommon. Development of gallstones (composed in part by protoporphyrin) occur in some patients as well as liver disease that can progress to cirrhosis (5–10%). The most serious complication is acute liver failure preceded by jaundice. There are no neurovisceral manifestations nor precipitating factors.

Diagnosis Elevated concentrations of free protoporphyrin in erythrocytes, plasma, and feces, with normal urinary porphyrins, are diagnostic.

Genetic Basis of the Disease The gene for ferrochelatase is assigned to chromosome 18 and contains 11 exons. Genetic defects are heterogeneous with missense and splicing mutations that frequently remove exon 2. Losses of exon 7 and 10 have also been described leading to unstable mRNA transcripts.

Management and Treatment Treatment is based on the avoidance of exposure to the sun, and the use of β-carotenes. Liver transplantation has not been successful because protoporphyrin production in the bone marrow leads to reaccumulation in the graft.

Porphyrias: Future Directions Three-dimensional and crystallographic studies of the proteins will help understand the mechanism of activity and the effect of different mutations. It will also be useful in establishing better genotype-phenotype correlations and identifying those patients at a higher risk of important complications.

Gene therapy for symptomatic patients is a possibility. Metabolic correction of the defect in cell lines derived from a patient with CEP using retroviral vectors carrying the URO III synthase gene has been shown. However, treatment strategies will be complicated because of the double synthesis and regulation of some of the enzymes of the pathway in the liver and in the bone marrow.

GALACTOSEMIA Inherited disorders of galactose metabolism are comprised of three diseases: classic galactosemia, galactokinase deficiency, and UDP-galactose-4-epimerase deficiency. They are characterized by the inability to catabolize galactose to carbon dioxide. Galactose metabolism fulfills two purposes: an energy source by the generation of glucose-1-phosphate and synthesis of galactosides (glycoproteins and glycolipids) using UDP-galactose as the galactosyl donor. Defects in the galactose metabolic pathway lead to accumulation of toxic metabolites, galactose-1-phosphate, and galactitol, and depletion of UDP-gal, both of which are potentially lethal.

Three enzymes are involved in galactose metabolism: galactokinase, galactose-1-P uridyl transferase (GALT), and UDP-galactose-4-epimerase (Fig. 42-3). Classic galactosemia derives from GALT deficiency and less frequently from severe epimerase deficit. Galactokinase deficit only produces galactitol, and the only pathological manifestation are cataracts.

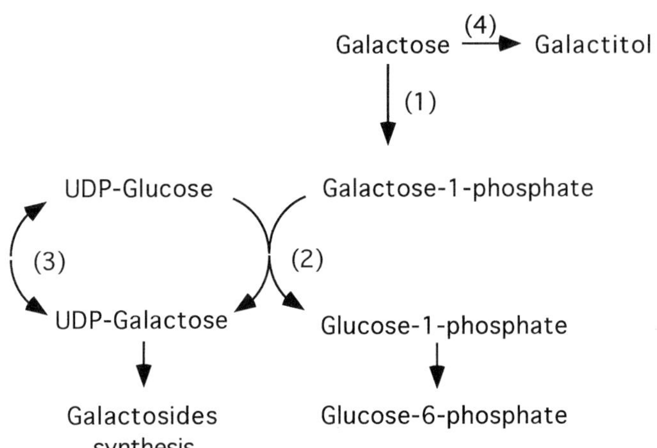

Figure 42-3 Galactose metabolism. Enzymes: (1) galactokinase, (2) galactose-1-phosphate uridyl transferase, (3) uridine diphosphate galactose-4-epimerase, (4) aldose reductase (nonspecific).

Table 42-5
Clinical Features of Galactosemia

Neonatal/early infancy period		*Chronic*	
Failure to thrive	(M)	CNS dysfunction	(TI)
Vomiting	(M)	Speech abnormality	
Diarrhea	(M)	Intellectual deficit	
Jaundice	(M)	Growth retardation	(TD)
Hemolysis	(M)	Ovarian dysfunction	(TI)
Hepatomegaly	(M)	Liver disease	(TD)
Cataracts	(M)		
Mental retardation	(M)		
Ascites	(S)		
Septicemia (*E. coli*)	(S)		
Renal failure	(S)		

CNS, central nervous system; M, mild disease; S, severe disease; TI, treatment independent (no improvement despite galactose withdrawal from the diet); TD, treatment dependent (not developed, if treatment is correct).

Clinical Manifestations (Table 42-5) Severely affected patients with the classic form of galactosemia, that are not quickly diagnosed and continue taking galactose with the diet, develop hepatic and kidney failure and die in few weeks resulting from septicemia. Milder forms are characterized by failure to thrive, vomiting, and diarrhea. Jaundice develops during the first few weeks of life and, if untreated, the liver disease may progress to cirrhosis. However, because of *in utero* exposure to toxic galactose metabolites, long-term outcome may include cataracts, speech defects, ovarian dysfunction, growth decline, and poor intellectual function, despite adequate treatment.

Diagnosis Diagnosis is made by demonstration of severe deficiency or lack of GALT activity in red cells, fibroblasts, or liver. Widespread screening of newborns for elevated blood galactose are effective, provided the newborns have been fed prior to the test. The test has allowed early identification of patients. The demonstration of a reducing sugar in urine that is not glucose has similar value. Prenatal diagnosis can be made by determination of GALT activity in cultured amniotic cells, biopsied chorionic villi, or determination of galactitol in amniotic fluid.

Genetic Basis of the Disease The galactose-1-P uridyl transferase gene is located at chromosome 9. Gene polymorphisms abound because of point mutations and changes in noncritical amino acid residues. The consequences are partial enzyme deficiencies that are usually asymptomatic. The most frequent gene defect is a Asn 314 to Asp mutation resulting in the Duarte variant of the enzyme. It is present in 4–14% of the population and produces a 50% decrease in enzymatic activity. Duarte/Normal allele heterozygotes show 75% activity, Duarte homozygotes 50%, and Duarte/Galactosemic heterozygotes 25%. The most frequent lethal mutation is Gln 188 to Arg in exon 6 (60% in overall patient population and 68% in Caucasians; only 16% in African Americans). This mutation is close to the catalytic active site and results in undetectable enzyme activity, as determined in yeast expression studies. In addition, several other point mutations including splice site mutations have been described, leading to instability of the protein or decrease in activity. Crossreacting immune protein may or may not be present indicating the heterogeneity of the genetic defects. Finally, the protein acts as a dimer, raising the possibility of the presence of mixed heterodimers in the case of heterozygotes. The prevalent Gln 188 to Arg mutation can be determined by PCR amplification, followed by restriction enzyme digestion with Hpa II that can cleave a newly created site resulting from the mutation.

Molecular Pathophysiology of Disease Galactose-1-P accumulation is probably responsible for the liver damage although the mechanism of toxicity is not clear. It could be related to energy depletion, as ATP used to phosphorylate galactose to galactose-1-P cannot be metabolized. Galactitol accumulation in the lens causes osmotic swelling and the formation of cataracts. UDP-galactose depletion has been correlated with ovarian dysfunction and probably mental impairment, but the mechanism is not completely understood.

Management and Treatment The only available treatment consists of a complete exclusion of galactose from the diet.

EPIMERASE DEFICIENCY This condition is inherited in an autosomal recessive pattern, and two forms have been described: one without clinical significance and one resembling classic galactosemia (described in only two patients). The gene is located on chromosome 1, but the defects have not been yet published. Clinical findings are indistinguishable from those derived from galactose-1-P uridyl transferase deficiency. Diagnosis is similar to classic galactosemia, but galactose-1-P uridyl transferase activity is present.

HEREDITARY FRUCTOSE INTOLERANCE This is an autosomal recessive disease caused by a defect in aldolase B, an enzyme responsible for the metabolism of the fructose present in sugar, juices, and fruit. Sucrose and sorbitol are also metabolized to fructose. Fructose-bisphosphate aldolase is the enzyme responsible for the conversion of fructose-1-phosphate into D-glyceraldehyde and dihydroxyacetone phosphate. It has three distinct isoforms: aldolase B is the isoform expressed in the liver, kidney, and intestinal mucosa; aldolase A is expressed ubiquitously and is the only one in the muscle, while aldolase C is characteristic of the brain.

Clinical Manifestations (Table 42-6) Symptoms typically start after cessation of breast feeding. Exposure to fructose leads to vomiting, diarrhea, and abdominal pain. Symptomatic hypoglycemia causes pallor and trembling in infants. Loss of consciousness can occur. Ingestion of large quantities can cause convulsions and coma. Continuous exposure leads to failure to thrive, jaundice, liver disease progressing to cirrhosis, metabolic acidosis, renal tubular disease, and growth retardation. Heavy administration causes hemorrhagic diathesis and death. Patients develop a protective aversion to fructose-containing foods.

Diagnosis Clinical suspicion together with demonstration fructosemia and fructosuria are the basis of the diagnosis. Enzyme activity can be determined in liver or intestinal biopsy, which demonstrates that leukocytes or fibroblasts in affected individuals do not contain aldolase B.

Genetic Basis of the Disease Aldolase B is a tetramer of 364 amino acids. The gene is located in chromosome 9 and contains nine exons, the first of which is not translated. The genetic defects are heterogeneous. The most frequent involves a point mutation causing Ala-149 to Pro (exon 5, 67% alleles), close to residues responsible for the binding to the substrate, followed by Ala-174 to Asp (exon 5, 16%). Several other missense mutations have been described, leading to amino acid change or frameshift and truncated protein, as well as deletions from a single base to 1.65 kb, stop codon mutations, and a translation codon mutation. An Ala-149 to Pro mutation was demonstrated by PCR followed by digestion with *Aha*II, as this novel restriction site was generated by the mutation. Most gene defects can be studied with a limited number of allele-specific oligonucleotides.

Table 42-6
Clinical Features of Hereditary Fructose Intolerance

Acute exposure	*Chronic exposure*	*Sequelae*
Sweating	Poor feeding	Cirrhosis
Pallor	Failure to thrive	Liver steatosis
Trembling	Vomiting	Aversion to sweets
Dizziness	Irritability	Peculiar feeding habits
Nausea	Apathy	
Vomiting	Jaundice	
Abdominal pain	Hepatomegaly	
Apathy, lethargy	Abdominal distention	
Coma	Edema, ascites	
Convulsions	Hemorrhage	
Growth retardation	Tremor, jerking	

Molecular Pathophysiology of Disease Fructose ingestion or intravenous administration in these patients leads to fructose-1-P accumulation. This induces hypoglycemia by inhibition of glycogenolysis and gluconeogenesis, and ATP depletion, used in the formation of high amounts of fructose-1-P. A small infusion of fructose lead to phosphorylation of fructose that can sequester up to 80% of the liver inorganic phosphate.

Management and Treatment Treatment consists of absolute removal of fructose, sorbitol, and sucrose from the diet. Contrary to galactosemia, in which some problems can remain despite strict adherence to the diet, recovery is complete, except when liver cirrhosis has already been established.

ACKNOWLEDGMENTS

This work was supported in part by a grant from the National Institutes of Health, NIH DK-42182 (GYW). Juan Ruiz is the recipient of a grant from Fundacion Ramon Arces (Spain).

SELECTED REFERENCES

Bacon BR, Tavill AS. Hemochromatosis and the iron overload syndromes. In: Zakim D, Boyer TD, eds. Hepatology: A Textbook of Liver Disease, 3rd ed. Philadelphia: WB Saunders, 1996; pp. 1439–1472.

Bothwell TH, Charlton RW, Motulsky AG. Hemochromatosis. In: Scriver CR, Beaudet AL, Sly WS, Valle D, eds. The Metabolic and Molecular Bases of Inherited Disease, vol 2, 7th ed. New York: McGraw-Hill, 1995; pp. 2237–2269.

Bull P, Thomas GR, Forbes J, Rommens JM, Cox DW. The Wilson disease gene is a putative copper transporting P-type ATPase similar to the Menke's disease gene. Nat Genet 1993;5:327–337.

Cox DW. α1-Antitrypsin Deficiency. In: Scriver CR, Beaudet AL, Sly WS, Valle D, eds. The Metabolic and Molecular Bases of Inherited Disease, vol 3, 7th ed. New York: McGraw-Hill, 1995; pp. 4125–4158.

Cox TM. Aldolase B and fructose intolerance. FASEB J 1994;8:62–71.

Danks DM. Disorders of copper transport. In: Scriver CR, Beaudet AL, Sly WS, Valle D, eds. The Metabolic and Molecular Bases of Inherited Disease, vol 2, 7th ed. New York: McGraHill, 1995; pp. 2211–2235.

Davis W, Chowrimootoo GFE, Seymour CA. Defective biliary copper excretion in Wilson's disease: the role of caeruloplasmin. Eur J Clin Invest 1996;26:893–901.

Feder JN, Gnirke A, Thomas W, et al. A novel MHC class I-like gene is mutated in patients with hereditary haemochromatosis. Nature Med 1996;13:399–408.

Goodman SI, Greene CL. Metabolic disorders of the newborn. Ped in Rev 1994;15:359–365.

Kappas A, Shigeru S, Galbraith RA, Nordmann Y. The porphyrias. In: Scriver CR, Beaudet AL, Sly WS, Valle D, eds. The Metabolic and Molecular Bases of Inherited Disease, vol 2, 7th ed. New York: McGraw-Hill, 1995; pp. 2103–2159.

Parkkila S, Waheed A, Britton, et al. Association of the transferrin receptor in human placenta with HFE, the protein defective in hereditary hemochromatosis. Proc Natl Acad Sci USA 1997;94: 13,198–13,202.

Perlmutter DH. Clinical manifestations of alpha-1-antitrypsin deficiency. Gastroenterology Clin N Am 1995;24:27–43.

Puy H, Deybach JC, Lamoril J, et al. Molecular epidemology and diagnosis of PBG deaminase gene defects in acute intermittent porphyria. Am J Hum Genet 1997;60:1373–1383.

Pyeritz RE. Genetic heterogeneity in Wilson disease: lessons from rare alleles. Ann Intern Med 1997;127:70–72.

Rothenberg BE, Voland JR. β2-Microglobulin knockout mice develop parenchymal iron overload: a putative role of the major histocompatibility complex in iron metabolism. Proc Natl Acad Sci USA 1996;93:1529–1534.

Santos M, Schilman MW, Rademakers LHPM, Marx JJM, Desousa M, Clevers H. Defective iron homeostasis in beta 2-microglobulin knockout mice recapitulates hereditary hemochromatosis in man. J Exp Med 1996;184:1975–1985.

Saudubray JM, Ogier H, Charpentier C. Clinical approach to inherited metabolic diseases. In: Fernandes J, Saudubray JM, van den Berghe G, eds. Inborn Metabolic Diseases, 2nd ed. Berling: Springer-Verlag, 1995; pp. 3–39.

Savransky E, Hytiroglou P, Harpaz N, Thung SN, Johnson EM. Correcting the PIZ defect in the α1-antitrypsin gene of human-cells by targeted homologous recombination. Lab Invest 1994;70:676–683.

Segal S, Berry GT. Disorders of galactose metabolism. In: Scriver CR, Beaudet AL, Sly WS, Valle D, eds. The Metabolic and Molecular Bases of Inherited Disease, vol 1, 7th ed. New York: McGraw-Hill, 1995; pp. 967–1000.

Sveger T, Eriksson S. The liver in adolescents with α1-antitrypsin deficiency. Hepatology 1995;22:514–517.

Tanner MS, Taylor CJ. Liver disease in cystic fibrosis. Archiv Dis Childhood 1995;72:281–284.

Tanzi RE, Petrukhin K, Chernov I, et al. The Wilson disease gene is a copper transporting ATPase with homology to the Menke's disease gene. Nat Genet 1993;5:344–350.

Teckman JH, Perlmutter DH. Conceptual advances in pathogenesis and treatment of childhood metabolic disease. Gastroenterology 1995; 108:1263–1279.

Thomas GR, Forbes JR, Roberts EA, Walshe JM, Cox DW. The Wilson disease gene: spectrum of mutations and their consequences. Nat Genet 1995;9:210–217.

Welsh MJ, Tsui LC, Boat TF, Beaudet AL. Cystic Fibrosis. In: Scriver CR, Beaudet AL, Sly WS, Valle D, eds. The Metabolic and Molecular Bases of Inherited Disease, vol 3, 7th ed. New York: McGraw-Hill, 1995; pp. 3799–3876.

Wu GY, Wu CH. Gene therapy by targeting nucleic acids to hepatocytes. In: Arias IM, Boyer JL, Fausto N, Jakoby WB, Schachter DA, Shafritz DA, eds. The Liver: Biology and Pathology, 3rd ed. New York: Raven, 1994; pp. 1537–1546.

Wu Y, Whitman I, Molmenti E, Moore K, Hippenmeyer P, Perlmutter DH. A lag in intracellular degradation of mutant α1-antitrypsin correlates with the liver disease phenotype in homozygous PiZZ α1-antitrypsin deficiency. Proc Natl Acad Sci USA 1994;91: 9014–9018.

43 Viral Hepatitis and Liver Disease

SANJEEV GUPTA AND MICHAEL OTT

DEFINITION

Viral hepatitis is characterized by necroinflammatory liver disease with asymptomatic, acute and chronic presentations. The "hepatitic" presentation refers to a significant rise in serum aminotransferases in the presence of normal or minimally increased serum alkaline phosphatase levels. Hepatitis viruses may be cleared with no lasting sequalae, persist indefinitely without causing apparent disease, or cause chronic hepatitis and multiple complications, including cirrhosis and hepatocellular carcinoma (HCC). Acute hepatitis usually refers to recent onset of virus infection with viral persistence for not longer than 6 months. The susceptibility to and consequences of viral hepatitis are determined by incompletely defined host factors, the size of the initial viral inoculum, and the presence or absence of infection with other hepatitis viruses. The diagnosis of specific viral etiologies requires laboratory testing because clinical presentations may be indistinguishable from one another.

INTRODUCTION

Even though hepatitis epidemics have been recorded from the ancient times, the nature of viral hepatitis remained obscure until after the Second World War. In the 1950s, based on epidemiological evidence, such as observations of the route of transmission, incubation period, case clustering, and so on, the existence of more than one hepatitis virus was surmised, and early investigators distinguished between the short-incubation or "infectious" (type A) and the long-incubation or "serum" (type B) hepatitis. The progress during the past three decades in isolating and characterizing commonly encountered hepatitis viruses has been truly remarkable. These advances could not have been made without the advent of molecular biology methods. In 1965, an important advance was made when serologic testing revealed the hepatitis B virus surface antigen (HBsAg) in Australian aborigines, so the antigen was initially called Australia antigen. This discovery provided means for diagnosing hepatitis B infection and paved the way for defining the biology of the hepatitis B virus (HBV). In 1973, the hepatitis A virus (HAV) was visualized. However, despite the ability to recognize HAV and HBV infection, a number of patients showed evidence for neither of these viruses, and such cases were classified as suffering from NonA, NonB viral hepatitis. Each succeeding decade brought forth implausible new discoveries and more hepatitis viruses have been identified. The hepatitis delta virus (HDV) was recognized in the mid 1970s, the hepatitis C virus (HCV), which is responsible for a large proportion of nonA, nonB hepatitis, was cloned in 1989, and in the 1990s, further additions have been made to this viral alphabet, with the cloning of the hepatitis E virus (HEV), the provisionally designated hepatitis G virus (HGV), and the hepatitis GB viruses (HGBVs). A tentatively designated hepatitis F virus turned out not to be a true viral isolate. Hepatitis may be a result of additional nonhepatotropic viruses, e.g., cytomegalovirus, herpes simplex virus-1, Epstein-Barr virus, and so on. Also, a "hepatitic" presentation may be encountered in disorders, such as autoimmune hepatitis, heavy metal accumulation, or drug-toxicity, which need to be carefully considered in differential diagnosis.

The applications of modern molecular genetics tools have unraveled some mysteries of the hepatitis viruses and provided novel insights into the biology of viral persistence and hepatic oncogenesis, although much further work is necessary to translate these insights into molecular therapies. Similarly, molecular immunology needs to generate insights into how circulating antibodies confer lifelong immunity against some viruses, e.g., HAV or HBV, but do not protect against others, e.g., HCV or HDV. Our goal here is to provide an overview of the molecular biology of hepatitis viruses and how this information helps to understand hepatic pathophysiology. The limited scope of this chapter precludes a full discussion of this rapidly advancing and broad area, which, fortunately, excites enormous interest among investigators worldwide.

GENOME STRUCTURES AND ORGANIZATION

The shared bond among hepatitis viruses is their proclivity for causing liver disease. However, the individual viruses themselves differ significantly in phylogenetic relationships, genome organization, replication strategy, and so on. For instance, HAV belongs to the picornavirus family, HBV to the hepadnavirus family (with other members infecting the woodchuck, Peking duck, ground squirrel, heron, and a tree shrew), HCV to a new genus in the flavivirus family, and so on (Table 43-1). Also, it is at times forgotten that virus replication is not necessarily restricted to the liver and individual viruses, e.g., HBV or HCV, may infect additional organs, including hematopoietic cells, pancreas, kidney, and spermatozoa, depending on which cell type offers permissive conditions for viral gene expression. The presence of extrahepatic virus reservoirs imposes limitations on therapies, e.g., orthotopic liver transplantation (OLT) is difficult in the presence of ongoing HBV

From: *Principles of Molecular Medicine* (J. L. Jameson, ed.), ©1998 Humana Press Inc., Totowa, NJ.

Table 43-1

Virus	*Family*	*Genome structure*	*Genome size*
HAV	Picornaviridae	Positive strand RNA	7.5 kb
HBV	Hepadnaviridae	Double stranded DNA with incomplete circle	3.2 kb
HCV	Flaviviridae	Positive strand RNA	9.5 kb
HDV	Viroid Deltaviridae	Negative strand RNA	1.7 kb derives envelope from HBV
HEV	Calciviridae	Positive strand RNA	7.5 kb
HGV and related HGBVs	Flaviviridae	Positive strand RNA	9 kb

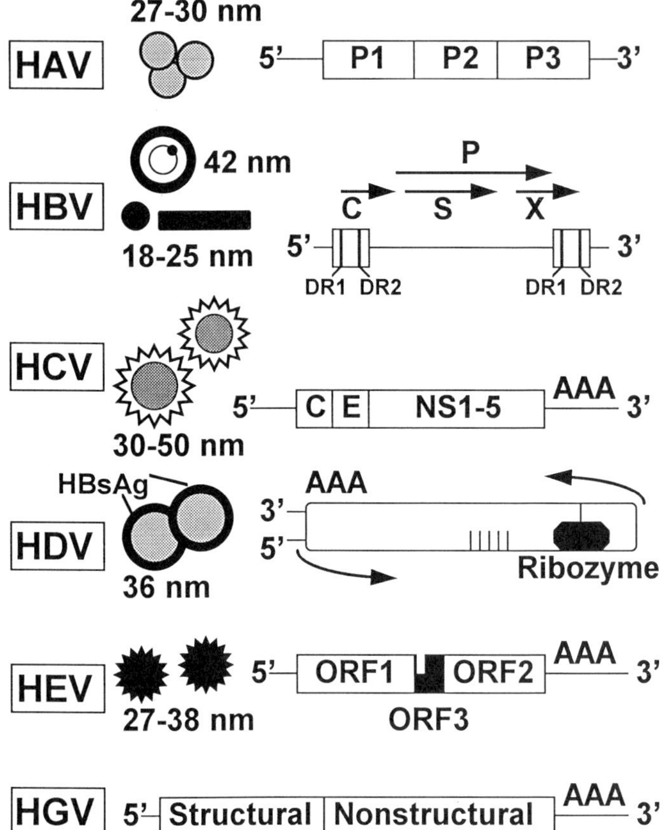

Figure 43-1 Schematic depiction of the structure of various hepatitis viruses and their general genomic organization. *See* the text for more detailed descriptions.

replication because the transplanted liver is virtually always reinfected with the virus leading to a peculiarly aggressive disease and rapid liver failure.

HEPATITIS A VIRUS In 1973, immunoelectron microscopy showed the virus in the stool of infected patients. Subsequently, development of immunoassays provided seroepidemiological insights, including ones for the existence of additional water-borne hepatitis viruses, such as HEV, and the ability to culture HAV in the 1980s led to the development of effective vaccines. The HAV is an important cause of acute water-borne hepatitis and afflicts enormous number of populations worldwide who have limited access to safe drinking water, specially in underdeveloped regions. However, the virus does not cause chronic disease. The infection most commonly affects children and may manifest with no or easily overlooked symptoms. Serological evidence indicates a rising level of immunity with age in hyperendemic areas, such that by the age of 40 years, approximately 50–60% of the population may be immune. On the other hand, acute HAV hepatitis in patients older than 40 years, e.g., in nonimmune travelers, could be severe and fatal.

The virion particles exhibit a smooth and round exterior with a protein shell (capsid) enclosing a single-stranded RNA of approximately 7.5 kb in size (Fig. 43-1). The genomic organization of HAV follows that of other picornaviruses. There are untranslated regions (UTR) at both the 5' and 3' ends of the genomic RNA extending to ~0.7 and ~0.06 kb in length, respectively. The open reading frames are designated P1, P2, and P3 regions. The P1 region encodes the capsid polypeptides termed VP1, VP2, VP3, and VP4. The P2 region encodes the nonstructural proteins designated P2A, P2B, and P2C, the functions of which are poorly defined, although viral protease and other enzymatic activities have been identified. The P3 region encodes for P3A, P3B, P3C, and P3D proteins, which are necessary for viral replication and serve as the genome-linked protein Vpg (P3B), a viral protease (P3C), and the viral RNA polymerase (P3D). The function of the P3A protein remains unknown. The virus uses a mucin-like glycoprotein of 451-amino acids on the cell surface as its receptor. In similarity with other RNA viruses, HAV exhibits differences in nucleotide sequences, which lead to altered genotypes (*see below*). However, the mutations do not alter the immunogenic epitopes encoded by the P1 region and immunity against the virus is not abrogated. During natural infection, the initial host response is manifested with IgM class antibody against capsid polypeptides followed by the protective IgG class antibody, which confers lifelong immunity against reinfection. An important recent advance has been the development of highly effective vaccines arising from the ability to propagate HAV in cell culture.

HEPATITIS B VIRUS One of the most important hepatitis viruses, HBV infection represents a major public health burden with an estimated 350 million cases worldwide. The virus is commonly acquired by exposure to contaminated blood or via sexual activity. The HBsAg carrier rates in low endemic areas (e.g., 0.1–0.2% in the United States, United Kingdom, and parts of Western Europe) contrast with areas of moderate endemicity (2.5% in Spain, Italy, Japan, and Greece) or high endemicity (11–15% in South Africa, Taiwan, and Hong Kong). In some geographically isolated communities, prevalence of HBV infection, as indicated by any serological marker, is very high, e.g., in Alaskan Eskimos. Very young age is a most important factor predisposing to persistent HBV infection and unless altered by immunization, infection is the rule in infants born to HBV carrier mothers (90–100% transmission). Persistent infection is increased in the immunocompromised and with small viral inoculum.

Much more is known about the molecular biology of HBV than the other hepatitis viruses, although even here critical aspects of

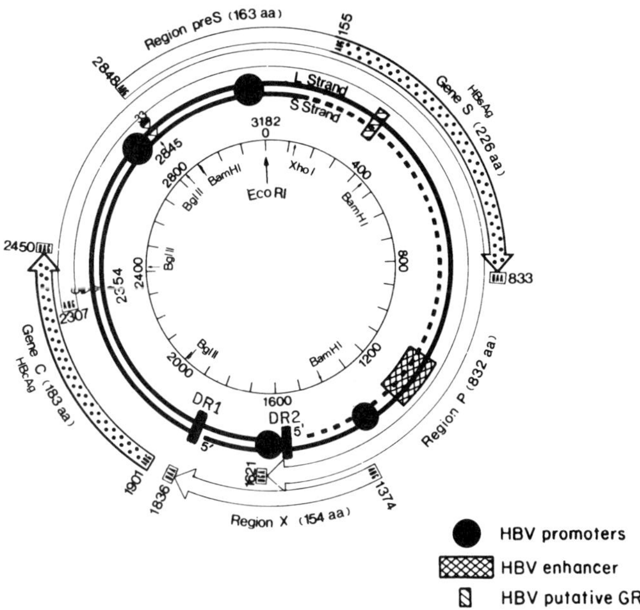

Figure 43-2 The genome of HBV is constituted by two circular DNA strands, of which the shorter one (S strand) is incomplete and constitutes the "sense" orientation. The positions of various regulatory sequences are as shown.

virus replication and other events have not been fully determined. The virus was physically demonstrated by electron microscopy more than 20 years ago and identified as the agent responsible for "serum hepatitis." The HBV primarily exists in the liver and serum. The infectious virion is represented by the "Dane particle," which has a diameter of 42 nm and contains an outer envelope of protein and membrane lipids with an inner nucleocapsid of 27-nm size (Fig. 43-1). However, the most abundant particles (10^3- to 10^6-fold excess) are 16- to 25-nm spherical particles and 22-nm diameter filamentous particles (up to 1000 nm long), which are devoid of viral nucleic acids and are noninfectious.

The HBV genome is a small circular DNA of 3.2–3.3 kb arranged in two strands (Fig. 43-2). The long DNA strand, also designated the minus (–) strand, is of full length and is complementary to viral mRNAs. This full-length strand is complete other than missing only one or a few nucleotides at 1800 nucleotides from the *Eco*RI restriction enzyme recognition site (which is arbitrarily used as 0 to map nucleotide positions). The other DNA strand is shorter, lacks from 15 to 50% of the sequence and is designated as the plus (+) strand. The 5' end of the short strand is located at nucleotide 1560, but its length and the 3' end differ considerably. The circular configuration of the genome is maintained by base pairing of the 5' termini of the two DNA strands with a "cohesive end" region constituted by 250–300 overlapping nucleotides. A viral DNA polymerase activity associated with the nucleocapsid repairs this single-stranded region of the (+) or short-strand DNA by adding nucleotides to its 3' end, although, despite formation of a complete circle, it is not covalently closed. The HBV genome shows additional asymmetries at the 5' ends with a covalently linked protein at the (–) or long strand and an oligoribonucleotide attached to the (+) short strand DNA. In addition, the cohesive end region contains 11 bp direct repeats, termed DR1 and DR2 regions, which serve important functions during virus replication.

Table 43-2
HBV Gene Products

Gene	*Protein product*	*Function*
pre S1	p39/p42[a] (large HBsAg)	Envelope
pre S2	P33[a]/p36[a] (middle HBsAg)	Envelope
S	p24/p27[a] (small HBsAg)	Envelope
C	15 kDa (HBcAg)	Nucleocapsid
pre C/C	16–25 kDa (HBeAg)	Unknown
P	70–90 kDa	DNA polymerase
X	15 kDa (HBxAg)	Unknown/cellular transactivator

[a]Glycosylated species.

The HBV contains four translational open reading frames (ORFs) on the (–) or long DNA strand (Table 43-2). The overlapping nature of these ORFs and transregulation by enhancer elements are one of the unique features of the complex genomic organization. The hepatitis B surface antigen (HBsAg) ORF spans map positions 833–2848 and constitutes the 3' portion of another larger coding region. An upstream reading frame (ORF pre-S) with two conserved initiating ATG codons directs transcription of the larger HBsAg-related envelope proteins, termed pre-Sl and pre-S2. The HBcAg (ORF C) is encoded by nucleotides spanning 1836–2450 bases and is preceded by another upstream ORF termed pre-C region, which could encode a larger HBcAg-related polypeptide. The viral polymerase is encoded by ORF P, map position 1621–2357. Finally, the HBxAg, which has transactivating properties, is encoded by a region overlapping the HBsAg and HBcAg ORFs that constitute the ORF X (map positions 1374–1818). The ORF X is the only one that is not well-conserved in all hepadnaviruses and is absent in duck HBV. The (+) or short DNA strand is not known to transcribe any viral gene product.

The HBV expresses 3.5 kb (genomic) and 2.4 or 2.1 kb (subgenomic) polyadenylated mRNA species. The 5' end of the 3.5 kb genomic mRNA arises from the pre-C region and the 3' end from the C gene, where a specific polyadenylation signal is located. The genomic mRNA contains an additional approximately 100 nucleotides beyond the genome, implying that the 3.5-kb genomic RNA is transcribed from the covalently closed double-stranded DNA and that the polyadenylation signal is skipped over during the first cycle around the genome. The 2.4-kb subgenomic mRNA encodes the pre-S1 protein, although it also transcribes pre-S2, S, and X proteins. The 5' end of the 2.1-kb RNA has been mapped to approximately 20 nucleotide pairs upstream of the pre-S2 region and this mRNA generates the pre-S2 and S proteins. The mRNAs encoding X or P have not yet been identified, although the pregenomic mRNA possibly is responsible for the DNA polymerase. In patients with chronic HBV infection, novel HBV mRNA species can be found and represent fusion transcripts of integrated viral DNA and flanking cellular sequences. The viral gene expression is regulated by several elements: Promoters have been found for pre-S1, pre-S2, HBcAg, and HBxAg; two enhancer elements designated HBEn I (map position 1080–1234) and HBEn II (in pre-C region) have been identified; a glucocorticoid responsive element is also present. Viral mRNA transcription is terminated by a conserved element in ORF C responsible for RNA cleavage and polyadenylation. The HBV enhancer and promoter sequences bind specific cellular transcription factors, among which the C/EBPs and HNFs-1 and -3 are most significant. The cell type-specificity of HBV expression is regulated by interactions among cellular transcription factors with both upregulatory and downregulatory effects, although more knowledge is necessary for understanding their interactions.

The viral gene products subserve somewhat expected functions but also have poorly understood effects upon the host cell. All virion particles are enclosed in HBsAg. The envelope HBsAg proteins produced by the ORF S are three: small HBsAg (226 amino acids), pre-S2 plus S or middle HBsAg (281 amino acids), and pre-S1 plus pre-S2 plus S or large HBsAg (389–400 amino acids). The small HBsAg is rapidly secreted from cells, whereas excess production of the large HBsAg leads to intracytoplasmic retention of HBsAg and development of so-called "ground-glass" hepatocytes seen in chronic HBV carriers. The HBsAgs are principally present in 22-nm particles that contain approximately 25% lipid derived from the host cytoplasm. The HBsAg proteins are generally resistant to proteases, heat, and chaotropic substances but not to detergents. The viral envelope is mostly composed of small HBsAg (~ 90%). The presence of pre-S2 in the envelope facilitates binding to serum albumin, whereas the preS1 domain is thought to be involved in receptor-mediated entry of virion particles into hepatocytes. The HBsAg contains a major serologic group-specific determinant termed "a" and subtype determinants d, y, w, and r, producing four main serotypes adw, ayw, adr and ayr. Each viral subtype shows differences in geographic distribution.

The nucleocapsid core contains a 21-kDa basic phosphoprotein termed the hepatitis B core antigen (HBcAg). The HBcAg may exist in multiple sizes because of posttranslational processing. Nucleocapsid cores are found in the nuclei of infected hepatocytes and are a marker of HBV replication. The nucleocapsids enclose the pregenomic mRNA and viral DNA polymerase during replication. The viral DNA polymerase is a putative 70–90-kDa protein with reverse transcriptase activity. An endogenous protein kinase activity is also present in hepadnaviral core particles, but the functional significance of core phosphorylation is unknown. The pre-C region of the virus contains an inphase sequence with an ATG codon approx 80 nucleotides upstream to the core ATG to serve as the HBeAg mRNA initiation site. Expression of the pre-C gene generates a 25-kDa HBe protein and this undergoes removal of several NH2-terminal amino acids to generate a 23-kDa protein (p23). The transmembranously located p23 is further modified for secretion as p16 to p20 unglycosylated and mature HBeAg. The HBeAg is found in serum during viral replication, although its function is unknown. The HBxAg is the smallest HBV protein at approximately 15 kDa. Although this protein is expressed during HBV infection and can be found in the infected liver, as well as serum, its precise function has been elusive. In vitro DNA transfection studies show that HBxAg can transactivate a variety of viral enhancer and promoter elements.

Viral replication occurs through a complex series of events with key steps requiring more information (Fig. 43-3). After entry into cells, the virion DNA undergoes conversion in the nucleus to covalently closed circular DNA (ccc DNA), although how this occurs is unknown. This is followed by transcription of the 3.5-kb pregenome mRNA from the (-) strand of the ccc DNA. The host RNA polymerase is used for generating the "pregenome" by reverse transcription within a nuclear core particle, which is then transported to the cytoplasm. The "genomic" RNAs are heterogeneous with several choices for 5' ends over a 31-bp region that includes the first ATG in the ORF C. Synthesis of the (-) strand DNA is initiated in the short DR1 sequence near either the 3' or 5' end with the participation of an unidentified protein primer. An RNAse H function of the polymerase degrades mRNAs as the (-) strand elongates. Why the (+) strand remains incomplete is unknown. Although the viral replication mechanism with the use of a reverse transcriptase step is similar to the replication strategies of retroviruses and cauliflower mosaic viruses, the viruses are fundamentally different. Nonetheless, use of reverse transcriptase comes with a greater likelihood of mutations in the viral genome at a frequency greater than DNA viruses, although the frequency of such errors may be less than that of RNA viruses (*see below*). The viral genomes isolated from a single patient are homogeneous, as determined by restriction enzyme mapping, and within a single HBV subtype only occasional differences are noted. However, different serological subtypes show considerable variation in nucleotide sequences, which may differ by up to 10%, with small additions or deletions scattered throughout the genome.

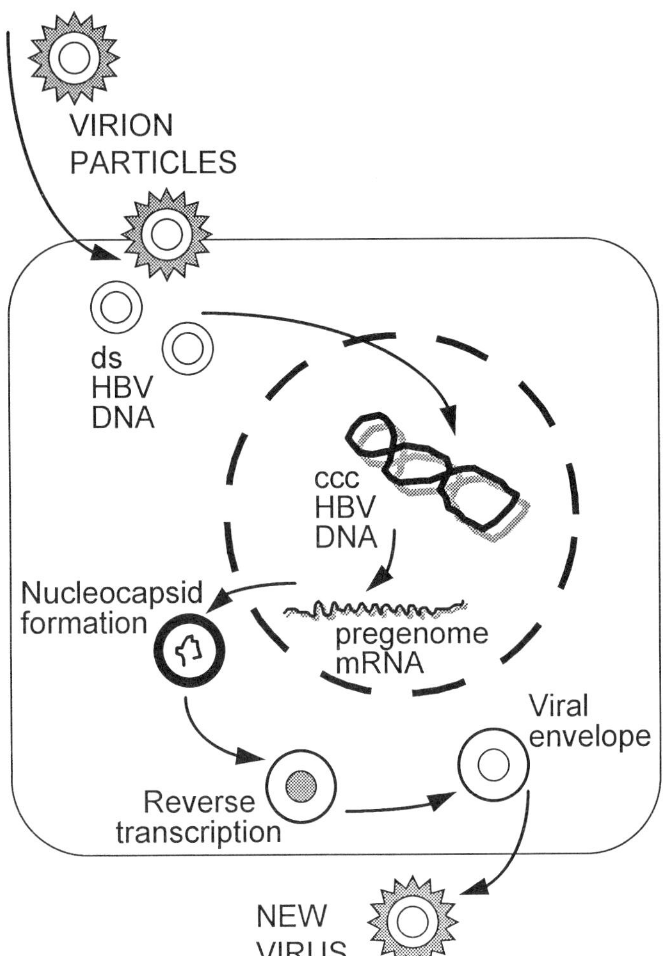

Figure 43-3 HBV replication steps include translocation of the double-stranded viral DNA into cell nucleus and conversion to covalently closed circular (ccc) DNA, transcription of the 3.4-kb pregenome mRNA and nucleocapsid formation. The genome is replicated by reverse transcription in nucleocapsids and packaged in the viral envelope constituted by the HBsAg proteins before secretion of virion particles.

After infection, serum HBsAg is the first marker to be detected followed by serum HBeAg and then virion particles containing HBV DNA and DNA polymerase. The serum HBV DNA best correlates with replicating and infectious HBV. Serum HBV DNA positivity beyond 4 weeks of acute hepatitis indicates delayed viral clearance and predisposition to chronic hepatitis. Anti-HBc directed against HBcAg appears before anti-HBs in patients with viral clearance and both persist for several years. Much of the anti-HBc is of the IgG class, although early on serum anti-HBc is of an IgM class and is helpful in diagnosing acute HBV infection. After clearance of HBV with anti-HBs, lifelong immunity may be developed. This protective capacity of anti-HBs is the basis for successful vaccination against HBV. Anti-HBs is primarily of "a" group specificity and protects against all HBV subtypes. However, vaccine-escape mutants have been recognized (*see below*).

HEPATITIS C VIRUS Despite recognition of posttransfusion nonA, nonB hepatitis in the early 1970s, cloning of HCV required ingenious use of molecular biology methods and was finally accomplished in 1989. Worldwide, HCV infection may be as prevalent, if not more, than HBV. Within the United States, HCV is responsible for more than one million cases with liver disease and for probably a far greater number of people with asymptomatic or silent infection. The risk factors include intravenous drug use (38%), sexual/household contact (10%), blood transfusion-related (4%), occupational exposure (2%), and renal dialysis (1%), although in most cases no obvious source is apparent. A minority may acquire the infection at birth (0–13% risk). The disease is particularly prevalent in Asia (25%) and subsaharan Africa and less so in Europe, United States, and Australia. The development of disease is poorly defined, though it may be related to the size of the viral inoculum, the titer of the virus, and possibly the viral genotype. Unlike HBV, which infrequently causes chronic infection (<1% after acute hepatitis), HCV far more frequently causes chronic hepatitis (approximately 50%).

The virion particles are 30–50 nm large and are sensitive to chloroform, formalin, heat, and ultraviolet light. Although HCV was deduced to be an RNA virus, its cloning proved difficult and required novel strategies. The ultimately successful strategy by a group in the United States used enriched HCV particles from a chimpanzee infected with NonA, NonB virus. Viral nucleic acids were extracted and cDNA expression libraries made in a bacteriophage system. This system allowed expression of recombinant viral proteins, which were screened with a panel of serum samples from chronic NonA, NonB virus carriers containing antibodies. Extensive screenings ($>1 \times 10^6$ clones) yielded five serum-reactive cDNA clones, of which one (clone 5-1-1) proved to be specific for viral sequences and hybridized only with viral RNAs. Using this 5-1-1 clone, three additional overlapping clones were then obtained, and to generate immunoassays, one clone (c100-3) was expressed as a superoxide dismutase fusion protein in yeast. Japanese workers also cloned HCV in 1989 from 100 L of pooled human serum. Of the 29 Japanese clones isolated, 12 were identical to the clone identified by the United States group. Despite enormous subsequent work in learning about HCV, knowledge of its molecular biology and replication mechanisms is limited.

The viral genome is encoded by an approximately 9.4 kb size single-stranded RNA of (+) sense orientation. The genome is organized with only one ORF in the center flanked at both the 5' and the 3' end with UTR regions of variable length (Fig. 43-1). The viral genome is subdivided into a domain transcribing structural genes (Core [C] and Envelope [E1 and E2]) toward the 5' end and

Table 43-3
HCV Gene Products

Gene	*Protein product*	*Function*
C	p22	Nucleocapsid
E1	gp33	Envelope
E2/NS1	gp70	Envelope
NS2	p23	Metalloproteinase
NS3	p72	Serine protease/helicase
NS4 (a/b)	p10/p27	Unknown
NS5 (a/b)	p58/p70	RNA-dependent DNA-polymerase

a large domain transcribing nonstructural genes (NS1-5) toward the 3' end. The 5' UTR region spans 324–341 nucleotides and contains up to five ORFs with the potential to transcribe small polypeptides, but no such proteins have been identified. The 5' region is also the most highly conserved area of the virus and contains a secondary stem-loop structure, which initiates 5' cap-independent polyprotein translation from the first AUG codon and thus serves as the viral internal ribosomal entry site (IRES). This mechanism of protein translation is also found in other viruses, such as picornavirus members (poliomyelitis virus, hepatitis A virus, and so on). The single ORF spanning virtually the entire genome encodes a large HCV polypeptide of approximately 3010 amino acid residues and gives rise to additional proteins *(see below)*. The 3' UTR region is downstream from the central ORF and spans 27–55 nucleotides. A single stem-loop structure precedes the stop codon in the NS5 region. A polyadenylated tail distal to the 3' UTR was present in the original viral isolate but has been absent in some other isolates. The overall genomic organization has led to classification of HCV as a distant member of flaviviridae (typical members: yellow fever virus, dengue fever virus, and so on), although a separate genus has been proposed for HCV.

The HCV polyprotein gives rise to multiple proteins by cotranslational or posttranslational processing using both viral and host proteases (Table 43-3). The structural proteins are thought to be processed by host-encoded signal peptidases. The core protein is highly basic, lacks N-glycosylation sites, shows RNA-binding capacity, and serves in nucleocapsid formation with roles possibly extending to a signal sequence function. Antibodies against the recombinant core protein are useful for demonstrating viral replication in cells or tissues. The E1 protein, as well as the E2/NS1 proteins, contribute to the viral envelope and contain N-glycosylation sites. These domains are hypervariable and provide one explanation for the lack of protective antibodies against the virus, as well as the difficulties in generating effective future vaccines. The E2/NS1 region corresponds to the first nonstructural protein of flaviviruses, but, unlike other viruses, the HCV protein is not secreted outside the cell. The NS2 protein is highly hydrophobic, and its function is unknown at present. The NS3 protein contains a nucleoside triphosphate-binding activity and serves as a helicase for unwinding the RNA genome during replication. In addition, the NS3 protein is involved in processing of nonstructural viral proteins via its protease activity. The NS4 protein is hydrophobic and binds to the membrane but its function is unknown. Finally, the NS5 protein serves as the viral RNA-dependent RNA polymerase and is necessary for viral replication.

No DNA intermediate is necessary for HCV replication, and it proceeds through an intermediate (–) RNA strand, which is

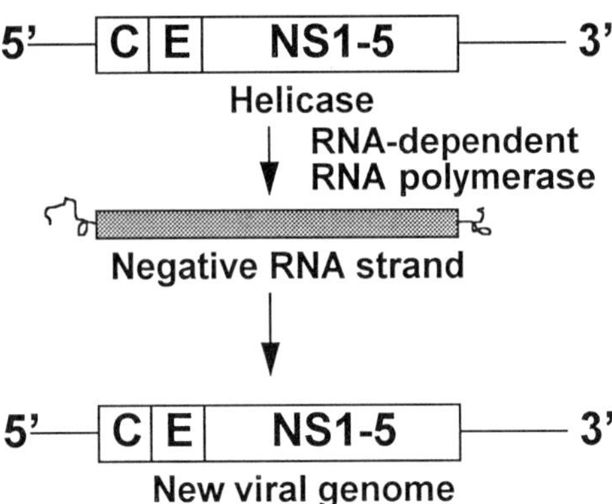

Figure 43-4 Replication of HCV does not require any DNA intermediate. The (+) strand polarity genomic RNA is transcribed by the NS5 region RNA-dependent RNA polymerase and the (–) strand RNA is transcribed again to generate new viral genomes.

reverse-transcribed to generate new viral genomes (Fig. 43-4). The presence of this (–) strand HCV RNA has been demonstrated during active viral replication. In addition, subgenomic RNA species have also been found in chronic HCV carriers, although the significance of this finding is unclear because subgenomic RNAs could simply represent defective RNAs or viral particles. During prolonged viral replication, proofreading errors may be common. In addition, selection pressures may lead to the emergence of mutated viruses. Among the hepatitis viruses, HCV shows the most extensive capability for mutating, as indicated by viral heterogeneity. As noted above, the 5' UTR region and the core region are most conserved. The least conserved portion of the virus appears to be the NS5 region between nucleotides 7400–7550. The HCV E1 and E2/NS regions are also poorly conserved.

During acute hepatitis, HCV RNA is detected in the blood within days after infection, although why the RNA should circulate without secretion of core particles is unclear. The overall level of HCV RNA may be low, although heavy viremia may be associated with 1×10^7 or more genome equivalents/mL. The diagnosis of active viral replication is usually based on demonstrating HCV RNA in serum with quantitative polymerase chain amplification reactions (PCR). The PCR systems most commonly utilize reverse transcription of the viral RNA with primers based on highly conserved 5'-end structural sequences. The reverse-transcribed cDNA is further amplified with a second set of primers representing sequences "internal" to the first set of primers and this is referred to as a "nested PCR." Modifications have been made to the PCR method by incorporation of enzymatically labeled oligonucleotides so that amplification of the oligonucleotides can be quantitated by chemical reactions. Such a branched DNA (bDNA) PCR offers greater convenience in quantitating the virus but may be 50- to 100-fold less sensitive than the nested PCR. Along with viral replication, antibodies against HCV (initially IgM class) also appear in the blood, although this may lag for several weeks. The anti-HCV is nonprotective, however, and its presence correlates with ongoing viral replication. Viral clearance is characterized by disappearance of both HCV RNA and anti-HCV.

HEPATITIS D VIRUS The presence of HDV in the liver of chronic HBV carriers was detected serendipitously during immunostaining analysis. Initially, it was thought that a new HBV antigen had been stained. However, further studies, including transmission in animals, soon showed that this was a novel, albeit defective, virus requiring HBV for some of its components. The HDV is a unique RNA virus related to plant viroids and satellite viruses, although with sufficient differences for proposed classification in a separate floating genus termed deltaviridae. Viroids contain nonencapsidated infectious RNA particles and are incapable of producing virions, whereas plant satellite viruses require a helper virus for replication and encapsidation. In similarity with these agents, HDV is unable to establish autonomous infection, requires a genetically unrelated virus (HBV), is smaller than all known animal viruses with a unique single-stranded circular structure, possesses ribozyme activity for self cleavage and ligation, and *in situ* analysis shows the presence of HDV RNA in the nucleus instead of the cytoplasm, which is a characteristic of RNA viruses. However, HDV is distinct from viroids in the ability to encode its own protein (HDAg).

The virus is prevalent worldwide, with significant endemicity in the Mediterranean basin, Middle East, South America, West Africa, and some South Pacific islands. Its significance derives from extensive worsening of disease in chronic HBV carriers, as well as its unique genetic mechanisms. Because HDV requires HBsAg for its assembly and virulence, its host range is the same, and it can infect primates, rodents, and ducks in the presence of appropriate hepadnaviruses. The virion particles are 36 nm in size with an outer envelope consisting of HBsAg, which surrounds an 1nm size nucleocapsid containing the hepatitis D antigen (HDAg), and an RNA genome of 1.7 kb (Fig. 43-1). The HDV RNA is a single-stranded circular molecule with a high G+C content (60%) and tendency for much intramolecular base pairing. In nondenaturing conditions, the RNA genome is folded into unbranched structures with terminal loops. The genomic RNA, as well as the replicative antigenomic RNA intermediate, contain multiple ORFs, but only a single HDV RNA domain is translated. The "viroid-like domain" encompasses 600–980 nucleotides toward the 5' end of the virus and includes a ribozyme sequence, whereas the remaining 75% of the ORF encodes for HDAg and constitutes the so-called "cellular domain."

Two HDV mRNA species have been identified and these contain the viroid and virusoid consensus sequences GAAAC and GAUUUU. The GAAAC sequence is essential for the ribozymal self-cleavage of virusoid RNA with similar implications for HDV. The HDV ribozyme occupies 150 nucleotides in the genome and cleaves between U and G at arbitrarily mapped 688/689 genomic positions. The HDV ribozyme shows unique properties, including remarkable efficiency and heat stability with retention of activity at up to 75°C.

The HDAg is a phosphoprotein with the capacity to bind RNA and exists as two polypeptides of 24- and 29-kDa sizes. The HDAg contains a leucine zipper-type domain, nuclear localization signal, HDV RNA-binding domain conferred by the middle one-third of the molecule, as well as a prenylation domain, which facilitates interactions with HBsAg. The HDAg is expressed in the nucleus, however, whereas HBsAg is localized in the cytoplasm. Despite this difference in their subcellular location, viral packaging is unimpeded, although it is a mystery as to how HDAg and HBsAg come together during virion assembly. During HDV replication in the nucleus of infected hepatocytes, a 0.8-kb antigenomic polyadenylated RNA appears in the cytoplasm. This RNA is 500 times less abundant than genomic RNA and is thought to encode HDAg. In vitro studies show that HDV replication does not require HBV and can occur in liver-, as well as non–liver-derived cells. Studies

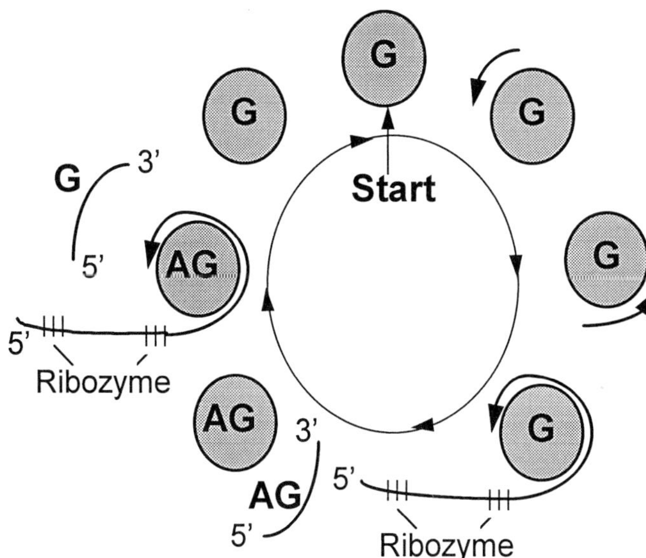

Figure 43-5 Replication of HDV proceeds through "rolling circle" mechanisms. The genomic (G) viral genome is transcribed by cellular polymerase activity and follows the circle with elongation of a linear sequence containing ribozyme domains. The endogenous ribozyme self cleaves the replicated antigenomic (AG) sequence, which circularizes. Repetition of a second rolling circle mechanism then gives rise to the genomic sequence with completion of the replication process.

in transgenic mice expressing HDV cDNA show that HDV is very well-expressed in the skeletal muscle, brain, testes, and kidney, and expressed relatively poorly in the liver. These findings are in contrast with HBV expression, which is most abundant in hepatocytes and not supported by cells of nonepithelial lineage, such as the skeletal muscle, brain, and testes, including in transgenic animals. The differences are most likely mediated by interactions between cellular transactivators and viral regulatory domains. It is interesting that HDV has not been found to replicate in extrahepatic locations in infected individuals, which must indicate its restricted distribution in the body dependent on the susceptibility of individual organs to HBV infection.

The replication of HDV utilizes a unique "double rolling circle" mechanism (Fig. 43-5). The circular HDV RNA genome serves as the initial template to generate an antigenomic RNA intermediate. The antigenome RNA is initially transcribed in a linear form and the completed transcript undergoes self-cleavage and ligation by the ribozyme activity. The circularized antigenome template is in turn transcribed to similarly originate a linear genomic RNA with cleavage by ribozyme and recircularization. In tissues supporting HDV replication, HDV RNA is present as monomers, dimers, and trimers of both strand polarities, consistent with this rolling circle model of replication. The RNA-dependent RNA replication most likely utilizes the cellular RNA polymerase II itself, because the virus does not contain any polymerase activity and can replicate independently of HBV. There is evidence to suggest that HDV usurps the cellular transcriptional machinery, such as by recruiting specific transcription factors with the aid of small HDAg, which allows the use of RNA polymerase II. In this way, the small HDAg occurs in great abundance during viral replication compared with the large HDAg. In contrast, the large HDAg serves as a dominant repressor of HDV replication by as yet poorly understood mechanisms and also helps package virions.

In acute infection, serum HDAg is often the first detectable marker, although its concentrations decline rapidly, and HDAg is rarely detected for more than 1–2 weeks. Molecular hybridization shows serum HDV RNA in approx 60% within the first week of illness. Persistence of serum HDV RNA beyond 3 weeks of the onset of acute hepatitis may predict chronicity. Antibodies to HDAg (anti-HD) appear in serum and may be either IgM or IgG class. In chronic HDV infection, IgM and IgG anti-HD are often detected for years, along with serum HDV RNA, which correlates with intrahepatic HDAg expression and viral replication. The anti-HDs are not neutralizing and similar to HCV, but unlike HAV, HBV, or HEV, development of anti-HD antibodies does not protect against reinfection.

HEPATITIS E VIRUS This is an important virus involved in epidemics of water-borne hepatitis. The first extensive epidemic ascribed to HEV was recognized in Delhi, India, in 1955, with >29,000 cases. Subsequent large epidemics have occurred elsewhere in Asia, Africa, and Central America, with the epidemic in Xinjiang region of China in 1986–1988 affecting >100,000 people. The HEV is transmitted via the feco-oral route with a high attack rate. Pregnant women suffer from severe or fulminant hepatitis E with high mortality rates, approaching 20%. The virus is encountered sporadically among travelers to endemic areas in the West, including the United States. Infection with HEV has not been identified in animals other than man, although cynomolgus macaques and tamarins are susceptible and provide valuable animal models of HEV infection. The virus does not cause chronic disease.

The HEV virions are spherical, nonenveloped particles with spikes and indentations on the surface (Fig. 43-1), which are characteristic of the calciviridae family, although HEV is thought to constitute a unique genus. The virus was first visualized by immunoelectron microscopy in stool from a patient and an experimentally infected cynomolgus macaque. The virus was subsequently cloned from RNA in infected bile and this utilized molecular hybridization screening of cDNA libraries. The HEV was found to have a 7.6-kb, single-stranded polyadenylated RNA genome. The viral genome contains three open reading frames with the ORF1 spanning 5079 bases in the 5' region and ORF2 spanning 1980 bases toward the 3' region with an additional 65 bases separating the ORF2 from the polyadenylated tail. The ORF3 spans 369 bases and overlaps the ORF1 by one nucleotide on its 5' end and ORF2 by 328 bases toward its 3' end. The ORF1 expresses nonstructural genes and contains a motif encoding an RNA-dependent RNA polymerase, as well as two well-conserved motifs associated with helicases. The structural genes are in the 3' end of the genome and expressed via subgenomic transcripts. The virus expresses two polyadenylated mRNAs of 2- and 3.7-kb sizes. These mRNAs can be detected by PCR in the liver, serum, and fecal extracts of patients with HEV.

The virus expresses type-specific epitopes, which are broadly reactive on immunotransblot analysis, in structural domains conferred by ORFs 2 and 3. There is evidence for significant regional variations in the ORF2 and 3 sequences in viral isolates obtained from different geographic parts of the world, although whether these differences are sufficient for molecular epidemiology studies needs further analysis. The hepatitis E antigen (HEAg) is recognized by immunostaining in the cytoplasm of infected hepatocytes and appears before the onset of clinically overt hepatitis. Serological tests have been developed by recombinant DNA technologies to assay for IgM and IgG class anti-HEV antibodies, although diagnosis can also be made by detecting HEV nucleic acid sequences by PCR.

HEPATITIS G VIRUS AND HEPATITIS GB VIRUSES The existence of patients with hepatitis and absence of markers for known hepatitis viruses generated ongoing interest in isolating additional viruses. In the early 1990s, three viruses were isolated from stored blood from a patient encountered in the 1950s with the initials GB. These viruses were designated GBV-A, GBV-B, and GBV-C, and assigned to the flaviviridae family. In 1995, a new RNA virus designated HGV was sequenced from the serum of a chronic HCV carrier by using an immunoscreening approach. The HGV was found to have an RNA genome of approximately 9.1 kb in size with an organization similar to flaviviridae, including HCV. The 5' end of the genome contains the structural genes and the 3' end the nonstructural genes. There are highly conserved sequence motifs for a helicase, two proteases, and an RNA-dependent RNA polymerase, although the polypeptides have not been extensively studied.

Interestingly, sequence analysis showed that HGV was essentially identical to GBV-C (95 and 86% homology at amino acid and nucleotide levels, respectively). The global homologies between HGV and GBV-A (45%), GBV-B (25%), and HCV (26%) were somewhat less striking, although similarities in their genome organization and specific regions of the genome indicated close phylogenetic relationships. The 5' UTR region was found to be highly conserved in HGV, although sequences of viral isolates in different geographic regions show differences in the capsid protein. The HGV polyprotein expressed in a recombinant vaccinia virus system was found to produce multiple peptides using protease activities, similar to that observed with HCV.

The HGV has been transmitted to chimpanzees, tamarins, and cynomolgus macaques with HGV RNA detected in serum by using reverse transcriptase-PCR. The HGV is prevalent in approximately 1–2% of volunteer blood donors in the United States, with increased prevalences in selected populations, such as polytransfused hemophiliacs (20%) and intravenous drug users (50%). However, although serum HGV RNA has been found for prolonged periods in patients with acute, fulminant, or chronic hepatitis, the significance of these findings is unclear because liver disease in HGV carriers can be blamed on other causes. By itself, HGV has not been found to cause liver disease. One view suggests that HGV is not actually pathogenic, and the issue of whether HGV and related HGBVs are even hepatitis viruses is presently under debate. The notion is that HGV is simply a harmless commensal virus.

MOLECULAR PATHOPHYSIOLOGY OF DISEASE

Interactions between virus and host factors are most important in determining whether viral persistence and chronic liver disease will occur. The significant differences in the outcomes of infection with various hepatitis viruses are summarized in Table 43-4. Anicteric hepatitis is extremely common in all cases, specially hepatitis A and E. The HAV and HEV cause only acute hepatitis and are cleared by neutralizing antibodies with lifelong immunity. Similarly, HBV may also be cleared by anti-HBs, although the situation may rarely be complicated by the emergence of "vaccine-escape" mutants *(see below)*. On the other hand, HCV and HDV induce nonprotective antibody responses. When the host immune response is impaired, e.g., organ transplant recipients, chronic renal failure, chemotherapy, and so on, viral persistence is more likely. Small viral inocula may be insufficient to elicit a vigorous immune response and also in this setting viruses may persist. The association of HBV and HCV with diseases involving circulating immune complexes (e.g., polyarteritis nodosa, membranoproliferative glomerulonephritis, aplastic anemia, cryoglobulinemias, and so on) is another example of how viral-host interactions may contribute to disease. Induction of chronic liver disease and disease exacerbations seen frequently in HBV and HCV infections are interlinked first and above all to the replicative states of the virus and the vigor of the host immune response. Both HBV and HCV are thought to cause chronic liver injury arising from activation of the cellular immune response. The injury is mediated by complex mechanisms involving both cytotoxic T lymphocytes (CTL) as well as secondary cytokine-mediated events. Additional mechanisms of cell injury involve expression of injurious viral proteins, although these need further characterization.

Replicating and Nonreplicating States of Viruses These states of HBV are defined by the presence of replicative virus (serum HBV DNA+, HBeAg+/anti-HBe–, HBV DNA polymerase+, IgM anti-HBc+) or its absence (serum HBV DNA–, IgM anti-HBc–, HBeAg–/anti-HBe+). During HBV replication, hepatocytes display HBsAg and HBcAg and are surrounded by a mononuclear infiltrate containing activated lymphocytes. The HBV replication may be intermittent or persistent, at high levels or at low levels, and liver disease rapidly progresses with patients being infectious. During the nonreplicative phase, HBV DNA is negative and HBcAg is not produced. Active liver inflammation is absent and histologic evidence of HBV may be limited to "ground glass" hepatocytes or inactive cirrhosis. However, the states of replicative quiescence and activity are interchangeable. Such a change may occur in response to pharmacological interventions, such as use of glucocorticoids or chemotherapeutic agents, which increase viral replication, or spontaneously in response to unidentified stimuli. Spontaneous reactivation of HBV replication approaches an annual incidence of up to 10–35% and may lead to fulminant hepatitis, a rapid downhill course, or worsening of chronic liver disease. Nucleotide sequence analysis of HBV DNA in patients with reactivations has suggested that some episodes of reactivation represent reinfection with mutated HBV. During viral replicative states, serum HBV DNA may be found as partially double-stranded DNA, although full-length genomes and DNA:RNA hybrids may also be found. Maternal transmission is most significant for HBV, and the risk correlates with the viral replication status for both HBV and HCV. A characteristic feature of HBV is related to its integration in the host genome. In the replicative phase, HBV DNA in hepatocytes is mainly in free virion or replicating forms, and integration into host genome is not evident. In the nonreplicating phase, random integrations occur, replicative forms of free virion DNA are not found, and HBV is not secreted. In other nonpermissive infections, clusters of HBsAg-producing cells with the appearance of a focal clonal growth have been noted. In these cases, HBV has been identified in liver DNA integrated into the host genome. A mixed type of persistent infection may also occur with features of both replicating and nonreplicating infection in the same liver. In cases with impaired or blocked secretion of HBV, replicative intermediates and extrachromosomal forms may accumulate, facilitating HBV DNA integrations. It has been suggested that the region between DR1 and DR2 may facilitate HBV DNA integrations, but no consistently satisfactory mechanism has yet been identified. No specific cellular sites have

Table 43-4
Comparison of the Clinical Features of Viral Hepatitis

Features	*A*	*B*	*C*	*D*	*E*	*G*
Incubation (days)	15–50	28–160	14–160	20–120	15–60	14–30
Fecal excretion	+	–	–	–	+	–
Viremia	Transient	Prolonged	Prolonged	Prolonged	Probably transient	Prolonged
Routes of transmission						
Oral	+	–	–	–	+	–
Percutaneous	Rare	+	+	+	–	Possible
Blood Transfusion	Rare	+	+	+	–	+
Sexual	+	+	–	–	Unknown	Unknown
Perinatal	–	+	±	–	Unknown	Unknown
Age at onset	Children and adolescents	All ages, neonatal in endemic areas	All ages	All ages	Mostly children and adolescents	Adult
Rash or arthralgia	Uncommon	May occur	Uncommon	Uncommon	May occur	–
Fever	Frequent	Uncommon	Uncommon	Uncommon	Frequent	–
Waxing and waning hepatitis	–	–	+	–	–	?+
Biphasic hepatitis	Rare	–	–	+	–	–
Cholestatic hepatitis	+	–	–	–	+	–
Diagnosis of acute infection	Serum IgM anti-HAV	Serum IgM anti-HBc	Serum HCV RNA; IgM anti-HCV	Serum IgM anti-HDV; HDV RNA	Serum anti-HEV; Serum or stool HEV RNA	Serum HGV RNA
Diagnosis of chronic infection	–	Serum HBsAg; serum HBV DNA	Serum HCV RNA; anti-HCV	Serum IgM and IcG anti-HDV: HDV RNA	–	Serum HGV RNA
Frequency of fulminant hepatitis	Rare	Moderate	Rare	Moderate to high	Very high in the pregnant	–
Chronic carrier state	–	+	+	+	–	+
Hepatocellular carcinoma	–	+	+	±	–	–
Mortality during acute hepatitis	Low, worse in >40 years of age	Low	Low	May be high in superinfected chronic HBV carriers	Low; very high during pregnancy	?None
Vaccine	Yes	Yes	No	No	No	No

been found to support preferential HBV DNA integrations, although topoisomerase I, which is a nuclear enzyme, was shown to cleave open ciruclar HBV DNA at preferred integration positions and to potentially mediate DNA integrations. Nonetheless, more information is necessary to define how HBV DNA integrations occur and what their precise significance might be.

During HBV replication, all viral proteins are expressed. The cellular immune response is thought to be induced most prominently by HBcAg expression. The preS1 and preS2 proteins are preferentially coexpressed with HBcAg during viral replication. Specific cellular immune responses against HBV antigens are well-recognized. Circulating lymphocytes from chronic HBV carriers show cytotoxicity against autologous hepatocytes in vitro, which can be blocked by anti-HBs. The HBV proteins are not usually cytopathic, and liver injury is mediated by activated cytolytic T lymphocytes sensitized by HLA-restricted HBcAg expression. In contrast, HBeAg can occupy lymphocyte receptors used for binding HBcAg and provide immunological escape to the virus by preventing clearance of infected hepatocytes despite HBcAg expression. The tolerance to HBV can indeed be broken in transgenic animals by administration of activated HLA-restricted CTL, which results in clearance of hepatocytes expressing HBV antigens, as well as decrease in viral gene expression because of cytokine release. In animals, extensive cell clearance has been associated with fulminant hepatitis, recreating the situation in patients with natural infection.

The outcomes of liver disease in patients with HBV and HDV show variability, although it is unclear whether it is a result of viral factors, altered host immune response, or both. In susceptible hosts, HDV is highly infectious, and compared with HBV, its infectivity may be greater by multiple orders of magnitude. When HDV and HBV infections occur simultaneously (coinfection), HDV suppresses HBV replication and may cause a biphasic hepatitis, with the initial hepatic injury caused by HDV replication. Similarly, HDV suppresses HCV replication as well. On the other hand, when HDV infection occurs in chronic HBV carriers (superinfection), the abundance of replicative HBV intermediates, as well as HBcAg, is reduced, and peripheral markers of HBV, including HBsAg, may disappear without actual virus clearance. In the setting of superinfection, even small HDV inocula that might not cause hepatitis in the setting of HBV and HDV coinfection, may be "rescued" and become pathogenic. Chronic HBV carriers are, therefore, at specially grave risk for acquiring HDV infection, when blood products negative for HBsAg could yet contain infectious HDV. Enhanced virulence of HDV during serial passages or because of unknown factors may cause severe or fulminant hepatitis. Although in vitro replication of HDV, as well as expression of HDAg in transgenic mice, does not necessarily lead to a cytopathic effect, when HDV is efficiently replicated, each cell may contain thousands of virion particles, and toxicity may potentially arise from hijacking of cellular resources. The exclusive use of RNA polymerase II by HDV may attenuate cellular gene expression. Also, evidence has been provided for sequence similarities between HDV RNA and the 7S signal recognition particle in cells for protein translocation, which may interfere with cellular protein synthesis. Finally, immune responses involving cytotoxic lymphocytes against HDV, similar to the host immune response against HBV, may be involved in cell clearance or cytokine-mediated cytotoxicity. In patients with HIV infection or immunosuppression, HDV replication is unchanged, suggesting that immunodeficiency does not influence HDV directly, which is in contrast with increased HBV replication in such settings.

Studies of HCV in experimentally infected chimpanzees showed that HCV could be cleared rapidly, persist indefinitely with continuous replication, or replicate intermittently with variable periods of quiescence. During infection with HCV, the liver is markedly infiltrated with mononuclear cell aggregates containing B lymphocytes in the center surrounded by a network of reticular cells and another zone of various subpopulation of lymphocytes. The lymphocytes from chronic HCV carriers are cytotoxic in vitro to autologous hepatocytes, although this is not HLA-restricted. The activated lymphocytes recognize multiple viral antigens, including core, E1, and E2/NS proteins. In some, manifestations of autoimmune liver disease (liver-kidney-microsomal hepatitis) have been ascribed to molecular mimicry with HCV antigens. Similar to HBV, when HCV replication is attenuated, liver disease may be minimal. Of greater significance perhaps is the host immune response. "Healthy carriers" have been identified in whom chronic HCV infection and replication are established but have no liver disease. Disease progression may be arrested in the fortunate few responsive to interferon-α (IFN-α) with subduing or clearance of HCV replication (Fig. 43-6).

Relationship with Hepatic Oncogenesis A number of epidemiologic studies clearly established relationships between chronic viral hepatitis and HCC. The relative risk for HCC in chronic HBV carriers may be increased by up to >200-fold. Similarly, hepadnavirus infection in woodchucks, and Peking ducks is associated with increased incidence of HCC. Observations in patients, as well as experimentally infected woodchucks indicate that simultaneous infection with HDV and HBV can accelerate the onset of HCC. The association between HCC and chronic HCV infection has also been confirmed by extensive epidemiological studies. For instance, in a large Japanese study, the relative risk for HCC in patients with chronic hepatitis was increased sevenfold in HBsAg+ patients and fourfold in patients with anti-HCV.

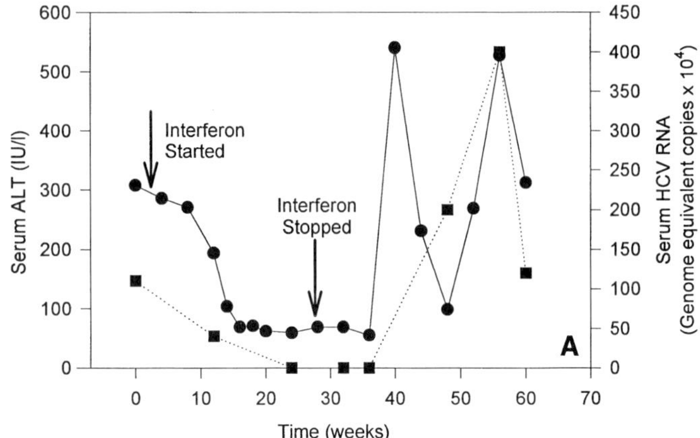

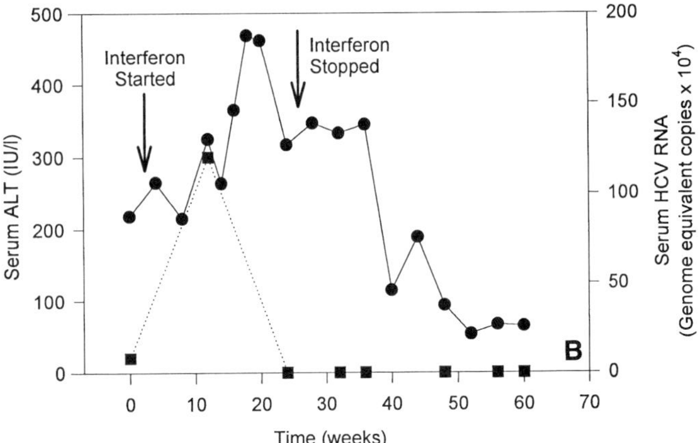

Figure 43-6 Representative responses in chronic HCV carriers treated with IFN-α. ●, serum ALT; ■, serum HCV RNA. **(A)** A patient who was found to respond to the drug during treatment but promptly relapsed with resumption of viral replication, as well as hepatic inflammation upon discontinuation of the drug. This is one of the most common responses to IFN-α treatment. **(B)** This patient showed less dramatic decrease in serum HCV RNA while on IFN-α, but the virus was cleared in a delayed manner. Most such patients clear virus temporarily, although in some sustained viral clearance may be associated with significant improvement in liver disease and decreased requirement for OLT.

The potential role of specific viral and cellular gene products in HCC has been subjected to extensive investigation. Whereas candidate genes have been identified for HBV, which integrates into the host genome, similar mechanisms have not been found for HCV, which does not integrate in the genome. The HBV DNA integrations were originally observed in HCC-derived cell lines and similar observations were subsequently made in patients. Most HBV DNA integrations occur during persistent infection in precancerous tissues. Although the majority of HBV integrations produce unique bands on DNA blot analysis, which indicates clonal expansion of cells containing integrated sequences, whether viral integrations contribute to cell transformation or clonal expansion has not been established. The integrated HBV DNA sequences vary from relatively simple to multiple rearrangements, deletions, inversions or duplications, and chromosomal translocations. Most integrations disrupt the viral genome organization, although some may contain greater than unit-length HBV DNA with apparently intact genomes. The HBV integrations have not been shown to induce insertional mutagenesis, although random HBV integrations have been found in or adjacent to specific genes, including the erb A protooncogene and cyclin A gene. Other HBV integrations have been responsible for translocations between chromosomes 17q22 and 18q11, chromosomes 17 and 7, and chromosomes 9 and 5. However, HBV does not contain an oncogene, and transfection with HBV DNA in general lacks mutagenic potential. Evidence concerning whether HBV could augment or activate specific proto-oncogenes by itself has been inconclusive, although increased c-*myc* expression has been shown in HCC in woodchucks. Alternative mechanisms concerning the loss of tumor suppressor genes, such as p53, have not provided incriminating evidence related to HBV.

Another way to examine the role of viral proteins in causing disease is by using transgenic mouse lines. In transgenic mice expressing only the small HBsAg molecule, no liver disease is observed. However, when large HBsAg is expressed in transgenic mice, the filamentous form of HBsAg is overproduced and entrapped in the cytoplasm. In the HBV transgenic mouse line designated 50-4, expression of large HBsAg leads to hepatic injury, ground glass hepatocytes, cellular degeneration, and Kupffer cell or hepatocyte hyperplasia, followed by aneuploidy, focal nodular hyperplasia or liver cancer. As ground glass hepatocytes are frequently observed in chronic HBV carriers, it is possible that similar pathophysiological mechanisms may be involved. The HBxAg has also been subjected to much study because this protein can transactivate cellular genes, which may be important in cell growth. However, evidence from three lines of transgenic mice expressing HBxAg showed that most animals did not develop HCC, although mild hepatitis, nuclear pleomorphism, focal necrosis, nodular hyperplasia, or increased mitotic activity were noted in some animals. In another transgenic line with more prolonged expression of HBxAg, there were progressive changes in the liver with eventual development of hepatic adenomas or carcinomas. Therefore, under certain circumstances, HBV gene products could interact with other cellular genes to induce oncogenesis.

Whether HDV has an impact at the cellular and molecular level in hepatic oncogenesis requires more study. One possibility is that the HDV ribozyme may alter transcriptional regulation despite a >10-fold lower affinity for heterologous DNA sequences. In addition, HDAg is a basic phosphoprotein with histone-like DNA-binding capacity, and this could also potentially modulate the activity of regulatory genes in infected hepatocytes. Additional possibilities by which HBV, as well as HCV, could induce HCC must include activation of specific cell populations under selection pressure induced by ongoing cell necrosis and regeneration and the responsiveness of emerging cell clones to specific growth factors. The evidence for the involvement of growth factors in HCC has begun to emerge. The transforming growth factor-alpha (TGF-α) may help transform liver cells by increasing cell proliferation and turnover rates, and TGF-α transgenic mice show increased incidence of HCC. In addition, coexpression of TGF-α along with c-*myc* or SV40 TAg accelerates both the onset and growth rate of HCC. Therefore, the current evidence is inconclusive with regard to any single viral gene being oncogenic for the liver. It may be that HCC arises mainly from increased cell turnover and attempt of newly emerged cells to evade virus infection. Repeated cycles of liver injury and cell proliferation could amplify selection events with the help of hepatic growth factors.

VIRAL MUTATIONS AND MUTANT PROTEINS

In general, RNA viruses are more prone to mutations because transcription with the RNA polymerase carries with it less fidelity. However, because HBV utilizes a reverse transcription step, it also shows significant mutations in its nucleotide sequence. Are there additional reasons for mutations to arise? Particularly, could mutations in viruses reflect evolutionary pressures or escape mechanisms? These tantalizing questions are unresolved, but viral mutations have been observed with greater frequency in patients with advanced liver disease, presumably related to active viral replication and robust immune responses, as well as in response to antiviral therapies, such as lamivudine treatment of chronic HBV carriers and IFN-α treatment of chronic HCV carriers.

HAV MUTATIONS Based on differences in the nucleic acid sequence, seven genotypes of HAV have been recognized and designated genotypes I–VII. The genotypes show nucleic acid diversity of 15% or more. Only four HAV genotypes are associated with human disease, with the rest being pathogenic for monkeys. The genotypes I and III have been subtyped with additional nucleic acid sequence differences (IA and B; III A and B) approaching approximately 7.5%. The value of genotyping at present concerns molecular epidemiology studies with certain genotypes being more prevalent in some geographic areas. For instance, the genotype IA is most commonly isolated in the United States. However, despite the genotype variability, HAV constitutes a single serotype and development of neutralizing antibodies after natural infection confers lifelong immunity. The neutralizing IgG class antibodies bind to a common region on the surface of the virus. Although the amino acid sequences of VP1, VP2, and VP3 regions may also exhibit differences in various substrains, these changes do not provide an immunological "escape" for reinfection in an immune host. Analysis of immunogenic domains of the virus, including the use of recombinant DNA technology, has been subject to major efforts because of its significance in the development of effective vaccines.

The HBV mutations identified involve the HBsAg, HBeAg, HBcAg, and possibly HBxAg, coding regions. The most commonly involved HBsAg region is responsible for conferring the "a" group-specific epitope, which is shared by all three small, middle, and large HBsAg molecules. The consequences of point mutations in HBsAg are substitutions in specific amino acids, such as at amino acid positions 122, 145, and others, which result in the loss of epitope conformation. As a result, the virus no longer can bind anti-HBs. The practical consequence is that in patients with anti-HBs, including after vaccination, reinfection with the mutated HBV could occur, along with chronic liver disease. A number of such cases termed "vaccine-escapes" have recently been identified with liver disease in previously immune patients. In addition, patients with mutations in the HBsAg region have been found to be younger and to present with more advanced disease, including cirrhosis, ascites, and HCC, albeit cirrhosis may be less active at such a presentation.

Mutations in the precore HBV region were found in patients that were replicating HBV without producing HBeAg. Analysis of HBV DNA purified and amplified by PCR from sera of such HBV DNA+, HBeAg–/anti-HBe+ patients showed mutations in two codons of the precore region of the ORF C, one of which leads to generation of a TAG translational stop signal. The result is a mutant HBeAg, which is no longer secreted and may be indirectly associated with liver disease of greater severity because HBeAg would no longer mask HBcAg from being recognized by activated CTL. In additional patients, precore mutant HBV has been identified in the setting of acute or fulminant hepatitis, although the evidence suggests that such mutant HBVs are not necessarily more likely to induce fulminant hepatitis in naive individuals. Nonetheless, patients with precore mutations may present more often with greater symptoms, jaundice, and hepatic inflammation. Mutations in the precore HBV regions have also been known to generate replication-incompetent viruses, which may function in a dominant negative fashion to suppress replication of the wild-type virus, and their potential use for gene therapy has recently been explored *(see below)*.

HCV MUTATIONS Genotyping by type-specific PCR; direct sequencing; restriction-fragment-length polymorphisms; DNA hybridization with type-specific probes or reverse hybridization with sub-type-specific probes; and serologic analysis with group-specific antibodies has identified multiple HCV variants. The substitution rate of HCV has been estimated at 0.9×10^{-3} per nucleotide per year. Proposals for genotype classifications are based on variations in the core region (four subtypes), NS3 region (two subtypes) and NS5 region (two subtypes). Six major genotypes are recognized with a series of subtypes. The original United States HCV isolate is designated HCV type I and is the commonest isolate (72%), followed by type II (14%), type III (6%), and type IV (1%). The type Ia HCV is most widespread in the United States, whereas type Ib is most prevalent worldwide. Mixed genotypes may also coexist (4%). The type I HCV is found in approximately 50% cases with posttransfusion HCV. Although patients with HCV types III and IV tend to be younger, viremia levels are in general similar in all genotypes, and no firm correlations have been established between genotype and disease activity. However, in Japan and Europe, type I HCV may be associated with greater viremia, compared with types 2 and 3. In addition, HCV types II and III may respond better to treatment with IFN-α as compared with type I HCV. Within individual patients, HCV may exist as a spectrum of closely related viral genomes, which is referred to as viral *quasi-species*. The development of HCV quasi-species appears to be related to increasing duration of carrier states, greater viremia, HCV type Ib, and a poor response to IFN-α treatment. The significance of viral quasi-species is unclear and this requires more analysis.

Finally, the genotypic variability in HDV has resulted in tentative identification of three genotypes. The majority of HDV infection is with the genotype I (80% nucleotide sequence similarity among strains). The genotype II was found in an isolate from Japan (75% sequence similarity with genotype I). Three viral isolates from South America constituting genotype III have shown only 60–65% sequence similarity with the other two genotypes and have been responsible for fulminant hepatitis. The presence of HDV quasi-species within individual patients have also been noted. Its RNA genome is consistent with poor fidelity during replication and a mutation rate has been estimated of 3×10^{-2} to 3×10^{-3} substitutions/nucleotide/year.

THERAPIES

The therapies are extremely limited. Patients with acute hepatitis are treated symptomatically because most cases resolve spontaneously. If fulminant hepatitis develops, intensive care management is necessary and orthotopic liver transplantation (OLT) may be lifesaving. The pharmacokinetics of drugs may be altered in the presence of liver disease and this needs careful consideration.

The availability of effective drugs to inhibit viral replication has been unsatisfactory. A variety of nucleoside analogs and other compounds have been ineffective. The largest experience has been with IFN-α, which inhibits the HBV DNA polymerase and also suppresses HCV replication. There are three kinds of interferons (α, β, and γ), which are endogenous, naturally occurring glycoproteins with antiviral, antiproliferative and immunomodulatory activities. IFN-α is derived from leukocytes, IFN-β from fibroblasts, and IFN-γ from T lymphocytes. Although IFN-α and -β are similar and share the same cell surface receptor, IFN-γ is a different molecule with a separate receptor. Most antiviral studies in HBV and HCV have been with IFN-α, as IFN-β is unstable. The mass of data concerning therapeutic trial of IFN-α in HBV and HCV is too large to discuss here. However, the drug benefits by decreasing viral replication, hepatic inflammation, and fibrosis. Patients with relatively low level of serum HBV DNA or serum HCV RNA, along with younger age, less advanced or prolonged disease, and possibly with HCV genotype other than type I are likely to benefit most. Despite the best circumstances, however, viral clearance is extremely rare, responses are most often temporary, side effects are multiple, and IFN-α therapy is expensive. Recently, lamivudine, a nucleoside analog, has shown promise in suppressing HBV replication, although rapid appearance of mutant strains in this situation is a limitation.

Searches for alternative therapies have continued and include consideration of gene therapy approaches. The use of antisense gene sequences to suppress transcription offers a novel therapeutic approach, which is most attractive because of its potential specificity. In principle, stretches of nucleotides in a reversed orientation to the native mRNA sequences will hybridize and inactivate mRNAs. The suggested mechanisms in antisense gene regulation include perturbations in splicing at exon/intron junctions, mRNA transport from nucleus to cytoplasm, initiation factor-binding for translation, assembly of ribosomal subunits at start codons, and interference with ribosome travel along coding mRNA sequences. Studies with synthetic oligonucleotides have identified potential targets for HBV antisense sequences. Recently, HBsAg expression has been inhibited in vitro with the use of antisense oligonucleotides against HBsAg coding regions. The use of receptor-mediated endocytosis to deliver oligonucleotides specifically to the liver may potentially increase local drug delivery. In addition, antisense oligonucleotides against early preS or DR2 regions were effective in vivo, although continuous infusions and very high doses were required. However, despite these successes, extensive body distribution of oligonucleotides and low cellular uptake and degradation of oligonucleotides pose problems in in vivo applications. An alternative could be to express antisense sequences using cDNAs introduced into infected cells. This has not been extensively tested because unless dominant negative targets could be identified, such antisense strategies could potentially be defeated by the stochastic requirements of inactivating each and every mRNA transcribed. It may be possible to use cDNA sequences to covalently target and repress transcriptionally active DNA domains, but this requires more study. The use of dominant negative HBcAg mutants that markedly inhibit wild-type HBV replication has also been proposed. Using cell lines supporting viral replication, expression of the inhibitory HBcAg mutants with retroviral or adenoviral vectors almost completely suppresses HBV replication.

Efforts have also been ongoing to identify suitable genetic targets for treating HCV. The conserved 5' structural sequences are particularly attractive for this purpose. If expression of HCV core antigen could be suppressed, virion assembly and replication should be significantly affected. Studies with antisense oligonucleotides complementary to the HCV core antigen have shown marked inhibition of viral replication. Similarly, if ribosomal attachment to the IRES could be inhibited, polyprotein translation should be affected, with major effects on all aspects of the virus.

Additional therapies could potentially be devised with better insights into mechanisms of viral persistence and molecular biology of specific viruses. The knowledge concerning the role of individual gene products is necessary for defining suitable genetic targets. The potential therapies could well involve novel antiviral compounds, such as the recently investigated BMS-200475, which is a proprietary guanosine analog. Whether immunological mechanisms could be harnessed for therapeutic purpose, such as by adoptive transfer or induction of antiviral CTL requires further work. Another potential mechanism could be to induce resistance in hepatocytes against viral infection. Similarly, intimate knowledge of the viral receptors would help develop novel drugs to block viral entry into cells. An understanding of viral transcriptional regulatory mechanisms would help develop novel drugs to block viral entry into cells. Also, it is clear that viruses are capable of infecting animals in a species-specific manner depending on the presence or absence of their receptors in cells. Although specific receptors responsible for internalizing hepatitis viruses into cells have not been fully characterized, further work could offer additional therapeutic targets. On the other hand, transplantation of cells or organs from another species resistant to viral hepatitis could offer means to treat patients in end-stage liver failure. Patients with chronic HCV are able to undergo OLT with meaningful survival despite reinfection of the transplanted liver, which is not the case in chronic HBV carriers. Starzl and colleagues proposed that transplantation of liver from baboons, which are not susceptible to HBV, will be successful if allograft rejection were prevented. However, in chronic HBV carriers that were subjected to OLT with baboon livers, survival was limited to only a few weeks, although the transplanted livers showed normal function. It was most likely that the baboon livers were rejected, and further work concerning xenograft tolerance is necessary if such an approach is to be seriously considered.

VACCINES Prevention is the most effective strategy for reducing the burden of viral hepatitis. Success in culturing HAV and HBV has led to the development of highly successful vaccines. The early HBV vaccines were prepared from inactivated virus or HBsAg purified from pooled plasma of HBV carriers. Recombinant HBsAg vaccines contain smaller nonglycosylated HBsAg particles (17–25 n*M*) compared with the natural vaccine and are produced commercially by expressing HBV cDNAs in yeast. The recombinant HBV vaccines have been proven to be safe and highly effective (90–95%), although adequate levels of anti-HBs require three doses during 6 months and additional boosters after several years. Similarly, effective vaccines have been developed for HAV (97% protection), although currently available vaccines use inactivated virus. Recombinant HAV vaccines based upon the P1 region or the simian HAV epitopes are under study.

Despite significant efficacy, conventional vaccines are disadvantaged by the requirement for multiple doses, several months to adequate immunity, boosters to sustain antibody response, and large amounts of antigens, which are expensive to produce. Recently, interest has developed in the use of genetic vaccines, whereby specific viral proteins are expressed by intramuscular injection of cDNAs. Such genetic vaccines against HBV and HCV have been shown in animals to efficiently express recombinant proteins and to rapidly generate high titer antibodies. The genetic vaccines have potential in converting nonresponders with no antibodies after HBV vaccination. In addition, repeated administration of genetic vaccines is being explored to induce antibody or CTL responses for clearing HBV in chronic carriers.

FUTURE DIRECTIONS AND CONCLUSIONS

Further advances in our understanding of the molecular biology of hepatitis viruses is critical for pathophysiological and therapeutic insights. The availability of effective cell culture systems for several viruses, including HCV, HDV, and HEV will greatly facilitate analysis of molecular mechanisms and vaccine development. Recent progress in culturing HCV and HEV has been encouraging. Similarly, the availability of convenient animal models will be helpful and further allow testing of novel therapies in vivo. Transgenic mouse models will be helpful in analyzing the role of individual viral gene products. Information is necessary to fill gaps in our knowledge of viral life cycles, host-virus interactions, and viral pathogenesis. Parallel advances in gene transfer vectors and mechanisms regulating expression of introduced genes will facilitate gene therapy strategies while appropriate genetic targets are identified. The current pace of molecular discoveries suggests that the next decade will bring forth enormously exciting novel tools for unraveling the pathophysiology of viral hepatitis, as well as revolutionary ways to treat infected individuals.

SELECTED REFERENCES

Alt M, Renz R, Hofschneider PH, Paumgartner G. Specific inhibition of hepatitis C viral gene expression by antisense phosphorothiote oligodeoxynucleotides. Hepatology 1995;22:707–717.

Blumberg B, Alter HJ, Visnich S. A "new" antigen in leukemia sera. JAMA 1965;191:541–546.

Bradley DW. Hepatitis E virus: a brief review of the biology, molecular virology, and immunology of a novel virus. J Hepatol 1995;22 (Suppl 1):140–145.

Chisari FV. Hepatitis B virus transgenic mice: insights into the virus and the disease. Hepatology 1995;22:1316–1325.

Dusheiko GM, Roberts JA. Treatment of chronic type B and C hepatitis with interferon alfa: an economic appraisal. Hepatology 1995;22: 1863–1873.

Feinstone SM, Kapikian AZ, Purcell RH. Hepatitis A: detection by immune electron microscopy of a virus like antigen associated with acute illness. Science 1973;182:1026–1029.

Goodarzi G, Gross SC, Tewari A, Watabe K. Antisense oligodeoxyribonucleotides inhibit the expression of the gene for hepatitis B virus surface antigen. J Gen Virol 1990;71:3021–3025.

Gupta S, Govindarajan S, Cassidy WM, Valinluck B, Redeker AG. Acute delta hepatitis: serological diagnosis with particular reference to hepatitis delta virus RNA. Am J Gastroenterol 1991;86:1227–1231.

Gupta S, Shafritz DA. Viral mechanisms in hepatic oncogenesis. In: Arias IM, Boyer J, Fausto N, Jacoby WR, Schachter D, Shafritz DA, eds. The Liver: Biology and Pathobiology. New York: Raven, 1994; pp. 1429–1453.

Guptan RC, Thakur V, Sarin SK, Banerjee K, Khandekar P. Frequency and clinical profile of precore and surface hepatitis B mutants in Asian-Indian patients with chronic liver disease. Am J Gastroenterol 1996;91:1312–1317.

Houghton M, Weiner A, Han J, et al. Molecular biology of the hepatitis C viruses-implications for diagnosis, development and control of viral disease. Hepatology 1991;14:381–388.

Howard CR. The structure of hepatitis B envelope and molecular variants of hepatitis B virus. J Viral Hepat 1995;2:165–170.

Ji W, St CW. Inhibition of hepatitis B virus by retroviral vectors expressing antisense RNA. J Viral Hepat 1997;4:167–173.

Lai MM. The molecular biology of hepatitis delta virus. Annu Rev Biochem 1995;64:259–286.

Linnen J, Wages J Jr, Zhang-Keck Z-Y, et al. Molecular cloning and disease association of hepatitis G virus: a transfusion-transmissible agent. Science 1996;271:505–508.

Offensperger W, Offensperger S, Walter E, et al. In vivo inhibition of duck hepatitis B virus replication and gene expression by phosphorothioate modified antisense oligodeoxynucleotides. EMBO J 1993;12:1257–1262.

Scaglioni P, Melegari M, Takahashi M, Roy Chowdhury J, Wands J. Use of dominant negative mutants of the hepadnaviral core protein as antiviral agents. Hepatology 1996;24:1010–1017.

Shafritz DA, Shouval D, Sherman ML, et al. Integration of hepatitis B virus DNA into the genome of the liver cells in chronic liver disease and hepatocellular carcinoma. New Engl J Med 1981;305: 1067–1073.

Starzl T, Fung J, Tzakis A, et al. Baboon to man liver transplantation. Lancet 1993;341:65–71.

van Doorn LJ. Molecular biology of the hepatitis C virus. J Med Virol 1994;43:345–356.

Wu GY, Wu CH. Specific inhibition of hepatitis B viral gene expression in vitro by targeted antisense oligonucleotides. J Biol Chem 1992; 267:12,436–12,439.

Zhang H, Chao SF, Ping LH, Grace K, Clarke B, Lemon SM. An infectious cDNA clone of a cytopathic hepatitis A virus: genomic regions associated with rapid replication and cytopathic effect. Virology 1995;212:686–697.

44 Pancreatic Exocrine Dysfunction

DAVID WHITCOMB AND JONATHAN COHN

INTRODUCTION

The pancreas is a retroperitoneal gland with both endocrine and exocrine functions. Pancreatic endocrine hormones are released by the islets into the circulation where they are essential for the regulation of intermediary metabolism (*see* Chapter 47). Pancreatic exocrine secretions (pancreatic juice), produced by the concerted action of pancreatic acinar and ductal cells, are delivered into the duodenum where they are essential for normal digestion. Different pancreatic enzymes promote the efficient digestion of complex carbohydrates, lipids, proteins, and other nutrients (Table 44-1). It is noteworthy that many of these digestive enzymes have the potential to digest components of the pancreas itself. Such autodigestion is normally prevented by several mechanisms. For example, many digestive enzymes exist in an inactive (proenzyme) form until they reach the duodenum. Other mechanisms either prevent activation of proenzymes inside the pancreas or inhibit the enzymes if they are inadvertently activated prematurely.

Pancreatic exocrine dysfunction can present clinically either as an acute illness (acute pancreatitis) or as a chronic process (pancreatic insufficiency with or without chronic pancreatitis). Inherited causes of pancreatic exocrine disease include hereditary pancreatitis and cystic fibrosis (CF). In both conditions, the responsible gene is now known and information is rapidly emerging concerning the role of the gene's protein product during normal pancreatic function and during the pathogenesis of pancreatic exocrine dysfunction.

ACUTE PANCREATITIS

BACKGROUND Acute pancreatitis is defined clinically as pancreatic inflammation characterized by the sudden onset of abdominal pain in association with elevation in blood or urine pancreatic enzyme levels. In about 80% of the cases, acute pancreatitis is mild and recovery is expected. However, in the remaining cases, acute pancreatitis is severe and can produce potentially life-threatening complications. The keys to clinical management are early recognition of severe acute pancreatitis, anticipation of complications, and prevention of recurrence.

CLINICAL FEATURES Acute pancreatitis usually causes epigastric abdominal pain of acute onset. The pain tends to be constant and may radiate to the mid-back. Vomiting occurs in 80% of cases and provides little pain relief. Abdominal tenderness with guarding occurs in half of cases but tends to be less severe than anticipated based on either the severity of reported pain or the degree of pancreatic inflammation (by abdominal CT or ultrasound), and this discrepancy results from the retroperitoneal location of the pancreas.

DIAGNOSIS In a patient presenting with typical abdominal pain, a serum amylase or lipase level more then 2.5 times the upper limit of normal strongly suggests the diagnosis of acute pancreatitis. CT with intravenous contrast is the most sensitive method of assessing the degree of pancreatic injury, pancreatic necrosis, and local extrapancreatic complications but is usually unnecessary in mild pancreatitis. In most cases, acute pancreatitis is associated with an identifiable cause, with gallstones and alcohol ingestion being the most common factors (Table 44-2). When the cause of pancreatitis is identified early, this may suggest strategies to prevent ongoing pancreatic injury and to prevent recurrence.

MOLECULAR PATHOPHYSIOLOGY A breakthrough in understanding the nature of acute pancreatitis came in 1896 when Chiari proposed that this condition represents autodigestion, rather than infection, of the pancreas. Autodigestion of the pancreas is a major threat because this organ normally produces enormous quantities of potentially dangerous digestive enzymes. To prevent autodigestion, three types of protective strategies are employed. In the first strategy, many enzymes (except amylase and lipase) are synthesized as proenzymes requiring enzymatic cleavage for activation. Activation normally occurs after the proenzymes are secreted by the pancreas into the intestinal lumen, where the intestinal brush border enzyme, enterokinase, cleaves trypsinogen activation peptide (TAP) from trypsinogen (the proenzyme) to generate trypsin (the active enzyme). Trypsin also activates trypsinogen and efficiently activates all other pancreatic digestive enzymes. Thus, the activation of trypsin in the duodenum is highly desirable as a key element in the rapid propagation of the digestive enzyme activation cascade.

In the pancreas, however, widespread activation of trypsin may be disastrous. This is especially important in humans because human trypsinogen has a propensity to autoactivate. Additional protective strategies are therefore necessary to prevent autoactivation of the digestive enzyme cascade in the pancreas. For example, within the acinar cell, autoactivation of trypsinogen and other digestive enzymes is limited by maintenance of low intracellular calcium, by maintenance of a neutral pH, and by the subcellular isolation of zymogen granules. Furthermore, because of a constant background of trypsinogen autoactivation, a limited amount of pancreatic secretory trypsin inhibitor (PSTI) is synthe-

From: *Principles of Molecular Medicine* (J. L. Jameson, ed.), ©1998 Humana Press Inc., Totowa, NJ.

Table 44-1
Pancreatic Digestive Enzymes

Proteinases
Trypsin(ogen),
Chymotrypsin(ogen),
(Pro)carboxypeptidases,
(Pro)elastases
Kalikreinogen
Pancreatic α-amylase
Pancreatic lipase
Other enzymes
(Pro)colipase I, II
(Pro)Phospholipase A2
Ribonuclease
Deoxyribonuclease I

Table 44-2
Causes of Acute Pancreatitis

Mechanical	Gallstones
	Biliary microlithiasis
	Post ERCP (multifactorial)
	Pancreatic cancer
	Anatomical predisposition
	Pancreas divisum
	Annular pancreas
	? sphincter of Oddi dysfunction
Toxins	Chronic alcohol abuse (multifactorial)
	Scorpion bite
	Medications
	Anticholinesterases
	L-asparaginase
	Azathioprine
	Dideoxyinosine (DDI)
	Estrogen
	6-Mercaptopurine
	Salicylates
	Thiazide-diuretics
	Valproic acid
	Vinca alkaloids
	Other (idiosyncratic reactions)
Hereditary	Trypsinogen gene mutation (? others)
Metabolic	Hyperlipidemia (triglycerides >1000)
	Hypercalcemia
Trauma	Blunt abdominal trauma
	Penetrating ulcer
	Postoperative/post-ERCP
Infections	Mycoplasma pneumonia
	Virus (mumps, coxsackie, CMV, HSV, HIV)
	Bacteria
	Mycobacterium avium-intracellular
Vascular	Vasculitis (e.g., connective tissue diseases)
	Hypotension (Postoperative: e.g., CABG)
	Infarction
Idiopathic	Unknown

sized with trypsinogen. If trypsin activity in the acinar cells exceeds the inhibitory capacity of PSTI, then a trypsin self-destruct mechanism is initiated in which the peptide chain connecting the two globular domains of trypsin is cut at arganine II (R117) by trypsin and mesotrypsin. Cleavage at this site permanently inactivates trypsin and other digestive enzymes with this design because the two halves of the molecule separate, thereby eliminating the active site of the enzyme. Finally, if active digestive enzymes escape from the pancreatic acinar cells into the intracellular space or plasma, they are inactivated by hepatocyte-derived α_2-macroglobulin and α_1-protease inhibitors. Thus, multiple protective strategies exist to prevent pancreatic autodigestion and acute pancreatitis.

The sequence of events initiating acute pancreatitis at the cellular level remains controversial, but several features are common to most models of experimental pancreatitis. Microscopically, zymogen granules accumulate at the apex of the acinar cells without being secreted. This functional block of secretion reflects the disruption of normal intracellular mechanisms, including the organization of microtubules and other proteins, which are necessary for exocytosis. The second feature is premature activation of digestive enzymes within the acinar cells. Although the intracellular site and mechanism responsible for digestive enzyme activation is uncertain, it seems clear that activation of these enzymes promotes "autodigestion" of pancreatic cells and initiates an inflammatory reaction.

Once an episode of acute pancreatitis is triggered, a characteristic inflammatory reaction occurs that is independent of the initiating factors. When acinar cells are damaged, they begin leaking activated digestive enzymes and other cellular elements into the interstitial space. This triggers an inflammatory response with the release of proinflammatory mediators, including interleukin-1 (IL-1), IL-2, IL-6, IL-8, tumor necrosis factor-α (TNF-α), and platelet-activating factor (PAF) (*see* Chapter 30). If pancreatic injury is mild, then the inflammatory response is self-limited and the process contained. However, if pancreatic injury is severe, then a more intense inflammatory response ensues. This inflammatory response is responsible for many of the local and systemic complications of acute pancreatitis. For example, the acute phase reaction and hypermetabolic state in severe acute pancreatitis with fever, decreased peripheral vascular resistance, and increased cardiac output are driven by cytokines. The pulmonary complications of hypoxia and adult respiratory distress syndrome (ARDS) largely develop because of the release of phospholipase A_2 from activated macrophages. Finally, the progression of pancreatic edema to pancreatic necrosis may be driven, in part, by TNF-α. In animal models of acute pancreatitis, when proinflammatory cytokines are inhibited (i.e., PAF inhibitors) or the anti-inflammatory cytokine IL-10 is given, the severity of pancreatic injury is reduced, and survival improves. Although clinical intervention at the initiation of acute pancreatitis is impossible in most cases, the severity of acute pancreatitis may be reduced by early administration of agents that modify the immune response. Specific PAF inhibitors, for example, show great promise in this regard. Thus, acute pancreatitis could be considered to progress through three general phases: an acute injury from a variety of causes, a characteristic inflammatory response that depends on the severity of injury, followed by a healing phase.

GENETIC PREDISPOSITION TO ACUTE PANCREATITIS Hereditary pancreatitis and familial hypertryglyceridemia predispose affected family members to acute pancreatitis. Hereditary pancreatitis represents a primary disorder of the pancreas, whereas patients with familial hypertryglyceridemia suffer from pancreatitis secondary to markedly elevated tryglycerides. Hereditary pancreatitis is a chronic, recurrent inflammatory disorder of the pancreas affecting family members in multiple generations. This disorder encompasses all features of acute pancreatitis and chronic pancreatitis. Thus, understanding the molecular basis of pancreatic injury in hereditary pancreatitis may provide insight into the pathogenesis of other forms of acute and chronic pancreatitis.

Hereditary pancreatitis is inherited as an autosomal dominant trait with 80% penetration and variable expression. Nearly 100 kindreds have been reported since the genetic nature of this disorder was recognized by Comfort and Steinberg in 1952. The cause of hereditary pancreatitis was determined after the gene was localized to chromosome VII and then identified by sequencing of candidate genes. This analysis showed that hereditary pancreatitis is caused by a mutation that was in a cationic trypsinogen gene, resulting in an arginine to histidine (R-H) substitution at residue 117. This R117H mutation was observed in all patients with hereditary pancreatitis and in all obligate carriers from five kindreds, but not in individuals who married into the families nor in 140 unrelated individuals.

The effect of the R117H mutation on trypsinogen regulation has been studied through the X-ray crystal structure, molecular modeling, and protein digest analyses. Taken together, these data suggest that R117 occurs in a trypsin-sensitive site in the chain connecting the two globular domains of trypsinogen, and that the R117H mutation eliminates the final control of excessive trypsin activity in the pancreas by removing the natural cleavage site of the trypsin-like enzymes (Fig. 44-1). This finding explains why hereditary pancreatitis is an autosomal-dominant disorder. Even if only half of the trypsinogen molecules resist proteolytic degradation, this is sufficient to initiate the digestive enzyme activation cascade in the pancreas and therefore express the phenotype. This also explains why attacks of acute pancreatitis occur episodically rather than continually: Attacks occur when the rate of intrapancreatic trypsinogen activation overwhelms the protective effects of PSTI.

The discovery of the hereditary pancreatitis gene has had important implications for understanding the pathogenesis of pancreatitis in general. First, it showed that intrapancreatic protease activation is sufficient to cause acute pancreatitis in humans. Second, it emphasizes the importance of trypsinogen autoactivation in humans and may explain why it has been difficult to study acute pancreatitis in animal models in which trypsinogen is more stable. Finally, it demonstrates a direct link between recurrent acute pancreatitis and chronic pancreatitis.

MANAGEMENT AND TREATMENT Mild pancreatitis tends to be a self-limited process. Treatment is supportive and includes pancreatic rest (nothing by mouth), intravenous hydration, and analgesics. Patients usually recover within 3 days and can be discharged from the hospital when oral intake is adequate to prevent dehydration.

By contrast, severe pancreatitis can result in life-threatening complications requiring aggressive management. Because these patients are at risk for sudden death, ICU admission is often indicated during the initial phase of severe acute pancreatitis. To predict which patients with acute pancreatitis are most likely to develop life-threatening complications, several prognostic schemes have been developed (*see* Table 44-3). These schemes remain useful for assisting in identification of the subset of patient with acute pancreatitis for whom intensive monitoring is most appropriate.

Early recognition is key to the management of the most common life-threatening complications of severe acute pancreatitis. Cardiovascular collapse and respiratory failure each may occur rapidly and require aggressive support. Multiorgan failure may develop as nutritional stores are depleted, and early nutritional support should be considered. Sepsis and infected pancreatic necrosis also are commonly occurring complications. Prophylactic broad spectrum antibiotics such as imipenem or cefuroxime may reduce the frequency of these serious infectious complications.

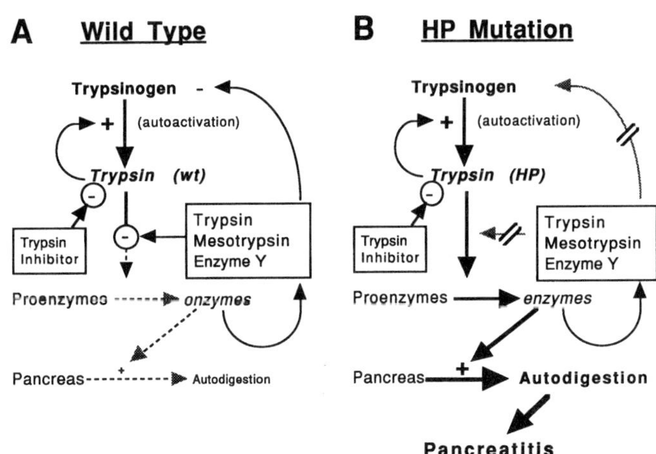

Figure 44-1 Model of trypsin self-destruct mechanism preventing pancreatic autodigestion. **(A)** Autoactivation and enzymatic activation of trypsinogen generate trace amounts of active trypsin within pancreatic acinar cells. Active trypsin is inhibited by a limited supply of trypsin inhibitor (PSTI). If trypsin activity exceeds the inhibitory capacity of PSTI, then proenzymes, including mesotrypsin and enzyme Y, are activated. These enzymes feed-back to inactivate wild-type (wt) trypsinogen, trypsin, and other zymogens. **(B)** Activation of mutant (HP) trypsin in amounts that exceed the inhibitory capacity of PSTI results in activation of proenzymes. Since the Arg 117 cleavage site for trypsin-like enzymes is replaced by His in the HP mutant trypsin, trypsin continues to activate trypsinogen and other zymogens unabated, leading to autodigestion of the pancreas and pancreatitis.

Table 44-3
Prognostic Criteria in Acute Pancreatitis

Ranson Criteria[a]	On admission
	Age >55 years
	Leukocyte count >16,000/mm^3
	Blood glucose >200 mg/dL
	Serum LDH >350 IU/L
	Serum GOT (SGOT/AST) >250 IU/dL
	At 48 h Hematocrit decreases >10%
	BUN rises >5 mg/dL
	Serum calcium <8 mg/dL
	Arterial PO2 <60 mmHg
	Base deficit >4 mEq/L
	Estimated fluid sequestration >6 L
Glasgow Criteria[b]	On Admission
	Age >55 years
	WBC count >15,000/μL
	Glucose > 180 mg/dL
	BUN >45 mg/dL
	PO2 <60 mmHg
	Albumin <3.2 g/dL
	Calcium <8 mg/dL
	LDH >600 IU/L

[a]Each factor is one point. Three or more points suggest severe acute pancreatitis

[b]Each factor is one point. Three or more points suggest severe acute pancreatitis

FUTURE DIRECTIONS Because the injury phase of acute pancreatitis is usually brief and early recognition is difficult, prevention is important. Understanding the sites and mechanisms of early enzyme activation, the factors controlling the inflammatory response, and the resulting pathologic events may be helpful in limiting pancreatic damage when pancreatic injury occurs. Now that the cause of hereditary pancreatitis is known and the gene has been cloned, transgene animal models can be developed to aid in the study of human pancreatitis, and strategies to prevent hereditary pancreatitis and other forms of pancreatitis can be developed.

Increasing knowledge of the cytokine networks are also important. PAF inhibitors that have been designed through computer simulations may be clinically useful in reducing the severity of severe acute pancreatitis if given within 24–48 hours. These advances offer new hope in the prevention and treatment of acute pancreatitis.

PANCREATIC INSUFFICIENCY

BACKGROUND Chronic pancreatitis differs from acute pancreatitis in that there is permanent loss of exocrine function, resulting in pancreatic insufficiency. This is often associated with persistent pancreatic inflammation, leading to fibrosis and atrophy of the pancreas and to dilatation and distortion of the ducts. In adults, the most common cause of chronic pancreatitis and of pancreatic insufficiency is alcohol. In children, CF is the most frequent cause of pancreatic insufficiency, and chronic pancreatitis rarely occurs.

CF is a common disease with an incidence of 1/2000 in the United States. Roughly 90% of patients with CF develop pancreatic insufficiency, and pancreatic dysfunction is such a prominent feature of CF that the disease was initially termed fibrocystic disease of the pancreas. This section will discuss pancreatic insufficiency with an emphasis on the molecular pathogenesis of pancreatic insufficiency in CF.

CLINICAL FEATURES The most important manifestations of pancreatic insufficiency result from malabsorption of incompletely digested nutrients. Malabsorption of fat and fat-soluble vitamins is usually prominent, leading to steatorrhea associated with delayed growth or weight loss. In patients with CF, meconium ileus or pulmonary symptoms often suggest the diagnosis before pancreatic insufficiency is evident. (The clinical features of CF are described further in Chapter 37.) In adults, the most common cause of pancreatic insufficiency is chronic pancreatitis resulting from alcoholism. Prominent symptoms include chronic midepigastric pain (often postprandial), weight loss (largely as a result of food avoidance), and steatorrhea. In addition, diabetes mellitus sometimes accompanies pancreatic insufficiency resulting from CF or advanced chronic pancreatitis.

DIAGNOSIS A diagnosis of pancreatic insufficiency is suggested by the combination of steatorrhea (malabsorption of more than 5% of ingested fat during a 24- or 72-h stool collection) with normal bowel mucosal morphology (by biopsy) and function (e.g., D-xylose absorption). The diagnosis is supported by a clear response to pancreatic enzyme replacement therapy. When the diagnosis is uncertain, the reference standard for documenting pancreatic insufficiency is the secretin test. In this test, the duodenum is intubated to measure the amount of HCO_3^- and fluid secreted by the pancreas in response to secretin. Pancreatic insufficiency can also be detected by noninvasive tests such as the dual-label Schilling test, benteromide test, or Sudan stain.

In children and young adults with pancreatic insufficiency, a diagnosis of CF is most commonly established by the sweat test (quantitative pilocarpine iontophoresis). When a child with pancreatic insufficiency has a normal sweat test, the differential diagnosis includes Shwachman's syndrome (an autosomal recessive condition associated with neutropenia) and rare enzyme deficiencies (e.g., congenital lipase deficiency).

In adults, pancreatic insufficiency most often results from chronic pancreatitis. The most common cause of chronic pancreatitis is alcohol, although other conditions causing recurrent episodes of acute pancreatitis may also lead to chronic pancreatitis, including hereditary pancreatitis. The diagnosis of chronic pancreatitis is usually supported by evidence of pancreatic atrophy, ductal dilatation or calcification, or a mass/pseudocyst, as detected by one or more imaging procedures (abdominal radiograph, sonogram, CT or ERCP). It is noteworthy that serum amylase, lipase and trypsinogen levels are elevated in acute pancreatitis, but that these tests are usually within or below normal limits in patients with pancreatic insufficiency or chronic pancreatitis.

GENETIC BASIS OF DISEASE The genetics of CF are presented in Chapter 37. Briefly, the inheritance pattern of CF is autosomal recessive, the gene causing CF was mapped to chromosome VII by linkage analysis, and this gene was identified by positional cloning. The protein product of this gene was named the CF transmembrane conductance regulator (CFTR), based on the anticipated function of the protein. The *CFTR* gene contains 27 exons, spans 250 kb, and encodes an integral membrane protein containing 1480 amino acids. In many types of epithelial cells, CFTR regulates ion fluxes across the plasma membrane by functioning as a cAMP-regulated Cl^- channel and as a regulator of other ion channels.

Much has been learned from mutational analyses of the *CFTR* gene. A single mutation, deletion of the phenylalanine normally in position 508 (ΔF508), accounts for roughly 70% of CF alleles. To date, over 700 additional mutations have been identified in other abnormal CF alleles, of which none account for more than 4% of CF alleles. CF patients vary widely with respect to the severity and progression of their pulmonary and pancreatic disease. In the case of CF pulmonary disease, it has been difficult to correlate subsets of CF-causing *CFTR* mutations with mild vs severe disease. This suggests that factors other than genotype play an important role in determining the progression of CF pulmonary disease. In the case of CF pancreatic disease, by contrast, clear genotype-phenotype correlations do exist. These correlations are so striking that they were recognized as part of the initial identification of the *CFTR* gene, in which it was noted that almost all ΔF508 homozygotes have pancreatic insufficiency. By contrast, pancreatic insufficiency is exceptional in compound heterozygotes with certain less common mutations (e.g., ΔF508/R117H). Thus, the *CFTR* genotype is the predominant factor determining the severity of CF pancreatic disease, whereas other factors play a greater role in determining the progression of CF lung disease.

Apart from CF, Shwachman's syndrome and hereditary pancreatitis are additional examples of inherited diseases in which a primary defect in pancreatic function leads to pancreatic insufficiency. It is not known whether genetic factors predispose to chronic pancreatitis or pancreatic insufficiency associated with other conditions such as alcoholism.

MOLECULAR PATHOPHYSIOLOGY OF DISEASE CF pancreatic disease is associated with characteristic pathologic and

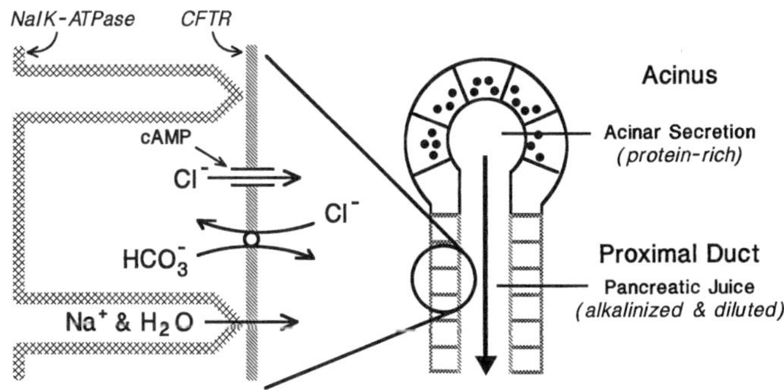

Figure 44-2 A model summarizing the role of the cystic fibrosis transmembrane conductance regulator, CFTR, during exocrine secretion by the pancreas. CFTR normally occurs at the apical membranes of the epithelial cells lining small pancreatic ducts. When activated by cAMP, CFTR allows CL^- ions to flow across the apical membrane into the duct lumen. Cl^- ions in the duct lumen lead to HCO_3^-/Cl^- exchange, and this tends to alkalinize the pancreatic juice. The secreted anions also draw Na^+ ions and H_2O into the lumen, thereby diluting the pancreatic juice. In cystic fibrosis, the absence of CFTR causes defective dilution and alkalinization of the pancreatic juice as it passes through the duct, leading eventually to obstruction of the ducts by inspissated secretions. (From Marino CR, Matovcik LM, Gorelick FS, Cohn JA. Localization of the cystic fibrosis transmembrane conductance regulator in pancreas. J Clin Invest 1991;88:712.)

physiologic abnormalities. Obstruction of the intralobular pancreatic ducts is an early pathologic event and impaired pancreatic secretion of bicarbonate is an early physiologic defect. These findings suggest that CFTR may normally function to prevent obstruction of the intralobular ducts and to promote bicarbonate secretion. These concepts are supported by available data concerning the localization of CFTR in human pancreas. The predominant site of CFTR mRNA and protein in pancreas is in the cells lining the proximal ductules. Within these duct epithelial cells, CFTR protein is predominantly detected as a component of the apical plasma membrane.

The distribution of CFTR in pancreas supports the model shown in Fig. 44-2, which postulates an important role for CFTR-associated Cl^- channels in the regulation of ductular secretion. According to this model, secretory stimuli act via cAMP to activate CFTR and thereby open Cl^- channels at the apical membrane of the duct cell. Because of the driving force provided by the Na^+/K^+–ATPase at the basolateral membrane, opening apical Cl^- channels results in Cl^- efflux across the apical membrane, leading to movement of Na^+ and water into the lumen and thereby diluting the pancreatic juice. Increased lumenal Cl^- also activates Cl^-/HCO_3^- exchange at the duct-cell apical membrane, and this alkalinizes the pancreatic juice. This model suggests that CFTR in the duct cell contributes to the normal dilution and alkalinization of pancreatic juice. In humans with CF, the ultimate result of the absence of CFTR at this site is a defect in the dilution and alkalinization of the protein-rich acinar secretions in the duct lumen, leading to the formation of protein plugs and thereby to pancreatic injury in CF.

Uncertainty remains concerning the precise mechanism by which pancreatic injury results from defective dilution and alkalinization of the pancreatic juice in CF. Dilution and alkalinization both may help to prevent precipitation of proteins as the pancreatic juice flows through the ducts. Beyond this, data from in vitro models suggest that alkalinization of the lumen of the pancreatic duct system may also be important for maintaining normal acinar cell function during exocytosis.

MANAGEMENT AND THERAPY Pancreatic enzyme replacement is the cornerstone of therapy for pancreatic insufficiency. Widely used enzyme preparations include a combination of lipase, amylase, and proteases. Because lipase is rapidly degraded at low pH, replacement enzymes are commonly administered either as enteric-coated microspheres or in combination with an H_2-receptor antagonist. Moderate enzyme doses are usually sufficient to achieve partial correction of steatorrhea with marked improvement in nutrition. Complete correction of steatorrhea is usually not possible even when very high enzyme doses are administered. High enzyme doses should be used with caution because they have been associated with colonic strictures.

Pain control is often the predominant issue in treating chronic pancreatitis. Structural causes for pain include ductal obstruction as a result of strictures, tumor, pseudocyts or stones, and a parenchymal compartment syndrome in which exocrine tissue is encased by fibrosis. Pain resulting from structural causes is typically intermittent and often occurs when serum cholecystokinin levels increase after a fat- or protein-rich meal. Medical therapy for this type of pain can include using gastric acid suppression, or pancreatic enzyme supplements. Narcotics may be added for more severe pain and may also reduce pancreatic exocrine secretion. Surgical options include procedures designed to relieve areas of ductal obstruction or fibrotic encasement of functional parenchyma. Chronic pancreatitis can also cause pain resulting from inflammation. This pain can be severe and unremitting, and surgical resection and celiac ganglion ablation are important management options.

FUTURE DIRECTIONS To date, the genes causing two forms of pancreatic insufficiency have been identified, hereditary pancreatitis and CF. For both diseases, exciting progress has been made in defining the mechanisms leading to pancreatic dysfunction. As these mechanisms become better understood, this knowledge may lead to new strategies for delaying the progression of pancreatic injury. Such strategies could benefit patients with hereditary pancreatitis or CF and might also be of benefit to patients with exocrine pancreatic injury resulting from other causes. More generally, it is noteworthy that, even though alcohol is the most common cause of chronic pancreatic dysfunction, this condition only develops in a small fraction (<5%) of alcoholics. It seems plausible that genetic factors may predispose to pancreatic disease among alcoholics, and testing this hypothesis will be an important goal of future work.

SELECTED REFERENCES

Durie PR. Inherited and congenital disorders of the exocrine pancreas. Gastroenterologist 1996;4:169–187.

Frey CF. Current management of chronic pancreatitis. Adv Surg 1995;28:337–370.

Gorry MC, Gabbaizedeh D, Furey W, Gates LK Jr., Preston RA, Aston CE, Zhang Y, Ulrich C, Ehrlich GD, Whitcomb DC. Multiple mutations in the cationic trypsinogen gene are associated with hereditary pancreatitis. Gastroenterology 1997;113:1063–1068.

Kingsnorth A. Role of cytokines and their inhibitors in acute pancreatitis. Gut 1997;40:1–4.

Kloppel G, Maillet B. A morphological analysis of 57 resection specimens and 9 autopsy pancreata. Pancreas 1991;6:266–274.

Kusske AM, Rongione AJ, Reber HA. Cytokines and acute pancreatitis [editorial]. Gastroenterology 1996;110:639–642.

Marino CR, Matovcik LM, Gorelick FS, Cohn JA. Localization of the cystic fibrosis transmembrane conductance regulator in pancreas. J Clin Invest 1991;88:712–716.

Ranson JHC, Rifkind KM, Roses DF, Fink SD, Eng K, Spencer FC. Prognostic signs and the role of operative management in acute pancreatitis. Surg Gynecol Obstet 1974;139:69–81.

Rinderknecht H. Pancreatic secretory enzymes. In: Liang V, Go W, et al., Eds. The Pancreas: Biology, Pathobiology, and Disease, 2nd ed. New York: Raven, 1993; pp. 219–251.

Sainio V, Kemppainen E, Puolakkainen P, et al. Early antibiotic treatment in acute pancreatitis. Lancet 1995;346:663–667.

Slaff J, Jacobson D, Tillman C, Curington C, Toskes P. Protease-specific suppression of pancreatic exocrine secretion. Gastroenterology 1984;87:44–52.

Whitcomb DC, Gorry MC, Preston RA, et al. Hereditary pancreatitis is caused by a mutation in the cationic trypsinogen gene. Nat Genet 1996;13:141–145.

Wyllie R. Hereditary pancreatitis. Am J Gastroenterol 1997;92:1079–1080.

45 Small- and Large-Bowel Dysfunction

DEBORAH C. RUBIN

BACKGROUND

In the past 10–15 years, the application of molecular biological and genetic techniques to research in the luminal gastrointestinal tract epithelium has led to exciting advances in several broad areas. Many enterocyte-specific genes that play critical roles in the digestion and absorption of luminal nutrients have been cloned and sequenced. Their chromosomal localization, structure, and regulation of expression have been at least partially characterized. These studies have provided the groundwork for understanding the pathophysiology of several rare but well-described genetic disorders of small intestinal transport and have begun to clarify the mechanisms underlying more common gastrointestinal problems, such as lactase deficiency. In addition, sophisticated genetic and molecular techniques are finally being applied to the study of complex, multifaceted disorders, such as the inflammatory bowel diseases (IBDs), providing novel animal models to be used to understand their pathophysiology and to design new therapies. Of great potential clinical importance are the identification of a disease-susceptibility locus for Crohn's disease and of very specific susceptibility loci for celiac sprue. This chapter will attempt to summarize the important molecular and genetic developments relevant to the study of inflammatory bowel disease, celiac sprue, lactase deficiency, glucose-galactose malabsorption, and abetalipoproteinemia as several prominent examples of how molecular techniques can help advance the practice of gastrointestinal medicine.

INFLAMMATORY BOWEL DISEASE

CLINICAL FEATURES The inflammatory bowel diseases (IBDs) include Crohn's disease and ulcerative colitis. These are chronic inflammatory disorders of the gastrointestinal tract that are manifested by symptoms of diarrhea and abdominal pain. Although the clinical presentation may be quite similar, important differences in their underlying pathophysiology result in unique complications and long-term sequelae. In ulcerative colitis, the colon is the primary organ that is affected, but Crohn's disease can occur in any part of the gastrointestinal tract from mouth to anus. Ulcerative colitis is characterized by a predominantly superficial mucosal inflammation. In Crohn's disease, the inflammatory process is transmural and granulomatous, affecting all layers of the gastrointestinal tract, from mucosa to serosa (Table 45-1).

From: *Principles of Molecular Medicine* (J. L. Jameson, ed.), ©1998 Humana Press Inc., Totowa, NJ.

The etiology of these disorders is presently unknown. Recent studies of mice with targeted disruption of several cytokine or T-cell receptor genes, or of chimeric transgenic mice with disruption of the N cadherin gene, have provided promising new models of inflammatory bowel disease. These novel systems may help clarify the etiology and pathogenesis of these disorders and aid in the design of new therapeutic agents.

EPIDEMIOLOGY There are marked geographic differences in the incidence of IBD. The highest incidence rates are found in northern Europe and North America among Caucasians, ranging from 2–10 per 100,000. IBD appears to be more common in Jews of European or Ashkenazic origin, but not of Sephardic (African and Mediterranean) origin. The peak age of onset is from 15–25 years, and a second peak between 55–65 years of age has been suggested. There is a slight female predominance in the prevalence of both disorders. Although the disease is most common in Caucasians, the incidence in African Americans appears to be increasing. Cigaret smoking increases the risk of Crohn's disease but appears to be protective in ulcerative colitis.

CROHN'S DISEASE

Location of Disease, Signs, and Symptoms Crohn's disease can affect any part of the gastrointestinal tract. The most frequently involved sites are the ileocolon (40%), the small intestine alone (30%), or the colon alone (25%). Other regions of the gastrointestinal tract may also be involved, including the mouth, esophagus, and stomach. Anal involvement is common. Inflammation may involve the bowel in a segmental fashion, with "skip" areas of normal small and large intestine intermixed with patches of inflamed mucosa. Symptoms resulting from the inflammatory process include abdominal pain (especially in the right lower quadrant as a result of to terminal ileal involvement) and diarrhea. Other frequent symptoms include fever, weight loss, and malaise. A variety of extraintestinal manifestations including arthritis, uveitis/iritis, and skin diseases, such as erythema nodosum and pyoderma gangrenosum, are associated with inflammatory bowel disease. Signs of active Crohn's disease include right lower quadrant abdominal fullness, mass or tenderness, and a chronically ill appearance.

There are multiple causes of diarrhea in Crohn's disease. Enhanced secretion occurs in the small bowel and colon resulting from inflammation. Patients with ileal disease or ileal resection may malabsorb bile salts, since specific receptors and transport proteins are expressed only in the ileum. Unabsorbed bile acids then enter the colon where they produce a secretory diarrhea. Extensive terminal ileal involvement or resection of greater than

Table 45-1
Comparison of Crohn's Disease and Ulcerative Colitis

Clinical feature	*Crohn's disease*	*Ulcerative colitis*
Site of involvement	Entire gastrointestinal tract	Colon only
Pathology	Transmural granulomas	Mucosal inflammation
Extraintestinal manifestations	Skin Eyes Joints	Skin Eyes Joints
Complications	Strictures, fistulas, abscesses	Strictures, colon cancer, toxic megacolon
Treatment	Surgical removal of diseased segments avoided because of disease recurrence	Surgical removal of diseased colon is curative

100 cm of ileum results in fatty acid diarrhea from excessive loss of bile salts that cannot be replaced by enhanced hepatic production. Fat malabsorption may also result from bacterial overgrowth because of strictures of the small bowel, leading to deconjugation of bile salts. Crohn's disease has also been associated with lactase deficiency, resulting in maldigestion of milk and milk products. Undigested lactose then produces an osmotic diarrhea.

Complications The transmural inflammatory process characteristic of Crohn's disease leads to many complications.

Fistulae Inflammation may lead to ulceration through all layers of the bowel, resulting in the formation of fistulous tracts. Fistulas can form between the gut and any neighboring organ. Enteroenteric, enterocolonic, and enterocutaneous fistulas are frequently found in Crohn's disease. Less common are enterovesicular and enterovaginal fistulae.

Strictures Strictures of the small or large bowel may result from chronic inflammation and can lead to intestinal obstruction. If severe and unremitting despite conservative management, strictures may require surgical resection to permit the continuation of normal enteral nutrition.

Perforations and Abscess Formation Perforation of the small bowel or colon may precipitate the onset of an acute abdomen requiring immediate surgical intervention. Alternatively, perforations and fistulas may produce intraabdominal abscesses, another common complication of Crohn's disease. Abscesses may occur anywhere in the peritoneal cavity and must be drained to control sepsis.

Malnutrition and Malabsorption Patients who have undergone surgical resection or who have extensive small bowel inflammation, fistulas, or strictures may suffer from short bowel syndrome with excessive diarrhea, volume loss, and malabsorption. These patients frequently require treatment with total parenteral nutrition (TPN) to maintain a normal nutritional and fluid and electrolyte status. As indicated above, loss of functional ileum may lead to fat malabsorption. Because of these complications, surgery is avoided whenever possible.

Nephrolithiasis Kidney stones are most frequently composed of oxalate and are found in patients with ileal disease and fat malabsorption. Calcium, which normally binds to oxalate to produce insoluble calcium oxalate, is instead bound by fatty acids. This leads to the formation of sodium oxalate, which is readily absorbed through the colon, leading to hyperoxaluria and stone formation.

ULCERATIVE COLITIS

Location of Disease, Signs and Symptoms Ulcerative colitis is characterized by a continuous mucosal inflammatory process affecting the colon. Inflammation may be confined to the rectum alone (ulcerative proctitis), may extend from the rectum to the left colon, or may involve the entire colon. Unlike Crohn's disease, at least part of the rectum is always involved, and the inflammatory process is continuous in affected areas (i.e., there are no skip regions). Abdominal pain, diarrhea, and gastrointestinal bleeding are common clinical presentations of this disorder. Anorexia and weight loss are occasionally present but are not common. Unlike Crohn's disease, which frequently follows a low-grade, chronic course, ulcerative colitis patients may present with fulminant colitis necessitating urgent colectomy. Physical findings include abdominal tenderness and grossly bloody stool on rectal examination. In fulminant cases, abdominal distention, massive hemorrhage, fever, and tachycardia may be present.

Complications Toxic megacolon may occur in patients with acute fulminant colitis. The colon becomes atonic and dilated because of severe inflammation and can perforate if untreated. Toxic megacolon requires emergent surgical consultation and in many cases, removal of the colon. Strictures may result from chronic inflammation. Colon cancer is an important complication of long-standing ulcerative colitis. Although the precise risk of colon cancer is not clear, it is increased in patients with disease for greater than 8–10 years and is higher in patients with pan-colitis compared to left-sided colitis alone. To prevent colon cancer, either prophylactic colectomy or yearly colonoscopic screening for dysplasia/cancer is recommended, depending on the patient's preference and disease activity. A recent important advance has been the development of the ileoanal anastomosis. Instead of an ileostomy, bowel continuity is maintained by creating an ileal reservoir in place of the rectum. This has led to greater acceptance of surgical options in the treatment of ulcerative colitis.

EXTRAINTESTINAL MANIFESTATIONS There are multiple extraintestinal manifestations of IBD, including arthritis, skin and ocular diseases, liver involvement, kidney stones, and osteoporosis. The arthritic complaints include colitic arthritis, ankylosing spondylitis, and sacroiliitis. The large joints are generally involved in colitic arthritis. Arthritic complaints generally respond to adequate treatment of the bowel disease. Symptoms resulting from ankylosing spondylitis and sacroiliitis may be severe and more refractory to treatment. Skin manifestations of IBD include pyoderma gangrenosum and erythema nodosum. Ocular diseases include uveitis and episcleritis. Liver involvement may manifest as sclerosing cholangitis or pericholangitis. Cholesterol gallstones occur in Crohn's disease if there is ileal involvement or after resection, resulting in bile salt malabsorption. Finally, kidney stones may form in patients with small intestinal Crohn's disease and fat malabsorption and are usually composed of calcium oxalate or urate. Osteoporosis may result from chronic fat malabsorption, leading to calcium and vitamin D deficiency, and from chronic corticosteroid therapy.

DIAGNOSIS

History and Physical Exam A history of bloody diarrhea, abdominal pain, and fever should lead to a strong suspicion for ulcerative colitis. Symptoms in Crohn's disease are frequently more indolent and chronic, including intermittent diarrhea and fevers, abdominal pain, and weight loss. Physical findings in ulcerative colitis may include abdominal tenderness, and in fulminant disease, distention, decreased bowel sounds, and an acute abdomen. In Crohn's disease, abdominal tenderness and an inflammatory abdominal mass may be present, particularly in the right lower quadrant. The perianal and perirectal regions should be examined for signs of fistulization and abscess. Signs of extraintestinal disease, including arthritis, ocular inflammation, and skin nodules or ulcers may be detected.

Laboratory and Pathologic Examinations There is no specific laboratory test that is diagnostic of ulcerative colitis or Crohn's disease. An elevated white blood cell count can be seen in active disease or may be an indicator of sepsis as a result of perforation or abscess formation in Crohn's disease. Anemia may result from gastrointestinal bleeding or nutrient deficiencies (e.g., vitamin B_{12} from ileal Crohn's disease, decreased iron absorption in duodenal Crohn's disease). Erythrocyte sedimentation rate may be elevated in active disease. Nutritional parameters such as blood total protein and albumin levels may also be deranged in Crohn's disease.

Pathologic specimens (endoscopic biopsies or surgical resection) may reveal evidence of active inflammation. A characteristic finding of colitis are crypt abscesses, in which neutrophils invade the crypts. Granulomas are more characteristic of Crohn's disease. Crypt atrophy and distortion are also seen, as is acute and chronic inflammation with lymphocytes and eosinophils, and mucin depletion. Ulceration of the mucosa occurs in ulcerative colitis, but the presence of transmural inflammation is most characteristic of Crohn's disease.

Radiological and Endoscopic Studies Evaluation of the mucosa for the presence of active disease can be achieved by endoscopic examination. In patients with symptoms of colitis, colonoscopy may aid in the initial diagnosis and is required to determine the extent of disease activity. The mucosal surface is observed for the presence of erythema, edema, granularity, friability, and ulceration. The extent of colonic involvement may help differentiate Crohn's disease from ulcerative colitis. The presence of skip areas, in which normal mucosa is intermixed with inflamed mucosa, is most characteristic of Crohn's disease, whereas, in ulcerative colitis, inflammation is continuous. During colonoscopy, the terminal ileum may be entered and evaluated for involvement by Crohn's disease. Direct visualization of the upper gastrointestinal tract by routine upper endoscopy or small-bowel enteroscopy may also help to establish the presence of Crohn's disease.

Radiological examination is an important part of the diagnostic evaluation of patients with IBD. Contrast studies are useful for detecting strictures and fistulas, as well as for assessing disease activity in regions of the small intestine that are inaccessible to routine endoscopy. Patients with ulcerative colitis may demonstrate typical findings on barium enema, including straightening and shortening of the colon, loss of normal haustrations, and inflammatory polyps or malignancy. Mucosal detail is more difficult to assess with radiography; endoscopic examination is generally preferred. In patients with very active colitis, radiographic examination is avoided because of the fear of inducing toxic megacolon as a result of the introduction of air and barium. Similarly, colonoscopic testing is performed with caution and usually in a limited manner. Computerized axial tomographic scanning is an important diagnostic modality, particularly for abscess detection in Crohn's disease. If accessible, CT-directed drainage of abscess collections may be performed.

Genetic Basis Genetic factors have been suggested to play a role in the pathogenesis of IBD because of an increased incidence in families, specific ethnic groups, and in twins. Approximately 10–20% of patients with IBD have a family history, and the risk for first-degree relatives to develop IBD is 2–5%. Twin studies indicate that monozygotic twins have a higher concordance rate than dizygotic twins. The complex clinical manifestations of these diseases suggest a heterogeneous genetic basis, confirmed by heterogeneity in HLA class II and antineutrophil cytoplasmic antibody markers in ulcerative colitis. Since inflammatory T cells appear to play a role in IBD pathogenesis, attention has focused on MHC class II genes. By using a PCR-sequence-specific oligonucleotide approach to type HLA class II DRB1, DRB3, DRB4, and DRB5 loci in patients and matched controls, a positive association was observed with the HLA-DRB3*0301 allele in Crohn's disease, but not in ulcerative colitis. Yet, a recent study of two families with Crohn's disease has identified a disease-susceptibility locus on chromosome 16, centered around loci D16S409 and D16S419. A nonparametric two-point sibling-pair linkage method was utilized. This region of the genome contains several genes that may be involved in the pathogenesis of Crohn's disease, including CD11 integrin cluster, CD19, sialophorin, and the IL-4 receptor. However, the relative risk for siblings of patients with Crohn's disease with this locus was estimated to be 1.3, indicating that surely there are other susceptibility loci.

Molecular Pathophysiology The etiology of the IBDs is presently unknown. One widely accepted hypothesis is that IBD results from an abnormal host immune response to normal gut components such as microflora, nutrients, or cellular constituents. This may also be accompanied by a primary defect in gut permeability that allows antigens to nonspecifically "leak" through the mucosa and thereby stimulate an inflammatory response. The possible role of an infectious agent such as Mycobacterium paratuberculosis has also been postulated.

The search for the underlying host immune defect(s) has been the subject of much research. A variety of immune abnormalities have been identified in patients with IBD but the molecular basis has not yet been clarified. However, recent studies using embryonic stem cell techniques to selectively delete immune mediator and other genes have produced novel animal models of IBD that have provided some insight into the molecular pathophysiology.

Disruption of Immunoregulatory Genes or N-cadherin Leads to IBD in Mice The specific role of a gene can be determined in the whole animal in "loss of function" experiments that utilize embryonic stem-cell techniques. Mutations in specific target genes can be created in these cells to delete the gene or produce a sequence that encodes a nonfunctional protein. The mutated stem cells are injected into a mouse blastocyst and grown in a host mouse. Heterozygous mice are then backcrossed to create homozygous mutants.

In this manner, targeted deletion of various immune mediator genes has been performed. Interestingly, when IL-2, IL-10, major histocompatibility class II or T-cell receptor α or β genes are deleted, gross inflammation of the bowel is produced in mice. Similarly, a dominant negative N-cadherin mutation, specifically targeted to intestinal cells by a gut-specific promoter, produced a marked depletion in E-cadherin expression in the crypt and villus and resulted in inflammation of the small bowel.

IL-2 is produced by activated T cells and is an important regulator of immune responses. It increases T cell proliferation, leads to differentiation of B cells, and activates macrophages, NK cells, and LAK cells. IL-10 is produced by T helper cell subset 2, macrophages, keratinocytes, Ly-1 B cells, and thymocytes. It increases MHC class II expression on B cells and suppresses macrophage activation in vitro. IL-10 inhibits IL-1, IL-6, and tumor necrosis factor-α (TNF-α) production by activated macrophages.

Deletion of the IL-2 or IL-10 gene produced inflammation of the intestine, but with different clinical features. Deletion of IL-2 led to colonic disease, with diarrhea, rectal prolapse, and bleeding. Pathological examination of the colon showed crypt abscesses, ulceration, goblet-cell depletion, and epithelial dysplasia. MHC class II expression, normally limited to the small intestine, was seen in the colon. In contrast, deletion of IL-10 led to a chronic enterocolitis affecting the entire gastrointestinal tract, with growth retardation and iron deficiency anemia. Mucosal inflammation, with villus loss, mucosal gastrointestinal erosions, and crypt hyperplasia were found in small intestine and colon. MHC class II expression was aberrantly enhanced in small bowel and colonic epithelium. The onset of disease in the majority of mice was relatively rapid; by 3–4 weeks, growth retardation was noted.

Interestingly, in both models, maintenance in a pathogen-free environment greatly diminished the intestinal inflammation. IL-10 mice had disease limited to the proximal colon only, and IL-2 mice were disease-free. A third model of inflammatory bowel disease was generated in T cell receptor α or β mutants, which lack αβ T cells. These mice developed colonic inflammation but no diarrhea or bleeding.

Not only can immune cell defects produce intestinal inflammation, but disruption of the protective epithelial barrier may also lead to IBD. Recent studies focused on the function of E-cadherin in the intestine. A dominant negative N-cadherin mutant was linked to an intestine-specific promoter and thus was selectively disrupted in the gut, in villus as well as crypt cells. This resulted in markedly decreased expression of E-cadherin, with gross disruption of the epithelial barrier and severe mucosal inflammation. The small intestine was selectively affected, with lymphoid hyperplasia, blunted villi, cryptitis and crypt abscesses, mucosal ulcerations, and eventually adenoma formation.

Although these models of IBD are diverse, they support several hypotheses regarding the etiology of these disorders. Disruption of the epithelial barrier can lead to intestinal inflammation, even in the presence of a normal immune system. Selective immune defects that lead to the unopposed action of B cells can produce inflammation of the gut. Also, the intestine is clearly vulnerable to inflammation because of constant external antigen exposure and the presence of luminal substances.

MANAGEMENT

Medical Therapy (Table 45-2) Since the underlying cause of IBD is still unknown, therapy is presently directed toward controlling the intestinal inflammatory response. One of the mainstays of treatment are oral and enema compounds containing 5 aminosalicylic acid (5-ASA), available in several different forms. These compounds are effective as single agents in the treatment of mild to moderate ulcerative or Crohn's colitis. They are used in conjunction with corticosteroids in the treatment of severe disease. Although their precise mechanism of action is unknown, these drugs are thought to inhibit leukotriene synthesis via their inhibition of neutrophil lipoxygenase, particularly LTB4. Sulfasalazine was the first of these agents and consists of 5-ASA bound to a sulfapyridine residue to prevent its premature absorption in the small intestine. Colonic bacteria are required to release the 5-ASA component. However, many side effects result predominantly from the sulfapyridine component, including dose-related effects, such as headache, nausea, vomiting, anorexia, fever, and rash. Idiosyncratic, hypersensitivity responses include rash, hemolytic and aplastic anemia, and agranulocytosis. Also, long-term usage in young men is frequently limited by its adverse effects on sperm count and morphology. Therefore, several compounds have been formulated containing 5-ASA alone, with various modifications to facilitate its delivery to the small intestine and colon, or preferentially to the ileum and colon, without excessive systemic absorption prior to reaching its preferred site. These include Pentasa, Asacol, and Dipentum. Pentasa and Asacol are released by pH-dependent mechanisms. Pentasa is an ethylcellulose-coated form of mesalamine (5-ASA) that is released throughout the small intestine and colon. Asacol is coated with an acrylic-based resin that dissolves at pH7.0 or greater, facilitating its release only at the terminal ileum and colon. Dipentum consists of two 5-ASA molecules linked by an azo bond that is cleaved in the colon. These newer formulations clearly have fewer side effects than sulfasalazine and thus have led to an expanded pharmacologic armamentarium. Mesalamine in enema form (Rowasa enemas) is a valuable treatment for ulcerative proctitis.

Table 45-2
Medical Therapy for IBD

5-Aminosalicylic acid compounds
Sulfasalazine (Azulfidine)
Mesalamine
Oral (Pentasa, Asacol, Dipentum)
Enema (Rowasa)
Suppository (Rowasa)
Glucocorticoids
Oral
Enema
Suppository
Intravenous
Antibiotics
Metronidazole
Immunosuppressive agents
Azathioprine
6-mercaptopurine
Cyclosporine
Oral
Enema
Intravenous
Methotrexate
Intramuscular
Oral

Corticosteroids are important in the therapy of moderate to severe IBD because of their broad anti-inflammatory actions. Corticosteroids are used in the treatment of active ulcerative colitis as well as Crohn's disease of the small and large bowel. Because of the numerous side effects attendant with chronic glucocorticoid usage, long-term therapy for IBD is avoided. There are no data supporting its use in maintaining disease remission, unlike 5-aminosalicylate-containing compounds in colitis.

Antibiotics are critical for the treatment of infectious complications of Crohn's disease, such as sepsis, abscess formation, and small-bowel bacterial overgrowth. Metronidazole has been used successfully to treat perianal disease and colonic Crohn's disease.

Immunosuppressive agents such as azathioprine and its metabolite, 6 mercaptopurine, are used in Crohn's disease, and to a lesser extent in ulcerative colitis, for steroid-dependent and poorly controlled patients. Treatment is generally begun in patients who cannot be tapered from corticosteroids because of recurrent symptoms and who have major side effects from them, such as osteoporosis, hypertension, cataracts, or glucose intolerance. Alternatively, immunosuppressive agents may be added to treat the patient with refractory disease inadequately treated with corticosteroid and 5-ASA compounds. Immunosuppressive agents are also used in patients with ulcerative colitis and refractory proctitis, but less commonly.

Less-well-studied, but presently being actively investigated for use in severe ulcerative colitis and Crohn's disease, are methotrexate and cyclosporine. There are data that support the use of intravenous cyclosporine for severe colitis as a last-ditch medical effort to avoid surgical intervention. Methotrexate may be used as an alternative medication for steroid-dependent patients, but its efficacy is still unproved.

Surgical Treatment In fulminant ulcerative colitis that is refractory to medical therapy, total colectomy may be unavoidable. In addition, surgical resection may be required for corticosteroid-dependent patients with ulcerative colitis who have major steroid-induced side effects. Colectomy may also be performed in patients with colonic dysplasia or carcinoma, or prophylactically to prevent colon cancer in patients with >10-year history of active ulcerative colitis. As an alternative to prophylactic colectomy, yearly colonoscopic screening for colon cancer may be performed after 8–10 years of disease. The major problems with this approach are that cancers in ulcerative colitis arise from flat mucosa and therefore may be missed, and accurate grading of dysplasia is difficult. Colectomy is curative in ulcerative colitis, and ileoanal anastomotic procedures eliminate the need for an ileostomy. This surgical procedure is not an option for patients with Crohn's disease, since there is a high incidence of recurrent disease in the ileal pouch leading to diarrhea, bleeding, pain, severe malfunction of the pouch, and, eventually, the need for revision. In addition, surgery is not curative in Crohn's disease since it recurs commonly, in all parts of the intestinal tract. Therefore, the approach to patients with Crohn's disease is very cautious, and surgical intervention is avoided whenever possible. However, limited resection is often performed to relieve obstruction as a result of strictures, to repair perforations, or for abscess drainage.

Future Directions Targeted gene knockout studies in mice and attempts to localize a susceptibility locus for Crohn's disease have been very exciting developments in the past several years. The novel mouse models should prove useful for elucidating the pathogenesis of these disorders and for designing more effective therapies. The identification of the gene(s) that are responsible for the familial risk of IBD will undoubtedly continue to be a major research focus.

CELIAC SPRUE

CLINICAL FEATURES Celiac sprue is a chronic disease of the small intestinal mucosa resulting from exposure to dietary proteins contained in wheat, rye, and barley. The alcohol-soluble component of wheat-derived gluten, or gliadin, and similar proteins derived from rye, barley, and oats, are toxic to the mucosa of susceptible individuals. In classic celiac sprue, the small bowel demonstrates complete villus atrophy and marked crypt hyperplasia, resulting in malabsorption and diarrhea. It is clear that specific host genetic factors are required in combination with exposure to gliadin to damage the epithelium. Linkage to histocompatibility antigen loci has been recognized for many years. Recent progress has been made in identifying specific peptide motifs in gliadin that are responsible for the adverse small bowel effects, in defining the features of the immune response, and in clarifying the genetic basis of celiac sprue.

CLINICAL PRESENTATION Patients with celiac sprue exhibit a broad spectrum of clinical presentations. In children, the disease tends to occur in the first 3 years of life. In adults, the peak incidence is in the third decade, but may occur at any age. In the classic clinical presentation, extensive loss of normal villi throughout the small intestine leads to gross malabsorption and steatorrhea, severe weight loss, wasting, multiple vitamin deficiencies, and abdominal distention. The vitamin deficiencies may lead to anemia (B12, folate, iron) or a bleeding diathesis (vitamin K). Neurologic symptoms such as peripheral neuropathy and paresthesias are also common. In other cases, patients may be asymptomatic or complain only of mild abdominal discomfort, malaise, bloating, and diarrhea. Those with more patchy proximal intestinal involvement may present simply with iron or folate deficiency or osteomalacia. Relatives of patients with celiac sprue who are screened for the disease often have mild illness or may be completely asymptomatic.

Celiac sprue is frequently associated with other disorders. Dermatitis herpetiformis is characterized by severely pruritic papulovesicular lesions of the skin. The majority of afflicted patients show intestinal biopsy findings characteristic of celiac sprue. These patients are often only mildly affected by the gut lesion and may even be asymptomatic. Isolated nutrient deficiencies may be the only clinical manifestation. Both the intestinal and skin lesions resolve with gluten withdrawal.

Other diseases that are associated with celiac sprue include insulin-dependent diabetes mellitus (50-fold higher incidence of celiac disease in patients with diabetes), thyroid disease, and selective IgA deficiency, which share similar HLA haplotypes. Complications of celiac sprue include the development of T-cell lymphoma or other gastrointestinal malignancies. Ulcerative jejunoileitis is a serious complication resulting in ulceration and stricture of the small bowel with bleeding, perforation, and obstruction. Finally, patients may become refractory to removal of gluten from the diet and may require treatment with corticosteroids or immunosuppressive agents.

EPIDEMIOLOGY Celiac sprue is most prevalent in Caucasians, particularly in Northern Europe. The highest prevalence has been reported in Ireland at a frequency of 1:300 but the more typical incidence in Europe is 1–2/10,000 population. Asians from India and Pakistan are also frequently affected, but the disease is rare in Japanese, Chinese, and African peoples. A study of Minnesota residents who were symptomatic and had celiac sprue documented by biopsy and response to a gluten-free diet revealed an incidence of celiac sprue of 1.2/100,000 person-years in the United States, with a prevalence of 21.8/100,000. Recent studies have indicated a decrease in the prevalence of childhood celiac sprue in several European countries, perhaps as a result of changes in feeding or other unidentified environmental factors.

DIAGNOSIS A valuable test for the diagnosis of celiac sprue is the small intestinal biopsy. Forceps biopsies of the duodenum or proximal jejunum can be obtained during routine upper endoscopy, or peroral capsule biopsy techniques may be used. Biopsy should be performed prior to the initiation of gluten withdrawal and can also be repeated after removal of gluten from the diet to document an adequate response. Typical findings on biopsy are absence or atrophy of villi, crypt elongation and hyperplasia, and increased immune cell infiltrate. There is a marked increase in intraepithelial lymphocytes and infiltration of the lamina propria with lymphocytes, eosinophils, and macrophages. Since the biopsy findings in celiac sprue are not unique and can be seen in tropical sprue, lymphoma, viral or eosinophilic gastroenteritis, common variable immunodeficiency, or parasitic infection, the clinical response to removal of gluten in conjunction with biopsy is critical for definitively making the diagnosis. Rechallenge with gluten and rebiopsy is rarely recommended (except in equivocal cases).

Antibody tests have also been used in conjunction with small bowel biopsy to confirm the diagnosis. Serum antigliadin antibodies are positive in approximately 90% of patients with untreated sprue but are also found in other disorders such as sarcoidosis and rheumatoid arthritis. Antiendomysial antibodies, which are directed against extracellular matrix components, are also elevated in patients with histologic abnormalities on biopsy, detecting >95% of untreated patients. Antireticulin antibodies may also be elevated, but are much less sensitive, although more specific than the antigliadin antibody.

GENETIC BASIS Genetics plays an important role in celiac sprue, but in conjunction with environmental and other factors. The evidence for a genetic basis comes from family and twin studies. Approximately 8–12% of family members of patients with celiac sprue are also affected, as determined by intestinal biopsy. Interestingly, only 50% of all family members with abnormal biopsies manifest symptoms of the disease. In identical twins, there is 70% concordance for celiac sprue, indicating that factors other than genetics play a role in disease susceptibility.

The linkage of celiac sprue with specific major histocompatibility complex genes has been recognized for many years. There is a very strong association with HLA Class II haplotypes. In Northern Europeans, the DR w17 and DQ w2 serologic specificities are very common. HLA DQ2 is present in 90% of patients with celiac sprue. Molecular analysis indicates that a specific DQ alpha and beta chain molecule encoded by DQA1*0501 and DQB1*0201 is found in 99% of Scandinavians with sprue. In Southern European populations, the same HLA-DQ molecule is expressed on an HLA-DR7 and DR5 (or DR11/DR7, DR12/DR7) haplotype, as opposed to HLA DR3, DQ2 (or HLA-DR17) in Northern Europeans. These molecules are necessary but not sufficient for developing the disease, since HLA identical siblings have only 40–50% concordance for this disease, and only a small percentage of the population that carries these alleles develops sprue. In addition, some populations do not demonstrate the same very high percentage of patients with HLA-DQ2, but instead are DR4-positive. Sequence analysis of the HLA DQ alleles from patients with celiac disease revealed no mutations when compared to normal individuals. This suggests that molecules encoded in regions outside of this HLA locus are required for generating the disease, and there may be different genetic subgroups.

MOLECULAR PATHOPHYSIOLOGY The biochemistry of gluten and gliadin has been intensively studied to identify the protein moieties that are responsible for toxicity. The alcohol-soluble component of gluten, gliadin, appears to be responsible for the disease. Gliadin and similar proteins derived from barley and rye contain many proline and glutamine residues, and intestinal injury is dependent on the presence of these amino acids. Oral or rectal challenge with purified oligopeptides, derived from various parts of the gliadins containing proline and glutamine residues, indicates that specific motifs produce mucosal damage. Oral challenge with oligopeptides showed a C-terminal peptide and one derived from amino acids 31–49 of A-gliadin produced histological changes consistent with sprue. Rectal challenge with gliadin leads to a mucosal inflammatory response, with an influx of intraepithelial lymphocytes and adhesion molecule expression.

Based on its sequence homology to A-gliadin, another environmental factor that may play a role in the pathogenesis of celiac sprue is a history of adenovirus 12 infection. There is a region of homology between the adenovirus serotype 12 E1b protein to A-gliadin that spans 12 amino acids, with 8 identical residues. In addition, almost 90% of patients with untreated celiac sprue had serologic evidence of prior adenovirus 12 infection, compared to only 17% of disease controls. These data suggest that mechanisms of molecular mimicry may be involved in the pathogenesis of this disorder, in which T cells recognize peptides in common to gliadin and viral proteins. However, adenovirus 12 DNA has not been detected in intestinal samples, and peptide challenge with an oligopeptide derived from the homologous region has not been shown to produce intestinal injury.

MANAGEMENT Removal of all gluten from the diet is the primary therapy for celiac sprue. Wheat, rye, oats, and barley-containing products must be eliminated from the diet, since gluten and other related prolamins can produce injury. This restricted diet must be maintained lifelong. Patients may initially exhibit lactose intolerance because of villus atrophy and brush border enzyme deficiency, but this should resolve with treatment.

DISORDERS OF SMALL INTESTINAL ABSORPTION AND TRANSPORT

The brush border of the small intestinal enterocyte contains disaccharidases, peptidases, and transport proteins that are responsible for the absorption of ingested nutrients. In the past several years, progress has been made in clarifying the molecular basis of several disorders characterized by selective malabsorption of carbohydrates or lipids. In this section, a summary of recent advances in understanding the pathophysiology underlying several of the more common of these defects is presented.

LACTASE DEFICIENCY

CLINICAL FEATURES AND EPIDEMIOLOGY Lactase is one of the best-studied of the brush border enzymes. It is responsible for the hydrolysis of lactose into glucose and galactose. Several clinical categories of lactase deficiency have been described. Congenital lactase deficiency is a rare autosomal recessive disorder, resulting in milk intolerance from birth. Much more common is the onset of diminished enzyme activity in childhood or adolescence and lasting into adulthood, also known as adult-onset hypolactasia. Loss of brush border lactase activity may also result from other small intestinal disorders, such as Crohn's disease, celiac sprue, viral illnesses, or other infections.

Loss of lactase activity beginning in childhood/adolescence occurs in the majority of humans throughout the world except for Caucasian populations. In particular, most white northern Europeans and their descendants in North America and Australia (populations that were traditionally cattle farmers and thus persistent milk drinkers) retain high lactase activity lifelong. The prevalence of lactase deficiency throughout the world supports the hypothesis that the decline in lactase activity with age is a "normal" event in response to weaning, common to all land mammals. Persistence of lactase activity has therefore been postulated to be the result of a genetic mutation that occurred in milk-drinking populations, leading to a survival advantage, since milk drinkers might be healthier. Alternatively, it was thought that milk-drinking past normal weaning from the breast might directly influence lactase activity, but this has been disproved.

Ingestion of milk and milk products in deficient individuals leads to abdominal pain, diarrhea, bloating, and excessive flatulence resulting from unabsorbed lactose in the lumen. This results in increased small-bowel fluid. Fermentation of lactose in the colon produces hydrogen, methane, and carbon dioxide gas. Removal of lactose-containing products in the diet leads to resolution of these symptoms.

DIAGNOSIS A lactose tolerance test may be performed, which consists of administering 50 g of lactose orally. If sufficient lactase activity is present, blood glucose levels will rise by >20 mg/dL over a 2-h period. Lactase deficiency is diagnosed by the lack of serum glucose elevation and, frequently, the onset of symptoms of malabsorption, with gas, diarrhea, bloating, and abdominal pain. If the serum glucose increases, yet symptoms also occur, one must consider occult diabetes mellitus. Alternatively, hydrogen breath testing a trial of dietary lactose avoidance may be attempted. After restriction of oral intake of milk and milk products, the patient is assessed for symptom resolution. Finally, small bowel biopsy allows for definitive diagnosis, but is unnecessary given the adequacy of the other two approaches.

GENETIC BASIS AND MOLECULAR PATHOPHYSIOLOGY As determined by population and family studies, adult-onset hypolactasia is an autosomal-recessive trait, and persistence of lactase activity is autosomal-dominant. The molecular basis for lactase persistence/nonpersistence has been the subject of intensive investigation. In the majority of studies, lactase-specific activity and protein levels correlate very well with mRNA concentrations, indicating transcriptional regulation of lactase expression. However, sequence analysis of the lactase cDNA and 1 kb of its promoter region has not revealed differences between sequences from persistent and nonpersistent patients. Yet, recent studies using known DNA marker polymorphisms in the exons of the lactase gene have suggested that *cis*-acting elements are responsible for the persistence/nonpersistence phenotype, based on differences in level of expression of lactase comparing one allele to the other. On the other hand, characterization of trans-acting factors that regulate lactase expression have revealed that levels of NF-LPH-1, an intestine-specific transactivator that binds to a sequence close to the TATA box, are high in newborn pigs with high lactase activity and low in adult pigs with low lactase activity. Still other data suggest that there is a second phenotype of lactase deficiency, in which posttranslational processing of lactase-phlorizin is altered. Thus, the precise molecular mechanisms underlying lactase persistence/nonpersistence are still controversial.

MANAGEMENT The treatment of symptomatic lactase deficiency consists of removal of lactose-containing nutrients from the diet and/or the use of oral enzyme replacement therapy. It is preferable to continue some milk and dairy food ingestion because of their rich calcium stores, especially in children and in women who are prone to osteoporosis. Lactase oral preparations are available in capsules or tablets and can be chewed. Replacement pills are taken with meals and titrated to diminish symptoms. Lactase may also be added directly to milk and ingested after an overnight incubation, or pretreated milk can be purchased.

FUTURE DIRECTIONS The ready availability of oral lactase capsules and the ease of treatment of symptoms by dietary avoidance or supplementation makes more sophisticated approaches to treatment, such as gene therapy, unnecessary. The major research interest still lies in determining how epidemiologic observations are linked to genetics; i.e., what are the genetic alterations that led to lactase persistence in the milk-drinking populations of the world, and are there differences among different ethnic or racial groups? These are questions of great interest to population and evolutionary geneticists.

GLUCOSE–GALACTOSE MALABSORPTION

CLINICAL FEATURES Glucose–galactose malabsorption is a rare congenital disorder in which enterocytic transport of glucose and galactose is absent, resulting from mutation of the gene encoding the Na^+/glucose cotransporter SGLT-1. This disease is characterized by the onset of profuse watery diarrhea in newborns that responds to the removal of dietary sources of glucose and galactose. Diarrhea usually develops within 4 d of birth. The diarrhea is so severe that dehydration is frequent. As in other diseases of carbohydrate absorption, the presence of unabsorbed sugars leads to an increased osmotic load in the small intestine with increased luminal fluid. Laboratory findings include an acidic stool pH because of colonic bacterial metabolism of unabsorbed sugar. In addition, sugar is found in the urine, consistent with the expression of SGLT-1 in the kidney. Oral monosaccharide tolerance tests reveal that absorption of glucose and galactose, but not fructose, is impaired.

GENETICS AND MOLECULAR PATHOPHYSIOLOGY Glucose galactose malabsorption is an autosomal recessive disease. The precise incidence of this disorder has not been determined, but it is clearly rare, as indicated by the few case reports in the literature. Frequently, there is a history of consanguineous marriage.

Expression cloning of the cDNA that encodes SGLT-1, the Na/glucose cotransporter, by Wright's group, provided a major breakthrough in understanding pathophysiology of this disorder. Specific mutations in SGLT-1 lead to loss of transporter function in humans, resulting in glucose and galactose malabsorption. Analysis of cDNA reverse-transcribed from RNA from intestinal biopsies of two affected sisters showed a single missense mutation, with a single base change from G to A at position 92, changing an aspartate to an asparagine. Their parents were heterozygous for this mutation. The autosomal recessive inheritance of this disorder was confirmed. The mutant SGLT1 mRNA was expressed in *Xenopus laevis* oocytes and compared to the normal SGLT1 mRNA for ability to transport a glucose analog, α-methyl d glucopyranoside. As anticipated, the mutant SGLT1 demonstrated no detectable transport activity.

Subsequently, 30 other patients have been screened for mutations in SGLT1. The mutations included missense, nonsense, and frame shift mutations, and some occurred in splice sites at intron-exon boundaries. Two areas were identified as "hot spots" for missense mutations, between residues 289–304 and 369–405. Analysis of the mutant proteins indicated that loss of transporter activity was a result of production of truncated or nonfunctional protein, defective trafficking of the transporter, or defects in the transport cycle. The SGLT1 gene has been localized to chromosome 22 on the distal q arm.

MANAGEMENT The treatment of glucose–galactose malabsorption is the immediate removal of lactose, glucose, and galactose-containing substances from the diet. Fructose is well-tolerated, and a fructose-based formula can be substituted, with rapid resolution of symptoms. There are reports of increasing tolerance to glucose and galactose with age. Rechallenge with small amounts of these sugars may be possible.

FUTURE DIRECTIONS The cloning of the SGLT-1 cDNA and the identification of naturally occurring mutations has already led to notable advances in our knowledge of the basic mechanisms of sugar transport. The regulation of expression of this and other cotransporters, their mode of insertion in the membrane, and structure–function correlation may be addressed in the research laboratory. With the identification of the SGLT1 gene, gene therapy may eventually be considered. However, in the near future, this is unlikely because of the relative ease of treatment by elimination diets, and the rarity of this disorder.

ABETALIPOPROTEINEMIA

CLINICAL FEATURES Abetalipoproteinemia is a rare disorder, characterized by the absence of apolipoprotein (apo) B containing lipoproteins in plasma. Patients present in infancy with diarrhea resulting from severe fat malabsorption, poor weight gain, and acanthocytosis. Atypical retinitis pigmentosa and spinocerebellar degeneration become apparent at older ages. Ocular symptoms include decreased night and color vision, and neurologic signs of ataxia, spastic gait and dysmetria, loss of deep tendon reflexes, and decreased vibratory and proprioceptive sense appear in the second decade. Spontaneous hemorrhage characteristic of a bleeding diathesis may occur because of vitamin K deficiency.

DIAGNOSIS The hallmark of this disorder is an abnormal plasma lipid profile, in association with signs of spinocerebellar degeneration and a pigmented retinopathy. Total cholesterol and triglyceride plasma levels are extremely low, and there is an absence of apo B-containing plasma lipoproteins, including chylomicrons, VLDLs, and LDLs. Most patients are anemic as a result of enhanced hemolysis of abnormal red blood cells (acanthocytes). Fat malabsorption leads to deficiency of fat soluble vitamins. In particular, vitamins E, K, and A are affected since they are transported in chylomicrons. Vitamin E deficiency is most severe, because its absorption from the intestine, transport to the liver, and circulation in the plasma are dependent on apo B-containing lipoproteins. Vitamin E deficiency is clinically important since it is thought to be responsible for the development of neurologic and retinal sequelae. Intestinal biopsy reveals lipid-laden enterocytes but normal villi and is useful for distinguishing this disorder from other intestinal illnesses associated with fat malabsorption.

GENETICS AND MOLECULAR PATHOPHYSIOLOGY Abetalipoproteinemia is a rare autosomal recessive disorder. Consanguinity is common in these families. An absence of plasma lipoproteins containing apo B led to the hypothesis that this disorder is a result of a defect in the apo B gene. However, linkage between apo B and abetalipoproteinemia in families has not been established by restriction fragment-length polymorphism analysis, and defects in the apo B gene have not been identified. Since assembly or secretion of apo B-containing lipoproteins were most likely defective in this disorder, the microsomal triglyceride transport (MTP) protein was examined in affected individuals. This gene, located on chromosome 4q22-24, encodes a protein that catalyzes the transport of triglyceride, cholesteryl ester, and phospholipid between membranes. It is a heterodimer composed of a protein disulphide isomerase, and an 88-kDa subunit that is responsible for the lipid transport activity. This larger subunit shares homology with lipovitellin 1, a member of the lipid-binding lipovitellin complex that serves as a source for lipid in the developing embryo. Wetterau and colleagues showed that MTP activity, and particularly the 88-kDa subunit, normally present in microsomes from liver and intestine, was absent in intestinal biopsies from patients. Sequence analysis of cDNA and genomic DNA from patients with abetalipoproteinemia revealed homozygous frameshift and nonsense mutations in the gene encoding the 88-kDa subunit, resulting in truncated proteins. Analysis of additional patients indicated frameshift and splice site mutations, most of which lead to the formation of a truncated protein. Transfection of Cos-1 cells with mutant MTP cDNAs lacking part of the carboxy-terminus show decreased lipid transfer activity, supporting the hypothesis that alterations of this protein are the primary cause of abetalipoproteinemia.

MANAGEMENT A low-fat diet and supplementation with high doses of vitamin E as well as vitamins A and K are required. In particular, it is critical to avoid vitamin E deficiency, since this appears to be the primary cause of the severe and irreversible neurologic and ocular changes characteristic of this disease.

FUTURE DIRECTIONS The cloning of the cDNA encoding the microsomal triglyceride transport protein raises the possibility of gene therapy in the future. Although many of the devastating neurologic and ocular sequelae may be avoided by high doses of vitamin E, there may be a role for gene replacement in refractory patients. Also, rapid, definitive diagnosis is crucial, so that prenatal screening of siblings may be useful. Finally, since patients with MTP deficiency have very low cholesterol and triglyceride levels, identification of selective inhibitors of its activity may prove to be a valuable addition to the treatment of hypercholesterolemia.

SELECTED REFERENCES

Boll W, Wagner P, Mantei N. Structure of the chromosomal gene and cDNAs coding for lactase-phlorizin hydrolase in humans with adult-type hypolactasia or persistence of lactase. Am J Hum Genet 1991;48:889–902.

Escher JC, de Koning ND, van Engen CGJ, et al. Molecular basis of lactase levels in adult humans. J Clin Invest 1992;89:480–483.

Evans L, Grasset E, Heyman M, Dumontier AM, Beau JP, Desjexu JF. Congenital selective malabsorption of glucose and galactose. J Ped Gastroenterol and Nutr 1985;4:878–886.

Goggins M, Kelleher D. Celiac disease and other nutrient related injuries to the gastrointestinal tract. Am J Gastroenterol 1994;89(Suppl): S2–S17.

Harvey CB, Wang Y, Hughes LA, et al. Studies on the expression of intestinal lactase in different individuals. Gut 1995;36:28–33.

Hediger MA, Coady MJ, Ikeda TS, Wright EM. Expression cloning and cDNA sequencing of the Na/glucose cotransporter. Nature 1987; 330:379–381.

Heresbach D, Alizadeh M, Dabadie A, et al. Significance of interleukin-1 beta and interleukin-1 receptor antagonist genetic polymorphism in inflammatory bowel diseases. Am J Gastroenterol 1997;92: 1164–1169.

Hermiston ML, Gordon JI. Inflammatory bowel disease and adenomas in mice expressing a dominant negative N-cadherin. Science 1995; 270:1203–1207.

Hugot JP, Laurent-Puig P, Gower-Rousseau C, Olson JM, Lee JC, et al. Mapping of a susceptibility locus for Crohn's disease on chromosome 16. Nature 1996;379:821–823.

Kagnoff MF, Harwood JI, Bugawan TL, Erlich HA. Structural analysis of the HLA-DR, -DQ, and -DP alleles on the celiac disease-associated-DR3 (Drw17) haplotype. Proc Natl Acad Sci USA 1989;86: 6274–6278.

Kuhn R, Lohler J, Rennick D, Rajewsky K, Werner M. Interleukin-10-deficient mice develop chronic enterocolitis Cell 1993;75:263–274.

Lloyd M, Mevissen G, Fischer M, et al. Regulation of intestinal lactase in adult hypolactasia. J Clin Invest 1992;89:524–529.

Marsh MN. Gluten, major histocompatibility complex, and the small intestine. A molecular and immunobiologic approach to the spectrum of gluten sensitivity ('celiac sprue'). Gastroenterology 1992;102: 330–354.

Martin MG, Turk E, Lostao P, Kerner C, Wright EM. Defects in Na/glucose cotransporter (SGLT1) trafficking and function cause glucose-galactose malabsorption. Nat Genet 1996;12:216–220.

Rader DJ, Brewer HB. Abetalipoproteinemia: new insights into lipoprotein assembly and vitamin E metabolism from a rare genetic disease. JAMA 1993;270:865–869.

Sadlack B, Merz H, Schorle H, Schimpl A, Feller AC, Horak I. Ulcerative colitis-like disease in mice with a disrupted interleukin-2 gene. Cell 1993;75:253–261.

Sharp D, Blinderman L, Combs KA, et al. Cloning and gene defects in microsomal triglyceride transfer protein associated with abetalipoproteinemia. Nature 1993;365:65–69.

Sollid LM, Markussen G, Ek J, Gjerde H, Vartdal F, Thorsby E. Evidence for a primary association of celiac disease to a particular HLA DQ alpha/beta heterodimer. J Exp Med 1989;169:345–350.

Stenson WF, Lobos E. Sulfasalazine inhibits the synthesis of chemotactic lipids by neutrophils. J Clin Invest 1982;69:494–497.

Strober W, Ehrhardt RO. Chronic intestinal inflammation: an unexpected outcome in cytokine or T cell receptor mutant mice. Cell 1993;75: 203–205.

Troelsen JT, Olsen J, Noren O, Sjostrom H. A novel intestinal trans-factor (NF-LPH-1) interacts with the lactase-phlorizin hydrolase promoter and co-varies with the enzymatic activity. J Biol Chem 1992; 267:20,407–20,411.

Turk E, Zabel B, Mundlos S, Dyer J, Wright EM. Glucose/galactose malabsorption caused by a defect in the Na+/glucose cotransporter. Nature 1991;350:354–356.

Wetterau JR, Aggerbeck LP, Bouma M, et al. Absence of microsomal triglyceride transfer protein in individuals with abetalipoproteinemia. Science 1992;258:999–1001.

Yang Y, Harvey CB, Ratt WS, et al. The lactase persistence/non-persistence polymorphism is controlled by a *cis*-acting element. Hum Molec Genet 1995;4:657–662.

ENDOCRINOLOGY VII

SECTION EDITORS:

MICHAEL J. MCPHAUL AND J. LARRY JAMESON

46 Mechanisms of Hormone Action

William L. Lowe, Jr., Richard G. Pestell, Laird D. Madison, and J. Larry Jameson

INTRODUCTION

Hormones provide a form of communication between different cells and from one organ to another. The dramatic effects of hormones on physiologic functions such as growth and metabolism have allowed relatively sophisticated studies to elucidate their sources of production, sites of action, and how they are controlled. Because hormones act by binding to specific receptors, studies that have defined their mechanisms of action have also provided important paradigms for how receptors activate intracellular signaling cascades that lead to altered cellular responses.

Endocrine disorders ultimately involve abnormalities of hormone production or action. A relatively large number of these diseases have a well-defined genetic basis. There are now many examples of mutations that occur in genes that encode hormones, their receptors, second messenger signaling pathways, and the transcription factors that transduce hormone signals. The purpose of this chapter is to review basic principles of hormone signaling through their receptors. There has been a remarkable expansion of knowledge in this area in recent years. The structures and signal transduction networks for membrane receptors are finally coming into focus; nuclear receptors were cloned within the last decade and have revealed an unexpectedly complex family of proteins that serve as direct regulators of gene expression. The impact of this new information on our understanding of the pathophysiology of disease is already being felt in terms of the ability to predict specific receptors or pathways that may harbor mutations in different disorders. In this chapter, we will cite selected examples of such mutations, and the reader is referred to other chapters in this section for more detailed discussions of these disorders.

CLASSIFICATION OF HORMONES AND RECEPTORS

Hormones can be divided generally into three major classes: (1) derivatives of amino acids (e.g., dopamine and catecholamines); (2) peptides and proteins (e.g., thyrotropin-releasing hormone or insulin); and (3) derivatives of steroids (e.g., estrogen or cortisol). For the most part, amino acid derivatives and peptide hormones interact with membrane receptors on the cell surface, whereas the steroid hormones act by crossing the plasma membrane to interact with intracellular receptors.

From: *Principles of Molecular Medicine* (J. L. Jameson, ed.), ©1998 Humana Press Inc., Totowa, NJ.

As described in detail below, membrane receptors can be divided into several distinct classes. After binding hormones, these receptors activate a complex array of second messenger signaling pathways that often involve cascades of kinases. Nuclear receptors, such as the glucocorticoid or progesterone receptors, bind hormones in the cytoplasm before translocation into the nucleus (Fig. 46-1). Other receptors in this family, such as the thyroid hormone receptor, bind hormone in the nucleus without a separate hormone-induced translocation step. In the nucleus, these receptors interact with DNA target sites to either stimulate or repress the expression of specific genes.

Regardless of the class of receptors, certain principles apply to hormone–receptor interactions. Hormones bind to receptors with high affinity and specificity to allow appropriate physiologic responses. Most receptors bind hormones with affinity constants that approach the circulating levels of hormones (usually $<10^{-9}$ *M*) to allow responses over a dynamic range of physiologically relevant changes in hormone levels. Receptor numbers vary greatly in different target tissues, providing one of the major determinants of specific cellular responses to widely circulating hormones. For example, luteinizing hormone (LH) receptors are located almost exclusively in the gonads. In contrast, insulin receptors are widely distributed, reflecting the need for insulin-induced metabolic responses in most tissues.

Receptor specificity is a reflection of differential affinities of the receptor for structurally related molecules. Although structurally similar, LH, follicle-stimulating hormone (FSH), and thyroid-stimulating hormone (TSH) are highly selective for their individual receptors. Similarly, steroids such as progesterone, estrogen, and glucocorticoid exhibit no physiologically significant crossreactivity among their receptors. There are important exceptions to these examples of specificity. Parathyroid hormone (PTH) and parathyroid hormone-related peptide (PTH-RP) appear to share a common receptor. Insulin, insulin-like growth factor-1 (IGF-I), and IGF-II crossreact to some degree with their respective receptors. This latter circumstance may explain why some malignancies that overproduce IGF-II can cause hypoglycemia because of inappropriate stimulation of insulin receptors by IGF-II.

FEEDBACK REGULATION IN ENDOCRINE AXES

Feedback regulatory systems are pervasive in the field of endocrinology. Each of the major hypothalamic–pituitary hormone axes are governed by negative feedback, which serves to maintain

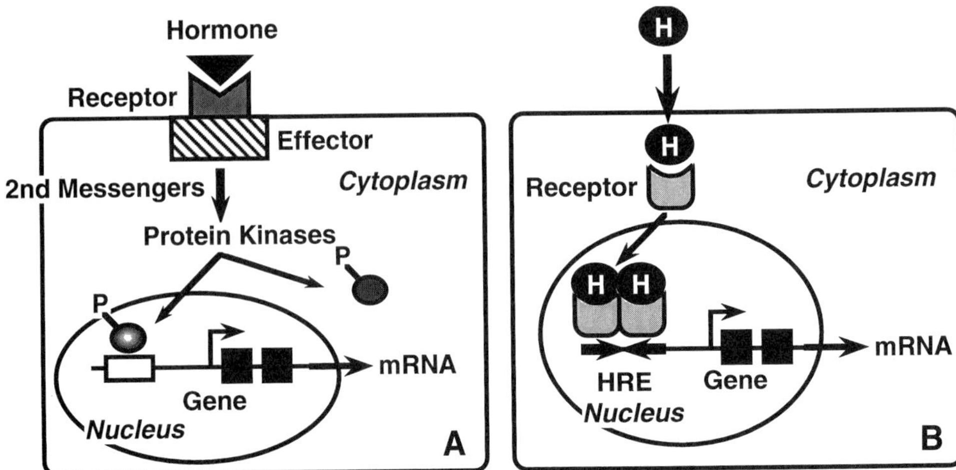

Figure 46-1 Membrane and nuclear receptors that mediate hormone action. A membrane receptor is shown on the left. Hormones and growth factors bind with high affinity to the extracellular domain of the receptors. Membrane receptors **(A)** communicate to intracellular signaling pathways, which typically include cascades of protein kinases. These kinases act on many different cellular targets, including other receptors, ion channels, the cytoskeleton, metabolic pathways, and transcription factors. Nuclear receptors **(B)** reside within the cytoplasm or the nucleus before hormone binding. Hormones traverse the plasma membrane and induce nuclear translocation and receptor activation. The activated receptors act as transcription factors to alter levels of gene expression. (After Jameson JL. Principles of hormone action. Oxford Textbook of Medicine, 1996. Reprinted with permission from Oxford University Press.)

hormone levels within a very narrow range. The principle of feedback control is well-illustrated by the example of the hypothalamic–pituitary–thyroid axis (Fig. 46-2). Thyrotropin-releasing hormone (TRH) stimulates TSH secretion from the pituitary. TSH stimulates the synthesis and secretion of thyroid hormone (T4 and T3), which in turn suppresses the production of hypothalamic TRH and pituitary TSH. A typical regulatory loop therefore has both positive (TRH, TSH) and negative (T4, T3) components, providing exquisite control over hormone levels and action.

In addition to classic endocrine feedback loops in which hormones are produced by one gland and act on a different gland, a variety of local regulatory systems have also been characterized (Fig. 46-3). These so-called autocrine and paracrine systems are used commonly during development and by most growth factors. Local control of growth factor production and action helps to restrict their sites of action. For example, circulating levels of activin are relatively low, but local production in the gonads and pituitary may permit localized biologic effects without a requirement for systemic exposure to high levels of hormone. In many cases, the distinction between endocrine and paracrine actions may become blurred. For example, IGF-I appears to act as both a true hormone and a paracrine factor. In the liver, growth hormone increases production of circulating IGF-I. However, in most other tissues, the production of IGF-I is also regulated locally.

The clinical practice of endocrinology is intimately linked to these principles of feedback control systems and hormone action. Using these concepts, one can often localize whether a disorder is caused by hormone excess or deficiency, or by an abnormality in tissue sensitivity to hormone action. Advances in molecular genetics are allowing these diagnostic algorithms to expand by another dimension. In addition to measuring hormone levels, it is now possible to test for enzyme deficiencies by identifying mutations in affected genes (e.g., 21-hydroxylase), or to predict genetic risk in inherited syndromes such as the multiple endocrine neoplasia syndromes.

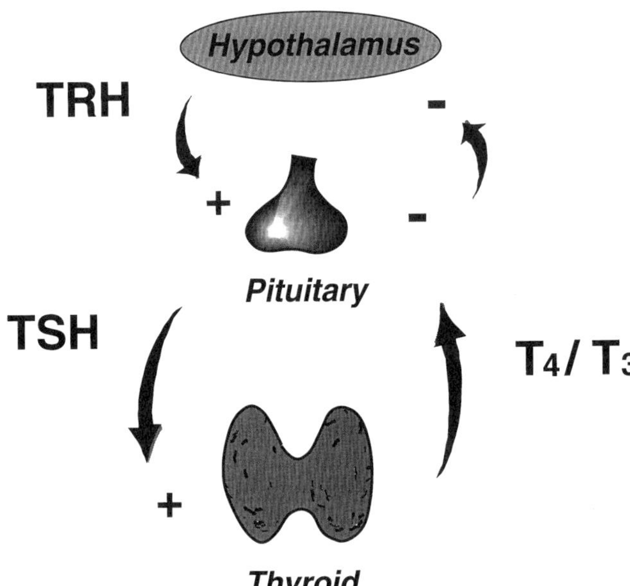

Figure 46-2 Positive and negative feedback regulation by hormones. The hypothalamic–pituitary–thyroid axis provides a prototypical example of feedback regulatory pathways in the endocrine system. Hypothalamic thyrotropin releasing hormone (TRH) stimulates thyroid stimulating hormone (TSH) secretion by the pituitary gland. TSH stimulates the biosynthesis and secretion of thyroid hormones (T4 and T3) from the thyroid gland. Thyroid hormones feed back to inhibit the production of TRH and TSH. Because the pituitary integrates both positive and negative regulation, it establishes a setpoint for TSH and consequently, thyroid hormone levels. (After Jameson JL. Principles of hormone action. Oxford Textbook of Medicine, 1996. Reprinted with permission from Oxford University Press.)

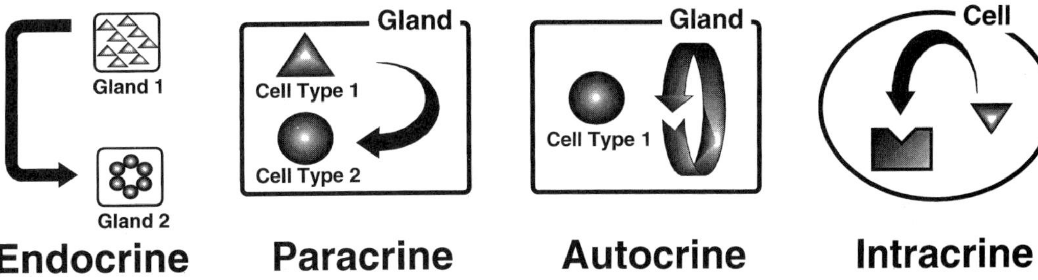

Figure 46-3 Hormones and growth factors can act at a distance or locally. Endocrine action refers to hormones that are secreted from one gland and enter the circulation to act on a different target gland. Paracrine action involves hormones or growth factors that are produced by one cell but act locally on an adjacent cell. In autocrine action, a growth factor acts on the same cell from which it is produced. Intracrine action suggests that some hormones act on intracellular receptors in the same cells in which they are produced. (After Jameson JL. Principles of hormone action. Oxford Textbook of Medicine, 1996. Reprinted with permission from Oxford University Press.)

MEMBRANE RECEPTORS

Receptors on the surfaces of cells provide an essential component of communication with extracellular ligands. These membrane receptors fall into three general classes based on their structure and mechanisms of signal transduction: (1) the single transmembrane domain receptors; (2) the seven transmembrane domain receptors; and (3) the four transmembrane domain receptors. The latter class functions as transmitter-gated ion channels and will not be described further in this chapter.

SINGLE TRANSMEMBRANE DOMAIN RECEPTORS

TYROSINE KINASE RECEPTOR FAMILY The tyrosine kinase receptors represent a large family of receptors that are involved in many facets of cell growth responses. As their name implies, members of this receptor family possess intrinsic tyrosine kinase activity. Although there are at least seven different subfamilies, certain generalizations can be made about the entire family of receptors (Fig. 46-4). With the exception of the insulin receptor family, these receptors consist of a single subunit and dimerize on ligand binding. Dimerization is followed by autophosphorylation, which actually occurs as a result of transphosphorylation (e.g., one cytoplasmic domain phosphorylates the other cytoplasmic domain in the dimer). The initial transphosphorylation reaction increases the tyrosine kinase activity of the receptor and results in phosphorylation of other specific tyrosines within the cytoplasmic domain. These phosphotyrosines then serve as recognition sites for a variety of intracellular signal transduction molecules. For example, binding to the phosphorylated receptor can occur via Src homology 2 (SH2) domains that are present in signal transduction adaptor molecules. SH2 domains are regions of ~100 amino acids that are folded to form a binding pocket for phosphotyrosine. Because the cytoplasmic domain of growth factor receptors is typically phosphorylated on multiple tyrosines, a variety of different SH2-containing molecules can bind to the receptor (Fig. 46-4). Another recently identified domain, the phosphotyrosine-binding (PTB) domain, also facilitates interactions between signaling molecules and receptors by binding to phosphotyrosine.

In addition to forming homodimers, receptor tyrosine kinases can also form heterodimers with other members of their family, greatly increasing the diversity of signal transduction molecules that are potentially activated by a single ligand. This phenomenon is illustrated by the epidermal growth factor (EGF) receptor family, which appears to be important in the growth of several different tumors, including breast and uterine cancers. One member of that family, ErbB3, has several repeats of a Tyr-X-X-Met (where X is any amino acid) motif in its cytoplasmic domain. When the tyrosine in this motif is phosphorylated, it is recognized by the SH2 domain of phosphoinositol-3-kinase (PI3-kinase). This amino acid motif is not present in the EGF receptor. EGF-induced heterodimerization of the EGF receptor and ErbB3 results, therefore, in activation of PI3-kinase activity, as well as pathways that are otherwise stimulated by homodimerization of the EGF receptor.

The insulin and IGF-I receptors represent an exception to the rule of ligand-induced dimerization of tyrosine kinase receptors. In the absence of ligand, these receptors form disulfide-linked homo- or heterodimers. Ligand binding presumably induces a conformational change in the receptor that stimulates activation and "autophosphorylation" (actually transphosphorylation as described above). Another difference exhibited by this subfamily of receptors is that the phosphotyrosines on the insulin and IGF-I receptor are poor binding sites for SH2 domains. Rather, these receptors phosphorylate insulin-related substrates 1 and 2 (IRS-1, IRS-2), which have at least 20 potential sites for tyrosine phosphorylation, and appear to serve as adaptors for the insulin family of receptors. A variety of proteins with SH2 domains have been shown to interact with IRS-1 and IRS-2.

Several different diseases involve alterations in the function of the insulin receptor. Distinct mutations affect multiple aspects of insulin receptor function, including receptor biosynthesis, processing of the proreceptor, transport of the receptor to the cell surface, affinity for insulin, and receptor tyrosine kinase activity. These mutations result in the syndrome of type A extreme insulin resistance (Online Mendelian inheritance of man number [OMIM] 147670). In many cases, the mutations cause more severe insulin resistance than would be anticipated for a 50% reduction in functional receptors. This phenomenon may result from the formation of a heterodimer between normal and mutated receptors with dominant negative inhibition of normal receptor function. Patients with leprechaunism (OMIM 246200), a syndrome that is characterized by intrauterine growth retardation and characteristic physical abnormalities, exhibit insulin resistance that is more severe than that seen in patients with the type A syndrome. This syndrome is inherited in an autosomal recessive manner and may be caused by the inheritance of two abnormal insulin receptor alleles. Although mutations in the insulin receptor are rare, the phenomenon of insulin resistance is quite common, and is the major cause of diabetes mellitus in adults. Few mutations have been identified in the

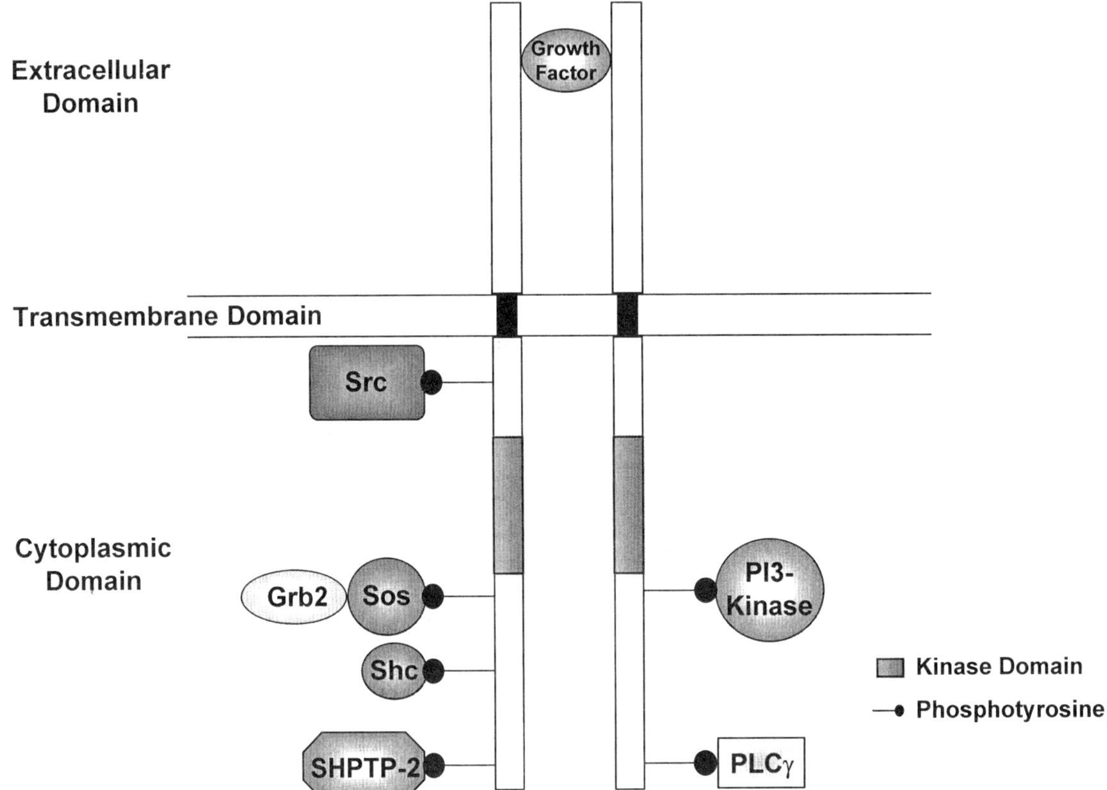

Figure 46-4 A tyrosine kinase receptor and interacting proteins. Different tyrosine kinases interact with an array of intracellular adaptor molecules such as Grb2, which serve as recognition sites for other cellular proteins. Phosphorylation of tyrosine kinases, often by a dimeric partner, creates recognition sites for proteins, such as Shc, Src, SOS, PI3-kinase, phospholipase C (PLC), and protein tyrosine phosphatases (PTP). The exact repertoire of adaptors and enzymes that interact with a tyrosine kinase is variable and provides a mechanism for generating diverse cellular responses.

insulin receptor in patients with this more common form of insulin resistance. Rather, this acquired form of insulin resistance presumably involves postreceptor defects in the insulin signaling pathway, although the exact steps that are affected remain to be delineated.

CYTOKINE RECEPTOR FAMILY Cytokines include traditional hormones, such as growth hormone (GH) and erythropoietin, as well as colony-stimulating factors and interleukins. In several cases, such as the interleukins, a variety of different endocrine, neural, hepatic, and hematopoietic systems are targets of the cytokines. The structural features of the cytokine receptors are similar to tyrosine kinase receptors except that the cytoplasmic domain does not contain motifs indicative of kinase activity. Moreover, although some of the cytokine receptors are monomers (e.g., growth hormone, prolactin, erythropoietin, leptin), others consist of several subunits, some of which are shared among different cytokine receptors. In addition, some members of this receptor family secrete soluble forms of the receptor that can bind circulating ligands. For example, in the case of the GH receptor, the extracellular domain is shed into the circulation and functions as a GH binding protein.

The mechanism of cytokine-induced signal transduction was poorly understood for many years in view of the lack of intrinsic enzyme activity in the cytoplasmic domain of these receptors. However, the cytokine receptors have now been shown to activate the Janus kinases (JAKs). The JAK kinase family members, which include JAK1, JAK2, JAK3, and Tyk2, are cytoplasmic protein tyrosine kinases that associate with the cytoplasmic domain of cytokine receptors via conserved receptor motifs. The activated JAKs phosphorylate tyrosines in the cytoplasmic domain of the cytokine receptors, which creates binding sites for signal transduction molecules that contain SH2 domains. In addition, the JAKs transmit intracellular signals by phosphorylating a family of latent transcription factors called the STAT proteins (signal transducers and activators of transcription). It is likely that each specific receptor elicits responses from a unique constellation of kinases and STAT proteins.

Endocrine diseases associated with mutations of cytokine receptors include alterations in growth. Patients with familial growth hormone resistance or Laron-type dwarfism (OMIM 245590) have proportionate short stature associated with elevated plasma growth hormone levels and do not respond to exogenous treatment with growth hormone. In most cases, the syndrome is inherited in an autosomal recessive fashion, and patients lack functional growth hormone receptors secondary to gene deletions or point mutations in the receptor. More recently, the growth hormone receptor from some patients with this syndrome was shown to have a point mutation in the extracellular domain that results in a small reduction in receptor affinity, but abrogates the ability of the receptor to dimerize, thus demonstrating the importance of receptor dimerization in signal transduction. Finally, in a selected group of children with idiopathic short stature, about one-third were found to have mutations in the growth hormone receptor that affected the level of receptor expression or its affinity for growth hormone.

SERINE-THREONINE KINASE RECEPTOR FAMILY A more recently described family of receptors contain endogenous serine-threonine kinase activity. These receptors bind to and transmit the signals of the transforming growth factor-β (TGF-β) family of ligands. These growth factors include the TGF-βs, activins, bone morphogenic proteins, and müllerian-inhibiting substance. The TGF-β and activin receptors are the prototypical and best characterized receptors in this family.

Activin and TGF-β receptor complexes are composed of two different subunits, the type I and type II receptors. Both of these receptors are transmembrane proteins with intrinsic serine-threonine kinase activity, and both are required for ligand-induced signal transduction. The type II receptors have high affinity for their ligands and a long cytoplasmic domain that possesses serine-threonine kinase activity. Multiple isoforms of the type II receptor subunit have been described, and, similarly, there are at least six different type I receptors. The type I receptors are similar in structure to the type II receptors, including the presence of the serine-threonine kinase domain. Unlike the type II receptors, these receptors appear to have no ability to bind ligand.

Ligand binding to the type II receptor recruits the type I receptor, resulting in the formation of a hetero-oligomeric complex that likely is a heterotetramer of two type I and two type II receptors. The type II receptor appears to phosphorylate the type I receptor after it is recruited into the complex by ligand binding. The type I receptor subsequently phosphorylates other downstream substrates, including the Smad proteins. At least eight different Smad proteins have now been identified. Interestingly, the gene encoding one of these proteins, Smad 4, is deleted in ~50% of pancreatic carcinomas. When tested, growth of these tumors was not inhibited by TGF-β. The diversity of signals that can be generated by the activins and TGF-βs is increased by the ability of multiple type II receptors to interact with multiple type I receptors, each of which may transmit selective signals. Different components of this receptor family have been knocked out in transgenic mice, confirming a pleomorphic role in development. In addition, mutations in the receptor for müllerian-inhibiting substance causes retained müllerian structure in males.

GUANYLYL CYCLASE RECEPTOR FAMILY The guanylyl cyclase family of receptors contains an extracellular ligand-binding domain and a single transmembrane domain. The cytoplasmic domain contains a catalytic cyclase domain that is responsible for ligand-induced conversion of guanosine triphosphate (GTP) to cyclic guanosine monophosphate (cGMP), which activates protein kinases, phosphodiesterases, and ion channels. To date, four different receptors with guanylyl cyclase activity have been cloned. The prototype for this family is the GC-A receptor for atrial natriuretic peptide (ANP) and brain natriuretic peptide. The ability of cGMP analogs to mimic the effect of ANP in cells confirms that cGMP generation mediates ligand-induced signal transduction by these receptors. In mice, disruption of the gene encoding the GC-A receptor results in salt-resistant hypertension. A second receptor, the GC-B receptor, binds type C natriuretic peptide, and another receptor with guanylyl cyclase activity (GC-C receptor) binds to guanylin, a recently identified peptide that is produced by epithelial cells.

PHOSPHOTYROSINE PHOSPHATASE FAMILY Although much work has focused on kinases, a series of protein tyrosine phosphatases (PTPs) have recently been cloned and play an important role in cellular function. Some of these proteins contain receptor-like structures that are characterized by an extracellular domain, a transmembrane domain, and a cytoplasmic domain that contains one or two catalytic domains.

CD45 was one of the first transmembrane protein tyrosine phosphatases to be recognized. It is required for T-cell function and activates two members of the Src family of protein tyrosine kinases, $p56^{lck}$ and $p59^{fyn}$, by dephosphorylating a phosphotyrosine at the C-terminus of these proteins. This phosphotyrosine inhibits the kinase activity of $p56^{lck}$ and $p59^{fyn}$. Another group of tyrosine phosphatases contains an extracellular domain that is similar to cell adhesion molecules. These proteins may be involved in cell–cell interactions, although regulated activity of these phosphatases has not been demonstrated. When gene targeting was used to knock out one member of this family, the LAR receptor-like protein tyrosine phosphatase, impaired terminal differentiation of breast alveoli was present, suggesting a role in breast development. PTPβ is representative of a final class of protein tyrosine phosphatases. The extracellular domain of PTPβ has the structure of a proteoglycan and is capable of interacting with the extracellular matrix protein tenascin.

SEVEN TRANSMEMBRANE DOMAIN RECEPTORS

The seven transmembrane domain family of receptors contain several hundred members. These receptors have a conserved structure that is characterized by seven hydrophobic domains that are inserted into the membrane (Fig. 46-5). These receptors bind a wide variety of ligands including: (1) small molecules such as biogenic amines (e.g., epinephrine and norepinephrine) and odorants; (2) ions such as Ca^{2+}; (3) small peptides like vasopressin and thyrotropin releasing hormone; and (4) large protein hormones such as parathyroid hormone and the glycoprotein hormones. These ligands bind to regions of the extracellular domain, and in some instances make contacts with the receptor within the transmembrane domain.

The seven transmembrane domain receptors are coupled to G proteins, which serve as effectors to initiate signal transduction. Although the composition and regulation of G proteins is rather complex, the components of this system are well-characterized and play an important role in several endocrine diseases. G proteins are heterotrimers that consist of an α-subunit and a combined β–γ-subunit. There are at least sixteen different α-subunit genes as well as several different β- and γ-subunits (Table 46-1). Within any given cell type, multiple different receptors, G proteins, and effectors are present. This diversity of G protein subunits requires specific interactions that appear to be mediated by the intracellular loops and C-terminus of the receptor.

In the absence of ligand, the α-subunit is bound to GDP and remains associated with the β–γ-subunits. Ligand binding to the receptor induces a conformational change in the receptor that promotes binding of a G protein to the receptor. After coupling to the receptor, guanosine diphosphate (GDP) is exchanged for GTP on the α-subunit and the β–γ-subunit is dissociated. These steps activate the G protein and initiate interactions with downstream effector molecules (e.g., adenylyl cyclase). The α-subunit contains an intrinsic GTPase activity that converts GTP to GDP, which restores the inactive state and allows reassociation with the β–γ-subunits. Regulation of GTPase activity therefore represents an important point of control of G protein function. The β–γ-subunits may also play a role in the activation of effector molecules. They appear to mediate tyrosine phosphorylation of the adaptor molecule Shc,

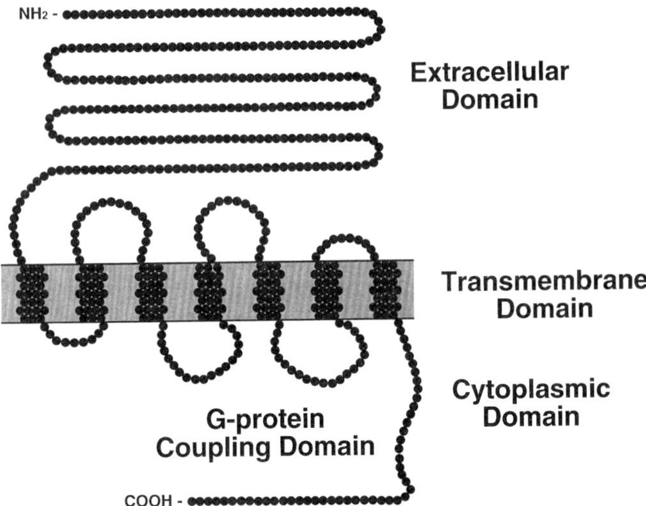

Figure 46-5 Structure of a seven transmembrane domain receptor. The G-protein coupled receptors share several structural features, including the characteristic seven transmembrane-spanning domains. The amino-terminal (NH_2) domain is located extracellularly and is involved in hormone interaction for some receptors. The seven transmembrane domains are connected by intra- and extracellular loops of amino acids. In three dimensions, the hydrophobic "barrels" are thought to be circularized when viewed from above. For many receptors, the ligands bind within the transmembrane domains. The intracellular loops and carboxy-terminal tail (COOH) are involved in coupling to G proteins and in intracellular signaling. Phosphorylation of the cytoplasmic tail and interactions with cellular proteins, such as arrestin, modulate receptor signaling, desensitization, and recycling. (After Jameson JL. Principles of hormone action. Oxford Textbook of Medicine, 1996. Reprinted with permission from Oxford University Press.)

which leads to activation of *Ras* and subsequently mitogen-activated protein kinase *(see below)* via a pathway that requires tyrosine kinases.

The relationship of G proteins to endocrine diseases was first postulated for Albright's hereditary osteodystrophy (OMIM 300800), which is characterized by variable resistance to a variety of hormones that are coupled to G proteins (e.g., PTH, TSH, glucagon). These patients have a variety of different mutations that affect the amount or function of Gsα-subunits. Although this provides a rational explanation for multiple hormone resistance, it remains unclear why some Gsα-coupled receptors are affected more severely than others. Remarkably, Albright also described a syndrome caused by activation rather than inactivation of the Gsα-subunit. This disorder, referred to as McCune-Albright syndrome (OMIM 174800), is characterized by polyostotic fibrous dysplasia, *cafe au lait* spots, hyperfunctioning ovarian cysts, and autonomous function in other glands, including the thyroid and pituitary glands. Patients with McCune-Albright syndrome have mutations in Gsα that inhibit the intrinsic GTPase. Consequently, the G protein cannot hydrolyze GTP, and it remains in an "activated" state, resulting in constitutive stimulation of downstream signaling pathways. In many ways, these mutations are analogous to those which occur in the structurally similar *Ras* proto-oncogene *(see below)*. *Ras* mutations also inhibit GTPase activity and are associated with constitutive signaling and enhanced cellular growth. The clinical manifestations of McCune-Albright syndrome reflect the activation of pathways that are normally stimulated by G-protein-coupled receptors. Thus, skin pigmentation likely mimics melanocyte stimulating hormone, bone dysplasia reflects overactivity of the PTH pathway, and ovarian cysts may reflect activation of gonadotropin pathways. The G-protein mutations in McCune-Albright syndrome are sporadic and postzygotic (all patients are mosaic for the mutation). It is presumed that germline mutations would be lethal.

The spectrum of known G-protein mutations has expanded considerably in recent years. On the basis of the observation that a subset of growth hormone-secreting pituitary adenomas had high levels of cyclic adenosine monophosphate (cAMP) production, it was discovered that Gsα mutations occur in 30–40% of cases with this type of pituitary tumor. These mutations are analogous to those in McCune-Albright syndrome. They occur in the same locations of the G protein and also result in constitutive activation. The primary difference is that the mutations are only found in the tumor tissue, and are therefore somatic in origin. G-protein mutations have now been found in other endocrine tumors, including hyperfunctioning adenomas of the thyroid, and a form of precocious puberty that results from activation of G proteins in Leydig cells of the testis (causing a premature increase in testosterone).

Activating mutations in seven transmembrane domain receptors have also been described and have cellular effects that are similar to those of Gsα mutations in the specific tissues in which the receptors are expressed (Table 46-2). For example, activating mutations of the TSH receptor have been identified in autonomously functioning thyroid nodules (*see* Chapter 50). These mutations, which are distributed throughout the transmembrane domain, result in constitutive activation of G-protein signaling. Constitutive activation of the cAMP pathway leads to cellular proliferation, as well as enhanced thyroid cell function. Analogous mutations have been identified in the LH receptor and cause precocious puberty in males. In the PTH receptor, activating mutations cause bone dysplasia. In the calcium receptor, activating mutations are responsible for familial hypocalcemia because they mimic feedback suppression of PTH by calcium. Given that a variety of different G-protein-coupled receptors have been shown to be activated by mutations, it is likely that the spectrum of diseases caused by this group of receptors will continue to expand.

Inactivating mutations of several G-protein coupled receptors have also been described (Table 46-2). These mutations are inherited in an X-linked or autosomal recessive manner and typically cause resistance to the hormone that normally activates the receptor. For example, vasopressin receptor mutations cause a form of nephrogenic diabetes insipidus that is unresponsive to exogenous vasopressin, and TSH receptor mutations cause resistance to TSH. In other cases, the phenotype is more complex, perhaps because receptor function is also required for normal development. Genotypic males with LH receptor mutations can present with pseudohermaphroditism, reflecting incomplete sexual differentiation. Heterozygous inactivating calcium receptor mutations cause the syndrome of familial hypocalciuric hypercalcemia (FHH) (OMIM 145980), and homozygous mutations cause severe neonatal hypercalcemia (*see* Chapter 51).

INTRACELLULAR SIGNALING PATHWAYS

As described above, membrane receptors represent a critical cellular link to the extracellular environment. Within the cell, an intricate set of signaling pathways communicate receptor

Table 46-1
Mammalian G-Protein α-Subunits

a-Subunit	*Expression*	*Effector molecule(s)*
G_s	Ubiquitous	Increases adenylyl cyclase and Ca^{2+} channel activity
G_{olf}	Olfactory	Increases adenylyl cyclase activity
G_{t1}	Rod photoreceptors	Increases cGMP phosphodiesterase activity
G_{t2}	Cone photoreceptors	Increases cGMP phosphodiesterase activity
G_{gust}	Taste cells	Unknown
G_{i1}	Neural > other	Decreases adenylyl cyclase and K^+ channel activity
G_{i2}	Ubiquitous	Decreases adenylyl cyclase and K^+ channel activity
G_{i3}	Other tissues > neural	Decreases adenylyl cyclase and K^+ channel activity
G_o	Neural, endocrine	Decreases Ca^{2+} channel activity
G_z	Neural, platelets	Unknown
G_q	Ubiquitous	Increases phospholipase C-β1 activity
G_{11}	Ubiquitous	Increases phospholipase C-β1 activity
G_{14}	Liver, lung, kidney	Increases phospholipase C-β1 activity
$G_{15/16}$	Blood cells	Increases phospholipase C-β1 activity
G_{12}	Ubiquitous	Unknown
G_{13}	Ubiquitous	Unknown

Table 46-2
Endocrine Disorders Associated with Mutations of Seven Transmembrane Domain Receptors and G Proteins

Mutated protein	*Disorder*	*OMIM no.*	*Type of mutation*
Gain of function mutations			
$G\alpha_s$	McCune-Albright syndrome	174800	Somatic
	Acromegaly-somatotroph adenomas		Somatic
	Hyperfunctioning thyroid adenomas		Somatic
$G\alpha_{i2}$	Adrenal cortical and ovarian neoplasms	139360	Somatic
LH receptor	Familial male precocious puberty	152790	Autosomal dominant
TSH receptor	Nonautoimmune hereditary hyperthyroidism	275200	Autosomal dominant
	Hyperfunctioning thyroid adenoma		Somatic
PTH receptor	Jansen metaphyseal chondrodysplasia	169468	Autosomal dominant
Calcium sensing receptor	Hypoparathyroidism; hypocalcemia	145980	Autosomal dominant
Loss of function mutations			
$G\alpha_s$	Albright hereditary osteodystrophy	300800	Autosomal dominant
ACTH receptor	Familial ACTH resistance	202200	Autosomal recessive
Vasopressin receptor	Nephrogenic diabetes insipidus	304800	X-linked
Calcium sensing receptor	Familial hypocalciuric hypercalcemia	145980	Autosomal dominant
	Neonatal severe hyperparathyroidism		Autosomal recessive
FSH receptor	Hypergonadotropic ovarian dysgenesis	136435	Autosomal recessive
LH receptor	Male pseudohermaphroditism	152790	Autosomal recessive
GHRH receptor	Dwarfism	139191	Autosomal recessive
TSH receptor	Congenital hypothyroidism	275200	Autosomal recessive
TRH	Congenital hypothyroidism	188545	Autosomal recessive

OMIM, Online Mendelian inheritance of man; LH, luteinizing hormone; TSH, thyroid stimulating hormone; PTH, parathyroid hormone; ACTH, adrenocorticotropic hormone; FSH, follicle-stimulating hormone; GHRH, growth hormone releasing hormone; TRH, thyrotropin releasing hormone.

responses to other receptors, as well as to the cytoplasmic and nuclear compartments. For the most part, these signaling pathways consist of enzyme cascades, although there are exceptions, including gases such as nitric oxide (NO), lipids, and transcription factors (such as the STAT proteins). In many cases, receptors activate several different signaling pathways. The strategy of using combinations of pathways provides an important mechanism for generating specific cellular responses. Another characteristic of signal transduction pathways is the potential for "crosstalk" in which one pathway may activate or inhibit another pathway. Again, this generates the potential for diverse responses. In the section below, specific examples are provided for some of the better studied signaling pathways that play a key role in endocrine responses.

p21*ras* AND MITOGEN-ACTIVATED PROTEIN KINASES

Because growth factors induce a variety of cellular responses, including proliferation, there has been great interest in delineating the pathways that mediate growth factor responses. Recently, there has been tremendous progress in the elucidation of numerous cytoplasmic and nuclear kinases involved in growth responses.

The number of different kinases is enormous, and they have been estimated to account for as many as 5–10% of transcribed genes. The family of mitogen-activated protein kinases (MAPKs) includes the extracellular signal-regulated kinases (ERKs), stress-activated or c-Jun N-terminal protein kinases (SAPKs on JNKs), and p38-kinases (Fig. 46-6). As noted above, tyrosine phosphorylation of growth factor receptors, such as EGF, creates a binding site for a variety of adaptor proteins. One adaptor, growth factor receptor-binding protein 2 (Grb-2), binds to tyrosine-phosphorylated proteins through its central SH2 domain. Grb-2 contains flanking SH3 domains that recruit proline-rich guanine nucleotide exchange factors, such as SOS (*Drosophila* son of sevenless). After growth factor treatment (e.g., EGF), the Grb-2–SOS complex associates with the tyrosine-phosphorylated receptor, which leads to the activation of p21*ras* and induction of downstream kinases.

The signal transduction pathways downstream of growth factor receptors involve a complex interplay of parallel, diverging, and converging pathways. The Ras proteins link growth factor receptor activation to protein phosphorylation and gene regulation through cascades of protein kinases. Induction of MAPKs requires dual phosphorylation on threonine and tyrosine residues by MAPK kinases (MAPKK) or MEKs. Several different protein kinases are capable of functioning as MEK kinases (MEKKs), including Raf-1 (Fig. 46-6). In some cell types, the SAPKs and p38 kinases are activated by cellular stresses, including specific stimuli such as tumor necrosis factor-α (TNF-α), UV irradiation, or genotoxic alkylating chemicals. The mechanisms by which one particular MAPK module is activated in response to a particular stimulus may depend on which combinations of kinases are present as well as interactions among various signaling cascades.

Transcription factors (e.g., c-Jun, c-Fos, ATF-2, Elk-1) are one of the targets of MAPK cascades and provide an important mechanism for altering patterns of gene expression in response to extracellular signals. Phosphorylation of the transcription factor can alter interactions with transcriptional partners, change DNA binding affinity for a particular DNA sequence, or affect the activation surfaces that interact with the basal transcription apparatus. As an example, c-Jun is phosphorylated by several different kinases, including ERKs and SAPKs. Amino-terminal phosphorylation of c-Jun by the SAPKs enhances transactivation function, whereas phosphorylation of c-Jun near its DNA binding domain enhances DNA binding.

As with hormone regulatory systems, negative feedback is critical for dampening signal transduction systems once they have been activated. Because most of these pathways involve reversible protein phosphorylation, protein phosphatases provide a mechanism for temporally modulating specific signals. It has been estimated that there may be as many as 1000 distinct protein phosphatase genes. The physiologic importance of these phosphatases is exemplified by the ability of SV40 small t antigen to exert its cellular transforming effects by inhibiting protein phosphatase 2A (PP2A), with consequent induction of MEK and ERK activity in the cell. Various growth factors induce phosphatases differentially. This may explain, in part, why treatment with one growth factor can result in sustained activation of ERK, whereas another factor causes transient stimulation of the kinase.

CALCIUM SIGNALING

Many cellular responses involve alterations in intracellular calcium as a mechanism for transmitting signals. There are two main pathways that initiate Ca^{2+} signaling. In nonexcitable cells, the slow inositol pathway (inositol 1,4,5-trisphosphate [IP_3]) predominates, initiated either by receptor tyrosine kinases or by G-protein-coupled receptors of the seven transmembrane domain class. Receptor tyrosine kinases stimulate phospholipase Cγ to produce IP_3, which acts as a second messenger to trigger the release of Ca^{2+} from the endoplasmic reticulum. The G-protein-coupled receptors can increase intracellular Ca^{2+} by activating phospholipase Cβ. In excitable cells, voltage-dependent Ca^{2+} channels trigger more dramatic Ca^{2+} fluxes. Calcium binds to calmodulin (CaM), which serves as an intracellular sensor of calcium concentration. CaM binds to a number of enzymes (CaM kinases 1–5) protein phosphatases, and adenylate cyclases. The p21*ras*–MAPK signaling pathway is also activated by alterations in intracellular Ca^{2+}.

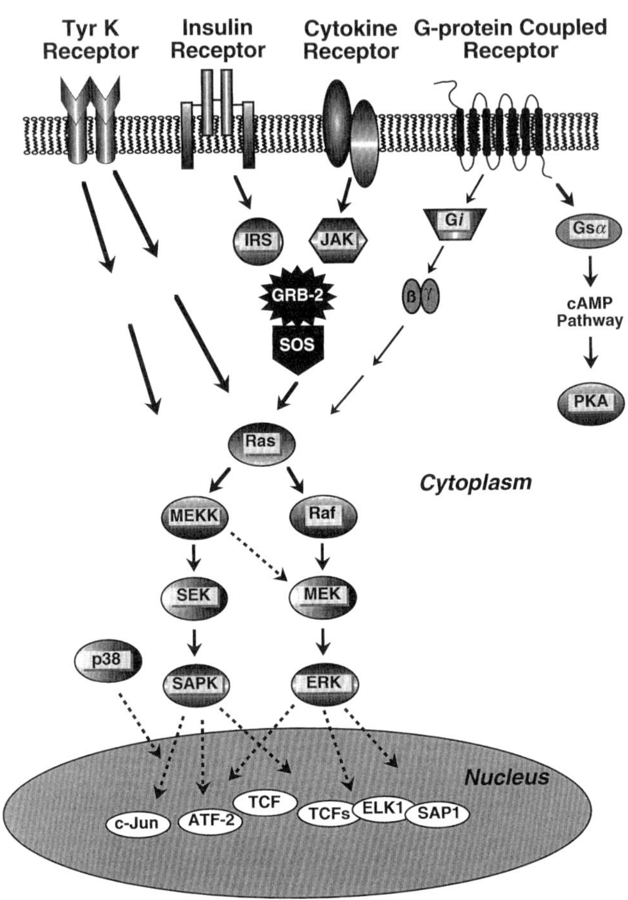

Figure 46-6 Signal transduction cascades. Most cells express a wide variety of different growth factor receptors. Each of these receptors can activate an array of signaling pathways, not all of which are shown. Tyrosine kinases induce the binding of SH2 domain proteins, such as Grb2. Grb2 binds to guanine nucleotide exchange factors, such as son of sevenless (SOS). This pathway can also be activated by the insulin receptor via insulin-related substrate (IRS) or by cytokine receptors via Janus-activated kinases (JAK). Although Gsα-coupled receptors act primarily through the cAMP pathway, they can also activate mitogen-activated kinases (MAPK) through their β–γ-subunits. This figure emphasizes the observation that different receptors can activate the *ras* pathway along with one or more downstream kinase cascades. *Ras* activates several downstream kinases in a cell type-specific manner. The preferential activation of a particular MAPK module, such as activation of the extracellular regulated kinase (ERK) rather than the SAPK pathway, provides a mechanism for specific responses. There are many cellular targets of these kinases, including a variety of transcription factors that are involved in cellular growth responses.

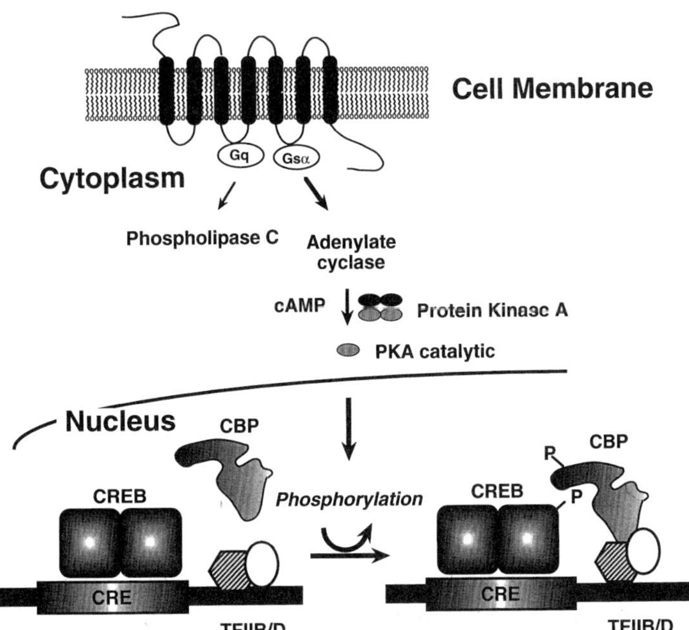

Figure 46-7 cAMP stimulation of transcriptional responses. G-protein-coupled receptors provide a major pathway for the generation of cAMP by adenylate cyclase. Increased cAMP levels within the cell cause dissociation of the tetrameric protein kinase A (PKA) holoenzyme leading to the release of the active catalytic subunit of PKA. The active catalytic subunit is translocated to the nucleus, where it phosphorylates transcription factor CREB, which binds as a homodimer to specific cAMP response elements (CREs) on target genes. The phosphorylation of CREB induces the binding of the coactivator, CREB-binding protein (CBP), which is also a substrate for phosphorylation. These transcription factors act by interacting with basal transcription factors such as TFIIB and TFIID. Several other kinases may phosphorylate CREB, including the calcium-regulated kinases.

Cyclic AMP response element binding protein (CREB) has been implicated as one of several transcription factors that can be activated by alterations in intracellular calcium. Ca^{2+}-induced phosphorylation of CREB requires a novel p21*ras*-dependent 105-kDa kinase. This novel kinase leads to phosphorylation of CREB at Ser 133, and thereby enhances transactivation function *(see below)*. Activation of these transcription factors by Ca^{2+} leads to the induction of temporally distinct immediate-early and delayed response genes.

cAMP-DEPENDENT SIGNALING

cAMP-dependent signaling cascades are typically initiated by the binding of peptide hormones to their membrane receptors. However, intracellular cAMP concentrations are also modulated by processes intrinsic to the cell, such as the cell cycle. The pleiotropic array of cellular effects of cAMP are primarily mediated by protein kinase A, which acts on a number of cellular substrates, including enzymes, the cytoskeleton, and transcription factors. As depicted in Fig. 46-7, cAMP binds to a regulatory subunit of protein kinase A, leading to dissociation of an active catalytic subunit that phosphorylates specific substrates.

In addition to receptors, ion channels, cytoskeletal proteins, and enzymes, a group of transcription factors are important targets of the protein kinase A pathway. These include the CREBs and activating transcription factors (ATFs) that are members of the B-Zip class of transcription factors. Posttranslational modification of CREB by phosphorylation at serine residues induces conformational changes that alter the affinity of CREB for coactivator proteins, such as CREB-binding protein (CBP) or the TATA box-binding protein coactivator TAF_{II} 110. CBP is thought to form a bridge between CREB and the basal transcription apparatus (Fig. 46-7). CBP also interacts with other B-Zip proteins, such as c-Jun and c-Fos, other transcription factors, including c-Myb, as well as specific kinases. In addition to a clear role in cAMP signaling, CBP has also been implicated in mitogenic signaling. Consistent with its role in multiple cell signaling pathways, mutations of CBP cause Rubinstein-Tabi syndrome (OMIM 180849), which is associated with mental retardation, multiple congenital anomalies, and predisposition to malignancy. The B-Zip dimerization structure of the CREB and ATF proteins provides the basis for numerous combinations of different members of this family. The closely related cAMP response element modulator (CREM) gene product can act as a transdominant negative regulator of CREB transcriptional activity, either by forming inactive heterodimers with CREB or by binding to the CRE as an inactive complex.

In addition to the canonical CRE, several other DNA regulatory elements and transcription factors are capable of stimulating gene transcription in response to cAMP. The transcription factor, activator protein 2 (AP-2), also functions in basal, phorbol ester, and cAMP-mediated transcriptional induction. The CAAT enhancer binding protein (C/EBP) induces transcription of the adipocyte protein 2 gene promoter (aP2 gene) and stearoyl acyl CoA desaturase (SCD-1) through a region that is also regulated by cAMP. cAMP-responsive regions of several genes appear to overlap with binding sites for nuclear receptors, some of which may also transduce cAMP effects.

CELL-CYCLE REGULATORY SIGNAL TRANSDUCTION PATHWAYS

Phosphorylation plays an essential regulatory role in the cell cycle, and a large array of cyclin-dependent kinases (CDKs) have been identified (*see* Chapter 6). The regulatory subunits of the

CDKs, known as cyclins, form complexes with their catalytic partners, to function as heterodimeric holoenzymes that phosphorylate specific proteins, including the tumor suppressor protein pRB (*see* Chapter 105). Phosphorylation of pRB blocks its critical inhibitory function, allowing cell-cycle progression and differentiation to occur. Several proteins capable of binding cyclins and inhibiting CDK activity have been identified and are referred to as CDKIs. The CDKIs inhibit cell-cycle progression and inhibit tumor formation. Translocation of the cyclin D1 gene has been associated with certain cases of hyperparathyroidism (*see* Chapter 51), and actually led to the identification of cyclin D1 in humans. In these cases, a somatic inversion of chromosome 11 brings cyclin D1 under the control of the PTH promoter. Consequently, cyclin D1 is overexpressed in the parathyroid cell and results in cellular proliferation.

NUCLEAR RECEPTORS

OVERVIEW OF NUCLEAR RECEPTOR ACTION The nuclear receptor superfamily consists of several hundred structurally related proteins that function by increasing or decreasing the rate of gene transcription (*see* Chapter 3). The nuclear receptors mediate the physiologic actions of small cell-permeable hormones, such as the sex steroid molecules (estrogen, testosterone, and progesterone), cortisol, aldosterone, and vitamin D, as well as retinoids that are derived from dietary vitamin A. There is also a large subfamily of nuclear receptors for which no ligand has been identified, or which may not require the binding of a ligand for functional activation. This group of receptors are referred to as orphan nuclear receptors. Nuclear receptors interact with specific DNA sequences, known as hormone response elements (HREs), that are typically located in the promoter regions of target genes. After the receptor binds to DNA, it is positioned to interact with other transcription factors to alter rates of gene transcription.

STRUCTURE AND CLASSIFICATION OF NUCLEAR RECEPTORS Although nuclear receptors can be classified based on their ligands, structural similarities and DNA recognition sites provide a particularly useful classification system because it allows predictions to be made for receptor members that have not been characterized extensively. The DNA-binding domain (DBD) is the most highly conserved region of nuclear receptors (Fig. 46-8). The DBD consists of two centrally located zinc fingers, the structure of which has been well characterized using X-ray crystallography and nuclear magnetic resonance studies. The amino acid sequence at the carboxyterminal base of the first zinc finger is the primary determinant of DNA binding specificity, and provides a convenient means for classifying subfamilies of receptors that bind to related DNA elements. Other domains of nuclear receptors have also been clearly delineated. The ligand-binding domain (LBD) is located in the carboxyterminus of the receptor. This region of nuclear receptors has several overlapping functional domains, including regions required for dimerization and for transcriptional activation and repression. The structure of the ligand-binding domain has also been solved by X-ray crystallography, and several lines of evidence indicate that ligand binding induces significant conformational changes in the receptor. The amino-terminal region of nuclear receptors is the most variable and the least characterized. In some cases, it has been shown to contain additional transcription-activating domains.

Nuclear receptors can generally be divided into two groups (Table 46-3). The classic steroid receptors share a similar DNA-binding domain and DNA recognition sequence. This group includes receptors for glucocorticoids, mineralocorticoid, progesterone, and testosterone. Of note, even though the estrogen receptor (ER) binds to a steroid hormone, it shares more in common with the second group of nuclear receptors *(see below)*. The steroid receptors often reside in the cytoplasm of the cell, complexed with proteins of the heat shock family. After ligand binds to the receptors, they disassociate from the heat shock proteins, translocate to the nucleus, and bind to hormone response elements in target genes. The steroid group of receptors bind to DNA only as homodimers, and their DNA binding sites reflect this twofold symmetry by being configured as palindromic pairs of monomeric "half-sites."

A second major group of nuclear receptors includes thyroid hormone receptor (TR), retinoic acid receptor (RAR), ER, and many others that share a similar DNA recognition sequence in the first zinc finger, and bind to a related DNA sequence, AGGTCA. This group of receptors also shows great flexibility in terms of dimerization. Many of these receptors can bind to DNA as monomers (particularly orphan receptors), but several bind to DNA as heterodimers as well as homodimers. The heterodimer partners typically include other members of this receptor subfamily. The retinoid X receptors (RXRs) serve as heterodimeric partners for several different nuclear receptors, including RARs, TRs, vitamin D receptor (VDR), and peroxisome proliferator-activating receptors (PPARs). The heterodimers typically bind to hormone response elements that are arranged as direct repeats rather than in a palindromic manner. The spacing between these half-sites, and variations in some of the contextual bases, provide specificity to different receptors, providing a partial explanation for how so many different receptors can share a common binding motif but elicit distinct cellular responses. Most members of this subfamily bind nonsteroid molecules and are located in the nucleus before ligand binding. They are able to bind to DNA in the absence of ligand, often with specific regulatory effects (e.g., gene silencing). Thus, the regulation of this group of receptors represents a complex interplay of receptor dimers, interactions with different DNA elements, and binding by specific ligands.

A subject of great interest is whether orphan receptors function without ligands, or whether the ligand remains to be identified. The RXRs were initially classified as orphan receptors, but are now known to bind 9-*cis* retinoic acid. The PPARγ receptors have been found to bind a variety of eicosanoids, as well as thiazolidinediones that are used to treat non–insulin-dependent diabetes. Other orphan receptors may be regulated by posttranslational modifications such as phosphorylation.

There has been rapid progress toward defining the mechanism by which nuclear receptors influence gene transcription. Several of the nuclear receptors have been found to physically interact with the basal transcription factor, TFIIB. Using in vitro transcription analysis, the nuclear receptors have been shown to facilitate the rate of assembly and stabilize basal transcription factors in the preinitiation complex that forms at the TATA box. An additional level of transcriptional control occurs through nuclear receptor interactions with "coactivator" or "corepressor" proteins, which in turn interact with proteins of the basal transcription factor complex. Several of these proteins have been identified on the basis of their ability to interact with nuclear receptors, but their role in transcriptional modulation is still being defined. Coactivators and corepressors may contribute to the development of specific diseases. Recently, a region of chromosome 20q that is often ampli-

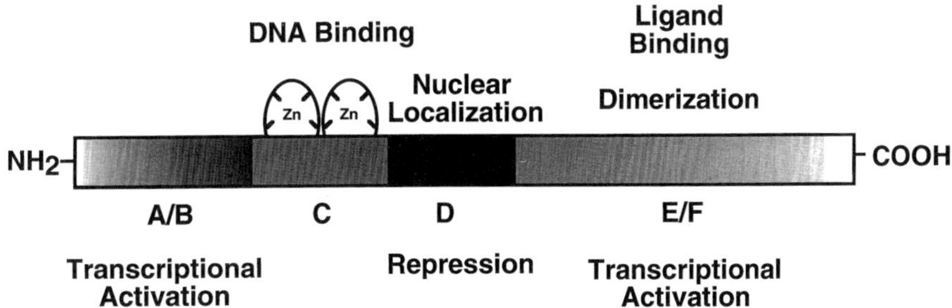

Figure 46-8 Nuclear hormone receptors. The nuclear receptors contain conserved modular functional domains. The central DNA-binding domain (C) is the most highly conserved region. Characteristic zinc finger domains are depicted. The carboxy-terminal region (E/F) contains several functional domains, including ligand binding, dimerization, and transcriptional activation region. A region (D) between the ligand-binding domain and the DNA-binding domain mediates nuclear localization and binds transcriptional corepressors. In most receptors, the amino-terminal domain (A/B) contains motifs involved in transcriptional activation.

Table 46-3
Ligands and Antagonists for Nuclear Receptors

Receptor	*Ligand*	*Antagonists*	*DNA response element*	*P box*
Glucocorticoid subfamily				
GR	Cortisol	RU-486	TGAACATGTTCT	GSCKV
PR	Progesterone	RU-486	TGAACATGTTCT	GSCKV
MR	Aldosterone, cortisol	Spironolactone	TGAACATGTTCT	GSCKV
AR	Dihydrotestosterone	Flutamide, cyproterone acetate	TGAACATGTTCT	GSCKV
ER/TR Family				
ER	Estrogen	Tamoxifen, clomiphene, ICI 164, 384	AGGTCAnnnTGACCT	EGCKA
TR	Triiodothyronine (T3)	None	AGGTCAnnnnAGGTCA	EGCKG
VDR	1,25-Dihydroxyvitamin D	None	AGGTCAnnnAGGTCA	EGCKG
RAR	All-*trans* retinoic acid	Ro 41-5253	AGGTCAnnnnnAGGTCA	EGCKG
RXR	9-*cis* Retinoic acid	None	AGGTCAnAGGTCA	EGCKG
PPARγ	Prostaglandin J_2, thiazolidinedione	None	AGGTCAnAGGTCA	EGCKG

PR, progesterone receptor; GR, glucocorticoid receptor; MR, mineralocorticoid receptor; AR, androgen receptor; ER, estrogen receptor; TR, thyroid hormone receptor; VDR, vitamin D receptor; RAR, retinoic acid receptor; RXR, 9-*cis* retinoic acid receptor; PPAR, peroxisome proliferator activated receptor. The P-box refers to a five-amino acid sequence (in single letter code) at the base of the first zinc finger in the DNA-binding domain of the nuclear receptors. The half-sites refer to a consensus nucleotide sequence recognized by the DNA-binding domains of the receptor subfamilies.

fied in breast cancers was shown to encode a steroid receptor coactivator, AIB1, that enhances estrogen-dependent transcription and is overexpressed in ~65% of breast cancers. The CBP gene is also translocated in a subset of treatment-induced cases of acute myelogenous leukemias. Another important aspect of nuclear receptor action is their ability to crosstalk with other regulatory pathways. For example, growth factor pathways can alter the function of some nuclear receptors, such as the ER and progesterone receptor (PR). Certain nuclear receptors, including the glucocorticoid receptor (GR), TR, and RAR, interact with c-Jun or c-Fos, resulting in mutual antagonism. There is also evidence for nuclear receptor interactions with CBP, providing another means to inhibit the pathways (e.g., CREB, c-Jun, c-Fos) that converge on the CPB integrator protein. Finally, several nuclear receptors have been found to alter the conformation of DNA and associated chromatin, and in this manner may be able to alter the access of other transcription factors to the regulatory regions of genes.

PHYSIOLOGIC EFFECTS OF NUCLEAR RECEPTORS

Nuclear receptors serve an important role in development, cell differentiation, metabolism, and reproduction. Some of these functions will be described briefly to provide examples of how nuclear receptors impact on physiology. The orphan receptor, steroidogenic factor-1 (SF-1) provides a good example of a receptor that plays a critical developmental role. SF-1 is selectively expressed in the adrenal gland and in reproductive tissues. Targeted disruption of SF-1 has been shown to prevent adrenal development and causes dysfunction at multiple levels of the reproductive axis. SF-1 appears to play dual role in cell viability and the direct regulation of a variety of steroidogenic enzyme genes.

The glucocorticoid receptor mediates the widespread effects of cortisol on blood pressure, blood glucose levels and insulin action, neuropsychiatric status, diurnal variation in body temperature, and immune responses. The closely related mineralocorticoid receptor binds aldosterone and regulates the renal handling of potassium and sodium.

The sex steroid receptors determine the phenotypic appearance of secondary sexual characteristics and control the production of oocytes and sperm. Testosterone itself binds relatively weakly to the androgen receptor, but it is converted to the more active metabolite, dehydrotestosterone, by the enzyme 5α-reductase,

Table 46-4
Disorders Caused by Mutations in Nuclear Receptors

Receptor	*Disorder*	*OMIM no.*	*Mechanism*	*Inheritance*
Androgen receptor	Androgen insensitivity	313700	Premature stop codon, DNA-binding domain mutation	X-linked
Androgen receptor	Prostate cancer		Point mutations	Somatic
Estrogen receptor	Estrogen resistance	133430	Point mutations, deletions	Autosomal recessive
Estrogen receptor	Breast cancer		? Postreceptor	Somatic
Glucocorticoid receptor	Glucocorticoid resistance	138040	Point mutations	Autosomal dominant
Thyroid hormone receptor β	Resistance to thyroid hormone	188570	Ligand-binding mutations	Autosomal dominant
Vitamin D receptor	Vitamin D-resistant rickets	277440	DNA-binding mutant, ligand-binding mutant	Autosomal recessive
Retinoic acid receptor	Promyelocytic leukemia	180240	Fusion protein lacking RAR DNA-binding domain	Somatic translocation

OMIM, Mendelian inheritance of man; RAR, retinoic acid receptor.

which is expressed at high levels in many androgen-responsive tissues. Therefore, tissue specific variation in 5α-reductase expression can influence the extent of androgen responsiveness. The reproductive nuclear receptors are also notable because of the existence of clinically useful receptor antagonists (Table 46-3). RU-486 binds with high affinity to the progesterone receptor ligand-binding domain (it also binds the glucocorticoid receptor) in such a manner that its transcriptional activating properties are blocked. Similarly, tamoxifen binds to the estrogen receptor ligand-binding domain but fails to convert the receptor to a transcriptionally active form. The development of specific receptor antagonists for reproductive and other nuclear receptors is an active area of investigation, and promises to provide a plethora of useful new drugs and experimental tools.

The nonsteroid nuclear receptors (e.g., thyroid hormone, retinoid, vitamin D, and the orphan receptors) mediate a variety of developmental and metabolic pathways. In several cases, multiple receptor isoforms provide an additional level of control. For example, there are two separate genes for TRs, three for all-*trans* RARs, and three for the retinoic 9-*cis* RXRs. In addition, many of these genes generate multiple receptor subtypes by virtue of alternate mRNA splicing or alternate promoter usage. The function of individual isoforms is not clear, but there is a complex pattern of overlapping tissue-specific expression. Receptor subtype expression is highly regulated during development, and there is striking tissue-specific expression of various nuclear receptor isoforms in adult organs. Therefore, like the peptide hormone receptors, tissue responsiveness to the hormone signal is regulated at its most fundamental level by selective expression of the nuclear receptor in responsive tissues.

Nuclear receptors have been found to play a prominent role in human disease, many of which are described in detail in subsequent chapters (Table 46-4). The most well-described disorders are those of resistance to nuclear hormone action, caused by deletion or mutation of the receptors. Such hormone-resistance syndromes have been described for the estrogen, glucocorticoid, androgen, vitamin D, and thyroid hormone receptors. As an example, androgen resistance is inherited in an X-linked fashion, reflecting the X-chromosomal location of the androgen receptor. More than 50 complete or partially inactivating mutations of the androgen receptor have been described (*see* Chapter 56). In the fully resistant form (testicular feminization), 46,X,Y individuals have female secondary sexual features, but milder cases of resistance can result in more subtle forms of feminization. Resistance to thyroid hormone is unusual because it is inherited in an autosomal dominant manner (*see* Chapter 50). In this disorder, the mutations are limited to the carboxy-terminal domain of the receptor, and result in loss of thyroid hormone binding or transactivation. However, because dimerization and DNA binding are preserved, the inactive mutant receptors can still bind to target genes and act as antagonists. This "dominant negative" property appears to explain the dominant pattern of inheritance. Another important example of nuclear receptor mutations causing human disease involves a translocation of the RAR receptor (t15; 17) in acute promyelocytic leukemia in which the RAR-α recombines with a putative tumor suppressor, PML. Treatment with high doses of retinoids causes the maturation of the leukemic cells and can result in clinical remission. Somatic mutations of other receptors (estrogen, androgen) are thought to play a role in hormonally responsive tumors, such as breast and prostate cancer. Recently, environmental toxins, such as DDT and halogenated aromatic hydrocarbons, have been found to interact with the nuclear receptors for androgens and estrogen. Finally, our knowledge of nuclear receptor biology will eventually allow a better understanding of conditions of nuclear hormone excess and deficiency states, such as Cushing's disease, adrenal insufficiency, hyperthyroidism, and hypothyroidism.

SELECTED REFERENCES

Anzick SL, Kononen J, Walker RL, et al. AIB1, a steroid receptor coactivator amplified in breast and ovarian cancer. Science 1997;277: 965–968.

Boguski MS, McCormick F. Proteins regulating Ras and its relatives. Nature 1993;366:643–654.

Chao MV. Neurotrophin receptors: a window into neuronal differentiation. Neuron 1992;9:583–593.

Clapham DE. Calcium signaling. Cell 1995;80:259–268.

Cobb MH, Goldsmith EJ. How MAP kinases are regulated. J Biol Chem 1995;270:14,843–14,846.

Collu R, Tang J, Castagne J, et al. A novel mechanism for isolated central hypothyroidism: inactivating mutations in the thyrotropin-releasing hormone receptor gene. J Clin Endocrinol Metab 1997;82:1561–1565.

Conklin BR, Bourne HR. Structural elements of G alpha subunits that interact with G beta gamma, receptors, and effectors. Cell 1993;73: 631–641.

Gammeltoft S, Kahn CR. Hormone signaling via membrane receptors. In: DeGroot LJ, ed. Endocrinology. Philadelphia: WB Saunders, 1995; pp. 17–65.

Ghosh A, Greenberg ME. Calcium signaling in neurons: molecular mechanisms and cellular consequences. Science 1995;268:239–247.

Glass CK, Rose DW, Rosenfeld MG. Nuclear receptor coactivators. Curr Opin Cell Biol 1997;9:222–232.

Habener JF. Cyclic AMP second messenger signaling pathway. In: DeGroot LJ, ed. Endocrinology. Philadelphia: WB Saunders, 1995; pp. 77–92.

Hahn SA, Schutte M, Hoque AT, et al. DPC4, a candidate tumor suppressor gene at human chromosome 18q21.1. Science 1996;271: 350–353.

Heldin CH. Dimerization of cell surface receptors in signal transduction. Cell 1995;80:213–223.

Hunter T. Protein kinases and phosphatases: the yin and yang of protein phosphorylation and signaling. Cell 1995;80:225–236.

Ihle JN. Cytokine receptor signalling. Nature 1995;377:591–594.

Ihle JN. STATs: signal transducers and activators of transcription. Cell 1996;84:331–334.

Insel PA. Seminars in medicine of the Beth Israel Hospital, Boston. Adrenergic receptors—evolving concepts and clinical implications. N Engl J Med 1996;334:580–585.

Jameson JL. Applications of molecular biology in endocrinology. In: DeGroot LJ, ed. Endocrinology. Philadelphia: WB Saunders, 1995; pp. 119–147.

Jameson JL. Principles of hormone action. In: Weatherall DJ, Ledingham JGG, Warrell DA, eds. Oxford Textbook of Medicine. Oxford: Oxford Medical Publishers, 1996; pp. 1553–1573.

Josso N, di Clemente N. Serine/threonine kinase receptors and ligands. Curr Opin Genet Dev 1997;7:371–377.

Karin M. The regulation of AP-1 activity by mitogen-activated protein kinases. J Biol Chem 1995;270:16,483–16,486.

Kishimoto T, Taga T, Akira S. Cytokine signal transduction. Cell 1994;76:253–262.

Malarkey K, Belham CM, Paul A, et al. The regulation of tyrosine kinase signalling pathways by growth factor and G-protein-coupled receptors. Biochem J 1995;309:361–375.

Mangelsdorf DJ, Thummel C, Beato M, et al. The nuclear receptor superfamily: the second decade. Cell 1995;83:835–839.

Marshall MS. Ras target proteins in eukaryotic cells. FASEB J 1995; 9:1311–1318.

Marshall CJ. Specificity of receptor tyrosine kinase signaling: transient versus sustained extracellular signal-regulated kinase activation. Cell 1995;80:179–185.

Massague J. Receptors for the TGF-beta family. Cell 1992;69:1067–1070.

Massague J, Weis-Garcia F. Serine/threonine kinase receptors: mediators of transforming growth factor beta family signals. Cancer Surv 1996;27:41–64.

Mathews LS. Activin receptors and cellular signaling by the receptor serine kinase family. Endocr Rev 1994;15:310–325.

McDonald NQ, Chao MV. Structural determinants of neurotrophin action. J Biol Chem 1995;270:19,669–19,672.

Pestell RG, Jameson JL. Transcriptional regulation of endocrine genes by second messenger signalling pathways. In: Weintraub BD, ed. Molecular Endocrinology: Basic Concepts and Clinical Correlations. New York: Raven, 1995; pp. 59–76.

Post GR, Brown JH. G protein-coupled receptors and signaling pathways regulating growth responses. FASEB J 1996;10:741–749.

Saltiel AR. Diverse signaling pathways in the cellular actions of insulin. Am J Physiol 1996;270:E375–E385.

Schlessinger J. How receptor tyrosine kinases activate Ras. Trends Biochem Sci 1993;18:273–275.

Spiegel AM. Defects in G protein-coupled signal transduction in human disease. Annu Rev Physiol 1996;58:143–170.

Spiegel AM, Weinstein LS, Shenker A. Abnormalities in G protein-coupled signal transduction pathways in human disease. J Clin Invest 1993;92:1119–1125.

Tsai MJ, O'Malley BW. Molecular mechanisms of action of steroid/thyroid receptor superfamily members. Annu Rev Biochem 1994;63:451–486.

van Biesen T, Luttrell LM, Hawes BE, Lefkowitz RJ. Mitogenic signaling via G protein-coupled receptors. Endocr Rev 1996;17:698–714.

Van Sande J, Parma J, Tonacchera M, Swillens S, Dumont J, Vassart G. Somatic and germline mutations of the TSH receptor gene in thyroid diseases. J Clin Endocrinol Metab 1995;80:2577–2585.

Wilks AF, Oates AC. The JAK/STAT pathway. Cancer Surv 1996;27: 139–163.

Woodgett JR, Avruch J, Kyriakis J. The stress activated protein kinase pathway. Cancer Surv 1996;27:127–138.

47 Diabetes Mellitus

William L. Lowe, Jr.

INTRODUCTION

Diabetes mellitus affects approximately 5% of the general population with its prevalence varying between ethnic groups and geographic regions. The majority of cases are accounted for by two different types of diabetes, type 1 and 2, which account for approximately 10 and 90% of cases of diabetes, respectively. Although these two disorders share a common phenotype, fasting and postprandial hyperglycemia, their etiology is distinct. Type 1 diabetes is characterized by pancreatic β-cell deficiency with a resulting absolute deficiency of insulin. The β-cell deficiency is most commonly secondary to autoimmune-mediated destruction. Type 2 diabetes, in contrast, is characterized by a deficiency of insulin action as a result of a combination of insulin resistance and β-cell dysfunction that is manifest as inadequate insulin secretion in the face of insulin resistance and hyperglycemia.

The familial clustering of both type 1 and 2 diabetes has long suggested a genetic contribution to the origin of the diseases. In the case of type 1 diabetes, the concordance rate among monozygotic twins is 25–50%, whereas the relative risk to an individual with a first-degree relative with type 1 diabetes is approximately 5–10% compared with the 0.4% risk in the general population. Although these data are consistent with a genetic contribution to the origin of the disease, the lack of 100% concordance in monozygotic twins suggests that environmental factors also make a significant contribution to the pathogenesis of the disease. These environmental factors have not been clearly defined, but seasonal variation in the onset of type 1 diabetes and its association with preceding episodes of specific viral infections suggest that viruses may be one of the important environmental factors. Familial clustering of disease is much more apparent in type 2 diabetes. The concordance rate among monozygotic twins has been shown to be 50–95%, whereas approximately 40% of siblings and approximately 30% of offspring of affected individuals develop either type 2 diabetes or impaired glucose tolerance. Again, these data are consistent with a significant genetic contribution to the development of type 2 diabetes but suggest that environmental influences are also important in its etiology.

With the advent of molecular genetics, significant progress has been made in defining the genetics of rare, monogenic forms of diabetes as well as more typical type 1 and 2 diabetes. This progress is reflected in the recent reclassification of diabetes that includes diagnostic categories of genetic defects in β-cell function and insulin action. This chapter will describe the recent advances in the genetics of both type 1 and 2 diabetes as well as monogenic forms of diabetes.

From: *Principles of Molecular Medicine* (J. L. Jameson, ed.), ©1998 Humana Press Inc., Totowa, NJ.

GENETICS OF TYPE 1 DIABETES MELLITUS

Type 1 diabetes often presents abruptly with marked hyperglycemia, polyuria, and ketoacidosis, which occur as a result of insulin deficiency. This dramatic presentation of the disease suggested initially that type 1 diabetes was the result of an acute event, but with an improved understanding of the pathogenesis of the disease, it is now clear that onset of the disease is a chronic process that can be divided into a series of stages. As will be discussed below, individuals have a genetic predisposition for diabetes. In certain of these individuals, an autoimmune process is initiated, presumably in response to some environmental exposure. There is then a period of active autoimmunity characterized by the presence of autoantibodies and progressive β-cell destruction but with maintenance of normal blood sugars and glucose tolerance. With sufficient β-cell destruction, impaired glucose tolerance, which is typically not clinically evident, and, subsequently, diabetes develop. Depending on the rate of decline of β-cell function, older patients may be presumed to have type 2 diabetes mellitus because of residual insulin secretion, albeit not sufficient insulin secretion to maintain euglycemia. As destruction of the residual β cells continues, a new stress, e.g., infection, often results in the acute presentation of diabetes. Ultimately, absolute insulin dependence develops because of total or near total β-cell destruction.

The autoimmune-mediated destruction of pancreatic β cells is characterized by two features, autoantibodies and insulitis. Autoantibodies present in type 1 diabetes mellitus are directed against a variety of β-cell antigens, including insulin, glutamic acid decarboxylase (GAD65 and 67), membrane proteins that are homologous to tyrosine phosphatases (ICA512 and IA-2), and islet neuroendocrine ganglioside. Although the presence of two or more of these antibodies is predictive of progression to diabetes in relatives of affected individuals, their role in the immune-mediated destruction of the islets cells is still unclear. Insulitis is characterized by inflammatory infiltrates in the islets consisting primarily of CD8 cells but also of CD4 cells, B cells, macrophages, and natural killer cells. The cause of type 1 diabetes mellitus, and, thus, the trigger for the autoimmune process, is complex and involves both a genetic predisposition and environmental factors. The genetics of type 1 diabetes mellitus are now being defined.

Type 1 diabetes does not follow a simple Mendelian pattern of inheritance. As demonstrated by studies in identical twins, there is not a 100% concordance between a susceptible genotype and disease presence. Presumably the penetrance of the disease genes is influenced by environmental factors that are, as yet, undefined. Moreover, studies in both mice and now humans clearly demonstrate that the disease is polygenic, suggesting that a sufficient complement of genes must be inherited to confer susceptibility to diabetes. Two approaches have been used to define genes that predispose to type 1 diabetes—identifying candidate genes by comparing the frequency of alleles of specific genes in diabetic and control populations (case-control or association studies) and genome scanning to identify chromosomal loci associated with disease susceptibility. Given the autoimmune origin of type 1 diabetes, the major histocompatibility locus (MHC) or human leukocyte antigen (HLA) region was examined initially as a candidate susceptibility locus. Association studies identified this region as a potential susceptibility locus, and this was confirmed in subsequent linkage studies. This locus is now referred to as *IDDM1*. The degree of family clustering of a disease is referred to as λ_s and can be estimated by comparing the disease risk in siblings of affected individuals to the prevalence of the disease in the general population. For type 1 diabetes, the λ_s is 15, whereas the λ_s for *IDDM1* is estimated to be 2.6, suggesting that *IDDM1* accounts for 35–40% of the familial inheritance of the disease.

Progress has been made in defining how *IDDM1* confers susceptibility to disease. The MHC is located on the short arm of chromosome 6 (6p21) and encodes proteins involved in the regulation of the immune process (*see* Chapter 31). The MHC consists of three major regions, A, B, and C, that encode class I genes, and the D region, which encodes class II genes. The class I molecules are highly polymorphic and present peptide fragments of foreign antigens to cytotoxic T lymphocytes. The class II molecules present foreign processed antigen to helper T cells and, thus, are involved in initiating the immune response. Class II molecules consist of an α and β chain that are encoded by different genes. There are two major classes of class II genes, the DR and DQ genes. The β but not the α chain in the DR molecules is polymorphic, whereas both the α and β chains are polymorphic in DQ molecules.

Initially an association between class I alleles and type 1 diabetes was demonstrated, but it is now clear that class II molecules are more important in conferring risk. The original association with class I molecules was likely caused by the nonrandom association of class I alleles with the class D alleles (linkage disequilibrium). Moreover, linkage disequilibrium of the DQ and DR alleles has created extended haplotypes (the presence of several genes on the same chromosome). Some of these class II alleles predict susceptibility to type 1 diabetes, whereas others either confer protection or are neutral. It is likely that both DR and DQ alleles are important in regulating susceptibility to type 1 diabetes. Interestingly, all of the DQ β chain alleles encoding a gene product with an aspartic acid at position 57 are either protective or neutral. In contrast, alleles with alanine or valine at position 57 confer susceptibility, whereas the one allele with serine at position 57 confers weak susceptibility. Position 57 of the DQ β chain is not, however, the sole determinant of risk; susceptibility and protection are also conferred by other residues in the DQ β chain and by different alleles of the other chains. The biologic consequences of these and other amino acid differences are still being defined, but changes in peptide-binding sites of these class II molecules may alter the specificity of the immune response to foreign or self-antigens by affecting the binding affinity of different peptide antigens for the class II molecules.

A second susceptibility locus that has been identified using a candidate gene approach is the insulin gene locus on chromosome 11p15.5. Linkage of this region, which is referred to as *IDDM2*, has also been demonstrated to type 1 diabetes. Among the polymorphisms in this region is the variable number of tandem repeats (VNTR) locus in the 5'-flanking region of the insulin gene. The VNTR consists of tandem repeats of a 14- to 15-bp core sequence. Three different alleles have been identified. The class I allele contains 34 to 45 repeats and is associated with a two- to fivefold increased risk of type 1 diabetes. The class III allele contains 141 to 209 repeats and has a dominant protective effect. The class II allele has approximately 80 repeats but is rare, and its association with disease susceptibility has not been defined. The λ_s for *IDDM2* is 1.3, and it accounts for 10% of the familial inheritance of type 1 diabetes.

Table 47-1
Susceptibility Loci for Type 1 Diabetes Mellitus

Susceptibility locus	*Chromosome*	*Linked markers*	λ_s
IDDM1[a]	6p21	HLA-DQB1, -DRB1	2.60
IDDM2[a]	11p15	Insulin VNTR	1.29
IDDM3	15q26	...	...
IDDM4[a]	11q13	FGF3, D11S1337	1.07
IDDM5[a]	6q25	D6S476-ESR-D6S448	1.16
IDDM7	2q31	D2S152	1.13
IDDM8[a]	6q27	D6S281	1.42
IDDM11	14q24.3–q31	D14S67	...
IDDM12[a]	2q33	CTLA-4	...
IDDM13	2q34	IGFBP-2, -5	...
	7q	GCK (glucokinase)	...

[a]Linkage confirmed in independent studies using independent data sets.
Adapted from Todd and Farrall (1996) and Cordell and Todd (1995).

IDDM2 is located within a 50-kbp region of chromosome 11 that contains the genes encoding tyrosine hydroxylase, insulin, and insulin-like growth factor-II (IGF-II). Multiple polymorphisms are present within this region, but an extensive series of genetic analyses mapped the *IDDM2* susceptibility locus to the VNTR in the 5'-flanking region of the insulin gene, suggesting that the variable number of repeats in some manner confers susceptibility to disease, perhaps because of effects on insulin gene expression. In vitro studies using the VNTR in reporter gene constructs have demonstrated that the VNTR modulates insulin gene expression, although conflicting data were obtained regarding the effect of the class III compared with class I allele on gene expression. In vivo studies have demonstrated that the class III allele is associated with decreased pancreatic insulin gene expression compared with transcription from the class I allele. A mechanism by which the VNTR could affect disease susceptibility via its effects on pancreatic expression of the insulin gene was not obvious. Subsequent studies, however, have examined effects of the VNTR on prenatal and postnatal expression of the insulin gene in the human thymus. Interestingly, the class III allele is associated with an approximately 2.5-fold increase in insulin gene expression in the thymus compared with the class I allele. Similarly, increased levels of proinsulin are present in thymi from class III/I heterozygotes compared with class I/I homozygotes. Increased expression of insulin in the thymus might facilitate tolerance to insulin by promoting deletion of insulin-specific T lymphocytes, and, thus, provide protection from type 1 diabetes.

Because *IDDM1* and *IDDM2* account for only approximately 50% of the familial clustering of type 1 diabetes, additional genes must be involved. To identify these genes, genome scans have been performed using DNA from sibling pairs affected by type 1 diabetes. The aim of genome scans using affected sib pairs is to scan the entire genome with a collection of genetic markers, calculate the degree of allele sharing at each marker or locus, and identify those chromosomal loci in which allele sharing by the affected siblings occurs with greater frequency than expected,

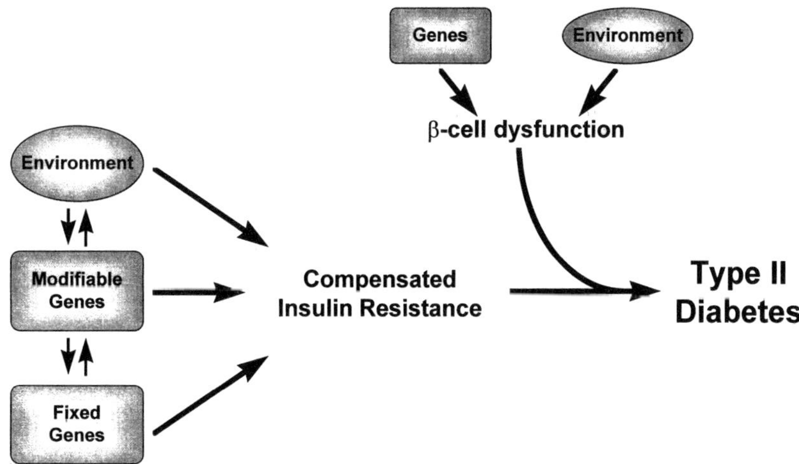

Figure 47-1 Schematic model of the origin of type 2 diabetes mellitus. Type 2 diabetes is secondary to both insulin resistance and inadequate insulin secretion secondary to β-cell dysfunction. With sufficient β-cell function, euglycemia or impaired glucose tolerance is maintained in the presence of insulin resistance at the expense of hyperinsulinemia (compensated insulin resistance). With concomitant β-cell dysfunction, however, inadequate insulin secretion to compensate for the insulin resistance results in the onset of type 2 diabetes. Similarly, a primary defect in β-cell function may result in type 2 diabetes in the presence of some degree of insulin resistance. Both insulin resistance and β-cell dysfunction are influenced by genetic and environmental factors. Type 2 diabetes is multigenic, and its penetrance is secondary to the expression of several different genes, some of which are likely fixed and act independently of environmental factors. Other predisposing genes might be modifiable in that their expression or action is influenced by environmental factors. Interactions between genes are also likely to contribute to insulin resistance and β-cell dysfunction.

based on the frequency of the allele in the population. Increased sharing of alleles at a specific locus suggests that a gene(s) within that chromosomal locus contributes to the pathogenesis of the disease. Genome scans have now identified additional type 1 diabetes susceptibility loci (Table 47-1). Some of these loci have been confirmed by replication using additional families, whereas others await replication. None of these loci has an effect of the magnitude of *IDDM1*, but each may confer risk similar to that conferred by *IDDM2*. The genes at these loci that are responsible for conferring susceptibility to type 1 diabetes still await definition. As an increasing number of susceptibility loci are identified, an additional question that is raised is whether these different loci are acting epistatically. Epistasis, or interaction, between loci, indicates that the genotype at one locus affects the contribution of another locus. One implication of this is that loci that act epistatically may be acting through the same or related pathways. In contrast to epistasis is genetic heterogeneity, which indicates that two loci confer disease susceptibility independently, implying that the two loci confer risk via their effects on separate biologic pathways. This lack of interaction would suggest that an alteration in either pathway is associated with susceptibility to disease. *IDDM1* and *IDDM2* appear to act epistatically, whereas the action of *IDDM1* and *IDDM4* best fits a model of genetic heterogeneity. The potential interaction, or lack thereof, of the other susceptibility loci awaits further study.

Definition of the genetic etiology of type 1 diabetes will have several clinical implications. Currently, the vast majority of affected individuals are identified subsequent to the onset of diabetes when nearly complete β-cell destruction has occurred. A relatively limited subset of individuals at risk for developing type 1 diabetes can be identified before the onset of disease based on a family history of type 1 diabetes and the presence of antibodies directed against islet cells. Not all such individuals develop type 1 diabetes, however, and the risk of developing diabetes in these individuals is defined by the degree of loss of first phase insulin secretion during an intravenous glucose tolerance test. This loss of first phase insulin secretion occurs secondary to β-cell destruction and indicates activity of the autoimmune process. Currently, treatment of at risk individuals with insulin before the onset of altered glucose homeostasis is being tested as a means of preventing or delaying the onset of diabetes. On the basis of studies in animal models of diabetes, "vaccination" with insulin or a peptide that contains the epitope against which the majority of anti-insulin antibodies are directed is also being considered. Because a significant decrease in first phase insulin secretion indicates that marked β-cell destruction has already occurred, if susceptible individuals can be identified earlier, based on their complement of susceptibility genes, and screening can be extended beyond those with a positive family history, it may be possible to intervene earlier, before the onset of β-cell destruction, and, thus, have a much greater impact on delaying or preventing the onset of type 1 diabetes. Second, as the pathways that are responsible for initiating the autoimmune process are identified, new therapies designed to interfere specifically with these pathways and prevent β-cell destruction can be developed. These therapies will likely be more efficacious in preventing the onset of diabetes than those that are currently available.

GENETICS OF TYPE 2 DIABETES MELLITUS

Type 2 diabetes mellitus is a heterogeneous disorder that develops in response to both genetic and environmental factors (Fig. 47-1). In contrast to type 1 diabetes, type 2 diabetes is often diagnosed during routine screening by the detection of hyperglycemia or because of mild symptoms of hyperglycemia, e.g., polyuria. Much like type 1 diabetes, individuals with type 2 diabetes pass through a series of phases before the onset of diabetes. Initially, plasma insulin levels are increased because of insulin resistance, but euglycemia is maintained. In the second phase, postprandial hyperglycemia is present despite persistent hyperinsulinemia. Finally, insulin secretion declines in the face of persistent insulin resistance, which results in diabetes. Thus, affected individuals demonstrate both insulin resistance, manifest as hyperinsulinemia and decreased insulin-stimulated glucose uptake into tissues, and abnormal β-cell function, manifest as altered glucose-induced insulin secretion. Obesity is an additional contributing factor to type 2 diabetes via its effects on insulin sensitivity. Obesity, in turn, is affected by both energy expenditure and intake. Energy expenditure is dependent to a large degree on resting metabolic rate, whereas energy intake is regulated by the central nervous system and behavioral regulation of eating and satiety. All of the above processes are in part heritable, but complex, and depend on a variety of different gene products, each of which may have the potential to contribute to the genetic predisposition to type 2 diabetes.

Consistent with the heterogeneity of type 2 diabetes and the multiple contributing factors described above, mathematical modeling has suggested that type 2 diabetes is a polygenic disease. Consequently, onset of the disease likely requires the simultaneous presence of a subset of genes that affect the above processes. Because different subsets of genes are probably sufficient to confer susceptibility to type 2 diabetes, susceptibility genes likely vary between and, possibly, within populations. Moreover, environmental factors that have still not been fully defined contribute to the development of type 2 diabetes. Thus, disease susceptibility genes may be present in unaffected individuals because they lack a required complement of disease susceptibility genes or needed environmental factors to induce diabetes. This has and will continue to complicate attempts to define susceptibility genes for type 2 diabetes. An additional complication in defining the genetics of type 2 diabetes is that it is of late onset. Typically, parents, especially affected parents who may have succumbed to the complications of diabetes, are not available for study, and offspring are unlikely to be affected. Thus, family studies of type 2 diabetes are difficult. Finally, although it is clear that type 2 diabetes is polygenic and genetically heterogeneous, it is still unclear whether there are two or three major variants of the disease with additional minor variants or whether type 2 diabetes is truly heterogeneous with multiple variants, each of which accounts for a small percentage of affected individuals.

Despite the above challenges, progress has been made in defining the genetics of late-onset type 2 diabetes. As with type 1 diabetes, the candidate gene approach and genome scanning have been used to identify genes that confer susceptibility to type 2 diabetes, but these studies have been complicated by all of the issues described above. Moreover, unlike *IDDM1*, which is a major susceptibility locus for type 1 diabetes, it is possible that there is not a major susceptibility gene for type 2 diabetes; rather, multiple genes that confer a limited degree of susceptibility may exist.

GENETICALLY DEFINED FORMS OF TYPE 2 DIABETES

Given the complexities of the genetics of type 2 diabetes, substantial effort has been applied using both candidate gene and positional cloning approaches to define the genetics of rare, but monogenic, forms of diabetes with the hope that this will provide insight into the genetics of type 2 diabetes.

Mitochondrial Diabetes Mellitus The role of mutations in mitochondrial DNA as a cause of disease is becoming increasingly appreciated (*see* Chapter 103). Mitochondrial DNA is inherited maternally and encodes 13 polypeptide subunits involved in oxidative phosphorylation and the respiratory pathway, 22 transfer RNAs (tRNAs), and 2 ribosomal RNAs. Mitochondrial DNA is vulnerable to mutation because it is composed almost exclusively of coding sequences, lacks protection by histones, has inefficient repair mechanisms, and is exposed to reactive oxygen species produced during oxidative phosphorylation. Mitochondrial DNA undergoes mutation 5–10 times faster than nuclear DNA. The possibility that mitochondrial DNA mutations might contribute to the pathogenesis of diabetes mellitus was suggested by the association of diabetes with several mitochondrial diseases and by the maternal inheritance of mitochondrial DNA, given the slight preference for maternal transmission of type 2 diabetes.

Initially, a syndrome of diabetes mellitus and deafness caused by sensorineural hearing loss was identified in two pedigrees. In both, an A/G exchange at nucleotide 3243 in the mitochondrial $tRNA^{Leu(UUR)}$ gene was noted. This particular mutation was located within a mitochondrial DNA-binding site for a protein that contributes to the termination of transcription at the boundary between the 16S ribosomal RNA and $tRNA^{Leu(UUR)}$ genes. Thus, this mutation alters both $tRNA^{Leu(UUR)}$ synthesis and mitochondrial protein synthesis in general. Interestingly, $tRNA^{Leu(UUR)}$ is a hot spot for mutations; 10 disease-related mutations have been identified within this gene, 4 of which are associated with diabetes mellitus.

Identification of these syndromes raised the question as to the role of mitochondrial DNA mutations in the pathogenesis of diabetes mellitus. A variety of studies have determined that of patients with type 1 and 2 diabetes mellitus, the A/G exchange in the $tRNA^{Leu(UUR)}$ gene is present in 0.5–1.5% of patients. If only those patients with a family history of diabetes are considered, the prevalence of the mutation is two to five times higher. Characterization of affected individuals and their siblings demonstrated that 48% presented with diabetes and deafness, 21% had diabetes alone, 15% had deafness alone, 3% had deafness associated with some neurologic changes, and 13% had diabetes, deafness, and the findings of the MELAS syndrome (mitochondrial myopathy, encephalopathy, lactic acidosis, and strokelike episodes). The phenotypic variation is presumably caused by variable numbers of mitochondria containing normal compared with abnormal mitochondrial DNA (heteroplasmy) between tissues. Heteroplasmy results from unequal separation of mitochondrial populations during mitosis and differential accumulation of subsequent mitochondrial mutations.

Although patients with mitochondrial DNA mutations were initially diagnosed as having either type 1 or 2 diabetes mellitus, there were differences between these patients and those with "typical" type 1 or 2 diabetes. Those diagnosed initially as having type 1 diabetes in general lacked anti–islet cell antibodies and did not typically have a history of diabetic ketoacidosis, whereas those initially diagnosed as having type 2 diabetes tended to be leaner and to be more likely to be treated with insulin compared with general populations with type 2 diabetes. Subsequent studies to define the etiology of diabetes in patients with mitochondrial mutations demonstrated decreased insulin secretion in response to an oral glucose tolerance test, whereas measures of glucose utilization demonstrated essentially normal insulin sensitivity. The above findings suggest that the primary defect in patients with mitochondrial mutations is in the pancreatic β cell. The pathway of glucose-induced insulin secretion is still being elucidated, but oxidative phosphorylation and ATP generation are thought to play an important role in insulin secretion (Fig. 47-2), so mutations in β-cell mitochondrial DNA would likely interfere with insulin secretion because of insufficient ATP generation.

In patients with diabetes accompanied by hearing loss, a diagnosis of mitochondrial DNA mutations as the cause of the diabetes should be considered. Patients with these mutations should be advised that they will be much more likely to require insulin therapy because of the insulin deficiency that develops. Moreover, family members need to be carefully screened for both diabetes and evidence of sensorineural hearing. Frequently, the hearing

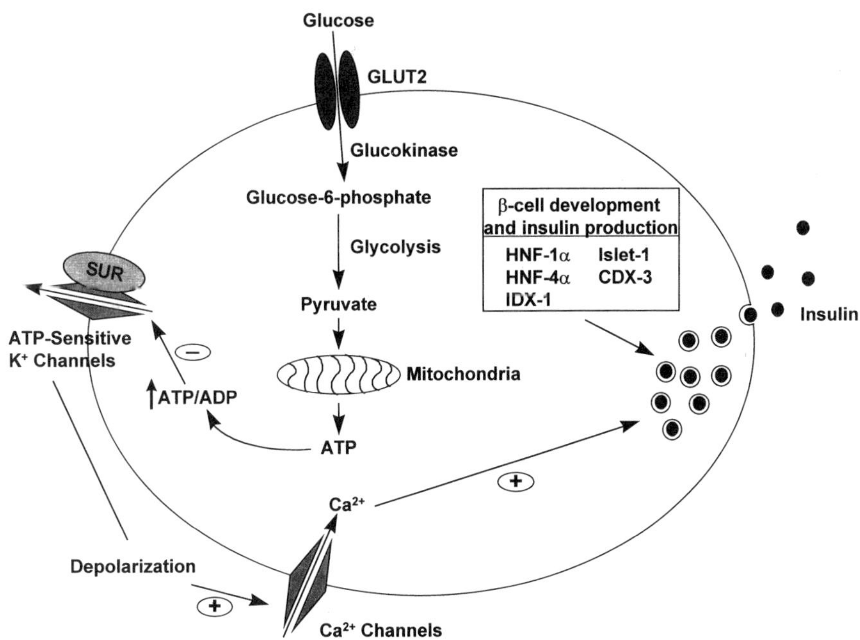

Figure 47-2 Schematic representation of glucose-stimulated insulin secretion by the pancreatic β cell. Glucose uptake is mediated by GLUT2, and glucose is phosphorylated by glucokinase to generate glucose-6-phosphate. Metabolism of glucose-6-phosphate via glycolysis yields pyruvate, which enters the tricarboxylic acid cycle in the mitochondria to generate ATP. The generation of ATP increases the ATP to ADP ratio in the cytoplasm, which inhibits activity of the ATP-sensitive K^+ channels. The ATP-sensitive K^+ channel is a complex of the sulfonylurea receptor (SUR) and an inwardly rectifying K^+-channel protein (KIR6.2). Inhibition of these channels results in membrane depolarization and opening of voltage-dependent Ca^{2+} channels. The resulting increase in the intracellular concentration of Ca^{2+} stimulates insulin secretion. β-cell development and insulin production are regulated by a variety of factors, including several different transcription factors.

loss develops after the onset of diabetes, so those patients with diabetes need to be examined over time for hearing loss.

Maturity Onset Diabetes of the Young (MODY) MODY is a subtype of diabetes that is monogenic and provides a model for studying the molecular genetics of type 2 diabetes. MODY is characterized by an early age of onset of diabetes and an autosomal dominant mode of inheritance that is based on the demonstration of a positive family history in three successive generations. Disease onset often occurs between 9 and 13 years of age and typically, although not universally, occurs before 25 years of age.

Characterization of MODY patients from different kindreds revealed phenotypic differences between patients suggesting heterogeneity, which molecular genetic analyses confirmed. Linkage to polymorphisms in the glucokinase gene on chromosome 7p was demonstrated in some patients, whereas in other patients positional cloning techniques demonstrated linkage to markers on either chromosome 20q or 12q. Subsequent genetic analyses demonstrated that the kindred described as having MODY1 had a mutation in the hepatocyte nuclear factor (HNF)-4α gene on chromosome 20q, whereas kindreds with MODY3 had mutations in HNF-1α on chromosome 12q. Mutations in the glucokinase gene were shown to cause diabetes in kindreds with MODY2. Finally, a kindred was described recently in which early-onset type 2 diabetes (MODY4) cosegregated with an inactivating mutation in the insulin promoter factoral (IPF-1) gene. Mutations in these genes do not account for all cases of MODY, suggesting that additional MODY genes await description.

The phenotypic differences between patients with the different forms of MODY provide some insight into the function of the responsible genes. Glucokinase is a key enzyme in glucose metabolism in β cells and hepatocytes and catalyzes the formation of glucose-6-phosphate from glucose. Glucokinase participates in glucose sensing and links glucose to insulin secretion. In patients with glucokinase mutations, the severity of enzyme impairment is correlated to the degree of hyperglycemia. Because of the decreased sensitivity of the β cells to glucose in these patients, the dose–response curve for glucose-induced insulin secretion is shifted to the right, but increased insulin secretion is observed with increasing degrees of hyperglycemia. Whether altered glucose metabolism in hepatocytes contributes to the hyperglycemia is not known. Because of the underlying origin of the hyperglycemia, patients with MODY2 typically present early in life, usually before puberty, with mild fasting hyperglycemia that does not worsen over time.

As noted, MODY1, MODY3, and MODY4 are caused by mutations in HNF-4α, HNF-1α, and IPF-1, respectively. HNF-4α is a transcription factor that is a member of the steroid–thyroid superfamily of nuclear receptors. Members of this receptor family are typically ligand-activated, but whether there is a ligand that activates HNF-4α is unknown. HNF-1α is a homeodomain transcription factor that functions either as a homodimer or as a heterodimer with the structurally related transcription factor HNF-1β. As their names imply, both of these factors are important for hepatic gene expression, but they are expressed in other tissues, including pancreatic islets. How mutations in these factors cause diabetes is unknown, although HNF-1α is known to be a weak *trans*-activator of the rat insulin I gene. HNF-4α is a positive regulator of HNF-1α expression and, thus, decreased HNF-1α production likely contributes to the cause of diabetes in patients with HNF-4α mutations. Little else is known about the function of HNF-1α and HNF-4α in pancreatic islets, but elucidation of their function will likely provide insight into islet cell development and function. IPF-1 is a transcription factor that regulates both pancreatic development and insulin gene transcription. The other issue that has not been resolved is why MODY1, MODY3, and MODY4 are autosomal dominant diseases, implying that mutation of one allele results in disease. It is unclear whether the product of the mutant allele functions in a dominant negative fashion and inhibits activity of the product of the wild-type allele or whether a reduction in the amount of active transcription factor causes disease (haploinsufficiency).

The phenotype of patients with MODY1 and MODY3 provides some insight into how mutations in HNF-1α and HNF-4α confer susceptibility to diabetes. The primary defect in patients with MODY1 and MODY3 is in the β cell. These patients have normal insulin sensitivity but demonstrate decreased insulin secretion in response to glucose. Unlike patients with MODY2, a progressive increase in insulin secretion with increasing hyperglycemia is not observed, suggesting a reduced capacity for insulin secretion. Similar defects, albeit not as severe, are present in individuals who have mutations in HNF-1α or HNF-4α but are not, as yet, diabetic. Thus, mutations in HNF-1α and HNF-4α appear to affect the regulation of insulin secretion or β-cell development.

As noted, patients with MODY2 typically have mild fasting hyperglycemia and are much less susceptible to the microvascular and macrovascular complications of diabetes compared with patients with type 2 diabetes. Patients with MODY1 and MODY3, in contrast, exhibit the microvascular and macrovascular complications associated with diabetes, but do not have the phenotype commonly associated with late-onset type 2 diabetes, obesity, hypertension, and hypercholesterolemia. These observations raise the issue of the contribution of mutations in the MODY genes to the etiology of late-onset type 2 diabetes. Although approximately 5% of women with gestational diabetes mellitus and a first-degree relative with diabetes have mutations in the glucokinase gene, neither linkage studies nor mutational analyses suggest that mutations in glucokinase account for significant numbers of cases of late-onset type 2 diabetes. Mutations in HNF-4α appear to be rare, since only a single kindred with MODY1 has been described. Moreover, the mutation in HNF-4α associated with MODY1 was not present in a large population of Japanese with late-onset type 2 diabetes. Similarly, there is no evidence for linkage of the HNF-4α locus to type 2 diabetes. Further studies need to be done, but to date, there are no data to suggest that HNF-4α mutations account for a significant number of cases of late-onset type 2 diabetes. Mutations in HNF-1α appear to be more common. In studies of patients with early onset diabetes (<40 years old) and a family history of diabetes, many of whom represent previously undescribed cases of MODY, mutations in HNF-1α have been found in 7–36% of patients, whereas in patients with more typical late-onset type 2 diabetes, mutations in HNF-1α are rare. More intriguing, however, is a recent study in an isolated population in Finland that examined people with late-onset type 2 diabetes (age of onset less than 60 years of age with a mean age of onset of 58 years), and a strong family history of diabetes. In the subgroup of patients with the lowest quartile of insulin secretion during an oral glucose tolerance test, linkage to the MODY3 locus on chromosome 12q was demonstrated. Mutations in HNF-1α have not yet been demonstrated in this population, but this study suggests that milder mutations in HNF-1α may contribute to a subset of late-onset type 2 diabetes. Weak linkage to the MODY3 locus was found in whites with late-onset type 2 diabetes complicated by diabetic nephropathy, but no evidence for linkage has been found in other populations, including African Americans and Mexican Americans. Thus, there is some evidence to suggest that mutations of HNF-1α contribute to late-onset type 2 diabetes in some subgroups of patients , but the exact role of HNF-1α still remains to be defined.

Now that the MODY genes have been defined, genetic testing will be available to family members from MODY kindreds. This will have implications for disease screening in these individuals, as well as institution of preventive measures, e.g., exercise, diet, and weight control, to minimize insulin resistance. Secondly, as the role of the hepatocyte nuclear factors in pancreatic development is elucidated, new therapeutic targets to enhance β-cell function may become available.

Insulin Gene Insulin is a primary hormone in the regulation of glucose homeostasis and, thus, represents a natural candidate gene for type 2 diabetes. Six different mutations that affect insulin processing and action have been described, but these mutations are rare. Three of these mutations alter the primary sequence of the A or B chain of insulin. These mutations affect insulin binding to its receptor and, thus, decrease the efficacy of insulin. Individuals with these mutations typically have mild hyperglycemia in association with hyperinsulinemia. Three mutations that affect proinsulin processing have also been described. These mutations have only a minimal effect on glucose homeostasis but result in hyperproinsulinemia. Because of their rarity, most individuals who bear insulin gene mutations are heterozygotes who have minimal impairment of glucose homeostasis, although this can be modified by obesity and increasing age. Insulin gene mutations are present in low prevalence in type 2 diabetes suggesting they do not make a major contribution to the disease. Moreover, linkage studies have not demonstrated linkage of the insulin gene locus to type 2 diabetes.

Because insufficient insulin secretion to compensate for insulin resistance contributes to the cause of type 2 diabetes, the role of mutations in the insulin gene promoter has also been examined. Promoter variants, including an 8-bp insertion in the promoter of some African Americans, have been described, but there is no evidence to suggest that insulin gene promoter variants contribute significantly to type 2 diabetes. Moreover, the role of the VNTR in the insulin gene promoter has also been examined. Again, no clear association of any of the alleles with type 2 diabetes has been demonstrated.

Insulin Receptor Gene As the most proximal site of insulin action, the insulin receptor is a second candidate gene for type 2 diabetes. The insulin receptor is a transmembrane receptor with tyrosine kinase activity that is activated on insulin binding (*see* Chapter 46 for details of signal transduction via tyrosine kinases). Normal tyrosine kinase activity is critical for transmission of a signal via the insulin receptor.

The potential role of insulin receptor mutations in diabetes mellitus was revealed by the demonstration that insulin receptor mutations were associated with specific syndromes of extreme insulin resistance, including leprechaunism, Rabson-Mendenhall syndrome, and type A extreme insulin resistance. These syndromes differ phenotypically because of different degrees of insulin resistance. Leprechaunism is associated with the greatest degree of insulin resistance and is characterized by intrauterine and postnatal growth retardation, dysmorphic facies, lipoatrophy, acanthosis nigricans (a cutaneous manifestation of insulin resistance), and death in early infancy. Rabson-Mendenhall presents in early childhood and is characterized by insulin-resistant diabetes mellitus, abnormal facies, dental dysplasia, thickened nails, hirsutism, precocious puberty, and acanthosis nigricans. Although these patients exhibit severe insulin resistance, they exhibit a lesser degree of insulin resistance than patients with leprechaunism. Finally, type A insulin resistance is characterized by extreme insulin resistance,

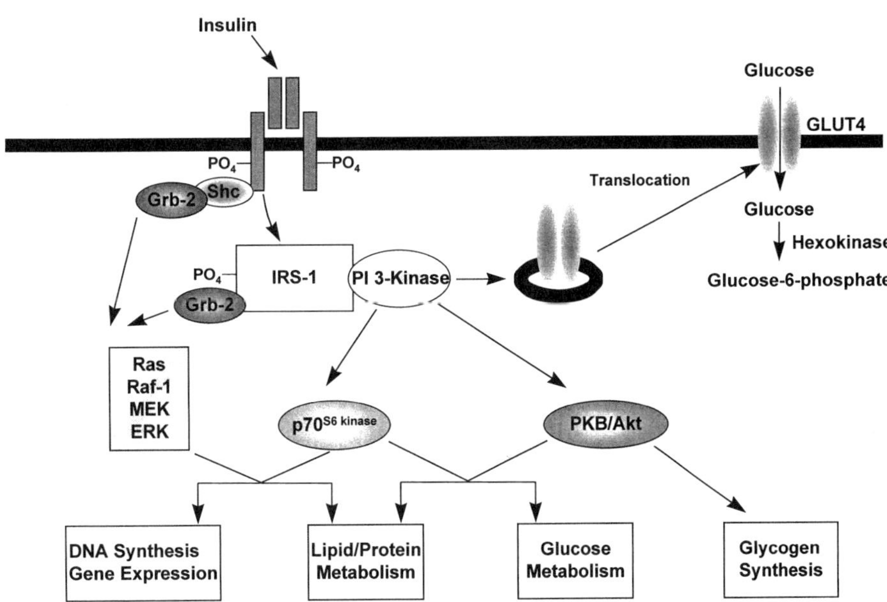

Figure 47-3 Schematic representation of insulin-induced signaling. Insulin signaling is initiated by insulin binding to the insulin receptor and activation of the receptor's intrinsic tyrosine kinase activity. Substrates for the tyrosine kinase include insulin receptor substrate-1 (IRS-1) and Shc. Through an interaction with Grb-2, both IRS-1 and Shc are able to activate a mitogen-activated protein kinase (MEK) and subsequently the mitogen-activated protein kinases (MAPKs), ERK1 and 2. Activation of phosphatidylinositol 3-kinase (PI 3-kinase), through its interaction with IRS-1, results in translocation of the insulin-responsive glucose transporter, GLUT4, to the plasma membrane and activation of two additional kinases, $p70^{S6\ kinase}$ and protein kinase B (PKB) or Akt. Activation of PKB has recently been shown to result in activation of glycogen synthase. Not shown are additional substrates of the insulin receptor, including IRS-2, pp60 (IRS-3), a novel 160-kDa protein that is phosphorylated in response to insulin (IRS-4), and the proto-oncogene c-Cbl, which is an adipocyte-specific substrate for the insulin receptor. The contribution of these and other signaling pathways to insulin-induced effects is still being elucidated, but the likely contribution of multiple pathways to these different effects is illustrated. The relative contribution of the different pathways probably varies in different cell types, and it is likely that additional pathways not shown here also contribute to insulin-induced effects. Alteration of any of the molecules in these different signaling pathways would be expected to have an effect on insulin sensitivity and contribute to the development of insulin resistance.

albeit of lesser degree than that seen in the above two syndromes, and is often associated with normal or only mildly impaired glucose homeostasis and acanthosis nigricans. Women with this syndrome typically exhibit hyperandrogenism, hirsutism, and polycystic ovaries. The varying degree of insulin resistance present in these different syndromes is determined by the number of mutant alleles inherited, as well as the severity of the mutations. Patients with leprechaunism typically inherit two mutant alleles, whereas patients with the Rabson-Mendenhall syndrome and type A insulin resistance inherit one or two alleles with mutations that confer different degrees of receptor dysfunction. To date, more than 40 mutations in the insulin receptor have been described. These mutations occur throughout the receptor with effects on receptor synthesis or processing, insulin binding, or tyrosine kinase activity.

The role of insulin receptor mutations as a causative factor in type 2 diabetes is not as clear. Receptor mutations that induce more subtle defects in receptor activity than those described above have been identified but are rare. It has been estimated that no more than 1–2% of patients with type 2 diabetes have mutations in the tyrosine kinase domain of the insulin receptor that affect receptor function. Studies designed to demonstrate association of restriction fragment length polymorphisms (RFLPs) in the insulin receptor with type 2 diabetes have been largely negative, and linkage of the insulin receptor to type 2 diabetes has not been demonstrated. Thus, there is no evidence to suggest that insulin receptor mutations contribute significantly to the pathogenesis of type 2 diabetes.

GENETICS OF LATE-ONSET TYPE 2 DIABETES Despite significant progress in defining the genetics of monogenic forms of diabetes, genetic abnormalities that contribute to the majority of cases of late-onset type 2 diabetes have yet to be identified using this approach. For that reason, both candidate gene and genome scanning and positional cloning approaches have been used to define the genetics of type 2 diabetes.

Candidate Genes for Late-Onset Type 2 Diabetes The candidate gene approach depends on the use of educated guesses to choose gene products that may have an effect on glucose homeostasis and, thus, predispose an individual to the development of type 2 diabetes. Logical candidates would include genes that affect insulin production, glucose metabolism in pancreatic β cells, insulin processing and secretion, insulin action and glucose metabolism in peripheral tissues, genes that regulate body weight, eating behavior, and satiety, and genes that encode inhibitors of insulin action (Figs. 47-2 and 47-3). Because of the frequent association of altered cholesterol and triglyceride metabolism with diabetes, genes that affect lipid metabolism have also been considered as candidate genes for type 2 diabetes. A summary of the results of studies using the candidate gene approach is presented in Tables 47-2 through 47-7.

An association of specific missense mutations or other polymorphisms with type 2 diabetes has been demonstrated for several genes, including the sulfonylurea receptor, glucagon receptor, prohormone convertase 2, insulin receptor substrate 1 (IRS-1), glycogen synthase, amylin, and Rad (Ras-related protein associated with diabetes) genes. In each case, however, other studies have been unable to replicate the findings in different populations or only a single study has been performed. Moreover, with the

Table 47-2
Candidate Genes for Type 2 Diabetes With Effects on Insulin Production, Processing, or Secretion

Candidate genes	*Findings*
Genes that regulate β-cell development and function	
Hepatocyte nuclear factor-1α	Mutations of this gene are responsible for MODY3. Linkage of the MODY3 locus on chromosome 12q to late-onset type 2 diabetes in Finnish population with low insulin secretion has been demonstrated. Role in late-onset type 2 diabetes otherwise has not been defined.
Hepatocyte nuclear factor-4α	Mutations in this gene are responsible for MODY1. Mutation responsible for MODY1 was not present in a population of Japanese with late-onset type 2 diabetes. Linkage of the MODY1 locus to type 2 diabetes has not been demonstrated.
Insulin promoter factor (IPF-1 or IDX1)	Homozygous mutation of this transcription factor that regulates β-cell development and insulin gene transcription results in pancreatic agenesis. Heterozygous state cosegregates with early-onset type 2 diabetes (MODY4).
Genes that regulate insulin gene transcription	
Islet-1 *(Isl-1)*	No association of polymorphisms with type 2 diabetes or evidence for linkage.
Caudal-type homeodomain 3 *(CDX3)*	No evidence for linkage with type 2 diabetes.
Genes with an effect on insulin secretion	
Inwardly rectifying K^+-channel subunit *(Kir6.2)*	No evidence for linkage with type 2 diabetes. No association of multiple missense mutations and silent polymorphisms with type 2 diabetes.
G-protein-coupled muscarinic potassium channel *(KCNJ3)*	No evidence for association of any alleles with type 2 diabetes or of linkage with type 2 diabetes.
G-protein-coupled inwardly rectifying potassium channel-2 *(KCNJ7)*	No mutations noted in patients with type 2 diabetes. No association of different alleles with type 2 diabetes. No evidence of linkage with type 2 diabetes.
Sulfonylurea receptor	Demonstration of association of a silent polymorphism with type 2 diabetes in two different populations. No evidence of linkage with type 2 diabetes in multiple populations.
Glucagon	No evidence for linkage with type 2 diabetes.
Glucagon receptor	Missense mutation associated with type 2 diabetes in two populations but this same missense mutation was not detected in other populations.
Glucagon-like peptide-1 receptor	No evidence for association of different alleles with type 2 diabetes. No evidence for linkage with type 2 diabetes.
Gastric inhibitory polypeptide receptor	No association between missense mutations and type 2 diabetes.
Glucokinase regulatory protein	No evidence for linkage with type 2 diabetes.
Amylin	Association of a missense mutation with type 2 diabetes but no evidence for linkage in multiple different populations.
Genes with an effect on insulin processing	
Prohormone convertase 2	Association of a specific allele defined with microsatellite markers with type 2 diabetes. No evidence for linkage with type 2 diabetes.

MODY, mature onset diabetes of the young.

Table 47-3
Candidate Genes for Type 2 Diabetes With an Effect on β-Cell Glucose Metabolism

Candidate genes	*Findings*
Mitochondrial FAD-linked glycerophosphate dehydrogenase *(GPD2)*	No evidence for association of specific alleles with type 2 diabetes. No evidence for linkage with type 2 diabetes.
Pyruvate kinase *(PKM)*	No evidence for linkage with type 2 diabetes.
Glucose transporter 2 *(GLUT2)*	No evidence for association of missense mutations with type 2 diabetes. No evidence for linkage with type 2 diabetes.
Hexokinase I *(HK1)*	No evidence for linkage with type 2 diabetes.

FAD, flavin adenine dinucleotide.

exception of IRS-1, which has shown weak linkage to the age of onset of type 2 diabetes but not to the disease itself, there is no evidence for linkage of any of these genes to type 2 diabetes. Linkage studies using candidate genes have also been of limited utility, although a few positive findings have been reported. Fatty acid binding protein 2 (FABP2) is not linked to type 2 diabetes, but linkage of this locus to fasting and insulin-stimulated glucose levels has been demonstrated. Moreover, association of a specific missense mutation in the FABP2 gene with fasting and glucose-stimulated insulin levels was demonstrated in Pima Indians, but this finding was not replicated in a white population. Weak evidence for linkage of the apolipoprotein A_2 gene was found in a single study that has not been replicated, whereas a trend toward linkage of the phosphoenolpyruvate carboxykinase (PEPCK) gene to type 2 diabetes in patients with an onset before 46 years of age was demonstrated in one study, but no evidence for linkage was found in another study. Thus, to date, a gene that makes a significant contribution to type 2 diabetes in a majority of cases has not been identified. Because type 2 diabetes appears to be a polygenic disorder with significant heterogeneity between affected individuals, however, a major "diabetogene" that is important in all affected individuals may not exist, and the importance of different "diabetogenes" in conferring risk for type 2 diabetes may vary between different populations. For these reasons, studies that fail

Table 47-4
Candidate Genes for Type 2 Diabetes With an Effect on Insulin Action and Glucose Metabolism

Candidate genes	*Findings*
Insulin receptor substrate 1 (IRS-1)	Multiple missense mutations have been identified with one, Gly972Arg, being found with increased prevalence in patients with type 2 diabetes in some studies but not others. No evidence for linkage of IRS-1 with type 2 diabetes in one study whereas another found possible weak linkage of IRS-1 with a gene affecting age of onset of type 2 diabetes.
Phosphatidylinositol 3-kinase (PI3-K)	No association of a missense mutation with type 2 diabetes, although in homozygous state the missense mutation was associated with decreased insulin sensitivity and glucose disappearance constant.
Glycogen synthase *(GYS1)*	Increased association of specific alleles identified by either microsatellite markers or RFLP with type 2 diabetes in some populations, but no mutations found in the gene. In other studies, no evidence for association of the same alleles with type 2 diabetes. No evidence for linkage with type 2 diabetes.
Inhibitor 2 of type 1 protein phosphatase *(PPP1R2)*	No evidence of mutations in coding sequence of the gene in insulin-resistant compared with insulin-sensitive Pima Indians.
Protein serine–threonine phosphatase 1β *(PPP1CB)*	No evidence for linkage with type 2 diabetes.
Glucose transporter 1 (GLUT1)	Association of an allele defined by RFLP analysis with type 2 diabetes in obese overweight women. No evidence for linkage with type 2 diabetes.
Glucose transporter 4 (GLUT4)	No association of RFLP or missense mutation with type 2 diabetes. No evidence of linkage to type 2 diabetes.
Hexokinase II	No evidence of association of multiple missense mutations with type 2 diabetes, except for possibly one missense mutation present in 2.7% of patients with type 2 diabetes but not in control subjects. No evidence for linkage to type 2 diabetes.
Fructose 1,6-bisphosphatase	No evidence for linkage with type 2 diabetes.
Hepatic phosphofructose kinase	No evidence for linkage with type 2 diabetes.
Phosphoenolpyruvate carboxykinase	Trend toward linkage in sib pairs diagnosed with type 2 diabetes before age 46, whereas no evidence for linkage in another family study.
Pyruvate kinase (PKL)	No evidence for linkage with type 2 diabetes

RFLP, restriction fragment length polymorphism.

Table 47-5
Candidate Genes for Type 2 Diabetes That Regulate Eating Behavior and Adiposity

Candidate genes	*Findings*
Leptin *(ob)*	No evidence for mutations in *ob* gene in patients with type 2 diabetes. No evidence for linkage with type 2 diabetes.
Tubby *(TUB)*	No evidence for linkage with type 2 diabetes.
Cholecystokinin receptor B	In sib pairs with type 2 diabetes diagnosed before age 45, suggestive evidence for linkage of locus on chromosome 11 where cholecystokinin B receptor is located with type 2 diabetes.

Table 47-6
Candidate Genes for Type 2 Diabetes That Are Inhibitors of Insulin Action

Candidate genes	*Findings*
Growth hormone	Weak evidence for linkage of growth hormone locus with type 2 diabetes.
Rad *(RAD1)*	Evidence for association of minor alleles of an intronic trinucleotide repeat with type 2 diabetes. No association of this polymorphism with type 2 diabetes found in a second study. No evidence for linkage with type 2 diabetes.
TNF-α	No evidence for linkage with type 2 diabetes.
TNF-β	No evidence for linkage between TNF-β and age of onset of type 2 diabetes.

Rad, Ras-related protein associated with diabetes; TNF, tumor necrosis factor.

to demonstrate association or linkage of a candidate gene to type 2 diabetes may be misleading, and larger studies or studies using specific at-risk populations may be required to document the role of specific candidate genes in the pathogenesis of type 2 diabetes.

Identification of Susceptibility Loci for Late-Onset Type 2 Diabetes Less information is available using genome scanning and positional cloning techniques to identify susceptibility loci for late-onset type 2 diabetes. An early approach to this problem was to examine for linkage of specific traits that are altered in affected individuals. In Pima Indians, linkage of a locus on chromosome 1 to the acute response of insulin to intravenous glucose was observed using microsatellite markers. Interestingly, this locus is close to the recently identified leptin receptor. Leptin has been shown to have an effect on insulin secretion, although neither linkage of the leptin receptor itself to the acute insulin response nor mutations in the leptin receptor in Pima Indians have been demonstrated. Studies examining linkage of loci on specific chromosomes to type 2 diabetes have yielded limited results. Suggestive evidence for linkage of a region of chromosome 11 with type 2 diabetes has been demonstrated in whites of Northern European descent, whereas two studies examining loci on chromosome 20 demonstrated evidence for linkage of a specific region of chromosome 20q, which is distinct from the MODY1 locus, to type 2 diabetes in white sib pairs. Interestingly, no evidence for linkage of this region was observed in African Americans, consistent with the idea of genetic heterogeneity between populations. Moreover, the IDDM loci described in Table 47-1 are not linked to type 2

Table 47-7
Candidate Genes for Type 2 Diabetes With an Effect on Lipid Metabolism

Candidate genes	*Findings*
Fatty acid binding protein 2 (FABP2)	No evidence for linkage with type 2 diabetes. Linkage of FABP2 locus to 2-h postglucose insulin level in Mexican American sib pairs. In Pina Indians, linkage of locus to maximal insulin-stimulated glucose uptakeand fat oxidation. In Finnish population, weak association of the missense mutation with fasting and glucose-stimulated insulin levels but not fat oxidation.
Hormone-sensitive lipase	No association of missense mutation with type 2 diabetes.
Lipoprotein lipase	No evidence for linkage with type 2 diabetes or age of onset of type 2 diabetes.
Hepatic triglyceride lipase	No evidence for association with type 2 diabetes.
Very-low-density lipoprotein receptor	No evidence for linkage with type 2 diabetes.
Apolipoprotein CII	No evidence for linkage with type 2 diabtetes. No evidence for association of alleles identified using microsatellite markers with type 2 diabetes.
Apolipoprotein A_2	Weak evidence for linkage with type 2 diabetes in a study of white families.
Apolipoprotein B	No evidence for linkage with type 2 diabetes.
Cholesterol ester-transfer protein	No evidence for linkage with type 2 diabetes.

diabetes. Finally, a genome scan that was designed to identify susceptibility loci for type 2 diabetes in Mexican American sib pairs demonstrated a single susceptibility locus on chromosome 2, now referred to as *NIDDM1*. In white French sib pairs, suggestive evidence for linkage of *NIDDM1* with type 2 diabetes was observed. Candidate genes within this region of chromosome 2 have not yet been identified. Genome scanning to identify susceptibility loci for type 2 diabetes is still in its early stages, but as methods for identifying susceptibility loci for complex diseases and for performing genome scans improve, additional susceptibility loci will be identified.

Clinical Implications Defining the genetics of type 2 diabetes will not only elucidate the molecular basis for the disease, but it will also have important clinical implications. First, understanding the molecular basis for the disease will facilitate the development of new therapeutic modalities. Second, as susceptibility genes are defined, the genetic burden of a given individual can be determined. In appropriate individuals, aggressive preventive measures might be instituted. Moreover, type 2 diabetes can be subclassified based on the predisposing genes present in a patient and that subclassification can be used to direct therapeutic interventions in that patient on the basis of the probable underlying pathophysiology.

SELECTED REFERENCES

Alcolado JC, Thomas AW. Maternally inherited diabetes mellitus: the role of mitochondrial DNA defects. Diabetic Med 1995;12: 102–108.

Atkinson MA, Maclaren NK. The pathogenesis of insulin-dependent diabetes mellitus. N Eng J Med 1994;331:1428–1436.

Bennett ST, Todd JA. Human type 1 diabetes and the insulin gene: principles of mapping polygenes. Annu Rev Genet 1996;30:343–370.

Cordell HJ, Todd JA. Multifactorial inheritance in type 1 diabetes. Trends Genet 1995;11:499–504.

Davies JL, Kawaguchi Y, Bennett ST, et al. A genome-wide search for human type 1 diabetes susceptibility genes. Nature 1994;371:130–136.

Fajans SS, Bell GI, Bowden DW, Halter JB, Polonsky KS. Maturity onset diabetes of the young (MODY). Diabetic Med 1996;13:S90–S95.

Frougel P. Glucokinase and MODY: from the gene to the disease. Diabetic Med 1996;13:S96,97.

Gerbitz K-D, Gempel K, Brdiczka D. Mitochondria and diabetes: genetic, biochemical, and clinical implications of the cellular energy circuit. Diabetes 1996;45:113–126.

Gerbitz K-D, van den Ouweland JMW, Maassen JA, Jaksch M. Mitochondrial diabetes mellitus: a review. Biochim Biophys Acta 1995;1271: 253–260.

Ghosh S, Schork NJ. Genetic analysis of NIDDM: the study of quantitative traits. Diabetes 1996;45:1–14.

Hanis CL, Boerwinkle E, Chakraborty R, et al. A genome-wide search for human non–insulin-dependent (type 2) diabetes genes reveals a major susceptibility locus on chromosome 2. Nat Genet 1996;13:161–166.

Kahn CR, Vicent D, Doria A. Genetics of non–insulin-dependent (type-II) diabetes mellitus. Annu Rev Med 1996;47:509–531.

Kaisaki PJ, Menzel S, Lindner T, et al. Mutations in the hepatocyte nuclear factor-1α gene in MODY and early-onset NIDDM: evidence for a mutational hotspot in exon 4. Diabetes 1997;46:528–535.

Lehto M, Tuomi T, Mahtani MM, et al. Characterization of the MODY3 phenotype: early-onset diabetes caused by an insulin secretion defect. J Clin Invest 1997;99:582–591.

Mahtani MM, Widen E, Lehto M, et al. Mapping of a gene for type 2 diabetes associated with an insulin secretion defect by a genome scan in Finnish families. Nat Genet 1996;14:90–94.

Moller DE, Bjorbaek C, Vidal-Puig A. Candidate genes for insulin resistance. Diabetes Care 1996;19:396–400.

Owerbach D, Gabbay KH. The search for IDDM susceptibility genes: the next generation. Diabetes 1996;45:544–551.

Pugliese A, Zeller M, Fernandez A Jr, et al. The insulin gene is transcribed in the human thymus and transcription levels correlate with allelic variation at the *INS* VNTR-*IDDM2* susceptibility locus for type 1 diabetes. Nat Genet 1997;15:293–297.

She J-X. Susceptibility to type 1 diabetes: HLA-DQ and DR revisited. Immunol Today 1996;17:323–329.

Slover RH, Eisenbarth GS. Prevention of type 1 diabetes and recurrent β-cell destruction of transplanted islets. Endocr Rev 1997;18:241–258.

Stoffers DA, Ferrer J, Clarke WL, Habener JF. Early-onset type II diabetes mellitus (MODY4) linked to IPF-1. Nat Genet 1997;17:138,139.

Taylor SI. Lilly Lecture: molecular mechanisms of insulin resistance. Lessons from patients with mutations in the insulin-receptor gene. Diabetes 1992;41:1473–1490.

Thompson DB, Janssen RC, Ossowski M, Prochazka M, Knowler WC, Bogardus C. Evidence for linkage between a region on chromosome 1p and the acute insulin response in Pima Indians. Diabetes 1995;44:478–481.

Todd JA, Farrall M. Panning for gold: genome-wide scanning for linkage in type 1 diabetes. Hum Mol Genetics 1996;5:1443–1448.

Turner RC, Hattersley AT, Shaw JTE, Levy JC. Type 2 diabetes: clinical aspects of molecular biological studies. Diabetes 1995;44:1–10.

Vafiadis P, Bennett ST, Todd JA, et al. Insulin expression in human thymus is modulated by *INS* VNTR alleles at the *IDDM2* locus. Nat Genet 1997;15:289–292.

Vionnet N, Hani EH, Lesage S, et al. Genetics of NIDDM in France: studies with 19 candidate genes in affected sib pairs. Diabetes 1997;46:1062–1068.

Yamagata K, Furuta H, Oda N, et al. Mutations in the hepatocyte nuclear factor-4α gene in maturity-onset diabetes of the young (MODY1). Nature 1996;384:458–460.

Yamagata K, Oda N, Kaisaki PJ, et al. Mutations in the hepatocyte nuclear factor-1α gene in maturity-onset diabetes of the young (MODY3). Nature 1996;384:455–457.

48 Pituitary Function and Neoplasia

SHLOMO MELMED

INTRODUCTION

The cell types of the mature adenohypophysis are derived embryologically from somatic ectoderm associated with Rathke's pouch. Highly specific trophic factors determine a precise temporal and spatial development of cells expressing unique gene products. The six hormones of the anterior pituitary gland are expressed by at least five distinct hormone-producing cell populations, including corticotrophs (pro-opiomelanocortin, POMC), somatotrophs (growth hormone, GH), lactotrophs (prolactin, PRL), thyrotrophs (thyroid-stimulating hormone, TSH), and gonadotrophs (follicle-stimulating hormone, FSH, and luteinizing hormone, LH) (Table 48-1). Each of these cells are identified by specific assays of polypeptide gene expression, including single-cell mRNA, immunoelectron microscopy, and immunocytochemical assays. The temporal ontogeny of these gene products is initially adrenocorticotropic hormone (ACTH) and α-subunit. After the appearance of Pit-1, a pou-domain transcription factor, mixed mammosomatroph products appear. Distinct GH- and PRL-expressing cells PRL-expressing cells follow and TSH, LH, and FSH are the final IPII types to mature at 12 weeks.

Each of the anterior pituitary trophic hormones is induced by a respective hypothalamic releasing hormone, and their transcription is regulated by negative feedback inhibition of their respective target hormone (Table 48-2).

CORTICOTROPH CELLS

The corticotrophs constitute between 15 and 20% of the adenohypophyseal cell population, and express strong granular cytoplasmic immunopositivity for ACTH and other POMC fragments.

Corticotrophin-releasing hormone (CRH) and glucocorticoids exert opposite effects on POMC gene transcription; CRH increases POMC mRNA and protein content via cyclic adenosine monophosphate (cAMP), whereas the glucocorticoid negative feedback effect is probably mediated through binding of the glucocorticoid receptor complex to *cis*-active POMC promoter sequences. Several enhancer elements have been identified on the POMC gene promoter. These appear to act synergistically in regulating POMC transcription. POMC transcription is also induced by β-adrenergic activation and insulin-induced hypoglycemia.

From: *Principles of Molecular Medicine* (J. L. Jameson, ed.), ©1998 Humana Press Inc., Totowa, NJ.

REGULATION OF ACTH

Ligand activation of the CRH receptor (Gs protein containing seven transmembrane domains) on the corticotroph stimulates ACTH synthesis as well as release. POMC transcriptional regulation is mediated by cAMP as well as indirectly by c-fos activation. Arginine vasopressin (AVP), physical stress, exercise, acute illness, and hypoglycemia all increase ACTH levels. Several cytokines mediating inflammatory and or immune responses, including tumor necrosis factor-α, interleukin-1 (IL-1), IL-6, and leukemia-inhibitory factor (LIF), also stimulate ACTH, whereas glucocorticoids and opiates inhibit ACTH transcription and release. This neuroimmune endocrine interface appears to occur directly at the level of POMC gene expression. ACTH secretion is pulsatile, with an endogenous circadian rhythm associated with a parallel diurnal pattern of glucocorticoid secretion. Both ACTH and cortisol are higher in the early morning and decline at night.

Hypercortisolism may be caused by pituitary corticotroph adenomas (Cushing's disease) (70%), ectopic ACTH production (12%), cortisol-producing adrenal adenomas, carcinoma and hyperplasia (18%), and, rarely, ectopic CRH production. Iatrogenic hypercortisolism caused by prolonged administration of glucocorticoids produces a similar clinical syndrome.

ACTH-CELL ADENOMA About 10–15% of all pituitary adenomas are ACTH-producing tumors that are usually well-differentiated microadenomas. About 5% are silent corticotroph adenomas. Secretory granules in tumor cells immunostain positively for ACTH, β-endorphin, β-LPH, and N-terminal peptide. Although these adenomas exhibit unrestrained ACTH secretion with resultant hypercortisolemia, they often retain suppressibility in the face of high doses of administered glucocorticoids.

ECTOPIC ACTH SECRETION ACTH production by small cell lung carcinomas and bronchial and thymic carcinoids may result in florid manifestations of Cushing's syndrome. The POMC mRNA transcript derived from nonpituitary ACTH-secreting tumors may be longer than the normal transcript or that detected in pituitary tumors. CLIP and β-MSH fragments may also be detected in ectopic tumors, indicating alternative POMC processing. Glucocorticoids do not suppress POMC mRNA expression in small cell lung cell lines, thus highlighting their unrestrained gene expression.

CUSHING'S SYNDROME Patients typically present with truncal obesity, hirsutism (also associated with a "moon facies" and "buffalo hump"), cutaneous striae, muscle weakness, osteoporosis, acne, hypertension, depression, and ovarian dysfunction. Because hypercortisolemia is associated with insulin resistance,

Table 48-1
Human Anterior Pituitary Hormone Gene Expression and Regulation

Cell	*Fetal appearance*	*Hormone*	*Chromosomal gene locus*	*Protein*	*Size, kDa*	*Amino acid number*
Corticotroph	6 wk	POMC	2p	Polypeptide	ACTH-4.5	266 (ACTH-39)
Somatotroph	8 wk	GH	17q	Polypeptide	22	191
Lactotroph	12 wk	PRL	6	Polypeptide	23	199
Thyrotroph	12 wk	TSH	α—6q; β—1p	Glycoprotein α-, β-subunits	28	211
Gonadotroph	12 wk	FSH LH	β—11p β—19q	Glycoprotein α-, β-subunits	34 28.5	210 204

Table 47-2
Regulation of Pituitary Hormone Secretion and Action

Hormones	*Stimulators*	*Inhibitors*	*Peripheral receptor*	*Target*	*Trophic effects*	*Normal range*
ACTH	CRH, AVP gp-130 cytokines	Glucocorticoids	GSTD	Adrenal	Steroid production	ACTH, 4–22 pg/L
GH	GHRH	Somatostatin, IGF-I, activins	Single transmembrane	Liver, other tissues	IGF-I production, growth induction, insulin antagonism	<0.5[a] μg/L
PRL	Estrogen, TRH	Dopamine	Single transmembrane	Breast, other tissues	Milk production	M, <15; F, <20 μg/L
TSH	TRH	T_3, T_4, dopamine Somatostatin, glucocorticoids	GSTD	Thyroid	T_4	0.1–5 mU/L
FSH/LH	GnRH, estrogen	Estrogen Inhibin	GSTD	Ovary, testis	Sex steroid, follicle growth, germ cell maturation	M, 5–20 IU/L; F(basal), 5–20 IU/L

GSTD, G_s protein coupled with seven transmembrane domains.
[a] = integrated over 24 hours.
(Adapted from Shimon I, Melmed S. In: Endocrinology, Conn P, Melmed S, eds. Totowa, NJ: Humana, 1996.)

patients may also have impaired glucose tolerance. Ectopic Cushing's syndrome associated with small cell lung carcinoma is usually more acute with relatively rapid onset of hypertension, edema, hypokalemia, glucose intolerance, and hyperpigmentation. The most direct way to demonstrate ACTH hypersecretion of pituitary origin is by catheterization of the inferior petrosal venous sinuses. ACTH measurements in petrosal and peripheral venous plasma before and after CRH stimulation may document a central-to-peripheral venous gradient of ACTH concentrations.

ACTH hypersecretion by a corticotroph adenoma is usually suppressible by high doses of dexamethasone, whereas ectopic ACTH secretion persists despite high doses of dexamethasone. High-resolution pituitary magnetic resonance imaging (MRI) with gadolinium enhancement with a sensitivity of 2 mm is useful in determining the location of corticotroph adenomas. The treatment of choice is trans-sphenoidal adenomectomy, with a cure rate as high as 80% in experienced centers.

GROWTH HORMONE

Somatotrophs comprise more than 40% of pituitary cells and reveal intense cytoplasmic immunopositivity for GH. The GH genomic locus consists of five highly conserved genes, including hGH (exclusively expressed in somatotrophs), whereas the others are also expressed in placental tissue. *Cis*-elements within 300 bp of 5' flanking DNA of the GH promoter mediate both pituitary-specific and hormone-specific signaling. These include Pit-1, a 33-kDa tissue-specific transcription factor, which binds to specific promoter sites on the GH, PRL, and TSH-β genes regulating their respective transcription. The T3 receptor may synergize with Pit-1 in stimulating GH transcription, although this effect may be species specific. Pit-1 also appears to be a determinant of growth hormone-releasing hormone (GHRH) receptor function, inasmuch as Pit-1 mutations may block GHRH-induced somatotroph proliferation.

Pulsatile GH secretion is associated with low or undetectable basal levels between peaks. In children, maximum GH secretory peaks occur within an hour of deep sleep onset. Somatostatin (SRIF) and GHRH interact to generate pulsatile GH release. GHRH stimulates GH synthesis and secretion, whereas SRIF, as well as the target hormone insulin-like growth factor-1 (IGF-I), inhibit GH secretion. GHRH signaling is mediated by cAMP, and several additional signals regulate GH gene expression, including glucocorticoids, IGF-I, activin, T3, and phorbol esters.

The GH receptor is expressed mainly in the liver and in other tissues. GH binding proteins are soluble short forms of the hepatic GH receptor and are identical to its cleaved extracellular domain. These proteins may prolong circulating GH half-life and may also competitively inhibit GH binding to peripheral surface receptors.

ACROMEGALY Tumor-derived GH hypersecretion leading to acromegaly may be caused by excess GHRH or excess GH elaboration. More than 95% of patients with acromegaly harbor a GH-secreting pituitary adenoma, two-thirds have pure GH-cell tumors, and the others have plurihormonal tumors, usually expressing PRL in addition to GH.

These patients have elevated GH and IGF-I levels and normal GHRH concentrations. Ectopic acromegaly may be central as a result of excess GHRH production by functional hypothalamic tumors, or peripheral as a result of rare extrapituitary GH-secreting tumors (pancreas) and the more common tumors secreting GHRH (carcinoid, pancreas, small cell lung cancer). Patients with ectopic acromegaly exhibit normal (central) or elevated (peripheral) GHRH levels. Interestingly, somatotroph hyperplasia and ultimately true GH-cell adenomas may develop in these latter patients.

The clinical manifestations of acromegaly include acral enlargement and visceromegaly. Tongue, salivary glands, thyroid, heart, and soft organs all enlarge. Skeletal overgrowth leads to mandibular prognathism, frontal bossing, increased hand, foot, and hat size, and wide incisor spacing. These features result in voice deepening, headaches, painful arthropathy and carpal tunnel syndrome, muscle weakness and fatigue, oily skin and hyperhydrosis, hypertension and left ventricular hypertrophy, and sleep apnea. Glucose intolerance because of insulin antagonism by GH commonly occurs. Overall mortality is increased in acromegaly because of an increased incidence of cardiovascular disorders, malignancy, and respiratory disease. Mortality rates correlate well with GH levels, and effective therapeutic suppression of GH may lead to normalized mortality outcomes. *Trans*-sphenoidal adenoma resection is the indicated treatment for GH-secreting pituitary adenoma. Octreotide, a long-acting somatostatin analog, significantly attenuates GH and IGF-I levels in most patients, and chronic administration of the long-acting octapeptide is also accompanied by marked clinical improvement.

PROLACTIN

The acidophilic lactotrophs contain PRL-immunostaining secretory granules and constitute 15% of adenohypophysial cells. PRL is highly homologous to GH and placental lactogen (PL), which may all have originally arisen from a common ancestral gene.

The PRL gene has two lactotroph-specific transcription activation regions, a proximal promoter (–422 to +33) and a distal enhancer element (–1831 to –1530), both containing specific binding sites for Pit-1. Dopamine, a potent inhibitor of PRL, acts through the D2 dopamine receptor to decrease intracellular cAMP and PRL gene transcription, synthesis, and release. Dopamine effects are mediated by the phosphoinositide-calcium pathway. Vasoactive intestinal polypeptide (VIP) induces, whereas glucocorticoids and thyroid hormones suppress, PRL transcription and secretion. Estrogens and TRH induce PRL transcription and secretion by either *trans*-activating an estrogen-responsive PRL enhancer element or by inducing the phosphoinositide–protein kinase C pathway. The estrogen receptor may in fact directly synergize with Pit-1 to induce PRL transcription.

Although PRL receptors are widely distributed, their hormonal regulation is tissue specific. High progesterone levels during pregnancy limit breast PRL receptor number, but early in lactation their numbers increase markedly. Prostatic PRL receptor levels are increased by testosterone and decreased by estrogens.

Prolactinomas are the most common hormone-secreting pituitary adenomas and, depending on their size, are classified as microprolactinomas (<10 mm, 90% of which affect women), or macroprolactinomas (>10 mm, 60% of which affect men). PRL serum levels greater than 200 μg/L are usually associated with a prolactinoma. Hyperprolactinemia presents as hypogonadism with amenorrhea and galactorrhea in women, and impotence and infertility in men. Patients harboring macroadenomas are usually males, and their clinical presentation may be associated with local mass effect signs of headaches and visual field disturbances. Most patients are successfully treated with dopamine agonists while trans-sphenoidal surgery is reserved for drug-resistant tumors, which comprise about 5–10% of patients.

THYROID-STIMULATING HORMONE

Thyrotrophs comprise 5% of the anterior pituitary cell population. TSH and the glycoproteins, LH, FSH, and human chorionic gonadotropin (hCG), are composed of two noncovalently linked subunits, a common α and a specific β. Although the α-subunit is expressed in pituitary thyrotrophs and gonadotrophs and in placental cells, cell-specific expression depends on different promoter regions. Tissue specificity is determined by the β-subunit despite their 75% structural homology. Although Pit-1 binds to the β-subunit promoter, it is not required for α-subunit expression. Both α- and β-subunit transcriptions are induced by TRH and inhibited by triiodothyronine(T_3) and dopamine. TSH secretion is stimulated by TRH, whereas thyroid hormones, dopamine, SRIF, and glucocorticoids suppress TSH.

TSH-producing pituitary adenomas comprise less than 1% of all pituitary tumors and secrete both TSH α- and β-subunits. The tumor-derived α-subunit is synthesized in excess of the β-subunit, a characteristic useful for differential diagnosis. TSH-secreting tumors fail to respond to thyroid hormone-negative feedback but are suppressed by somatostatin. Clinical presentation usually includes hyperthyroidism and diffuse goiter, with elevated or inappropriately normal TSH levels in the presence of elevated thyroid hormones. Tumors are usually large and often invasive with commonly observed local mass effects. Trans-sphenoidal pituitary surgery is the preferred initial therapeutic approach, but surgical cure is elusive and most patients require adjuvant medical or radiation therapy. The somatostatin analog, octreotide, suppresses TSH and may attenuate further tumor growth. Thyroid ablation to cure hyperthyroxinemia is not recommended because of the potential risk of pituitary tumor expansion as a result of disinhibition of the thyrotroph cells from negative feedback.

FOLLICLE-STIMULATING HORMONE AND LUTEINIZING HORMONE

Gonadotrophs represent up to 10% of anterior pituitary cells and express both FSH and LH-β-subunits. Gonadotropin-releasing hormone (GnRH) induces the transcription of all three gonadotropin subunits, whereas estrogen attenuates their transcription, in part by inhibiting hypothalamic GnRH. However, estrogen may exert positive pituitary feedback and may actually increase LH-β mRNA under several physiologic conditions. A novel gonadotroph-specific protein (SF-1) appears to regulate pituitary α-subunit gene expression distinct from placental regulation of this gene.

GONADOTROPH CELL TUMORS Gonadotroph adenomas are among the most common pituitary adenomas. These "nonsecreting" adenomas are clinically nonfunctional because the gonadotropins and their subunits are either not released or are inefficiently secreted and usually do not produce a distinct clinical syndrome. These tumors result in elevated α- and FSH-β-subunit and, rarely, LH-β serum levels. Some adenomas secrete α-subunits but not intact FSH or LH. TRH administration usually induces secretion of gonadotropins or their subunits, in patients harboring these non-functional adenomas, unlike the absent TRH response seen in normal subjects. Most nonsecreting adenomas immunostain positively for intact FSH and LH, or α-, FSH-β-, and LH-β-subunits. Excessive secretion of FSH or LH may occasion-

Table 48-3
Pituitary Failure Associated with Pit-1 Mutations

Mutation	*Clinical phenotype*	*Autosomal inheritance*
DNA binding domain		
143Arg→Gln	Growth retardation	Recessive
158Ala→Pro	Hypothyroid; growth retardation	Recessive
172Arg→Stop	Hypothyroid	Recessive
271Arg→Trp	Growth retardation; impaired thyroid reserve	Dominant
135Phe→Cys	Growth retardation; hypothyroidism	Recessive
Activation domain		
^{24}Pro→Leu	Growth retardation	Dominant

Table 48-4
Classification of Pituitary Adenomas[a]

Adenoma cell origin	*Hormone product*	*Clinical syndrome*
Lactotroph	PRL	Hypogonadism, galactorrhea[b]
Gonadotroph	FSH, LH, subunits	Silent or hypogonadism
Somatotroph	GH	Acromegaly, gigantism
Corticotroph	ACTH	Cushing's disease
Mixed growth hormone and prolactin cell	GH, PRL	Acromegaly, hypogonadism
Other plurihormonal cell	Any	
Acidophil stem cell	PRL, GH	Hypogonadism, acromegaly
Mammosomatotroph	PRL, GH	Hypogonadism, acromegaly
Thyrotroph	TSH	Hyperthyroidism
Null cell	None	Pituitary failure
Oncocytoma	None	Pituitary failure

[a]Hormone-secreting tumors are listed in decreasing order of frequency. All tumors may cause local pressure effects, including visual disturbances, cranial nerve palsy, and headache.

[b]Females present with amenorrhea and infertility and males present with impotence or infertility.

ally downregulate the reproductive axis resulting in clinical hypogonadism. Mass effects, including optic chiasm pressure and other neurologic symptoms, may be the initial symptoms of large gonadotroph tumors. Surgical excision is the most effective therapy and pharmacologic agents are largely ineffective in shrinking these tumor masses.

ANTERIOR PITUITARY FAILURE As discussed above, Pit-1 appears to be a critical transcription factor in determining tissue-specific expression of GH, PRL, and TSH. Studies in dwarf mice indicate that intact Pit-1 is required to sustain these functional anterior pituitary cell types. Several transgenic mice models expressing dysfunctional GH transcriptional regulation exhibit markedly attenuated or absent GH gene expression. For example, the snell dwarf mouse has a Pit-1 point mutation. In humans, sporadic and familial cases of Pit-1 mutation have recently been described exhibiting varying degrees of combined GH, PRL, and TSH basal deficiency, or impaired reserve. Some of those patients may exhibit a hypoplastic pituitary gland (Table 48-3). The autosomal dominant or recessive Pit-1 mutations associated with this heterogenous clinical syndrome include dysfunctional point mutations with defective binding to pituitary gene promoters (e.g., 158 A to P), and dominant negative missense mutations (e.g., 271 Arg to Trp). Once Pit-1 function and regulation are clarified, further genetic disorders associated with combined pituitary hormone deficiency or possibly hyperfunction should become apparent.

A missense mutation (77 Cys → Arg) in the GH molecule also leads to short stature. This mutant GH has weakened signal-transducing capacity, and may also function as a dominant negative inhibitor of wild-type GH.

PATHOGENESIS OF PITUITARY TUMORS

Each of the anterior pituitary cell types may give rise to monoclonal benign neoplasms that are either hormonally functional or nonfunctional (Table 48-4). Functional tumors are characterized by autonomous trophic hormone secretion, leading to clinical hormone excess syndromes, including hyperprolactinemia, acromegaly or Cushing's disease. Nonfunctioning pituitary adenomas secrete clinically inactive glycoprotein hormones or their free subunits. True pituitary carcinomas are extremely rare, and less than 40 cases have been unequivocally documented.

CLONAL ORIGIN OF PITUITARY ADENOMAS Complete resection of well-circumscribed pituitary adenomas often results in a cure of unrestrained or paradoxical hormone hypersecretion. This observation prompted the question as to whether these tumors were clonal expansions of a single disordered cell. Disordered hypothalamic regulation would likely give rise to a generalized polyclonal cellular hyperplasia, as is seen in patients harboring extrapituitary tumors elaborating hypothalamic releasing hormones (e.g., GRH, CRH). Alternatively, an intrinsic genetic defect within the pituitary would likely be associated with clonal proliferation.

Using X-chromosomal inactivation analysis of female patients heterozygous for sex-linked genes, several groups have confirmed the monoclonal origin of functional and nonfunctional pituitary tumors. When clonal analysis was performed on tumor DNA for hypoxanthine phosphoribosyl transferase (HPRT) or phosphoglycerate kinase (PGK) in heterozygous patients with acromegaly, Cushing's disease, prolactinomas, and nonfunctioning tumors, a preferential loss of the inactive X-chromosome allele was observed after digestion with methylation-sensitive enzymes. The monoclonal origin of these tumors has been confirmed by the high allelic cleavage ratio of the visualized demethylated vs nondemethylated DNA restriction bands.

These observations have prompted the quest for unraveling an intrinsic pituitary genetic defect resulting in either activation of a cell stimulator or inactivation of an inhibitor of cell proliferation.

HYPOTHALAMIC ORIGIN OF PITUITARY ADENOMAS Hypothalamic hormones regulate expression of the respective pituitary hormone genes by binding to specific cell surface receptors. In addition, these peptides may also induce DNA synthesis and enhanced mitotic activity in their target pituitary cells. Thus, mice expressing a GHRH transgene will exhibit somatotroph hyperplasia and ultimately adenoma. Patients harboring tumors elaborating ectopic GHRH or CRH may also present with GH-cell or ACTH-cell hyperplasia or adenomas, in addition to the hormone hypersecretory syndrome. Recently pituitary tumor-derived GHRH, SRIF, and TRH have been characterized by in situ or reverse transcriptase polymerase chain reaction (RT-PCR) techniques. These observations of intrapituitary peptide expression may in fact imply a paracrine role for the hypothalamic peptides in pituitary tumorigenesis.

***gsp* MUTATIONS** Peptide hormone signal transduction involves coupling of activated cell surface receptors with membrane G proteins, consisting of three polypeptides: an α-chain that binds to guanine nucleotide, and a β- and γ-chain. Ligand-induced activation of the receptor induces the binding of GTP, which causes a conformational change in G protein, releasing the α-subunit from βγ, allowing it to interact with target proteins. Hydrolysis of bound GTP to GDP by the intrinsic GTPase activity of the α-subunit terminates the ligand-induced signal (Fig. 48-1). GHRH, by binding to its somatotroph receptor coupled to G proteins, uses cAMP as a second messenger to stimulate GH secretion and somatotroph proliferation. A subset of GH-secreting pituitary tumors contains elevated intracellular cAMP levels and increased in vitro GH secretion, and is not responsive to further GHRH stimulation. Intratumoral adenylyl cyclase levels are constitutively enhanced about 10-fold compared with levels in unaffected patients. The GHRH-independent induction of cAMP in these tumors could conceivably occur as a result of either constitutive activation of GHRH receptor or the catalytic domain of adenylyl cyclase or the stimulatory subunit of G protein. In fact, point mutations of Gsα were identified in about a third of these tumors. These missense mutations occur either in Arg-201 (Arg → Cys or His) or in Gln-227 (Gln → Arg), in a region of the Gsα that is involved in GTP hydrolysis. Thus, these *gsp* mutations activate Gsα by inhibiting its intrinsic GTPase activity. In the cAMP-responsive somatotroph cells, therefore, conversion of Gsα into an activating oncogene, *gsp*, may explain the pathogenesis of unrestrained cell proliferation and GH hypersecretion in these tumors. Gsα activation also induces both the Pit-1 promoter and serine phosphorylation of the cAMP response-protein (CREB) in acromegalic tissue, thus promoting somatotroph cell proliferation. In fact, CREB phosphorylation appears to be a universal finding in GH-cell adenomas, and is significantly lower in clinically silent gonadotroph cell adenomas. Interestingly, the *gsp* mutation is detected at a negligible frequency in Japanese patients, implying a geographic selection for the mutation. Unfortunately, no significant clinical phenotype is associated with *gsp* mutations, and ultimate tumor behavior and response to therapy is not altered in these patients. It would therefore appear that additional cAMP-associated signaling genes are involved in GH-cell tumorigenesis.

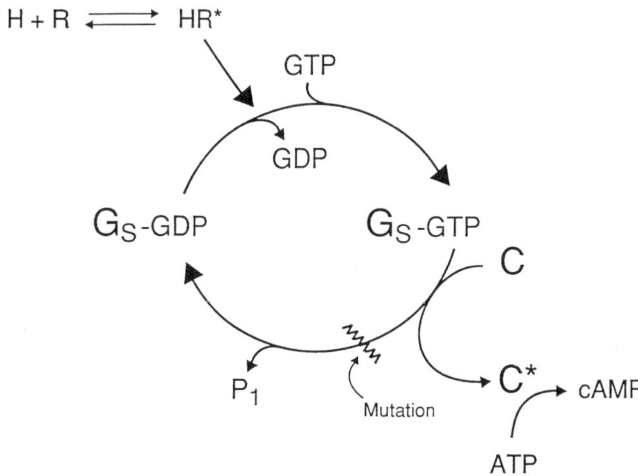

Figure 48-1 Inhibition of GTPase results in constitutively elevated cAMP and, consequently, enhanced growth hormone (GH) secretion. (Adapted from Spada.)

ras Transduction of intrapituitary hypothalamic, peripheral hormonal, and paracrine growth factor signals uses pathways other than those coupled to G proteins. The product of the protooncogene *ras* plays an important role in growth factor signal transduction. There are three functional *ras* genes, H-, N-, and K-*ras*, that encode a 21-kDa protein, $p21^{ras}$. The guanine nucleotide-binding protein $p21^{ras}$ possesses intrinsic GTPase activity and is associated with the plasma membrane. Downstream *ras* signaling involves protein kinase cascades that transduce the incoming signal to the nucleus. Point mutations of the *ras* gene can convert it to a constitutively active oncogene that has been implicated in the development of a variety of tumors, and represents one of the most common mutations detected in human neoplasia. *Ras* gene mutations, however, occur very rarely in pituitary tumors. Only a single invasive prolactinoma was found to harbor a missense *ras* mutation. *Ras* mutations were also detected in metastatic deposits of pituitary carcinomas, but not in the respective primary pituitary tumors. These findings suggest that activation of *ras* is not an initial event in pituitary tumorigenesis; however, point mutations of *ras* may be important for the development or growth of metastases originating from rarely occurring pituitary carcinomas.

Recently, an activating transforming gene *(PTTG)* was isolated from rat and human pituitary tumors and is located on chromosome 5q33. This locus has been implicated as a marker for several other malignances.

TUMOR SUPPRESSOR GENES Studies of the *MEN-I* gene locus surprisingly yielded evidence for tumor suppressor gene participation in pituitary tumorigenesis. Loss of heterozygosity of chromosome 11q13 is present not only in hereditary pituitary tumors associated with *MEN-I*, but also in up to 20% of sporadically occurring pituitary adenomas, including GH-, PRL-, and ACTH-cell adenomas, as well as some nonfunctional tumors. Several of these tumors exhibiting 11q13 loss of heterozygosity

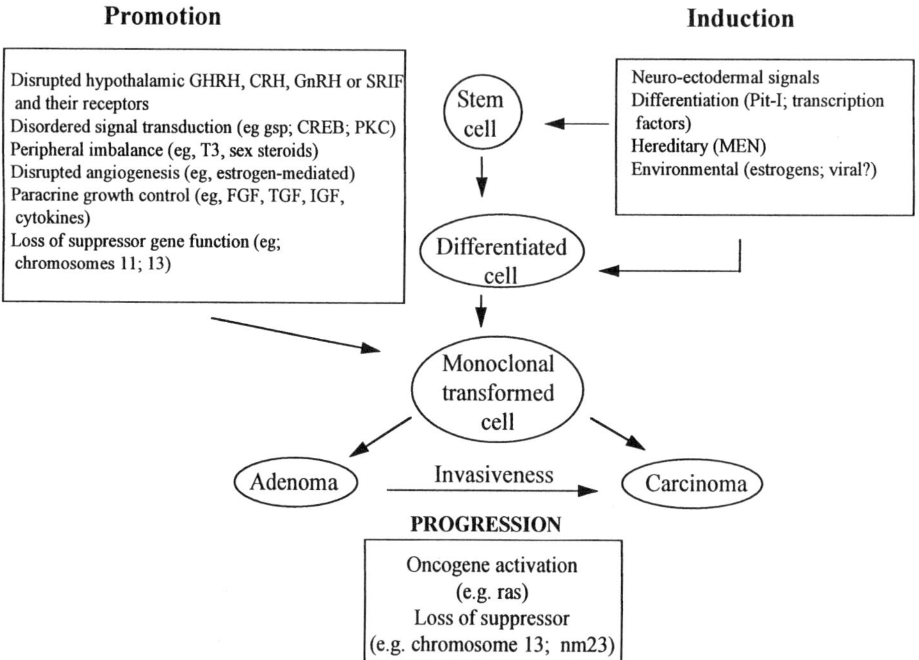

Figure 48-2 Summary of known subcellular events leading to pituitary tumor formation. (Adapted from Melmed et al. J Clin Endocrinol Metab 1995;80:3395–3402.)

concurrently were shown to harbor a *gsp* mutation, lending further credence to a multistep cause of pituitary tumors. Recently, the gene for *MEN-1 (menin)* has been cloned. However, it appears that sporadic pituitary tumors do not manifest mutations of this tumor suppressor gland, even in the presence of chromosone II LOH.

The retinoblastoma susceptibility gene *(RB)* is inactivated in a variety of human tumors. Individuals with germline mutations on one *RB* allele have >90% chance of developing a childhood retinoblastoma. The *RB* gene maps to chromosome 13ql4, and loss of heterozygosity at this locus is seen in retinoblastoma cells. The *RB* gene product is a major determinant of cell cycle control and acts as a signal transducer interfacing the cell cycle with specific transcriptional activation. The RB protein is phosphorylated in a cell cycle-dependent manner, being maximal at the start of the S phase and low after mitosis and entry into G1, and its activity appears regulated by the state of phosphorylation. Loss of RB protein function deprives the cell of an important mechanism for restraining cell proliferation.

The role of the *RB* gene in pituitary tumor formation was initially suggested by observations made in transgenic mice, in which one allele of the *RB* gene was disrupted. Although homozygous *RB* mutations are lethal early in fetal life, mice heterozygous for the *RB* gene mutation are not predisposed to retinoblastoma, but interestingly demonstrate pituitary tumors at a high frequency. These tumors originate from the pars intermedia of the pituitary, and express POMC immunoreactive products. The wild-type *RB* allele is absent in these pituitary tumors, whereas the mutant allele is retained. Pituitary tumor tissue derived from these mice also expresses a truncated dysfunctional RB protein.

In benign human pituitary microadenomas no loss of heterozygosity at the *RB* locus has been detected. However, in invasive pituitary macroadenomas and in pituitary carcinomas, allelic deletions at the *RB* locus were observed. Therefore, loss of heterozygosity at the *RB* locus is unlikely to be an initiating event in pituitary tumorigenesis, but rather *RB* or an associated tumor suppressor gene may play a role in progression of benign tumors to more invasive and malignant phenotypes. Since immunoreactive RB protein appears to be present in these tumors, it is likely that another tumor suppressor gene is located on chromosome 13 in close proximity to the *RB* locus and might be involved in pituitary tumor progression.

nM23, a disphosphate kinase gene associated with suppression of breast cancer and melanoma metastases, has been shown to be highly expressed in small noninvasive pituitary adenomas. Pituitary *nM23* expression correlates inversely with cavernous sinus invasiveness and is markedly attenuated in large invasive tumors.

Interestingly, although *p53* tumor suppressor gene mutations have been detected in a wide variety of human tumors, no *p53* mutation has been detected in a comprehensive screening of pituitary tumors.

INTRAPITUITARY PARACRINE GROWTH FACTORS

Several intrapituitary growth factors and cytokines are expressed in normal and tumorous tissue. Their paracrine or autocrine regulation of specific pituitary function involves several trophic hormones either singly or in combination. These factors include epidermal growth factor (EGF), nerve growth factor (NGF), IGF-I, activin, and endothelin. Cytokines, including IL-6, IL-2, and LIF, also participate in paracrine regulation of trophic hormones. Although several in vitro and in vivo rat models have demonstrated growth factor-mediated pituitary mitogenesis, most of the information yielded from studies of human pituitary tumors is largely descriptive. The paucity of human tissue, as well as the failure of human pituitary cells to proliferate in vitro, has largely limited the subcellular regulatory studies required to establish a direct tumorigenic link for these growth factors.

The most compelling evidence in favor of a growth factor role in pituitary pathogenesis is that derived from studying the fibroblast growth factor (FGF) family. Basic FGF (bFGF) is abundantly expressed in the pituitary, regulates PRL and TSH secretion, and also may stimulate human pituitary cell mitogenesis in vitro. Interestingly, circulating bFGF, as well as bFGF auto-antibodies, is detectable before pituitary tumor resection in patients with *MEN I*, and bFGF levels fall after surgery. These observations imply that at least in MEN-I, the pituitary adenoma may be a source of this mitogen. FGF-4, which may behave as a transforming proto-oncogene is expressed in human prolactinomas and has recently also been shown to induce PRL transcription. The FGF family may also mediate estrogen-induced pituitary angiogenesis, thus lowering portal concentrations of dopamine and facilitating lactotroph proliferation.

Other paracrine growth factors that have been implicated in pituitary tumorigenesis include EGF, transforming growth factor-α (TGF-α) and -β, and IGF-I. The gp-130 family of cytokines, including IL-6 and LIF, are expressed in functional pituitary adenomas, regulate POMC transcription, and may in fact be inhibitory for pituicyte mitogenesis.

In summary, the molecular pathogenesis of pituitary adenomas appears multifactorial (Fig. 48-2). Clearly early proximal DNA-altering events may occur. These may involve transcription factor dysregulation (e.g., Pit-1), hereditary mutations (e.g., MEN), or possible viral insults. Multiple promoting influences may subsequently impinge on the previously "initiated" cell and determine clonal expansion. These factors include disordered hypothalamic hormone receptor signaling (e.g., *gsp*); overstimulation by ectopic (or paracrine?) hypothalamic hormones (e.g., GRH, CRH); disordered paracrine growth factor action (e.g., FGF-4, bFGF); disordered signal transduction (e.g., PKC); loss of negative feedback inhibition (e.g., hypothyroidism or hypogonadism); estrogen-mediated or paracrine angiogenesis (e.g., vascular endothelial growth factor; LIF); and loss of tumor suppressor activity (e.g., chromosomes 11 and 13). Once the cell has been transformed, its ultimate growth characteristics and neoplastic behavior appear to be determined by several genes acting relatively distally, including *ras* and *nm23*.

SELECTED REFERENCES

Alexander J, Klibanski A. Gonadotropin-releasing hormone receptor mRNA expression by human pituitary tumors in vitro. J Clin Invest 1994;93:2332–2339.

Alexander JM, Biller BM, Bikkal H, Zervas NT, Arnold A, Klibanski A. Clinically non-functioning pituitary tumors are monoclonal in origin. J Clin Invest 1990;86:336–340.

Alexander JM, Swearingen B, Tindall GT, Klibanski A. Human pituitary adenomas express endogenous inhibin subunit and follistatin messenger ribonucleic acids. J Clin Endocrinol Metab 1995;80:147–152.

Bates AS, Farrell WE, Bicknell EJ, et al. Allelic deletion in pituitary adenomas reflects aggressive biological activity and has potential value as a prognostic marker. J Clin Endocrinol Metab 1997;82: 818–824.

Bertherat J, Chanson P, Montminy M. The cyclic adenosine 3'5'-monophosphate-responsive factor CREB is constitutively activated in human somatotroph adenomas. Mol Endocrinol 1995;9:777–783.

Boggild MD, Jenkinson S, Pistorello M, et al. Molecular genetic studies of sporadic pituitary tumors. J Clin Endocrinol Metab 1994;78:387–392.

Clayton RN, Boggild M, Bates AS, Bicknell J, Simpson D, Farrell W. Tumour suppressor genes in the pathogenesis of human pituitary tumours. Horm Res 1997;47:185–193.

Cohen LE, Wondisford FE, Salvatoni A, et al. A "hot spot" in the pit-1 gene responsible for combined pituitary hormone deficiency: clinical and molecular correlates. J Clin Endocrinol Metab 1995;80:679–684.

Eyde Theill L, Karin M. Transcriptional control of GH expression and anterior pituitary development. Endocr Rev 1993;14:670–689.

Greenman Y. Melmed S. Heterogenous expression of two somatostatin receptor subtypes in pituitary tumors. J. Clin Endocrinol Metab 1994;78:393–403.

Herman V, Fagin J, Gonski R, Kovacs, Melmed S. Clonal orgin of pituitary andenomas. J Clin Endocrinol Metab 1990;71:1427–1433.

Melmed S, Ho K, Klibanski A, Reichlin S, Thorner M. Recent advances in pathogenesis, diagnosis and management of acromegaly. J Clin Endocrinol Metab 1995;80:3395–3402.

Nowakowski BE, Maurer RA. Multiple Pit-1 binding sites facilitate estrogen responsiveness of the prolactin gene. Mol Endocrinol 1994;8:1742–1749.

Orth DN. Cushing's Syndrome. N Engl J Med 1995;332:791–802.

Pei L, Melmed S, Scheithauer B, Kovacs K, Benedict WF, Prager D. Frequent loss of heterozygosity at the retinoblastoma susceptibility gene (RB) locus in aggressive pituitary tumors: evidence for a chromosome 13 tumor suppressor gene other than RB. Cancer Res 1995;55:1613–1616.

Ray D, Melmed S. Pituitary cytokine and growth factor expression and action. Endocr Rev 1997;18:206–228.

Shimon I, Melmed S. Genetic basis of endocrine disease: pituitary tumor pathogenesis. J Clin Endocrinol Metab 1997;82:1675–1681.

Spada A, Faglia G. G protein dysfunction in pituitary tumors. In: Melmed S, ed. Oncogenesis of pituitary tumors. Basel: Karger, 1995.

Melmed S, ed. The Pituitary. Cambridge, MA: Blackwell Science, 1995.

Voss JW, Rosenfeld MG. Anterior pituitary development: short tales from dwarf mice. Cell 1992;70:527–530.

Zimering MB, Riley DJ, Thakker-Varia S, et al. Circulating fibroblast growth factor-like autoantibodies in two patients with multiple endocrine neoplasia type1 and prolactinoma. J Clin Endocrinol Metab 1994;79:1546–1552.

49 Growth Hormone Deficiency Disorders

Joy D. Cogan and John A. Phillips III

INTRODUCTION

Growth hormone (GH) is a multifunctional hormone produced in the pituitary that promotes postnatal growth of skeletal and soft tissues through a variety of effects (Fig. 49-1). Controversy remains about the relative contribution of direct and indirect actions of GH. On the one hand, the direct effects of GH have been demonstrated in a variety of tissues and organs and GH receptors have been documented in a number of cell types. On the other, a substantial amount of data indicates that a major portion of the effects of GH are mediated through the actions of GH-dependent insulin-like growth factor I (IGF-I). IGF-1 is produced in many tissues, primarily the liver, and acts through its own receptor to enhance the proliferation and maturation of many tissues, including bone, cartilage, and skeletal muscle. In addition to promoting growth of tissues, GH has also been shown to exert a variety of other biologic effects, including lactogenic, diabetogenic, lipolytic, and protein anabolic effects, as well as sodium and water retention.

At the cellular level, a single GH molecule binds two GH receptor molecules (GHR) causing them to dimerize (*see* Chapter 46). Dimerization of the two GH-bound GHR molecules is believed to be necessary for signal transduction, which is associated with the tyrosine kinase JAK-2. It has been suggested that the diverse effects of GH may be mediated by a single type of GHR molecule that can possess different cytoplasmic domains or phosphorylation sites in different tissues. When activated by JAK-2, these differing cytoplasmic domains can lead to distinct phosphorylation pathways, one for growth effects and others for various metabolic effects.

The frequency of GH deficiency (either isolated or concomitant with other pituitary hormone deficiencies) is estimated to range from 1/4,000 to 1/10,000 in various studies. Most cases are sporadic and are assumed to arise from cerebral insults or defects that include cerebral edema, chromosomal anomalies, histiocytosis, infections, radiation, septo-optic dysplasia, trauma, or tumors affecting the hypothalamus or pituitary. Magnetic resonance imaging examinations detect hypothalamic or pituitary anomalies in about 12% of patients who have isolated GH deficiency (IGHD).

Interestingly, estimates of the proportion of GH-deficient cases having an affected parent, sib, or child range from 3 to 30% in different studies. This occurrence of familial clustering suggests that a significant proportion of cases may have a genetic basis. The genetics and molecular pathophysiology of familial IGHD and panhypopituitary dwarfism will be discussed in the following sections.

From: *Principles of Molecular Medicine* (J. L. Jameson, ed.), ©1998 Humana Press Inc., Totowa, NJ.

CLINICAL FEATURES Adequate amounts of GH are needed throughout childhood to maintain normal growth. Newborns with GH deficiency are usually of normal length and weight. Some may have micropenis or fasting hypoglycemia in addition to their low linear growth, which becomes progressively retarded with age. In those with IGHD, skeletal maturation is usually delayed in proportion to their retardation height. Truncal obesity, facial appearance younger than expected for their chronologic age, delayed secondary dentition, and high-pitched voice are often present. Puberty may be delayed until the late teens but normal fertility usually occurs. Fine, wrinkled skin appearing similar to that of premature aging is seen in affected adults. Concomitant deficiencies of other pituitary hormones—e.g., luteinizing hormone (LH), follicle-stimulating hormone (FSH), thyroid-stimulating hormone (TSH), and adrenocorticotropin hormone (ACTH)—in addition to GH, is called panhypopituitary dwarfism. With these additional hormone deficiencies, the retardation of growth and skeletal maturation is often more severe and spontaneous puberty may not occur.

Laron syndrome is an autosomal recessive disorder caused by target resistance to the action of GH (Online Mendelian inheritance of man number [OMIM] 245590). Subjects with Laron syndrome are similar in clinical appearance to those with severe isolated GH deficiency. At the biochemical level, Laron syndrome subjects have low levels of IGF-I, despite increased circulating levels of GH. This contrasts with the low levels of both IGF-I and GH that are seen in GH deficiency. Molecular analyses have identified heterogeneous exon deletions and base substitutions in the GHR genes of a large number of Laron syndrome patients. Although treatment with exogenous GH is ineffective in those with GHR dysfunction, replacement therapy with recombinant IGF-I has been shown to be effective.

DIAGNOSIS Although short stature, delayed growth velocity, and delayed skeletal maturation are all seen with GH deficiency, none of these is specific for this disorder. Patients should be evaluated for other systemic diseases before provocative tests of GH deficiency. These provocative tests include postexcercise, L-Dopa, insulin-tolerance, arginine, insulin-arginine, clonidine, glucagon, and propranolol. Inadequate GH peak responses (usually <7–10 ng/mL) differ from test to test. Testing for concomitant deficiencies of LH, FSH, TSH, ACTH should be done to obtain a more accurate diagnosis and to plan optimal treatment.

FAMILIAL ISOLATED GH DEFICIENCY

GENETIC BASIS AND MOLECULAR PATHOPHYSIOLOGY OF DISEASE Familial IGHD is associated with at least

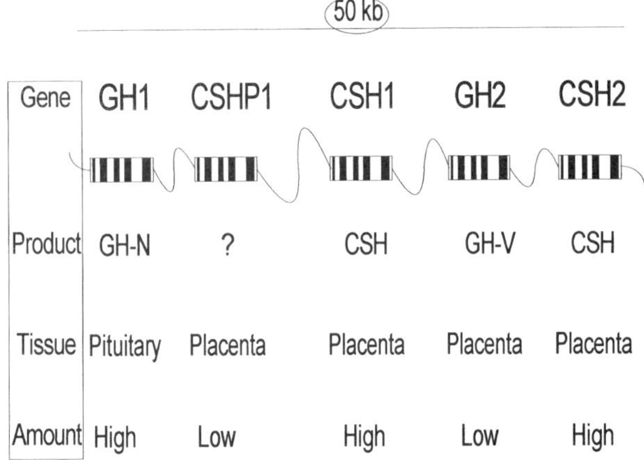

Figure 49-1 Schematic overview of the GH gene cluster, including the protein products and expression patterns of its component genes.

four Mendelian disorders (OMIM 139250 and 307200). These include two forms that have autosomal recessive (IGHD IA and IB) inheritance, as well as autosomal dominant (IGHD II) and X-linked (IGHD III) forms. Recently, a variety of molecular defects have been detected that cause these disorders (*see* Table 49-1). These defects will be reviewed on the basis of the type of inheritance (IGHD I–III) that they cause.

IGHD IA The most severe form of IGHD, called IGHD IA, has an autosomal recessive mode of inheritance. Affected individuals occasionally have short lengths at birth and hypoglycemia in infancy, but uniformly develop severe dwarfism by 6 months of age. In response to replacement therapy with exogenous GH, IGHD IA subjects have a strong initial anabolic and growth response that is frequently followed by the development of anti-GH antibodies in sufficient titer to block the response to GH replacement.

Deletions Initially, all individuals with IGHD IA were found to be homozygous for GH1 gene deletions and developed anti-GH antibodies with treatment. Subsequently, additional cases with GH1 gene deletions have been described who also have complete GH deficiency, but respond well to GH replacement. Thus, the clinical outcomes of subjects with the same molecular findings vary, making the presence of anti-GH antibodies an inconsistent finding in IGHD IA cases.

At a molecular level, Southern blot analysis showed deletions of approximately 6.7, 7.0, or 7.6 kb, with most (approximately 75%) being 6.7 kb. DNA sequence analysis of the fusion fragments associated with GH1 gene deletions have shown that homologous recombination between sequences flanking the GH1 gene cause these deletions (Fig. 49-1). Currently, GH1 gene deletions are detected using polymerase chain reaction (PCR) amplification of the homologous regions flanking the GH1 gene and the fusion fragments associated with GH1 gene deletions (*see* Fig. 49-2). Because the fusion fragments associated with 6.7-kb deletions differ in the size of fragments produced by certain restriction enzymes (*see Sma*I sites indicated by solid circle in Fig. 49-2), homozygosity or heterozygosity for these deletions can easily be detected by enzyme digestion of PCR products. A variety of studies suggest that 13–15% of subjects with severe IGHD (>–4.5 SD in height) have GH1 gene deletions. Recently, frameshift and nonsense mutations have also been found in subjects with the IGHD IA phenotype, such that this disorder may best be described as complete GH deficiency as a result of GH1 gene defects, rather than gene deletions alone.

Deletion and Frameshift Mutations Two affected sibs diagnosed with IGHD IA have been reported who are compound heterozygotes for deletion and frameshift mutations of the GH1 gene. Southern blot analysis showed the patients to be heterozygous for the 6.7-kb GH gene deletion. DNA sequence analysis of the retained GH1 gene showed it had a cytosine deleted in the 18th codon of the prohormone sequence. This single base deletion results in a frameshift within the signal peptide coding region that prevents the synthesis of any mature GH protein. These patients presented with severe growth failure, and after an initial growth response to treatment with exogenous GH, had high titers of anti-GH antibodies.

Nonsense Mutations A G→A transition in the 20th codon that converts a Trp codon (TGG) to a Stop codon (TAG) of the GH-N signal peptide has been reported in a consanguineous Turkish family with IGHD IA. This results in the termination of translation after residue 19 of the signal peptide and no production of mature GH. Patients homozygous for this mutation have no detectable GH and produce anti-GH antibodies in response to exogenous GH treatment. Interestingly, this mutation generates a new *Alu*I site that can be readily screened for by PCR amplification of the GH gene followed by *Alu*I digestion and gel electrophoresis (Fig. 49-3).

IGHD IB Patients with IGHD IB are characterized by low, but detectable levels of GH, stature more than 2 SD below the mean for age and sex, an autosomal recessive mode of inheritance, and a positive response and immunologic tolerance to treatment with exogenous GH. Some patients clinically diagnosed as IGHD IA because of an apparent lack of endogenous GH are actually type IB. In these patients, their GH gene defects result in a mutant GH protein that cannot be effectively measured by radioimmunoassay (RIA). The presence of this protein may explain their good response to GH therapy and lack of anti-GH antibodies. A diagram showing all of the IGHD IA and IB mutations is shown in Fig. 49-4.

Splicing Mutations A G→C transversion in the first base of the donor splice site of intron IV has been detected in a consanguineous Saudi Arabian family. The effect of this mutation on mRNA splicing was determined by transfecting the mutant gene into cultured mammalian cells and DNA sequencing of the resulting GH cDNAs. The mutation was found to cause the activation of a cryptic splice site 73 bases upstream of the exon IV donor splice site. This altered splicing results in the loss of amino acids 103→126 of exon IV and creates a frameshift that alters the amino acid encoded for by exon V. Such changes in the amino acids encoded by exons IV and V may not only affect the stability and biologic activity of the mutant GH protein, but as studies with bovine GH mutants have shown, also derange intracellular targeting of GH protein products to the secretory granule.

A G→T transversion has been identified at the same site in another consanguineous Saudi family. Analysis of GH mRNA transcripts from the lymphoblastoid cells of affected patients confirmed that the G→T transversion had the same effect on splicing as the G→C transversion. Both of these mutations destroy an *Hph*I site that enables their detection by restriction digestion of GH gene PCR products followed by gel electrophoresis. Patients homozygous for these defects responded well to exogenous GH treatment and did not make anti-GH antibodies.

A G→C transversion of the fifth base of intron IV was identified in a highly consanguineous family diagnosed with IGHD I. This mutation created a new *Mae*II site that was used to screen all

Table 49-1
Mutations in the GH Genes of GH-Deficient Subjects

IGHD type	Location	Nucleotide change[a]	Effect of mutation	References
IA		Deletion	7.6-kb deletion of GH gene	Vnencak-Jones et al. (1990)
		Deletion	7.0-kb deletion of GH gene	Vnencak-Jones et al. (1990)
		Deletion	6.7-kb deletion of GH gene	Vnencak-Jones et al. (1990)
	Exon II	5536 del C	Frameshift after 17th aa of signal peptide	Duquesnoy et al. (1990)
	Exon II	5543 G→A	Stop codon after 19th aa of signal peptide	Cogan et al. (1993)
IB	Intron IV	6242 G→C	Donor splice site mutation; frameshift	Cogan et al. (1994)
	Intron IV	6242 G→T	Donor splice site mutation; frameshift	Miller-Davis et al. (1993)
	Intron IV	6246 G→C	Donor splice site mutation; frameshift	Abdul-Latif (1995)
	Exon III	5938-39 del AG	Frameshift after 55th aa of mature GH	Igarashi et al. (1993)
II	Intron III	5955 G→A	Donor splice site mutation; exon 3 skip	Cogan et al. (1995)
	Intron III	5955 G→C	Donor splice site mutation; exon 3 skip	Binder et al. (1995)
	Intron III	5960 T→C	Donor splice site mutation; exon 3 skip	Cogan et al. (1994)
	Intron III	5982-99 del	Splicing mutation; exon 3 skip	Cogan et al. (1997)
	Intron III	5982 G→A	Splicing mutation; exon 3 skip	Cogan et al. (1997)

[a]Nucleotide numbering according to Chen et al., 1989.

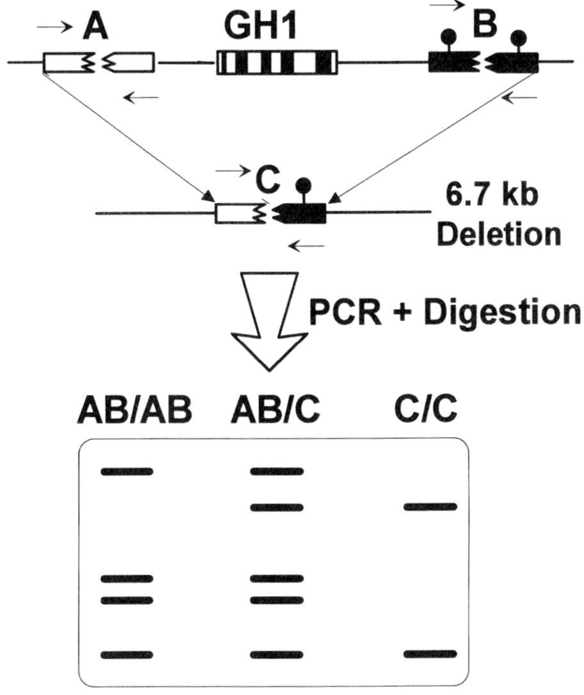

Figure 49-2 PCR amplification of homologous sequences flanking the GH1 gene. Flanking sequences are distinguished from GH-deletion fusion fragments by restriction enzyme digestion (●), shown above, and gel electrophoresis, shown below.

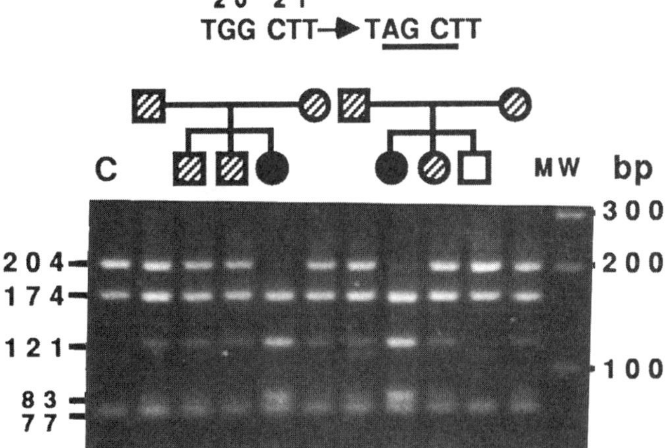

Figure 49-3 Detection of the GH G→A codon 20 (Trp→Stop) mutation by restriction enzyme digestion with *Alu*I and gel electrophoresis. Note when this mutation is present a new *Alu*I recognition site occurs and the normal 204-bp fragments are cleaved to 121 and 83 bp.

family members for the mutation. Reverse transcriptase-polymerase chain reaction (RT-PCR) analysis of GH mRNA transcripts from the lymphoblastoid cells of an affected patient demonstrated that the mutation destroyed the intron IV donor splice site and had the same overall effect on splicing as the +1G→C transversion described above.

Deletion and Frameshift An IGHD patient with severe growth retardation was found to have two GH gene defects. The first GH allele was a 6.7-kb deletion and the second had a 2-bp deletion in exon III. This 2-bp deletion results in a frameshift within exon III and generates a premature stop codon at the position of amino acid residue 132 in exon IV. The patient had a positive response to GH replacement therapy and did not produce anti-GH antibodies, again suggesting that some GH-related protein is produced.

IGHD II IGHD II has an autosomal dominant mode of inheritance. Patients diagnosed with IGHD II have a single affected parent, vary in clinical severity between kindreds, and respond well to GH treatment. All IGHD II patients with GH gene defects reported to date have mutations in intron III that alter splicing of GH transcripts resulting in skipping of exon III (*see* Fig. 49-5A). The mechanism by which the mutant, truncated GH protein inactivates the normal GH protein is not proven, but is thought to be through disruption of normal intracellular protein transport or the formation of GH heterodimers (Fig. 49-5B).

Dominant-Negative Mutations A T→C transition of the 6th base of the donor splice site of intron III was the first mutation associated with IGHD II. The mutant GH gene was transfected

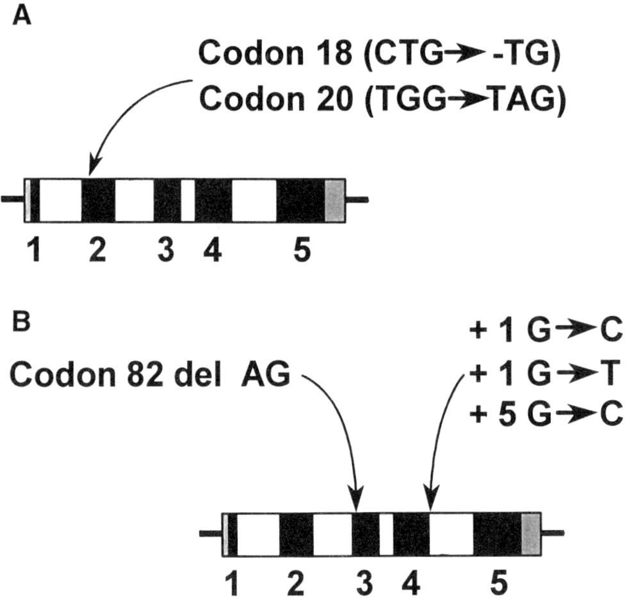

Figure 49-4 Schematic representation of the GH1 gene showing the locations of various IGHD IA **(A)** and IB **(B)** mutations.

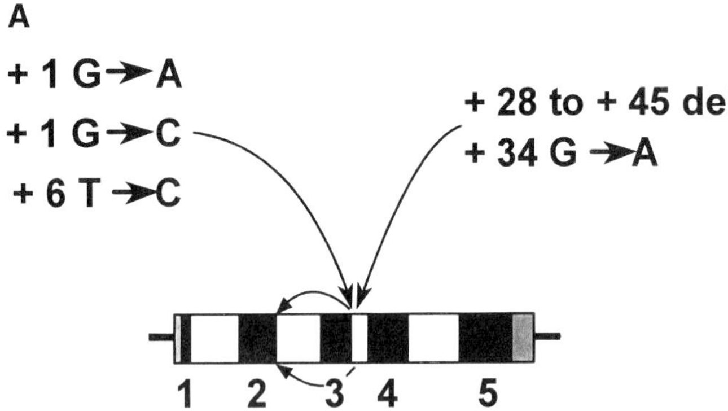

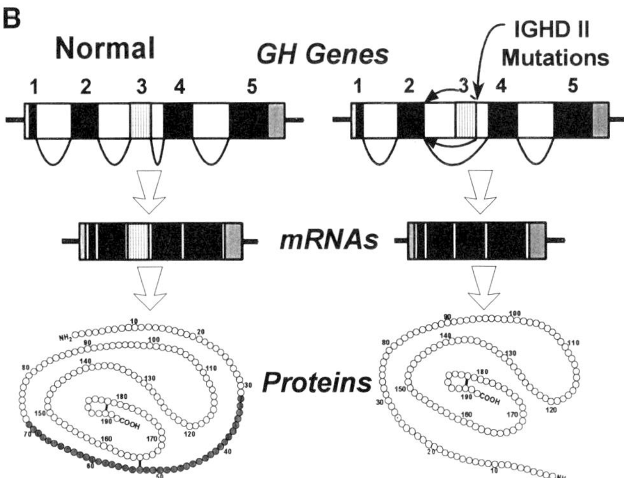

Figure 49-5 Schematic representation of **(A)** the GH1 gene showing the locations of various IGHD II mutations and **(B)** the mRNA splicing patterns of the normal GH and IGHD II mutant GH genes. Note that the deleted amino acids corresponding to exon III are shaded in the normal peptide (left) and absent in the mutant peptide (right).

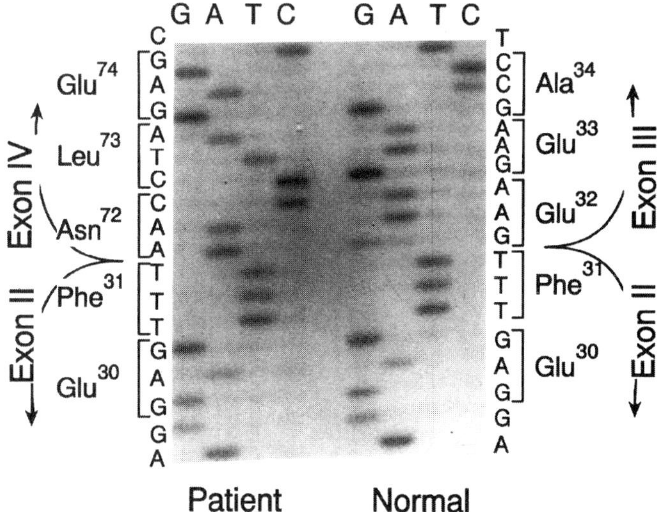

Figure 49-6 DNA sequence analysis of normal (right) and IGHD II mutant (left) GH cDNAs showing exon III skipping in the latter.

into cultured mammalian cells and the GH mRNA transcripts analyzed by direct sequencing of their corresponding cDNAs. The mutation was found to inactivate the intron III donor splice site causing deletion or skipping of exon III and the loss of amino acids 32→71 from the corresponding mature GH-N protein products (*see* Fig. 49-6). All of the affected patients in this family were heterozygous for the intron III +6T→C change and had low, but measurable, GH levels after provocative stimulation. Affected subjects responded well to treatment with exogenous GH without forming significant levels of anti-GH antibodies.

Two additional IGHD II mutations have been identified that both alter the first base of the intron III donor splice site. One is a G→C transversion and the other is a recurring G→A transition. The latter has been identified in three nonrelated kindreds and is believed to arise because of the high mutation frequency of CpG dinucleotides. Both mutations were shown to cause exon III skipping in lymphoblastoid cells and transfection studies, respectively.

Two intron III mutations that alter splicing and do not occur within the branch consensus, donor, or acceptor sites have been recently identified. The first deletes 18 bp, del+28→45, and the second is a G→A transition of the 28th base of intron III. Transfection studies and sequencing of the GH RT-PCR products demonstrated that the overall effect on splicing was the same as the other IGHD II donor splice site mutations. The mechanism by which these two mutations alter splicing is unknown, but may involve secondary structure or a protein-binding site.

IGHD III IGHD III has an X-linked mode of inheritance, but distinct clinical findings in different families. Affected individuals in some kindreds have agammaglobulinemia associated with their IGHD, but others do not. This suggests that contiguous gene defects of Xq21.3→q22 may occur in some cases. Interestingly, other cases of IGHD have been found to have an interstitial deletion of Xp22.3 or duplication of Xq13.3→q 21.2 suggesting that multiple loci may cause IGHD III.

BIODEFECTIVE GH Kowarski et al. studied two unrelated boys, with growth retardation, delayed bone ages, and low levels of somatomedin (but normal GH levels) after stimulation. Treat-

Table 49-2
Mutations in the Pit-1 Genes of Subjects with CPHD

Mode	*Codon*[a]	*Nucleotide change*	*Effect of mutation*	*References*
AR		Deletion	Deletion of Pit-1 gene	Wit et al. (1989)
	135	T→G	Amino acid change (Phe→Cys)	Pelligrini et al. (1996)
	143	G→A	Amino acid change (Arg→Gln)	Ohta et al. (1992)
	158	G→C	Amino acid change (Ala→Pro)	Wit et al. (1989)
	172	C→T	Generates a stop codon	Tatsumi (1992)
	250	G→T	Generates a stop codon	Irie et al. (1995)
AD	24	C→T	Amino acid change (Pro→Leu)	Ohta et al. (1992)
	271	C→T	Amino acid change (Arg→Trp)	Radovick et al. (1992) Cohen et al. (1995)

[a]Codon number from the translation start site.

ment with exogenous human GH induced normal levels of somatomedin and a significant increase in growth rate. While the family data did not support a specific mode of inheritance, a mutation resulting in a biologically ineffective GH molecule was speculated. Valenta et al. described a similar case and confirmed a structural abnormality of the GH molecule: 60–90% of circulating GH was in the form of tetramers and dimers (normal, 14–39% in plasma) and the patients' GH polymers were abnormally resistant to conversion into monomers by urea.

Subsequently, Takahashi et al. reported a boy who was short at birth (39 cm at 41 weeks' gestation) and –6.1 SD below the mean at 4.9 years when his bone age was 2 years. He had normal body proportions, but a prominent forehead and saddle nose. His IGF-I was 34 ng/mL (normal 35–293). Basal GH levels were 7–14 ng/mL and peak levels after insulin induced hypoglycemia; arginine and levodopa administration were 38, 15, and 35 ng/mL, respectively. Serum IGF-I was unchanged after 3 days of daily subcutaneous injections of 0.1 U of recombinant human GH/kg body weight (0.035 mg/kg). During prolonged treatment with GH (0.18 mg/kg/wk), his serum IGF-I was 200 ng/mL and his rate of linear growth increased to 6.0 cm/yr from 3.9 cm/yr before treatment. Assay of the bioactivity of his GH was below the normal range, and isoelectric focusing of his serum showed an abnormal GH peak in addition to a normal peak, whereas serum from his father and normal controls contained only one peak. The affected son was heterozygous for a C→T transition that encodes an Arg→Cys substitution at codon 77 (Arg77Cys) of his GH1 gene. Inexplicably, his father, also heterozygous for this mutation, was of normal height, had a peak GH level of 23.7, and normal isoelectric focusing results.

GHRH RECEPTOR MUTATIONS Lin et al. demonstrated that the molecular basis for the "little" (lit) mouse phenotype, characterized by a hypoplastic anterior pituitary gland, is a point mutation in the growth hormone-releasing factor receptor (GHRHR) gene that results in an Asp→Gly substitution at residue 60 (Asp60Gly). Anterior pituitaries of mutant mice showed spatially distinct proliferative zones of GH-producing stem cells and mature somatotrophs, each regulated by a different trophic factor.

Wajnrajch et al. found a nonsense mutation in the human GHRHR gene in two first cousins, a boy and a girl, of a consanguineous Indian Moslem family with profound GH deficiency. The phenotypes of the 3.5-year-old girl and her 16-year-old cousin were poor growth since infancy and both were extremely short. They were prepubertal with frontal bossing and predominantly truncal obesity. While both failed to produce GH in response to standard provocative tests and to repetitive stimulation with GHRH, they responded to administration of GH. The affected individuals were homozygous for a G→T transversion at position 265 of their GHRHR genes, resulting in a premature termination mutation (Glu72Stop). The mutation introduced a *Bfa*I restriction site into the amplified GHRHR gene fragment which could be used to detect the mutation in DNA samples from family members. Wajnrajch et al. noted that, since both GH releasing peptide (a synthetic hepapeptide) and nonpeptidyl benzamines can stimulate GH release without involvement of the GHRH receptor, they might be useful in therapy of this disorder. Subsequently, Maheshwari et al. found the same GHRHR mutation in an isolate from the Indus valley of Pakistan.

FAMILIAL COMBINED PITUITARY HORMONE DEFICIENCY

GENETIC BASIS AND MOLECULAR PATHOPHYSIOLOGY OF DISEASE Familial combined pituitary hormone deficiency (CPHD) is characterized by deficiency of one or more of the other pituitary trophic hormones (ACTH, FSH, LH, or TSH) in addition to GH deficiency (OMIM 262600). Whereas the great majority of cases are sporadic, there are Mendelian forms with autosomal recessive, autosomal dominant, or X-linked modes of inheritance. Mutations of the Pit-1 and Prop-1 genes are associated with CPHD in humans. Both of these genes are members of the POU (Pit-1, Oct-1, Unc-86) homeodomain family of transcription factors and they each play an important role in pituitary development.

Pit-1 The Pit-1 gene (OMIM 173110) encodes a protein that binds to and transactivates promoters of the GH1 and PrL genes and is required for differentiation and proliferation of somatotropes, lactotropes, and thyrotropes. At least eight different Pit-1 mutations have been found in humans in a subtype of CPHD associated with GH, PrL, and TSH deficiency (*see* Table 49-2).

Autosomal Recessive Pit-1 Mutations The first and second Pit-1 mutations reported were found in two consanguineous Japanese families. In one family, a C→T transition in codon 172 converted a CGA (arginine)→TGA (stop). Both parents were heterozygous and the affected child was homozygous for the mutation. In the second family, an A→G transition in codon 143 changing a CGA (arginine)→CAA (glutamine) was found. The patient was shown to be homozygous for this mutation, while the parents and two unaffected siblings were shown to be heterozygous. Both mutations occur in the POU-specific domain and are believed to affect binding of the Pit-1 protein to the DNA.

The third and fourth Pit-1 mutations were found in two Dutch families who had postnatal growth failure with complete deficiencies of GH and PrL, while the T4 levels were low or normal prior to or following GH replacement. Subjects in one family who had normal T4 levels were homozygous for a G→C substitution in codon 158 changing GCA (alanine)→CCA (proline). This mutation interferes with formation of Pit-1 homodimers and dramatically reduces the altered Pit-1's ability to activate transcription. Subjects in the second family with low T4 levels were found to have one deleted Pit-1 gene and one Pit-1 gene with the previous mutation. These cases emphasize the importance of determining PrL levels and TSH responses to TRH in evaluating CPHD. Since GH and TSH deficiency often occur together, finding a low PrL level and absent TSH responses should raise the question of their having Pit-1 gene defects.

A fifth Pit-1 mutation was identified in a Thai patient with deficiency of GH, TSH, and PrL. Both parents were healthy and found to be heterozygous for a G→T transversion in codon 250, which converted a GAA(Glu)→TAA(Stop) codon. The CPHD patient was found to be homozygous for the mutation. This mutation resulted in complete loss of the POU-homeodomain, which is necessary for DNA binding.

A sixth Pit-1 mutation has been reported in a consanguineous family of Tunisian descent. All four affected sibs were found to be homozygous for a T→G transversion in codon 135 converting a TTT(Phe)→TGT(Cys) in the POU-specific domain of Pit-1. The patients were found to have pituitary hypoplasia and deficiencies of GH, TSH, and PrL.

Autosomal Dominant Pit-1 Mutations The first dominant-negative mutation identified in the Pit-1 gene was a G→T substitution in codon 271 converting a GGG (arginine)→TGG (tryptophan). This mutation is located in the POU-homeodomain and does not affect binding of the mutant Pit-1 protein to DNA but functions as a dominant inhibitor of Pit-1 action by some, as of yet unknown mechanism. Three unrelated patients have been reported to be heterozygous for this mutation. Two of the patients were evaluated as adults and found to have pituitary hypoplasia and deficiencies of GH, PrL, and TSH. The third patient was identified at only 2 months of age and found to have a normal pituitary and normal basal levels of TSH but a delayed TSH response in a TRH stimulation test. The authors suggest that, since Pit-1 may be necessary for anterior pituitary cell survival, the affected patient will develop hypolasia and TSH deficiencies with age.

The second dominant-negative Pit-1 gene mutation was a T→C transition in the 24th codon, converting a CCT (proline)→CTT (leucine). This proline residue resides within the major transactivating domain of Pit-1 and is highly conserved in different species. The mechanism by which this mutation exerts its dominant-negative effect is also not known.

Prop-1 Ames dwarf (df/df) mice have CPHD and hypocellular anterior pituitaries that lack somatotropes, lactotropes, thyrotropes, and GH transcripts. Since df/+ but not df/df mice expressing the hGHRH transgene have somatotrope hyperplasia, the df gene product is thought to be required before e16.5 of development. The genetic defect associated with the Ames dwarf phenotype has recently been found in the gene called Prophet of Pit-1 (Prop-1) (OMIM 601538) that encodes a pituitary specific homeodomain factor. Sequence analysis of the Prop-1 cDNA in the df/df mouse revealed a T→C transition in codon 83 that causes a Ser→Pro amino acid change in the first helix of its homeodomain. While Prop-1 is required for expression of Pit-1, the mechanism of its action remains uncertain.

Wei et al. recently reported finding three human Prop-1 gene defects in studies of four families with familial autosomal recessive CPHD. In addition to the GH, PrL, and TSH deficiency seen with Pit-1 defects, Prop-1–deficient subjects also have LH and FSH deficiency, which prevents the onset of spontaneous puberty. Family I had three affected sibs, all homozygous for a C→T transition in codon 120 of the Prop-1 gene. This mutation encoded a TGC(Arg)→CGC(Cys) substitution in the third helix of the homeodomain, which greatly reduced the protein's DNA-binding and transactivating abilities. Families II and III were found to have the same 2-bp AG deletion in codon 101 that causes a frameshift that results in a premature stop at codon 109. The truncated protein product was found to have no DNA binding or transactivating abilities. The patient in family IV had two different Prop-1 gene mutations (compound heterozygosity). One allele had the 2-bp AG deletion described above and the second allele had a T→A transversion that encodes a TTC(Phe)→ATC(Ile) substitution at codon 117. The resulting protein product exhibited both greatly reduced DNA-binding and transactivating abilities.

CURRENT TREATMENT

Recombinant derived GH is available worldwide and is administered by subcutaneous injection. To obtain an optimal outcome, children with GHD should be started on replacement therapy as soon as their diagnosis is established. The initial dosage of recombinant GH is based on body weight, but the exact amount used and the frequency of administration may vary between different protocols. The dosage increases with increasing body weight to a maximum during puberty and is usually discontinued by approximately 17 years of age.

Conditions that are treated with GH include (1) those in which it has proven efficacy and (2) a variety of others in which its use has been reported but its use is not accepted as standard practice. Disorders in which GH treatment is of proven efficacy include GH deficiency, either isolated or in association with CPHD and Turner's syndrome. The clinical responses of individuals with the first two disorders to GH replacement therapy varies depending on (1) the severity and age at which treatment is begun, (2) recognition and response to treatment of associated deficiencies such as thyroid hormone deficiency, and (3) whether treatment is complicated by the development of anti-GH antibodies. The outcome of Turner's syndrome subjects varies with the severity of their short stature, chromosomal complement, and age at which treatment was begun.

Additional disorders in which the use of GH has been reported but for which its efficacy is not accepted as standard practice include treatment of (1) selected skeletal dysplasias such as achondroplasia, (2) Prader-Willi syndrome, (3) growth suppression secondary to exogenous steroids such as chronic autoimmune diseases, (4) chronic renal failure, (5) extreme idiopathic short stature, (6) Silver-Russell syndrome, and (7) intrauterine growth retardation. There is, in general, insufficient data to establish the efficacy of GH replacement therapy in treating these disorders because of the limited number of subjects and lack of use of standardized protocols.

FUTURE DIRECTIONS

Several problems contribute to incomplete ascertainment of affected individuals, which in turn can result in less than optimal outcomes. These problems in ascertainment include the spectrum of severity, lack of a single provocative test that is both very sensitive and specific, and lack of an assay to test for qualitative changes in endogenous GH. Improvements in techniques that address these problems could facilitate the detection of and improve the outcome of treated patients in the future.

A number of genetic defects in GH biosynthesis have been documented that prevent some affected individuals from secreting GH. These include those defects that result in the synthesis of truncated GH molecules, lack of GHRH receptor function, and mutant GH products that have dominant-negative effects on the normal GH products that are present. In the future, agonists of GH secretion, for example, that complement the function of GHRH, may be found that can enhance release of the stored GH that is found in some of these cases. The efficacy of IGF-I in treating Laron dwarfism and IGHD patients who are resistant to exogenous GH because of anti-GH antibodies has been proven. Additional uses of IGF-I or perhaps isoforms of IGF-I that have prolonged half-lives may provide improved efficacy in the future.

Although potential applications of gene therapy to somatic cells are feasible, targeted and regulated expression that is pituitary specific remains impractical. Thus, potential applications of gene therapy to achieve appropriate hormonal regulation less dangerously than with exogenous GH replacement seem remote.

SELECTED REFERENCES

Abdul-Latif HD, Brown MR, Parks JS, et al. Mutation of intron 4 of the GH-1 gene causes GH deficiency. Endocrine Society Programs & Abstracts 1995;470.

Binder G, Ranke MB. Screening for growth hormone (GH) gene splice-site mutations in sporadic cases with severe isolated GH deficiency using ectopic transcript analysis. J Clin Endocrinol and Metab 1995;80:1247–1252.

Binder G, Brown M, Parkas JS. Mechanisms responsible for dominant expression of human growth hormone gene mutations. J Clin Endocrinol Metab 1996;81:4047–4050.

Cogan JD, Phillips III JA, Sakati N, Frisch H, Schober E, Milner RDG. Heterogeneous growth hormone (GH) gene mutations in familial GH deficiency. J Clin Endocrinol Metab 1993;76:1224–1228.

Cogan JD, Phillips JA III, Schenkman SS, Milner RDG, Sakati N. Familial growth hormone deficiency: a model of dominant and recessive mutations affecting a monomeric protein. J Clin Endocrinol and Metab 1994;79:1261–1265.

Cogan JD, Prince MA, Lekhakula S, et al. A novel mechanism of aberrant pre-mRNA splicing in humans. Hum Mol Genet 1997;6:909–912.

Cogan JD, Ramel B, Lehto M, et al. A recurring dominant negative mutation causes autosomal dominant growth hormone deficiency—a clinical research center study. J Clin Endocrinol Metab 1995; 80:3591–3595.

Cohen LE, Wondisford FE, Salvantoni A, et al. A hot spot in the Pit-1 gene responsible for combined pituitary hormone deficiency: clinical and molecular correlates. J Clin Endocrinol and Metab 1995;80:679–684.

Cohen LE, Wondisford FE, Radovick S. Role of Pit-1 in the gene expression of growth hormone, prolactin, and thyrotropin. Endocrinol Metab Clin North Am 1996;25:523–540.

Duquesnoy P, Amselem S, Gourmelen M, LeBouc Y, Goossens M. A frameshift mutation causing isolated growth hormone deficiency type 1A. Am J Hum Genet 1990;47:A110.

Herington AC. New frontiers in the molecular mechanisms of growth hormone action. Mol Cell Endocrinol 1994;100:39–44.

Igarashi Y, Ogawa M, Kamijo T, et al. A new mutation causing inherited growth hormone deficiency: a compound heterozygote of a 6.7 kb deletion and two base deletion in the third exon of the GH-1 gene. Hum Mol Genet 1993;2:1073,1074.

Irie Y, Tatsumi K, Ogawa M, et al. A novel E250X mutation of the PIT1 gene in a patient with combined pituitary hormone deficiency. Endocr J 1995;42:351–354.

Lin SC, Lin CR, Gukovsky I, Lusis AJ, Sawchenko PE, Rosenfeld MG. Molecular basis of the little mouse phenotype and implications for cell type-specific growth. Nature 1993;364:208–213.

Maheshwari H, Silverman BL, Dupuis J, Baumann G. Dwarfism of Sindh: a novel form of familial isolated GH deficiency linked to the locus for the GH releasing hormone receptor. Endocrine Society Program & Abstracts 1996;OR46-2.

Miller-Davis S, Phillips JA III, Milner RDG, Al-Ashwal A, Sakati NA, Summar ML. Detection of mutations in GH genes and transcripts by analysis of DNA from dried blood spots and mRNA from lymphoblastoid cells. The Endocrine Society Program and Abstracts 1993;333.

Neely EK, Rosenfeld RG. Use and abuse of human growth hormone. Annu Rev Med 1994;45:407–420.

Ohta K, Nobukuni Y, Mitsubuchi H, et al. Mutations in the Pit-1 gene in children with combined pituitary hormone deficiency. Biochem Biophys Res Comm 1992;189:851–855.

Pelligrini-Bouiller I, Belicar P, Barlier A, et al. A new mutation of the gene encoding the transcritption factor Pit-1 is responsible for combined pituitary hormone deficiency. J. Clin. Endocr. Metab 1996;81d:2790–2796.

Pfaffle RW, DiMattia GE, Parks JS, et al. Mutation of the POU-specific domain of Pit-1 and hypopituitarism without pituitary hypoplasia. Science 1992;257:1118–1121.

Pfaffle R, Kim C, Otten B, et al. Pit-1: clinical aspects. Horm Res 1996;45:25–28.

Phillips JA III. Inherited defects in growth hormone synthesis and action. In: Scriver CR, Beaudet AL, Sly WS, Valle D, eds. The Metabolic and Molecular Basis of Inherited Disease, 7th ed. New York: McGraw-Hill, 1995; vol 3, pp. 3023–3044.

Phillips JA III, Cogan JD. Molecular basis of familial human growth hormone deficiency. J Clin Endocrinol and Metab 1994;78:11–16.

Radovick S, Nation M, Du Y, Bergh LA, Weintraub BD, Wondisford FE. A mutation in the POU-homeodomain of Pit-1 responsible for combined pituitary hormone deficiency. Science 1992;257:1115–1118.

Ranke MB. Growth hormone therapy in children: when to stop? Horm Res 1995;43:122–125.

Rosen T, Johannsson G, Johansson JO, Bengtsson BA. Consequences of growth hormone deficiency in adults and the benefits and risks of recombinant human growth hormone treatment. Horm Res 1995;43:93–99.

Rosenfeld RG, Rosenbloom AL, Guevara-Aguirre J. Growth hormone (GH) insensitivity due to primary GH receptor deficiency. Endocr Rev 1994;15:369–390.

Sobrier ML, Dastot F, Duquesnoy P, et al. Nine novel growth hormone receptor gene mutations in patients with Laron syndrome. J Clin Endocrinol Metab 1997;82:435–437.

Sornson MW, Wu W, Dasen JS, et al. Pituitary lineage determination by the Prophet of Pit-1 homeodomain factor defective in Ames dwarfism. Nature 1996;384:327–333.

Strasburger CJ. Implications of investigating the structure-function relationship of human growth hormone in clinical diagnosis and therapy. Horm Res 1994;41:113–120.

Strobl JS, Thomas MJ. Human growth hormone. Pharmacol Rev 1994;46:1–34.

Takahashi Y, Kaji H, Okimura Y, Goji K, Abe H, Chihara K. Brief report: short stature caused by a mutant growth hormone. New England J Med 1996;334:432–436.

Tatsumi K, Miyai K, Notomi T, et al. Cretinism with combined pituitary hormone deficiency caused by a mutation in the PIT1 gene. Nature Genet 1992;1:56–58.

Vnencak-Jones CL, Phillips JA III, De-fen W. Use of polymerase chain reaction in detection of growth hormone gene deletions. J Clin Endocrinol and Metab 1990;70:1550–1553.

Wajnrajch MP, Gertner JM, Harbison MD, Chua SC Jr, Leibel RL. Nonsense mutation in the human growth hormone-releasing hormone receptor causes growth failure analogous to the little (lit) mouse. Nature Genet 1996;12:88–90.

Wit JM, Drayer NM, Jansen M, et al. Total deficiency of growth hormone and prolactin, and partial deficiency of thyroid stimulating hormone in two Dutch families: a new variant of hereditary pituitary deficiency. Hormone Res 1989;32:170–177.

Wyatt DT, Mark D, Slyper A. Survey of growth hormone treatment practices by 251 pediatric endocrinologists. J Clin Endocrinol and Metab 1995;80:3292–3297.

Wu W, Cogan JD, Pfaffle RW, et al. Mutations in PROP1 cause familial combined pituitary hormone deficiency. Nature Genet (in press).

50 Thyroid Disorders

PETER KOPP AND J. LARRY JAMESON

INTRODUCTION

The thyroid is controlled by a classic hormonal feedback system, the hypothalamic–pituitary thyroid axis (Fig. 50-1). The hypothalamic peptide, TRH (thyrotropin-releasing hormone), stimulates the production and secretion of the glycoprotein hormone TSH (thyroid-stimulating hormone) in the pituitary. TSH in turn stimulates growth and function of thyroid follicular cells resulting in the production of the thyroid hormones, thyroxine (T4) and triiododothyronine (T3). Thyroid hormone has multiple effects on differentiation, growth, and metabolism of peripheral tissues. At the level of the cell, thyroid hormone action is primarily mediated by nuclear receptors that regulate gene transcription.

After the characterization of thyroid disorders at the clinical and biochemical level, the cloning of many key genes responsible for thyroid hormone synthesis and action provides the tools for unraveling underlying molecular defects (Table 50-1). These findings continue to broaden our insights into the mechanisms governing thyroid cell growth and function under physiologic conditions, as well as in thyroid disease.

Disorders affecting thyroid function result either in hypothyroidism or hyperthyroidism. The cardinal clinical characteristics of these hormonal states are summarized in Table 2. Hypothyroidism is the most common disorder of thyroid function and, besides iodine deficinecy, it is most frequently caused by chronic autoimmune Hashimoto's thyroiditis. The most frequent cause of hyperthyroidism is also an autoimmune disorder, Graves' disease, followed in prevalence by toxic multinodular goiters and toxic adenomas. All other causes of decreased or elevated thyroid function are rare. Congenital hypothyroidism, which affects 1 in 3000 to 4000 newborns, may occur sporadically or as an inherited disorder. The sporadic form of congenital hypothyroidism is caused by thyroid agenesis or dysgenesis. The molecular causes underlying sporadic thyroid dysgenesis have not been elucidated. Besides environmental factors, alterations in thyroid-specific transcription factors involved in thyroid embryogenesis are likely candidates. Thyroid hypoplasia may be caused by inherited loss-of-function mutations in the TSH receptor. In hereditary congenital hypothyroidism, there are defects in one or more steps in thyroid hormone biosynthesis. Dyshormogenesis is much rarer than thyroid dysgenesis. The cloning of many of the genes encoding the involved proteins will allow further characterization of these disorders at the molecular level.

From: *Principles of Molecular Medicine* (J. L. Jameson, ed.), ©1998 Humana Press Inc., Totowa, NJ.

Defects resulting in hyperthyroidism or hypothyroidism have been localized at all levels of the hypothalamic–pituitary–thyroid axis. Deficiency in hypothalamic TRH and mutations in the pituitary-specific transcription factor, Pit-1, or in the gene encoding TSH-β, lead to congenital central hypothyroidism. TSH-secreting pituitary adenomas result in hyperthyroidism. At the level of the thyroid gland, insensitivity to TSH or defects in hormone synthesis and secretion cause hypothyroidism. Autosomal dominant, non–autoimmune familial hyperthyroidism caused by constitutively activating mutations in the TSH receptor (TSHR) gene has been recognized as a new pathophysiologic entity. Congenital hyperthyroidism is rare and usually caused by transplacental passage of autoantibodies from a hyperthyroid mother, but may also occur through sporadic TSHR mutations in the germline. Somatic mutations in the TSHR, or in the α-subunit of the stimulatory G protein (Gsα), can result in hyperfunctioning adenomas.

The transport of T4 is altered by a variety of defects in binding proteins. At the level of the target organs, mutations in the nuclear thyroid hormone receptors may cause the syndrome of resistance to thyroid hormones.

Although the molecular defects underlying the pathogenesis of thyroid nodules as well as papillary, follicular, and anaplastic thyroid cancers, are far from being completely understood, the tools of molecular biology are providing important new insights. A majority of thyroid nodules are of monoclonal origin, making somatic mutations in growth-controlling genes a likely cause for their development. Defects in proto-oncogenes or tumor suppressor genes have been implicated in all forms of benign and malignant thyroid tumors (*see* Chapter 7). Among other important insights, the detection of certain molecular defects has already impacted the clinical management of patients with multiple endocrine neoplasia type 2 (MEN2) (*see* Chapter 54).

Although this chapter does not review all thyroid disorders comprehensively, it provides an overview of the genetic defects affecting thyroid function and growth at all levels of the axis.

THYROTROPIN-RELEASING HORMONE DEFICIENCY

TRH is a hypothalamic tripeptide (Glu-His-Pro) generated from a large prohormone of 27 kDa. Besides its role as a stimulator of the pituitary gland, where it releases thyrotropin (TSH) and prolactin (PRL), TRH is found in numerous areas of the brain and in some peripheral organs.

A few patients with congenital hypothyroidism have isolated TRH deficiency in the absence of apparent destructive hypotha-

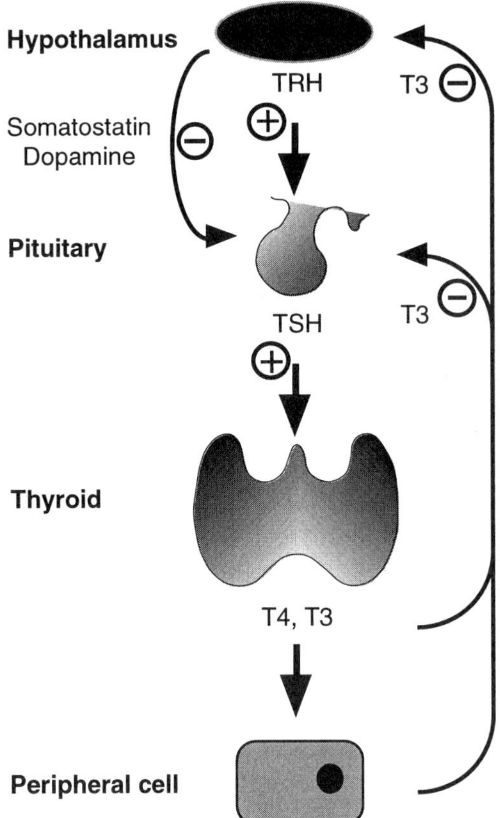

Figure 50-1 The hypothalamic–pituitary–thyroid axis. The hypothalamic hormone, thyrotropin-releasing hormone (TRH), enhances production and secretion of the pituitary hormone, thyroid-stimulating hormone (TSH), which then stimulates thyroid hormone synthesis in follicular cells. Thyroid hormones act on multiple target genes in peripheral cells through nuclear receptors that regulate gene transcription. T3 regulates TSH and TRH through a negative feedback mechanism.

lamic lesions. The diagnosis of central hypothalamic hypothyroidism is made on the basis of the constellation of low basal TSH that increases after administration of exogenous TRH. The molecular defect underlying these cases remains elusive, but could result from a defect in the synthesis or secretion of TRH, or from abnormal development of hypothalamic TRH-producing neurons.

AUTONOMOUS PRODUCTION OF TSH

TSH is a heterodimeric glycoprotein hormone. It shares a common α chain with the pituitary hormones, follicle-stimulating hormone (FSH) and luteinizing hormone (LH), as well as the placental hormone choriogonadotropin (CG). Each of these hormones has a unique β chain; the gene for the TSH-β–subunit has been localized to chromosome 1p22, the α chain is encoded on chromosome 6.

Hypersecretion of TSH by thyrotroph pituitary adenomas is a rare cause of hyperthyroidism. Biochemically, these patients are characterized by an inappropriate secretion of TSH and hyperthyroxinemia. Typically, there is also excessive secretion of free α-subunit, and this feature can help to make the diagnosis. In about 20%–30% of cases, there is cosecretion of growth hormone (GH). Magnetic resonance imaging or computed tomograph scan can be used to confirm the diagnosis.

The molecular defects that result in autonomous growth and function of the thyrotrophs have not been elucidated yet. Clonal analysis with the X-inactivation technique in a small number of tumors showed that they are of monoclonal origin, suggesting a somatic mutation or the loss of tumor suppressor genes. Screening of several candidate genes *(Gsα, Gqα, G11α, TRH receptor)* in nine tumors did not show alterations in these genes.

In most cases, therapy consists of trans-sphenoidal removal of the pituitary adenoma. The somatostatin analog, octreotide, can suppress TSH in some patients. Preoperatively, hyperthyroid patients should be controlled with antithyroid drugs. Adjunctive radiation therapy is required in most patients with pituitary macroadenomas.

DEFECTIVE BIOSYNTHESIS OF TSH

TSH deficiency may occur in the setting of panhypopituitarism, most commonly because of a pituitary adenoma. Rare causes include familial panhypopituitarism and familial pituitary agenesis, which likely involve defects in pituitary development, but specific genes have not been identified yet. Two well-characterized defects that cause TSH deficiency include mutations in the Pit-1 gene and in the gene encoding the β-subunit of TSH. Isolated central hypothyroidism has also been described in a boy who was a compound heterozygote for inactivating mutations in the TRH receptor.

PIT-1 MUTATIONS Pit-1 (also referred to as growth hormone factor 1, GHF-1) is a pituitary-specific transcription factor of 33 kDa that regulates the development of somatotrophs, lactotrophs, and thyrotrophs, as well as expression of the *growth hormone, prolactin,* and *TSH-β subunit* genes. It is a member of the POU family of transcription factors, an eponym that was created after the identification of the first three members of this group, Pit-1, Oct-1, and Unc-86. Pit-1 contains two main functional domains, an activation domain and a DNA-binding domain that is formed by a POU-specific domain and a homeodomain. The homeodomain is similar to the homeobox-containing genes in *Drosophila* that control development of specific body segments. DNA sequences that bind the transcription factor are found in the promoters of the *GH, PRL, TSH-β,* and *Pit-1* genes. Several splice variants with different activation domains have been reported (Pit-1β, Pit-1T).

Pit-1 mutations were initially identified in strains of dwarf mice with hypoplastic pituitaries and lack of somatotrophs, lactotrophs, and thyrotrophs. The Jackson mouse has a genomic rearrangement of Pit-1 that results in a truncated protein. The Snell mouse has a point mutation resulting in an amino acid substitution in the homeodomain (tryptophan 261 to cysteine).

In humans, a variety of Pit-1 mutations have now been described. The first mutation was a homozygous point mutation that results in a truncated protein lacking the entire POU-homeodomain. The affected girl presented with cretinism and deficiency of thyrotropin, growth hormone, and prolactin. The parents, who were second cousins, were both heterozygous and had no hormonal abnormalities. This report was followed by further descriptions of Pit-1 mutations in different locations of the gene in patients with GH, PRL, and TSH deficiencies. Mutant proteins that cannot bind to DNA are inherited as autosomal recessive traits, whereas the mutations that lose transactivation, but retain DNA binding capacity, are inherited in an autosomal dominant manner. The latter mutants inhibit the function of the normal Pit-1 protein and, therefore, display a dominant-negative effect.

Table 50-1
Molecular Defects in Thyroid Disease[a]

Gene/protein	*Disease*	*Pathophysiology*	*Molecular defect*	*Inheritance*	*Chromosome*
TRH	Hypothalamic hypopituitarism	Isolated TRH deficiency	Unknown	AR	3
TRH-receptor	TSH-deficient hypothyroidism	Unresponsiveness to TRH	Inactivating mutations	AR	8q23
TSH	TSH-deficient hypothyroidism	TSH-β–subunit mutation, bioinactive TSH	Mutations in β chain	AR	α chain:6p21
	TSH-secreting adenomas/hyperthyroidism	Oversecretion of TSH, molecular defect unknown	Unknown	Sporadic	β chain:1p22
Pit-1	Combined pituitary hormone deficiency (GH, PRL, TSH); mouse: Snell, Jackson dwarf mice	Abnormal pituitary development; diminished GH, PRL, TSH synthesis and secretion	Mutation in *Pit-1* gene	AD, AR	3p11
TSH-receptor	Familial and sporadic congenital non-autoimmune hyperthyroidism	Constitutive activation with increased basal secretion of cAMP	Activating mutation	AD, sporadic	
	Toxic adenomas			Somatic	14q31
	Hypothyroidism, euthyroid hyperthyrotropinemia	Unresponsiveness to TSH	Inactivating mutations	AR	
Gsα (α-subunit of stimulatory G protein)	Toxic adenoma	Activation of cAMP cascade: enhancement of growth/function	Activating point mutations	Sporadic	
	McCune-Albright syndrome			Sporadic (mosaicism)	20q.13.2
	Pseudohypoparathyroidism Ia	Resistance to stimulus of G-protein-coupled receptors, incl. mutations TSH receptor	Inactivating point mutations	AD	
Thyroid hormone synthesis					
Sodium/iodide symporter	Congenital hypothyroidism, goiter	Defective iodine uptake	Inactivating point mutations	AR	19p12–13.2
Thyroperoxidase	Congenital hypothyroidism, goiter	Defective organification of iodide point mutations	Insertions, frameshift, stops,	AR	2p25
Pendred's syndrome	Sensorineural deafness, goiter	Partial organification defect	Inactivating mutations	AR	7q21–34
Thyroglobulin	Goiter; hypothyroidism, subclinical hypothyroidism, or euthyroidism; several animal models with goiter	Defective organification of iodide because of qualitative or quantitative Tg defects	Mutation in splice donor site; premature stop/alternate splicing; nonsense mutation	AR (AD in one kindred)	8q24
Dehalogenase	Congenital hypothyroidism, goiter	Loss of iodine through secretion of DIT, MIT	Unknown	AR	Unknown
Binding proteins					
Thyroxine-binding globulin	Decreased total T4 levels, euthyroidism	TBG deficiency	Deletions, frameshifts, premature stops, point mutations	X-linked recessive	Xq11–q23
	Increased total T4 levels, euthyroidism	TBG excess	Unknown	Probably X-linked recessive	
Transthyretin	Hyperthyroxinemia; familial amyloidotic polyneuropathy	Increased affinity for T4, T3	Point mutations	AD	18
Albumin	Familial dysalbuminemic hyperthyroxinemia	Increased affinity for T4, T3	Point mutations	AD	4q11–13
Nuclear thyroid hormone receptors/transcription factors					
Thyroid hormone receptor	Resistance to thyroid hormone; goiter, variable degrees of hypo- and hyperthyroidism	Elevated peripheral hormones with elevated TSH because of impaired peripheral hormone action coding region of TRβ)	Point mutations, deletions, frameshifts (one kindred with total deletion of of coding region of TRβ)	AD, sporadic (AR in one kindred with total deletion (no mutations detected in TRα)	TRβ 3p24.3 TRα17q11.2
TTF-1	Congenital goiter, thyroglobulin deficiency	Absence of TTF-1 expression	Unknown	AR (?)	14q12–q21
TTF-2	...	...	...	... (indirect evidence)	9q
Pax-8	...	...	...	...	2q12–q14

[a]Abbreviations: TRH, thyrotropin-releasing hormone; TRH-receptor, thyrotropin-releasing hormone receptor; TSH, thyroid-stimulating hormone; Pit-1, pituitary-specific transcription factor 1; TSH-receptor, thyroid-stimulating hormone receptor; Gsα, G protein stimulatory α-subunit; TTF-1, thyroid transcription factor 1; TTF-2, thyroid transcription factor 2; PAX-8, paired domain transcription factor 8; GH, growth hormone; PRL, prolactin; T4, thyroxine; CAMP, cyclic AMP; DIT, diiodothyronine; MIT, monoiodothyronine; TBG, thyroxine-binding globulin; AR, autosomal recessive; AD, autosomal dominant; TR, thyroid hormone receptor.

Table 50-2
Main Clinical and Biochemical Findings in Hyper- and Hypothyroidism

Hyperthyroidism	*Hypothyroidism*
Signs	
Hyperactivity	Lethargy
Tachycardia/arrhythmia	Bradycardia
Hyperthermia	Cold intolerance
Increased perspiration	Dry skin
Hyperreflexia	Hyporeflexia
Muscle weakness	Myxedema
Tremor	Hoarseness
Weight loss	Weight gain
Eyelid retraction	
Exophthalmos (Graves' disease)	
Diffuse or nodular goiter	
Intrauterine/neonatal	Intrauterine/neonatal
Mental retardation possible	Mental retardation
Advanced bone age	Neurologic deficit
	Retarded bone age/growth
Symptoms	
Nervousness	Fatigue, sleepiness
Weakness	Depression
Palpitation	Constipation
Increased appetite	Decreased appetite
Irregular menses	Irregular menses
	Paresthesia
Laboratory	
Primary	
T4 ↑, T3 ↑, TSH ↓	T4 ↓, T3 ↓, TSH ↑
Central	
T4 ↑, T3 ↑, TSH ↑	T4 ↓, T3 ↓, TSH ↓

An unusual case of Pit-1 deficiency because of a heterozygous, dominant-negative point mutation in a mother and her fetus led to severe fetal hypothyroidism with delays in respiratory, cardiovascular, neurologic, and bone maturation. The absence of Pit-1 and the ensuing hypoprolactinemia in the mother resulted in puerperal alactogenesis. This case illustrates the importance of Pit-1 in the control of different endocrine axes and the importance of prenatal thyroid hormone for normal fetal maturation.

TSH-β MUTATIONS Congenital hypothyroidism caused by isolated hereditary TSH deficiency is rare and results from autosomal recessive mutations in the TSH-β chain. The disorder is characterized by low T4 and low TSH that is not increased by administration of TRH. In one Japanese family, two sisters presented with cretinism. The parents were second cousins, and two other families from the same island were reported to harbor the same defect. A homozygous mutation (glycine 29 to alanine) affecting the so-called CAGYC region of TSH-β was identified in these Japanese families and in a family of Portuguese origin living in France. This amino acid sequence is highly conserved among all glycoprotein hormone β-subunits, and it is essential for normal heterodimerization with the α chain. The heterozygous members of these families had normal thyroid function.

In two related Greek families with congenital TSH-deficient hypothyroidism, a mutation in the *TSH-β* gene resulted in a truncated peptide including only the first 11 amino acids. A frameshift mutation was also reported in a Brazilian family. These mutants are unable to dimerize with the α-subunit and TSH was undetectable in affected family members. A mutation in the carboxy-terminal part of the TSH-β subunit (cysteine 105 to valine) affected a cysteine that is involved in the formation of a disulfide bond (cysteine 19 with cysteine 105). This conformational change results in inefficient hormone synthesis and loss of bioactivity.

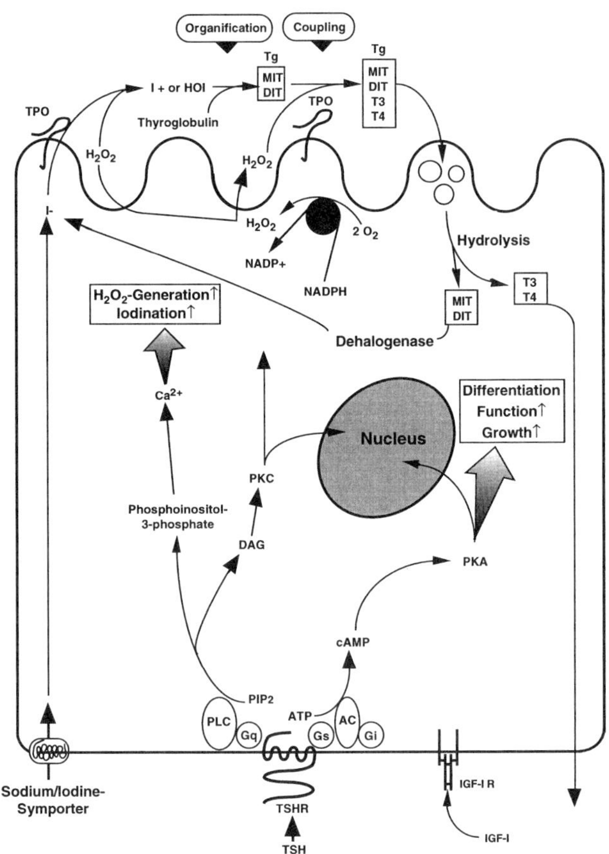

Figure 50-2 Thyroid hormone synthesis in a follicular cell. (For details, *see text.*) (TPO, thyroperoxidase; Tg, thyroglobulin; MIT, DIT, mono- and diiodothyronine; AC, adenylyl cyclase; PKA, protein kinase A; PKC, protein kinase C; PLC, phospholipase C; IGF-I, IGF-I R, insulin-like growth factor I [receptor]).

AUTONOMOUS FUNCTION OF THE TSHR

TSH exerts its effects on thyroid follicular cells through the TSHR, a member of the G-protein-coupled seven transmembrane domain receptors (Figs. 50-2 and 50-3). Together with the receptors for FSH and LH, it forms a distinct subfamily defined by a large amino-terminal extracellular domain involved in binding of the hormone. The 744-amino acid receptor is encoded by a gene containing 10 exons. The TSHR is coupled to Gsα and thus to the adenylyl cyclase cascade, which is the predominant signaling pathway for growth and function of the thyrocyte. It is, however, also coupled to Gq and also activates the inositol phosphate pathway.

Recently, mutations in several G-protein-coupled seven transmembrane domain receptors were found to confer constitutive activation to these receptors, a mechanism that defines an important new pathophysiologic entity. This type of activating mutation has been found in rhodopsin as a cause of retinitis pigmentosa, in the LH-CG receptor in male-limited precocious puberty, and in the TSHR, causing hyperthyroidism. Furthermore, point mutations in the Ca^{2+}-sensing receptor lead to familial hypocalciuric hypercalcemia and in the PTH receptor to metaphyseal chondrodysplasia.

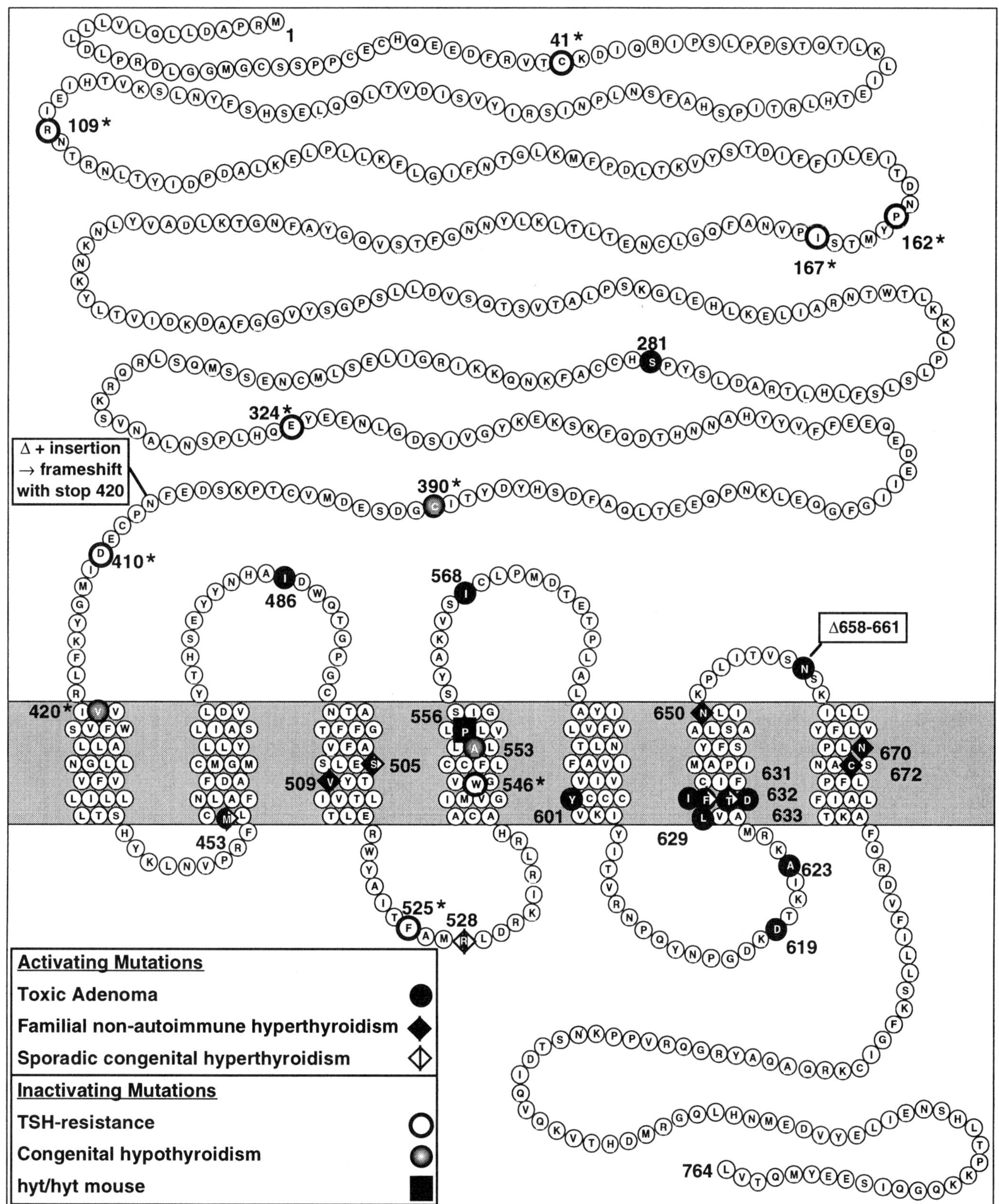

Figure 50-3 The thyroid-stimulating hormone receptor (TSHR) is a member of the G-protein-coupled seven transmembrane domain receptors. Naturally occurring activating mutations lead to enhanced growth and function and result in non–autoimmune hyperthyroidism. Inactivating mutations lead to compensated or overt hypothyroidism. *Compound heterozygote mutations.

Somatic mutations in the TSHR have been found in a number of toxic adenomas. In one series, they were present in 9 of 11 tumors, suggesting that most toxic adenomas contain mutations in this receptor (Fig. 50-3). In other studies, however, they were only present in a minority of tumors. This apparent discrepancy might be explained by differences in the prevalence in various geographic regions, selection of the tumors, or differences in the technical approach. Functionally, these mutations increase basal cAMP levels, and some of the mutants also activate the phospholipase C cascade. In contrast to activating mutations in other seven transmembrane domain receptors, there is a striking diversity in the affected residues, which are scattered over virtually the entire transmembrane domain of the TSHR, and they even occur in the extracellular domain (Fig. 50-3).

TSHR mutations occurring in the germline give rise to non–autoimmune familial hyperthyroidism. Gain-of-function mutations are by definition dominant and one mutated allele is thus sufficient to result in disease. The subsequent activation of the adenylyl cyclase pathway increases function and growth of thyroid follicular cells, resulting in hyperplasia and hyperthyroidism. The typical signs associated with autoimmune hyperthyroidism, such as exophthalmos, myxedema, stimulating autoantibodies, and lymphocytic infiltration of the thyroid gland, are absent. Five families with non–autoimmune familial hyperthyroidism and documented TSHR mutations have been reported (Fig. 50-3). Interestingly, the onset of hyperthyroidism may vary in carriers of the same mutation in a given kindred, suggesting that other factors (genetic background, iodine intake) can modify the phenotypic expression of the activated receptor. *De novo* germline mutations in the TSHR have been found in a few patients as a cause of sporadic non–autoimmune congenital hyperthyroidism.

Activating mutations in the TSHR have been found in a few cases of well-differentiated thyroid carcinomas, but they seem to be rare in these tumors. These naturally occurring mutations in the TSHR provide important new insights into receptor structure–function. It has been hypothesized that these mutations result in conformational changes converting the receptor from a "repressed" state into an activated state that couples to signal transduction pathways. The recognition of this new cause of hyperthyroidism also has clinical implications in that these patients often require a more aggressive therapeutic approach (surgery, ablative radiotherapy), and in families with non–autoimmune hyperthyroidism, molecular diagnostics allows early diagnosis and treatment.

INSENSITIVITY TO TSH AND INACTIVATING MUTATIONS OF THE TSHR

TSH insensitivity results in reduced synthesis and secretion of thyroid hormones and a small thyroid gland. It has been described in a kindred in which two affected individuals had normal thyroid hormone levels but high levels of TSH. In this family, the disorder was transmitted in an autosomal recessive mode and the patients were compound heterozygotes. The patients inherited a missense mutation in the TSHR from the father (asparagine 167 to isoleucine) and a distinct mutation from the mother (proline 162 to alanine), both affecting the extracellular, TSH-binding domain of the receptor (Fig. 50-3). In a few cases with congenital hypothyroidism and a normally located, hypoplastic gland, loss-of-function mutations have been found in the affected patients. Remarkably, these patients seem to have a normal or elevated thyroglobulin. However, inactivating mutations in the *TSH receptor* gene probably account for a minority of cases with congenital hypothyroidism. A study of 23 kindreds with familial congenital hypothyroidism did not find any evidence of linkage to the TSHR locus.

Severe congenital hypothyroidism caused by an inactivating mutation in the fourth transmembrane domain of the TSHR has been reported in the congenitally hypothyroid hyt/hyt mouse. The disorder is transmitted in an autosomal recessive manner, and thyroid tissue from homozygous mice shows unresponsiveness to TSH in vivo and in vitro. The mutation (proline 556 to leucine) eliminates TSH binding and receptor function, but the membrane localization of the receptor is preserved.

ACTIVATING AND INACTIVATING MUTATIONS IN Gsα

Analogous to the mutations in the TSHR, gain-of-function mutations in the α-subunit of the stimulatory G protein (Gsα), referred to as *gsp* mutations, lead to constitutive activation of the cAMP pathway, resulting in increased function and growth of thyroid follicular cells. In the thyroid, somatic mutations in *gsp* have been found with variable frequencies in nonfunctioning adenomas, toxic adenomas, and differentiated thyroid carcinomas. The most commonly affected amino acids are arginine 201 and glutamine 227. These mutations impair the hydrolysis of GTP to GDP, resulting in persistent activation of adenylyl cyclase. The same Gsα mutations are found in 35%–40% of somatotroph tumors in acromegalic patients. Gsα mutations also cause other endocrine syndromes (*see* Chapter 46). Sporadic mutations in Gsα that occur early in development cause the McCune-Albright syndrome.

In pseudohypoparathyroidism (PHP) type Ia, also referred to as Albright's hereditary osteodystrophy (AHO), the affected subjects show resistance to a variety of hormones that couple to G-protein coupled receptors (e.g., parathyroid hormone [PTH], TSH). Multiple hormone resistance is caused by reduced expression of the stimulatory Gsα-subunit, and a variety of loss-of-function mutations have been identified.

DEFECTIVE THYROID HORMONE SYNTHESIS

The major steps involved in thyroid hormone synthesis are summarized in Fig. 50-2. Iodide is actively transported into the thyroid follicular cell by a recently cloned sodium-iodide symporter, and it is then transferred to the apical side of the cells that faces the follicular lumen. Thyroperoxidase (TPO), which is localized in the apical membrane, oxidizes iodide and subsequently iodinates tyrosyl residues of the intrafollicular thyroglobulin (organification or iodination) in the presence of hydrogen peroxide. The iodotyrosines, mono- and diiodotyrosyl (MIT, DIT), are coupled to form T4 or T3 in a reaction that is also catalyzed by TPO (coupling). Thyroglobulin (Tg) molecules that contain T4, T3, and iodotyrosines are internalized into the follicular cell by pinocytosis and are digested in lysosomes. The thyronines, T4 and T3, are released into the circulation, whereas MIT and DIT are deiodinated by a dehalogenase and the released iodide is recycled.

Disorders resulting in congenital hypothyroidism have been identified at all major steps involved in hormonogenesis. The vast majority of disorders are caused by defects in Tg or TPO. Traditionally, organification defects are distinguished from coupling defects. Although this distinction is valuable, it is important to note that several proteins or cofactors (TPO, Tg, H_2O_2 generation) are involved in both steps. In other words, an abnormal TPO may be capable of iodinating Tg, but unable to couple MIT and DIT to T3 and T4. Similarly, Tg defects may result in an inability to organify iodine or, alternatively, they may only impede the coupling of iodotyrosines.

DEFECTS OF IODIDE TRANSPORT More than 20 cases suggestive of a defect of iodide uptake have been reported. There is a positive family history in about half of these cases, and consanguinity was present in about one-fourth of cases, suggesting an autosomal recessive trait. The clinical features include goiter, primary hypothyroidism, and little or no uptake of radioiodide. The salivary and gastric glands are also unable to concentrate iodide.

The recent cloning and characterization of a cDNA encoding the thyroid sodium-iodide symporter *(NIS)* will be useful for further defining the molecular defects in these disorders. This perchlorate-sensitive sodium-iodide symporter was cloned after functional screening of a rat cDNA library in *Xenopus laevis* oocytes. The isolated cDNA encodes a 618-amino acid protein and the secondary structure predicts that it contains 12 transmembrane domains. The human homolog has been cloned and mapped to chromosome 19p12–13.2. A homozygous missense mutation (threonine 354 to proline) in the *NIS* gene has been reported in a patient with congenital hypothyroidism as a result of an iodide transport defect. The parents of the patient were consanguineous and heterozygous for the defect.

Autoantibodies reacting with rat NIS have been detected in patients with autoimmune thyroid disease. Thus, it is likely that the NIS can be added to the list of thyroidal autoantigens, which includes TPO, Tg, and the TSHR.

THYROPEROXIDASE TPO, a glycosylated hemoprotein, catalyzes several pivotal reactions required for thyroid hormone synthesis: oxidation of iodide, the iodination of tyrosine residues in thyroglobulin, and the coupling of iodinated tyrosines to generate T4 and T3. The gene encoding TPO has been assigned to 2pter–p12, and it contains 17 exons. A number of polymorphisms result in restriction fragment length polymorphisms (RFLP), providing a convenient tool for linkage studies. Two cDNAs are generated by alternative splicing and result in two functional forms of the protein (105 and 110 kDa). TPO is historically referred to as the microsomal antigen in autoimmune thyroid disease. It is anchored in the membrane and its catalytic site is exposed to the follicular lumen.

TPO defects are believed to be the most frequent cause of inborn abnormalities of thyroid hormone synthesis. The first mutation in the *TPO* gene was reported in a hypothyroid boy with an iodide organification defect and congenital goiter. A homozygous duplication of four basepairs (GGCC) was found in exon eight. This insertion causes a frameshift and predicts a severely truncated protein. Analysis of the transcripts revealed, however, the presence of a cryptic splice site that restores the reading frame further downstream. Thus, the insertion leads to the substitution of amino acids in the middle of the protein without truncating the carboxy-terminal portion. Further mutations have been found in the *TPO* gene in nine families with a total organification defect. Besides various frameshift mutations (20-bp insertion in exon 2, 4-bp duplication in exon 8, C insertion at position 2505 in exon 14), point mutations are also found in scattered locations resulting in premature stops, substitutions of single residues, and alteration of splicing (border of exon 10 and intron 10). In four families, the patients were homozygous for one of these mutations, and there were compound heterozygotes in five families.

PENDRED'S SYNDROME In 1896, Pendred described a kindred with four sisters and a brother in which two of the girls were deaf-mutes and had large goiters. The association of goiter with deafness, together with a positive perchlorate discharge test, is now known as Pendred's syndrome. Metabolically, these patients present with mild hypothyroidism or euthyroidism. Tg levels are usually elevated because of chronic TSH stimulation. The deaf-mutism in Pendred's syndrome is associated with a defect in the cochlea, referred to as Mondini's cochlea, in which there is a single cavity consisting of only two turns instead of the normal three coils. The syndrome is inherited in an autosomal recessive pattern. Iodide is trapped by the thyroid gland, but its organification is impaired. This feature can be demonstrated by a positive perchlorate test after the administration of radiolabeled iodine. Normally, the trapped iodide is organified and bound to Tg; after the administration of perchlorate, which blocks iodide transport, only unbound iodide is released from the thyroid. A loss of iodide after perchlorate administration is thus indicative of an organification defect.

It has been postulated that both the goiter and deafness are related to a pleiotropic effect of a mutated gene in homozygous individuals. After demonstrating absence of linkage to the *TPO* and *Tg* genes, two groups established linkage of Pendred's syndrome with a locus on the long arm of chromosome 7 (7q21–34). Using a positional cloning strategy, the Pendred syndrome gene *(PDS)* has been identified very recently. It encodes a putative sulfate transporter, pendrin, which is expressed predominantly in the thyroid gland. Its exact role in the development and function of the inner ear and the thyroid remains to be defined.

HYDROGEN PEROXIDE GENERATION H_2O_2 is an essential factor in the iodination and coupling reactions. Although the ability of follicular cells to produce H_2O_2 has been known for more than three decades, the nicotinamide adenine dinucleotide phosphate (NADPH)-dependent oxidoreductase remains ill-defined. Deficiency in H_2O_2 generation may impede the organification of iodide. Two cases of euthyroid goiter and abnormal iodide organification associated with defective H_2O_2 generation have been reported. Addition of an H_2O_2-generating system to thyroid homogenates restored normal organification in vitro.

THYROGLOBULIN Tg is produced by thyroid follicular cells and is secreted into the follicular lumen. Some of its tyrosine residues are iodinated by TPO (organification and iodination), and the iodinated tyrosines, MIT and DIT, are subsequently coupled to form T3 and T4. Tg is, therefore, considered to be a thyroid hormone precursor. Besides its importance for hormone synthesis, Tg allows storage of iodine and thyroid hormone, which can be important under conditions of scarce iodine supply.

Tg is a large glycosylated protein of 2748 amino acids with a molecular mass of 330 kDa and a sedimentation rate of 12 S. The mature protein is formed by two noncovalent subunits (19 S thyroglobulin). Glycosylation plays an important role in the structure of the protein and accounts for 10% of total weight. The Tg monomer contains 20 glycosylation sites and there is extensive microheterogeneity in the composition of carbohydrates.

The *Tg* gene is one of the largest mammalian genes known to date, and it spans more than 300 kb. It has been mapped to chromosome 8q24 and contains 42 exons. Most exons are small (100 to 200 bp) with the exception of exons 9 and 10, which contain 1101 and 588 bp, respectively. The mature transcript contains an open reading frame of 8301 bp. The promoter has been well characterized and contains regulatory elements for the thyroid-specific transcription factors 1 and 2 *(see below)*, a ubiquitous factor, and cAMP response element binding proteins. TSH, the main regulator of the thyroid, acts via the cAMP signaling pathway.

Tg contains 67 tyrosines, but only a minority of these residues, localized in the carboxy- and amino-terminus, are hormonogenic sites. Complete hydrolysis of iodinated Tg yields only two to four molecules of the iodothyroxines, T4 and T3.

Defects of Tg synthesis or secretion have been studied extensively in animals and man. Tg abnormalities have been classified as quantitative or qualitative defects. Qualitative defects encompass structurally defective Tg, defective export from thyroid follicular cells, and defects in glycosylation. In individuals with structurally abnormal Tg, the coupling of iodotyrosines may be impaired. Thus, the majority of iodine bound to Tg is present in the form of MIT and DIT.

Clinically, these patients present with goiter and a metabolic status that may be hypothyroid, subclinically hypothyroid, or euthyroid. Tg defects are transmitted in an autosomal recessive manner, and in most cases, there is a history of consanguinity. However, RFLP analysis clearly demonstrated an autosomal dominant mode of inheritance in one kindred. Based on screening for neonatal hypothyroidism, the prevalence has been estimated to be 1 in 40,000 newborns. Goiter is typically present in early childhood. Thyroid radioiodine uptake is invariably elevated.

Tg can now be measured by radioimmunoassay (RIA); low or borderline Tg may indicate a quantitative defect, whereas patients with qualitative defects have normal or even an elevated Tg. After stimulation with TSH, no increase of Tg is observed in quantitative defects. The presence of abnormal iodoproteins in the serum is also suggestive of abnormal Tg synthesis. In the absence of sufficient Tg, albumin as well as other proteins are iodinated, generating iodotyrosines and iodohistidines. Ion-exchange chromatography after administration of iodine/125 results in elution of low T3 and T4, normal MIT and DIT, and high iodoproteins.

Although it is possible to diagnose Tg defects at the molecular level, this is not a trivial task considering the extremely large size of the gene. Further studies of patients with Tg abnormalities will be important for a more detailed understanding of the structure–function relationships in Tg.

The first models of Tg variants to be studied at the molecular level were the Afrikander cattle and the Dutch goat. The Afrikander cattle are characterized by large goiters and euthyroid metabolic status. The disorder is autosomal recessive. A mutation in exon 9 (arginine 697) leads to a premature stop codon. An alternative splice mechanism allows rescue to some degree by producing a misspliced 7.3-kb message missing exon 9. The original reading frame is maintained in this transcript and it is translated into a functional protein missing the part encoded by exon 9. Both transcripts are, however, present at much lower levels than normal. The Dutch goat is goitrous as well and, provided that the iodine intake is high, euthyroidism can be maintained. A nonsense mutation (tyrosine 296 to stop) in exon 8 results in a truncated protein. The fact that the goats can remain euthyroid despite this truncation is indirect evidence that the major hormonogenic sites are in the amino-terminal part of the protein.

Other animal species with Tg defects include the South Australian merino sheep (goiter, hypothyroidism, no normal intrathyroidal Tg), the bongo antelope (goiter, euthyroidism, absence of 660-kDa Tg), a cattle strain in Serbia (goiter, euthyroidism, decrease in 19 S Tg, increase in 12 S monomer), and the cog/cog mice (goiter, hypothyroidism, marked Tg deficiency).

In a well-studied human pedigree with congenital goiter and consanguineous parents, an RFLP in the *Tg* gene was found to segregate with the disease. Subsequently, a deletion of exon 4 because of a C to G transversion at position –3 in the acceptor splice site of intron 3 was found. This deletion removes one of the potential hormonogenic sites (tyrosine 130) from the Tg molecule. A family with two affected siblings revealed a point mutation creating a stop codon at position 1510; however, analogous to the Afrikander cattle, the mutation is removed by differential splicing that generates an mRNA shortened by 171 nucleotides. Recently, a quantitative Tg defect was found to be caused by the absence of thyroid-specific transcription factor (TTF-1) in a patient with congenital goiter *(see below)*.

DEHALOGENASE DEFECTS After entering the follicular cell, Tg is hydrolyzed, and T4 and T3 are secreted into the blood. The iodotyrosines, MIT and DIT, which are much more abundant in the Tg molecule, are deiodinated by an intrathyroidal dehalogenase and recirculated for hormone synthesis. In case of a defective dehalogenase system, MIT and DIT leak into the circulation and are excreted in the urine. This leads to severe iodine loss, and if the iodine supply is scarce, goiter and hypothyroidism ensue.

Clinically, patients with a deiodinase defect present with congenital hypothyroidism and a goitrous gland. The diagnosis is established by administration of radiolabeled DIT. Normally, DIT will be deiodinated, whereas in the case of a defective dehalogenase, the majority will be secreted unaltered in the urine. Administration of iodide in sufficient amounts to compensate for the increased loss, will reestablish a euthyroid metabolic state. The disorder is inherited in an autosomal recessive fashion. Biochemical testing in heterozygotes demonstrates an increased secretion of labeled DIT in the urine. The gene for the intrathyroidal dehalogenase has not been cloned.

SERUM-BINDING PROTEIN DEFECTS

Thyroid hormones circulate bound to plasma proteins. The three major binding proteins are thyroxine-binding globulin (TBG), transthyretin (TTR, formerly referred to as thyroxine-binding prealbumin), and albumin. Under physiologic conditions, only 0.03% of T4 and 0.3% of T3 circulate as free hormone.

Abnormalities in transport proteins can lead to either a decrease or an increase in total T4 levels. However, free hormone levels are within the normal range and the patients are clinically euthyroid. Failure to recognize these entities results in inappropriate treatment aimed at normalizing the total thyroid hormone levels. TTR variants are of additional clinical importance because some are associated with a form of amyloidosis.

THYROXINE-BINDING GLOBULIN TBG, which carries about 75–80% of T4, is an acidic glycoprotein synthesized in the liver. The mature protein contains 395 amino acids with four heterosaccharide chains with five to nine sialic acids. It contains a single T4-binding site. Like corticosteroid-binding globulin, it shows high homology with α1-antichymotrypsin and α1-antitrypsin proteases. The carbohydrates play a minor role in T4 binding, but have important effects on TBG stability and hepatic clearance rate. An increase in sialylation (e.g., induced by estrogens) lowers the hepatic clearance and thus increases TBG levels. Multiple other drugs either increase or decrease TBG concentrations by altering the synthesis rate or the degree of sialylation. The single copy gene encoding TBG is localized on the X-chromosome (Xq11–q23).

Inherited TBG abnormalities are classified into complete or partial deficiencies, or as TBG excess. Complete TBG-deficiency (TBG-CD) is defined as absence of TBG in the serum of hemizygous (XY) individuals. The heterozygous females in these kindreds have about half the normal amount of TBG because random X-inactivation results on average in a 50% reduction of the protein. The prevalence of complete deficiency has been estimated at 1:15,000. Partial deficiency is the most common form of TBG deficiency. In white and mixed populations, it is found with a frequency of 1:4,000. About 50% of Australian Aborigines have an abnormal TBG (TBG-A), and slow TBG (TBG-S) is found in African and Pacific island populations. Some of these TBG-variants have a reduced affinity for T4 (TBG-A, TBG San Diego). In some variants, an accelerated rate of degradation is responsible for low serum concentrations. The mutations in the *TBG* gene characterized so far are caused by deletions of single nucleotides resulting in frameshift and early termination or single base substitutions that alter the amino acid sequence.

TBG excess is not as frequent as TBG deficiency, and has an incidence of about 1 in 25,000 births. TBG and T4 levels are elevated three- to fivefold in hemizygotes and two- to threefold in heterozygous females. Because no mutations have been found in the coding sequence of the *TBG* gene in these cases, a defect in the promoter region has been postulated.

TRANSTHYRETIN TTR is a homotetramer formed of subunits containing 127 amino acids. It contains two T4 binding sites, but negative cooperativity allows occupancy of only one site at a given time. The *TTR gene* contains four exons and is localized on chromosome 18. TTR is predominantly synthesized in the liver, but also in the choroid plexus. Although the exact role of TTR in the brain is not known, it has been postulated that T4 binds to TTR in the epithelial cells of the choroid plexus and is then released into the cerebrospinal fluid.

A large number of TTR variants have been reported, and their impact on T4 affinity is highly variable. Many of the point mutations have been associated with distinct forms of amyloidosis. The inheritance is autosomal dominant in most instances. Although the clinical manifestations vary, most have polyneuropathy, and are sometimes referred to as familial amyloidotic polyneuropathy (FAP).

ALBUMIN Albumin is a monomer of 69 kDa and transports a wide variety of endogenous and exogenous hydrophobic compounds. About 5–10% of T4 is bound to albumin. Familial dysalbuminemic hyperthyroxinemia (FDH) is the most frequent form of euthyroid hyperthyroxinemia. The disorder is inherited in an autosomal dominant fashion and characterized by an albumin with an increased affinity for T4. After the demonstration of tight linkage between the FDH phenotype and the albumin gene, a point mutation at nucleotide 653 causing a substitution of arginine by histidine was identified in all cases reported so far.

PERIPHERAL MONODEIODINATION

T4 and T3 are generally thought to enter the peripheral tissues as unbound hormones. T4 is metabolized into the more active compound, T3, by intracellular 5'-monodeiodination, or into the inactive metabolite, reverse T3 (rT3), by 5-monodeiodination. Because roughly 80% of T3 is generated by monodeiodination, T4 is sometimes considered a prohormone. Several selenoenzymes with different tissue distributions are involved in 5'-monodeiodination. 5'-monodeiodinase type I is expressed primarily in liver, muscle, kidney, and skin. Type II 5'-monodeiodinase is expressed in the anterior pituitary, the brain cortex, brown adipose tissue, and, at high levels, in the thyroid gland. The type III deiodinase catalyzes the conversion from T4 and T3 into inactive metabolites by 5-monodeiodination. This selenoprotein is abundant in the placenta and regulates circulating fetal thyroid hormone concentrations during gestation. cDNAs have been cloned for each of the enzymes.

Defects in deiodination are very rare. A description of six females of three generations with hyperthyroidism and high T4 and T3, but unsuppressed TSH, was suggested to be caused by an inherited 5'-deiodinase type II defect. In two instances, high T4 and rT3, but normal T3, concentrations were reported and may be explained by a 5'-deiodinase defect.

RESISTANCE TO THYROID HORMONE

The thyroid hormones, T4 and T3, exert their multiple cellular effects through nuclear thyroid hormone receptors (TR), transcription factors that act by altering patterns of gene expression. The TRs were cloned on the basis of their relationship to other members of the steroid receptor superfamily, which share a characteristic central DNA-binding domain and a carboxy-terminal ligand-binding domain. In the TR, the carboxy-terminus of the receptor also contains nuclear localization signals, dimerization domains, and transactivation functions. The functional properties of the amino-terminal region of the receptor are not well-characterized, but it also seems to be involved in transactivation.

There are two thyroid hormone receptors, TRα and TRβ, that are encoded by separate genes located on chromosomes 17 and 3, respectively. They each bind thyroid hormones with high affinity, but TRα and TRβ differ in their developmental patterns of expression, tissue distribution, and the patterns of splicing to create additional isoforms. The TRs act in conjunction with thyroid receptor accessory proteins (TRAPs), like retinoid X receptor (RXR), that dimerize with the TR and enhance their binding to DNA. The TR binds as a monomer, or with greater affinity as homodimers or heterodimers, to thyroid hormone response elements (TREs) in specific target genes. Moreover, several factors that act as nuclear corepressors, such as SMRTs (silencing mediators for retinoid and thyroid hormone receptors) or NCoRs (nuclear receptor corepressors), have been cloned recently (*see* Chapter 3). The first cDNA encoding a nuclear receptor corepressor (NCoR 270 kDa) mediates ligand-independent inhibition of gene transcription by TR and other receptors. In genes regulated positively by thyroid hormones, the corepressor is proposed to interact with unliganded TR to inhibit transcription; this interaction is disrupted by T3, allowing putative coactivators to interact with the TR and activate gene transcription (Fig. 50-4).

Although there is considerable heterogeneity in the TREs of different target genes, most TREs contain two or more "half-sites" that correspond to the minimal recognition motif for a receptor monomer. The consensus TRE half-site consists of the DNA sequence, AGGTCA. These half-sites can be arranged as a palindrome, a direct repeat spaced by four nucleotides, or as an inverted repeat, also called lap (a term created by inversion of palindrome). Remarkably, TRs can bind to these TREs with different orientations as homodimers or heterodimers with RXRs, indicating flexibility in the determinants of the protein–protein interface.

Resistance to thyroid hormone (RTH) was first reported in 1967 by Refetoff, DeWind, and DeGroot, who described two sibs of a

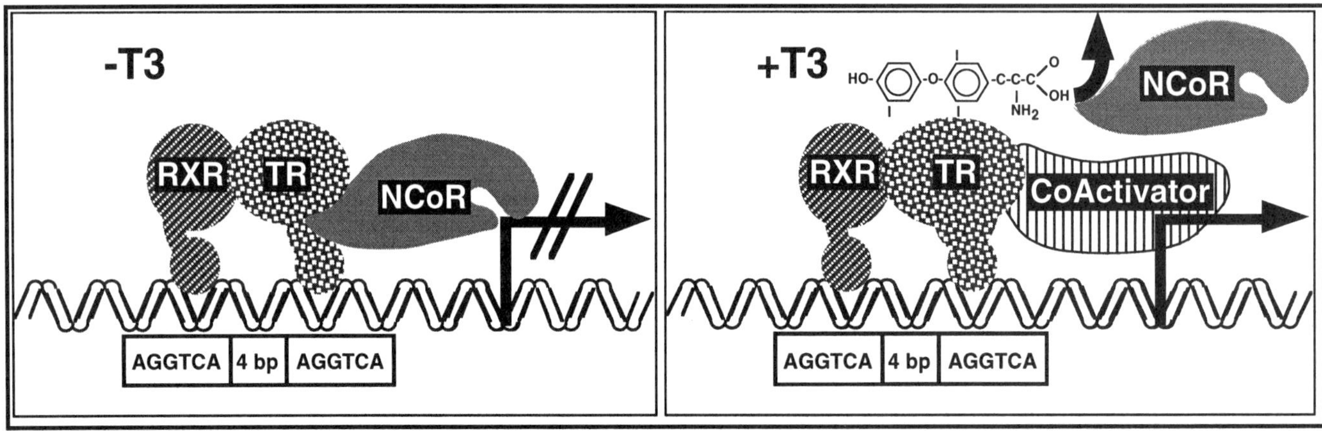

Figure 50-4 Model of thyroid hormone action on a positively regulated gene. In the absence of thyroid hormone, corepressors interact with thyroid hormone receptor (TR) homo- or heterodimers and silence transcription. Thyroid hormone causes displacement of corepressors and recruitment of coactivators and factors of the basal transcription apparatus to initiate gene expression.

consanguineous marriage presenting with goiter, high levels of protein-bound iodine, deaf-mutism, delayed bone age, and stippled epiphyses, but without signs of hyperthyroidism. It was postulated that hormone resistance in peripheral tissues was the explanation for the absence of signs and symptoms of thyrotoxicosis. After the cloning of the TRs, linkage analysis demonstrated that the *TRβ gene* is tightly linked to RTH, whereas no association could be demonstrated for *TRα*. The ultimate proof that a defect in the receptor is the cause of RTH was provided in 1989 by the demonstration of mutations in the *TRβ* gene, a finding that has been confirmed in multiple reports. Although the true incidence of RTH is unknown, it is a relatively rare disorder and approximately 400 patients have been reported. With the growing awareness of the existence of the disorder and the availability of genetic testing, this list is continuing to increase.

Biochemically, RTH is defined by elevated circulating levels of free thyroid hormones as a result of reduced target tissue responsiveness and normal, or elevated, levels of TSH. This "inappropriate" TSH level contrasts with the situation in hyperthyroidism, in which the pituitary secretion of TSH is suppressed. Patients with RTH typically present with goiter and a euthyroid or mildly hypothyroid metabolic state. Thus, pituitary resistance results in hypersecretion of TSH that compensates, at least partially, for hormone resistance in peripheral tissues. Despite this compensation, the clinical signs of RTH can include short stature, delayed bone maturation, hyperactivity and learning disabilities, and hearing defects, as well as variable degrees of hyperthyroidism and hypothyroidism.

With the exception of a single family harboring a deletion of the entire coding sequence of the entire *TRβ gene* and a recessive pattern of inheritance, all other reports of RTH demonstrate autosomal dominant inheritance. The mutant receptors act in a dominant-negative fashion to block the activity of normal TRα and TRβ receptors. It is striking that, with a few exceptions, the mutations are clustered within two domains in the carboxy-terminal region of the receptor between amino acids 310 and 347 (domain I) and amino acids 438–461 (domain II) (Fig. 50-5). Many mutations occur in CpG dinucleotide sequences, and in most cases, these nucleotide substitutions result in single amino acid changes. No mutations have been found within the DNA-binding domain or in the amino-terminus. In general, the mutations preserve critical receptor functions such as dimerization and DNA binding, while inactivating other activities such as T3 binding and transcriptional activation. The mechanism underlying the dominant-negative activity of mutant TRs seems to be caused predominantly by competition at the level of DNA binding.

These defects continue to provide important insights into the mechanisms of thyroid hormone action and the structure–function relationship of the TRs, as well as the molecular mechanisms of dominant-negative activity. The study of the recently developed murine knockout models and transgenic mice bearing mutant thyroid hormone receptors provide additional insights into the molecular basis of thyroid hormone action and RTH. For example, TRβ –/– mice display defective maturation of auditory function, demonstrating that TRβ is essential for the development of hearing.

TRANSCRIPTION FACTORS

THYROID TRANSCRIPTION FACTOR-1 (TTF-1) TTF-1 is a 38-kDa nuclear protein that mediates thyroid-specific gene transcription. The human gene contains a homeobox domain and a motif that is found in the NKX2 family of transcription factors. The gene has been localized to chromosome 14q12–q21. TTF-1 is involved in thyroid development and it stimulates thyroglobulin, and to a lesser degree, thyroperoxidase gene transcription. Besides the thyroid, TTF-1 is also expressed in brain tissues and in the lung. A murine knockout model of TTF-1, which is also known as T/EBP (thyroid-specific enhancer protein), led to severe alterations of forebrain, lung, and thyroid development.

Absence of TTF-1 expression has been found to cause defective thyroglobulin synthesis and congenital goiter. The disorder is probably recessive. Pax8 mRNA levels were normal in this patient and there was very little thyroglobulin mRNA. Thyroperoxidase mRNA was more abundant than in control tissues. In two recent studies, no alterations in the *TTF-1* gene were found in a large number of patients with congenital hypothyroidism. This suggests that TTF-1 mutations are unlikely to be an important cause of thyroid dysgenesis or agenesis.

THYROID TRANSCRIPTION FACTOR-2 (TTF-2) TTF-2 is a forkhead domain-containing transcription factor that binds to both the *Tg* and the *TPO* gene promoters. It is transiently expressed in the developing thyroid and anterior pituitary gland. In the thy-

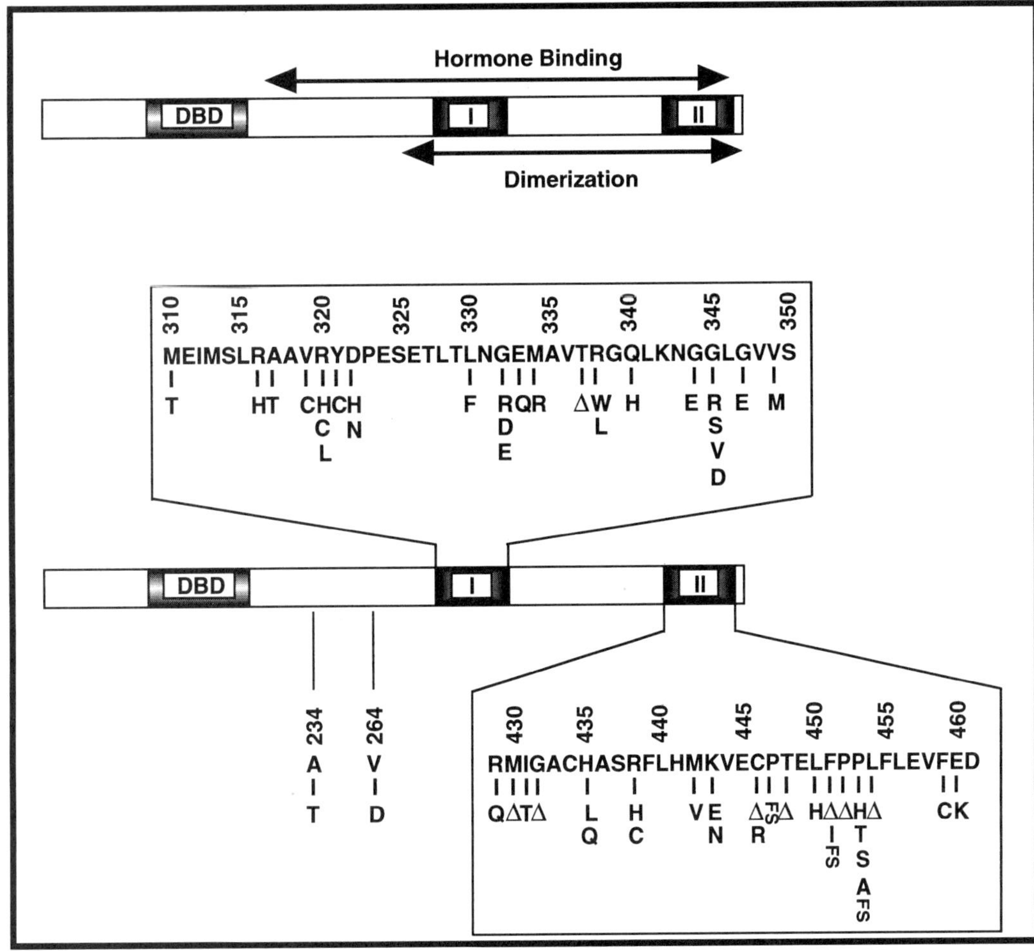

Figure 50-5 Structure of TRβ receptor and synopsis of mutations in TRβ in patients with resistance to thyroid hormone. With a few exceptions, the mutations are clustered in two domains in the carboxy-terminus of the receptor flanking the dimerization domain. (DBD, DNA-binding domain.)

roid, TTF-2 expression is downregulated just before the onset of *Tg* and *TPO* gene expression, suggesting that this transcription factor is a negative regulator of thyroid-specific gene expression during development. At later stages, IGF-I modulates the level of TTF-2 and results in increased expression of the *Tg* gene in vitro. TTF-2 expression is lost in cell lines transformed with Ki-*ras*, Ha-*ras* and polyoma middle-T oncogenes. So far, no human thyroid disease is known to be caused by defects or absence of TTF-2.

PAX-8 Pax-8 is a paired domain thyroid-specific transcription factor responsible for thyroid development and for *Tg* and *TPO* gene expression. In contrast to TTF-1, Pax-8 binds predominantly to the TPO promoter and, with less affinity, to the *Tg* promoter.

AUTOIMMUNE DISORDERS

Autoimmune thyroid disorders, such as Hashimoto's thyroiditis and Graves' disease, are by far the most common diseases affecting the gland. Both disorders are found more frequently in women than in men (4:1 to 10:1), a difference that is most commonly explained by influences of sex steroids on immunoregulatory mechanisms. The incidence of Graves' disease in the general population has been estimated at 0.2–1%. Autoimmune thyroiditis has been reported to occur in 3–4.5% of women. Thyroid autoantibodies are found in up to 15% of elderly women. Both disorders are familial and are thought to be polygenic. However, environmental factors probably modulate their phenotypic expression.

GRAVES' DISEASE The hereditary predisposition to Graves' disease has been addressed in many studies. Graves' disease occurs in about 3–9% of dizygotic and 30–60% of monozygotic twins. As in other autoimmune diseases, associations have been established between the disease and the presence of certain constellations of human leukocyte antigens (HLA). The activation of T cells requires interaction of T-cell receptors with an antigen and the HLA molecules of the major histocompatibility complex (MHC) I and II on the antigen-presenting cell (*see* Chapter 31). Subsequently, the T cell releases lymphokines and stimulates the production of (auto)antibodies in B cells. Graves' disease was one of the first autoimmune disorders with documented associations with certain HLA types, predominantly DR3 and B8 in whites, B17 in blacks of West Africa and African Americans, and B35 in Japanese. There are, however, many variations in these associations. The frequency of HLA-DR5 seems to be reduced in patients with Graves' disease.

Because stimulating autoantibodies against the TSHR (TSAb) are the cause of Graves' disease, their assessment can be helpful for establishing the diagnosis and they are potentially helpful in follow-up. The cloning of the *TSHR* led to the development of new bioassays that allow the measurement of TSAb. In these new assay systems, the *TSHR* has been stably transfected into cell lines and measurement of cAMP in response to a patient's serum allows a bioassay for thyroid autoantibodies. These assays allow distinction between TSab from antibodies that block the receptor (TBAb); these blocking antibodies may also be present in autoimmune thyroid disease. Several regions of the extracellular domain have been identified as possible epitopes for TSab, but so far no unifying model has been established.

HASHIMOTO'S THYROIDITIS Molecular biology established that the microsomal antigen in autoimmune thyroiditis is in fact TPO. The epitopes within the TPO enzyme that are the targets of autoantibodies are, however, still a matter of debate. Recombinant TPO is now used for assays of autoantibodies.

HLA correlations differ in part from those reported for Graves' disease and include primarily HLA-DR3, DR4, and DR5 haplotypes. It is noteworthy that members of the same family can be affected by either Graves' or Hashimoto's disease, suggesting that the immunogenetic predisposition for both entities is closely related.

THYROID CANCER

Thyroid cancers account for about 0.6–1.6% of all malignancies, and the incidence is 1 to 10 per 100,000 in most countries. The most common thyroid malignancies are papillary thyroid carcinomas (PTC) and follicular thyroid carcinomas (FTC), both originating from follicular cells, and accounting for about 60–90% of tumors. Their relative distribution is variable, but papillary carcinoma is generally 5–10 times more common. The incidence of FTC increases in regions with iodine deficiency. Besides the clinically relevant forms of papillary thyroid cancer, occult papillary thyroid cancer (<1 cm) is found in up to 25% of autopsies. The highly malignant anaplastic carcinoma (ATC) and several unusual variants of thyroid cancers (Hürthle cell carcinoma, insular thyroid carcinoma, primary squamous carcinoma, and lymphoma of the thyroid) are much rarer forms of thyroid malignancies. ATC is thought to arise from pre-existing well-differentiated carcinomas.

Radiation is a major risk factor for the development of benign and malignant thyroid neoplasms. This was recognized after the use of external radiation for medical treatment of benign and malignant conditions of the head and neck and more dramatically after releases of ionizing radiation from atomic explosions and accidents in nuclear facilities.

Papillary thyroid cancer, which presents with several distinct histologic subtypes, may occur in the setting of some rare autosomal dominant syndromes with disseminated neoplasias: familial adenomatous polyposis and Gardner's syndrome, as well as Cowden's syndrome, a condition characterized by multiple hamartomas with benign and malignant breast tumors, gastrointestinal polyps, ovarian cysts, and mucocutaneous papulae. In the latter case, germline mutations in the *PTEN* gene, a protein tyrosine–dual-specificity phosphatase, have been identified in four of five families. In some instances, the familial accumulation of PTC may, however, be the result of exposure to a shared risk factor rather than a familial disease in the strict sense. Also, familial aggregation of FTC seems to occur in some families with dyshormonogenesis. Cytogenetic alterations have been identified in some cases of papillary thyroid cancer (chromosome 1, unbalanced rearrangement with trisomy 5 and monosomy 16, 10, 17). The inversions on chromosome 10 prompted the discovery of the papillary thyroid cancer and *ret* rearrangement *(see below)*.

Several molecular mechanisms involved in the development of thyroid neoplasms have been elucidated during the last decade. By analogy to colon cancer, in which a multistep progression from polyclonal hyperplastic lesion to monoclonal adenoma and to carcinoma seems to occur, a stepwise linear model has also been proposed for thyroid malignancies (*see* Chapter 7). Although some features are consistent with such a scenario, the picture is far from being complete and further efforts are needed to fully understand thyroid oncogenesis.

CLONAL ANALYSIS Analysis of clonality has been performed in thyroid nodules, adenomas, and cancers using the X-inactivation technique in females. Studies of clonality of thyroid neoplasms revealed that the majority of thyroid nodules are monoclonal in origin, i.e., true adenomas. In multinodular goiters, polyclonal nodules coexist with monoclonal nodules, and the latter may have distinct clonal origins within the same gland. As expected, cancers are of monoclonal origin. The few reported exceptions are probably caused by contributions by stromal tissue.

Besides clonal analysis by means of the X-inactivation approach, loss of heterozygosity (LOH) has been demonstrated in follicular thyroid cancer (chromosome 3p; chromosome 11q13, harboring the gene linked to multiple endocrine neoplasia type 1, menin, and others). Taken together, these results suggest that somatic mutations in growth-related genes or loss of tumor suppressor genes occur in most of these tumors.

GROWTH FACTORS AND ONCOGENES Many growth factors are expressed abnormally in benign and malignant thyroid tumors (Table 50-3). In part, these alterations are probably secondary events because no structural abnormalities have been detected in the involved genes or the respective chromosomal locations.

Amplification of the *met* gene, encoding a heterodimeric tyrosine kinase whose ligand is the hepatic growth factor (HGF), has been reported in 70% of papillary thyroid cancer and undifferentiated thyroid cancer and in 25% of follicular cancer, and it is associated with an aggressive clinical and histologic phenotype. The expression of transcription factor c-*myc* increases in less differentiated thyroid tumors, and c-*myc* mRNA may correlate inversely with that of the TSHR.

Mutations in the three *ras* genes, Ha-*ras*, K-*ras*, and N-*ras*, which encode closely related 21-kDa proteins involved in signal transduction, have been found in numerous human tumors, including thyroid neoplasms. The most frequently mutated codons are 12, 13, and 61, and these mutations lead to a reduction of the GTPase activity, resulting in constitutive activation of the protein. Although mutations have been detected in both benign and malignant thyroid tumors, there is considerable variation in the reported prevalence of these mutations. This might be in part because of geographic differences or the techniques used to detect the mutations. *Ras* mutations appear to be most frequent in follicular cancer.

Rearrangements of the *ret* locus were found on the basis of characterization of an inversion in chromosome 10 in several papillary cancers. Ret is a transmembrane tyrosine kinase. Its ligand, glia-derived neurotrophic factor (GDNF) has been identified very recently. Normally, the ret proto-oncogene is not expressed in thyroid follicular cells but it is found in calcitonin-producing thyroid C cells. Several distinct types of translocations place different promoters upstream of the ret tyrosine kinase domain. Ret-papillary thyroid cancer rearrangements seem to be relatively specific for papillary thyroid cancer and occur in about 10–40% of cases.

Table 50-3
Molecular Alterations in Benign and Malignant Thyroid Tumors[a]

Gene	*Chromosomal location*	*Molecular Defect*	*Tumor*
TSHR	14q31	Point mutations	Toxic adenoma, differentiated carcinoma
Gsα	20q13.2	Point mutations	Adenoma, toxic adenoma, differentiated carcinomas
ret/PTC	10q11.2	Rearrangements PTC1: (inv(10)q11.2q21); PTC2: (t(10;17)(q11.2;q23)); PTC3: *ele1/TK*	PTC
ret	10q11.2	Point mutations	MEN, MTC
Trk	1q23–24	Rearrangements: *NTRK1/ TPM3;* *NTRK1/TPR;* *NTRK1/TAG*	MNG, PTC
ras	H-*ras* 11p15.5 K-*ras* 12p12.1 N-*ras* 1p13.2	Point mutations	Adenoma, differentiated thyroid carcinoma
p53	17p13	Point mutations, deletion, insertion	Differentiated carcinoma, anaplastic carcinoma
Rb	13q14.1–14	mRNA variants	Differentiated carcinoma, anaplastic carcinoma
p16 (MTS1, CDKN2A)	9p21	Deletions	Cell lines of differentiated carcinomas
p21/WAF	6p21.2	Overexpression	ATC, FTC, PTC
met	7q31	Overexpression	FTC
c-*myc*	8q24.12.–13	Overexpression	Differentiated carcinoma
PTEN	10q23	Point mutations	PTC in Cowden's syndrome
Loss of heterozygosity	3p 11q13 and other loci		FTC

[a]Abbreviations: *TSHR*, thyroid-stimulating hormone receptor; *Gsα*, G-protein stimulating α-subunit; *ret/PTC*, *ret* proto-oncogene/papillary thyroid carcinoma; *ret*, *ret* (rearranged during transfection) proto-oncogene; *Trk*, rearrangement of neurotrophic tyrosine kinase receptor type 1; and nonmuscle tropomyosin; *ras*, *ras* (rat sarcoma) proto-oncogene; *p53*, *p53* tumor antigen; *Rb*, retinoblastoma gene; *p16 (MTS1, CKN2a)*, tumor suppressor *p16* (multiple tumor suppressor1, cyclin-dependent kinase inhibitor-2A); *p21/WAF*, tumor suppressor *p21* (cyclin-dependent kinase inhibitor-1A, wild-type *p53*-activated fragment 1); *met*, *met* proto-oncogene (hepatocyte growth factor receptor); c-*myc*, c-*myc* (myelocytomatosis virus) proto-oncogene; *PTEN*, phosphatase and tensin homolog; *ele1/TK*, *ret*-activating gene *ele1*; *NTRK*, neurotrophic tyrosine kinase receptor; *TPM3*, tropomyosin 3; *TPR*, translocated promoter region; *TAG*, tyrosine kinase receptor-activating gene; MEN, multiple endocrine neoplasia; MTC, medullary thyroid carcinoma; MGN, multinodular goiter; ATC, anaplastic thyroid carcinoma; FTC, follicular thyroid carcinoma.

A second type of chimeric oncogene has been described in papillary thyroid cancer. The *TRK* gene, encoding a receptor for the nerve growth factor (NGF), can come under the control of several unrelated sequences through intrachromosomal rearrangements on chromosome 1q23–24: the tropomyosin gene, the *TPR* gene, and a gene referred to as *TAG* (TRK-activating gene).

Somatic *gsp* mutations, activating mutations in the α-subunit of the stimulatory G protein, occur in toxic adenomas *(see above)*. In comparison to toxic adenomas where they occur in up to 20% of all cases, *gsp* mutations are relatively uncommon in papillary thyroid cancer and FTC.

The tumor suppressor genes that have been studied in thyroid malignancies include the retinoblastoma susceptibility gene *(Rb)*, the *p53* gene, and *P16*. *Rb* maps to chromosome 13q14 and encodes a 110-kDa protein that regulates cell cycle control. When studied at the genomic or protein level, no *Rb* abnormalities have been found in thyroid carcinomas. This contrasts with a report on mRNA abnormalities in 55% of thyroid carcinomas.

P16, also referred to as *MTS1*, is an inhibitor of cyclin-dependent kinases (CDK) involved in the phosphorylation of *Rb* (*see* Chapter 6). The recent demonstration of homozygous deletions of *P16*, localized on chromosome 9p21, in two of three FTC and two of four papillary thyroid cancer cell lines suggests that *P16* might be an important tumor suppressor gene involved in the pathogenesis of thyroid malignancies.

The *p53* gene plays an important role in the development and progression of several human cancers. It exerts its function as a tumor suppressor by arresting cells in the G1 phase of the cell cycle, thus enabling repair of DNA damage. The *p53* gene is localized on chromosome 17p13. Germline mutations of *p53* are found in the Li-Fraumeni syndrome, familial breast cancer (*see* Chapter 7), and a wide variety of other human malignancies. As in other malignancies, mutations in *p53* are also thought to be involved in the progression of thyroid carcinomas and to play an important role in the process of dedifferentiation. Although they are more frequently found in anaplastic carcinomas, they may also occur in some follicular adenomas and differentiated carcinomas. Mutations occur predominantly at CpG dinucleotides, with positions 248 and 273 representing mutational hot spots.

MEDULLARY THYROID CANCER AND MULTIPLE ENDOCRINE NEOPLASIA Multiple endocrine neoplasia (MEN), familial and sporadic medullary thyroid cancer (FMTC/MTC) are more thoroughly reviewed in Chapter 54. MEN 2A is an autosomal dominant disease characterized by the association of MTC, parathyroid adenomas, and pheochromocytoma. In MEN 2B, parathyroid disease is absent, but the patients have mucocutaneous ganglioneuromas and some have a marfanoid habitus. FMTC is a familial cancer syndrome without other manifestations of the MEN complex.

Several mutations in the *ret* tyrosine kinase receptor have been identified as the cause of MEN 2A and FMTC. Most of these mutations affect conserved cysteines in the cysteine-rich domain that is thought to be involved in receptor dimerization and activation. In MEN 2B, a mutation at position 918, substituting methionine to threonine, has been found in 95% of the patients.

Although genetic testing for the diagnosis of cancer predisposition remains controversial, the recognition of mutations in the *ret* gene as cause of MEN 2A and FMTC has profound clinical implications. Before the availability of genetic testing, families with MEN 2A and FMTC were evaluated on a regular basis by measuring calcitonin levels after stimulation with pentagastrin or calcium. This test is hampered, however, by relatively low specificity and a requirement for repeated testing. The possibility of identifying genotype by mutational analysis allows accurate detection of affected and unaffected family members. Consequently, thyroidectomy can be performed in early childhood to prevent the development of MTC that occurs in about 90% of affected patients. This procedure is, therefore, likely to be associated with improved diagnostic accuracy, better cure rates, and reduced long-term costs.

RECOMBINANT HUMAN TSH AS DIAGNOSTIC TOOL IN THE FOLLOW-UP OF DIFFERENTIATED THYROID CARCINOMA After surgical procedures, patients with differentiated carcinomas of the thyroid are routinely evaluated by means of radioiodine scans and measurements of thyroglobulin. To achieve high sensitivity, these tests are traditionally performed after withdrawal of the suppressive treatment with thyroxine to achieve an increase in TSH to allow a high uptake of radioiodine in residual tissue. Withdrawal of thyroxine leads to hypothyroidism. Moreover, the increase in TSH may potentially lead to proliferation of residual tumor cells. To avoid these problems, exogenous TSH has been successfully administered during uninterrupted treatment with thyroxine before performing radioiodine scans and thyroglobulin measurements. These procedures were initially performed with bovine TSH or human TSH from autopsies, sources that are no longer acceptable because of the possibility of anaphylactic reactions and the transmission of infectious diseases (e.g., Jakob-Creutzfeld). After the cloning of the α- and β-subunits of human TSH, the production of recombinant TSH is now possible. Administration of recombinant human TSH is being evaluated in controlled protocols for the follow-up of patients with differentiated thyroid cancer and is likely to become a standard procedure.

TRANSGENIC MODELS

Important new insights into the pathophysiologic mechanisms controlling goiter and thyroid tumor formation have been gained using transgenic mice as models. The characterization of the Tg promoter has allowed tissue-specific expression of several transgenes in the thyroid. A first model expressed the chloramphenicol acetyltransferase (CAT) in the thyroid; CAT activity was detected only in thyroid tissue indicating that the *cis* regulatory elements present in the first 2000 bp of the promoter are sufficient for thyroid-specific expression.

Overexpression in the thyroid of the large T antigen of *SV40*, one of the most potent known viral oncogenes, resulted in rapidly growing undifferentiated goiters with progressive dedifferentiation with increasing age. The loss of differentiation was accompanied by marked hypothyroidism. Most of these animals died early, primarily from tracheal compression. The *E7* oncogene on the human papillomavirus type 16 inactivates the Rb tumor suppressor protein. Transgenic mice expressing *E7* develop hyperplastic goiters with large follicles and well-differentiated follicular cells.

By overexpression of the *herpes virus thymidine kinase 1* gene and treatment with the antiviral drug ganciclovir, thyroid follicular cells have been selectively ablated. Expression of the adenosine A2a receptor, a constitutive activator of the adenlylyl cyclase pathway, resulted in severe hyperthyroidism, tachyarrhythmias, and premature deaths as a result of congestive heart failure. These transgenic animals develop huge goiters, which are initially diffuse but develop nodules later in development, and provide an interesting model for hyperthyroidism and formation of nodular goiters. Other models have studied the oncogenic potential of targeted overexpression of mutated Ki-*ras*, Ha-*ras*, Gsα, the cholera toxin A1 subunit, and a mutated α1β-adrenergic receptor. In the latter case, the expression of the transgene resulted in the activation of both the cAMP and the phospholipase C pathways. This dual stimulation led to enhanced growth, hyperfunction, the development of invading malignant thyroid tumors, and, in older animals, differentiated metastases.

The targeted expression of the *ret*-papillary thyroid cancer 1 oncogene in a transgenic model led to carcinomas that resemble human papillary cancers. Targeted expression of the *ret* gene altered by an MEN 2A mutation in C cells under the control of the calcitonin gene-related peptide and calcitonin promoter led to overt bilateral C-cell hyperplasia and multifocal and bilateral MTC. These results provide evidence that the mutated *ret* gene is indeed oncogenic in parafollicular C cells.

SELECTED REFERENCES

Abramowicz M, Duprez L, Parma J, Vassart G, Heinrichs C. Familial congenital hypothyroidism due to inactivating mutation of the thyrotropin receptor causing profound hypoplasia of the thyroid gland. J Clin Invest 1997;15:3018–3024.

Bartalena L. Recent achievements in studies on thyroid hormone-binding proteins. Endocr Rev 1990;11:47–64.

Berry M, Banu L, Larsen P. Type I iodothyronine deiodinase is a selenocysteine-containing enzyme. Nature 1991;349:438–440.

Croteau W, Davey J, Galton V, St. German D. Cloning of the mammalian type II iodothyronine deiodinase: a selenoprotein differentially expressed and regulated in human and rat brain and other tissues. J Clin Invest 1996;98:405–417.

Croteau W, Whittemore S, Schneider M, St Germain D. Cloning and expression of a cDNA for a mammalian type III iodothyronine deiodinase. J Biol Chem 1995;270:16,569–16,575.

Dai G, Levy O, Carrasco N. Cloning and characterization of the thyroid iodide transporter. Nature 1996;379:458–460.

Damante G, DiLauro R. Thyroid-specific gene expression. Biochim Biophys Acta 1994;1218:255–266.

DeGroot L. Congenital defects in thyroid hormone formation and action. In: DeGroot L, ed. Endocrinology, 3rd ed. Philadelphia: WB Saunders, 1994; pp. 871–892.

Everett LA, Glaser B, Beck JC, et al. Pendred syndrome is caused by mutations in a putative sulphate transporter gene (PDS). Nature Genet 1997;17:411–422.

Farid N. Genetic factors in thyroid disease. In: Braverman L, Utiger R, eds. The Thyroid. Philadelphia: Lippincott, 1991; pp. 588–602.

Farid N, Shi Y, Zou M. Molecular basis of thyroid cancer. Endocr Rev 1994;15:202–232.

Forrest D, Golarai G, Connor J, Curran T. Genetic analysis of thyroid hormone receptors in development and disease. Recent Prog Horm Res 1996;51:1–22.

Fujiwara H, Tatsumi K, Miki K, et al. Congenital hypothyroidism caused by a mutation in the Na+/I– symporter. Nat Genet 1997;16:124,125.

Haugen B, Ridgway C. Transcription factor Pit-1 and its clinical implications: from bench to bedside. Endocrinologist 1995;5:132–139.

Jameson J, DeGroot L. Mechanisms of thyroid hormone action. In: DeGroot L, ed. Endocrinology, 3rd ed. Philadelphia: WB Saunders, 1994; pp. 583–601.

Kopp P, van Sande J, Parma J, Duprez L, Gerber H, Joss E, Jameson JL, Dumont JE, Vassart G. Congenital hyperthyroidism caused by a mutation in the thyrotropin-receptor gene. N Engl J Med 1995;332:150–154.

Lazar MA. Thyroid hormone receptors: multiple forms, multiple possibilities. Endocr Rev 1993;14:184–193.

Lazar MA. Thyroid hormone receptors: update 1994. In: Braverman, LE, Refetoff S, eds. Clinical and molecular aspects of diseases of the thyroid. Endocr Rev Monographs 3. 1994; pp. 280-283.

Ledent C, Parmentier M, Vassart G, Dumont J. Models of thyroid goiter and tumors in transgenic mice. Mol Cell Endocrinol 1994;100:167–169.

Medeiros-Neto G, Stanbury J. Inherited Disorders of the Thyroid System. Boca Raton, FL: CRC, 1994.

Medeiros-Neto G, Targovnik H, Vassart G. Defective thyroglobulin synthesis and secretion causing goiter and hypothyroidism. Endocr Rev 1993;14:165–183.

Petersen C, Scottolini A, Cody L, Mandel M, Reimer N, Bhagavan N. A point mutation in the human serum albumin gene results in familial dysalbuminaemic hyperthyroxinaemia. J Med Genet 1993;31:355–359.

Refetoff S. Inherited thyroxine-binding globulin abnormalities in man. Endocr Rev 1989;10:275–293.

Refetoff S. Inherited thyroxine-binding globulin abnormalities in man: update 1994. In: Braverman, LE, Refetoff S, eds. Clinical and molecular aspects of diseases of the thyroid. Endocr Rev Monographs 3. 1994; pp. 162–164.

Refetoff S, Weiss RE, Usala SJ. The syndromes of resistance to thyroid hormone. Endocr Rev 1993;14:348–399.

Sunthornthepvarakul T, Angkeow P, Weiss R, Hayashi Y, Refetoff S. An identical missense mutation in the albumin gene results in familial dysalbuminemic hyperthyroxinemia in 8 unrelated families. Biochem Biophys Res Commun 1994;202:781–787.

Sunthornthepvarakul T, Gottschalk M, Hayashi Y, Refetoff S. Resistance to thyrotropin caused by mutations in the thyrotropin-receptor gene. New Engl J Med 1995;332:155–160.

Van Sande J, Parma J, Tonacchera M, Swillens S, Dumont J, Vassart G. Somatic and germline mutations of the TSH receptor gene in thyroid disease. J Clin Endocrinol Metab 1995;9:2577–2585.

Vassart G, Dumont J. The thyrotropin receptor and the regulation of thyrocyte function and growth. Endocr Rev 1992;13:596–611.

Vassart G, Dumont J, Refetoff S. Thyroid disorders. In: Beaudet AL, Seriver CR, Sly WS, Vale D, eds. The Metabolic Basis of Inherited Disease, 7 ed. New York: McGraw-Hill, 1995; pp. 2883–2928.

Vassart G, Parma J, van Sande J, Dumont J. The thyrotropin receptor and the regulation of thyrocyte function and growth: update 1994. In: Braverman, LE, Refetoff S, eds. Clinical and molecular aspects of diseases of the thyroid. Endocr Rev Monographs 3. 1994; pp. 77–80.

Volpé R. Autoimmune thyroiditis. In: Braverman L, Utiger R, eds. The Thyroid, 6th ed. Philadelphia: Lippincott, 1991; pp. 921–933.

Wynford-Thomas D. Origin and progression of thyroid epithelial tumours: cellular and molecular mechanisms. Horm Res 1997; 47:145–157.

51 Disorders of the Parathyroid Gland

ANDREW ARNOLD AND ANDREW F. STEWART

INTRODUCTION

PARATHYROID HORMONE STRUCTURE, BIOSYNTHESIS, AND SECRETION The parathyroid hormone (PTH) gene is located on the short arm of chromosome 11. Its 3 exons encode mature PTH (84 amino acids), as well as its signal (25 amino acids) and "pro" (6 amino acids) peptides. The study of the structure and regulation of the PTH gene and the intricacies of PTH biosynthesis, posttranslational processing, and intracellular targeting have led to the accrual of a body of information that is as complete as that for any other peptide hormone. In the sections that follow, these areas are briefly reviewed as an introduction to the molecular disorders of the parathyroid gland. The reader is referred to several up-to-date extensive reviews at the end of this chapter for a more detailed treatment of the subject.

The Extracellular Calcium-Sensing Receptor Increases in the serum ionized calcium inhibit the secretion of PTH. Conversely, reductions in serum ionized calcium stimulate the cascade of events that lead to the secretion of PTH. This inverse sigmoidal relationship between serum calcium and PTH secretion is precisely controlled, is the key physiologic feature of the parathyroid gland, and accounts for the tight minute-to-minute regulation of PTH secretion and the strict maintenance of serum calcium. Recently, the cloning of a parathyroid calcium receptor has been reported (Fig. 51-1). The calcium receptor is expressed in a restricted number of tissues (including the parathyroid gland, the thyroid C cell, the renal tubule, and the central nervous system [CNS]), is present on the surface of parathyroid cells, and is coupled by G proteins to the cytosolic calcium–inositol phosphate–phospholipase C intracellular signaling pathways. The receptor also has the structural features of a seven transmembrane spanning G-protein coupled receptor with a large extracellular domain and has been demonstrated using cRNA injection into *Xenopus* oocytes to serve as a receptor for calcium in that it can recognize extracellular calcium in physiologic concentrations and can couple extracellular calcium signals to appropriate intracellular signals. The gene encoding the calcium receptor has been localized to chromosome 3q.

Transcriptional and Posttranscriptional Control PTH gene transcription is subject to both positive and negative regulation primarily through the combined regulatory effects of serum calcium concentration and of $1,25(OH)_2D$, the active form of vitamin D. Reductions in serum calcium and reductions in circulating $1,25(OH)_2D$ lead to activation of PTH gene transcription. Conversely, increases in serum calcium and in circulating $1,25(OH)_2D$ inhibit PTH gene transcription. These effects occur during a period of hours to days and are viewed as being important in the long-term or tonic regulation of PTH secretion.

From: *Principles of Molecular Medicine* (J. L. Jameson, ed.), ©1998 Humana Press Inc., Totowa, NJ.

PTH Biosynthesis PTH synthesis requires translation of the PTH mRNA on ribosomes, entry of the nascent preproPTH into the cistern of the endoplasmic reticulum (ER), cleavage of the signal peptide cotranslationally by signal peptidase on the lumenal side of the ER, passage of the immature peptide through the lamellae of the Golgi apparatus, targeting of the peptide into the secretory granules of the regulated secretory pathway, and cleavage of the "pro" segment of the peptide, presumably within the Golgi compartment. In addition, the quantity of stored hormone within secretory granules appears to be subject to regulation through degradation of mature PTH within secretory granules or within phagolysosomes, a process referred to as "crinophagy."

Control of Secretion During the short term, PTH secretion is regulated by the serum ionized calcium concentration. Changes in serum calcium concentration lead to immediate (minutes) and opposite changes in PTH secretion. The key features of this acute regulation appear to be those observed in other neuroendocrine peptide secretory systems (i.e., storage of preformed, completely processed hormone in dense core secretory granules, with secretory granule fusion to the cell membrane leading to immediate secretion) with one important difference: in most neuroendocrine cell types, fusion of secretory granules with the cell membrane is triggered by an increase in cytosolic calcium. The reverse is true in the parathyroid. The cellular mechanisms governing this inverse secretion–stimulus coupling in the parathyroid gland are incompletely understood.

FAMILIAL HYPOCALCIURIC HYPERCALCEMIA AND NEONATAL SEVERE HYPERPARATHYROIDISM

Familial hypocalciuric hypercalcemia (FHH, also referred to as familial benign hypercalcemia or FBH) is a disorder that is typically discovered incidentally on routine serum calcium screening. The hypercalcemia is usually mild (i.e., in the 10.5–12.0 mg/dL range), is lifelong, is generally not associated with the symptoms of hypercalcemia, and is associated with a reduction in the urinary excretion of calcium. Historically, patients with FHH were confused with patients with primary hyperparathyroidism, with the unfortunate consequence that affected patients underwent unsuccessful partial parathyroidectomy or complete parathyroidectomy with the development of surgical hypoparathyroidism. Since the initial description of the

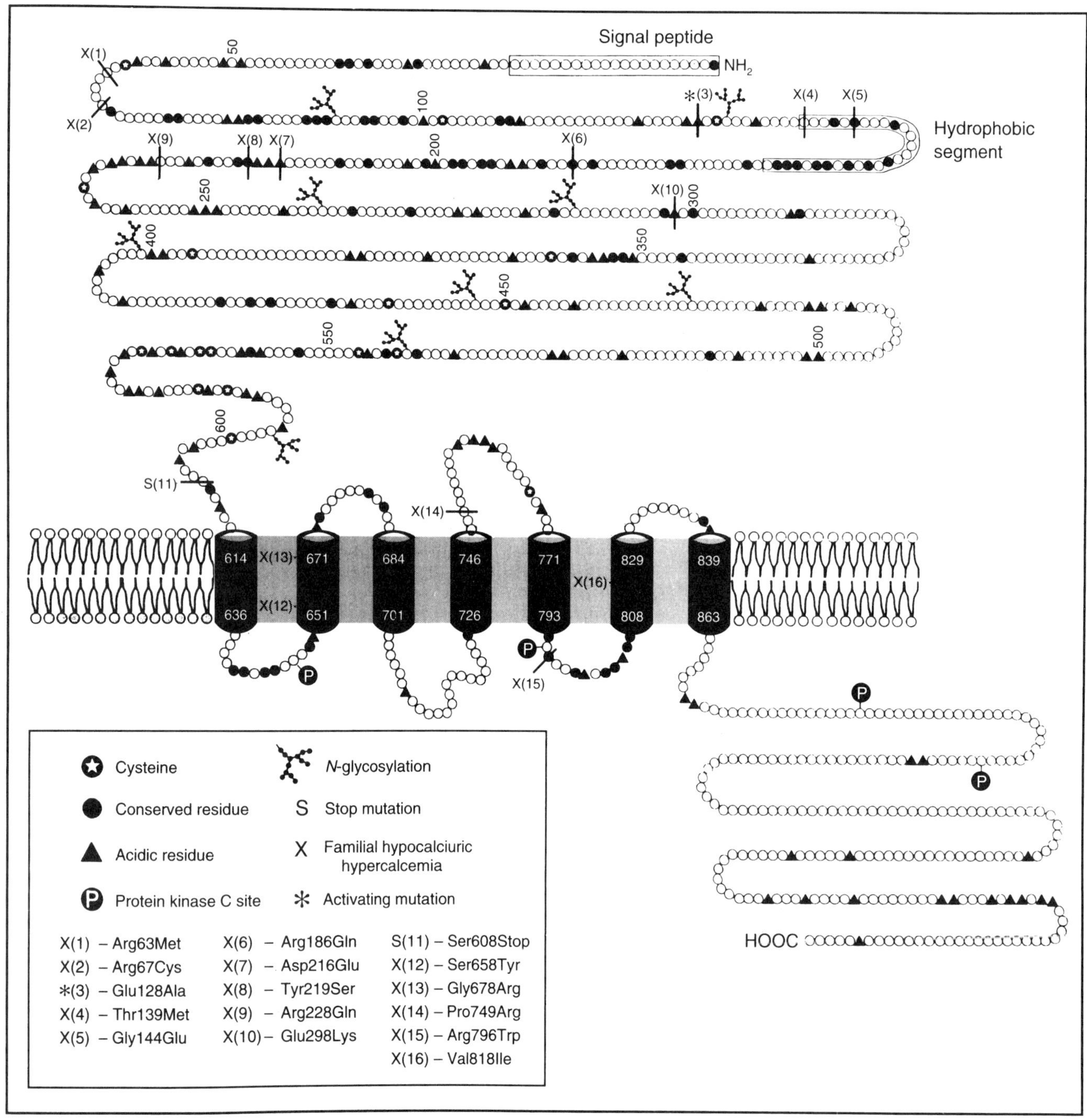

Figure 51-1 The structure of the calcium receptor. This figure shows the structure of the bovine calcium receptor or sensor. The important structural features are the seven putative transmembrane-spanning domains, the extracellular amino-terminal domain, and the cytoplasmic carboxy-terminus. As can be seen from the key within the figure, both activating (causing hypoparathyroidism) and inactivating (causing familial hypocalciuric hypercalcemia) mutations can occur. (Reproduced with permission from Brown et al. N Engl J Med 1995;333:234–240.)

syndrome in the 1970s, it has become clear that these patients do have a mild form of primary hyperparathyroidism with slightly elevated or inappropriately normal serum PTH concentrations, that they have inappropriately efficient renal reabsorption of calcium, that the parathyroid glands appear to have a defective ability to sense the hypercalcemia, and that multiple family members are typically involved, usually in an autosomal dominant fashion.

Recently, several groups have demonstrated that inherited inactivating mutations in the parathyroid cell surface calcium receptor appear to be responsible for the features of the syndrome in most affected kindreds (Fig. 51-1). The responsible mutations generally involve either the extracellular domain (presumably adversely influencing calcium binding to the receptor) or one of the transmembrane loops (presumably interfering with conformational changes that in turn lead to the activation of signal transduction pathways). In general, affected patients have been heterozygous for the mutant calcium receptor allele. Interestingly, however, infants have been described who appear to have a particularly malignant form of the syndrome, characterized by severe hypercalcemia (sometimes in the 20-mg/dL range) and prominent parathyroid hypercellularity. This form of the syndrome has been referred to as neonatal severe hyperparathyroidism (NSHPT). The syndrome in some of these infants has now been reported to result from a double dose of the mutant, inactivated calcium receptor gene, events that resulted in turn from consanguineous parentage.

In support of the concept that inactive mutant forms of the calcium receptor are responsible for the syndrome, it has been reported that expression in *Xenopus* oocytes of calcium receptors containing the same mutations as those encountered in humans with the disease results in impaired ability to sense extracellular calcium Also, an FHH-like phenotype is found in mice whose extracellular calcium receptor gene has been heterozygously knocked out, and a more severe phenotype similar to NSHPT is seen in mice with no functional copy of the gene. At the time of this writing, 15 mutations have been described in the calcium receptor in families with FHH (Fig. 51-1). In addition, other FHH families who map to the 3q region have been defined that do not display mutations in the coding region of the calcium receptor gene. These findings suggest that mutations in the intronic or regulatory regions of the calcium receptor gene may explain additional kindreds. Further, it is important to note that mutations in other genes will undoubtedly be demonstrated in the future; for some families with what appears to be standard FHH, the disease locus maps to chromosome 19p or other locations distinct from chromosomes 19 or 3. It is presumed that the genes at these other loci encode other proteins that play a role in the calcium sensing machinery.

HEREDITARY FORMS OF HYPOPARATHYROIDISM

The majority of patients with hypoparathyroidism have surgical or acquired autoimmune hypoparathyroidism. In contrast to these acquired forms of hypoparathyroidism, familial forms of congenital and acquired hypoparathyroidism have been described. These can be subdivided into familial syndromes in which hypoparathyroidism is accompanied by abnormalities in multiple other organ systems, and familial forms of hypoparathyroidism that are unaccompanied by other abnormalities (Table 51-1). These various syndromes are discussed below.

FAMILIAL VARIETIES OF HYPOPARATHYROIDISM ASSOCIATED WITH MULTIPLE ORGAN SYSTEM ABNORMALITIES These syndromes are of interest in that they represent genetic syndromes associated with hypoparathyroidism, but given their multisystem abnormalities, it is intuitive that the parathyroid gland abnormalities are not intrinsic to defects within the parathyroid gland but are in some fashion secondary to other developmental or regulatory abnormalities.

Hypoparathyroidism Associated With the Polyglandular Failure Syndrome This syndrome is composed of at least two subtypes. Hypoparathyroidism is most often associated with the pediatric variant of the syndrome, termed the HAM syndrome, an acronym for the hypoparathyroidism, Addison's disease, mucocutaneous candidiasis syndrome. The syndrome is an autoimmune disease that is associated with autoimmune destruction of the parathyroid glands and the adrenal glands, and is coupled with T-cell abnormalities that lead to mucocutaneous candidiasis. It is inherited in an autosomal recessive fashion, and is linked to chromosome 21q22.3. Circulating antibodies directed against parathyroid surface antigens have been difficult to demonstrate. One recent preliminary report suggests that a cell surface target of circulating autoimmune antisera in some affected patients is the calcium receptor.

Table 51-1
Hereditary Forms of Hypoparathyroidism

Familial hypoparathyroidism associated with multiple organ system abnormalities
Polyglandular failure type I or HAM syndrome
DiGeorge syndrome
Renal dysgenesis/sensorineural deafness syndromes
Autosomal recessive
Autosomal dominant
Isolated familial hypoparathyroidism syndromes
X-linked hypoparathyroidism
Autosomal recessive syndromes
PTH gene intron splice site mutation
Others
Autosomal dominant syndromes
Parathyroid hormone signal peptide mutation
Constitutively activating calcium receptor mutations
Others

The DiGeorge Syndrome The DiGeorge syndrome (*see* Chapter 120) is a complex of developmental disorders centered on the third and fourth branchial pouches that includes: (1) cardiac and conotruncal defects (such as ventricular septal defects, tetralogy of Fallot); (2) T-cell deficiency as a result of partial or incomplete development of the thymus gland; (3) craniofacial abnormalities; and (4) partial or complete hypoparathyroidism as a result of congenital absence or hypoplasia of the parathyroid glands. It may occur in both sporadic and inherited forms. The pattern of inheritance in the latter is consistent with an autosomal dominant mode of transmission. The vast majority of inherited and sporadic cases display deletions or translocations in the 22q11 region. The broad spectrum of abnormalities in patients with the DiGeorge syndrome together with the large region of DNA typically affected by these deletions and rearrangements suggests that defects in multiple adjacent genes at 22q11 may collectively account for the abnormalities observed. Candidate genes include *DGCR2/LAN*, which appears to encode a membrane-bound adhesion molecule; the *CTP* (human citrate transporter protein) gene; and *DGCR3*, which encodes what appears to be a DNA-binding protein. The last of these is particularly interesting for it appears to span the region of a 22q11 rearrangement breakpoint, and therefore its disruption seems likely to be functionally important.

Hypoparathyroidism Associated With Renal Dysgenesis and Sensorineural Hearing Loss This syndrome has been reported by several groups. Both autosomal dominant and autosomal recessive patterns of inheritance have been described. Linkage studies defining chromosomal locations for the putative responsible gene or genes have not been described.

FAMILIAL ISOLATED HYPOPARATHYROIDISM In contrast to the syndromes described above, several forms of familial hypoparathyroidism have been described in which hypoparathyroidism is the sole abnormality. These syndromes will certainly prove to represent a group of several disorders with differing molecular pathogenesis. Some are still poorly defined in molecular terms such as most autosomal recessive forms of the disorder and certain autosomal dominant forms. Others are partially defined in molecular terms, such as the X-linked form of the syndrome, which has recently been mapped to the Xq26–q27 region. Still others, including an autosomal dominant form, are well-understood in genetic and biochemical terms. In this situa-

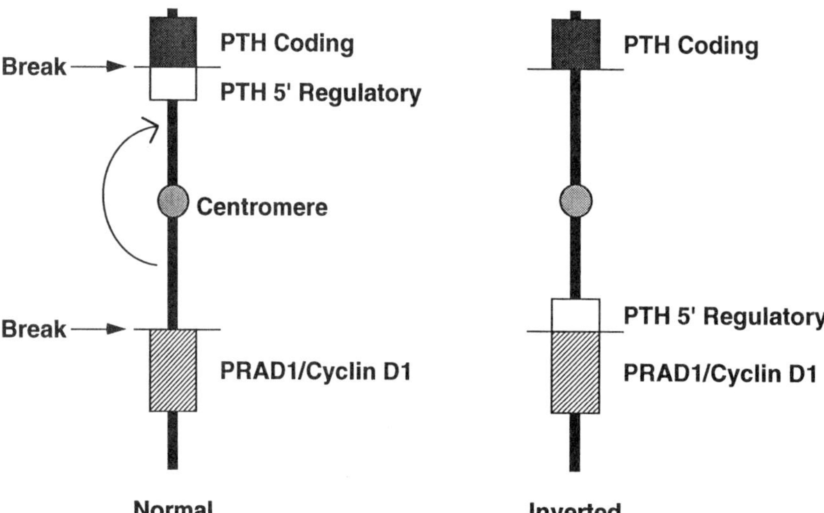

Figure 51-2 Schematic diagram illustrating the pericentromeric inversion of chromosome 11 deduced to have caused the observed rearrangement involving the *PTH* gene and the *PRAD1* gene in a subset of parathyroid adenomas. The tumor's other copy of chromosome 11, which contains an intact *PTH* gene, is not shown. (Reproduced with permission from Arnold A. Genetic basis of endocrine disease 5: molecular genetics of parathyroid gland neoplasia. J Clin Endocrinol Metab 1993;77:1108-1112.)

tion hypoparathyroidism results from a mutation that causes a Cys to Arg substitution in the middle of the hydrophobic core of preproPTH's signal peptide. The resultant mutant form of preproPTH is unable to be processed with normal efficiency. One curious aspect of this disorder is the question as to why a disabling mutation in only one allele of the PTH gene should lead to hypoparathyroidism. It is possible that accumulation of bound but poorly processed mutant preproPTH molecules in the endoplasmic reticulum might deny access of the normal allele's product to the processing apparatus, or otherwise interfere with the function of the parathyroid cell. Interestingly, this preproPTH mutation was the first signal peptide mutation reported to cause human disease, and signal peptide mutations have subsequently been found in preprovasopressin (causing diabetes insipidus) and in Factor X (causing a coagulopathy).

A family has been described with autosomal recessive hypoparathyroidism that appears to be caused by a splice junction mutation in intron 2 of the PTH gene. The resulting mRNA would have the sequences derived from exon 2, which contains the signal peptide, spliced out, and thereby lead to the production of a PTH species that could not enter the secretory pathway.

Recently, another mechanism underlying familial isolated hypoparathyroidism has been described. With the demonstration that familial hypocalciuric hypercalcemia may result from inactivating mutations in the extracellular calcium-sensing receptor (discussed above), it was logical to speculate that some cases of hereditary hypoparathyroidism might result from activating mutations in the calcium receptor. This type of syndrome has now been reported (Fig. 51-1). As would be expected, this kindred displays an autosomal dominant pattern of inheritance, and expression of the mutant calcium receptor in oocytes leads to constitutive activation of the inositol phosphate signal transduction pathway. The host parathyroid cell, therefore, behaves as though it were being exposed to higher than normal concentration of extracellular calcium and appropriately fails to secrete PTH. Similar mutations have also been identified in cases of sporadic hypoparathyroidism.

MOLECULAR GENETICS OF PARATHYROID GLAND NEOPLASIA

Primary hyperparathyroidism is caused by excessive secretion of PTH, resulting in hypercalcemia. Patients with primary hyperparathyroidism have both an excessive parathyroid cell mass and a resetting of the setpoint by which PTH secretion is tightly coupled to the parathyroid cell's ambient calcium level. In the large majority (>80%) of patients with primary hyperparathyroidism, a single benign parathyroid tumor (adenoma) is responsible, whereas multiple hypercellular glands are present in about 15% (primary hyperplasia). Parathyroid carcinoma is extremely rare, as is the ectopic secretion of PTH from nonparathyroid tumors. A comprehensive molecular description of parathyroid tumorigenesis will eventually need to fully explain the development of these types of tumors, as well as a variety of other special features such as the increased incidence of parathyroid tumors after exposure to neck irradiation and the disease's epidemiologic weighting toward postmenopausal women. Detailed molecular understanding will likely yield information of diagnostic, prognostic, preventative, or therapeutic importance, and recent progress gives cause for optimism in this regard.

CLONALITY IN PARATHYROID TUMORIGENESIS The monoclonality or polyclonality of human tumors is an informative reflection of their underlying pathogenetic mechanism. Early data measuring isoforms of the X-chromosome-encoded protein G6PD in parathyroid adenomas in heterozygous women had indicated that apparently single parathyroid adenomas were polyclonal growths, likely to result solely from a generalized growth stimulus. These results, however, proved to be misleading, since modern molecular methods have now solidly established the monoclonality of typical parathyroid adenomas, both by X-chromosome inactivation analysis and by the direct demonstration of monoclonal genetic alterations in parathyroid adenomas *(see below)*. Monoclonality highlights the concept that parathyroid adenomas are true neoplasms, consistent with clinical experience that surgical removal of the enlarged gland is generally curative. Neoplasia is a genetic disease, with most relevant DNA damage occurring somati-

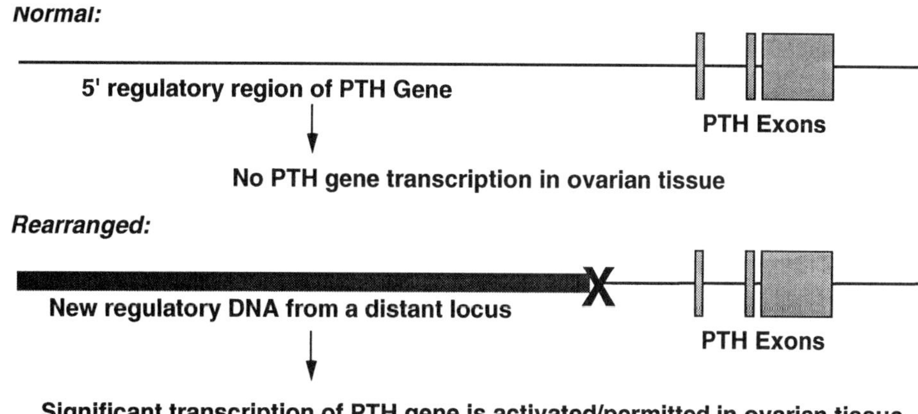

Figure 51-3 Molecular pathology of the ectopic production of PTH by an ovarian cancer. Schematic diagram of the normal PTH gene region (top) and the rearranged, amplified PTH gene region (bottom) in a PTH-secreting ovarian tumor. The bold **"X"** represents the breakpoint of the DNA rearrangement. (Reproduced with permission from Arnold A. Genetic basis of endocrine disease 5: molecular genetics of parathyroid gland neoplasia. J Clin Endocrinol and Metab 1993;77:1108–1112.)

cally. Monoclonality implies that the necessary accumulation of multiple mutations in a tumor progenitor cell occurs only rarely in a large population of cells within a tissue, conferring a selective growth advantage critical in tumor outgrowth or clonal evolution. The search is now on for the specific oncogenes and tumor suppressor genes that are clonally activated or inactivated, respectively, in parathyroid tumors. Two notable successes and several important leads, described below, have already emerged in this search.

The clonal status of parathyroid tumors other than adenomas has also been investigated. As expected, parathyroid carcinomas, like all cancers, are monoclonal. Much more surprisingly, however, a substantial percentage of parathyroid tumors in the setting of primary hyperplasia and severe secondary hyperparathyroidism of uremia has recently been shown to be monoclonal, indicating that clonal somatic mutations have given selected cells a growth advantage over their already hyperplastic neighbors. Monoclonality in the majority of MEN-1–associated parathyroid tumors examined suggests a similar process in this syndrome. It is quite conceivable that the "conversion" from polyclonality to monoclonality may be a key factor in the increasing autonomy of PTH secretion that develops in many hemodialysis patients, making them refractory to standard medical therapy. Future identification of the specific molecular culprits in such clonal outgrowths may lead to rational new therapy or preventative measures for this important clinical problem.

GENETIC DERANGEMENTS IN BENIGN PARATHYROID TUMORS

THE CYCLIN *D1/PRAD1* ONCOGENE Cyclin *D1/PRAD1*, to date the only oncogene implicated in sporadic parathyroid neoplasia, was discovered by virtue of its proximity to a clonal chromosomal breakpoint in a subset of parathyroid adenomas. Fig. 51-2 is a diagram of this chromosomal inversion, which causes overexpression of the cyclin *D1/PRAD1* gene by placing it in proximity to the strong tissue-specific enhancer of the *PTH* gene.

Cyclin *D1/PRAD1* is recognized to have a crucial role in regulating progression through the G1 phase of the cell division cycle. To do so, the cyclin D1 protein is believed to act as an activating regulatory subunit for its partner cyclin-dependent kinase(s), cdk4 or cdk6. One action of active cdk4 or cdk6 may be phosphorylation of the retinoblastoma gene product pRB, moving the cell toward S phase, but this mechanism has not yet been established in parathyroid tissue. A still-uncertain fraction of parathyroid adenomas contain an activated form of the cyclin *D1/PRAD1* oncogene; one recent study showed overexpression of the cyclin D1 protein in about 20% of adenomas. Cyclin D1 activation has also been incriminated in a variety of other human tumors, including B-cell lymphoma, breast, and esophageal cancers.

PUTATIVE TUMOR SUPPRESSOR GENES Inactivation of both alleles of a tumor suppressor gene is typically necessary to sufficiently eliminate its antioncogenic product, and somatic deletion of a sometimes large stretch of DNA that includes the relevant gene is a common inactivating mechanism. Thus, identification of genomic regions that are clonally and nonrandomly lost in parathyroid adenomas can point to the locations of putative parathyroid tumor suppressor genes. A growing proportion, now more than 70%, of parathyroid adenomas can be shown to bear at least one such clonal chromosomal defect.

The most common molecular defect described to date in parathyroid tumors is allelic loss on chromosome arm 1p, found in about 40% of adenomas; the putative tumor suppressor gene in this region has not yet been isolated. About 25% of adenomas contain allelic losses of chromosome 11 DNA, the region to which the *MEN-1* gene has been mapped. The gene responsible for *MEN-1* has been cloned using positional cloning techniques. The gene product, menin, is a 610-amino acid protein that lacks both a signal sequence and nuclear localization signal. Mutations in the affected individuals predict loss of function of the protein, suggesting that the *MEN-1* gene is a tumor suppressor gene. In a recent study of parathyroid tumors not associated with MEN-1, somatic mutations in *MEN-1* were present in 4 of 24 adenomas. All of the tumors with mutations in *MEN-1* exhibited loss of heterozygosity on 11q13 at the *MEN-1* locus. Thus, the tumors were hemizygous for the mutant allele. Still other regions of nonrandom clonal allelic loss in parathyroid adenomas, highlighting the locations of novel tumor suppressor genes, have been found on chromosome arms 1q, 6q, 9p, and 15q. These data emphasize the molecular heterogeneity underlying parathyroid adenomatosis.

OTHER GENETIC ASPECTS Some genes responsible for rare inherited predispositions to certain tumors have also proved important in more common, sporadic forms of the same tumors. The *MEN-1* gene, as mentioned above, is an example. The recent discovery of *Ret* proto-oncogene germline mutation in MEN-2A made this gene a candidate for involvement in nonfamilial hyperparathyroidism. However, studies have so far failed to document somatic *Ret* mutations in sporadic parathyroid adenomas. Similarly, inactivating mutations of the extracellular calcium-sensing receptor have been sought but not found in sporadic adenomas. It remains possible that somatic mutation in other genes involved in the calcium-sensing pathway may contribute to adenoma development, with the primary clonal setpoint defect driving the proliferative response. Finally, the gene responsible for an autosomal dominant predisposition to recurrent parathyroid adenomas and benign jaw tumors has been mapped to the long arm of chromosome 1; its ultimate identification may also provide insight into more common forms of hyperparathyroidism.

MOLECULAR PATHOGENESIS OF PARATHYROID CARCINOMA

The discovery that the cell-cycle regulator cyclin *D1*/PRAD1 can be involved in parathyroid tumorigenesis has raised the possibility that other cell-cycle regulatory genes may also contribute to parathyroid neoplasia. One example, the *RB* tumor suppressor gene implicated in retinoblastoma and a narrow spectrum of often aggressive malignancies, may be a key factor in the pathogenesis of many parathyroid carcinomas, although a neighboring gene on 13q might be the target of the frequent DNA deletions in this region. Genetic lesions that are confirmed to be enriched in malignant as opposed to benign parathyroid tumors could be clinically useful in molecular diagnosis, given the difficulties in making such distinctions histopathologically.

ECTOPIC SECRETION OF PTH

The ectopic secretion of PTH by nonparathyroid tumors is a rare cause of primary hyperparathyroidism. The molecular basis of ectopic PTH production in one such case, an ovarian carcinoma, was found to be a DNA rearrangement in the regulatory region of the tumor's PTH gene (Fig. 51-3). Similar detailed molecular pathology has yet to be described in other examples of human ectopic hormone excess, and might involve analogous DNA rearrangements or, alternatively, a change in the tumor tissue's characteristic DNA-binding proteins.

SELECTED REFERENCES

Aaltonen J, Bjorses P, Sandkuijl L, Perheentupa J, Peltonen L. An autosomal locus causing autoimmune disease: autoimmune polyglandular disease type I assigned to chromosome 21. Nat Genet 1994;8:83–87.

Agarwal SK, Kester MB, Debelenko LV, et al. Germline mutations of the MEN1 gene in familial multiple endocrine neoplasia type 1 and related states. Hum Mol Genet 1997;6:1169–1175.

Ahn TG, Antonarakis SE, Kronenberg HM, Igarashi T, Levine MA. Familial isolated hypoparathyroidism: a molecular genetic analysis of 8 families with 23 affected persons. Medicine 1986;65:73–81.

Arnold A. The cyclin D1/PRAD1 oncogene in human neoplasia. J Invest Med 1995;43:543–549.

Arnold A. Genetic basis of endocrine disease 5: molecular genetics of parathyroid gland neoplasia. J Clin Endocrinol Metab 1993;77:1108–1112.

Arnold A, Brown MF, Urena P, Gaz RD, Sarfati E, Drueke TB. Monoclonality of parathyroid tumors in chronic renal failure and in primary parathyroid hyperplasia. J Clin Invest 1995;95:2047–2053.

Arnold A, Horst SA, Gardella TJ, Baba H, Levine MA, Kronenberg HM. Mutation of the signal peptide-encoding region of the preproparathyroid hormone gene in familial isolated hypoparathyroidism. J Clin Invest 1990;86:1084–1087.

Baron J, Winer KK, Yanovski JA, et al. Mutations in the Ca (2+)-sensing receptor gene cause autosomal dominant and sporadic hypoparathyroidism. Hum Mol Genet 1996;5:601–606.

Bilous RW, Murty G, Parkinson DB, et al. Brief report: autosomal dominant familial hypoparathyroidism, sensorineural deafness, and renal dysplasia. N Engl J Med 1992;327:1069–1074.

Bjorses P, Aaltonen J, Vikman A, et al. Genetic homogeneity of autoimmune polyglandular disease type I. Am J Hum Genet 1996;59:879–886.

Brown EM, Gamba G, Riccardi D, et al. Cloning and characterization of an extracellular Ca^{2+}-sensing receptor from bovine parathyroid. Nature 1993;366:575–580.

Brown EM, Pollak M, Seidman CE, et al. Calcium-sensing cell-surface receptors. N Engl J Med 1995;333:234–240.

Budarf ML, Collins J, Gong W, et al. Cloning a balanced translocation associated with DiGeorge syndrome and identification of a disrupted candidate gene. Nat Genet 1995;10:269–278.

Chandrasekharappa SC, Guru SC, Manickam P, et al. Positional cloning of the gene for multiple endocrine neoplasia-type 1. Science 1997;276: 404–407.

Cryns VL, Yi SM, Tahara H, Gaz RD, Arnold A. Frequent loss of chromosome arm 1p DNA in parathyroid adenomas. Genes Chromosomes Cancer 1995;13:9–17.

Dotzenrath C, The BT, Farnebo F, et al. Allelic loss of the retinoblastoma tumor suppressor gene: a marker for aggressive parathyroid tumors? J Clin Endocrinol Metab 1996;81:3194–3196.

De Luca F, Ray K, Mancilla EE, et al. Sporadic hypoparathyroidism caused by *de novo* gain-of-function mutations of the Ca^{2+}-sensing receptor. J Clin Endocrinol Metab 1997;82:2710–2715.

Glover TW. CATCHing a break on 22. Nat Genet 1995;20:257,258.

Heppner C, Kester MB, Agarwal SK, et al. Somatic mutation of the MEN1 gene in parathyroid tumours. Nat Genet 1997;16:375–378.

Ho C, Conner DA, Pollak MR, et al. A mouse model of human familial hypocalciuric hypercalcemia and neonatal severe hyperparathyroidism. Nat Genet 1995;11:389–394.

Kronenberg HM, Bringhurst FR, Segre GV, Potts JT. Parathyroid hormone biosynthesis and metabolism. In: Bilezikian JP, Marcus R, Levine MA, eds. The Parathyroids. New York; Raven, 1994; pp. 125–138.

Li Y, Song YH, Rais N, et al. Autoantibodies to the extracellular domain of the calcium sensing receptor in patients with acquired hypoparathyroidism. J Clin Invest 1996;15:910–914.

Motokura T, Bloom T, Kim HG, et al. A novel cyclin encoded by a *bcl1*-linked candidate oncogene. Nature 1991;350:512–515.

Parkinson DB, Thakker RV. A donor splice site mutation in the parathyroid hormone gene is associated with autosomal recessive hypoparathyroidism. Nat Genet 1992;1:149–153.

Pearce SH, Williamson C, Kifor O, et al. A familial syndrome of hypocalcemia with hypercalciuria due to mutations in the calcium-sensing receptor. N Engl J Med 1996;10:1115–1122.

Pollak MR, Brown EM, Chou Y-HW, et al. Mutations in the human Ca^{2+}-sensing receptor gene cause familial hypocalciuric hypercalcemia and neonatal severe hyperparathyroidism. Cell 1993;75:1297–1303.

Pollak MR, Brown EM, Estep HL, et al. Autosomal dominant hypocalcaemia caused by a Ca^{2+}-sensing receptor gene mutation. Nat Genet 1994;8:303–307.

Potts JT, Bringhurst FR, Gardella T, Nussbaum S, Segre GV, Kronenberg HM. Parathyroid hormone: physiology, chemistry, biosynthesis, secretion, metabolism, and mode of action. In: DeGroot LJ, ed. Endocrinology, 3rd ed. Philadelphia: WB Saunders, 1995; pp. 920–966.

Thakker RV. Molecular genetics of hypoparathyroidism. In: Bilezikian JP, Marcus R, Levine MA, eds. The Parathyroids. New York: Raven, 1994; pp. 765–779.

Szabo J, Heath B, Hill VM, et al. Hereditary hyperparathyroidism-jaw tumor syndrome: the endocrine tumor gene HRPT2 maps to chromosome 1q21–q31. Am J Hum Genet 1995;56:944–950.

52 Congenital Adrenal Hyperplasia

ROBERT C. WILSON AND MARIA I. NEW

INTRODUCTION

The disorder congenital adrenal hyperplasia (CAH) is an autosomal recessive disease caused by mutations in genes that encode enzymes involved in various steps of adrenal steroid synthesis (Table 52-1). These defects result in the absence or decreased synthesis of cortisol from cholesterol. The anterior pituitary secretes excess adrenocorticotrophic hormone (ACTH) because of the loss of feedback regulation by cortisol, which results in overstimulation of the adrenals and causes hyperplasia.

Symptoms caused by CAH can vary from mild to severe depending on the degree of the enzymatic defect. In the classic forms of CAH, defects in the cytochrome P450 21-hydroxylase (21-OH) or 11β-hydroxylase (11β-OH) cause varying degrees of genital ambiguity in females owing to shunting of excess cortisol precursors to the androgen synthesis pathway (Fig. 52-1). Prenatal adrenal androgen excess causes virilization of female genitalia and postnatally results in advanced bone age and puberty in both females and males. Abnormalities in androgen synthesis as a result of defects in 3β-hydroxysteroid dehydrogenase (3β-HSD)–Δ^5, 4-isomerase, in 17α-hydroxylase (17α-OH)/17,20-lyase, and in the steroidogenic acute regulatory protein (StAR) result in inadequate prenatal virilization of males and depressed puberty in both sexes. Less severe, nonclassic forms of CAH present postnatally as signs of androgen excess.

ADRENAL STEROIDOGENESIS

Aldosterone, cortisol (compound F), and testosterone are derived from cholesterol and use many of the same enzymes for their synthesis in the adrenal cortex (Fig. 52-1). Therefore, defects in any of the enzymes that are common to the synthesis pathway of these hormones can result in the loss of a combination of some or all of these products.

Cortisol and aldosterone are synthesized in distinct zones of the adrenal cortex called the zona fasciculata (ZF) and zona glomerulosa (ZG), respectively. In addition, regulation of cortisol and aldosterone synthesis is controlled by different mechanisms. Cortisol synthesis is regulated by a negative feedback loop in which high serum levels of cortisol inhibit the release of ACTH from the pituitary, whereas low serum levels of cortisol stimulate the release of ACTH. This defines the hypothalamo–pituitary–adrenal axis (Fig. 52-2).

From: *Principles of Molecular Medicine* (J. L. Jameson, ed.), ©1998 Humana Press Inc., Totowa, NJ.

Aldosterone is required for the regulation of sodium reabsorption across the tight epithelium of the renal distal tubule, which indirectly controls fluid volume. Aldosterone synthesis is regulated by the renin-angiotensin system and serum potassium. Angiotensin II (a potent vasoconstrictor) directly stimulates the secretion of aldosterone by the ZG when there is a reduction in renal perfusion because of an increase in plasma renin. Serum potassium also regulates the synthesis of aldosterone, though independently of volume status.

21-HYDROXYLASE DEFICIENCY

More than 90% of classic CAH is caused by 21-hydroxylase deficiency (21-OHD). The syndrome is divided into three forms: classic salt-wasting, classic simple virilizing, and nonclassic.

CLASSIC SIMPLE VIRILIZING Fetal adrenocortical function begins in the third month of gestation. At this time reduction or loss of 21-hydroxylase activity will result in the build-up of 17α-hydroxyprogesterone (17-OHP). Because 17-OHP is a precursor of testosterone, elevated levels of 17-OHP are shunted to the androgen pathway, thus producing excess androgens. This excess adrenal androgen production coincides with the time of sexual development of the fetus and will result in varying degrees of genital ambiguity in newborn females. In extreme cases, the urethra extends the full length of the phallus and cannot be distinguished from that of a normal male. In most cases, however, the excess androgens result in an enlarged clitoris with fusion of the labioscrotal folds; it can also result in a urogenital sinus. For these females, the internal genitalia are normal with normal development of ovaries and Müllerian structures.

Males affected with 21-OHD are born with normal genitalia. After birth, both females and males develop signs of androgen excess, such as precocious development of pubic and axillary hair, acne, phallic enlargement, rapid growth, and musculoskeletal development. Though initial growth in these patients is rapid, potential height is reduced and short adult stature results because of premature epiphyseal fusion. Diagnosis may be delayed in males, because the genital ambiguity that leads to diagnosis at birth in females is absent in males. Even if diagnosis is not delayed and adrenal androgen excess is controlled, patients do not generally achieve their target height.

CLASSIC SALT-WASTING Salt-wasting 21-OHD makes up approximately 75% of classic 21-OHD. Depending on the severity of the loss of 21-hydroxylase function, adrenal aldosterone secretion may not be sufficient for regulating sodium reabsorption by distal renal tubules. Patients with insufficient aldosterone can suf-

Table 52-1
Forms of Adrenal Hyperplasia

Deficiency	*Syndrome*	*Ambiguous genitalia*	*Postnatal virilization*	*Salt metabolism*	*Steroids increased*	*Steroids decreased*	*Chromosomal location*
Steroidogenic acute regulatory protein (StAR)	Lipoid hyperplasia	Males		No salt wasting	None	All	8p11.2
3β-Hydroxysteriod dehydrogenase	Classic	Males	Yes	Salt wasting	DHEA, 17-OH-pregnenolone	Aldo, T, cortisol	1p13.1
	Nonclassic	No	Yes	Normal	DHEA, 17-OH-pregnenolone	—	?
17α-Hydroxylase	—	Males	No	Hypertension	DOC, corticosterone	Cortisol, T	10q24-25
21-Hydroxylase	Salt wasting	Females	Yes	Salt wasting	17-OHP, Δ^4-A	Aldo, cortisol	6p21.3
	Simple virilizing	Females	Yes	Normal	17-OHP, Δ^4-A	Cortisol	6p21.3
	Nonclassic	No	Yes	Normal	17-OHP, Δ^4-A	—	6p21.3
11β-Hydroxylase	Classic	Females	Yes	Hypertension	DOC, 11-deoxycortisol	Cortisol, ± aldo	8q21-22
	Nonclassic	No	Yes	Normal	11-deoxycortisol, ± DOC	—	8q21-22
Corticosterone methyl oxidase type II	Salt wasting	No	No	Salt wasting	18-OH-corticosterone	Aldo	8q21-22

Aldo, aldosterone; T, testosterone; Δ^4-A, Δ^4-androstenedione; DHEA, dephydropeiandrosterone; DOC, 11-deoxycorticosterone; 17-OHP, 17α-hydroxyprogesterone.

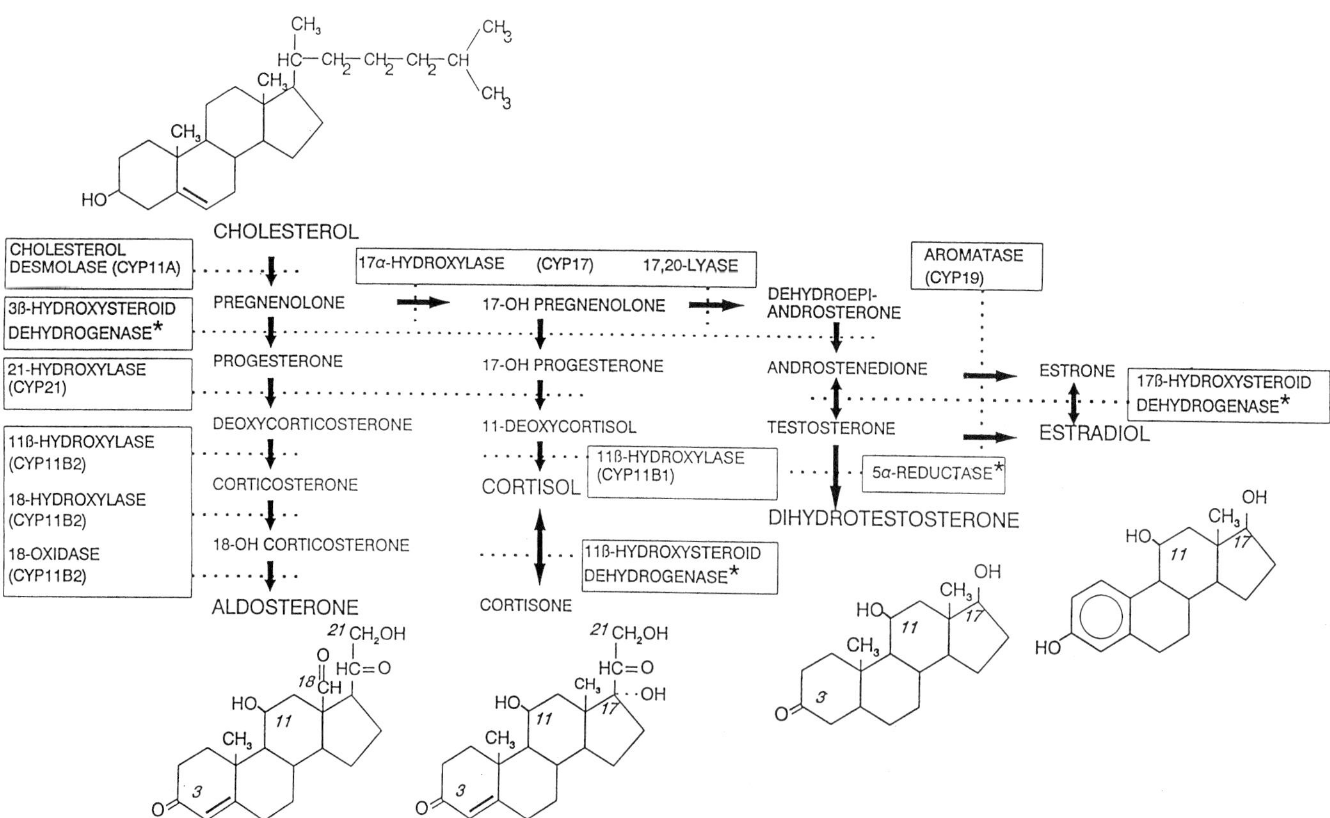

Figure 52-1 Pathways of steroid biosynthesis. Enzymatic activities catalyzing each bioconversion are enclosed in boxes. For those activities mediated by specific P450 cytochromes, systematic names of the enzymes (CYP followed by number) are listed in parentheses. Other bioconversions (marked with an asterisk) are mediated by different enzymes in various tissues. The planar structures of cholesterol, aldosterone, cortisol, dihydrotestosterone, and estradiol are placed near the corresponding labels.

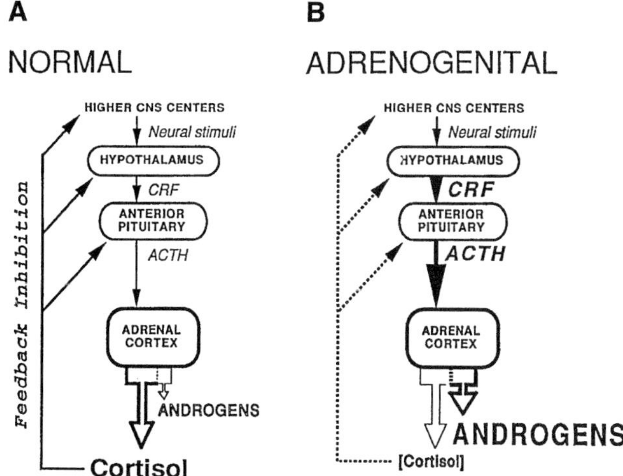

Figure 52-2 Feedback in the hypothalamic–pituitary–adrenal axis in **(A)** the normal individual and **(B)** the patient with classic congenital adrenal hyperplasia (CAH), formerly known as "adrenogenital syndrome."

fer from salt-wasting 21-OHD. These patients exhibit the same symptoms as those with simple virilizing 21-OHD but with the potential of adrenal crisis (azotemia, vascular collapse, shock, and death) because of renal salt-wasting. Adrenal crisis can occur as early as in the first 1–4 weeks of life. Although salt-wasting 21-OHD females may be diagnosed at birth because of ambiguous genitalia, affected males are at high risk of salt-wasting adrenal crisis since their normal genitalia do not make the condition obvious.

NONCLASSIC Nonclassic 21-OHD (NC21-OHD) may present at any time, in childhood, adolescence, or adulthood. Symptoms of NC21-OHD may be acne, premature development of pubic hair, advanced bone age, accelerated linear growth velocity, and as in classic 21-OHD, reduced adult stature as a result of premature epiphyseal fusion.

Females affected with NC21-OHD are born with normal genitalia, though postnatal symptoms may include hirsutism, temporal baldness, severe cystic acne, delayed menarche, menstrual irregularities, and infertility. A subset of female patients with NC21-OHD develop polycystic ovaries.

Boys manifesting NC21-OHD may have early beard growth, acne, early growth spurt, premature pubic hair, and an enlarged phallus. Proportionately small testes as compared with the size of the phallus is a reliable indication of adrenal androgen excess as opposed to testicular androgen excess. Adrenal androgen excess in men is not easily detectable and may only be manifested by short stature or oligozoospermia and diminished fertility.

No clinical signs are present in a limited number of males and females who are affected with NC21-OHD, as discovered during family studies. However, they are biochemically similar to affected patients.

EPIDEMIOLOGY The estimated worldwide frequency of classic 21-OHD is 1/13,000 live births. However, in two isolates the frequency is much higher (Yupik Eskimos in Alaska, 1/282, and the inhabitants of La Réunion island in France, 1/2141). Neonatal screening for 21-OHD has been initiated in 13 states in America.

It has been suggested that NC21-OHD is the most common autosomal recessive disorder. In some ethnic populations, the frequency of NC21-OHD is so high as to be the most frequent autosomal recessive defect. The disease frequency is 1/27 for Ashkenazi Jews, 1/53 for Hispanics, 1/63 for Yugoslavs, 1/100 in a heterogeneous white New York City population, and 1/333 for Italians.

MOLECULAR GENETICS In 1977, molecular genetic studies of 21-OHD showed linkage with certain human leukocyte antigens (HLA), in the human major histocompatibility complex, on the short arm of chromosome 6. For many years HLA linkage was used for establishing the affected status in family studies. However, in some cases in which the parents shared the same HLA antigens or if intra-HLA recombination occurred, HLA typing was not diagnostic.

It was not until 1984 that the gene for 21-hydroxylase was cloned. The gene for 21-hydroxylase is termed *CYP21*, after the nomenclature for cytochrome P450. Southern blot analysis determined that the *CYP21* gene was located within the serum complement component C4. This region of chromosome was duplicated, resulting in two isoforms of C4 (C4A and C4B) and what initially looked like two isoforms of *CYP21*. Sequence analysis of the two *CYP21* genes revealed that one of the isoforms contained a sequence that on translation would result in a truncated nonfunctional protein, and it was therefore termed *CYP21P* for pseudogene. The nonfunctionality of *CYP21P* was confirmed in families without any hormonal abnormalities in which the *CYP21P* gene was completely missing.

CYP21 and *CYP21P* are 96% to 98% homologous (Fig. 52-3) and are arranged in tandem within C4A and C4B, separated by approximately 30 kb. The duplication of the locus containing *CYP21* allows for misalignment of chromatids during meiosis, resulting in unequal crossing over. This results in a high frequency of deletions of the *CYP21* and *C4B* genes. Duplications also occur, but without any clinical consequence. Deletions of *CYP21* are found in approximately 20% of the patients with classic 21-OHD.

CYP21 and *CYP21P* consist of 10 exons spanning approximately 5 kb. Most of the 21-OHD patients carry mutations found in *CYP21P* (Fig. 52-4). The generally accepted mechanism by which these deleterious mutations are transferred to the active *CYP21* gene from the homologous position in *CYP21P* is through gene conversion. There are nine of these mutations that can be transferred to the active *CYP21* gene (Table 52-2). Four of these mutations result in truncated proteins as a result of premature termination of translation and are associated with the salt-wasting phenotype: (1) a point mutation in the second intron near the 3' splice site results in aberrant splicing 19 nucleotides upstream of the normal splice site; (2) in the third exon, an 8-base deletion can occur, resulting in nonsense amino acids and the occurrence of a stop codon 20 amino acids toward the carboxy-terminus; (3) in exon 7, one T nucleotide can be inserted into a run of seven T nucleotides, resulting in a frameshift that produces five aberrant amino acids and premature termination; and (4) a point mutation in exon 8 in codon 318 changes a glutamine to a stop codon. The five other mutations that can be transferred from *CYP21P* to *CYP21* result in amino acid substitutions: (1) A point mutation in exon 1 causes a substitution of proline by a leucine at codon 30 (P30L). This mutation has 60% of the activity of normal 21-hydroxylase when expressed in cell culture. The P30L mutation has been found to be associated with the nonclassic phenotype; (2) A point mutation in exon 4 causes a substitution of isoleucine by an asparagine at codon 172 (I172N) and is most often associated with the simple virilizing phenotype. This mutation results in less than 2% of normal 21-hydroxylase activity in in vitro expression studies; (3) A

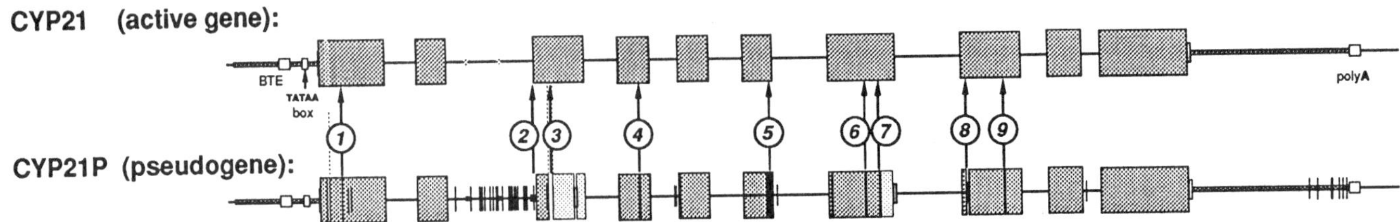

Figure 52-3 The two homologs: *CYP21* (the active gene) and *CYP21P* (the pseudogene). Noncorrespondent bases number less than 90 over a distance of 5.1 kb of DNA. Numbered are the pseudogene base changes that are frequently identified on mutant *CYP21* genes responsible for 21-hydroxylase deficiency through an apparent process termed gene conversion. (1) Missense mutation Pro-30 to Leu. (2) Point mutation in intron 2 causes new acceptor 3' site to be recognized by intron splicing mechanism. (3) Eight-basepair deletion shifts the reading frame. (4) Missense mutation Ile-172 to Asn. (5) Cluster of 3 nonconservative amino acid substitutions. (6) Conservative amino acid substitution Val-281 to Leu. (7) Single-base T insert shifts reading frame. (8) Nonsense mutation Gln to TAG. (9) Radical amino acid substitution (Arg-356 to Trp). KEY: BTE, basic transcriptional element; large boxes/line spaces, exons/introns (to scale); light shading, out-of-frame coding; half-height open boxes, stop codons; vertical lines not numbered, neutral amino acid polymorphisms; half-height vertical lines, silent mutations.

CYP21

7b. C to T transition at base 398--but may be neutral as it is 9 bases past splice site (may fall outside donor consensus sequence for this intron).

+

7. AA substitution at conserved position (four animal species): **Gly$_{291}$** to **Ser**.

SW

14b. AA substitution at non-conserved position: **Pro$_{105}$** to **Leu** (secondary).

+

14. AA substitution at conserved position: **Pro$_{453}$** to **Ser**.

NC

1. Missense mutation causing AA substitution **Pro$_{30}$** to **Leu**.

NC

4. AA substitution of lower hydrophobicity (destabilizes anchor in smooth ER membrane): **Ile$_{172}$** to **Asn**.

SV

6. AA substitution/helix-forming (change in folding slows insertion of heme group): **Val$_{281}$** to **Leu**.

NC

12. AA substitution: **Arg$_{356}$** to **Trp**.

SW/SV

11. AA substitution: **Arg$_{339}$** to **His**.

NC

2. Point mutation (A [var:C] to G) near end of intron activates cryptic acceptor site (AG pair just upstream) and the early splicing leaves 19 intronic bases in transcript: **aberrant 11 AA+ stop.**

SW/SV

14c. C to T transition at base position -4: corresponding C to U in mRNA may slightly slow start of translation (minor).

9. Point mutation G to C at beginning of intron 7: loss of GT dinucleotide (splicing donor site).

SW

13. Stop mutation: **Trp$_{405}$** to TAG

SW

SW

10. Stop mutation: **Gln$_{318}$** to TAG

SW

3. Deletion of 8 nt: frameshifted transcript following encodes **aberrant 20 AA + stop**.

(SW)

8. Single-base (T) insert in 7T run in codons 305-7: frameshift encodes **aberrant 5 AA + stop** after **Phe$_{306}$**.

SW

Codon 483. 15. Compound frameshifting mutation (GG to C) resulting in aberrant **56 AA sequence** (extends 45 AA beyond normal end of translation at codon 494). 16. G to C transversion*: AA substitution **Arg$_{483}$** to **Pro**. (*This could be the first step of a possible two-step process generating mutation 15.)

SW

5. Cluster of three point mutations in space of 10 bases causing three radical AA substitutions in region of protein with many charged residues:

Ile$_{236}$ (nonpolar) to **Asn** (polar/neutral)
Val$_{237}$ (nonpolar) to **Glu** (polar/negative)
Met$_{239}$ (nonpolar) to **Lys** (polar/positive).

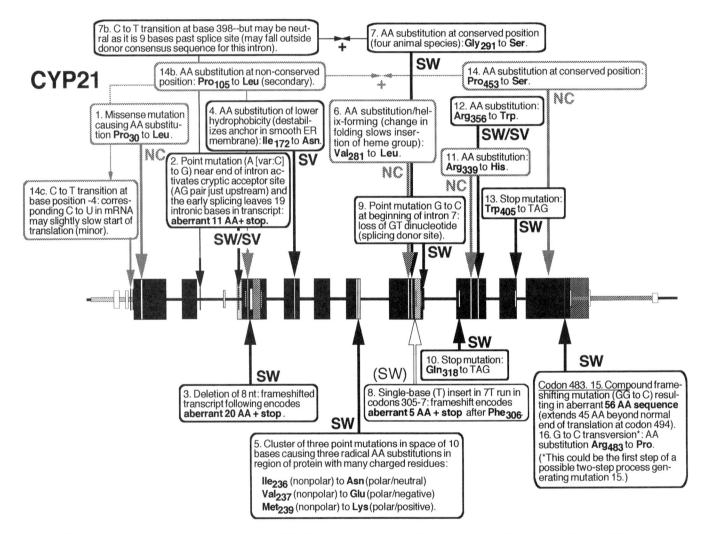

Figure 52-4 Mutations in the 21-hydroxylase gene *(CYP21)*. CAH phenotypes: SW, salt-wasting; SV, simple virilizing; NC, nonclassical.

cluster mutation in exon 6 as a result of the exchange of four nucleotides results in three amino acid substitutions and one polymorphism (the change codes for the original amino acid); (4) A point mutation in codon 281 substitutes a valine with a leucine (V281L). This mutation is associated with the nonclassic phenotype. Expression studies of the V281L mutation show 20–50% of normal 21-hydroxylase activity; and (5) A point mutation in exon 8 results in the substitution of arginine with tryptophan (R356W). This mutation is associated with the salt-wasting phenotype. Assignment of a phenotype to each of the individual mutations was done with patients that were either homozygous for the mutation or hemizygous for the mutation (the other allele had undergone a deletion). In addition to the nine mutations found in the pseudogene, several other mutations have been described in patients affected with 21-OHD.

HORMONAL DIAGNOSIS Baseline serum concentrations of 17-OHP are diagnostic of classic 21-OHD. The best method for hormonal diagnosis of 21-OHD is comparing baseline serum 17-OHP concentration and serum 17-OHP concentrations after adrenal stimulation by administration of synthetic ACTH (Cortrosyn). In NC21-OHD, diagnosis is made during the diurnal peak of cortisol production because serum 17-OHP concentrations are elevated, though random basal serum concentrations may not differ from that of normal. Nomogram plots of baseline vs stimulated 17-OHP concentrations result in three distinguishable groups (Fig. 52-5): Patients with classic 21-OHD have the highest coordinates, followed by patients with NC21-OHD, followed by plots of heterozygotes and genetically unaffected individuals, which overlap and cannot be distinguished.

Newborn diagnostic screening for classic 21-OHD has been instituted in about 12 states. Blood from a heel-prick is spotted onto filter paper and is tested for 17-OHP levels by radioimmunoassay. NC21-OHD can also be screened by measuring morning salivary 17-OHP, which correlates well with serum concentrations. It should be noted that serum 17-OHP may be elevated in premature infants and infants under stress, which can result in false-positive results.

PRENATAL DIAGNOSIS AND TREATMENT Prenatal diagnosis of 21-OHD has been performed for several decades. Originally, second trimester amniotic fluid was tested for elevated 17-OHP levels. However, in most cases when the fetus is a non–salt-waster (simple virilizer, or nonclassic), amniotic fluid 17-OHP levels are not elevated.

When HLA was found to be linked to 21-OHD, prenatal diagnoses using HLA serotyping of cultured fetal cells from amniocytes were performed. This procedure resulted in errors because of recombination or haplotype sharing between parents.

After mutations in the *CYP21* gene were found to be the cause of 21-OHD, prenatal diagnosis by direct molecular analysis was initiated. Fetal DNA is obtained from either cultured amniocytes or cultured cells obtained by chorionic villus sampling (CVS) and is used for specific amplification of the *CYP21* gene using the polymerase chain reaction (PCR). The PCR products are dot-blotted, followed by hybridization with radiolabeled allele-specific probes. However, this method is time consuming. We recently developed a method that only requires PCR with allele-specific primers, which reduces the time for prenatal diagnosis from about 2 weeks to only a few days, thus allowing unnecessary prenatal treatment to be terminated promptly *(see below)*.

It has been shown that the prenatal treatment (Fig. 52-6) of female fetuses affected with 21-OHD can greatly reduce or prevent virilization of external genitalia, preventing the need for later genital surgery. For this outcome, prenatal treatment must be initiated before 10 weeks of gestation. Dexamethasone (20 μg/kg) given orally to at-risk mothers, blind to the status of the fetus, suppresses fetal adrenal androgen secretion. Depending on which procedure is available, either CVS (10–12 weeks of gestation) or amniocentesis (15–18 weeks of gestation) is performed. Fetal cells are cultured for karyotyping and DNA analysis. If the fetus is male or the fetus is an unaffected female, prenatal treatment is terminated. Prenatal treatment is continued to term for affected female fetuses.

Prenatal treatment for the fetus with low doses of dexamethasone does not appear to have any side effects. Some patients have been followed in excess of 10 years of age without reported side effects. This is in spite of the findings in rodents that high doses of dexamethasone resulted in cleft palate formation *in utero* and placental degeneration with fetal death.

Maternal side effects as a result of prenatal dexamethasone treatment can include mood changes, weight gain, pedal and leg edema, striae, elevated blood pressure, and general discomfort. All complications disappeared on discontinuation of treatment, and because of the positive genital outcome of their prenatally treated daughters, all women with complications reported that they would undergo dexamethasone treatment again if they became pregnant. Therefore, the risk–benefit ratio is highly in favor of prenatal dexamethasone treatment of female fetuses affected with 21-OHD.

11β-HYDROXYLASE DEFICIENCY

Patients with 11β-hydroxylase deficiency (11β-OHD) are unable to convert 11-deoxycortisol (compound S) to cortisol. 11β-OHD is the second most common cause of CAH. The frequency of 11β-OHD is in the order of 1 in 100,000 births in the white population. As with 21-hydroxylase deficiency, cases of mild, late-onset forms of 11β-OHD also have been reported.

As in 21-OHD, 11β-OHD results in shunting of excess 17-OHP to the androgen pathway, causing prenatal virilization of external genitalia in affected females at birth. Also, as in 21-OHD, both males and females undergo premature virilization, resulting in precocious adrenarche and premature epiphyseal closure.

Patients with 11β-OHD also have a defective 17-deoxysteroid pathway. In 11β-OHD, 11-deoxycorticosterone (DOC) cannot be converted to corticosterone, which is eventually converted to aldosterone. In most cases, because of their mineralocorticoid activity, elevated serum levels of DOC and its metabolites induce hypokalemia with metabolic alkalosis and hypertension. High levels of serum S and DOC, and their corresponding urinary tetrahydrometabolites, are diagnostic of 11β-OHD.

MOLECULAR GENETICS There are two known isoforms of 11β-hydroxylase in humans. The genes that encode these isoforms are *CYP11B1* and *CYP11B2*, located on chromosome 8, region q21–22, and separated by 30 kb. These isozymes have 93% identity between their amino acid sequences. *CYP11B1* is highly expressed in all zones of the adrenal cortex and is regulated by ACTH. *CYP11B2* is expressed in the zona glomerulosa under the control of angiotensin II and potassium ion. Mutations in the *CYP11B1* gene are responsible for 11β-OHD.

Mutations in the *CYP11B2* gene cause a less frequently inherited disease (CMO II) in which aldosterone cannot be synthesized. This isoform is now termed aldosterone synthase. Aldosterone synthase, in addition to 11β-hydroxylase activity, also was found in vitro to have 18-hydroxylase and 18-oxidase activities.

CYP11B1 (11β-HYDROXYLASE) Mutations found in the *CYP11B1* gene causing 11β-OHD are shown in Fig. 52-7. The first mutation in the *CYP11B1* gene was found in families from Israel. A single point mutation in exon 8 was found in many of these families, resulting in a substitution of the arginine at codon 448 with a histidine. This mutation in these families was traced back to Moroccan Jewish settlements. A 2-base insert in exon 7 resulting in a frameshift was identified in a Turkish Jewish pedigree. This mutation completely altered the heme-binding domain,

Table 52-2
Steroidogenic Enzymes: Gene Mutation

Gene	*Exon*	*Mutation name/type*	*NT*	*AA*	*Comments*	
CYP21	1	Missense mutation (conversion)	CCG→CTG	P30L	Nonclassic (NC) phenotype	
	—	Aberrant splicing of intron 2 (conversion)	a [or c] →g	b656	Part of intron (end 19 bases) retained in mRNA processing: frameshift	Seen in more than 20% of nondeleted alleles
	3	Eight-base deletion (conversion)	(/G--) GAGACTAC (/T)	(Δ8)	Frameshift: 20-AA + stop	
	4	Missense mutation (conversion)	ATC→AAC	I172N	Affects anchoring in membrane	
	6	Cluster (conversion)	ATC→AAC	I236N		
			GTG→GAG	V237E#	#2 More charges added in region with multiple charged residues	
			ATG→AAG	M239K#		
	7	Missense mutation (conversion)	(C/)GTG →(C/)TTG	V281L	Prevalent NC mutation; HLA association (haplotype B14;DR1)	Ashkenazic Jews; many whites
	7	Missense mutation (phenotype: salt-wasting)	(C/)GGT →(C/)AGT (@C→T)	G291S @b398	AA substitution at conserved position @ at position +9 of intron (2° effect?)	
	7	Single base insertion (conversion)	→/T/→ (8th T in a 7T run)	Codon 305–307	(Frameshift: 5-AA + stop)	
		Loss of splice donor site	(AG)gt→ct -	b1785		
	8	Nonsense mutation (conversion)	(G/) CAG →(G/) TAG	Q318X		
	8	NC mutation		R339H		
	8	Missense mutation (conversion)	(G/) CGG →(G/) TGG	R356W	Radical AA substitution	
	9	Nonsense mutation		W405X		
	10	New NC allele	(G/) CCC →(G/) TCC CCG → CTG	P453S^{+} plus P105L	AA substitution of conserved (P453) and nonconserved (P105) residue	
	10	Compound frameshift mutation	GC→C	56-AA	Replaces last 11 AA and extends protein by a further 45 AA	
	10	Missense mutation	(CCC/) CGG →CCG (/GGG)	R483P	Possible 1st step of 2-step mechanism generating No. 15	
CYP11B1	1	Single base deletion	[C]	Codon 32	Frameshift (%other mutation not found; in intron?)	het%
	2	Nonsense mutation	TGG→TAG	W116X	Japanese (consanguineous)	hom
	2	Five-base duplication	AGA/CAA→/A GACA/	Codon 121–2	Frameshift Asian (Kenya)	hom
	3	Nonsense mutation	AAG→TAG	K174X	Premature termination	cmpd het
	5	Missense mutation	ACG→ATG	T318M	Parents Yemenite (first cousins)	(hom) x2
	6	Nonsense mutation	(G/)CAG→ (G/)TAG	Q338X	Parents both Indian Sikh	(hom) x2
	6	Nonsense mutation	CAG→TAG	Q356X	Number of other genetic defects; African American	(hom)
	6	Missense mutation	CGgt-- agG→ CAgt--agG	R374Q	Split codon (exon 6–7) Lebanese	(hom)
	7	Missense mutation	CGA→CAA	R384Q		cmpd het
	7	Missense mutation	CGA→GGA	R384G	Japanese	(hom)
	7	Two-base insert (frameshift)	-AG/A--→ /AG/	77-AA	Turkish Jewish	
	8	Missense mutation	GTG→GGG	V441G		(hom)
	8	Missense mutation	CAG→CGC	R448H	In heme-binding region; Moroccan Jewish/Berber	

(continued)

Table 52-2 *(continued)*

Gene	*Exon*	*Mutation name/type*	*NT*	*AA*	*Comments*	
CYP11B2	1	Five (four+one)-bp deletion	GTGCTGCCG → G----G-CG	Codons 12–14	North American family	hom (x3)
	3, 7	Double missense mutation (CMO II)	(C/)CGG →TGG GTG→GCG	R181W and V386A	In Iranian Jews	
CYP17	1	Nonsense mutation	TGG→TGA	W17X	Japanese	hom (x1)
	1	Deletion of 1 of 2 adjacent identical codons	TTCTTC →TTC	F53 or F54	Japanese	hom (x1)
	1	Missense mutation[a]		Y64S	White	cmpd het
	2	Missense mutation		S106P	Guamanian	hom (x2)
	2	Insert[a] (codon duplicated)		I112	White	cmpd het
	2	Seven-base duplication	-GCGCACA-	Codon 120+37-AA	Japanese	hom (x1)
	2	Extensive internal deletion and foreign (viral) DNA insert[a]	518-bp del and 469-pb insert	Exon 2 to exon 3	Italian	hom (x3)
	3	Nonsense mutation	(T/)GAG →(T/)TAG	E194X	White	cmpd het
	4	Nonsense mutation	CGA→TGA	R239X	White	cmpd het
	6	Missense mutation[a]	CCA→ACA	P342T	White	cmpd het
	6	Missense mutation[a]		H373L	Japanese	hom (x1)
	8	Single-base deletion	A/GGA GA	Codon 438	Japanese (Okinawan)	Hom
	8	Missense mutation[a]	CGC→CAC	R440H	German (heme-binding region)	hom (x1)
	8	Nonsense mutation[a]	CAG→TAG	Q461X	Swiss	cmpd het
	8	Four-base duplication	$[CATC]_2$	Codon 480	Frisian/Mennonite sect (New World)	hom (x9)
	8	Nine-base deletion[a]		Del: D487 S488 F489	Thai	hom (x1)
	8	Missense mutation	CGC→TGC	R496C	Swiss	cmpd het
HSD3B2	3	Missense mutation	GCC→ACC	A82T	In two remote kindreds (Brazil and Scotland)	hom (x4)
		Point mutation in intron 3[a]	G→A	Base 6651	US (mild form)	cmpd het
	4	Missense mutation[a]	GGG→AGG	G129R	US (mild form)	cmpd het
	4	Missense mutation	GAA→AAA	E142K		het
	4	Nonsense mutation	TGG→TAG	W171X	Unrelated kindreds (US, Switzerland)	hom, het
	4	Missense mutation	CTA→CGA	L173R	Subj:MPH but ident. sister no sympt (UK)	hom
	4	Single-base insert	[C]	Codon 186/7	Unrelated kindreds (US, Switzerland)	het
	4	Missense mutation[a]	AGT→GGT	S213G	US (mild form)	cmpd het
	4	Missense mutation[a]	AAG→GAG	K216E	US (mild form)	cmpd het
	4	Missense mutation[a]	GCC→CCC	A245P		het
	4	Compound missense/ frame-shift mutation	GTC/CG→ AAC/T [..AG]	V248N	US	
	4	Missense mutation	(C/)TAT →(C/)AAT	Y253N		het
	4	Missense mutation	(T/)TAC →(T/)GAC	Y254D		het
	4	Two-base deletion (frameshift mutation)[a]	Δ[AA]	Codon 273		
StAR	3	Frameshift mutation	1 bp deletion	238ΔA	Japanese	cmpd het (x1)
	—	Aberrant splicing in intron 4	T→A		11bp from splice acceptor	hom (x1)
	5	Frameshift mutation	629ΔCT			cmpd het (x1)
	5	Nonsense mutation	CGA→CTA	R193X	White	hom (x1)
	6	Missense mutation		A218V		
	7	Nonsense mutation	CAG→TAG	Q258X	Three unrelated kindreds: Korean (x1), Japanese (x2)	hom (x1); cmpd het (x2)
	7	Missense mutation		L260P		cmpd het (x1)
	7	Missense mutation		L275P		hom (x1)

[a]These mutations are not shown on the figures.

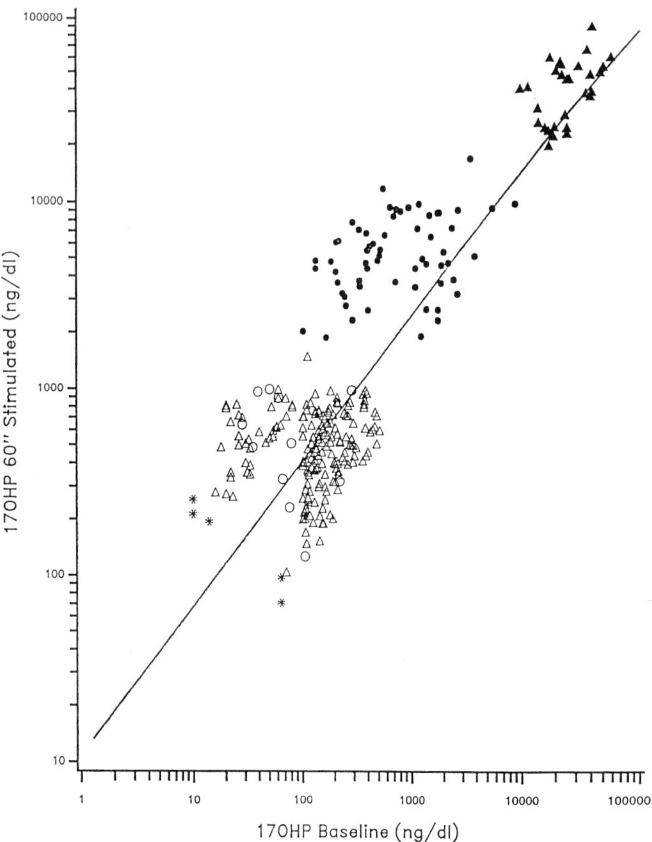

Figure 52-5 Nomogram relating baseline to adrenocorticotrophic hormone (ACTH)-stimulated serum concentrations of 17-hydroxyprogesterone (17-OHP). The scales are logarithmic. A regression line for all data points is shown. *, Genetically unaffected. Patients with: ▲, classical congenital adrenal hyperplasia; ●, nonclassical congenital adrenal hyperplasia. Heterozygotes for: △, classical congenital adrenal hyperplasia; ○, nonclassical congenital adrenal hyperplasia. (The data for this nomogram was collected between 1982 and 1991 at the Department of Pediatrics. The York Hospital–Cornell Medical Center, New York, NY 10021.)

resulting in an inactive enzyme. Within a heterogeneous population, eight other mutations have been identified: four missense mutations, a frameshift mutation (a single base deletion), and three point mutations. A mutation in codon 116 in exon 2, found in a Japanese patient, resulted in a substitution of tryptophan with a stop codon. Recently another mutation, a 5-base duplication, was found in exon 2.

CYP11B2 (ALDOSTERONE SYNTHASE) Defects in the last two steps of aldosterone synthesis result in salt-wasting syndromes (CMO I, 18-hydroxylation; CMO II, 18-oxidation) in infancy. Two homozygous mutations were identified in patients with CMO II in seven kindreds of Iranian-Jewish origin, a substitution of arginine with tryptophan at codon 181 (R181W), and a substitution of valine with an alanine at codon 386 (V386A). Three other Iranian-Jewish families also had the same mutations. Family members homozygous for either of the mutations alone were asymptomatic. In vitro studies of the individual mutations showed that the R181W mutation was deficient in 18-oxidase activity with reduced 18-hydroxylase activity and intact 11β-hydroxylase, whereas the V386A mutation had reduced 18-hydroxylase activity only.

Recently a 5-base deletion in exon 1 of *CYP11B2* was identified in a patient that had the biochemically CMO I phenotype. This frameshift mutation results in early termination at the end of exon 1 with complete lack of enzymatic activity in homozygous individuals.

CYP11B1–CYP11B2 CHIMERA A form of aldosteronism known as dexamethasone-suppressible or glucocorticoid-remediable hyperaldosteronism (DSH or GRH) is caused by the fusion of *CYP11B1* and *CYP11B2* (in addition to a normal copy of each). The chimeric gene contains the 5' end of *CYP11B1* and the 3' end of *CYP11B2*. Therefore, the regulation of this chimeric gene is under the control of ACTH, resulting in high levels of 18-oxocortisol from cortisol and abnormal 17α,18-hydroxysteroids. One copy of this chimeric gene is sufficient to produce the syndrome, hence this disorder is autosomal dominant. Dexamethasone treatment results in a prompt and sustained reduction of aldosterone. Patients with GRH have abnormal serum and urinary elevations of 18-hydroxy and 18-oxocortisol steroids.

PRENATAL DIAGNOSIS AND TREATMENT In 1996, the first case of prenatal treatment of a female fetus affected with 11β-OHD was reported. As with 21-hydroxylase deficiency, treatment of this fetus was initiated before a diagnosis could be completed. The molecular diagnosis revealed a homozygous missense mutation in *CYP11B1* identical to the mutation of her two affected sisters, who were both severely virilized at birth. However, prenatal dexamethasone treatment of this fetus resulted in normal genitalia at birth.

3β-HYDROXYSTEROID DEHYDROGENASE DEFICIENCY

A rare deficiency in the 3β-hydroxysteroid dehydrogenase/$\Delta^{5,4}$-isomerase (3β-HSD) enzyme results in a high ratio of Δ^5 to Δ^4 steroids, characterized by elevated serum Δ^5-steroids pregnenolone, 17-hydroxypregnenolone, and dihydroepiandrosterone (DHEA), with increased urinary Δ^5 metabolites pregnenetriol and 16-pregnenetriol. Because 3β-HSD is required for both adrenal and gonadal steroidogenesis, affected males may have incomplete genital development, resulting in sexual ambiguity at birth. Affected females may have very high levels of circulating DHEA with some peripheral conversion to more potent androgens, which leads to limited clitoral enlargement. A complete deficiency of 3β-HSD results in impaired aldosterone synthesis, causing salt wasting.

As with 21-hydroxylase and 11β-hydroxylase deficiencies, there is a spectrum of the level of 3β-HSD deficiency. The variations include a nonclassic form with postadrenarchal or peripubertal onset.

MOLECULAR GENETICS Two human isoforms of 3β-HSD have so far been identified by cloning of cDNA (several isoforms have been identified in rodents). Type I enzyme is expressed in the placenta, skin, and adipose tissue, and type II is expressed in the adrenal gland and the gonads.

The gene *HSD3B1* encodes the type I isoenzyme, and *HSD3B2* encodes the type II isoenzyme. Classically affected patients have mutations in the *HSD3B2* gene, of which several missense mutations have been found (Fig. 52-8). Patients with impaired aldosterone synthesis carry nonsense or frameshift mutations, or missense mutations that were shown to destroy enzymatic activity completely, when mutant cDNA was expressed in cultured cells. So far, no mutations have been found in the gene for type I. It is not yet known whether nonclassic 3β-HSD deficiency is caused by allelism of type II or whether a defect in another 3β-HSD is responsible for this phenotype. Genomic blot analysis suggests that there are as many as six *HSD3B* genes in humans.

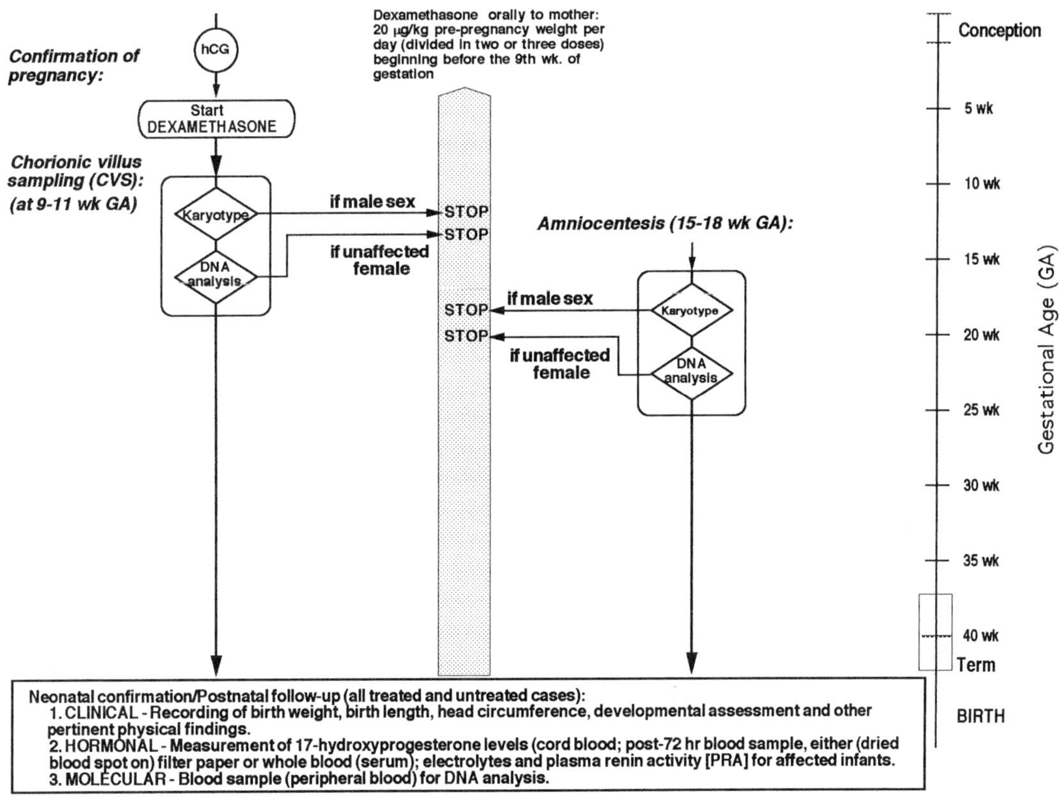

Figure 52-6 Algorithm depicting prenatal management of pregnancy in families at risk for a fetus affected with 21-hydroxylase deficiency.

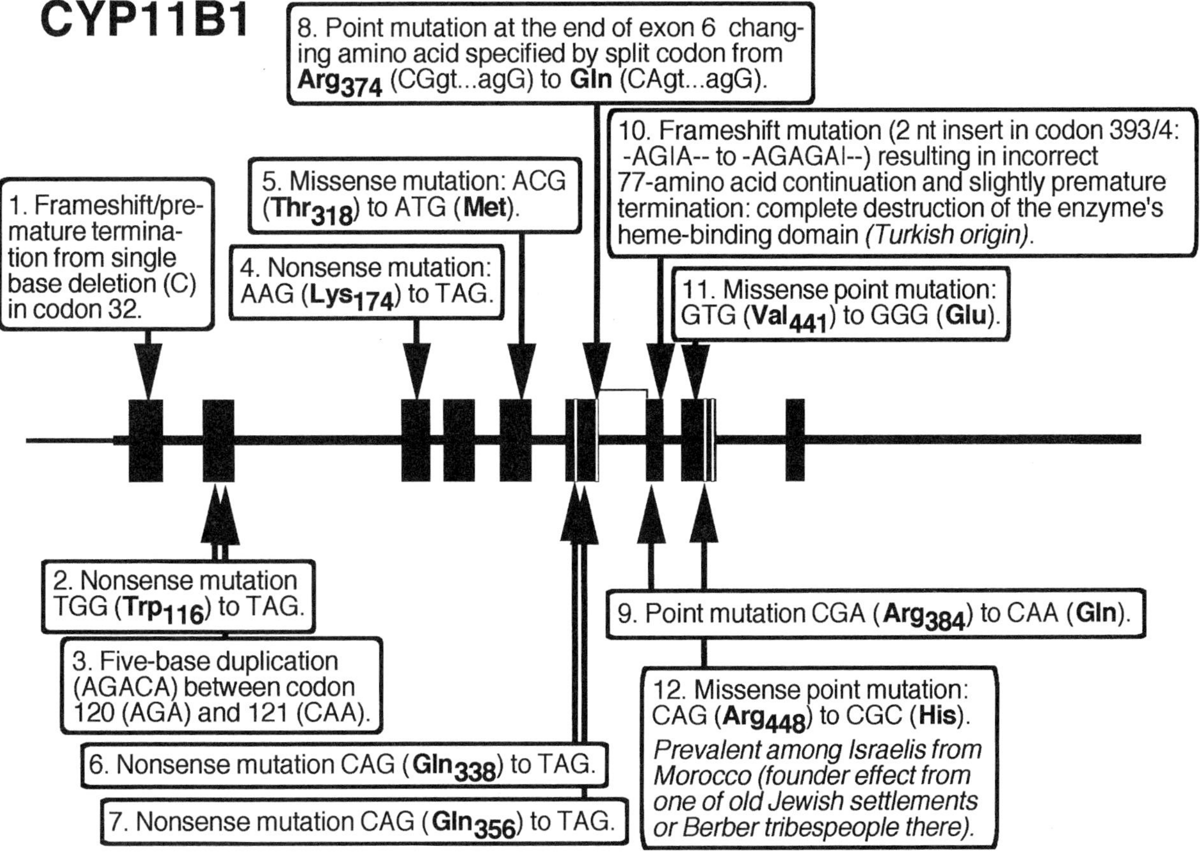

Figure 52-7 Mutations in the 11β-hydroxylase gene *(CYP11B1)*.

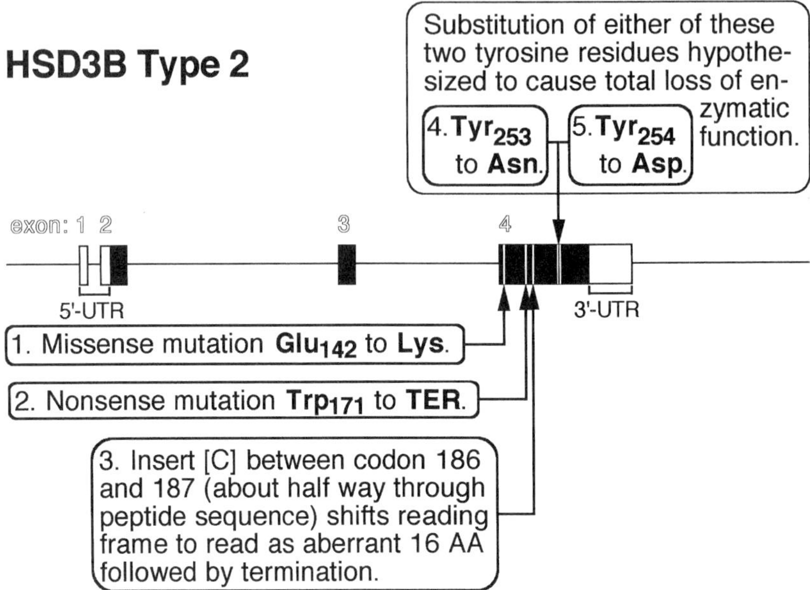

Figure 52-8 Some mutations in the type II 3β-HSD gene *(HSD3B2)*, producing salt-wasting and non–salt-wasting forms of 3β-HSD deficiency.

17α-HYDROXYLASE/17,20-LYASE DEFICIENCY

Defects of the *CYP17* gene produce 17α-hydroxylase deficiency CAH, which is a combined 17α-hydroxylase/17,20-lyase deficiency. Patients with 17α-hydroxylase deficiency are unable to convert pregnenolone and progesterone to 17α-hydroxypregnenolone and 17-OHP, respectively, and subsequently are unable to convert these hormones to DHEA and Δ^4-androstenedione, respectively, by 17,20-lyase activity. With a decreased ability to synthesize cortisol, elevated ACTH increases serum levels of DOC and especially corticosterone. Both adrenal glucocorticoids and sex steroids are diminished. Isolated 17,20-lyase has also been observed, which results in deficient C19 sex steroids in the adrenals and gonads. Patients with defective 17,20-lyase activity have increased levels of pregnanetriolone, a metabolite of 17-OHP.

A deficiency in 17α-hydroxylase activity results in low-renin hypertension, hypokalemia, and metabolic alkalosis. Affected females have normal genitalia at birth, but at pubertal age present with primary amenorrhea, lack of axillary and pubic hair, and no pubertal development, leading to hypoplastic breasts in adolescence. Affected males can be born with external female genitalia because of their deficient gonadal testosterone production, though a uterus and fallopian tubes do not develop because anti–Müllerian hormone secretion by Sertoli cells inhibits Müllerian duct development. The Wolffian ducts, however, are incompletely developed as well.

Steroid 17α-hydroxylase deficiency is a relatively rare cause of CAH, accounting for about 1% of cases overall. Between 100 and 120 cases of 17α-hydroxylase deficiency have been described, and only about 20 cases of 17,20-lyase deficiency have been reported.

MOLECULAR GENETICS A single gene, *CYP17*, encodes the 17α-hydroxylase enzyme (also a cytochrome P450); it exists in a single active copy and is identically transcribed in both adrenal and testis. *CYP17* is located on chromosome 10, region q24–q25, and to date about 17 mutations have been described (Fig. 52-9). These mutations appear to be random and hence do not appear to be caused by a predisposing mechanism.

Both compound heterozygotes and homozygotes have been described. Although homozygosity for a rare mutation is often taken to suggest consanguinity, an exception to this (an insertion mutation of four nucleotides in codon 480) was found in the homozygous state in several Mennonites, a small Anabaptist sect found in a number of communities across North America. The same mutation was also identified in patients from Friesland, the region in the Netherlands where the Mennonites first formed, suggesting an earlier founder effect.

Partial deficiencies are associated with missense mutations or, in one case, deletion of a single codon (ΔF53 or 54) maintaining the reading frame of translation. Complete deficiency of *CYP17* has also been found and is associated with frameshifts and nonsense mutations.

LIPOID CONGENITAL ADRENAL HYPERPLASIA

Lipoid congenital adrenal hyperplasia (LCAH) is extremely rare. The biochemical defect responsible for LCAH resides in the cholesterol side-chain cleavage system, causing a deficiency in the conversion of cholesterol to pregnenolone and resulting in profoundly impaired synthesis of all steroids. The term "lipoid" refers to the abnormal appearance of the adrenals at autopsy, now known to be the result of massive accumulations of cholesterol and cholesterol esters. Males are born with female-appearing external genitalia but have undescended testes, and females have a normal genital phenotype at birth but remain sexually infantile without treatment.

If not detected and treated, LCAH is fatal in newborn infants; death can occur within days to weeks of birth. Severe fluid and electrolyte disturbances, low levels of all steroids in plasma and urine and addisonian pigmentation are present. Very poor stress response and great susceptibility to infection are also seen.

MOLECULAR GENETICS It was originally thought that a defect in the cholesterol side-chain cleavage enzyme, cytochrome P450scc, was responsible for this disease, because P450scc produces pregnenolone from cholesterol. However, this enzyme was shown to be normal in patients with LCAH. Recently a new enzyme

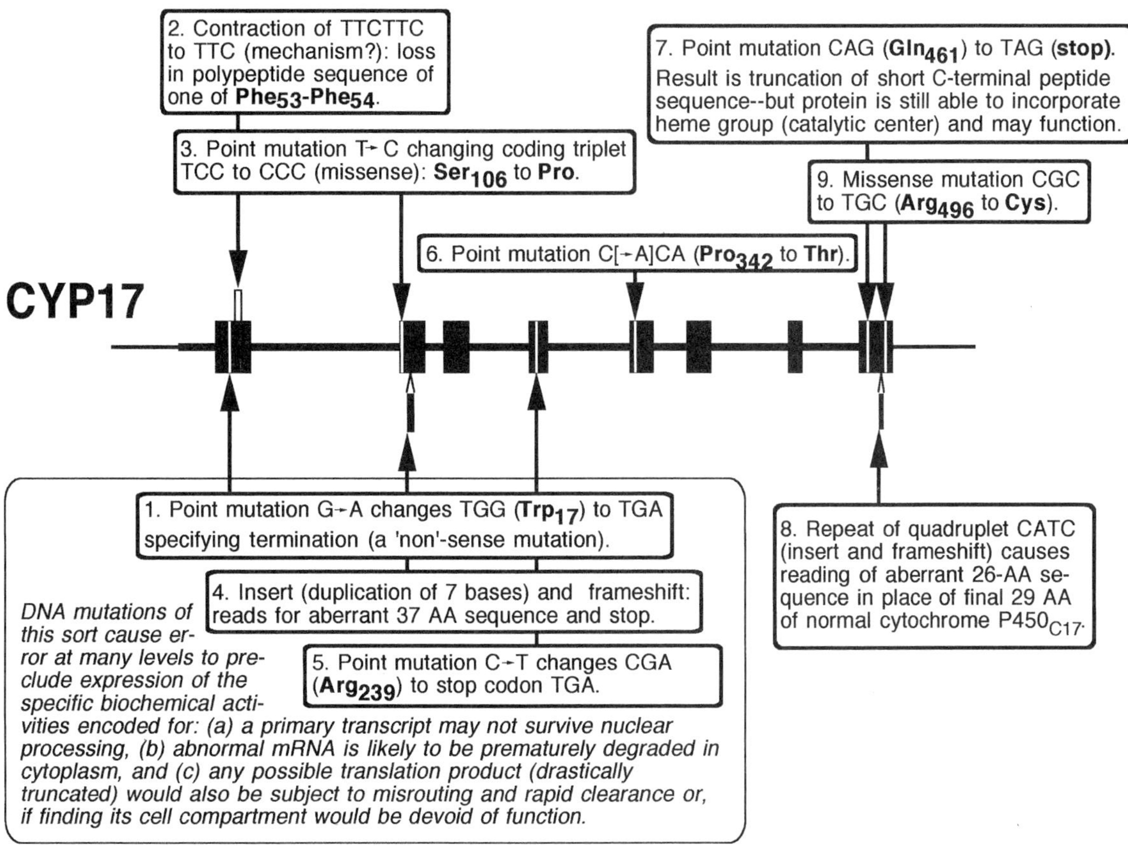

Figure 52-9 Mutations in the 17α-hydroxylase/17,20-lyase deficiency gene *(CYP17)*.

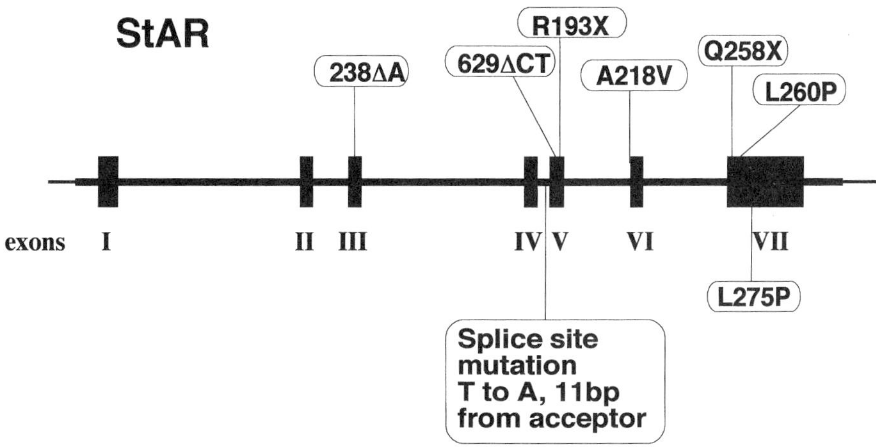

Figure 52-10 Mutations in the steroidogenic acute regulatory protein gene *(StAR)*.

has been discovered that is required for steroidogenesis, steroidogenic acute regulatory protein (StAR). StAR is involved in the transfer of cholesterol from the outer to the inner mitochondrial membrane, where it is then converted to pregnenolone. The gene encoding StAR is on chromosome 8, region p11.2, and a StAR pseudogene is located on chromosome 13. Mutations found in the gene encoding StAR were found to cause LCAH (Fig. 52-10). In three patients, a C-to-T transition in this gene resulted in premature termination. This was confirmed by Western analysis and in vitro studies, showing that these mutations produced completely inactive. In another report, a patient was found to have a splice site mutation caused by a T-to-A transversion in intron 4, resulting in the elimination of 185 nucleotides from the StAR mRNA. Six other mutations in the gene encoding StAR were reported from four patients in 1996.

TREATMENT

Treatment of CAH as a result of 21-hydroxylase deficiency has been ongoing since 1950. Glucocorticoid replacement therapy not only replaces the deficient hormone but also reduces the overstimulation of the adrenal cortex by reducing the release of ACTH, thereby suppressing the overproduction of adrenal androgens. Hydrocortisone (cortisol) is the compound most often used for replacement therapy for 21-OHD, 11β-OHD, and 17α-hydroxylase deficiency. Proper replacement therapy in 21-OHD and 11β-OHD ameliorates the effects of oversecretion of adrenal androgens, thus preventing further virilization, slowing accelerated growth and bone age advancement to a more normal rate, and allowing a normal onset of puberty. In 11β-OHD and 17α-hydroxylase deficiency, glucocorticoid treatment suppresses the oversecretion of DOC leading to the remission of hypertension. Excessive glucocorticoid administration can cause cushingoid facies, growth retardation, and inhibition of epiphyseal maturation.

Hydrocortisone is the physiologic hormone and therefore, minimizes complications. Oral administration is the usual mode of treatment, conventionally given daily in divided doses. It is believed that divided doses better suppress the production adrenal androgens. Hydrocortisone given in two equally divided doses of 10–20 mg/m^2 daily is adequate for the otherwise healthy child. The dosage may have to be increased for a few days to two to three times that of the normal daily dosage during times of non–life-threatening illness or stress. Families are given injection kits of hydrocortisone (50 mg for young children; 100 mg for older patients) for times of emergency. Up to 5–10 times the daily dosage may be required during surgical procedures.

Patients who show a poor response to the standard dosage of hydrocortisone may have their dosage increased to 20–30 mg/m^2 per day or their regimen may have to be changed to a synthetic hormone analog such as prednisone or dexamethasone. The use of these analogs requires critical dosage adjustment since they are more potent and longer acting.

Patients with salt-wasting CAH may also require mineralocorticoid replacement. A cortisol analog, 21-acetyloxy-9α-fluorohydrocortisone (Florinef: 9α-FF), is used for its potent mineralocorticoid activity. A combination of hydrocortisone and Florinef has proven to be quite effective in treatment of patients with salt-wasting 21-OHD.

In simple virilizing patients, it is common to find elevated plasma renin activity (PRA) because of the interaction of the renin–angiotensin–aldosterone system and the hypothalamo–pituitary–adrenal axis. Florinef given in these cases reduces the PRA, which in turn lowers ACTH levels further, resulting in better control of androgens without increased glucocorticoid dose.

Patients with NC21-OHD and nonclassical 3β-HSD deficiency are treated with low doses of dexamethasone. Excess ovarian androgen production may have to be suppressed by the use of progestational and estrogenic agents, which suppress the release of gonadotrophin. Other antiandrogen agents that may help include spironolactone and cyproterone acetate, and the androgen receptor blocker, flutamide. The aim of treatment in these patients is to minimize symptoms without giving rise to glucocorticoid side effects.

In lipoid congenital adrenal hyperplasia, because all steroidogenic enzymes are normal, a substrate for steroidogenesis can be used for effective treatment of patients. Freely diffusible 20α-hydroxycholesterol is recommended, which must be implemented as a lifelong treatment plan. Successful continuing management of a patient for 18 years was reported in 1985 using replacement glucocorticoids and mineralocorticoids in physiologic doses, and estrogen replacement induced a pubertal growth spurt.

FUTURE DIRECTIONS

For many diseases that are reasonably well-defined at a clinical, genetic, and molecular level, there remains the enigma of genotype not strictly correlating with phenotype, in which variation exists in the clinical phenotype associated with the same disease-producing mutation as defined by molecular techniques. Steroid 21-hydroxylase provides an example of this phenomenon. More than 200 patients were assessed for phenotypic characteristics by: (1) genital status with respect to virilization in females, (2) ACTH stimulation tests to evaluate secretion of androgens and 17-hydroxyprogesterone, and (3) salt-deprivation studies when safe to assess aldosterone deficiency and salt wasting. After dividing patients into 26 mutation-identical groups, it was found that half the groups did not conform to the genotype.

Because the mechanism for this phenomenon remains elusive, future studies should include investigation of the promoter and regulatory areas of the 21-hydroxylase gene. The surrounding genes may play a role in altering gene expression, though the different phenotypes of mutation-identical sibs cast doubt on this explanation. Activity of transcription factors, transport proteins, and other modifiers must also be studied.

ACKNOWLEDGMENTS

We wish to express our appreciation to Laurie Vandermolen for her editorial assistance. Significant sections of the work reported herein were supported by funding from USPHS Grant HD00072 and GCRC Grant RR 06020.

SELECTED REFERENCES

Andersson S, Geissler WM, Wu L, et al. Molecular genetics and pathophysiology of 17 beta-hydroxysteroid dehydrogenase 3 deficiency. J Clin Endocrinol Metab 1996;81:130–136.

Bongiovanni AM Congenital adrenal hyperplasia due to 3beta-hydroxysteroid dehydrogenase deficiency. In: New MI, Levine LS, eds. Adrenal Disease in Childhood, Pediatric and Adolescent Endocrinology, vol 13. Basel: S Karger, 1984; pp. 72–82.

Bose HS, Sugawara T, Strauss JF 3rd, Miller WL. The pathophysiology and genetics of congenital lipoid adrenal hyperplasia. International Congenital Lipoid Adrenal Hyperplasia Consortium. N Engl J Med 1996;335:1870–1878.

Forest MG, David M, Morel Y. Prenatal diagnosis and treatment of 21-hydroxylase deficiency. J Steroid Biochem Mol Biol 1993;45:75–82.

Fujieda K, Tajima T, Nakae J, et al. Spontaneous puberty in 46, XX subjects with congenital lipoid adrenal hyperplasia. Ovarian steroidogenesis is spared to some extent despite inactivating mutations in the steroidogenic acute regulatory protein (StAR) gene. J Clin Invest 1997;99:1265–1271.

Kater CE, Biglieri EG. Disorders of steroid 17α-hydroxylase deficiency. Endocrinol Metab Clin North Am 1994;23:341–357.

Mercado AB, Wilson RC, Cheng KC, Wei J-Q, New MI. Extensive personal experience with prenatal diagnosis of congenital adrenal hyperplasia owing to steroid 21-hydroxylase deficiency. J Clin Endocrinol Metab 1995;80:2014–2020.

Mornet E, Crete P, Kuttenn F, et al. Distribution of deletions and seven point mutations on CYP21B genes in three clinical forms of steroid 21-hydroxylase deficiency. Am J Hum Genet 1991;48:79–88.

New MI. Congenital adrenal hyperplasia. In: Degroot L, ed. Endocrinology, 3rd ed. Philadelphia: WB Saunders, 1995; pp. 1813–1835.

New MI, Crawford C. Molecular genetics of steroid 21-hydroxylase deficiency. Chapter 17. In: Wachtel S, ed. Molecular Genetics of Sex Determination. New York: Academic, 1994; pp. 399–438.

New MI, Crawford C, Wilson RC. Genetic disorders of the adrenal gland. In: Rimoin DL, Connor JM, Pyeritz RE, eds. Emery and Rimoin's Principles and Practice of Medical Genetics. In: Emery AEH, Rimoin

D, eds. Principles and Practice of Medical Genetics, 3rd ed. New York: Churchill, Livingstone, 1996; pp. 1441–1476.

New MI, White PC. Genetic disorders of steroid metabolism. In: Thakker R, ed. Genetic and Molecular Biological Aspects of Endocrine Disease. London: Bailliere Tindall, 1995; pp. 525–554.

Pang S, Clark A Congenital adrenal hyperplasia due to 21-hydroxylase deficiency: newborn screening and its relationship to the diagnosis and treatment of the disorder. Screening 1993;2:105–139.

Saenger P. New developments in congenital lipoid adrenal hyperplasia and steroidogenic acute regulatory protein. Pediatr Clin North Am 1997;44:397–421.

Sparkes RS, Kilsak I, Miller WL. Regional mapping of genes encoding human steroidogenic enzymes: P450scc to 15q23–q24, adrenodoxin reductase to 17q24–q25; and P450c17 to 10q24–q25. DNA Cell Biol 1991;10:359–365.

Speiser PW, Dupont J, Zhu D, et al. Disease expression and molecular genotype in congenital adrenal hyperplasia due to 21-hydroxylase deficiency. J Clin Invest 1992;90:584–595.

Stocco DM, Clark BJ. Role of the steroidogenic acute regulatory protein (StAR) in steroidogenesis. Biochem Pharmacol 1996; 51:197–295.

Wilson RC, Mercado AB, Cheng KC, New MI. Steroid 21-hydroxylase deficiency: genotype may not predict phenotype. J Clin Endocrinol Metab 1995;80:2322–2329.

White PC, Curnow KM, Pascoe L. Disorders of steroid 11beta-hydroxylase isozymes. Endocr Rev 1994;15:421–438.

White PC, New MI. Congenital adrenal hyperplasia. N Engl J Med 1987;316:1519–1524, 1580–1586.

White PC, New MI, Dupont J. Structure of human steroid 21-hydroxylase genes. Proc Natl Acad Sci USA 1986;83:5111–5115.

Yanase T, Simpson ER, Waterman MR. 17α-hydroxylase/17,20-lyase deficiency: from clinical investigation to molecular definition. Endocr Rev 1991;12:91–108.

Zerah M, Schram P, New MI. The diagnosis and treatment of nonclassical 3beta-HSD deficiency. Endocrinologist 1991;1:75–81.

53 Adrenal Diseases

CONSTANTINE A. STRATAKIS AND GEORGE P. CHROUSOS

INTRODUCTION

The adrenal glands became known as *gladulae renis incumbentes* through the work of Bartolommeo Eustachio, nearly five centuries ago. These anatomic structures, however, did not enter the realm of clinical medicine until the middle of the 19th century, when T. Addison described the first patients with adrenal insufficiency. In the years that followed, the three zonae of the adrenal cortex were defined and several clinical and pathologic abnormalities were described. Recently, a number of adrenocortical disorders have had their pathophysiology elucidated at the physiologic and molecular levels. This chapter reviews diseases associated with adrenocortical dysfunction, whose molecular pathogenesis is either known or under investigation. These include primary glucocorticoid and corticotropin resistance (hereditary isolated glucocorticoid deficiency, triple A syndrome), adrenal hypoplasia congenita, pseudohypoaldosteronism, adrenoleukodystrophy and adrenomyeloneuropathy, the apparent mineralocorticoid excess syndrome, and Carney complex. Adrenocortical cancer is discussed separately, since in its inherited forms (Li-Fraumeni and Beckwith-Wiedemann syndromes) the molecular pathogenesis has been elucidated to some extent, whereas little is known about the molecular mechanisms leading to sporadic carcinomas. The congenital adrenal hyperplasia syndromes and Liddle syndrome and other causes of hypertension are described elsewhere.

PRIMARY FAMILIAL OR SPORADIC GENERALIZED GLUCOCORTICOID RESISTANCE

BACKGROUND Primary familial or sporadic generalized glucocorticoid resistance (FGR or GGR, respectively—OMIM 138040) is a rare hereditary disorder characterized by hypercortisolism and the absence of stigmata of Cushing's syndrome. Glucocorticoids are crucial regulators of affect and behavior, metabolism, cardiovascular function, inflammation, and immunity. Complete inability of glucocorticoids to exert their effects on target tissues would be incompatible with life in primates. Thus, only syndromes of partial or incomplete glucocorticoid resistance exist and are caused by defects of the ubiquitous, classic glucocorticoid receptor (GR) (type II), which mediates most of glucocorticoid (GC) actions. GGR was the penultimate nuclear hormone resistance syndrome to be described, as late as 1976, and to date has been reported in several unrelated kindreds and, recently, in individual subjects.

From: *Principles of Molecular Medicine* (J. L. Jameson, ed.), ©1998 Humana Press Inc., Totowa, NJ.

CLINICAL FEATURES AND DIAGNOSIS The daily production of GC is tightly controlled by an elaborate feedback system, in which GC exert negative feedback on hypothalamic secretion of corticotropin-releasing hormone (CRH) and arginine vasopressin (AVP) and on pituitary secretion of corticotropin (ACTH). In states of resistance, this complex system is insensitive to concentrations of cortisol considered normal for the general population and the hypothalamic–pituitary–adrenal (HPA) axis is reset to a higher level because of compensatory increases of ACTH and cortisol secretion. Because the defect of the receptor is partial, adequate compensation for the end-organ insensitivity appears to be achieved by the elevated circulating cortisol; however, the excess ACTH secretion results in increased production of adrenal steroids with salt-retaining or androgenic activity. Because in GGR the peripheral tissues are presumably normally sensitive to mineralocorticoids and androgens, the clinical characteristics of the condition reflect the increased production of these hormones. Corticosterone, deoxycorticosterone, and even cortisol, through their interaction with the mineralocorticoid receptor, cause symptoms and signs of mineralocorticoid excess, such as hypertension or hypokalemic alkalosis. The excess androgens, such as Δ4-androstenedione, dehydroepiandrosterone (DHEA), and DHEA-sulfate (DHEA-S), on the other hand, lead to signs and symptoms of hyperandrogenism. The latter in women include cystic acne, hirsutism, male pattern baldness, menstrual irregularities, anovulation, amenorrhea, and infertility. In children, the excessive and early prepubertal adrenal androgen secretion can cause sexual precocity. Finally, the interference of adrenal androgens with the regulation of pituitary secretion of follicle-stimulating hormone (FSH) or ACTH-induced intratesticular growth of adrenal rests appears to be responsible for abnormal spermatogenesis and infertility in men with GGR. These clinical manifestations were not reported in all patients with FGR, and presentation varied even within families, including asymptomatic members.

The diagnosis of GGR is made by demonstrating a high cortisol production rate, i.e., high plasma total and free cortisol, elevated 24-hour urinary free cortisol (UFC) or 17-OH-corticosteroid excretion, resistance to dexamethasone suppression, and maintenance of the circadian and stress-induced patterns of GC secretion, albeit at higher levels, along with absence of Cushing's syndrome stigmata.

GENETIC BASIS OF DISEASE Inherited or spontaneous mutations of the GR gene causing quantitative or qualitative alterations in the function of the receptor protein had been suspected in this syndrome, because receptor studies in cells from affected

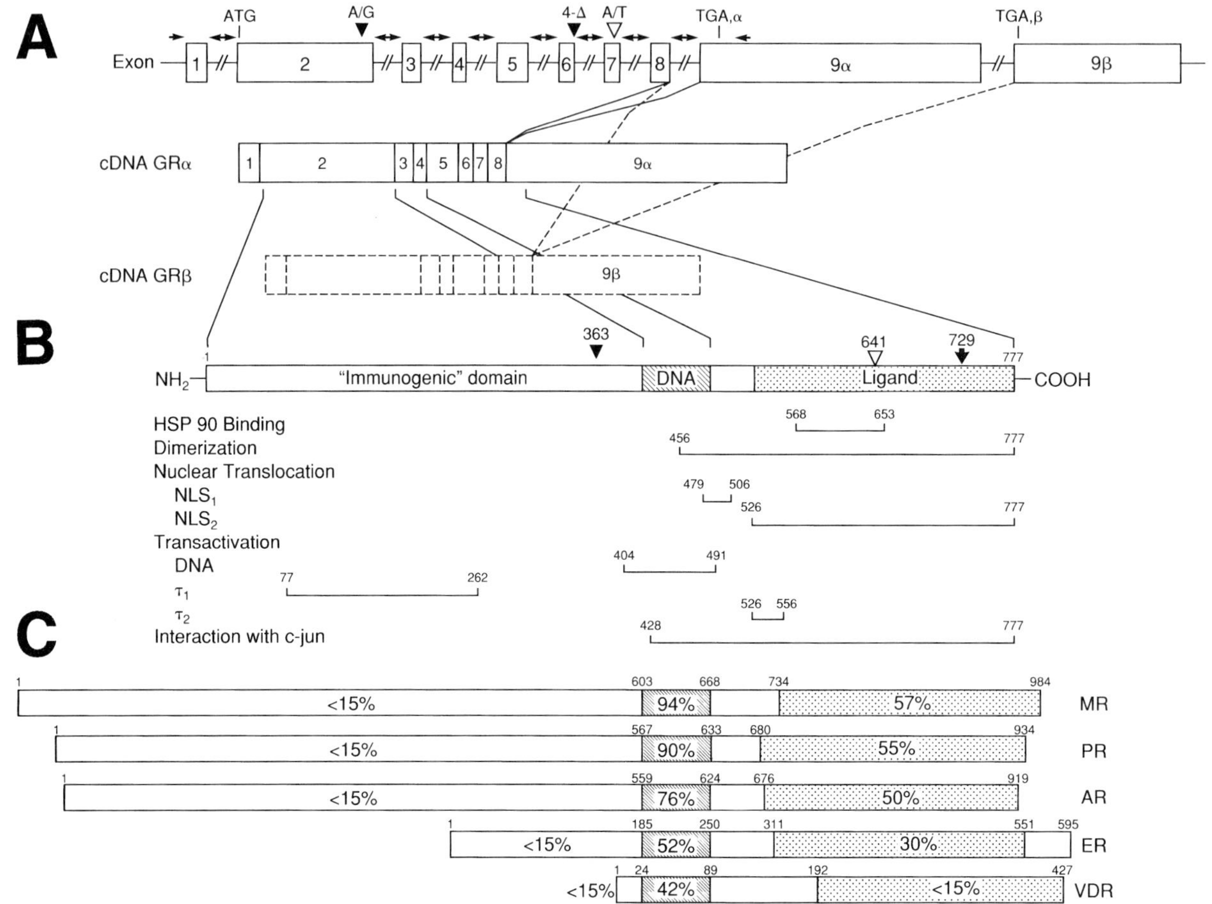

Figure 53-1 Genomic, cDNA, and protein structure of the human glucocorticoid receptor (hGRα): **(A)** The gene consists of 10 exons of variable length. The hGRβ is the product of alternative splicing and does not bind glucocorticoids. **(B)** The main domains of the hGR are represented in a linear model and the three identified mutations in kindreds-A and -B *(see text)* and the one reported by Malchoff et al. are shown at positions 641, 363, and 729 of the hGR protein, respectively. (HSP, heat shock protein; NLS, nuclear localization sequences.) **(C)** Homologies of the five other classes of steroid and sterol receptors to the hGR expressed as percent identity in primary sequence (MR, PR, AR, ER, and VDR are mineralocorticoid, progesterone, androgen, estrogen, and 1,25$(OH)_2$-vitamin D3 receptor, respectively.) (Modified from Stratakis et al. Ann NY Acad Sci 1994;746:362–376.)

individuals and their relatives had shown decreases in the receptor concentration and ligand-binding affinity, thermolability, and abnormal interactions with DNA. The cloning of the complementary DNA (cDNA) of the human GR in 1985 allowed the deduction of its primary structure, definition of its functional domains, and cloning of its gene, and permitted further studies on the molecular mechanisms of glucocorticoid resistance (Fig. 53-1). The GR gene is located on chromosome 5 and consists of 10 exons. The 777-amino acid GR has three main functional domains: the ligand-binding domain in the carboxy-terminus of the protein, the DNA-binding domain in the middle, and the amino-terminal domain, which was originally characterized by its property of providing antigenic epitopes for the generation of antireceptor antibodies and, hence, was called the "immunogenic domain." The first family in which the molecular basis of GGR was investigated was a large kindred (kindred-A), in which the propositus had no features of Cushing's syndrome despite a sevenfold elevation of free cortisol in serum. Less severe but unequivocal cortisol excess and dexamethasone resistance were found in one brother and a son. Borderline cortisol excess was detected in 6 of 27 additional relatives from three generations consistent with an autosomal codominant mode of inheritance, in which heterozygotes were affected either mildly or only biochemically. Studies of the GR in intact mononuclear leukocytes and cultured skin fibroblasts from the patients showed normal concentrations of the GR with diminished affinity for the hormonal ligand. The GR of Epstein-Barr virus (EBV)-transformed lymphoblast lines from the propositus and his mildly affected relatives, on the other hand, showed GR mRNA of the expected size but decreased ligand-binding affinity, increased thermolability, and reduced binding to DNA-cellulose after thermal activation. It was concluded from these studies that the most likely molecular defect was a mutation of the GR gene affecting the ability of the receptor to bind efficiently with the ligand.

The 2,3-kb coding region of the GR cDNA from the EBV-transformed lymphoblast lines established from three patients of kindred-A was amplified by PCR and sequenced. There was complete concordance with the published normal GR cDNA nucleotide sequence for all three patients, except at position 2054, where a thymidine (T) residue was present in place of the normal adenosine (A), resulting in a nonconservative amino acid substitution at position 641 of the GR protein and changing the aspartic acid codon (GAC) to the valine codon (GTC). The propositus was homozygous for the Val-641 mutation, whereas the amplified GR cDNAs from the mildly affected son and nephew contained both A and T residues at position 2054, suggesting heterozygosity. The functional significance of the identified mutation was tested by its introduction into the wild-type GR by PCR site-directed mutagenesis and use in transient cotransfection assays. Despite its normal expression, the mutant GR was not able to bind ligand and transactivate a GC-responsive gene in vitro.

A second family (kindred-B) was then investigated, in which the propositus was an adult woman with symptoms and signs of hyperandrogenism and elevated plasma cortisol concentrations. She, her father, and two brothers were biochemically affected to the same degree, with cortisol production indices within the Cushing's syndrome range; the male members, however, were completely asymptomatic. Glucocorticoid binding analysis in circulating mononuclear leukocytes from affected members demonstrated a 50% decrease of receptor concentrations and normal binding affinity for dexamethasone. The GR gene of the proband, her two affected brothers, and two unaffected siblings was studied also by PCR amplification and sequencing. A 4-bp deletion (Δ4) was identified at the 3' boundary of exon and intron 6 in all three affected subjects studied. The deletion removed a donor splice site in one allele, affecting the last two bases of the exon and the first two nucleotides of intron 6. This deletion segregated with the presence of glucocorticoid resistance, and all three affected members of the kindred were heterozygous for it. The Δ4 allele was not transcribed in vitro, a finding that was compatible with the reduction of the GR number by 50% in the patients' cells.

In a third family, a guanine-to-adenine point mutation was found in GR cDNA position 2317, leading to an amino acid substitution at position 729 of the GR protein within the ligand-binding domain. The mutation also led to decreased affinity and apparently compromised the functional ability of the GR. The propositus in this family is the only patient with FGR reported to present with isosexual precocious puberty, adding not only genetic but also clinical variability to the syndrome.

CLINICAL MANAGEMENT Patients with FGR are easily managed with high doses of synthetic glucocorticoids, such as dexamethasone, with no mineralocorticoid activity, which should be carefully titrated per individual. Monitoring of clinical and biochemical parameters is essential to avoid glucocorticoid excess.

FUTURE DIRECTIONS Glucocorticoid resistance may be more prevalent than previously believed and may have important implications for human pathophysiology. The variety of phenotypes and abnormal receptor studies described so far, as well as the complexity of the GR structure and its multitude of interactions within the cell, can with certainty predict that many more genetic defects will be identified as causes of glucocorticoid resistance in humans. The latter may include not only alterations of the GR gene structure and function, but also of other molecules that are important for defining glucocorticoid responsiveness of target tissues, including the β-isoform of the GR (GRβ), which does not bind ligand but has dominant negative activity on the classic isoform; the heat shock protein (hsp)-90 and hsp-70 and the immunophilins, which coexist as heteroligomers with the cytosolic GR; and several transcription factors, which physically and functionally interact with the receptor, such as c-*jun*, c-*fos*, and NFκB, as well as coactivator and corepressor molecules. GGR appears to be relatively frequent among women with hyperandrogenism and should be ruled out in these cases. States of GGR may also include local tissue unresponsiveness to GC, such as that observed in lymphoid and corticotroph neoplasia, autoimmune and allergic diseases, and, probably, psychiatric disorders.

HEREDITARY ISOLATED GLUCOCORTICOID DEFICIENCY AND THE TRIPLE A SYNDROME

BACKGROUND Hereditary isolated glucocorticoid deficiency (IGD—OMIM 202200) is a rare autosomal recessive disorder characterized by primary adrenal insufficiency without mineralocorticoid deficiency. Affected children usually have recurrent hypoglycemia, convulsions, or coma, which may result in death within the first 2 years of life. Unless recognized and treated early, this condition may lead to cachexia and failure to thrive. The disorder is occasionally associated with alacrima and achalasia of the esophagus (adrenal insufficiency, alacrima, achalasia, the "triple-A" or Allgrove syndrome), a disorder which is familial and inherited in an autosomal recessive manner (OMIM 200440).

CLINICAL FEATURES AND DIAGNOSIS Patients with IGD have adrenocortical resistance to ACTH, which presents in early infancy with hypoglycemia, hyperpigmentation, low urinary 17-hydroxycorticosteroids (17-OHCS), and absence of a cortisol, aldosterone and 17-OHCS response to ACTH stimulation. They retain, however, normal aldosterone responses to activation of the renin–angiotensin axis by salt restriction, orthostasis, and furosemide-induced diuresis. Accordingly, the zonae fasciculata and reticularis in these patients are atrophic, reduced to a narrow band of fibrous tissue, whereas the zona glomerulosa is relatively well-preserved.

GENETIC BASIS OF DISEASE The adrenocortical unresponsiveness to ACTH that underlies the pathogenesis of isolated glucocorticoid deficiency suggests that the defect responsible could be anywhere in the signaling cascade, from the membrane-bound G-protein-coupled ACTH receptor to the kinases stimulating steroidogenesis. Recently, the human ACTH receptor gene was cloned and its sequence was determined. It encodes a 297-amino acid protein, which, together with the melanocyte-stimulating hormone receptors, constitute a class of G-protein-coupled seven transmembrane domain (TMD) receptors whose genes are intronless. Abnormalities of the ACTH receptor (melanocortin receptor-2 *[MC2R]*) gene, which has been localized to chromosome 18p11.2, were found in four families with hereditary IGD. In one kindred, a G-to-T substitution was found at codon 74 of the MC2 gene, within TMD-II of the protein. The proband, a Scottish boy who was born to nonconsaguineous parents and exhibited hypoglycemia and hyperpigmentation early in infancy, was homozygote for this mutation, which was later described in two other apparently unrelated families from Scotland. In another kindred, the proband was a 5-year-old African-American boy with generalized hyperpigmentation and history of severe hypoglycemia since infancy, who was studied in our laboratory. This patient had two different point mutations in the coding region of the MC2 gene, each in either of the two alleles. The first mutation was a substitution of C by T at the first position of codon 201, normally encoding arginine, introducing the stop codon TGA. The site of this mutation corresponds to the beginning of the third intracellular loop of the ACTH receptor protein. The second mutation was a substitution of C by G at the third position of codon 120, causing a nonconservative amino acid substitution from serine to arginine in TMD-III of the receptor, thus disrupting ligand binding. The proband's asymptomatic parents and grandparents were carriers for each of the two mutations.

Although mutations of the MC2 gene appear to be responsible for the IGD syndrome in several families, in others the genetic defect remains elusive. In fact, genetic heterogeneity was recently demonstrated for this disease by the exclusion of the chromosome 18p11.2 locus of the MC2 gene with the use of an informative dinucleotide repeat marker *(D18S40)* in three families with IGD. In two additional families, the MC2 gene was sequenced and no mutations were found. In one of these, peripheral blood lymphocytes from the two affected siblings failed to respond to ACTH with an increase of adenylate cyclase levels. On the other hand, the *D18S40* marker segregated with the disease in four newly studied families with the syndrome. Thus, it appears that a little less than half of the cases of IGD may not be caused by mutations of the MC2 gene coding region.

Patients with the triple A syndrome have also been investigated and found not to have any genetic changes of the MC2 gene. Because adrenocortical insufficiency in this disorder is associated with alacrima and autonomic and other neurologic abnormalities, a contiguous gene deletion has been suggested for the etiopathogenesis of this disorder. The gene(s) was (were) recently mapped to human chromosome 12q13.

CLINICAL MANAGEMENT Patients with IGD are treated with replacement doses of hydrocortisone (12–15 mg/m^2/d) or equivalent doses of other glucocorticoids. They achieve normal growth and intellectual development if diagnosed and treated early, in contrast to patients with the triple A syndrome, who demonstrate progression of their neurologic deficits with age independently of the time of onset of glucocorticoid replacement and the number of hypoglycemic episodes.

ADRENAL HYPOPLASIA CONGENITA

BACKGROUND Adrenal hypoplasia congenita (AHC—OMIM 300200) is a developmental disorder of the adrenal gland that results in severe adrenal insufficiency and death in early infancy if left untreated. Two distinct forms, the autosomal recessive miniature (OMIM 240200) and the X-linked cytomegalic form have been described. The first reports of familial adrenal hypoplasia were published in the 1950s, when several pedigrees of affected male siblings and their maternal uncles were described, indicating X-linked inheritance. The autopsies in these patients showed structural disorganization and absence of the normal zonae of the adrenal glands. The biochemical profile of these patients was remarkable for low or absent serum levels of glucocorticoids and mineralocorticoids, low serum androgens, and failure of adrenal steroids to respond to ACTH. Several patients had ambiguous genitalia or cryptorchidism and were found to have hypogonadotropic hypogonadism (HHG) of pituitary or hypothalamic origin, and occasionally, other abnormalities, including glycerol kinase deficiency (GKD), hearing loss, and Duchenne's muscular dystrophy (DMD). The autosomal recessive form of the disease, on the other hand, is not associated with HHG or the other abnormalities seen in the X-linked form.

CLINICAL MANIFESTATIONS Both forms of AHC usually present in infancy as failure to thrive, vomiting, feeding difficulties, neonatal cyanosis and apnea, and seizures. Hypoglycemia, hyponatremia, and hyperkalemia are caused by the extremely low cortisol and aldosterone levels that fail to respond to endogenous or exogenous ACTH. Although ambiguous genitalia or cryptorchidism may be present in the autosomal recessive form also, HHG with no or minimal response of gonadotropins to gonadotropin-releasing hormone (GnRH) administration is only present in the X-linked form. The latter may also be associated with progressive high-frequency hearing loss and other neurologic abnormalities; however, association of the autosomal recessive AHC with anencephaly or isolated pituitary abnormalities has also been reported. The histologic findings differ in the X-linked and autosomal recessive forms of AHC. In the former, which is referred to as the "cytomegalic" type, the adrenal cortex shows disorganization with poor differentiation of cortical zones and presence of scattered clumps of eosinophilic cells. In the latter, which is called the miniature adult type, there is absence or near-absence of both fetal and permanent cortex.

GENETIC BASIS OF DISEASE The description of patients with the X-linked type of AHC and/or HHG, GKD, hearing loss, and DMD pointed to a contiguous gene deletion syndrome. Indeed, in 1992 an AHC locus was mapped to Xp21 in proximity to the DMD locus on the basis of the identification of several patients with deletions of this region. The region encompassing the DMD, GKD, and AHC loci was cloned, and the AHC locus mapped to a 250- to 500-kb region, telomeric to the GKD locus. Subsequently, the X-linked locus DSS (dosage-sensitive sex reversal) was mapped to Xp21 by microscopic duplications found in 46, XY phenotypically female patients, narrowing the AHC region to approximately 160 kb. The *DAX-1* (DSS-AHC critical region on the X chromosome) gene was then cloned from a phage contig spanning the region. It encodes a new member of the nuclear hormone receptor superfamily that has a novel DNA-binding domain, and acts as a dominant-negative regulator of transcription mediated by the retinoic acid receptor. The gene contains a single, long open reading frame, and its coding sequence is interrupted by a single, 3-kb-long intron. The *DAX-1* mRNA is only found in steroidogenic tissues (testes, ovaries, adrenals) as a single 1.9-kb RNA species and has been highly preserved in all species tested. Mutations of the *DAX-1* gene (nonsense, missense, and frameshift mutations and a single amino acid deletion) were found in patients with both X-linked AHC and HHG, who had no other genetic abnormality of the chromosome Xp critical region. On the other hand, patients with AHC and DMD or GKD had contiguous gene deletions, from which the following gene order was deduced for this portion of the short arm of chromosome X:Xpter-*AHC-GKD-DMD*-cen. No mutations in *DAX-1* were found in five other AHC patients, including one with histologically confirmed cytomegalic type of the disease. Thus, genetic heterogeneity exists even for the X-linked AHC. The genetic locus or the gene for the autosomal recessive type of AHC remains elusive.

CLINICAL MANAGEMENT Patients with AHC are given replacement glucocorticoids, fludrocortisone (0.1–0.4 mg/d), and salt supplementation in infancy and early childhood (1–2 g/d). Serum testosterone levels and a GnRH stimulation test are indicated in patients with AHC and normal testicular descent, because the absence of bilateral or unilateral cryptorchidism does not preclude HHG.

FUTURE DIRECTIONS As patients with AHC demonstrate, disruption of *DAX-1* does not prevent the initial stages of gonadal development in the human male but inhibits maturation of the hypothalamic–pituitary–gonadal axis and prevents differentiation of the adrenal gland beyond the fetal stage. Thus, *DAX-1* plays the role of a late developmental regulator of adrenal and gonadal steroidogenesis and, perhaps, pituitary function, that is comparable to that played by another orphan nuclear receptor protein, steroidogenic factor-1 (SF-1) in earlier developmental stages (*see* Chapter 57). Indeed, a putative SF-1 response element was recently identified in the *DAX-1* gene promoter region, indicating a coordination of expression of the two factors. Because genetic heterogeneity exists even for the X-linked AHC cases, other genes with similar roles in the regulation of steroidogenesis are expected to be found in the near future on the X and other chromosomes.

ADRENOLEUKODYSTROPHY AND ADRENOMYELONEUROPATHY

BACKGROUND Adrenoleukodystrophy (ALD, OMIM 300100) was first reported as an X-linked syndrome of Addison's disease and cerebral sclerosis in the 1960s. A decade later, it was found that cholesterol esters in the brain and adrenal tissue of these patients contained an excess amount of fatty acids with a chain length of 24–30 carbon atoms. The clinical phenotype varied considerably leading to the description of four different forms based on the age of onset and clinical severity. A defective peroxisomal β-oxidation system was found in skin fibroblasts from the patients in the early 1980s. Genetic studies in patients with ALD and other defects led to the recent (1993) identification of the *ALDP* gene.

CLINICAL MANIFESTATIONS ALD is a progressive, degenerative neurologic disorder with spastic paraplegia, peripheral neuropathy, limp and truncal ataxia, slurred speech, blindness, and cognitive hearing loss, associated with primary adrenal insufficiency and hypogonadism. Four distinct phenotypes have been recognized: a neonatal form that is manifested by severe neurologic deficits in infancy and leads to death in early childhood; classic ALD that affects young children, who usually die before they reach adulthood; adrenomyeloneuropathy (AMN), which is usually first manifested by adrenal insufficiency during the second and third decade of life, affects primarily the spinal cord, and gradually leads to severe neurologic deficits; and adult ALD that is present in female heterozygote carriers and is manifested by progressive spinal cord disease and ataxia. Patients with adrenal insufficiency only, or a form limited to the cerebrum, have also been described. As in the nervous system and elsewhere, the adrenal pathology of ALD is characterized by the accumulation of lipid inclusions. Plasma levels of very long chain fatty acids (VLCFA, C26:0) are elevated and there are abnormal C26:0/C22:0 and C24:0/C22:0 ratios. The determination of circulating hexahecosanoate can be used not only for the diagnosis of ALD, but also for the prenatal detection of the disease and for the identification of female carriers. An ACTH stimulation test is essential in every patient with ALD to identify the extent of impaired adrenal reserve, so that replacement therapy can be instituted promptly.

GENETIC BASIS OF DISEASE The earlier linkage of the ALD gene to the chromosome X locus of the glucose-6-phosphate dehydrogenase (G-6-PD) gene in women heterozygous for both ALD and electrophoretic variants of G-6-PD was confirmed by linkage analysis through the use of the *DXS52* DNA probe. Linkage to the Xq28 locus of this probe was established with a lod score of 13.76 with no recombinations ($\theta = 0$). By positional cloning and the use of structural deletions of the Xq chromosome found in patients who had both ALD and color blindness, the putative ALD gene was mapped in close proximity to and at the 5' end of the color gene cluster. The identification, in 1993, of a transcript from this genomic region designated ALDP (ALD protein) was followed by the report of several deletions and other mutations of the *ALDP* gene in patients with ALD or AMN. Comparison with the amino acid sequences of known genes suggests that ALDP is a member of the ATP-binding cassette (ABC) transmembrane transporter protein superfamily. Thus, ALDP appears to be a peroxisomal membrane transporter directly involved in the import of the peroxisomal enzyme lignoceroyl-CoA synthetase (VLCFA synthetase), the enzyme whose activity appears defective in ALD. The ALDP transcript has a 38.8% homology with that of the peroxisomal protein PXMP 1. Although there is no direct proof that ALDP is located in the peroxisomal membrane, and the peptide has no homology to any of the other known peroxisomal proteins or fatty acid CoA synthetases, it is postulated that mutations of the ALDP have an indirect effect on the β-oxidation of VLCFA by affecting VLCFA synthetase activity. In a recent study of 28 unrelated kindreds, defects of the ALDP gene were found in all of the patients, mostly nonsense or missense mutations.

CLINICAL MANAGEMENT Patients with ALD have multiple neurologic problems that are treated symptomatically. If adrenal insufficiency is present, replacement with hydrocortisone and fludrocortisone is needed. Accordingly, treatment with gonadal steroids may be needed if hypogonadism is present. There is no known improvement of the endocrine manifestations of ALD with the administration of "Lorenzo's oil," although a substantial decrease of serum VLCFA levels has been documented with its use and additional dietary therapy. Bone marrow transplantation was recently tried in patients with ALD and a multicenter study is now in progress.

FUTURE IMPLICATIONS The cloning of the ALDP gene provided a significant molecular insight into the function and structure of the peroxisomes, organelles that contain many enzymes and are involved not only in fatty acid oxidation, but also in prostaglandin degradation and amino acid metabolism, the formation of bile acids, and the biosynthesis of cholesterol and plasmalogens. Research is ongoing to further elucidate the role of the peroxisomes in steroidogenesis and other endocrine functions.

PSEUDOHYPOALDOSTERONISM

BACKGROUND Cheek and Perry first reported pseudohypoaldosteronism (PHA) in an infant with a severe salt-wasting syndrome in 1958. The syndrome was subsequently reported in more than 70 patients. Approximately one-fifth of these cases were familial. The disease is inherited in an autosomal recessive manner, although dominant inheritance cannot be excluded in several pedigrees. It is referred to as PHA type-I (OMIM 264350) to distinguish it from Gordon syndrome or hyporeninemic hypoaldosteronism (PHA-type II, OMIM 145260), which is characterized by renal tubular unresponsiveness to the kaliuretic, but not the sodium and chloride reabsortive, effect of aldosterone. The latter is inherited in an autosomal dominant manner.

CLINICAL MANIFESTATIONS Type-I PHA is manifested early in infancy with salt wasting, vomiting, and feeding difficulties that lead to severe dehydration and death if untreated. Hyponatremia, hyperkalemia, and acidosis are present despite marked renin excess and hyperaldosteronemia, and normal 17-hydroxysteroid excretion. Unresponsiveness to aldosterone may be limited to the renal tubule or generalized, in which case sodium excretion is increased not only in the urine, but also in sweat, saliva, and stool.

The sweat chloride test is positive. The symptoms improve with age and older patients with PHA require smaller doses of salt supplements and salt-retaining steroids.

GENETIC BASIS OF DISEASE A number of reports suggested that quantitative or qualitative defects of the mineralocorticoid receptor (MR) might be responsible for PHA, on the basis of studies that reported absent or decreased [^{3}H]-aldosterone binding to circulating leukocytes from patients with the disorder. The human MR was cloned in 1987 and its chromosomal locus was mapped to chromosome 4q31.1–2. A number of patients with type-I PHA have been studied for mutations of the coding and 5' regulatory regions of the human MR and no changes have been identified, with the exception of polymorphisms in the immunogenic domain of the receptor that did not segregate with the disease. Recently, the chromosome 4q31.1–2 locus of the human MR was excluded by homozygosity mapping of 10 inbred families with one or more affected individuals with type-I PHA. Subsequent genome scans for type-I PHA genes using DNA from 11 consanguineous families with PHA1 demonstrated linkage to a locus on chromosome 16, 16p12.2–13.11, in 6 families and to 12q13.1–pter in 5 families. These chromosomal regions contain the genes that encode the β-, γ-, and α-subunits of the amiloride-sensitive epithelial sodium channel (ENaC), *SCNN1B* and *SCNN1G* on chromosome 16 and *SCNN1A* on chromosome 12. Activating mutations of *SCNN1B* and *SCNN1G* cause Liddle's syndrome, which is characterized by hypertension associated with vascular expansion, hypokalemia, and alkalosis. This is essentially the converse phenotype of type-I PHA. Inactivating mutations in the different subunits of ENaC in patients with type-I PHA have now been reported. Two kindreds with premature termination of the α-subunit of ENaC have been identified. A missense mutation, substitution of serine for glycine at residue 37 (G37S), has also been identified in the β-subunit of ENaC. This missense mutation apparently changes the channel open probability (P_o) and results in a channel characterized by short open times and long closed times. Finally, a G-to-A substitution in a 3' acceptor splice site has been identified in mRNA encoding the γ-subunit. This mutation results in production of one of two aberrant proteins, either a truncated protein or a protein that lacks three highly conserved amino acids adjacent to the first transmembrane domain.

CLINICAL MANAGEMENT Patients with type-I PHA are aggressively treated in early infancy with salt supplementation (0.5–1.5 g/kg/d in four to six divided doses). Close monitoring of the sodium balance is needed especially during infancy, when plasma renin activity is not useful because of the large variation of this parameter in the first year of life. After the age of 2 years, the reduction of sodium supplement is often possible with gradual improvement of the symptoms and decrease of the dehydration crises. Recently, carbenoxolone, an inhibitor of 11-β-hydroxysteroid dehydrogenase (11-β-HSD), was used successfully in the treatment of type-I PHA.

FUTURE DIRECTIONS The identification of the responsible genes for type-I PHA undoubtedly offer significantly to the understanding of aldosterone physiology. Indeed, the genetic defects in PHA may involve postreceptor mechanisms in aldosterone action, such as the transport of sodium by the mineralocorticoid-responsive amiloride-sensitive sodium channel subunits. New therapeutic regimens for the patients with this disease are expected to be developed based on identification of the responsible genetic defects.

SYNDROME OF APPARENT MINERALOCORTICOID EXCESS

BACKGROUND The syndrome of apparent mineralocorticoid excess (AME—OMIM 218030) was first described in 1977 as a syndrome of hypertension, hypokalemia, and low plasma renin activity associated with normal cortisol, and subnormal aldosterone levels. Through the 1980s, the disease was investigated in several children and few adults; an abnormal cortisol-to-cortisone ratio was described in all these patients, suggesting that the defect was related to the oxidation of cortisol to its inactive metabolite. This reaction is mediated through the action of 11-β-hydroxysteroid dehydrogenase (HSD), an enzyme that is inhibited by licorice (glycyrrhetinic acid) and carbenoxolone. Licorice induces a clinical and biochemical syndrome that mimics that of AME when chronically ingested. Mutations of one of the two isoforms of this enzyme were recently found to be responsible for congenital AME, which is inherited in an autosomal recessive manner. So far, 25 patients with AME have been reported worldwide. A normal cortisol-to-cortisone ratio, however, has been identified in few of these patients, who do not appear to have an HSD defect (AME-type II, OMIM 207765).

CLINICAL MANIFESTATIONS Both types of AME present in early childhood (1–5 years of age) with severe hypertension, hypokalemic alakalosis, low plasma renin activity, and low to normal aldosterone levels. If left untreated, long-standing hypertension may lead to left ventricular hypertrophy, strokes, and retinopathy before the teenage years, although adult patients with milder manifestations of the syndrome have also been described. Type-I AME can readily be diagnosed by determination of the urinary tetrahydrocortisol and tetrahydrocortisone or serum cortisol-to-cortisone ratios.

GENETIC BASIS OF DISEASE HSD is a microsomal enzyme complex responsible for the interconversion of cortisol and cortisone. Two isoforms, encoded by two different genes, have been described; the type I isoform (HSD11B1) has two separate enzymatic activities: 11-β-dehydrogenase (which converts cortisol to cortisone) and 11-oxoreductase (which converts cortisone to cortisol). The type II isoform (HSD11B2) has only the first activity. Aldosterone is normally a much stronger mineralocorticoid than cortisol in vivo, yet both steroids have identical affinities in vitro for the aldosterone receptor. *In vivo*, certain tissues with this receptor are aldosterone selective (e.g., kidney and parotid), whereas others with the same receptor are not (e.g., hippocampus and heart). Thus, the dehydrogenase activity of HSD11B2, by converting cortisol to the inactive cortisone, is thought to be necessary to protect the renal mineralocorticoid receptor from the circulating cortisol (which has normally manyfold higher serum levels than aldosterone), allowing aldosterone to regulate sodium homeostasis in the renal tubule. The gene for HSD11B1 on chromosome 1 was first investigated for mutations in patients with AME, with negative results. The HSD11B2 gene was then cloned and mapped to chromosome 16q22. The HSDK gene shares only 14% homology with that of HSD11B1, has a total length of 6.2 kb, and consists of five exons. Defects of this gene were recently reported in eight kindreds with AME. All of the mutations were in or close to the catalytic domain of the enzyme, and resulted in decreased activity when tested in vitro. Partial correlation between phenotype and genotype was evident in these studies because patients with no detectable enzymatic activity of the in vitro mutant protein had the highest tetrahydrocortisol and tetrahydrocortisone ratio. Interestingly, intrauterine growth retardation (IUGR), a previously unrecognized manifestation of AME, was seen in the majority of the patients. Because HSD11B2 is highly expressed in the placenta, IUGR in AME patients was attributed to the placental deficiency of the enzyme. One of the investigated kindreds did not harbor mutations of the *HSDK* gene demonstrating genetic heterogeneity for the disease.

CLINICAL MANAGEMENT Patients with congenital AME respond to treatment with spironolactone (50–200 mg/d) and low sodium diet. Early diagnosis and treatment are essential to avoid complications of hypertension.

IMPLICATIONS FOR FUTURE AND PATHOPHYSIOLOGY The finding that patients with AME and mutations of the *HSDK* gene have IUGR correlates well with the observation that low-birth-weight infants are at increased risk for developing essential hypertension in later life. It is possible that genetic variations of HSD11B2 enzymatic activity have significant effects on fetal growth and on subsequent risk of hypertension. The *HSDK* gene may, thus, be one of the polygenes that cause essential hypertension.

CARNEY COMPLEX

BACKGROUND Carney complex (CC, OMIM 160980) is a familial multiple neoplasia (endocrine tumors and myxomas) and lentiginosis syndrome that is inherited in an autosomal dominant manner. Although the existence of the complex as an unrecognized, inherited syndrome was first suggested in 1985, combinations of several components of the syndrome and their familial occurrence had been reported earlier. Thus, the characteristic pathologic findings of the adrenal glands (primary pigmented nodular adrenocortical disease [PPNAD])—multiple, small, pigmented, adrenocortical nodules and internodular cortical atrophy—and a pituitary-independent, primary adrenal form of hypercortisolism were described in children and young adults with Cushing's syndrome as early as 1949. In the late 1970s, several familial cases of cutaneous and cardiac myxomas associated with lentigines (lentigo simplex) or ephelides and blue nevi of the skin and mucosae had been described under the acronyms, NAME (for nevi, atrial myxoma, myxoid neurofibromata, and ephelides) and LAMB (for lentigines, atrial myxoma, mucocutaneous myxoma, blue nevi) syndromes. The presence of "adrenal-stimulating immunoglobulins" leading to corticotropin-independent adrenocortical nodular hyperplasia in affected subjects was suggested in 1989.

CLINICAL MANIFESTATIONS Carney complex is manifested in children and young adults with at least two of the following: (1) PPNAD that can lead to Cushing's syndrome; (2) lentigines, ephelides, and blue nevi of the skin and mucosae; and (3) a variety of nonendocrine and endocrine tumors. The latter include myxomas of the skin, heart, breast, and other sites, psammomatous melanotic schwannoma, growth hormone-producing pituitary adenoma, testicular Sertoli cell tumor, and possibly other benign and malignant neoplasms, including tumors of the thyroid gland and ductal adenoma of the breast.

GENETIC BASIS OF DISEASE The chromosomal loci, where the genes for Carney complex reside were recently mapped by linkage analysis on chromosomes 2 and 17 (Fig. 53-2). Eleven kindreds with the disease were investigated with the use of highly polymorphic markers from areas of the human genome likely to be involved. Because telomeric translocations of chromosome 2 had been observed in cardiac myxomas and the gene that codes for POMC is located on the short arm of chromosome 2 (2p), this chromosome was examined for linkage. A maximal two-point lod score greater than 3 was obtained for three markers on the short arm of chromosome 2. The markers CA-5, CA-2, and *D2S123* produced lod scores of 3.26 ($\theta = 0.07$), 5.97 ($\theta = 0.03$), and 3.73 ($\theta = 0.04$), respectively. The *D2S123* locus has been linked to hereditary non–polyposis colorectal cancer (HNPCC) and a detailed map of this area of the short arm of chromosome 2p is available. A polymorphic marker from within the coding sequence of the POMC gene excluded the latter as a candidate gene for this disorder. Another gene located in the area, the *hMSH2* gene, responsible for DNA stability and tumor suppression, which was found mutated in HNPCC, was also excluded by the recombination events observed in chromosomes of patients with the disease. Multipoint linkage analysis defined a region approximately 4 cM long bordered by the CA-2 and *D2S378* markers as the most likely area harboring the responsible gene(s). The absence of other polymorphic markers from the area precluded a more refined mapping at the time. An additional genetic locus was recently identified, indicating that Carney complex is genetically heterogeneous.

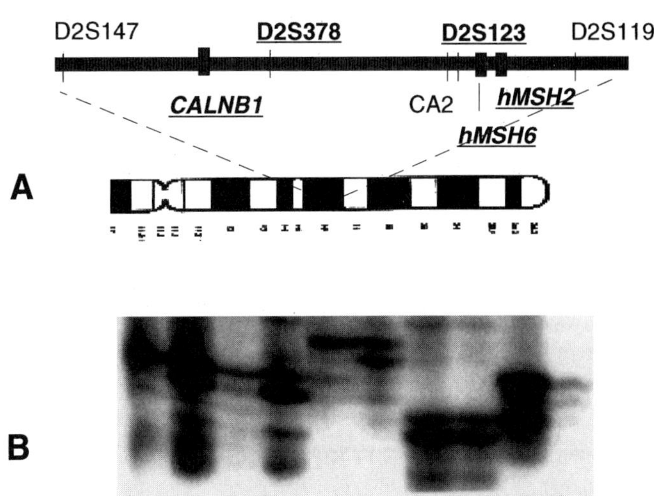

Figure 53-2 **(A)** Cytogenetic map of chromosome 2p16 with the corresponding genetic map. The genetic distances are expressed in centiMorgans (cM). The Carney complex critical region is bordered by markers D2S123 and D2S378. The gene responsible for microsatellite stability in dividing human cells *hMSH2* was excluded as a potential candidate for Carney complex, although it is located in close proximity to the disease locus. **(B)** Loss of heterozygosity and other changes in tumors from patients with Carney complex. B, blood; T, tumor. The disease is genetically heterogeneous.

CLINICAL MANAGEMENT Patients with the diagnosis of Carney complex need to undergo extensive and frequent monitoring for the detection and early treatment of the multiple tumors that are associated with this condition. Heart myxomas, if undiagnosed, can lead to sudden death, strokes, or peripheral embolization; thus, annual screening by echocardiography is recommended in patients with the complex and their families. If PPNAD is diagnosed, then bilateral adrenalectomy and lifelong glucocorticoid and mineralocorticoid replacement are recommended.

IMPLICATIONS FOR FUTURE The lesions associated with the complex originate from cells of mesenchymal (myxomas) or neural crest origin (spotty skin pigmentation, endocrine tumors). These features suggest that the genetic defects leading to Carney complex are involved in early development, growth, and proliferation of affected cells. Thus, candidate genes include those involved in tumor suppression and the control of the cell cycle, as well as those with specific effects on the function and growth of mesenchymal and zona fasciculata cells and melanocytes. Because there is considerable overlap between Carney complex and the familial lentiginosis syndromes (Peutz-Jeghers syndrome and others), it is expected that the Carney complex genes will contribute to the identification of the as-yet-unknown genetic defects responsible for the various lentiginoses.

ADRENAL CORTEX NEOPLASMS

BACKGROUND Cushing's syndrome because of adrenocortical tumors was reported at the turn of the century, almost a decade before the description of the syndrome and homonymous disease by Harvey Cushing. Since then, a great deal about adrenocortical tumors has been learned, although the treatment of adrenocortical malignancies has remained an utter frustration for the clinician. Hope for new treatments, however, recently sprang from the identification of at least two genetic defects leading to adrenal cancer. Somatic and germline mutations of the *p53* tumor suppressor gene are responsible for sporadic and inherited adrenal cancer, respectively. The latter is part of Li-Fraumeni syndrome (LFS, OMIM 151623), a familial multiple neoplasia syndrome that is inherited in an autosomal dominant manner. Another genetic condition associated with adrenal carcinoma and other tumors is the Beckwith-Wiedemann syndrome (BWS, OMIM 130650), which has been mapped to chromosome 11p15.5, and its inheritance is autosomal dominant but influenced by genomic imprinting and uniparental disomy.

CLINICAL MANIFESTATIONS Small benign adrenocortical tumors are present in up to 7% of adults older than 50 years of age. Usually, they are discovered incidentally, in the context of abdominal computed tomography (CT) or magnetic resonance imaging (MRI) scans performed for other reasons. The vast majority of these tumors are hormonally silent. Hormone-secreting benign adrenal adenomas are rare, and equally rare are hormonally silent or hormone-secreting adrenocortical carcinomas. Malignant neoplasias of the adrenal cortex account for 0.05–0.2% of all cancers. They occur in all ages, from early infancy to the seventh and eighth decades of life, although a bimodal age distribution has been reported with the first peak occurring before 5 years of age, and the second in the fourth to fifth decade. The most common syndrome associated with adrenal tumors is Cushing's syndrome, which is present in 30–40% of adult patients with adrenal cancer. Virilization, on the other hand, is present in 20–30% of adults, but is the most common clinical syndrome encountered in children with adrenocortical carcinoma. It is caused by hypersecretion of DHEA and its sulfated derivative (DHEA-S), as well as other adrenal androgens and steroid precursors, by the tumor. Feminization and hyperaldosteronism are rare clinical syndromes associated with hormonally active adrenal tumors. Hormonally silent tumors are either found incidentally or present with abdominal pain and fullness or by the symptoms of metastatic disease, which can involve locally the kidneys and inferior vena cava, and distally the liver, lungs, and bones.

GENETIC BASIS OF DISEASE Adrenal neoplasms were recently found to be monoclonal, like most other tumors, by X-chromosome inactivation analysis. Components of the G protein signaling pathway and the receptors coupled to it have been considered good candidate genetic defects leading to adrenal cancer. However, mutations of the ACTH receptor (MC2) or the Gs and Giα2 genes are not present in large series of sporadic adrenal tumors that have been investigated, although mutations of the Gsα gene cause macronodular adrenal disease and can lead to ACTH-independent Cushing's syndrome in McCune-Albright syndrome. A single case of an activating mutation of the MC2 gene leading to adrenal macronodular disease and Cushing's syndrome has also been reported.

Mutations of the *p53* tumor suppressor gene have been found in patients with LFS and many sporadic adrenal carcinomas. These are genetic defects that lead to loss of the normal inhibitory function of the p53 protein on the cell cycle and are concentrated in a highly conserved region of the gene between exons 5 and 8. The *p53* gene is located on chromosome 17p13.1; loss of heterozygosity (LOH) at this locus in a cell that has either undergone a somatic mutation or carries a germline genetic defect of the *p53* gene in the remaining allele leads to tumorigenesis ("two hit" or Knudson's hypothesis) (*see* Chapter 7). A locus on chromosome 11p15.5 has been implicated in BWS. One of the genes in this region encodes $p57^{KIP2}$, which is a potent inhibitor of several of the G1 cyclin/Cdk complexes and a negative regulator of cell proliferation. Like other genes in this region, $p57^{KIP2}$ is imprinted, and the maternal allele is expressed. In a series of nine patients with BWS, two were heterozygous for mutations in $p57^{KIP2}$. One was a missense mutation that resulted in a severely truncated protein, whereas the other was a frameshift mutation that would alter protein function. In the case of the missense mutation, transmission of the mutated allele from the mother was documented; thus the single allele expressed in the patient was the mutant allele. Whether the other patients have reduced expression of $p57^{KIP2}$ or involvement of another locus has not yet been determined. Consistent with a role of $p57^{KIP2}$ in BWS, knockout of the $p57^{KIP2}$ gene in mice results in a syndrome with phenotypic features seen in BWS, including adrenocortical hyperplasia.

CLINICAL MANAGEMENT The treatment of all primary adrenal tumors is surgical. Adrenal adenomas should be removed with the whole ipsilateral adrenal gland, and the contralateral gland should be examined for tumor. Complete resection of the tumor is the treatment of choice for adrenal carcinoma. If the patient does not have surgically curable disease, therapy with o,p'-DDD (mitotane) is usually initiated. o,p'-DDD, an adrenocytolytic agent given at maximally tolerated oral doses (up to 10 $g/m^2/d$), ameliorates the endocrine syndrome in approximately two-thirds of patients. Tumor regression or arrest of growth has been observed on as many as one third of patients. However, mean survival does not appear to be altered, although there are patients with unresectable carcinomas who achieved long-term survival. The prognosis of primary adrenal adenomas is excellent, but that of adrenal carcinomas generally poor, with a mean survival of approximately 18 months, although cures have been achieved for patients operated on early, while the tumor was still encapsulated.

CONCLUDING REMARKS

In addition to the diseases discussed, the genes for a number of genetic conditions that involve the adrenal glands or their targets have been cloned during the last decade. These include the genes for multiple endocrine neoplasia (MEN)-2A and -2B (*RET* proto-oncogene) and Von Hippel-Lindau's disease, which are associated with pheochromocytoma, the genes for other phacomatoses, such as neurofibromatosis -I and -II and tuberous sclerosis, which are associated with tumors of primarily the adrenal medulla and sympathetic ganglia, and the gene for MEN-1, which is associated with adrenal benign nodules. The genetic locus for multiple autoimmune endocrinopathy type-I (MAE-I), which is associated with autoimmune Addison's disease and failure of other endocrine glands, has been mapped to chromosome 21p, and was just cloned (the APECED gene). Additionally, new genes have been identified that appear to play an important role in adrenal development and physiology in transgenic animal studies, although a human disease has not been reported to be caused by them as yet. The most important appears to be a cell-specific orphan nuclear receptor, designated steroidogenic factor 1 (SF-1), which is a key regulator of the steroidogenic enzymes in the adrenal glands and elsewhere. Targeted disruption of the *Ftz-F1* gene, which encodes SF-1 in mice, caused congenital absence of the adrenal glands and gonads in both sexes, and gender reversal of the male animals. It has been suggested that mutations of the human SF-1 gene will also result in adrenal hypoplasia or aplasia and gonadal dysgenesis. Since the era of molecular medicine continues unabated, many new exciting discoveries are expected in the molecular medicine of the adrenal glands in the years to come.

SELECTED REFERENCES

Arai K, Tsigos C, Suzuki Y, et al. No apparent mineralocorticoid receptor defect in a series of sporadic cases of pseudohypoaldosteronism. J Clin Endocrinol Metab 1995;80:814–817.

Arai K, Tsigos C, Suzuki Y, et al. Physiological and molecular aspects of mineralocorticoid receptor action in pseudohypoaldosteronism: a responsiveness test and therapy. J Clin Endocrinol Metab 1994; 79:1019–1023.

Bamberger CM, Schulte HM, Chrousos GP. Molecular determinants of glucocorticoid receptor function and tissue sensitivity to glucocorticoids. Endocr Rev 1996;17:245–261.

Beuschlein F, Reincke M, Karl M, et al. Clonal composition of human adrenocortical neoplasms. Cancer Res 1994;54:4927–4932.

Carney JA, Young WF. Primary pigmented nodular adrenocortical disease and its associated conditions. Endocrinologist 1992;2:6–21.

Chang SS, Grunder S, Hanukoglu A, et al. Mutations in subunits of the epithelial sodium channel cause salt wasting with hyperkalaemic acidosis, pseudohypoaldosteronism type 1. Nat Genet 1996; 12:248–253.

Chung E, Hanokoglu A, Rees M, et al. Exclusion of the locus for autosomal recessive pseudohypoaldosteronism type-I from the mineralocorticoid receptor gene region on human chromosome 4q by linkage analysis. J Clin Endocrinol Metab 1995;80:3341–3345.

Chrousos GP. The hypothalamic–pituitary–adrenal axis and immune-mediated inflammation. N Engl J Med 1995;332:1351–1362.

Clark AJL, Weber A. Molecular insights into inherited ACTH-resistance syndromes. Trends Endocrinol Metab 1994;5:209–214.

Flack M, Chrousos GP. Neoplasms of the adrenal cortex. In: Holland R etal., ed. Cancer Medicine, 4th ed. Baltimore, MD: Williams & Wilkins, 1996; pp. 1563-1570.

Funder JW. Glucocorticoid and mineralocorticoid receptors: biology and clinical relevance. Annu Rev Med 1997;48:231–240.

Guo W, Mason JS, Stone CG Jr, et al. Diagnosis of X-linked adrenal hypoplasia congenita by mutation analysis of the DAX-1 gene. JAMA 1995;274:324–330.

Hatada I, Ohashi H, Fukushima Y. An imprinted gene p57KIP2 is mutated in Beckwith-Wiedemann syndrome. Nat Genet 1996;14:171–173.

Hurley DM, Accili D, Stratakis CA, et al. Point mutation causing a single amino acid substitution in the hormone-binding domain of the glucocorticoid receptor in familial glucocorticoid resistance. J Clin Invest 1991;5:229–233.

Lichtenberg MJL, Kemp S, Sarde C-O, et al. Spectrum of mutations in the gene encoding the adrenoleukodystrophy protein. Am J Hum Genet 1995;56:44–50.

Monder C, White PC. 11β-hydroxysteroid dehydrogenase. Vitam Horm 1993;47:187–271.

Mosser J, Douar A-M, Sarde C-O, et al. Putative X-linked adrenoleukodystrophy gene shares unexpected homology with ABC transporters. Nature 1993;361:726–730.

Mune T, Rogerson FM, Nikkila H, Agarwal AK, White PC. Human hypertension caused by mutations in the kidney isozyme of 11β-hydroxysteroid dehydrogenase. Nat Genet 1995;10:394–399.

Mune T, White PC. Apparent mineralocorticoid excess: genotype is correlated with biochemical phenotype. Hypertension 1996;27:1193–1199.

Parker KL, Schimmer BP. Steroidogenic factor 1: a key determinant of endocrine development and function. Endocr Rev 1997;18:361–377.

Penning TM. Molecular endocrinology of hydroxysteroid dehydrogenases. Endocr Rev 1997;18:281–305.

Reincke M, Karl M, Travis W, et al. p53 mutations in human adrenocortical neoplasms: immunohistochemical and molecular studies. J Clin Endocrinol Metab 1994;78:790–794.

Stratakis CA, Carney JA, Lin J-P, et al. Carney complex, a familial multiple neoplasia and lentiginosis syndrome: analysis of 11 kindreds and linkage to the short arm of chromosome 2. J Clin Invest 1996;97:699–705.

Stratakis CA, Jenkins RB, Pras E, et al. Cytogenetic and microsatellite alterations in tumors from patients with the syndrome of myxomas, spotty skin pigmentation, and endocrine overactivity (Carney complex). J Clin Endocrinol Metab 1996;81:3607–3614.

Stratakis CA, Karl M, Schulte HM, Chrousos GP. Glucocorticoid resistance in humans: elucidation of the molecular mechanisms and implications for pathophysiology. Ann N Y Acad Sci 1994;746:362–376.

Stratakis CA, Lin JP, Pras E, Rennert OM, Bourdony CJ, Chan WY. Allgrove (triple-A) syndrome in Puerto Rican kindreds maps to chromosome 12 (12q13). Proc Assoc Am Physician 1997;109(5):478–482.

Strautnieks SS, Thompson RJ, Gardiner RM, Chung E. A novel splice-site mutation in the gamma subunit of the epithelial sodium channel gene in three pseudohypoaldosteronism type 1 families. Nat Genet 1996;13:248–250.

Tsigos C, Arai K, Hung W, Chrousos GP. Hereditary isolated glucocorticoid deficiency associated with abnormalities of the adrenocorticotropin receptor gene. J Clin Invest 1993;92:2458–2461.

Tsigos C, Arai K, Latronico A-C, DiGeorge A, Rapaport R, Chrousos GP. A novel mutation of the ACTH-receptor (ACTH-R) gene in a family with the syndrome of isolated glucocorticoid deficiency but no ACTH-R abnormalities in two families with triple-A syndrome. J Clin Endocrinol Metab 1995;80:2186–2189.

White PC, Mune T, Agarwal AK. 11 β-Hydroxysteroid dehydrogenase and the syndrome of apparent mineralocorticoid excess. Endocr Rev 1997;18:135–156.

Zanaria E, Muscatelli F, Bardoni F, et al. An unusual member of the nuclear hormone receptor superfamily responsible for X-linked adrenal hypoplasia congenita. Nature 1994;372:635–641.

Zhang P, Liegeois NJ, Wong C, et al. Altered cell differentiation and proliferation in mice lacking p57KIP2 indicates a role in Beckwith-Wiedemann syndrome. Nature 1997;387:151–158.

54 Multiple Endocrine Neoplasia Type 2

ROBERT F. GAGEL, SARAH SHEFELBINE, AND GILBERT COTE

BACKGROUND

Less than four decades ago, John Sipple first described components of the clinical syndrome that now bears his name. Recognizing the association of thyroid cancer and bilateral pheochromocytomas in a patient at autopsy he reported this case along with several others in a 1961 article. Others more clearly defined the type of thyroid carcinoma and separated the clinical features of this syndrome, defined as multiple endocrine neoplasia type 2 (MEN-2), from multiple endocrine neoplasia type 1 (OMIM 131100) (Table 54-1).

CLINICAL FEATURES

MEN-2 consists of medullary thyroid carcinoma (MTC), pheochromocytoma, and hyperparathyroidism inherited as an autosomal dominant trait. The nomenclature for this disease syndrome has evolved during the decades since its initial description; a current classification system that reflects the clinical features and molecular causes is shown in Table 54-1. The syndrome originally described by Sipple has been classified as MEN-2A (OMIM 171400). It consists of MTC in nearly all gene carriers, pheochromocytoma in one-half, and hyperparathyroidism in 10–20% (Table 54-1). Characteristics of all neoplastic components associated with MEN-2 are bilaterality and multicentricity. This is especially important for MTC in which surgical cure is possible only by removal of all thyroid tissue.

There are three variants of MEN-2A: familial medullary thyroid carcinoma (FMTC); MEN-2A with cutaneous lichen amyloidosis (MEN-2A/CLA); and MEN-2A with Hirschsprung disease (Table 54-1). Medullary thyroid carcinoma in FMTC is inherited as an autosomal dominant trait without other features of MEN-2A. The MTC associated with FMTC tends to be less aggressive and is most likely to be confused with sporadic MTC because other manifestations of MEN-2A are not present, and many affected family members may be asymptomatic. A diagnosis of FMTC should be made only in large, multigenerational families because of the incomplete penetrance (50% or less) for other manifestations of MEN-2A. The MEN-2A/CLA variant, found in approximately 18 kindreds worldwide, is the association of MEN-2A with a characteristic pruritic skin lesion located over the central upper back. The clinical features, other than the skin lesion, are identical to classic MEN-2A, although hyperparathyroidism appears to be less common. Finally, a handful of families have been described with MEN-2A and Hirschsprung disease. The penetrance of the Hirschsprung phenotype is variable, ranging from complete penetration to a single affected member.

MEN-2B (OMIM 162300) is characterized by MTC and pheochromocytoma, as well as a unique phenotype of marfanoid habitus and mucosal, oral, and intestinal ganglioneuromatosis (Table 54-1). This disorder is transmitted as an autosomal dominant trait, although the majority of cases represent *de novo* mutations; the mutant allele is inherited from the father and the mutation is thought to occur during spermatogenesis. Medullary thyroid carcinoma associated with MEN-2B is more aggressive than that observed in MEN-2A. Development of carcinoma during the first year of life is common, and early death from metastatic MTC occurs in 30–40% of patients. The prognosis, however, is not universally poor. A number of multigeneration families suggests considerable variability in the outcome.

DIAGNOSIS

MEN-2 is a clinical syndrome that affects multiple endocrine organs. Medullary thyroid carcinoma and pheochromocytoma are the most common causes of morbidity and death. Hyperparathyroidism and its associated findings of hypercalcemia, nephrolithiasis, and bone loss are less commonly a clinical problem.

The C cell, the cell type comprising MTC, produces a small peptide hormone, calcitonin. The circulating concentration of this peptide is normally less than 10 pg/mL. In patients with MTC, serum calcitonin values are characteristically elevated and secretion may be stimulated 3- to 20-fold higher by intravenous pentagastrin, calcium, or a combination of the two. Prospective studies using provocative testing with pentagastrin or the combination of calcium and pentagastrin have been used successfully to identify MTC early in the course of the disease. Prospective pentagastrin screening and thyroidectomy have improved survival and quality of life in these kindreds, although not all children or young adults are cured with this approach. As many as 10–15% of these patients have evidence of recurrent disease in long-term follow-up studies. Whether earlier or more complete thyroidectomy based on genetic testing (to be discussed in the next section) will improve outcome is not certain and is currently under investigation.

Pheochromocytoma occurs in approximately 50% of family members with MEN-2. These tumors cause palpitations, headaches, and attacks of nervousness early in the course of tumor development; hypertension is infrequently found at this stage. In patients with large or bilateral tumors, hypertension and cardiac

From: *Principles of Molecular Medicine* (J. L. Jameson, ed.), ©1998 Humana Press Inc., Totowa, NJ.

Table 54-1
The Multiple Endocrine Neoplasia Syndromes

Multiple endocrine neoplasia type 1 (MEN-1)
Pituitary tumors
Parathyroid neoplasia
Islet cell neoplasia
Multiple endocrine neoplasia type 2 (MEN-2)
Multiple endocrine neoplasia type 2A (MEN-2A)
Medullary thyroid carcinoma 100%
Pheochromocytoma 50%
Parathyroid neoplasia (10–20%)
Variants of MEN-2A
Familial medullary thyroid carcinoma (FMTC)
MEN-2A with cutaneous lichen amyloidosis (MEN-2A/CLA)
MEN-2A with Hirschsprung disease
Multiple endocrine neoplasia type 2B
Medullary thyroid carcinoma (100%)
Pheochromocytoma (50%)
No parathyroid disease
Marfanoid habitus (nearly 100%)
Intestinal ganglioneuromatosis and mucosal neuromas (nearly 100%)

arrhythmias may occur. Before the recognition of this syndrome in 1961 at least one-half of the deaths in MEN-2 kindreds occurred suddenly and were attributed to cardiac disease; many were no doubt related to pheochromocytoma. The goal of screening for pheochromocytoma in kindreds with MEN-2 is to identify an adrenal tumor before it causes significant or life-threatening manifestations of catecholamine excess. One successful approach is the routine annual collection of a 12- or 24-h urine for catecholamines or metanephrines. Symptomatic patients will frequently have an elevation of either the plasma or urine catecholamines or metanephrine. Patients with abnormal values should have imaging studies. Computerized tomography provides better definition of the adrenal medulla and is less expensive. Magnetic resonance imaging provides greater specificity if the adrenal medulla lights up on T2-weighted images.

The major diagnostic problems occur at the transition between the normal and slightly abnormal state. Patients may have symptoms suggestive of pheochromocytoma with normal catecholamine measurements and imaging studies. In this situation the differentiation between intermittent abnormal catecholamine secretion and an anxiety disorder can be difficult. A trial of adrenergic blockade or inhibition of catecholamine synthesis with α-methyltyrosine may help separate these two possibilities. If the patient is improved by pharmacologic intervention and surgery is contemplated, the choice of which adrenal to remove may be difficult. Two approaches have been applied in this situation. The first is to continue adrenergic blockade or catecholamine synthesis inhibition for 1–2 years, during which time a radiologic abnormality may appear; second, octreotide or met iodobenzylguanidine scanning may occasionally identify the abnormal adrenal medulla.

GENETIC BASIS OF MEN-2

MAPPING THE CAUSATIVE GENE The identification of polymorphic DNA sequences throughout the human genome in the late 1970s led to a resurgence of interest in genetic linkage approaches to the identification of disease genes. A well-defined phenotype and large families made MEN-2 an ideal syndrome in which to apply this new technology. Progress was slow because of the lack of evenly spaced polymorphic markers throughout the genome and the necessity to use Southern blotting techniques rather than the current polymerase chain reaction techniques. The gene was mapped to centromeric chromosome 10 in 1987. Subsequent work by many groups narrowed the region containing the MEN-2 gene, leading to the identification of mutations of the c-*ret* proto-oncogene (OMIM 164760) in 1993 (Fig. 54-1).

The c-*ret* proto-oncogene was first discovered in 1985 when a rearranged form of this gene was shown to cause transformation. The c-*ret* proto-oncogene encodes a tyrosine kinase receptor. A naturally occurring rearrangement was subsequently identified in 10–35% of papillary thyroid carcinomas and named the papillary thyroid carcinoma or PTC oncogene. Three different PTC variants exist, each resulting from a chromosome 10 rearrangement that places the tyrosine kinase domain of the c-*ret* proto-oncogene under the transcriptional control of another constitutively expressed gene (OMIM 164761 and 188550). There is compelling evidence that the c-*ret* rearrangement causes transformation of the thyroid follicular cell in animal models of papillary thyroid carcinoma.

THE RET/GLIAL CELL-DERIVED NEUROTROPHIC FACTOR RECEPTOR SYSTEM A remarkable series of studies during the past 3 years have defined a tyrosine kinase receptor signaling system important for the development of the gastrointestinal neuronal system, the kidney, and several components of the sympathetic nervous system. The first important discovery was the development of profound gastrointestinal and renal abnormalities in mice in which the c-*ret* proto-oncogene was inactivated. Detailed studies in these animals showed gastrointestinal neuronal features analogous to those found in Hirschsprung disease with incomplete development of the enteric nervous system. There was also a complete lack of renal development in these animals. Components of the sympathetic nervous system, including the superior cervical ganglion, were also underdeveloped. The second important discovery was the finding that mice in which the gene for glial cell-derived neurotrophic factor (GDNF; OMIM 600837) had been inactivated demonstrated a phenotype analogous to that seen in the animals with a c-*ret* proto-oncogene knockout. These studies also illuminated the mechanism by which GDNF and Ret interact to promote normal renal development (Fig. 54-2). The ureteric bud (the developing renal ureteral collecting system) normally penetrates the metanephric blastema and branches to form the collecting system (Fig. 54-3). Recent studies have shown that the peptide GDNF is expressed in the developing metanephric blastema and interacts with the Ret receptor in the ureteric bud to promote normal interaction and branching of the ureteric bud into the developing kidney. Available facts suggest a similar pattern of interaction between Ret and GDNF in the developing enteric neuronal system. What is clear is that Ret is expressed in neural crest cells associated with somites 1–5. These Ret-positive cells migrate into the spinal cord and into the developing gastrointestinal tract during embryonic life. The finding of incomplete neuronal development in both the Ret and GDNF knockouts provides compelling evidence for an interaction between the ligand–receptor system of importance in neuronal innervation of the intestine (Fig. 54-3).

In an independent series of experiments, researchers discovered a receptor for GDNF, termed GDNFR-α, and showed it to complex with the Ret tyrosine kinase receptor to form a receptor for GDNF (OMIM 601496). This receptor system is unique because GDNFR-α is an extracellular protein that complexes with the Ret receptor, although specific details are sketchy (Fig. 54-2).

Clinical Syndrome	Codon of Ret Mutated
MEN 2A FMTC	609 611 618 620 634
FMTC	768 804
MEN2A/ CLA	634
MEN 2A/ Hirschsprung	609 618 620
MEN 2B	918

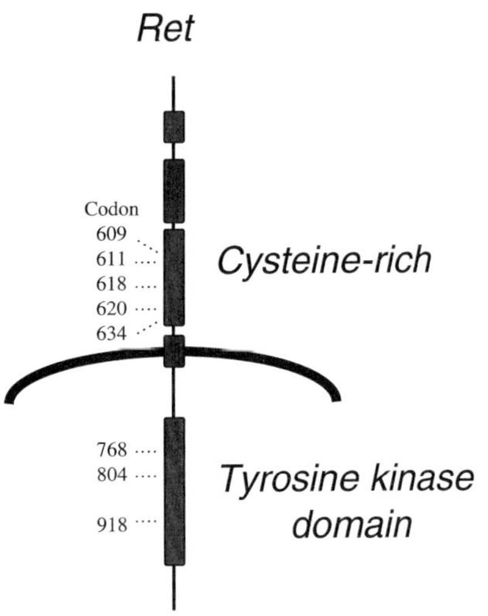

Ret

Codon 609 611 618 620 634

Cysteine-rich

768 804 918

Tyrosine kinase domain

Figure 54-1 Mutations of the c-*ret* proto-oncogene associated with hereditary medullary thyroid carcinoma. The most common mutations affect two regions of the Ret tyrosine kinase. Mutations of an extracellular cysteine domain (codons 609, 611, 618, 620, 630, 634), important for dimerization of the receptor, cause MEN-2A and its variants. Mutations of the tyrosine kinase domain are found in MEN-2B (codons 918, 883) and a few families with FMTC (768, 804, 891). Mutations of codons 790 and 791 have been identified in MEN-2A. MEN-2A, multiple endocrine neoplasia type 2A; FMTC, familial medullary thyroid carcinoma; MEN-2A/CLA, MEN-2A/cutaneous lichen amyloidosis; MEN-2A/Hirschsprung, MEN-2A/Hirschsprung disease variant; and MEN-2B, multiple endocrine neoplasia type 2B.

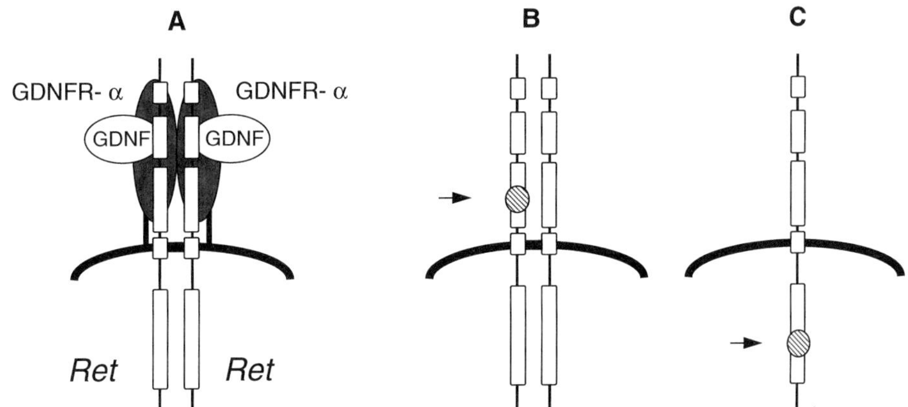

Figure 54-2 The Ret/GDNFR-α signaling system and the effect of c-*ret* proto-oncogene mutations on signaling. **(A)** Proposed model for the Ret/GDNFR-α receptor system. It is known that GDNF will bind to GDNFR-α. It is hypothesized that GDNFR-α transmits the signal to Ret to effect autophosphorylation and phosphorylation of downstream effector proteins. **(B)** Effect of a codon 634 mutation on Ret activation. Mutation of the extracellular domain results in dimerization of Ret, autophosphorylation, and phosphorylation of downstream substrates in the absence of GDNF. There is currently no evidence for or against participation of GDNFR-α in this process. **(C)** Effect of a codon 918 mutation on Ret activation. Mutation of the tyrosine kinase domain causes autophosphorylation and phosphorylation of a different set of downstream substrate proteins in the absence of Ret dimerization. There is currently no knowledge of GDNFR-α participation.

In the broader perspective these studies provide insight into an important neural crest development pathway. Studies of Ret expression in developing embryos have shown Ret expression in neural crest derived from somites one to five. Between days 9 and 10.5 there is migration of Ret-positive cells from the neural crest into the developing spinal cord and gastrointestinal tract (Fig. 54-4). It is possible to envision a trophic effect of GDNF interaction with Ret (and possibly GDNFR-α) to entice neural crest cells into their normal developmental location. Further studies of this system will lead to a greater understanding of these pathways.

MUTATIONS OF THE c-*ret* PROTO-ONCOGENE ASSOCIATED WITH MTC The mutations of c-*ret* in MEN-2 affect two domains within the Ret tyrosine kinase receptor. Mutations of a cysteine-rich region of the extracellular domain are the most common mutations found in MEN-2 and its variants (Fig. 54-1). Each of these point mutations convert a conserved cysteine at codons 609, 611, 618, 620, or 634 to another amino acid. A single mutation, Cys634Arg, accounts for more than 50% of all mutations associated with hereditary MTC, and more than 75% of all mutations affect codon 634. Genotype–phenotype correlation shows that a codon 634 mutation is most commonly associated

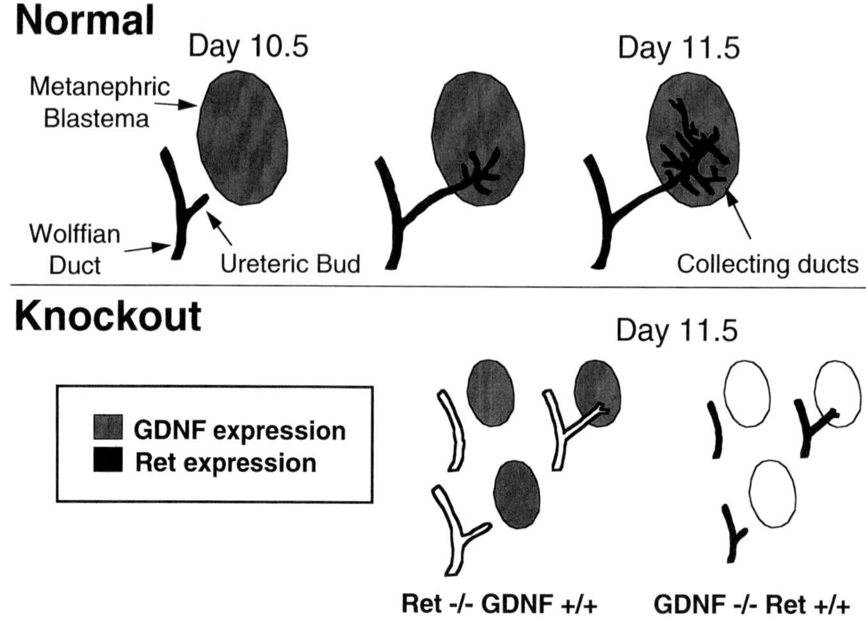

Figure 54-3 Schematic view showing mouse embryonic kidney development. The ureteric bud, derived from the Wolffian duct, normally migrates into the developing metanephric blastema to form the collecting system. In either Ret (Ret –/–) or GDNF (GDNF –/–) knockouts there is a defect in migration of the ureteric bud into the metanephric blastema resulting in a failure of normal kidney development.

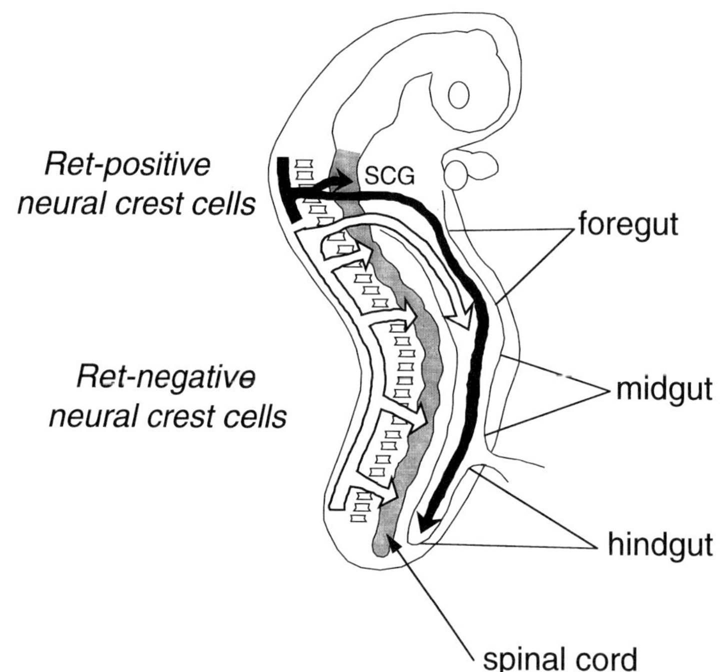

Figure 54-4 Migration of neural crest cells expressing the Ret tyrosine kinase into the developing spinal cord and gastrointestinal tract. Ret-expressing cells form the superior cervical ganglion (SCG), parts of the dorsal root of the spinal cord, and the enteric neuronal plexus of the gastrointestinal tract.

with classic MEN-2A or Sipple's syndrome. Mutations of the codons found in exon 10 (609, 611, 618, 620) are most commonly found in FMTC. Despite these correlative efforts, any of the extracellular cysteine mutations can be associated with MEN-2A or FMTC, a point of importance in the clinical management of kindreds with these mutations. More recently, codon 790 and 791 mutations have been identified in MEN-2A and FMTC. A clinician should not conclude that an individual with an exon 10 mutation will not develop a pheochromocytoma unless there are multiple generations within a family that have not developed pheochromocytoma. All patients with the MEN-2A/CLA syndrome have codon 634 mutations.

Germline mutations of the tyrosine kinase domain are found in MEN-2B (Met918Thr) and FMTC (Glu768Asp and Val804Leu) (Fig. 54-1). Two families with FMTC and germline codon 891 mutations have been identified. Ninety-five percent of patients with MEN-2B have the Met918Thr substitution or a mutation at codon 883 (Fig. 54-1); the mutation in the remaining 5% has not been identified. In the handful of kindreds with the codon 768 and 804 mutations the only clinical phenotype is familial MTC (Fig. 54-1).

Additional evidence for the oncogenicity of these mutations came from studies in which expression of mutant c-*ret* proto-oncogene in NIH-3T3 cells caused transformation. These studies showed that codon 634 mutation resulted in dimerization of the Ret tyrosine kinase receptor in the absence of its ligand, leading to autophosphorylation and phosphorylation of downstream proteins (Fig. 54-2). Transfection of the c-*ret* cDNA containing the Met918Thr mutation also causes transformation, although dimerization of the receptor does not occur and a different set of substrate proteins are phosphorylated (Fig. 54-2). Although not described, mutations of GDNF or GDNFR-α may be found in the small percentage of kindreds in whom mutations of the c-*ret* proto-oncogene have not been identified.

MUTATIONS OF THE c-*ret* PROTO-ONCOGENE ASSOCIATED WITH HIRSCHSPRUNG DISEASE Two independent lines of analysis led to the identification of mutations of the c-*ret* proto-oncogene in patients with Hirschsprung disease (OMIM 142623). The identification of a chromosome 10 deletion in a child with Hirschsprung disease led to mapping studies in familial Hirschsprung disease, which localized the causative gene to proximal chromosome 10q. Subsequent investigations identified inactivating and presumed activating mutations of the Ret tyrosine kinase in Hirschsprung disease. Analyses of kindreds in which MEN-2A and Hirschsprung disease cosegregate (Table 54-1) have identified codon 609, 618, or 620 mutations of the c-*ret* proto-oncogene. Mutations of the endothelin-B receptor gene (OMIM 131244) and its ligand, endothelin-3 (OMIM 131242), have also been identified in Hirschsprung disease. There are preliminary reports of mutations of the GDNF gene in Hirschsprung disease, although their significance is unclear; it seems likely that mutations of the GDNFR-α gene will be identified in this disorder.

Mutation analysis is readily available from several commercial sources.* Several techniques have been applied to detection of mutations, including direct DNA sequencing and restriction analysis for specific mutations, denaturing gradient gel electrophoresis, and reverse dot-blot analysis. All of these techniques are reproducible and performed on a whole blood sample from the patient. There are a few caveats. Genetic testing, like most other forms of laboratory analysis, will be associated with a small error rate caused by sample mixup, contamination of the PCR reaction, failure of specific primers to amplify the mutant allele, or technician copying errors, collectively estimated in the range of 5%. Before a decision is made to consider surgical intervention in a gene carrier or to eliminate an MEN-2 kindred member with a normal analysis from further screening, the test should be performed on a separately obtained and independently analyzed blood sample.

MUTATIONS OF THE c-*ret* PROTO-ONCOGENE IN SPORADIC MTC Somatic Met918Thr mutations of the c-*ret* proto-oncogene have been identified in approximately 25% of sporadic MTCs. There is suggestive but incomplete evidence that suggests that tumors with this particular mutation may pursue a more aggressive clinical course. It is important to consider c-*ret* proto-oncogene analysis in patients with apparent sporadic MTC because a compilation of available information suggests that 5–7% of patients with apparent sporadic MTC have germline mutations of the c-*ret* proto-oncogene.

MANAGEMENT AND TREATMENT

MANAGEMENT OF MEDULLARY THYROID CARCINOMA Negative Genetic Test Results The availability of reliable genetic testing makes it possible to identify gene carriers with near certainty. Children with negative test results in a kindred in which a c-*ret* mutation has been identified can be excluded from further screening studies. It is important to repeat the analysis on more than one blood sample to be certain of the test results. This is especially true of individuals who have a normal Ret analysis and will receive no further screening.

Positive Genetic Test Results There is incomplete agreement on how gene carriers should be managed. One approach is to continue pentagastrin testing on an annual basis with removal of the thyroid gland at the time of a first abnormal test. A 25-year experience with prospective screening using calcitonin measurements after pentagastrin stimulation indicates that 85–90% of children with MEN-2A can be cured by early thyroidectomy performed at the time of first positive pentagastrin or calcium-pentagastrin test. However, 5–15% of children with abnormalities detected by pentagastrin testing have developed probable metastatic MTC at a later date, suggesting either undetected metastatic spread at the time of thyroidectomy or incomplete thyroidectomy with subsequent transformation of residual C cells. This issue and the identification of a 6-year-old child with metastatic MTC in the context of MEN-2A has led a large percentage of clinicians who deal with this disease to recommend thyroidectomy based solely on genetic testing. The age of 5 years has been somewhat arbitrarily chosen as an appropriate age at which to perform thyroidectomy for several reasons: the child is old enough to understand the procedure; the surgical anatomy of the neck is easily delineated; and parents have less anxiety about performance of a thyroidectomy at this age. The belief is that early and complete thyroidectomy will improve the cure rate beyond the earlier reported figures of 85–90%, a rationale for which there is no current proof.

The completeness of thyroidectomy may be important. It is difficult to perform a total thyroidectomy without damage to the posterior capsule of the thyroid gland, leading to a higher incidence of hypoparathyroidism, a situation most surgeons choose to avoid. A few normal C cells in residual thyroid tissue attached to the posterior capsule may be of little concern in a 40- to 50-year-old patient, but there is the real possibility that a few normal cells expressing mutant Ret in a 5-year-old child may transform during a several decade follow-up. This concern has led some clinicians to recommend a total thyroidectomy, including the posterior capsule, central lymph node dissection, and transplantation of parathyroid tissue to the nondominant arm. Whether this approach will improve the already excellent long-term cure rate for this disease is unclear but seems worthy of investigation.

Another reason to consider thyroidectomy based on genetic testing is the relative insensitivity of pentagastrin testing. Thyroidectomy based on genetic testing has identified microscopic or macroscopic MTC in approximately one-half of patients with normal pentagastrin or calcium-pentagastrin tests. These results indicate that pentagastrin or combined calcium-pentagastrin testing is an insensitive technique for detection of early MTC in MEN-2A or FMTC, leaving open the possibility that metastasis may already have occurred in some patients at the time of thyroidectomy. When one combines all of these factors, performance of a thyroidectomy at the earliest possible age seems the most prudent course.

Children with MEN-2B should have a thyroidectomy performed during the first months of life because of the high probability of early metastasis. Whether early intervention will alter the long-term course of this disease is not currently known.

MANAGEMENT OF PHEOCHROMOCYTOMA The advent of genetic testing will have little impact on the management of pheochromocytoma in MEN-2 other than to exclude 50% of family members with normal genetic tests from further screening. Patients with pheochromocytomas should have unilateral or bilateral adrenalectomy. The issues related to unilateral or bilateral adrenalectomy in this disease have been discussed in detail elsewhere and will not be reviewed in this chapter. Patients with abnormal catecholamine secretion should have adrenal surgery performed before consideration of thyroidectomy.

MANAGEMENT OF HYPERPARATHYROIDISM Hyperparathyroidism occurs infrequently in children who have received prophylactic thyroidectomy for MTC. In one series there have been no cases of hyperparathyroidism in children who received thyroidectomy at a mean age of 13 years with a mean follow-up period in excess of 20 years. There is debate about the appropriate management of parathyroid neoplasia in older patients. Either subtotal parathyroidectomy or total parathyroidectomy with transplantation of parathyroid tissue to the nondominant forearm has been advocated.

FUTURE DIRECTIONS

Hereditary MTC is a rare disorder, but the specific molecular defect that causes this neoplastic syndrome provides a useful model in which to study strategies for inactivation of mutant Ret tyrosine kinase activity. The fact that a single gene defect causes three different neoplastic manifestations makes it an interesting model for study. Future strategies for prevention or treatment of this disease could include preimplantation screening with selection of embryos for implantation that do not carry the mutant Ret allele or strategies to inactivate or modify the mutant Ret mRNA. Although the cost of preimplantation screening is currently high, it seems likely that these costs would be recovered in a single generation with positive effects extending into future generations.

SELECTED REFERENCES

Angrist M, Bolk S, Halushka M, Lapchak PA, Chakravarti A. Germline mutations in glial cell-derived neurotrophic factor (GDNF) and RET in a Hirschsprung disease patient. Nat Genet 1996;14:341–344.

Angrist M, Kauffman E, Slaugenhaupt SA, et al. A gene for Hirschsprung disease (megacolon) in the pericentromeric region of human chromosome 10. Nat Genet 1993;4:351–356.

Asai N, Iwashita T, Matsuyama M, Takahashi M. Mechanisms of activation of the ret proto-oncogene by multiple endocrine neoplasia 2A mutations. Mol Cell Biol 1995;15:1613–1619.

Borst MJ, Van Camp JM, Peacock ML, Decker RA. Mutational analysis of multiple endocrine neoplasia type 2A associated with Hirschsprung's disease. Surgery 1995;117:386–391.

Carlson KM, Bracamontes J, Jackson CE, et al. Parent-of-origin effects in multiple endocrine neoplasia type 2B. Am J Hum Genet 1994;55: 1076–1082.

Carney JA, Go VL, Sizemore GW, Hayles AB. Alimentary-tract ganglioneuromatosis. A major component of the syndrome of multiple endocrine neoplasia, type 2b. N Engl J Med 1976;295:1287–1291.

Donis-Keller H, Shenshen D, Chi D, et al. Mutations in the RET proto-oncogene are associated with MEN 2A and FMTC. Hum Molec Genet 1993;2:851–856.

Durbec P, Marcos-Gutierrez CV, Kilkenny C, et al. GDNF signalling through the ret receptor tyrosine kinase. Nature 1996;381:789–793.

Edery P, Lyonnet S, Mulligan LM, et al. Mutations of the RET proto-oncogene in Hirschsprung's disease. Nature 1994;367:378–380.

Eng C, Clayton D, Schuffennecker I, et al. The relationship between specific *RET* proto-oncogene mutations and disease phenotype in multiple endocrine neoplasia type 2: international *RET* consortium analysis. JAMA 1996;276:1575–1579.

Evans DB, Lee JE, Merrell RC, Hickey RC. Adrenal medullary disease in multiple endocrine neoplasia type 2. Appropriate management. Endocrinol Metab Clin North Am 1994;23:167–176.

Farndon JR, Leight GS, Dilley WG, et al. Familial medullary thyroid carcinoma without associated endocrinopathies: a distinct clinical entity. Br J Surg 1986;73:278–281.

Gagel RF, Cote GJ, Martins Bugalho MJG, et al. Clinical use of molecular information in the management of multiple endocrine neoplasia type 2A. J Intern Med 1995;238:333–341.

Gagel RF, Levy ML, Donovan DT, Alford BR, Wheeler T, Tschen JA. Multiple endocrine neoplasia type 2a associated with cutaneous lichen amyloidosis. Ann Intern Med 1989;111:802–806.

Gagel RF, Tashjian AH, Jr., Cummings T, et al. The clinical outcome of prospective screening for multiple endocrine neoplasia type 2a: An 18-year experience. N Engl J Med 1988;318:478–484.

Grieco M, Santoro M, Berlingieri MT, et al. PTC is a novel rearranged form of the ret proto-oncogene and is frequently detected in vivo in human thyroid papillary carcinomas. Cell 1990;60:557–563.

Hennessey JF, Wells SA, Ontjes DA, Cooper CW. A comparison of pentagastrin injections and calcium infusion as provocative agents for the detection of medullary carcinoma of the thyroid. J Clin Endocr Metab 1974;39:487.

Hofstra RM, Osinga J, Tan-Sindhunata G, et al. A homozygous mutation in the endothelin-3 gene associated with a combined Waardenburg type 2 and Hirschsprung phenotype (Shah-Waardenburg syndrome). Nat Genet 1996;12:445–447.

Jing S, Wen D, Yu Y, et al. GDNF-induced activation of the Ret protein tyrosine kinase is mediated by GDNFR-a, a novel receptor for GDNF. Cell 1996;85:1113–1124.

Komminoth P, Kunz EK, Matias-Guiu X, et al. Analysis of RET proto-oncogene point mutations distinguishes heritable from nonheritable medullary thyroid carcinomas. Cancer 1995;76:479–489.

Lairmore TC, Howe JR, Korte JA, et al. Familial medullary thyroid carcinoma and multiple endocrine neoplasia type 2B map to the same region of chromosome 10 as multiple endocrine neoplasia type 2A. Genomics 1991;9:181–192.

Lee JE, Curley SA, Gagel RF, Evans DB, Hickey RC. Cortical-sparing adrenalectomy for patients with bilateral pheochromocytoma. Surgery 1996;120:1064–1071.

Lin LF, Doherty DH, Lile JD, Bektesh S, Colline F. GDNF: a glial cell line-derived neurotrophic factor for midbrain dopaminergic neurons. Science 1993;260:1130–1132.

Lips CJ, Landsvater RM, Hoppener JW, et al. Clinical screening as compared with DNA analysis in families with multiple endocrine neoplasia type 2A. N Engl J Med 1994;331:828–835.

Lyonnet S, Bolino A, Pelet A, et al. A gene for Hirschsprung disease maps to the proximal long arm of chromosome 10. Nat Genet 1993;4:346–350.

Mathew CG, Chin KS, Easton DF, et al. A linked genetic marker for multiple endocrine neoplasia type 2A on chromosome 10. Nature 1987;328:527,528.

Moley JF. The molecular genetics of multiple endocrine neoplasia type 2A and related syndromes. Annu Rev Med 1997;48: 409–420.

Moore MW, Klein RD, Farinas I, et al. Renal and neuronal abnormalities in mice lacking GDNF. Nature 1996;382:76–79.

Mulligan LM, Kwok JBJ, Healey CS, et al. Germline mutations of the RET proto-oncogene in multiple endocrine neoplasia type 2A (MEN 2A). Nature 1993;363:458–460.

Norum RA, Lafreniere RG, ONeal LW, et al. Linkage of the multiple endocrine neoplasia type 2B gene (MEN2B) to chromosome 10 markers linked to MEN2A. Genomics 1990;8:313–317.

Nunziata V, di Giovanni G, Lettera AM, D'Armiento M, Mancini M. Cutaneous lichen amyloidosis associated with multiple endocrine neoplasia type 2A. Henry Ford Hosp J 1989;37:144–146.

Pachnis V, Mankoo B, Costantini F. Expression of the c-ret proto-oncogene during mouse embryogenesis. Development 1993;119:1005–1017.
Pichel JG, Shen L, Sheng HZ, et al. Defects in enteric innervation and kidney development in mice lacking GDNF. Nature 1996;382:73–76.
Puffenberger E, Hosoda K, Washington S, et al. A missense mutation of the endothelin-B receptor gene in multigenic Hirschsprung's disease. Cell 1994;79:1257–1266.
Puliti A, Covone AE, Bicocchi MP, et al. Deleted and normal chromosome 10 homologs from a patient with Hirschsprung disease isolated in two cell hybrids through enrichment by immunomagnetic selection. Cytogenet Cell Genet 1993;63:102–106.
Robertson K, Mason I. The GDNF-RET signalling partnership. Trends Genet 1997;13: 1–3.
Romeo G, Ronchetto P, Luo Y, et al. Point mutations affecting the tyrosine kinase domain of the RET proto-oncogene in Hirschsprung's disease. Nature 1994;367:377,378.
Samaan NA, Draznin MB, Halpin RE, Bloss RS, Hawkins E, Lewis RA. Multiple endocrine syndrome type IIb in early childhood. Cancer 1991;68:1832–1834.
Salomon R, Attie T, Pelet A, et al. Germline mutations of the RET ligand GDNF are not sufficient to cause Hirschsprung disease. Nat Genet 1996;14:345–347.
Sanchez M, Silos-Santiago I, Frisen J, He B, Lira S, Barbacid M. Newborn mice lacking GDNF display renal agenesis and absence of enteric neurons, but no deficits in midbrain dopaminergic neurons. Nature 1996;382:70–73.
Santoro M, Carlomagno F, Romano A, et al. Activation of RET as a dominant transforming gene by germline mutations of MEN 2A and MEN 2B. Science 1995;267:381–383.
Schuchardt A, D'Agati V, Larsson-Blomberg L, Costantini F, Pachnis V. Defects in the kidney and enteric nervous system of mice lacking the tyrosine kinase receptor Ret. Nature 1994;367:380–383.
Schuchardt A, D'Agati V, Larsson-Blombert L, Costantini F, Pachnis V. RET-deficient mice: an animal model for Hirschsprung's disease and renal agenesis. J Intern Med 1995;238:327–332.
Simpson NE, Kidd KK, Goodfellow PJ, et al. Assignment of multiple endocrine neoplasia type 2A to chromosome 10 by linkage. Nature 1987;328:528–530.
Sipple JH. The association of pheochromcytoma with carcinoma of the thyroid gland. Am J Med 1961;31:163–166.
Sizemore GW, Carney JA, Gharib H, Capen CC. Multiple endocrine neoplasia type 2B: eighteen-year follow-up of a four-generation family. Henry Ford Hosp J 1992;40:236–244.
Takahashi M, Cooper GM. ret transforming gene encodes a fusion protein homologous to tyrosine kinases. Mol Cell Biol 1987; 7:1378–1385.
Takahashi M, Ritz J, Cooper GM. Activation of a novel human transforming gene, ret, by DNA rearrangement. Cell 1985;42:581–588.
Treanor JJS, Goodman L, de Sauvage F, et al. Characterization of a multicomponent receptor for GDNF. Nature 1996;382:80–83.
Trupp M, Arenas E, Falnzilber M, et al. Functional receptor for GDNF encoded by the c-ret proto-oncogene. Nature 1996;381:785–788.
van Heerden JA, Sizemore GW, Carney JA, Brennan MD, Sheps SG. Bilateral subtotal adrenal resection for bilateral pheochromocytomas in multiple endocrine neoplasia, type IIa: a case report. Surgery 1985; 98:363–366.
Vistelle R, Grulet H, Gibold C, et al. High permanent plasma adrenaline levels: a marker of adrenal medullary disease in medullary thyroid carcinoma. Clin Endocrinol 1991;34:133–138.
Wells SA, Jr., Baylin SB, Linehan WM, et al. Provocative agents and the diagnosis of medullary carcinoma of the thyroid gland. Ann Surg 1978;188:139–141.
Wells SA, Chi DD, Toshima K, et al. Predictive DNA testing and prophylactic thyroidectomy in patients at risk for multiple endocrine neoplasia type 2A. Ann Surg 1994;220:237–250.
Wells SA, Jr., Ellis GJ, Gunnells JC, Schneider AB, Sherwood LM. Parathyroid autotransplantation in primary parathyroid hyperplasia. N Engl J Med 1976;195:57–62.
Williams ED, Brown CL, Doniach I. Pathological and clinical findings in a series of 67 cases of medullary carcinoma of the thyroid. J Clin Pathol 1966;19:103–113.
Wohllk N, Cote GJ, Bugalho MMJ, et al. Relevance of RET proto-oncogene mutations in sporadic medullary thyroid carcinoma. J Clin Endocrinol Metab 1996;81:3740–3745.
Wohllk N, Cote GJ, Evans D, Goepfert H, Ordonez N, Gagel RF. Application of genetic screening information to the management of medullary thyroid carcinoma and multiple endocrine neoplasia. Endocrinol Metab Clin North Am 1996;25:1–25.
Xing S, Smanik PA, Oglesbee MJ, Trosko JE, Mazzaferri EL, Jhiang SM. Characterization of ret oncogenic activation in MEN2 inherited cancer syndromes. Endocrinology 1996;137:1512–1519.
Zedenius J, Wallin G, Hamberger B, Nordenskjold M, Weber G, Larsson C. Somatic and MEN 2A de novo mutations identified in the RET proto-oncogene by screening of sporadic MTCs. Hum Mol Genet 1994;3:1259–1262.

55 Molecular Mechanisms of Hypoglycemia Associated with Increased Insulin Production

PAMELA M. THOMAS, GILBERT J. COTE, AND ROBERT F. GAGEL

BACKGROUND

The differential diagnosis of hypoglycemia in the pediatric age group is broad (Table 55-1). In the neonatal period, transient hypoglycemia caused by hyperinsulinemia is common. It is, however, the rare newborn who presents with profound and prolonged hypoglycemia requiring substantial glucose replacement. When this is detected, it most commonly is caused by hyperinsulinism.

Persistent hyperinsulinemic hypoglycemia of infancy (PHHI), also known as familial hyperinsulinism or nesidioblastosis, is characterized by severe pancreatic islet β-cell dysfunction, which is manifest by secretion of insulin in an unregulated fashion despite life-threatening hypoglycemia. It is the most common cause of prolonged and severe hypoglycemia associated with hyperinsulinism in children. Description of this disorder as a unique clinical syndrome began 25 years ago with the association of nesidioblastosis, defined as the budding of isolated endocrine cells and islets from pancreatic duct cells, and severe infantile hypoglycemia. Recent findings have elucidated the molecular cause for hyperinsulinism in some families with this disorder and provided additional insight into the regulation of insulin secretion.

CLINICAL FEATURES

PHHI occurs in the setting of a normal pregnancy and the absence of maternal diabetes or blood type incompatibility. Presenting signs and symptoms of hypoglycemia include jitteriness, hypotonia, poor feeding, cyanosis, seizure, and sudden death. In addition to the symptoms and signs of hypoglycemia, increased adiposity may be noted during an otherwise normal examination. Approximately one-third of the children with clinical features of Beckwith-Wiedemann syndrome have hyperinsulinemic hypoglycemia. The relationship between PHHI and the Beckwith-Wiedemann syndrome, if any, is unknown. The incidence of PHHI has been estimated at 1/50,000 live births annually in a randomly mating Western European population. However, in a Saudi Arabian population, in which 50% of marriages were consanguineous, the incidence of this disorder was established as 1/2,675.

From: *Principles of Molecular Medicine* (J. L. Jameson, ed.), ©1998 Humana Press Inc., Totowa, NJ.

DIAGNOSIS

The diagnostic features of PHHI, listed in Table 55-2, are all attributable to the presence of hyperinsulinemia, which usually presents within the first year of life. The degree and persistence of hyperinsulinemia in PHHI are not seen in transient forms of hyperinsulinism. Histopathologic diagnosis is based on the presence of ductuloinsular complexes, islet hypertrophy, or islet cell proliferation.

GENETIC BASIS OF DISEASE

Recognition of familial forms of PHHI occurred after reports of affected siblings. Inheritance is in an autosomal recessive pattern. The increased incidence present in inbred populations is consistent with autosomal recessive inheritance.

The availability of well-characterized families allowed use of genetic linkage analysis for mapping of this disease gene. Glaser et al. reported linkage in 15 independent families, of which 12 were Ashkenazi Jewish, to the 6.6-cM interval between markers D11S926 and D11S928 on chromosome 11p. Subsequent analysis revealed evidence for a founder effect in the Ashkenazi Jewish ethnic population.

Using the homozygosity gene mapping strategy, we confirmed and narrowed the assignment of Glaser et al. The homozygosity gene mapping strategy is based on the premise that a rare disease in the affected progeny of a consanguineous mating is caused by inheritance of two identical copies of the disease gene from the common ancestor, a situation termed "homozygosity by descent." In addition, regions flanking the disease gene, calculated to be of a median length of 28 cM in first-cousin matings, will be homozygous by descent in most cases. Other regions of the genome will also be homozygous by descent, but such regions will vary among affected children. For an informative, tightly linked marker, the calculations of Lander and Botstein revealed that three first-cousin matings, each with a single affected offspring, will provide a LOD score >3.0, the accepted threshold for linkage. Ten or more nonrelated nuclear families with affected pairs of siblings would be required to generate a similar score. Study of progeny of five consanguineous families of Saudi Arabian origin, using the homozygosity mapping approach, allowed placement of PHHI to a 5-cM interval on chromosome 11p14–15.1, between markers D11S1334 and D11S899 (Fig. 55-1).

Table 55-1
Differential Diagnosis of Hypoglycemia in Children

Transient hypoglycemia
- Prematurity
- Small for gestational age
- Infants with systemic disease
- Infants of diabetic mothers
- Infants with erythroblastosis fetalis

Persistent hypoglycemia
- Hyperinsulinemia
  - Persistent hyperinsulinemic hypoglycemia of infancy
  - β-Cell adenoma
  - Beckwith-Wiedemann syndrome
  - Leucine sensitivity
  - Exogenous insulin abuse
  - Sulfonylurea use
- Hormone deficiency
  - Growth hormone
  - Cortisol
  - Glucagon
  - Panhypopituitarism
- Inborn error of metabolism
  - Glycogen storage diseases
  - Fat metabolism disorders
  - Amino acid metabolism disorders

Table 55-2
Characteristics of Persistent Hyperinsulinemic Hypoglycemia of Infancy

- Inappropriate elevation of serum insulin despite the presence of hypoglycemia
- Nonketotic hypoglycemia
- Increased glucose utilization rate (requires glucose infusion >15 mg · kg^{-1} · min^{-1} to maintain euglycemia)
- Glycemic response to glucagon

In vitro studies of PHHI have suggested a defect of glucose-regulated insulin secretion in pancreatic islet β cells. Assignment of the PHHI locus to chromosome 11p excluded known genes involved in β-cell function, including the glucokinase, islet glucose transporter, and glucagon-like peptide-1 receptor loci, as candidates for PHHI. Current models of insulin secretion propose that, as a result of glucose metabolism, increases in the intracellular ATP/ADP ratio in pancreatic β cells inhibit ATP-sensitive potassium (K_{ATP}) channels leading to β-cell membrane depolarization, opening of voltage-gated calcium channels, and ultimately an increase in exocytosis of insulin (Fig. 55-2). Therefore, candidate genes for PHHI included those involved in the β-cell glucose sensing mechanism and insulin secretion.

The high-affinity sulfonylurea receptor (SUR1), a subunit of the β-cell K_{ATP} channel, was considered as a candidate for the PHHI gene on the basis of its role as a modulator of insulin secretion. The human homolog of the SUR1 gene was localized to chromosome 11p15.1, the previously defined site of the PHHI locus, by fluorescent *in situ* hybridization, and this provided the impetus to begin mutational analysis.

Because of the presence of two nucleotide-binding fold (NBF) consensus sequences, the SUR1 is classified as a member of the ATP-binding cassette superfamily. Contained within the NBF regions are highly conserved phosphate-binding loops, termed "Walker motifs," that form intimate contact with the phosphates of bound nucleotide triphosphates. In other superfamily members, NBF-1 and NBF-2 have functional importance in the control of channel activity, through their interaction with cytosolic nucleotides. This class of molecules is involved in selective transport of substrate across the cell membrane against a concentration gradient using ATP hydrolysis as an energy source. Although each transporter is specific for a given substrate, the spectrum of substrates pumped by family members is diverse and includes amino acids, sugars, inorganic ions, polysaccharides, and peptides. The substrate for the SUR1 has not been elucidated. Other well-known members of this family include the multidrug resistance proteins, and the cystic fibrosis transmembrane conductance regulator (CFTR). Mutations in the CFTR have been shown to cause the autosomal recessive disorder cystic fibrosis, and the more frequent and severe disease alleles are located in the regions of the two NBFs.

A search for mutations in the SUR1 gene in a group of Saudi Arabian individuals affected with PHHI revealed two separate point mutations in splice sites of the NBF-2 region (Fig. 55-3). The first of these mutations, G1400D(23)X, causes skipping of exon 35 of the SUR mRNA transcript with inclusion of a premature stop 24 codons later. The second mutation (3992–9 G→A) was identified in the 3' splice site sequence of exon 33, the first exon of the NBF-2 region. In the presence of this splice site mutation, three cryptic 3' splice sites were used in place of the wild-type splicing pattern, resulting in a 7-bp addition, a 20-bp deletion, or a 30-bp deletion to exon 33.

Mutation of the NBF-1 region of SUR1, like disruption of the NBF-2 region, leads to the PHHI phenotype. Three mutations of the NBF-1 region of SUR1, including one point mutation that disrupts the Walker A motif (G716V), and two that alter RNA processing in the region (1672–20 A→G and 2552–1G→A), have been associated with familial PHHI. These additional mutations establish that both NBF regions of SUR1 are required for normal function, because mutation of either completely voids the ability of SUR1 to regulate insulin secretion and results in the PHHI phenotype.

Two additional mutations have been described in SUR1 in those affected with PHHI. The first is an in-frame deletion within the NBF-2 region (ΔF1388); the combination of the 3992–9 G→A and ΔF1388 mutations accounted for 88% of the PHHI chromosomes in the cohort of 25 Ashkenazi Jews studied. The second is a point mutation, again within the NBF2 region (G1479R) of SUR1, described in a single patient of unestablished ethnic origin; this mutation has been demonstrated to alter the sensitivity of SUR1 to MgADP. A summary of the published SUR1 mutations, depicting their relative locations within the NBF regions of the SUR1 gene, appears in Fig. 55-3.

When expressed individually, SUR1 is unable to produce the β-cell ATP-sensitive potassium current I_{KATP}. However, I_{KATP} can be reconstituted by coexpression of the inward rectifier Kir6.2 with SUR1. Because the Kir6.2 locus is within 5 kb of the SUR1 gene on chromosome 11p15.1 and it is a necessary member of the β-cell K_{ATP} channel, we considered Kir6.2 as an additional candidate gene for PHHI. A homozygous point mutation (L147P), located in the conserved α-helical second transmembrane domain of Kir6.2, was identified in the genomic DNA of a severely affected child from a consanguineous Iranian family. No phenotypic dif-

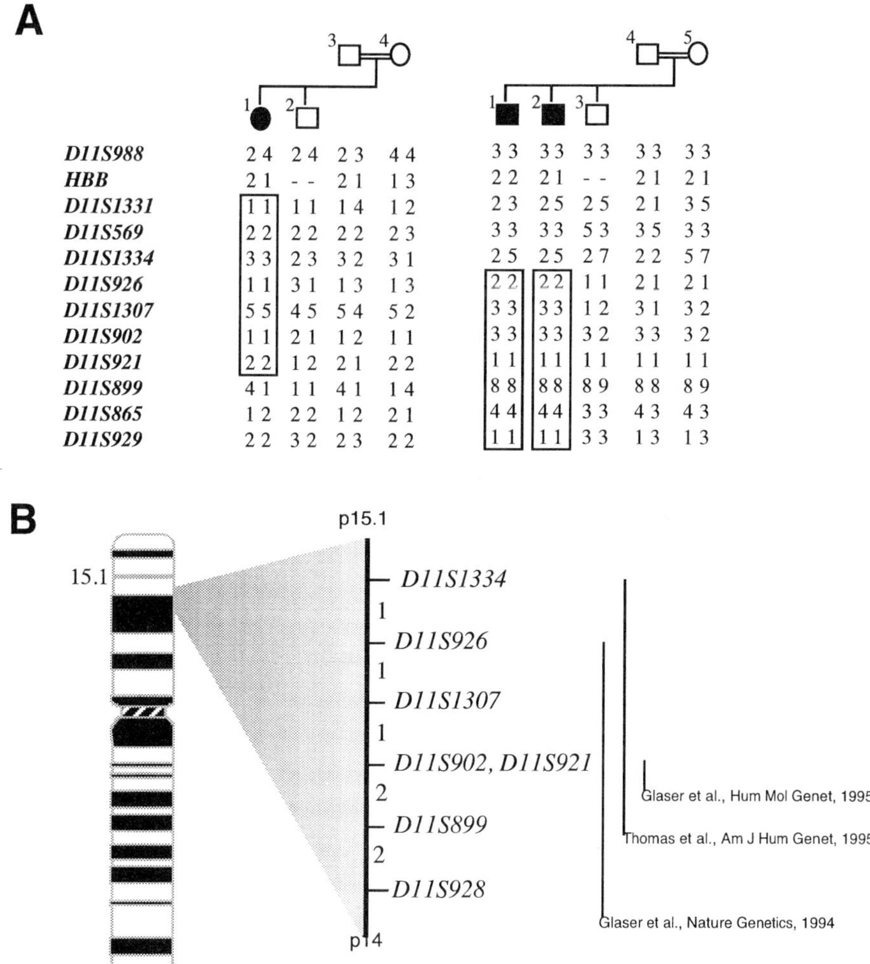

Figure 55-1 Linkage of persistent hyperinsulinemic hypoglycemia of infancy (PHHI) to chromosome 11p15. (**A**) Linkage of PHHI to the interval between the chromosome 11 markers D11S1334 and D11S899 using the homozygosity gene mapping strategy. Shown are simplified pedigrees and genotypes in the region of homozygosity on chromosome 11 of members of two informative families affected with PHHI. Regions of homozygosity in affected children are boxed. In both families the parents are second cousins. Note that within each family the parents share the same disease allele haplotype, which presumably is derived from their common ancestor. (**B**) Summary of linkage data assigning PHHI to chromosome 11p15.1. Polymorphic repeat markers in the 11p15 region are detailed. The numbers between markers are approximate distances in centiMorgans. The vertical lines at the right represent the progressively narrowed regions to which PHHI was linked.

ference was discernible between this family and those with mutations of either the first or second NBF regions of SUR1. The identification of a mutation in Kir6.2 in those affected with PHHI demonstrates genetic heterogeneity for this disorder. In addition, demonstration that loss of function of either Kir6.2 or SUR1 leads to unregulated secretion of insulin and the PHHI phenotype supports the model that these two subunits cooperate in the formation of I_{KATP}.

The identified mutations do not represent the full spectrum of mutations in individuals affected with PHHI, because we are aware of many families that exhibit linkage to chromosome 11p15.1, yet demonstrate none of the mutations now described. By analogy to individuals affected with cystic fibrosis and adrenoleukodystrophy, both of which are caused by mutations in ATP-binding cassette superfamily members, the spectrum of mutations in familial PHHI may be very large. Except in those cases that may be attributed to founder effects, like the Saudi Arabian and Ashkenazi Jewish populations studied, the mutations found to date appear to be of low frequency in the general PHHI population. In addition, the majority of those affected with PHHI exhibit sporadic, rather than familial, forms of the disease. Although sporadic forms of the disease are also associated with loss of K_{ATP} channel activity, it remains to be proven whether mutations of either SUR or Kir6.2 are responsible for these cases; it is possible that further genetic heterogeneity may be present and that additional genes with function related to K_{ATP} channel activity may be identified as responsible for sporadic forms of PHHI. Further comparison of phenotype and genotype status in those affected with PHHI is needed to ascertain whether a correlation may be made between specific mutations of K_{ATP} channel subunits and clinical course. Before prenatal diagnosis or genetic counseling may considered for clinical use for this disorder, further study to answer such questions is needed.

MOLECULAR PATHOPHYSIOLOGY OF DISEASE

The resting membrane potential of pancreatic islet β cells is set by potassium channels. A link between the metabolic state of the cell and membrane electrical events is created by the inhibition of

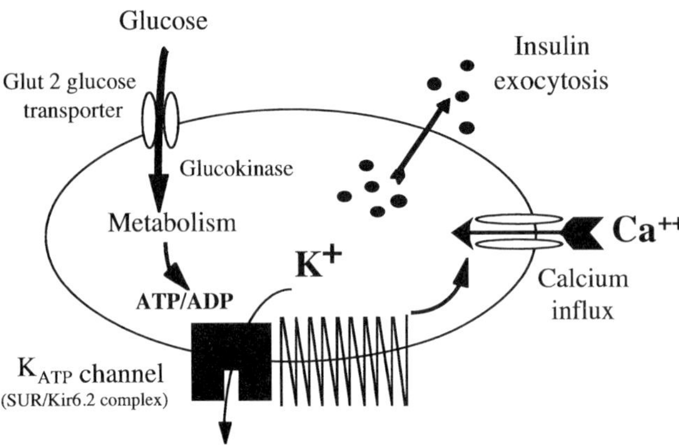

Figure 55-2 A schematic drawing of events leading to insulin secretion by pancreatic islet β cells. Alterations in intracellular ATP level leads to closure of ATP-sensitive potassium (K_{ATP}) channels, which are composed at least of the sulfonylurea receptor (SUR) and the inward rectifier Kir6.2. Subsequent membrane depolarization, opening of voltage-gated calcium channels, and exocytosis of insulin follows. In the presence of mutations in either the SUR or Kir6.2, K_{ATP} channels are unresponsive to alterations in intracellular ATP levels, leading to inappropriate closure, membrane depolarization, elevated intracellular calcium levels, and, ultimately, unregulated exocytosis of insulin.

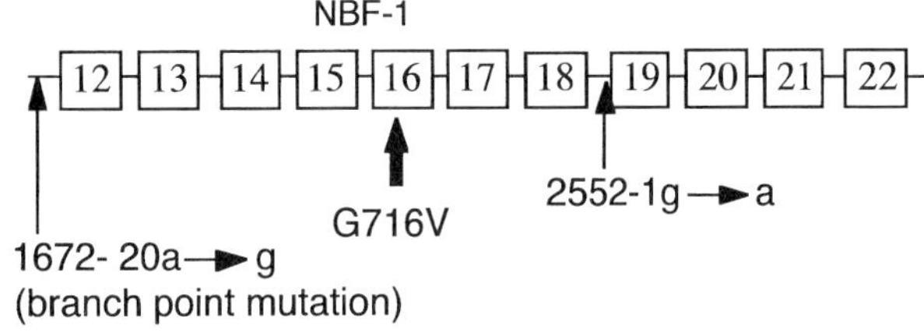

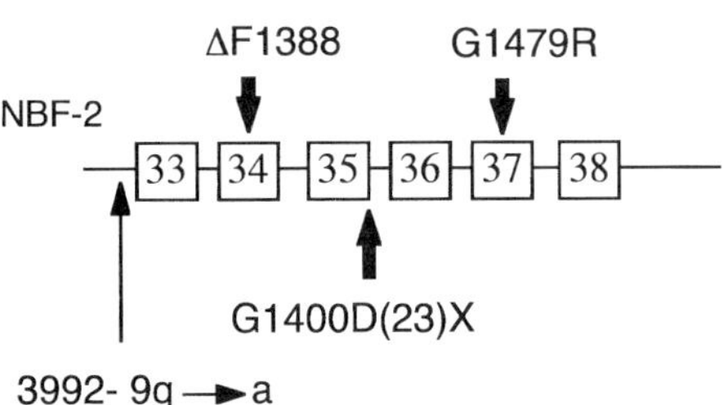

Figure 55-3 Mutations of SUR1 associated with persistent hyperinsulinemic hypoglycemia of infancy (PHHI). The SUR1 gene is composed of 39 exons. The nucleotide-binding fold regions (NBF-1 and -2) are diagrammed here, with NBF-1 in the upper, and NBF-2 in the lower, portion. Exons are represented as boxes and individual exon numbers are included.

K_{ATP} channels by ATP. As intracellular ATP level increases, inhibition of K_{ATP} channels progressively increases, leading to cell depolarization. The model for the molecular basis of PHHI, based on the molecular genetic data, predicts that disruption of either SUR1 or Kir6.2 results in both inappropriate closure of K_{ATP} channels and membrane depolarization, and subsequently to excessive unregulated insulin secretion. Direct support for this model has been obtained by patch-clamp analysis of primary cultured human islet cells obtained from a group of five infants affected with PHHI. All evaluated pancreatic specimens lacked K_{ATP} channel activity. Furthermore, the PHHI β cells were found to be spontaneously electrically active and to exhibit high basal cytosolic calcium concentrations as a result of calcium influx. Therefore, it can be conclusively stated that the pathogenesis of PHHI, as predicted by genetic evidence and supported by direct electrophysiologic measurements of patient pancreatic samples, is caused by abnormalities of the pancreatic islet K_{ATP} channel.

MANAGEMENT AND TREATMENT

For individuals affected with PHHI, prompt recognition and treatment, with rapid resolution of hypoglycemia, is imperative to prevent permanent damage to the developing central nervous system. Treatment involves use of intravenous solutions of glucose and drugs, such as diazoxide and somatostatin analogs, which inhibit insulin secretion. These medical regimens are often not feasible for long-term use because of lack of treatment success, side effects, and practical problems with drug delivery. Near-complete (95%) pancreatectomy is frequently required for resolution of hypoglycemia. The need for additional treatment strategies remains apparent. Although patients who have undergone 95% pancreatectomy have demonstrated few ill effects during the short term, endocrine pancreatic insufficiency and growth failure is a significant problem affecting the majority of those examined for longer periods.

The elucidation of the molecular basis for PHHI may allow the development of more effective therapy for this difficult management situation. One potentially promising recent addition to the therapeutic options for treatment of PHHI is the use of the calcium channel blocking agent verapamil, as proposed by Lindley et al. The trial use of this drug was based on the molecular pathophysiology of PHHI, which includes inappropriate activation of voltage-gated calcium channels and elevated intracellular calcium levels. In a single affected child, with persistent hypoglycemia despite treatment with glucagon, somatostatin, diazoxide, and 95% pancreatectomy, blood glucose levels and duration of fasting time increased after treatment with nifedipine. Studies of the resected pancreatic specimen from this child demonstrated that the excess spontaneous electrical activity present was reversibly blocked by verapamil. Further study of this treatment approach is needed to define the role for calcium channel blockade in the management of PHHI.

FUTURE DIRECTIONS

Study of PHHI has demonstrated that this is a genetically heterogeneous disorder of pancreatic islet K_{ATP} channel dysfunction. Before PHHI may reasonably be considered as a candidate disease for gene replacement therapy, an understanding of the phenotype of specific mutations is required because with time, spontaneous abatement of clinical symptoms occurs in some cases. Further understanding of the molecular basis for PHHI, and the associated aberrant regulation of insulin secretion, may provide additional insight into effective therapeutic options for this and other disorders of pancreatic function and glucose metabolism.

SELECTED REFERENCES

Aguilar-Bryan L, Nichols CG, Wechsler SW, et al. Cloning of the β-cell high-affinity sulfonylurea receptor: a regulator of insulin secretion. Science 1995;268:423–426.

Ashcroft FM. Adenosine 5'-triphosphate-sensitive potassium channels. Annu Rev Neurosci 1988;11:97–118.

Aynsley-Green A, Polak JM, Bloom SR, et al. Nesidioblastosis of the pancreas: definition of the syndrome and the management of the severe neonatal hyperinsulinaemic hypoglycaemia. Arch Dis Child 1981;56:496–508.

Glaser B, Chiu KC, Anker R, et al. Familial hyperinsulinism maps to chromosome 11p14-15.1, 30 cM centromeric to the insulin gene. Nature Genet 1994;7:185–188.

Haymond MW. Hypoglycemia in infants and children. Endocrinol Metabol Clin North Am 1989;18:211–252.

Higgins CF. ABC transporters: from microorganisms to man. Annu Rev Cell Biol 1992;8:67–113.

Higgins CF. The ABC of channel regulation. Cell 1995;82:693–696.

Inagaki N, Gonoi T, Clement JP, et al. Reconstitution of I-KATP: an inward rectifier subunit plus the sulfonylurea receptor. Science 1995;270:1166–1170.

Kane C, Shepherd RM, Squires PE, et al. Loss of functional KATP channels in pancreatic β-cells causes persistent hyperinsulinemic hypoglycemia of infancy. Nat Med 1996;2:1344–1347.

Kuvuvitis A, Deal C, Arbour L, Polychronakos C. An autosomal dominant form of familial persistent hyperinsulinemic hypoglycemia of infancy, not linked to the sulfonylurea receptor locus. J Clin Endocrinol Metab 1997;82:1192–1194.

Lander ES, Botstein D. Homozygosity mapping: a way to map human recessive traits with the DNA of inbred children. Science 1987; 236:1567–1570.

Leibowitz G, Glaser B, Higazi AA, Salameh M, Cerasi E, Landau H. Hyperinsulinemic hypoglycemia of infancy in clinical remission: high incidence of diabetes mellitus and persistent β-cell dysfunction at long-term follow-up. J Clin Endocrinol Metab 1995, 80:386–392.

Lindley KJ, Dunne MJ, Kane C, et al. Ionic control of β cell function in nesidioblastosis. A possible therapeutic role for calcium channel blockade. Arch Dis Child 1996;74:373–378.

Nestorowicz A, Wilson BA, Schoor KP, et al. Mutations in the sulfonylurea receptor gene are associated with familial hyperinsulinism in Ashkenazi Jews. Hum Mol Genet 1996;5:1813–1822.

Nichols CG, Shyng SL, Nestorowicz A, et al. Adenosine diphosphate as an intracellular regulator of insulin secretion. Science 1996;272: 1785–1787.

Rorsman P. The pancreatic beta-cell as a fuel sensor: an electrophysiologist's viewpoint. Diabetologia 1997;40:487–495.

Shilyansky J, Fisher S, Cutz E, Perlman K Filler RM. Is 95% pancreatectomy the procedure of choice for treatment of persistent hyperinsulinemic hypoglycemia of the neonate? J Pediatr Surg 1997, 32:342–346.

Thomas PM, Cote GJ, Hallman DM, Mathew PM. Homozygosity mapping, to chromosome 11p, of the gene for familial persistent hyperinsulinemic hypoglycemia of infancy. Am J Hum Genet 1995;56:416–421.

Thomas PM, Cote GJ, Wohllk N, et al. Mutations in the sulfonylurea receptor gene in familial persistent hyperinsulinemic hypoglycemia of infancy. Science 1995;268:426–429.

Thomas PM, Wohllk N, Huang E, et al. Inactivation of the first nucleotide-binding fold of the sulfonylurea receptor, and familial persistent hyperinsulinemic hypoglycemia of infancy. Am J Hum Genet 1996;59:510–518.

Thomas P, Ye Y, Lightner E. Mutation of the pancreatic islet inward rectifier Kir6.2 also leads to familial persistent hyperinsulinemic hypoglycemia of infancy. Hum Mol Genet 1996;5:1809–1812.

56 Regulation of Reproduction

MICHAEL J. MCPHAUL

INTRODUCTION

Reproduction involves the integration of biologic processes as diverse as behavior and specialized cell divisions. This integration is accomplished by a complex web of interrelated hormonal and neural circuits that employ a variety of signaling molecules and pathways. The goal of this overview is to introduce the major effectors and pathways that participate in this regulation. A basic tenet of this summary is that these pathways can be viewed as a cascade comprised of several different levels. Although many differences exist in this cascade between men and women, the general features and overall hierarchical organization are similar.

HYPOTHALAMUS

Early in embryogenesis, the cells destined to become gonadotropin-releasing hormone (GnRH)-secreting neurons migrate from the olfactory placode and became localized to specific regions of the preoptic and medial basal hypothalamus. Terminals of these neurons terminate on the long portal vessels, which carry the secreted GnRH to the gonadotropin-secreting cells of the anterior pituitary.

Although unique in many ways, one of the important characteristics of these GnRH-secreting neurons is the rhythmicity of their secretory patterns. For this reason, the complex of GnRH-secreting neurons has been collectively termed the "pulse generator." Episodic secretion of GnRH gives rise to measurable pulses of GnRH secretion approximately once each hour. Many influences that alter the secretion of gonadotropins can be traced to their effects on the pattern and amplitude of pulsatile GnRH release. This pattern of episodic secretion determines the activity of the other levels in the cascade below.

GnRH is an ancient molecule and its structure has been highly conserved in vertebrate species, from teleost fishes to humans. The mature GnRH molecule is a decapeptide and is derived from a precursor 82 amino acids in length that is processed into the mature GnRH peptide by specific endoproteases (Fig. 56-1). Of interest, in contrast to the high degree of evolutionary conservation of the structure of the GnRH decapeptide itself, surrounding regions of the GnRH precursor are less conserved. Although adjacent segments of the prohormone (e.g., the carboxy-terminal fragment known as GAP) may serve a distinct function, the sequences encoding this polypeptide are much less conserved between species. This lesser degree of conservation suggests that although it may play a distinct role in vertebrate physiology (one that has not yet been defined), its principal function may simply be its participation in the folding and processing of the mature hormone.

From: *Principles of Molecular Medicine* (J. L. Jameson, ed.), ©1998 Humana Press Inc., Totowa, NJ.

PITUITARY

SECRETION OF LUTEINIZING HORMONE AND FOLLICLE-STIMULATING HORMONE The anterior pituitary is derived from the pharyngeal epithelium and comprises of five cell types that secrete six polypeptide hormones. Unlike the other cell types of the pituitary, gonadotrophs secrete both follicle-stimulating hormone (FSH) and luteinizing hormone (LH). This departure from the "one cell, one hormone" rule that characterizes the other cell types of the anterior pituitary poses an apparent paradox, because FSH and LH can have different secretory patterns. Although the mechanisms by which this is accomplished have not been completely defined, it seems likely that the documented morphologic and functional heterogeneity of gonadotrophs is sufficient to account for the differential regulation of these hormones.

After delivery to the pituitary via the long portal vessels, GnRH binds to a specific receptor on the surface of the gonadotropin-secreting cells. This receptor is a member of a large gene family of membrane receptors that is predicted from its primary amino acid sequence to span the plasma membrane seven times and is most closely related to receptors from the same gene family that bind oxytocin and vasopressin (Fig. 56-2). In addition to those on the surface of the pituitary gonadotrophs, GnRH receptors have been detected in the gonads, prostate, and within selected regions of the brain (particularly GnRH-secreting cells of the hypothalamus). Although signal transduction is likely to involve a number of second messenger signaling pathways, the principal pathway appears to be via the G-protein-mediated stimulation of phospholipase C, rises in inositol 1,4,5-trisphosphate (IP_3), and changes in intracellular calcium levels. Activation of the mitogen-activated protein kinase (MAPK) cascade by GnRH has also been demonstrated. An important feature of this step in the hypothalamic–pituitary–gonadal (HPG) axis is that the episodic secretion of GnRH by the GnRH-secreting neurons causes GnRH to be presented to the receptor in an intermittent fashion. Furthermore, it is clear that this pulsatile binding of GnRH to its receptor on gonadotrophs is a critical attribute of this signaling pathway. Binding of GnRH to the GnRH receptor in a manner that is not pulsatile will lead to the induction of a state of tachyphylaxis and result in the cessation of LH and FSH secretion.

The principal effect of GnRH binding to its receptor on the surface of gonadotrophs is to stimulate the synthesis and release of

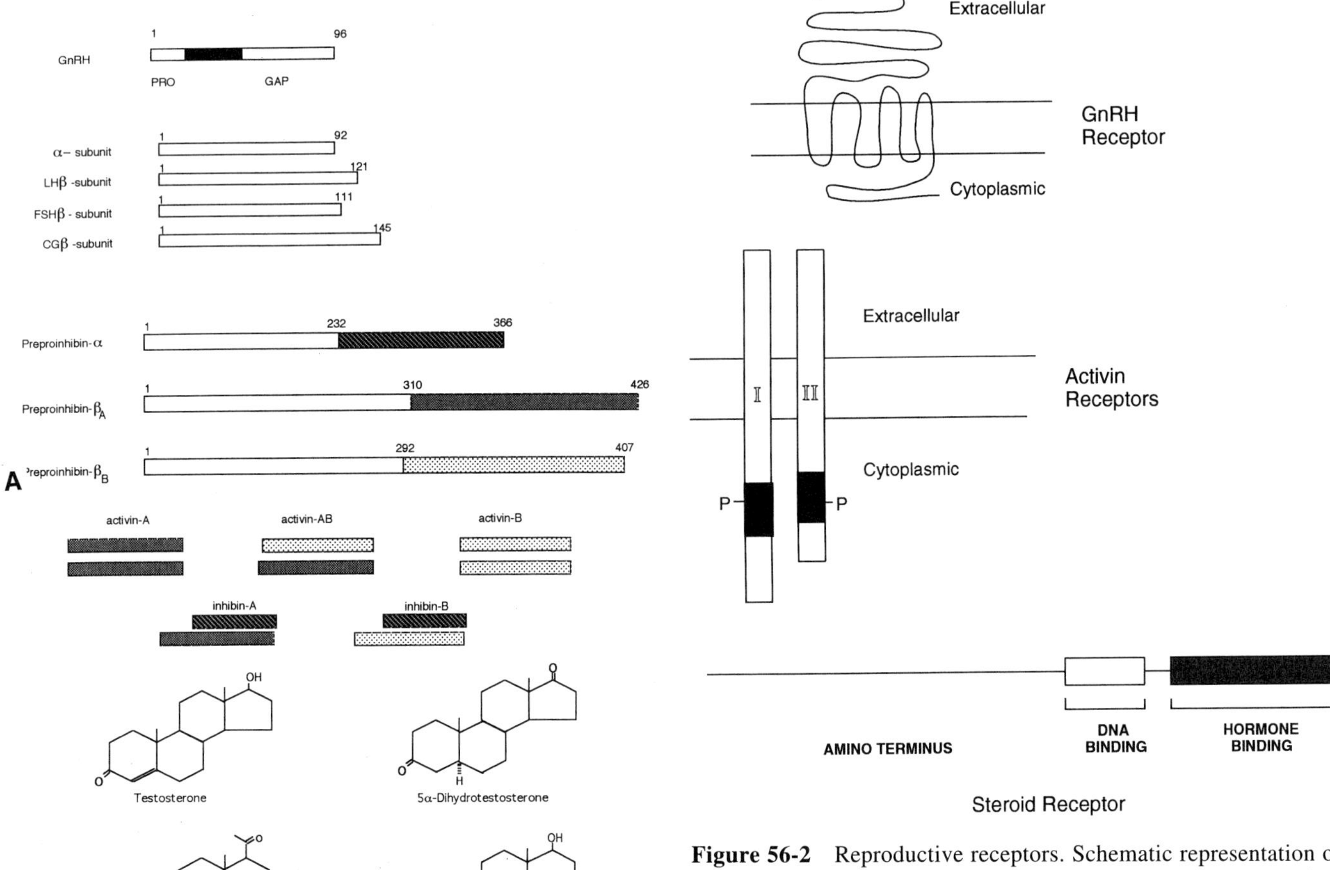

Figure 56-1 Reproductive hormones. The structures of the major classes of peptide involved in the process of reproduction are depicted. (Upper Panel) The positions of the pro- and GAP peptides are shown relative to the positions of the mature gonadotropin-releasing hormone (GnRH) molecule (shown as a dark bar). Luteinizing hormone (LH), follicle-stimulating hormone (FSH), and chorionic gonadotropin (CG) are heterodimeric glycoprotein hormones composed of a common α-subunit and a β-subunit that is unique for each hormone. (Middle panel) The structures of the hormones and subunits of inhibin and activin are presented. The two β-subunits and the single α-subunit are processed from larger precursors. As shown, combinations of these subunits give rise to a number of different heterodimeric (inhibins) and homodimeric combinations. (Lower panel) The structures of three of the major steroid hormones are shown. Each of the hormones is synthesized from cholesterol by the action of steroidogenic P450s and specific oxidoreductases.

LH and FSH. LH and FSH are heteromeric glycoprotein hormones that are structurally related and that likely evolved from a single ancestral precursor (Fig. 56-1). Both the common α-subunit and the unique β-subunits are processed from larger precursors that are cleaved by specific endoproteases to their mature forms. Glycosylation of both the α- and β-subunits occurs and has significant biologic effects, both in terms of the biologic activity and half-lives of these molecules. Because of the pulsatile nature of GnRH secretion, serum levels of FSH and LH also vary in a pulsatile fashion and protocols for the measurement of serum gonadotropin levels should take this moment-to-moment variation into account.

Figure 56-2 Reproductive receptors. Schematic representation of three major classes of receptor that transduce signals in the reproductive axes. (Above) GnRH , LH, and FSH receptors belong to a large family of transmembrane receptors that are coupled to G-protein-signaling pathways. The structures predicted for members of this large gene family include an extracellular domain that binds ligand, seven transmembrane-spanning segments, and cytoplasmic loops of varying lengths. The LH and FSH receptors are closely related to one another, whereas the GnRH receptor is more distant member of this gene family. (Middle) Activin receptors are composed of two nonidentical subunits that have been designated as type I and II (based on their molecular sizes and by analogy to the type I and II transforming growth factor-β receptors). Each comprises an extracellular domain, membrane-spanning segment, and cytoplasmic domain. The intracellular domain encodes a protein kinase that phosphorylates specific serine and threonine residues of target proteins. Signal transduction occurs only when ligand is bound to both type I and II subunits forming an active heteromeric complex. (Below) Structure of a prototypic member of the steroid hormone–thyroid hormone–retinoic acid family of nuclear receptors. Essential features include a DNA-binding domain that recognizes specific sequences within regulated genes, a hormone-binding domain that binds ligand with high affinity, and an amino-terminal segment that is of variable length, but that is important for the maximal regulation of responsive genes. This same general structure is applicable to additional members of this gene family (termed "orphan receptors") for which a ligand has not been identified. Some orphan receptors (such as DAX and SF-1) have been shown to play critical roles in the development and function of the hypothalamic–pituitary–gonadal axis.

GONADS

Although the patterns of hormone secretion may differ substantially between men and women at the level of the pituitary and hypothalamus, many of the components of this axis are similar.

This is not true of the gonads themselves. Both the testes and ovary are complex organs comprising a number of specialized cell types (discussed in Chapters 61 and 62). The focus of this section is to provide a partial description of the factors and receptors that have been shown to participate in the regulation of the gonadal axis.

SITES OF ACTION OF LH AND FSH—TESTES LH is delivered to the testes via the blood and exerts its effects by binding to a high-affinity receptor expressed on the surface of Leydig cells. Characterization of cDNAs encoding this receptor predicts that the LII receptor is approximately 670–680 amino acids long (depending on the species) and is predicted to encode seven segments that span the plasma membrane. The activation of this G-protein-associated receptor has been correlated with increased intracellular levels of cAMP, which is viewed as an integral part of the second messenger pathway. Results from some investigators suggest that additional second messenger pathways, such as activation by phospholipase C, also contribute to gene regulation effected by LH receptor activation.

In the testes, the FSH receptor is localized exclusively to the Sertoli cells. The isolation of cDNAs encoding the FSH receptor revealed it to be highly related to the LH receptor, both in terms of size, predicted amino acid composition, and structural organization. As with the LH receptor, it is also believed to be coupled to G-protein-dependent signaling pathways. Stimulation of adenylate cyclase appears to be a critical signaling pathway and modulation of intracellular calcium levels may also be important. Via these mechanisms, FSH is believed to modulate processes important for both Sertoli cell growth and differentiation and for Sertoli cell function in the regulation of spermatogenesis.

SITES OF ACTIONS OF LH AND FSH—OVARY As in the testes, LH and FSH receptors are distributed in a cell-type-specific fashion in the ovary. The FSH receptor is localized exclusively to the surface of granulosa cells. Stimulation of this receptor in granulosa cells activates cyclic AMP-dependent signaling mechanisms. This activation promotes granulosa cell growth and differentiation and stimulates the gene encoding the aromatase P450, the rate-limiting step in estrogen biosynthesis.

In contrast to the FSH receptor, the LH receptor is not confined to a single cell type within the ovary, but instead is expressed in both theca and granulosa cells. The levels of LH receptor detected in these cell types varies, depending on the developmental stage of the follicle. LH receptors are present only on the theca cells in immature follicles, but are detected on both theca and granulosa cells of mature antral follicles. In theca cells, LH is believed to stimulate the level of androgen synthesis via cyclic AMP-dependent pathways.

STEROID HORMONE SYNTHESIS Testes The bulk of steroid hormone synthesis in the testes is confined to the Leydig cells, which in adult males synthesize approximately 5 mg of testosterone daily. As noted above (and depicted schematically in Fig. 56-3), substantial variations in serum testosterone occur moment to moment, owing to the pulsatility of LH secretion. Only small quantities of estradiol and 5α-dihydrotestosterone (5α-DHT) are secreted directly by the testes and the remainder of these hormones are derived from metabolic conversion in nongonadal tissues.

Ovary Steroidogenesis in the ovary is complex and changes markedly during the follicular and luteal phases of the ovarian cycle. During early follicular development, enzymes early in the steroidogenic pathway (side-chain cleavage, 17-hydroxylase) are localized to the thecal cells and aromatase is detected in the granulosa cells ("two compartment" model of ovarian steroidogenesis, *see* Chapter 62). Following ovulation, the cells of the corpus luteum continue to express high levels of side-chain cleavage P450 and 17-hydroxylase, but the levels of expression of aromatase drop.

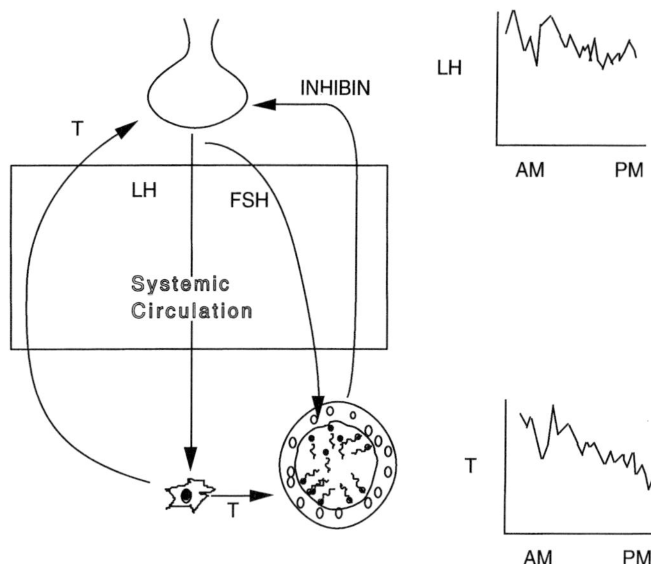

Figure 56-3 Integration of signals in the male reproductive axis. The pulses of GnRH secreted by neurons of the GnRH pulse generator are delivered via the long portal vessels to the cells of the anterior hypophysis. This signal leads to the pulsatile secretion of LH and FSH into the blood (shown at the upper right for LH). LH acts at the level of the Leydig cells within the interstitium of the testes to stimulate the pulsatile secretion of testosterone. The secreted testosterone acts within the testes to stimulate spermatogenesis and systemically to effect a number of physiologically processes, including the feedback regulation of LH secretion. FSH binds to the membranes of Sertoli cells, where it acts to promote the process of spermatogenesis. Inhibin secretion by the Sertoli cell (particularly inhibin-B) acts as a component of the feedback loop that regulates the secretion of FSH.

INHIBINS, ACTIVINS, AND FOLLISTATIN The development of assays to measure pituitary gonadotropin levels led to the identification of nonsteroidal activities of gonadal origin that could suppress FSH release in castrate animals. This activity, termed inhibin, was ultimately purified and found to be composed of heterodimeric molecules composed of α- and β-subunits. Subsequent cloning studies revealed the existence of genes encoding a single α-subunit and two distinct β-subunits (β_A and β_B), as shown in Fig. 56-1.

During studies to characterize the inhibins, it was noted that selected fractions of follicular fluid exhibited a distinctive activity. When used in appropriate bioassays, it was found that instead of inhibiting FSH release, these fractions led to a stimulation of FSH release. Purification of this activity, collectively termed activins, revealed that the active proteins were dimeric molecules composed of combinations of the same β-subunits that participate in the formation of inhibin heterodimers. Owing to its dimeric structure, three different activin molecules are possible: activin A, activin AB, and activin B, as shown in Fig. 56-1.

Studies by Ueno and coworkers established the existence of yet a third molecule capable of regulating FSH release in bioassays, termed follistatin. Analysis of the structure of cDNAs encoding follistatin have demonstrated that this molecule is unrelated to either inhibin or activin. Current models suggest that a large portion of the biologic activity of this molecule is believed to derive from its ability to bind (and sequester) biologically active activins.

Testes During embryonic development, the sites of α- and β-subunit expression vary, but become localized to the seminiferous tubule by the end of gestation. There is little question that Sertoli cells produce both inhibin and activin, although the mechanisms by which the production of these molecules by Sertoli cells are regulated is still unsettled. Available evidence suggests that the expression of inhibin subunits may vary in relation to the stage of development of the adjacent seminiferous tubule epithelium. Sertoli cells produce predominantly α-β_B inhibin (inhibin-B), which appears to be regulated (directly or indirectly) by FSH, and likely by other paracrine factors as well. It is presumably through the production of inhibin-B that the testes effects a negative regulatory influence on FSH secretion by the pathway. The regulation of production of activin expression by Sertoli cells has been less completely defined.

Ovary A number of studies have examined the identity of cell types that express α- and β-subunits in the ovary. Although some variation in the sites of subunit expression is evident in some studies, certain features are constant. First, it is clear that both α-subunit protein and α-subunit mRNA can be detected in the granulosa cells of growing follicles. Although patterns of β-subunit expression are more variable, it is detected in the thecal cells of dominant follicles in the human ovary.

Nongonadal Sites of Expression A great surprise resulting from the development of assays for inhibin and activin was the recognition that many tissues outside the reproductive tract could be shown to express activin and inhibin subunits. The expression patterns reported for the different subunits suggests that activins are made in a variety of tissues and are likely to subserve a number of functions. The expression of inhibins, on the other hand, is more restricted and appears to play a central role in the modulation of FSH. Although the expression of follistatin often parallels the expression of inhibin and activin subunits, additional sites of expression have been described that imply functions beyond those related solely to the modulation of inhibin or activin.

Mechanisms of Action The receptor that mediates the actions of activins is an area of active investigation. Specific proteins that bind activin have been identified and classified descriptively based on their physical properties. In crosslinking experiments, activin was shown to bind to two classes of membrane proteins (termed type I and type II receptors by analogy to the receptors for transforming growth factor [TGF]-β) having molecular weights of approximately ~50 and 70 kDa, respectively.

The detailed characterization of the activin receptors awaited the isolation of cDNAs encoding these proteins. The first such cDNA was isolated by expression cloning methods based on its capacity to confer on transfected cells the capacity to bind ^{125}I-labeled activin with high affinity. Analysis of the cDNA sequence predicted a transmembrane protein that contained motifs that suggested it employed a serine and threonine kinase as its intracellular signaling mechanism. The size of this receptor protein revealed it to be a type II activin receptor (Act RII). Subsequent studies revealed the existence of additional related members of the same gene family.

When antibodies directed at the type II activin receptors (such as Act RII) were used to precipitate the protein complexes crosslinked with ^{125}I-activin, the precipitates could be shown to contain proteins distinct from the type II receptors themselves. Screening strategies to isolate cDNAs encoding these proteins employed polymerase chain reaction (PCR)-based methods to identify cDNAs encoding novel transmembrane serine–threonine kinases. Subsequent crosslinking studies demonstrated that novel receptors isolated in this fashion (the activin type I receptors) could bind activin, but only in the presence of a type II activin receptor. The available evidence suggests that at least two distinct activin type I receptors exist. Thus, the combination of type I and type II receptors expressed in a given cell type is likely to afford an additional level at which differences in tissue responsiveness could be modulated.

To date, receptors have not been described that specifically bind either inhibin or follistatin. In the case of inhibin, owing to its distinct biologic properties, it is likely that such specific receptors exist. In the case of follistatin, however, it is believed that many, if not all, of its biologic properties can be accounted for on the basis of its capacity to bind and sequester activin with high affinity and the existence of a specific follistatin receptor seems less likely.

Insights From the Studies of Mice Carrying Targeted Disruptions of the Genes Encoding Inhibin, Follistatin, Activins, and the Activin Receptors The study of the physiologic roles of inhibins, activins, and follistatin have been complicated by the intricacies of the systems being studied. Investigators have attempted to unravel these intricate systems by deleting the functional genes in living animals. Such studies have provided a number of interesting insights.

Inhibin Matzuk and coworkers disrupted the functional α-subunit gene that is a component of both the inhibin-A and inhibin-B genes (*see* Fig. 56-1). As would be expected on the basis of the assays used to define the inhibins as regulators of pituitary FSH production, animals homozygous for the disrupted allele displayed elevated levels of serum FSH (*see* Chapter 10). Although the male and female homozygous mice were phenotypically normal, fertility was not normal in crosses with wild-type mice. Examination of the gonads revealed that the testes and ovaries of the homozygotes developed gonadal stromal tumor cells in a very high proportion of animals. These findings suggest that in addition to its role in the regulation of FSH, that in the cells of the gonadal stroma, inhibin—either directly or indirectly—also acts as a tumor suppressor. The basis for this capacity to antagonize the development of gonadal tumors remains to be elucidated. However, it is notable that gonadotropins are required for the development of activin-dependent tumors as crossbreeding with gonadotropin-deficient (hpg) mice prevents ovarian tumors. These findings indicate that gonadotropins are essential modifiers for tumor development in this model, perhaps reflecting their effects on follicle development.

Activins Owing to the subunit composition of the activin molecules, testing the functional relevance of the different forms of activin via the generation of knockout mice was considerably more complex. The first information was from studies of mice in which the β-B subunit was disrupted. Mice homozygous for a β-B mutant allele demonstrated normal viability. The most marked abnormalities were abnormalities of eyelid development and female reproduction. Mesoderm formation and neurulation were normal.

Considerably different phenotypes were noted in mice in which the β-A subunit was disrupted. Although mice homozygous for the deleted β-A allele progressed to term normally, the mice died within 24 hours of birth. These mice also displayed several consistent phenotypic abnormalities, particularly defects in whisker and tooth development. A variable number displayed abnormalities of palatal development.

When mice carrying the β-B and β-A mutant alleles were bred to produce compound homozygotes, it was observed that the phenotype of the resulting animals was additive. That is, the defects that were present were those observed in the animals carrying either mutant allele. This observation permitted two important conclusions. The first is that the molecules composed of the individual activin subunits (i.e., β-A and β-B homodimers) are not functionally compensating for one another. Second, these studies suggest that β-A/β-B heterodimers do not have a unique function during embryogenesis.

Activin Receptor Type II The study of mice carrying targeted deletions of the activin receptor II provided a number of interesting contrasts to the results obtained in studies of mice carrying disruptions of the β-A or β-B genes. Male mice were delayed in reaching fertility and female mice were infertile. In male mice, these functional changes were traced to a decrease of seminiferous tubule diameter and total volume. In females, frequent follicular atresia was seen and corpora lutea were rare, consistent with abnormalities of the estrous cycle in the mutant mice. Investigations of mice homozygous for the deleted Act RII gene documented reduced FSH levels in both male and female animals, compared with wild-type animals, permitting the authors to conclude that the reproductive defects observed were a consequence of the reduced FSH levels caused by the absence of Act RII signaling.

Although many of the phenotypic abnormalities were consistent with the findings of the activin subunit gene disruptions (particularly the effects on the pituitary and gonadal function), other major effects were noted that were specific for the Act RII disruption. In particular, mice carrying a disruption of this gene demonstrated defects of the first brachial arch (reminiscent of Pierre-Robin syndrome). These defects suggested that the Act RII receptor is involved in the transduction of signals that are involved in the formation of the first brachial arch. The nature of this signal (apparently distinct from the activins themselves since these features were not observed in the activin "knockouts" themselves) remains to be identified.

Follistatin Follistatin was originally defined on the basis of its capacity to antagonize the actions of activins. The targeted disruption of the murine follistatin gene permitted an examination of the physiologic impact of this molecule. Mice with the homozygous deletion died rapidly and displayed a number of defects, some of which suggested an alteration of activin function and many of which were specific for the follistatin gene disruption. Whisker development was abnormal, suggesting that follistatin may be an important modulator of the action of activin β-A. The shiny, taut skin resembled the skin of transgenic animals in which TGF-β overexpression had been directed using the keratin promoter. In addition, a number of additional defects were observed in the development of the musculoskeletal system, including changes in the number of ribs and vertebrae, as well as defects in the development of the palate. These results suggested that in addition to the role played in the modulation of activin function, follistatin may well play additional roles in the modulation of the function of other TGF-β related proteins or that it may possess functions that are independent of its role in the modulation of activins.

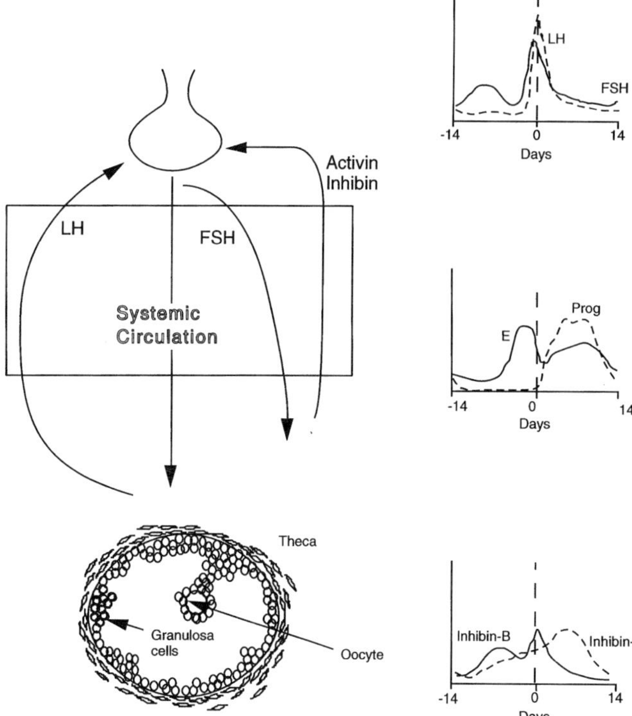

Figure 56-4 Integration of signals in the female reproductive axis. The pulsatile secretion of GnRH stimulates the pulsatile release of LH and FSH in to the blood by the gonadotropes (shown at upper right). Unlike the male, the levels of FSH and LH vary dramatically at different points in the menstrual cycle. FSH binds to the FSH receptor (localized to the plasma membranes of granulosa cells), where it acts to stimulate the growth of granulosa cells of the dominant follicle, as well as the levels of aromatase that they express. The sustained increased estradiol levels that result in the late follicular phase trigger the midcycle surge of LH and FSH that is required for ovulation. In the early portion of the menstrual cycle, LH acts principally at the levels of the ovarian stromal cells and stimulates the secretion of androstenedione, the substrate for granulosa cell estrogen synthesis (two-compartment model of ovarian hormonogenisis). After ovulation, the vascularization of the corpus luteum makes increased quantities of cholesterol—in the form of low-density lipoprotein—available for steroidogenesis, accounting for the increased progesterone secretion characteristic of the corpus luteum. If fertilization and implantation do not occur, the function of the corpus luteum declines, and progesterone and estradiol levels fall. As indicated (lower right), the regulation of serum inhibin-A and inhibin-B levels differ markedly at different points in the menstrual cycle.

INTEGRATION OF THE SIGNALS

Each component of the hypothalamic–pituitary–gonadal axis is coordinated in a hierarchical fashion after puberty in men and women. In men, although levels of the gonadotropins and testosterone can be shown to vary minute by minute and to display some diurnal variation, large-scale changes do not occur (Fig. 56-3).

In women, interplay between the ovary, hypothalamus, and pituitary results in the cyclic changes that characterize the menstrual cycle. A schematic representing the hormonal changes that occur during the menstrual cycle are depicted in Fig. 56-4.

MODULATION OF THE HYPOTHALAMIC–PITUITARY–GONADAL AXIS

INHIBITION OF GONADAL FUNCTION **Female Contraception** The most common intervention affecting the function of the HPG axis is use of oral contraceptives. In the United States, these preparations include small doses of estrogen (ethinyl estradiol) and one of several progestational agents (norethindrone, norethindrone acetate, norethynodrel, norgestrel, ethynodiol diacetate, norgestimate, or desogestrel). The administration of these estrogen and progestogen combinations in low doses serves to inhibit the normal midcycle surge and to prevent ovulation. In addition to a large number of different combinations of these agents, contraceptives containing only progestational agents are available as oral agents and as depot preparations.

As would be expected from their mechanisms of action, the inhibition of ovulation that is achieved using such agents is readily reversible and normal ovulatory cycles resume within 6 months in more than 95% of women after cessation of contraceptive use.

Male Contraception The success achieved in the development of oral contraceptives for women stimulated interest in developing similar methods for male contraception. These efforts have employed the parenteral administration of various androgen preparations. Protocols using weekly injections of testosterone enanthate have been the most widely studied and have been found to reproducibly induce a state of azoospermia or oligospermia. Using such protocols, contraception rates have been estimated at 0.8 pregnancies per 100 person-years in those patients whose sperm counts fall into the azoospermic range. Although this rate is comparable to other reversible methods of contraception, the failure to induce azoospermia in as many as 50% of subjects in some studies is unacceptable and is a major impediment to the broader application of such methods. The development of effective, reversible hormonal forms of male contraception have focused on the identification of regimens (e.g., the combination of testosterone injections and oral progestogens) that will lead to a higher frequency of azoospermia.

GnRH Analogs Attempts to deliver GnRH chronically to stimulate gonadal function led to the recognition that the pulsatile delivery of GnRH to the gonadotrophs was essential for normal gonadotroph function. As noted above, the continuous delivery of GnRH to the pituitary leads to the induction of a form of reversible secondary hypogonadism. The mechanism of this tachyphylaxis has been traced to a downregulation of GnRH receptors on the gonadotroph and an uncoupling of postreceptor pathways.

These observations have led to the development and application of GnRH agonists to induce a state of reversible hypogonadism. These agents have been widely used to achieve a functionally castrate state by pharmacologic means. Such regimens are effective in both men and women and have been employed in the treatment of a wide range of conditions.

STIMULATION OF GONADAL FUNCTION **Female** The techniques available to modulate the female reproductive tract and stimulate fertility have undergone explosive growth since the advent of successful in vitro fertilization (IVF) techniques in the late 1970s. Although the techniques and methodologies employed are quite varied, all rely on the use of agents to modulate the maturation of oocytes in a precise fashion, permitting the harvesting of ova for fertilization in vitro.

The simplest of such protocols employ the modulation of endogenous gonadotropin production using agents such as clomiphene citrate. This agent acts as an antiestrogen and acts to augment the secretion of endogenous gonadotropins. In some protocols, these effects are further augmented by the administration of exogenous gonadotropins.

Although somewhat more cost-effective, overall pregnancy rates using such stimulation protocols are lower than those using more conventional IVF treatment regimens. In these latter protocols, GnRH agonists are used to downregulate the production of endogenous gonadotropins so that ovarian follicular development can be regulated under circumstances in which the effect of endogenous gonadotropins are negligible. When suppression of ovarian function is achieved using these protocols, ovarian stimulation is achieved using exogenous gonadotropins for 9–10 days until follicular development is achieved. When follicular maturity is reached (assessed by ultrasonography and estradiol measurements), human chorionic gonadotrophin (hCG) is administered (to simulate the LH surge of a normal ovarian cycle), and oocytes are retrieved by a laparoscopic procedure.

Male In men, primary and secondary hypogonadism is treated most frequently with transdermal or injectable depot preparations of testosterone, owing to the rapid metabolism and inactivation of unsubstituted forms of testosterone and the hepatotoxicity associated with the oral administration of the more stable 17-substituted androgens.

The systemic administration of testosterone—although providing hormone sufficient to support normal potency and secondary sexual characteristics—does not result in intratesticular concentrations of androgen that are capable of supporting normal spermatogenesis. For this reason, when fertility is desired by men with secondary forms of hypogonadism, different hormonal regimens must be employed that incorporate stimuli that mimic the trophic influences of gonadotropins on the testes. In men that have never undergone normal pubertal maturation (and as such have never established normal spermatogenesis), replacement regimens that supply stimuli that mimic the effects of both LH and FSH must be employed. By contrast, the administration of hCG may suffice to reestablish fertility in individuals that have developed an acquired form of secondary hypogonadism as adults.

SUMMARY

Increasingly detailed information has been amassed regarding the molecules, the receptors and the mechanisms by which the function of the gonads are controlled. In some instances, this knowledge has permitted the definition of the pathophysiology causing specific disease entities. In other instances (e.g., polycystic ovarian disease), the use of this knowledge has not yet permitted a complete understanding of the disease entity to emerge.

ACKNOWLEDGMENTS

This work was supported by NIH grants DK03892 and DK52678.

SELECTED REFERENCES

Coerver KA, Woodruff TK, Finegold MJ, Mather J, Bradley A, Matzuk MM. Activin signaling through activin receptor type II causes cachexia-like symptoms in inhibin-deficient mice. Mol Endocrinol 1996;19:534–543.

Cummings DE, Bremner WJ. Prospects for new hormonal male contraceptives. Endocrinol Metab Clin North Am 1994;23:893–922.

Danforth DR. Endocrine and paracrine control of oocyte development. Am J Obstet Gynecol 1995;172:747–752.

Erickson GF, Danforth DR. Ovarian control of follicle development. Am J Obstet Gynecol 1995;172:736–747.

Evans RM. The steroid and thyroid hormone receptor superfamily. Science 1988;240:889–895.

Gaddy-Kurten D, Tsuchida K, Vale W. Activins and the receptor serine kinase superfamily. Recent Prog Horm Res 1995;50:109–129.

Hillier SG, Whitelaw PF, Smyth CD. Follicular oestrogen synthesis: the 'two-cell, two-gonadotrophin' model revisited. Mol Cell Endocrinol 1994;100:51–54.

Kumar TR, Wang Y, Lu N, Matzuk MM. Follicle stimulating hormone is required for ovarian follicle maturation but not male fertility. Nat Genet 1997;15:201–204.

Kumar TR, Wang Y, Matzuk MM. Gonadotropins are essential modifier factors for gonadal tumor development in inhibin-deficient mice. Endocrinology 1996;137:4210–4216.

Mangelsdorf DJ, Thummel C, Beato M, et al. The nuclear receptor superfamily: the second decade. Cell 1995;83:835–839.

Matzuk MM, Kumar TR, Bradley A. Different phenotypes for mice deficient in either activins or activin receptor type II. Nature 1995;374:356–360.

Matzuk MM, Kumar TR, Vassalli A, et al. Functional analysis of activins during mammalian development. Nature 1995;374:354–356.

Matzuk MM, Lu N, Vogel H, Sellheyer K, Roop DR, Bradley A. Multiple defects and perinatal death in mice deficient in follistatin. Nature 1995;374:360–363.

Moley KH, Schreiber JR. Ovarian follicular growth, ovulation and atresia. Endocrine, paracrine and autocrine regulation. Adv Exp Med Biol 1995;377:103–119.

Moore A, Krummen LA, Mather JP. Inhibins, activins, their binding proteins and receptors: interactions underlying paracrine activity in the testis. Mol Cell Endocrinol 1994;100:81–86.

Saez JM. Leydig cells: endocrine, paracrine, and autocrine regulation. Endocr Rev 1994;15:574–626.

Stojilkovic SS, Catt KJ. Expression and signal transduction pathways of gonadotropin-releasing hormone receptors. Recent Prog Horm Res 1995;50:109–129.

Vassalli A, Matzuk MM, Gardner HA, Lee KF, Jaenisch R. Activin/inhibin beta B subunit gene disruption leads to defects in eyelid development and female reproduction. Genes Dev 1994;8:414–427.

Woodruff TK, Mather JP. Inhibin, activin and the female reproductive axis. Ann Rev Phys 1995;57:219–244.

57 Disorders of Sex Determination and Differentiation

CHARMIAN A. QUIGLEY

THE BASIS OF NORMAL SEX DETERMINATION AND DIFFERENTIATION

Sex determination and differentiation are distinct, consecutive processes that follow the establishment of chromosomal sex at the time of fertilization. The term "sex determination" refers to the development of gonadal sex—a process that occurs at approximately 6–7 weeks' gestation in the human male fetus, and around 10–11 weeks' gestation in the female fetus. Male sex determination is synonymous with testis determination. This process (alternatively called primary sex differentiation) results from a coordinated series of exquisitely regulated, but as yet incompletely understood, events. As generally used, the term "sex differentiation," refers to the processes downstream of gonadal development—the processes that are regulated by gonadal secretions or lack thereof (also called secondary sex differentiation). In essence, the sex chromosome complement endowed at fertilization determines gonad type and the latter determines the pattern of differentiation seen in the genital ducts and external genitalia.

THE EMBRYOLOGY OF GONADAL AND GENITAL DEVELOPMENT In the first few weeks of gestation the primordial gonads develop from the condensation of a ridge of mesenchymal tissue located medial to the mesonephros (the forebear of the kidney), accompanied by thickening and proliferation of the coelomic epithelium, which penetrates the underlying mesenchyme. These primitive gonadal or genital ridges initially contain no germ cells. Between the 5th and 6th weeks of gestation (embryonic day 10.5–12 in the mouse) primordial germ cells migrate by ameboid movement from the endoderm of the yolk sac along the dorsal mesentery of the hindgut and into the indifferent gonad, where they invade the developing primary sex cords. Despite this, germ cells are not required for the processes of testis development to occur. At this stage the gonad comprises an outer cortex and inner medulla, and there is still no morphologic difference between the gonads of male and female fetuses. After the arrival of the germ cells, the gonad begins to differentiate: in the 46,XX fetus the cortex develops and the medulla regresses; in the 46,XY fetus the reverse occurs. The first discernible event in testis development is the appearance of primordial Sertoli cells, which differentiate from somatic cells of the coelomic epithelium. Soon after their appearance in the gonadal ridge, Sertoli cells proliferate, aggregate around the primitive germ cells, and align into cordlike structures, which subsequently become the seminiferous tubules. The seclusion of germ cells within the tubules prevents meiosis and commits the germ cells to spermatogenic development. This organizational process appears to be regulated by the Sertoli cells themselves. About 1 week later (around 8 weeks), steroidogenic Leydig cells differentiate from primitive interstitial cells of mesonephric origin. This process too may be controlled by paracrine influences from Sertoli cells, possibly anti-Müllerian hormone (AMH).

In contrast with the germ cell-independent development of the testes, the presence of germ cells is a prerequisite for normal ovarian differentiation. Without the germ cell seeding of the gonadal primordium, the tissue degenerates into a nonfunctional, mainly fibrous "streak." Before week 10 of gestation the only feature that distinguishes an ovary is the absence of testicular features. Thereafter, ovarian structure becomes distinguishable, with the development of the primary medullary sex cords. Secondary cortical sex cords provide the supporting structure for the arriving germ cells. These break up into clusters, becoming the primordial follicles at about week 16. The primordial follicles contain the diploid oocytes, which remain quiescent until puberty. Follicular cells arise from the same cell lineage as Sertoli cells. Theca cells represent the ovarian counterpart of Leydig cells.

There is a notable difference in the chronology of testicular versus ovarian development, the process of testis formation being completed by 8 weeks' gestation, at which time the process of ovarian development has not yet begun. In fact, morphologic ovarian development is not completed until after most of the processes of phenotypic sex differentiation, described in the following section, have occurred. This, and the fact that phenotypic development is normal even in complete absence of the ovary, highlights the lack of involvement of the ovary in this process. The embryologic development of the testis and ovary are summarized in Fig. 57-1.

The primitive internal genital tracts are also indistinguishable between the sexes until 7 weeks' gestation (Fig. 57-2). The fetus is endowed with two sets of internal duct structures: the paramesonephric (Müllerian) ducts, and the mesonephric (Wolffian) ducts. From the 8th week of gestation hormonal secretions from the fetal testes induce masculinization of the internal genital structures. Initially the Wolffian ducts are stabilized by the action (mainly local) of testosterone and thereafter undergo differentiation into the epididymides, vasa deferentia, and seminal vesicles; these pro-

From: *Principles of Molecular Medicine* (J. L. Jameson, ed.), ©1998 Humana Press Inc., Totowa, NJ.

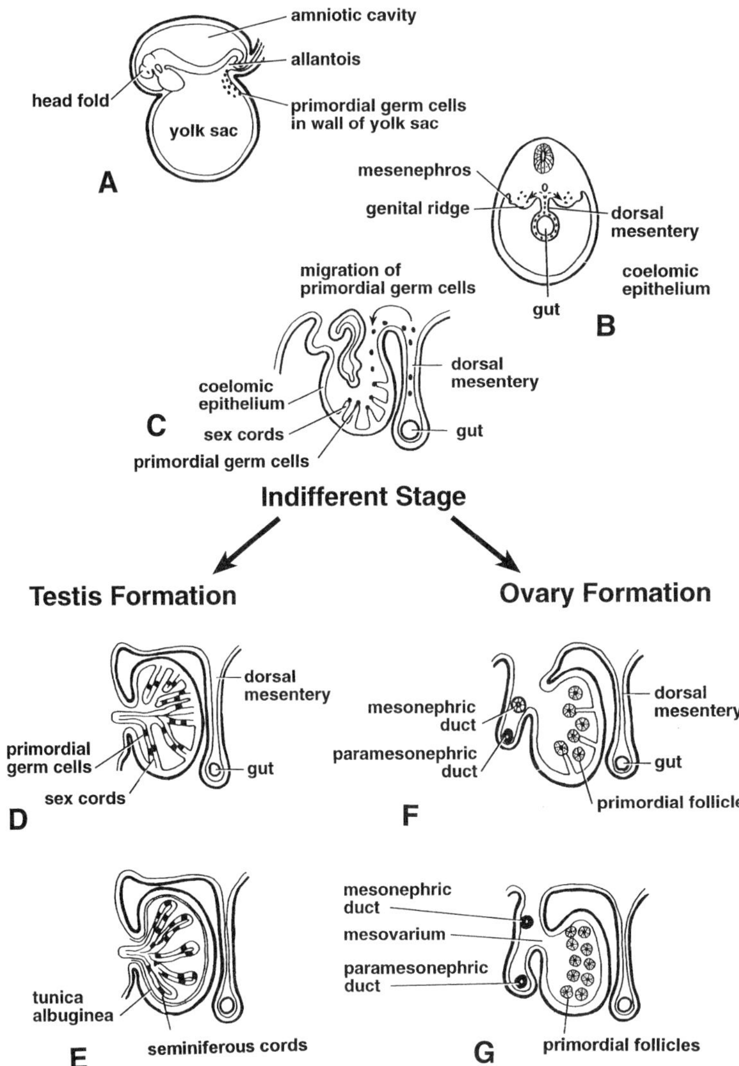

Figure 57-1 Embryologic development of the gonads. **(A)** The primordial germ cells are located in the wall of the yolk sac in early embryogenesis. **(B)** At about the 5th–6th week of human gestation, germ cells migrate by ameboid movement from the coelomic epithelium, along the dorsal mesentery of the hindgut, to the genital ridge, the site of the future gonad. **(C)** During formation of the indifferent (bipotential) gonad, the primordial germ cells infiltrate the primary sex cords, which subsequently become the seminiferous tubules of the testis, or the primordial follicles of the ovary. **(D,E)** Formation of the testis continues after arrival of the germs cells, although these are not required for the process to occur. Probably under the direction of the newly differentiated Sertoli cells, the sex cords differentiate as the seminiferous tubules, in which germ cells are embedded. Morphologic development of the testis is complete by 8 weeks' gestation. **(F,G)** Formation of the ovary occurs later than that of the testis, at around week 10 of gestation, and does require the presence of germ cells. The primary sex cords develop into primordial follicles at about week 16 of gestation.

cesses occur between approximately 8 and 13 weeks' gestation. Dihydrotestosterone does not appear to mediate these processes, since the enzyme required for its production is not expressed in Wolffian tissues at the time of their differentiation. In parallel to the masculinization of the internal genitalia represented by Wolffian development, a process of "defeminization" of the genital ducts occurs as the Müllerian ducts regress under the influence of locally acting AMH secreted by testicular Sertoli cells, at around 8–10 weeks. The Müllerian ducts are obliterated by the 11th week of gestation, the only remnant of their existence in the 46,XY fetus being the prostatic utricle. Absence of one testis results in retention of the Müllerian structures and only limited Wolffian development on that side, indicating that the effects of AMH and testosterone are mediated to some extent in a paracrine fashion.

In the absence of testicular secretions, as in the normal 46,XX fetus, the inverse set of genital tract developmental processes occurs. Without local androgen action, the Wolffian ducts regress between about weeks 9 and 13. Similarly, in the absence of AMH the Müllerian ducts are permitted to develop. Their upper portions form the Fallopian tubes. The lower sections fuse and differentiate as the uterus and upper part of the vagina. The lower portion of the vagina derives from the urogenital sinus, which remains patent in the absence of androgen action.

Just as the gonads and internal genitalia are indistinguishable between the sexes for the first few weeks of life, so it is for the external genital primordia (Fig. 57-3). In the 4th week of gestation the external genitalia of both karyotypic sexes are represented simply by a midline protuberance—the genital tubercle. By week

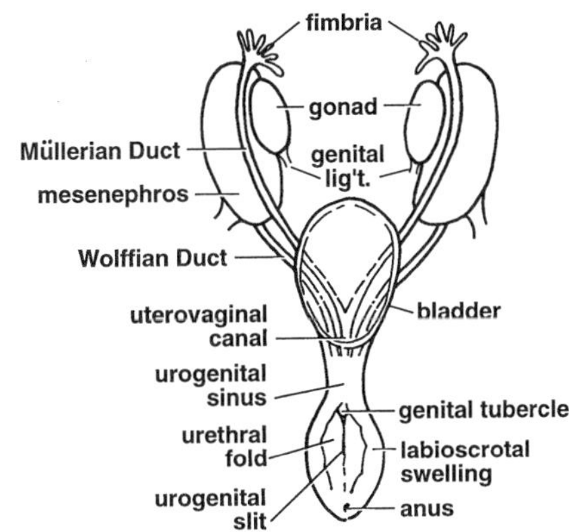

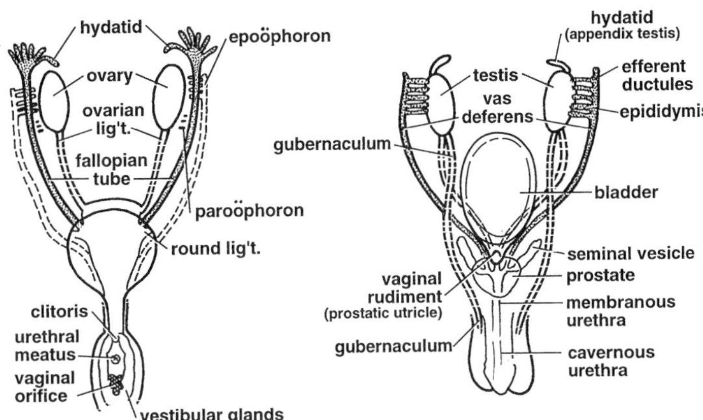

Figure 57-2 Embryologic development of the internal genitalia. **(Indifferent Stage)** The primitive internal genitalia at 7 weeks' gestation, showing the presence of both paramesonephric or Müllerian (female) and mesonephric or Wolffian (male) duct systems. **(Female Development)** In the female fetus between weeks 9 and 13 of gestation there is regression of the Wolffian ducts (shown with broken lines) with differentiation and development of the Müllerian ducts (shaded). The upper portions of the Müllerian ducts form the Fallopian tubes; the lower portions fuse to form the uterus, cervix, and upper part of the vagina. The urogenital sinus remains patent in the absence of androgen action, forming the lower part of the vagina. **(Male Development)** Differentiation of the Wolffian ducts in the male fetus occurs under the influence of testosterone between 9 and 13 weeks of gestation. These develop as the epididymis, vas deferens, and seminal vesicles (shaded). By week 11, the Müllerian ducts are obliterated by a process of apoptosis that occurs under the direction of AMH secreted by Sertoli cells (broken lines).

6 (still indifferent) two medial folds, the urethral folds, flank the urogenital groove, and two larger folds, the labioscrotal folds, are present laterally. Under the influence of androgen action (primarily dihydrotestosterone), the genital tubercle elongates to form the body of the penis, and the urethral folds fuse ventrally from behind forward, to form the penile urethra. The labioscrotal swellings or folds grow toward each other, fusing in the midline to form the scrotum. Dihydrotestosterone (DHT) also induces the urogenital sinus to differentiate as the prostate, and inhibits the formation of the vesicovaginal septum. These processes are completed by week 12 of gestation.

The testes migrate from their original lumbar location to the level of the internal inguinal ring above the scrotum, between 12 and 24 weeks' gestation. Descent of the testes through the inguinal ring and into the scrotum begins around week 28, and in most infants is completed by term.

In the absence of significant androgen action, such as in the normal female fetus, the genital tubercle elongates only slightly to form the clitoris (Fig. 57-3). The urogenital sinus remains open and the vesicovaginal septum forms between the genital and urinary portions of the urogenital sinus, so that the urethra opens anteriorly and the vagina posteriorly. The vestibule of the urogenital sinus is bordered laterally by the urethral folds, which fail to fuse and instead develop as the labia minora. Further laterally, the labioscrotal swellings enlarge somewhat but also remain unfused, forming the labia majora. There is minor fusion posteriorly, forming the posterior commissure, and anteriorly, producing the mons pubis. These events occur from about week 7 to week 12 of gestation. The timetable of gonadal and genital differentiation is shown in Fig. 57-4.

GENETIC AND HORMONAL CONTROL OF SEX DETERMINATION AND DIFFERENTIATION A complex interplay of genes, hormones, transcription factors, and receptors is required for normal sex determination and differentiation (Fig. 57-4; Table 57-1). The primary event governing the path down which morphologic sex differentiation proceeds is the development of

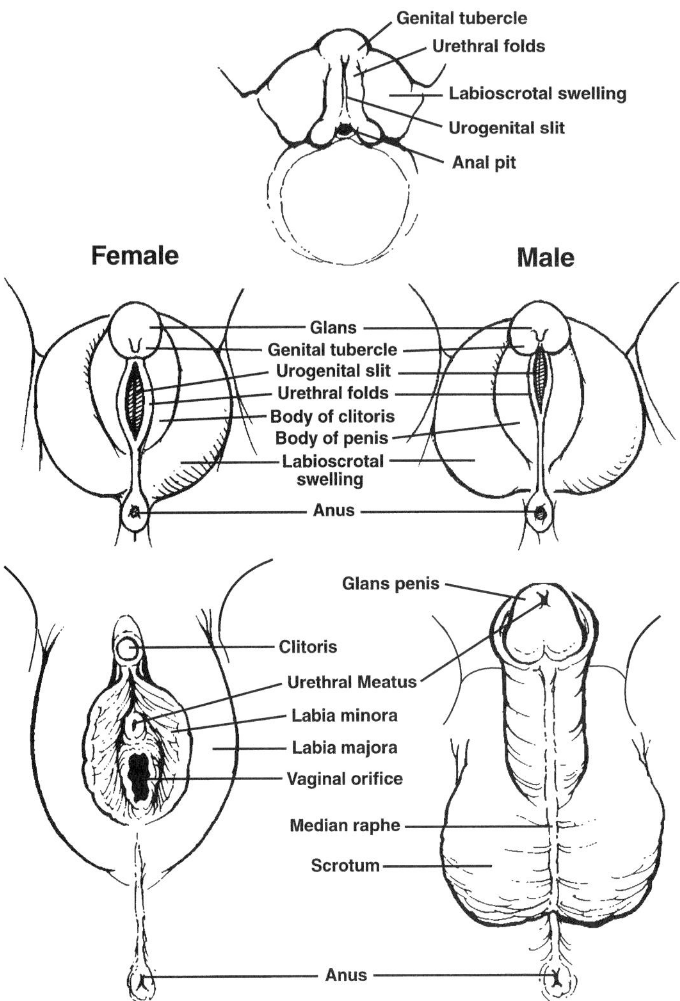

Figure 57-3 Differentiation of the external genitalia. **(Top)** At week 6 of gestation the external genitalia are undifferentiated, consisting of the midline genital tubercle, two medial urethral folds flanking the urogenital slit, and two larger labioscrotal swellings laterally. **(Left)** In the absence of androgen action the genital tubercle becomes the clitoris and the urogenital sinus remains patent. The vesicovaginal septum forms to separate the urethra from the vagina, located posteriorly. The urethral folds develop as the labia minora, whereas the labioscrotal folds enlarge slightly, remaining unfused, as the labia majora. **(Right)** In the male fetus in the presence of androgens (mainly DHT), the genital tubercle elongates to become the body of the penis, and the urethral folds fuse in the midline to form the penile urethra. The labioscrotal swellings fuse and enlarge to become the scrotum. These processes are completed approximately between weeks 8 and 12 of gestation.

the testis. In the 1930s the elegant experiments of Jost determined that maleness was a state imposed on the fetus that would otherwise develop as a female, because development of the ovary and female phenotype occur when the fetus is not exposed to the influences of specific "maleness-determining" genes.

SEX AND TESTIS DETERMINATION The process of testis development appears to be controlled by a switchlike mechanism that involves the Y chromosomal *SRY* gene and its encoded protein, and, no doubt, other genes and proteins that either regulate or are regulated by SRY. However, for SRY to function, it must have a target—that is, there must first be development of the gonadal primordium. A candidate gene that may regulate the very earliest stages of gonadal development is the orphan nuclear receptor or transcription factor, steroidogenic factor 1 *(SF-1)*. Although its exact role is still being elucidated, SF-1 appears to be a key factor in development of the reproductive tract, at least in rodents. Analysis of studies in mice with deletions for the murine homolog of the *SF-1* gene reveals that *SF-1* is required in both sexes for development of the bipotential primordial gonads and the embryologic adrenal glands, and for development and function of pituitary gonadotrophs. SF-1 appears to be one of the earliest-acting factors in the sex determination cascade and likely regulates genes encoding factors acting further down the pathway of gonadal development, such as AMH, WT1, DAX-1, LHb, P450scc, and perhaps even SRY itself, either directly or indirectly, via intermediate steps. Colonization of the bisexual gonad by germ cells is one of the earliest events in gonadal development, occurring before any morphologic distinction between the gonads of males and females is detectable. In mice, and probably in other mammals, the c-*Kit*/steel receptor–ligand system directs migration of germ cells from the yolk sac to the gonad and may also be responsible for their survival in their new milieu.

Once development of the primordial gonadal and genital structures has occurred, the next steps diverge between the sexes. In the karyotypic male a primary "switch" that initiates specific testicular development is the Y chromosome-encoded transcrip-

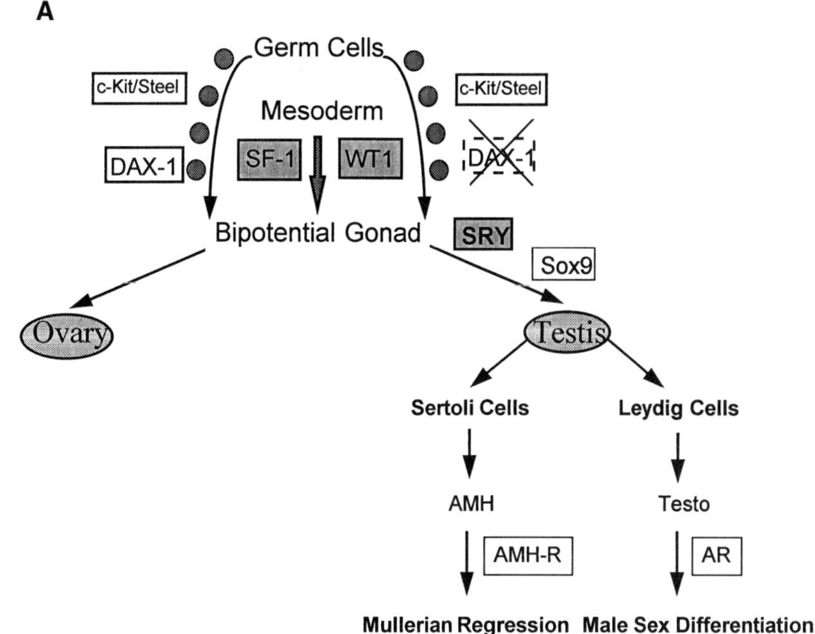

Figure 57-4 Control and timing of gonadal and sexual differentiation. **(A)** Hypothetical scheme for genetic control of sex determination. The genetic determinants of gonadal and genital differentiation are shown in approximate sequence. c-Kit receptor and steel factor are involved in germ cell migration, one of the earliest events in gonad formation. SF-1 and WT-1 appear to be required for normal formation of the primordial bipotential gonad. SRY directs differentiation of the bipotential gonad as a testis, probably with interaction of other genes such as *SOX9*. It is presumed that *DAX-1* (or a nearby gene) is repressed in male development, since duplication of the locus suppresses testis development. After definitive testis formation has occurred, the testicular hormones AMH and testosterone direct the processes of Müllerian regression and masculinization of internal and external genitalia, each acting via a specific receptor (AMH receptor and androgen receptor). **(B)** Timetable. In both male and female development the first event of sex differentiation is the migration of germ cells, at around 5–6 weeks' gestation. This is followed by testicular development in the male. After onset of AMH and testosterone secretion at approximately 7–8 weeks' gestation, the Müllerian ducts regress and Wolffian ducts differentiate. The pattern of development is parallel, but essentially opposite, and somewhat delayed for female fetuses. In particular, there is a marked lag between testicular and ovarian development.

Table 57-1
Factors Involved in Sex Determination and Differentiation

Gene name	*Locus*	*Protein name*	*Protein type*	*Action*	*Possible targets*
SRY	Yp11.3	SRY	HMG box-type ligand-independent transcription factor	Bends DNA	AMH SOX9 $P450_{arom}$
SOX9	17q24–25	SOX9	HMG box-type ligand-independent transcription factor	Sertoli cell development Transcription regulation	DAX-1 Unknown
WT1	11p13	WT1	Ligand-independent transcription factor Tumor repressor	Transcription regulation	Unknown
DAX-1	Xp21	DAX-1	Orphan nuclear receptor	Inhibits SOX9 Regulation of gonadotropes Development of adrenals	SOX9
SF-1/Ftz-F1	9q33	SF1	Orphan nuclear receptor	Development of hypothalamic nucleus Development of gonads/adrenals Regulation of steroidogenesis	$P450_{scc}$ LHβ DAX-1 AMH
c-Kit	4q12	c-Kit	Transmembrane tyrosine kinase receptor	Migration/proliferation of stem cells ? Suppresses apoptosis	—
slf	12q22	Steel factor	Membrane-bound and soluble peptides Ligand for c-Kit receptor	As for c-Kit	c-Kit receptor
LH/CGR	2p21	LH/CG receptor	Seven transmembrane-spanning G protein-coupled peptide hormone receptor	Transduces LH signal Activates cAMP production	—
StAR	8p11.2	StAR	Mitochondrial protein transport factor	Mediates cholesterol transport to inner mitochondrial membrane	Unknown
AMH	19p13.2–13.3	AMH (MIS)	Glycoprotein homodimer, member of TGF-β family	Müllerian duct regression ? Regulates testicular descent	AMHR
AMHR	12q13	AMH Receptor	Transmembrane serine–threonine kinase receptor of TGF-β receptor type	Müllerian duct regression ? ? Regulates testicular descent	—
SRD5IA	5p15	5α-Reductase 2	Microsomal enzyme	Converts testosterone → DHT	—
AR	Xq11–12	AR	Ligand-dependent nuclear transcription factor	Transcription regulation	AMHR ?P450arom

tion factor, SRY. SRY appears to direct the process of seminiferous tubule organization by Sertoli cells and to regulate transcription of the Sertoli cell glycoprotein AMH; AMH in turn may play a role in directing undifferentiated interstitial cells to develop as Leydig cells. Once testicular differentiation is established, other Y-encoded genes are required to maintain spermatogenesis. A number of other genes have been identified as having involvement in testis development; however, their exact positions in the path of testis development, their functions, and the factors that they regulate or by which they are regulated remain to be elucidated. These include the *SRY*-related gene *SOX9*, the Wilms tumor suppressor gene *WT1*, and the gene encoding the orphan nuclear receptor or transcription factor DAX-1. X-chromosomal sequences are also likely to affect testis development, since the presence of one or more additional X chromosomes (in Klinefelter syndrome and its variants) causes reduced testicular size.

At present, the factors directing ovarian development are poorly characterized; however, there is presumably an equally complex network of controls guiding this process. One such gene likely resides on the X chromosome and is probably a dosage-sensitive locus, as evidenced by girls and women with Turner syndrome, whose ovaries regress in the absence of two functional copies of the X chromosome. A candidate for this role is *DAX-1*. Duplication of the region of the X chromosome containing this gene results in development of streak ovaries in 46,XY individuals. In addition, the murine homolog of *DAX-1* is expressed in developing ovary at a time consistent with a regulatory role. Another ovarian determinant is likely autosomal, evidenced by the characterization of familial ovarian dysgenesis. The current hypothesis to explain the control of ovarian development is that it occurs when there is active function of as yet unidentified genes that repress testis-determining genes.

SEX DIFFERENTIATION Differentiation of the internal and external genitalia along male or female lines depends on the presence or absence of functional testicular tissue. Once function of the testis is established, at around 8 weeks of human gestation, development of the male sexual phenotype is under control of fetal hormones and the receptors that mediate their action. These include fetal luteinizing hormone (LH), the luteinizing hormone-chorionic gonadotropin (LH/CG) receptor, at least five steroidogenic enzymes involved in testosterone biosynthesis, steroid 5α-reductase 2 required for conversion of testosterone to dihydrotestosterone, the androgen receptor, AMH, and the AMH receptor.

Development of Wolffian structures requires testosterone, which is produced by testicular Leydig cells after activation of their cell surface receptor, the LH/CG receptor, a member of the seven transmembrane domain G-protein coupled class of receptors. During the first trimester of gestation the ligand for this receptor is probably CG, produced in large quantity by the placenta. Subsequently, endogenous fetal LH is the primary ligand. The lack of dependence on fetal LH during genital morphogenesis is evidenced by the normal penile development of male infants with hypopituitarism; however, the subnormal penile size of these infants highlights the role of LH and testosterone action in the penile growth that occurs in the third trimester. Action of CG or LH at the Leydig cell LH/CG receptor stimulates testicular steroidogenesis. Sertoli cells may also help regulate Leydig cell secretion in a paracrine fashion. The biochemistry and molecular biology of the steroidogenic enzymes is described in further detail below. The outcome of this multistep process is a high local, and to a lesser extent systemic, concentration of testosterone.

Testosterone action is mediated by the androgen receptor (AR), a nuclear receptor-transcription factor found in high concentration in the tissues of the Wolffian ducts and external genitalia. Activation of AR by androgen binding results in interaction of the receptor–ligand complex as a dimer with the promoter regions of target genes, to regulate their transcription. The exact targets of the AR in genital development remain to be determined; however, the gene for the AMH receptor may be one of them. In external genital tissues testosterone (T) is converted by steroid 5α-reductase 2 to dihydrotestosterone, which has greater affinity for the AR. The same molecular events occur after interaction of either T or DHT with AR. In the absence of high androgen concentration, as in the female or androgen-deficient fetus, there is insufficient activated AR to induce transcription of target genes required for stabilization and development of the Wolffian system and for masculinization of the external genitalia. The female fetus bears the same AR as the male; thus, it is primarily the available concentration of androgens that is the major determinant of morphogenesis. AR function is described in further detail in Chapter 60.

Müllerian duct regression is induced by the Sertoli cell glycoprotein hormone, AMH, a member of the transforming growth factor β (TGF-β) class. The stimuli for AMH secretion by Sertoli cells are largely unknown, although there is evidence for regulation by both SRY and SF-1. The actions of AMH require a specific receptor, the AMH type II receptor (AMHR), a member of the serine–threonine kinase group of transmembrane proteins. Action of AMH at its receptor, which localizes in the mesenchyme surrounding the Müllerian ducts, results in involution of Müllerian structures by apoptosis. Expression of the AMH receptor may be regulated in part by AR.

Analysis of gene expression in wild-type and transgenic mice has led to the formation of a number of hypotheses to address the complex mechanisms of sex determination. Although these hypotheses are continually changing as more is learned about the timing and patterns of gene expression, and as new genes are discovered, the following represents a working hypothesis: *SF-1* and *WT1* are required to induce development of the primordial, bipotential gonad in both sexes; once this rudimentary structure is formed, specific sex-determining genes come into play; *SOX9* is required for Sertoli cell development and testis differentiation. However, in the female, *SOX9* is suppressed by *DSS/DAX-1*. In the male, *SRY* represses *DSS* (which is in single copy in the normal male), allowing expression of *SOX9* and subsequent testis differentiation (Fig. 57-4).

Estrogens and their receptor do not appear to play a significant role in mammalian sex determination and differentiation in either sex. This is evidenced by the fact that during normal fetal development males and females are exposed to equally high levels of maternal estrogens. Similarly, there is no phenotype associated with estrogen deficiency or inability to respond to estrogen *in utero*: transgenic mice with targeted disruption of the estrogen receptor, both males and females, are phenotypically normal at birth. Their fertility is, however, reduced.

DISORDERS OF SEX DETERMINATION AND DIFFERENTIATION

GENERAL BACKGROUND AND MOLECULAR PATHOPHYSIOLOGY Abnormalities of sex determination and differentiation comprise two major clinical groups: disorders of gonadal development, with secondary effects on genital development, and defects of genital morphogenesis in the presence of normal gonads. The terminology is sometimes confusing: sex reversal refers to the condition in which the individual's genetic sex opposes the gonadal (and therefore generally the phenotypic) sex. These are individuals with 46,XY karyotype who have no testes (in their place usually are streak gonads) and have a female (or ambiguous) phenotype, and those with 46,XX karyotype who have testes and male (or ambiguous) phenotype. Pseudohermaphroditism (either male or female) refers to conditions in which karyotype and gonad are congruous; however, there is a discrepancy between the gonadal and the phenotypic sex: individuals with 46,XY karyotype and testes whose phenotype is female or ambiguous and those with 46,XX karyotype and ovaries whose phenotype is male or masculinized. Infants of either karyotypic sex with these latter disorders have phallic development that ranges from a completely formed penis to a diminutive clitoris; the labioscrotal region may be fully fused and rugose, or bifid and smooth; the internal structures may be mainly Müllerian (in the absence of AMH action), mainly Wolffian (in the presence of local androgen action), or a combination of the two. The genital morphology essentially reflects fetal production of, and response to, androgens and AMH during the critical period of gestation.

In contrast to disorders of testicular development and function, disturbance of ovarian development or function does not adversely affect fetal development of the normal female internal or external genital phenotype. However, exposure to supranormal androgen levels during gestation can induce masculinization of a female fetus, but has no detrimental effect on male fetal development. The disorders of sex determination and differentiation are summarized in Table 57-2. Approach to diagnosis and management is discussed at the conclusion of the chapter.

Because of the multiplicity of enzymes, hormones, receptors, and transcription factors involved, there are numerous opportunities for the usually well-coordinated processes of sex determination and differentiation to go awry. Hormones have no intrinsic action and must act via specific receptors. Thus hormone deficiencies are expressed by lack of function of the corresponding receptor. In general, steroid hormone deficiencies, resulting from defects of genes encoding biosynthetic enzymes, are manifest only in the presence of two defective gene alleles and are inherited as autosomal recessive traits. Compound heterozygosity occurs when the two alleles encoding an autosomal recessive trait each carry a different mutation. The functional outcome depends on the severity of the mutations independently, as well as on their interaction.

Table 57-2
Disorders of Sex Determination and Differentiation

Sex determination disorders
46,XY sex reversal (46,XY karyotype with ovaries or streak gonads)
SRY deletion/mutation
SOX9 mutation
DSS duplication
WT1 deletion/mutation
46,XX sex reversal (46,XX karyotype with testes)
XX^{Y+}—*SRY* translocation
XX^{Y-}—probable mutation of downstream regulator of testis development
True hermaphroditism (various karyotypes with ovotestes)
Chromosomal anomalies[a]
Sex differentiation disorders
46,XY pseudohermaphroditism (46,XY karyotype with testes and female or ambiguous internal or external genitalia)
Impaired testosterone production
LH/CG receptor defect (Leydig cell hypoplasia)
Defects of testosterone biosynthesis
Defect of steroidogenic acute regulatory protein (StAR)
3β-Hydroxysteroid dehydrogenase deficiency
17α-Hydroxylase deficiency
17,20-Lyase deficiency
17β-Hydroxysteroid dehydrogenase deficiency
Impaired androgen response
5α-Reductase deficiency
Androgen insensitivity syndromes
Impaired anti-Müllerian hormone production or action
46,XX pseudohermaphroditism (46,XX karyotype with ovaries and male or ambiguous internal or external genitalia)
Fetal androgen excess
Congenital adrenal hyperplasia
21-hydroxylase deficiency
11-β hydroxylase deficiency
3-β hydroxysteroid dehydrogenase deficiency
Aromatase deficiency
Maternal androgen excess[a]
Drugs
Adrenal/ovarian tumors

[a]Not discussed in this chapter.

Receptors that mediate peptide hormone action, such as membrane-associated receptors like the LH/CG receptor, act as transducers of the hormone signal, setting off an intracellular signal cascade. Mutations of transducer-type receptors cause either an increase or a decrease in the activity of the system, depending on whether the mutation is an activating or an inhibitory one: this is illustrated by the contrasting effects of mutations in the LH/CG receptor, inhibitory mutations being associated with the syndrome of Leydig cell hypoplasia *(see below)*, whereas activating mutations are associated with the syndrome of familial male precocious puberty (*see* Chapter 59). Defects of these receptors are expressed only in the presence of two defective gene alleles.

Nuclear transcription factor receptors, such as those for steroid hormones, interact directly with target genes to modify their transcription, usually in a ligand-dependent fashion. Absence of ligand or defective ligand binding translates to absent or reduced activity of the ligand-dependent transcription factors; complete absence of a transcription factor (such as occurs when the encoding gene is deleted) not surprisingly results in lack of transcription of target genes. A second class of transcription factors appears to be ligand independent (e.g., SRY, WT1). Mutations that alter protein–DNA interactions between transcription factors and their target genes may result in decreased, increased, or sometimes promiscuous transcriptional activation, the latter being caused by loss of DNA-binding specificity. In the case of a heterozygous mutation, the abnormal protein produced from the mutant gene may interfere with the action of the normal protein produced from the wild-type allele of the gene, a process referred to as the "dominant-negative" effect. In this situation, the mutant protein impairs the action of the normal one, either by blocking access of the normal factor to its target DNA, by forming inactive dimers that are unable to bind the target DNA sequence, or by sequestering other critical transcription factors because of disturbed protein–protein interactions. Defects in genes encoding intracellular receptors and transcription factors are usually considered dominant conditions, as generally only one mutant allele is required for detrimental effect. An exception is the AR, defects of which are inherited in an X-linked recessive fashion.

DISORDERS OF SEX DETERMINATION: SEX REVERSAL AND TRUE HERMAPHRODITISM This section describes disorders of genes known or thought to be involved in development of the gonads. Syndromes associated with sex chromosome aneuploidy are detailed in Chapter 58. Two major classes of disorders will be discussed—those involving genes located on the sex chromosomes, and those involving autosomal genes. The general clinical features of sex reversal and true hermaphroditism are described

Table 57-3
Disorders of Sex Determination

Disorder	*Frequency*	*Phenotype*	*Gonad type*	*Karyotype*	*SRY*
XX male	1:20,000	Male Ambiguous (20%)	Testis	46,XX	*SRY*+ (90%) *SRY*–
True hermaphrodite	1:20,000	Ambiguous	Ovotestis	46,XX (70%) 46,XX/46,XY (20%) Other (46,XY rare)	*SRY*– *SRY*+ (few)
XY gonadal dysgenesis	1:100,000			46,XY	SRY normal (90%)
Partial		Ambiguous	Testis (dysgenetic)		*SRY* mutation
Complete (Swyer syndrome)		Female	Streak		*SRY* deletion

initially and are summarized in Table 57-3. Clinical features unique to specific gene defects are described in the relevant subsections.

General Clinical Features of Disorders of Sex Determination The archetypal and most common form of sex reversal is 46,XX maleness. Approximately 1:20,000 men has a 46,XX karyotype. The phenotype of most affected individuals with 46,XX maleness is similar to that seen in Klinefelter syndrome (47,XXY): structurally normal testes are present (sometimes cryptorchid) and the internal and external genitalia are male. Testicular size and histology are normal in infancy. Pubertal virilization occurs to a greater or lesser degree, but like those with Klinefelter syndrome, affected postpubertal individuals have small testes and are azoospermic, presumably because of the detrimental effect of the extra X chromosome. Histologically the testes have atrophic, hyalinized seminiferous tubules and Leydig cell hyperplasia. Up to 20% of 46,XX individuals with testes have subnormal masculinization, manifest by cryptorchidism, hypospadias, or frank genital ambiguity. 46,XX males are taller than average for females, but shorter than 46,XY males, presumably because of absence of stature-determining genes located on Yq.

True hermaphroditism defines the condition in which there is coexistence of ovarian and testicular tissue in the same individual, usually in the same gonad (ovotestis), less often in opposite gonads. Approximately 70% of affected individuals have a 46,XX karyotype and some cases may represent a variant form of 46,XX maleness. Without thorough histologic evaluation of the gonads it may be impossible to distinguish undervirilized 46,XX males from 46,XX true hermaphrodites. In addition, true hermaphroditism and complete sex reversal can coexist within the same family. Approximately 20% of individuals with true hermaphroditism have chromosomal mosaicism for 46,XX/46,XY or less commonly 46,XX/47XXY; a small number of cases have a pure 46,XY karyotype and a few with 47,XXY karyotype have been reported. Notably, the testicular portions of the gonads are dysgenetic, with interstitial fibrosis and rare or absent spermatogonia, although the ovarian portions are histologically normal. Malignant degeneration of the gonad is reported in approximately 5% of cases. Most affected individuals with true hermaphroditism have ambiguous genitalia; however, the phenotypic spectrum is broad: for example, one case of a fully masculinized boy with bilaterally descended ovotestes has been reported. A hallmark, although not universal feature is asymmetric genital development—Müllerian structures (which may include a full or hemiuterus) on one side, and Wolffian structures on the other; a gonad-containing hemiscrotum on one side (more often the right) with a flat, empty labium majorum on the other. In general the pattern of development reflects the predominant functional nature of the gonad on the ipsilateral side. In association with an ovotestis, the internal genitalia may show elements of both Müllerian and Wolffian origin on the same side. The pattern of pubertal development reflects the function of the gonads, and fertility is not uncommon.

The disorder that represents the converse of 46,XX maleness is complete gonadal dysgenesis in a 46,XY female (Swyer syndrome; XY gonadal dysgenesis); however, it is much less common than the former condition, occurring in only 1:100,000 females. Affected individuals have streak gonads with female internal and external genitalia, although significant phenotypic variation is found within affected families. There is a high incidence of gonadal neoplasia (gonadoblastomas and germinomas) in the streak gonads. Because of deficient estrogen production, breast development is poor and these individuals often present with delayed puberty or primary amenorrhea; gonadotropin concentrations are in the castrate range. Pubic hair is usually present. Probably because of the presence of Y chromosomal stature-determining genes, affected women are of normal to tall stature compared with 46,XX females. They have no physical stigmata of Turner syndrome. However, individuals with deletion of the short arm of the Y chromosome (including the *SRY* locus), in addition to the general features described above, have certain features of Turner syndrome, such as lymphedema. The disturbances of testicular development (complete or partial gonadal dysgenesis) are associated with genital development that essentially reflects the functional state of the gonads at the critical period of sex differentiation.

In contrast to the numerous disorders of testicular development, clearly defined disorders of ovarian development (other than Turner Syndrome) are rare. One example of abnormal ovarian development likely resulting from a single gene defect is 46,XX gonadal dysgenesis. This disorder does not cause sex reversal, internal and external genitalia being those of a normal female. Affected young women present with failure of normal pubertal development, without phenotypic features of Turner syndrome; they are of normal height for females, and shorter than those with 46,XY gonadal dysgenesis, highlighting the role of Y chromosomal genes in stature determination. Their gonads are streaks;

however, in contrast to those with 46,XY gonadal dysgenesis, no increase in incidence of gonadal neoplasia has been found. Gonadotropins, particularly follicle-stimulating hormone (FSH), are markedly elevated. A familial form of 46,XX gonadal dysgenesis, in which affected individuals also have sensorineural deafness, is known as Perrault syndrome. In a large Finnish study of familial, apparently autosomal recessive, cases, the disorder is associated with mutations of the gene encoding the FSH receptor.

DISORDERS OF SEX DETERMINATION INVOLVING LOCI ON THE SEX CHROMOSOMES **Sex-Determining Region of the Y Chromosome—SRY Gene** The existence of a Y chromosomal "maleness-determining" gene was postulated in the 1930s, and in the 1960s was designated the "testis-determining factor" (TDF). Many candidates were proposed and rejected over the years. In 1990 the existence of such a gene was confirmed, with the discovery of the *SRY* gene (*Sry* in the mouse).

Genetic and Molecular Pathophysiology The study of individuals with the syndromes of 46,XY gonadal dysgenesis and 46,XX maleness was the catalyst for the eventual localization and characterization of the *SRY* gene. The human *SRY* gene is a 1.0-kb intronless gene located just centromeric to the pseudoautosomal region of Yp (Yp11.3). The encoded protein acts as the dominant inducer of testis development in mammals. However, despite its preeminent role in testis determination, other Y-encoded sequences appear to regulate *SRY* expression.

Expression of *Sry* occurs in the gonadal tissue of fetal mice in the earliest period of specific testis formation, being first detected at embryonic day 10.5 in pre–Sertoli cells in the developing gonadal ridge. This finding suggests that these cells are integral to the process of testis development; indeed, one of the primary events in testis development appears to be induction of Sertoli cell differentiation. *Sry* expression peaks at day 11.5 and declines once testicular development is established, at day 12.5. Notably *Sry* expression is quite restricted to the urogenital ridge, with no evidence for expression in any other tissue at this critical time. *Sry* expression and Sertoli cell differentiation are followed by testis differentiation, most notably, Sertoli cell-regulated organization of seminiferous tubules and Leydig cell differentiation.

The human *SRY* gene comprises a single coding exon that predicts a 203-amino acid protein. Approximately the middle one-third of the protein represents the HMG (high-mobility group) domain, which endows SRY with its sequence-specific binding to a target nucleotide sequence—5'-AACAAAG-3'. The presence of the HMG box places SRY within a family of DNA-binding, transcription-regulating proteins, the HMG box proteins. The target genes of SRY are largely unknown, but may include those encoding AMH and the steroidogenic enzyme CYP11. Nuclear magnetic resonance spectroscopy analysis of the interaction between the SRY protein and the *AMH* gene promoter reveals that SRY binds in a sequence-specific manner in the minor groove of the DNA helix, intercalating the isoleucine residue at position 68 between the DNA strands, causing some unwinding of the strands and 70–80° bending of the DNA. In addition, SRY displays sequence-independent binding at four-way DNA junctions, which are intrinsically bent. Despite the absence of an activation domain, SRY–DNA interaction mediates transcriptional regulation, perhaps by bringing together distant DNA sequences or by facilitating access of other important transcription-regulating proteins to regulator sequences within specific testis-inducing target genes. It has been suggested that the spatial arrangement of the nucleoprotein complex organized by SRY is critical for the expression of these genes.

There are two main subtypes of 46,XX maleness and 46,XX true hermaphroditism—XX^{Y+} and XX^{Y-}. The majority of patients with complete 46,XX maleness are XX^{Y+}, resulting from translocation of all or part of the distal end of the Y chromosome, containing *SRY*, to the short arm of one X chromosome during paternal gamete meiosis (Fig. 57-6). In contrast, the majority of patients with 46,XX true hermaphroditism are XX^{Y-}. The molecular-phenotypic inference from these findings is that the presence of Y chromosome material results in a greater degree of masculinization. Two specific hot spots for Yp-Xp recombination within areas of high X-Y sequence homology have been reported to account for more than 50% of such recombination events. The presence of *SRY* in the genome of a 46,XX male can be confirmed by Southern blot or polymerase chain reaction (PCR) analysis. 46,XX males with unambiguous masculinization, more than 90% are *SRY* positive, whereas the converse holds for 46,XX males with genital ambiguity, approximately 5–10% of whom are positive for *SRY*. A small number of 46,XX true hermaphrodites have been found to be *SRY* positive. Nonrandom inactivation of the *SRY*-bearing X chromosome is the postulated explanation for the presence of ovarian and testicular tissue in the same gonad in individuals with *SRY*-positive true hermaphroditism. The coexistence of 46,XX complete maleness and 46,XX true hermaphroditism in a number of families is also postulated to reflect variations in the pattern of inactivation of the *SRY*-bearing X chromosome between affected individuals, affecting *SRY* expression. 46,XX maleness and true hermaphroditism are clearly genetically heterogeneous conditions. The finding that approximately 5–10% of 46,XX males with testes are completely negative for all Y-encoded sequences (XX^{Y-}) indicates that non-Y sequences must be responsible for testis determination in these cases, as discussed below. The absence of spermatogenesis in 46,XX males has been attributed to two factors, the presence of the extra X chromosome, and the absence of Y chromosomal genes involved in spermatogenesis.

In parallel to the finding of *SRY* sequences in the majority of 46,XX males, it would be predicted that most sex-reversed 46,XY females would have defects of the *SRY* gene. However, in general this has not proven to be the case; 85–90% of 46,XY females do not have demonstrable defects within the coding region of *SRY*. Suggested explanations for this finding include the theoretical presence of mutations located outside the HMG box-encoding region of the gene, such as in sequences important for regulation of *SRY* expression, of inactivating mutations in (as yet uncharacterized) upstream regulators of *SRY*, or of mutations that induce constitutive activity in genes usually negatively regulated by *SRY*.

SRY mutations are more common in 46,XY sex-reversed females with complete rather than partial gonadal dysgenesis. In the minority of individuals in whom an *SRY* defect can be detected, a variety of cytogenetic and molecular abnormalities have been reported. Phenotypic variation between individuals harboring the same mutation, both within and between kindreds, has been described. Variable penetrance is suggested as the explanation for the finding of the same *SRY* gene mutation in both affected and unaffected 46,XY individuals in certain families. Germline mosaicism for the *SRY* mutation may be associated with fertility in the fathers of affected individuals. Reported defects include deletion of Yp, isolated deletion of *SRY*, and at least 20 single-base mutations within the HMG box-encoding region of the *SRY* gene

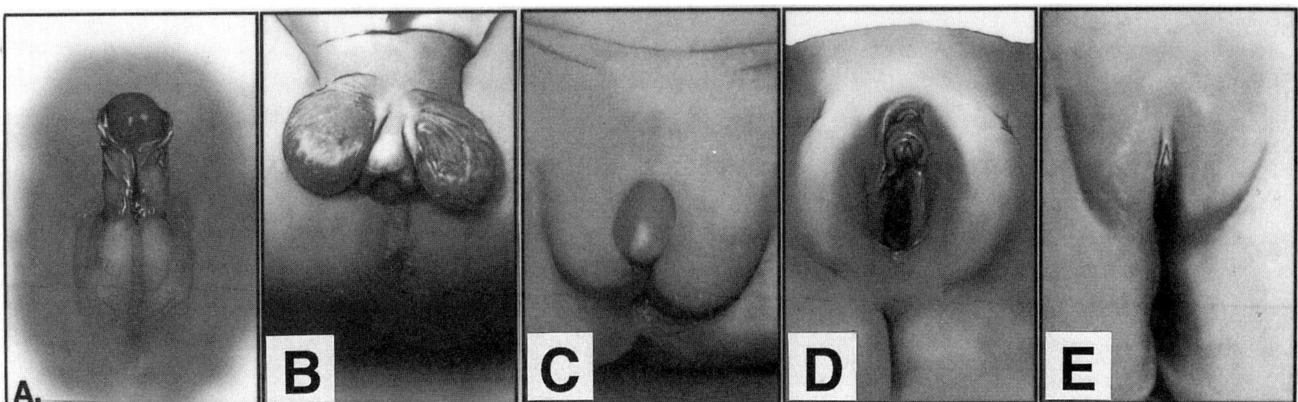

Figure 57-5 Clinical examples of male pseudohermaphroditism. These infants all have 46,XY karyotype and show varying degrees of subnormal masculinization, more severe moving from left to right. **(A)** This baby has a mild androgen receptor defect. The defect of androgen action is manifest by failure of fusion of the urethra, resulting in penile hypospadias. There is also cryptorchidism with subnormal scrotal development. **(B)** This infant has a small penis with perineoscrotal hypospadias and a completely bifid scrotum. **(C)** This child has marked genital ambiguity: the phallic structure is intermediate between a clitoris and a penis, and the labioscrotal folds are smooth and unfused. Nevertheless, the testes are present in the labioscrotal folds. **(D)** The only evidence of androgen action in this 46,XY child is the mildly enlarged clitoris. **(E)** Complete lack of androgen action in a 46,XY individual (complete androgen-insensitivity syndrome; a patient with Leydig cell LH receptor defect would have a similar appearance).

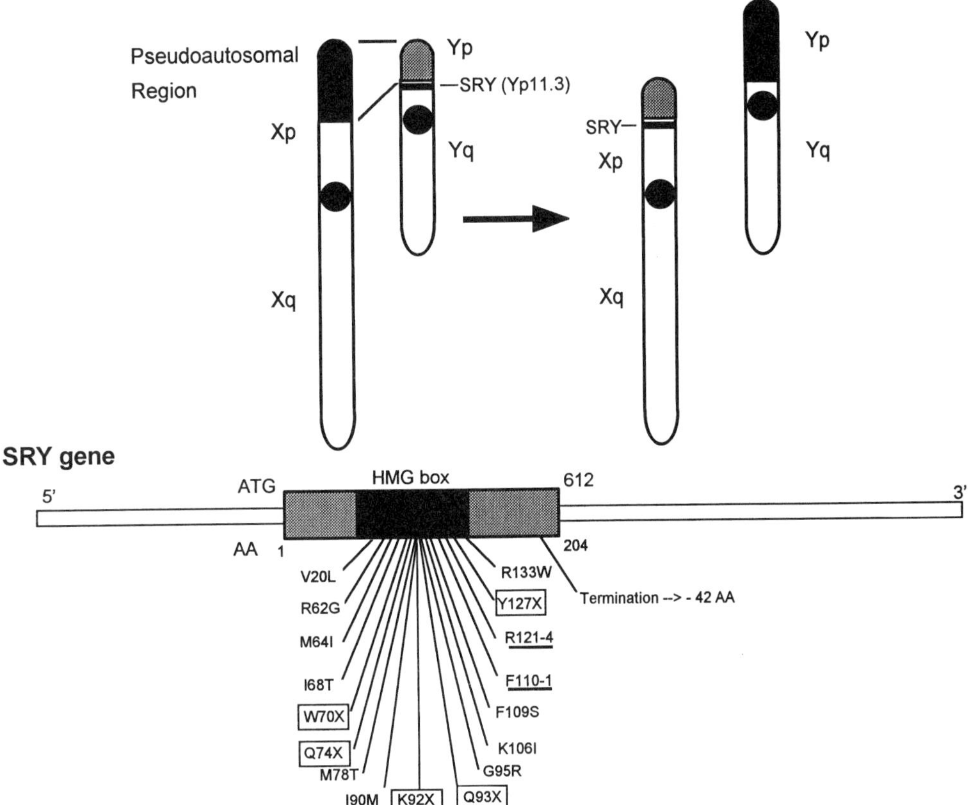

Figure 57-6 The *SRY* gene. **(Upper)** Mechanism of translocation of the *SRY* gene onto the X chromosome. During paternal gamete meiosis there is pairing of the X and Y chromosomes in their pseudoautosomal regions (shaded) located on their short arms, with obligatory crossing over of homologous sequences. Genes in this region escape X inactivation. The *SRY* gene is located just proximal to the pseudoautosomal boundary; therefore, an unequal crossover between the Y and X chromosomes could result in translocation of Y chromosomal material (shown here as the whole of the pseudoautosomal region), including the *SRY* gene, to the distal X chromosome. These recombination events occur with increased frequency at two hot spots that contain areas of high X-Y sequence homology. **(Lower)** Mutations in the human *SRY* gene. There are many missense mutations in the *SRY* gene, all occurring within the region encoding the conserved HMG box. These are shown below the gene, using the single letter amino acid code designation (*see* Fig. 8B). Nonsense mutations introducing premature termination codons are boxed; frameshift mutations are underlined. Only one mutation has been reported outside the HMG box-encoding region. This was a nonsense mutation predicting truncation of the SRY protein by 42 amino acids.

(Fig. 57-6). Severe *SRY* gene mutations resulting in failed protein expression include a frameshift because of a 4-bp deletion, and a nonsense mutation introducing a premature termination codon into the message. Only one mutation has been reported outside the *SRY* HMG box-encoding region, this being a nonsense mutation in the 3' region of the gene resulting in loss of 42 amino acids from the carboxyl-terminus of the protein.

The majority of *SRY* mutations reported to date produce nonconservative amino acid substitutions at highly conserved sites within the HMG domain. In vitro analysis of mutant SRY proteins containing amino acid substitutions reveals abnormal DNA binding and bending: some mutant SRY proteins bind DNA less avidly but bend DNA normally, whereas others bind with near-normal affinity but bend the DNA to a different angle. The most severe defects appear to arise *de novo*, whereas the milder ones are compatible with fertility and thereby transmission to offspring. This is further evidenced by the fact that less dramatic missense mutations cause partial, rather than complete, gonadal dysgenesis, indicating that the mutant SRY protein likely retains some transcription-activating function. *SRY* gene mutations have also been reported in a few cases of 46,XY true hermaphroditism. One example was a postzygotic somatic mutation, because the affected individual had only the wild-type *SRY* sequence in leukocyte DNA but had both wild-type and mutant alleles in DNA derived from the gonads.

Although SRY is probably the key positive regulator of testis determination, there are clearly other upstream and downstream factors that must be activated or repressed to allow testis development to occur. This is implied by the following: (1) the majority of 46,XY females with gonadal dysgenesis have an intact *SRY* gene; and (2) some 46,XX males with testes are completely Y negative, indicating that non-Y sequences must be responsible for testis determination in these cases. Furthermore, the tight ontogeny of *Sry* expression during embryogenesis in the mouse suggests the presence of a "controller," that is, at least one upstream regulator of expression of the critical switch gene. In this regard, it is notable that a potential binding site for the early growth response-Wilms tumor 1 family of transcription factors has been reported upstream of the *SRY* open reading frame.

Dosage-Sensitive Sex Reversal–Adrenal Hypoplasia Congenita Critical Region on the X Chromosome, Gene 1—*DAX-1* The *DAX-1* gene is implicated in development of the reproductive tract by its involvement in two unusual X-linked syndromes: dosage-sensitive sex reversal (DSS) and adrenal hypoplasia congenita-hypogonadotropic hypogonadism (AHC/HHG).

Clinical Features Karyotypic males with a duplication of the region of the X chromosome containing the *DAX-1* gene have typical features of 46,XY sex reversal, with streak gonads and a female phenotype. In contrast, individuals with deletion of this region have normal testes and normal male genitalia, although cryptorchidism has occasionally been reported. These males have congenital hypoplasia of the adrenal glands and many die unexpectedly in infancy or early childhood of undiagnosed adrenal failure, generally ascribed to "Addison disease." Those who, with replacement therapy, survive childhood also commonly have hypogonadotropic hypogonadism resulting in failure of pubertal virilization. This compound syndrome is known as adrenal hypoplasia congenita–hypogonadotropic hypogonadism (AHC/HHG) (*see* Chapter 59). One report also describes late development of high-frequency hearing loss in affected individuals. Female carriers of AHC/HHG have no clear abnormality of either adrenal gland development or gonadotropin secretion; however, the author has received some reports of menstrual irregularity and early menopause.

Genetic and Molecular Pathophysiology The occurrence of sex reversal in the presence of two copies of sequences in the Xp21 region led to the designation of this locus as the dosage-sensitive sex reversal region (DSS). Subsequently it was determined that this same region was deleted in individuals with adrenal hypoplasia congenita (AHC). The *DAX-1* gene (DSS adrenal hypoplasia congenita locus on the X chromosome, gene 1) was cloned by analysis of this region in such patients. A well-described cytogenetic microdeletion syndrome encompassing the Xp21 region includes deletions of *DAX-1*, the dystrophin *(DYS)* gene (deletions of which cause Duchenne muscular dystrophy), and the gene encoding glycerol kinase (GK). The 5.0-kb *DAX-1* gene located at Xp21.3–21.2 encodes a new, although probably rather primitive, orphan member of the nuclear hormone receptor superfamily of transcription factors. The gene demonstrates evolutionary conservation, homologous sequences being detected in an X-linked pattern of distribution in many species. It comprises two exons and one intron that encode a 470-amino acid protein. The amino-terminal region of the protein, encoded by the first exon of the gene, contains a novel DNA-binding domain that has little homology with that of other members of the family. However, the ligand-binding domain, encoded in part by the first and in part by the second exon of the gene, has strong similarities with those of the retinoic acid and retinoid X receptors.

Expression of the homologous gene in the mouse occurs in the first stages of gonadal and adrenal differentiation and in the developing hypothalamus. In human studies, *DAX-1* is expressed in adult testis and adrenal cortex, in the hypothalamus and pituitary gland, and at low level in adult ovary and liver. The expression of *DAX-1* at all levels of the hypothalamic–pituitary–adrenal and gonadal axes supports its role in the coordinated development of the adrenal and reproductive systems and suggests that the DAX-1 protein may be directly or indirectly involved in gonadal regulation of hypothalamic–pituitary function. The promoter region of the *DAX-1* gene contains a binding site for SF-1, linking the two transcription factors in the control of development of steroidogenic tissues and suggesting that SF-1 may directly regulate *DAX-1*. Furthermore, the fact that disruption of *SF-1* inhibits development of gonads and adrenals *(see below)*, whereas deletion of *DAX-1* disturbs only adrenal development, suggests that *DAX-1* is downstream of *SF-1* in this cascade.

Duplication of the *DAX-1*-containing region of the X chromosome (DSS) results in classic sex reversal, with ovarian development in 46,XY individuals. Overexpression of this region impairs testis formation despite the presence of a functional *SRY* gene; suggesting a "toxic" effect on testicular development. In contrast, carrier females with duplication of this region may be fertile, indicating that double dosage of this locus does not impair normal ovarian differentiation. Whether the sex-reversing gene is *DAX-1* itself awaits analysis in transgenic animals. Recently, a cluster of potential candidates for the role of sex-reversal gene has been isolated from a region within 50 kb of *DAX1*, including *MAGE-Xp* or *MAGEL1* (melanoma associated antigen gene), *DAM6*, and *DAM10 (DSS/AHC* critical interval genes belonging to the *MAGE* superfamily). These genes are expressed in adult testis and the latter two are expressed in lung tumors. Their developmental roles remain to be characterized.

Although adrenal development does not proceed beyond the fetal stage, disruption of *DAX-1* does not prevent testicular development in males, indicating that this gene does not appear to play a role in normal testis differentiation. However, potential interactions between DAX-1 and the primary testicular switch, SRY in testis formation remain to be examined. Deletion of *DAX-1* has been reported in a number of patients with isolated AHC, whereas frameshift, premature termination, codon deletion, and missense mutations have been found in *DAX-1* genes of individuals with combined AHC/HHG, suggesting a possible dominant-negative effect of a retained but structurally abnormal protein on hypothalamic–pituitary function.

If *DAX-1* is indeed the sex-reversal gene, it may represent a link between normal ovarian and testicular differentiation pathways. Different genes must be activated or repressed to allow differentiation of ovary rather than testis or vice versa. It is conceivable that DAX-1 (or a related locus) may act as a repressor of a gene or genes involved in testis determination; thus, absence of the gene product is inconsequential for testis development, but excess is detrimental. Loss of one allele likely has minimal effect on ovarian function because there is an active locus on the other X chromosome. It has been suggested that this locus may be a remnant of an ancestral sex-determining system that operated by dosage before the process of X-chromosome inactivation evolved.

SEX DETERMINATION DISORDERS INVOLVING LOCI ON THE AUTOSOMES Analysis of a number of informative families with 46,XX^{Y-} maleness, true hermaphroditism, or both reveals transmission patterns consistent with an autosomal dominant trait. One postulated mechanism to explain sex reversal in such cases is the presence of an upregulatory mutation in an as yet uncharacterized downstream regulator of testis determination.

SRY Homeobox-like Gene 9—*SOX9* After the discovery of the *SRY* gene, many related genes were soon identified. Those that encode proteins with more than 60% similarity to the *SRY* HMG box region have been termed *SOX* genes. One such gene, *SOX9*, is significantly involved in the process of testis formation.

Clinical Features The syndrome of campomelic dysplasia features a distinctive form of skeletal malformation that is present in 75% of 46,XY individuals affected by sex reversal (ovaries or streak gonads, and female internal and external genitalia). Affected 46,XX individuals have normal ovarian and external genital development. In most cases death occurs in infancy or early childhood because of respiratory compromise. The syndrome is uncommon, estimates of its frequency ranging from 1/5,000–1/200,000 live births.

Genetic and Molecular Pathophysiology *SOX9* was identified by cloning of a chromosomal translocation breakpoint from a sex-reversed patient with camptomelic dysplasia. The gene is located at 17q24–25, in a region termed sex-reversal autosomal 1 (SRA1); its cDNA is approximately 3.9 kb in size. The *SOX9* gene displays strong sequence conservation throughout mammalian evolution. Furthermore, the sequence similarity between *SOX9* and *SRY* suggests a possible evolutionary relationship between the two that may represent evolution from a dosage-dependent sex-determination system to a dominant system. Notably, dosage sensitivity is a feature of many regulatory genes.

In the human fetus, *SOX9* mRNA is detectable by Northern analysis in brain, liver, and kidney; by *in situ* hybridization, *SOX9* expression is detectable in the testis at week 18 of gestation in the area of the rete testis and seminiferous tubules. In the adult, *SOX9* message is expressed most strongly in testis. It is also highly expressed in pancreas, prostate, kidney, brain, and the skeleton and at low level in most other adult tissues. In the mouse, the homologous *Sox9* gene is highly expressed in fetal skeletal tissues, as well as neural, cardiac, and other tissues. Its expression can be detected in mRNA isolated from whole embryos at day 8.5. Consistent with a role in testis determination, *Sox9* expression parallels Sertoli cell differentiation.

SOX9 encodes a 509-amino acid protein with features of a transcription regulator: it contains a putative DNA-binding HMG box domain and a proline- and glutamine-rich domain in its carboxy-terminal third, similar to activation domains of other transcription factors. In vitro deletion of this latter region destroys the transactivating function of the protein. SOX9 activates transcription via the nucleotide motif recognized by other HMG domain transcription factors, 5'-AACAAAG-3', and may represent another switchlike mechanism, because it appears to act in a dominant fashion, similar to SRY. SOX9 may be acting just downstream of SRY and may represent a target for SRY; however, this remains speculative, because the appropriate HMG box binding motif has not been identified within the *SOX9* gene promoter. One postulated relationship between the two transcription factors in testis determination is that *SOX9* expression in another cell type is required to complement *SRY* expression by Sertoli cells. Analysis of this hypothesis will require information regarding the comparative ontogeny of *SOX9* and *SRY* expression.

Inactivating mutations in one *SOX9* allele have been identified in a number of 46,XY individuals with camptomelic dysplasia and sex reversal. No patient has been reported with mutations in both *SOX9* alleles. In general *SOX9* mutations appear to occur *de novo*, providing further evidence of the autosomal dominant nature of the disorder. Mutations reported to date likely destroy protein function; these include frameshifts and nonsense mutations that lead to premature chain termination and loss of large portions of the protein. Thus the phenotype of individuals with these mutations appears to be caused by loss of function of the encoded transcription factor (haploinsufficiency), rather than resulting from a dominant-negative or gain-of-function effect. Missense mutations have not yet been reported. Affected sibling pairs with normal parents have been reported, likely as a result of gonadal mosaicism for the mutant gene.

Recently, a number of patients with autosomal sex reversal and campomelic dysplasia have been found to have chromosome 17 breakpoints at least 50–130 kb from the *SOX9* locus, suggesting the presence of other genes responsible for the same phenotype, or perhaps a disturbance of *SOX9* expression because of mutation of an upstream regulator. Positional cloning of the chromosome 17q breakpoint in one patient with sex reversal in the absence of campomelia (so-called acampomelic camptomelic dysplasia) identified a 3.5-kb cDNA that is expressed in testis but appears not to be translated. It was suggested by the authors that the mRNA itself has a functional role in sex determination.

Wilms Tumor 1—WT1 The Wilms tumor 1 *(WT1)* gene product, a member of the early growth response (EGR) family of transcription factors, is implicated in gonadal and genital development by analysis of human mutations and transgenic mice with a deletion of the gene.

Clinical Features Two clinical syndromes are associated with defects of the Wilms tumor 1 gene *(WT1)*. The Denys-Drash syndrome comprises a triad of gonadal dysgenesis, congenital nephropathy, and subsequent development of Wilms tumor. Patients with Denys-Drash syndrome have heterogeneous disorders of gonadal and genital development. The gonads range from streak gonads or ovotestes in either 46,XX or 46,XY individuals, to rudimentary or dysgenetic testes in 46,XY patients, or normal ovaries (in a 46,XX patient). Perhaps because of an ascertainment bias, the majority of patients (about 90%) have 46,XY karyotype. Their external genitalia are usually ambiguous, sometimes female, occasionally male. The internal genitalia are often incongruous with respect to the external genital phenotype: Wolffian structures may be present in phenotypic females, Müllerian structures in phenotypic males. Even in 46,XX females, there may be anomalous internal genital development, and one 46,XY patient with dysgenetic testes had neither Müllerian nor Wolffian structures. Gonadoblastomas and granulosa cell tumors have been reported in some cases. The congenital nephropathy (caused by diffuse or focal mesangial sclerosis) generally presents with proteinuria and hypertension in the first year of life, with progression to renal insufficiency and death by 2 years of age. Wilms tumor is reported in more than 50% of cases, most presenting with an abdominal mass in the second year of life. The incidence would probably be higher if the patients survived longer, and in fact most are found to have persistent intralobar renal blastema, which may be the precursor of Wilms tumor. Of interest, the incidence of hypospadias and cryptorchidism is 10-fold higher in patients with bilateral Wilms tumor (distinct from the Denys-Drash syndrome) than in the general population.

In the WAGR syndrome, affected individuals, in addition to Wilms tumor and genitourinary abnormalities or gonadoblastoma, have aniridia and mental retardation. This disorder appears to be a contiguous gene defect, caused by heterozygous deletion of the 11p13 region that contains the *WT1* gene. Thus, other genes located in this region may also be involved in pathogenesis.

Genetic and Molecular Pathophysiology The *WT1* gene located in chromosomal region 11p13 is approximately 50 kb in size, contains 10 exons, encoding four distinct mRNA species (of approximately 3 kb), generated by the presence or absence of two alternative splice sites. The fact that all transcripts are expressed at a similar level suggests that each encoded protein makes a significant contribution to normal function. Interactions between the four proteins, each of which may have distinct targets and functions, may be important in the control of cellular proliferation and differentiation exerted by WT1. *WT1* expression occurs at a similar time to that of *SRY*, *WT1* mRNA being detectable in pronephric and mesonephric tissues on embryonic day 10.5 in the mouse, at which time *SRY* expression is detectable in pre–Sertoli cells. By embryonic day 11.5 the nephrogenic cord, condensing metanephric tissue, and urogenital ridge display high levels of *WT1* message. In the developing gonad *WT1* expression is localized to the stromal cell components, and in mature gonads it is confined to the Sertoli cells of the testis and granulosa and epithelial cells of the ovary. Expression also has been detected in abdominal and lung mesothelium.

The WT1 protein is a putative 45- to 49-kDa tumor suppressor with four contiguous Cys2-His2 zinc finger domains (encoded by exons 7–10) and an amino-terminus rich in proline and glutamine, consistent with a role as a transcription factor. WT1 has been shown to have separate domains that subserve transcriptional repression and transcription activation: residues 85–124 encompass the repressor domain, and 181–250 the activator domain. These regions are distinct from the DNA-binding domain and their activities are probably mediated by protein–protein interaction. The WT1 protein shows homology to the early growth response-1 *(EGR-1)* gene product and has similar binding sites (5'-CGCCCCCGC-3'). These proteins are expressed early in the cell cycle, at G0 to G1 transition. The target genes for WT1 are at present unknown; however, it is suggested that the normal role of WT1 during embryologic development is to initiate a transcriptional program that controls differentiation of glomerular epithelial cells and gonadal primordium. The absence of both sets of internal genital duct anlagen in one patient would be compatible with a primary role of WT1 in early development of the bipotential internal duct systems. In renal tissue it acts as a tumor suppressor.

Examination of transgenic mice homozygous for a knockout mutation of *WT1* established a crucial role for WT1 in early urogenital development, with mutant embryos displaying failure of renal and gonadal development. Specifically, at day 11 of gestation, the cells of the metanephric blastema underwent apoptosis, the ureteric bud failed to grow out from the Wolffian duct, and the formation of the metanephric kidney did not occur. The mice were nonviable, probably because of abnormal development of the mesothelium, heart, and lungs.

The Denys-Drash syndrome in humans is associated with heterozygous germline mutations in *WT1* in approximately 95% of cases examined to date. The mutations cluster within or near the zinc finger (ZF) coding region (exons 7–10, particularly exon 9), most producing amino acid substitutions in ZF2 and ZF3. One mutation, encoding an arginine to tryptophan substitution at position 394 in the third zinc finger, has occurred recurrently, being present in approximately half of the cases reported to date. Other reported mutations include a variety of nonconservative missense, nonsense, frameshift, and splice-junction mutations, most of which appear *de novo*, since parental *WT1* genes are normal. In one case, however, the normal father of an affected child was found to be heterozygous for the mutant allele, a finding that suggested either mosaicism or reduced penetrance of the mutant gene. The disorder is genetically dominant, because no patients have been described with mutations in both alleles of the gene. The WAGR syndrome likely results from heterozygous loss of contiguous genes within the 11p13 region including the *WT1* gene, accounting for the aniridia and mental retardation that accompany the Wilms tumor and genitourinary abnormalities in WAGR cases. In patients in whom it has been examined, the mutant allele appears to have arisen in the paternally derived chromosome 11. The dominant phenotype associated with the null mutation indicates dosage sensitivity at this locus—that is, two functional copies of the gene are required to prevent the abnormalities associated with the syndrome.

The molecular pathophysiology of *WT1* mutations appears to be lack of normal DNA binding by the WT1 protein, because mutant WT1 proteins containing nonconservative amino acid substitutions within the zinc finger region do not bind to the EGR-1 consensus-binding sequence bound by wild-type WT1. Mutations that affect zinc-coordinating cysteine or histidine residues likely prohibit DNA binding by disrupting proper spatial organization of the zinc finger. WT1 appears to play a dominant-positive role in renal and gonadal development. Formation of inactive mutant–wild-type dimers could theoretically produce a dominant-negative effect, presumably via heterodimerization with wild-type WT1 protein. Interestingly, complete deletion of the *WT1* gene produces milder genital abnormalities (cryptorchidism and/or hypospadias), than does a mutation that encodes expression of an abnormal WT1 protein, again suggesting a dominant-negative mechanism of action of mutant WT1. Although *WT1* mutations are heterozygous at the germ cell level, tissue from the Wilms tumors of these patients generally demonstrates loss of heterozygosity for *WT1*, indicating that two mutant *WT1* alleles may be required for loss of tumor suppressor function of WT1 ("two-hit" hypothesis). A role for interaction between WT1 and the ubiquitous tumor suppressor, p53, is suggested by an interaction between the two factors in transfected cells. The two may interact by direct protein–protein interaction or via an intermediate, and there is evidence that the tumor suppressor function of WT1 may be dependent on such an interaction, rather than be intrinsic to the protein itself.

Steroidogenic Factor 1—SF-1 Defects of steroidogenic factor 1 (SF-1) have not yet been reported in humans; however, the phenotype of transgenic mice with targeted disruption of the homologous gene (*fushi tarazu* factor-1 *[Ftz-F1]*) is well-characterized, and provides important insights into aspects of mammalian gonadal development.

SF-1 (also referred to as adrenal 4-binding protein [Ad4BP]), appears to hold a strategic position in inducing the development of the reproductive tract. Not only does SF-1 regulate gonadal and adrenal development, it also appears to control development of an important hypothalamic nucleus, and of pituitary gonadotropin-secreting cells. Furthermore, SF-1 regulates expression of the genes encoding three key steroidogenic enzymes: cholesterol side-chain cleavage enzyme, steroid 21-hydroxylase, and the aldosterone synthase isozyme of steroid 11β-hydroxylase.

The human gene encoding SF-1 is located at 9q33 and its murine homologue is on mouse chromosome 2. Two distinct proteins—SF-1 and ELP (embryonal long terminal repeat)—are produced by alternative promoter usage and splicing; however, the critical protein with respect to reproductive tract development is SF-1. SF-1 is an orphan nuclear receptor or transcription factor that contains the typical two central zinc fingers and a carboxy-terminal ligand-binding domain. *SF-1* is expressed in the urogenital ridge of male and female mice at embryonic day 9–9.5, the earliest stage of organogenesis of the gonads (still indifferent, and before *SRY* expression); it is subsequently expressed in fetal Sertoli cells and in the primordial cells of the adrenal glands. Consistent with its role in regulation of steroidogenesis, it is expressed before expression of the first enzyme of steroidogenesis, $P450_{scc}$. Expression in fetal ovaries is quite low, and disappears between embryonic days 13.5 and 16.5, in keeping with the lack of ovarian steroidogenic activity at that time. *SF-1* mRNA is detectable in the developing mouse pituitary at embryonic day 13.5–14.5 and can be specifically detected in gonadotrophs. In adult mice *SF-1* is expressed in all primary steroidogenic tissues, including all zones of the adrenal cortex, testicular Leydig and Sertoli cells, ovarian theca and granulosa cells, and corpus luteum. There is sexually dimorphic expression of *SF-1* postnatally. In male rats testicular *SF-1* mRNA levels decline markedly after the first week of life, whereas ovarian *SF-1* expression increases in females.

The expression of *SF-1* appears to be regulated by another factor, probably a helix-loop-helix protein similar to *c-Myc*, that binds to a region in the promoter of the rat *Ftz-F1* gene (homologous to *SF-1*), designated the *E box*. Expression of the binding factor precedes that of *SF-1*. This fact, and its tissue-specific pattern of expression, is consistent with a role as a regulator of *SF-1* expression. This factor may be the earliest member of the gonadal development cascade as yet identified.

SF-1 functions differently from most other members of the nuclear receptor family, because it appears to bind as a monomer, rather than as the more usual dimer, to a nonpalindromic DNA steroid response element half-site, 5'-AGGTCA-3'. Potential targets for SF-1 include the genes encoding $P450_{scc}$, DAX-1, LHβ, AMH, and oxytocin, because SF-1 binding sites have been located within the promoter regions of these genes.

The functional importance of *SF-1* and *Ftz-F1* is addressed by studies in transgenic animals. Both male and female mice lacking a functional *Ftz-F1* gene had phenotypically female internal and external genitalia and died in the neonatal period of adrenal insufficiency. They failed to develop steroidogenic tissues, having neither gonads nor adrenal glands (the steroidogenic components of adrenal glands and gonads likely have a common embryologic origin in the urogenital ridge). Interestingly, these mice did display mesenchymal thickening in the gonadal ridge area at the earliest stages of gonadal development (embryonic day 10.5), but thereafter the cells of this region underwent apoptosis (programmed cell death), suggesting that the role of SF-1 and Ftz-F1 may be in maintaining rather than initiating gonadal development. These mice also had abnormal development of the ventromedial hypothalamic nucleus, a region important in control of pituitary gonadotropin secretion. Expression of proteins specific to gonadotroph cells, LHβ, FSHβ (follicle-stimulating hormone), and gonadotropin-releasing hormone (GnRH) receptor was absent, implicating SF-1 in gonadotrope development and LH and FSH expression.

The presence of female internal genitalia in the null animals of both sexes indicates that the Müllerian ducts did not regress as expected in the males, reflecting lack of AMH action, because of absence of Sertoli cells. In females, expression of *SF-1* during the critical period of genital development would be detrimental to normal sex differentiation. SF-1 induction of *AMH* expression would likely induce Müllerian regression and failure of oviduct and uterine development. The fact that SF-1 expression in developing ovaries is low supports this hypothesis. Interestingly, although SF-1 binds to the promoter of the *AMH* gene, it is unable to regulate *AMH* gene expression in cotransfection assays using a heterologous cell line, unless its ligand-binding domain is deleted. This finding suggests a role for a possible ligand for SF-1 in its regulation of *AMH* expression in vivo, perhaps a Sertoli cell-specific factor. Such a factor could prove to be critical in the sex determination cascade.

In evaluating the role of SF-1 in reproductive tract development, a key question arises regarding the possible interactions between SRY and SF-1. The fact that the *Ftz-F1* null mice have no gonadal tissue at all, whereas individuals with *SRY* mutations develop gonads that more or less resemble ovaries suggests that normal *SF-1* or *Ftz-F1* expression must occur before *SRY* can be effective in inducing testis determination. Furthermore, expression of the two genes is temporally dissociated, *SF-1* being expressed in mouse testis at embryonic day 9–9.5, before transient gonadal *SRY* expression at day 10.5. However, in the older embryo expression of *SRY* correlates with sexually dimorphic expression of *SF-1*. In males SRY promotes upregulation of *SF-1*; absence of SRY in females results in reduced *SF-1* expression. In view of the discordant timing of expression of these proteins, this is likely an indirect effect. In this context it has been suggested that SRY could act by silencing a repressor of *SF-1*, thus facilitating *SF-1* expression.

In summary, SF-1 has multiple key roles in reproductive tract development, controlling development of the gonads and adrenal glands themselves, a hypothalamic center that regulates gonadal function, gonadotropin expression, and production of the two hormones essential for male sex differentiation—testosterone (by regulation of key steroidogenic enzymes) and AMH.

c-*kit* Receptor and Steel Factor In the mouse, the steel factor *(Slf)* and its receptor, c-*kit*, represent a growth factor–receptor system that is involved in development of three major cell lineages: hemopoietic cells, melanocytes, and germ cells. Mice with mutations at either the *Slf* or c-*kit* locus have white coat color, sterility, and anemia, attributable to failure of stem-cell populations (melanoblasts, primordial germ cells, and pluripotent hemopoietic stem cells) to migrate and/or proliferate effectively during development.

The mouse c-*kit* gene is a proto-oncogene whose product is a 145- to 160-kDa transmembrane tyrosine kinase receptor of the same family as a number of growth factor receptors (such as insulin-like growth factor I and platelet-derived growth factor). The human c-*kit* gene is located at 4q12, spans more than 70 kb of DNA, and includes 21 exons, which are alternatively spliced. The longest transcript is approximately 5.2 kb. In mouse, Kit protein is expressed in primordial germ cells, spermatogonia, Leydig cells, and growing oocytes. Expression can be detected in primordial germ cells as early as mouse embryonic day 7.5, ceasing as germ cell proliferation is completed, after arrival at the gonadal ridge on day 13.5–15.5, and returning during the postnatal maturation of oocytes and spermatogonia.

The Kit receptor appears to be active in a homodimer form. Thus, mutations of a single allele at the c-*kit* locus may cause defective receptor activity by combination of mutant receptor with wild-type, inhibiting the action of the normal receptor (dominant-negative effect).

The ligand for the c-kit receptor, known as steel factor (Slf), stem cell factor (SCF), or Kit ligand (KL), is encoded by the Steel *(Slf)* locus. The gene maps to human chromosome 12q22. By alternative splicing the *Slf* gene codes for two different peptides, a membrane-bound form and a soluble form. In the testis, steel factor is produced primarily by the Sertoli cell. Deletion of the entire *Slf* gene is lethal in mice, whereas a mutation that allows production of only the soluble form of steel factor, while resulting in abnormal germ cell migration and spermatogenesis, is nevertheless compatible with life. These facts are interpreted as indicating that the membrane-bound form of Slf is crucial for differentiation of tissues. Slf and c-kit may in fact have their primary role as survival factors, because they appear to suppress apoptosis.

Although c-kit and Slf are crucial for the development and migration of primordial germ cells in rodents, understanding of their role in human testicular development is still evolving. In normal human testicular development Kit protein is detectable up to 15 weeks of gestation. However, in fetal testes of individuals with intersex conditions Kit was detectable at a later stage, suggesting disturbance of the timing of germ cell development. Notably, individuals with intersex conditions are at increased risk for development of germ cell tumors, and Kit is expressed at high level by seminomas, one type of germ cell tumor. In adult testicular tissue Kit protein is detectable in undifferentiated spermatogonia, whereas Slf/SCF is found on the membrane of the seminiferous tubules and on the surface of Sertoli cells, suggesting that the c-kit and Slf system may act in a paracrine fashion. SCF is also expressed in human ovary and cultured granulosa/luteal cells, in which it is downregulated by gonadotropins. Interestingly, both proteins are also expressed in the human central nervous system, particularly in the cerebellum, in addition to a wide variety of other fully differentiated tissues, suggesting that this system may have roles that extend well beyond fetal life. Despite the known role of c-kit in migration and proliferation of germ cells (in addition to hemopoietic stem cells and melanoblasts) in the mouse, human c-*kit* mutations have not been associated with reduced fertility in humans, but have been found only in association with piebaldism and in a human mast cell leukemia cell line.

In summary, in the mouse the c-kit–steel receptor–ligand system plays a crucial role in migration, differentiation, and survival of primordial cells destined to become germ cells, and there is evidence for a role for these factors in human testicular development and carcinogenesis. It has been hypothesized that c-kit and SCF may have a regulatory function in normal testicular tissue by providing environmental factors necessary for spermatogenesis. The relevance of this system to human fertility is yet to be addressed.

DISORDERS OF SEX DIFFERENTIATION: 46,XY AND 46,XX PSEUDOHERMAPHRODITISM These disorders represent abnormalities of genital morphogenesis, in the presence of gonads that are appropriate for karyotype.

46,XY Pseudohermaphroditism Male (46,XY) pseudohermaphroditism describes the condition in which an individual with male karyotype and normally formed testes has abnormal masculinization of the internal and/or external genitalia. The causes are numerous, but in essence there are two major classes—defects of production or response to testosterone, and defects of production or response to AMH. The causes of male pseudohermaphroditism are summarized in Table 57-2. Clinical examples are provided in Fig. 57-5.

Disorders of Testosterone Production or Action: General Clinical Features The genital phenotype in these conditions generally reflects the severity of the defect at the functional level. 46,XY individuals with profound deficiency of androgen production or action have an entirely female phenotype. Those in whom some degree of androgen production and action is retained have a wide spectrum of genital phenotypes, including minor degrees of posterior labial fusion or clitoral enlargement; ambiguous genitalia characterized by incomplete labioscrotal fusion and a clitoris-like phallus; and more significant masculinization with reasonable penile size accompanied by urethral hypospadias, penile chordee, and cryptorchidism. The testes may be located anywhere from the abdomen to the inguinal canals or the labioscrotal region. Internal genital structures range from fully feminized, separate vaginal and urethral structures in cases in which there is minimal androgen action, to more masculinized structures, such as a urogenital sinus with ectopic vaginal orifice, in milder cases in which a moderate degree of androgen production and action has occurred. The development of Wolffian duct structures (epididymis and vas deferens) is also variable, depending on the degree of local testosterone secretion and action in early gestation. The vaginal pouch is blind and Müllerian duct structures are absent or diminutive because AMH is secreted normally by the Sertoli cells.

Disorders of Testosterone Production or Action: Specific Disorders—Leydig Cell Hypoplasia *Clinical Features and Diagnosis.* Leydig cell hypoplasia (LCH) is a rare cause of male pseudohermaphroditism, in which Leydig cell differentiation and testosterone production are impaired because of absence or defective function of LH/CG receptors on Leydig cell progenitors. This condition is generally inherited in a male-limited, autosomal recessive pattern. Inability to respond to CG or LH because of absence of the appropriate receptor results in inadequate testosterone production *in utero* and thereafter. The genital phenotype is generally female; however posterior labial fusion, a small vagina, or a urogenital sinus may be present, and occasional patients with small penis are reported, suggesting significant T production in the first trimester. Minimal development of either male or female secondary sexual characteristics occurs at puberty, a feature that distinguishes this condition from the androgen insensitivity syndromes, in which high estrogen production at puberty results in excellent breast development in most cases.

In postpubertal individuals the testes are slightly small. Although Sertoli cells are normal there is hyalinization of the seminiferous tubules and interrupted spermatogenesis and absent or reduced Leydig cells. The latter finding indicates that LH is required for development and survival of Leydig cells. Testicular membrane preparations do not bind labeled hCG, a fact that, until recently, has served as the primary evidence of a defect of the LH/CG receptor.

The diagnosis of Leydig cell hypoplasia would be suggested by low testosterone levels, despite high serum LH, in a 46,XY infant with female or ambiguous external genitalia; this hormonal profile should allow diagnostic differentiation from the androgen insensitivity syndromes, because in these latter conditions, at least theoretically, testosterone concentrations are high. Unlike infants with a testosterone biosynthetic defect, who may also have low serum testosterone and high LH, there is no elevation of testosterone precursors. In addition, there is no increase in testosterone or its precursors in response to hCG administration. Failure of pubertal development in a phenotypic female with high serum LH and no measurable sex steroids would also suggest this diagnosis.

Genetic and Molecular Pathophysiology. LCH is an apparently rare autosomal recessive disorder with an estimated prevalence of approximately 1:1,000,000, although this low prevalence may in part reflect lack of ascertainment. The 60-kb gene encoding the LH/CG receptor (CH/CG-R) is located at chromosomal position 2p21 and comprises 11 exons and 10 introns. The encoded receptor is a member of the seven transmembrane domain class of G-protein-coupled receptors in which ligand binding induces increased intracellular production of cyclic AMP, the principal mediator of hormone action in this system. Exons 1–10 encode the major portion of the amino-terminal extracellular domain, containing a leucine-rich repeat, whereas exon 11 codes for a small part of the extracellular domain, as well as all 7 transmembrane loops and the carboxy-terminal intracellular region. The LH/CG receptor has significant homology with the FSH and thyroid-stimulating hormone (TSH) receptors.

Testicular Leydig cells constitutively express LH/CG receptor in the absence of hormone. Interestingly, the receptor appears to be regulated by its ligand (LH or CG) via two processes: uncoupling (a fairly immediate process that results in reduced cAMP production in response to ligand, without reducing receptor number) and downregulation (a slower, biphasic process resulting in reduced receptor number because of internalization and degradation of already formed receptors, followed by reduced receptor mRNA transcription, via a cAMP-mediated process). These regulatory events are believed to contribute to the phenomenon of desensitization that occurs in the presence of continuous hormonal stimulation. In contrast to the constitutive receptor expression seen in Leydig cells, ovarian cells require hormonal stimulation for receptor expression: in the preovulatory follicle estrogen and FSH synergystically induce receptor mRNA expression in rat granulosa cells, also via cAMP-mediated events. Subsequently, the high levels of LH that occur at ovulation downregulate receptor expression. There appears to be some constitutive expression of LH/CG receptor in theca cells, in addition to hormonal regulation similar to, though less tight than, that seen in granulosa cells.

To date, reports of inactivating mutations in the *LH/CG-R* gene are scarce. In a pair of phenotypic female 46,XY siblings with Leydig cell hypoplasia a nonsense mutation was found in exon 11 of one allele of the *LH/CG-R* gene, introducing a premature termination codon that predicts truncation of the protein within the 5th transmembrane domain. Interestingly, the mutation was also present heterozygously in the phenotypically normal father and was absent in the mother. The affected siblings were therefore presumed to be compound heterozygotes, harboring a second undetected mutation on the other allele of the gene. In vitro studies of this mutant receptor revealed reduced cell surface expression of mutant receptor protein compared with the normal protein. In addition, hCG stimulation of cAMP production was impaired. In another family, three phenotypically female 46,XY siblings who had lack of breast development and primary amenorrhea, high serum LH, and absent Leydig cells on testicular histology, were found to be homozygous for a nonsense mutation that predicts protein termination in the third cytosolic loop of the receptor. Interestingly, their 46,XX sister, who had undergone menarche at 20 years of age, thereafter developing secondary amenorrhea, and who also had increased serum LH concentration, was homozygous for the same mutation. Another pair of affected siblings, born to consanguineous parents, were found to have a homozygous missense mutation resulting in an alanine to proline change at amino acid 593 in the 6th transmembrane domain of the receptor. In vitro studies revealed that although the receptor had normal affinity of binding for CG, the ligand-bound state did not induce cAMP production. The impaired cAMP production by Leydig cells harboring this mutant receptor explains the lack of hormonal action, since transduction of the hormonal signal requires cAMP-mediated events. The final patient whose mutation has been identified to date is a phenotypically male child with subnormal penile size, whose testes were normally descended. His serum LH was at the upper limit of normal for age during childhood. Analysis of genomic DNA revealed a missense mutation that converted the native serine to tyrosine at position 616 in the seventh transmembrane domain of the receptor. Surprisingly, in view of the normal masculinization of the affected child, in vitro studies of the mutant receptor revealed absent LH binding and cAMP production. This apparent paradox suggest either that testosterone secretion during the first trimester of gestation, when external genital morphogenesis occurs, is not LH or CG dependent, or that the in vitro finding of a nonfunctional LH/CG receptor does not reflect its activity in vivo. In contrast, penile growth during the third trimester is clearly dependent on function of the LH/CG receptor.

Defects of Testosterone Biosynthesis A defect in any of the enzymatic steps of testosterone biosynthesis can cause ambiguous genitalia because of insufficient testosterone production during male sexual differentiation. Depending on the location of the enzymatic defect in the steroidogenic pathway, these disorders may also affect glucocorticoid and mineralocorticoid biosynthesis by the adrenal gland (Fig. 57-7). Five defects of testosterone biosynthesis have been described; however, they are relatively uncommon causes of male pseudohermaphroditism. Because all of the genes encoding these enzymes are located on autosomes, these disorders are inherited as autosomal recessive traits. Table 57-4 summarizes molecular information regarding enzymes of steroidogenesis.

The molecular and biochemical heterogeneity within each defect and the consequent variability of the testosterone biosynthetic defect makes it impossible to distinguish these enzyme disorders on clinical grounds. Internal and external genital development is variable, covering the full gamut of features described above. Wolffian derivatives also may be normal or hypoplastic, depending on the severity of the testosterone deficit.

Congenital Lipoid Adrenal Hyperplasia: Steroidogenic Acute Regulatory Protein—StAR; P450 Side-Chain Cleavage Enzyme—P450$_{scc}$ The first and rate-limiting step in gonadal and adrenal steroidogenesis (Fig. 57-7) is the transfer of cholesterol from the outer mitochondrial membrane to the inner membrane, mediated by a recently discovered protein, steroidogenic acute regulatory protein (StAR). Thereafter, conversion of cholesterol to pregnenolone involves three distinct biochemical reactions: 20α-hydroxylation, 22-hydroxylation, and side-chain cleavage (the C20—C22 bond). These reactions are mediated by a mitochondrial mixed function oxidase, cytochrome P450$_{scc}$ (previously known as 20,22-desmolase), located on the inner mitochondrial membrane. A defect in the conversion of cholesterol to pregnenolone causes congenital lipoid adrenal hyperplasia (CLAH), the rarest and most severe form of congenital adrenal hyperplasia. In this condition, neither the gonads nor the adrenals have steroidogenic capability.

Clinical Features and Diagnosis. Infants with this disorder usually present in the first few weeks of life with hyponatremia, hyperkalemia, and metabolic acidosis reflecting severe salt-wasting adrenal insufficiency, often resulting in neonatal death. Affected 46,XY infants usually have completely female external genitalia although minimal masculinization has been reported. Other features are typical for a defect of androgen production, as described above. 46,XX infants have normal female internal and external genital development. Computed tomography or magnetic resonance imaging scan of the abdomen reveals very large, lipid-laden adrenal glands as a result of the accumulation of cholesterol and cholesterol esters. Interestingly, the testes contain normal Leydig cells without lipid accumulation. Serum concentrations of adrenocorticotropic hormone (ACTH) are markedly increased (causing increased skin pigmentation in some cases), as is plasma renin activity, whereas serum and urinary concentrations of all adrenal and gonadal steroids and their metabolites, even after ACTH or hCG stimulation, are profoundly low. Adrenal and gonadal tissues from these patients are unable to convert cholesterol to pregnenolone in vitro. The disease has been said to be extremely rare in European populations; however, this may result in part from failure of ascertainment and early neonatal death precluding the diagnosis in many cases. In contrast, it is thought to be the second most common form of adrenal hyperplasia in Japan and more than 50% of cases reported to date are of Japanese or Korean heritage. Unlike other forms of congenital adrenal hyperplasia (CAH), heterozyotes display normal steroid responses to ACTH stimulation, since the defect is caused by absence or dysfunction of the StAR protein and not to a steroidogenic enzyme deficiency.

Genetic and Molecular Pathophysiology. The cholesterol transport protein *StAR* is encoded by an 8-kb gene located at 8p11.2 that comprises seven exons and six introns and contains an 855-bp open reading frame. A related pseudogene maps to chromosome 13. *StAR* mRNA expression is stimulated by trophic hormones, such as LH and ACTH, via cyclic AMP-mediated events. In addition, the promoter of the *StAR* gene contains binding sites for SF-1 and the estrogen receptor, implicating these important transcription factors in regulation of *StAR* expression. *StAR* mRNA expression in the human is limited to the ovary, testis, adrenal cortex, and kidney. Interestingly, although the placenta is an abundantly steroidogenic tissue, *StAR* is not expressed there, nor in brain, reflecting the fact that these tissues do not exhibit acute regulation of steroidogenesis. *StAR* is not expressed in any nonsteroidogenic tissues. The StAR protein comprises 285 amino acids and contains a hydrophobic amino-terminal region typical of a mitochondrial targeting sequence. It is produced as a 37-kDa cytosolic precursor that is imported to the mitochondria, where it is processed to four mature 30-kDa forms. The acute response of steroidogenic cells to stimulation is the transport of cholesterol to the inner mitochondrial membrane and the cholesterol side-chain cleavage enzyme. The mechanism of action of StAR in this process is thought to involve formation of contact sites between the inner and outer mitochondrial membranes.

In three apparently unrelated Asian patients, homozygous mutations have been detected in the gene encoding StAR: perhaps because of a founder effect, two individuals (one Japanese, one Korean) had the same mutation converting the codon for glutamine at position 258 to a termination codon. The third subject had a similar nonsense mutation, converting arginine 193 to a termination codon. One further patient with CLAH was found to have a mutation that disturbed mRNA splicing, resulting in deletion of the 185 bp of sequence corresponding to exon 5 of the gene. The deleterious effect of these mutations is presumably caused by absence of a functional protein and subsequent cellular damage because of the accumulation of cholesterol esters.

P450 Side-Chain Cleavage Enzyme—P450$_{scc}$ The first enzyme of steroidogenesis, P450$_{scc}$, is encoded by the 20-kb *CYP11A* gene localized to the q23–q24 region of chromosome 15. The gene is expressed in steroidogenic tissues, such as adrenal cortex, ovarian granulosa cells, testicular Leydig cells, and placenta. Expression of the P450$_{scc}$ gene is enhanced by ACTH, gonadotropins, cAMP, and SF-1, which may be acting via other factors. Expression patterns are tissue-specific and involve the use of alternate promoter sequences. The P450$_{scc}$ protein complex is located on the inner mitochondrial membrane. Electrons are transferred from NADPH to adrenodoxin reductase, a membrane-bound flavoprotein, then to adrenodoxin, a soluble iron-sulfur protein,

---

Figure 57-7 *(continued on next page)* Pathway of steroid biosynthesis and defects in steroidogenesis. The first step in steroidogenesis is the transport of cholesterol across the mitochondrial membrane, mediated by the transport protein StAR. The remaining steps in adrenal and gonadal steroidogenesis are accomplished by a number of enzymes. Most are of the P450 cytochrome family. However, 3β-hydroxysteroid dehydrogenase and 17β-hydroxysteroid dehydrogenase are of the short-chain alcohol dehydrogenase family.

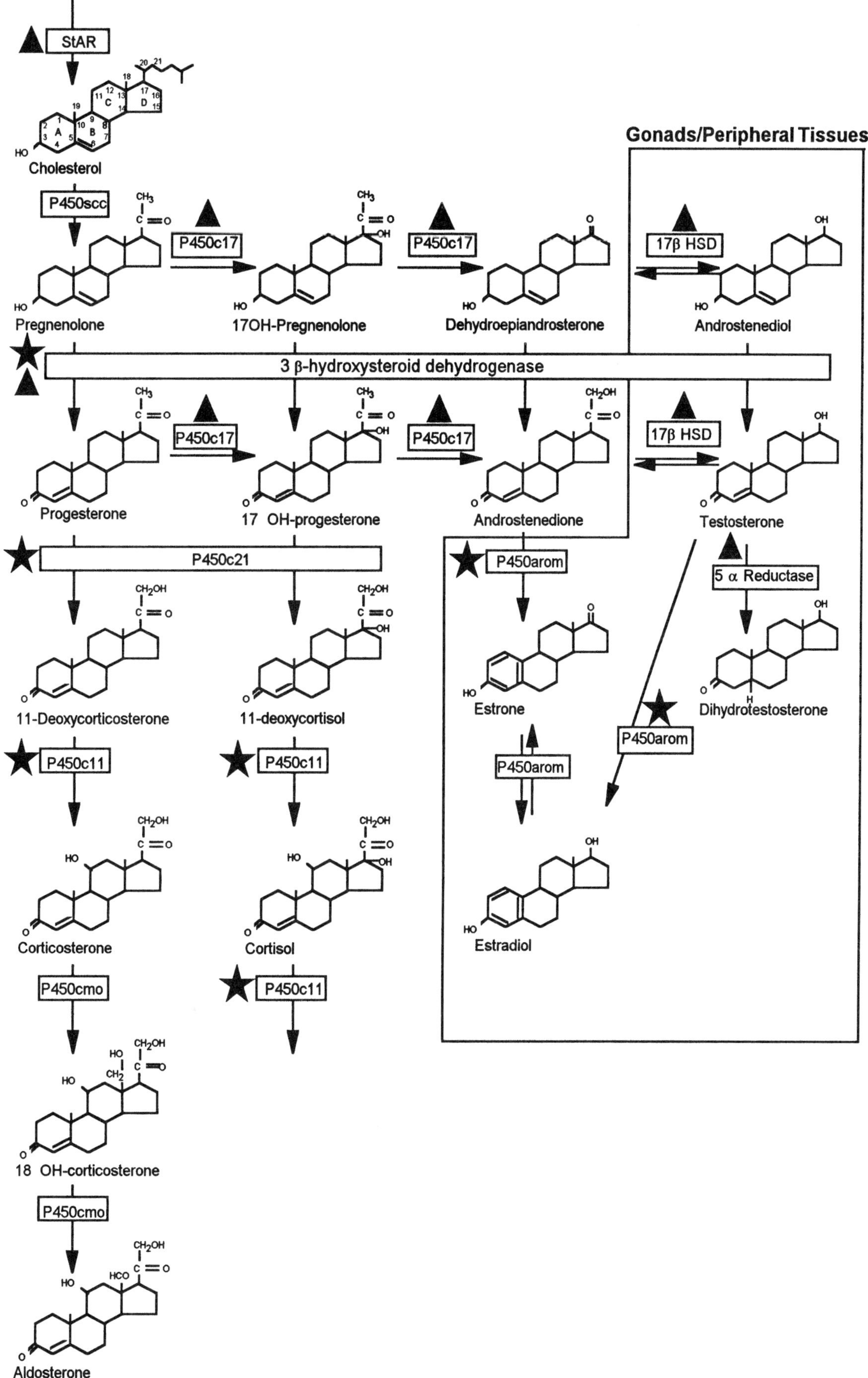

Fig. 57-7 *(continued)*. Molecular defects that cause male pseudohermaphroditism are designated by triangles. Defects that cause female pseudohermaphroditism are designated with stars. 3β-Hydroxysteroid dehydrogenase deficiency can cause either male or female pseudohermaphroditism.

Table 57-4
Enzymes Involved in Steroidogenesis, Their Encoding Genes, and Chromosomal Loci

Gene name	*Locus*	*Enzyme name*	*Enzyme type/location*	*Tissue*	*Action*	*Cofactors*
CYP11A	15q23–24	P450scc	Cytochrome P450 mixed function oxidase Mitochondria	Adrenals, gonads	20α-Hydroxylation 22α-Hydroxylation 20–22 Side-chain cleavage	NADPH Adrenodoxin Adrenodoxin Reductase
HSD3B2	1p13–11	3βHSD	Dehydrogenase Membrane bound	Adrenals, gonads	Conversion of 3β-hydroxy-Δ^5-steroids to 3-keto-Δ^4-steroids	NAD^+
CYP21	6p21.3	P450C21	Ctyochrome P450 Mitochondria	Adrenals, gonads	21-Hydroxylation	NADPH
CYP11B1	8q22	P450C11	Cytochrome P450	Fascic, glomerulosa	11-Hydroxylation	NADPH
CYP11B2	8q22	P450cmo	Ctyochrome P450	Glomerulosa only	11 Hydroxylation, 18-Hydroxylation 18-Oxidation	
CYP17	10q24.3	P45017α	Cytochrome P450 Endoplasmic reticulum	Adrenals, gonads	17α-Hydroxylation 17-20 Side-chain cleavage (lyase)	NADPH
HSD17 (EDH17B1)	17q12–21	17βHSD	Dehydrogenase isozoymes	Gonads, placenta, other tissues	Interconversion androstenedione/ testosterone; esterone/estradiol	NADPH
HSD17B2 (EDH17B2)	16q24.1–24.2	17βHSD2	Membrane bound			
HSD17B3 (EDH17B2)	9q22	17βHSD3				
CYP19	15q21.1	P450arom	Cytochrome P450 Endoplasmic reticulum	Gonads, placenta	Conversion C19–C18 steroids	NADPH Reductase
SRD5A1	5p15	5α-reductase 1		Liver, skin	Reduction C19 and C21 steroids	NADPH
SDR5A2	2p23	5α-reductase 2	Microsomes	Liver, external genitalia		

and finally to the enzyme $P450_{scc}$ itself. No molecular defects in *CYP11A* have been found to date, despite extensive molecular studies; limited studies of adrenodoxin and adrenodoxin reductase mRNAs have also been normal in individuals with CLAH.

3β-Hydroxysteroid Dehydrogenase Deficiency The 3β-hydroxysteroid dehydrogenase/Δ^5–Δ^4 isomerases (3β-HSD1 and 3β-HSD2) are two highly homologous noncytochrome, membrane-bound short chain alcohol dehydrogenases that require NAD^+ as a cofactor. Both have two separate enzymatic activities: dehydrogenase activity and isomerase activity (conversion of Δ^5-steroids to Δ^4-steroids), the net result of which is the conversion of 3β-hydroxy-Δ^5-steroids (pregnenolone, 17-hydroxypregnenolone, and dehydroepiandrosterone) to the 3-keto-Δ^4-steroids (progesterone, 17-hydroxyprogesterone, and Δ^4-androstenedione, respectively). This is an essential step in the biosynthesis of all classes of steroid hormones; deficiency of 3β-HSD activity in steroidogenic tissues impairs both adrenal and gonadal (testicular and ovarian) steroidogenesis and is reported to be the second most common cause of congenital adrenal hyperplasia.

Clinical Features and Diagnosis. Affected 46,XY individuals have variable impairment of internal and external genital masculinization resulting from inadequate fetal testosterone biosynthesis because of defective function of the testicular isozyme, 3β-HSD2. In some cases there is also salt wasting adrenal insufficiency as a result of reduced synthesis of aldosterone and cortisol. Less severe "late-onset" forms of 3β-HSD present with more complete masculinization and without salt-wasting, reflecting genetic heterogeneity within this disorder. Because of lack of estrogen production, there is no breast enlargement at puberty, either in 46,XX or 46,XY individuals. The classic hormonal profile is a markedly increased concentration of the Δ^5-steroids (pregnenolone, 17-hydroxypregnenolone, and dehydroepiadrosterone) and their metabolites in the serum and urine. However, somewhat confusingly, Δ^4-steroids may also be increased, because of peripheral conversion of Δ^5-steroids to Δ^4-steroids resulting from 3β-HSD1 activity in peripheral tissues. Nevertheless, despite peripheral conversion, the ratio of Δ^5- to Δ^4-steroids and their metabolites is generally elevated. The peripheral Δ^5- to Δ^4- steroid conversion explains the paradoxical finding of ambiguous genitalia in conjunction with apparently normal Δ^4-steroid levels in some of these patients. Although Δ^4- steroid concentrations may be normal peripherally, it is probable that they were inadequate at the tissue level in the developing genitalia, and that specific activity of the testicular isoform, 3β-HSD2, is required to generate adequately high androgen levels during embryogenesis.

Genetic and Molecular Pathophysiology. There are two highly homologous human genes encoding isoenzymes responsible for 3β-HSD activity—*HSD3B1* and *HSD3B2*, encoding 3β-HSD1 and 3β-HSD2, respectively. The genes are approximately 7–8 kb in size and contain 4 exons and 3 introns. There is evidence for tight linkage between these genes, which are both located within band p13.1 on chromosome 1. Three pseudogenes containing stop codons or deletions have also been identified. The *HSD3B1* gene is the predominant form expressed in nonsteroidogenic tissues, such as liver and kidney, and encodes a 371-amino acid (42-kDa) protein. No mutations have yet been detected in the type I gene in individuals with 3β-HSD deficiency. The type II isoform of 3β-HSD has the same enzymatic activities but is expressed almost exclusively in the steroidogenic cells of the adrenals and gonads. In bovine adrenocortical cells the enzyme colocalizes with $P450_{scc}$ at the inner mitochondrial membrane, suggesting a possible functional association between the two enzymes in regulation of steroidogenesis. Studies in cultured human adrenal cells reveal regulation of 3β-HSD mRNA and protein levels by ACTH and angiotensin II. In Leydig cells there is some evidence from rodent studies that 3β-HSD activity is regulated by LH/CG.

More than 20 different mutations have been reported in the *HSD3B2* genes of individuals with 3β-HSD deficiency, including 14 different single-base mutations in one study. Other mutations include a single-base insertion resulting in a frameshift, an intronic mutation causing aberrant splicing, and single-base mutations causing either premature termination (nonsense mutations) or amino acid substitutions (missense mutations). Gene conversion events (transfer of deleterious mutations from associated pseudogenes) have been suggested to underlie some of the mutations in *HSD3B2*. In vitro studies using site-directed mutagenesis to recreate a number of mutant 3β-HSDs, reveal significantly reduced enzyme affinity and specific activity for the substrates pregnenolone and dehydroepiandrosterone, and in some cases for the enzyme cofactor NAD^+. The finding of a specific abnormality of NAD^+ binding associated with substitution of aspartic acid for glycine at position 15 raises the speculation that this region may contribute to the NAD-binding domain of the enzyme.

Although absence of salt losing in some patients with severe undermasculinization suggests that impairment of enzyme activity may differ between gonads and adrenals, molecular data indicate that the enzyme is similarly dysfunctional for either of its two main substrates, pregnenolone (adrenal) and dehydroepiandrosterone (gonad). These data suggest that the absence of salt wasting in some individuals results from weak residual enzyme activity sufficient to prevent salt loss, but insufficient to produce the testosterone levels required for male sex differentiation. The clinical heterogeneity of affected individuals (i.e., salt losing vs non–salt losing, varying degrees of masculinization) is at least in part explained by the genetic heterogeneity. Not surprisingly, mutations that completely destroy enzyme activity are associated with a more severe syndrome than are those that allow retention of some enzyme function. In general patients with non–salt wasting disease have up to 10% retained enzyme activity; however, there is no clear correlation between the molecular defect, enzyme activity, and clinical phenotype. The gene is located on an autosome and affected individuals are generally homozygous for the mutant allele; consanguinity has been reported in a number of pedigrees. Compound heterozygosity for two different mutations has been reported in a number of classically affected patients, and minor manifestations of simple heterozygosity have been described, including mild overproduction of Δ^5-steroids and mild ovarian dysfunction.

17α-Hydroxylase Deficiency and 17,20-Lyase Deficiency A single microsomal enzyme, cytochrome P450c17, catalyzes two consecutive oxidation reactions, the 17α-hydroxylase and 17,20-lyase (17,20-desmolase) reactions of adrenal and gonadal steroidogenesis. The 17α-hydroxylase reaction converts pregnenolone to 17-hydroxypregnenolone and progesterone to 17-hydroxyprogesterone, respectively (Fig. 57-7). This reaction is the rate-limiting step in androgen biosynthesis. The 17,20-lyase reaction cleaves the C17,20 bond to convert the C21 steroid 17-hydroxypregnenolone to the C19 steroid dehydroepiandrosterone (DHEA) and likely also catalyzes the equivalent conversion of 17OH-progesterone to Δ^4-androstenedione, although this latter is somewhat controversial, with discrepant findings in various studies. DHEA and androstenedione are the major precursors of testosterone and estradiol.

Clinical Features and Diagnosis. 17α-Hydroxylase is required for cortisol, androgen, and estrogen synthesis and the enzyme is expressed in adrenal cortex and gonads. 17α-Hydroxylase deficiency may be characterized by deficiency of either or both of this enzyme's activities; however, the molecular basis for this differential expression of the defect is at present unclear. Because of fetal androgen deficiency, 46,XY individuals with 17α-hydroxylase deficiency in the adrenals and gonads have female external genitalia, although a few individuals with limited masculinization have been described. In 46,XX individuals the external genitalia are normal; however, there is failure of development of secondary sexual characteristics at puberty (breast development, pubic and axillary hair) because of deficiency of both adrenal androgens and ovarian estrogen (*see* Chapter 37).

Deficiency of 17α-hydroxylase activity also impairs adrenal cortisol production, and the resultant compensatory ACTH hypersecretion stimulates synthesis of progesterone, deoxycorticosterone (DOC), corticosterone, and 18-hydroxycorticosterone. The excess of the latter three compounds causes salt and water retention, hypertension, and hypokalemia because of their mineralocorticoid activity. Renin activity is therefore suppressed and aldosterone production reduced. Despite impaired cortisol production, evidence of glucocorticoid deficiency is unusual, perhaps because corticosterone has weak glucocorticoid activity.

In addition to catalyzing the 17α-hydroxylation reaction in the adrenals and gonads, $P450_{17\alpha}$ also catalyzes the 17,20-lyase reaction resulting in conversion of 17-hydroxypregnenolone to DHEA, and probably 17-hydroxyprogesterone to androstenedione (Fig. 57-7). Thus, deficiency of the lyase activity in the gonads prohibits synthesis of DHEA, Δ^4-androstenedione, testosterone, and estrogen. Glucocorticoid and mineralocorticoid production are retained because the enzymatic defect is distal to these pathways. hCG stimulation produces an increased ratio of 17-hydroxy-C21-steroids (17-hydroxyprogesterone and 17-hydroxypregnenolone) to C19-steroids (DHEA and Δ^4-androstenedione).

Genetic and Molecular Pathophysiology. CYP17 is a single 6.6-kb, 8 exon, 7 intron gene located on chromosome 10 at band q24.3. The *CYP17* gene is very similar to *CYP21* (encoding the 21-hydroxylase enzyme), and the two may have originated from a common ancestral gene. $P450_{17\alpha}$ is expressed in human adrenal, testis, and ovarian theca cells, but not in ovarian granulosa cells or placenta. $P450_{17\alpha}$ mRNA is upregulated by ACTH via cAMP, and cAMP regulatory regions have been identified in the 5'-flanking region of the bovine $P450_{17\alpha}$ gene; expression is also regulated by the inhibin-activin system in the ovary. Gene transcription is inhibited by activators of protein kinase C. The *CYP17* gene encodes cytochrome $P450_{17\alpha}$ a 508-amino acid, 57-kDa protein that is part of the $P450_{17\alpha}$ complex anchored to the smooth endoplasmic reticulum of steroidogenic cells. The complex includes a 78-kDa flavoprotein reductase termed P450 reductase, containing binding domains for nicotinamide adenine dinucleotide phosphate (NADPH), flavin mononucleotide (FMN), and flavin adenine dinucleotide (FAD); and the cytochrome $P450_{17\alpha}$ enzyme itself, which contains heme-binding and steroid-binding regions, accepts electrons from NADPH via the P450 reductase, and catalyzes the overall oxidation reaction. The ratio of 17α-hydroxylase to 17,20-lyase activity differs between adrenal and testis and is developmentally regulated at adrenarche, an increase in the ratio of lyase to hydroxylase activity occurring at this time. Site-directed mutagenesis has elucidated specific amino acid residues critical for either the 17α-hydroxylase or the 17,20-lyase activity; however, the basis for the time- and tissue-specific differential regulation of the enzyme's two main activities is not yet fully understood. There is evidence that serine phosphorylation of the enzyme increases lyase activity, whereas dephosphorylation eliminates this activity. Other regulatory features may include variation in the ratio of the NADPH P450 reductase to the $P450_{17\alpha}$ enzyme itself, resulting in alterations of electron transfer to the enzyme. The presence of specific endoplasmic reticulum membrane lipids in certain cell types has also been suggested as a factor involved in the differential activity of this enzyme's functions.

A variety of molecular defects has been described in the $P450_{17\alpha}$ genes of at least 15 individuals with 17α-hydroxylase deficiency. These include large deletions or insertions, small deletions and duplications, and single-base mutations causing frameshifts, premature termination, or amino acid substitutions. In vitro studies of a recreated mutant $P450_{17\alpha}$, in which histidine at position 373 was replaced by leucine, revealed that the mutant enzyme failed to bind the heme moiety critical for catalytic activity. Other mutations, however, are located distant from the critical heme-binding region or the active site, suggesting that the enzyme is sensitive to structural change. Interestingly, one specific mutation, a 4-base duplication that alters the reading frame of the *CYP17* gene, was found in six Dutch families and two families of Canadian Mennonites, suggesting that a founder mutation had presumably occurred in the Dutch antecedents of the Mennonites. Compound heterozygosity has been reported in this form of congenital adrenal hyperplasia, as well as in the more common forms. Individuals heterozygous for a single 17α-hydroxylase mutation are clinically normal; however, ACTH stimulation produces increased serum concentrations of DOC, corticosterone, and 18-hydroxycorticosterone.

A number of cases of 17,20-lyase deficiency have been reported in which 17α-hydroxylase activity was said to have been normal. Theoretically, different mutations in the $P450_{17\alpha}$ gene could result in either 17α-hydroxylase deficiency, 17,20 lyase deficiency, or both. However, in vitro protein expression of mutant genes of individuals with the clinical diagnosis of isolated 17α-hydroxylase deficiency has revealed the presence of combined enzyme deficiencies in all cases studied thus far and there is no clear molecular explanation for the apparently retained 17α-hydroxylase activity in vivo. In vitro analysis of mutant $P450_{17\alpha}$ enzymes predicted from the mutations detected in one compound heterozygote 46,XY patient with ambiguous genitalia reveals that retention of 20% of normal 17,20-lyase activity is adequate for some degree of masculinization.

17β-Hydroxysteroid Dehydrogenase 3 Deficiency The 17β-hydroxysteroid dehydrogenases (17β-HSDs, also known as 17β-ketosteroid reductases and as estradiol 17β-dehydrogenases) are NAD^+/NADPH-dependent, membrane-bound enzymes not of the cytochrome P450 type, which catalyze the only reversible steps in the steroid biosynthetic pathway: interconversion of Δ^4-androstenedione⇔testosterone, DHEA⇔Δ^5-androstenediol and estrone⇔estradiol) (Fig. 57-7) by oxidation or reduction of C-18 and C-19 steroids. There are at least three or four tissue-specific isozymes with differing specificity for either the oxidative or the reductive reaction. The isozymes are encoded by at least three distinct genes. 17β-HSD3 is the testicular isozyme, responsible for the final step in testosterone synthesis, reduction of androstenedione to testosterone. Deficiency of this enzyme is the most common defect of androgen production.

Clinical Features and Diagnosis. Interestingly, although 46,XY individuals with deficiency of testicular 17β-HSD3 activity have female or mildly masculinized external genitalia, their internal genitalia are well-masculinized, with normally formed epididymis, vas deferens, and seminal vesicles. Reduced activity of testicular 17β-HSD3 is inferred by the finding of elevated ratios of androstenedione to testosterone and estrone to estradiol in spermatic venous samples. In addition, testicular tissues of affected individuals demonstrate impaired conversion of labeled Δ^4-androstenedione to testosterone in vitro. This defect is isolated to the gonads—the site of expression of 17β-HSD3. Other tissues have normal 17β-HSD activity because of normal function of the type 1 and 2 isozymes. The relatively normal masculinization of internal structures may result from activity of 17β-HSD isozymes other than 17β-HSD3 in the proximity of the Wolffian ducts producing adequate local testosterone by conversion of testis-derived androstendione. In contrast there is insufficient testosterone at the level of the external genital primordia to act as substrate for 5α-reductase conversion to dihydrotestosterone.

A striking feature of this disorder is the marked virilization that occurs at puberty. Affected 46,XY individuals develop a male body habitus with abundant body and facial hair, enlargement of the penis and testes to normal adult size, and pigmentation and rugation of the labioscrotal folds. Gynecomastia is variably present. Many affected individuals spontaneously adopt the male gender role, with apparently adequate sexual function, but with infertility. These clinical observations correlate with normalization of peripheral and spermatic vein testosterone levels. Part of this effect appears likely to be related to increased LH secretion and Leydig cell hyperplasia, because Δ^4-androstenedione levels remain markedly elevated, indicating persistent enzyme dysfunction. Peripheral testosterone production as a result of retained extragonadal 17β-HSD activity may also contribute. The phenotype and clinical course of individuals with 17β-HSD deficiency is similar to that of individuals with 5α-reductase deficiency (described below).

The diagnosis of 17β-HSD3 deficiency is suggested by a 10- to 15-fold elevation of the ratios of Δ^4-androstenedione to testosterone and of estrone to estradiol in the perinatal period, after hCG stimulation in childhood, or after puberty. Because of a secondary increase in 3β-HSD activity, DHEA may be normal or only mildly elevated. Glucocorticoid and mineralocorticoid synthesis remain normal because the enzymatic defect is distal to these pathways.

Genetic and Molecular Pathophysiology. There are at least four HSD17B enzymes encoded by separate genes and expressed in a tissue-specific fashion, some being expressed predominantly in estrogenic or androgenic tissues and others more widely. The nomenclature of this group of genes and enzymes is quite daunting: the type 1 enzyme, 17β-HSD I, is also known as estradiol-17β dehydrogenase II. This isozyme is encoded by a gene located at 17q11–12, referred to as *HSD17B1* or *EDH17B2*. This locus in fact contains two genes in tandem: *h17b-HSDI* and *II*. The active gene is *h17b-HSDII*; *h17b-HSDI* is a pseudogene, also referred to as *EDH17BP1*, which is 89% homologous to the active gene. 17b-HSD I appears to be the isozyme responsible for ovarian 17β-HSD activity. The type 2 isoform, 17β-HSDII, is encoded by *HSD17B2*, located at 16q24. This isozyme, which is a 387-amino acid, approximately 43-kDa progestin-regulated protein, is responsible for 17β-HSD activity in placenta and endometrium. Located predominantly in the endometrium, placenta, liver, and small intestine, this isozyme has a preference for NAD^+ as its cofactor in oxidation of estradiol and testosterone to estrone and androstenedione, respectively. The testicular isoform, 17β-HSD3 (III), which is the isozyme implicated in male pseudohermaphroditism as a result of 17β-HSD deficiency, is encoded by *HSD17B3 (EDH17B3)*, which shares 23% sequence homology with the *HSD17B1* and *2* genes. The gene spans 60 kb, contains 11 exons, and is located at 9q22. This isozyme preferentially uses NADPH as its cofactor in the reduction of androstendione to testosterone. In addition to being found in ovary, testis, and placenta, significant levels of various 17β-HSD mRNAs are found in peripheral sites, such as uterus, breast, prostate, and adipose tissue. In these peripheral locations 17β-HSD may play a major role in regulating the levels of active androgens and estrogens, by using either their oxidative or reductive functions. The 17β-HSDs are not expressed in the adrenals.

Mutations have been identified in the *HSD17B3* genes of approximately 20 individuals with 17β-HSD deficiency. These include single-base mutations causing amino acid substitutions, frameshift mutations, and splice junction mutations causing abnormal mRNA splicing and thereby disturbed protein structure and enzyme function. One 46,XY phenotypic female was found to have compound heterozygosity for two distinct amino acid substitutions and another had compound heterozygosity for a splice acceptor mutation and a missense mutation. When expressed in cultured mammalian cells in vitro the mutant enzymes displayed impaired enzyme activity. The unusual finding of normal Wolffian structures in these 46,XY phenotypic females is potentially explained by activity of 17β-HSD isozymes other than 17β-HSD3 converting testis-derived androstenedione to testosterone in the local area of the internal genital structures. Mutations have not been reported in the *HSD17B1* or *HSD17B2* genes to date. 17β-HSD deficiency is inherited in an autosomal recessive fashion and a number of extensive inbred Arab kindreds with numerous affected individuals have been reported.

Disorders of Androgen Action 5α-REDUCTASE DEFICIENCY The 5α-reductases are microsomal enzymes that catalyze the 5α-reduction of many C19 and C21 steroids, using NADPH as a cofactor. In the context of disorders of sexual differentiation, the most critical of these reactions is the conversion of testosterone to DHT, mediated by the isozyme 5α-reductase 2 (II). Deficiency of this enzyme results in a form of male pseudohermaphroditism previously referred to as pseudovaginal perineoscrotal hypospadias. This disorder is described in greater detail in Chapter 60.

Clinical Features and Diagnosis. Deficiency of 5α-reductase 2 in the tissues of the bipotential fetal external genitalia and urogenital sinus results in inadequate local DHT concentrations. As in other forms of defective androgen production or action, there is subnormal masculinization of these structures, generally presenting as ambiguous external genitalia. The genital phenotype varies widely between and even within affected kindreds, the most consistent findings being underdevelopment of the penis and prostate. It is on the basis of these clinical findings that the requirement for DHT in external genital masculinization has been inferred. Because differentiation of the gonads and Wolffian ducts is not dependent on DHT, the testes, epididymides, vasa deferentia, and seminal vesicles develop normally.

One of the most intriguing and well-documented features of this disorder is the striking virilization, including increased muscularity and deepening of the voice, that occurs at puberty in many affected individuals. In addition, the testes often enlarge and descend; however, spermatogenesis is absent or severely impaired. Whether this virilization is mediated by improved DHT levels or by supranormal T levels remains unclear. Acne, facial hair, temporal hair recession, and prostatic enlargement do not develop, presumably because these events require higher concentrations of DHT. In contrast to patients with androgen insensitivity syndromes, described below, gynecomastia does not develop because there is no increase in testicular estrogen production. Many affected individuals initially raised as females change their gender role to male around the time of puberty, for reasons that have not been fully elucidated, but likely include cultural as well as biologic factors.

Reduced conversion of T to DHT in the target tissues results in the marked increase in the ratio of T to DHT diagnostic of 5α-reductase 2 deficiency. In normal infants (2 weeks to 6 months of age), the hCG-stimulated T:DHT ratio is approximately 5 ± 2 (mean ±SD). Affected infants have markedly increased T:DHT ratios, in the 20–60 range or higher. Serum concentrations of LH may be mildly increased. 5α-Reductase 2 deficiency can be differentiated from 17β-HSD deficiency by the characteristic increase of serum androstenedione in the latter condition. A more direct, but more invasive diagnostic method is the in vitro demonstration of decreased 5α-reductase activity in genital skin fibroblasts; however, because post-hCG serum T:DHT concentrations are diagnostic, this procedure is not required to verify the diagnosis.

Genetic and Molecular Pathophysiology. There are two isozymes of 5α-reductase encoded by separate genes. 5α-Reductase 1 is encoded by the *SRD5A1* gene located at 5p15, and 5α-reductase 2, the enzyme defective in the clinical syndrome of 5α-reductase deficiency, is encoded by the *SRD5A2* gene located at 2p23. The genes are structurally similar, with five coding exons and four introns each. The two enzymes share approximately 50% amino acid identity. Androgen binding is mediated by the ends of the enzyme molecule and binding of NADPH, required as the cofactor for the reduction reaction, by the carboxy-terminal half. The 5α-reductase isozymes have differential expression patterns. The type 1 isozyme is not detectable in the fetus, but is transiently expressed in newborn skin and scalp, and permanently expressed in the liver, and in skin after puberty. The type 2 isozyme is expressed in the liver and in androgen target tissues, including the external genitalia, accessory sex organs, and prostate. The ontogeny of 5α-reductase 2 expression is incompletely characterized; however, the enzyme is not expressed in the Wolffian ducts at the time of their differentiation, a finding that supports the contention that T rather than DHT is the critical androgen involved in this process. Its expression is upregulated by androgens, as demonstrated by the marked increase in 5α-reductase 2 mRNA level in the prostate of castrate animals after testosterone administration. Expression appears to be regulated in the opposite fashion in the liver. Interestingly, 5α-reductase activity has also been detected in neurons.

5α-Reductase 2 deficiency is inherited in an autosomal recessive fashion, and there is a high frequency of consanguinity within affected kindreds. A wide variety of mutations has been identified in affected families from more than 20 different ethnic groups. Mutations range from complete deletion of the *SRD5A2* gene in a Papua New Guinea kindred, to single-base mutations distributed throughout the *SRD5A2* gene that result in gene-splicing defects, amino acid substitutions, or premature termination. A number of affected kindreds demonstrate compound heterozygosity for different mutations. In vitro expression of mutant proteins reveals a variety of causes of deficient enzyme activity: deletions, premature termination codons, and splice junction defects prevent expression of a functional enzyme; whereas amino acid substitutions impair binding of testosterone or produce an unstable enzyme. Alterations in both androgen and NADPH binding may be produced by such mutations. Differences in enzyme stability and affinity for testosterone and NADPH between kindreds reflect the genetic heterogeneity of the enzyme defect. There is no abnormality of the isozyme 5α-reductase 1 in individuals with the clinical syndrome of 5α-reductase deficiency, a fact that may in part explain the marked pubertal virilization of affected individuals.

Androgen Insensitivity Syndromes (Androgen Receptor Disorders) The androgen receptor (AR) is a nuclear transcription factor that is activated by binding of androgen to a conformation capable of binding to elements in the promoter regions of androgen regulated genes to regulate their transcription. Defective function of this transcription factor results in resistance to the effects of androgens—the well-characterized androgen insensitivity (or resistance) syndromes. These conditions are described in greater detail in Chapter 60.

Clinical Features and Diagnosis. The syndromes of androgen insensitivity (AIS), referred to by some authors as testicular feminization, are believed to comprise the most common definable cause of male pseudohermaphroditism. Affected individuals display variable degrees of defective masculinization. In the complete form of AIS not only is the genital phenotype unequivocally female, the labia minora and majora and clitoris in fact may be underdeveloped. Individuals with partial forms of AIS, who have some retained AR activity, have external genital phenotypes ranging from female with pubic hair at puberty, to almost completely masculinized. The complete form of AIS has a prevalence of approximately 1:20,000 male births. The prevalence of the partial forms of AIS is unknown.

Diagnosis of AIS in infancy currently relies on clinical features, because there have been no definitive hormonal studies in infants. Preliminary data in a few infants with complete AIS (CAIS) suggest absence of the typical postnatal LH and T surge seen at around 6–12 weeks of age in normal male infants. Diagnosis of CAIS is generally based on the classic clinical findings of 46,XY karyotype, testes, and absent uterus in an otherwise normal phenotypic female. The only condition with which complete AIS could be confused in infancy is Leydig cell hypoplasia (described above). However, the brisk T response to hCG in patients with CAIS should clearly differentiate these two conditions.

Diagnosis of partial forms of AIS in infancy is notoriously difficult, because there is no clear hormonal profile; however, a few case reports have noted increased concentrations of LH and T. Lack of suppression of sex hormone-binding globulin after androgen administration may aid in the diagnosis of these conditions; however, such studies have been undertaken in only a limited number of cases to date. The diagnosis of AIS should be suspected in a 46,XY infant with female or ambiguous genitalia if either the baseline or the hCG-stimulated concentrations of T and DHT are normal or exaggerated without disproportionate excess of T precursors. Demonstration of abnormal androgen binding in cultured genital skin fibroblasts or identification of a mutation in the AR gene of an affected individual confirms the diagnosis, but is impractical outside of research institutions. Furthermore, measured receptor levels and androgen binding affinity often correlate poorly with the degree of masculinization. Depending on the severity of the androgen resistance, varying degrees of virilization and/or feminization occur at puberty. At and beyond puberty, LH, T, and DHT increase to supranormal levels and serum estrogen concentrations are also enhanced, because of testicular estrogen secretion (driven by LH) and peripheral aromatization of T.

Genetic and Molecular Pathophysiology. The approximately 90-kb gene encoding the AR contains eight coding exons and seven introns and is localized to the q11–12 region of the human X chromosome. AIS is thus inherited in an X-linked fashion. The AR is expressed in a wide array of genital and nongenital tissues, reflecting its role as a fairly ubiquitous transcription factor. The *AR* gene encodes a 110-kDa protein that is a member of the steroid receptor superfamily, comprising of three major functional domains: amino-terminal (transcription-regulating), central DNA-binding (zinc finger), and carboxy-terminal steroid-binding. After binding androgen, the AR, as a homodimer, interacts with androgen response element (ARE) DNA sequences in the promoter regions of target genes to regulate their transcription.

Molecular analysis of the *AR* genes of more than 100 hundred unrelated individuals with various forms of AIS has revealed a highly heterogeneous genetic basis for the spectrum of clinical disorders. Defects include rare complete and partial gene deletions, insertions and deletions of a few basepairs, and single-base mutations that disrupt splice junctions, introduce premature termination codons, or cause amino acid substitutions. Complete and subtotal deletions of the *AR* gene, as well as frameshift and nonsense mutations, result in absence of a functional AR protein. In contrast, missense mutations resulting in amino acid substitutions, of which at least 150 have now been described, allow production of a structurally normal protein. The majority of missense mutations (approximately 80%) are located in the five exons encoding the steroid-binding domain, with almost all of the remainder occurring in the two exons encoding the DNA-binding domain. The function of many mutant receptors has been analyzed in vitro: when the mutation affects the steroid-binding domain androgen binding may be absent, reduced (affinity or capacity or both), or qualitatively abnormal (thermolability of binding, increased ligand dissociation, or altered binding specificity). Mutations located within the zinc finger DNA-binding domain are generally associated with normal (occasionally increased) androgen binding; however, there is altered affinity, capacity, or specificity of receptor binding to appropriate DNA sequences. In vitro studies indicate that the underlying abnormality of defective ARs, whether the mutation affects DNA or androgen binding, is loss of transcriptional competence of the mutant receptor—reduced ability to regulate transcription of androgen-dependent target genes.

Disorders of Anti-Müllerian Hormone Production or Action—The Persistent Müllerian Duct Syndrome—Types I and II DISORDERS OF ANTI-MÜLLERIAN HORMONE PRODUCTION Anti-Müllerian hormone ([AMH] or Müllerian inhibiting substance [MIS]) is a glycoprotein product of testicular Sertoli cells that mediates regression of the Müllerian duct structures during normal male embryogenesis. Deficiency of this hormone or abnormality of its receptor results in persistence of the Müllerian ducts, resulting in the mildest form of male pseudohermaphroditism.

Clinical Features and Diagnosis. Karyotypic males with deficiency of AMH have normal male external genitalia, normal testicular histology, and normal Wolffian duct differentiation. The two specific defects found in these individuals are persistence of the Müllerian ducts, and abnormalities of testicular descent (the persistent Müllerian duct syndrome—PMDS). The typical case is that of a phenotypically normal male infant with bilateral cryptorchidism (normal testicular histology) and inguinal hernias, who is found, at the time of hernia repair, to have a uterus, cervix, and fallopian tubes in the inguinal canal. Serum concentrations of AMH, which is readily measurable in the serum of normal males until puberty, are reduced in most affected individuals with PMDS, referred to as type I. In some, AMH concentrations are normal, suggesting either bioinactivity of the hormone (not yet reported), or an AMH receptor defect (discussed below), referred to as PMDS type II. A recent study determined that mutations of AMH and AMHR each account for approximately 50% of cases of PMDS.

Genetic and Molecular Pathophysiology. The human gene encoding AMH contains five exons and is located on chromosome 19, at position p13.3–13.2. Persistent Müllerian duct syndrome is therefore inherited in an autosomal recessive, male-limited, pattern. After *SRY*, *AMH* is the first molecular marker specific for testis differentiation. Its expression in developing mouse testis begins significantly later than that of *SRY*, at about day 13.5. In fact, *SRY* may regulate *AMH* production in males, because the *AMH* gene contains a regulatory element within its promoter that likely binds SRY. Notably however, the 48-h temporal dissociation between the expression of these two proteins suggests involvement of one or more intermediate factors. *AMH* expression is also regulated by SF-1, which binds to the *AMH* gene promoter, likely using a cofactor for optimal gene regulation. After puberty, AMH production is downregulated by androgens (a feature absent in individuals with AIS). *AMH* is not expressed prenatally in the ovary. However low amounts of AMH are released into the follicular fluid by mature granulosa cells in normal postpubertal females, who do not express SRY.

AMH, a member of the TGF-β family of growth factors, is a 560-amino acid, approximately 70-kDa glycoprotein that forms a 140-kDa homodimer. AMH is produced by Sertoli cells not only during the critical period, when it induces regression of the Müllerian ducts (weeks 9–11 of human gestation), but also in late gestation, after birth, and even in adulthood (at a reduced level), suggesting that AMH may have physiologic roles other than its control of Müllerian duct regression. In its role as the inducer of Müllerian duct regression in males during embryogenesis, AMH acts in a paracrine fashion, mediating only the regression of the ipsilateral Müllerian duct. Given the fact that the testes are invariably undescended in PMDS, one postulated role for AMH in the latter part of gestation is in the regulation of testicular descent. However, this speculation is tempered by the finding of variable AMH levels in boys with simple cryptorchidism. A postulated role of AMH in postpubertal females is to inhibit oocyte meiosis, allowing for enhanced oocyte maturation before selection for ovulation. AMH acts via the type II AMH receptor at target sites.

Mutations of the *AMH* gene have been identified in approximately 20 patients with the PMDS type I phenotype who have low or undetectable serum AMH. These include premature termination codons, frameshift mutations, and missense mutations present in the homozygous or compound heterozygous state. Surprisingly, the first exon of the *AMH* gene appears particularly mutation-prone although it codes for an amino-terminal part of the AMH protein, which is not essential to bioactivity. The deleterious effect of *AMH* gene mutations reflects loss of function of the encoded peptide, presumably because of the markedly abnormal structure created by protein truncation, the predominant form of mutation reported to date.

Disorders of Anti-Müllerian Hormone Action The clinical features of this disorder are identical to those of the originally described PMDS. Since the availability of bioassay and radioimmunoassay and techniques for measurement of AMH, this group of patients has been identified by the finding of normal or increased serum concentrations of bioactive AMH (PMDS type II).

Genetic and Molecular Pathophysiology. The gene encoding human AMH receptor contains 11 exons and is located at 12q13. Surprisingly, the expression of *AMHR* is not detected until mouse embryonic day 15, substantially later than that of its ligand AMH (day 13.5). If this is a true biologic phenomenon, rather than a methodologic artifact, its basis remains to be explained. It is similarly enigmatic that expression of *AMHR* is regulated by androgens; however, androgens are not produced until after the onset of AMH secretion, in the hiatus between *AMH* and *AMHR* expression, suggesting that initial regulation of AMHR is not by androgens or AR. In mouse *AMHR* is expressed in mesenchymal cells adjacent to the Müllerian ducts, suggesting that AMH may alter some aspect of the mesenchyme surrounding the Müllerian ducts, which in turn induces duct regression. The receptor protein is a membrane-bound serine–threonine kinase similar to those for TGF-β and activin, containing a single transmembrane domain. Although it binds ligand directly, it requires the presence of a type I receptor for signal transduction.

Since its recent cloning, mutations in the human *AMHR* gene have been elucidated. The first reported case had a homozygous mutation at the splice donor site of intron 2, resulting in a downstream amino acid substitution and insertion of four new residues. In a study of 16 *AMHR* mutations, 10 patients had a 27-bp deletion in exon 10. Four patients were homozygous for this mutation, which predicts the loss of nine amino acids from the protein, and 6 patients were compound heterozygotes, having missense mutations on their other allele.

46,XX Pseudohermaphroditism Essentially, disorders of female sex differentiation (female pseudohermaphroditism) represent the converse of male pseudohermaphroditism, in general resulting from excessive androgen exposure. Although intuitively likely, exaggerated response to normal androgen levels has not yet been described as a cause of female pseudohermaphroditism. There are far fewer causes of virilization of a female fetus than there are of undermasculinization of a male fetus. Abnormalities of Müllerian development, such as the Mayer-Rokitansky-Küster-Hauser syndrome, represent the mildest form of female pseudohermaphroditism. Lack of fetal estrogen effect does not affect gonadal or genital development, clearly evidenced by the fact that transgenic mice deleted for the estrogen receptor are phenotypically normal.

Disorders Producing Excessive Fetal Androgenization The most common cause of excess fetal androgen production is congenital adrenal hyperplasia (of the 21-hydroxylase, 11β-hydroxylase, or 3β-hydroxysteroid dehydrogenase deficiency types). Molecular defects in these disorders are summarized in Figs. 57-8 and 57-9. A much rarer cause of female pseudohermaphroditism is aromatase deficiency in which fetal virilization results from high levels of testosterone and androstenedione because of the inability to convert these precursors to estrogens (Fig. 57-10). Female pseudohermaphroditism as a result of maternal androgen excess will not be discussed here.

Disorders Producing Excessive Fetal Androgenization: General Clinical Features Virilization of a karyotypic female can produce variable genital phenotypes, depending primarily on the timing, duration, and degree of androgen excess. The phenotype ranges from limited clitoromegaly and posterior labial fusion in the milder cases, to intermediate degrees of virilization with labioscrotal fusion, a urogenital sinus, and significant clitoral enlargement, to severely virilized genitalia that are indistinguishable from those of a cryptorchid male infant. The gonads are normal ovaries and Müllerian duct derivatives develop normally, reflecting absence of AMH. Even in the most virilized infants, Wolffian development does not occur, perhaps because of differences in timing of adrenal versus gonadal androgen production or the presence of less significantly increased androgen concentrations in the vicinity of the Wolffian ducts.

Disorders Producing Excessive Fetal Androgenization: Specific Disorders—Congenital Adrenal Hyperplasia

21-Hydroxylase Deficiency Steroid 21-hydroxylase is a microsomal cytochrome P450 enzyme (P450c21), located on the smooth endoplasmic reticulum, that catalyzes the hydroxylation of progesterone to deoxycorticosterone and 17-hydroxyprogesterone to 11-deoxycortisol, using an NADPH-dependent cytochrome reductase as a cofactor. Deficiency of this enzyme is the most common cause of congenital adrenal hyperplasia in both sexes (*see* Chapter 52).

Clinical Features and Diagnosis. Hydroxylation is impaired in the zona fasciculata of the adrenal glands of those with 21-hydroxylase deficiency, so that 17-hydroxyprogesterone (17-OHP) is not converted to 11-deoxycortisol, the immediate precursor of cortisol. Cortisol deficiency leads to a compensatory increase in ACTH secretion that in turn drives the adrenal gland, resulting in overproduction of cortisol precursors, particularly 17-OHP. These steroids are shunted down the remaining functional steroidogenic pathway, producing a surfeit of androgens (mainly testosterone) that results in virilization of 46,XX fetuses but has no untoward effect on the male fetus. In more than half of cases, 21-hydroxylase is also deficient in the zona glomerulosa and there is failure of conversion of progesterone to 11-deoxycorticosterone, resulting in deficiency of aldosterone. Shock or death may result from severe salt wasting and resultant hypovolemia.

There are four major clinical forms of 21-hydroxylase deficiency: salt wasting (which accounts for approximately 75% of cases), simple virilizing, nonclassic "late onset" (also called attenuated or acquired), and cryptic (asymptomatic). Only the two most severe forms, which produce genital ambiguity, will be discussed. Female infants with the classic virilizing form of 21-hydroxylase deficiency have variable masculinization of the genitalia as described above.

The virilizing form of 21-hydroxylase deficiency is the most likely diagnosis in an infant with genital ambiguity in the presence of 46,XX karyotype. This should be suspected in any partially virilized infant in whom gonads can not be located, either by palpation or by ultrasonography. The presence of a uterus enhances the likelihood of this diagnosis. Increased serum concentrations of 17-hydroxyprogesterone, often as high as 40,000–60,000 ng/dL, are invariably present in infants with enzyme deficiency severe enough to cause virilization; this is accompanied by hyponatre-

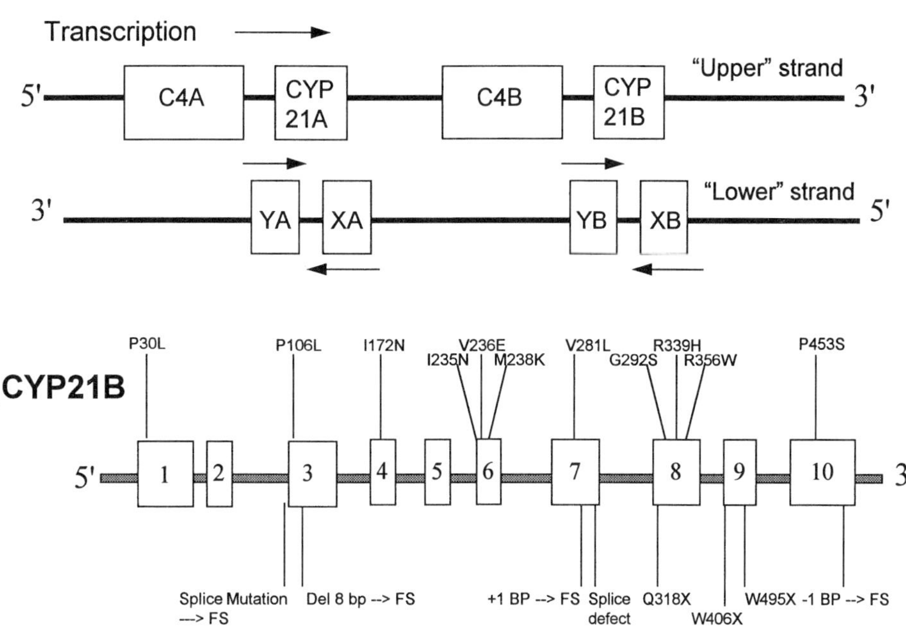

Figure 57-8 Genomic organization and molecular defects of *CYP21B* (encoding steroid 21-hydroxylase). **(A)** Genomic organization. *CYP21B*, the gene that encodes 21-hydroxylase, is located in complex a region of chromosome 6 that has undergone a duplication event. There are thus a number of pairs of tandemly arranged genes in this region. On the upper DNA strand, reading from the 5' direction, the arrangement is as follows: *C4A* (pseudogene for the 4th component of complement), *CYP21A* (the so-called pseudogene of *CYP21*), *C4B* (the active gene encoding the 4th component of complement), *CYP21B* (the gene encoding P450c21). On the lower strand the arrangement is even more complex: two genes (*XB* and *XA*) that overlap the 3' ends of *CYP21B* and *CYP21A*, respectively, are transcribed from the 5' to 3' direction. Two contiguous genes (*YB* and *YA*), which likely also arose by gene duplication, are transcribed in the opposite direction, using promoter sequences in the 5' region of *CYP21A*. The orientation of transcription is indicated by the arrows. **(B)** Molecular defects of *CYP21B*. Missense mutations, resulting in amino acid substitutions, are shown above the gene structure. The standard single letter amino acid code has been used. Other deleterious mutations, including nonsense mutations, splicing defects, and nucleotide deletions causing frameshifts, are shown below the gene. (Single letter amino acid code: A, alanine; C, cysteine; D, aspartic acid; E, glutamic acid; F, phenylalanine; G, glycine; H, histidine; I, isoleucine; K, lysine; L, leucine; M, methionine; N, asparagine; P, proline; Q, glutamine; R, arginine; S, serine; T, threonine; V, valine; W, tryptophan; Y, tyrosine. X denotes a nonsense mutation introducing a termination codon.)

mia, hyperkalemia, and hyperreninemia in those with the salt-wasting form. An ACTH stimulation test is not necessary to make the diagnosis of CAH in a virilized female infant.

Genetic and Molecular Pathophysiology. P450c21 is encoded by the *CYP21* gene *(CYP21B)* located on chromosome 6 at position p21.3, within about 2 centiMorgans of the HLA complex, with which it has tight linkage. *CYP21* and *CYP17* (encoding $P450_{17\alpha}$) are thought to have arisen from a common ancestor gene. *CYP21* contains 10 exons and its 2.0-kb cDNA encodes a 55-kDa protein. There is a homologous gene, generally considered a pseudogene, designated *CYP21P* (or *CYP21A*), located 30-kb upstream. This gene contains three deleterious mutations: an 8-bp deletion in exon 3, a T insertion in exon 7, and a stop codon in exon 8, such that it does not encode P450c21. However, the finding that sequences within this gene are transcribed has led to speculation that it may not in fact be a pseudogene. The gene encoding the fourth component of complement *(C4B)*, is located centromeric to *CYP21* and it too has a homologous pseudogene *(C4A)* near the *CYP21* pseudogene. These two gene-pseudogene pairs are believed to have arisen through a duplication event. The genetic arrangement is further complicated by the presence of two additional genes, termed *XB*, and *YB*, that overlap *CYP21* on the complementary DNA strand. *XB* is transcribed in the opposite direction to produce an extracellular matrix protein termed tenascin-X; the product of *YB* is unclear. A homologous pair of genes, *XA* and *YA*, overlap *CYP21A* on the complementary DNA strand. *CYP21* expression is regulated by ACTH via cAMP, using a specific cAMP-responsive sequence in the 5'-flanking region of the gene that binds a putative adrenal-specific nuclear protein (ASP). In addition, SF-1 activates the P450c21 promoter, as does another homologous orphan nuclear receptor nerve growth factor-induced gene-B (NGFI-B). Expression of this latter transcription factor increases dramatically in the adrenal cortex in response to stress. Interestingly, expression of P450c21 has recently been demonstrated in skin.

Inheritance of 21-hydroxylase deficiency is autosomal recessive and the incidence of the disorder ranges from 1:15,000 (some white populations) to 1:700 (Yupik Eskimo tribe), the general incidence being reported as approximately 1:5,000. Molecular defects in *CYP21* have been elucidated in approximately 100 patients with 21-hydroxylase deficiency. These almost all appear to have arisen as a result of recombination events between *CYP21* and its homologous pseudogene, *CYP21P*, and result in either deletion of *CYP21*, or transfer of mutations from the pseudogene to the functional gene (a process termed "gene conversion"). This phenomenon has been suggested to account for the predominance of 21-hydroxylase deficiency over other forms of CAH. Complete deletion of *CYP21* occurs in about 20% of cases of the classic salt-wasting form. In a few cases the deletion has included the neigh-

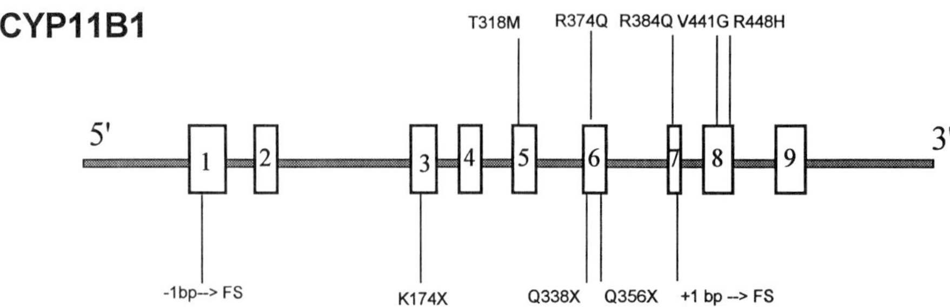

Figure 57-9 Molecular defects of *CYP11B1*. Mutations in *CYP11B1* causing 11β-hydroxylase deficiency and female pseudohermaphroditism have been reported in a number of individuals. Missense mutations are shown above the gene; frameshift (FS) and nonsense mutations are shown below the gene. Mutation R448H is found commonly in Moroccan Jews. This residue is probably required for heme binding. The majority of mutations have been found in exons 6–8.

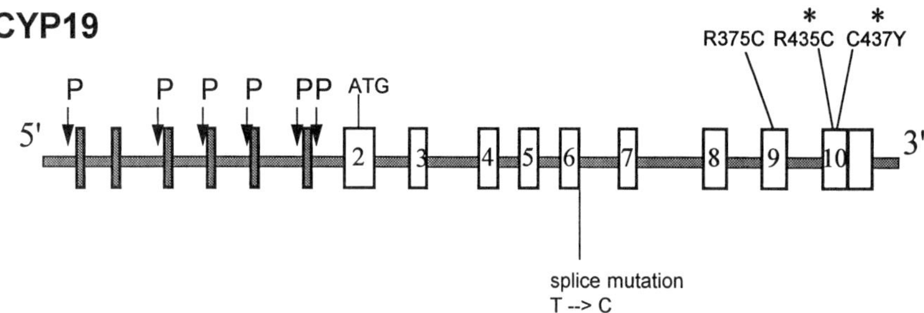

Figure 57-10 Molecular defects of *CYP19* gene. The *CYP19* gene (encoding the aromatase enzyme, P450arom) has a complex structure in its 5' region: there are six untranslated exons (shaded boxes, locations not clearly known) and six alternate promoters used in different tissues (designated "P"); translation begins within exon 2. Rare mutations causing female pseudohermaphroditism have been reported. The two missense mutations shown above the gene denoted with asterisks were present in the same patient, who was therefore a compound heterozygote. Because of its role in heme binding, cysteine 437 is highly conserved. A splice junction mutation resulting in an 87-bp insertion is depicted below the gene. The patient was homozygous for this mutation.

boring *C4* gene. However, as in most other genetic disorders, single-base mutations are common, and cause truncation, aberrant splicing, or amino acid substitutions. In a comprehensive study of 88 families, Speiser et al. determined that the most common mutation was an A-G change in the second intron affecting mRNA splicing (26%); large deletions had occurred in about 21% of affected individuals; substitution of isoleucine 172 by asparagine was found in 16%; and replacement of valine 281 by leucine in 11%. Homozygosity for severe mutations is present in about 50% of those with classic salt-wasting 21-hydroxylase deficiency. Correlations between enzyme activity (phenotype) and mutation (genotype) were noted, although some patients' enzymatic phenotypes were not as predicted from their genotype. Compound heterozygosity for different *CYP21* mutations is common. The clinical and enzymatic findings of such patients results from the combined effect of different mutations in each allele.

In vitro analysis of mutant 21-hydroxylase enzymes has been performed in a number of cases. A mutant containing threonine at position 428 in place of cysteine has complete loss of enzymatic activity and heme binding. Of note, cysteine 428 is invariant among all P450 enzymes and is believed to be the heme-binding site. Other amino acid substitutions depress enzyme activity to varying degrees.

11β-Hydroxylase Deficiency 11β-Hydroxylase is a cytochrome P450 enzyme that catalyzes the final step in cortisol synthesis, 11β-hydroxylation of 11-deoxycortisol to cortisol in the zona fasciculata of the adrenal gland. A related isozyme in the zona glomerulosa, aldosterone synthase, catalyzes the final three steps in aldosterone synthesis, hydroxylation and dehydrogenation (oxidation) of 11-deoxycorticosterone to aldosterone (these latter activities are also referred to as corticosterone methyl oxidase types I and II [CMO I; CMO II]). Deficiency of 11β-hydroxylase results in a relatively common form of congenital adrenal hyperplasia, accounting for approximately 5% of cases, depending on ethnic background. This enzyme is not involved in gonadal steroidogenesis.

Clinical Features and Diagnosis. There is a relatively high frequency of 11β-hydroxylase deficiency in Saudi Arabia and in Moroccan and Iranian Jews because consanguinity in these families is common. Affected female (46,XX) infants present with variable genital virilization, similar to those with 21-hydroxylase deficiency. In a number of kindreds, affected females have been so severely virilized that they have been reared as males, the diagnosis delayed until puberty, when breast development and menses occurred. 11-Deoxycortisol is massively elevated and serum concentrations of 11-deoxycorticosterone, adrenal androgens, testosterone (by conversion from androstenedione), and ACTH are also increased. The distinguishing clinical feature of this condition is the presence of hypertension, induced by increased secretion of 11-deoxycorticosterone, the mineralocorticoid activity of which causes sodium retention and suppression of plasma renin activity. Hypokalemia resulting from the mineralocorticoid excess is variably present. There is minimal correlation between the severity of the virilization and the hypertension. Precocious pseudopuberty and advanced skeletal maturation occurs in untreated cases of both sexes.

Genetic and Molecular Pathophysiology. There are two genes encoding 11β-hydroxylase isozymes. The 6.5-kb, 9-exon *CYP11B1* gene encoding P450C11*(P450XIB1)* is localized to 8q21. A contiguous gene, *CYP11B2*, located approximately 40 kb away within the same chromosomal locus, encodes a second 11β-hydroxylase isozyme (P450cmo) that displays 93% amino acid homology with the first. *CYP11B1* and *CYP11B2* are structurally homologous to *CYP11A*, the gene that encodes $P450_{scc}$, and the trio represent a subfamily within the P450 superfamily.

CYP11B is expressed in the zona fasciculata of the adrenal cortex, under regulation by ACTH via cAMP. Like genes encoding other steroidogenic enzymes, the *CYP11B* promoter also contains a binding site for SF-1. P450C11 is a mitochondrial protein predicted to contain 479–503 amino acids, including an amino-terminal mitochondrial signal sequence. P450C11 catalyzes 11β-hydroxylation of 11-dexoxycortisol to cortisol in the zona fasciculata of the adrenal gland. It also has limited 18-hydroxylase activity. *CYP11B2*, the gene expressed in the zona glomerulosa, encodes the isozyme P450cmo (P450aldo; P450XIB2), which catalyzes the three-step conversion of 11-deoxycorticosterone to aldosterone (11-hydroxylation, 18-hydroxylation, and 18-oxidation). Its expression is regulated by angiotensin II.

Mutations in *CYP11B1* have been reported in at least 12 individuals with 11β-hydroxylase deficiency. Reported mutations include a 2-bp insertion and a 1-bp deletion (both of which cause a frameshift, deleting the enzyme's heme-binding domain); single-base mutations introducing termination codons (nonsense mutations), and a number of missense mutations causing amino acid substitutions. Substitution of arginine by histidine at position 448 is the predominant defect in P450C11 in Moroccan Jews, suggesting a founder effect. This amino acid is highly conserved and believed to be required for heme binding. Transient transfection studies reveal that this mutation abolishes enzymatic activity. Despite this, individuals heterozygous for this mutation have no demonstrable hormonal abnormalities, indicating that approximately 50% of enzyme activity is adequate for normal steroidogenesis. Hydroxylase activity is also abolished in other mutant enzymes containing different amino acid substitutions. The majority of mutations cluster in exons 6–8 of the *CYP11B1* gene, suggesting that this region encodes residues critical for enzymatic activity. Notably, clinical variation has been observed between individuals with the same mutation.

The mutations reported to date are *de novo* point mutations. The relatively high frequency of mutations in this gene is suggested to result from its high frequency of CpG dinucleotides, a well-recognized mutational hot spot in the human genome, rather than from recombination between *CYP11B1* and *CYP11B2* (as occurs between *CYP21* and its adjacent pseudogene *CYP21A*). Mutations in *CYP11B2* cause aldosterone synthase deficiency, which can present in infancy with hyponatremic, hypovolemic shock, but does not affect sexual differentiation in either sex.

3β-Hydroxysteroid Dehydrogenase Deficiency 3β-Hydroxysteroid dehydrogenase (3β-HSD) is a noncytochrome, membrane-bound enzyme that requires NAD^+ as a cofactor to catalyze the conversion of 3β-hydroxy-Δ^5-steroids (pregnenolone, 17-hydroxypregnenolone, and dehydroepiandrosterone) to the 3-keto-Δ^4-steroids (progesterone, 17-hydroxyprogesterone, and Δ^4-androstenedione; Fig. 57-7). Deficiency of 3β-HSD, which is less common than 21-hydroxylase deficiency, impairs steroidogenesis in the adrenals and gonads, resulting in reduced synthesis of cortisol, aldosterone, and gonadal steroids.

Clinical Features and Diagnosis. Deficiency of 3β-HSD produces significant genital ambiguity in males, as described in detail above. However, in karyotypic females 3β-HSD deficiency is associated with only mild genital virilization (mild clitoromegaly or posterior labial fusion) not of sufficient severity to suggest genital ambiguity. Further clitoral enlargement and premature development of pubic and axillary hair may occur during childhood in untreated patients. The androgenization in females results from exaggerated levels of the relatively weak androgen dehydroepiandrosterone. Some cases have associated salt wasting because of reduced synthesis of aldosterone and cortisol.

Genetic and Molecular Pathophysiology. Details of the genetics and molecular biology of this gene are provided in the preceding section on 3β-HSD deficiency as a cause of male pseudohermaphroditism and will not be reviewed here. One affected female without genital ambiguity was found to be homozygous for a nonsense mutation that produced a truncated protein of 169 amino acids, compared with the usual 371 amino acids. Compound heterozygosity for a missense mutation and an intronic mutation likely causing a splicing defect was found in another female with normal genitalia, whose affected brother had ambiguous genitalia. Other mutations in affected females will likely be similar to those found in affected males and their effect on genital development will probably reflect the nature and severity of the mutation.

Aromatase Deficiency The conversion of androgens to estrogens is controlled by aromatase (P450arom), a cytochrome P450 enzyme located in the endoplasmic reticulum of estrogen-producing cells. Using NADPH-cytochrome P450 reductase as a cofactor, this microsomal enzyme catalyzes conversion of C19 steroids (androstenedione and testosterone) to C18 estrogens (estradiol, estrone, estriol), by modification of the steroid A ring to a phenolic ring.

Clinical Features and Diagnosis. Androgens produced by the fetal adrenal gland and then desulfated and aromatized by the placenta are the major source of circulating estrogens during pregnancy. An apparently rare cause of female pseudohermaphroditism is the inability to convert fetal androgens to estrogens because of lack of placental aromatase activity. Three cases of aromatase deficiency have been described. In two cases, the mothers developed progressive virilization in the latter part of pregnancy, which resolved after delivery; serum androgens were high and estrogens low. Despite this, growth and development of the fetuses and placentas throughout gestation were normal. In the first case in vitro assays of the placenta after delivery revealed negligible aromatase activity. Absence of maternal virilization in the third case suggested that some aromatase activity was retained.

The 46,XX affected infants in each case had male-appearing or ambiguous external genitalia with marked clitoral enlargement, rugation and fusion of labioscrotal folds, and a single meatus at the base of the phallic structure. The virilization results from conversion of dehydroepriandrosterone sulfate (DHEAS) to androstenedione and testosterone by the placenta; its inability to aromatize these steroids to estrogens results in massive elevations of these compounds. Most recently, a pair of affected 46,XX and 46,XY siblings have been reported. The female had ambiguous genitalia, similar to those described above; the male was normally masculinized.

The two affected 46,XX subjects who are now postpubertal exhibited features of androgen excess from puberty onwards. Clitoral enlargement and development of facial acne were noted, in addition to absence of breast development, attributed to deficiency of ovarian aromatase. Gonadotropins were modestly elevated, accompanied by high adrenal androgen concentrations, high plasma testosterone, low estradiol concentrations, and ovarian cysts on pelvic ultrasound. Because estrogens are the hormones primarily responsible for skeletal maturation, this was delayed, resulting in tall stature. There was also significant osteoporosis in the affected adult male.

These cases, as well as the single reported case of an estrogen receptor (ER) mutation and the evidence from ER-deleted transgenic mice, indicate that contrary to long-standing beliefs, estrogens are not required for fetal survival.

Genetic and Molecular Pathophysiology. Aromatase (P450arom) is a cytochrome P450 enzyme encoded by a 9-exon, 70-kb gene designated *CYP19*, whose chromosomal locus is 15q21.1. P450arom is expressed in a wide variety of human tissues, including the granulosa and luteal cells of the ovary, testicular Sertoli and Leydig cells, the placenta, adipose tissue, brain, muscle, and liver and in the preimplantation blastocyst. Expression levels and transcript sizes are quite different in these various tissues and expression is regulated in part by the use of tissue-specific alternative promoters, in ovary, placenta, brain, and adipose tissue. However, because the translational start site is conserved in the various mRNA species, the same protein is expressed in all tissues. Like that of other steroidogenic enzymes, the aromatase gene promoter contains a binding site for SF-1, and it appears that this site is involved in the cAMP-mediated regulation of gene expression. The expressed protein is similar to other P450 enzymes, containing a carboxy-terminal heme-binding region encoded by the 9th exon.

The defects in the above cases were inherited in an autosomal recessive pattern and there was known parental consanguinity in one case. In the first case described, the affected girl was homozygous for a splice junction point mutation that resulted in translation of an abnormal peptide containing an extra 29 amino acids. In vitro analysis revealed that the mutant enzyme retained only a minimal level of activity. In the second case, the affected individual was found be a compound heterozygote for two single-base mutations that introduced two separate amino acid substitutions into the enzyme: arginine to cysteine at position 435 and cysteine to tyrosine two residues downstream, at amino acid 437. In vitro analyses of the mutant enzymes revealed extremely low activity in the presence of the R435C substitution, and complete absence of activity with the C437Y defect. Cysteine 437 is very highly conserved, and is apparently involved in heme binding, hence the destructive effect of the mutation on enzyme function. In the final case, the mutation replaces a highly conserved arginine residue with cysteine at position 375 of the peptide. The mutant protein expressed in vitro had only 0.2% of the activity of wild-type P450arom. The region of the protein in which arginine 375 is located is postulated to be involved in anchoring the enzyme to the cell membrane. Molecular defects in *CYP19* are summarized in Fig. 57-10.

Disorders of Müllerian Development MAYER-ROKITANSKY-KÜSTER-HAUSER (MRKH) SYNDROME Although individuals with this disorder clearly are phenotypic females, the condition technically represents the mildest form of female pseudohermaphroditism, in parallel with PMDS in the male. This developmental abnormality appears to result from defective Müllerian duct fusion in early gestation; however, the exact nature of the defect remains unclear. Affected girls usually present in their teens with primary amenorrhea in the presence of otherwise normal secondary sexual development. Examination reveals absence or severe hypoplasia of the vagina; uterine agenesis is usual; however, some uterine development (uni- or bicornuate uterus), or occasionally a normal uterus, may be present. The ovaries are normally developed. There appear to be two subtypes of the disorder—the typical (isolated) and atypical forms, frequency of each being approximately equal. The typical form is characterized by the laparoscopy or laparotomy findings of symmetric muscular buds (the Müllerian remnants) and normal Fallopian tubes. The atypical form has asymmetric hypoplasia of one or both buds, with or without dysplasia of the Fallopian tubes. The atypical form has associated anomalies including renal defects (agenesis or ectopia in about 30–50% of patients) and skeletal abnormalities (vertebral malformations; Klippel-Feil anomaly) of varying severity. The MURCS association comprises Müllerian duct aplasia, renal agenesis or ectopia, and cervical somite dysplasia (Klippel-Feil). This represents the most severe form of the disorder and may represent a mesodermal malformation spectrum. Laparoscopy is required to distinguish the typical from the atypical form of the MRKH syndrome. Because of these associated anomalies, all patients with vaginal atresia should have skeletal radiographs and renal and pelvic ultrasound performed.

The MRKH syndrome occurs in 1 in 4000–5000 females. Most cases are sporadic; however, a genetic defect likely underlies familial cases (approximately 5%), which have been reported in patterns consistent with sex-limited autosomal dominant or autosomal recessive inheritance. Galactose-1-phosphate uridyl transferase activity is reduced in some patients and may represent a candidate gene for MRKH syndrome.

DIAGNOSIS AND MANAGEMENT OF DISORDERS OF SEX DETERMINATION AND SEX DIFFERENTIATION

DIAGNOSIS Abnormalities of sexual development require evaluation by an experienced team, including a pediatric endocrinologist, urologist, and geneticist. In the newborn period, rapid but careful diagnosis and early, appropriate sex assignment are essential to optimize parental adjustment to the child's apparently incongruous genital appearance and to minimize subsequent psychosocial problems for the child. The principal aims of the diagnostic evaluation are to determine (1) presence of potentially life-threatening adrenal steroid deficiencies and electrolyte derangements; (2) chromosomal sex; (3) type and functional status of the gonads; (4) internal genital anatomy; and (5) most appropriate sex-of-rearing.

Consanguinity between parents is suggestive of autosomal recessive conditions, such as CAH and 5α-reductase deficiency. Likewise, the presence of similarly affected siblings or a family history of ambiguous genitalia, infertility, amenorrhea, lack of pubertal development, or sudden death in infancy is suggestive of a genetically determined defect. A history of genital abnormalities, severe gynecomastia, or infertility in maternal relatives suggests an X-linked condition, such as androgen insensitivity. A history of maternal virilization during pregnancy could suggest aromatase deficiency.

Clinical, ultrasound, and radiographic examination should define the following features:

1. External genital anatomy. Specifically, the size of the phallic structure (stretched penile length, excluding foreskin,

Table 57-5
Steroid Profiles in Disorders of Sex Differentiation

Disorder	*Prog*	*DOC*	*Aldo*	*17OHPreg*	*17OHP*	*11-Deoxycortisol*	*Cortisol*	*DHEA*	*Δ4A*	*Testo*	*DHT*
LCH	N	N	N	N	N	N	N	N	N	↓↓	↓↓
CLAH (StAR)	↓	↓	↓	↓	↓	↓	↓	↓	↓	↓	↓
3β-HSD	N or ↑	↓	↓	↑↑	N or ↑	↓	↓	↑↑	N or ↑	N or ↑	N or ↓
17α-OH	↑	↑	↓	↓	↓	↓	↓	↓	↓	↓	↓
17β-OH	N	N	N	N	N	N	N	N or ↑	↑	↓	↓
5α-Red	N	N	N	N	N	N	N	N	N	↑	↓
AIS	N	N	N	N	N	N	N	N	N	N or ↑	N or↑
21-OH	↑	↓	↓	↑	↑↑↑	↓	↓	↑	↑	↑↑	NA
11β–OH	N	↑	↓	N or ↑	N or ↑	↑↑↑	↓	↑	↑	↑	NA
Aromatase deficiency	N	N	N	N	N	N	N	↑↑↑	↑↑↑	↑↑↑	↑↑↑

LCH, leydig cell hypoplasia; CLAH, congenital lipoid adrenal hyperplasia; StAR, steroidogenic acute regulator protein; 3β-HSD, 3β-hydroxysteroid dehydrogenase deficiency; 17α-OH, 17α-hydroxylase deficiency; 17β-OH, 17β-hydroxylase deficiency; 5α-red, 5α-reductase deficiency; AIS, androgen insensitivity syndrome; 21-OH, 21-hydroxylase deficiency; 11β-OH, 11β-hydroxylase deficiency. Prog, progesterone; DOC, deoxycorticosterone; Aldo, aldosterone; 17OHPreg, 17α-hydroxypregneneolone; 17OHP, 17α-hydroxyprogesterone; DHEA, dehydroepiandrosterone; Δ4A, androstenedione; Testo, testosterone; DHT, dihydrotestosterone.

and diameter at midshaft), location of the urethral meatus, presence of a separate vaginal orifice, size, and fusion and rugation of labioscrotal folds provide information regarding the degree of fetal androgenization. Hyperpigmentation of the genitalia represents evidence of ACTH excess as a result of some form of CAH.

2. Location of gonads. Gonads in the inguinal region are highly likely to be testes (ovarian herniation occurs exceptionally rarely), suggesting that the infant is probably a genotypic male (or much less likely, another karyotype with presence of *SRY*). If no gonads are palpable in a partially masculinized infant, ultrasound examination is required to locate the gonads (which may be anywhere from the inguinal ring to the abdomen) and to examine for associated developmental abnormalities of the renal tract.
3. Presence or absence of a uterus. Because of exposure to maternal estrogens, the uterus is enlarged and readily detectable by rectal examination or ultrasonography in newborn females. Presence of a uterus reflects absence of AMH effect during gestation, generally indicating that the gonads are not testes (or, if testes are present, that AMH action was absent during gestation).
4. Internal genital anatomy. Cystoscopy or voiding cystourethrogram is required to define the anatomy of the lower urogenital structures, including type of urethra (long, male-type vs short, female-type), presence of a vagina or more rudimentary structure such as a prostatic utricle, and presence and location of the vaginal orifice (perineal vs urethral). The longer the urethra, smaller the vaginal structure, and higher its entry to the urethra, the greater the degree of androgenization that occurred *in utero*.
5. Presence of other dysmorphic features or intrauterine growth retardation. These findings may suggest that the genital defect is part of a more generalized disturbance of morphogenesis.

Despite careful examination, it is almost impossible to differentiate between many of the disorders of sex determination and differentiation on clinical grounds alone. Detailed laboratory evaluation is urgent if dealing with an infant with ambiguous genitalia in whom the sex of rearing is yet to be determined. Hormone secretion in the immediate postnatal period is dynamic, with hormone concentrations changing rapidly over the first few days of life. Therefore, optimally, blood should be drawn within the first 36 h of life for hormone analysis. Primary care institutions should be instructed that for any infant with a concern regarding genital development, 10 mL of blood should be drawn immediately and the serum frozen for later use. The following studies should be undertaken urgently on fresh blood:

1. Karyotype. In all cases a formal karyotype is required. A buccal smear is inadequate because of frequent false-negative results.
2. Electrolytes and adrenal steroids for evidence of congenital adrenal hyperplasia. 17-Hydroxyprogesterone (for 21-hydroxylase deficiency); 11-deoxycortisol (for 11-hydroxylase deficiency); 17-hydroxypregnenolone and dehydroepiandrosterone (for 3β-hydroxysteroid dehydrogenase deficiency); pregnenolone; progesterone; 17-hydroxypregnenolone; and 17-hydroxyprogesterone (for 17-hydroxylase deficiency); and in most cases, plasma renin activity should be measured on the initial blood sample. Other more discriminating steroids can be measured on the stored, frozen serum once the karyotype and initial critical values are obtained. Normal electrolytes in the immediate postnatal period do not exclude congenital adrenal hyperplasia, and until definitive results are obtained, these should be monitored for development of hyponatremia and hyperkalemia.
3. Testosterone (T), dihydrotestosterone (DHT), and T precursors to determine the presence of a defect of T biosynthesis or 5α-reductase deficiency in karyotypic males (Table 57-5). Serum T is high (>200 ng/dL) in cord blood, but plummets to become almost undetectable at the end of the first week of life, rising from about 2–3 weeks, to peak at >200 ng/dL at around 8–12 weeks of age. Serum T falls

again from 12 to 16 weeks, finally becoming essentially unmeasurable by 6 months of age. Steroid analysis should therefore be performed during periods of maximal testicular activity, or, if this is not possible, after testicular stimulation with hCG (gonadal steroids and DHT are measured before, and 24 h after, administration of 1500 IU hCG every other day for three doses). Normal infants respond with T values >200 ng/dL, often much higher. An increased ratio of T to DHT (>20:1) during periods of active testicular steroidogenesis or after hCG is found in 5α-reductase deficiency. Hormonal profiles found in defects of T biosynthesis are summarized in Table 57-5. T and DHT concentrations are probably within normal limits in AIS; however, increased concentrations have been reported in a few infants with partial AIS. Minimal data are available for infants with complete AIS.

4. LH and FSH. LH concentration should be markedly increased in infants with Leydig cell hypoplasia and may also be increased in infants with partial AIS. FSH is increased in those with gonadal dysgenesis, but may not be elevated in early infancy.
5. ACTH stimulation test. This is required to characterize steroidogenic defects that affect the adrenals as well as the gonads (CLAH, 3β-hydroxysteroid dehydrogenase deficiency, and 17-hydroxylase deficiency). In virilized karyotypic females, an ACTH stimulation test is not required for diagnosis of 21-hydroxylase deficiency, but may aid diagnosis of other forms of CAH by exaggerating precursor steroid levels.
6. Gonadal biopsy. This may be required in cases of suspected gonadal dysgenesis.

If concentrations of testosterone, DHT, and steroid precursors are normal in a karyotypic male with abnormal masculinization, the differential diagnosis then likely rests between a partial form of AIS and the perplexing "black box" of undiagnosable forms of male pseudohermaphroditism.

MANAGEMENT Sex of Rearing Although an accurate diagnosis is important, sex assignment is based primarily on gonadal and genital morphology rather than diagnosis. It has been usual practice to assign female sex-of-rearing to any infant with ovaries, no matter how virilized, since she is potentially fertile. The converse principle has not generally been applied for infants with testes, since it has been argued that successful functional outcome after reconstruction of severely undermasculinized genitalia is unlikely. This is clearly a vital area of management, and one that is currently undergoing re-examination. Unfortunately, a detailed discussion of the principles, practice, and outcome of sex assignment of infants with disorders of sex determination and differentiation is beyond the scope of this chapter.

Gonadectomy Gonadectomy is required for all individuals reared as females who have testes or gonadal dysgenesis and a Y-bearing cell line. However, opinion regarding the optimal timing of this procedure varies. For individuals with 46,XY or mosaic forms of gonadal dysgenesis, gonadectomy is advisable at the time of diagnosis, because of the high risk of malignancy. In those reared as females who have retained production of and responsiveness to testosterone, gonadectomy should be undertaken at the time of initial genital reconstructive surgery to prevent potential virilization at puberty. In those with complete AIS (therefore no response to T), the timing of gonadectomy is the subject of debate. Some physicians recommend early gonadectomy for psychological reasons; others prefer to defer this until after puberty to take advantage of the excellent spontaneous feminization that results from endogenous testicular estrogen secretion. In following the latter course it is important that the young woman be made aware in early adolescence that the gonads will need to be removed at the completion of puberty because of the risk of malignancy. If inguinal hernia repair is required in early childhood, simultaneous gonadectomy is considered advisable, to obviate the need for a second surgical procedure.

Hormone Replacement Therapy Gonadectomized individuals and females with CLAH or aromatase deficiency require estrogen supplementation at the appropriate time for puberty and thereafter, to induce and maintain feminization. The addition of cyclic progesterone is generally recommended once feminization is established, and is mandatory for those with a uterus. For partially virilized infants reared as male, testosterone therapy is usually required in infancy to enhance penile size before surgery, and may be beneficial at puberty to optimize virilization. Certain individuals with partial forms of AIS may require and respond to high-dose testosterone therapy. Despite the enzymatic defect in conversion of testosterone to DHT, this therapy may also normalize serum DHT concentrations and improve virilization in some men with 5α-reductase deficiency.

Affected individuals of either sex with any form of congenital adrenal hyperplasia require standard replacement therapy with glucocorticoids and mineralocorticoids. Treatment with physiologic doses of glucocorticoids suppresses ACTH production, thus reducing levels of precursor steroids that otherwise produce detrimental effects, such as virilization, advanced skeletal maturation, and, in the 17-hydroxylase and 11-hydroxylase deficiency forms of CAH, hypertension. The addition of antiandrogens to the standard therapy for CAH is currently under investigation.

Prenatal Diagnosis and Treatment of CAH Prenatal diagnosis and treatment of female fetuses affected by virilizing 21-hydroxylase deficiency has been undertaken successfully in a number of cases. This procedure requires that the molecular defect has been characterized in a prior affected sibling. Dexamethasone treatment is initiated as soon as pregnancy is confirmed. At 10 weeks' gestation, a chorionic villus biopsy is performed and karyotype determined. If the karyotype is 46,XY, dexamethasone is suspended because masculinization is normal in affected males. If the karyotype is 46,XX, dexamethasone is continued until the status of the fetus is determined by molecular analysis of *CYP21*. If the 46,XX fetus is determined to be unaffected, dexamethasone treatment is suspended; if affected, the treatment is continued until term. Although not yet reported, this procedure would also be applicable in other forms of CAH, provided the molecular defect has been determined in an older sibling. Maternal complications of dexamethasone treatment are not insignificant (often quite severe Cushingoid changes), and such management should be undertaken only under the guidance of a team experienced with this therapy.

SELECTED REFERENCES

Andersson S, Geissler WM, Wu L, et al. Molecular genetics and pathophysiology of 17 beta-hydroxysteroid dehydrogenase 3 deficiency. J Clin Endocrinol Metab 1996;81:130–136.

Andersson S, Bishop RW, Russell DW. Expression cloning and regulation of steroid 5alpha-reductase, an enzyme essential for male sex differentiation. J Biol Chem 1989;264:16,249–16,255.

Bose HS, Pescovits OH, Miller WL. Spontaneous feminization in a 46, XX female patient with congenital lipoid adrenal hyperplasia due to a homozygous frameshift mutation in the steroidogenic acute regulatory protein. J Clin Endocrinol Metab 1997;82:1511–1515.

Cramer DW, Goldstein DP, Fraer C, Reichardt JK. Vaginal agenesis (Mayer-Rokitansky-Kuster-Hauser syndrome) associated with the N314D mutation of galactose-1-phosphate uridyl transferase. Mol Hum Reprod 1996;2:145–148.

Curnow KM, Slutsker L, Vitek J, et al. Mutations in the CYP11B1 gene causing congenital adrenal hyperplasia and hypertension cluster in exons 6, 7 and 8. Proc Natl Acad Sci USA 1993;90:4552–4556.

Foster JW, Dominguez-Steglich MA, Guioli S, et al. Campomelic dysplasia and autosomal sex reversal caused by mutations in an SRY-related gene. Nature 1994;372:525–530.

Goodfellow PN, Lovell-Badge R. *SRY* and sex determination in mammals. Annu Rev Genet 1993;27:71–92.

Ingraham HA, Lala DS, Ikeda Y, et al. The nuclear receptor steroidogenic factor 1 acts at multiple levels of the reproductive axis. Genes Dev 1994;8:2302–2312.

Josso N. AntiMullerian hormone: new perspectives for a sexist molecule. Endocr Rev 1986;7:421–433.

Labrie F, Luu-The V, Lin SX, et al. The key role of 17 beta-hydroxysteroid dehydrogenases in sex steroid biology. Steroids 1997;62:148–158.

Lin D, Sugawara T, Strauss JF III, et al. Role of steroidogenic acute regulatory protein in adrenal and gonadal steroidogenesis. Science 1995;267:1828–1831.

Luo X, Ikeda Y, Parker KL. A cell-specific nuclear receptor is essential for adrenal and gonadal development and sexual differentiation. Cell 1994;77:481–490.

Luu-The V, Labrie C, Simard J, et al. Structure of two in tandem human 17beta-hydroxysteroid dehydrogenase gene. Mol Endocrinol 1990;4: 268–275.

MacLean HE, Warne GL, Zajac JD. Intersex disorders: shedding light on male sexual differentiation beyond SRY. Clin Endocrinol 1997;46: 101–108.

McPhaul MJ, Marcelli M, Zoppi S, Wilson CM, Griffin JE, Wilson JD. Mutations in the ligand-binding domain of the androgen receptor gene cluster in two regions of the gene. J Clin Invest 90:2097–2101.

Morishima A, Grumbach MM, Simpson ER, Fisher C, Qin K. Aromatase deficiency in male and female siblings caused by a novel mutation and the physiological role of estrogens. J Clin Endocrinol Metab 1995;80: 3689–3698.

Morrison-Graham K, Takahashi Y. Steel factor and c-Kit receptor: from mutants to a growth factor system. Bioessays 1993;15:77–83.

Muscatelli F, Strom TM, Walker AP, et al. Mutations in the *DAX-1* gene give rise to both X-linked adrenal hypoplasia congenita and hypogonadotropic gonadism. Nature 1994;372:672–676.

Newfield RS, New MI. 21-Hydroxylase deficiency. Ann N Y Acad Sci 1997;17:219–229.

Pelletier J, Bruening W, Kashtan CE, et al. Germline mutations in the Wilms tumor suppressor gene are associated with abnormal urogenital development in Denys-Drash syndrome. Cell 1991;67:437–447.

Penning TM. Molecular endocrinology of hydroxysteroid dehydrogenases. Endocr Rev 1997;18:281–305.

Quigley CA, De Bellis A, Marschke KB, El-Awady MK, Wilson EM, French FS. Androgen receptor defects: Historical, clinical and molecular perspectives. Endcocr Rev 1995;16:271–321.

Ramkissoon T, Goodfellow P. Early steps in mammalian sex determination. Curr Opin Genet Dev 1996;6:316–321.

Segaloff DL, Ascoli M. The lutropin/choriogonadotropin receptor...4 years later. Endocr Rev 1993;14:324–347.

Shen W-H, Moore CCD, Ikeda Y, Parker KL, Ingraham HA. Nuclear receptor steroidogenic factor 1 regulates the Mullerian inhibiting substance gene: a link to the sex determination cascade. Cell 1994;77:651–661.

Shozu M, Akasofu K, Harada T, Kubota Y. A new cause of female pseudohermaphroditism: placental aromatase deficiency. J Clin Endocrinol Metab 1991;72:560–566.

Simard J, Rheaume E, Sanchez R, et al. Molecular basis of congenital adrenal hyperplasia due to 3-beta hydroxysteroid dehydrogenase deficiency. Mol Endocrinol 1993;7:716–728.

Simpson ER, Mahendroo MS, Means GD, et al. Aromatase cytochrome P450, the enzyme responsible for estrogen biosynthesis. Endocr Rev 1994;15:342–355.

Simpson ER, Zhao Y, Agarwal VR, et al. Aromatase expression in health and disease. Recent Prog Horm Res 1997;52:185–213.

Speiser PW, Dupont J, Zhu D, et al. Disease expression and molecular genotype in congenital adrenal hyperplasia due to 21-hydroxylase deficiency. J Clin Invest 1992;90:584–595.

Wagner T, Wirth J, Meyer J, et al. Autosomal sex reversal and campomelic dysplasia are caused by mutations in and around the *SRY*-related gene *SOX9*. Cell 1994;79:1111–1120.

Waterman MR. A rising StAR: an essential role in cholesterol transport. Science 1995;267:1780,1781.

Wilson JD, Griffin JE, Russell DW. Steroid 5alpha-reductase 2 deficiency. Endocr Rev 1993;14:577–593.

Yanase T, Simpson ER, Waterman MR. 17alpha-hydroxylase/17,20-lyase deficiency: from clinical investigation to molecular definition. Endocr Rev 1991;12:91–108.

58 Sex Chromosome Disorders

ANDREW R. ZINN

INTRODUCTION

Because sex chromosome disorders frequently result in abnormalities of sexual differentiation, the two subjects are usually discussed together in medical texts. The biology of human sexual differentiation and the pathophysiology of associated defects were discussed in the previous chapter. This chapter examines sex chromosome disorders from a genetic perspective, emphasizing unique features, such as X inactivation and dosage compensation, X-Y recombination, and male-specific functions of the Y chromosome. Table 58-1 summarizes karyotype, genotype, and phenotype data for selected disorders included in this chapter. The reader should consult an endocrinology textbook for more information about the clinical features of the various disorders.

STRUCTURE AND FUNCTION OF HUMAN SEX CHROMOSOMES

The structures of the human X and Y chromosomes and the approximate positions of some genes of interest are depicted in Fig. 58-1. The X chromosome is about 160 Mb in length. It contains probably thousands of genes, encoding a variety of enzymes and structural and regulatory proteins. A distinguishing feature of most of these genes is that males have only one copy, accounting for X-linked recessive inheritance of many genetic diseases (*see* Transmission of Human Genetic Diseases, Chapter 4). By contrast, the much smaller Y chromosome is believed to contain a paucity of genes. The Y chromosome is divided into two parts. The euchromatic portion is about 30 Mb in length and contains all known Y-linked genes. The heterochromatic portion on the long arm can vary in length among normal men, averaging approximately 20 Mb. This region is composed of simple repetitive sequences and probably does not contain any genes. Because females do not require any Y-specific gene products, the Y chromosome has generally been regarded as functioning only in sexually dimorphic processes, such as testis formation and male gametogenesis. This notion is incorrect. As the discussion of Turner's syndrome will show, the Y chromosome also contains genes involved in general viability, growth, and morphogenesis.

Normally there is no recombination between the X and Y chromosomes except in the most distal regions, where the chromosomes pair and recombine during male meiosis. This pairing may be important for proper chromosome segregation. It is important to note that the X and Y chromosomes bear identical copies of these recombining regions, and therefore genetic markers in these "pseudoautosomal" regions do not show strictly sex-linked inheritance. The short arm (p) pseudoautosomal region spans about 2.6 Mb and appears to be gene-rich. The region is known to contain genes for two cytokine receptor α-subunits (*CSF2RA*, *IL3RA*), an adenine nucleotide translocase *(ANT3)*, two lymphocyte cell surface antigens (*CD39*, *MIC2*), the enzyme acetylserotonin methyltransferase *(ASMT)*, a nuclear protein of unknown function *(XE7)*, and the 5' part of the gene for a red blood cell antigen *(Xg)*. Thus far, the only gene assigned to the 0.4-Mb long arm (q) pseudoautosomal region is *IL9R*, which encodes another cytokine receptor.

Only a handful of genes have been discovered in the strictly sex-linked portion of the Y chromosome. Known Y-specific genes encode the testis-determining factor *(SRY)*, a zinc-finger protein of unknown function *(ZFY)*, a ribosomal protein *(RPS4Y)*, a homolog of the tooth-bud protein amelogenin *(AMELY)*, the male transplantation antigen H-Y *(SMCY)*, and several testis-specific proteins that may function in spermatogenesis (*TSPY*, *RBM*, and *DAZ*). Interestingly, the *ZFY*, *RPS4Y*, *AMELY*, and *SMCY* genes all have closely related X homologs, perhaps reflecting divergence of the sex chromosomes from an ancestral autosome pair. Alternatively, these X-Y homologous genes may be the result of subsequent transposition events. Data on the origin of X-Y genes from evolutionary comparisons of other species are equivocal.

X INACTIVATION AND DOSAGE COMPENSATION

Unlike the genes just mentioned, the vast majority of X-linked genes do not have Y homologs. Thus males have only one copy of most X-linked genes, whereas females have two. This gender difference in the dosage of X-linked genes is balanced at the level of expression by the inactivation of one X chromosome in females during early embryogenesis, first postulated in the early 1960s by Mary Lyon. The choice of which X chromosome undergoes inactivation in each embryonic cell is normally random, but the pattern of inactivation propagates to daughter cells. Thus normal women are mosaic with regard to which X chromosome is active. The inactive X chromosome becomes hypermethylated and late-replicating, and in most tissues it condenses into the Barr body or sex chromatin. This process is irreversible except in oocytes, in which the inactive X is reactivated just before meiosis.

Cytogenetic studies of X deletions and translocations indicate that a *cis*-acting region of the proximal long arm must be present for a chromosome to undergo X inactivation. The process appar-

From: *Principles of Molecular Medicine* (J. L. Jameson, ed.), ©1998 Humana Press Inc., Totowa, NJ.

Table 58-1
Features of Selected Sex Chromosome Disorders

Disorder	*Karyotype*	*Molecular cytogenetics*	*Sexual phenotype*	*Gonads*	*Extragonadal features*	*Molecular defect*
XY gonadal dysgenesis (Swyer syndrome, XY female, MIM 306100)	46,XY	Usually normal	Female	Streak gonads; risk of gonadoblastoma	Tall stature	*SRY* mutation in some cases
XYp– Turner female	46,XY; 46,XYp–	Small Yp deletion, often with Xp;Yp translocation	Female	Streak gonads; risk of gonadoblastoma	Turner-like, especially lymphedema	Deletion of *SRY* and nearby gene(s)
XX male (MIM 278850) gene	46,XX	Y;X or Y;autosome translocation in most cases	Male	Testes with azoospermia	Klinefelter-like	Presence of *SRY* in most cases
Dosage-sensitive sex reversal (MIM 600191)	46,XY; 46,XY,dup(X); unbalanced X translocation	Xp21.2 disomy	Female	Streak gonads	No specific features	Overexpression of *DAX1* gene?
Camptomelic dysplasia with sex reversal (MIM 211970)	46,XY, sometimes abnormality involving 17q24.3-q25.1		Female	Streak gonads	Severe skeletal abnormalities, extraskeletal defects	Haploinsufficiency of *SOX9* gene
Klinefelter's syndrome	47,XXY and variants		Male	Hyalinized testes; azoospermia	Poor to normal virilization; gynecomastia; long legs	Not known
Turner's syndrome	45,X and variants		Female	Streak gonads	Short stature, webbed neck, aortic coarctation, cubitus valgus, others	Not known
45,X/46,XY mosaicism (including mixed gonadal dysgenesis)	45,X/46,XY mosaic		Male, female, or ambiguous genitalia	Streak gonads or dysgenetic testis with risk of gonadoblastoma; normal testes in some cases	Turner-like (variable)	
Gonadoblastoma (MIM 424500)	46,XY, 46,XYp–, 45,X/46,X,+mar	Presence of Y material	Female	Dysgenetic gonad	Variable	Not known
Syndrome associated with small ring X chromosomes	45,X/46,X,r(X) mosaic	Ring X lacking X inactivation center in Xq13.2	Female	Streak ovaries	Mental retardation, multiple congenital anomalies	Functional disomy of unknown X-linked genes
$46,XY_{Xq}$ syndrome	46,XYq–	Yq;Xq translocation	Male	Not reported	Mental retardation, microcephaly, other anomalies	Functional disomy of unknown X-linked genes
Azoospermia (MIM 415000)	46,XY or 46,XYq-	Yq11.23 deletion	Male	Azoospermia; variable histology	Sometimes short stature	Deletion of *DAZ* gene?

MIM numbers from Online Mendelian Inheritance in Man, OMIM™, January 1996.

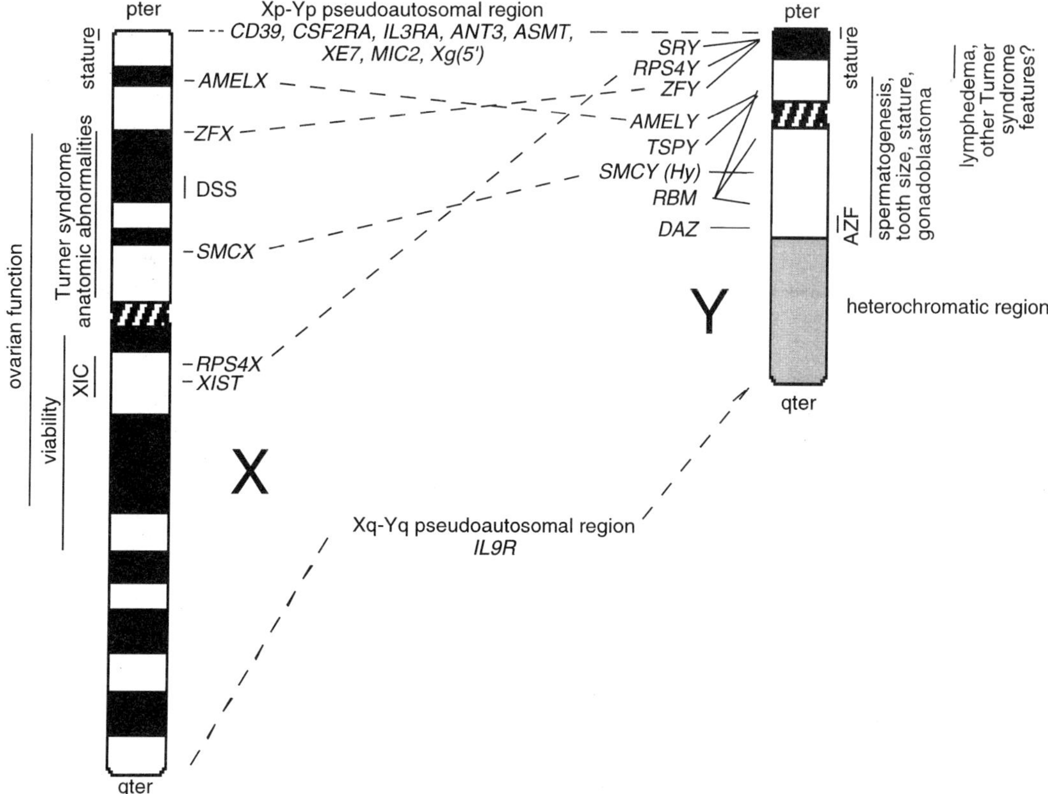

Figure 58-1 Structure and function of the human sex chromosomes. Cloned genes are italicized. Dashed lines indicate functional X-Y homologs. Vertical lines indicate loci not yet defined molecularly. pter, qter = telomores.

ently initiates within this region, termed the X inactivation center *(XIC)*, and then spreads to the rest of the chromosome. A gene discovered fortuitously in the *XIC* region termed *XIST* (X-inactive specific transcript) has been implicated in the initiation of X inactivation. The *XIST* expression pattern is unique: the gene is transcribed only from the inactive X chromosome. Expression of *XIST* precedes chromatin condensation and transcriptional inactivation of other X-linked genes. The gene is transcribed as a >15-kb polyadenylated, alternatively spliced RNA that does not appear to encode any protein. The RNA is localized within the nucleus to the Barr body, where it may serve a structural function. Once *XIST* is expressed and X inactivation has occurred, the inactive state of the chromosome is maintained by DNA methylation and chromatin condensation.

Although X inactivation is a chromosome-wide phenomenon, some specific genes escape X inactivation, i.e., they are transcribed from both the active and inactive X chromosomes. These genes are not dosage compensated. In some instances, Y-linked copies may serve instead to equalize the levels of gene products in males and females. For example, it appears that all short arm pseudoautosomal genes escape X inactivation. The X-linked homologs of the Y-linked genes *ZFY*, *RPS4Y*, and *SMCY* also escape X inactivation. However, some genes that escape X inactivation have no functional Y-linked homologs. Why such X-specific genes should escape inactivation is unclear (indeed, in most cases mouse orthologs undergo X inactivation). The signals that determine whether a gene is subject to X inactivation are unknown. Some genes that escape X inactivation are clustered, and local chromatin structure is likely to be important.

DISORDERS OF SEX DETERMINATION

Classic studies indicated that phenotypic sex in the fruit fly *Drosophila melanogaster* is determined by the numerical ratio of X chromosomes to autosomes; the *Drosophila* Y chromosome is genetically inert with regard to sex determination. It was once thought that the same mechanism of sex determination would be true for mammals. However, karyotyping studies in the late 1950s showed that XO and XX humans are female, whereas XY and XXY individuals are male. These data established the Y chromosome's primacy in human testis determination. Further cytogenetic and molecular genetic studies of rare "sex reversed" XX males and XY females culminated with the report in 1990 by Peter Goodfellow and colleagues of the single Y-linked gene, *SRY* (sex-determining region Y), that directs the differentiation of the bipotential gonad into testes. The human *SRY* gene encodes a protein of 204 amino acids that belongs to the high-mobility group (HMG) family of DNA-binding proteins. The gene is expressed in adult testis (where its function is unknown) and transiently in the gonadal ridge during embryogenesis. In all likelihood *SRY* acts by regulating transcription of other genes. The SRY protein binds to the minor groove of the double helix at specific sequences, and its binding induces a bend in the target DNA. It is not yet known which genes are regulated by *SRY*, nor is it certain whether SRY binding activates or inhibits transcription. One gene that might be activated by SRY binding is *MIS*, which encodes the Müllerian inhibiting substance that causes regression of the presumptive female reproductive tract.

The discovery of *SRY* has clarified the etiology of most cases of XX sex reversal. The *SRY* gene and adjacent Y chromosome

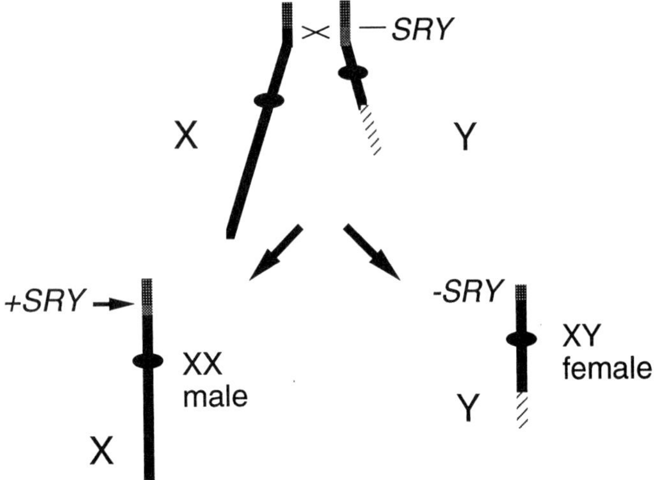

Figure 58-2 Aberrant Xp-Yp interchange.

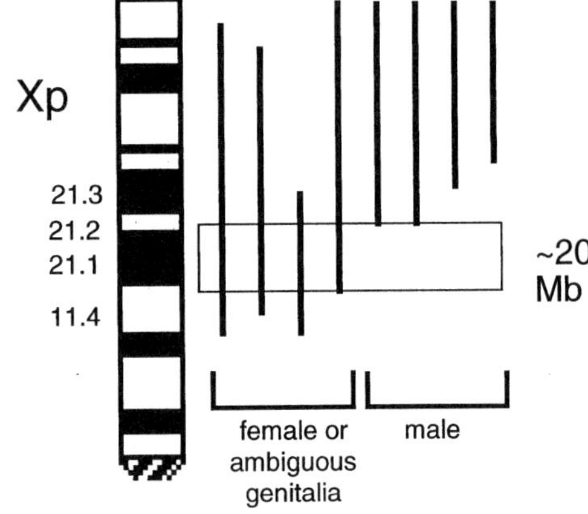

Figure 58-3 Sexual phenotype of XY individuals with various Xp duplications.

sequences can be detected in most XX males by DNA hybridization or polymerase chain reaction (PCR) assays. The most frequent location of *SRY* sequences in these males is the short arm of the X chromosome. *SRY*'s propensity to be translocated from Yp to Xp can be explained by the gene's proximity to the pseudoautosomal region. The mechanism of transposition involves aberrant X-Y interchange during male meiosis (Fig. 58-2).

The translocated *SRY* gene is probably subject to X inactivation. Some cases of incomplete sex reversal, e.g., XX true hermaphroditism (presence of both testicular and ovarian tissue), may be due to mosaic *SRY* expression as a result of stochastic X inactivation.

Mutations that eliminate *SRY* or affect the region of the protein involved in DNA binding cause XY sex reversal. However, only about 10% of XY females have detectable *SRY* mutations. The remaining 90% remain unexplained and are presumably caused by environmental factors or mutations in other genes required for testis determination.

One such gene has already been identified because of its similarity to *SRY*. This gene, denoted *SOX9* (SRY box), was cloned as a member of the *SRY* subfamily of HMG proteins. Lesions in one copy of the *SOX9* gene, which maps to chromosome 17, have been discovered in several patients with camptomelic dysplasia, a rare skeletal disorder associated with XY sex reversal. The other copy of the gene in these patients is apparently normal. The mechanism by which half-normal dosage, or haploinsufficiency, of *SOX9* causes both skeletal malformations and sex reversal is not yet known. Expression studies of the mouse homolog are consistent with the direct involvement of *SOX9* in both abnormalities.

Still another gene has been implicated in sex determination by studies of sex chromosome disorders. A number of XY females have been reported with partial X chromosome duplications that include band Xp21.1 of the short arm (Fig. 58-3). Because, in the absence of a second X chromosome, the duplicated X is not inactivated, sex reversal is thought to be caused by twofold increase in expression of a gene or genes within the duplication.

Using molecular markers to study these subjects and 27 other unexplained 46,XY females, Bardoni et al. identified a submicroscopic Xp duplication in one subject and delimited the critical region of Xp21.1 associated with sex reversal to just 160 kb. They designated the Xp locus causing sex reversal *DSS* (dosage-sensitive sex reversal). An attractive candidate gene for *DSS* known to lie within the critical region is *DAX1*, a member of the nuclear hormone receptor gene superfamily. Loss of function mutations in *DAX1* cause congenital adrenal hypoplasia and hypogonadotropic hypogonadism but do not prevent testis determination. An interesting notion is that *DSS* may represent an ovary determining gene. Whether the *DAX1* gene is indeed *DSS* should become clear from experiments using transgenic mice.

SEX CHROMOSOME ANEUPLOIDIES

XY sex reversal associated with *SOX9* haploinsufficiency or *DSS* duplication illustrates the critical importance of proper gene dosage. Abnormal gene dosage also plays a role in the phenotypes of numerical sex chromosome disorders, or aneuploidies. The most common sex chromosome aneuploidy is Klinefelter's syndrome (47,XXY; 46,XY/47,XXY; and variants), with an incidence of about 1 in 500 male births. The extra X chromosome is usually the result of meiotic nondisjunction during paternal or maternal gametogenesis. The phenotype is variable but is characterized by small, firm testes, azoospermia, tall stature, eunuchoid habitus, gynecomastia, and elevated gonadotropin levels (Fig. 58-4). Azoospermia is caused by loss of spermatogenic cells. Animal studies suggest that this loss is somehow caused by the presence of an unpaired X chromosome at the pachytene stage of meiosis. Hyalinization of seminiferous tubules and impaired Leydig cell testosterone production follows loss of germ cells. Exogenous androgen is the treatment of choice for testosterone deficiency, whereas treatment of severe gynecomastia is surgical.

The phenotype of Klinefelter's syndrome is mild compared to disorders involving an extra autosome, for example trisomy 21 (Down's syndrome). The reason for the milder phenotype in XXY men is that the additional X chromosome undergoes inactivation, whereas extra autosomes in other aneuploidy syndromes remain active. For this same reason, XXX females are usually normal, although they may be subfertile. Individuals with greater degrees of X aneuploidy (e.g., 48,XXXY; 48,XXXX; 49,XXXXY; or 49,XXXXX karyotypes) often show more severe abnormalities, even though all the supernumerary chromosomes undergo X inactivation. These abnormalities, which include mental retardation and skeletal malformations, are presumably caused by increased dosage of genes that escape X inactivation. Interestingly, some

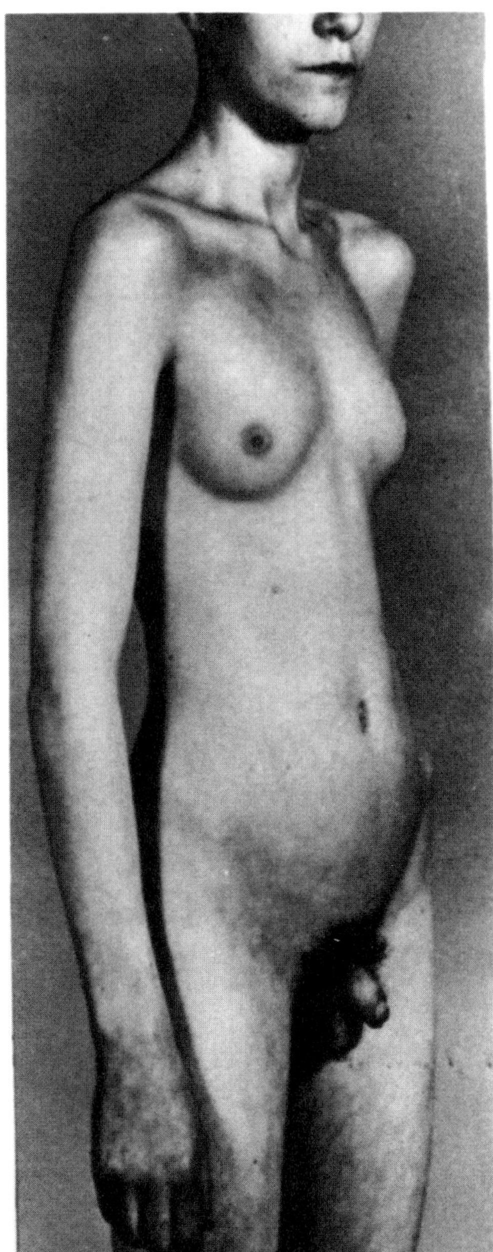

Figure 58-4 Klinefelter's syndrome. (Used with permission from Blackwell Science.)

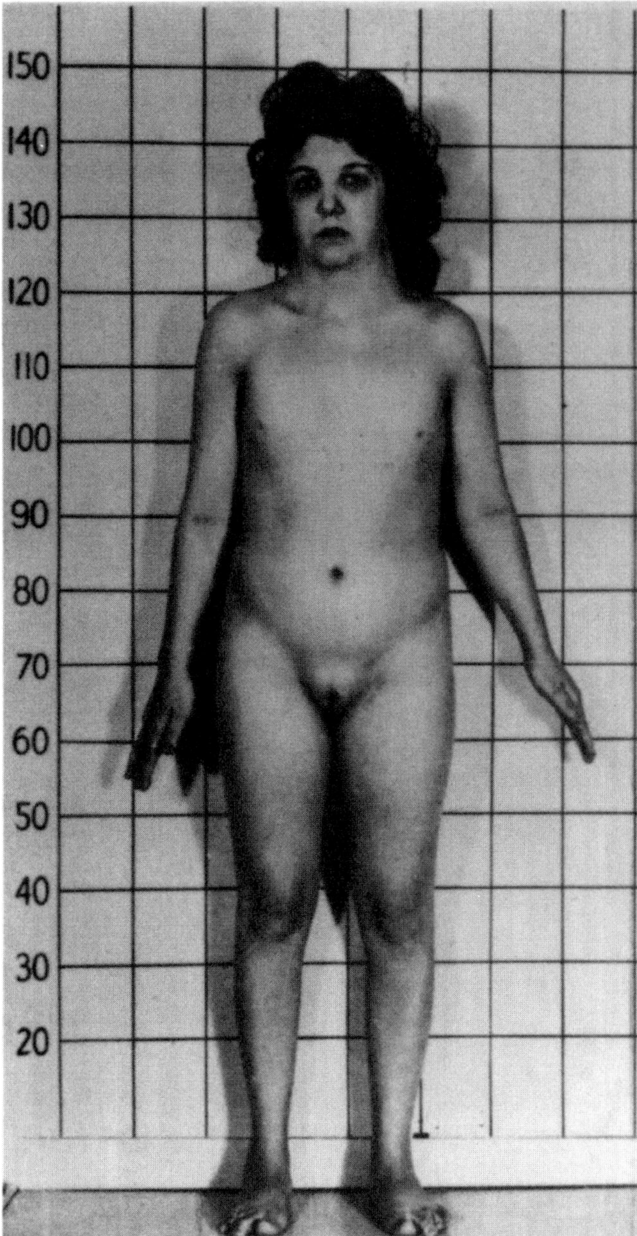

Figure 58-5 Turner's syndrome. (Used with permission from Blackwell Science.)

similar features have been noted in men with severe Y aneuploidy, such as 48,XYYY or 49,XYYYY karyotypes, suggesting that the culprit genes may be X-Y homologous or pseudoautosomal.

By contrast to Klinefelter's syndrome, the loss of one sex chromosome, or monosomy X, causes the more severe disorder known as Turner's syndrome. Partial or complete monosomy X (45,X karyotype) is found in about 1 in every 3000 liveborn girls. The prenatal incidence is much greater: as many as 2% of all human conceptuses are estimated to be 45,X, but fewer than 1% survive to term. Paradoxically, liveborns with monosomy X have only modestly reduced life expectancy. An adult woman with Turner's syndrome is shown in Fig. 58-5. As with Klinefelter's syndrome, the phenotype is variable. Characteristic features include growth retardation, ovarian failure, and specific physical abnormalities, such as webbed neck, aortic coarctation, increased carrying angle of the elbows (cubitus valgus), lymphedema, horseshoe kidney, and others. Metabolic and endocrine abnormalities are also frequent, including hypertension, glucose intolerance, and autoimmune thyroid disease. Girls with Turner's syndrome are not typically mentally retarded, although as a group they show selective impairment of nonverbal cognitive skills such as visual-spatial abilities.

The pathophysiology of Turner's syndrome is poorly understood. Growth retardation is not caused by growth hormone deficiency, although administration of pharmacologic doses during childhood accelerates growth and may increase final stature. Ovarian failure reflects rapid oocyte loss beginning around 6 months of gestation. Usually by early infancy there are few or no remaining oocytes, and the ovaries become fibrous streaks. Infertility is the rule, with rare exceptions. Ovarian sex steroid production is usually deficient, and most girls with Turner's syndrome require hormonal replacement therapy to induce puberty and to maintain cyclic menses. Some extragonadal manifestations, such as webbed neck, lymphedema of the extremities, and perhaps aortic coarctation, may be caused by delayed or defective lymphatic vessel development.

The mechanism of chromosome loss in Turner's syndrome is not known. Meiotic nondisjunction probably accounts for only a minority of cases. The single X chromosome is maternal in about three-fourths and paternal in about one-fourth of 45,X patients. There are no imprinting effects, i.e., the parental origin of the X does not appear to influence the phenotype. Many patients with Turner's syndrome have karyotypic variants of monosomy X, most commonly mosaicism, the presence of two or more cell lines with different karyotypes (e.g., 45,X/46,XX). Mosaicism results from mitotic errors after conception. The second cell line often contains a structurally aberrant X chromosome. Mosaicism for a cell line with two or more copies of the X chromosome long arm enhances viability as compared with the nonmosaic 45,X constitution.

Mosaicism for a Y-bearing cell line, most often 45,X/46,XY karyotype, deserves particular mention. The phenotype varies depending upon the proportion of XY cells and their tissue distribution. Bilateral testes may be present, or there may be unilateral testicular tissue with a contralateral streak gonad, a condition termed mixed gonadal dysgenesis (*see* Chapter 57). Regardless of the sexual phenotype, the presence of a Y chromosome confers a high risk of gonadoblastoma, a malignant tumor arising in the dysgenetic gonad. Prophylactic removal of streak gonads or histologically abnormal testes is recommended in any patient whose karyotype includes Y material. The Y-linked gene(s) predisposing to gonadoblastoma appears to be distinct from *SRY*, because XY females with *SRY* deletions or mutations are still at risk. Some studies using sensitive PCR assays have reported an alarmingly high prevalence of cryptic Y sequences in Turner's syndrome patients. However, in the absence of testes or virilization, the clinical significance of low levels of Y material detected by PCR but not by karyotype is uncertain.

Several genetic mechanisms underlie the phenotype of Turner's syndrome. Oocyte loss may be caused in part by the effects of an unpaired X chromosome during meiosis, analogous to spermatogonia loss in Klinefelter's syndrome. Haploinsufficiency, or half-normal dosage of X-linked genes, may also contribute to ovarian failure. As previously noted, the inactive X chromosome is reactivated in oocytes; diploid expression of certain X-linked genes may be required for normal oocyte function. Consistent with this hypothesis, small deletions of Xq have been observed in some otherwise normal women with premature menopause.

Anatomic abnormalities, such as lymphedema associated with Turner's syndrome, suggest that diploid dosage of certain X-linked genes is important not only for ovarian function, but also for extragonadal development. Yet, after early embryogenesis, only one X chromosome is active in somatic tissues of normal women. This apparent contradiction can be explained if the genes responsible for extragonadal Turner features escape X inactivation. How then do we explain normal development in males, who have only one X chromosome? One possibility is male-specific upregulation of X-linked gene expression, the mechanism of dosage compensation in *Drosophila*. However, there is no evidence for such upregulation in mammals. Another possibility is that in addition to its role in sex determination, the Y chromosome supplies a second copy of certain genes whose dosage is critical for normal somatic development.

Present data, although not definitive, favor the latter hypothesis. Deletions of either the Xp or Yp pseudoautosomal region are associated with short stature, suggesting that at least part of the growth retardation in Turner's syndrome is caused by haploinsufficiency of one or more pseudoautosomal genes. A strong candidate called *SHOX* (short stature homeobox-containing gene) was discovered by Rao and colleagues. Other evidence that X-Y homologous genes play a role in Turner's syndrome comes from studies of Y deletions associated with sex reversal. Rare XY females with *SRY* deletions can arise by the same mechanism of aberrant Xp-Yp interchange that causes XX males (Fig. 58-2). In addition to streak gonads, these XYp– females almost invariably display extragonadal Turner's syndrome features, most commonly lymphedema. By contrast, XY females with *SRY* point mutations or intragenic deletions have streak ovaries but no extragonadal manifestations of Turner's syndrome. These data imply that there is at least one Y-linked Turner's syndrome gene near *SRY*. David Page and colleagues have identified two candidate genes in this region, *ZFY* and *RPS4Y*. Both genes have X-linked homologs that escape X inactivation, as predicted for Turner's syndrome genes. The *ZFX* and *ZFY* genes encode highly similar zinc finger proteins of unknown function that may be transcription factors. The *RPS4X* and *RPS4Y* genes encode isoforms of S4, a ubiquitous ribosomal small subunit protein. The S4X and S4Y proteins have been shown to function interchangeably in ribosomes, consistent with the hypothesis that *RPS4Y* serves to provide a second dose of S4 in males. However, the amount of S4Y in ribosomes is only about 10% that of S4X, and no biochemical consequences of S4 haploinsufficiency have been demonstrated. Thus the role of either *RPS4X/RPS4Y* or *ZFX/ZFY* in Turner's syndrome is speculative. Interestingly, the mouse *Zfx* and *Rps4* genes are both subject to X inactivation. Moreover, there do not appear to be functionally interchangeably mouse Y homologs. Even though the overall complement of X-linked genes in humans and mice is very similar, the XO mouse has good viability, is fertile, and is anatomically normal. Species differences in X inactivation and X-Y homology may explain the striking contrast in the phenotype of monosomy X in mice versus humans.

OTHER SEX CHROMOSOME DISORDERS

One variant of Turner's syndrome that has received much attention involves mosaicism for a ring X chromosome, or 45,X/46,X,r(X) karyotype. The associated phenotype varies dramatically. Some individuals have typical Turner's syndrome, whereas others show more severe abnormalities such as mental retardation and multiple congenital anomalies. The severity of the phenotype correlates inversely with the size of the ring; larger rings tend to be associated with a milder phenotype.

It is remarkable that a partial deletion, e.g., a ring, can be more deleterious (at least in liveborns) than the complete absence of one X chromosome. The explanation may lie with X inactivation and dosage compensation. Some small ring X chromosomes lack the *XIC* region; others retain *XIC* but fail to express the *XIST* gene (Fig. 58-6).

The absence of *XIST* expression correlates with the severity of the phenotype. Barbara Migeon and coworkers have shown that

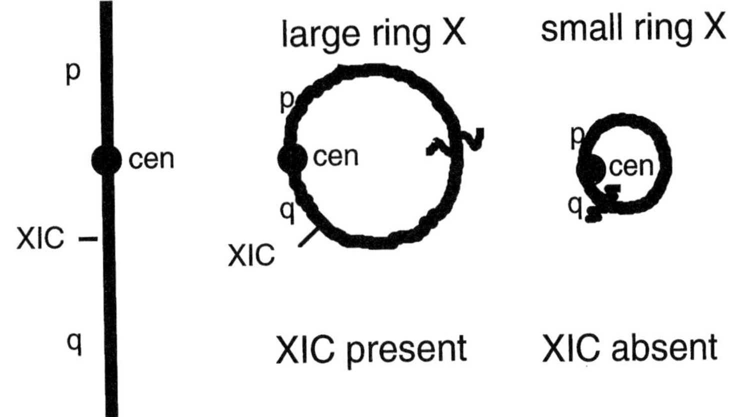

Figure 58-6 Two types of ring X chromosomes.

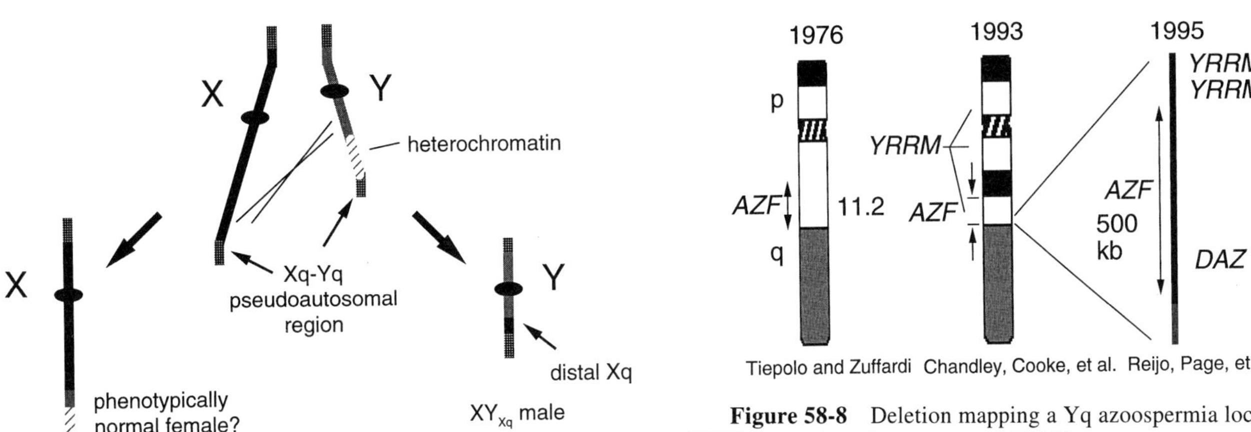

Figure 58-7 Aberrant Xq-Yq interchange.

Figure 58-8 Deletion mapping a Yq azoospermia locus. (*YRRM* genes have been renamed *RBM*.)

rings that fail to express *XIST* express some genes that are normally X inactivated. Thus the severe phenotype associated with mosaicism for a small ring X chromosome is probably caused by overexpression of one or more X-linked genes, as yet unidentified.

The importance of dosage compensation is also illustrated by another sex chromosome disorder. About one in every 1000 males lacks a portion of Yq, including the heterochromatic region. Men with the 46,XYq– karyotype are often normal, consistent with the absence of genes in this region. Deletions extending into the Yq euchromatic region are sometimes associated with short stature or infertility. In rare cases there are severe abnormalities, such as mental retardation, microcephaly, and other dysmorphic features. The severity of the phenotype does not generally correlate with the extent of the deletion.

After the discovery of long arm pseudoautosomal region, David Page and colleagues speculated that aberrant Xq-Yq interchange might be one cause of Yq deletions, just as aberrant Xp-Yp recombination causes Yp deletions (Fig. 58-2). To test this hypothesis, they studied ten 46,XYq– males and found evidence of aberrant Xq-Yq recombination in three subjects. All three had severe phenotypes. The other seven subjects in whom there was no evidence of abnormal X-Y recombination showed only mild or moderate abnormalities. In the three severely affected subjects, portions of distal Xq as large as 10 Mb were translocated to the Y chromosome, resulting in partial X disomy (Fig. 58-7).

One X-linked gene within the translocated portion, *G6PD* (glucose-6-phosphate dehydrogenase), was shown to be expressed from both the normal X and the translocated portion, leading to a twofold increase in enzyme activity. Page et al. concluded that diploid dosage of one or more genes in distal Xq caused the severe phenotypes of the three severely affected subjects. They termed this disorder the "XY_{Xq} syndrome."

Molecular characterization of Yq deletions has also yielded insight into the function of the Y chromosome in male reproduction. As noted above, some men with cytogenetically visible Yq deletions have azoospermia (the absence of sperm in semen), suggesting that the euchromatic portion of Yq contains one or more genes important in spermatogenesis. This Yq locus is denoted *AZF* (azoospermia factor) (Fig. 58-8).

Several groups have found using DNA assays that up to 10% of men with unexplained azoospermia bear *de novo* Yq microdeletions. Two candidates for *AZF* have been identified by positional cloning. The first is a family of Y-specific genes originally called *YRRM* (Y RNA recognition motifs), discovered by Ann Chandley, Howard Cooke, and colleagues. These genes, now designated *RBM,* are members of a larger family of RNA-binding proteins. There are at least three functional genes and numerous Y-linked pseudogenes. Most *RBM* sequences are clustered near the *AZF* region of distal Yq, but related sequences are also present near the centromere on both Yp and Yq. One of the functional genes is absent in most normal Japanese men and thus appears to represent a normal polymorphism. The *RBM* genes are expressed specifically in germ cells, where they may play a role in RNA splicing or packaging during spermatogenesis. The presence of multiple *RBM* genes, at least some of which are polymorphic, makes it difficult to infer their importance from naturally occurring deletions.

The second *AZF* candidate, termed *DAZ* (deleted in azoospermia), was discovered by Rene Reijo, David Page, and colleagues. Like the *RBM* genes, *DAZ* encodes an RNA recognition motif and shows testis-specific expression. Reijo et al. found that *DAZ* but not *RBM* was deleted in 12 of 89 azoospermic men with *de novo* Yq deletions. Interestingly, testicular biopsies from some of these men showed variable defects, even among adjacent seminiferous tubules in some instances. The defects ranged from the complete absence of germ cells (Sertoli-cell-only syndrome) to meiotic arrest with occasional mature condensed spermatids. *DAZ* is a strong candidate for *AZF*, the locus whose frequent deletion is associated with azoospermia, but this does not rule out a role for the *RBM* genes as well in spermatogenesis. Understanding the precise functions of these male-specific genes is the subject of active investigation.

SUMMARY

The study of human sex chromosome disorders has been richly rewarding. Classic chromosome studies of Klinefelter's syndrome, Turner's syndrome, and mixed gonadal dysgenesis revealed the mechanism of mammalian testis determination. Genetic studies are now yielding molecular explanations for disorders of sex determination. Identification of genes responsible for other phenotypes associated with sex chromosome disorders, such as the ring X syndrome, the XY_{Xq} syndrome, and Turner's syndrome, should be forthcoming. Molecular studies of these "experiments of nature" will also provide further insight into the unique biology of the mammalian sex chromosomes.

SELECTED REFERENCES

Online Mendelian Inheritance in Man, OMIM™. 1996. Center for Medical Genetics, Johns Hopkins University, Baltimore, MD, and National Center for Biotechnology Information, National Library of Medicine, Bethesda, MD. World Wide Web URL: http://www3.ncbi.nlm.nih.gov/omim/

Affara NA, Lau YF, Briggs H, et al. Report and abstracts of the first international workshop on Y chromosome mapping 1994. Cytogenet Cell Genet 1994;67:359–402.

Anonymous [editorial]. SOX9 and the switch hitting genes. Nat Genet 1995;9:1,2.

Bardoni B, Zamaria E, Guioli S, et al. A dosage sensitive locus at chromosome Xp21 is involved in male to female sex reversal. Nat Genet 1994;7:497–501.

Bogan JS, Page DC. Ovary? Testis?—a mammalian dilemma. Cell 1994;76:603–607.

Cooke HJ, Elliott DJ. RNA-binding proteins and human male infertility. Trends Genet 1997;13:87–89.

Foresta C, Ferlin A, Garolla A, Rossato M, Barbaux S, De Bortoli A. Y-chromosome deletions in idiopathic severe testiculopathies. J Clin Endocrinol Metab 1997;82:1075–1080.

Herzing LB, Romer JT, Horn JM, Ashworth A. Xist has properties of the X-chromosome inactivation centre. Nature 1997;386:272–275.

Lahn BT, Ma N, Breg WR, Sratton R, Surti U, Page DC. Xq-Yq interchange resulting in supernormal X-linked gene expression in severely retarded males with 46,XYq– karyotype. Nat Genet 1994; 8:243–250.

Migeon BR. X-chromosome inactivation: molecular mechanisms and genetic consequences. Trends Genet 1994;10:230–235.

Pevny LH, Lovell-Badge R. Sox genes find their feet. Curr Opin Genet Dev 1997;7:338–344.

Rao E, Weiss B, Fukami M, et al. Pseudoautosomal deletions encompassing a novel homeobox gene cause growth failure in idiopathic short stature and Turner syndrome. Nat Genet 1997;16:54–63.

Reijo R, Lee TY, Salo P, et al. Diverse spermatogenic defects in humans caused by Y chromosome deletions encompassing a novel RNA-binding protein. Nat Genet 1995;10:383–393.

Schwartz ID, Root AW. The Klinefelter syndrome of testicular dysgenesis. Endocrinol Metab Clin North Am 1991;20:153–163.

Skuse DH, James RS, Bishop DV, et al. Evidence from Turner's syndrome of an imprinted X-linked locus affecting cognitive function. Nature 1997;387:705–708.

Willard HF, Cremers F, Mandel JL, Monaco AP, Nelson DL, Schlessinger D. Report and abstracts of the fifth international workshop on human X chromosome mapping 1994. Cytogenet Cell Genet 1994;67: 295–358.

Zinn AR. Growing interest in Turner syndrome. Nat Genet 1997;16:3,4.

Zinn AR, Page DC, Fisher EMC. Turner syndrome—the case of the missing sex chromosome. Trends Genet 1993;9:90–93.

59 Disorders of Pubertal Development

KAREN D. BRADSHAW AND CHARMIAN A. QUIGLEY

INTRODUCTION

Puberty is a complex developmental process that culminates in sexual-maturity. This transitional period begins in late childhood and is characterized by maturation of the hypothalamic–pituitary–gonadal axis, the appearance of secondary sexual characteristics, acceleration of growth, and ultimately the capacity for fertility. Significant endocrinologic changes accompany these developmental events. This chapter reviews the physiologic changes of normal puberty and examines the causes of precocious and delayed sexual maturation.

NORMAL PUBERTAL DEVELOPMENT

The age at which the somatic changes of puberty begins is variable. In industrialized countries, pubertal changes usually begin between 8 and 13 years of age in girls, and between 9 and 14 years of age in boys. This variability in the time of onset is likely a reflection of the number of distinct influences that can affect the time at which it begins, both genetic and environmental. Approximately 5% of a given population will have the onset of puberty at an age outside of this range and will be considered to have either precocious or delayed puberty.

In girls, the first somatic change that occurs is usually the beginning of breast development (thelarche), although in a minority of instances, pubic hair growth (pubarche) is the initial event. Thelarche and pubarche occur at mean ages of 10.9 and 11.2 years, respectively. Although the process of pubertal development is in fact a continuum, for descriptive purposes it is usually described in terms of a series of distinct stages, the five stages of breast and pubic hair development outlined by Marshall and Tanner being the most commonly employed scheme (Table 59-1). In parallel with the somatic changes of puberty, the volume of the ovaries and uterus enlarges, and the mucosa of the vagina thickens and becomes keratinized, evidenced clinically by lightening of the color of the mucosa from a deep red to a pale pink. After a variable period, averaging a little less than 2 years from the onset of breast development, most of the processes of pubertal maturation are complete, and menarche (the first menstrual period) occurs. Although most girls achieve menarche a little before their 13th birthday, the timing of this event is variable, and may occur as late as 14½ years in normal girls.

From: *Principles of Molecular Medicine* (J. L. Jameson, ed.), ©1998 Humana Press Inc., Totowa, NJ.

As in girls, puberty in boys is often described as a series of five distinct stages, based on testicular size, penile development, and distribution and character of pubic hair. In boys, the first physical evidence of puberty is an increase in testicular size. Measurement of the testes (length and width) or estimation of testicular volume using a Prader orchidiometer allows for early detection of pubertal onset. Testicular volume of 4.0 mL (or length of 2.5 cm), representing the onset of puberty, is noted at an average age of about 11½ years. Testicular enlargement is followed by scrotal thinning, development of pubic hair, and penile enlargement. Adult testicular volumes and penile dimensions are generally achieved by about 16 years of age; however, there is quite marked individual variation, with young men completing their sexual maturation anywhere between the ages of 14 and 18 years.

In addition to the appearance and development of secondary sexual characteristics in both boys and girls, puberty represents a period during which marked changes in body size and composition occur. Before the onset of puberty, the bodies of boys and girls are composed of similar proportions of adipose tissue and muscle. By the end of puberty, boys have a higher percentage of muscle and a lower percentage of fat relative to girls. It is during this period that the most rapid increases in bone mineralization occur.

PHYSIOLOGY OF PUBERTY

HORMONES AND PUBERTY Puberty is a period during which many dramatic hormonal changes occur. Of these, it is clear that changes in the axes controlling the secretion of growth hormone and gonadal steroids play central roles in this process.

Growth hormone (GH) is produced by the somatotrophs of the anterior pituitary gland. Although its control is complex, its synthesis and release is under the principal control of growth hormone releasing hormone (GHRH), which is released by the nerve endings of the hypothalamic GHRH neurons into the hypophyseal portal circulation. In response to pulses of GHRH, the pituitary releases pulses of GH into the systemic circulation. GH exerts its effects by binding to high-affinity receptors on the surfaces of responsive cells.

Although GH certainly modulates some biologic processes directly, in many tissues the actions of GH are modulated indirectly through the action of growth factors that are produced in response to the action of GH, specifically insulin-like growth factor-1 (IGF-I, previously known as somatomedin C) and its complex series of binding proteins. Serum levels of IGF-I rise with age in concert with age-related increases in mean GH levels.

Table 59-1
Stages of Development of Secondary Sexual Characteristics

Boys: genital (penis) development	
Stage 1	Prepubertal: testes, scrotum, and penis of about same size and proportion as in early childhood.
Stage 2	Enlargement of scrotum and testes. Skin of scrotum reddens and changes in texture.
Stage 3	Enlargement of penis, at first mainly in length. Further growth of testes and scrotum.
Stage 4	Increased size of penis with growth in breadth and development of glans. Testes and scrotum larger; scrotal skin darkened.
Stage 5	Genitalia adult in size and shape.
Girls: breast development	
Stage 1	Prepubertal: elevation of papilla only.
Stage 2	Breast bud stage: elevation of breast and papilla as small mound. Enlargement of areola diameter.
Stage 3	Further enlargement and elevation of breast and areola, with no separation of their contours.
Stage 4	Projection of areola and papilla to form a secondary mound above level of breast.
Stage 5	Mature stage: projection of papilla only, related to recession of areola to general contour of breast.
Both sexes: pubic hair	
Stage 1	Prepubertal: vellus over pubes is not further developed than over abdominal wall.
Stage 2	Sparse growth of long, slightly pigmented, downy hair, straight or slightly curled, chiefly at base of penis or along labia.
Stage 3	Considerably darker, coarser, and more curled hair. Hair spreads sparsely over junction of pubes.
Stage 4	Hair now adult in type, but area covered is still considerably smaller than in adult. No spread to medial surface of thighs.
Stage 5	Adult in quantity and type with distribution of horizontal (or classically "feminine") pattern.
Stage 6	Spread up linea alba (male-type pattern).

At the onset of puberty, increased activity of the gonadotropin releasing hormone (GnRH) pulse generator causes a progressive rise in mean concentrations of gonadotropins, resulting from an increase in the frequency and amplitude of GnRH pulses *(see below)*. These increases are first detected as nocturnal gonadotropin pulses, but as puberty progresses gonadotropin pulses also increase during daytime, until adult mean gonadotropin levels are achieved.

More recently, a role for leptin, the recently described hormone produced by adipose tissue, in the onset of puberty has been described. In leptin-deficient ob/ob mice, treatment with leptin restores puberty and fertility. Subsequent studies have demonstrated that treatment of normal prepubertal mice with leptin accelerates maturation of the reproductive tract and results in earlier reproduction. Similarly, in prepubertal boys, leptin levels increase several months before the onset of puberty, as determined by the initial rise in testosterone.

Concentrations of a variety of other hormones also change with onset and progression of puberty. As a result of increased sex steroid concentrations, sex hormone-binding globulin is lower during puberty than in childhood. The gonadal peptide inhibin, structurally related to transforming growth factor-β (TGF-β), is regulated by and involved in regulation of follicle-stimulating hormone (FSH). This product of Sertoli and granulosa cells shows a progressive increase in mean concentration with advancing puberty in both sexes. Concentrations of the glycoprotein anti-Müllerian hormone (AMH) show quite marked sexual dimorphism. AMH is produced in Sertoli cells and is relatively high in newborn boys, but undetectable in girls. In contrast, the hormone becomes very low in boys during puberty, at which time AMH concentrations increase in girls.

The role of estrogens in the process of skeletal maturation in both boys and girls had been postulated for some time. As an example, effective suppression of the rapid skeletal maturation seen in boys with gonadotropin-independent forms of precocious puberty requires inhibition of aromatase activity to reduce serum estradiol concentrations, in addition to antiandrogens to interfere with androgen action. Furthermore, a female patient with a genetic deficiency of aromatase activity had no pubertal growth spurt and exhibited delayed skeletal maturation, indicating that estrogens are required for these events.

Inferences drawn from such cases regarding the importance of estrogen in promoting skeletal maturation in both sexes are reinforced by contrasting the patterns of pubertal development in syndromes of androgen and estrogen resistance. Studies of patients with complete testicular feminization (complete androgen insensitivity) have documented that a normal pubertal growth spurt is observed with the onset of pubertal gonadal function. Such findings suggest that the effects of gonadal steroids in male pubertal development are not mediated via the androgen receptor, but are instead exerted indirectly after the conversion of testosterone to estrogen.

The study of a male patient with estrogen resistance, in whom estrogens are unable to exert their effects at the tissue level, confirms these deductions. In this patient with estrogen resistance, an inactivating mutation of the estrogen receptor was shown to have several discernible physiologic consequences. First, the epiphyseal growth plates of this man demonstrated no evidence of epiphyseal fusion. Consequently, at the time of diagnosis (age 28) the patient was still growing. In addition to these effects on bone maturation, skeletal mineralization was also abnormal. At age 28, the patient's mineral bone density was markedly decreased, even when corrected for his retarded bone age of 15 years.

These considerations emphasize the complex hormonal interactions that characterize the process of normal puberty. It is clear that the normal functioning of each of these components is necessary for normal pubertal development to occur. As described below, abnormalities at many levels can disrupt normal pubertal growth, development and maturation.

MATURATION OF THE HYPOTHALAMIC–PITUITARY–GONADAL AXIS Maturation of the reproductive system occurs in a phasic manner in humans and in higher primates, and can be viewed as occurring in several distinct stages.

The first stage, which begins during fetal life and lasts until late infancy, is characterized by development of the neuroendocrine systems responsible for regulation of the reproductive system. The area in the arcuate nucleus of the hypothalamus destined to become the GnRH pulse generator develops intrinsic and unregulated pulsatile activity by about 11 weeks of gestation. During this stage the reproductive system appears to be fully active, with gonadotropin and sex steroid hormone concentrations being measurable in fetal plasma. Concentrations of luteinizing hormone (LH) and FSH peak at about 4–5 months' gestational age. Later in gestation, negative feedback from gonadal steroids begins to regulate the unrestrained pulsatile activity of the hypothalamic pulse generator and by term, gonadotropin levels (and by inference the activity of the GnRH pulse generator) are low.

At the time of delivery the infant is separated from the dominant source of sex steroids, the placenta, and owing to the withdrawal of this negative feedback, the levels of gonadotropins rise. This increase is responsible for a transient secondary stimulation of the infant's gonads occurring in the first months after birth. Although occurring in both boys and girls, this is observed most readily in female infants in whom there may be prolonged neonatal breast budding.

By 6 months of postnatal age, gonadotropin and sex steroids concentrations in plasma have again declined to low levels and the third stage of maturation begins. This stage lasts throughout childhood, and is characterized by low plasma concentrations of LH, FSH, and sex steroids.

From a physiologic perspective, the prepubertal stage of development presents apparent contradictions. Measurements of gonadotropins and sex steroids during fetal development suggest that the hypothalamic–gonadal axis has completely developed *in utero* and that it is regulated by steroid hormones during the latter stages of pregnancy. Despite this, during the prepubertal period, gonadotropins remain low even when sex steroid concentrations are extremely low, such as in patients with Turner's syndrome or in castrate children. That serum gonadotropin concentrations remain low under such conditions suggests that additional inhibitory mechanisms in the central nervous system or hypothalamus have developed. Early studies to explain these different regulatory behaviors focused on examining the sensitivity of the hypothalamus and pituitary to feedback inhibition by gonadal steroids. Such investigations demonstrated that the levels of estrogen and androgen required to inhibit LH and FSH secretion in young prepubertal animals and in humans are consistently lower than those required to suppress gonadotropin levels to an equivalent extent in adult castrate animals. Such differences in the sensitivity of regulation of gonadotropin secretion in young prepubertal and adult animals have been described in a number of different species. Although such observations have substantial power in explaining the prepubertal quiescence of gonadotropin secretion, other observations suggest that additional mechanisms might also be operative. Although mean serum concentrations of gonadotropins are low during the prepubertal period, the reproductive system is not completely inhibited during this stage, because small spontaneous LH pulses occur at a low frequency in normal children.

The fourth stage, puberty itself, occurs as the result of reactivation of the reproductive axis. Although a great deal of effort has been expended to identify the signals that control the onset of puberty, it appears that the mechanisms responsible for the initiation of pubertal events are extremely complex and likely involve the integration of numerous different signals, including attainment of a certain body mass or composition and perhaps neural signals derived from centers within the central nervous system that serve as a biologic clock.

The onset of puberty is heralded by striking increases in nocturnal LH secretion, manifest by an increase in amplitude and frequency of LH pulses. These increases of LH precede rises of sex steroid concentrations and the development of secondary sex characteristics. As pubertal maturation progresses, the amplitude and frequency of gonadotropin pulses also increase during the day, in a pattern similar to that seen at night, until the final stage of sexual maturation, adulthood, is reached. In this period, regular pulses of GnRH establish the mature pattern of gonadal steroid secretion. In females, this results in the regular cyclical variations of gonadotropins, estrogen, and progesterone characteristic of the menstrual cycle. In males, the same regular pulses of GnRH establish a pattern characterized by relatively constant levels of testosterone and gonadotropins, with minimal diurnal variation.

VARIATIONS OF NORMAL PUBERTY

EARLY Fairly common forms of partial premature pubertal development are the isolated development of pubic hair (premature pubarche) and the isolated development of breasts (premature thelarche). Although these are benign conditions, such patients must be followed closely to monitor for progression to constitutional precocious puberty (CPP).

Precocious pubarche is most often a benign condition secondary to early adrenarche. Balducci et al. studied 171 subjects with isolated precocious pubarche. Mild abnormalities of steroidogenesis (nonclassic forms of 21-hydroxylase or 3-β hydroxysteroid deficiency) were present in 12% of patients as diagnosed by adrenocorticotropic hormone (ACTH) stimulation tests. In the majority of those, basal 17α-hydroxyprogesterone (17α-OHP) levels were higher than in pubertal norms and were thought to be a good screening test to determine which patients should undergo ACTH stimulation testing. In some patients premature pubarche may predict the development of functional hyperandrogenism in the mid-teenage years associated with polycystic ovarian syndrome in girls.

Premature thelarche is typically associated with a degree of FSH secretion, antral follicular development, and ovarian function that is greater than that measured in age-matched prepubertal control subjects. The prevalence of ovarian microcysts detected by ultrasonography is increased in these girls; however, plasma estradiol is commonly unmeasurable despite genitourinary cytology that shows evidence of estrogenization. Premature thelarche usually occurs in the first 2 years of life and regresses before puberty. Children who present with breast development later are more likely to have some degree of continued breast development, representing an early stage of precocious puberty. Once breast development is stimulated much beyond the breast-bud stage and reaches early adolescent proportions, breast contour generally does not regress. Occasionally (approximately 10–15%) girls go on to develop complete precocious puberty, but in the majority of patients the breast bud is a transient event that warrants only close follow-up for the appearance of other pubertal signs.

PRECOCIOUS PUBERTAL DEVELOPMENT

The development of isosexual secondary sexual characteristics before the age of 8 years in girls and before the age of 9 years in boys is termed precocious puberty. Precocious puberty is characterized by early and progressive sexual development accompanied by advancement of skeletal maturation as measured by bone age. The rapid linear growth that characterizes precocious puberty is

Table 59-2
Causes of Gonadotropin-Dependent (Central) Precocious Puberty[a]

Idiopathic precocious puberty
CNS tumors
Craniopharyngioma
Hypothalamic hamartoma
Optic glioma, astrocytoma, and others
Other CNS disorders
Static encephalopathy (secondary to infection, hypoxia, trauma, etc.)
Low-dose cranial radiation
Hydrocephalus
Arachnoid cyst
Septo-optic dysplasia
Secondary central precocious puberty
After late treatment of congenital adrenal hyperplasia
Hypothyroidism

[a]An overview of the causes of gonadotropin-dependent precocious puberty.

Table 59-3
Gonadotropin-Independent Precocious Puberty[a]

Boys
Testicular disorders
Familial male precocious puberty (testotoxicosis)
McCune-Albright syndrome
Leydig-cell adenomas
Human chorionic gonadotropin-secreting tumors
Androgen-secreting teratomas
Girls
Ovarian disorders
McCune-Albright syndrome
Granulosa or theca-cell tumors
Simple follicular cyst
Other estrogen-secreting tumors (teratomas, dysgerminomas)

[a]An overview of the causes of gonadotropin-independent precocious puberty. This term is used interchangeably with the term peripheral precocious puberty.

associated with premature and rapid skeletal maturation and fusion of the epiphyses, in most cases resulting in short adult stature compared with genetic height potential.

There are two major classes of precocious puberty: disorders that result from early reactivation of the hypothalamic–pituitary–gonadal axis (generally referred to as gonadotropin-dependent or central precocious puberty, Table 59-2) and those that do not (referred to as gonadotropin-independent precocious puberty, Table 59-3). Most girls and approximately half of boys who present with precocious puberty have central, gonadotropin-dependent precocious puberty which results from the secretion of GnRH from the hypothalamus. Although central precocious puberty is much more common among females than males, boys with this form of precocious puberty are more likely to be found to have an underlying central nervous system (CNS) abnormality. By contrast, the majority of girls have no discernible structural CNS lesion and are thus said to have an "idiopathic" form of the disorder. The overall incidence of gonadotropin-dependent precocious puberty has increased in both sexes because of the survival of children who have received CNS irradiation for brain tumors or leukemia.

GENERAL EVALUATION Evaluation of patients with early pubertal development should begin with a detailed history focused on the occurrence of prior CNS trauma, radiation, or seizure activity, exposure to exogenous sex steroids in cosmetics or food, or a positive family history. In girls, physical examination should focus on determining whether the development reflects androgen action, estrogen action, or both. Girls with isolated androgenization most likely have premature adrenarche or congenital adrenal hyperplasia, whereas those with estrogenization or evidence of both androgen and estrogen action are more likely to have precocious puberty. In boys, the presence of isolated androgenization most likely represents premature adrenarche, whereas the finding of testicular volumes of more than 4.0 mL is diagnostic of precocious puberty. Diagnostic evaluation should begin with an X-ray to assess bone age as a marker for sex steroid hormone action. In general establishing that skeletal age is concordant with chronological age allows for continued observation.

When secondary sexual characteristics are associated with an advanced bone age, measurements of estradiol, testosterone, and thyroid hormone should be obtained, and a GnRH stimulation test is indicated to differentiate between central (gonadotropin-dependent) and peripheral (gonadotropin-independent) causes of precocious puberty. In most cases, the diagnosis of gonadotropin-dependent precocious puberty, particularly in younger children, warrants obtaining a magnetic resonance imaging (MRI) or computerized tomography head scan.

GONADOTROPIN-DEPENDENT PRECOCIOUS PUBERTY

IDIOPATHIC PRECOCIOUS PUBERTY In girls, most cases of precocious puberty are central (gonadotropin-dependent) in origin, and are believed to be caused by premature maturation of the hypothalamic–pituitary–ovarian axis. In perhaps two-thirds of cases, no recognizable cause of the disorder can be found. In these cases, the pattern of development and progression parallels that of normal pubertal development, although the onset is at an early age.

CNS DISORDERS Lesions of the CNS are well-recognized as causing central precocious puberty. Common causes include static encephalopathy as a result of infection, hypoxia, trauma, or irradiation during infancy or early childhood. A less common, but nonetheless important, cause of central precocious puberty is a CNS tumor. These tumors can be viewed as causing precocious puberty by one of two distinct mechanisms. Hypothalamic hamartomas are benign tumors that have been shown to contain measurable GnRH. As such, they may be considered to be acting as ectopic GnRH pulse generators that have escaped from the normal inhibitory influences exerted in the prepubertal period on the centers that normally secrete GnRH. These small tumors are more frequently diagnosed in boys than in girls and are most easily visualized using MRI, as some may be only 2 or 3 mm in size. These tumors tend to grow slowly—if at all—and rarely cause neurologic symptoms.

The chance of finding CNS pathology in either sex is inversely proportional to the age of the child, with the greatest yield in children younger than 4 years old. Kappy found that in girls whose pubertal development began after 6 years of age, any CNS pathology was already known or clinically evident, suggesting that routine MRI in these children will less likely have positive findings. In contrast, Pescovitz and coworkers reported that in a series of 4000 children referred to the National Institutes of Health, about one-third of the girls and more than 90% of the boys had an identifiable lesion of the

CNS visible on computed tomography or MRI scans. This high prevalence of CNS lesions reflects the referral population.

Cranial irradiation has dose-dependent effects on many hypothalamic–pituitary functions. Although doses of cranial irradiation exceeding 50 g to the hypothalamic–pituitary axis may render a child gonadotropin deficient, lesser doses of irradiation have been associated with early puberty in both sexes. Low-dose cranial irradiation (18–24 g) used in the CNS prophylactic treatment of acute lymphoblastic leukemia is associated with a downward shift in the distribution of ages at pubertal onset and menarche in girls. Central precocious puberty is rare in boys treated in this manner.

The pathophysiology of central precocious puberty in nonhamartomatous lesions of the CNS is not yet established. It is possible that neural defects located near the hypothalamus cause precocious puberty by interfering with tonic central nervous system inhibition of the hypothalamic–pituitary–gonadal axis. It is also possible that focal derangements of the cellular environment in the vicinity of GnRH neurons may be causally related to the premature activation of GnRH secretion. Junier and Ojeda have speculated that neurotrophic or mitogenic activities produced locally in response to brain injury may be involved in the process. They suggest that the response of GnRH neurons to hypothalamic injury comprises three phases: an initial stage during which some of the neurons lose mature morphologic characteristics, reverting to a presumably more immature condition; an intermediate phase in which morphologic differentiation is reestablished and an increased synthesis of TGF-β by reactive astrocytes enhances GnRH release without affecting GnRH gene expression through a process that may involve glial release of prostaglandins; and a third phase in which the rise in sex steroids caused by the GnRH-dependent increase in basal LH release activates GnRH neurons to secrete gonadotropins in an episodic nature.

TREATMENT OF GONADOTROPIN DEPENDENT PRECOCIOUS PUBERTY Historically, medroxyprogesterone and cyproterone acetate were used to attempt to suppress activation of the hypothalamic–pituitary–gonadal axis. Neither of these agents was satisfactory, because they were not fully effective in inhibiting pubertal or skeletal maturation or in improving adult height.

The recognition that the continuous, nonpulsatile presentation of GnRH to the pituitary gonadotrophs induced a state of secondary hypogonadism led to the development and use of potent GnRH agonists in the therapy of precocious puberty. These gonadotropin-releasing hormone analogs (GnRHa; *see also* Chapter 34) represent the first truly effective treatment for central precocious puberty. Significant reductions in basal and peak (GnRH-stimulated) serum FSH and LH concentrations occur within the first month of GnRHa therapy. In parallel with these changes, a reduction in plasma concentrations of estradiol (in girls) and testosterone (in boys) occurs after the first month and persists while the drug is administered. Importantly, the effects of these drugs are reversible. After withdrawal of GnRHa therapy, gonadotropin and gonadal steroid concentrations return to their pretreatment levels.

Institution of GnRHa therapy results in a decrease in growth velocity, usually within a range that is appropriate for the child's skeletal maturation. The slowing of linear growth is accompanied in most cases by slowing of skeletal maturation—one of the primary aims of such treatment. Preservation of, or an increase in, adult height can be achieved in some children with gonadotropin-dependent precocious puberty treated with GnRHa. Most investigators, using the tables of Bayley and Pinneau, reported increases in the predicted final height of patients during the course of GnRHa therapy with a mean increase of 5 cm. Most studies suggest that the greatest improvement in predicted adult height is obtained in children whose bone ages are relatively young at the onset of treatment, indicating the need for early diagnosis and intervention. The length of time that such therapy is continued depends on bone age and estimates of final height in individual cases. Although concern has been raised regarding the possible effect of pubertal suppression on skeletal mineralization, an important feature of normal puberty, evidence available to date indicates no significant problem. Baens et al. evaluated the bone mineral density (BMD) in female patients treated with GnRHa for gonadotropin-dependent precocious puberty who had completed therapy and had subsequently attained a bone age of greater than 14 years. They found that BMDs were not different from those of a control population of girls with the same bone ages.

The physical effects of pubertal suppression are not limited to the effects on bone development. The majority of girls experience no increase in breast development, and a third show regression to an earlier Tanner stage, correlating with a reduction in ovarian and uterine size. Some girls experience transient vaginal bleeding approximately 2–4 weeks after initiation of GnRHa therapy because of estrogen withdrawal. Effects on pubic hair are less predictable, although most children show either no progression or a minor degree of regression. Some children show an increase in pubic hair that correlates with normal adrenarche.

GONADOTROPIN-INDEPENDENT PRECOCIOUS PUBERTY

Gonadotropin-independent forms of precocious puberty are about one-fifth as common as gonadotropin-dependent forms of precocious puberty. Gonadotropin-independent precocious puberty is characterized by increased production of gonadal steroids, causing the typical physical changes of puberty, in the absence of reactivation of the hypothalamic–pituitary axis (Fig. 59-1). This form of precocious puberty includes conditions that mimic the effect of pituitary gonadotropins on gonadal function, such as those in which there is secretion of gonadotropins from nonpituitary sources. Table 59-3 lists conditions associated with gonadotropin-independent precocious puberty. Molecular mechanisms underlying two forms of gonadotropin-independent precocious puberty, familial Leydig-cell hyperplasia and McCune-Albright syndrome, have recently been described.

McCUNE-ALBRIGHT SYNDROME McCune-Albright syndrome (MAS) is characterized classically by the clinical triad of cutaneous hyperpigmentation, polyostotic fibrous dysplasia, and endocrine dysfunction. Although it is stated that at least two of the features of the triad must be present to make the diagnosis, this guideline should be interpreted with caution, since the features may develop over time. The condition occurs distinctly less frequently in boys than in girls, who comprise 90% of affected patients. In contrast to those with central precocious puberty, these girls not uncommonly present with vaginal bleeding as the first sign of their sexual development. A pattern of variable involvement of hormone-secreting cells occurs in subjects with MAS, and the endocrine abnormalities are characterized by excessive function of these cells. The most common endocrine manifestation of MAS is precocious puberty, often associated with ovarian cysts. A waxing and waning course of the precocious puberty is not uncommon. Depending on the specific cell types affected, a variety of

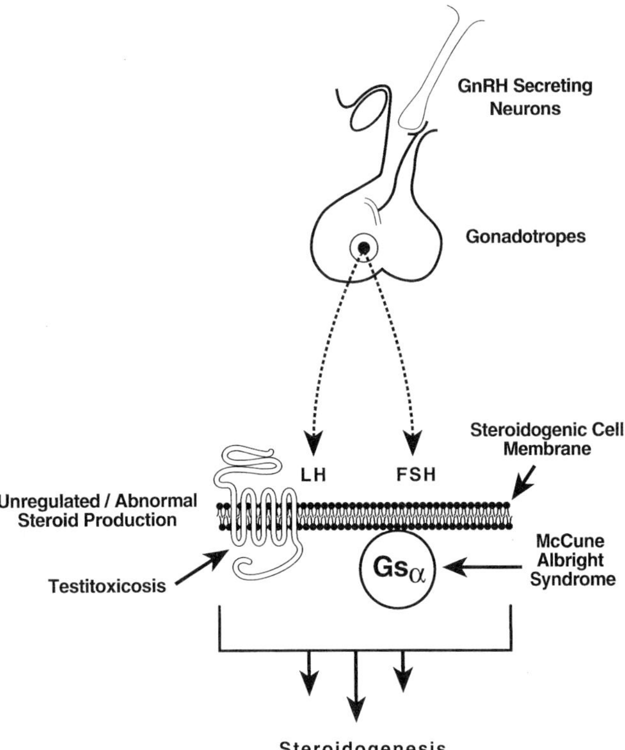

Figure 59-1 A schematic representation of the hypothalamic–pituitary–gonadal axis indicating the levels disturbed in selected forms of precocious puberty. Testitoxicosis (familial male precocious puberty, FMPP) is caused by amino acid substitution mutations in the membrane receptor for luteinizing hormone (LH) that result in its constitutive, ligand-independent activation. The gonadotropin-independent gonadal function that is observed in individuals with McCune-Albright syndrome is caused by mutations in a component of the FSH-regulated signaling cascade in granulosa cells of the ovary. In these individuals, replacement of one of two critical amino acid residues in a G protein subunit (Gsα) results in the constitutive activation of adenylate cyclase, mimicking the effect of FSH receptor activation in stimulating steroidogenesis in granulosa cells.

other endocrine disturbances may occur, including hyperthyroidism (caused by nodular or follicular thyroid hyperplasia) in 20–40% of patients, hypercortisolism (caused by nodular adrenal hyperplasia), and growth hormone- or prolactin-secreting pituitary adenomas.

The peculiar bone lesion of MAS (polyostotic fibrous dysplasia) may occur in any bone, including long bones, the skull, and pelvis, and result in pathologic fracture or severe disfigurement. Malignant degeneration occurs in up to 4% of lesions. The usually large, pigmented cutaneous lesions (*café-au-lait* patches) have irregular, "serrated" outlines. Their distribution, like the variable involvement of endocrine tissues, reflects an underlying genetic mosaicism that results from a postzygotic somatic cell mutation occurring after a number of cell divisions have taken place. Common sites of occurrence of the *café-au-lait* patches include the forehead, the neck or upper back, the shoulder and upper arm, the lumbosacral region, and the buttocks. They often follow a distribution that is not dermatomal, but in fact relates to the lines of Blaschko, which are thought to represent the patterns of dorsal and ventral outgrowth of two different cell populations during early embryogenesis. The hyperpigmentation is present in the basal epidermis; the number and size of melanocytes is normal, but the melanosomes are enlarged. The skeletal and cutaneous involvement in MAS is commonly asymmetrical and the skin lesions often stop abruptly at the midline.

The diverse clinical abnormalities of MAS have in common the involvement of cells that respond to extracellular signals through activation of the hormone-sensitive adenylate cyclase system, the membrane-bound enzyme that catalyzes the formation of the intracellular second messenger cyclic adenosine monophosphate (cAMP). However, these endocrine disturbances are not accompanied by increased plasma concentrations of the relevant trophic or stimulatory hormones. Thus, girls with precocious puberty caused by MAS have ovarian enlargement and follicular hyperplasia but have low serum levels of LH and FSH and a prepubertal response of LH to administration of GnRH.

The basis of the gonadotropin-independent nature of the precocious sexual development in MAS was elucidated by the identification of mutations that activate the intracellular second messager pathways by which the trophic hormones such as gonadotropins and thyrotropin signal. The activity of the hormone-sensitive adenylate cyclase system is primarily regulated by two guanine-nucleotide binding proteins (G proteins)—one inhibitory and the other stimulatory (*see* Chapter 46). Schwindinger et al. identified a mutation in the gene encoding the α-subunit of the stimulatory G protein that regulates adenylate cyclase activity. A heterozygous guanine to adenine transition was found in exon 8 of the gene encoding the α-subunit of Gs, predicting the replacement of arginine by histidine at position 201 of the mature protein. This amino acid is located within a critical region of the Gsα protein and the substitution causes a marked decrease in the intrinsic GTPase activity of Gsα, prolonging the survival of the active conformation of the enzyme and resulting in constitutive activation of adenylate cyclase activity. The consequent increased production of cAMP explains the increases in endocrine organ function typical of this disease, since this system mediates the stimulatory effects of many hormones (gonadotropins, thyrotropin, adrenocorticotropin, and GH-releasing hormone). In addition, cAMP modulates cellular proliferation in certain tissues, providing a basis for the hyperplasia seen in some tissues in MAS. Subsequent work by Weinstein and coworkers confirmed and extended these findings. Using PCR and allele-specific hybridization, these investigators identified two types of mutation at the same position implicated by Schwindinger (the codon encoding amino acid residue 201), resulting in substitution of either a histidine or a cysteine residue for the native arginine at this position. In the pathologic specimens from each of four patients with MAS studied by Weinstein, the mutant allele was found to be present in greatest abundance, relative to the normal allele, in the tissues histologically most affected, but in low levels in most of the tissues examined. The mutation has been found within the dysplastic bone lesions of affected patients, and may produce these lesions by inducing proliferation of mesenchymal progenitor cells. The mutation has also been detected in the hyperpigmented skin lesions, which commonly colocalize with the bone lesions, but its role in their pathogenesis remains unclear. Inactivating mutations of Gsα are associated with pseudohypoparathyroidism.

The findings reported above are consistent with the hypothesis that a spontaneous mutation early in gestation produced an abnormal monoclonal cell population and that the variable clinical presentation of MAS is caused by the varying degrees of somatic mosaicism of this genetic alteration that would otherwise represent an autosomal dominant lethal defect. Because of this mosaicism, MAS is not inherited.

FAMILIAL MALE PRECOCIOUS PUBERTY Although the endocrine disturbances are confined to the testes, a similar mechanism characterizes another GnRH-independent form of precocious puberty, familial male precocious puberty (FMPP, familial testotoxicosis). This disorder is inherited in an autosomal dominant, male-limited pattern and is characterized by the onset of puberty (testicular enlargement) before 4 years of age. Testosterone production and Leydig cell hyperplasia occur autonomously, in the context of low, prepubertal levels of LH. The clinical hallmark of this disorder is the relatively modest enlargement of the testes for the degree of virilization. Affected adult men are often short because of early epiphyseal fusion; however, they are otherwise healthy and have normal fertility. Although LH concentrations are low in childhood, they are normal in adulthood, indicating that normal maturation of the hypothalamic–pituitary–gonadal axis occurs. The disorder is not expressed in heterozygous females, since estrogen production by ovarian follicles requires coordinated stimulation by both LH and FSH; thus, activation of the LH pathway alone has no significant effect.

The pathogenesis of this gonadotropin-independent form of precocious puberty has been traced to heterozygous mutations within specific segments of the gene encoding the receptor for luteinizing hormone and chorionic gonadotropin (the LH/CG receptor). The LH/CG receptor is a member of the seven transmembrane domain family of G-protein coupled receptors. Unlike the inactivating mutations of the LH receptor, which can occur in many parts of the molecule, most of the activating mutations of the LH receptor have resulted in amino acid substitutions within the fifth and sixth transmembrane helices and the cytoplasmic loop that connects them. Shenker et al. found a mutation that resulted in replacement of the native aspartate with glycine, at position 578, in the sixth transmembrane helix of the protein. In vitro studies of the mutant receptor containing the Asp 578 to Gly substitution demonstrated marked increase in cyclic AMP production in the absence of ligand. It is presumed that the structural changes induced in the LH receptor by these amino acid substitutions shift these portions of the receptor to a conformation that mimics the conformation of the normal LH receptor activated by LH. This conformation of the mutant LH receptor leads to the agonist-independent production of cAMP, and thereby to autonomous testosterone production by the Leydig cells of affected boys. The presence of the Asp 578 to Gly mutation in most affected kindreds studied to date is believed likely to reflect a common genetic ancestry in many cases. However the finding of this same mutation in a number of ethnically diverse individuals suggests the occurrence of fresh mutations in some cases. Other less common mutations include replacement of alanine 572 by valine, threonine 577 by isoleucine, aspartate 582 by glycine, and methionine 575 by isoleucine. This latter amino acid is located in the sixth transmembrane domain of the receptor, close to a region important for binding of G proteins. Recently, a mutation that converts methionine 398 to threonine has been reported. In contrast with the majority of mutations in this disorder, this amino acid is located in the second transmembrane domain of the receptor. Notably, there was phenotypic heterogeneity associated with this mutation, since one boy carrying the mutant allele had no evidence of precocious puberty.

ECTOPIC HORMONE PRODUCTION Human chorionic gonadotropin (hCG)-secreting germ cell tumors have been thought to cause precocious puberty exclusively in boys. Because of the extensive structural homology of the β-subunits of hCG and LH, the excess hCG acting through the LH receptor stimulates Leydig cell production of testosterone.

Non-CNS tumors causing gonadotropin-independent precocious puberty in females have also been described. In such instances, the pubertal development is most often traced to the presence of a granulosa cell ovarian tumor or an adrenal tumor that produces excess estrogen.

Although the cell types and hormones differ in the different tumors described above, they do share a common characteristic. That is, in each instance a hormone that is normally produced by specific cell types and regulated in a very precise fashion is expressed by the neoplastic cells in an inappropriate or unregulated fashion. Although not well-studied, it appears that the genetic events leading to the genesis of the neoplasms in some way mimic the signals controlling hormonogenesis.

Although not strictly a cause of precocious puberty, congenital adrenal hyperplasia, most commonly because of deficiency of 21-hydroxylase, is another cause of early virilization. It is distinguished by absence of testicular enlargement in boys (hence the designation "pseudopuberty"), and virilization without feminization in girls.

TREATMENT OF GONADOTROPIN-INDEPENDENT FORMS OF PRECOCIOUS PUBERTY Because patients with these forms of precocious puberty demonstrate pubertal development that is independent of pituitary gonadotropin secretion, GnRH agonist therapy is ineffective, at least as part of initial management. As such, even though the molecular lesions are different, treatments for FMPP and MAS are instead focused on directly inhibiting the synthesis or action of sex steroids.

In boys with FMPP, this has been approached through administration of inhibitors of steroidogensis, such as the antifungal agent ketoconazole. This compound inhibits the enzyme that catalyzes the cleavage of the 20,22 bond of the cholesterol molecule, and thus inhibits the synthesis of both androgens and estrogens. An alternative approach has been to employ drugs that block the actions of androgen at the level of the androgen receptor itself. Although more potent drugs are now available, published reports have used spironolactone, a drug that has demonstrated modest activity as a competitive inhibitor of androgen receptor function. Results using this drug have been somewhat disappointing, but have been more encouraging when coupled with testolactone. This compound is an aromatase inhibitor that blocks the enzyme (P450 aromatase) that catalyzes aromatization of testosterone, the rate-limiting step in estrogen biosynthesis, thereby reducing the high estrogen concentrations responsible for the accelerated skeletal maturation typical of this condition. Of note, the early maturation of the hypothalamus induced by exposure to high levels of sex steroids may result in the activation of the endogenous GnRH pulse generator, leading to the development of central, gonadotropin-dependent precocious puberty, secondary to the preexisting gonadotropin-independent precocious puberty. In such instances, the addition of GnRHa therapy is required to prevent progression of pubertal development and skeletal maturation.

Treatment of girls with precocious puberty because of MAS uses drugs that inhibit the synthesis of estrogen (aromatase inhibitors). The longest-term studies of this type have used testolactone.

Although demonstrating some efficacy, the benefits were minimal and were likely caused by imperfect patient compliance (because of side effects of the drug) and the relatively low potency of testolactone itself in inhibiting aromatase activity. The availability of more potent aromatase inhibitors (e.g., arimidex) may improve the effectiveness of such approaches in the future. The approach to inhibition of testosterone synthesis in boys with precocious puberty caused by MAS is similar to that employed in the treatment of patients with FMPP. Addition of a GnRH analog is required for those patients with MAS who develop secondary central precocious puberty.

CONTRASEXUAL DEVELOPMENT

Contrasexual (or heterosexual) development refers to feminization in males or virilization in females, and can occur at any age, either prepubertally or postpubertally. These disorders are not forms of puberty. Evaluation consists of careful history and physical examination followed by measurement of gonadal and adrenal steroids, and in more subtle cases, ACTH stimulation testing to identify cryptic or atypical forms of congenital adrenal hyperplasia. Depending on the pattern of steroid hormone excess detected, imaging of the adrenals, gonads, or liver may be required. Gynecomastia is the most common manifestation of feminization and in pubertal boys is usually a benign self-limited condition; however, gynecomastia in a prepubertal boy is clearly pathologic. When associated with hypogonadism, Klinefelter's syndrome should be considered and a karyotype obtained. In most cases, estrogen concentrations are not increased. However, in those patients in whom there is measurably high estrogen concentration, the source of excess estrogen may be a neoplasm (e.g., adrenal, hepatic, or testicular), an abnormality of steroid metabolism, or increased extraglandular conversion of C-19 steroids to C-18 estrogens, such as occurs in the presence of significant obesity (gynecomastia is more common in obese boys). Exposure to exogenous estrogens is another uncommon cause of feminization in males.

Females with virilization may have adrenal or gonadal sources of androgen excess, causing development of sexual hair, clitoromegaly, acne, and hirsutism. The most common cause of virilization in prepubertal girls is congenital adrenal hyperplasia (CAH) because of deficiency of 21-hydroxylase activity ("late-onset" or "attenuated" CAH). Other virilizing forms of CAH include 3β-hydroxysteroid dehydrogenase and 11-hydroxylase deficiency. Severely advanced skeletal maturation is a common accompaniment of the virilization in affected girls, and these conditions can be further complicated by the development of secondary central precocious puberty. A variety of molecular defects underlie these enzyme deficiencies, as described in Chapter 57. Virilizing adrenal adenoma or ovarian neoplasms are associated with elevated levels of dehydroepiandrosterone sulfate, androstenedione, or testosterone. β-hCG and α-fetoprotein may also be increased and should be measured as markers for ovarian, testicular, and hepatic tumors in virilized girls and feminized boys.

DELAYED PUBERTAL DEVELOPMENT

Delayed puberty is defined by lack of physical changes of sexual maturation at a chronological age that is two standard deviations above the mean age of onset of puberty. In the United States, the ages of 12 years in girls and 14 years in boys serve as practical guidelines to determine the need for evaluation. Diagnostic evaluation should differentiate between constitutional delay, hypogonadotropic hypogonadism, and hypergonadotropic hypogonadism. Causes of delayed puberty are listed in Table 59-4.

Table 59-4
Causes of Delayed Pubertal Development

Constitutional delay
Hypogonadotropic hypogonadism
- Isolated gonadotropin deficiency
- Kallmann's syndrome and variants
- Functional gonadotropin deficiency
  - Chronic systemic disease and malnutrition
  - Anorexia nervosa
  - Exercise-induced amenorrhea
- CNS disorders
  - Tumors
  - Radiation therapy
  - Anatomic defects (e.g., septo-optic dysplasia)
- Miscellaneous disorders
  - CHARGE association
  - Noonan's syndrome
  - Aarskog syndrome
  - Prader-Willi syndrome
  - Laurence-Moon-Biedl or Bardet-Biedl syndromes

Hypergonadotropic hypogonadism
- Klinefelter's syndrome
- Primary testicular failure
- Gonadal dysgenesis and variants
- Primary ovarian failure

VARIATIONS OF NORMAL PUBERTY—DELAYED (CONSTITUTIONAL DELAY) Constitutional delay of puberty is a common, benign condition that represents a variant of normal puberty. The pattern of pubertal progress in affected children is quite normal; however, its time of onset is delayed with respect to the population as a whole. Boys are referred for evaluation of this condition significantly more often than are girls. In conjunction with their delayed pubertal development, these children generally have mildly short stature, approximately two to three standard deviations below the mean for age throughout childhood. Their short stature is accompanied by delayed skeletal maturation (2–4 years behind chronological age) and these children generally demonstrate sexual maturation that is more commensurate with their bone age than their chronological ages. Adult height and sexual maturation are achieved significantly later, many young men reporting continued linear growth in their late teens or early 20s. Final height is generally appropriate for the genetic background, but is commonly in the low normal range. The family history often reveals other affected individuals in the family, most often males.

HYPOGONADOTROPIC HYPOGONADISM

Hypogonadotropic hypogonadism describes the deficiency of pulsatile release of gonadotropins, which may result from a variety of hypothalamic or pituitary disorders. In the presence of a hypothalamic defect, or absence of GnRH-secreting neurons, failure of GnRH secretion results in lack of stimulation of pituitary gonadotropin secretion. In contrast, pituitary disorders, such as tumors or hypophysitis, cause direct failure of pituitary gonadotropin secretion.

During embryogenesis, the olfactory nerves and terminal nerve develop from the olfactory placode in the nose. The olfactory sensory neurons have short dendrites that terminate at the olfcatory epithelium in dendritic knobs with cilia that contain G-protein coupled, seven transmembrane domain, odorant receptors. The olfactory nerves associate with the terminal nerve and vomeronasal nerve to produce a bridge between the olfactory epithelium and the forebrain. The cells that will become GnRH-synthesizing neurons arise within the region of the olfactory placodes and migrate from the nasal epithelium, through the cribriform plate of the nose and then along the olfactory tract–forebrain axis to reach the preoptic and hypothalamic areas, where they differentiate to become the GnRH-secreting neurons. The exact cellular origin of the GnRH neurons has yet to be established; however, there is evidence in studies of embryonic chicks that they in fact derive from an embryonic precursor in the region that will become the nasal epithelium, rather than the olfactory placode itself. These GnRH-secreting neurons, which are dispersed through the medial basal hypothalamus rather than being located in a discrete nucleus, transduce neural signals into a hormonal signal—the periodic secretion of GnRH. Given the developmental connection between olfactory and GnRH neurons, it is of particular interest to note the relationship between olfactory acuity and reproduction in animals, evidenced by the importance of pheromones in sexual attraction.

KALLMANN'S SYNDROME AND VARIANTS Isolated gonadotropin deficiency may occur sporadically or in a familial pattern. In contrast to patients with delayed puberty because of CNS tumors or constitutional delay, those with gonadotropin deficiency usually have appropriate or tall stature for their age. Untreated adults and individuals of pubertal age commonly have eunuchoid proportions.

Kallmann's syndrome was first described in 1856. It is uncommon, occurring with approximately one-tenth the frequency of Klinefelter's syndrome (approximately 1:10,000 in males and 1:50,000 in females). As originally described, it comprised the association of hypogonadotropic hypogonadism with anosmia or hyposmia resulting from agenesis or hypoplasia of the olfactory bulbs and tracts. The disorder results from failure of fetal GnRH secretory neurons to migrate from the olfactory placode, where they arise, to the medial basal hypothalamus. Three modes of transmission have been described: X-linked, autosomal recessive, and autosomal dominant.

Typical clinical features of Kallmann's syndrome include delayed puberty, eunuchoid habitus, gynecomastia, and reduced sense of smell (often unknown to the patient). Cryptorchidism and a small penis are present in infancy in some affected individuals. Carrier females may display partial defects, such as reduced sense of smell, delayed menarche, or irregular menses, but are normally fertile. Other clinical features of Kallmann's syndrome include unilateral renal agenesis in up to 40% of patients; midline facial anomalies, such as cleft lip, high-arched or cleft palate, or other forms of imperfect facial fusion; short metacarpals; talipes cavus; cerebellar ataxia; sensorineural deafness; epilepsy; and synkinesia (mirror movements of the hands). Variant forms of Kallmann's syndrome manifest varying combinations of these features. MRI scans may demonstrate hypoplasia of the olfactory gyri and absent olfactory bulbs and tracts. When analyzed histologically, the olfactory epithelium of a patient with Kallmann's syndrome was thinner than normal and contained fewer neurons. Those that were present lacked cilia, were immature, or showed signs of degeneration.

The X-linked form of Kallmann's syndrome has been most extensively studied. Positional cloning studies by Legouis et al. led to the isolation and characterization of the gene defective in this form of Kallmann's syndrome. The Kallmann gene *(KAL1* or *KALIG1)*, which is located at Xp22.3, and (at least partially) escapes X inactivation, encodes a 680-amino acid protein that is apparently extracellular in location. An inactive homologous pseudogene *(KALP)* is located on the Y chromosome at Yq11. The derived amino acid sequence of KAL1 predicts a protein that contains a leader peptide and no transmembrane or anchoring regions are present. The protein contains four fibronectin type III motifs (FNIII), suggesting a role in cell adhesion. Its general structure is similar to that of known neural-cell adhesion molecules (NCAMs) that mediate neurite outgrowth or axon–axon interactions. Such a function would be consistent with the well-characterized defect of embryonic neuronal migration in patients with Kallmann's syndrome. In addition to these motifs, the protein sequence also contains a region (the WAPS domain, or whey acidic protein core domain) that has been associated with proteinase inhibitor activity in a number of proteins. This association of domains in the predicted amino acid sequence of the *KAL1* gene suggests that this protein may also play a role in the tissue remodeling that accompanies this neuronal migration. Examination of the pattern of expression of the gene during embryogenesis demonstrates that it can be detected in various neuronal populations of the central nervous system, including cells of the olfactory bulbs. These findings have suggested that the KAL1 protein might be involved both in directing neuronal migration, as well as influencing the differentiation of specific cell types. KAL is conserved in other mammals, including monkey, cow, rabbit, and sheep, and in xenopus, zebra fish, and chicken, in which it is expressed in a wide range of tissues. Of note, it is not conserved in mice or rats, a fact that has hampered its characterization.

Studies of patients with the X-linked form of Kallmann's syndrome indicate heterogeneity at the genetic level, although all but one of the mutations reported to date predict the absence or marked truncation of the encoded protein. In a study of 21 male patients with the X-linked form of the disorder, Hardelin and coworkers detected a range of abnormalities within the *KAL1* gene, including large deletions in two families, and nine different point mutations in other affected individuals, resulting in introduction of premature termination codons into the sequence. These findings support the involvement of the *KAL1* gene in the pathogenesis of Kallmann's syndrome. It is suggested that defects of *KAL1* gene expression may underlie the varied clinical findings in Kallmann's syndrome. The relationship of KAL1 to disorders such as epilepsy or synkinesia is suggested by knowledge of its role in neuronal migration. The role of KAL1 in events such as kidney formation and migration is more obscure; however, KAL is expressed in the Wolffian duct, which is involved in renal development by interaction with the metanephric mesenchyme.

To date, the genetic causes of the other forms of Kallmann's syndrome (i.e., non-X-linked) have not been defined. However, studies of individuals with Kallmann's syndrome associated with cytogenetic abnormalities have suggested possible loci for genes responsible for the autosomal dominant form of Kallmann's syndrome *(KAL2)* at 1q, 7q, and 12q. It is likely that the genetic defects will be traced to other genes that participate in the pathways affecting migration of the GnRH-secreting neurons.

Treatment of individuals with Kallmann's syndrome with supplemental testosterone will induce virilization, whereas intranasal GnRH or intramuscular chorionic gonadotropin can stimulate endogenous sex steroid production and even reproductive capability.

ISOLATED GONADOTROPIN DEFICIENCY A number of families have been reported in which affected individuals have isolated gonadotropin deficiency without the features of Kallmann's syndrome. The inheritance pattern is autosomal recessive. Although not yet reported in humans, it is likely that this defect results from GnRH deficiency as a result of mutations in the gene encoding GnRH, as has been observed in the hypogonadal (Hpg) mouse.

ISOLATED FSH DEFICIENCY A small number of patients have been reported to have isolated deficiency of FSH. A woman with isolated deficiency of FSH who presented with primary amenorrhea and infertility was found to have a mutation in the gene encoding the β-subunit of FSH. The 2-bp sdeletion caused a frameshift in the coding sequence, predicting the formation of a truncated protein that lacks regions required for association with the α-subunit of FSH and for binding to the FSH receptor.

FUNCTIONAL GONADOTROPIN DEFICIENCIES Severe systemic and chronic disorders and malnutrition are associated with delayed puberty or failure to progress through the stages of puberty. In general, when body weight is less than 80% of ideal weight for height a functional gonadotropin deficiency may occur. Examples include the functional gonadotropin deficiencies associated with anorexia nervosa and exercise-induced amenorrhea. In such instances, normal hypothalamic–pituitary–gonadal function accompanies restoration of normal body mass.

CNS DISORDERS

Mass lesions, such as sellar or suprasellar tumors (e.g., craniopharyngioma), commonly disturb the processes of pubertal development, causing either precocious puberty (as described *above*) or pubertal delay. Such tumors cause pubertal delay by impairing hypothalamic or pituitary function. In addition to abnormalities of pubertal development, growth failure, polydipsia, polyuria, and visual disturbances may also be part of the presentation of children with craniopharyngioma.

HYPERGONADOTROPIC HYPOGONADISM

Primary gonadal failure is associated with elevated gonadotropins because of the absence of negative feedback effects of gonadal sex steroids. The most common causes of hypergonadotropic hypogonadism are associated with karyotypic and somatic abnormalities, but isolated gonadal failure can also present with delayed puberty without other abnormal physical findings.

MUTATIONS OF THE LH AND FSH RECEPTORS The receptors for the gonadotropins LH/CG and FSH are both members of the seven transmembrane domain family of G-protein coupled receptors. Selective defects in the gonadal response to gonadotropins have been traced in several pedigrees to mutations of the genes encoding the FSH and LH/CG receptors. In males, rather than being associated with delayed puberty, mutations in the gene encoding the LH/CG receptor are classically associated with a form of male pseudohermaphroditism termed Leydig-cell hypoplasia (LCH). This disorder is characterized by female phenotype in the presence of a 46,XY karyotype, low serum testosterone, increased serum LH, and lack of testosterone secretion in response to hCG administration. Mutations in the LH/CG gene, particularly in the transmembrane regions of the receptor protein, causing this phenotype include those that result in premature termination or amino acid replacement.

The discovery of inactivating mutations in the LH receptor in patients with LCH and defective fetal masculinization is to be expected. Several interesting aspects of LH receptor mutations deserve comment. First is that a 46,XX sibling of two patients with LCH was a phenotypically normal adult female with amenorrhea and cystic ovaries, suggesting that such a defect was consistent with normal pubertal development, but impairment in the normal ovarian cycle. Second, the identification of a missense mutation of the LH receptor in a phenotypic male infant evaluated for a small but normally formed penis suggests that the range of altered phenotypes associated with abnormalities of the LH receptor may be broader than those initially identified.

An uncommon form of hypergonadotropic hypogonadism is 46,XX gonadal dysgenesis. Affected girls, who typically present with pubertal failure, are of normal stature and have no phenotypic features of Turner's syndrome. The condition appears to be genetically heterogeneous and both sporadic and familial cases have been reported. One familial variant—Perrault syndrome—has sensorineural hearing loss associated with the hypogonadism. A candidate recessive gene on chromosome 2, the *ODG1* gene (ovarian dysgenesis 1) was identified by analysis of a large cohort of affected Finnish patients. The disorder is common in this population (1: 8300 females) and is inherited in an autosomal recessive manner. Aittomaki et al. have recently discovered a missense mutation in the gene encoding the FSH receptor in affected families. The FSH receptor gene is located at 2p21, coinciding with the *ODG1* locus. A limited number of families with such defects have been described to date. The mutation in the FSHR gene in this group is an arginine to valine substitution at amino acid 189, located in the extracellular ligand-binding domain of the receptor. The mutation segregated with the affected phenotype and had a dramatic effect on the binding of ligand and the stimulation of cAMP production. Of interest, the affected males in the pedigrees were phenotypically normal and half were fertile, suggesting that variable defects in spermatogenesis might be the only discernible effect in males with the disorder.

KLINEFELTER SYNDROME The most common form of primary testicular failure is Klinefelter's syndrome (47,XXY karyotype), which occurs with an incidence of 1:1000 males. Male sexual differentiation is normal; testicular function remains relatively normal until about the age of puberty, declining thereafter. Patients with Klinefelter's syndrome do not usually present with delayed puberty, although affected patients may demonstrate a slowing or arrest of pubertal development as testicular function declines. Supplemental testosterone is then required. Klinefelter's syndrome and its variants are described in Chapters 57 and 58.

TURNER'S SYNDROME Turner's syndrome, 45,X gonadal dysgenesis, is associated with short stature, female phenotype, and delayed or absent pubertal development. Patients have "streak" gonads consisting of fibrous tissue without germ cells (germ cells may be present in infancy). Other classic but variable phenotypic features include ptosis, low-set ears, micrognathia, a short "webbed" neck, a broad shieldlike chest, hypoplastic areolae, short fourth or fifth metacarpals, cubitus valgus, structural anomalies of the kidney, extensive pigmented nevi, hypolastic, hyperconvex fingernails and toenails, and left-sided cardiovascular anomalies, coarctation of the aorta being the most common.

Disordered growth is a major clinical feature of this syndrome, beginning *in utero* and worsening progressively from early childhood onward. Patients have no pubertal growth spurt and reach a mean final height approximately 20 cm shorter than that of the reference population. Although short stature is a classic feature of Turner's syndrome, it is not a feature of other forms of hypergonadotropic hypogonadism that occur without karyotypic abnormalities. Because growth hormone secretion is usually normal in Turner's syndrome, it is likely that the short stature is related to a subtle form of skeletal dysplasia, reflecting imbalances of gene expression caused by the absent X chromosome segments. Growth hormone treatment improves growth rates and the adult height of many affected patients.

Pubic hair may appear late and is usually sparse in distribution. Serum gonadotropin concentrations in Turner syndrome are high between birth and 4 years of age. They decrease toward the normal range in prepubertal patients and then rise to castrate levels after 9 or 10 years of age.

Variant forms of gonadal dysgenesis are associated with a variety of mosaic phenotypes, usually including a 45,X line, in addition to more complex X chromosomal rearrangements. Girls and women with these karyotypes may have phenotypic features typical of those with the classic syndrome of 45,X gonadal dysgenesis, or may have fewer manifestations. Patients with Swyer syndrome (46,XY complete gonadal dysgenesis) have streak gonads and pubertal delay similar to those with Turner's syndrome. They do not, however, have the short stature typical of Turner's syndrome and, in most cases, do not have the other phenotypic features. Gonadal dysgenesis and other sex chromosome defects are outlined in Chapters 57 and 58.

Other causes of primary ovarian failure include radiation therapy, chemotherapy, and premature menopause. Patients with Addison's disease may have autoimmune oophoritis and other features of autoimmune disease, in addition to their adrenal failure. Primary amenorrhea is a common presenting feature of women with androgen-insensitivity syndrome (phenotypic females with 46, XY genotype and androgen resistance). A sex steroid biosynthetic defect as a result of 17α-hydroxylase deficiency will be manifested by delayed puberty and primary amenorrhea in a phenotypic female (regardless of genotype) with hypokalemia and hypertension.

Breast development in female patients with pubertal delay may be induced by estrogen replacement therapy using either a conjugated equine estrogen (such as Premarin) or synthetic estrogen (such as ethinyl estradiol) at slowly increasing doses until feminization is achieved. Thereafter, a progestin is required to induce uterine endometrial cycling, and for convenience, an appropriate relatively low-dose combined oral contraceptive pill may be used. Estrogen replacement therapy in Turner's syndrome is more complex, requiring coordination of timing with respect to growth hormone therapy to optimize adult height achievement.

SELECTED REFERENCES

Ahima RS, Dushay J, Flier SN, Prabakaran D, Flier JS. Leptin accelerates the onset of puberty in normal female mice. J Clin Invest 1997;99:391–395.

Aittomäki K, Lucena JLD, Pakarinen P, et al. Mutation in the follicle-stimulating hormone receptor gene causes hereditary hypergonadotropic ovarian failure. Cell 1995;82:959–968.

Burstein S. Editorial: growth disorders after cranial radiation in childhood. J Clin Endocrinol Metab 1994;78:1280,1281.

Balducci R, Boscherini B, Mangiantini A, Morellini, Toscano V. Isolated precocious pubarche: an approach. J Clin Endocrinol Metab 1994;79: 582–589.

Chehab FF, Mounzih K, Lu R, Lim ME. Early onset of reproductive function in normal female mice treated with leptin. Science 1997;275:88–90.

Clayton RN. Molecular genetics, hypogonadism and luteinizing hormone. Clin Endocrinol 1992;34:201,202.

Duke VM, Winyard PJ, Thorogood P, Soothill P, Bouloux PM, Woolf AS. KAL, a gene mutated in Kallmann's syndrome, is expressed in the first trimester of human development. Mol Cell Endocrinol 1995;110:73–79.

Furui K, Suganuma N, Tsukahara S-I, et al. Identification of two point mutations in the gene coding luteinizing hormone (LH) β-subunit, associated with immunologically anomalous LH variants. J Clin Endocrinol Metab 1994;78:107–113.

Feuillan PP, Foster CM, Pescovitz OH, et al. Treatment of precocious puberty in the McCune-Albright syndrome with the aromatase inhibitor testolactone. N Engl J Med 1986;315:1115–1119.

Georgopoulos NA, Pralong FP, Seidman CE, Seidmen JG, Crowley WF Jr, Vallejo M. Genetic heterogeneity evidenced by low incidence of KAL-1 gene mutations in sporadic cases of gonadotropin-releasing hormone deficiency. J Clin Endocrinol Metab 1997;82:213–217.

Hardelin JP, Levilliers J, Blanchard S, et al. Heterogeneity in the mutations responsible for X chromosome linked Kallman syndrome. Hum Mol Genet 1993;2:373–377.

Hardelin JP, Petit C. A molecular approach to the pathophysiology of the X-linked Kallman's syndrome. Baillieres Clin Endocrinol Metab 1995;9:489–507.

Holland FJ, Fishman L, Bailey JD, Fazekas AT. Ketoconazole in the management of precocious puberty not responsive to LHRH analogue therapy. N Engl J Med 1986;312:1023–1027.

Jameson JL. Inherited disorders of the gonadotropin hormones. Mol Cell Endocrinol 1996;125:143–149.

Junier MP, Hill DF, Costa ME, Felder S, Ojeda SR. Hypothalamic lesions that induce female precocious puberty activate glial expression of the epidermal growth factor receptor gene: differential regulation of alternatively spliced transcripts. J Neurosci 1993;13:703–713.

Kappy MS, Ganong CS. Advances in the treatment of precocious puberty. Advances in Pediat 1994;41:223–261.

Kawate N, Kletter GB, Wilson BE, Netzloff ML, Menon KMJ. Identification of constitutively activating mutation of the luteinizing hormone receptor in a family with male limited gonadotrophin independent precocious puberty (testotoxicosis). J Med Genet 1995;32:553,554.

Kosugi S, Van Dop C, Geffner ME, et al. Characterization of heterogeneous mutations causing constitutive activation of the luteinizing hormone receptor in familial male precocious puberty. Hum Mol Genet 1995;4:183–188.

Kraaij R, Post M, Kremer H, et al. A missense mutation in the second transmembrane segment of the luteinizing hormone receptor causes familial male-limited precocious puberty. J Clin Endocrinol Metab 1995;80:3168–3172.

Latronico AC, Anasti J, Arnhold IJ, et al. A novel mutation of the luteinizing hormone receptor gene causing male gonadotropin-independent precocious puberty. J Clin Endocrinol Metab 1995;80:2490–2494.

Latronico AC, Anasti J, Arnhold IJP, et al. Testicular and ovarian resistance to luteinizing hormone caused by inactivating mutations of the luteinizing hormone. N Engl J Med 1996;334:507–512.

Laue L, Chan WY, Hsueh AJ, et al. Genetic heterogeneity of constitutively activating mutations of the human luteinizing hormone receptor in familial male-limited precocious puberty. Proc Natl Acad Sci USA 1995;92:1906–1910.

Laue L, Jones J, Barnes KM, et al. Treatment of familial male precocious puberty with spironolactone, testolactone, and deslorelin. J Clin Endocrinol Metab 1993;76:151–155.

Laue L, Wu SM, Kudo M, et al. A nonsense mutation of the human luteinizing hormone receptor gene in Leydig cell hypoplasia. Hum Mol Genet 1995;4:1429–1433.

Lee PA. Advances in the management of precocious puberty. Clin Pediatr 1994;33: 54–61.

Legouis R, Cohen-Salmon M, Del Castillo I, Petit C. Isolation and characterization of the gene responsible for the X chromosome-linked Kallmann syndrome. Biomed Pharmacother 1994;48:241–246.

Matthews CH, Borgato S, Beck-Peccoz P, et al. Primary amenorrhoea and infertility due to a mutation in the β-subunit of follicle-stimulating hormone. Nat Genet 1993;5:83–86.

Mantzoros CS, Flier JS, Rogol AD. A longitudinal assessment of hormonal and physical alterations during normal puberty in boys. V. Rising leptin levels may signal the onset of puberty. J Clin Endocrinol Metab 1997;82:1066–1070.

Nachtigall LB, Boepple PA, Pralong FP, Crowley WF Jr. Adult-onset idiopathic hypogonadotropic hypogonadism—a treatable form of male infertility. N Engl J Med 1997;336:410–415.

Neely EK, Bachrach LK, Hintz RL, et al. Bone mineral density during treatment of central precocious puberty. J Pediatr 1995;127:819–822.

Ogilvy-Stuart AL, Clayton PE, Shalet SM. Cranial irradiation and early puberty. J Clin Endocrinol Metab 1994;78:1282–1286.

Paul D, Conte FA, Grumbach MM, Kaplan SL. Long term effect of gonadotropin-releasing hormone agonists therapy on final and near-final height in 26 children with true precocious puberty treated at a median age of less than 5 years. J Clin Endocrinol Metab 1995;80:546–551.

Pescovitz OH, Comite F, Hench K, et al. The NIH experience with precocious puberty: diagnostic subgroups and response to short-term luteinizing hormone releasing hormone analogue therapy. J Pediatr 1986;108:47–54.

Plant TM. Puberty in primates. In: Knobil E, Neill JD, eds. The Physiology of Reproduction, 2nd ed. New York: Raven, 1994; pp. 453–485.

Rao E, Weiss B, Fukami M, et al. Pseudoautosomal deletions encompassing a novel homebox gene cause growth failure in idiopathic short stature and Turner syndrome. Nat Genet 1997;16:54–63.

Schwindinger WF, Francomano CA, Levine MA. Identification of a mutation in gene encoding the subunit of the stimulatory G protein of adenylyl cyclase in McCune-Albright syndrome. Proc Natl Acad Sci USA 1992;89:5152–5156.

Shankar RR, Pescovitz OH. Precocious puberty. Adv Endocrinol Metab 1995;6:55–89.

Shenker A. G protein-coupled receptor structure and function: the impact of disease-causing mutations. Baillieres Clin Endocrinol Metab 1995;9:427–451.

Shenker A, Laue L, Kosui S, Merendino JJ Jr, Minegishi T, Cutler GB Jr. A constitutively activating mutation of the luteinizing hormone receptor in familial male precocious puberty. Nature 1993;365:652–654.

Smith EP, Boyd J, Frank GR, et al. Estrogen resistance caused by a mutation in the estrogen-receptor gene in a man. N Engl J Med 1994;331:1056–1061.

Styne DM. New aspects in the diagnosis and treatment of pubertal disorders. Pediatr Clin North Am 1997;44:505–529.

Tapanainen JS, Aittomaki K, Min J, Vaskivuo T, Huhtaniemi IT. Men homozygous for an inactivating mutation of the follicle-stimulating hormone (FSH) receptor gene present variable suppression of spermatogenesis and fertility. Nat Genet 1997;15:205,206.

Weinstein LS, Shenker A, Gejm an PV, Merino MJ, Friedman E, Spiegel AM. Activating mutations of the stimulatory G protein in the McCune-Albright syndrome. N Engl J Med 1991;325:1688–1695.

Weiss J, Axelrod L, Whitcomb RW, Harris PE, Crowley WF, Jameson JL. Hypogonadism caused by a single amino acid substitution in the β subunit of luteinizing hormone. N Engl J Med 1992;326:179–183.

Whitney EA, Layman LC, Chan PJ, Lee A, Peak DB, McDonough PG. The follicle-stimulating hormone receptor gene is polymorphic in premature ovarian failure and normal controls. Fertil Steril 1995;64: 518–524.

Winter JSD, Hughes IA, Reyes FI, Faiman C. Pituitary-gonadal relations in infancy: Patterns of serum gonadal concentrations in man from birth to two years of age. J Clin Endocrinol Metab 1976;42:679–686.

Winters SJ. Expanding the differential diagnosis of male hypogonadism. N Engl J Med 1992;326:193–195.

Yano K, Hidaka A, Saji M, et al. A sporadic case of male-limited precocious puberty has the same constitutively activating point mutation in luteinizing hormone/choriogonadotropin receptor gene as familial cases. J Clin Endocrinol Metab 1994;79:1818–1823.

Yano K, Kohn LD, Saji M, Kataoka N, Okuno A, Cutler GB Jr. A case of male-limited precocious puberty caused by a point mutation in the second transmembrane domain of the luteinizing hormone choriogonadotropin receptor gene. Biochem Biophys Res Commun 1996; 220:1036–1042.

Yano K, Saji M, Hidaka A, et al. A new constitutively activating point mutation in the luteinizing hormone/choriogonadotropin receptor gene in cases of male-limited precocious puberty. J Clin Endocrinol Metab 1995;80:1162–1168.

Zachman M, Prader A, Sobel EH, et al. Pubertal growth in patients with complete androgen insensitivity: indirect evidence for the importance of estrogen in girls. J Pediatr 1986;108:694–697.

60 Defects of Androgen Action

MICHAEL J. MCPHAUL

INTRODUCTION

Since 1935 it has been recognized that the principal androgen secreted by the testes is testosterone. The seminal observations of Bruchovsky and Wilson and of Anderson and Liao, however, led to the recognition that although testosterone is the most abundant circulating androgen, 5α-dihydrotestosterone is the predominant hormone found complexed to the androgen receptor (AR) in the nuclei of target cells, such as the prostate. This finding opened a new perspective on androgen physiology and focused attention on the enzyme that mediated this conversion, 5α-reductase, as a potential modulator of androgen action in selected tissues. As described below, this inference has been confirmed by the later recognition that in selected patients abnormalities in male development are caused by defects in the conversion of testosterone to 5α-dihydrotestosterone.

STRUCTURE AND MECHANISM OF ACTION OF THE ANDROGEN RECEPTOR

Abundant biochemical and genetic data demonstrated that the actions of androgen were mediated by a single receptor that was encoded on the X-chromosome, and that defects in this receptor protein, the AR, could present as a range of abnormalities of male phenotypic sexual development. The isolation of cDNAs encoding the AR revealed it to be a member of a large group of related transcription factors, the steroid-thyroid hormone-retinoid family of nuclear receptors. This family includes members that are ligand responsive and others that are believed to be constitutively active or modulated by other influences, such as phosphorylation. All exhibit a modular structure (displayed for the AR in Fig. 60-1) comprising a highly conserved DNA-binding domain, a less highly conserved carboxy-terminal hormone-binding domain, and an amino-terminal segment that is poorly conserved between individual family members, both in terms of primary amino acid sequence and length. The DNA-binding domain is composed of two elements (termed "zinc fingers") that mediate the sequence-specific DNA binding of the AR. This segment is the most highly conserved region between members of this gene family. The carboxy-terminus is approximately 250 amino acids long and encodes the portion of the protein that binds androgens with high affinity. Of note, the amino-terminus of the AR is somewhat atypical in that it contains three segments composed of repeated amino acids (one of repeated glutamine residues, one of repeated proline residues, and one of repeated glycine residues). Polymorphisms of these regions appear to have little effect on AR function in normal individuals, but expansions of the glutamine repeat have been implicated in the pathogenesis of spinal and bulbar muscular atrophy (Kennedy's syndrome, *see below*).

The non–ligand-bound AR is believed to exist in the cell in association with a number of ancillary proteins, particularly members of the heat shock protein family. After the binding of hormone, the receptor dissociates from these proteins and binds to specific DNA sequences within or adjacent to androgen-responsive genes. This ligand-activated receptor is believed to interact with components of the transcriptional apparatus to stimulate formation of active transcription complexes. In some models, the AR appears to modulate genes in a negative fashion or to alter mRNA stability, but these phenomena have been less-well-characterized.

ANDROGEN RECEPTOR DEFECTS

CLINICAL FEATURES A spectrum of phenotypes can result from defects of AR function (Table 60-1). Patients completely unresponsive to the actions of androgen (referred to as complete testicular feminization or complete androgen insensitivity) have a 46,XY karyotype, but an external phenotype that is completely female in appearance, despite normal or elevated levels of circulating androgens. Owing to the secretion and action of Müllerian-inhibiting substance (MIS) by the functional testes present in these patients, the uterus and fallopian tubes are absent. Such individuals are usually raised as females and may first seek attention for evaluation of primary amenorrhea. Gonadectomy is often performed, because the intra-abdominal testes show an increased rate of malignant tumor development. With estrogen replacement, these individuals often lead completely normal lives as women, although they are infertile.

The term incomplete testicular feminization has been applied to individuals with nearly complete forms of androgen resistance who demonstrate only slight evidence of virilization (such as clitoromegaly). These patients are usually managed in a fashion similar to that of patients with complete testicular feminization.

Partial androgen resistance or Reifenstein's syndrome is a constellation of features that includes severe defects of male urogenital development (perineal or penoscrotal hypospadias) and gynecomastia. Reifenstein's syndrome represents a far more difficult clinical problem. As noted, the developmental abnormalities are substantial and the surgical correction of these defects often requires multiple separate surgical sprocedures. Such efforts are hampered by the small size of the genitalia of affected children. After

From: *Principles of Molecular Medicine* (J. L. Jameson, ed.), ©1998 Humana Press Inc., Totowa, NJ.

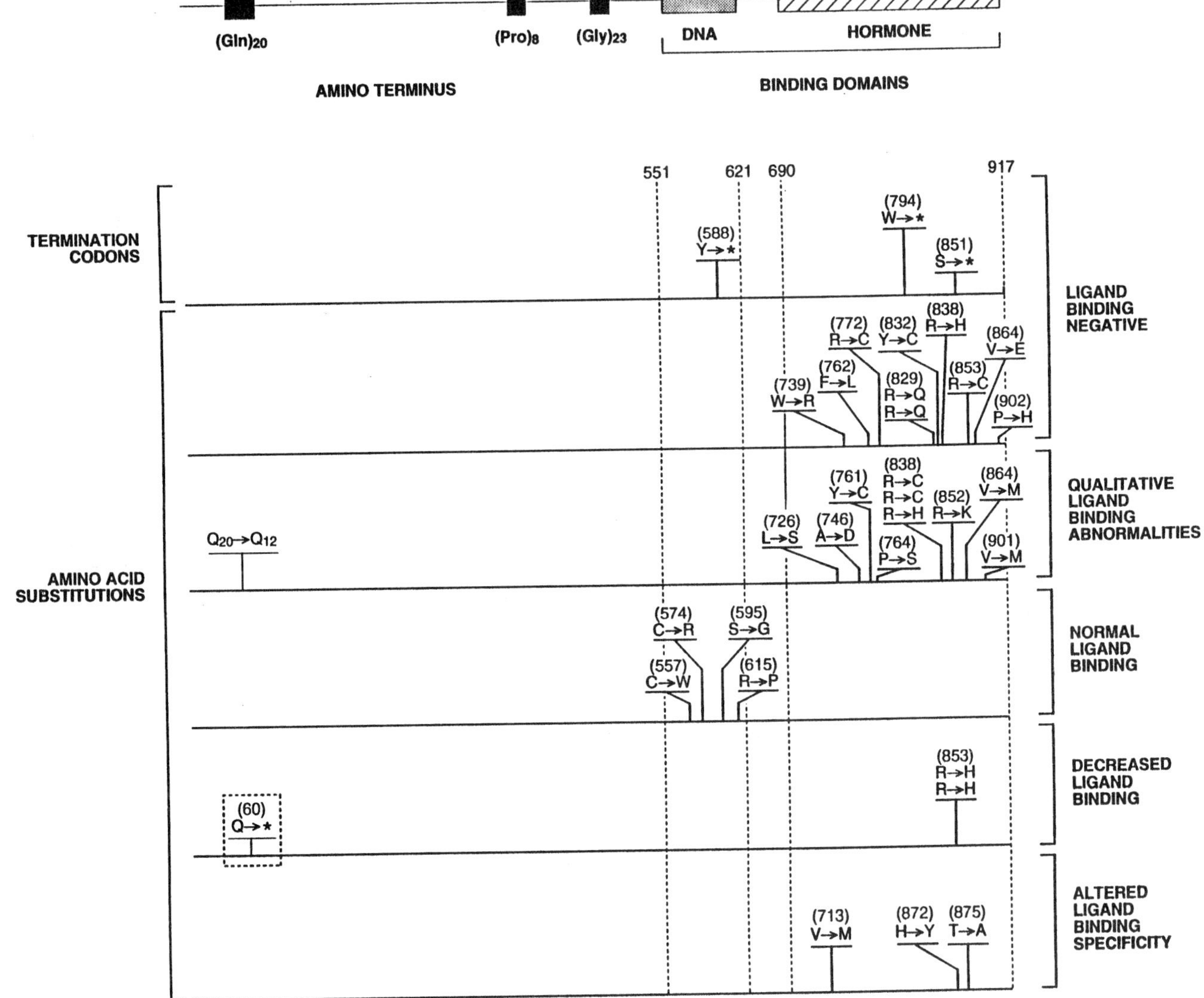

Figure 60-1 Mutations of the human androgen receptor that cause abnormalities of androgen receptor function. A schematic representation of the human androgen receptor (AR) is shown. The approximate boundaries of the DNA- and hormone-binding domains are indicated, as are the locations of the repeated stretches of glutamine, proline, and glycine residues within the amino terminus. (Below) The mutations causing androgen resistance are grouped according to the type of genetic lesion (amino acid substitution or premature termination codon, left margin) or the effect that mutation has on receptor function (right margin). Also included in this figure are three mutations reported in the literature detected in prostate cancer specimens that appear to alter the binding characteristics and activities of the mutant ARs. Not depicted in this summary are deletions and insertions of AR gene segments that account for 5–10% of AR mutations. Expansions of the glutamine repeat that causes spinal and bulbar muscular atrophy are also not represented. (Adapted from McPhaul et al, J Clin Endocrinol Metab 1993;76:17–23.)

surgical correction, most individuals with this phenotype are raised as males, although many exhibit difficulty with gender identity.

At the mildly affected end of the spectrum, a small number of individuals have been described in which normal development of the external genitalia has occurred, but in which some degree of undervirilization is clinically evident. In some, this phenotype has been associated with azoospermia and infertility without undervirilization, whereas in others normal sperm density and fertility occur in undervirilized men. Patients with these phenotypes have been identified as having AR defects on the basis of a family history and abnormalities of in vitro ligand-binding assays of the androgen receptor. Although specific AR defects have now been reported in association with these syndromes, it is not clear how frequently such phenotypes are caused by AR defects in the general population.

An unusual variation of the undervirilized phenotype is that presented by patients with spinal and bulbar muscular atrophy (SBMA, Kennedy's syndrome) (*see* Chapter 100). Patients with this syndrome have normal male development and normal male secondary sexual characteristics throughout much of their lives but develop signs of clinical androgen resistance beginning in middle age. Although these signs of androgen resistance that they display are unmistakable (usually gynecomastia), the difficulties presented by the symptoms of anterior motor neuron degeneration pose a far more serious threat to the health of such patients and represent the usual cause of death in affected individuals.

ANDROGEN RECEPTOR MUTATIONS AND DEFECTIVE AR FUNCTION Molecular defects of the AR that cause the syndromes of androgen resistance have been studied by a number

Table 60-1
Phenotypes Associated with Defects in the Genes Encoding the Androgen Receptor and 5α-Reductase II

Gene	*Syndrome*	*External genitalia*	*Wolffian duct derivatives*	*Müllerian duct derivatives*
AR	Complete testicular feminization Complete androgen insensitivity	Completely female	Not virilized	Absent
	Incomplete testicular feminization	Predominantly female; some clitoromegaly, closure of the posterior fourchette	Usually partially virilized	Absent
	Reifenstein syndrome	Substantial phallic development, but with severe forms of hypospadias	Variable defects	Absent
	Under-virilized, fertile male	Male phenotype with small phallus	Male	Absent
	Infertile male	Male phenotype	Male	Absent
5α-Reductase II	5α-Reductase deficiency	Can be variable: ranging from female external genitalia at birth to a predominantly male phenotype with hypospadias	Normal male	Absent

of groups. The causative mutations have been identified in more than 100 pedigrees and now include all of the major clinical syndromes. A database listing the mutations causing androgen resistance is accessible via the Internet.

Deletions or insertions of the AR gene have been found to occur with a frequency of approximately 5–10% of patients with androgen resistance and range in size from single or multiple nucleotides to deletions of the entire gene. Because such mutations disturb the open reading frame of the AR, patients with this type of mutation do not express an intact receptor protein and, with few exceptions, lack detectable androgen binding in their cells and tissues. In addition, because the intact AR is not present in the tissues of such patients, AR function is absent and affected individuals always demonstrate the phenotype of complete testicular femininization.

In contrast to the frequency of deletions and insertions in the AR gene, single nucleotide substitutions are much more frequent and account for the bulk of patients with androgen resistance as a result of AR mutations. In some cases, such substitutions result in large changes of receptor structure, as when they result in alterations of AR mRNA splicing or introduction of premature termination codons within the AR open reading frame. These instances, as with gene deletion or insertion mutations that interrupt the primary sequence of intact AR protein, are usually associated with a lack of detectable androgen binding in tissues and a phenotype of complete testicular feminization.

Single nucleotide substitutions that result in single amino acid changes within the AR protein are the most frequent type of mutation in the AR. To this point, these defects have been found to fall into two large categories: those within the DNA-binding domain and those that have been localized to the hormone-binding domain of the receptor. Unlike the other mutation categories described above (deletions, insertions, premature termination), the effect of these substitutions on AR function can be quite variable, and thus the entire spectrum of androgen-resistant phenotypes has been traced to single amino acid substitutions within the AR protein. In most instances, the principal effect of the amino acid substitution is on AR function, whereas major effects on the level of AR abundance, as measured in patient fibroblasts, are uncommon.

Amino acid substitutions in the DNA-binding domain have little effect on the binding of ligand by the mutant receptor. Despite the capacity of these mutant ARs to bind ligand normally, receptor function is reduced after ligand stimulation, compared with the activity of the normal AR. This reduced function can be shown to be caused by a decreased capacity of the mutant AR to bind to target sequences within responsive genes. In this category of mutation, the degree of impairment of receptor binding to DNA appears to have a direct relationship to the degree that receptor function is reduced. Similar conclusions hold true for larger alterations of receptor structure occurring within the DNA-binding domain that maintains the reading frame of the receptor (e.g., deletions of single amino acid residues within the DNA-binding domain or the single reported instance caused by in-frame deletion of exon 3).

Amino acid substitutions in the hormone-binding domain (HBD) can result in a variety of changes in the capacity of the AR to bind its ligand. In a surprisingly small proportion of cases, the amino acid replacement renders the receptor completely unable to bind ligand. Under these circumstances, it is presumed that the alteration of the HBD structure is distorted. This conformational change blocks the capacity of the AR to bind its ligand and the mutant receptor is thus "locked" into an inactive conformation. This type of mutant AR is functionally equivalent to mutations that result in the synthesis of truncated forms of the AR, because even pharmacologic doses of potent synthetic androgens are unable to restore receptor function in vivo or in functional assays performed in vitro.

More frequently, however, amino acid substitutions in the HBD lead to the synthesis of mutant ARs that exhibit ligand-binding properties that are abnormal compared with the binding properties of the normal AR (e.g., bind ligand with a reduced affinity or stability). Although the exact type of ligand-binding abnormality differs depending on the nature and location of the amino acid substitution within the hormone-binding domain, it appears that the formation and stability of the hormone–receptor complex is the final determinant of the degree of impairment of mutant AR function. In vitro studies of such mutant receptors demonstrate that the use of multiple high doses of physiologic ligands (testosterone or dihydrotestosterone) or the use of potent nonmetabolizable androgen agonists can overcome the defective function of many mutant ARs of this type. In addition to its mechanistic implications, this finding may have substantial clinical implications as well, since it suggests that the pharmacologic manipulation of many mutant ARs may be possible.

Studies have now been performed to study the levels of expression and the function of normal and mutant ARs. It seems clear that the major effect of most mutations in the AR is not at the level of AR abundance, but at the level of AR function. This is not true in all cases, however, with the most obvious exceptions being mutations that result in truncation of the receptor protein (e.g., termination codons or alterations of mRNA splicing). There also appears to be a relationship between the level of mutant AR function and the phenotype observed in the patient: mutant ARs devoid of function being associated with complete testicular feminization, those with partial activity associated with incomplete forms of androgen resistance. This relationship is most clearly seen using assays that measure the level of AR function in fibroblasts established from the patient under study (e.g., delivery of an androgen-responsive reporter gene directly into the cultured fibroblasts).

ANDROGEN RECEPTOR MUTATIONS—SPECIAL CASES The androgen-resistance syndrome described above is caused by mutations that impair receptor function to various degrees. Two additional types of AR mutation have been identified that result in an alteration of AR responsiveness or an apparent "gain" of function.

The first example of a "gain of function" mutation in the androgen receptor is the genetic defect causing Kennedy's syndrome. The pathogenesis of this extraordinary disease was traced to the expansion of a triplet nucleotide repeat (CAG) encoding a repeated sequence of glutamine residues within the amino-terminus of the receptor (*see* Fig. 60-1). The expansion of this glutamine repeat, the first of an increasing number of similar diseases that have also traced to the expansion of trinucleotide repeats (*see* Chapter 100), is believed to have two different effects on AR function. First, it is clear that the expansion of this segment of the AR diminishes the capacity of the AR to activate responsive genes after androgen stimulation. This diminished AR function can be demonstrated using a variety of functional assays and is presumably the cause of the subtle signs of androgen resistance observed in affected individuals. It is clear from the study of rare patients with complete deletions of the AR that the SBMA phenotype (progressive death of motor neurons in bulbar nuclei and in the spinal cord) is not caused by a simple lack of functional AR. Instead, this disease appears to be caused by some type of toxic "gain of function" that is caused by the expression of androgen receptors containing the expanded glutamine repeats in specific cell types. Analogy to results obtained from the study of the Huntington disease gene (also caused by a glutamine repeat expansion) would suggest that the glutamine expansion may permit interaction of the mutant AR with intracellular targets in spinal motor neurons that somehow mediate the observed cell-type-specific toxicity. Studies have also raised the possibility that a lower number of CAG repeats may correlate with the age of onset of prostate cancer.

The second type of AR mutation that causes a gain or alteration of receptor function are the mutations that have been identified in human prostate cancer specimens. First identified in a prostate tumor cell line, LNCaP, amino acid substitutions have been identified in a number of clinical prostate cancer specimens. Although a number of these mutations have been identified, fewer have been completely studied as to the effect that they have on the ligand responsiveness of the mutated AR. In those instances in which detailed studies have been performed, tests of receptor function using androgen-responsive reporter genes demonstrate that the mutant ARs can be stimulated by ligands that cannot ordinarily activate the normal unmutated AR. Such ligands include adrenal androgens and even compounds (such as hydroxyflutamide) that normally act to antagonize the function of the unmutated AR. It is not yet possible to conclude how important these mutant receptors are in the progression of prostate cancers toward the androgen-independent phenotype.

5α-REDUCTASE DEFICIENCY

PHYSIOLOGIC AND CLINICAL STUDIES The observation that 5α-dihydrotestosterone was the principal hormone bound to the AR in the nuclei of target cells suggested the potential importance of 5α-reductase in androgen physiology. The subsequent identification of rare patients with specific defects of virilization who formed reduced quantities of 5α-reduced androgen metabolites served to emphasize the importance of this metabolic step. The normal virilization of other tissues, such as the epididymis in patients with clinical 5α-reductase deficiency, led to the concept that the action of testosterone was sufficient to effect the actions of androgen in selected tissues, but that the formation of 5α-dihydrotestosterone was crucial in others, such as the prostate, a dichotomy that as yet is still unexplained mechanistically.

CLINICAL PHENOTYPE The clinical features of infants with a deficiency of 5α-reductase are consistent with a marked defect of androgen action (Table 60-1). The external genitalia are characterized by a microphallus, severe hypospadias, and a bifid scrotum. A blind vaginal pouch is present and opens either directly onto the perineum or onto a urogenital sinus. Owing to the production of MIS by the functional testes, no Müllerian structures are present. It is of interest that at puberty, several changes take place in the phenotype of affected individuals. The phallus enlarges and some male secondary sexual characteristics appear, such as changes in voice and muscle mass. Notably, this increase in testosterone has not been reported to result in acne, prostate growth, or male pattern baldness. It has also been reported that in such individuals, raised initially as females, gender identity may change after the pubertal rise in androgen levels.

5α-REDUCTASE STRUCTURE AND MECHANISM OF ACTION Attempts to purify 5α-reductase using classic techniques of protein purification failed and its structure remained elusive until Anderson and colleagues employed expression cloning in *Xenopus* oocytes to isolate a cDNA encoding a steroid 5α-reductase from rat prostate in 1992. This advance permitted a number of studies by this same group and resulted in the isolation of cDNAs encoding two related isozymes (Fig. 60-2) encoded by two distinct, related genes from humans and from all vertebrate species examined to date. Inspection of the structures of the cDNAs indicate substantial sequence divergence between the two isozymes, both within and between different species (Fig. 60-2). Both enzymes are extremely hydrophobic and are believed to be imbedded in the nuclear membrane of cells, accounting for the failure of extensive efforts to purify the enzyme in an active form. Structural differences between the two isozymes confer substantial differences in their physical properties that have been exploited to develop compounds that inhibit one or the other isozyme preferentially.

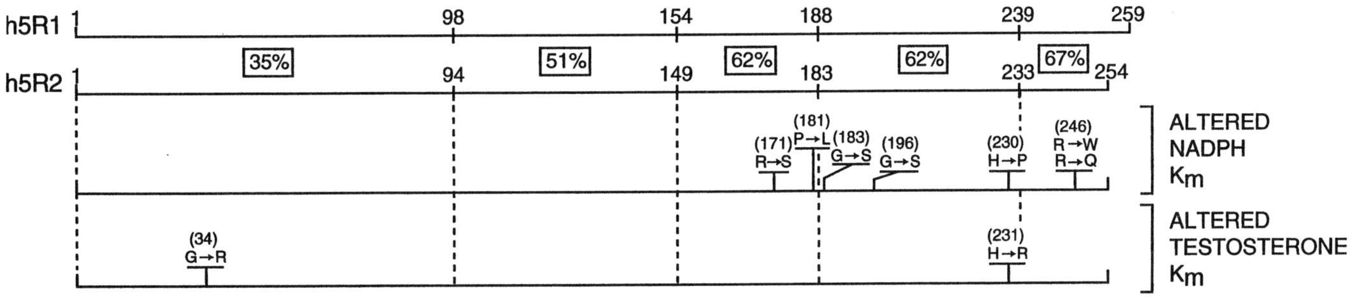

Figure 60-2 Comparison of the structures of human steroid 5α-reductase I and II and mutations that alter the binding of testosterone and NADPH. (Above) Alignment of the predicted protein sequences for steroid 5α-reductase I (259 amino acids) and steroid 5α-reductase II (254 amino acids). The degree of sequence identity is shown for each of the five coding exons (boxed percentages). (Below) Mutations identified within the coding sequence of steroid 5α-reductase deficiency. Although mutations have been detected in each coding exon that result in 5α-reductase II deficiency, only mutations that cause alterations in the binding of testosterone or NADPH are indicated. (Drawn after Russell et al, Annu Rev Biochem 1994;63:25–61.)

Studies of the distribution of the two isozymes (Table 60-2) have demonstrated that the patterns of expression of these two proteins differ, both in terms of tissue, cell type, and stage of development. These differences suggest substantially different physiologic roles for the two enzymes.

GENETIC DEFECTS OF STEROID 5α-REDUCTASE II The genetic lesions causing clinical 5α-reductase deficiency have now been identified in a number of families from around the world. In all instances, when a genetic defect has been detected, it has been traced to a mutation within the 5α-reductase II gene. Unlike the AR gene, the gene encoding 5α-reductase II is autosomal and each individual possesses two copies of the 5α-reductase II gene. For this reason, mutations causing clinical 5α-reductase deficiency are recessive and the inheritance of two defective 5α-reductase II gene alleles is required for the defects to be manifest. 5α-Reductase II deficiency is infrequently caused by deletions or insertions in the gene. More often, defects in the gene are caused by mutations that result in premature termination of the protein or single amino acid substitutions within the open reading frame. Identification of the locations of these substitutions and determination of the physical properties of the mutant enzymes have permitted the identification of amino acid residues important for binding of steroid substrates and for the binding of nicotinamide adenine dinucleotide phosphate (NADPH), a cofactor required for the reduction reaction. Of interest, these studies have also identified sites that have been mutated repeated in apparently unrelated pedigrees. These sites are apparently more susceptible to mutation.

As a consequence of the recessive nature of clinical 5α-reductase II deficiency, it would be expected that the genetic basis of this rare trait would be traced most frequently to homozygosity for a single defective allele (e.g., consanguinity). Surprisingly, a high proportion of patients (40%) have been found to be compound heterozygotes, suggesting either an unexpectedly high mutation rate of the 5α-reductase II gene or a high frequency of individuals in the general population that carry single defective alleles.

GENETIC DEFECTS OF STEROID 5α-REDUCTASE I An abnormal phenotype caused by a deficiency of 5α-reductase I has not yet been described in humans. The differential expression of steroid 5α-reductase I in selected tissues (*see* Table 60-2) suggests that specific phenotypes in humans that result from lesions in this gene may well be identified in the future.

Table 60-2
Distribution of 5α-Reductase I and II Expression in Rat and Human Tissues

	Rat		*Human*	
	Type I	*Type II*	*Type I*	*Type II*
Skin	—	—	+*	+[a]†
Testes	D*	1+*	ND†	
Epididymis	D*[e]	5+*[e]	ND†	+[b]†,*
Vas deferens	D*	1+*	—	—
Seminal vesicle	D	1+*	ND†	+†
Ventral prostate	D[d]*	D[d]*		
Prostate			ND†,*	+[c]†,*
Ovary	2+*	ND*		
Adrenal	3+*	D*		
Brain	3+*	ND*		
Colon	3+*	D*		
Heart	ND*	ND*		
Intestine	3+*	D*		
Kidney	3+*	ND*		
Liver	4+*	ND*	+†,*	+†,*
Lung	2+*	ND*		
Muscle	ND*	ND*		
Spleen	D*	ND*		
Stomach	D*	ND*		
Pons	—	—	ND	+
Cerebral	—	—	ND	+
Hypothalamus	—	—	ND	+

Summary of studies measuring 5α-reductase I and II expression using measurements of the corresponding RNA (*) or protein (†) are derived from published studies of Russell and coworkers. The rating scales (1+ least, 5+ highest) used in this summary are designed to convey a sense of the relative abundance of the 5α-reductase isozymes in the two species—rat and human—that have been studied most carefully. Because the rat and human measurements have been conducted separately, they can only be compared with one another in a qualitative fashion. D is detectable (i.e., at the limits of detection). ND, is not detected; —, values not reported. In addition to the results tabulated here, the studies of Thigpen et al. clearly indicate that in the human substantial changes in abundance can be demonstrated in the expression of the type I and type II isoenzymes in a tissue at different times in development.

[a]Histochemical studies indicate that the expression of 5α-reductase II is localized to the cells of the dermal papilla.

[b]Staining localized to epithelial cells in histochemical studies.

[c]Staining localized to basal epithelial and stroma cells.

[d]Type I is detected in basal epithelial cells and type II in stroma cells in *in situ* hybridization studies of the regenerating rat central prostate.

[e]Type I and II are localized to the epithelial cells using *in situ* hybridization.

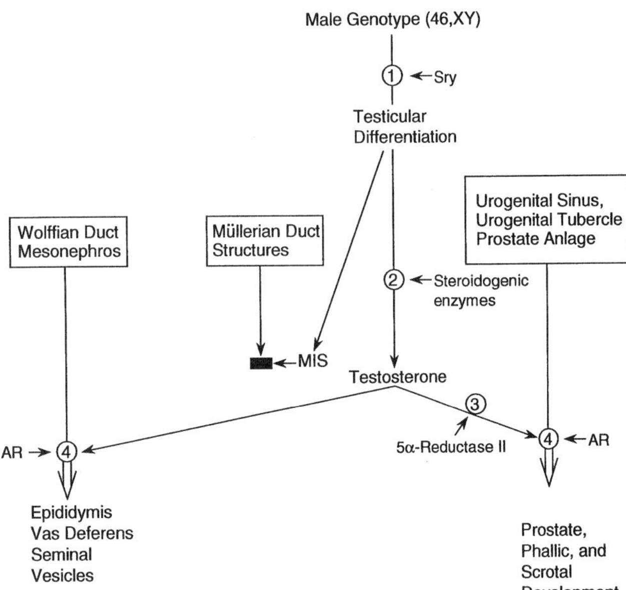

Figure 60-3 Schematic the pathways controlling the development of the normal male phenotype. Male sexual development is a complex cascade of events that can be affected by lesions in a number of genes. Some, such as lesions in the *AR* or *SRY*, can cause disturbances of virilization of all androgen-responsive tissues. The effects of defects in other genes, however (such as mutations of 5α-reductase II), are manifest only in selected tissues. It is likely that defects in other genes can contribute to defects in virilization, as a large proportion of the subjects with abnormalities of male phenotypic development cannot be accounted for by defects in the genes most carefully studied to date, such as the AR and steroid 5α-reductase II.

Owing to the lack of mutations in the human population, the first insights into the nature of defects that may be expected in humans have come from experiments in mice in which steroid 5α-reductase I gene has been disrupted by homologous recombination. Male mice homozygous for this targeted null allele develop normally, both prenatally and postnatally. Unexpectedly, although female mice homozygous for this same null allele develop normally into adulthood, when pregnant, such mice fail to initiate parturition normally. Experiments in which different steroids were administered to these steroid 5α-reductase I-deficient mice suggested that the synthesis and actions of 5α-reduced androgens were important elements of the normal parturition process in mice. Although the mechanisms and generality of these findings remain to be determined, such results suggest that 5α-reductase I may play important—and even unexpected—roles in human physiology as well.

SUMMARY

The development of the male phenotype is a complicated process that involves the active participation of genes involved at many levels, from gonadal differentiation to the androgen receptor itself. Defective virilization can be caused at defects anywhere along the pathway displayed schematically in Fig. 60-3. Taking into account the clinical syndromes caused by known defects of genes such as steroid 5α-reductase II and the androgen receptor, the pathogenesis of a large proportion of defects in virilization remains unexplained. It is conceivable that some may represent defects in genes required for normal AR function or at steps beyond the site of action of the AR itself (e.g., coactivators, or defects in genes activated by the AR).

ACKNOWLEDGMENTS

This work was supported by NIH grants DK03892 and DK52678.

SELECTED REFERENCES

Giovannucci E, Stampfer MJ, Krithivas K, et al. The CAG repeat within the androgen receptor gene and its relationship to prostate cancer. Proc Natl Acad Sci USA 1997;94:3320–3323.

Gottlieb B. Androgen Receptor Gene Mutation Data Base MC33@musicamcgill.ca

Hardy DO, Scher HI, Bogenreider T, et al. Androgen receptor CAG repeat lengths in prostate cancer: correlation with age of onset. J Clin Endocrinol Metab 1996;81:4400–4405.

Hiort O, Sinnecker GH, Holterhus PM, Nitsche EM, Kruse K. The clinical and molecular spectrum of androgen insensitivity syndromes. Am J Med Genet 1996;63:218–222.

Imperato-McGinley J. 5 Alpha-reductase-2 deficiency. Curr Ther Endocrinol Metab 1997;6:384–387.

Lumbroso S, Lobaccaro JM, Vial C, et al. Molecular analysis of the androgen receptor gene in Kennedy's disease. Report of two families and review of the literature. Horm Res 1997;7:23–29.

Marcelli M, Zoppi S, Wilson CM, Griffin JE, McPhaul MJ. Amino acid substitutions in the hormone-binding domain of the human androgen receptor alter the stability of the hormone receptor complex. J Clin Invest 1994;94:1642–1650.

McPhaul MJ, Marcelli M, Zoppi S, Griffin JE, Wilson JD. Genetic basis of endocrine disease 4. The spectrum of mutations in the androgen receptor gene that causes androgen resistance. J Clin Endocrinol Metab 1993;76:17–23.

Quigley CA, DeBellis A, Marschke KB, El-awady MK, Wilson EM, French FS. Androgen receptor defects: historical, clinical, and molecular perspectives. Endocr Rev 1995;16:271–321.

Mahendroo MS, Cala KM, Russell DW. 5α-Reduced androgens are required for parturition in mice. Mol Endocrinol 1996;10:380–392.

Russell DW, Wilson JD. Steroid 5α-reductase: two genes/two enzymes. Annu Rev Biochem 1994;63:25–61.

Thigpen AE, Silver RI, Guileyardo JM, Casey ML, McConnell JD, Russell DW. Tissue distribution and ontogeny of steroid 5α-reductase isozyme expression. J Clin Invest 1993;92:903–910.

Wilson JD, Griffin JE, Russell DW. Steroid 5α-reductase 2 deficiency. Endocr Rev 1993;14:77–93.

61 Testicular Diseases

MARCO MARCELLI

TESTICULAR EMBRYOGENESIS

Between 1947 and 1952 Alfred Jost formulated the concept that sexual differentiation is an ordered process in which chromosomal sex determines gonadal sex, and gonadal sex in turn directs the development of phenotypic sex. Since 1959 it has been known that in humans and other mammals the Y chromosome determines maleness. These insights led to the postulate of a gene or genes on the Y chromosome that would act as a "master switch" to set in motion the cascade of events that leads to the development of the male gonads. The discovery and the roles played by the genes involved in testicular embryogenesis and their involvement in human diseases and experimental models characterized by abnormal testicular development are discussed in Chapter 57.

BASIC ENDOCRINOLOGY OF THE TESTIS

MICROSCOPIC ORGANIZATION From a functional point of view, the microscopic architecture of the testis consists of two regions, the interstitial and tubular compartments, which are separated by the basal lamina. The interstitial compartment contains loose connective tissue with interspersed epithelial cells, the Leydig cells, which are specialized for the synthesis and secretion of testosterone. The tubular compartment consists of cylindrical structures, the seminiferous tubules, which are lined with Sertoli and germinal cells. Sertoli cells create support for the germ cells by resting on the basal membrane of the tubule and extending apically, and are believed to produce several growth factors affecting the process of testicular development and sperm maturation. In addition, they offer a critical contribution to the process of male sexual differentiation through the production of anti-Müllerian hormone (AMH), which causes regression of the Müllerian ducts. The growth and maturation of the germinal epithelium into mature spermatozoa is a highly synchronized process. According to the degree of maturation, germ cells can broadly be classified as spermatogonia, primary spermatocytes, secondary spermatocytes, spermatids, and spermatozoa. However, in post pubertal individuals more than a dozen different stages of germinal cell maturation have been described on the basis of subtle histologic differences.

Cytoplasmic projections originating from the Sertoli cells between spermatogonia and primary spermatocytes are connected by tight junctions, and divide the tubule into the basal compartment (containing the Leydig cells, the basal lamina, the myoid cells, and the spermatogonia) and the adluminal compartment (containing primary and secondary spermatocytes, spermatids, and mature spermatozoa). Diffusion of protein, ions, or steroid hormones between the adluminal and basal compartments is impossible, since, similar to the blood–brain barrier, the tight junctions between these two compartments of the testis create an environment that is impermeable to macromolecules.

From: *Principles of Molecular Medicine* (J. L. Jameson, ed.), ©1998 Humana Press Inc., Totowa, NJ.

PHASES OF SPERMATOGENESIS The germinal epithelium undergoes continuous replication to regenerate multipotent stem cells, as well as to produce cells that can proceed through subsequent maturative changes that result in the formation of mature spermatozoa. The mechanisms regulating sperm maturation are largely unknown; however, it is well-established that spermatogenesis occurs only in the presence of androgens and a functional androgen receptor, and that Sertoli cells have a dual role of providing physical support for the maturing germinal cells and of producing, under the stimulation of follicle-stimulating hormone (FSH) and testosterone, factors important for the stimulation of germ-cell maturation. Two human conditions, congenital hypogonadotropic hypogonadism (HH) and men after hypophysectomy, have been very instructive in understanding the role played by the two gonadotropins in inducing sperm maturation. In congenital HH, the administration of human chorionic gonadotropin (hCG), a luteinizing hormone (LH)-like molecule that induces high intratesticular level of testosterone, is followed by the induction of germ-cell maturation from spermatogonia to spermatids. To obtain the full maturation of spermatids to spermatozoa, however, the simultaneous administration of FSH is required. Similarly, replacement with both gonadotropins is necessary to restore spermatogenesis after hypophysectomy, although once spermatogenesis is restored, it can be maintained by injecting hCG alone. Hence, the actions of both gonadotropins are necessary for normal spermatogenesis to occur. Three main events are necessary for the completion of spermatogenesis: (1) stem-cell renewal by mitosis, (2) reduction of chromosomal number by meiosis, and (3) transformation of conventional cells into specialized elements that can reach and fertilize the egg.

Spermatogonial Stem-Cell Renewal The most primordial cells of the germinal lineage are called spermatogonia, of which three types are usually recognizable morphologically. The type A dark spermatogonium, which is thought to be the most primordial, is characterized by a densely stained chromatin containing a centrally located pale area, known as the nuclear vacuole. The type A pale spermatogonium, has a palely staining chromatin and one or two nucleoli. The type B spermatogonium is smaller, has coarse granules of heavily stained chromatin, and is believed to represent a more advanced level of maturation when compared with the type A cells.

Meiotic Maturation A minority of type B spermatogonia commit themselves to further differentiation, and, by responding to unknown stimuli, divide and detach from the basement membrane of the tubule to form the primary spermatocytes. These cells undergo a complex maturation process involving two meiotic divisions: the first from primary spermatocytes into secondary spermatocytes and the second from secondary spermatocytes to spermatids. When primary spermatocytes reach the time of the first meiotic division, they have already engaged in DNA synthesis, and each of their chromosome pair consists of four chromatids. Hence, when the first meiotic division occurs, the resulting secondary spermatocytes contain a haploid number of chromosomes, but each is composed of a pair of chromatids (haploid number of chromosomes and diploid DNA content). Only after the second meiotic division do the developing germ cells (at this level of maturation termed spermatids) have both haploid chromosomal number and haploid DNA content.

Spermiogenesis In the final phase of germ-cell maturation spermatids undergo a number of morphologic changes, and are transformed into specialized cells that can reach and fertilize the ovum. These can be conveniently followed in five phases, consisting of (1) nuclear changes, (2) acrosome formation, (3) flagellum development, (4) redistribution of cytoplasm, and (5) spermiation. During the final phases of sperm maturation the nuclear chromatin condenses, the nucleus becomes progressively smaller and more peripheral, and is positioned in close contact with the cell membrane (nuclear changes), from which it is separated by the acrosomal cap. The latter is formed from large vacuoles produced by the Golgi complex, and contains enzymatic activities important for the penetration of the ovum during fertilization (acrosomal formation). The next most important change observed during this phase consists in the development of the sperm tail (flagellar development), the structure capable of generating the motion of mature spermatozoa. Its architecture is highly conserved among species, and consists of nine peripheral doublet microtubules (known as subfibers A and B), surrounding an additional central pair of microtubules, and is arranged in pattern termed the "9 + 9 + 2" structure. Connections between each peripheral doublet are provided by dynein arms, which project from subfibers A toward subfibers B, and by nexin links. Dynein arms are made of dynein, a protein with ATPase activity that is vital to the generation of flagellar motility. Other connections between each peripheral doublet and the two central microtubules are provided by radial spikes. The intimate connections between the central and peripheral tubular structures of the sperm tail are critical for the achievement of the typical wavelike motion necessary for the propulsion of the mature spermatozoa. Diseases associated with absence of the dynein arms, and with sperm immotility, have been described, and are discussed in Table 61-1.

The eccentric migration of the nucleus toward the acrosomal cap occurs simultaneously with the caudal migration of the cytoplasm toward the developing tail (redistribution of the cytoplasm). The latter is facilitated by a system of cytoplasmic filaments, which extend from the nuclear membrane close to the acrosome to the caudal end of the developing sperm. The seminiferous tubules empty into a network of ducts called the rete testis. By the time the spermatids reach the rete testis, they have been shed of almost the entire cytoplasm, which at this stage is termed the residual body, and is phagocytosed and degraded by the surrounding Sertoli cells (spermiation).

FINAL PHASES OF SPERM MATURATION The interval from the beginning of spermatogenesis to the delivery of sperm into the rete testis is approximately 74 days. During the next 12 days, spermatozoa transit through the epididymis and vas deferens, undergo a number of final morphologic and functional changes, and acquire motility and full capacity to fertilize an ovum.

PHYSIOLOGY OF TESTICULAR FUNCTION A discussion of the hormonal regulation of testicular function, of the synthesis and mechanism of action of testicular steroids, and of the feedback mechanisms regulating the hypothalamic–pituitary–testicular axis is presented in Chapter 56.

MALE HYPOGONADISM

Disorders of testicular function result from abnormalities involving the endocrine (Leydig cells) or reproductive (germ-cell maturation) compartments of the testis. If low testosterone production is present, it is usually accompanied by infertility, because normal spermatogenesis requires normal production of testicular androgens (hypogonadism with undervirilization and infertility). However, there are situations in which hypogonadism is restricted to the germinal compartment (hypogonadism with infertility and normal virilization).

The serum levels of gonadotropins indicate at what site within the hypothalamic–pituitary–gonadal (HPG) axis the defect is localized. In those instances in which gonadal function is abnormal (hypergonadotropic or primary hypogonadism), gonadotropin levels are elevated. In those instances in which the hypothalamopituitary structures are defective (hypogonadotropic or secondary hypogonadism), gonadotropin levels are inappropriately normal or low. Depending on the serum level of gonadotropins, hypogonadism can be classified as hypergonadotropic or hypogonadotropic (if caused by testicular or hypothalamic-pituitary disorders, respectively) and eugonadotropic (if the abnormality lies only in the germinal cells) (Tables 61-1 through 61-3).

Both congenital and acquired forms of Leydig cell dysfunction have been described, and the clinical picture that results when testosterone synthesis is impaired is different depending on whether androgen deficiency developed prenatally, before puberty, or after puberty (Table 61-4). If the developing fetus was not exposed to adequate level of androgen as a result of testicular failure during fetal development, the infant will be affected with pseudohermaphroditism, characterized by a large spectrum of potential abnormalities, including ambiguous genitalia, micropenis, and rudimentary testes (Table 61-4). If reduced testosterone production developed before puberty, but testicular function was normal during embryogenesis, androgen-related somatic changes that are observed at puberty are absent or incomplete and the patient develops an eunuchoid habitus because of failure of closure of the epiphyses and poor development of the skeletal muscles and body hair (Table 61-4). If reduced testosterone production developed after puberty, the first symptom of the patient is impotence, whereas loss of secondary sexual characteristics may take 5–10 years to become complete (Table 61-4).

Hypogonadism manifested by abnormal sperm production (Table 61-1 and 61-3) can be associated with normal virilization, since many infertile men produce normal or only minimally abnormal amounts of testosterone. However, in other cases infertility is associated with a reduced production of testosterone and clinical signs of androgen deficiency (infertility from hypergonadotropic or hypogonadotropic disorders [Table 61-2]). In such cases, infertility is a direct consequence of the reduced testosterone production.

Table 61-1
Eugonadotropic Germinal Cell Failure

	Clinical features and causes	*Treatment*
Ductal obstruction	*See text.*	*See text.*
Varicocele	Most frequently recognized cause of infertility; however, infertility is not always associated with its presence. It is still debated why varicocele causes infertility.	Surgical removal is indicated in adult with infertility of unknown cause, and in adolescent with testicular growth failure. Whether surgical removal improves sperm quality or not is still controversial.
CAH (congenital adzenal hyperplasia)	Suppression of LH and FSH by supraphysiologic production of androgens.	Exogenous glucocorticoid.
Infections	The microorganisms most frequently detected are *Ureaplasma urealyticum* and *Chlamydia trachomatis*. They are thought to induce infertility by impairment of germ-cell maturation, inflammatory occlusion of the ejaculatory ducts, induction of autoimmune phenomenon, and dysfunction of ejaculated sperm.	Doxycycline.
Immotile cilia syndrome	Sperm of normal number and morphology, but with no motility. Associated with bronchiectasis and sinopulmonary infections because of immotility of respiratory cilia. Kartagener's syndrome is the association of immotile cilia syndrome and situs inversus. Immotile cilia syndrome is caused by deletion or shortening of dynein arms and absence of central microtubules.	Microinjection in the perivitelline space or into the oocyte of the recovered sperm.
Autoimmunity	Autoantibodies can be detected against the basement membrane of the seminiferous tubule or against the sperm in 5–10% of men evaluated for infertility.	Steroids (however not always useful to improve sperm quality).
Environmental factors	Lead, mercury, cadmium, dibromochlorpropane (DBCP), 1,1,12-trichloro-2,2-*bis*(*p*-chlorophenyl-ethane) (DTT), *p,p*'-DDE	Remove toxin.
Drugs and radiation	Chemotherapeutic agents, anabolic steroids, cocaine, marijuana, ethanol, radiation >1.0 gy, ^{131}I treatment >100 mCi, high scrotal temperature.	Remove toxin.
Retrograde ejaculation	Associated with diabetes, transurethral prostatectomy. Typically with an ejaculate of <1.3 mL.	α-Adrenergic agonists or intraoperative recovery of sperm from vas deferens or epididymis.
Failure of emission	Associated with spinal cord injury, multiple sclerosis, diabetes.	Electroejaculation, recovery of sperm from vas deferens or epididymis.

HYPERGONADOTROPIC DISORDERS

Hypergonadotropic disorders of the testes are caused by primary testicular failure, and, as shown in Table 61-2, they can be grouped in two main categories, congenital and acquired abnormalities. Some congenital syndromes lead to primary hypogonadism as a result of chromosomal abnormalities, enzymatic defects, or receptor defects. Others are congenital multiorgan diseases with associated hypogonadism. Acquired diseases causing primary hypogonadism result from the direct exposure of the testis to a large variety of exogenous toxic agents. The typical endocrine abnormalities found in these patients consist of decreased to undetectable serum levels of testosterone and an elevation of the two gonadotropins above the normal range owing to the absence of the negative feedback inhibition exerted by testosterone.

HYPERGONADOTROPIC HYPOGONADISM CAUSED BY CHROMOSOMAL ABNORMALITIES

KLINEFELTER'S SYNDROME Background This syndrome was initially described in 1942, at a time when no techniques to study hormone levels or chromosomal banding were available. Its frequency is about 1/500 males at conception, but only 1/1000 live male newborns. Therefore, even if the Klinefelter phenotype is perceived as benign, half of all 47,XXY fetuses are lost before birth. In the large majority of cases this syndrome is associated with a 47,XXY chromosomal pattern; however 46,XY/47,XXY mosaicism is detected in approximately 10% of patients. Less frequently it is found in 46,XX males, or in individuals with Xq trisomy, X-autosome translocations, or poly-X (48XXXY, 49XXXXY).

Clinical Features Prepubertal diagnosis of this disorder is possible in the cases in which microphallus or cryptorchidism are part of the prepubertal phenotype, or when a determination of the karyotype is requested if mental retardation or multiple congenital anomalies are detected by the physician.

The features of undervirilization are most often detected in the postpubertal patient and include bilateral gynecomastia, small testes, azoospermia, decreased muscular mass, and abnormal skeletal proportions suggestive of eunuchoid habitus. Small testicular size because of the absence of germ cells is a consistent clinical abnormality. In addition, progressive hyalinization and fibrosis of the seminiferous tubules results in increased testicular consistency.

Mild mental retardation and personality disorders are identified more frequently in patients with Klinefelter's syndrome than in the general population, and these abnormalities are usually more evident in the group of patients with polysomic-X conditions. Other conditions that have been detected with increased frequency in patients with Klinefelter's syndrome include thyroid abnormalities, diabetes mellitus, and breast and other types of cancer.

Table 61-2
Hypogonadotropic and Hypergonadotropic Disorders

Hypergonadotropic disorders	*Hypogonadotropic disorders*
Congenital	**Congenital**
Chromosomal abnormalities	**Associated with gonadotropin deficiency**
Klinefelter's syndrome	Kallmann's syndrome
46,XX males	Fertile eunuch syndrome
46,XY pure gonadal dysgenesis (Swyer syndrome)	Associated with biologically inactive LH
Multiorgan diseases	**Mutations of the LH gene**
Myotonic dystrophy	
Alströmis syndrome	**Associated with central nervous system disorders**
Ullrich Noonan syndrome	Prader-Lahart-Willi syndrome
Bilateral anorchia	Laurence-Moon-Biedl syndrome
Down's syndrome	Möbius's syndrome
Niemann Pick disease	Börjeson-Forssman-Lehman syndrome
Receptor defects	LEOPARD syndrome
LH-resistant testis	Rud's syndrome
Syndromes of androgen resistance	Lowe's syndrome
Defects of steroidogenesis	Carpenter's syndrome
Lipoid CAH	**Associated with adrenal insufficiency**
3β-Hydroxysteroid	Adrenal hypoplasia congenita
Dehydrogenase/Δ^5-Δ^4-isomerase (3β-HSD) deficiency	
17α-Hydroxylase/17,20-lyase deficiency	**Acquired**
17β-Hydroxysteroid dehydrogenase (17β-HSD) deficiency	**Associated with anatomic disorders**
Type 2 5α-reductase deficiency	Pituitary apoplexy
Acquired	Primary or metastatic tumors of pituitary or adjacent structures
Viral	Infection
Medications	Infiltrative disorders (hemochromatosis, sarcoidosis, histiocytosis, lymphocytic hypophysitis)
Trauma	Empty sella
Environmental	**Functional**
Autoimmunity	Secondary to Cushing's syndrome
Ionizing radiation	to ethanol
	to exercise
	to empty sella
	to hyperprolactinemia
	Associated with systemic diseases
	AIDS
	Liver diseases
	Renal diseases
	Hemochromatosis
	Neurologic diseases

From a clinical standpoint, patients affected by 46,XY/47,XXY mosaicism manifest less serious phenotypic abnormalities, and can be fertile. However, other variants of this disease, including 48,XXXY, 48,XXYY, and 49,XXXXY individuals, are associated more frequently with cryptorchidism, growth retardation, mental deficiency, antisocial behavior, facial dysmorphism, and skeletal abnormalities.

The endocrine features of these patients show a typical evolution that becomes evident when they are examined for a period of years. Usually basal FSH, LH, and testosterone are normal in virtually all subjects studied before age 12; however, by age 14 LH and FSH are elevated. At these early states, the secretion of testosterone is kept within the normal range by the increased production of gonadotropins. By the time the patient has reached his middle 20s, however, primary gonadal failure is evident and testosterone levels will be low or in the low range of normal, despite elevated gonadotropins.

Diagnosis Final diagnostic confirmation of this syndrome is obtained by analyzing the karyotype and by detecting one of the many chromosomal abnormalities described above.

Genetic Basis of Disease The most common cause of Klinefelter's syndrome is nondisjunction during the first or second meiotic division. The extra X chromosome can be of paternal or maternal origin with approximately the same frequency. Most of the maternal cases are associated with impaired disjunction during the first meiotic division, and maternal age is a factor in these cases. A second possible mechanism, occurring in 3% of the cases, is nondisjunction after the first postzygotic mitosis. A third potential mechanism was described in an Italian family, in which the mother had a 46,XX/47,XXX mosaicism, possibly because of a nondisjunctional event during her zygotic development, and three of her children were affected by the classic Klinefelter karyotype 47,XXY.

The origin of the 46,XY/47,XXY mosaicism derives from nondisjunctional events in mitosis during zygotic development.

Table 61-3
Causes of Hypergonadotropic and Eugonadotropic Germinal Cell Failure

Hypergonadotropic	*Eugonadotropic*
Undescended testis (cryptorchidism)	Ductal obstruction
Germinal cell aplasia (Sertoli cells only syndrome)	Varicocele
Idiopathic seminiferous tubular failure with hyalinization	Congenital adrenal hyperplasia
Androgen resistance	Heat
	Infections
	Radiation
	Drugs
	Autoimmunity
	Impairment of sperm transport
	Immotile cilia syndrome

Table 61-4
Manifestations of Leydig Cell Dysfunction

Prenatal Leydig cell dysfunction
External genitalia: female, ambiguous; male, hypoplastic
Wolffian duct derivatives: absent; rudimentary
Müllerian duct derivatives: absent
Gonads: small; rudimentary testes, which can be located intra-abdominally, inside the inguinal canal, or in the scrotum
Prepubertal Leydig cell dysfunction
External genitalia: small penis <3–4 cm, small testis <5 mL, lack of rugal folds, and pigmentation in the scrotum
Accessory sex organs: small prostate and seminal vesicles
Hair growth: no development of terminal facial hair, no recession of scalp line, decreased body hair, female escutcheon
Linear growth: eunuchoidal skeletal proportions
Bone development: delayed bone age, predisposition to osteoporosis
Voice: voice remains high-pitched
Muscle mass: absent; reduced development of muscle mass
Psyche: decreased libido
Postpubertal Leydig cell dysfunction
External genitalia: softening and decreased volume of the testes
Psyche: decreased libido, sexual potency, and aggressivity
Bone: predisposition to osteoporosis
Hair growth: decreased growth and amount of facial, pubic, and axillary hair
Spermatogenesis: impaired
Muscle mass: decreased

Patients with mosaicism have a lesser degree of gynecomastia and androgen deficiency. Normal testicular size has been described in these patients, and this is particularly true when the normal stem cell line 46,XY is present in the testis.

The additional sex chromosomes in patients with 48,XXYY karyotype derive from successive nondisjunctional events in the first and second meiotic division in the father. In contrast, the additional X chromosomes in 49,XXXXY patients are maternally derived, and originate from sequential nondisjunctional events in both the first and second meiotic divisions.

Whether development of the Klinefelter phenotype requires the entire extra X chromosome remains an open question. One study looking at phenotype–karyotype correlations has associated the development of the Klinefelter phenotype with genes mapping to region Xq11–Xq22. However this observation was not confirmed by other investigators in a patient with a 47,X,del(X)(pter–p11),Y karyotype.

Therapy The main complaints of these patients are the symptoms of hypogonadism, particularly gynecomastia, infertility, and reduced libido, and several psychosocial problems. Standard treatment for these problems is replacement with testosterone, which should be started immediately after puberty. Gynecomastia is usually unresponsive to treatment with testosterone, and many of these patients will require surgical removal of the enlarged breasts. Infertility is not improved by the treatment with testosterone, and in most cases a further reduction in the sperm count will be observed. Because this disease is associated with an increased risk of developing breast cancer that may approach 20 times that for normal men, some authors have advocated yearly screening mammography, but it is not clear whether this is a useful measure.

46,XX MALES Background and Clinical Features This is a variant of Klinefelter's syndrome, occurring in approximately 1/20,000 male births. The phenotype resembles that of patients with Klinefelter's syndrome, with the major difference being short stature, because of the absence of Y sequences that are important for normal somatic growth, and normal intellectual development. The testes are small and firm, androgen production is compromised, and gynecomastia is a frequent abnormality present in adolescent patients. Germ cells are absent, and serum levels of gonadotropins elevated. Affected individuals have male psychosexual identification.

Diagnosis These patients are usually referred to a physician to investigate the typical phenotypic abnormalities that become evident after puberty. Some of these patients are referred at an earlier stage of their life, since at times this entity is associated with hypospadias, particularly in the subgroup of patients in whom no Y sequences are detected. The identification of a 46,XX karyotype associated with a male phenotype and endocrine studies showing hypogonadism and infertility permit the successful diagnosis of this condition.

Genetic Basis of Disease The presence of Y material containing *SRY* can be demonstrated in the X chromosome of approximately 80% of these patients. This event is caused by X-Y recombination occurring outside the pseudoautosomal segments in which X-Y pairing normally occurs, resulting in the transfer of *SRY* from the Y to the X chromosome. The consensus is that *SRY* translocated to the X chromosome is sufficient to trigger testicular differentiation and the development of a male phenotype. The remainder of these patients (approximately 20%) do not carry any identifiable Y sequence and have larger incidence of ambiguous genitalia. As yet, no mechanism has been identified to account for the male phenotypic development observed in these patients. One possibility could be an activating mutation of a factor normally induced by *SRY* in the cascade of events leading to the differentiation of the male gonad.

The pathogenesis of infertility in these patients is probably caused, as in Klinefelter's syndrome, by the presence of two X chromosomes in the germ cells and the lack of regions of the Y chromosome that are essential for spermatogenesis. Management of these patients is the same as that for patients with Klinefelter's syndrome.

46,XY PURE GONADAL DYSGENESIS (SWYER SYNDROME) Background and Clinical Features 46,XY pure gonadal dysgenesis, of which a complete and an incomplete form have been described, occurs both in sporadic and familial forms.

The complete form of this disease is associated with an impairment of testosterone and AMH production that begins in the initial phase of fetal development, and results in a female phenotype characterized by sexual infantilism with bilateral streak gonads, Müllerian duct development, and female internal organs.

In the incomplete form of the disease the virilization of the phenotype depends on the degree of differentiation achieved by the gonads, which varies from streak gonads to dysgenetic testes, and on their residual capacity to produce testosterone and AMH. In the incomplete form of the disease virilization is never normal. Therefore the characteristics of the internal and external genitalia of these patients are more ambiguous than in the complete form. The presence of spontaneous gynecomastia is associated with an estrogen-secreting neoplasm, which in these patients can frequently be a gonadoblastoma. Unlike 46,XX males, this entity is associated with normal stature because of the presence of most of the Y chromosome.

Diagnosis 46,XY pure gonadal dysgenesis is a form of primary hypogonadism that is typically associated with increased levels of gonadotropins. Testosterone levels are almost undetectable in patients with the complete form, and decreased but detectable in patients with the incomplete form. The diagnosis should be suspected in individuals presenting with primary hypogonadism, a 46,XY karyotype, and with the phenotype and pattern of inheritance discussed above.

Genetic Basis of Disease This disease is associated with a remarkable degree of genetic heterogeneity. It has been associated with abnormalities occurring in the Y-linked *SRY* gene, with an X-linked pattern of inheritance, and with a sex-limited autosomal dominant inheritance. Defects of *SRY* (deletions of the *SRY* gene and most frequently point mutations) have been detected in approximately 10–15% of the sporadic cases and in three kindreds with the familial form. Other X-linked and autosomal genes that could be involved with this syndrome, including *AMH*, *SF-1*, *WT1*, *DSS*, and *SOX-9*, are discussed in Chapter 57.

Molecular Pathophysiology of Disease The association of this disease with alterations in the sequence of *SRY*, and potentially with other autosomal or X-linked genes, is leading to a more sophisticated understanding of the complex cascade of events required for normal testicular differentiation. The sequence of events, and the precise mechanism of interaction among these factors is not completely clear and currently is under investigation.

Treatment The sex of rearing should be based on the degree of genital ambiguity. When this critical dilemma has been properly addressed and skeletal growth is complete, the rudimentary gonads should be prophylactically removed, since they may undergo malignant degeneration. At this point testosterone or estrogen replacement should be started to ensure the development of the secondary sexual characteristics and the prevention of osteopenia.

HYPERGONADOTROPIC HYPOGONADISM FROM MULTIORGAN DISEASES

ALSTRÖM SYNDROME Clinical Features This rare entity, described in 1959 by Alström, is characterized by autosomal recessive inheritance, and by multifactorial disorders including retinal pigment degeneration, obesity, diabetes mellitus, acanthosis nigricans, sensorineural deafness, chronic nephropathy, and metabolic abnormalities such as hyperuricemia and hypertriglyceridemia. Hypogonadism is typically a clinical feature of affected men, but not women. It is a primary form of hypogonadism, associated with low testosterone and high gonadotropin levels. Alström's syndrome is usually associated with normal secondary sexual characteristics; however, the small testes demonstrate hyalinized tubules and thickening of the lamina propria.

Genetic Basis of Disease The pathophysiology of Alström's syndrome is unknown. Because it is expressed only in the homozygous state, a single-gene abnormality, as yet undefined, is responsible for this multisystem involvement. Recently, the disease gene was localized to chromosome 2p.

NOONAN SYNDROME (MALE TURNER'S SYNDROME) Background and Clinical Features This disease was once classified as the male Turner's syndrome, because of the association of primary testicular failure with many of the clinical stigmata of Turner's syndrome. The incidence is estimated to be between 1:1000 and 1:5000 live male births. Approximately half of the cases are familial and the pattern of inheritance is autosomal dominant with variable penetrance. The typical clinical picture includes webbed neck, ptosis, hypertelorism, down-slanting palpebral fissures, low set of posteriorly rotated ears, congenital heart disease, short stature, low hairline, shield chest, cubitus valgus, and hypogonadism because of primary testicular failure. The most frequently occurring cardiac malformation is pulmonic stenosis, followed by atrial septal defect. The testes are frequently hypoplastic and intra-abdominal. The endocrine function of the testes can be normal, or consistent with primary Leydig cells dysfunction (high gonadotropins and low testosterone). Although some affected individuals are fertile, infertility is present in the majority of patients and is associated with germinal cell aplasia.

Diagnosis The diagnosis is suspected in 46,XY individuals presenting with the clinical features described above and with a normal karyotype.

Genetic Basis of Disease The genetic abnormality accounting for this rare disorder has recently been localized on chromosome 12q22–qter by genome linkage analysis of a three-generation Dutch family with the disease, and 20 smaller two-generation families from Great Britain. The biologic and biochemical characteristics of the gene product are currently unknown.

Treatment The treatment is directed toward the cardiac complications of the disease. At puberty, affected males can require replacement with testosterone.

MYOTONIC DYSTROPHY Background and Clinical Features Myotonic dystrophy (MD) is an autosomal dominant disorder that expresses remarkable variability in its clinical manifestations. It becomes apparent in adulthood, and is characterized by progressive weakness and atrophy of the facial, neck, hand, and lower extremities muscles. Myotonia can manifest in several muscles and is characterized by prolonged muscle contraction with inability to relax. Other features include cataracts, cardiac arrhythmias, baldness, primary hypothyroidism, mental retardation, and, in as many as 80% of these patients, primary testicular failure.

Diagnosis Hypogonadism in MD is a primary testicular disease, as suggested by the presence of testosterone levels ranging from modestly decreased to low normal and slightly elevated gonadotropins that hyperrespond to LH-releasing hormone (LHRH) stimulation. Testicular atrophy is usually noted during adulthood. There is good correlation between the circulating levels of testosterone and the clinical signs of androgen deficiency, which usually are mild. Most patients maintain normal facial and body hair growth and normal libido. The histology of the testes varies from normal to marked tubular atrophy or peritubular hyalinization, with or without loss of the interstitial cells. Testicular size is frequently decreased in association with complete germinal cell destruction. Infertility is reported in as many as 44% of the cases in a recent series.

Genetic Basis of Disease This disease has been associated with expansion of a highly polymorphic GCT repeat located in the sequence of the myotonin-protein kinase gene, which has been mapped on chromosome 19q13.2–13.3. In the normal population, the GCT tract length ranges from 5 to 30 repeats. In patients affected by MD the size of the GCT tract expands dramatically, up to 2000–3000 copies. The mechanism responsible for the association between the expansion of the GCT repeat located in the myotonin-protein kinase gene and hypogonadism has not yet been defined.

Therapy Replacement therapy with testosterone has been advocated for patient with low testosterone not only to correct the hypogonadism, but also to increase and maintain muscular size and strength.

BILATERAL ANORCHIA (VANISHING TESTES SYNDROME) Background This syndrome is also known as "congenital anorchia" or "testicular agenesis." Bilateral anorchia is found in approximately 1% of boys receiving surgery for bilateral cryptorchidism. It is found in approximately 1 of every 20,000 male newborns.

Clinical Features The phenotype detected in these patients correlates with the time of embryologic development at which testicular function became deficient. Individuals in which testicular function became abnormal before 8 weeks of gestation have female internal and external genitalia. Individuals developing abnormal testicular function between 8 and 10 weeks of gestation exhibit an intermediate phenotype, with ambiguous genitalia and variable masculinization of the internal structures. Loss of testicular function after 10 weeks of gestation is associated with the development of a normal male phenotype. In each instance, no histologic or hormonal evidence for the presence of a functioning testis is available. Hormonal studies are compatible with primary gonadal failure, with high gonadotropin and low testosterone level.

Diagnosis The diagnosis of this disorder should be suspected in patients with anorchia in whom intra-abdominal gonads cannot be demonstrated by provocative testing or during explorative surgery.

Genetic Basis of Disease The pathogenesis for the degeneration and disappearance of the testes is controversial because it could potentially result from trauma, vascular insufficiency, or infection. Several sibships with multiple affected individuals have been reported. In one case there was parental consanguinity, suggesting a possible autosomal recessive transmission of the disease.

HYPERGONADOTROPIC HYPOGONADISM FROM RECEPTOR DEFECTS

LH-RESISTANT TESTIS (LEYDIG CELL HYPOPLASIA) Clinical Features Leydig cell hypoplasia is a rare condition. In 46,XY individuals it is associated with primary testicular failure and a spectrum of phenotypic abnormalities of the internal and external genitalia. It is inherited as an autosomal recessive disorder.

In male patients the main clinical features of this syndrome consist of ambiguous external genitalia, ranging from extreme forms that present as 46,XY females to milder forms in which normal phallic development is observed. The internal genitalia consist of a blind-ending, rudimentary vagina, owing to the absence of Müllerian derivatives and the presence of Wolffian duct-derived structures. The histologic features of the testis consist of a drastic reduction in the number of Leydig cells, which in some instances are completely absent, and in limited germ-cell maturation.

Although virilization of the external genitalia is very limited in these patients, Wolffian duct-derived structures, such as the vas deferens and the epididymis, undergo normal embryologic development. This implies that during fetal development the Leydig cells of these patients are able to produce androgens despite the inactivating mutations of the LH receptor, suggesting that during early fetal development Leydig cell maturation and androgen production may be independent of LH stimulation.

Diagnosis These patients manifest a resistance to LH, as shown by the elevated level of LH and low level of testosterone. FSH has been reported to be normal in most cases, and abnormally elevated in a minority of patients. Testosterone precursors such as dihydroepiandrosterone (DHEA), 17α-progesterone, progesterone, and androstenedione are low compared with normal males. As would be anticipated, the LHRH stimulation test is associated with an LH hyperresponse.

A clinical picture of abnormal virilization associated with low testosterone and testosterone precursors in the presence of high LH is virtually diagnostic of this syndrome. Alternatives to consider in the differential diagnosis are androgen resistance because of defects in the androgen receptor, type 2 5α-reductase deficiency,

Table 61-5
46,XY Patients with Inactivating Mutations of the LH Receptor Gene Causing LH Resistance

	Ethnic background	*Familial consanguinity*	*Clinical phenotype*	*Mutation*	*Functional characterization of the receptor*
Family 1	Brazilian	+	Development of testis, epididymis, and vas deferens. External phenotype: female	Ala593→Pro	Lack of hCG-dependent cAMP production
Family 2	Brazilian	–	Testicular development. External phenotype: female	Arg554→Stop	Presumed completely inactive
Family 3	Puerto Rican	+ (four generations earlier)	Micropenis, otherwise normal male phenotype	Ser616→Tyr	Lack of ligand binding

and defects of testosterone biosynthesis. Each defect can be differentiated on the basis of the clinical phenotype and hormonal data.

Genetic Basis of Disorder The association of Leydig cell hypoplasia with an abnormal binding activity of the LH receptor and with the endocrine features described above led to the identification of the LH receptor as the culprit in this syndrome. Although the cDNA encoding this molecule has been available since 1990, this hypothesis has only recently been confirmed by the molecular analysis of the LH receptor gene in three unrelated families with the disorder. The clinical features, LH-receptor mutations and functional abnormalities of the LH-receptor gene in these families, are described in Table 61-5.

Molecular Pathophysiology of Disease Mutations in the coding sequence of the LH receptor have the potential to affect any of the functions performed by this molecule, including LH binding, G-protein activation with subsequent production of cyclic adenosine monophosphate (cAMP), posttranslational modifications or postsynthesis transport. The Ala593Pro mutation is localized to the sixth transmembrane domain of the LH receptor gene. Binding analysis of this mutant receptor using ^{125}I-hCG has shown only minor changes in ligand binding (normal kDa, and decreased B_{max} caused largely by decreased transfection efficiency of the mutated receptor in HEK293 cells). When compared with the wild-type receptor, however, it is clear that this mutation completely prevents cAMP production, indicating that the region of the gene containing residue 593 is important for normal intracellular signal transduction. The molecular analysis of the missense mutation Ser616Tyr causes a total loss of ligand binding, and consequently of cAMP production, indicating that this amino acid, which is located in the seventh transmembrane domain of the receptor, is critical for normal ligand binding. The third mutation identified, Arg554→Stop, causes premature interruption of the translation process of the LH receptor mRNA, eliminates a large part of the receptor, and presumably prevents transduction of the hormonal signal. The molecular analysis of more patients affected by this disorder will be useful in dissecting the structure–function correlation of the LH receptor gene.

Treatment Androgen or estrogen replacement therapy is indicated depending on gender selection. The final choice as to how these patients should be raised depends on the same criteria established for patients with other forms of male pseudohermaphroditism. The intra-abdominal gonads should be surgically removed at the time of the diagnosis to prevent neoplastic degeneration. In most instances it is recommended that pediatric patients affected by micropenis should receive a course of testosterone treatment to normalize the size of the phallus.

SYNDROMES OF ANDROGEN RESISTANCE Hypogonadism because of androgen receptor defects is associated with a wide spectrum of clinical phenotypes, ranging from 46,XY women with the syndrome of complete testicular feminization to phenotypically normal men affected by infertility. The clinical features, endocrinology, biochemistry, and molecular biology of these syndromes are discussed in Chapter 60.

HYPERGONADOTROPIC HYPOGONADISM CAUSED BY DEFECTS IN THE SYNTHESIS OF TESTOSTERONE IN 46,XY INDIVIDUALS

(20,22-DESMOLASE, 3β-HYDROXYSTEROID DEHYDROGENASE, 17α-HYDROXYLASE/17,20-DESMOLASE, 17β-HYDROXYSTEROID DEHYDROGENASE DEFICIENCY) The pathway for steroid biosynthesis shown in Table 61-6 is responsible for the conversion of cholesterol to testosterone, and consists of five well-characterized enzymatic steps.

Genetic diseases associated with impaired activity of each of these enzymes have been described. Because normal production of testosterone by the developing testis is critical for the development of a normal male sexual phenotype, abnormalities of these enzymes in 46,XY individuals are associated with different degrees of male pseudohermaphroditism. Three of these enzymes (20,22-desmolase, 3β-Hydroxysteroid dehydrogenase, and 17α-hydroxylase) are involved in both cortisol and testosterone biosynthesis; hence, individuals with abnormalities of these enzymes are affected by a combination of male pseudohermaphroditism and hypoadrenalism. Some of these congenital abnormalities can be partial, and may become clinically evident only at puberty.

CONGENITAL LIPOID ADRENAL HYPERPLASIA (CHOLESTEROL SIDE-CHAIN CLEAVAGE DEFICIENCY, $P450_{scc}$ DEFICIENCY) Background Congenital lipoid adrenal hyperplasia (lipoid CAH) is a rare autosomal recessive defect in which the synthesis of all steroid hormones (estrogens, glucocorticoids, mineralocorticoids, and androgens) is impaired. This syndrome has recently been associated with genetic abnormalities of the StAR (steroidogenic acute regulatory) protein, the factor that mobilizes cholesterol from the outer mitochondrial membrane into the inner mitochondrial membrane.

Clinical Features Newborn patients with this disease have female external genitalia irrespective of karyotype, exhibit a severe form of salt-losing congenital adrenal hyperplasia (CAH), and accumulate lipids in the gonads and adrenals, which are grossly enlarged. Male infants with this syndrome present with male pseudohermaphroditism, characterized by female external genitalia with a blind-ending hypoplastic vagina, absent uterus and fal-

Table 61-6
Pathway of Testosterone Synthesis

CHOLESTEROL		
$P450_{scc}$ ↓ 20,22-Desmolase		
	3β-Hydroxysteroid dehydrogenase (3β-HSD)	
PREGNENOLONE	→	PROGESTERONE
$P450_{c17}$ ↓ 17α-Hydroxylase		$P450_{c17}$ 17α-Hydroxylase ↓
17-OII-PREGNENOLONE	→	17-OH-PROGESTERONE
$P450_{c17}$ ↓ 17,20-Desmolase		$P450_{c17}$ 17,20-Desmolase ↓
DHEA	→	ANDROSTENEDIONE
↓ 17β-Hydroxysteroid dehydrogenase		17β-Hydroxysteroid dehydrogenase ↓
ANDROSTENEDIOL	→	TESTOSTERONE
	3β-Hydroxysteroid dehydrogenase (3β-HSD)	

lopian tubes, hypoplastic Wolffian derivatives, and cryptorchid testes. Heterozygous parents of affected siblings develop normally. Their condition is not unmasked by provocative testing.

Diagnosis This disease should be suspected at birth in patients with a salt-losing crisis and the phenotype discussed above. Further aid to a correct diagnosis is obtained by showing the typical enlargement of the adrenals and testes, which is visible using magnetic resonance imaging (MRI) or computed tomographic scanning. Typically the serum levels of cortisol, aldosterone, and testosterone are undetectable adrenocorticotropic hormone (ACTH), FSH, and LH are elevated, and no response is evident after stimulation with ACTH or β-hCG. At puberty a minimal degree of virilization can occur in 46,XY individuals.

Genetic Basis of Disease For a long time this disease has been ascribed to defects of the $P450_{scc}$ system, which consists of the cholesterol side-chain cleavage enzyme and two electron transfer proteins, termed adrenodoxin reductase (AR) and adrenodoxin (AD). This conclusion was based on hormonal studies of affected patients who were unable to produce adrenal and gonadal steroids, and on the inability of mitochondria from affected tissues to convert cholesterol to pregnenolone. However, a role for $P450_{scc}$ has been ruled out in molecular studies of affected individuals, in which abnormalities in the coding sequence of this gene have never been detected. In addition, $P450_{scc}$, AR, and AD are normally transcribed and translated in the steroidogenic tissue of affected individuals, suggesting that the lesion responsible for lipoid CAH is located elsewhere. When the role of the StAR protein became clear, this factor appeared immediately to be the candidate gene responsible for lipoid CAH. Molecular analysis of the StAR protein, now performed in at least 22 families, has confirmed that this factor has a central role in the etiology of lipoid CAH. Mutations affecting both alleles of the *StAR* gene have been detected in 95% of the patients. Most families have homozygous mutations, and a minority appear to be compound heterozygotes. The importance of these mutations in the etiology of lipoid CAH has also been demonstrated by showing that *StAR* cDNAs carrying these mutations lack the ability to promote pregnenolone synthesis in transfected cells.

Therapy Glucocorticoid and mineralocorticoid replacement is the first therapeutic step for these patients. Given the sexual phenotype, most patients are raised as females. Prophylactic orchidectomy followed by estrogen replacement should be performed to prevent the neoplastic degeneration of the retained gonads and to avoid any possible virilization at the time of puberty.

3β-HYDROXYSTEROID DEHYDROGENASE (3β-HSD) Δ^5,Δ^4-ISOMERASE DEFICIENCY **Background** 3β-HSD regulates the conversion of Δ^5-3β-hydroxysteroids (pregnenolone, 17-OH pregnenolone, dehydroepiandrosterone, and androstenediol) into the corresponding Δ^4-3-ketosteroids (progesterone, 17-OH-progesterone, androstenedione, and testosterone, respectively). Absent or reduced activity of this enzyme is potentially associated with impaired formation of all steroid hormone classes, including progesterone, mineralocorticoids, glucocorticoids, androgens, and estrogens.

Clinical Features There is a remarkable heterogeneity in the clinical presentation of 46,XY individuals affected by this disease. The two major clinical features of these patients are incomplete virilization and salt-wasting. The degree of salt-wasting is heterogeneous, and ranges from life threatening to clinically inapparent syndromes. In a similar fashion, the defects of virilization can range from the development of various genital ambiguities (including hypospadias, micropenis, and presence of a blind-ending vagina) to, in rare cases, the development of normal external genitalia. In most instances, the Wolffian duct derivatives develop normally, suggesting that although the prenatal testes were capable of some androgen production, these quantities were insufficient to permit normal development of the sexual phenotype. The Müllerian duct derivatives involute normally indicating normal production of AMH by the Sertoli cells. At puberty these patients have typical hypergonadotropic hypogonadism with high gonadotropin and low testosterone. These endocrine abnormalities are associated with gynecomastia, spermatogenic arrest, and phenotypic features of undervirilization. Interestingly, no correlation has been made between the degree of salt-wasting and of impairment of male sexual differentiation, suggesting that 3β-HSD mutations can affect the different steroidogenic pathways differentially.

Diagnosis The diagnosis of this disorder should be suspected in patients presenting with adrenal and gonadal insufficiency. An elevated ratio of Δ^5- to Δ^4-steroids is characteristic of this disorder; however, the interpretation of the endocrine data can be complicated by the increased level of some Δ^4-steroids, including serum 17-OH-progesterone and Δ^4-androstenedione, and urinary pregnanetriol. This is caused by the presence of two 3β-HSD enzymes, of which only one is mutated (*see* Genetic Basis of Disease).

Genetic Basis of Disease This disease is transmitted as an autosomal recessive character, and the gene is located in the region p11–p13 of chromosome 1. Two isoenzymes with 3β-HSD activity have been cloned, and have been designated type I and type II 3β-HSD. Their structural organization consists of four exons and three introns, which are included in a genomic DNA fragment of about 7.8 kb. The type I 3β-HSD mRNA is transcribed in the breast, placenta, and skin, and to a much lower degree in the gonads. The type II isoenzyme is transcribed exclusively in the adrenals, testis, and ovary. The identification of two isoenzymes with the same activity and with a different pattern of expression has the potential of explaining the presence of normal to elevated serum levels of some Δ^4-3-ketosteroids in the patient population with 3β-HSD deficiency. Since the disease causes salt-wasting and ambiguous genitalia, it would be expected that the type II isoenzyme (which is exclusively transcribed in the adrenals and gonads) is the mutated gene and the type I isoenzyme (which is transcribed in the periphery) would maintain its activity and would be responsible for the residual conversion of Δ^5-3β-hydroxysteroids to Δ^4-3-ketosteroids. In agreement with this expectation, the molecular abnormalities causing clinical 3β-HSD deficiency have so far been localized exclusively to the type II isoenzyme. Numerous mutations in the coding region of the 3β-HSD gene have been identified by sequence analysis of SSCP (single-strand conformational polymorphism) variants detected in genomic DNA obtained from these patients. They include missense, nonsense, and frameshift mutations, and have been detected in homozygous or compound heterozygous patients. Their functional characterization has been very useful in defining the functionally important regions of the 3β-HSD gene.

Molecular Pathophysiology There is a reproducible correlation between the impairment of the enzymatic activity caused by each mutation and the clinical abnormalities of the patients. This is particularly true with regard to the presence of salt-wasting forms of the disease in which no residual enzymatic activity is detected. Molecular analysis of the 3β-HSD gene of these patients has shown the presence of nonsense mutations (causing the synthesis of prematurely truncated proteins) and missense mutations (causing the replacement of critical amino acids) (Table 61-7). The only identified patient of this group with minimal residual enzymatic activity (0.1–0.3%) is a compound heterozygote carrying two missense mutations (Leu108Trp and Pro186Leu). The presence of such low level of activity is most likely inadequate to prevent the development of salt-wasting.

In patients with non–salt-wasting forms of the disease, there is residual 3β-HSD activity that ranges from 1 to 10%, a level that appears to permit sufficient mineralocorticoid synthesis to prevent salt-wasting. Interestingly, in patients with this milder form of the disease premature stop codons have not been described, which completely abolish 3β-HSD activity, rather only missense or splicing mutations have been found (Table 61-8).

Of note is the observation that the amino acid residues that are mutated are conserved in all members of the vertebrate 3β-HSD isoenzymes described to date.

It is not yet clear why the clinical abnormalities of genital development and salt-wasting do not correlate. A potential explanation for this phenomenon is that different mutations affect C_{21} and C_{19} steroidogenesis in different ways. Future molecular investigations of more patients with 3β-HSD deficiency should help to clarify this point.

Therapy Therapy involves replacement with glucocorticoids and, if required, mineralocorticoids. Sufficient androgens should be given early in life to correct the microphallus and allow surgical treatment of hypospadias. Normal replacement doses should be given at the time of puberty.

Table 61-7
Mutations of the Type II 3β-HSD Gene Detected in 46,XY Patients with the Salt-Wasting Form of 3β-HSD Deficiency

Origin	*Karyotype*	*Mutation*
Spain/Portugal	46,XY	Leu108Trp
		Pro186Leu
United States	46,XY	Glu124Lys
		Trp171Stop
Holland	46,XY	1-bp insertion at 186
		Tyr253Asn
United States	46,XY	Trp171Stop
		1-bp insertion at 186
Afghanistan/Pakistan[a]	46,XY	2-bp deletion at 273
Algeria	46,XY	Gly15Asp

[a]This mutation was detected in three families originating from the same region in northwest Pakistan.

Modified from Simard J, et al. J Steroid Biochem Mol Biol 1995; 53:127–138.

Table 61-8
Mutations Detected in the Type II 3β-HSD Gene in 46XY Patients with the Non–Salt-Wasting Losing Form of 3β-HSD Deficiency

Origin	*Karyotype*	*Mutation*
United States[a]	46,XY	Gly129Arg
		G-A 6651 (new splice site)
Algeria	46,XY	Asn100Ser
United States[a]	46,XY	Tyr254Asp
		No mutations in the second allele
Scotland[b]	46,XY	Leu173Arg
Brazil	46,XY	Ala82Thr

[a]This mutation was detected in two siblings of the same family.

[b]This mutation was detected in two members of the same family.

Modified from Simard J, et al. J Steroid Biochem Mol Biol 1995; 53:127–138.

17α-HYDROXYLASE/17,20-LYASE DEFICIENCY Background Two important steps of the steroidogenic pathway are regulated by the enzyme 17α-hydroxylase/17,20-lyase ($P450_{c17}$). The first reaction consists of the 17α-hydroxylation of pregnenolone and progesterone into 17-hydroxypregnenolone and 17-hydroxyprogesterone. These C_{21} steroids undergo cleavage of the C-17,20 carbon bond via the 17,20-lyase reaction to yield the C_{19} steroids dehydroepiandrosterone and androstenedione.

To date, more than 120 cases with $P450_{c17}$ deficiency have been described in the worlds literature. The large majority of these patients are affected by complete 17α-hydroxylase deficiency; however, about 20 cases with a partial form of this disease have been described. There is clear evidence that $P450_{c17}$ catalyzes both the 17α-hydroxylase and 17,20-lyase reactions, but the description of 14 patients with only 17,20-lyase deficiency indicates that a complete understanding of this disorder has not yet been achieved.

Clinical Features Of the enzymatic activities catalyzed by $P450_{c17}$, 17α-hydroxylase is critical for the production of both glucocorticoid and sex steroids, whereas 17,20-lyase, which is located one step downstream in the steroidogenic pathway, is critical for the production of sex steroids only. In theory, defects of $P450_{c17}$ activity could occur as isolated deficiencies of 17α-hydroxylase or 17,20-lyase or as combined 17α-hydroxylase/17,20-lyase deficiency. In practice it is almost impossible to differentiate between combined 17α-hydroxylase/17,20-lyase and isolated 17α-hydroxylase deficiencies on clinical and biochemical grounds. However, isolated 17,20-lyase deficiency has been described as an independent entity in 14 patients, and two types of enzymatic defects have been proposed for this syndrome. In the first one there is an incomplete defect of the Δ^4 and Δ^5 pathways, whereas in the second type, associated with normal serum levels of DHEA, there is a complete defect only in the Δ^4 pathway.

The deficient production of cortisol observed in these patients is associated with a compensatory overproduction of ACTH, which stimulates the production of large amounts of corticosterone, usually found at concentrations 50- to 100-fold higher than normal. Although corticosterone has a lower affinity for the glucocorticoid receptor (GR) than does cortisol, its activity is sufficient to prevent the development of overt adrenal insufficiency. As a result of the increased production of deoxycorticosterone (DOC), corticosterone, and 18-hydroxycorticosterone, affected patients develop retention of water and salt, hypokalemic alkalosis, and hypertension. Suppression of renin and aldosterone production is a feature of most patients; however, a few individuals with normal or elevated aldosterone have been reported in the Japanese literature, and this finding has still not been adequately explained.

Deficient production of sex steroids is associated in these patients with hypogonadism and a compensatory overproduction of gonadotropins. Since normal levels of testosterone synthesis are necessary during fetal life for the development of the normal male sexual phenotype, affected patients manifest different abnormalities of the external genitalia, ranging from an apparent female phenotype with a blind-ending vagina to hypospadias and male-appearing genitalia with micropenis. The Wolffian derivatives can be hypoplastic or normal, the Müllerian derivatives are normally involuted, and the hypoplastic testes may be located intra-abdominally, in the inguinal canal, or in the scrotum. There is lack of correlation between the severity of hypertension and hypokalemia and that of hypogonadism, again suggesting that the various mutations of $P450_{c17}$ can affect the C_{21} and C_{19} steroidogenic pathways in different ways.

Diagnosis 17α-Hydroxylase/17,20-lyase deficiency should be considered in every 46,XY patient with a family history of pseudohermaphroditism that suggests an autosomal recessive inheritance. It is usually recognized in young adults with hypertension, hypokalemia, and ambiguous genitalia. The diagnosis of 17α-hydroxylase deficiency can be confirmed by demonstrating increased serum concentrations of pregnenolone, progesterone, corticosterone, 18-hydroxy-DOC, and DOC, associated with increased urinary excretion of their respective glucoronidate metabolites. Plasma renin activity, serum cortisol, and aldosterone are usually suppressed and ACTH is elevated. Affected males have low testosterone and elevated gonadotropins. The response to hGC and ACTH stimulation tests are impaired. This steroid pattern applies to patients with combined 17α-hydroxylase/17,20-lyase deficiency. In patients with 17,20-lyase deficiency the clinical symptoms are usually limited to the sexual phenotype. An important feature of this latter group of patients is the presence of normal serum level of cortisol and DOC and of their urinary metabolites. However, because of the presence of 17,20-lyase deficiency, these patients have been found to have increased serum level of progesterone, 17OH-progesterone, and OH-pregnenolone, increased urinary level of pregnanetriolone, and decreased serum level of testosterone and its precursors.

Genetic Basis of Disease The human $P450_{c17}$ gene *(CYP17)* is a single copy gene, located on chromosome 10q24–25. It consists of eight exons and seven introns spanning 6569 bases. Full-length cDNA clones have been isolated from adrenal and testicular sources and have the same nucleotide sequence. When the cDNA clones encoding this enzyme are expressed in cultured cells, the expressed protein displays both 17α-hydroxylase and 17,20-lyase activities. The molecular and functional analyses of 20 mutations of the *CYP17* gene have been published (Table 61-9). They show that the genetic lesions of 17α-hydroxylase deficiency are random events, and that there are no structural features of the gene predisposing to specific abnormalities. The functional analyses of these mutations have shown that they impair both 17α-hydroxylase and 17,20-lyase activities, giving further demonstration that this gene encodes a protein possessing both enzymatic activities. Only a limited number of mutations have been reported more than once and were detected in unrelated individuals from Guam and of German-Dutch descent, indicating that this disorder is genetically heterogeneous, unless associated with a specific ethnic group.

Molecular Pathophysiology ***Introduction*** The description of the molecular defects and functional abnormalities affecting patients with the complete and incomplete forms of 17α-hydroxylase deficiency and with isolated 17,20-lyase deficiency have elucidated several new aspects of this disease. The biochemical events associated with 17α-hydroxylase activity consist of a chain of events involving proper anchorage of the enzyme into the microsomal membrane, heme binding, substrate binding, transfer of electrons from NADPH to cytochrome P450 reductase, and O_2 binding. Mutations specifically affecting heme and substrate binding have been identified. Targeted site-directed mutations of the rat *CYP17* have been very informative in dissecting the amino acids of this protein that contribute to the 17α-hydroxylase and 17,20-lyase activities and showed the importance of residues Arg346 and Arg363 in inducing 17,20-lyase and 17α-hydroxylase activities, respectively.

Complete Combined 17α-Hydroxylase and 17,20-Lyase Deficiency Fifteen mutations resulting in loss of 17α-hydroxylase and 17,20-lyase activity have been identified in the *CYP17* gene. They include insertion of premature termination codons, amino acid replacements, or small deletions. Premature termination codons resulting from nonsense mutations or from other abnormalities of the open reading frame (including deletions or insertions of DNA) lead to truncated forms of the P450c17 protein, which, by being deprived of the C-terminal heme-binding domain, become functionally inactive. Complete loss of enzymatic function in three patients with missense mutations has identified residues Ser106, His373, and Arg440 as critical for both 17α-hydroxylase and 17,20-lyase activities. Of note is the speculation that the mutation occurring in amino acid residue 106 may affect substrate binding, whereas the two other mutations (His373 and Arg440) affect heme binding.

Partial Combined 17α-Hydroxylase and 17,20-Lyase Deficiency Partial deficiency of 17α-hydroxylase and 17,20-lyase has been studied in two patients. One of these two patients was a boy with ambiguous genitalia, carrying two different *CYP17* mutant alleles: one resulting in an Arg239Stop nonsense mutation

Table 61-9
Mutations of the CYP17 Gene in 46,XY Patients with 17α-Hydroxylase/17,20-Lyase Deficiency

Origin	*Karyotype*	*Sex of Rearing*	*Mutation*
Canada[a] Netherlands[a]	46,XY	F	4 bp duplication
Switzerland	46,XY	F	Gln461→Stop Arg496→Cys
Italy	46,XY	F	Deletion and insertion in exons 2 and 3
Guam[b]	46,XY	F	Ser106→Pro
Caucasian	46,XY	F	Tyr64→Ser Duplication of Ile112
Canada	46,XY	M	Arg239→Stop Pro342→Thr

[a]This mutation was described in two unrelated Canadians of German origin and in 6 unrelated families residing in the Friesland region of the Netherlands.

[b]This mutation was described in two unrelated individuals from Guam.

Modified from Yanase T. J Steroid Biochem Mol Biol. 1995;53:153–157.

and the other causing a Pro342Thr missense mutation. The residual activity of these two alleles was respectively 0 and 20% of normal. These data, together with the functional analysis of a 46,XY female with homozygous premature termination codons (with residual functional activity of 0%) and of her normally virilized heterozygous father (thought to have a residual functional activity of 50%), have been very useful in understanding the amount of 17α-hydroxylase activity that is necessary for the development of the male sexual phenotype. Because the boy with ambiguous genitalia had a residual activity of 20% and the normally virilized individual described above was thought to have a residual activity of 50%, it would appear that the threshold activity necessary to change the sexual phenotype from female to ambiguous male is between 0 and 20%, and to change from ambiguous to normal is between 20 and 50%.

Isolated 17,20-Lyase Deficiency Only one patient with this form of the disorder has been analyzed at the molecular level. This patient was found to be a compound heterozygote, with one allele containing an Arg496Cys missense mutation and the other allele containing a Glu461Stop nonsense mutation. In contrast to the clinical study, both alleles of this patient showed a dramatically reduced activity of both 17α-hydroxylase and 17,20-lyase. This finding prompted a clinical reevaluation of the patient, who was found to have deficient activity of both 17α-hydroxylase and 17,20-lyase when reexamined at age 25 years. These results led to speculation that the levels of $P450_{c17}$ activity expressed in vivo were affected by unknown age-dependent factors or that a modifying effect had been exerted by the estrogen replacement that had been initiated in the interim.

Treatment Treatment consists of replacement with cortisol, which accomplishes suppression of ACTH followed by the normalization of DOC, corticosterone, and 18-hydroxycorticosterone, and by the normalization of renin and aldosterone levels. Adult 46,XY individuals reared as females require estrogen replacement and removal of the abdominal gonads to prevent their malignant degeneration. Adult 46,XY individuals raised as males require androgen replacement, surgical correction of their external genitalia, and, if necessary, orchiopexy.

17β-HYDROXYSTEROID DEHYDROGENASE DEFICIENCY (17β-HSD DEFICIENCY) **Background** The enzyme 17β-hydroxysteroid dehydrogenase (17β-HSD) catalyzes the conversion of androstenedione and estrone into testosterone and estradiol, respectively. As such, it converts two weak precursors, androstenedione and estrone, into two potent hormones, testosterone and estradiol, that, on interacting with high affinity with their receptors, induce their biologic effects. The reaction catalyzed by 17β-HSD is reversible. The reduction of the 17-keto group is believed to occur mainly in the testis and ovary, where it is required for the synthesis of testosterone and estradiol. The oxidation reaction, which is believed to occur in several peripheral tissues, is important for the inactivation of these two hormones.

Five different isoenzymes with 17β-HSD activity have been isolated and designated 1 through 5 according to the chronological order of their identification. These isoenzymes have different biochemical features, and are expressed in different tissues (Table 61-10). Interestingly, the isoenzymes 1 and 3 favor the reduction reaction, whereas the type 2 and 4 isoenzymes favor the oxidation reaction. The isoenzymes 2 and 4 have ubiquitous tissue distribution, whereas the isoenzymes 1 and 3 are expressed in a more selective way. The mRNA of the type 1 isoenzyme is present in the ovary and placenta, whereas the type 3 mRNA has been detected almost exclusively in the testis. Information concerning the type 5 isoenzyme is at present less detailed. Mutations of the type 3 isoenzyme have recently been associated with 17β HSD deficiency.

Clinical Features Approximately 42 patients from 23 families with classic 17β-HSD deficiency have been reported. This number probably does not reflect the high incidence of this syndrome in the Gaza strip, where it is estimated that 1 in 100–150 individuals is affected by this disorder. The pattern of inheritance is autosomal recessive. At birth these patients present with female external genitalia, absent Müllerian and normal Wolffian duct derivatives, and undescended testes. Based on this phenotype, gender assignment is female in almost every case. At puberty, both virilization (developing a deep voice, large phallus, and various degree of body and facial hair) and feminization (developing variable degree of gynecomastia) occur. Some of these individuals have undergone a change in gender role behavior in parallel with the virilization occurring at the time of puberty. Impaired 17β-HSD activity explains the abnormal virilization of the external genitalia at birth, the elevated serum level of androstenedione and decreased testosterone, and the enhancement of pituitary gonadotropin production. A milder form of late-onset 17β-HSD deficiency has recently been identified in 3 adult patients with gynecomastia and hypogonadism in a study of 48 subjects with idiopathic pubertal gynecomastia. The frequency of this syndrome is unknown. It is

Table 61-10
Features of Five Isoenzymes with 17β-HSD Activity

17β-HSD deficiency	*Amino acid size*	*Exons*	*Chromosome localization*	*Tissue localization*	*Cellular localization*	*Preferred substrate*	*Preferred cofactor*	*Catalytic preference*
Normal	327	6	17q21	Ovary, placenta	Cytosol	Estrogens	NADPH	Reduction
Normal	387	5	16q24	Endometrium, placenta, liver	Microsomes	Androgens, estrogens, progestogens	NAD^+	Oxidation
Mutated	310	11	9q22	Testis	Microsomes	Androgens, estrogens	NADPH	Reduction
	736			Ubiquitous	Peroxisomes	Estrogens	NAD^+	Oxidation
	323	9	10p14–15					Reduction

Modified from Andersson S, et al. Trends Endocrinol Metab 1996;7:121–126.

equally unclear whether these patients are heterozygous for an inactivating mutation of type 3 17β-HSD or whether they are homozygous for a mutation of type 3 17β-HSD causing a milder enzymatic defect.

Endocrine Features and Diagnosis The diagnosis should be considered in 46,XY patients presenting with pseudohermaphroditism inherited with an autosomal recessive pattern. Plasma androstenedione, estrone, and gonadotropin levels are elevated, whereas testosterone and dihydrotestosterone are decreased or in the low normal range. Steroid hormone metabolism has been studied in the testes of several affected subjects. In these tissues it was found that the conversion of androstenedione to testosterone was consistently abnormal. However, other authors have found that the oxidative reaction catalyzed by 17β-HSD was normal in cultured fibroblasts obtained from one patient.

Most of these patients are diagnosed at puberty, when they are referred for failure to menstruate, or because they develop a mixed pattern of virilization and feminization. The diagnosis of 17β-HSD deficiency is more challenging in the newborn. However, the correct interpretation of the endocrine tests should permit the diagnosis of this disorder in any age group.

Genetic Basis of Disease Because of its biochemical characteristics and tissue distribution, type 3 17β-HSD was considered to be a good candidate to cause the clinical abnormalities of 17β-HSD deficiency. Subsequent analysis has identified 14 mutations of this gene in 17 families with the typical phenotypic, endocrine, and genetic features of the syndrome. The mutations detected include 10 missense mutations, 3 splice junction abnormalities and 1 small deletion resulting in a frameshift. Patients with the syndrome were most frequently homozygous (12), but heterozygotes (1) and compound heterozygotes (4) have been described as well (Table 61-11). The mutation Arg80Gln has been detected in three unrelated families, including a member of the large kindred from the Gaza strip and two Brazilian families. Considering the high incidence of 17β-HSD deficiency in the Gaza strip, screening programs for this mutation may be worthwhile in that part of the world to detect heterozygosity or for prenatal diagnosis. The real frequency of this mutation in the entire Arab population of the Gaza strip could be very high, if one considers that homozygous females are asymptomatic, have normal internal and external genitalia, undergo normal sexual development, and have unimpaired fertility.

The frequency of compound heterozygosity underscores the possible high frequency of heterozygous carriers, a potentially important fact, considering the recent identification of individuals with partial deficiency of testicular 17β-HSD activity that was reported in a group of patients with gynecomastia.

Molecular Pathophysiology of Disease Nine of the ten substitution mutations described in Table 61-11 have been recreated in vitro, and the activity of the mutated enzyme was studied in transfected cells. Eight of the nine mutations are completely inactivating. However, in agreement with biochemical studies performed in cultured genital skin fibroblasts, the ninth mutation (Arg80Gln) retains a small amount of activity. Detailed analysis of the enzymatic activity of this mutant has revealed a 100-fold decreased affinity for the cofactor NADPH, localizing at least a portion of the NADPH-binding domain to the region surrounding residue 80.

These recent developments in the molecular biology of 17β-HSD deficiency have permitted understanding of why these patients undergo virilization at the time of puberty. The consensus is that androstenedione, which is produced by the testes in supraphysiologic concentrations at the time of puberty, provides the substrate for the extraglandular production of testosterone by one of the four 17β-HSD isoenzymes that are not impaired in this disorder. However, two clinical features of 17β-HSD deficiency await adequate explanation. It is not clear why inadequate virilization is more complete during embryonic development, when the external genitalia do not virilize at all, than at the time of puberty, when a substantial masculinization of the phenotype occurs. In addition, it is not clear why the embryonic structures of the developing male genitalia respond to the hormonal abnormalities created by 17β-HSD deficiency in a different way. In this disorder the Wolffian derivatives undergo almost normal virilization during embryogenesis, whereas the external genitalia do not virilize at all. Further studies of subjects affected by 17β-HSD deficiency should help to answer these important biologic questions.

Treatment Patients are usually raised as females and treatment consists of gonadectomy followed by estrogen replacement at the time of expected puberty. When the diagnosis is correctly identified in early infancy and gender reassignment is possible, the patients should receive testosterone treatment at pediatric doses and genitoplasty early in infancy and be replaced with adult doses of testosterone at the time of expected puberty. The basic enzymatic defect persists, and impaired spermatogenesis is present during adulthood.

TYPE 2 5α-REDUCTASE DEFICIENCY The enzyme 5α-reductase is involved in the conversion of testosterone into the powerful 5α-reduced metabolite dihydrotestosterone (DHT). Two isoenzymes have been isolated that share this enzymatic activity, and have been designated types 1 and 2 5α-reductase. The clinical syndrome is associated with mutations of the type 2 isoenzyme.

Table 61-11
Summary of the Mutations Detected in Type 3 17β-HSD

Ethnic background	*Family history*	*Mutation*	*Comment*
Homozygous patients			
Lebanese	Yes	Arg80Gln	Residual enzymatic activity
Brazilian	Yes	Arg80Gln	Residual enzymatic activity
Syrian	No	655-1, G-A	Disrupt splice acceptor
Greek	Yes	655-1, G-A	Disrupt splice acceptor
American	No	325+4, A-T	Disrupt splice donor
American	No	325+4, A-T	Disrupt splice donor
German	No	325+4, A-T	Disrupt splice donor
German	No	Phe208Ile	Inactivates enzyme
Iranian	No	Ser65Leu	Inactivates enzyme
Polish	No	Δ 777–783	Frame shift truncates protein
Brazilian	No	Ala203Val	Inactivates enzyme
Brazilian	Yes	Glu215Asp	Inactivates enzyme
Compound heterozygous patients			
American	No	Ser232Leu Met235Val	Both inactivate enzyme
American	Yes	325+4, A-T Pro282Leu	Disruption of splice donor; inactivates enzyme
Brazilian	Yes	Arg80Gln 326-1, G-T	Residual enzyme activity; disrupts splice acceptor
Italian German-Irish	No	325+4, A-T Gln176Pro	Disrupt splice donor
Heterozygous patients			
American	No	Val205Glu	Inactivates enzyme

Modified from Andersson S, et al. J Clin Endocrinol Metab 1996;81:130–136.

ACQUIRED CASES OF HYPERGONADOTROPIC HYPOGONADISM

None of these conditions of primary hypogonadism has a genetic basis. They are listed according to their etiology in Table 61-12.

HYPOGONADOTROPIC DISORDERS

Several congenital and acquired disorders (listed in Table 61-2) account for HH. Their common denominator consists of the impaired production of LHRH or of gonadotropins by the hypothalamus or pituitary gland. This in turn results in failure to stimulate the correct production of gonadal steroids and in a spectrum of clinical manifestations that vary depending on whether the abnormality developed before birth, before puberty, or after puberty (Table 61-4).

HYPOGONADOTROPIC DISORDERS ASSOCIATED WITH ISOLATED GONADOTROPIN DEFICIENCY

KALLMANN'S SYNDROME Background The first description of Kallmann's syndrome (KS) dates back to 1856 by Maestre de San Juan, but it was not until the original description by Kallmann in 1944 that the disease was recognized as an inherited entity.

It is found in 1 of every 10,000 newborn males, and in 1 of every 50,000 newborn females, and occurs in both sporadic (in up to 50% of the cases) and familial forms. Because of its predominance in the male sex, it was initially thought that KS is an X-linked disorder. However, there is now convincing evidence that additional forms exist that demonstrate autosomal recessive and autosomal dominant forms of transmission. In agreement with this heterogeneous inheritance, chromosomal abnormalities have been detected both in the X chromosome and, in patients with the autosomally inherited form, in autosomes. Within the X chromosome, the KS gene has been located in the Xp22.3 region. At least five different syndromes are caused by abnormalities involving this region of the X chromosome, including short stature, chondrodysplasia punctata, mental retardation, ichthyosis, and KS. The location of the gene(s) responsible for the autosomally transmitted KS is not yet known.

Embryology of the LH-RH Neurons The molecular events associated with the migration of the LHRH-secreting neurons during embryogenesis are intimately connected with the pathogenesis of KS. These neurons originate in the epithelium of the olfactory placode, from which they migrate into the brain by the 12th week of gestation along the pathway of the developing olfactory tract, represented by the olfactory, terminalis, and vomeronasal nerves. The LHRH neurons enter the brain through the nervus terminalis and vomeronasal, and thence into the septal-preoptic area and the hypothalamus. The normal migration of the LHRH neurons depends on genes located in Xp22.3, the same area of the X chromosome that is deleted in patients with KS. This was demonstrated by Schwanzel-Fukuda in a fetus with KS and a deletion of Xp22.3, in whom LHRH-expressing neurons were not found in the hypothalamus, but were instead identified beneath the forebrain, within the dural layers of the meninges and on the cribriform plate. When the migration is completed, there are fewer LHRH neurons in the brain (approximately 1500), than there were in the nose at the beginning of this process, probably because during the migration many cells die or differentiate into other cell types. Only after reaching their final destination in the brain do the LHRH-containing neurons acquire the capacity to secrete LHRH.

Table 61-12
Acquired Causes of Hypergonadotropic Hypogonadism

Viral orchitis
Sixty percent of postpubertal individuals with mumps orchitis exhibit damage to the germinal epithelium or both the germinal and interstitial epithelia
Drugs causing hypergonadotropic hypogonadism grouped according to their mechanism of action
Competition with the androgen receptor
Spironolactone
Cimetidine
Flutamide
Nilutamide
Bicalutamide
Cyproterone
Direct toxic effect on Leydig cells
Antineoplastic drugs
Cyclophosphamide
MOPP combination chemotherapy (mechlorethamine, vincristine, procarbazine, and prednisone)
ABVD combination chemotherapy (doxorubicin, bleomycin, vinblastin, and dacarbazine)
Ethanol
Inhibitors of testosterone synthesis
Ketoconazole
Spironolactone
Cyproterone
Tetracycline
Ethanol
Stimulators of estradiol synthesis or activity
Estrogenic compounds
Digoxin
Spironolactone
Environmental toxins
Lead
DDT (1,11,1-trichloro-2,2-*bis*(*p*-chlorophenyl)ethane)
p,p'DDE (1,1-dichloro-2,2-*bis*(*p*-chlorophenyl)ethylene)
Radiation
15 rads: transient germinal epithelium damage causing ↑ FSH
>600 rads: permanent germinal damage
2000–3000 rads: permanent germinal and interstitial damage
Autoimmunity
As part of the autoimmune polyglandular syndrome type II
Trauma
Frequent acquired cause of hypogonadotropic hypergonadism because of the relatively unprotected intrascrotal position of the testes

Clinical Features Individuals affected by KS can sometimes be recognized before puberty because of the presence of microphallus or cryptorchidism. Most patients, however, are recognized at puberty when they present with delayed appearance of the secondary sex characteristics or for the development of eunuchoid features. Abnormalities observed in KS other than those related to hypogonadism include hyposmia, anosmia, cleft lip, or cleft palate. Other symptoms occasionally described with the disease are sensory neural deafness, ocular motor abnormalities, abnormal spatial visual attention, cerebellar dysfunctions, talipes cavus deformity, and unilateral renal aplasia. It should be kept in mind that anosmia, which is considered one of the cardinal symptoms of KS, is not present in every patient, and that in some large series this feature is absent in up to 50–60% of the cases. In addition, some KS patients also manifest other diseases, like chondrodysplasia punctata, mental retardation, ichthyosis, short stature, and ocular albinism, which are associated with the deletion of the distal short arm of the X chromosome.

The hypogonadism of KS is caused by reduced secretion of LHRH by the hypothalamus, as shown by the observation that in almost every KS individual there is adequate response of LH and FSH after sufficient priming of the pituitary with exogenous LHRH. The decreased secretion of LHRH results in an abnormal secretory pattern of LH pulses, ranging from decreased or absent amplitude to diminished frequency. In the complete form of LHRH deficiency, LH and FSH deficiency is severe, and no evidence of sexual maturation is evident. In the incomplete form (known as the fertile eunuch syndrome), there is either normal FSH and low LH, or partial defects in both, with some degree of germ cell maturation. Although it is widely believed that this syndrome represents a continuum with the complete form of KS, the genetic studies to establish whether the fertile eunuch syndrome is a variable manifestation of KS or a separate genetic entity have not been performed. Microphallus and olfactory disturbances appear to be less common in this variant. Another variant form of isolated gonadotropin deficiency has been described in men with isolated FSH deficiency.

Laboratory tests reveal low serum FSH and LH levels and low testosterone. However, a large degree of heterogeneity in the serum levels of FSH and LH can be observed.

Diagnosis The diagnosis is suggested by the typical clinical picture and laboratory tests that demonstrate hypogonadotropic hypogonadism. The most challenging differential diagnosis is with delayed puberty. Important criteria are the ability to show the presence of anosmia or hyposmia, any other associated congenital defect or positive family history for KS. However, the separation of these two entities may require a prolonged period of observation.

Genetic Basis of Disease Using positional cloning techniques, two independent groups have isolated a candidate gene for KS *(KAL)* that is located at the Xp22.3 interval. Evidence that this gene is responsible for KS comes from the observation that in some affected patients it contains extensive deletions, or point mutations. The presence of a highly conserved *KAL* homolog in the Y chromosome has somehow delayed the development of mutation scanning strategies; however, point mutations within the 14 exons of the gene have been detected in at least 14 patients.

Molecular Pathophysiology Sequence analysis of the *KAL* cDNA has provided interesting insights into the pathogenesis of Kallmann's syndrome. The predicted protein is 680 amino acids long. Owing to the lack of a transmembrane domain or a phosphatidyl inositol anchorage site, it is believed to be an extracellular matrix molecule. Search for homologies has shown the presence of two important motifs. The first is a 4-disulfide core domain, found in a number of proteins with protease inhibitory activity, that is located in the N-terminal part of the molecule. The second is a region of similarity with the fibronectin type III repeat, found in numerous adhesion molecules involved in axon to axon interaction or in neuronal migration. Based on these sequence homologies, the KAL protein may represent an extracellular matrix factor that possesses both antiprotease and adhesion (or antiadhesion) functions. This protein may play a critical role in the migration process involving the olfactory and LHRH neurons during embryogenesis. Its absence or abnormal function in Kallmann's syndrome may help to explain the double clinical defect (hypogonadism, anosmia) observed in many of these patients. In addition, abnormalities of the KAL protein could also explain some of the other, less frequent, manifestations of the disease. RNA *in situ* hybridization studies have demonstrated *KAL* mRNA expression in the Purkinje cells of the cerebellum, the nucleus of the oculomotor nerve, the mesonephros, and the facial mesenchyme, which correlates with the presence in some KS patients of cerebellar dysfunctions, eye movement defects, unilateral renal aplasia, and cleft palate.

Despite these important new developments, there are still a number of unanswered questions. The *KAL* gene does not explain the autosomal types of KS, which is probably caused by abnormalities of autosomal genes that influence the migration of the LHRH neurons to the hypothalamus. In addition, it is not clear what the defect is in patients with hypogonadotropic hypogonadism without anosmia or in patients affected by the sporadic form of KS. If the sense of smell of patients without anosmia is normally developed, one can hypothesize that their olfactory bulb has developed normally and that their *KAL* gene may be normal, or that they represent a group with variable penetrance of the LHRH migratory defect, with mutations that do not completely impair function of the *KAL* gene product. In patients affected by the sporadic form of KS there is no supportive family history of an X-linked trait. Initial reports in abstract form suggest that the *KAL* gene is mutated only in a minority of these patients. Therefore the sporadic form of KS seems to be a heterogeneous disorder, arising in part from *de novo* mutations of the *KAL* gene, and in part from mutations of an unidentified autosome.

HYPOGONADOTROPIC HYPOGONADISM FROM BIOLOGICALLY INACTIVE LH

HYPOGONADISM CAUSED BY MUTATIONS IN THE GENES OF THE HPG AXIS Abnormalities occurring in the sequences of the genes encoding LHRH, the LHRH receptor, LH, or FSH have the potential of explaining some cases of idiopathic hypogonadotropic hypogonadism (HH) or infertility in males. However only a few such patients have been identified. It is likely that heterozygous patients with these mutations are subfertile; therefore, one can speculate that patients carrying homozygous mutations in the genes of the HPG axis are very rare because they would be the product of two subfertile individuals.

Evidence supporting the possibility that mutations of the LHRH gene are associated with hypogonadotropic hypogonadism is illustrated by the hpg mouse, an animal model with hypogonadism and infertility as a result of a deletion of the LHRH gene. Two studies have investigated the sequence of gonadotropin-releasing hormone (GnRH) in patients with idiopathic HH. Weiss et al. studied the coding region, the promoter, and the 3' untranslated tract of the GnRH gene in three male patients. No mutations were detected in this study. In another investigation reported in abstract form, Layman and collaborators identified a homozygous A-to-G transition 85 bp downstream from the splice donor site of intron 2 in 1 of 117 patients with HH. These authors speculated that this mutation could create a potential alternate donor splice site or affect transcription of the GnRH gene; however, no data have been presented in this regard.

Mutations of the FSH gene have not been reported in men, but are known to account for hereditary hypergonadotropic ovarian failure in women. Individuals of male sex with mutations of the FSH receptor have been identified in these pedigrees. These individuals are predicted to have a spectrum of abnormalities ranging from azoospermia to normospermia; however, the characteristics of their sexual phenotype have not yet been described in detail. The FSH receptor can also undergo activating mutations, as recently described by Gromoll and collaborators in a man who was able to sustain spermatogenesis despite being hypophysectomized.

HYPOGONADOTROPIC HYPOGONADISM CAUSED BY MUTATIONS OF THE LH GENE In males, only one case of hypogonadism with infertility has been associated with mutations of the LH gene. The propositus of this study was a 17-year-old patient with a hormonal profile showing low testosterone, high immunoreactive LH, and normal FSH. A testicular biopsy specimen revealed arrest of spermatogenesis and the absence of Leydig cells. When this patient was treated with exogenous hCG, a normal increase in testosterone secretion occurred, which was in contrast with the initial diagnosis of primary hypogonadism. Subsequently, the LH of this patient was found to be devoid of biologic activity using a dispersed Leydig cell bioassay, suggesting the production of an immunologically active but biologically inactive LH molecule. Sequence analysis of the coding sequence of the LH β gene revealed the patient to be homozygous for a missense mutation, Gln to Arg at amino acid residue 54. Functional experiments have shown that this mutation impairs the ability of the resulting LH to bind and activate its receptor. This study was extended to other

Table 61-13
Syndromes Associated With Central Nervous System Disorders

	Clinical and genetic features
Prader-Willi syndrome	*See text*
Möbious syndrome	*See text*
Laurence-Moon-Biedl syndrome	*See text*
Börjeson-Forssman-Lehman syndrome	X-linked mental retardation (XLMR) syndrome, mapped to Xq26–27. Associated with supraorbital ridges, ptosis, hypotonia, mental retardation, hypogonadism
LEOPARD syndrome	Lentigenes, ECG conduction defects, ocular hypertelorism, pulmonic stenosis, retarded growth, deafness, hypogonadism
Rud's syndrome	Mental retardation, epilepsy, hypogonadism, ichthyosis
Lowe's syndrome	XLMR syndrome mapped to Xq26. Associated with cataracts, renal tubular acidosis, hypogonadism, hypotonia, mental retardation
Carpenter's syndrome	Obesity, acrocephaly, craniosynostosis, agenesis of the hands and feet

members of the family, including three maternal uncles and the mother of the propositus, and has elucidated how heterozygous carriers of both sexes manifest clinically. The mother of the patient, an obligate heterozygote, underwent normal puberty and was fertile. The three heterozygous maternal uncles underwent normal puberty, reported normal libido and sexual performance, and had a normal physical examination. However, their serum testosterone concentration was low in several measurements, and at the time of the study they were childless. Therefore, given the limited nature of the pedigree, it would appear that heterozygous mutations of the LH gene do not manifest with important clinical abnormalities in the female sex, but may be associated with infertility in males.

Although mutations of the LH gene causing hypogonadism and infertility have only been detected in one male patient, the description of this case report has permitted a better understanding of the physiologic role played by LH during the embryologic development of the male sexual phenotype. The proband of this study was born with normal masculinization of his genitalia and with descended testes. Thus one can argue that LH is not critical for normal male sexual development, and that during embryogenesis adequate amounts of androgens from the adrenals or the testes are produced, probably under the stimulation of placental hCG.

HYPOGONADOTROPIC HYPOGONADISM ASSOCIATED WITH CENTRAL NERVOUS SYSTEM DISORDERS

Several congenital syndromes have been described in which central nervous system (CNS) disorders are associated with hypogonadotropic hypogonadism (Table 61-13). One hypothesis is that these disorders may be the consequence of a spectrum of congenital abnormalities disrupting at the same time the neuronal pathways leading the LHRH neurons into the hypothalamus and the normal development of the CNS. The identities and function of the gene(s) responsible for this group of syndromes are unknown.

PRADER-WILLI SYNDROME (PWS) Introduction PWS is an unusual condition occurring in 1 of every 25,000 newborns that is associated in about 50% of the cases with an interstitial deletion of chromosome 15, involving 15q11–q13. It is generally sporadic, although 10 families with more than one case have been described. The origin of the deleted chromosome 15 is paternal in almost all the individuals investigated by cytogenetic and DNA studies, making PWS one of the best examples for parental imprinting in humans.

Clinical Features The PWS phenotype is characterized by childhood obesity, carbohydrate intolerance, short stature, mental deficiency, infantile hypotonia, small hands and feet, a characteristic face, and hypogonadism. The latter is present in 95% of the cases, is mostly caused by GnRH deficiency, and is associated with cryptorchidism, micropenis, and scrotal hypoplasia. The response of serum gonadotropin concentrations to a single GnRH bolus is usually attenuated; however, long-term treatment with clomiphene or GnRH may stimulate gonadotropin secretion.

Genetic Basis of Disease The large size of the 15q11–q13 deletion has hampered the identification of candidate PWS genes in this region; however, the identification of two atypical PWS deletions, which greatly reduces the common region of deletion, has helped in focusing the quest for candidate genes to a smaller portion of 15q11–q13. As a result, three genes displaying paternal allele-specific expression have been recently identified in the area commonly deleted in PWS. One of these genes is the small nuclear ribonucleoprotein-associated polypeptide N gene *(SNRPN)*, a molecule involved in mRNA splicing, that is transcribed only from the paternal allele. The two other candidate genes are *PAR-5* and *PAR-1*, which were isolated from a YAC contig of the region deleted in PWS, and cluster together with *SNRPN* to a roughly 250-kb subregion of 15q11–q13.

Molecular Pathophysiology of Disease Whether any of these three genes is directly involved in the phenotype of PWS is currently under investigation. Considering the role played by *SNRPN* in mRNA splicing and the complex phenotype of PWS, one is tempted to speculate that a malfunctioning *SNRPN* contributes to PWS by altering the expression of several different and unrelated genes. This theory awaits confirmation in the years to come.

LAURENCE-MOON-BIEDL SYNDROME This entity has traditionally been considered as the association of retinitis pigmentosa, obesity, mental retardation, polydactyly, spastic paraparesis and hypogonadism. Currently two syndromes with slightly different manifestations are recognized: the Laurence-Moon syndrome, in which spastic paraparesis dominates and polydactyly is very rare; and the Bardet-Biedl syndrome, with very rare neurologic complications and frequent occurrence of dystrophic extremities and renal disease. Hypogonadism is present in both entities, and it manifests with microphallus, hypospadias, and undescended testes in prepubertal boys. There is disagreement on the origin of testicular failure as cases of both primary and secondary hypogonadism have been reported in the literature. The dis-

Table 61-14
Functional Causes and Systemic Diseases Associated with Hypogonadotropic Hypogonadism

Functional causes

Hyperprolactinemia: Patients affected by hyperprolactinemia can develop HH because of either the direct effect of hyperprolactinemia, which impairs the hypothalamic release of LHRH, or the mass effect of the adenoma.

Cushing's syndrome: Increased cortisol impairs normal production of LHRH.

Exercise: In men strenuous exercise can associate with decreased testosterone levels, without any change in LH and Testesterone Binding Globulin (TeBG) production. Usually without clinical signs.

Melatonin: One case of HH with increased melatonin production has been described, in which spontaneous normalization of melatonin hypersecretion was associated with reversal of HH.

Systemic diseases

AIDS: Frequent association between AIDS and HH (observed in 30% of HIV-positive patients in one study). In addition, preliminary data suggest that hypogonadism is probably associated with the wasting syndrome frequently observed in these patients.

Obesity: associated with ↓ TeBG, ↓ total testosterone, normal free testosterone, and ↑ estradiol (the latter because of increased peripheral conversion of aromatizable compounds).

Liver diseases: Multifactorial hypogonadism, with primary and secondary components, characterized by ↓ testosterone, ↑ estradiol, and gonadotropin levels from normal to moderately elevated.

Renal failure: Multifactorial hypogonadism with primary and secondary components. Hyperprolactinemia, a cause of HH, is present in 25% of men with chronic renal insufficiency undergoing dialysis.

Hemochromatosis: Multifactorial hypogonadism, with primary and secondary components. The secondary form of hypogonadism is predominant and it is caused by accumulation of iron in the pituitary gland. It is associated with diabetes, liver cirrhosis, and congestive heart failure.

ease is transmitted in an autosomal recessive manner, as indicated by a consanguinity rate of 48% among parents of affected patients in one series, and by a male to female ratio of 47:41 by combining two large studies.

MÖBIOUS SYNDROME This entity is also known as congenital oculofacial paralysis and is associated with multiple cranial nerve paralyses involving the 3rd, 4th, 5th, 9th, 10th, and 12th nerves, mental retardation, gait disturbances, peripheral neuropathy, and hypogonadism. Gonadotropin deficiency has been documented in several patients; however, considering the normal gonadotropin response to GnRH, GnRH deficiency is likely to constitute the primary defect. It is transmitted as an autosomal dominant trait, although sporadic cases have also been described. The clinical characteristics of the remaining syndromes belonging to this group of diseases are summarized in Table 61-13.

HYPOGONADOTROPIC HYPOGONADISM ASSOCIATED WITH ADRENAL INSUFFICIENCY

ADRENAL HYPOPLASIA CONGENITA Background Adrenal hypoplasia congenita (AHC) is a rare congenital disorder in which hypogonadotropic hypogonadism is associated with adrenal insufficiency. Two forms of this disorder have been described, the miniature adult form, secondary to ACTH deficiency transmitted as an autosomal recessive character, and the X-linked primary, or cytomegalic form.

Clinical Features ACH usually manifests with symptoms of adrenal insufficiency early in infancy. Gonadotropin deficiency is commonly associated with the X-linked primary form of AHC, and is noted at the expected time of pubertal maturation. The nature of the hypogonadotropic hypogonadism reported in these patients may be caused by pituitary gland dysfunction, based on lack of gonadotropin responses to prolonged pulsatile stimulation with synthetic GnRH.

Genetic Basis of Disease The gene for AHC has been mapped to chromosome Xp21 based on the deletion of this region in patients with a contiguous gene syndrome that includes AHC, glycerol kinase deficiency, and Duchenne muscular dystrophy. The gene responsible for this syndrome, designated *DAX-1*, has recently been isolated. It is a new member of the nuclear hormone receptor superfamily, and has been found to be deleted in some AHC patients or to have point mutations in patients with AHC, but no evidence of a deletion. The exact role played by this gene in the pathogenesis of the hypogonadotropic hypogonadism observed in AHC is currently under investigation.

ACQUIRED FORMS OF GONADOTROPIN DEFICIENCY FROM FUNCTIONAL CAUSES OR SYSTEMIC DISEASES

A brief discussion of these diseases, none of which has a genetic etiology, is presented in Table 61-14.

ANATOMIC DISORDERS ASSOCIATED WITH HYPOGONADOTROPIC HYPOGONADISM

A large number of anatomic disorders are associated with HH (Table 61-2). Infiltrations of the pituitary by inflammatory lesions, as in the case of lymphocytic hypophysitis, or by granulomatous diseases, such as in sarcoidosis, tuberculosis, and histiocytosis X, are well-described causes of gonadotropin deficiency. Other disorders consist of tumors developing in the hypothalamic–pituitary region. They act by the local compression and destruction of the gonadotroph. They include nonsecretory or secretory pituitary adenomas, craniopharyngiomas, dysgerminomas, metastases, meningiomas, hamartomas, or hypothalamic tumors.

Panhypopituitarism can also be the consequence of pituitary apoplexy. This condition has been described in patients affected by pituitary tumors or diabetes mellitus, in patients harboring lesions producing increased intracranial pressure, and in the setting of radiotherapy and anticoagulation. Residual LH and FSH deficiency after pituitary apoplexy has been described in 76 and 58% of the patients, respectively, and diminished testosterone secretion in 85% of the subjects investigated in a large study. The mechanism is believed to reflect the direct destruction of the adenohypophysis by the apoplexy.

Table 61-15
Systemic Disorders Associated With Infertility

Diseases impairing fertility	*Mechanism*
Infections	
Gonorrhea	Obstruction of the seminal pathway
Syphilis	Orchitis
Tuberculosis	Obstruction of the seminal pathway
Infectious parotitis	Orchitis
Chlamydial epididymitis	Obstruction of the seminal pathway
Brucellosis	Orchitis
Filariasis	Obstruction of the seminal pathway
Typhoid	Orchitis
Endocrine Disorders (other than hypogonadism)	
Thyrotoxicosis	Increased estrogen level
Diabetes	Impotence and ejaculatory disturbances
Systemic illnesses	
Renal failure	Hypogonadism
Hepatic failure	Hypogonadism
Sickle cell anemia	Impaired sexual maturation
Neurologic diseases	
Paraplegia	Impotence, ejaculatory dysfunctions, decreased testosterone level
Chronic respiratory tract diseases	
Bronchiectasis	Associated with immotile cilia syndrome or with Young's syndrome
Chronic sinusitis	
Chronic bronchitis	

GERMINAL CELL FAILURE

INTRODUCTION Infertility is usually defined as lack of conception after 1 year of adequate and unprotected intercourse. In many Western countries, approximately 15% of couples are unable to conceive within 12 months. Female and male factor disorders are equally distributed, and each are present in about 50% of the cases. Significant abnormalities are found in the male alone in one-third of the cases, while in an additional 20% of cases abnormalities are found in both members of the couple. Therefore, given the high incidence of concomitant disease in both partners, basic evaluation is warranted in both the man and the woman.

In the male partner it is useful to proceed in a stepwise way, starting with (1) a careful medical history, which is then followed by (2) a physical exam, (3) a semen analysis, and, if useful, (4) a testicular biopsy.

By questioning the patient, one should always keep in mind that a group of treatable causes of infertility are associated with decreased testosterone production as a result of a hypothalamic or pituitary cause. To ascertain this the patient should be asked whether he underwent normal puberty, and whether he is affected by symptoms of impotence or decreased libido. If this is the case, an appropriate work-up, including measurement of LH, FSH, testosterone, and prolactin and imaging of the pituitary, is warranted. In addition to hypogonadotropic disorders, numerous systemic disorders should be considered a possible secondary cause of male infertility (Table 61-15).

Another possible cause of infertility is caused by a direct anatomic damage to the testis or seminal pathways. Consequently it is important to investigate whether the patient has a history of testicular trauma or torsion or of genitourinary or testicular infections, and whether he underwent genitourinary surgery. Finally, it is important to ascertain whether the patient has been taking medications or illicit drugs or has been exposed to environmental factors known to affect normal gonadal function (Table 61-1).

It is useful to classify disorders of the germinal compartment of the testes according to the serum FSH level. Based on this, male infertility can be of the hypogonadotropic, hypergonadotropic, or eugonadotropic type. Hypogonadotropic disorders fall in the group of diseases discussed in Table 61-2. Patients with a hypogonadotropic disorder are affected by the simultaneous failure of the interstitial and germinal cells and belong to a group of infertile patients for which successful treatments are available.

Hypergonadotropic and eugonadotropic disorders represent categories of infertility that are characterized by increased or normal levels, respectively, of FSH (Table 61-3). In such states, the interstitial compartment is usually not affected by the disease, and therefore infertility will be the only symptom. Although a large number of conditions have been associated with male infertility, specific etiologies have been defined for only a small percentage of the conditions recognized. In many series, 60–80% of the infertile population consists of individuals with varicocele or idiopathic disease (Table 61-16). Since the exact mechanism causing infertility in men with varicocele is not understood, one can conclude that the etiology of infertility has not been defined in as many as 80% of patients. It is reasonable to assume that a better understanding of the basic biology of male infertility will permit a more successful treatment of these patients in the future.

EUGONADOTROPIC GERMINAL CELL DYSFUNCTION

OBSTRUCTION OF THE SEMINAL PATHWAY Introduction Acquired or congenital obstruction of the epididymis, vas deferens, or ejaculatory duct leads to azoospermia in up to 6% of infertile men. Up to 40% of men with azoospermia are eventually found to have an obstruction at some level of the seminal pathways, which is typically associated with normal testicular development, normal FSH, and normal histology of the testicular biopsy specimen. A classification based on the findings at explor-

Table 61-16
Relative Frequency of Diseases Associated with Male Infertility

Idiopathic	38.9%
Varicocele	40.3%
Cryptorchidism	6.4%
Epididymal or vas deferens obstruction	4.1%
Klinefelter's syndrome	1.9%
Mumps orchitis	1.6%
Hypogonadotropic hypogonadism	0.6%
Nonmotile sperm	0.6%
Irradiation/chemotherapy	0.5%
Coital disorders	0.5%
Other	4.5%

Modified from Baker HGW, et al. Relative incidence of etiological disorders in male infertility. In: Santen RJ, Swerdloff RS, eds. Male Reproductive Dysfunction: Diagnosis and Management of Hypogonadism, Infertility and Impotence. New York: Marcel Dekker, 1986; pp. 341–372.

atory scrototomy in 365 patients with azoospermia and normal serum FSH levels is shown in Table 61-17. Of these entities, only those with a genetic etiology will be discussed in detail. The others are grouped in Table 61-18.

CONGENITAL BILATERAL ABSENCE OF THE VAS DEFERENS (CBAVD) Background The most frequent genetic abnormality causing ductal obstruction is known as congenital bilateral absence of the vas deferens, or CBAVD, an autosomal recessive condition associated with azoospermia, which accounts for at least 1–2% of infertility cases in men. A similar abnormality, known as congenital unilateral absence of the vas deferens (CUAVD) has also been described, and it is believed to be an incomplete form of CBAVD. Recently, both these entities have been shown to be a genital form of cystic fibrosis (CF).

Clinical Features The typical patients with CBAVD presents with infertility as a result of absence of the vas deferens, and with a low-volume (<1 mL), acidic (pH <7.0) ejaculate, which consists predominantly of prostatic fluid. The seminal vesicles of these patients are often anatomically and functionally abnormal, as shown by the fact that only a small percentage of men with CBAVD have completely normal seminal vesicles on transrectal ultrasonography, and by the observation that CBAVD is associated with agenesis or dysplasia of the seminal vesicles in up to 75% of patients. Testicular anatomy and function are otherwise normal, as shown by their normal size and consistency on physical exam, the normal level of testosterone and FSH, and the normal histology of the biopsy specimen. Therefore, apart from azoospermia, the typical patient with CBAVD is healthy, and, unlike patients with CF, is not affected by disease of the respiratory system and pancreas.

Diagnosis On physical exam, the scrotal vasa are frequently not palpable, and the epididymal remnants are firm and enlarged. As stated above, further support for the diagnosis of CBAVD comes from the association of azoospermia with a low-volume ejaculate and normal testicular size and function.

Genetic Basis of Disease Absent or rudimentary vasa deferentia are not unique to CBAVD, but are noted also in 95% of males with CF. Since the ductal abnormalities of these two entities are very similar, it was postulated that CF and CBAVD could be related disorders. This possibility was confirmed once the gene responsible for cystic fibrosis was isolated and identified as the cystic fibrosis transmembrane-conductance regulator *(CFTR)* gene, and mutations of this molecule were detected both in CF and CBAVD. As a consequence, the general consensus is that CBAVD is a primarily genital form of cystic fibrosis, and that CF and CBAVD are extremes of a clinical spectrum. Studies performed on patients representing the entire clinical spectrum of CF have shown that the minimal amount of residual normal *CFTR* mRNA that is compatible with a normal phenotype is between 8 and 12% of normal. In patients with severe cystic fibrosis this amount is reduced to less than 1–3% of normal, whereas in those with an intermediate level of normal *CFTR* mRNA, a phenotype of mild cystic fibrosis develops. Hence, since CBAVD patients have an even milder form of CF that is uniquely localized in the vas deferens, the level of normal *CFTR* mRNA transcribed in this syndrome should be only slightly below the minimal amount necessary for a normal phenotype.

Molecular Pathophysiology of Disease A recent study, analyzing a large number of patients with CBAVD and CUAVD, has permitted a better understanding of the genetic lesions responsible for this condition (Table 61-15). In this series, mutations in the open reading frame (ORF) of both *CFTR* alleles were present in 19% of patients (group A); 33% of patients had the combination of one *CFTR* allele mutated in the ORF and one *CFTR* allele carrying the 5T variant (group B). The latter is a form of *CFTR* associated with 5 thymidines in the sequence known as "polyT sequence," which is located in intron 8 and is associated with reduced levels of *CFTR* mRNA. Thus, when the 5T allele is present together with an ORF mutation in the other allele, the amount of correctly transcribed *CFTR* is minimal, and the patient exhibits CBAVD. Mutations in the ORF of only one *CFTR* allele were present in 19% of patients (group C), suggesting that in this group other, but still undetected, *CFTR* abnormalities must be present in the second allele outside the ORF. The 5T allele and a normal second allele were present in 7% of patients (group D), also suggesting that the second allele must carry other still undetected abnormalities. Finally, 22% of patients did not carry ORF mutations or the 5T allele of *CFTR* (group E), suggesting either that CBAVD is a heterogeneous syndrome caused by genes other than *CFTR*, or that other undetected mutations are present in both alleles outside the ORF.

CUAVD and the *CFTR* Gene The presence of ORF mutations of the *CFTR* gene in patients with CUAVD is well established. In addition 25% of such patients were found to carry a 5T allele in the study by Chillón et al., suggesting that CUAVD could very well be an incomplete form of CBAVD.

Therapy Until recently patients with CBAVD were considered untreatable. However, the combination of in vitro fertilization with direct microsurgical aspiration of sperm (MESA) from the proximal ductal system has been successful in achieving pregnancies.

OTHER EUGONADOTROPIC DISORDERS CAUSING GERMINAL CELL FAILURE These disorders are discussed in Table 61-1.

HYPERGONADOTROPIC GERM-CELL FAILURE

IDIOPATHIC GERMINAL CELL FAILURE Background and Clinical Features This is a heterogeneous and large group, accounting for 60–80% of all patients with infertility. In the large majority of cases these patients are normally virilized, and the only clinical finding may be the presence of atrophic gonads. Some of

Table 6-17
Relative Frequency of Conditions Associated With Obstructive Azoospermia

Abnormality	*Percentage of patients*	*Cause*	*Other features*
Empty epididymis	13	Defective spermatogenesis, immune orchitis	Associated with abnormal testicular biopsy and abnormal spermatogenesis
Capital epididymal blocks	29	Young's syndrome, caused by inspissated secretion	Obstruction between ductuli efferentes and ductuli epididymis
Caudal epididymal blocks	19	Postinfective (epididymitis, after tuberculosis or gonorrhea)	
Blocked vas	11	Postinfective or postsurgery	Vasectomy is the most frequent cause of vasal obstruction
CBAVD *See text*	18	Associated with mutations of CFTR	
CUAVD *See text*	5	Associated with mutations of CFTR	
Ejaculatory duct blocks	14	Congenital, traumatic, or neoplastic (local extension of prostate cancer)	Diagnosed preoperatively, based on features of ejaculate

Modified from Hendry WF, et al. Ann R Coll Surg Engl 1990;72:396–407.

Table 61-18
CBAVD Patients Classified According to Genetic Abnormalities of CFTR

Mutation in ORF of both alleles (19%)
Mutation in ORF of one allele, and 5T variants in second allele (33%)
Mutation in ORF of one allele (19%)
5T variant in one allele (7%)
No detectable abnormalities of CFTR (22%)

Modified from Chillon M, et al. N Engl J Med 1995;332:1475–1480.

these patients may have normal FSH levels, and therefore are classified as eugonadotropic, whereas others have increased FSH levels and, consequently, are classified as hypergonadotropic. The histologic abnormalities detected in the testes of these patients are heterogeneous and consist of germinal cell aplasia (also known as Sertoli-cell-only syndrome [SCOS] of which two types have been described depending on whether germinal cell aplasia is present in each [type I] or most [type II] testicular tubules), arrest of germinal cell maturation at the spermatogonia or spermatocyte stage, or hyalinization of the seminiferous tubules with hypospermatogenesis. In these patients semen analysis may encompass the entire spectrum of sperm abnormalities, ranging from azoospermia to oligospermia, astenospermia, and presence of a stress pattern of sperm morphology. A careful medical history can help in detecting the minority of cases caused by infection, cytotoxic drugs, immunologic factors, or cryptorchidism; however, the mechanism leading to most of the cases is unknown. A genetic component has long been suspected, and autosomal or X-linked inheritance has been detected in a number of pedigrees. In addition, a genetic abnormality arising as a *de novo* mutation of an elusive "azoospermia factor" in the Y chromosome has been theorized since 1976.

Identification of a Putative Azoospermia Factor of the Y Chromosome A systematic approach to the identification of the azoospermia factor (AZF) has recently produced some important developments. Using genomic DNA extracted from 89 men in whom semen analysis had revealed azoospermia and testicular biopsy specimens showed a range of abnormalities ranging from SCOS to maturation arrest, Reijo and colleagues have performed a detailed deletion map of a 30-Mb fragment of the Y chromosome, which included proximal Yq, the centromere, and Yp. A deletion of an area called the AZF region was detected in 12 of 89 azoospermic men in a portion of Yq, which appeared to be a new event, since no such deletion was present in the genomic DNA of 7 male relatives that was tested as a control. By using exon trapping, these investigators were able to identify a novel gene within the AZF region. This molecule, named *DAZ* (deleted in azoospermia), is a single-copy gene that is transcribed only in the testes and bears an RNA recognition motif, suggesting that it is an RNA-binding protein. The frequency by which the AZF region is deleted is high. According to the study of Reijo et al., 1 of every 8 men with azoospermia has a deletion of the AZF region. Thus, since approximately 1 in 1000 men is azoospermic because of severe spermatogenic defects, it appears that the AZF region is deleted at the rate of 1 in every 10,000 newborn males.

Absence of Correlation Between *DAZ* Deletion and Biopsy Findings The histology of the testes that was available in 9 of the 12 men carrying a deletion of the AZF region was very heterogeneous. Five patients were affected by SCOS and four by maturation arrest at the level of spermatogonia or premeiotic spermatogenic cells. In addition, in two of the patients with maturation arrest, the biopsy specimen revealed the presence of occasional mature, condensed spermatids. This finding was quite unexpected, since the general consensus has always been that the azoospermia factor regulates some specific step in the process of sperm maturation, and therefore its absence should have been associated with a specific histologic abnormality.

Current Status of Knowledge The information generated by these new findings can be condensed in four major points. First, germ cells can persist, at least in some men, even when an intact AZF region is not present. Second, the AZF region is not absolutely required for the production of mature, condensed spermatids, and it is not essential for progression of male germ cells through meiosis. Third, SCOS and testicular maturation arrest are not distinct disorders, at least when associated with Yq deletions, but appear to represent different manifestations of the same underlying defect. Finally, despite these considerations, the AZF region contains a gene, *DAZ*, which may represent the elusive azoospermia factor. As an RNA-binding protein, DAZ has all of the features of a potentially important regulatory molecule and could regulate some basic phenomenon required for sperm maturation. In addition, *DAZ* was found to be deleted in 12 azoospermic patients, and because it is transcribed only in the testes, it is expressed in a location that seems directly tied to spermatogenesis. Further evidence supporting an important role for the AZF region in spermatogenesis comes from the observation that this segment of the Y chromosome is also deleted in a minority of patients (2 of 35) affected by oligospermia (i.e., <15–10,000,000 sperm/mL). In addition, loss of the *Drosophila* gene *boule*, which has remarkable similarity to *DAZ*, results in azoospermia in fruit flies.

Even if the evidence provided to date is convincing, more concrete proof, for example in the form of inactivating point mutations in nondeleted azoospermic and oligospermic patients, will be necessary to establish that the *DAZ* transcript is critical for spermatogenesis.

Unsolved Issues The identification of *DAZ* does not exclude that other genes within AZF may be important for gametogenesis, or that genes essential for spermatogenesis may be present elsewhere in the human Y chromosome. One such factor could belong to the *RBM* (RNA-binding-motif) family of genes, which were previously reported by Ma and collaborators as putative AZF candidates, and do not map within the AZF region identified by Reijo et al. Further evidence for the presence of other Y-derived factors important for spermatogenesis comes from two recent deletion studies of the Y chromosome in azoospermic and oligospermic patients. In the study of Najmabadi et al., microdeletions were detected in 11 of 60 patients. In 4 of these 11 patients the deletion did not correspond to the AZF region. In the study of Vogt and collaborators, microdeletions were found in 13 of 370 patients. Interestingly, this study has identified two additional segments of Yq, besides the AZF region of Reijo et al., that are deleted in azoospermic patients. These regions of the Y chromosome have been named AZF-a, -b, and -c. According to the data of Vogt et al., and in contrast to the finding of Reijo et al., the deletion of each of the three potential AZF regions is associated with a specific histologic abnormality of the testis. Deletion of AZF-c, which coincides with the segment defined as the AZF region by Rejio et al., is associated with type II SCOS. Deletions of AZF-a and -b are associated with type I SCOS and spermatogenic arrest at the spermatocyte stage, respectively. A candidate spermatogenesis gene for segment AZF-b is *RBM1*, which is absent in patients lacking this fragment of chromosome Y. Candidate spermatogenesis genes for segment AZF-c are *DAZ* and *SPGY* (the latter is a new gene, isolated by Vogt's group, which is localized in this area of chromosome Y and has 85% sequence similarity to *DAZ*). No candidate spermatogenesis genes for segment AZF-a have yet been identified.

Extension of these studies to a larger number of patients should help to understand more details on the role played by Yq in controlling spermatogenesis.

Therapy Since the understanding of the basic mechanisms causing idiopathic germinal cell failure is poor, the medical treatments available are mostly empirical or based on uncontrolled trials. The rationale is to use hormonal therapy with the aim to stimulate sperm production. Treatments include administration of clomiphene citrate, tamoxifene, testolactone, testosterone, bromocriptine, gonadotropins, and gonadotropin-releasing factor. There is no clear data indicating whether these treatments result in increased pregnancy rate or improved semen quality.

New hope for some of these patients is offered by the development of new techniques in assisted reproduction, including subzonal sperm microinjection and intracytoplasmic injection of spermatozoa retrieved from the epididymis. Some of these techniques are becoming increasingly more effective in improving the prognosis of severe male factor infertility.

CRYPTORCHIDISM **Background and Clinical Features** Cryptorchidism is a common anomaly detected in humans and many animal species, consisting of the failure of one or both testes to reach their final destination inside the scrotum at the end of the process of testicular migration from the abdominal cavity. It is a condition occurring with increasing frequency, found in 3–5% of newborn males. Many undescended testes will spontaneously reach the scrotal cavity during the initial 3 months of life, and consequently the incidence of cryptorchidism will drop to 0.8% at 1 year of age. Spontaneous testicular descent is unlikely to occur after the 12 month of age. Bilateral cryptorchidism is observed in 15% of the cases.

The clinician should be aware of other conditions mimicking cryptorchidism, such as pseudocryptorchidism, in which the gonad at times occupies a scrotal position and at times retracts in the inguinal canal, and the ectopic testes, in which the testes migrate through an ectopic pathway and eventually will occupy a pubic, femoral, perineal, or superficial inguinal position.

Etiology Many cryptorchid testes will eventually be unable to fulfill their reproductive role because of abnormalities occurring in their germinal compartment. In this regard, it is controversial whether the failure to descend into the scrotum is the cause or the consequence of the abnormalities present in a cryptorchid testis. Although there is not a unifying theory for all cases of cryptorchidism, failure to migrate inside the scrotum could be, at least in some cases, the consequence of blunted gonadotropin production during the third trimester of gestation. Migration of the testes inside the scrotum is thought to be regulated by the shortening of the gubernaculum, an androgen-dependent process requiring both maternal hCG and fetal LH, which stimulate the fetal testes to produce testosterone. The importance of testosterone in this process is also indirectly underscored by the observation that antiandrogen treatment of pregnant dams blocks testicular descent in rat pups. There is still considerable disagreement as to whether cryptorchidism should be considered a genetic disease or not, and evidence in favor of and against such a possibility has been presented. However, many genetic diseases associated with impairment of androgen synthesis or action, and with conditions predisposing to inadequate intra-abdominal pressure, like the prune belly syndrome, cause bilateral cryptorchidism. Additional information on the genes responsible for the intrascrotal migration of the testes during sexual differentiation is offered with increasing frequency by the study of mice models carrying targeted deletion of factors thought to be active during urogenital embryogenesis. One such factors is the *Hoxa10* gene, a member of the *HOX* gene family of transcription factors, whose absence is associated with developmental abnormalities, including bilateral cryptorchidism resulting in severe defects in spermatogenesis and increasing sterility with age. Progress in the identification of the network of genes involved in regulating testicular descent during embryogenesis should help in understanding the cause, and in directing a proper treatment of cryptorchidism.

Treatment The first step in the treatment of these boys is using hCG or LHRH alone or in combination. hCG should be given at a total dose of 10,000 IU for 2–3 weeks, after 6 months of age. LHRH can be given as a nasal spray at the dose of 20 μg/d. The success of this treatment, which can be inflated if the treated patient population includes boys with retractile testis, varies and ranges between 10 and 35% among the different studies. Subjects who do not respond to medical treatment should undergo orchiopexy and should be operated on between ages 6 and 18 months. Another important consideration in favor of early surgery is that intra-abdominal positioning of a testis is associated with an increased risk of malignant degeneration. Despite this, there is no clear-cut evidence that demonstrates that placing the retained testis inside the scrotum reduces the risk of neoplastic degeneration.

ANDROGEN RESISTANCE The infertile man syndrome is one of the phenotypes described in patients with androgen resistance. A study published in 1982 suggested that at least 40% of patients with idiopathic azoospermia were affected by a form of androgen resistance causing decreased ^{3}H-DHT binding of the receptor, as assessed by monolayer binding assay of genital skin fibroblasts cultured from these patients. No abnormalities of the pituitary–testicular axis were detected in these individuals. Although an interesting possibility, there is significant controversy as to whether 40% of infertile patients are indeed affected by androgen resistance as this study implies. Molecular analysis of the androgen receptor in this group of patients has not been performed in a systematic way; however, a partial gene deletion in one of seven azoospermic men was detected by PCR and Southern analysis in one study.

SELECTED REFERENCES

Andersson S, Geissler W, Wu L, et al. Molecular genetics and pathophysiology of 17β-hydroxysteroid dehydrogenase 3 deficiency. J Clin Endocrinol Metab 1996;81:130–136.

Andersson S, Russel D, Wilson J. 17β-Hydroxysteroid dehydrogenase deficiency. Trends Endocrinol Metab 1996;7:121–126.

Baker H, Burger H, de Kretser D, et al. Relative incidence of etiological disorders in male infertility. In: Santen R, Swerdloff R, eds. Male Reproductive Dysfunction: Diagnosis and Management of Hypogonadism, Infertility and Impotence. New York: Marcel Dekker, 1986; pp. 341–372.

Ballabio A, Andria G. Deletions and translocations involving the distal short arm of the human X chromosome. Hum Mol Genet 1992;1:221–227.

Ballabio A, Zoghbi H. Kallmann Syndrome. In: Scriver CR, Beaudet AL, Sly WS, Valle D, eds. The Metabolic Bases of Inherited Disease. New York: McGraw Hill, 1995; pp. 4549–4557.

Burris TP, Guo W, McCabe ER. The gene responsible for adrenal hypoplasia congenita, DAX-1, encodes a nuclear hormone receptor that defines a new class within the superfamily. Recent Prog Horm Res 1996;51:241–259.

Castro-Magnana M, Angulo M, Uy J. Male hypogonadism with gynecomastia caused by late-onset deficiency of 17-ketosteroid reductase. N Engl J Med 1993;328:1297–1301.

Chillòn M, Casals T, Mercier B, et al. Mutations in the cystic fibrosis gene in patients with congenital absence of the vas deferens. N Engl J Med 1995;332:1475–1480.

Collin GB, Marshall JD, Cardon LR, Nishina PM. Homozygosity mapping at Alstrom syndrome to chromosome 2p. Hum Mol Genet 1997;6:213–219.

Cooke HJ, Elliot DJ. RNA-binding proteins and human male infertility. Trends Genet 1997;13:87–89.

Eberhart C, Maines J, Wasserman S. Meiotic cell cycle requirement for a fly homologue of human deleted in azoospermia. Nature 1996; 381:783–785.

Ferguson-Smith MA, Goodfellow PN. SRY and primary sex-reversal syndromes. In: Scriver CR, Beaudet AL, Sly WS, Valle D, eds. The Metabolic Bases of Inherited Disease. New York: McGraw-Hill, 1995; pp. 739–748.

Franco B, Guioli S, Pragliola A, et al. A gene deleted in Kallmann's syndrome shares homology with neural cell adhesion and axonal pathfinding molecules. Nature 1991;353:529–536.

Geissler WM, Davis DL, Wu L, et al. Male pseudohermaphroditism caused by mutations of testicular 17β-hydroxysteroid dehydrogenase 3. Nat Genet 1994;7:34–39.

Georgopoulos NA, Pralong FP, Seidman CE, Seidman JG, Crowley WF Jr, Vallejo M. Genetic heterogeneity evidenced by low incidence of KAL-1 gene mutations in sporadic cases of gonadotropin-releasing hormone deficiency. J Clin Endocrinol Metab 1997;82: 213–217.

Hendry W, Levison D, Parkinson C, Parslow J, Royle M. Testicular obstruction: clinico-pathological studies. Ann R Coll Surg Engl 1990;72:396–407.

Husmann D, McPhaul M. Time-specific androgen blockade with flutamide inhibits testicular descent in the rat. Endocrinology 1991; 129:1409–1416.

Jamieson C, van-der-Burgt I, Brady A, et al. Mapping a gene for Noonan syndrome to the long arm of chromosome 12. Nat Genet 1994;8: 357–360.

Kremer H, Kraaij R, Toledo SPA, et al. Male pseudohermaphroditism due to a homozygous missense mutation of the luteinizing hormone receptor gene. Nat Genet 1995;9:160–164.

Krumlauf R. Hox genes in vertebrate development. Cell 1994;78:191–201.

Latronico A, Anasti J, Arnhold I, et al. Brief report: testicular and ovarian resistance to luteinizing hormone caused by inactivating mutations of the luteinizing hormone-receptor gene. N Engl J Med 1995;334:507–512.

Legouis R, Hardelin J-P, Levilliers J, et al. The candidate gene for the X-linked Kallmann syndrome encodes a protein related to adhesion molecules. Cell 1991;67:423–435.

Lin D, Sugawara T, Strauss J, et al. Role of steroidogenic acute regulatory protein in adrenal and gonadal steroidogenesis. Science 1995;267: 1828–1831.

Ma K, Inglis J, Sharkey A, et al. A Y chromosome gene family with RNA-binding protein homology: candidates for the azoospermia factor controlling human spermatogenesis. Cell 1993;75:1287–1295.

Mason A, Hayflick I, Zoeller R. A deletion truncating the GnRH gene is responsible for hypogonadism in the hpg mouse. Science 1986; 234:338–340.

Muscatelli F, Strom T, Walker A, et al. Mutations in the DAX-1 gene give rise to both X-linked adrenal hypoplasia congenita and hypogonadotropic hypogonadism. Nature 1994;372:672–676.

Najmabadi H, Huang V, Yen P, et al. Substantial prevalence of microdeletions of the Y-chromosome in infertile men with idiopathic azoospermia and oligozoospermia detected using a sequence-tagged site-based mapping strategy. J Clin Endocrinol Metab 1996;81: 1347–1352.

Özcelik T, Leff S, Robinson W, et al. Small nuclear ribonucleoprotein polypeptide N (SNRPN), an expressed gene in the Prader-Willi syndrome critical region. Nat Genet 1992;2:265–269.

Reijo R, Alagappan R, Patrizio P, Page D. Severe oligozoospermia resulting from deletions of azoospermia factor gene on Y chromosome. Lancet 1996;347:1290–1293.

Reijo R, Lee T-Y, Salo P, et al. Diverse spermatogenic defects in humans caused by Y chromosome deletions encompassing a novel RNA-binding protein gene. Nat Genet 1995;10:383–393.

Rheaume E, Simard J, Morel Y, et al. Congenital adrenal hyperplasia due to point mutations in type II 3 beta-hydroxysteroid dehydrogenase gene. Nat Genet 1992;1:239–245.

Satokata I, Benson G, Maas R. Sexually dimorphic sterility phenotypes in Hoxa10-deficient mice. Nature 1995;374:460–463.

Schwanzel-Fukuda M, Bick D, Pfaff D. Luteinizing hormone-releasing hormone (LHRH)-expressing cells do not migrate normally in an inherited hypogonadal (Kallmann) syndrome. Mol Brain Res 1989; 6:311–326.

Schwanzel-Fukuda M, Pfaff D. Origin of luteinizing hormone-releasing hormone neurons. Nature 1989;338:161–164.

Simard J, Rheaume E, Mebarki F, et al. Molecular basis of human 3β-hydroxysteroid-dehydrogenase deficiency. J Steroid Biochem Mol Biol 1995;53:127–138.

Simard J, Rheaume E, Sanchez R, et al. Molecular basis of congenital adrenal hyperplasia due to 3β-hydroxysteroid dehydrogenase deficiency. Mol Endocrinol 1993;7:716–728.

Tapanainen JS, Aittomaki K, Min J, Vaskivuo T, Huhtaniemi IT. Men homozygous for an inactivating mutation of the follicle-stimulating hormone (FSH) receptor gene present variable suppression of spermatogenesis and fertility. Nat Genet 1997;15:205,206.

Vogt P, Edelman A, Kirsch S, et al. Human Y chromosome azoospermia factor (AZF) mapped to different subregions in Yq11. Hum Mol Genet 1996;5:933–943.

Waldstreicher J, Seminara SB, Jameson JL, et al. The genetic and clinical heterogeneity of gonadotropin-releasing hormone deficiency in the human. J Clin Endocrinol Metab 1996;81:4388–4395.

Weiss J, Axelrod L, Whitcomb R, Harris P, Crowley W, Jameson J. Hypogonadism caused by a single amino acid substitution in the β subunit of luteinizing hormone. N Engl J Med 1992;326: 179–183.

Yanase T. 17α-Hydroxylase/17,20-lyase defects. J Steroid Biochem Mol Biol 1995;53:153–157.

Yanase T, Simpson ER, Waterman MR. 17α-Hydroxylase/17,20-lyase deficiency: from clinical investigation to molecular definition. Endocr Rev 1991;12:91–108.

Zachmann M. Defects in steroidogenic enzymes. Discrepancies between clinical steroid research and molecular biology results. J Steroid Biochem Mol Biol 1995;53:159–164.

Zanaria E, Muscatelli F, Bardoni B, et al. An unusual member of the nuclear hormone receptor superfamily responsible for X-linked adrenal hypoplasia congenita. Nature 1994;372:635–641.

62 Ovarian Diseases

ELIZABETH A. MCGEE AND NICHOLAS A. CATALDO

INTRODUCTION

The primary function of the human ovary, the production of fertilizable gametes, is essential to the survival of the human species. Traditionally, ovarian gametogenesis has been viewed as intricate and delicately balanced, but recent information suggests that, although intricate, this process may be governed by multiple parallel, redundant systems, which evolved by enhancing reproductive success. Knowledge of ovarian physiology derived from disciplined studies at the molecular level is just beginning to be applied clinically, and the application of molecular biology to the prevention and treatment of ovarian disease is still in its infancy. This chapter will outline some aspects of current research on the molecular physiology of both the normal and abnormal ovary.

OVARIAN FUNCTION

OVARIAN ONTOGENY In the third week after fertilization, germ cells arise in the yolk sac endoderm at the caudal aspect of the embryo and begin to migrate to the gonadal ridge, which at this stage consists of coelomic epithelial mesenchyme and elements of the mesonephros. At this stage presumptive ovaries are indistinguishable from presumptive testes. The factors that govern formation of the gonadal ridge are not known, but the expression of the orphan nuclear receptor SF1, the *DAX* gene product (which may be regulated by SF1), and the nuclear receptor WT1, that is the product of the Wilms' tumor gene, are all required early in this process. Although *SRY* plays a key role in testicular differentiation in the male, genes that play a similar role in directing ovarian development have not been identified. Differentiation of the ovary is generally believed to begin approximately 2 weeks later than testes become identifiable in males and to proceed by default when testis-determining factors are absent. Unlike the testis, which can form in the absence of germ cells, formation of a functional ovary requires the interaction of germ cells with the gonadal ridge and mesonephros; if germ cells do not reach the presumptive ovary, it degenerates into a fibrous streak.

The regulation of germ cell migration to the gonadal ridge is not clearly defined, but adhesion molecules, including fibronectin, laminin, and the integrins, likely play a role. However, a more clearly understood pair of molecules in this process, extensively studied in the mouse, is the receptor c-kit and its ligand. A transmembrane protein with tyrosine kinase activity encoded by the dominant white spotting (W) locus, c-kit is expressed by primordial germ cells. The kit ligand, called stem cell factor (SCF) or mast cell growth factor, is encoded by the steel (Sl) locus and is expressed by cells along the germ cell migration pathway from the yolk sac to the genital ridge. There are two splice variants of the transmembrane form of SCF, one of which can be cleaved to form a soluble form (Fig. 62-1). Mutations in cell surface SCF, such as Steel-dickie and Steel-panda, result in the decreased ability of germ cells to migrate to the genital ridge and decreased survival of the cells that do arrive. Many W mutations result in female sterility or decreased numbers of primordial follicles, but some mice with these mutations are fertile, even in the face of reduced receptor kinase activity or reduced c-kit mRNA expression. Though c-kit and its ligand are thought to have a critical role in germ cell migration and proliferation, the lack of a uniform phenotype in these mutants suggests a more complex system with other modulating factors involved. Transforming growth factor-β (TGF-β) has been suggested to be a chemotactic factor released by the genital ridge, whereas tumor necrosis factor (TNF)-α has been suggested as an early germ cell mitogen that along with leukemia inhibitory factor (LIF) could prevent premature differentiation during migration. Future investigations will likely clarify the roles of growth and chemotactic factors and adhesion molecules in the process of germ cell migration.

After reaching the genital ridge, the primordial germ cells, now called oogonia, must continue to both proliferate and survive. Oogonia become invested by a single layer of flat, pregranulosa cells derived from the rete ovarii to form primordial follicles. If they fail to be surrounded by these pregranulosa cells, oogonia die spontaneously, apparently by apoptosis. The receptor c-kit and its ligand, SCF, may play a role in oogonial survival, since apoptosis can be blocked in vitro by added SCF. Other factors implicated in the regulation of oogonial apoptosis include LIF and related molecules oncostatin M and ciliary neurotropic factor, as well as interleukin (IL)-4 and basic fibroblast growth factor (bFGF). The role of these factors in human germ cell migration, proliferation, and survival has not been defined. Few studies have been performed on human embryonic tissue, but in one such study c-kit was localized to human oogonia.

In the human embryo, germ cells reach the gonadal ridge by the 7th week of gestation. Oogonia increase their number by mitosis from approximately 10,000 by the 6th week to 6 million by 20 weeks' gestation, at which time their number peaks and mitosis ceases. By 11–12 weeks, some oogonia have begun their transformation into oocytes by entering meiosis; they remain arrested at

From: *Principles of Molecular Medicine* (J. L. Jameson, ed.), ©1998 Humana Press Inc., Totowa, NJ.

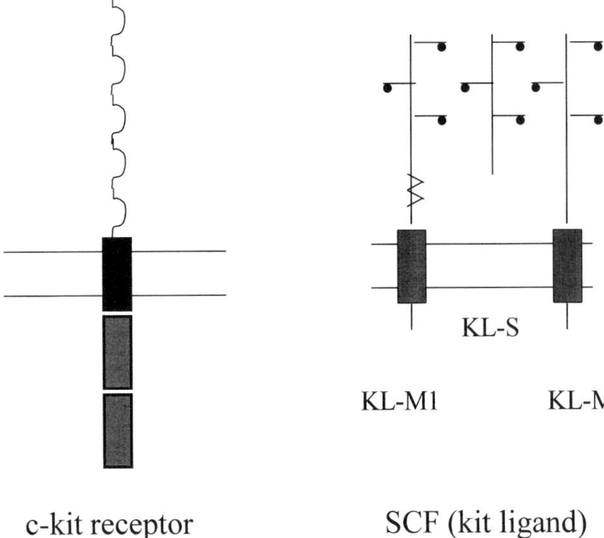

Figure 62-1 **(Left)** The c-kit receptor is a member of the PDGF branch of the tyrosine kinase family of receptors, with a large extracellular domain containing five IgG-like domains. Its intracellular tyrosine kinase region is separated by a kinase insert. **(Right)** SCF, the c-kit ligand, has two forms (KL-M1 and KL-M2) that can be generated by alternate splicing of the same gene. The KL-M1 form can be proteolytically cleaved to form a soluble KL-S. (Modified from Donovan, 1994.)

the dictyotene stage of the first meiotic prophase until they are ovulated. Oocytes that do not enter meiosis are lost by the time of birth. Formation of primordial follicles (Fig. 62-2A) begins at about 16 weeks' gestation and is complete by 6 months after birth.

Factors other than those mentioned may also play a role in follicle formation. Involvement of gonadotropins or other pituitary factors in the process of follicle formation is suggested by one study showing that this process occurs inefficiently and to variable degrees, with a poorly organized rete ovarii, in monkeys that were hypophysectomized *in utero*. Other genetically but not physiologically defined factors regulate follicle formation in the fetal sheep ovary: the Booroola Merino and Inverdale strains, studied because of their tendency to have large litters, have also been noted to have delayed or defective follicle formation. Homozygotes for the Booroola mutation $FecB^{B}$ show delayed follicular formation and growth, whereas homozygotes for the Inverdale mutation $FecX^{I}$ show a total failure of development past the primary stage. Genes in humans homologous to the sheep $FecB^{B}$ and $FecX^{I}$ have not yet been identified.

Some germ cell tumors in women are believed to arise from germ cells that failed to migrate successfully to the gonad. These tumors can be found at many sites near the normal germ cell migration path, including the mediastinum, adrenal, and both the small and large intestinal mesenteries, as well as in more remote sites such as the pineal gland. The incidence of germ cell tumors has been increasing, leading some investigators to conclude that environmental and intrauterine toxic exposures may affect germ cell migration. Further study of these tumors, as well as of the migration of germ cells in animal models, may give additional insight into the processes of germ cell migration, proliferation, survival, and tumorigenesis.

FOLLICULAR DEVELOPMENT Primordial follicles (Fig. 62-2A) can begin further development at any time after their formation, or they may remain dormant for more than 50 years. As a primordial follicle begins to mature, the granulosa cells become cuboidal and divide to form several layers around the oocyte (Fig. 62-2B). The zona pellucida, a mucoid glycoprotein layer around the oocyte that is formed by both granulosa cells and the oocyte, appears as the granulosa cells differentiate. A distinct theca layer begins to condense around the follicle and becomes vascularized. Since the theca is separated from the avascular granulosa by a basement membrane, access of serum proteins to the granulosa and oocyte is functionally limited. As both the granulosa and theca cells continue to divide and the oocyte increases in size, an antrum develops within the granulosa layer, filled with fluid that is a transudate from the thecal vasculature (Fig. 62-2C). Follicular fluid also contains proteins secreted by granulosa cells, many of which are paracrine factors important for continued follicular development.

How primordial follicles are maintained in a relatively static condition for decades and then induced to grow and differentiate is still poorly understood. Static primordial follicles do not demonstrate differentiated function, suggesting that they either express suppressors, or fail to express activators, of the genes that induce follicular differentiation. One candidate suppressor of granulosa cell differentiated function is the product of the Wilms' tumor gene WT1, a zinc-finger transcription factor. In rodents, high levels of WT1 are expressed in the gonadal ridge and in the granulosa cells of primordial follicles and lower levels in primary and early secondary follicles, but minimal levels in more developed follicles. WT1 represses the expression of inhibin-α, insulin-like growth factor (IGF)-II, IGF-I receptor, early growth response gene *(EGR)*-1, *PAX-2*, platelet-derived growth factor (PDGF)-A, colony-stimulating factor (CSF)-1, and TGF-α. It has been hypothesized that by suppressing the expression of growth and differentiation genes, WT1 can act on early follicles as a "stasis factor," and as the level of WT1 falls, the rate of follicular development increases. Further studies should elucidate the regulation of WT1 expression, as well as the interaction of WT1 with other genes involved in follicular development.

A second factor that may play a role as an activator of human folliculogenesis is growth and differentiation factor (GDF)-9, a member of the TGF-β superfamily. In the mouse, GDF-9 is expressed in oocytes at the primary through preovulatory follicle stages, and it is necessary for follicular development past the early secondary stage. Female mice deficient in GDF-9 are infertile and resistant to gonadotropin stimulation, despite the expression of gonadotropin receptors in their ovaries.

Early follicular growth can occur in the absence of gonadotropin stimulation, as evidenced by the presence of preantral follicles in the ovaries of anencephalic infants as well as in gonadotropin-deficient patients. Although larger antral follicles are clearly dependent on gonadotropin for further mitosis and differentiation as well as protection from apoptosis, several in vitro studies of rodent follicles have suggested a role for follicle-stimulating hormone (FSH) in earlier follicle development as well, perhaps in conjunction with activin or other factors. The initial stimulus to follicular growth and the exact role of FSH in preantral follicle development are still not clearly understood, nor is the molecular basis of the induction of granulosa cell FSH receptors. An interaction of granulosa and oocyte factors is likely to regulate early follicle growth and development.

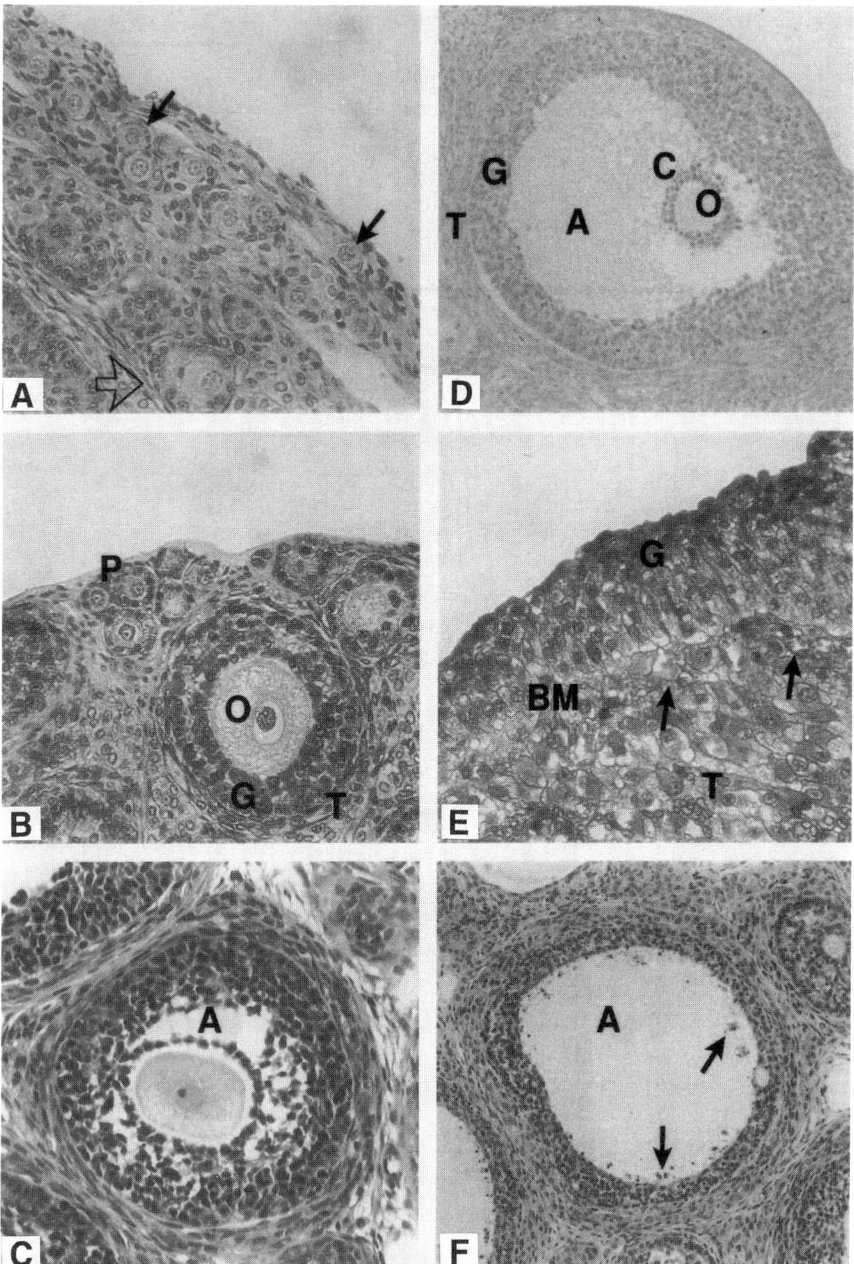

Figure 62-2 **(A)** Primordial follicles just below the epithelium of the ovary (dark arrows) with clusters of transitional and primary follicles (open arrow). **(B)** Primary follicles (P) and a secondary follicle with an oocyte (O) surrounded by granulosa cells (G) with an external theca layer (T). **(C)** A slightly larger follicle that is beginning to develop an antrum (A). **(D)** A maturing Graafian follicle, with a large antrum (A), a cumulus (C) surrounding the oocyte (O), with well-developed granulosa and theca layers. **(E)** Higher magnification of the follicular wall of a preovulatory follicle. The granulosa layer is separated from the thickened theca layer by the basement membrane (B). Just beneath the basement membrane, a rich vascular network (dark arrows) is developing. **(F)** An atretic follicle, with cellular debris or apoptotic bodies (dark arrows) visible in the antrum.

THE OVARIAN CYCLE Cyclic ovarian function, which leads to the maturation of usually a single dominant follicle per ovulatory cycle, its transformation into a corpus luteum, and then the regression of the corpus luteum in the absence of pregnancy, is dependent on the pulsatile secretion of FSH and luteinizing hormone (LH), which begins at puberty. The ovarian cycle is normally 26–30 days in length and has been classically divided into a follicular phase and a luteal phase, each of roughly 14 days, separated by ovulation at midcycle (Fig. 62-3). For reference, the first day of menstrual bleeding is designated Cycle Day 1. The follicular phase, which begins with the onset of menses, is characterized by the selection of one member of a cohort of developing follicles as the dominant follicle. This follicle becomes the largest follicle in either ovary, reaching a diameter of 20 mm or more before ovulation, and secretes increasing amounts of estrogen, principally 17-β-estradiol. The dominant follicle can be identified by vaginal sonography by cycle day 6 and it has established an estrogen-dominant follicular microenvironment by cycle day 8.

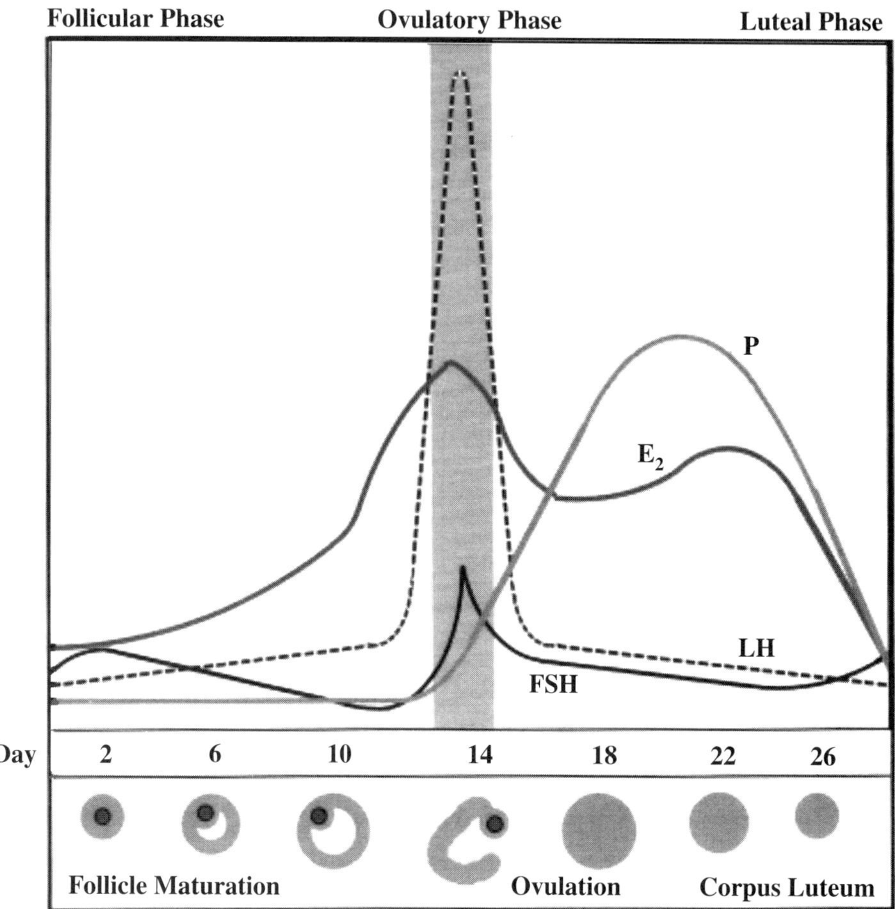

Figure 62-3 The serum levels of estrogen (E), progesterone (P), FSH, and LH throughout the follicular and luteal phases of the ovarian cycle. (Modified from Carr BR The ovary, in Textbook of Reproductive Medicine.)

The luteal phase, which begins at the time of ovulation, is characterized by the organization of the corpus luteum from the remaining granulosa and theca cells of the dominant follicle. The corpus luteum produces the large quantities of progesterone necessary to sustain an early pregnancy.

FOLLICULAR STEROIDOGENESIS Only healthy, dominant follicles produce significant quantities of estrogen. Follicular steroidogenesis requires the cooperation of both granulosa and theca cells and the stimulation of these cells by FSH and LH, respectively. FSH and LH are heterodimeric glycoprotein hormones produced by the pituitary, which share a similar α-subunit but contain distinct but related β-subunits. The receptors for FSH and LH are also distinct but homologous proteins, each of which is a member of a family of receptors that have seven membrane-spanning regions and transmits its signal by activating a guanosine triphosphatase (GTPase) designated G_s (Fig. 62-4). Binding of gonadotropin to its receptor thereby activates adenylate cyclase and increases generation of cyclic adenosine monophosphate (cAMP), an activator of the protein kinase A pathway of signal transduction. Although the role of FSH and LH receptors in steroidogenesis is well established, LH has been suggested to have additional functions resulting from the activation of the phosphoinositol or protein kinase C pathways.

Because all of the enzymes required for estrogen synthesis from cholesterol are not present in significant quantities in either the granulosa or theca alone, both cell types must participate in this process. Theca cells, which have receptors for LH but not FSH, respond to LH stimulation by producing the enzymes P450 cholesterol side-chain cleavage ($P450_{scc}$) and 17α-hydroxylase/17,20-lyase ($P450_{c17}$), as well as cholesterol transport proteins. Cholesterol is metabolized to pregnenolone by $P450_{scc}$ and then to dehydroepiandrosterone (DHEA) by $P450_{c17}$ (Fig. 62-4). DHEA is converted to androstenedione by the action of 3β-hydroxysteroid dehydrogenase (3β-HSD). Androstenedione diffuses out of the theca cell, across the follicular basement membrane, and into granulosa cells, where it is converted into estradiol through the action of the enzymes P450 aromatase ($P450_{arom}$) and 17β-hydroxysteroid dehydrogenase, both stimulated by FSH. This cooperation in estrogen biosynthesis between theca and granulosa cells has been termed the two-cell model of ovarian steroidogenesis.

FOLLICULAR SELECTION AND DOMINANCE In a spontaneous cycle, usually only one follicle is selected to become dominant and eventually ovulate, while the remaining antral follicles undergo atresia. How a follicle escapes the fate of atresia and assumes dominance is not well-understood. Our understanding of this process has been considerably enhanced in the last few decades by observing the results of ovulation-induction treatment in infertile women. Such therapies work by increasing circulating FSH, of either exogenous or endogenous origin, and thereby often result in multiple dominant follicles in a single cycle. Greater than

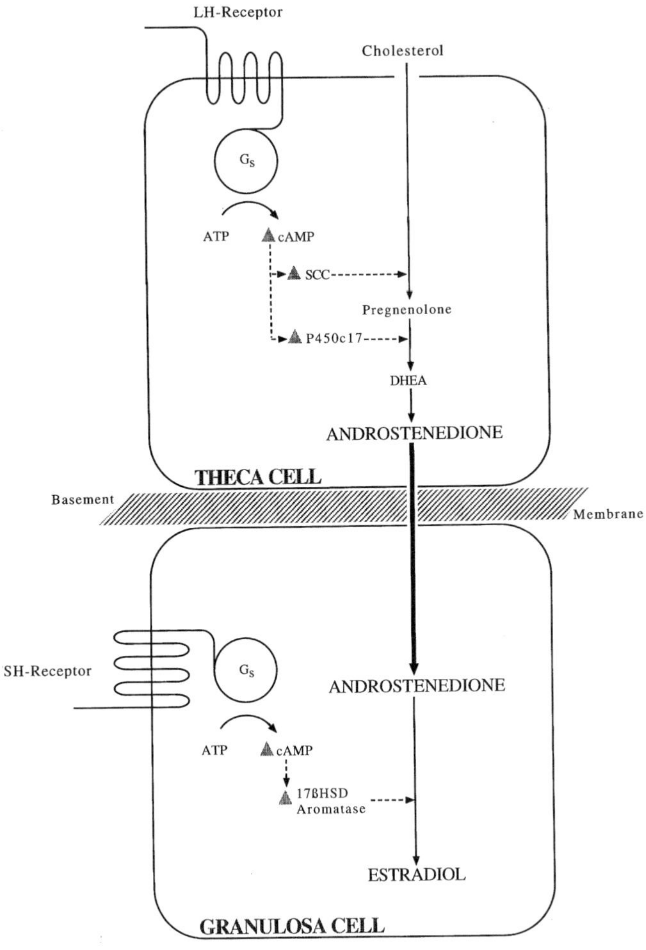

Figure 62-4 The cooperation of the granulosa and the theca cells in the production of estrogen from cholesterol.

normal FSH levels appear to "rescue" follicles in a developing cohort that might otherwise have undergone atresia, lending credence to the concept that FSH plays a critical role in this process. In a natural ovulatory cycle, circulating FSH begins to rise at the end of the luteal phase, in association with decreasing serum levels of estrogen and inhibin, a granulosa-derived protein that inhibits pituitary FSH release. This FSH increase advances the growth of the leading cohort of follicles. By cycle day 6, the estrogen and inhibin secreted by these growing follicles lead in turn to a decrease in serum FSH (Fig. 62-4), which coincides with a slowing of growth and the eventual atresia of the nondominant follicles. The role of FSH in preventing follicular atresia is supported by studies of granulosa cell apoptosis in vitro.

FSH stimulates granulosa cell expression of several proteins that could function in a positive feedback loop to promote development of the dominant follicle. Foremost of these is the LH receptor. The induction of LH responsiveness in the granulosa is critical to allow the dominant follicle to ovulate in response to the midcycle LH surge and subsequently to develop into a corpus luteum. It also may allow intracellular cAMP levels to be maintained in the face of declining FSH stimulation. FSH also induces granulosa cells to increase production of other proteins that modulate follicular function. Among these are inhibin, which acts on the theca to augment androstenedione biosynthesis as well as on the pituitary to decrease FSH output, thereby slowing the development of nondominant cohort follicles; and IGFs, which augment FSH-induced growth and steroidogenesis in granulosa cells as well as LH-induced steroidogenesis in the theca.

How the dominant follicle is selected from among its cohort of recruited follicles is still a mystery. Current research into this question has focused on the regulation of LH receptors, the process of angiogenesis in growing follicles, the role of cytokines and growth factors in the synergistic regulation of follicle growth and steroidogenesis, and the regulation of aromatase by steroid metabolites. The role of the balance in intracellular second messenger pathways and receptor crosstalk is also being investigated.

Numerous putative autocrine and paracrine ovarian regulatory factors have been investigated extensively in the last few years. Much information has accumulated on the action of such factors on ovarian tissues in vitro (Table 62-1), and clearly such proteins have a role in modulating gametogenesis and steroidogenesis. The ability of a factor to elicit a response in an isolated in vitro system does not necessarily imply that it can elicit the same response in a dynamic organism with multiple modulatory influences. The role of individual factors in vivo has been technically more difficult to establish, because many of these factors exist in families of multiple receptors and ligands that can potentially compensate for another factor rendered inactive, for instance with genetic knockout techniques. Such genetic knockouts can also produce systemic effects that prevent the demonstration of a clear ovarian role of the nonfunctional gene. Targeted transgenic studies in which the alteration of gene expression can be limited both developmentally and anatomically will likely aid in clarifying the intraovarian role of many substances. The difficulties encountered in identifying the roles of each ovarian paracrine factor suggest that the redundancy in the reproductive system has evolutionary significance in that it reduces the dependence of the reproductive process on any single gene product.

FOLLICULAR ATRESIA Atresia is a fate that can befall a follicle at any stage of development, from primordial to antral. Once a primordial follicle leaves the quiescent state and enters the growth phase, it must progress inevitably to either ovulation or loss through atresia. The majority of ovarian follicles are lost through atresia. Atresia of antral follicles has been well-studied in several animal models and has been shown to involve granulosa cell apoptosis. Apoptosis thus plays a major role during folliculogenesis and dominant follicle selection, in addition to its role in the reduction of oocyte number in the fetal ovary. Apoptosis is usually associated with degradation of chromosomal DNA into oligonucleosomal fragments by the activation of a Ca^{2+}/Mg^{2+}-dependent endonuclease. This degradation of granulosa cell DNA thus serves as a biochemical marker of follicular atresia and has allowed the study of this process in some detail. Studies have identified endonuclease activity and DNA fragmentation in the granulosa cells of rat follicles induced to become atretic by gonadotropin withdrawal. DNA fragmentation has been found in granulosa cells from atretic follicles in a number of species, including primates.

The regulation of antral follicular apoptosis has been extensively studied in an immature, pregnant mare serum gonadotropin (PMSG)-treated rat model. PMSG stimulates the development of numerous healthy antral follicles, which can be dissected from the ovary and either cultured intact or punctured to obtain granulosa cells for monolayer culture. In both models, apoptosis is induced by culture in serum-free medium, and can be prevented by adding

Table 62-1
Growth Factor Actions

Growth factor	*Action*
Tyrosine kinase receptors	
Insulin/IGF-I/IGF-II	Possibly increase early follicle growth; enhance gonadotropin-stimulated steroidogenesis; enhance LHR expression
EGF/TGF-α	Stimulate GC proliferation; inhibit FSHR(GC) and LHR(TC) expression; inhibit steroidogenesis and inhibin secretion
FGF	Stimulate GC proliferation; inhibit TC steroidogenesis; stimulate angiogenesis
SCF	Germ cell migration, proliferation, and survival; oocyte growth?; meiosis inhibition?
PDGF	Enhance TC proliferation; inhibit TC steroidogenesis
VEGF	Stimulate angiogenesis
NGF	Possible role in early follicle development
KGF	GC mitogen; suppress apoptosis
HGF	GC mitogen
Serine–threonine kinase receptors	
inhibin[a]	Augment thecal steroidogenesis
activin	Augment progesterone production; enhance FSH action
MIS	Promote meiosis, follicle growth
TGF-β	Follicle growth; inhibit thecal $P450_{c17}$; inhibit differentiation
GDF-9[a]	Initiation of follicle development?
7-TM G-protein linked receptors	
GnRH	Promote meiosis; promote apoptosis
VIP	Early follicle growth and differentiation
PACAP	Early follicle growth and differentiation
Cytokines	
IFN-γ	Decrease granulosa steroidogenesis; promote apoptosis
TNF-α	Decrease granulosa steroidogenesis; induce LIF/IL-1 expression
IL-1	Increase prostaglandins; decrease progesterone; prevent premature follicle rupture?
IL-2	Suppress ovulation; augment progesterone production
IL-6/IL-11/OSM/LIF	Promote germ cell survival; suppress FSH action

[a]Inhibin and GDF-9 are included with the serine–threonine kinases because of homology. Their receptors have not yet been described.
GC, granulosa cell; TC, theca cell.

to this medium FSH, LH/human chorionic gonadotropin (hCG), epidermal growth factor (EGF), or bFGF. IGF-I prevented granulosa cell apoptosis only in intact follicles, not in dispersed granulosa cells, suggesting that it acts on the theca. Growth hormone-induced IGF-I secretion also blocks apoptosis in preovulatory follicles. IL-1 also decreases apoptosis in intact follicles, apparently through nitric oxide acting as a mediator to raise intracellular cyclic guanosine monophosphate.

Other work has suggested a role for activin in follicular atresia and hence granulosa cell apoptosis. Activin is a protein product of granulosa cells, originally identified for its pituitary FSH-stimulatory action, that also affects steroidogenesis and other differentiated functions of granulosa and theca cells. In primates, systemic activin-A administration in the early follicular phase appears to cause the demise of the dominant follicle despite a rise in serum FSH. In vitro activin treatment of primate mature granulosa and luteal cells inhibits steroidogenesis and decreases the number of steroidogenic cells, but the role of cell death in these effects is uncertain. In an immature, PMSG-primed rat model, activin-A injected into the ovarian bursa promoted the atresia of antral follicles. Another study in which activin was subcutaneously administered to immature rats resulted in enhanced growth of smaller follicles, but increased atresia of granulosa cells within larger follicles. Also, an in vitro study of early antral follicles in culture demonstrated modest activin inhibition of apoptosis. Activin may have different roles in small secondary and early antral than in large antral and preovulatory follicles. Further studies are needed to clarify the role of activin in follicle growth and apoptosis.

A number of molecules have been implicated as intracellular mediators of apoptosis in granulosa cells. Members of the Bcl-2 family of apoptosis regulatory proteins, which includes Bcl-2, Bax, Bcl-x-long, and Bcl-x-short, are expressed by granulosa cells of humans and other species. In the immature rat model described above, Bax mRNA expression by granulosa cells was decreased by in vivo PMSG treatment and increased in serum-free follicle culture, but Bcl-2 expression was unaffected. The tumor suppressor p53, which can promote apoptosis, was localized to granulosa cells only in atretic follicles, and its expression was decreased by PMSG and increased in serum-free follicle culture.

Another mediator of apoptosis is a cell-surface protein homologous to the TNF-α receptor, known as Fas, APO-1, and CD95. Fas can be activated to transduce an apoptotic signal by either a natural ligand (Fas ligand, a TNF-α homolog) or anti-Fas antibody. In women, Fas is expressed by luteinizing granulosa cells, with stimulation by interferon-γ (IFN-γ), and anti-Fas antibody triggers apoptosis. The intracellular events resulting from activation of Fas appear to involve activation of an acidic sphingomyelinase that can generate ceramide, an intracellular second messenger known to be capable of transducing an apoptotic signal. The action of Fas may be mediated in part through the Bcl-2 system.

Apoptosis may occur because of the presence of specific signals leading to cell death or may occur by default if positively regulating systems are not activated. The exact role of atresia in the dynamics of follicle growth and dominant follicle selection has not been clearly determined.

OVULATION As the dominant follicle matures, it produces increasing amounts of estrogen, thereby effecting positive feedback on the pituitary gonadotrophs to produce the midcycle gonadotropin surge. The LH surge begins about 36 h and peaks about 10 h before ovulation; it triggers the major events of ovulation, including resumption of meiosis, cumulus expansion, cumulus-oocyte expulsion, and luteinization. The underlying regulation of these seemingly independent events has been studied intensively by those interested in both fertility control and infertility treatment. The duration of the LH surge has been found to be critical in triggering the events of ovulation: in primates, LH levels must be maintained for 18–24 h for oocyte maturation to occur, but for 34–48 h for optimal granulosa luteinization and corpus luteum function. Surge levels of LH are also necessary for the expression of prostaglandin-related genes in the rodent ovary.

In the developing follicle, resumption of meiosis is apparently inhibited by a signal to the oocyte originating in cumulus cells. In vitro, meiosis resumes in oocytes from antral follicles if the cumulus is removed or in response to cAMP. Atretic follicles of some species may exhibit meiosis briefly, as the granulosa cells lose function. Follicular fluid and granulosa cell-conditioned media both can inhibit meiosis of oocytes in vitro. These findings have led to the suggestion that granulosa cells produce an oocyte maturation inhibitor (OMI) under gonadotropin regulation. The identity of OMI has remained elusive. Hypoxanthine, a purine derivative, can inhibit meiosis in vitro and has been suggested to be the physiologic OMI. Other candidate OMIs have included inhibin and Müllerian inhibitory substance (MIS). Alternatively, the inhibition of meiosis may be a result of the functional relationship between the granulosa and the oocyte, and maturation may follow its physical disruption. This issue has not been resolved.

During the process of ovulation, the cumulus-oocyte complex loses its connection to the mural granulosa cells and probably briefly floats freely in the follicular fluid. At this time the follicular circumference is expanding, but the intrafollicular pressure does not increase. For the oocyte to be ovulated and reach the fallopian tube, it must pass through the mural granulosa layer, the follicular basement membrane, the theca layer, the ovarian stroma, and the surface epithelium of the ovary. This process is simplified because the enlarging follicle migrates (or expands) to the periphery of the ovary, adjacent to the surface epithelium.

Prostaglandins of the E and F series are elevated in follicular fluid before ovulation; and in rats prostaglandin synthetase is regulated by LH. The exact function of prostaglandins in ovulation is not known, but high doses of prostaglandin synthetase inhibitors have been reported to interfere with ovulation in humans.

The process of ovulation has been compared to the inflammatory response of wound healing. As in wound healing, plasminogen activators (PA) have been shown to play a role in the tissue remodeling that occurs during ovulation and formation of the corpus luteum. The regulation of the PA system at the time of ovulation has been recently characterized in the rat. Tissue plasminogen activator (tPA) is secreted by rat granulosa cells and produced but not secreted by the theca. Production of both tPA and an inhibitor, called plasminogen activator inhibitor (PAI), are stimulated by the gonadotropin surge; but PAI mRNA expression peaks about 6 h after rats are given hCG as a surrogate LH surge, while tPA expression does not peak until 12 h after hCG; thus the inhibitor is likely present before the production of the activator. Before ovulation, tPA mRNA and protein are expressed at high levels by the granulosa, while PAI is expressed strongly by the preovulatory theca and surrounding interstitium. After hCG, follicles enlarge rapidly and protrude from the ovarian surface. At 12 h after hCG, thecal expression of PAI in the portion of the follicle closest to the ovarian surface is lower than in the rest of the follicle. Granulosa expression of tPA in this region is greater than in the rest of the follicle. This temporal and spatial differential expression of tPA and its inhibitor could allow plasmin, which is generated from plasminogen from both serum and follicular fluid, to thereby activate collagenases only at the site of the stigma, where the cumulus-oocyte complex escapes from the follicle. The localized follicular expression of interstitial and Type IV collagenases and their inhibitors also appears to be regulated by LH.

Experimental disruption of the components of the PA system by several methods decreases the efficiency of ovulation, but seldom results in complete ovulatory suppression. Transgenic mice lacking either tPA or urokinase (uPA) gene function are fertile and have no obvious reproductive phenotype. Animals derived from these lines and lacking both functional genes have impaired wound healing. Although they are still fertile, early studies suggest that they ovulate at a decreased rate. The lack of clear inhibition of ovulation in the absence of plasminogen activators suggests that, as with follicle growth, the process of ovulation is also governed by redundant regulatory systems.

THE LUTEAL TRANSITION After the release of the oocyte, the follicle begins its transition to the corpus luteum, the endocrine organ of pregnancy. The factors regulating this metamorphosis are not entirely understood, but the quality of luteal function is correlated with the adequacy of the follicular phase of the cycle. Studies of human granulosa and luteal cells cultured in vitro implicate the absolute level of intracellular cAMP in driving the cellular events of luteinization. The relatively lower levels of cAMP generated by FSH induce cell growth and replication, but the higher levels generated in response to LH lead to cessation of cell division and increased steroidogenesis. This cAMP effect may be augmented by other second messenger pathways activated by LH. Recently, a 43-kDa cAMP response-element binding protein (CREB) was shown to be expressed in growing primate follicles, but not in corpora lutea, and was correlated with expression of proliferating cell nuclear antigen. Differential expression of CREB may be another mechanism by which cAMP can exert different responses in the same tissue at different times.

Another key step in the formation of the corpus luteum is angiogenesis, the growth of numerous small vessels into the previously avascular granulosa. Vascular endothelial growth factor (VEGF), which stimulates proliferation of capillary endothelial cells, is expressed by human granulosa-luteal cells under positive regulation by LH. Other angiogenic factors, including bFGF and PDGF, may also be involved in this process. Vascularization allows the granulosa direct access to serum-derived growth factors and hormones, as well as to LDL-cholesterol used as a precursor for progesterone synthesis.

Progesterone, the principal product of the corpus luteum, is necessary both to prepare the endometrium for implantation and to maintain early gestation. The LH surge induces large increases in granulosa cell steroid acute regulatory protein (StAR), $P450_{scc}$, and 3β-HSD expression, which lead to more efficient synthesis of progesterone. The human corpus luteum, unlike that of some other mammals, continues to secrete estrogen in addition to progesterone, particularly during the mid-luteal phase (Fig. 62-3). The human corpus luteum is also distinctive, in that 17-hydroxyprogesterone is not a substrate for the lyase function of $P450_{c17}$, as it is in many other species. Therefore the metabolism of pregnenolone either to progesterone by 3β-HSD or to androstenedione (an estrogen precursor) by $P450_{c17}$ is a key branch point in luteal steroid production and the regulation of these enzymes could be a critical determinant of luteal steroid products.

LUTEAL REGRESSION In the absence of pregnancy, the corpus luteum begins to degenerate spontaneously after 2 weeks. This process, like follicular atresia, involves apoptosis, since both spontaneous and experimentally induced luteal regression are associated with morphologic apoptosis or oligonucleosomal DNA fragmentation. DNA fragmentation also occurs in luteinized human granulosa cells obtained during oocyte retrieval for in vitro fertilization.

Although prostaglandins have been implicated in spontaneous luteal regression in nonprimate species, the mediators of luteolysis in primates have not been definitively identified. A role for macrophages, lymphocytes, and their secretory products (cytokines), as well as prostaglandins, has been proposed. Macrophages and lymphocytes invade the corpus luteum and become more numerous as the corpus luteum ages. Cytokines, including IFN-γ of lymphocyte origin and TNF-α of macrophage origin, decrease steroidogenesis by luteal cells from human, rat, and cow. Fas antigen has been localized to the human corpus luteum, suggesting its involvement in luteal regression. The possible role of locally produced IFN-γ and lymphocyte-derived Fas ligand in mediating apoptosis during luteolysis is being investigated further.

OVARIAN SENESCENCE Menopause refers to the permanent cessation of menses. Ovarian function generally follows a gradual decline, with cyclical bleeding becoming increasingly irregular; only about 10% of women experience an abrupt natural cessation of menses. Women may ovulate during the menopausal transition, but bleeding during this interval is often the result of fluctuations in estrogen levels not related to ovulation and luteal demise. Therefore, a patient's memory of the timing of her last menstrual period may not be an accurate estimation of the cessation of ovulatory function. Several prospective studies of ovarian function during the menopausal transition are currently under way.

Primordial follicles are believed to enter the growth phase at a relatively constant rate and are subject to loss through atresia at any stage of their development. There is excellent evidence, however, that their rate of loss increases as menopause approaches. This accelerated loss, predicted to begin on the average at age 38 years, is associated with a decrease in inhibin and an increase in FSH serum levels. It is not understood why the rate of follicular loss increases at this age, but it may be dependent on the mass of the declining primordial follicle pool. Ongoing studies of unilaterally ovariectomized women, who have a decreased follicle pool, may shed light on this question.

SUMMARY Human ovarian tissue has been difficult to obtain for regulatory studies of folliculogenesis, luteinization, and luteolysis, and significant differences exist between humans and nonprimate animal models. Primate models will continue to be important in the study of these processes. However, the use of new technologies, which allow the evaluation of smaller amounts of tissue, as well as the development of cell lines and long-term tissue culture techniques, are allowing more in-depth studies of human tissues involving the regulation of follicular growth and atresia, ovulation, luteinization, and steroidogenesis.

OVARIAN DYSFUNCTION

DISORDERS OF INCREASED OVARIAN FUNCTION

McCune-Albright syndrome McCune-Albright Syndrome (MAS), or polyostotic fibrous dysplasia, is caused by a postzygotic mutation in the *GNAS1* gene encoding the α-subunit of $G_{s\alpha}$, a G protein that stimulates adenylate cyclase. The resulting sporadic activation of G-protein-linked processes throughout the body leads to diverse manifestations, including bony lesions, *café-au-lait* skin lesions, and endocrine dysfunction. In the ovary, the activating mutation of the adenylate cyclase system leads to the premature development of relatively normal-appearing follicles, which include a thecal component and can secrete estrogen, independent of gonadotropin stimulation. As a result, approximately half of girls affected with MAS will exhibit signs of isosexual precocity, often presenting with vaginal bleeding. Follicles grow and regress, causing relapsing and remitting manifestations of precocity. Normal pregnancies have been reported in women with MAS who had developed isosexual precocity, but infertility and subfertility have also been noted. Long-term evaluation of larger numbers of these patients will be needed to accurately evaluate their fertility potential. It is possible that some cases of idiopathic gonadotropin-independent sexual precocity may be localized manifestations of mutations similar to that in MAS, but this has not yet been demonstrated.

Granulosa Cell Tumors Granulosa cell tumors represent 5–10% of all ovarian neoplasms and can be divided into two types, juvenile and adult, on the basis of histology and age of occurrence. Juvenile tumors are diagnosed in the first three decades of life, whereas adult-type tumors often present after menopause. About 5% of all granulosa cell tumors are diagnosed before the normal age of puberty. These tumors are generally multicystic and only rarely malignant. When these tumors occur prepubertally, about 80% produce sufficient estrogen to result in isosexual precocity; they account for about 10% of isosexual precocity in girls. Some of these tumors also produce inhibin, indicative of differentiated granulosa cell function; serum inhibin levels have been measured as a marker of tumor recurrence. Currently being sought are possible mutations in the genes encoding the inhibin subunits and gonadotropin and growth factor receptors that might promote granulosa cell replication and tumorigenesis.

In the adult-type granulosa cell tumor, mutations have been identified in the G_i subunit of regulatory G proteins, although the physiologic significance of these mutations has not been established. It is uncertain why the inability to turn off a normally transcribed stimulatory signal, as with the G_i mutation described above, should be manifested as tumor in later life, whereas the uncontrolled activation of the same signal, in MAS, is manifested as a relatively normal-appearing follicle earlier in life. Further studies will be necessary to elucidate the regulatory events involved in the stimulation of follicular growth by cAMP.

Multifollicular Ovulation Twin and higher-order multiple gestations have long been a source of general curiosity and scientific interest. Monozygotic twinning results from the division of a single zygote after fertilization and is believed to be primarily related to zygote factors, with possible contributions from uterine and implantation factors. The incidence of monozygotic twinning has been relatively constant over time and among diverse ethnic groups. By contrast, the incidence of dizygotic twinning, which results from the separate fertilization of two ovulated eggs, varies among ethnic groups and has fluctuated over time. Although the study of genetically identical monozygotic twins has been of great interest to both psychiatrists and geneticists because of the ability to examine the effect of different environments on the same genetic background, ovarian physiologists are understandably more interested in dizygotic twinning as a resource to evaluate the mechanisms determining the ovulatory quota. In every species there is a relatively constant number of oocytes released each cycle, the ovulatory quota, and hence an average litter size. In humans, usually only a single fertilizable egg is produced per cycle, though this control can be overridden by agents that increase gonadotropin stimulation of the ovary.

Variations in the incidence of dizygotic twinning has fueled discussion of the possibility of the underlying molecular mechanisms involved. Dizygotic twins have been noted to occur with a frequency as high as 1 in 8 pregnancies in some African populations and as low as 1 in 400 in some Pacific Rim countries. The incidence of twinning varies over the reproductive life span, with a higher frequency noted in the later reproductive years. Twinning also occurs with a high frequency within some families. Pharmaceutical agents to induce and augment spontaneous ovulation are associated with increased rates of multifollicular ovulation and multifetal pregnancy. One of these, clomiphene citrate, acts as a partial estrogen antagonist, thereby decreasing the negative feedback of estrogen on pituitary FSH secretion. This increase in FSH secretion presumably promotes ovulation by rescuing some recruited follicles that would otherwise have undergone atresia. Injections of FSH, as either human menopausal gonadotropins or purified or recombinant FSH, similarly stimulate development of increased numbers of follicles. The ability to induce superovulation pharmacologically and produce large numbers of mature oocytes in a single cycle has been critical in the development of in vitro fertilization and other assisted reproductive technologies. The introduction of these therapies for the infertile couple has fueled the study of the control of follicular growth, selection, dominance, and atresia.

Is there a molecular explanation for the increased ovulatory quota in families or population clusters with high rates of twinning? Mothers of twins have been studied in search of hormonal differences that could result from a genetic mutation and would be reflected in increased FSH action on the ovary. Some studies have shown higher levels of both estrogen and FSH in the follicular phase in mothers of twins, while inhibin levels may be either normal or elevated. Examination of familial twin clusters has revealed no mutations in the FSH-β, GnRH, LH-β, and FSH receptor genes. No other mutation has yet been found in humans which could account for the apparent increased gonadotropin activity and enhanced follicular survival, although studies of the GnRH receptor, inhibin-α, and the IGF system are ongoing.

More intriguing in understanding the molecular basis of the ovulatory quota have been genetic studies of two strains of sheep with large litter size, the Booroola Merino and the Inverdale. The Booroola gene mutation, designated $FecB^B$, is autosomal and is associated with an increased number of ovulations in the heterozygous state and a further increase in the homozygote. The altered physiology is not well-understood, but appears to result in maturation of larger numbers of follicles of a smaller size, with no net difference in total granulosa cell mass compared with wild-type Booroolas. Serum FSH is slightly elevated, but no other abnormalities in the hypothalamic–pituitary–ovarian axis are detectable. The Inverdale mutation, $FecX^I$, is X-linked. $FecX^I$ heterozygotes, like $FecB^B$ heterozygotes and homozygotes, show increased number of antral follicles, but homozygotes display failure of ovarian development and have streak gonads. Several groups are currently studying fecundity-related genes in sheep, but the relationship of these genes to twinning in humans has not yet been established.

DISORDERS OF DIMINISHED OVARIAN FUNCTION A number of disorders lead to diminished ovarian function. The spectrum of ovarian phenotypes of these disorders, which can include lack of estrogen production, menstrual acyclicity, and infertility, often overlaps, leading to confusion both in classifying these disorders and in determining their molecular basis. Diminished ovarian function is traditionally classified by its time of onset relative to menarche, but many disorders may have their origin in fetal life or childhood and remain unrecognized until clinical presentation when a girl fails to exhibit estrogen-induced secondary sexual characteristics at the time of expected puberty. A developmental approach to the classification of diminished ovarian function may be more helpful in understanding and recognizing these naturally occurring functional ovarian defects.

Ovarian Dysgenesis Absolute ovarian failure can result from improper ovarian development during embryogenesis. As discussed above, ovarian development depends on complex interactions between germ cells and components of the gonadal ridge, and interference with either component will result in ovarian dysgenesis, with fibrous streaks devoid of germ cells replacing the ovaries. Patients with streak ovaries are sexually infantile and generally have elevated serum gonadotropins by the time of expected puberty, because they lack normal negative feedback from ovarian estrogen and inhibin.

The most common cause of gonadal dysgenesis is Turner's syndrome, or monosomy X. The lack of a second X chromosome results in streak gonads and numerous characteristic somatic features, including shield chest, widely spaced nipples, and lymphatic abnormalities. In Turner's syndrome, germ cells apparently migrate normally to the ovaries, but primordial follicles are not formed efficiently and germ cells are lost. Gonadal dysgenesis in girls with Turner's syndrome could potentially result from a defect at any of the stages of follicle formation, including the entry of oocytes into meiosis and the association of oocytes with granulosa cells.

Gonadal dysgenesis also occurs in women with two apparently normal X chromosomes. Several disorders that include craniofacial abnormalities are associated with ovarian dysgenesis, including an interstitial deletion of chromosome 2q found in a girl with ovarian dysgenesis, mental retardation, craniofacial abnormalities, and cardiac defects. Deletions of chromosome 3q have also been associated with gonadal dysgenesis and ovarian failure. It is possible that large chromosomal deletions interfere with the process of pairing in meiosis, resulting in early germ cell loss. However, gonadal dysgenesis also occurs with apparently normal karyotypes. In Denys-Drash syndrome, a mutation in the *WT1* gene is associated with renal malformations, Wilms' tumor, and gonadal dysgenesis. Most cases of this syndrome are in genetic males, but a few have been reported in genetic females. Sensorineural deafness and blepharophimosis have also been associated with lack of ovarian function. Further study of the cause of the associated disorders, many of which occur in midline structures, is likely to reveal common systemic molecular defects that have consequences for both the ovary and other organs during early development.

Failure of Ovarian Function In another group of disorders, the ovaries may be formed normally but still not function adequately. This might result from deficiency of specific factors regulating the initiation of follicle growth, such as GDF-9. Alternatively, normally formed but unresponsive ovaries have been shown to result from mutations affecting gonadotropin function.

An FSH receptor mutation was recently found among a group of Finnish women selected because of primary or early secondary amenorrhea. Initial study of these women suggested a recessive pattern of inheritance, and linkage analysis of multiplex families mapped the trait to chromosome 2p, the known location of the FSH receptor (FSHR) gene. Sequencing the FSHR gene in affected individuals revealed a mutation in exon 7, which encodes a portion of the extracellular domain of the receptor. In expression studies, this mutant receptor was unable to stimulate cAMP production in response to FSH. Further analysis of the receptor in the expression system demonstrated apparently normal ligand binding affinity but extremely low levels of receptor expression. The authors concluded that the recessive disorder leading to amenorrhea resulted from either abnormal FSH receptor trafficking or increased receptor degradation.

Though LH receptor (LHR) defects have long been recognized as a cause of testicular Leydig cell hypoplasia, recently an inactivating mutation of LHR was associated with anovulation in a woman who apparently exhibited secondary sexual characteristics at puberty but had a small uterus and never had regular cyclic menses. Three of her sisters were XY pseudohermaphrodites with normal female external genitalia and absent Leydig cells on gonadal histology. The LHR in all four of these patients contained a homozygous mutation that created a stop codon in the third intracellular loop, resulting in a nonfunctional receptor. The index patient's history demonstrates that LHR function is not essential for estrogen production in quantities sufficient for breast development, despite being necessary for ovulation and luteinization.

There are also isolated reports of mutations associated with gonadotropin subunit defects. Hypergonadotropic hypogonadism has been reported in a woman with a homozygous mutation in the FSH-β gene that results in an FSH molecule unable to bind to its receptor. Her fertility was restored with exogenous FSH treatment. In contrast to female heterozygotes with the FSHR mutation described above, who often have large families, this patient's mother, an obligate heterozygote, was subfertile and had ovulatory dysfunction. It is possible that the presence of a defective FSH molecule interfered with the function of the normal protein, thereby reducing the efficiency of follicle growth and ovulation.

Defects in the enzymes necessary for estrogen biosynthesis can also result in sexual infantilism, but ovarian stimulation and in vitro fertilization have been performed successfully in some patients with estrogen deficiency, indicating that estrogen is not necessary for human preovulatory follicle development.

Premature Ovarian Failure Premature ovarian failure (POF), also called premature menopause, is clinically defined as the loss of ovarian function before the age of 35 years despite adequate gonadotropin stimulation. Generally this term is applied to women who have undergone normal pubertal sexual maturation and have experienced some degree of cyclic ovarian function. Premature ovarian senescence can result from either an abnormally small endowment of primordial germ cells or increased germ cell loss with time.

A number of X-linked conditions are associated with POF. Although Turner's syndrome usually results in severe early germ cell loss and gonadal dysgenesis, some germ cell survival can occur in ovaries of women with X-chromosome mosaicism or partial deletions, allowing for short-lived ovarian function including normal puberty and even, rarely, fertility. Two X-chromosome loci have been linked to POF by the study of translocations in affected families: POF1, at Xq26–q28, and POF2, at Xq13.3–q21.1. The specific genes at these loci responsible for this phenotype have not yet been identified.

Another X-chromosome locus that may be associated with ovarian senescence is the fragile X gene, *FMR-P*, which maps to Xq28. The fragile X syndrome is caused by a lack of FMR-P protein resulting from an amplification of CCG triplet nucleotide repeats within the promoter region of this gene. Males with fragile X syndrome exhibit mental retardation, facial dysmorphism, and macroorchidism. Female fragile X carriers show an increased rate of premature menopause and an increased rate of dizygotic twinning, which may be an epiphenomenon of the increase in gonadotropins as ovarian senescence approaches. It is presently unclear how these observations are related to the fragile X genotype. Although it has been suggested that FMR-P plays a role in germ cell proliferation in the testis, its role in the ovary has not been demonstrated. If it affects the efficiency of primordial follicle formation, a mutation at this locus might lead to a decrease in the overall follicular complement and thus an earlier cessation of cyclic ovarian function.

Any defect that decreases the efficiency of formation of primary follicles, resulting in a smaller starting pool of follicles, could potentially lead to POF, even if follicles were depleted at a normal rate. Increased atresia of oocytes in primordial follicles in the fetus or of small follicles at a later time could also lead to POF. Dysregulation of the complex mechanisms that regulate ovarian apoptosis could be a factor, although no such defects have been demonstrated in women to date. Further studies of familial POF clusters may reveal defects in factors regulating cell–cell interaction, cell growth, or apoptosis.

Progressive Ovarian Damage Galactosemia is an autosomal recessive metabolic disorder characterized by a deficiency of galactose-1-phosphate uridylyltransferase, leading to an inability to metabolize galactose and the accumulation of potentially toxic galactose-1-phosphate in tissues. Treatment with dietary galactose restriction improves or prevents the development of abnormalities of the liver, kidney, eye, and central nervous system. Women with this disorder develop ovarian failure nearly without exception. The time of its onset is variable and appears to depend on the age of institution of dietary treatment. Both primary amenorrhea and rare pregnancies have been observed. Ovarian failure develops over several years in association with follicular depletion, and once established is irreversible. The gonadotropins produced by these women are biologically active, despite the fact that galactose is present in the carbohydrate moiety of normal gonadotropins; gonadotropin receptors are probably also normal, since ovulation can occur and testicular function in males with galactosemia is normal. The molecular basis for the accelerated depletion of ovarian follicles in galactosemia is unknown. It is hoped that dietary intervention begun early enough, perhaps *in utero* after prenatal diagnosis in offspring of known carriers, will be successful in reversing this process.

Autoimmune disorders may also cause progressive ovarian damage and lead to POF. POF may occur as an isolated autoimmune endocrinopathy, or it may be associated with other known autoimmune diseases of the endocrine system, including Hashimoto's thyroiditis, insulin-deficient diabetes, and Addison's disease. Histologic examination of the ovaries in women with autoimmune POF often reveals a lymphoplasmacytic infiltrate involving growing but not primordial follicles. Abnormal ovarian monocytes and fibroblasts have been reported, as well as altered serum cytokine profiles. Although antiovarian antibodies have been described in some cases of POF, they are not consistently directed against any single antigen. Ovarian failure often follows a relapsing and remitting course and pregnancies can occur, occasionally after prolonged absence of ovarian function. Further investigation will define the relative roles of cell-mediated and humoral immunity in this form of ovarian failure.

POLYCYSTIC OVARY SYNDROME Polycystic ovary syndrome (PCOS) was first described by Stein and Leventhal in 1935 as the association of enlarged, cystic ovaries with amenorrhea and hirsutism. Since then, PCOS has been the subject of much study leading to few definitive answers. Central to the frustration involved in the study of PCOS is the lack of agreement on a definition of the syndrome, along with probable variations in phenotypes among patient populations. These differences lead to difficulties in comparing studies of PCOS.

The definition of PCOS most often accepted in the United States is that of ovulatory dysfunction associated with ovarian hyperandrogenism. Other features that have been used in various combinations as inclusion criteria are the sonographic appearance of many small subcapsular ovarian cysts and increased stroma, an elevated LH/FSH ratio, elevated androstenedione or testosterone, hirsutism, and truncal obesity. Generally excluded or considered as a distinct subset of PCOS is hyperthecosis, a severe form of progressive androgenization beginning just after puberty and resulting from a proliferation of ovarian theca.

Though the lesions responsible for PCOS have not been established, the interaction of inappropriate signals from the central nervous system and the ovary is thought to perpetuate what has been called a vicious cycle (Fig. 62-5). Excess androgen is aromatized to estrogen in the periphery, a process more pronounced in obesity. Tonic estrogen levels enhance pituitary LH secretion, while suppressing FSH secretion. Elevated LH continues the cycle by stimulating excessive thecal androgen production. What initiates this cycle in PCOS is not known, but other disease processes can also result in tonic estrogen levels, anovulation, and hirsutism, including Cushing's syndrome, thyroid dysfunction, adult-onset adrenal hyperplasia, and steroid-producing ovarian tumors. PCOS may therefore be viewed as a final common pathway resulting from any of a number of metabolic derangements.

According to one theory, PCOS results from exaggerated adrenarche in obese girls, leading to increased peripheral conversion of adrenal androgens to estrogens. Prospective studies of young girls are underway to test this hypothesis.

Another possible cause of the PCOS phenotype is an abnormality of the hypothalamic gonadotropin-releasing hormone (GnRH) pulse generator. Increased LH pulse frequency and amplitude have been found in some PCOS patients, suggesting an underlying increased GnRH pulse frequency. As shown in Fig. 62-5, possible causes of abnormal GnRH pulse generation include alteration of central dopaminergic tone, central progesterone resistance, and alterations in the feedback response to steroids.

At the ovarian level, abnormalities in the response to gonadotropins have been suggested. Follicles from PCOS ovaries have decreased numbers of granulosa cells with low aromatase activity in vivo, yet they can respond to FSH in culture by increasing aromatase activity. Furthermore, follicle growth and ovulation can be stimulated with low doses of exogenous FSH in these patients. Also suggested, but not yet conclusively demonstrated, as intraovarian abnormalities responsible for PCOS are the presence of an intrafollicular FSH antagonist, such as an IGF-binding protein; dysfunctional regulation of paracrine growth factors; and alterations in the regulation of steroidogenic enzyme activity.

It has also been hypothesized that PCOS results from an overproduction of inhibin by granulosa cells. Inhibin is a dimeric protein product of granulosa cells, which acts both to decrease pituitary FSH release and to increase thecal androgen production. However, inhibin α- and β-subunit expression in PCOS ovaries does not differ from that in normal ovaries.

In summary, it is uncertain whether the events that initiate the pathophysiology of the hypothalamic–pituitary–ovarian axis in PCOS originate centrally or within the ovary, or indeed if the same abnormality is responsible in all women with this syndrome.

Hyperinsulinemia and PCOS Many women with PCOS, both obese and lean, show peripheral insulin resistance and compensatory hyperinsulinemia. The ovary in PCOS escapes insulin resistance, and hyperandrogenism may thus result from excessive insulin-stimulated thecal androgen production. In addition to a direct action on androgen production, high serum levels of insulin inhibit hepatic production of IGF-binding protein-1, resulting in increased bioavailability of IGF-I to the theca.

Although the role of insulin resistance in the pathogenesis of PCOS has not been established, its molecular basis has been studied, and treatments that ameliorate insulin resistance are showing promise in correcting the reproductive abnormalities. Though the association of polycystic ovaries and hyperandrogenism was first described in syndromes associated with insulin receptor (IR) mutations, such structural mutations have generally not been identified in PCOS, but rather insulin resistance appears to result from postreceptor defects in signal transduction. On binding insulin, the IR activates protein kinase cascades which mediate both the metabolic (e.g., glucose and amino acid uptake, lipogenesis) and endocrine (e.g., stimulation of gonadal steroidogenesis) actions of insulin. Studies of adipocytes from both obese and lean women with PCOS demonstrate a postreceptor defect in insulin-stimulated glucose uptake that appears intrinsic rather than acquired, in that it is associated with decreased content of the insulin-dependent glucose transporter GLUT4. Compared with normal cycling women, PCOS subjects show a greater degree of serine phosphorylation of the IR on adipocytes, a mechanism postulated to inhibit tyrosine phosphorylation and thereby retard signal transduction. Functionally significant genetic polymorphisms in proteins of the insulin signaling system have been demonstrated in insulin resistance associated with non–insulin-dependent diabetes, and similar polymorphisms might be anticipated in women with insulin resistance and PCOS. In support of a functional rather than direct genetic origin of insulin resistance, insulin sensitivity is improved by metformin and troglitazone, drugs that act by facilitating postreceptor events.

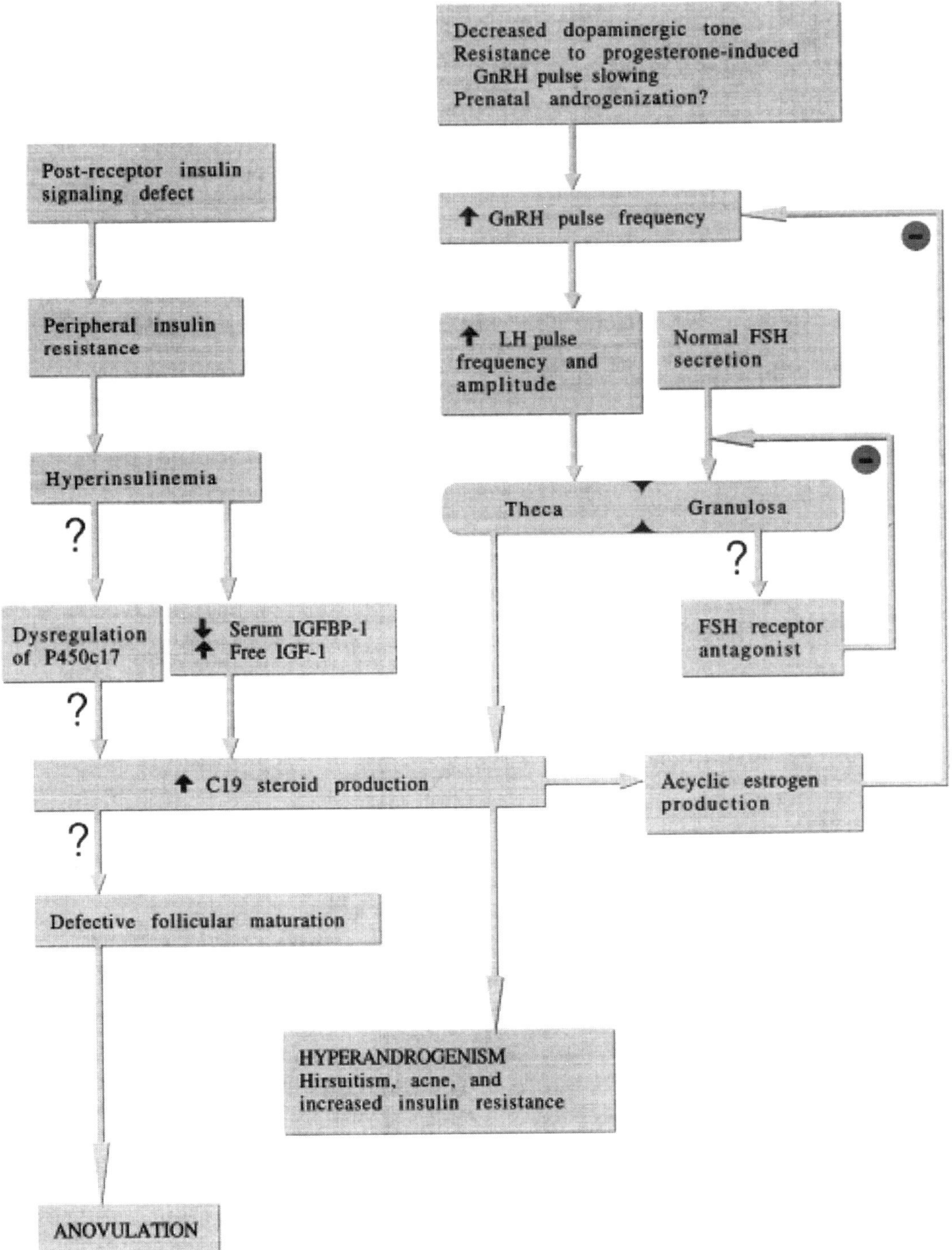

Figure 62-5 The pathophysiology of the polycystic ovary syndrome. Shown are the influences on the hypothalamic–pituitary–ovarian axis that have been postulated to result in the phenotypic abnormalities shown in the shaded boxes at the bottom. Uncertain relationships are also noted, including the stimulation of LH secretion by insulin and the impact of dysregulation of $P450_{c17}$ activity on androgen production by the theca.

Genetic Studies Although no single molecular abnormality is common to all women with PCOS, pedigree studies have suggested either polygenic inheritance or incomplete penetrance of a dominant mutation. Several associated genetic markers have been found; they include genes encoding a dopamine receptor expressed in the hypothalamus, enzymes involved in steroid biosynthesis, and major histocompatibility complex (HLA) antigens. A mutation in the D3 dopamine receptor was found with increased frequency in hyperandrogenic, dysovulatory Hispanic women and was associated with resistance to ovulation induction with clomiphene; a deficiency of dopamine action has been postulated to elevate circulating LH in PCOS. A potentially activating point mutation in the promoter of the gene encoding the androgen synthetic enzyme $P450_{c17}$ was associated with PCOS in women and with premature male-pattern baldness in men. This mutation did not cosegregate with either of these disorders, however, excluding a causal relationship. Mutations in the steroid biosynthetic enzymes 21-hydroxylase, $P450_{arom}$, 17β-HSD, and 3β-HSD have all been associated with hyperandrogenic anovulatory syndromes resembling PCOS, but steroidogenesis in ovarian tissue from women with PCOS is not defective in vitro. Association of PCOS with HLA DR and DQ, but not A, B, or C, alleles has also been reported in women with negative screens for 21-hydroxylase deficiency, which is closely linked to HLA. More recently, an association of the VNTR (variable number of tandem repeats) locus, which is present in the 5'-flanking region of the insulin gene, with an increased risk of PCOS was demonstrated. Interestingly, the genotype associated with PCOS is also associated with decreased insulin gene expression in the process.

PCOS: Summary In summary, PCOS exhibits many common but not universal features, including disordered folliculogenesis, ovarian hyperandrogenism, pituitary hypersensitivity to GnRH and exaggerated LH release, and peripheral insulin resistance. Despite these common features, molecular and genetic evidence does not point to a single defect in the majority of affected women. The PCOS phenotype is likely the final common expression of a number of other defects, perhaps of single gene origin, that have yet to be elucidated. Ongoing studies using animal models with PCOS-like syndromes, as well as prospective human studies, may increase our understanding of the pathogenesis of this complex syndrome.

SUMMARY

The mechanisms that direct germ cells in the yolk sac to migrate to the gonadal ridge and become enclosed in a follicular apparatus, and then direct these follicles to begin to grow in controlled cohorts during 50 or more years, are far from being completely identified. More is known about the effects of gonadotropins and growth factors on cohorts of follicles recruited to the final steps of preovulatory development, but the exact molecular mechanisms governing dominance, ovulation, and luteinization also remain to be clarified. Tissue remodeling is clearly of prime importance in the cycling ovary, but it is apparently regulated by multiple redundant systems. As knowledge of these processes advances, a more precise picture of the myriad causes of ovarian dysfunction will become apparent.

SELECTED REFERENCES

Aittomaki K, Lucena JL, Pakarinen P, et al. Mutation in the follicle-stimulating hormone receptor gene causes hereditary hypergonadotropic ovarian failure. Cell 1995;82:959–968.

Barbieri RL, Smith S, Ryan KJ. The role of hyperinsulinemia in the pathogenesis of ovarian hyperandrogenism. Fertil Steril 1988;50:197–212.

Chandrasekher YA, Hutchison JS, Zelinski-Wooten MB, Hess DL, Wolf DP, Stouffer RL. Initiation of periovulatory events in primate follicles using recombinant and native human luteinizing hormone to mimic the midcycle gonadotropin surge. J Clin Endocrinol Metab 1994;79:298–306.

Chenevix-Trench G, Healey S, Martin NG. Reproductive hormone genes in mothers of spontaneous dizygotic twins: an association study. Hum Genet 1993;91:118–120.

Clark BJ, Soo SC, Caron KM, Ikeda Y, Parker KL, Stocco DM. Hormonal and developmental regulation of the steroidogenic acute regulatory protein. Mol Endocrinol 1995;9:1346–1355.

Cunniff C, Jones KL, Benirschke K. Ovarian dysgenesis in individuals with chromosomal abnormalities. Hum Genet 1991;86:552–556.

Davis JS. Mechanisms of hormone action: luteinizing hormone receptors and second-messenger pathways. Curr Opin Obstet Gynecol 1994;6:254–261.

Donovan PJ. Growth factor regulation of mouse primordial germ cell development. Curr Top Dev Biol 1994;29:189–225.

Dunaif A, Scott D, Finegood D, Quintana B, Whitcomb R. The insulin sensitizing agent troglitazone improves metabolic and reproductive abnormalities in the polycystic ovary syndrome. J Clin Endocrinol Metab 1996;81:3299–3306.

Faddy MJ, Gosden RG. A mathematical model of follicle dynamics in the human ovary. Hum Reprod 1995;10:770–775.

Gharani N, Waterworth DM, Batty S, et al. Association of the steroid synthesis gene CYP11a with polycystic ovary syndrome and hyperandrogenism. Hum Mol Genet 1997;6:397–402.

Gordon JD, Shifren JL, Foulk RA, Taylor RN, Jaffe RB. Angiogenesis in the human female reproductive tract. Obstet Gynecol Surv 1995;50: 688–697.

Gudermann T, Birnbaumer M, Birnbaumer L. Evidence for dual coupling of the murine luteinizing hormone receptor to adenylyl cyclase and phosphoinositide breakdown and Ca^{2+} mobilization. Studies with the cloned murine luteinizing hormone receptor expressed in L cells. J Biol Chem 1992;267:4479–4488.

Gulyas BJ, Hodgen GD, Tullner WW, Ross GT. Effects of fetal or maternal hypophysectomy on endocrine organs and body weight in infant rhesus monkeys *(Macaca mulatta)*: with particular emphasis on oogenesis. Biol Reprod 1977;16:216–227.

Hillier SG, Whitelaw PF, Smyth CD. Follicular oestrogen synthesis: the "two-cell, two-gonadotrophin" model revisited. Mol Cell Endocrinol 1994;100:51–54.

Hoek A, van Kasteren Y, de Haan-Meulman M, Hooijkaas H, Schoemaker J, Drexhage HA. Analysis of peripheral blood lymphocyte subsets, NK cells, and delayed type hypersensitivity skin test in patients with premature ovarian failure. Am J Reprod Immunol 1995;33:495–502.

Horie K, Fujita J, Takakura K, et al. The expression of c-kit protein in human adult and fetal tissues. Hum Reprod 1993;8:1955–1962.

Hsu SY, Kubo M, Chun SY, Haluska FG, Housman DE, Hsueh AJ. Wilms' tumor protein WT1 as an ovarian transcription factor: decreases in expression during follicle development and repression of inhibin-alpha gene promoter. Mol Endocrinol 1995;9:1356–1366.

Hsueh AJ, Eisenhauer K, Chun SY, Hsu SY, Billig H. Gonadal cell apoptosis. Rec Prog Horm Res 1996;51:433–456.

Kaufman FR, Donnell GN, Roe TF, Kogut MD. Gonadal function in patients with galactosaemia. J Inher Metab Dis 1986;9:140–146.

Kim JG, Moon SY, Chang YS, Lee JY. Autoimmune premature ovarian failure. J Obstet Gynaecol Res 1995;21:59–66.

Kol S, Adashi EY. Intraovarian factors regulating ovarian function. Curr Opin Obstet Gynecol 1995;7:209–213.

Latronico AC, Anasti J, Arnhold IJ, et al. Brief report: testicular and ovarian resistance to luteinizing hormone caused by inactivating mutations of the luteinizing hormone-receptor gene. N Engl J Med 1996;334:507–512.

Legro RS. The genetics of polycystic ovary syndrome. Am J Med 1995;98:9S–16S.

Leonardsson G, Peng XR, Liu K, et al. Ovulation efficiency is reduced in mice that lack plasminogen activator gene function: functional redundancy among physiological plasminogen activators. Proc Natl Acad Sci USA 1995;92:12,446–12,450.

Leung PC, Steele GL. Intracellular signaling in the gonads. Endocr Rev 1992;13:476–498.

Luoh SW, Bain PA, Plakiewicz RD, et al. Zfx mutation results in small animal size and reduced germ cell number in male and female mice. Development 1997;124:2275–2284.

Lyons J, Landis CA, Harsh G, et al. Two G protein oncogenes in human endocrine tumors. Science 1990;249:655–659.

Matthews CH, Borgato S, Beck-Peccoz P, et al. Primary amenorrhoea and infertility due to a mutation in the beta-subunit of follicle-stimulating hormone. Nat Genet 1993;5:83–86.

McGrath SA, Esquela AF, Lee SJ. Oocyte-specific expression of growth/differentiation factor-9. Mol Endocrinol 1995;9:131–136.

McNatty KP, Smith P, Hudson NL, et al. Development of the sheep ovary during fetal and early neonatal life and the effect of fecundity genes. J Reprod Fertil Suppl 1995;49:123–135.

Morales A, Laughlin G, Butzow T, Maheshwari H, Baumann G, Yen SSC. Insulin, somatotropic, and luteinizing hormone axes in lean and obese women with polycystic ovary syndrome: common and distinct features. J Clin Endocrinol Metab 1996;81:2854–2864.

Nagata S, Golstein P. The Fas death factor. Science 1995;267:1449–1456.

Nestler JE. Role of hyperinsulinemia in the pathogenesis of the polycystic ovary syndrome, and its clinical implications. Semin Reprod Endocrinol 1997;15:111–122.

New MI. Nonclassical congenital adrenal hyperplasia and the polycystic ovarian syndrome. Ann NY Acad Sci 1993;687:193–205.

Powell CM, Taggart RT, Drumheller TC, et al. Molecular and cytogenetic studies of an X;autosome translocation in a patient with premature ovarian failure and review of the literature. Am J Med Genet 1994;52:19–26.

Rabinovici J, Blankstein J, Goldman B, et al. In vitro fertilization and primary embryonic cleavage are possible in 17 alpha-hydroxylase deficiency despite extremely low intrafollicular 17 beta-estradiol. J Clin Endocrinol Metab 1989;68:693–697.

Richards JS. Hormonal control of gene expression in the ovary. Endocr Rev 1994;15:725–751.

Roberts VJ, Barth S, El-Roeiy A, Yen SSC. Expression of inhibin/activin system messenger ribonucleic acids and proteins in ovarian follicles from women with polycystic ovarian syndrome. J Clin Endocrinol Metab 1994;79:1434–1439.

Shi H, Segaloff DL. A role for increased lutropin/choriogonadotropin receptor (LHR) gene transcription in the follitropin-stimulated induction of the LHR in granulosa cells. Mol Endocrinol 1995;9: 734–744.

Somers JP, Benyo DF, Little-Ihrig L, Zeleznik AJ. Luteinization in primates is accompanied by loss of a 43-kilodalton adenosine 3',5'-monophosphate response element-binding protein isoform. Endocrinology 1995;136:4762–4768.

Talbot JA, Bicknell EJ, Rajkhowa M, Krook A, O'Rahilly S, Clayton RN. Molecular scanning of the insulin receptor gene in women with polycystic ovarian syndrome. J Clin Endocrinol Metab 1996;81:1979–1983.

Tilly JL. Ovarian follicular atresia: a model to study the mechanisms of physiological cell death. Endocr J 1993;1:67–72.

Tsafriri A. Ovulation as a tissue remodelling process. Proteolysis and cumulus expansion. Adv Exp Med Biol 1995;377:121–140.

Waterworth DM, Bennett ST, Gharani N, et al. Linkage and association of insulin gene VNTR regulatory polymorphism with polycystic ovary syndrome. Lancet 1997;349:986–990.

Weinstein LS, Shenker A, Gejman PV, Merino MJ, Friedman E, Spiegel AM. Activating mutations of the stimulatory G protein in the McCune-Albright syndrome [see comments]. N Engl J Med 1991;325: 1688–1695.

Young RH, Scully RE. Endocrine tumors of the ovary. Curr Top Pathol 1992;85:113–164.

Zhang LH, Rodriguez H, Ohno S, Miller WL. Serine phosphorylation of human P450c17 increases 17,20-lyase activity: implications for adrenarche and the polycystic ovary syndrome. Proc Natl Acad Sci USA 1995;92:10,619–10,623.

63 Breast Cancer

MELORA D. BERARDO, D. CRAIG ALLRED, AND PETER O'CONNELL

INTRODUCTION

Breast cancer is the second leading cause of cancer death affecting women in the United States, with more than 180,000 new cases each year. Even with recent advances in breast cancer treatment, approximately one-half of breast cancer patients will eventually die of this disorder. The high mortality of breast cancer has focused attention on prevention and on identifying breast cancer precursors. Invasive breast cancer may develop gradually from specific microscopically defined precursor lesions. However, these lesions are relatively common and only a small proportion of the proposed precursor lesions appear to progress to invasive breast cancer, emphasizing that progression is nonobligatory. Identifying biologic and genetic abnormalities that herald progression to invasive breast cancer may enable us to intervene before progression occurs.

BREAST CANCER EVOLUTION

Invasive breast cancer probably evolves from normal epithelium of the terminal duct or lobular unit through a series of increasingly abnormal proliferative lesions including typical and atypical hyperplasia and noninvasive *(in situ)* carcinoma. Typical hyperplasia, or proliferative disease without atypia (PDWA), is composed of myoepithelial and epithelial cells growing in an irregular pattern of slitlike lumina and papillations. Atypical ductal hyperplasia (ADH) is composed primarily of epithelial cells and has a more regular growth pattern. Both typical and atypical "hyperplasias" are misnomers in the sense that recent genetic evidence demonstrates that they are really benign neoplasms. Ductal carcinoma *in situ* (DCIS) is a malignant neoplasm with low-grade and high-grade types. The low-grade "noncomedo" type of DCIS is composed of relatively small regular epithelial cells that typically grow in a perforated microglandular pattern. The high-grade "comedo" variant of DCIS is characterized by large irregular epithelial cells usually growing in solid sheets with prominent central necrosis. Examples of each of these lesions are shown in Fig. 63-1. There are also lobular, as opposed to ductal, variants of atypical hyperplasia and *in situ* carcinoma, but so little is known about their biologic characteristics that they will not be emphasized in this chapter.

Epidemiologic studies support this model of breast cancer evolution (Table 63-1). Studies of previously excised breast lesions show progressively increasing relative risks (RR) of later developing invasive breast cancer in women with typical hyperplasia (RR = 1.5–2), atypical hyperplasia (RR = 4–6), and noninvasive carcinoma (RR = 10–12). These results are consistent with the notion that incomplete excision and residual disease progresses to invasive breast cancer, or alternatively, with the notion that these lesions are markers for other abnormalities left behind with the capacity to progress. Similar evidence is provided by studies of *in situ* carcinoma treated by lumpectomy, which show local recurrence rates of 10–75%, with half the recurrences being invasive cancer. Postmortem studies of women dying of causes other than breast cancer show that typical hyperplasia, atypical hyperplasia, and *in situ* carcinoma are present in about 30, 2, and 2% of random breasts, respectively. The precursor-product concept is supported by histopathologic studies that find these same lesions in a very high proportion (50–90%) of breasts containing invasive breast cancer, consistent with the idea that they may be precursors.

This model represents a reasonable working hypothesis in the design of studies to investigate the biologic mechanisms underlying the development and progression of human breast cancer. Table 63-2 summarizes biologic abnormalities known to be associated with these putative precursor lesions when they are not accompanied by invasive breast cancer. Table 63-3 summarizes abnormalities in morphologically similar lesions when they are found in breasts already containing invasive cancer. Nearly all the biologic characteristics studied so far were first described in invasive breast cancer, and have only recently been reevaluated in premalignant and preinvasive breast disease. Tables 63-2 and 63-3 summarize many of the findings discussed in this chapter. Several interesting studies have not been included because they used ambiguous terminology for premalignant disease, or their results were descriptive rather than quantitative and difficult to tabulate.

GENETIC FACTORS PARTICIPATING IN THE PROGRESSION TO CANCER

Whatever mechanisms are behind the overall growth imbalance in breast cancer evolution, measurement of biologic parameters governing proliferation itself may eventually prove to be useful prognostic factors in the clinical management of this disease. In the next section, genetic factors that potentially participate in the progression from premalignant lesions to breast cancer will be reviewed. These include genes involved in signal transduction, such as hormone receptors, oncogenes, growth factors, and their receptors, which are frequently upregulated in malignancies. Also covered are overall parameters of cell growth, such as proliferation rate and DNA content. Finally, we review genes that are specifically inactivated in malignancies, the tumor suppressor genes, which have been implicated in studies of breast cancers and hereditary breast cancer families. Development of an understanding of the genes that control cell proliferation, either alone or in combination with other factors, may be found to enhance our ability to more appropriately match treatment to risk in patients who already have breast cancer or its antecedents.

HORMONE RECEPTORS

ESTROGEN RECEPTOR (ER) Estrogen is an important hormone involved in regulating the differentiation and proliferation of normal breast epithelial cells. Its effects are manifold and incompletely understood. It influences cells by interacting with the estrogen receptor (often referred to as ER) in the nucleus, eliciting a cascade of transcriptional regulatory activity. Prolonged estrogen exposure has been demonstrated to be the most significant risk factor for developing invasive breast cancer. This increased

From: *Principles of Molecular Medicine* (J. L. Jameson, ed.), ©1998 Humana Press Inc., Totowa, NJ.

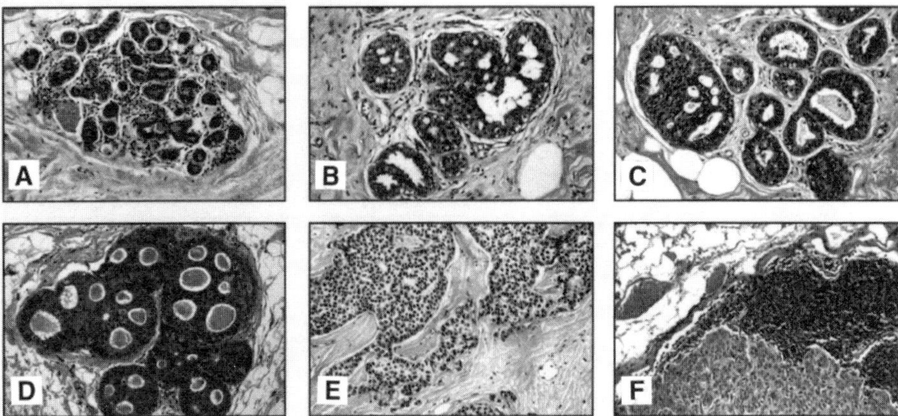

Figure 63-1 Representative photomicrographs of putative precursor lesions and malignant invasive breast cancers. **(A)** Normal terminal duct lobular unit (TLDU), where many breast cancers are thought to arise. **(B)** Proliferative disease without atypia (PDWA, or typical hyperplasia) is composed of myoepithelium and epithelium growing in an irregular pattern of slitlike lumina and papillations. **(C)** Atypical ductal hyperplasia (ADH) is composed primarily of epithelial cells and has a more regular growth pattern. **(D)** Ductal carcinoma *in situ* (DCIS) is an unequivocal malignant neoplasm with two particularly common morphologic phenotypes. The low-grade or "noncomedo" type of DCIS (ncDCIS) is composed of relatively small regular epithelial cells that typically grow in a perforated microglandular pattern (shown here). The high-grade "comedo" variant of DCIS (cDCIS) is characterized by large irregular epithelial cells growing in solid sheets with prominent central necrosis (not shown). **(E)** Invasive breast cancers break down and escape from the duct. Note the lighter staining stromal elements. **(F)** Breast cancer metastasis in a lymph node. The metastasis is the lighter staining tissue at the bottom of the picture growing inside the darker staining lymphoid tissue.

risk may be partially caused by the mitogenic effect of estrogen on breast epithelium, which may permit the accumulation of random genetic damage taking place in replicating cells. The ER gene maps to chromosome 6q25.1, and is overexpressed in 60–70% of invasive breast cancers. Overexpression of ER is associated with lower risk of relapse, prolonged overall survival, and enhanced response to endocrine therapy relative to ER-negative tumors.

ER expression appears to be generally low in normal breast epithelium, with the exception of a small peak during the first week of the menstrual cycle. Immunohistochemical (IHC) studies show that expression is usually restricted to 1–2% of normal cells, but that nearly all breasts contain at least a few ER-positive cells. There are only a few small IHC studies of ER in hyperplastic breast disease, and they show that ER is significantly overexpressed relative to normal epithelium in these lesions. About a third of typical hyperplasias, and all atypical hyperplasias, contained a significant proportion (>20%) of ER-positive cells, and virtually all hyperplastic lesions contained at least a few positive cells. A relatively large number of studies have evaluated ER expression in noninvasive carcinomas. On average, about 20% of comedo DCIS express ER, compared with about 70% of noncomedo DCIS. The rate of ER overexpression for *in situ* carcinomas reported as mixed or not-otherwise-specified (NOS) ranges from 40 to 90%. ER expression of noninvasive cancer appears to be about the same whether or not they are associated with invasive breast cancer. The data regarding this issue for hyperplastic lesions is too sparse to evaluate.

PROGESTERONE RECEPTOR (PR) PR expression in normal breast epithelium is regulated by ER. Similar to ER, PR is overexpressed in a significant proportion of invasive breast cancers (50–60%), and such tumors have a relatively better prognosis and response to antihormonal therapy than PR-negative tumors. The PR gene is mapped to chromosome 11q22–23, but PR expression has not yet been studied in hyperplastic breast disease. There is a single study reporting very low (0%) and high (80%) rates of ER-positive comedo and noncomedo DCIS, respectively.

PROLIFERATION RATE

Cell-cycle kinetics provides a very strong prognostic factor in invasive breast cancer. Proliferation has been measured by light microscopic mitotic index, S-phase fraction (SPF), by flow cytometry, thymidine-labeling index (TLI), and IHC for cell-cycle related proteins such as Ki67. Regardless of the methodology used, rapidly proliferating tumors are consistently associated with significantly shorter disease-free and overall survival.

The proliferation of normal breast epithelium is regulated by the menstrual cycle, with maximum rates seen during the follicular phase. Absolute proliferation rates of normal cells are usually quite low—1 to 2% or less. The little information available regarding proliferation in hyperplastic breast disease suggests that rates are relatively higher in atypical than typical hyperplasia, but still very low in absolute terms in both types of lesions. For noninvasive carcinomas median TLIs of 5.2 and 1.8 have been measured in comedo and noncomedo DCIS, respectively. The trend was similar in a small study measuring median SPF in comedo (SPF = 12.3) and noncomedo (SPF = 6.5) lesions. The proliferation rates of hyperplasias and *in situ* carcinomas from breasts containing invasive cancer may be substantially higher than morphologically similar lesions unassociated with invasive disease.

DNA CONTENT

DNA content is diploid in normal breast epithelium. Although ploidy has apparently not been evaluated in typical hyperplasia of the breast, two small studies of atypical hyperplasia report that 30% of these lesions are aneuploid. DNA content has been more thoroughly investigated in noninvasive carcinomas. Several studies have shown that 60–85% of comedo DCIS are aneuploid, compared with 30–50% for noncomedo DCIS. DNA content has not been evaluated in premalignant or preinvasive lesions in breasts containing invasive cancer.

The majority of invasive cancers (60–70%) contain abnormal amounts of DNA (aneuploidy), which is thought to be a crude reflection of major clonally selected chromosomal gains or losses. Aneuploidy in invasive breast cancer is modestly associated with reduced disease-free and overall survival in patients with invasive breast cancer.

ONCOGENES AND GROWTH FACTOR RECEPTORS

Many oncogenes and/or growth factors have been shown to be activated or inappropriately expressed in invasive breast cancer (*see* Chapter 7). A few of these have also been evaluated in premalignant and preinvasive breast disease.

ERBB2 The most thoroughly studied gene in breast cancers is *ERBB2* (also known as c-*erbB2 HER2*, or c-*neu*). The *ERBB2* gene resides on chromosome 17q11.2–12 and codes for a 185-kDa transmembrane glycoprotein with tyrosine kinase activity. It is a member of the type 1 growth factor receptor family, and its ligand is unknown. The gene is amplified or overexpressed in 20–30% of invasive breast carcinomas,

Table 61-1
Morphologic Model of Breast Cancer Evolution and Epidemiologic Evidence Supporting It

Model	*Relative risk of developing invasive breast cancer*	*Incidence in random breasts*	*Rate of concurrence with invasive breast cancer*
Normal epithelium	1	—	—
Typical hyperplasia	2[a]	30%	50–90%
Atypical hyperplasia	4–6[a]	1–2%	50–90%
In situ carcinoma	10–12[b]	1–2%	50–90%
Invasive carcinoma	—	1–2%	—

[a]Bilateral relative risk; [b]Ipsilateral relative risk.

and this activation is associated with many unfavorable prognostic factors and poor clinical outcome.

IHC has been used to detect overexpression of *ERBB2* in premalignant or preinvasive breast disease relative to normal epithelium. A small number of typical and atypical hyperplasias have been evaluated for *ERBB2* and, with rare exception, no overexpression has been detected. Several studies have addressed *in situ* carcinomas. In studies involving more than 100 combined cases, very high rates of overexpression (60–100%) were found in comedo DCIS. Equally comprehensive studies of noncomedo DCIS found much lower rates (0–50%). Additional studies of mixed or NOS DCIS reported intermediate rates of c-*erbB2* overexpression ranging from 30 to 80%. No overexpression was observed in the less than 50 cases of *in situ* lobular carcinoma that have been evaluated. Studies evaluating *ERBB2* in premalignant and preinvasive lesions from breasts containing invasive cancer find about the same rates of overexpression and amplification as when invasive cancer is not present.

The weight of evidence suggests that activation of *ERBB2* is an important early event in malignant transformation leading to *in situ* carcinoma. Given the overall high rates of *ERBB2* activation associated with *in situ* carcinomas, contrasted with the much lower rates observed in invasive cancer, many cases of *in situ* carcinoma stop overexpressing this oncogene as they evolve to invasive disease; alternatively, a significant proportion of invasive lesions must arise *de novo* by mechanisms independent of *ERBB2*.

EPIDERMAL GROWTH FACTOR RECEPTOR (EGFR) EGFR (c-*erbB1*) is a 170-kDa transmembrane glycoprotein encoded by a gene on chromosome 7p12. It is a type 1 growth factor receptor with tyrosine kinase activity that binds several known ligands, including epidermal growth factor and transforming growth factor-α. This gene is rarely amplified, but is overexpressed in about 40–50% of invasive breast cancers. This expression is associated with many unfavorable biologic characteristics and relatively poor clinical outcome. EGFR appears to be present at low levels in most normal breast epithelial cells. In one small report, expression was observed in 25% of DCIS. Otherwise, EGFR has not been evaluated in premalignant or preinvasive breast disease.

***ras* GENE FAMILY** The *ras* family of oncogenes (designated N-*ras*, H-*ras*, and K-*ras*) encodes highly similar proteins with molecular weights of about 21 kDa. The *ras* genes map to chromosomes 1p13, 11p15, and 12p12.1, respectively. They are involved in the intracellular transduction of external stimulation of growth factor receptors coupled to the GTPase-activator proteins RASA, NF1, and others. The RAS proteins become activated on stimulation, and transduce these signals to other effector molecules, and subsequently are inactivated. Mutated RAS proteins are expressed but appear to have lost the ability to be inactivated. Mutations of *ras* genes are common in some types of cancer, but the incidence and significance of mutations in breast cancer is unclear. Expression rates varying from 30 to 80% have been reported in invasive breast cancer, depending on the assay.

Using IHC, rates of *ras* expression in normal breast epithelium have been reported to range from 0 to 100%, suggesting that there are significant technical inconsistencies between studies. A handful of studies have evaluated *ras* expression in precursor lesions of invasive breast cancer, but, to date, have made no definitive attempt to correlate expression and mutation. One study of typical hyperplasias reported variable rates of RNA expression for H-*ras* (4.5%), K-*ras* (22%), and N-*ras* (30%). IHC studies of *ras* expression in typical hyperplasias report rates of 80–100%. A single small IHC study observed *ras* expression in 100% of atypical hyperplasias and noninvasive carcinomas. These results, while incomplete, suggest that *ras* expression may gradually increase during the transition from hyperplastic to malignant breast disease. The issue of comparing levels of *ras* activation in premalignant disease from breasts with and without cancer is unexplored. However, a provocative preliminary study found a relatively elevated rate of *ras* expression in hyperplasias from women who later developed invasive breast cancer (15 years follow-up), compared with hyperplasias from women who did not (40 vs 20%, respectively).

***Myc* GENE FAMILY** The *myc* family of cellular oncogenes encode nuclear DNA-binding phosphoproteins, which play important but as yet incompletely understood roles in the regulation of cell growth and differentiation. MYC proteins form heterodimeric complexes with basic helix-loop-helix-leucine zipper transcription factors whose activity is regulated by a number of positive (MAX) and negative (MAD, MXI1) regulators. The best characterized members of this multigene family, *myc*, *mycn*, and *mycl*, map to chromosomes 8q24, 2p22–24, and 1p32, respectively. The prototypical member of this family, *myc*, is activated by gene rearrangement, amplification, or overexpression. Estimates of the frequency of *myc* activation range from 1 to 56% of invasive breast cancers studied, and such activation is modestly associated with an aggressive biologic phenotype and poor clinical outcome.

IHC studies show *myc* expression in the epithelium of 0–60% of normal breasts, again suggesting that technical inconsistencies may be confounding this issue. A single study measuring RNA expression found *myc* in 18% of typical hyperplasias. A few studies evaluating mixed or NOS DCIS found a 100% incidence of MYC protein expression by IHC, and an 11% rate of *myc* amplification by Southern blotting. In an interesting preliminary report, the rate of *myc* expression was higher in patients with "benign" biopsies who later exhibited invasive breast cancer than in patients who did not (53 vs 17%, respectively).

GROWTH FACTORS

Growth factors regulate cellular proliferation through receptor mediated autocrine or paracrine mechanisms. Disruption of these peptide–receptor interactions may be involved in the development and progression of many types of cancer. A few have been evaluated in precursors of invasive breast cancer.

TRANSFORMING GROWTH FACTOR-α (TGF-α) TGF-α maps to chromosome 2p13. TGF-α, and its receptor EGFR, are reported to be overexpressed in up to 50% of invasive breast cancers, and in most studies both are associated with increased proliferation, other aggressive biologic features, and relatively poor clinical outcome. Preliminary IHC studies find low rates (0–8%) of TFG-α expression in normal breasts. In the few cases examined, the majority (87–100%) of both hyperplastic lesions and noninvasive carcinomas overexpress TGF-α; other studies noted increased immunostaining for TFG-α in normal epithelium adjacent to rapidly proliferating epithelium, suggesting a possible juxtacrine effect.

Table 63-2
Biomarker Phenotypes of Precursor Lesions From Breasts Without Invasive Cancer

		Ductal hyperplasia		*Ductal carcinoma* in situ		
Biomarker assay	*Normal*	*Typical*	*Atypical*	*Comedo*	*Noncomedo*	*Mixed/NOS*
Hormone receptors (% positive)						
Estrogen receptor						
IHC[a]		30	100	20–54	60–89	65
Progesterone receptor						
IHC (H score >40)[a]				0	80	
Proliferation rate (n)						
Mitoses/lobule	0.22					
TLI (% + cells)	0.98			5.2	1.8	3.2
MI (per 40 HPF)		3.5	6.7			26.5
Flow (median SPF)				12.3	6.5	6.9
IHC (%Ki67 + cells)	0.91					4.6
DNA content (% aneuploid)						
IA (signal > 5n)			30	82–85	46–53	30–67
Flow (DI > 1.0)				55–61	27–39	44
Oncogenes/growth factor receptors (% positive)						
c-*erbB2*/*HER2 neu*						
IHC (> 0% + cells)	0	0	0–10	62–100	0–50	42–78
SB (DNA amplif.)						40%
c-*erbB1*/epidermal growth factor receptor						
IHC (> 0% + cells)						25
EIA (any + signal)	100					
ras						
NB (any + H-*ras*)		4.5				
NB (any + K-*ras*)		22				
NB (any + N-*ras*)		30				
IHC (> 0% + cells)	50–100	81–100	100			100
myc						
NB (any + *myc*)		18				
IHC (> 0% + cells)	0–62					100
Growth factors (% positive)						
TGF-α						
IHC (mean score > 0)[a]	8	100	87			100
TGF-β						
IHC (score ≥ 4)[a]	0					0
IGF-1						
IHC (score ≥ 4)[a]	0					0
Tumor suppressor genes (% positive)						
p53						
IHC (> 0% + cells)	0		0	33–67	0–25%	16–33
Sequencing (DNA mut.)						20

[a]DCCA, dextran-coated charcoal assay; IHC, immunohistochemistryl; EIA, enzyme immunoassay, TLI, thymidine labeling index; MI, mitotic index; HPF, high-power field; Flow, flow cytometery; SPF, S phase fraction; IA, image analysis; DI, DNA index; SB, Southern blotting; RA, radioactive ligand uptake; NB, Northern blotting; WB, Western blotting.

TRANSFORMING GROWTH FACTOR-β (TGF-β) TGF-α is a member of a family of closely related peptides with growth inhibitory properties. The prototypical member of this family, TGF-β1, maps to 19q13. In the normal breast, the subtypes of TGF-β are expressed in both epithelial and stromal cells. By IHC, the patterns of TGF-β expression suggest that it participates in the regulation of differentiation and growth inhibition by both autocrine and paracrine mechanisms. Paradoxically, TGF-β appears to be expressed in the majority of invasive breast cancers, suggesting that malignant cells may have lost the ability to respond to its inhibitory effects. Very little information is available regarding TGF-β expression in precursor lesions of invasive breast cancer. One study found no evidence of expression by IHC in a few noninvasive carcinomas. In contrast, another small descriptive IHC study reported appreciable expression in normal, premalignant, and invasive malignant lesions.

INSULIN-LIKE GROWTH FACTOR 1 (IGF-I) IGF-I (formerly called somatomedin C) is a member of a family of growth factors homologous to insulin, but has distinct receptor binding and biologic effects. This gene maps to chromosome 12q22–24. It is a physiologic mediator and stimulator of normal cell growth. Most invasive breast cancers appear to express receptors for IGF-I, and are stimulated to grow in vitro in response to exogenous IGF-I and IGF-II. Preferential expression of IGF-I and -II by stromal cells suggests that they may function in a paracrine fashion. As with most growth factors, very little is known about IGF-I or -II expression in premalignant breast disease. There is a single report involving a handful of cases finding no expression of IGF-II in DCIS. Descriptive studies of "fibrocystic disease," which may harbor hyperplastic lesions, have observed expression of IGF-I in 50% of cases.

TUMOR SUPPRESSOR GENES AND HEREDITARY BREAST CANCER GENES

In contrast to the genes discussed in the previous sections, which increased gene expression stimulates neoplastic transformation, the tumor suppressor genes (TSG) lead to malignant transformation primarily by loss of function. Genetic studies of rare families predisposed to specific cancers or patterns of cancers have lead to the identification of a number of TSGs (*see* Table 63-4) by positional cloning techniques. Hereditary cancer families are rare, and the function of many of the TSGs are unknown. However, loss of heterozygosity (LOH) events at these loci are frequently seen in many cancer

Table 63-3
Biomarker Phenotypes of Precursor Lesions From Breasts with Invasive Cancer

		Ductal hyperplasia		*Ductal carcinoma* in situ			
Biomarker assay	*Normal*	*Typical*	*Atypical*	*Comedo*	*Noncomedo*	*Mixed/NOS*	*Invasive breast cancer*
Hormone receptors (% positive)							
Estrogen receptor							
IHC				0	80	72–92	57–90
Proliferation rate							
MI/40 HPF		14.6				51.3	
IHC (% Ki67 + cells)						6	11
DNA content (% aneuploid)							
IA (signal > 4n)						88	69
Oncogenes/growth factor receptors (% positive)							
c-erbB2/HER2 neu							
SB (DNA amplif.)						29	17
IHC (> 0% + cells)	0	0	0	61–75	7–11	17–78	11–45
ras							
IHC (> 0% + cells)	83						100
myc							
SB (DNA amplif.)						11	4
Growth factors (% positive)							
TGF-α							
IHC (mean score > 0)						100	100
Tumor suppressor genes (% positive)							
p53							
Sequencing (DNA mut.)						0	32

IHC, immunohistochemistryl; MI, mitotic index; HPF, high-power field; IA, image analysis; SB, Southern blotting.

types, including sporadic breast cancers. These observations suggest that both inherited and somatic mutations are targeting the same genes.

RB The *RB* gene is perhaps the archetypal TSG, and was originally characterized as a cancer predisposition gene in a childhood ocular tumor, retinoblastoma. Statistical analysis of retinoblastoma epidemiology suggested two forms of this disorder, a unilateral, unifocal presentation with no clear hereditary basis, and a bilateral, multifocal, hereditary form. These data led Knudson, on the basis of studies of the kinetics of tumor formation in the hereditary versus sporadic forms of retinoblastoma, to propose the "two-hit" model of genetic predisposition to cancer. Knudson proposed that the RB phenotype segregated in families as an apparent autosomal dominant trait, with affected individuals inheriting only a single functional copy of the *RB* gene. The tumors appearing in affected individuals resulted from the loss of the remaining functional allele of the *RB* gene in retinal cells. The unifocal development of retinoblastoma in sporadic cases is also caused by loss of both functional *RB* alleles, but in this circumstance reflected the low statistical probability of damage to both copies of the same gene during retinal development. The *RB* gene has proved to be a nuclear phosphoprotein of 110 kDa. RB undergoes cyclic phosphorylation and dephosphorylation during the cell cycle. Current models suggest that the unphosphorylated form of RB complexes with RB-associated proteins that are essential for cell division, and that on phosphorylation, RB releases these factors, permitting entry into the cell cycle. LOH of the *RB* locus is found at relatively high frequency in breast cancers, but interpretation of these deletion events are complicated by the discovery of the nearby *BRCA2* gene. Interestingly, carriers of inherited *RB* gene mutations are not at greatly increased risk of breast cancer, suggesting that although *RB* gene mutations may promote breast cancer evolution, these mutations are not themselves sufficient to cause breast cancer.

TP53 *TP53 (p53)* is a tumor suppressor gene located on chromosome 17p13. It encodes a 53-kDa nuclear phosphoprotein that functions as a transcription factor and is involved in the regulation of cell proliferation. Mutated *TP53* is very common in many types of cancer. Although wild-type *TP53* is undetectable by IHC, many *TP53* mutations are missense point mutations resulting in an inactive protein with a prolonged half-life, which accumulates to very high concentrations in the cell nucleus. For this reason, measuring TP53 protein expression is a relatively easy and accurate surrogate assay for detecting mutations. Up to 50% of invasive breast cancers contain mutated or overexpressed *TP53*, which is associated with many other aggressive biologic factors and poor clinical outcome.

There are very few studies regarding *TP53* alterations in normal and hyperplastic breast epithelium. In IHC studies involving less than 50 samples of normal breast epithelium, no expression of *p53* was observed, consistent with wild-type gene structure and function. The "normal" epithelium of patients with Li-Fraumeni syndrome, who have inherited *p53* mutations, often overexpress *TP53*. One study has evaluated nine cases of atypical hyperplasia, and found no evidence of expression. Noninvasive carcinomas have been evaluated more thoroughly. Investigations involving more than 100 cases of comedo DCIS observed rates of *TP53* overexpression ranging from 33 to 67%, approaching that of invasive breast cancer. These same studies also examined an appreciable number of noncomedo DCIS, and found much lower rates ranging from 0 to 25%. Other studies evaluating mixed or NOS DCIS report intermediate rates of overexpression or mutation ranging from 16 to 33%. Currently, there is no substantial information regarding the *TP53* status of premalignant or preinvasive diseases in breasts also containing cancer.

OTHER POTENTIAL BREAST CANCER TSG Other TSGs that have been identified are involved in diverse functions, including check point control, such as *MTS1* (p16), transcriptional repression *(WT1)*, signal transduction modulation (*RASA*, *NF1*), and DNA repair (*MSH2*, *MLH1*, *ATM*), suggesting that mutations in genes regulating cell proliferation, genetic stability, and cell death could all drive the process of clonal evolution.

GENES MUTATED IN HEREDITARY FORMS OF BREAST CANCER Because of the high prevalence of breast cancer in the population, clustering of breast cancer in families is not unusual. Therefore, the etiology of families with multiple cases of breast cancer may reflect chance and environmental factors, as well as heredity. Approximately 5–10% of breast cancer is now thought to have a hereditary basis. Hereditary breast cancers are inherited in an autosomal dominant fashion, and, as in *RB* and other inherited cancers, breast cancer gene heterozygotes only form tumors in breast epithelial cells that lose the remaining, normal copy of the gene. Germ line mutations in three genes, *TP53 (see above)*, *BRCA1*, and *BRCA2*, have been detected in hereditary breast cancer families.

Table 63-4
Cloned TSGs with LOH in Breast Cancers

Gene (HGM symbol)	*Location*	*Gene product*
Bacterial mutS homolog *(MSH2)*	2p22–21	DNA mismatch repair mutant in HNPCC
Bacterial mutL homolog *(MLH1)*	3p23–22	DNA mismatch repair mutant in HNPCC
Von-Hippel Lindau *(VHL)*	3p25–26	Cell membrane protein
ras p21 GTPase activator *(RASA)*	5q13	*ras*-GTPase activator protein
Adenomatous polyposis coli *(APC)*	5q21	Cytoplasmic protein (unknown function)
p16 (MTS1)	9p21	Inhibitor of cyclin-dependent kinase 4
Ataxia telangiectasia *(ATM)*	11q23	DNA repair
Breast cancer 2 *(BRCA2)*	13q13	Unknown function
Retinoblastoma *(RB)*	13q14	Nuclear phosphoprotein regulating entry into cell cycle
p53 (TP53)	17p13	Transcription factor regulating entry into cell cycle
Neurofibromatosis 1 *(NF1)*	17q11.2	*ras*-GTPase activator protein
Breast cancer 1 *(BRCA1)*	17q21	Nuclear protein of unknown function—transcription factor?

LI-FRAUMENI SYNDROME Inherited *TP53* mutations result in the Li-Fraumeni syndrome, a very rare, familial association of childhood sarcomas, early onset breast cancer in females, and other malignant neoplasms. The high frequency of somatic mutations of *TP53* in sporadic cancers and mutations of *TP53* in Li-Fraumeni syndrome is evidence supporting the common genetic pathways in the evolution of inherited and acquired breast cancer.

BRCA1 In contrast, the relationship of between mutations of *BRCA1*, the most common hereditary breast cancer predisposition gene, and sporadic breast cancer is less clear. The *BRCA1* gene was first mapped by genetic linkage studies of breast cancer families, and the gene was eventually identified by positional cloning studies. This gene encodes a 220-kDa protein. Its nuclear localization and the identification of two zinc-finger DNA domains near the amino-terminus of the protein have led to speculation that BRCA1 may function as a transcription factor. Mutant *BRCA1* gene carriers are at a very high risk of exhibiting breast cancer at a young age and also show increased risk of having ovarian cancer. Germ line mutations in *BRCA1* account for 50% of all hereditary breast cancers, and may account for 2% of all breast cancers. Although LOH of the 17q21 region is frequently seen in sporadic breast cancers, somatic mutations of *BRCA1* are absent in sporadic breast cancers. The LOH of the *BRCA1* region may be associated with downregulation of this gene in developing breast cancers, and gene transfer experiments indicate that expression of wild type *BRCA1* protein inhibits the growth of breast cancers in vitro and in vivo. Other recent studies of indicate that the BRCA1 protein is aberrantly localized to the cytoplasm in breast cancer cell lines. Thus, in sporadic breast cancers, faulty BRCA1 localization because of mutation of a putative chaperone protein might have the same effect as mutation of *BRCA1* itself.

BRCA2 A third breast cancer susceptibility locus, designated *BRCA2*, was also mapped by genetic linkage studies of breast cancer families. Positional cloning studies recently isolated *BRCA2*, and characterization of this gene is in progress. Gene carriers are at high risk of developing breast cancer, breast cancer of the male breast, and potentially, other cancers. No clues to the apparent function of *BRCA2* have yet emerged from DNA sequence analysis, except for reports of distant homology to part of the *BRCA1* gene. Germline mutations have been detected in *BRCA2*, and the LOH events found in breast and other cancers from *BRCA2* gene carriers always delete the normal *BRCA2* allele. Studies of the relationship of *BRCA2* to sporadic breast cancers are complicated by the nearby *RB* gene because most tumors studied lose both genes within the LOH region, it is unclear which gene is involved in the clonal evolution process. One report indicates that a breast cancer cell with chromosome 13q LOH maintained heterozygosity for *RB*, but was homozygous for markers around *BRCA2*, suggesting that *BRCA2* is responsible for the putative LOH event.

OTHER POTENTIAL INHERITED BREAST CANCER GENES Epidemiologic studies have suggested that other genes are associated with increased risks of breast cancer, albeit at a much smaller magnitude than the genes discussed above. Studies of a highly polymorphic markers in the *HRAS* gene on chromosome 11p15 have associated particular alleles of *HRAS* with elevated risk of breast cancer and other cancers.

It is well established that homozygotes for mutations in the ataxia-telangiectasia *(ATM)* gene are at extremely high risk of cancer, particularly lymphoma and leukemia. Studies linking excess cancer risk in *ATM* mutation heterozygotes are more controversial. These studies suggest that female relatives of patients with ATM have excess risk of breast cancer; with the estimated relative risk of breast cancer to ATM heterozygotes of 3.9-fold. These results suggest that *ATM* heterozygotes could account for 3.8% of breast cancer cases.

Two new genes involved in DNA repair, designated *MSH2* and *MLH1*, have been identified at chromosome 2p22–21, and 3p23–22, respectively. Mutations in these genes lead to hereditary nonpolyposis colon cancer (HNPCC). A consequence of mutations in genes is microsatellite instability, or destabilization of the polymorphic alleles found at simple sequence repeat polymorphisms (microsatellites). This phenomenon is thought to result from impaired DNA repair, and is characteristic of the colon cancers found in HNPCC patients. DCIS, lobular carcinoma *in situ* (LCIS), invasive, and metastatic breast cancers have been evaluated for microsatellite instability. Microsatellite instability is observed in about 20% of invasive breast cancers, and was observed at moderate frequency *in situ* breast cancers. All chromosomal loci investigated demonstrated low levels of microsatellite instability. Microsatellite instability was significantly correlated with the lobular histotype, and with lymph node involvement. A trend was also observed associating microsatellite instability and large tumor size, implying that tumors with microsatellite instability may be more aggressive.

ALLELIC IMBALANCE OR LOSS-OF-HETEROZYGOSITY (LOH) Loss-of-heterozygosity (LOH) refers to the disappearance of polymorphic marker alleles when constitutional DNA and tumor DNA from a cancer patient are genotyped. The LOH events are genomic deletions that discard the normal copies of TSGs, or uncover existing TSG mutations. Breast cancers have been extensively studied for LOH events, which have been detected on almost every chromosome arm. Breast cancer LOH regions coincide with known TSG loci. However, it remains to be determined whether the LOHs are related to mutations in the known TSGs or in as yet unknown genes in the vicinity. The availability of large numbers of highly polymorphic segments of the human genome that can be easily amplified in formalin-fixed, paraffin-embedded archival breast tumors by polymerase chain reaction (PCR) should allow breast cancer researchers to precisely map the LOH loci, and either implicate known TSGs or identify new ones.

The concept that invasive breast cancer arises from certain precursor lesions has been based primarily on epidemiologic and histopathologic evidence. More recent studies provide genetic evidence supporting this model of breast cancer evolution. For instance, LOH analysis in a series of hyperplasias, noninvasive, invasive, and metastatic carcinomas were carried out. LOH was evaluated by PCR amplification of 13 highly polymorphic gene loci that had shown high rates of loss (>25%) in previous studies of invasive breast cancer. DNA was extracted from precursor or cancer lesions microdissected from formalin-fixed, paraffin-embedded tissue from breasts with and without invasive cancer. Hyperplasias and *in situ* carcinomas from breasts without invasive cancer showed at least 1 LOH (for the 13 loci tested) in 29 and 66% of lesions, respectively. Such accumulation or selection of allelic losses is unequivocal evidence that most (probably all) of these lesions are true neoplasms. The incidence of LOH in hyperplasias and *in situ* carcinomas from breasts with invasive cancer was even higher (52 and 80%, respectively). At least 1 LOH was also found in 95% of invasive cancers and 97% of metastatic cancers evaluated. The majority of LOH-positive hyperplasias (53%) and *in situ* carcinomas (79%) from breasts containing invasive cancer shared their LOH phenotypes with a more "advanced" lesion present in the same breast, consistent with the idea that there are precursor–product relationships between them. Invasive cancer shared its LOH phenotype with metastatic cancer from the same patient 85% of the time.

PROPERTIES OF ESTABLISHED MALIGNANCIES

INVASION AND METASTATIC SPREAD OF BREAST CANCER Dysregulation of genes involved in the control of cell growth results in the establishment of an *in situ* malignancy; however, alterations in the expression of new classes of genes fuel the processes of invasion and metastasis that result in evolution of breast cancer towards systemic disease. This novel gene expression changes the binding relationships of the breast cancer cells to extracellular matrix (ECM) components of the basement membrane, such as fibronectin, laminin, and collagen. In the case of breast cancers, particular attention has been focused on the expression of the laminin receptors, because the interactions of breast cancer cells to basement membrane laminin are much greater than those of normal breast tissue. Another class of cell adhesion proteins under scrutiny in breast cancer invasion are the integrins, which comprise a large family of transmembrane glycoproteins involved in cell–matrix and cell–cell interactions by functioning as receptors to extracellular matrix proteins, and also as adhesion molecules.

This change in binding relationships between breast cancer cells and the ECM components are a prelude to release of proteolytic enzymes that lead to the destruction of the basement membrane and subsequent invasion of the breast cancer into the surrounding tissue. These include serine proteinases, collagenases, and cysteine proteinases that specifically degrade ECM components. In breast cancers, capthepsin B, a lyzosomal cysteine proteinase with a broad spectrum of action against many proteins, including all the ECM components mentioned above, has been extensively studied. Results from these studies indicate that breast tumors that expressed high levels of capthepsin D had a negative prognostic impact for ultimate tumor spread or recurrence.

After invasion, malignant cells may spread to distant sites through the process of metastasis. Malignant cells penetrate lymphatic or vascular channels and ultimately arrest in small lymphatics or capillaries, although less than 0.01% survive in the circulation. Most cancers seem to respond to the local environment in response to growth factors produced by the host tissue. In a permissive environment, cancers can reverse the process of escape from the primary tumor and invade back across the basement membrane into the surrounding tissue. Ultimately, these micrometastases must release growth factors to stimulate the production of new blood vessels. This process, referred to as angiogenesis, must take place to continue growth at the new site. Invasive breast cancers usually spread to local and regional lymph nodes, particularly to the axillary, mammary, and superclavicular nodes. Distant sites of breast cancer metastasis include bone, lung, liver, pleura, adrenals, skin, and brain.

BREAST CANCER PROGNOSTIC FACTORS By far the most important prognostic factor for breast cancer is the stage at the time of diagnosis. Breast cancers are categorized as stage I–IV on the basis of tumor size and evidence of metastatic spread. Stage I refers to tumors 2 cm or less without direct extension or nodal metastases. Stage II refers to tumors 2–5 cm without nodal metastases, or with homolateral axillary metastases with no evidence of fixation to surrounding structures. Stage III refers to tumors larger than 5 cm with or without nodal metastases, or any tumor with axillary metastases sufficiently extensive to cause fixation of the affected nodes to adjacent structures, or any tumor with fixation to adjacent muscle or fascia that does not include the chest wall. Stage IV refers to any tumor with fixation to the chest wall or skin of the breast; any tumor with metastasis to regional nodes outside the axillary region, or other more distant metastases.

The histologic grade of the primary tumor is another useful prognostic indicator. The degree of glandular differentiation (the extent to which the tumor still resembles normal breast structures) and the extent of nuclear atypia in terms of size, irregularity of shape, and prominence of nucleoli are noted. Poor levels of differentiation and cells with large, irregularly shaped nuclei with prominent nucleoli are indicators of poor prognosis.

The level of proliferation is another useful prognostic factor. Proliferation can be assessed histologically by the mitotic index; or by immunohistochemical evaluation of proteins associated with proliferation, such as Ki-67 or PCNA; or by measurement of the number of cells in the S phase of the cell cycle by flow cytometry. High levels of cell division are associated with poor prognosis.

ESTROGEN RECEPTORS AND BREAST CANCER Estrogen and progesterone are implicated in the development of breast cancer by a number of epidemiologic observations, including increased risk for breast cancer with either early menarche or delayed menopause, and by exogenous administration of estrogens after menopause. In contrast, ovariectomy confers a protective effect against developing breast cancer. Taken together, these observations suggest that breast cancers are dependent on these hormones for their growth and evolution. Estrogen is a powerful mitogen for both normal breast epithelium and breast cancer cells; endogenous estrogen stimulates cell proliferation and tumor progression. This mitogenic signal is mediated by the estrogen receptor, a member of the nuclear receptor family. Stimulation of the ER upregulates expression of the PR. Therefore, measurement of the status of both ER and PR by ligand-binding analysis has become an important tumor marker. In general, ER-positive tumors are better differentiated, show lower mitotic activity, and are less aneuploid than ER-negative tumors, although ER-negative DCIS may have progressed beyond hormonal dependence, but these popular speculations may be an oversimplification. For example, in one recent study, proliferation was measured in DCIS and normal terminal duct lobular units (TDLUs) in the same breasts from a large number of patients dichotomized on the basis of menopausal status. Proliferation rates in TDLUs were much lower in postmenopausal compared with premenopausal women, consistent with the well-known mitogenic effect of estrogen on normal breast epithelium. In contrast, there was no difference in proliferation between the two groups in DCIS, suggesting that replication may be relatively independent of hormonal control, regardless of ER status. However, much remains to be studied in this important area of breast cancer research.

The "good" histopathologic features of ER-positive tumors translate into improved disease-free survival and better overall survival for patients with ER-positive tumors. ER status may eventually be shown to be useful as a prognostic factor in the clinical management of patients who already have DCIS or cancer, either alone or in combination with other factors such as histology and proliferation rate. However, its most promising role relates to its ability to mediate the effects of antihormonal drugs, such as tamoxifen, that might be used in future chemoprevention trials. These agents inhibit the recruitment of cells into the cell cycle by estrogen, resulting in diminished proliferation of breast cancer cells.

Overall, about 70% of primary breast cancers are ER-positive, and approximately 60% of these patients respond to antiestrogen therapy. Several studies have shown that tamoxifen can prolong disease-free survival in patients with ER-positive invasive breast cancer, probably by binding ER and suppressing cell division. Other studies have shown that the relative risk of developing a second breast cancer in patients initially treated with tamoxifen may be reduced by as much as half. These favorable effects may be as biologically relevant to premalignant lesions and carcinoma *in situ* (CIS) as they are to invasive breast cancer, and this type of reasoning has already provided theoretical support for a few ongoing chemoprevention trials in patients at high risk for developing invasive breast cancer. Unfortunately, prolonged tamoxifen therapy fails in most patients because of acquired resistance to its antiestrogenic effects. Tamoxifen resistance probably arises as a result of tumor-specific alterations ER gene structure or expression.

BREAST CANCER TREATMENT With increased public awareness of breast cancer, combined with expanded use of screening mammography, 70% of breast cancers now present with stage I disease. Approximately 70% of these patients will be cured by surgery, with about 30% recurring within 5 years. Primary breast cancer surgery ranges from total mastectomy to more breast-conserving approaches such as lumpectomy. Although the chances of surviving breast cancer are approximately the same with either mastectomy or lumpectomy with radiation therapy, local failure rates remain higher after the latter procedure, ranging from 2 to 40%. This wide range of local recurrence is probably caused by differences in surgical or radiotherapeutic techniques, such as definition of surgical margins and doses of radiation delivered. The 30% of patients presenting with stage II or greater disease, and those patients with stage I disease who recur, derive significant benefit from adjuvant chemotherapy, such as systemic chemotherapy with cyclophosphamide, methotrexate, and fluorouracil. So far, the benefit of adjuvant chemotherapy for women with stage I breast cancers is marginal, and not without morbidity. Much of current breast cancer research is dedicated to identifying tumor biologic factors that predict recurrence in order to tailor specific treatments to the patient's needs.

SUMMARY

The majority of invasive breast cancers most likely evolve from precursor lesions. However, the putative precursor lesions are common relative to invasive breast cancer, emphasizing that progression is not obligatory, and that many biologic abnormalities underlying tumor progression are morphologically silent at the light microscopic level. Identifying these abnormalities may provide the ability to diagnose premalignant lesions at high risk for progression to invasive breast cancer, and allow for some type of intervention before progression occurs. Many studies are beginning to investigate the biologic characteristics of putative precursor lesions, such as hyperplasias and *in situ* carcinoma. Most such studies have retrospectively looked at features first described in invasive breast cancer. To date, very little is known with certainty about the biology of hyperplastic breast disease. *In situ* carcinomas have been more thoroughly studied, and there is considerable but still incomplete information regarding ER, proliferation rate, ploidy, *ERBB2*, and *TP53* status in such lesions. With the exception of these few biomarkers, however, very little else is known with certainty about the biology of preinvasive breast cancer. Based on recent genetic evidence supporting a precursor–product relationship between precursor lesions and invasive cancer in the same breast, future studies might benefit from evaluating the biologic phenotypes of putative precursors taken from breasts with and without invasive cancer. Comparison of phenotypes in these contrasting settings may emphasize biologic events that are critical in breast cancer evolution.

ACKNOWLEDGMENTS

This work was supported by NIH/NCI grants CA54174, CA30195, and CA58183.

SELECTED REFERENCES

Allred DC, Clark GM, Elledge R, et al. Association of p53 protein expression with tumor cell proliferation and clinical outcome in node-negative breast cancer. J Natl Cancer Inst 1993;85:200–206.

Allred DC, O'Connell P, Fuqua SAW. Biomarkers in early breast neoplasia. J Cell Biochem 1993;17G:125–131.

Alpers CE, Wellings SF. The prevalence of carcinoma in situ in normal and cancer-associated breasts. Hum Pathol 1985;16:796–807.

Bartow SA, Pathak DR, Black WC, Key CR, Teaf SR. Prevalence of benign, atypical, and malignant breast lesions in populations at different risk for breast cancer: a forensic autopsy study. Cancer 1987;60:2751–2760.

Bodian CA, Perzin KH, Lattes R, Hoffmann P, Abernathy TG. Prognostic significance of benign proliferative breast disease. Cancer 1993;71:3896–3907.

Bos JL. ras oncogenes in human cancer: a review. Cancer Res 1989;49:4682–4689.

Carter CL, Corle DK, Micozzi MS, Schatzkin A, Taylor PR. A prospective study of the development of breast cancer in 16,692 women with benign breast disease. Am J Epidemiol 1988;128:467–477.

Casey G. The BRCA1 and BRCA2 breast cancer genes. Curr Opin Oncol 1997;9:88–93.

Catzavelos C, Bhattacharya N, Ung YC, et al. Decreased levels of the cell-cycle inhibitor p27Kip1 protein: prognostic implications in primary breast cancer. Nat Med 1997;3:227–230.

Dupont WD, Page DL. Risk factors for breast cancer in women with proliferative breast disease. N Engl J Med 1985;3:146–151.

Dupont WD, Parl FF, Hartmann WH, et al. Breast cancer risk associated with proliferative breast disease and atypical hyperplasia. Cancer 1993;71:1258–1265.

Easton D, Ford D, Peto J. Inherited susceptibility to breast cancer. Cancer Surv 1993;18:95–113.

Frykbert ER, Masood S, Copeland EM, Bland KI. Ductal carcinoma in situ of the breast. Surg Gynec Obstet 1993;177:425–440.

Henderson BE, Ross R, Bernstein L. Estrogens as a cause of human cancer: the Richard and Hindau Rosenthal Foundation Award Lecture. Cancer Res 1988;48:246–253.

Hurlin PJ, Ayer DE, Grandori C, Eisenman RN. The Max transcription factor network: involvement of Mad in differentiation and an approach to identification of target genes. Cold Spring Harb Symp Quant Biol 1994;59:109–116.

Kintanar EB, Raju U. Further delineation of patterns of atypical ductal hyperplasia (ADH): an analysis of ADH patterns associated with intraductal and invasive breast carcinoma. Mod Pathol 1991;4:12A.

Knudson AG. Hereditary cancer, oncogenes, and anti-oncogenes. Cancer Res 1985;45:1437–1443.

Krontiris TG, Devlin B, Karp DD, Robert NJ, Risch N. An association between the risk of cancer and mutations in the HRAS1 minisatellite locus. N Engl J Med 1993;329:517–523.

Levine AJ, Momand J, Finlay CA. The p53 tumor suppressor gene. Nature 1991;351:453–456.

London SJ, Connolly JL, Schnitt SJ, Colditz GA. A prospective study of benign breast disease and the risk of breast cancer. JAMA 1992;267:941–944.

Ludwig T, Chapman DL, Papaioannou VE, Efstratiadis A. Targeted mutations of breast cancer susceptibility gene homologs in mice: lethal phenotypes of Brca1, Brca2, Brca1/Brca2, Brca1/p53, and Brca2/p53 nullizygous embryos. Genes Dev 1997;11:1226–1241.

McDivitt RW, Stevens JA, Lee NC, Wingo PA, Rubin GL, Gersell D. Histologic types of benign breast disease and the risk for breast cancer. Cancer 1992;69:1408–1414.

NSABP Protocol P-1. A clinical trial to determine the worth of tamoxifen for preventing breast cancer. Pittsburgh, PA: National Surgical Adjuvant Breast and Bowel Project, 1992.

O'Connell P, Pekkel V, Fuqua SAW, Osborne CK, Allred DC. Molecular genetic studies of early breast cancer evolution. Breast Cancer Res Treat 1994;32:5–12.

Osborne CK, Clark GM, Ravdin PM. Adjuvant systemic therapy of primary breast cancer. In: Harris JR, Lippman ME, Morrow M, Hellman S., eds. Diseases of the Breast. Philadelphia: Lippincott-Raven, 1996; pp. 487–547.

Osborne CK. Receptors. In: Harris JR, Hellman S, Henderson IC, Kinne DW, eds. Breast Diseases. Philadelphia: JB Lippincott, 1991; pp. 301–325.

Porter PL, Malone KE, Heagerty PJ, et al. Expression of cell-cycle regulators p27Kip1 and cyclin E, alone and in combination, correlate with survival in young breast cancer patients. Nat Med 1997;3:222–225.

Powles TJ, Jones AL, Ashley SE, et al. The Royal Marsden Hospital Pilot tamoxifen chemoprevention trial. Breast Cancer Res Treat 1994;31:73–82.

Rutqvist LE, Cedermark B, Glas U, et al. Contralateral primary tumors in breast cancer patients in a randomized trial of adjuvant tamoxifen therapy. J Natl Cancer Inst 1991;83:1299–1306.

Sharan SK, Morimatsu M, Albrecht U, et al. Embryonic lethality and radiation hypersensitivity mediated by Rad51 in mice lacking Brca2. Nature 1997;386:804–810.

Swift M, Reitnauer PJ, Morrell D, Chase CL. Breast and other cancers in families with ataxia-telangiectasia. N Engl J Med 1987;316:1289–1294.

Suzuki A, de la Pompa JL, Hakem R, et al. Bcra2 is required for embryonic cellular proliferation in the mouse. Genes Dev 1997;11:1242–1252.

NEPHROLOGY VIII

SECTION EDITOR:
DENNIS AUSIELLO

64 Renal Development

VIKAS P. SUKHATME

INTRODUCTION

This overview begins with a review of key concepts in developmental biology as they apply to the kidney. Molecules of demonstrated importance in nephrogenesis are then discussed. Finally, the focus is on implications of this work for basic science and clinical nephrology.

DESCRIPTION OF KIDNEY DEVELOPMENT

In mammals, the urogenital system develops sequentially in three stages: the first two stages, that is, formation of the pronephros and mesonephros, are transient. The last stage, development of the metanephros, represents the final kidney in reptiles, birds, and mammals; whereas, in fish and amphibians, the mesonephros is the final kidney. Importantly, all three steps in kidney development are characterized by induction of mesenchyme to epithelium. Here we shall focus only on metanephric development. Ureteric bud epithelium, an out-pouching of the Wolffian duct, invades metanephric mesenchyme, initiating "induction" of mesenchyme at its tip. Based on histologic features, the subsequent process has been divided into various steps: condensation, vesicle formation, comma and S-shaped body formation, glomerular cleft formation with angiogenesis, and then nephron formation (proximal and distal segments). In turn, as part of a reciprocal interaction, mesenchyme causes ureteric bud to branch sequentially, with mesenchymal condensates surrounding each new tip, thereby leading to differentiation in a centrifugal manner. The bifurcating ureteric bud structures ultimately form the collecting duct. Though this description of embryonic kidney development owes much to the classic work of Grobstein and Saxen, only recently have there been substantial advances in defining some of the critical underlying regulatory molecules.

CONCEPTS AND METHODOLOGIES IN STUDYING DEVELOPMENT AND THEIR APPLICATION TO THE KIDNEY Developmental biologists of the past were embryologists and anatomists. Their primary work consisted initially of detailed observations. Later, many effectively utilized a "cut-and-paste" approach. These ablation and/or transposition experiments—for example, those of Spemann—led to many key developmental principles, especially the concept of induction. The next wave of developmental biologists were geneticists, who generated a host of developmental mutants in lower organisms such as Drosophila. Finally, molecular genetics invaded the field, and descriptions at the level of molecules—transcription factors, matrix proteins, extracellular and intracellular signals—have emerged. This fusion of embryology, classical genetics, and molecular and cell biology has invigorated the field.

We begin with some general concepts in developmental biology. The first notion is that of mosaic vs regulative development. Vertebrate embryos display regulative development: removal of a blastomere or even an entire half of an embryo still leads to the formation of a normal embryo. In contrast, development in Caenorhabditis elegans is mosaic, that is, cell fate is more rigidly determined. Regulative development is largely a result of morphogens, molecules influencing various processes; for example, cell movement, polarization, or differentiation. These morphogens may be diffusible or cell-surface-bound. The effect of these morphogens is to set up (an) inductive event(s), a process whereby one cell influences another cell's development. In turn, a cascade of events can occur, the key mediators being transcription factors, growth and differentiating factors, cell adhesion molecules, and extracellular matrix.

Several approaches can be utilized to identify these molecules. Two broad schemes emerge: the phenotype-to-genotype approach and vice versa. The former is best exemplified by the use of positional cloning. Advantages are that the cloned gene is obviously of developmental importance and no prior knowledge of the protein is required for its identification. The disadvantage is that this methodology is demanding (albeit getting easier) and only a few mouse and human models exist; that is, the underlying genes may represent a small subset of developmentally critical genes. To circumvent this difficulty, zebrafish may be a suitable organism in which to perform a saturation mutagenesis analysis. In the phenotype to genotype approach, the initial goal is to identify candidate genes of developmental importance. A useful starting point is homology screening, either through low-stringency nucleic acid hybridization or through polymerase chain reaction (PCR)-based methodologies, or consider homologs of genes with demonstrated importance in lower organisms. A focus on growth factors or their receptors, adhesion molecules, proto-oncogenes, transcription factors, or intracellular signaling molecules is likely to yield the most useful information. Moreover, ± screening from cells at different developmental stages could be intersected with the above approaches. A narrowed list of clones could then be analyzed by *in situ* hybridization and/or Northern analysis to check for tissue-restricted and stage-specific expression. Ultimately, one could use

From: *Principles of Molecular Medicine* (J. L. Jameson, ed.), ©1998 Humana Press Inc., Totowa, NJ.

either forced ectopic expression in transgenic mice or in lower organisms (of the wild-type gene or a dominant negative construct) or knockout studies including conditional knockouts in cell culture or animals to analyze the function of the candidate gene. Less definitive results, but at considerably less cost, could be obtained utilizing antisense oligonucleotides or antibodies in kidney organ culture.

A useful framework for thinking about development is to divide events into three sequential categories: those involving patterning, those relating to cell differentiation and commitment, and those concerning morphogenesis. Patterning refers to regional specification, that is, the establishment of a body plan. It usually has to precede cell differentiation, in which cells start from a pluripotent or multipotent state and progressively assume specific differentiated fates that bring them closer to their final function in the developed organism. It is important to distinguish cell differentiation from commitment or determination. Commitment is the narrowing of the phenotypic possibilities open to a cell; differentiation is the actual enactment of that limited capability. As a result, commitment usually precedes differentiation. Morphogenesis refers to the creation of form—that is, the shaping of new structures—and therefore usually occurs after some differentiation has begun. Thus, these three, often sequential events—patterning, cell differentiation and commitment, and morphogenesis—form a logical paradigm in which to view development.

It is important to recognize that diverse molecular and cellular processes underlie these three steps. These processes include: cell growth and death (usually apoptosis rather than necrosis), cell motion, cell adhesion, imprinting, and cytoplasmic segregation. To delineate these processes, what they are and where and when they occur during a given developmental process is the challenge to the cell and molecular biologist.

How Does This Developmental Paradigm Relate to Kidney Development? With regard to patterning, it is noteworthy that the formation of the metanephric kidney occurs only after the two earlier kidneys (the pronephros and the mesonephros) have formed. Nothing is known about the critical morphogen(s) that govern(s) the timing, location, or orientation of these structures. Regarding cell commitment and differentiation, cell lineages in the kidney have been delineated for many cell types with the exception of mesangial cells and endothelial cells of the glomerular capillary tuft: metanephric mesenchyme gives rise to the epithelial glomerular components, as well as to proximal and distal nephron. Ureteric bud epithelium develops into the mature collecting duct. These fate-mapping data arise from chimeric embryos and through the use of β-galactosidase transducing retroviruses to mark cells. Some of the more interesting questions relating to cell differentiation are the nature of the inducing signal from the ureter that leads to conversion of mesenchyme to polarized epithelium, the nature of the reciprocal interaction (mesenchyme to ureteric bud signaling), the development of the mesangial cell, the formation of the basement membrane, and the process of angiogenesis. Many excellent reviews are available that cite the changes in gene expression of various molecules during these steps. Additional candidates may be identified by educated guesswork from other tissues showing mesenchyme to epithelium conversion or through methodologies mentioned above, such as homology screening. Moreover, the availability of better cell culture systems (for example, cells arrested at different stages of differentiation, which can be differentiated in culture by change in matrix or serum components) will also serve as useful starting reagents. Below, we only cite data that provide definitive proof of the importance of a select subset of potential critical molecules. Finally, with regard to morphogenesis in the kidney, diverse questions arise: What causes the formation of the cleft in the glomerulus? What is responsible for the complex branching that occurs in the nephron? How does the collecting system reshape after its initial formation? Few answers are currently available to these problems.

GENETIC CASCADES Based on studies in lower organisms, a particularly fruitful approach to defining the elaborate genetic program that regulates kidney development is to focus on transcription factor genes expressed in the embryonic kidney, perhaps identified initially by homology screening. That a candidate gene is critical for nephrogenesis can then be established by the generation of a knockout mouse. Subsequently, efforts to identify downstream targets as well as upstream events—that is, *cis* elements and transfactors regulating expression of these transcription factor genes—can be utilized to start building a database of gene–protein interactions. Another useful starting point to identify potential critical transcription factors is to focus on the regulation of genes whose products play physiologic roles in the adult kidney. After ascertaining that transcriptional control plays a role in their expression, a search for factors regulating their expression will undoubtedly provide clues to tissue-specific regulation and define critical events occurring earlier in developmental time. Alternatively, genes essential for nephrogenesis, whether transcription factors or not, as ascertained by knockout or ectopic expression studies in transgenic mice, can form the starting point for such "upstream" studies.

CLONED GENES CRITICAL FOR NEPHROGENESIS We shall not discuss here many candidate genes—based on their stage-specific expression—of possible importance in kidney development. Rather we cite only data from in vivo "experiments" (in mouse or man) that clearly establish the importance of a candidate gene for nephrogenesis.

WT-1 (Wilms' tumor gene-1) is a tumor suppressor gene involved in the genesis of Wilms' tumor. The protein functions as a transcription factor with a DNA binding domain consisting of four zinc fingers, three of which are similar to those of the EGR gene family. Human mutations in the DNA binding region of WT1 have been characterized and are present in 10–20% of Wilms' tumors. Importantly, the best correlation of these mutations is in the rare Denys-Drash syndrome. During embryogenesis, WT1 expression is tissue-restricted. It is most strikingly expressed in induced metanephric mesenchyme and subsequently in podocytes. Persistent expression is noted in mesothelial tissues: pericardium, pleural, and peritoneal cells. WT1 knockout mice display no metanephric kidney, no gonads, and an abnormal mesothelium, leading to hypoplastic lungs and heart. The homozygotes die at embryonic day 13–15. Curiously, formation of the mesonephric kidney is largely unaffected, though the number of nephrons is decreased two- to threefold and ureteric bud fails to grow. The latter result was unexpected since WT1 is minimally expressed in uninduced mesenchyme and is not detectable in ureteric bud or Wolffian duct. Blastemal cells in the knockout mouse undergo apoptosis. Pax 2 *(see below)* is expressed on the ureteric bud side in WT1 (–/–) embryos but not in blastema, suggesting that WT1 expression is a prerequisite for Pax 2 expression in blastema.

Of the Pax gene family, Pax 2 and Pax 8 are expressed in developing kidney. These genes encode transcription factors and are related to the Drosophila segmentation genes in a region referred to as the paired box. Pax 2 expression occurs in the collecting system and in condensed mesenchyme, comma and S-shaped structures, but not in mature glomeruli, whereas Pax 8 expression differs from that of Pax 2 in that it is absent in the ureteric bud. Little Pax expression is seen in the adult. Increased Pax 2 expression has been formed in the hyperproliferative dysplatic epithelia of tubuler of children with dysplastic kidneys. When Pax 2 expression was constituently expressed in a transgenic mouse, including epithelial cells of the glomerulus, marked developmental anomalies resulted, reminiscent of those seen in the Finnish congenital nephrotic syndrome. Also, in Danforth's short tail mouse, Pax 2 expression is absent in mesenchyme. These mice show renal agenesis. Pax 2 stimulates the WT-1 promoter, and it may play a role in tissue-specific expression of WT-1.

The N-myc proto-oncogene belongs to the myc family of basic helix-loop-helix/leucine-zipper transcription factors. N-myc expression during nephrogenesis is similar to that of Pax 2 except that no expression is seen in the ureteric bud. N-myc knockout mice die at 11.5 days of gestation, precluding study of metanephric development. The mesonephros shows a decreased number of tubules and hypoplasia.

OP-1, also known as BMP-7, is a member of the TGF-β family, which shows striking expression in induced mesenchyme and early epithelial structures of the glomerulus with lesser expression in the ureteric duct. OP-1 knockouts display severe defects in the developing kidney. Though some comma and S-shaped bodies are present, the extensive formation of tight condensates is markedly reduced, resulting in a highly disorganized structure with much loose interstitial tissue. These data indicate a critical role for OP-1 in the survival and growth of both epithelium and mesenchymal components of the developing kidney. However, it is possible that even earlier defects in nephrogenesis might be noted if effects of maternal transfer of OP-1 to the embryo could be negated.

Wnt-4, a secreted glycoprotein, is part of the Wnt gene family, whose members play diverse developmental roles. During nephrogenesis, Wnt-4 expression is detected in condensing mesenchyme, comma and S-shaped bodies, and later restricted transiently to the region of epithelial fusion between the S-shaped bodies and collecting duct. Mice deficient in Wnt-4 activity fail to form pretubular aggregates, thus exhibiting a block in epithelial transformation of metanephric mesenchyme. Initial expression of WT1 in Wnt-4 knockout mice is normal. N-myc and Pax 2 expression is also normal except none is present in tubules. Pax 8 expression is, however, completely absent. These findings indicate that Wnt-4 activity plays no role in the development of ureteric epithelium.

Bcl-2, an oncogene described first in a B-cell lymphoma, functions by blocking programmed cell death or apoptosis. Apoptotic cells have been noted in the corticonephrogenic zone as well as in the papilla and may account for 3% of the cells in the developing kidney. As a first approximation, Bcl-2 expression is widespread in the developing kidney: in branching ureteric bud, metanephric cap tissue, and early tubular structures, and persists at lower levels in glomeruli, tubules, and collecting duct. Bcl-2 knockout mice develop polycystic kidneys with dilated tubules and hyperproliferative glomerular epithelial cells. The interstitium also contains immature cells.

The mouse limb deformity (ld) locus was identified as a result of transgene insertion. Several proteins (termed formins), the result of alternative splicing of the ld transcript, have been identified; they encode nuclear proteins expressed in the apical ectodermal ridge, a structure critical for limb development, as well as in epithelial cells of the pronephros and mesonephros (in the chicken). The human kidney is the major site of expression among several fetal tissues analyzed. Insertional mutagenesis at the ld locus in the mouse gives rise to a recessively inherited characteristic limb deformity (reduction and fusion of the distal bones and digits) and a renal aplasia phenotype, findings consistent with the pattern of expression of the ld transcript.

Defects in the PKD1 gene, identified recently by positional cloning, account for approximately 85% of mutations in autosomal dominant polycystic kidney disease (ADPKD). The gene product is a transmembrane protein expressed primarily on the ureteric bud side. It is most prominent in mature tubules, with lower levels in Bowman's capsule and the proximal ureteric bud. PKD1 is also expressed in hepatic bile ductules and pancreatic ducts (sites of cystic changes in ADPKD) and in skin (not known to be affected ADPKD). Based on the characterized human mutations in the PKD1 gene, it is clear that this gene product is of obvious import in nephrogenesis, though little mechanistic insight is currently available to account for the complex phenotypic changes noted in cells from PKD patients. A second gene (PKD2) for ADPKD has been identified by positional cloning. The PDK2 gene shares homology with PKD1 and appears to be a member of the family of voltage-activated calcium channels.

The PDGF family consists of three homo/heterodimeric members: AA, AB, and BB. The PDGF-α receptor binds both A and B chains, whereas the PDGF-β receptor only binds the B chain. The PDGF-α receptor is expressed in mesagnial structures in early glomeruli, but it declines as glomeruli mature. Since PDGFs mediate chemotaxis, differentiation, and growth, and affect production of extracellular matrix, they are prime candidates to be key developmentally important molecules. Mice deficient for PDGF B chain activity show renal, cardiovascular, and hematologic abnormalities and die perinatally. Importantly, no glomerular tuft forms, perhaps because of the absence of mesangial cells. A single or a few widened capillary loops are present. In addition, PDGF-β receptor knockout mice exhibit a similar glomerular defect. These findings are consistent with earlier data that mesangial cells respond mitogenically to PDGF (BB and AB more than AA) primarily through the PDGF-β receptor. Furthermore, they also suggest that mesangial cell development depends on a well-developed capillary network or vice versa.

c-Ret, a receptor protein tyrosine kinase, is normally expressed at the advancing tip of the ureteric bud, in the Wolffian duct, as well as in the developing central and peripheral nervous systems. Mice lacking c-Ret activity die postnatally because of complete or partial failure of renal development, with histology of rudimentary kidneys showing marked disorganization and decrease in tubules (proximal and distal), glomeruli, and vessels, as well as reduced ureteric bud branching. Moreover, large regions of undifferentiated mesenchyme are also present. These findings suggest that the c-Ret receptor transduces a critical signal presumably derived from metanephric mesenchyme involved in ureteric bud branching and growth.

FUTURE PROSPECTS

Though the pace of developmental biology research, as it pertains to the kidney, has clearly accelerated in recent years, many gaps remain in our understanding. What implications might this new knowledge have? From the basic science standpoint, nephrogenesis shares many features with other developmental systems such as the mammary gland, lung, and pancreas: inductive interactions, angiogenesis, branching morphogenesis, and so on. Thus, insights gained in one system will aid in the other. New families of growth factors or receptors may be identified, or novel members of pre-existing families might emerge. From a clinical standpoint, there is the emerging belief that mechanisms involved in development play a role, not only in primary renal genetic disorders, but also in the response of the kidney to injury, both acute and chronic. Introduction of growth factors such as HGF or IGF-I or blockade of ICAM-1 may prevent acute renal failure. Chronic injury caused by overexuberant production of TGF-β1, PDGF, or FGF might be amenable to therapy, either by preventing action of these molecules or, potentially, by transdifferentiating the resident cells that produce them. Both protein-based and gene therapy approaches could be envisioned. In this vein, one might be able to differentiate blastemal cells in a Wilms' tumor, thereby decreasing production of IGF-II, a factor that likely functions in an autocrine fashion to promote blastemal cell growth. Such differentiating agents might include peptide factors or other molecules by analogy with the use of all *trans*-retinoic acid in the treatment of acute promyelocytic leukemia. Finally, though it is hard to envision because of the complex architecture of the kidney, introduction of a suitable stem-cell population might lead to new nephron formation. Interestingly, adult fish, for example, do generate new functioning nephrons in response to toxic injury. Thus, many and varied opportunities for novel interventions will undoubtedly present themselves in the years ahead, fueled by a better understanding of kidney development.

SELECTED REFERENCES

Abboud HE, Bhandari B, Choudhury GG. Cell biology of platelet-derived growth factor. In: Schlondorff D, Bonventrer JV, eds. Molecular Nephrology: Kidney Function in Health and Disease. New York: Marcel Dekkar, 1995; pp. 573–590.

Burrow CR, Wilson PD. A putative Wilms' tumor-secreted growth factor activity required for primary culture of human nephroblasts. Proc Natl Acad Sci USA 1993;90:6066–6070.

Clapp WL, Abrahamson DR. Developmental and gross anatomy of the kidney. In: Tisher CC, Brenner BM, eds. Renal Pathology, 2nd ed. Philadelphia: Lippincott-Raven, 1994.

Consortium AP. Analysis of the genomic sequence for the autosomal dominant polycystic kidney disease (PKD1) gene predicts the presence of a leucine rich repeat. Hum Mol Genet 1995;4:575–582.

Consortium TEPKD. The polycystic kidney disease 1 gene encodes a 14 kb transcript and lies within a duplicated region on chromosome 16. Cell 1994;77:881–894.

Consortium TIPKD. Polycystic kidney disease: the complete structure of the PKD1 gene and its protein. Cell 1995;81:289–298.

Dressler GR. Developmental control genes. In: Schlondorff D, Bonventre JV, eds. Molecular Nephrology: Kidney Function in Health and Disease. New York: Marcel Dekkar, 1995; pp. 1–13.

Dressler GR, Wilkinson JE, Rothenpieler UW, Patterson LT, Williams-Simons L, Westphal H. Deregulation of Pax-2 expression in transgenic mice generates severe kidney abnormalities. Nature 1993;362:65–67.

Dudley AT, Lyons KM, Robertson EJ. A requirement for Bone Morphogenetic Protein-7 (BMP-7) during development of the mammalian kidney and eye. Genes Dev 1995;9:2795–2807.

Edelman GM. Topobiology. New York: Basic Books, 1988.

Floege J, Hudkins KL, Seifert RA, Francki A, Bowen-Pope DF, Alpers CE. Localization of PDGF alpha-receptor in the developing and mature human kidney. Kidney Int 1997;51:1140–1150.

Gashler AL, Sukhatme VP. Egr-1: prototype of a zinc finger family of transcription factors. In: Cohen WE, Moldave K, eds. Progress in Nucleic Acid Research and Molecular Biology, vol. 50. New York: Academic, 1995; pp. 191–224.

Geng L, Segal Y, Peissel B, et al. Identification and localization of polycystin, the PKD1 gene product. J Clin Invest 1996;98:2674–2682.

Haber DA. Wilms' Tumor. In: Schlondorff D, Bonventre JV, eds. Molecular Nephrology: Kidney Function in Health and Disease. New York: Marcel Dekker, 1995; pp. 1–13.

Herzlinger D, Koseki C, Mikawa T, Al-Awqati Q. Metanephric mesenchyme contains multipotenet stem cells whose fate is restricted after induction. Development 1992;114:565–572.

Karp SL, Ortiz-Arduan A, Li S, Neilson EG. Epithelial differentiation of metanephric mesenchymal cells after stimulation with hepatocyte growth factor or embryonic spinal cord. Proc Natl Acad Sci USA 1994;91:5286–5290.

Kelly KJ, Williams WW, Jr., Colvin RB, Bonventre JV. Antibody to intercellular adhesion molecule 1 protects the kidney against ischemic injury. Proc Natl Acad Sci USA 1994;91:812–816.

Kreidberg JA, Saiola H, Loring JM, et al. WT-1 is required for early kidney development. Cell 1993;74:679–691.

Lawrence PA. The Making of a Fly. Oxford, UK: Blackwell Scientific, 1993.

Lefebvre P, Thomas G, Gourmel B, et al. Pharmacokinetics of oral all-trans retinoic acid in patients with acute promyelocytic leukemia. Leukemia 1991;5:1054–1058.

Leveen P, Pekny M, Gebre-Medhin S, Swolin B, Larsson E, Betsholtz C. Mice deficient for PDGF B show renal, cardiovascular, and hematological abnormalities. Genes Dev 1994;8:1875–1887.

Luo G, Hofmann C, Bronckers ALJJ, Sohoki M, Bradley A, Karsenty G. BMP 7 is an inducer of nephrogenesis, and is also required for eye development and skeletal patterning. Genes Dev 1995;9:2808–2820.

Maas RL, Jepeal LI, Elfering SL, et al. A human gene homolous to the formin gene residing at the murine limb deformity locus: chromosomal location and RFLPs. Am J Hum Genet 1991;48:687–695.

McConnell MJ, Cunliffe HE, Chua LJ, Ward TA, Eccles MR. Differential regulation of the human Wilms tumour suppressor gene (WT1) promoter by two isoforms of PAX2. Oncogene 1997;14:2689–2700.

Miller SB, Martin DR, Kissane J, Hammerman MR. Hepatocyte growth factor accelerates recovery from acute ischemic renal injury in rats. Am J Physiol 1994;266:F129–F134.

Miller SB, Martin DR, Kissane J, Hammerman MR. Insulin-like growth factor I accelerates recovery from ischemic acute tubular necrosis in the rat. Proc Natl Acad Sci USA 1992;89:11,876–11,880.

Mochizuki T, Wu G, Hayashi T, et al. PKD2, a gene for polycystic kidney disease that encodes an integral membrane protein. Science 1996; 272:1339–1342.

Onuchic L, Wilson P, O'Sullivan E, Hebert R, Germino G. Polycystin is developmentally regulated and increased in human cystic epithelium. J Am Soc Nephrol 1995;6:705.

Phelps DE, Dressler GR. Aberrant expression of Pax-2 in Danforth's short tail (Sd) mice. Dev Biol 1993;157:251–258.

Reimschussel R, Bennett RO, May EB, Lipsky MM. Development of newly formed nephrons in the goldfish kidney following hexachlorobutadiene-induced nephrotoxicity. Toxicol Pathol 1990;18:32–38.

Saito A, Yamazaki H, Nakagawa Y, Arakawa M. Molecular genetics of renal diseases. Intern Med 1997;36:81–86.

Saxen L. Organogenesis of the Kidney. Cambridge University Press, Cambridge, UK 1987.

Schuchardt A, D'Agati V, Larsson-Blomberg L, Costantini F, Pachnis V. Defects in the kidney and enteric nervous system of mice lacking the tyrosine kinase receptor Ret. Nature 1994;367:380–383.

Schuchardt A, D'Agati V, Pachnis V, Costantini F. Renal agenesis and hypodysplasia in ret-k-mutant mice result from defects in ureteric bud development. Development 1996;122:1919–1929.

Soriano P. Abnormal kidney development and hematological disorders in PDGF β-receptor mutant mice. Genes Dev 1994;8:1888–1896.

Stanton BR, Perkins AS, Tessarollo L, et al. Loss of N-myc function results in embryonic lethality and failure of the epithelial component of the embryo to develop. Genes Dev 1992;6:2235–2247.

Stark K, Vainio S, Vassileva G, McMahon AP. Epithelial transformation of metanephric mesenchyme in the developing kidney regulated by Wnt-4. Nature 1994;372:679–683.

Trumpp A, Blundell PA, de la Pompa ZL, Zeller R. The chicken limb deformity gene encodes nuclear proteins expressed in specific cell types during morphogenesis. Genes Dev 1992;6:14–28.

Veis DJ, Sorenson CM, Shutter JR, Korsmeyer SJ. Bcl-2 deficient mice demonstrate fulminant lymphoid apoptosis, polycystic kidneys, and hypopigmented hair. Cell 1993;75:229–240.

Ward CJ, Turley H, Ong AC, et al. Polycystin, the polycystic kidney disease 1 protein, is expressed by epithelial cells in fetal, adult and polycystic kidney. Proc Natl Acad Sci USA 1996;93:1524–1528.

Winyard PJ, Risdon RA, Sams VR, Dressler GR, Woolf AS. The PAX2 transcription factor is expressed in cystic and hyperproliferative dysplastic epithelia in human kidney malformations. J Clin Invest 1996;98:451–459.

Zeller R, Jackson-Grusby L, Leder P. The limb deformity gene is required for apical ectodermal ridge differentiation and anteroposterior limb pattern formation. Genes Dev 1989;3:1481–1492.

65 Mechanisms of Leukocyte Extravasation

M. Amin Arnaout

INTRODUCTION

The recruitment of leukocytes from the blood stream into tissues is a key step in immune surveillance and host defense against pathogens. It is also an essential factor in acute and chronic inflammation. Therefore, elucidation of the molecular events that underlie leukocyte emigration into tissues in physiologic and pathologic states is important in understanding mechanisms of disease and in devising new therapies. In this concise review, current understanding of the molecular basis of leukocyte emigration into tissues is presented.

ANATOMIC FEATURES OF LEUKOCYTE EXTRAVASATION

STAGES IN TRANSENDOTHELIAL MIGRATION OF PHAGOCYTES The transition of leukocytes from the blood into tissues involves a series of interactions between leukocytes and the vascular endothelium. Some of these interactions were elegantly described in the late 19th century by Cohnheim. In classic ex vivo studies using the mesentery and the tongue of frogs, Cohnheim found that as these tissues became irritated by manipulation under the microscope, the vessels dilated, and the blood flow increased transiently, then slowed down. Polymorphonuclear leukocytes (largely neutrophils) began to contact the vessel wall and to roll, with some adhering firmly, and then slowly crept across the endothelium into the extravascular space (Fig. 65-1). Refinements to the technique of intravital video microscopy has since allowed better monitoring and quantitative analysis of these interactions. As leukocytes enter postcapillary venules, they are pushed toward the endothelium by the faster moving (at 1–3 mm/s) red blood cells. In tissues continuously exposed to mechanical and/or chemical stress (such as the skin and gut), a significant proportion of polymorphonuclear leukocytes establish unstable interactions (contact) with endothelium, which, under flow conditions (shear stresses varying between 3 and 20 dyne/cm^2), force a rotational motion of the leukocyte (rolling). The slower speed of rolling leukocytes (approx. 20–60 μm/s) permits some to stick or firmly adhere to endothelium (i.e., become stationary for several seconds) as a prelude to emigration, a process that takes few minutes to complete. Whereas rolling appears to be a necessary precursor to neutrophil extravasation in mesenteric and skin postcapillary venules, it may not be a prerequisite for emigration in other vascular beds. In rabbit lung, for example, neutrophil extravasation occurs in capillaries, not postcapillary venules. The geometric dimensions of such capillaries give little room for neutrophils to roll prior to adhesion and emigration.

The earliest leukocytes present at an inflammatory site tend to be neutrophils. This can be shown experimentally by the intradermal injection of the bacterial-derived product lipopolysaccharide (LPS). This elicits rapid influx of neutrophils peaking within approximately 4 h and soon followed by a mononuclear cell infiltration, which becomes predominant by 48 h. Other types of inflammation are accompanied by the predominance of other leukocyte cell types. For example, parasitic diseases are associated with an inflammatory influx where eosinophils predominate, whereas chronic inflammation is usually accompanied by a predominance of mononuclear cells.

PATTERNS OF LYMPHOCYTE EMIGRATION (HOMING) INTO TISSUES **Homing of Naive Lymphocytes** In contrast to phagocytic cells, most lymphocytes (with the exception of some terminally differentiated cells, such as γδ intraepithelial cells and plasma cells) that cross the endothelial cell barrier into tissues, migrate back to the blood and then again into tissues (i.e., they recirculate). Less than 1:100,000 lymphocytes is specific for a certain antigen, and hence the need for these cells to continuously circulate through the potential ports of "foreign" antigen entry (lungs, skin, and gastrointestinal tract [GI], and their draining lymph nodes) for efficient immune surveillance. Blood to lymph recirculation can be demonstrated experimentally by injecting labeled lymphocytes intravenously and monitoring their appearance in the cannulated thoracic duct and in the spleen, for example. Approximately 40% of injected lymphocytes are recovered from spleen after 1 h, making it the predominant organ through which lymphocytes circulate. An additional 10% of lymphocytes circulate through the rest of secondary lymphoid organs in humans. Under normal conditions, recirculation of naive lymphocytes (those that have not encountered antigen) through secondary lymphoid organs takes place through histologically distinct postcapillary venules called high endothelial venules (HEV), with no significant migration across normal "flat" venular endothelium (Fig. 65-2A). Recirculation through the spleen takes place through blood sinusoids. Extravasated lymphocytes then leave the lymph nodes through the efferent lymphatic vessels. Recirculation of lymphocytes through peripheral and mucosal secondary lymphoid organs is not random: distinct subpopulations target either one or the other

From: *Principles of Molecular Medicine* (J. L. Jameson, ed.), ©1998 Humana Press Inc., Totowa, NJ.

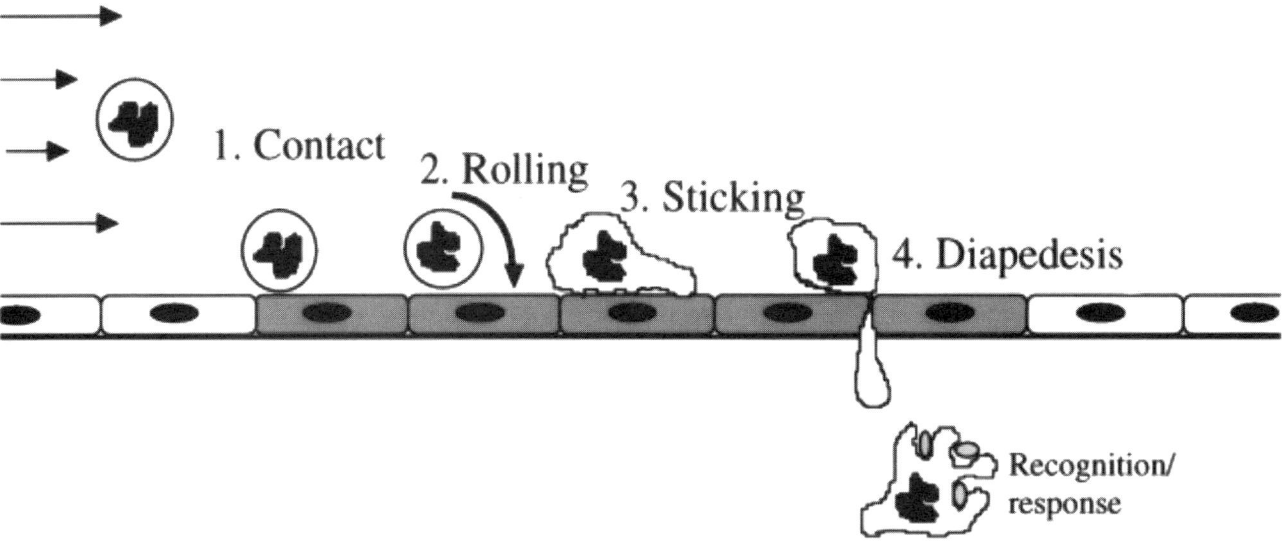

Figure 65-1 Stages in the extravasation of a leukocyte into the extravascular interstitium. Activated endothelial cells are shaded. (*See text* for details.)

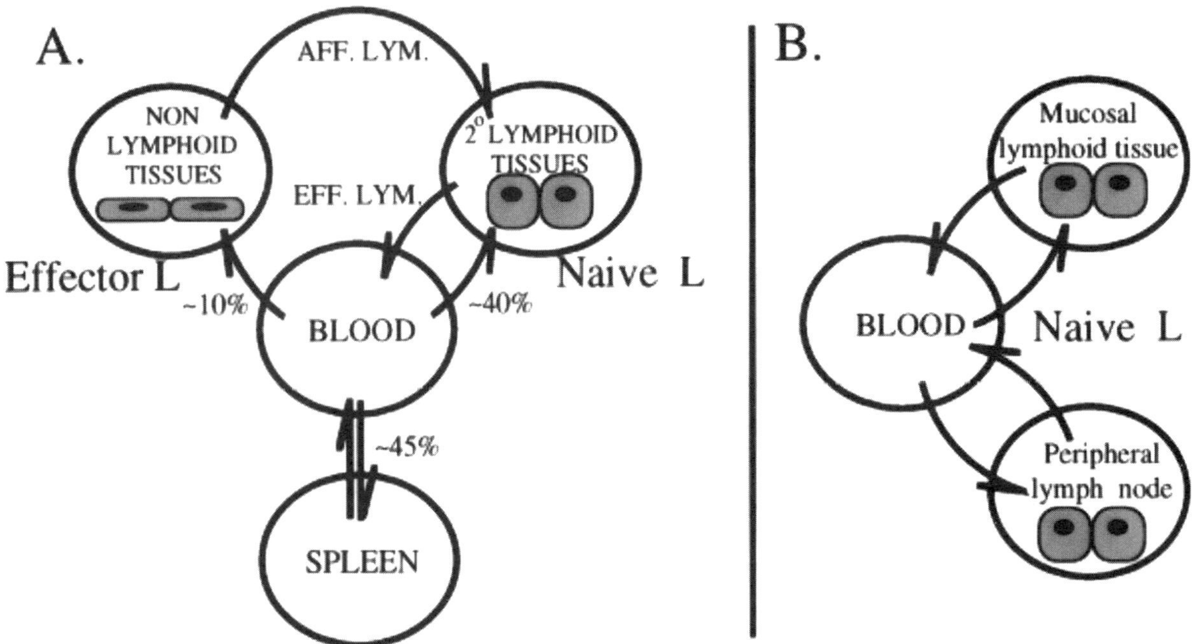

Figure 65-2 Recirculation routes of naive and effector lymphocytes. **(A)** Approximately 40% of naive lymphocytes move between the blood and secondary lymphoid tissues—mucosal lymphoid tissues and peripheral lymph nodes—with subpopulations migrating through either one or the other **(B)**. Naive cells migrate across cuboidal specialized venular endothelium (HEV). Effector lymphocytes extravasate through flat endothelium in nonlymphoid tissues and reach back to mucosal or lymph nodes through afferent lymphatics. (*See text* for details.)

(Fig. 65-2B). Important features of the cuboidal-shaped HEV that may be important in facilitating large-scale migration of lymphocytes include discontinuous intercellular junctions; synthesis of sulfated glycotopes that are unique to this endothelium; and a prominent glycocalyx, which facilitates retention of normally secreted growth factors and adhesion molecules, and of matrix proteins including laminin and fibronectin. HEV endothelium is normally restricted to secondary lymphoid tissues, with the exception of the spleen.

Homing of Activated Lymphocytes Once a naive lymphocyte encounters its antigen, usually on the surface of a dendritic antigen-presenting cell (APC), the lymphocyte is held at this site for several days, in close contact with APC, during which time it is activated by ligation of its antigen receptor in the presence of costimulatory signals, and begins to divide. Its progeny then re-enter the circulation via the efferent lymphatics and through the thoracic duct into the blood. These effector/memory cells, in contrast to their predecessors, acquire the ability to selectively home in on the organs where they first encountered antigen. For example, lymphocytes activated in mucosal intestinal lymphoid tissues (which include organized structures such as Peyer's patches and tonsils) or in the peripheral lymph nodes (PLN) preferentially home back to the gut and PLN, respectively. Their migration into these sites, however, does not normally follow the same path that their predecessors followed: The activated cells preferentially migrate across "flat" endothelium of the nonlymphoid tissues and not through HEV endothelium—their access to the secondary lymphoid organs takes place through the afferent lymphatics draining into this organ (Fig. 65-2A). These distinct migration routes ensure the continuous delivery of naive lymphocytes to sites of antigen exposure, of activated cells to nonlymphoid tissues for antigen elimination, and contribute to the rapid recall and faster responses characteristic of secondary immune reactions.

These "normal" leukocyte migratory patterns can be altered in pathologic states: Effector lymphocytes can extravasate across "flat" and HEV endothelium in acute inflammation. In addition, chronically inflamed extra lymphoid tissues (such as rheumatoid synovium, pancreas in diabetes mellitus, and the thyroid gland in autoimmune thyroiditis), can acquire HEV-like properties, thus facilitating large-scale migration of lymphocytes into these sites.

Table 65-1
Leukocyte and Endothelial Cell Adhesion Molecules Involved in Leukocyte Extravasation

Leukocyte receptor	*Endothelial ligand*
CD62L (L-selectin)	GlyCAM-1; CD34; MadCAM-1; ?[a]
PSGL-1	CD62P (P-selectin); ?
PSGL-1; ESL-1; ?	CD62E (E-selectin)
CD49d/β7 (α4β7)	MadCAM-1; VCAM-1 (CD106); Fibronectin
CD49d/CD29 (α4β1)	CD106; Fibronectin
CD51/CD61 (αVβ3)	CD31 (PECAM-1)
CD11a/CD18 (αLβ2)	ICAM-1 (CD54) ICAM-2 (CD102)
CD11b/CD18 (αMβ2)	CD54; CD102; Fibrinogen; ?
CD11c/CD18 (αXβ2)	Fibrinogen, ?
CD44	?; Hyaluronate; Fibronectin
?	VAP-1[b]
?	VAP-2
?	CD49f/CD29[c] (α6β1, EA-1)

[a]? indicates ligands or receptors that remain to be identified.
[b]VAP-1, VAP-2, vascular adhesion proteins 1 and 2. Their functional significance in vivo is not established.
[c]CD49f/CD29, a laminin receptor that may be involved in lymphocyte adhesion to endothelium and in targeting thymocyte progenitors to the thymus, an area not further discussed in this concise review.

MOLECULAR BASIS OF LEUKOCYTE EXTRAVASATION

Genetic and molecular cloning studies unraveled the major receptor/ligand systems involved in leukocyte extravasation (Table 65-1). These belong to five cell adhesion molecule families, the integrins, selectins, immunoglobulin-like, proteoglycans, and mucins.

The first indication that leukocyte recruitment into tissues is mediated by specific surface receptors came from understanding the pathophysiology of a genetic deficiency in leukocyte-adhesion-dependent functions called leukocyte adhesion molecule (LeuCAM) deficiency (LAD). In this disease, leukocyte contact and rolling on vascular endothelium are intact, but the sticking and diapedesis components of extravasation are defective. Biochemical and immunochemical studies identified the defective leukocyte proteins as CD11/CD18 (β2 integrins), members of the integrin family.

ADHESION MOLECULES MEDIATING EXTRAVASATION OF PHAGOCYTIC CELLS **Contribution of Selectins to Neutrophil Influx** In neutrophils, selectins expressed on leukocytes (L-selectin) and on vascular endothelium (P- and E-selectin) mediate the initial neutrophil contact and rolling on mesenteric venular endothelium. The slower speed of rolling enables leukocytes to sense and react to the local microenvironment. Many inflammatory mediators (presented by endothelia in free or proteoglycan-bound forms) are recognized by G-protein-coupled leukocyte surface receptors belonging to the seven-membrane spanner family, members of which include the IL-8-, C5a-, MCP-1-, and PAF receptors. Ligation of these receptors triggers leukocyte activation. This leads to rapid switching of leukocyte integrins from inactive to active states, that are able to mediate firm adhesion and cell migration (Fig. 65-3). This activation-dependency, which is sensitive to pertussis toxin, a G-protein αi inhibitor, distinguishes firm adhesion from contact and rolling activities. Rolling followed by firm adhesion and neutrophil emigration may proceed in an integrin-dependent but selectin-independent manner when blood flow is reduced or stopped, conditions that prevail in many inflammatory states such as ischemia-reperfusion injury, sepsis, and occlusive vascular diseases.

Each of the three selectins can mediate early contact and neutrophil rolling. Studies in selectin knockout mice reveal complementary roles for P- and L- selectin but overlapping roles for P- and E-selectins in neutrophil contact and rolling. Early contact and rolling caused by surgical exposure of venules is P-selectin-mediated, whereas rolling on cytokine-activated endothelium is L-selectin-dependent. Neutrophil extravasation into the peritoneal cavity of P- or L-selectin-deficient mice is significantly reduced but is normal in E-selectin-deficient mice. Thioglycolate-induced neutrophil accumulation in the peritoneal cavity of E-selectin deficient mice is significantly reduced by anti–P-selectin monoclonal antibodies (MAbs), although this treatment is ineffective in reducing influx in normal mice. Thus, optimal neutrophil extravasation, at least in the peritoneum, is mediated by P- and E-selectin working in concert, in combination with L-selectin. While neutrophil accumulation into the peritoneal cavity is reduced in P-selectin knockout mice, it is unaffected in the lung, emphasizing the important role of vascular hemodynamics as well as tissue-specific endothelial-cell adhesion profiles in recruitment of inflammatory cells in different vascular beds.

Structural and Physical Factors Contributing to Selectin-Mediated Neutrophil Adhesion Selectins project a significant distance from the cell surface (approximately 15–43 nm depending on the number of short concensus complement repeats (SCR) (Fig. 65-3). This provides one likely explanation for their utility in mediating the initial contact between leukocytes and endothelium. The shorter length of L-selectin (only two SCRs) is compensated for by its preferential expression on membrane microvilli. Selectins bind to several ligands in a calcium-dependent manner.

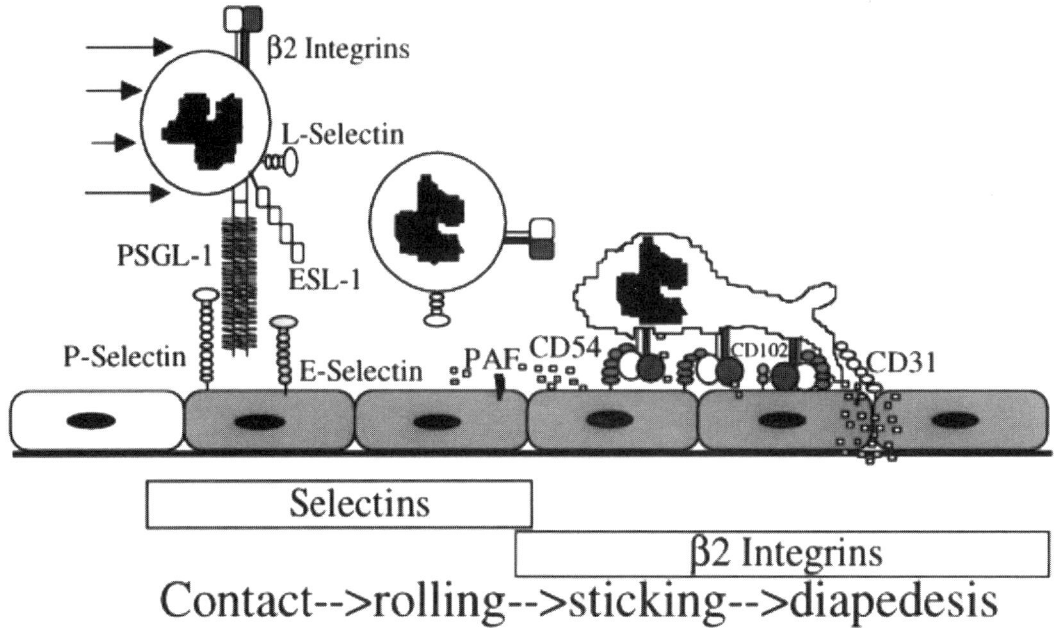

Figure 65-3 Adhesion molecules mediating neutrophil extravasation. Selectins act early in mediating contact and rolling, with integrins mediating sticking and emigration. P-selectin consists of an N-terminal globular lectin domain (~4× 2.5 × 2.5 nm), followed by an EGF-like region (small rectangle in figure), and nine SCRs arranged as rod-shaped structures, with each SCR aligned as a bead fitted into the proposed triple loop structure. The homologous E- and L-selectins contain six and two SCRs, respectively. Alternative spliced forms of selectins have been reported. PSGL-1 is a disulfide-linked dimeric transmembrane glycoprotein having a large mucin ectodomain depicted as a rod-like structure with arbitrary-based carbohydrate branches. ESL-1 contains multiple cysteine-rich repeats with an N-terminal putative ligand binding region. The vascular ligand(s) for neutrophil L-selectin remains to be identified. Integrins, heterodimers of an α-subunit noncovalently associated with a β-subunit, are drawn to accommodate the head and tail morphology revealed by EM studies. Dimensions of the combined head and each tail are 8 × 10 nm and 15 nm, respectively, with the N-terminal halves drawn as squares (low-affinity forms) or as circles (high-affinity forms). Inflammatory mediators are shown as small white boxes, released from the subendothelium and/or surface expressed (as in the case of platelet activating factor, PAF, and others). Integrin ligands CD54, CD102, and CD31 (a ligand for αvβ3) are transmembrane glycoproteins and members of the immunoglobulin (Ig) family (characterized by the presence of the Ig domain with dimensions 4 × 2.5 nm, depicted here as ellipsoidal). CD54, CD102, and CD31 contain five, two, and six Ig domains respectively.

SELECTIN LIGANDS Most selectin ligands carry sialylated or sulfated fucosylated structures, normally expressed on the termini of O- or N-linked oligosaccharides or glycolipids. A common prototype of a selectin ligand is Lewis X (Le^x), a lactosamine (Galβ1-3GlcNAc or Galβ1-4GlcNAc) backbone in an α1-3 linkage to a fucose, and an α2-3 linkage to a sialic acid (sialylated Le^x) or to sulfate (sulfo-Le^x). The affinity of monovalent sLe^x to selectins is low (micromolar to millimolar range). Proper presentation of such monovalent carbohydrates is therefore essential for promoting contact and rolling in vivo. The dense patches of O-linked oligosaccharides, presented by cell surface mucins, may explain why many physiologic selectin ligands belong to this class of glycoproteins. Mucins also assume rigid extended structures (Fig. 65-3), projecting several nanometers from the cell surface, thus providing ample opportunity for the Ca^{2+}-dependent high on-rate, high off-rate interaction that characterizes selectin-ligand interactions.

Neutrophil L-selectin and vascular P-selectin bind to mucin-type ligands. None of the three cloned L-selectin ligands, GlyCAM-1, CD34, or MadCAM-1 (Table 65-1) appear to be involved in promoting neutrophil contact and rolling in post-capillary venules: expression of GlyCAM-1 is limited to HEV endothelium. Although CD34 is expressed by nonlymphoid "flat" endothelium, it does not contain the sulfated oligosaccharides required for recognition by L-selectin. Furthermore, its expression is downregulated by inflammatory cytokines such as IL-1 and tumor necrosis factor-α (TNF-α), which normally promote neutrophil extravasation. MadCAM-1 expressed on "flat" endothelium also lacks L-selectin-binding carbohydrates. These observations suggest that L-selectin-mediated neutrophil contact and rolling in postcapillary venules is mediated by yet to be characterized carbohydrate-based ligands.

The P-selectin ligand on neutrophils is a cell surface mucin dimer called PSGL-1 (Table 65-1, Fig. 65-3). PSGL-1 is expressed on neutrophils, monocytes, NK cells, and lymphocyte subsets. PSGL-1 can also be recognized by E-selectin, accounting perhaps for the functional overlap between P- and E-selectins. Another P-selectin ligand was recently isolated from mouse neutrophils and HL60 cells, and appears to be a sialylated glycoprotein of 160 kDa (80 kDa reduced). Its structure is unknown at present. E-selectin also binds to ESL-1, a nonmucin leukocyte glycoprotein that is identical to fibroblast growth factor receptor (FGFR) type 3. ESL-1 is ubiquitous, but is only sialylated and fucosylated in myeloid cells, and therefore serves as an E-selectin ligand in these cell types. The contribution of ESL-1 to neutrophil contact and rolling in vivo remains to be established.

Regulated Expression of Selectins L-selectin is constitutively expressed in leukocytes, but is rapidly shed when cells are activated. P-selectin is expressed within few minutes on the endothelial cell surface as a result of mobilization of intracellular vesicles (Weibel-Pallade bodies) by thrombin or histamine. Other stimuli such as oxygen-free radicals and TNF-α can maintain this expression for longer periods by preventing the normal endocytosis of expressed P-selectin and through increased synthesis, respectively. E-selectin is newly synthesized and expressed within 1–4 h in response to lipopolysaccharides or cytokines such as interleukin-1 (IL-1) and TNF-α, with the level of expression returning to baseline by 24–48 h in vitro. The rapid expression of P-selectin makes it an ideal candidate for rapid neutrophil contact and rolling observed on venular endothelium. Expression of both P- and E-selectin at later time points may explain the observations that P-selectin can compensate for E-selectin deficiency, and that loss of contact and rolling is incomplete in P-selectin knockout mice.

Mechanisms of Integrin-Mediated Neutrophil Adhesion Integrin-mediated firm adhesion occurs through β2 integrins, the predominant integrins expressed in neutrophils. β2 integrins bind to ligands expressed on vascular endothelium such as CD54 (ICAM-1) and CD102 (ICAM-2) and others that remain to be identified (Fig. 65-3). Transendothelial migration (across tight junctions) is also integrin-mediated. Both firm adhesion and transendothelial migration are energy-dependent processes requiring cell activation and the transformation of integrins from low- to high-avidity states. Although integrins are essential in emigration, the counter receptors involved and the events that facilitate this transition are not clearly defined at present. CD31, a heavily glycosylated Ig member, which is preferentially expressed at endothelial tight junctions, can serve as a counter-receptor for integrin αVβ3. The migrating neutrophil induces endothelial cell retraction through an increase in endothelial cell intracellular Ca^{2+}, thus transiently loosening the tight junctions while squeezing through. A homophilic interaction between neutrophil and endothelial CD31 may be involved in this process. Migration through the basement membrane and subendothelial tissues, rich in matrix proteins and hyaluronate, may involve CD44, an abundant neutrophil proteoglycan, in addition to leukocyte integrins.

Factors Contributing to the Influx of Other Phagocytic Cells In contrast to neutrophils, where β2 integrins predominate, eosinophils and monocytes express additional members of the integrin family, including β1, β3, and β7, which may play complementary or overlapping roles in the emigration of these cells. Thus, the nature and kinetics of appearance of leukocyte subpopulations at an inflammatory site (for example, the early appearance of neutrophils in infected regions, or the accumulation of eosinophils at allergic sites) are determined in part by the intrinsic adhesion profile of leukocytes. In addition, the type of inflammatory mediators present and the nature and kinetics of the endothelial and leukocyte adhesion responses to these mediators are crucial. Some mediators are cell-specific (e.g., monocyte chemotactic protein 1 [MCP-1] and IL-5 for monocytes and eosinophils, respectively); IL-4 selectively upregulates expression of CD106 (VCAM-1) on endothelial cells, thus facilitating the influx of eosinophils and mononuclear cells that express α4 integrins (the receptors for CD106). Other mediators induce the influx of leukocyte subtypes by increasing expression of a number of endothelial CAMs (e.g., the monokines IL-1 and TNF-α induce expression of CD54, CD106, E-, and P-selectins) and/or by activating leukocytes (e.g., C5a, IL-8, platelet activating factor, GM-CSF, and TNF-α activate neutrophils and monocytes). Inflammatory mediators may act additively, synergistically, or antagonistically. For example, interferon-γ (INF-γ), together with LPS or TNF-α (but not IL-1), prolongs expression of E-selectin. TGF-β and IL-4, either alone or in combination, inhibit cytokine-induced E-selectin expression. Finally, differences exist in the adhesive phenotype of endothelium from different vascular beds, and in its response to mediators. IL-1 and TNF-α are poor inducers of CD54 on cultured synovial-derived endothelium, in contrast to umbilical vein-derived endothelium. TNF-α can upregulate expression of CD54 and E-selectin on both arterial and venous-derived endothelium, but the inducible expression of CD106 by TNF-α is restricted to venular endothelium. Other agonists, such as oxidized LDL or lysophosphocholine (that are associated with atherogenesis), can induce CD106 (and CD54) expression on cultured arterial endothelium and likely contribute to the inflammatory origins of atherosclerosis.

ADHESION MOLECULES MEDIATING LYMPHOCYTE EXTRAVASATION As in the case of transendothelial emigration of phagocytes, endothelial- and leukocyte-adhesion molecules and mediators orchestrate the trafficking of lymphocyte subpopulations into lymphoid and nonlymphoid organs.

Migration of Naive Lymphocytes Recirculation of naive cells through HEV in PLN and in mucosal lymphoid tissues, such as Peyer's patches (PP), is largely mediated by L-selectin and by L-selectin and α4β7 integrin, respectively (Fig. 65-4). P-selectin is not involved, since most lymphocytes lack P-selectin ligands. Migration into both tissues requires β2 integrins. Supporting evidence comes from knockout mice, in which L-selectin deficiency leads to loss of naive cell recirculation through PLN nodes but only to a 50% reduction in recirculation through PP. Expression of the sulfated L-selectin ligands CD34 and GlyCAM-1, but not MadCAM-1 on PLN HEV, is in large part responsible for the fact that lymphocyte recruitment to PLN is L-selectin-mediated. Although GlyCAM-1 is not an integral membrane protein, it may still be involved in adhesion through an association with the thick glycocalyx of HEV. MadCAM-1 expression on PP and the lack of GlyCAM-1 expression in this tissue are important determinants in directing lymphocyte trafficking to PP. MadCAM-1 binds L-selectin through its mucin domain and integrin α4β7 through its N-terminal Ig-domain, thus accounting for the limited dependency of lymphocyte trafficking to PP on L-selectin (Fig. 65-4), and for the fact that mucosal lymphoid tissues in L-selectin knockout mice are populated by lymphocytes. Lymphocyte contact and rolling on PP HEV can be mediated by L-selectin or by α4β7, with the latter also contributing to firm adhesion. The selective expression of α4β7 on microvilli (as in the case of selectins) may in part explain its ability to mediate lymphocyte contact and rolling. β2 integrins also contribute to the pertussis-sensitive firm adhesion and emigration (Fig. 65-4). Their partial role in lymphocytes is predicted by the nearly normal lymphocyte extravasation and functions in Leu-CAM deficiency (LAD). The nature of the "physiologic" mediators involved in integrin activation during lymphocyte recirculation is undetermined at present.

Emigration of Effector/Memory Cells The phenotype of the leukocyte and receptive endothelium are also largely responsible for the predominant migration of effector lymphocytes through "flat" endothelium. Effector lymphocytes are largely L-selectin-negative but display preactivated integrins (Fig. 65-5). In addition,

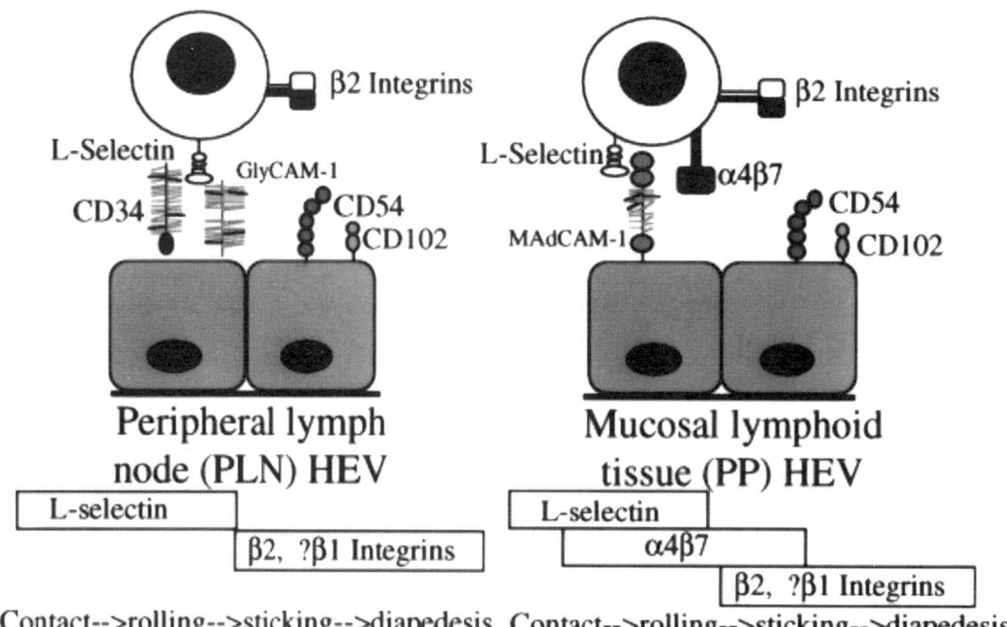

Figure 65-4 Major adhesion molecules mediating recirculation of naive lymphocytes. The L-selectin ligands CD34 and GlyCAM-1 on PLN HEV have mucin domains, as well as sulfated moieties (shown as black branches). MadCAM-1 is also sulfated on PP HEV (but not on "flat" endothelium) and is composed of a mucin domain as well as three Ig domains. (*See text* for details.)

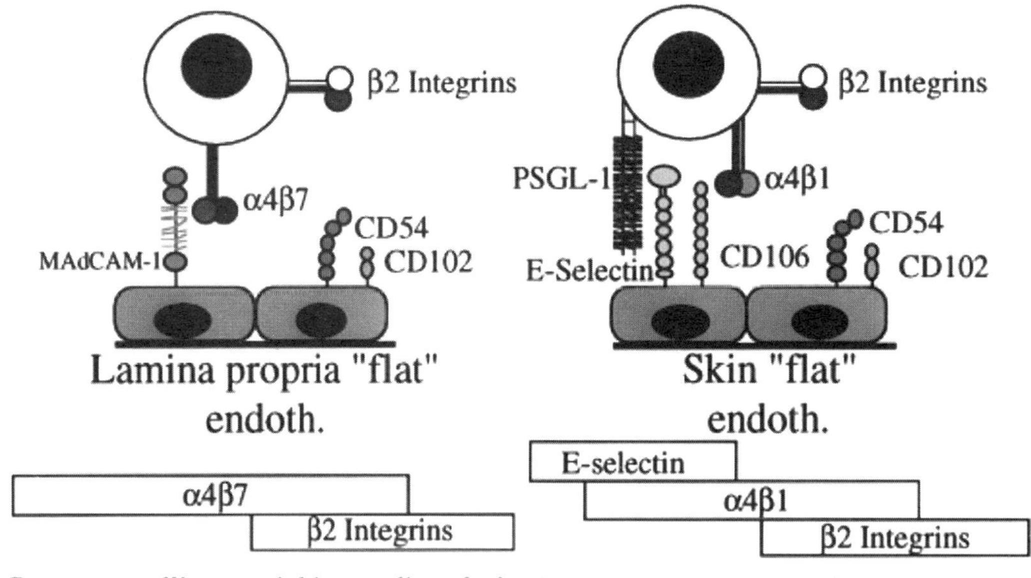

Figure 65-5 Major adhesion receptors mediating recirculation of effector lymphocytes. CD106, an Ig member with seven Ig domains (and alternatively spliced forms) serves as a ligand for α4 integrins in inflamed endothelium. (*See text* for details.)

MadCAM-1 is expressed in lesser amounts on flat endothelium compared to HEV, and is not properly sulfated, ensuring a predominance of α4β7 and α4β1 integrins in mediating contact, rolling, and firm adhesion in nonlymphoid tissues of the gut and inflamed organs, respectively. Effector lymphocytes (with preactivated integrins) also tend to arrest rapidly after very brief (or no) rolling. β2 integrins also contribute to firm adhesion and emigration (Fig. 65-5). High expression of CD44 on effector/memory cells may facilitate lymphocyte migration through the subendothelium.

Lymphocyte Homing to Other Nonlymphoid Tissues L-selectin plays minimal roles in targeting lymphocyte subsets to the skin, since venular endothelium generally lacks the glycotopes required for recognition by L-selectin. This, together with the fact that most lymphocytes do not express functional P-selectin ligands, may explain why contact and rolling are mediated by the vascular

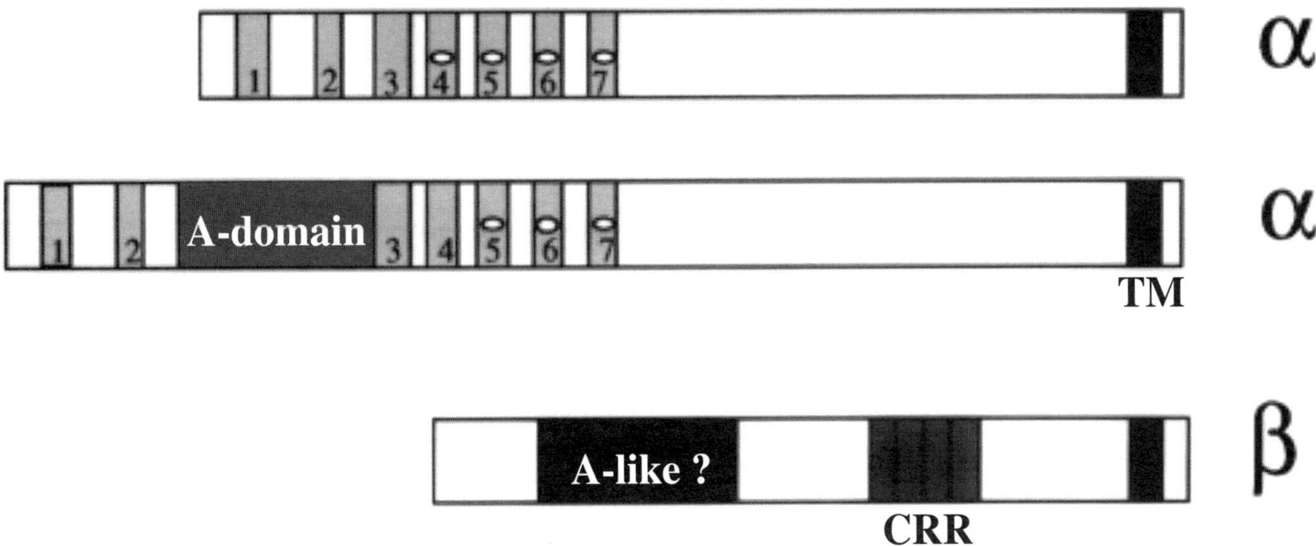

Figure 65-6 Schematic diagram showing the primary structural features of integrin α- and β-subunits. Three or four of the seven repeats in the ectodomain of the α chains (generally repeats 4–7 and 5–7 in integrins lacking and containing the α A-domain, respectively) contain consensus metal binding sites (indicated by closed circles). The position of the A-domain, present in the α chains of all four β2 integrins, as well as those of α1β1, α2β1, and αEβ7, is shown. The β chain contains a C-terminal, four cysteine-rich repeats (CRR), and a putative A-like domain. Both the α and β chains span the plasma membrane once and contain, with the exception of β4, short cytoplasmic tails.

E-selectin, which is constitutively expressed in this tissue (Fig. 65-5). Vascular E-selectin binds to a cutaneous lymphocyte antigen (CLA) that is identical to a modified form of PSGL-1. Lymphocytes targeted to skin are α4β1-positive but α4β7-negative, and are therefore likely to utilize α4β1 integrin to mediate contact and rolling in an analogous manner to mucosal-targeted lymphocytes. As in most other tissues, β2 integrins contribute to lymphocyte firm adhesion and emigration. It remains unclear if novel organ-specific receptor/ligands or combinations of already known adhesion molecules are responsible for selective lymphocyte emigration to other organs such as lung, central nervous system, joints, or pancreas in disease states. The acquisition of the HEV phenotype in chronic inflammatory disorders affecting these organs (e.g., rheumatoid arthritis, multiple sclerosis, diabetes mellitus) and the anti-inflammatory effects of MAbs directed against selectins and/or integrins in animal models of these diseases, argue that already known receptors/ligand pairs are involved in lymphocyte emigration in these pathologic states.

STRUCTURAL ANALYSIS OF THE SELECTIN AND INTEGRIN LIGAND-BINDING SITES

SELECTIN LIGAND-BINDING DOMAIN The crystal structure of the C-type lectin-EGF domains of human E-selectin was recently solved. The lectin domain, which contains the ligand-binding site, is ovoid in shape, consisting of five β strands, two α-helices, and an extended number of loops. It contains a Ca^{2+} ion, well-coordinated by the side chains of E80, N82, N105, D106, the main chain carbonyl of D106, and two water molecules, forming the typical pentagonal bipyramid coordination sphere. The side chains of the conserved amino acids essential for ligand binding (Y48, N82, N83, E92, Y94, K11, and K113) lie on the same face as the bound Ca^{2+}, forming a single binding site, which can coordinate a monovalent carbohydrate ligand such as sLe^x. How such an arrangement allows selectin–ligand interactions with rapid on/off rates and of sufficient affinities to withstand the forces applied by the blood flow is unclear at present. One hypothesis proposes that affinity of a selectin-monovalent saccharide pair may be significantly enhanced by receptor clustering, as in other receptor-ligand interactions. Another view contends that side-chains from separate but clustered saccharide units (displayed by a mucin or a proteoglycan) would bind with higher affinity to an individual receptor lectin domain.

INTEGRIN LIGAND-BINDING DOMAINS Integrins bind to structurally unrelated ligands, including immunoglobulins, proteoglycans, cadherins, complement proteins, coagulation factors, and a large number of matrix proteins. Despite the structural complexity and diversity of these ligands, one common feature that is essential for recognition by integrins is a short and surface-accessible sequence containing a negatively charged aspartic acid or glutamic acid residue. Integrin binding to most ligands is also dependent on divalent cations and requires rapid switching of integrins from a low- to a high-avidity state in response to cell activation signals. Increased affinity appears to be a result of activation-dependent conformational changes in integrins. Such changes are suggested by certain MAbs that react with integrins after, but not before, cellular activation. The best candidates for integrin activation in the vasculature are chemokines acting through their G-protein-coupled receptors. The nature of the conformational changes that lead to a change in integrin affinity is not known.

Chemical crosslinking, mutagenesis, peptide inhibition and/or direct ligand binding studies using isolated integrin domains have identified three potential ligand binding regions (Fig. 65-6). One major site is located in a von Willebrand factor (vWF) A-type domain present in the extracellular region of the α-subunit of seven integrins. This domain undergoes conformational changes in response to activation in whole cells and binds directly to several integrin ligands in a divalent-cation–dependent manner. A second metal-dependent ligand binding site is located in a proposed A-like domain present in all integrin β-subunits. Identification of this site was based on chemical crosslinking, peptide inhibition studies, and mutagenesis of single amino acids that block integrin ligand binding. No direct binding studies have so far been carried out using the isolated A-like β domain. It is important to recognize that this domain is also involved in the noncovalent association of the integrin β-subunits to their α-subunit counterparts. A third putative ligand binding region has been mapped to the EF-hand-like calcium binding domains 5 and 6 of the α-subunits (Fig. 65-6).

Crystal structure of the A-domain from integrin CD11b revealed that it adopts the common "dinucleotide-binding" α/β fold, with seven amphipathic α-helices surrounding a mostly parallel centrally located hydrophobic β-sheet. A single divalent cation binding site—metal ion-dependent adhesion site (MIDAS)—is located in a crevice at the top of the β-sheet, explaining the divalent-cation-dependent binding of this domain to several ligands. The MIDAS motif comprises a DxSxS sequence (residues 140–144 in CD11b, D, aspartic acid, S, serine x = any amino acid) from the βA-α1 loop, threonine (T)209 from the α3-α4 loop, and D242 from the βD-α5 loop. The two serines and the threonine make strong bonds to the metal via their sidechain hydroxyl oxygen atoms; two water molecules also bind directly to the metal, and the two aspartates make indirect contacts via water molecules. In the crystal, the side chain of a glutamate residue from a neighboring molecule completes the metal coordination. This arrangement may be a mimic of a natural integrin–ligand interaction and may explain the essential role of acidic residues in integrin ligands. The DxSxS motif is present in the β conserved region, which also assumes a similar hydropathy profile, forming the basis for the proposal that a modified A-like domain is also present in all integrin β-subunits. Recent studies show that the integrin A-domain also exists in a second conformation, suggesting a structural basis for the conformational changes observed at integrin activation.

LEUKOCYTE ADHESION AS A TARGET OF ANTI-INFLAMMATORY THERAPEUTICS

Since excessive accumulation of activated leukocytes in extravascular tissues contributes to several acute and chronic inflammatory disorders, targeting the responsible receptors to prevent injury has been a major therapeutic goal. Blocking MAbs to selectins, β2 and α4 integrins, and some of their ligands (e.g., CD54, CD31) have been found to markedly attenuate the parenchymal and microvascular dysfunctions observed in several animal models of inflammation, including ischemia-reperfusion injury, allograft rejection, antigen-induced arthritis, diabetes mellitus, immune complex-induced alveolitis, and glomerulonephritis. The inhibitory effects of anti-β2 integrin/ligand MAbs in these models is understandably incomplete, as patients with β2 integrin deficiency display near-normal functions of mononuclear cells. As discussed above, mononuclear leukocytes display and use multiple integrins in mediating cell adhesion, in contrast to neutrophils, which predominantly express β2 integrins. In these, as well as other models of immunologic injury, use of anti-α4 MAbs has significant anti-inflammatory effects. As expected *(see above)*, a combination of anti-β2 and α4 integrin antibodies was found to almost completely inhibit mononuclear leukocyte recruitment in the majority of the inflammation models tested. Since integrins not only mediate extravasation but also several potentially harmful functions in the extravascular interstitium (e.g., bystander damage to healthy tissues, associated with phagocytosis, exocytosis of toxic compounds, and target cell killing), some of the beneficial effects of anti-β2 and anti-α4 integrin MAbs can also alleviate injury despite little or no inhibitory effects on extravasation.

Blocking MAbs directed against L-, P- or E-selectins also reduce inflammation in several models of ischemia-reperfusion injury, immune-complex diseases, and acute inflammation. The protective effects observed using single anti-selectin MAbs have been partial, and may require targeting all three selectins simultaneously, as suggested by the gene knockout studies described above.

SUMMARY

Significant progress has been made in understanding the molecular basis of the migration of various leukocytes from the blood stream into tissues under physiologic and pathologic states. Specific adhesion molecules on leukocytes and the vascular endothelium intertwine in response to locally released inflammatory signals to generate selective migration patterns, which ensure efficient surveillance of the body compartments by immune and inflammatory cells. While the identity of some adhesion and signaling molecules involved in leukocyte extravasation remains to be defined (Table 65-1), the therapeutic potential of targeting some of the already known key receptors has been amply documented in animal models of inflammatory diseases, and more recently in phase II and III clinical trials. Structural and biochemical studies are beginning to unravel the fine details of receptor–ligand interactions and should help in reconstructing the structural basis for the dynamic interaction between receptors and ligands during leukocyte emigration. These approaches will likely lead to more specific small molecule-based therapeutics.

ACKNOWLEDGMENTS

We thank Colleen Loiselle for secretarial help. The author's work is supported by grants from the National Institutes of Health.

SELECTED REFERENCES

Albelda SM, Smith CW, Ward PA. Adhesion molecules and inflammatory injury. FASEB J 1994;8:504–512.

Allport JR, Ding HT, Ager A, Steeber DA, Tedder TF, Luscinskas FW. L-selectin shedding does not regulate human neutrophil attachment, rolling, or transmigration across human vascular endothelium in vitro. J Immunol 1997;158:4365–4372.

Arbones ML, Ord DC, Ley K, et al. Lymphocyte homing and leukocyte rolling and migration are impaired in L-selectin (CD62L) deficient mice. Immunity 1994;1:247–260.

Arnaout MA. Leukocyte adhesion molecule deficiency: its structural basis, pathophysiology and implications for modulating the inflammatory response. Immunol Rev 1990;114:145–180.

Arnaout MA. Structural diversity of cell adhesion molecules and their role in inflammation. (Chapter 20) In: Kelley WN, Harris ED, Ruddy S, Sledge CB, eds. Textbook of Rheumatology. 1997; pp. 303–322.

Bargatze RF, Butcher EC. Rapid G protein-regulated activation event involved in lymphocyte binding to high endothelial venules. J Exp Med 1993;178:367–372.

Bargatze RF, Jutila MA, Butcher EC. Distinct roles of L-selectin and integrins α4β7 and LFA-1 in lymphocyte homing to Peyer's patch-HEV in situ: the multistep model confirmed and refined. Immunity 1995;3:99–108.

Baumhueter S, Dybdal N, Kyle C, Lasky LA. Global vascular expression of murine CD34, a sialomucin-like endothelial ligand for L-selectin. Blood 1994;84:2554–2565.

Bullard DC, Qin L, Lorenzo I, et al. P-selectin/ICAM-1 double mutant mice show a complete block in peritoneal emigration of neutrophils. J Clin Invest 1995;95:1782–1788.

Butcher EC, Picker LJ, Butcher EC. Lymphocyte homing and homeostasis. Science 1996;272:60–66.

Carlos TM, Harlan JM. Leukocyte-endothelial adhesion molecules. Blood 1994;84:2068–2101.

Clark RA, Erickson HP, Springer TA. Tenascin supports lymphocyte rolling. J Cell Biol 1997;137:755–765.

Cohnheim J. Lectures in General Pathology, 2nd ed., vol. 1 (translated from the 2nd German ed.) London: The New Sydenham Society; 1889.

Downey GP, Worthern GS, Henson PM, Hyde DM. Neutrophil sequestration and migration in localized pulmonary inflammation. Am Rev Resp Dis 1993;147:168–176.

Frenette PS, Mayadas TN, Rayburn H, Hynes RO, Wagner DD. Susceptibility to infection and altered hematopoiesis in mice deficient in both P- and E-selectins. Cell 1996;84:563–574.

Frenette PS, Wagner DD. Insights into selectin function from knockout mice. Thromb Haemost 1997;78:60–64.

Fuhlbrigge RC, Kieffer JD, Armerding D, Kupper TS. Cutaneous lymphocyte antigen is a specialized form of PSGL-1 expressed on skin-homing T cells. Nature 1997;389:978–981.

Gaboury JP, Kubes P. Reductions in physiologic shear rates lead to CD11/CD18-dependent, selectin-independent leukocyte rolling in vivo. Blood 1994;83:345–350.

Gailit J, Clark RAF. Wound repair in the context of extracellular matrix. Curr Opin Cell Biol 1994;6:717–725.

Labow MA, Norton CR, Rumberger JM, et al. Characterization of E-selectin-deficient mice: demonstration of overlapping function of endothelial selectins. Immunity 1994;1:709–720.

Lazaar AL, Albelda SM, Pilewski JM, Brennan B, Pure E, Panettieri RA Jr. T lymphocytes adhere to airway smooth muscle cells via integrins and CD44 and induce smooth muscle cell DNA synthesis. J Exp Med 1994;180:807–816.

Lee J-O, Rieu P, Arnaout MA, Liddington R. Crystal structure of the A-domain from the α-subunit of β2 integrin complement receptor type 3 (CR3, CD11b/CD18). Cell 1995;80:631–638.

Lesley JR, Hyman R, Kincade PW. CD44 and its interaction with the extracellular matrix. Adv Immunol 1994;54:271–335.

Mayadas TN, Johnson RC, Rayburn H, Hynes RO, Wagner DD. Leukocyte rolling and extravasation are severely compromised in P-selectin-deficient mice. Cell 1993;74:541–554.

Michishita M, Videm V, Arnaout MA. A novel divalent cation-binding site in the A domain of the β2 integrin CR3 (CD11b/CD18) is essential for ligand binding. Cell 1993;72:857–867.

Muller WA, Weigl SA, Deng X, Phillips DM. PECAM-1 is required for transendothelial migration of leukocytes. J Exp Med 1993;178:449–460.

Mulligan MS, Warren JS, Smith CW, et al. Lung injury after deposition of IgA immune complexes. J Immunol 1992;148:3086–3092.

Rosen SD, Bertozzi CR, Leukocyte adhesion: two selectins converge on sulphate. Curr Biol 1996;6:261–264.

Ross R. The pathogenesis of atherosclerosis: a perspective for the 1990s. Nature 1993;362:801–809.

Rossiter H, Alon R, Kupper TS. Selectins, T-cell rolling and inflammation. Mol Med Today 1997;3:214–222.

Salmi M, Granfors K, MacDermott R, Jalkanen S. Aberrant binding of lamina propria lymphocytes to vascular endothelium in inflammatory bowel diseases. Gastroenterology 1994;106:595–605.

Salmi M, Jalkanen S. Human vascular adhesion protein 1 (VAP-1) is a unique sialoglycoprotein that mediates carbohydrate-dependent binding of lymphocytes to endothelial cells. J Exp Med 1996;183:569–579.

Schmid-Schonbein GW, Usami S, Skalak R, Chien S. The interaction of leukocytes and erythrocytes in capillary and postcapillary vessels. Microvasc Res 1980;19:45–70.

Springer, TA. Traffic signals for lymphocyte recirculation and leukocyte emigration: the multistep paradigm. Cell 1994;76:301–314.

Varki A. Selectin ligands. Proc Natl Acad Sci USA 1994;91:7390–7397.

66 Ischemic Acute Renal Failure

Joseph V. Bonventre

INTRODUCTION

Acute renal failure (ARF) is a clinical syndrome characterized by a deterioration of renal function over hours to days, with associated failure of the kidney to excrete nitrogenous waste products and to maintain fluid and electrolyte homeostasis. This clinical entity was defined in the seminal works of Bywaters, who characterized it in victims of aerial bombings during World War II. Bywaters described tubular cell necrosis and intratubular pigmented casts in the kidneys of these patients.

ARF can result from decreased delivery of oxygen and nutrients to renal tubular cells, a toxic or obstructive insult to the renal tubule, a tubulointerstitial process with inflammation and edema, or a glomerular disease resulting in a primary reduction in glomerular filtration. If the defect in clearance is related to obstruction of urinary outflow, the ARF is termed "postrenal." ARF is "prerenal" if the kidney itself is functionally normal or near-normal, so that kidney function is abnormal because of decreased renal blood flow. If the reduction in total organ or local blood flow becomes severe enough to cause tubular cell injury, prerenal ARF has progressed to "ischemic" ARF with tubular necrosis, loss of concentrating ability, and loss of ability of the kidney to conserve sodium. Prerenal azotemia and ischemic ARF are responsible for most episodes of ARF. Nephrotoxins are responsible for the next largest category of causes of ARF. Radiocontrast agents and various drugs including aminoglycosides are the most common toxic causes of ARF.

Since ischemia is the primary cause of ARF, most of what we know about the cellular and molecular features of ARF have been established using ischemia as the model insult in animals and as the focus of studies in humans. We will devote this chapter primarily to ischemic ARF. One should recognize, however, that many of the features of postischemic ARF are likely to be applicable to toxic ARF, where the pathological features of tubular injury are quite similar to those seen in the postischemic state.

The pathophysiology of ischemic renal injury is relevant not only to the acute setting associated with reduction in total renal perfusion but also to diseases such as hemolytic uremic syndrome, thrombotic thrombocytopenic purpura (TTP), acute vasculitis, and acute atheroembolic disease. In addition, many chronic diseases of the kidney result in ischemic injury to this organ. These include renal vascular disease, diabetic and hypertensive nephropathy, collagen vascular diseases, and chronic tubulointerstitial diseases.

There are vascular and tubular components to the pathophysiology of ischemic ARF. In this chapter, we will review the vascular, cellular, and molecular features of the pathophysiology of tubular cell injury. We will then discuss the molecular response of cells to hypoxia and relate this to gene induction in the kidney in response to ischemia. Finally, the important features of the repair process of the kidney after an ischemic insult will be presented.

VASCULAR COMPONENT OF ARF

The pathophysiology of ischemic acute renal failure is complex. There is clearly an important vascular component to the injury, not only at the level of total renal perfusion but also at the microvascular level where heterogeneity of blood flow, arteriolar vasoconstriction, and capillary obstruction limit oxygen delivery to renal tubular cells, whose oxygen needs are quite high. At a systemic level, inadequate blood flow to the kidney may result from hypotension, decreased cardiac function, renal artery stenosis, or occlusion. Within the kidney, small vessel disease secondary to atherosclerosis, atheroemboli, or vasculitis can result in ischemia. In addition, ischemia may result from local vasoconstriction due to an imbalance between vasoconstrictive and vasodilatory factors. These changes in vasoconstrictive forces may result from systemic vasoactive agents that are active locally on the small vessels of the kidney. Alternatively, damage to the endothelium, or alteration in endothelial function, may result in decreased production of vasodilatory substances, such as nitric oxide. With ischemia and reperfusion, there is preglomerular vasoconstriction that results in a primary reduction in glomerular filtration rate (GFR). Vasodilatory responses to agents such as acetylcholine are decreased in the postischemic tissue. There also is loss of autoregulation, with ischemic renal failure interfering with the normal vasodilatation that occurs in response to lowering of intraluminal pressure at the microvascular level.

There have been therapeutic attempts in animals as well as in humans to counter the vasoconstriction that occurs with ischemic acute renal failure. The renal vasculature is quite sensitive to endothelin, which reduces renal blood flow and glomerular filtration rate (GFR). Intraarterial injection of antibodies into a branch of the rat renal artery results in preservation of postischemic glomerular blood flow and single-nephron GFR in the region of the kidney supplied by the branch artery. Dopamine has been administered for both prevention and treatment of ARF in critically ill

From: *Principles of Molecular Medicine* (J. L. Jameson, ed.), ©1998 Humana Press Inc., Totowa, NJ.

patients. Clinical studies, however, do not support the routine use of dopamine for either prophylaxis or established ARF. Furthermore, the benefit of dopamine may be outweighed by its potential side effects, such as tachyarrhythmias, pulmonary shunting, and gut or digital necrosis.

Because calcium within vascular smooth muscle cells increases vascular tone and contributes to vasoconstriction, calcium channel blockers have been used as renovascular vasodilators. Their utility in ARF has been demonstrated in renal allografts, where calcium antagonists reduce the incidence of tubular necrosis and delayed graft function. Furthermore, in other conditions in which vasoconstriction is prominent, such as cyclosporine therapy and radiocontrast-induced ARF, calcium channel blocking agents have been reported to be effective in prevention of ARF. The use of these agents is limited, however, by their potential to cause systemic hypotension and therefore worsen ARF.

In animals, atrial natriuretic peptides (ANPs) attenuate the severity and potentiate the recovery of renal function even when administered after the ischemic insult in experimental ARF. This effect is presumed to be a result of the vasodilatory actions of ANPs, although these agents are also natriuretic and diuretic. Preliminary results from a multicenter prospective study indicate that these agents do not have a beneficial role in patients with ARF.

Heterogeneity of blood flow plays an important role in the pathophysiology of ischemic renal failure. Differences in the distribution of blood flow contributes to the heterogeneous nature of the tubule lesions seen with ischemia. Vascular congestion in the outer medulla and decreased blood flow to this region are features of experimental ischemic acute renal failure in rats. This vascular congestion may result in part from swelling of endothelial or tubular epithelial cells, resulting in interference with flow through the vasa recta.

The vulnerability of the tubules in the outer medulla is also enhanced by the vasa recta countercurrent exchange of oxygen, which results in a marked drop-off in oxygen tension, with increasing distance into the medulla from the cortex. The S3 segment, pars recta, of the proximal tubule, traverses this region and is more sensitive to ischemic injury than is the S1 or S2 segment. This vulnerability results from the imbalance between metabolic demand and oxygen delivery in this nephron segment. While many medullary cells increase their rates of glycolysis in an anaerobic environment, S3 proximal tubule cells in the outer medulla are not able to preserve their ATP levels using the glycolytic pathway, despite their ability to utilize glucose as an energy source to a greater extent than can S1 and S2 proximal cells.

Ischemia also results in primary changes in the glomeruli. The major morphological change in glomeruli of postischemic kidneys is capillary loop collapse, which is probably secondary to mesangial and vascular smooth muscle cell contraction. There is also flattening of the visceral epithelial cell bodies with increased permeability.

TUBULAR COMPONENT OF ARF

A pathological hallmark of ischemic and toxic ARF is tubular necrosis. With ischemia and reperfusion there are structural, biochemical, and vascular changes in the kidney that result in desquamation of viable and nonviable tubular cells, intraluminal tubular obstruction, and transtubular backleak of the glomerular filtrate.

STRUCTURAL CHANGES Early morphological changes observed with ischemia include disruption of the microtubular and actin cytoskeletal networks and blebbing of proximal tubule cell apical membranes with loss of the brush border. Proximal tubule cells lose their polarity and the integrity of their tight junctions, perhaps as a consequence of alterations in the actin cytoskeleton. Within 15 min of ischemia, Na^+-K^+-ATPase redistributes from the basolateral to the apical membrane, interfering with Na^+ and Na^+-coupled vectorial transport in the proximal tubule. There is loss of adhesion of viable epithelial cells, perhaps because of redistribution of integrins to the apical surface. Live and dead cells slough into the tubular lumen, contributing to cast formation. Tubular obstruction results in increased intratubular pressure and a reduction in GFR. Arg-Gly-Asp (RGD) peptides are partially protective against ischemic injury in animals. These peptides are proposed to act by interfering with cell–cell adhesion in the tubular lumen, thus preventing the increase in proximal tubular pressure normally observed in ischemic acute renal failure in animals. Loss of the epithelial cell barrier and the tight junctions between viable cells results in backleak of the glomerular filtrate, further reducing effective GFR. RGD peptide binding sites have also been identified along the intimal surface of blood vessels in ischemic kidneys.

Given the importance of intratubular obstruction to the pathophysiology of ARF, a potential approach to therapy would be to increase intratubular flow rate in an attempt to decrease the formation of obstructing casts. Furosemide and bumetanide have been used with this rationale. While these diuretics have been shown in experimental animal models to partially protect the kidney against ischemic injury, many studies in humans have failed to demonstrate effectiveness of these agents to prevent or treat postischemic ARF.

VOLUME REGULATION With energy store depletion and cell injury, cell swelling occurs. This may be of particular significance in the outer medulla, where endothelial cell swelling into the lumen of the capillary, together with extrinsic pressure resulting from tubular cell swelling, may compromise capillary patency. Mannitol has been administered to animals and patients with the rationale that prevention of cell swelling and increase in intratubular flow might decrease intratubular obstruction and mitigate renal dysfunction. Mannitol and other osmotic agents have been demonstrated to have a protective effect in the preservation of transplanted kidneys and prevention of delayed graft function, which is most often ischemic in etiology. Mannitol is also likely effective in the prevention of myoglobinuric ARF and is recommended, along with vigorous fluid replacement and $NaHCO_3$, for the prevention and treatment of early myoglobinuric ARF.

CALCIUM In addition to the role that calcium plays in vasoconstriction mediated by the vascular smooth muscle cell, calcium may have a primary toxic intracellular action in the renal tubular cell as a consequence of ischemia. Under normal conditions, extracellular $[Ca^{2+}]$ is 10,000-fold greater than cytosolic $[Ca^{2+}]$. ATP-dependent mechanisms are responsible for maintenance of this large gradient. ATP depletion leads to an increase in $[Ca^{2+}]$ in tubular epithelial cells. This increase in $[Ca^{2+}]$ results in part from an increase in intracellular $[Na^+]$, which occurs secondary to energy depletion and consequent inhibition of the Na^+/K^+ ATPase. The decrease in the transmembrane $[Na^+]$ gradient potentiates Ca^{2+} entry into the cell via the Na^+/Ca^{2+} exchanger. There is inhibition of Ca^{2+} extrusion by Ca^{2+} ATPases because of decreased ATP. Thus, Ca^{2+} accumulates within ischemic cells. There are a number of Ca^{2+}-activated enzymes, such as proteases and phospholipases, which can be toxic to cells. In addition, uptake into mitochondria may interfere with ATP generation and ultimately lead to mitochondrial destruction. In addition, increased levels of cytosolic [Ca^{2+}] can lead to disruption of the cytoskeleton. While increases in cytosolic [Ca^{2+}] occur soon after hypoxia in experimental systems, there remains some controversy as to the extent to which increased cytosolic [Ca^{2+}] causes the ischemic tubular cell injury.

ACIDOSIS Kidney ischemia stimulates glycolysis, thus increasing the generation of protons and leading to a decrease in cellular pH. Although severe acidosis has been proposed to be detrimental to the kidney, mild acidosis (pH 6.9) protects cells and the isolated perfused kidney against hypoxia and substrate deprivation in vitro. The mechanism of protection by mild degrees of acidosis is not known. The protection is not dependent on preservation of cellular ATP levels. Reduction in pH protects tubules exposed to ionomycin or mitochondrial inhibitors despite the fact that the tubules have increases in [Ca^{2+}]$_i$ equivalent to those changes observed in unprotected tubules. Acidosis has been reported to stabilize cell membranes and may decrease transmembrane calcium flux.

It is possible that the protection afforded by reduced pH results from inhibition of an enzymatic process that would otherwise be detrimental to the cells, such as phospholipase A_2 activity. When blood flow and oxygen delivery are re-established, the extracellular pH rapidly returns to normal. With the increase in intracellular pH upon reperfusion, activation of phospholipase A_2 would be enhanced. This might lead to further alteration in membrane structure and secondarily to enhanced Ca^{2+} permeability, which in turn will further enhance phospholipase A_2 activation. The increase in pH that occurs as a consequence of reperfusion may contribute in an important way to "reperfusion injury."

REACTIVE OXYGEN SPECIES Reactive oxygen species are partially reduced species of oxygen that can cause marked tissue injury. With restoration of oxygen after a period of ischemia, there is a rapid burst of oxidant formation. Reactive oxygen species react with cell membranes to form lipid peroxides, which are generated at high levels during reperfusion. Sources of these oxidants in the kidney include mitochondrial electron transport, endoplasmic reticulum mixed function oxidases, cyclooxygenases, lipoxygenases, the xanthine oxidase system, autooxidation of catecholamines, and neutrophil NADPH oxidase. Reactive oxygen species are toxic to cells in vitro via complex mechanisms involving lipid peroxidation of plasma and mitochondrial membranes, increases in cytosolic calcium concentration, reduction in cellular ATP levels, and activation of phospholipases and endonucleases. The fact that some animal studies show protection against functional tissue damage with antioxidants or reactive oxygen species scavengers, while other studies show no such protection, has resulted in disagreement regarding the extent to which reactive oxygen species contribute to the functional deficits associated with ARF.

By their action to increase phospholipase A_2 activity and enhance arachidonic acid availability, reactive oxygen species increase the production of vasoactive eicosanoids. In the glomerulus, the net effect of production of these eicosanoids is an increase in arteriolar resistance and a decrease in glomerular ultrafiltration coefficient. Another way in which reactive oxygen species may cause local vasoconstriction in the microvasculature of the kidney is by the degradation of the vasodilator nitric oxide.

PURINE DEPLETION With ischemia and reperfusion, there is ATP utilization, without the normal savage mechanisms that are responsible for the regeneration of ATP from ADP, AMP, and their nucleoside and base breakdown products. As a result, these purine breakdown products accumulate in cells. Unlike nucleotides (ATP, ADP, AMP, IMP), adenosine and hypoxanthine leak out of cells. Adenosine can constrict both afferent and efferent arterioles. Hypoxanthine is converted by xanthine oxidase to uric acid, a process that generates reactive oxygen species. Whereas some animal experiments have indicated that intravenous administration of ATP and magnesium protected against ischemic injury, other investigators have found that ATP can cause direct injury to oxygenated proximal tubules and is vasoconstrictive. The loss of adenine nucleotide precursors during the ischemic period limits the ability of the postischemic kidney to regenerate ATP upon reoxygenation.

PHOSPHOLIPASES The phospholipase A_2 (PLA_2) family of enzymes hydrolyze phospholipids to generate free fatty acids and lysophospholipids. Membrane lipid peroxidation associated with ischemia/reperfusion enhances the susceptibility of membranes to PLA_2. PLA_2 activation may adversely affect cell viability by direct actions on membranes or indirectly because of metabolic products. PLA_2 can cause membrane degradation and changes in plasma and mitochondrial membrane bioenergetics and permeability. PLA_2 acts synergistically with reactive oxygen species to confer these toxicities. In addition, the PLA_2-induced production of lysophospholipids, arachidonic acid, eicosanoids, and platelet activating factor, results in destructive cellular processes in the kidney. The toxic products of PLA_2-induced phospholipid degradation alter cell and mitochondrial membrane permeability, resulting in an alteration of the bioenergetic capacity of the cell. In addition, eicosanoids are vasoconstrictive and chemotactic for neutrophils.

INFLAMMATION, LEUKOCYTES, AND ADHESION MOLECULES

Leukocytes have been implicated in the pathophysiology of ischemic ARF. Adherence of the leukocyte to the vascular endothelium is an essential step for extravasation of the cell into ischemic tissue. Complement activation, a consequence of ischemia/reperfusion, is chemotactic for neutrophils. Adherent and activated leukocytes release reactive oxygen species, proteases, elastases, myeloperoxidase, leukotrienes, and other enzymes that damage the ischemic tissue directly, enhance additional inflammatory cell infiltration, and increase vasoconstriction. These mediators, together with leukotriene B4 and platelet activating factor, generated by the infiltrating cells, increase vascular permeability and upregulate adhesion molecule expression promoting further inflammation. In addition, interactions of neutrophils by endothelium may cause capillary plugging that can interfere with restitution of blood flow to areas of the kidney upon reperfusion, even though total renal blood flow is restored.

Neutrophil CD11/CD18 adhesion molecules play important roles in neutrophil-endothelial interactions. These heterodimeric molecules are composed of a common β chain (CD18) and distinct α chains: CD11a (lymphocyte function-associated antigen-1, LFA-1), CD11b (Mac-1 or Mo1), and CD11c (p150,95). LFA-1 and Mac-1 bind to intercellular adhesion molecule 1 (ICAM-1) on endothelial cells. ICAM-1 is a member of the immunoglobulin supergene family. Postischemic kidneys sustain increased injury when perfused with activated neutrophils. The administration of a monoclonal antibody directed against ICAM-1 protects animals from ischemic ARF, even when this antibody is administered 2 h after the ischemic period. Furthermore, ICAM-1-deficient mice are protected against acute renal failure.

APOPTOSIS

It has generally been considered that the cell death that accompanies ischemia/reperfusion represents a passive response of the cell to a depletion of energy stores in the setting of high metabolic demand with pathobiological consequences as described above. It may be, however, that there are certain circumstances postischemia when the cell contributes to its own demise actively, perhaps programmed to commit suicide so that the organ is better positioned to repair itself, an "altruistic cell death." There is a great deal of evidence that a form of programmed cell death or "apoptosis" occurs in the postischemic animal brain and some evidence that it also occurs in postischemic heart and kidney. When the kidney is made chronically ischemic by partially occluding the renal artery, both necrosis and apoptosis of renal epithelial cells is observed over the next 2–8 days. From 10–28 days after clip placement, during the time when there is marked reduction in renal mass, there is continued cell death, but only apoptosis is observed. In studies where the renal artery is completely occluded and the kidney is then reperfused, there is morphological and biochemical evidence for apoptosis, including DNA fragmentation and endonuclease activation. Apoptosis has also been described in clinical ARF in man, particularly in post-transplant ARF, where it coexists with necrosis.

Cell death and cell survival genes have been identified in the nematode, *Caenorhabditis elegans*, and mammalian homologs have recently been identified. The *bcl-2* gene product inhibits apoptosis in many mammalian systems. Increased Bcl-2 protein levels have been found in viable neurons after ischemia/reperfusion. Overproduction of Bcl-2 in transgenic mice resulted in a reduction in brain infarction volume in response to ischemia and reperfusion. After renal injury, Bcl-2 expression is increased in regenerating proximal tubule cells; Bcl-2 knockout mice manifest congenital renal hypoplasia and develop multicystic kidney disease.

GENES WHOSE EXPRESSIONS ARE ALTERED BY HYPOXIA

Oxygen deprivation is common in biology. Prokaryotes are well-adapted to this "stress" and have developed special defense mechanisms to deal with it. Some vertebrate species, for example, the Western painted turtle, can survive long periods of anoxia with minimal adverse consequences. These vertebrates are exceptions, however, since compromised oxygen delivery with resultant hypoxia is highly detrimental to brain, cardiac, kidney, and liver function in most vertebrates. Nevertheless, mammals may have evolved mechanisms to respond to hypoxia, to limit injury and to potentiate recovery of damaged tissue.

Hypoxia in tissue culture increases expression of a number of genes resulting in increased production of various types of proteins (Table 66-1). Some of these proteins may prevent or mitigate injury, although if and how this might occur remains speculative at the present time. Probably the most well-studied mammalian gene in which oxygen exerts control of expression is the erythropoietin gene, which responds to hypoxia with increased gene transcription. This hypoxic response appears to be mediated by two *cis* elements, the dominant of which is the 3' enhancer. A 5' element works in combination with this 3' element to give a maximal response. A hypoxia-inducible factor (HIF) has been identified which specifically binds to the 3' enhancer element.

Table 66-1
Mammalian Genes Whose Expressions Are Modified by Hypoxia in Cell Culture

Gene	
Erythropoetin	↑
HSP-70	↑
Tyrosine hydroxylase	↑
Platelet-derived growth factor A and B	↑
Interleukin-1α	↑
c-*jun*	↑
c-*fos*	↑
Vascular endothelial growth factor	↑
TGF-β1	↑
Placental growth factor	↓
Lactate dehydrogenase	↑
Phosphoglycerate kinase 1	↑
Phosphoenolpyruvate carboxykinase	↓

A number of other genes have been found to be induced with hypoxia in tissue culture. Genes encoding the glycolytic enzymes, lactic dehydrogenase and phophoglycerate kinase-1, are upregulated. Although the control of glycolysis is primarily at the level of posttranslational modifications of glycolytic enzymes, upregulation of these genes might enhance energy production from glycolysis in the hypoxic cell.

Hypoxia also results in upregulation of other genes which may serve in the injury or repair process or induce vasodilatation. These include genes encoding growth factors such as PDGF-A and B, TGF-β1, vascular endothelial growth factor (VEGF), and endothelin. These proteins have been implicated in regulation of vascular tone, wound healing, angiogenesis, proliferation, antiproliferation, and embryonic development. Interleukin 1α, tyrosine hydrolase, and HSP70 are also upregulated. By contrast, hypoxia results in a decrease in placental growth factor mRNA levels. It has been reported that hypoxia responsive transcription-activating cis elements are present in the 5' flanking region of the VEGF, LDH, and phosphoglycerate kinase-1 genes. Hypoxia increases the mRNA levels of VEGF, as it does tyrosine hydrolase, by increased transcription as well as increased RNA stability.

Another mechanism by which an organism can protect itself against hypoxia and reoxygenation or potentiate cell death is to increase or decrease its defense against reactive oxygen species. Catalase and superoxide dismutase are induced in procaryotes during shifts from anaerobic to aerobic environments. By contrast, in the postischemic kidney, there are reduced mRNA levels of superoxide dismutase. In neuronal cells, it has been shown that downregulation of superoxide dismutase causes apoptotic cell death.

Exposure of eukaryotic cells to a variety of stresses, including ischemia and reperfusion, thermal and oxidative stress, viruses, calcium ionophores, and heavy metals induces a remarkably conserved "heat shock response." This response is highly conserved in evolution and is seen with hypoxia and reoxygenation in *Drosophila* larvae. The "heat-shock response" includes the preferential synthesis of "heat-shock proteins" (HSPs), while generalized cellular protein synthesis is suppressed. With ischemia and reperfusion, there is activation of heat-shock transcription factor and increase in mRNA levels of members of the HSP-70 gene family. The postischemic early localization of HSP-72 to the apical part of the proximal cell positions this protein at the site of the cell undergoing rapid changes during the early period of ischemia.

It has been reported that the postischemic kidney becomes relatively resistant to a subsequent ischemic insult. It has been proposed that the heat-shock response may confer this protection. The heat-shock response protects cultured neurons against amino acid excitotoxicity, which is believed to be the effector mechanism of ischemic injury to the brain in vivo. It remains controversial, however, whether the heat-shock response confers protection of the kidney against tubular cell injury.

RECOVERY FROM ACUTE RENAL FAILURE

In contrast to the heart and brain, where ischemia results in permanent cell loss, the kidney, severely damaged by ischemia or toxins, has the ability to completely restore structure and function. The tubular epithelium can completely regenerate and differentiate. Active mitotic activity is characteristic of ischemic ARF in humans, and epithelial cell regeneration has been recognized as a hallmark of tubular necrosis since the descriptions by Bywaters. Postischemic recovery recapitulates certain aspects of renal development. Proteins normally expressed only in early nephron development are expressed in the recovering kidney epithelium. Likewise, other proteins, which are normally expressed in the adult kidney but at low levels or not at all in the embryonic kidney, such as Kid-1, preproEGF, and Tamm Horsfall protein, are downregulated in the postischemic kidney.

Epithelial morphogenesis in renal development depends on soluble and nonsoluble factors including growth factors and matrix components. It is possible that the developmental hierarchy of gene expression is repeated in the repair process postischemia. After ischemia proliferating cell nuclear antigen (PCNA), a marker, albeit not specific, for the G_1-S transition in the cell cycle and hence mitogenesis, was detected primarily in the S3 segment of the proximal tubule. PCNA was maximally expressed at 2 days postischemia. Most, if not all, of the surviving epithelial cells in the damaged tubule have the capacity to undergo a mitogenic response. Thus, restoration of the epithelium does not rely on a small population of "stem cells." This participation of a large percentage of parenchymal cells in the tissue repair process is similar to what is seen in liver regeneration after partial hepatectomy, where more than 95% of remaining hepatocytes of the young rat progress through the cell cycle. In the liver, the hepatocytes do not dedifferentiate, either morphologically or functionally, during this process of regeneration. More than 70 immediate-early genes have been identified to be induced after partial hepatectomy. Many of these genes do not have known functions.

Vimentin, normally present in mesenchymal cells but not in epithelial cells, and hence a marker for the state of differentiation, is prominently expressed in the S3 segment 2–5 days postischemia, whereas it is undetectable in epithelial cells from either sham-operated control kidneys or contralateral kidneys from experimental animals. Cells in the S3 segments in the outer stripe of the medulla that stain positively for PCNA also stain positively for vimentin. Vimentin staining is also positive in kidneys that are chronically ischemic as a result of imposed renal artery stenosis.

IMMEDIATE-EARLY GENES AND PROTO-ONCOGENES

A number of immediate-early genes and protooncogenes are induced in the postischemic period (Table 66-2). Since many of these same genes are induced when cells are exposed to growth factors, it becomes of interest to know whether the induction of these genes is involved in the proliferative response postischemia. Some of the encoded proteins are transcription factors. Transcription factors play critical roles in the regulation of cell growth and differentiation and the processes by which embryonic cells become spatially organized to form differentiated tissues in the process termed "pattern formation." Genes induced with ischemia and reperfusion include c-*fos*, *Egr-1* (*zif-268*), c-*jun*, c-*myc*, *KC*, and *JE*. The signals for induction of these genes have not been clearly defined. In some cases, hypoxia itself may play a role, but other genes are likely induced in response to injury or in response to cytokines, oxidant stress, or other mediators that are present in the postischemic tissue. It is clear that expression of these genes is not equivalent to mitogenesis, since many of the cells in which these genes are expressed, for example, the thick ascending limbs, are not the cells undergoing proliferation. Thus the induction of these genes may play a role in protection of cells against ischemic injury or in mounting a response that will help regenerate other cells in the kidney. Since the products of these genes are localized to cells that do not undergo necrosis or apoptosis, they are not marking cell death. Immediate-early gene expression may reflect a cellular response to the dedifferentiating influences of ischemic injury. If the damage is not severe enough to kill the cell, the cell may respond to the insult with a "differentiation" response that is mediated in part by the expression of these immediate-early or protooncogenes.

Table 66-2
Genes Whose Kidney Expression Is Modulated with Ischemia/Reperfusion

Immediate-early genes, transcription factors	
Kid-1	↓
Egr-1	↑
c-*Fos*	↑
JC	↑
KE	↑
Growth Factors	
PDGF	↑
TGF-β	↑
IGF-1 binding protein	↓
IGF-1	↓
Growth hormone	↓
prepro EGF	↓
Heparin binding EGF-like growth factor	↑
HGF	↑
c-*met*	↑
Others	
Clusterin	↑
Lipocortin (annexin 1)	↑
HSP-70	↑
Actin	↑
Vimentin	↑
Histone H_{2b}	↑
Superoxide dismutase	↓
renin	↓
E-selectin	↑
Calcyclin	↑
bcl-2	↑
bax	↑
Receptor for activated c-kinase	↑
Osteopontin	↑

In evaluating the potential consequences of increased production of a protein such as c-Jun in the postischemic kidney it is also necessary to understand what regulates the function of the protein. *Trans*-acting activity of c-Jun is positively regulated by phosphorylation of two serine residues in the amino-terminus. The stress-activated protein kinases (SAPKs), also called p54 MAP and JNK kinases, are a subfamily of the extracellular signal-regulated kinase (ERK) family of serine/threonine kinases, which are upregulated in response to the inflammatory cytokine, tumor necrosis factor α (TNF-α), UV irradiation, and cellular stresses, including heat shock and inhibitors of protein synthesis. The SAPKs are markedly activated in response to renal ischemia and reperfusion. This activation of SAPKs, resulting in increased transactivation of c-Jun, may function in cytoprotection, differentiation, apoptosis, and/or repair.

Another important implication of the above described pattern of immediate early gene response is that two of these genes, *JC* and *KE*, encode proteins that are chemotactic. Thus the generation of these proteins may recruit neutrophils and other inflammatory cells to the site of injury with consequent adverse effects as described previously. In addition to these adverse effects, however, it is possible that the infiltrating inflammatory cells may produce factors that act in a paracrine manner to enhance survival, increase regeneration, and/or increase apoptosis in an effort to eliminate cells irreversibly injured. Ischemia also alters the antigenic characteristics of the tubular epithelial cell. These modifications may cause a cell-mediated immune response which, if prolonged, can lead to chronic tubulitis and interstitial inflammation.

The proto-oncogene, c-*myc*, is induced during regeneration after folic-acid-induced injury to the kidney. Members of the myc family are also expressed in the developing kidney and have been implicated in both the control of mitogenesis as well as differentiation.

OTHER GENES WHOSE EXPRESSIONS ARE MODIFIED WITH ISCHEMIA In addition to the above genes there are a number of other genes whose expressions are modified with ischemia/reperfusion. These include clusterin, a gene that is also upregulated in the prostate when testosterone withdrawal induces apoptosis. Kidney lipocortin 1 (annexin 1) levels are also increased in the postischemic kidney. Since this protein binds to phospholipids, it may act to protect lipids against phospholipase attack. E-selectin expression is upregulated with ischemia. This may enhance leukocyte-endothelial adhesion. Other genes whose expression is primarily in the kidney, such as *renin* and *Kid-1*, are downregulated in the postischemic organ.

GROWTH FACTORS

An important component of the repair process in the kidney may involve the local induction of genes encoding growth factors, which then act in a paracrine or autocrine manner to enhance epithelial cell regeneration. mRNA levels of the gene that encodes the platelet-derived growth factor-B (PDGF-B) increase in response to hypoxic exposure of endothelial cells. While PDGF likely does not directly enhance the growth of kidney epithelial cells, this growth factor may induce fibroblasts to release factors that may act on the epithelial cell to enhance proliferation and potentiate tubulogenesis.

Another growth factor that may be important for the recovery of the kidney after an ischemic insult is epidermal growth factor (EGF). EGF is a potent mitogen for kidney epithelial cells. Infusion of EGF into the rat enhances mitogenesis and potentiates recovery from ischemic acute renal failure. With ischemia, however, there is a marked reduction in levels of preproEGF mRNA along with reduced urinary excretion of EGF, although binding of EGF increases in both cortical and medullary tissue. By contrast to the fall in EGF levels postischemia, there is marked induction of heparin-binding EGF-like growth factor (HB-EGF) mRNA in the kidney after ischemia and reperfusion. HB-EGF, like EGF, is mitogenic for kidney epithelial cells. The mRNA of HB-EGF is localized to the distal nephron, suggesting it may exert a paracrine function on the proximal nephron where mitogenesis predominates postischemia.

Transforming growth factor-α (TGF-α) is a 50-amino acid peptide that exerts its biological effects via the EGF receptor. Developing mesonephric tubules, renal cell carcinomas and other human tumors produce TGF-α. TGF-α may derive from infiltrating macrophages in the postischemic tissue and then act on epithelial cells to promote mitogenesis. TGF-α is more important than EGF in the fetus, where mRNA for EGF is not detectable prenatally. It is possible that TGF-α may play an important role in the kidney undergoing repair. TGF-β is also increased in regenerating tubules following ischemic injury and is localized primarily to tubules of the outer medulla.

There are increased amounts of insulin-like growth factor I (IGF-1) receptors after renal ischemia. There is also a decrease in IGF-1 binding protein mRNA. Thus IGF-1 bioavailability is increased in the postischemic kidney. Administration of IGF-1 accelerates recovery of rat serum creatinine levels after an ischemic insult, and its effects are being evaluated in human trials. IGF-I is produced in the mesonephros and promotes organogenesis of the kidney. These effects on renal development support the view that factors important for repair of the kidney are recapitulating roles played during renal development. IGF-1 likely has effects other than its action as a growth factor, which may contribute to its protective effect in the postischemic kidney. It increases GFR in normal and postischemic kidneys and is anabolic, decreasing protein breakdown. IGF-1 has been shown to prevent apoptosis in differentiated cells, acting as a survival factor, without stimulating proliferation. In addition, IGF-1 is a potent inducer of nitric oxide release from endothelial cells and through this action may decrease neutrophil adherence to the postischemic endothelium. PDGF and TGF-β, present in increased amounts in the postischemic kidney, are also chemoattractants and may contribute to the inflammatory response.

Hepatocyte growth factor has also been shown to enhance recovery of the kidney after ischemic and mercuric chloride-induced renal injury. mRNA levels of HGF and its receptor for this growth factor, c-met, are markedly increased, particularly in the outer medulla, in the postischemic period.

CONCLUSIONS AND SPECULATION

It is clear that, while we have come a long way in the last 15 years in our understanding of the biochemical and pathophysiological determinants of renal cell injury postischemia, much remains unknown. In addition, while we have come to recognize the important parallels between renal development and postischemic repair, we know little about the factors responsible for the remarkable ability of the kidney to regenerate and restore morphological and functional integrity. We do not understand why this process of repair is delayed in many of our patients.

In order to understand the recovery process from ischemic ARF it will be necessary to understand how cell cycle signals and effectors are integrated. How do growth factors and cell-matrix interactions influence the process? Are novel growth factors involved, factors that remain to be discovered? Perhaps a better understanding of the hierarchy of gene activation that occurs in renal development will provide critical insight into the normal repair process and how to best influence it therapeutically. A better understanding of how tubulogenesis is controlled ex vivo in artificial matrices may provide important insight into the role played by matrix factors and may further our progress in an ultimate quest to "create" a functional tubule in vivo.

ACKNOWLEDGMENTS

The author is supported in part by NIH Grants DK39773, DK38452, and NS 10828.

SELECTED REFERENCES

Abuelo JG. Diagnosing vascular causes of renal failure. Ann Int Med 1995;123:601–614.

Bacallao R, Fine LG. Molecular events in the organization of renal tubular epithelium: from nephrogenesis to regeneration. Am J Physiol 1989;257:F913–F924.

Badr KF. Novel mediators of sepsis-associated renal failure. Semin Nephrol 1994;14:3–7.

Basile DP, Liapis H, Hammerman MR. Expression of bcl-2 and bax in regenerating rat renal tubules following ischemic injury. Am J Physiol 1997;272:F640–F647.

Basile DP, Rovak JM, Martin DR, Hammerman MR. Increased transforming growth factor-beta 1 expression in regenerating rat renal tubules following ischemic injury. Am J Physiol 1996; 270:F500–F509.

Better OS, Stein JH. Early management and prophylaxis of acute renal failure in traumatic rhabdomyolysis. N Engl J Med 1990; 322:825–828.

Bonventre JV. Mechanisms of ischemic acute renal failure. Kidney Int 1993;43:1160–1178.

Bonventre JV, Weinberg JM. Kidney preservation ex vivo for transplantation. Annu Rev Med 1992;43:523–553.

Brady HR, Singer GG. Acute renal failure. Lancet 1995;346: 1533–1540.

Brezis M, Rosen S. Hypoxia of the renal medulla—its implications for disease. N Engl J Med 1995;332:647–655.

Bywaters EG, Beall D. Crush injures with impairment of renal function. Br Med J 1941;1:427–432.

Conger JD. Interventions in clinical acute renal failure: What are the data? Am J Kid Dis 1995;26:656–576.

Fish EM, Molitoris BA. Alterations in epithelial polarity and the pathogenesis of disease states. N Eng J Med 1994;330:1580–1588.

Franklin SC, Moulton M, Sicard GA, Hammerman MR, Miller SB. Insulin-like growth factor I preserves renal function postoperatively. Am J Physiol 1997;272:F257–F259.

Gleadle JM, Ebert BL, Firth JD, Ratcliffe PJ. Regulation of angiogenic growth factor expression by hypoxia, transition metals, and chelating agents. Am J Physiol 1995;268:C1362–C1368.

Granger DN, Korthuis RJ. Physiologic mechanisms of postischemic tissue injury. Annu Rev Physiol 1995;57:311–332.

Kelly KJ, Williams WW, Colvin RB, Bonventre JV. Antibody to intercellular adhesion molecule-1 protects the kidney against ischemic injury. Proc Natl Acad Sci USA 1994;91:812–816.

Lazarus JM. Acute renal failure. New York: Churchill Livingstone, 1993.

Miller SB, Martin DR, Kissane J, Hammerman MR. Insulin-like growth factor I accelerates recovery from ischemic acute tubular necrosis in the rat. Proc Natl Acad Sci USA 1992;89: 11,876–11,880.

Noiri E, Romanov V, Forest T, et al. Pathophysiology of renal tubular obstruction: therapeutic role of synthetic RGD peptides in acute renal failure. Kidney Int 1995;48:1375–1385.

Oliver J, MacDowell M, Tracy A. The pathogenesis of acute renal failure associated with traumatic and toxic injury. Renal ischemia, nephrotoxic damage and the ischemuric episode. J Clin Invest 1951; 30:1307–1351.

Pombo CM, Bonventre JV, Avruch J, Woodgett JR, Kyriakis JM, Force T. The stress activated protein kinases are major c-jun amino-terminal kinases activated by ischemia and reperfusion. J Biol Chem 1994;269:26,545–26,551.

Romanov V, Noiri E, Czerwinski G, Finsinger D, Kessler H, Goligorsky MS. Two novel probes reveal tubular and vascular Arg-Gly-As (RGD) binding sites in the ischemic rat kidney. Kidney Int 1997;52:93–102.

Safirstein RL, Bonventre JV. Molecular response to ischemic and nephrotoxic acute renal failure. In: Schlöndorff D, Bonventre JV, eds. Molecular Nephrology. New York: Marcel Dekker, 1995; pp. 839–854.

Sorenson CM, Padanilam BJ, Hammerman MR. Abnormal postpartum renal development and cystogenesis in the bcl-2 (-/-) mouse. Am J Physiol 1996;271:F184–F193.

Toback FG. Regeneration after acute tubular necrosis. Kidney Int 1992;41:226–246.

Weinberg J. The cell biology of ischemic renal injury. Kidney Int 1991;39:476–500.

Witzgall R, Brown D, Schwarz C, Bonventre JV. Localization of PCNA, vimentin, clusterin and c-Fos in post-ischemic kidneys. Evidence for a heterogeneous genetic response among nephron segments, and a large pool of mitotically active and dedifferentiated cells. J Clin Invest 1993;93:2175–2188.

67 Potassium Secretory Channels in the Kidney

STEVEN C. HEBERT

INTRODUCTION

The regulation of urinary potassium excretion depends on the coordinated function of potassium transporters (cotransporters and exchangers), ion pumps, and specialized channels in apical and basolateral membranes of distinct cell types along the distal nephron of the mammalian kidney. This chapter focuses on recent molecular and functional information about these potassium secretory channels in the thick ascending limb of Henle (TAL) cells and principal cells in the cortical collecting duct (CCD).

Ion channels are integral membrane proteins that span the lipid bilayer to form narrow hydrophilic (water-like) pores through which ions move passively in accord with electrochemical driving forces. Fluxes of ions as high as 1 million per second can be achieved through these pores. Channels open or close rapidly in response to biological signals by switching between conducting and nonconducting conformations of the protein subunits forming a single ion channel. This mechanism of control of the channel by biological stimuli is referred as "gating." Ion channels can also distinguish or discriminate among ions, an important characteristic called "selectivity": e.g., potassium may permeate a channel pore at a rate 10^4-fold higher than that for Na^+, despite being smaller than the K^+.

Based on these properties, K^+ channels can be classified into five broad groups:

1. Voltage-gated K^+ channels can open or close in response to changes in membrane potential.
2. Calcium-activated K^+ channels are modulated by changes in the intracellular calcium concentration.
3. Ligand-gated K^+ channels are controlled by neurotransmitters (serotonin), hormones (norepinephrine and acetylcholine), cyclic nucleotides (cyclic GMP), or extracellular nucleotides (purinogenic or purinoceptors).
4. ATP-sensitive K^+ (KATP) channels are regulated by the intracellular concentration of ATP.
5. Stretch-regulated channels are modulated by mechanical forces (e.g., stretch).

Ion channels can vary considerably in their electrophysiological and pharmacological properties, even within a single class. Thus, K^+ channels can also be categorized, based on the characteristics of their ionic current profile, as delayed or outward rectifiers and inward rectifiers (Fig. 67-1).

RENAL K^+ SECRETORY CHANNELS

Potassium channels involved in K^+ secretion by distal segments of the nephron belong to the class of channels referred to as inward rectifiers. Inwardly rectifying K^+ (IRK) channels are characterized by a lack of significant voltage-gating and by their ability to transport potassium more readily in the inward (absorptive) than outward (secretory) direction. This ability to conduct better in one than the opposite direction is called *rectification* and is defined by plotting channel current against holding potential (called an I-V or current-voltage curve) and observing the slope (conductance) of the I-V curve (Fig. 67-1). Inward rectifiers exhibit a higher conductance at hyperpolarized membrane potential, where the K^+ current is in the influx direction, than during depolarization, where the current becomes outward. IRK channels exhibit either a "strong" or a "weak" type of inwardly rectification. The strongly rectifying channels exhibit little or no conductance above a certain threshold potential (usually at or near the resting membrane potential of the cell), making them well-suited to function in maintaining the resting membrane potential and in regulating cell excitability (e.g., in muscle cells). On the other hand, the weakly rectifying channels show a reduced, but significant, conductance at depolarizing potentials. Moreover, these latter channels open and close in response to cellular metabolic events (via nucleotide [or ATP]-mediated inhibition of channel activity), and thereby may serve important roles in some cells during ischemia (e.g., in heart and brain). This latter characteristic of nucleotide sensitivity has given these channels the name *ATP-sensitive* or K_{ATP} channel.

Renal K^+ Secretory Channels in TAL and Principal Cells are K_{ATP} Channels In the kidney, secretory K_{ATP} channels have been characterized in apical membranes of thick ascending limb (TAL) cells and principal cells of the cortical collecting duct (CCD). In both medullary (MTAL) and cortical (CTAL) segments of the TAL, K_{ATP} channels are the dominant conductance in apical plasma membranes and provide the crucial K^+ efflux pathway for potassium entering cells via the apical Na^+:K^+:$2Cl^-$ cotransporter (Fig. 67-2). This apical recycling of potassium ensures that an adequate supply of luminal potassium is provided for efficient function of the Na^+:K^+:$2Cl^-$ cotransporter. In addition, this channel mediates the apical component of a transcellular (basolateral-

From: *Principles of Molecular Medicine* (J. L. Jameson, ed.), ©1998 Humana Press Inc., Totowa, NJ.

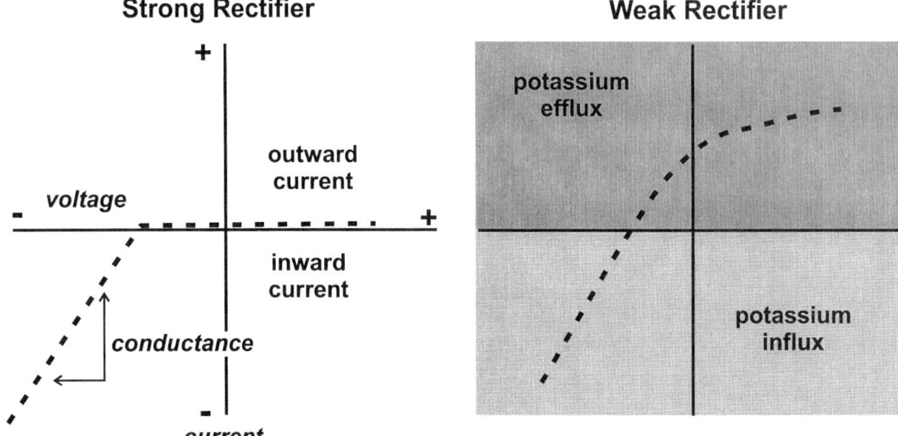

Figure 67-1 Differences in strong and weak inward rectifying channels. The dashed lines represent current-voltage (I-V) plots for both types of rectifiers. Positive current (the upper half of the I-V plot) represents potassium efflux from cells (secretion), while negative current is potassium influx into cells. The slope (arrows) of the I-V curve is the conductance. Note that the conductance for strong rectifiers goes to zero for positive currents. In contrast, the weak rectifiers exhibit significance conductance at positive currents.

to-apical) current flow that returns to the basolateral side via the paracellular pathway predominantly as a cation current carrying Na^+, Ca^{2+}, and Mg^{2+}. This paracellular current is sufficient to account for one-half of the net transepithelial movement of sodium, making this system of Na^+ absorption about twice as efficient (moles Na^+ absorbed/mole Ox_2 consumed) as cells utilizing sodium channels, where all of the Na^+ absorbed traverses the transcellular pathway (e.g., the principal cell). In fact, the apical K^+ channels are so important for net transepithelial Na^+ transport in the TAL that blockade of these channels virtually abolishes salt absorption in this nephron segment.

The conductive properties of the apical membranes of TAL cells are almost entirely because of potassium. Two types of inwardly rectifying and ATP-sensitive K^+ channels have been identified on apical membranes of TAL segments by patch clamp: a *low-conductance* (20–35 pS) channel and an *intermediate-conductance* (70 pS) channel. Both channels exhibit a high open probability (P_o), are inhibited by m*M* MgATP ($K_{1/2} \approx 0.6$–1 m*M*), and are exquisitely sensitive to reductions in cytosolic pH (~50% reduction in P_o by a 0.2-pH unit decrease). The activity of the intermediate conductance K_{ATP} channel can be significantly reduced by tetraethylammonium (TEA) or quinine, whereas these agents have no effect on the low-conductance channel. In contrast, the low, but not intermediate, conductance channel is inhibited by high concentrations (~250 μ*M*) of gliburide. In the rat TAL, the intermediate conductance K_{ATP} channel makes up about 65–70% of the total apical K^+ conductance. A low conductance K_{ATP} channel with nearly identical properties has been identified in apical membranes of principal cells in the CCD where it mediates K^+ secretion into urine (Fig. 67-2).

The K_{ATP} channel in rat TAL and principal cells is highly regulated by hormones, metabolism, and changes in acid-base state (Fig. 67-3). Metabolic-related changes in ATP dually modulated channel activity: high MgATP concentrations (within the normal range of ATP; 2–3 m*M*) reversibly block channel activity ($K_{1/2} \approx 0.6$–1.0 n*M*) while lower concentrations of MgATP (50–100 μ*M*) are required to maintain channel activity. The stimulatory effect of low ATP concentration, however, clearly relates to regulation of channel activity by phosphorylation-dephosphorylation processes (Fig. 67-3):

1. Channel activity rapidly diminishes (called channel "run-down") on patch excision unless the cytosolic face is exposed to low concentrations of MgATP.
2. Generally, the catalytic subunit of cAMP-dependent protein kinase, PKA, is also required for channel maintenance, and PKA, together with MgATP, can restore channel activity after run-down.
3. Nonhydrolyzable ATP analogs cannot maintain or restore channel activity.
4. In patches in which channel activity is maintained by MgATP alone, the PKA inhibitor (PKI) reversible reduces channel activity, providing evidence for an important role for endogenous PKA.
5. PKC reversibly inhibits channel activity and antagonizes the stimulatory effect of PKA, a process that is Ca^{2+}-dependent.

The ratio of cellular ATP:ADP may be more important than ATP concentration, since low concentration of ADP can reverse the MgATP-mediated inhibition of these channels. Cytosolic pH is also an important regulator of the low-conductance K_{ATP} channel in the apical membranes of principal cells; cellular acidification within the physiologically achievable range leads to channel inhibition. Finally, K_{ATP} channel activity in rat principal cells is also inhibited by activation of protein kinase C or calcium-calmodulin-dependent kinase II, arachidonic acid (or its metabolites), and by actin cytoskeleton.

What is the evidence that these K_{ATP} channels mediate K^+ secretion into tubular urine? Large-conductance (maxi-K) channels (a type of voltage-gated channel) and K_{ATP} channels are the only potassium channels observed on patch clamping apical membranes from TAL and principal cells. Whereas either channel could, in principle, mediate potassium secretion, maxi-K channels are normally quiescent at normal resting cell voltages (but can be activated by μ*M* cytosolic Ca^{2+} or cell swelling), making them a less likely candidate for K^+ secretion. Moreover, maxi-K channels are inhibited by TEA while $K^+(Rb^+)$ secretion and the transepithelial voltage in the CCD are not blocked by luminal TEA. This provides strong evidence that the low-conductance K_{ATP}, and not the maxi-K^+ channel, is involved in K^+ secretion by principal (and TAL) cells.

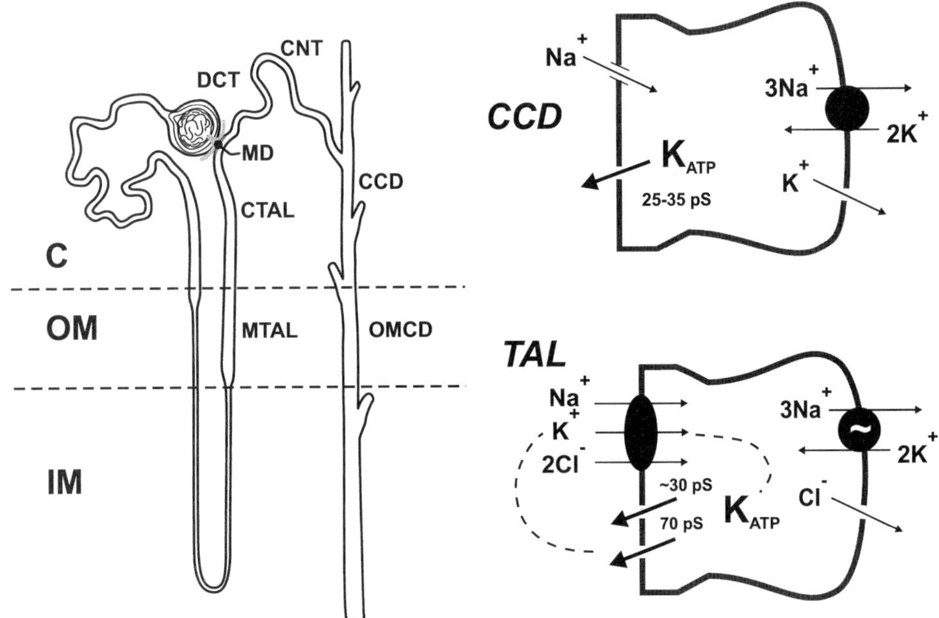

Figure 67-2 Schematic representation of the apical secretory potassium channels in thick ascending limb (TAL) cells and in principal cell from the cortical collecting duct (CCD). In CCD, Na^+ passively enters principal cells through apical membranes via the amiloride-sensitive channel and is actively extruded across basolateral membranes via the Na^+-K^+-ATPase. The K^+ entering cells via this latter pump is either secreted across apical membranes by the low-conductance secretory K_{ATP} channel or recycles across basolateral membranes by one of several potassium channels. In TAL, two types of K^{ATP} channels (the **low** conductance –30 pS and the **intermediate** conductance –70 pS channels) mediate apical recycling of potassium entering cells via the Na^+-K^+-Cl^- cotransporter. (*See text* for discussion.)

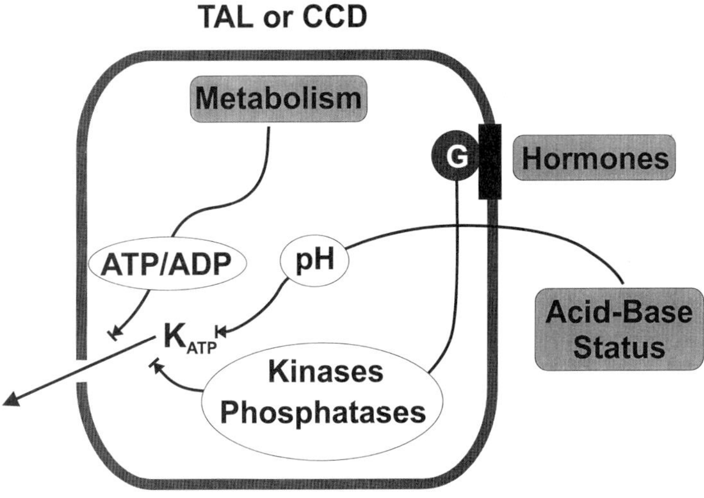

Figure 67-3 The activity of the apical, potassium secretory K_{ATP} channels in TAL and principal cells are regulated by hormones, acid-base status, and metabolic state of the cell. (*See text* for discussion and further details.)

Finally, it is somewhat curious that inward rectifiers should be used at all in renal cells for potassium secretion since the outward (and in this case the lower) conductance is what determines the magnitude of potassium secretion at any given electrochemical driving force (Fig. 67-1). While the answer to this question may never be known with certainty, the intrinsic high open probability of these channels, together with its sensitivities to pH and the metabolic state of the cell (Fig. 67-3), do provide for a level of regulation that may offer distinct advantages for a channel involved in modulation of K^+ secretion.

A MOLECULAR MODEL FOR INWARD-RECTIFYING CHANNELS

A candidate for the renal secretory inward-rectifier potassium channel was recently cloned from rat kidney (ROMK1). ROMK1 encodes a ~45-kDa protein having only two potential membrane-spanning helices (M1 and M2); (Fig. 67-4) bracketing an H5-like region (thought to form part of the pore in voltage-gated channel). This predicted topology makes ROMK1 quite distinct from voltage-gated (*Shaker* family) potassium or ligand-gated ion channels (Fig. 67-4). Subsequent to the cloning of ROMK1, other inwardly

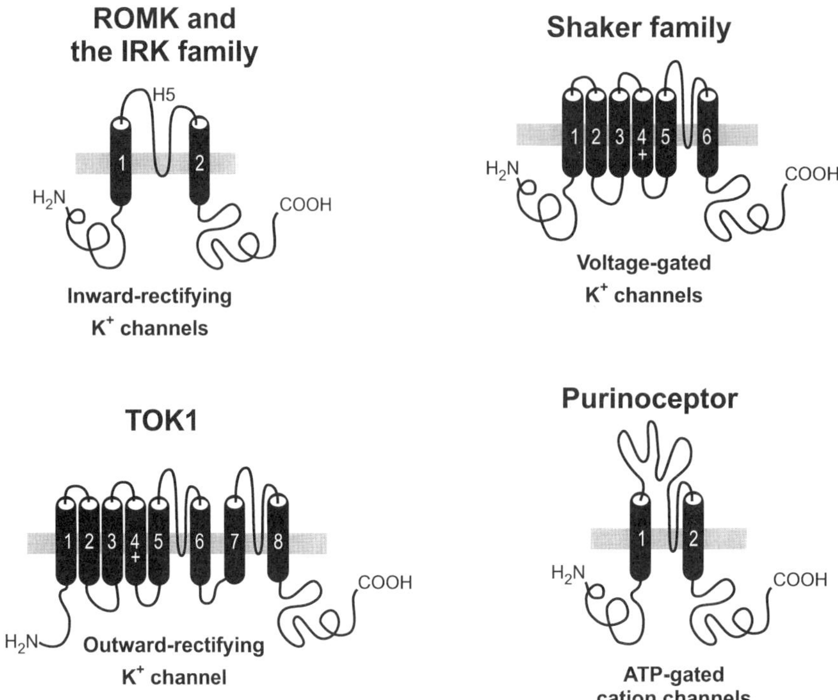

Figure 67-4 The proposed topology of renal potassium channels. The cylinders represent putative membrane spanning α-helices and are numbers 1–6 from the amino (NH_2)-terminus to the carboxy (COOH)-terminus. (*See text* for discussion.)

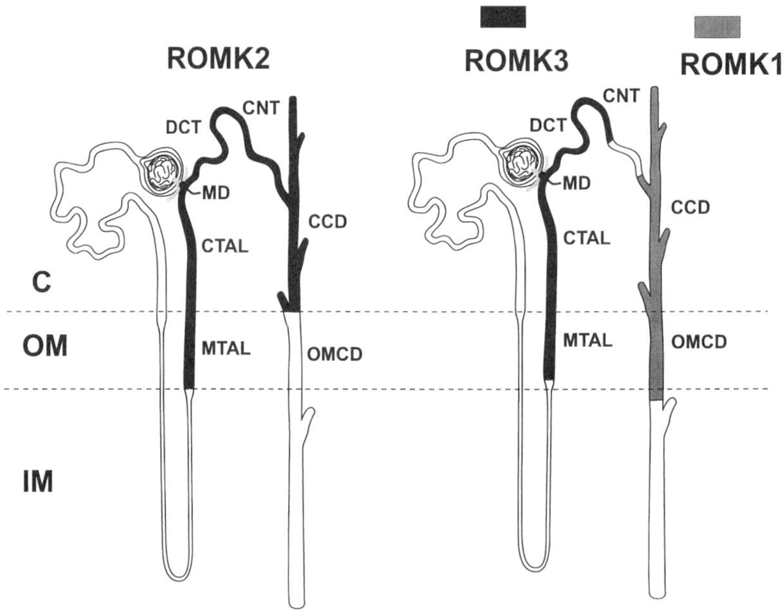

Figure 67-5 Distribution of ROMK channel isoforms along the rat nephron. MTAL and CTAL, medullary and cortical thick ascending limb of Henle, respectively; MD, macula densa; CNT, connecting tubule; CCD, cortical collecting duct; OMCD, outer medullary collecting duct. (*See text* for discussion.)

rectifying K^+ channels have been isolated from kidney and a number of other tissues, and all exhibited a similar general topology. These genes and their channel protein products form a new family of potassium channels called the inwardly rectifying K^+ (IRK) family. More recently, other cation channels have been cloned that exhibit the two-membrane spanning domain type of topology: a novel channel found in *Saccharomyces cerevisiae*, in which this domain is in a tandem combination with a six-membrane-spanning domain typical of the *Shaker* family; P_{2x}-type purinoceptor channels activated by binding extracellular ATP and expressed in nerve cells; and the amiloride-sensitive Na^+ channel expressed in kidney principal cells. Whether there is a common evolutionary thread among these distinctive channel families remains to be elucidated.

Molecular diversity in ROMK is achieved by alternative splicing (the isoforms are designated ROMK1, ROMK2a, ROMK2b,

Table 67-1
Characteristics of ROMK and K_{ATP} Channels in Kidney

	ROMK	*Intermediate conductance*	*Low conductance*
Single channel conductance, γ(pS)	30–45	70	25–35
Inward rectifier	Yes	Yes	Yes
Open probability, P_o	High	High	High
ATP inhibits	Yes	Yes	Yes
↓ P_o by ↑ ATP or ↑ (ADP/ATP)	$K_i \approx 2.5$ n*M*	At (m*M*)	$K_i \approx 0.5$–1 m*M*
Inhibited by glyburide	No	No	Yes High υ*M*
Ion selectivity	$K^+ >> Na^+$	$K^+ = Rb^+ = NH_4 = Cs^+ >> Na^+$	$K^+ >> Na^+$ (20:1)
pH_i-dependence (↑ pH_i reduces P_o)	Yes	Yes	Yes

and ROMK3); these spliced isoforms are both functional as channels and alternatively expressed along the mammalian nephron. The finding that the ROMK gene contains introns within the coding region is an unusual feature for a mammalian K^+ channel, suggesting that these splicing events may serve some important role in altering channel function or regulation (or both). ROMK1–ROMK3 isoforms are produced by alternative splicing at the 5' end of the transcripts, which alters both the length and amino acid sequence of the encoded channel at initial segment of the NH_2-terminus. The role of the NH_2-terminal variations on the ROMK isoforms in altering channel function and regulation by phosphorylation-dephosphorylation processes is currently under active investigation.

As shown in Fig. 67-5, ROMK isoforms are differentially expressed along the nephron, with the overall distribution of ROMK being consistent with this IRK, representing the low-conductance secretary K_{ATP} channel observed in TAL and principal cells. ROMK2, which encodes the channel with the shortest NH_2-terminus, is the most widely distributed of the ROMK transcripts. In contrast, the ROMK1 transcript is only expressed in collecting ducts (CCD, OMCD, and initial IMCD), whereas ROMK3 is expressed only in the earlier nephron segments (MTAL, CTAL, and DCT). Thus, all of these nephron segments, except the OMCD, apparently express at least two different ROMK isoforms: ROMK2 and one of the isoforms (ROMK1 or ROMK3) encoding a channel protein with a longer NH_2-terminus. Do ROMK isoforms associate to form heteromultimeric complexes in some of these nephron segments? Would such heteromultimeric channels exhibit distinctive functional and regulatory properties? While these important questions are being actively pursued in several laboratories, other inward-rectifying K^+ channels have recently been shown to heteromultimeric complexes: the G-proteingated cardiac atrial K^+ channel formed from two IRK subunits and the pancreatic β-cell K_{ATP} formed from an IRK and the sulfonylurea receptor, which is a member of the P-glycoprotein family. The latter is quite interesting, since ROMK lacks significant sensitivity to glyburide, while the native low-conductance K_{ATP} in TAL or principal cells is inhibited by high micromolar concentrations of this potent sulfonylurea (Table 67-1). Could ROMK associate with a p-glycoprotein which would, like the β-cell K_{ATP}, impart sulfonylurea sensitivity? Mutations in ROMK1 cause the antenatal variant of Bartter syndrome.

FUNCTION OF ROMK CHANNELS AND CORRELATION WITH STRUCTURE ROMK K+ channels expressed in *Xenopus laevis* oocytes have been shown to exhibit many of the ion permeation and regulatory properties of the native low-conductance K_{ATP} channels observed on patch clamping of apical membranes of thick ascending limb and principal cells. These ROMK channels have the following basic properties: a unitary conductance of 30–45 pS in symmetrical 140–150 m*M* KCl; high K^+:Na^+ selectivity ($K^+ > Rb^+ > NH4^+ > Na^+$, Li^+); weak inward rectification resulting from block by internal Mg^{2+} and/or a polyamine such as spermine or spermidine; marked sensitivity to "cytosolic" side reductions in pH; modulation by arachidonic acid; run-down or loss of channel activity in excised patches in the absence of MgATP that involves dephosphorylation by a protein phosphatase; reactivation of channels after run-down by re-exposure to MgATP and the catalytic subunit of protein kinase A; and sensitivity (inhibition) by higher concentrations of MgATP.

Importantly, ROMK channels exhibit no reduction in channel activity with addition of millimolar concentrations of TEA^+ to extracellular media. This lack of sensitivity to TEA^+ is in K^+ secretion in kidney since both K^+ secretion by the CCD and the low-conductance K_{ATP} channel found in principal cells are characteristically unaffected by TEA^+. The aromatic amino acid, phenylalanine, at position 148 within the H5 region on ROMK1, could impart significant sensitivity to external TEA^+ in ROMK channels, since site-directed mutagenesis studies in *Shaker* channels have shown that aromatic amino acids at a similar position confers a high sensitivity to external TEA^+. It is plausible that the positively charged arginine, at position 147 in ROMK1, might interfere with TEA^+ binding, and explain the lack of high TEA^+ sensitivity in the ROMK1 channel. In this regard, recall that the intermediate conductance K_{ATP} channel found in rat TAL is sensitive to block by external TEA^+. This pharmacological difference, together with the differences in single channel conductance and sensitivities to glyburide, provide strong evidence that ROMK does not, by itself, encode the –70 pS K_{ATP} channel. However, the similarity in many of the properties of the low- and intermediate-conductance channels suggest that these IRKs may be structurally similar. The possibility remains, however, that the intermediate conductance channel could be a heteromultimer of ROMK and some other IRK.

As discussed earlier in this chapter, inward rectification is also a characteristic of the apical secretary K_{ATP} channels in kidney as well as other members of the IRK family of channels. Recent studies have begun to identify important amino acid residues or segments critical for both types of rectification. The COOH-, but not NH_{2-}, terminus appears to be important in determining inward rectification. Moreover, a single negatively charged amino acid residue (aspartic acid) in the second membrane-spanning helix of the strong inward rectifiers like IRK1 appears to be important in imparting this type of rectification. Importantly, ROMK lacks this charged amino acid residue, consistent with its weak type of inward rectification.

As discussed above, the secretory K^+ channels in distal nephron segments are ATP-sensitive or K_{ATP} channels. A segment following the second membrane-spanning region contains a Walker A site motif (GXG[H in ROMK]XXGK) within a so-called $P0_4$-binding or P loop that has been linked to ATP binding in many other proteins. In fact, a 27-amino acid region containing the Walker type A site exhibits significant similarity to the catalytic subdomain I of ERBB3, a member of the epidermal growth factor (EGF) receptor tyrosine kinase family. Based on this potential ATP-binding segment and the presence of several potential protein kinase A and protein kinase C phosphorylation sites in the COOH-terminus of ROMK channel proteins, we have suggested that this region forms a regulatory domain. Recent studies are consistent with the role of this COOH-terminal domain in regulation by nucleotides and protein serine-threonine kinases.

In summary, molecular cloning has begun to identify important ion channels in the mammalian kidney. One of these, ROMK, appears to form the ion permeation pore of the ATP-sensitive inwardly rectifying K^+ channel that mediates potassium secretion into tubular urine of TAL and CCD. Future studies will clearly provide new information on the function and regulation of this channel and provide new insights into renal potassium handling.

ACKNOWLEDGMENT

This work was supported in part by a grant from the National Institutes of Health (DK37605) to SCH.

SELECTED REFERENCES

Ashcroft FM. Adenosine 5'-triphosphate-sensitive potassium channels. Annu Rev Neurosci 1988;11:97–118.

Ashcroft SJH, Ashcroft FM. Properties and functions of ATP-sensitive K-channels. Cell Signalling 1990;2:197–214.

Boim MA, Ho K, Shuck ME, et al. The ROMK inwardly rectifying ATP-sensitive K^+ channel. II. Cloning and intrarenal distribution of alternatively spliced forms. Am J Physiol (Renal Fluid Electrolyte Physiol) 1995;268:F1132–F1140.

Gebremedhin D, Kaldunski M, Jacobs ER, Harder DR, Roman RJ. Coexistence of two types of $Ca^{(2+)}$-activated K^+ channels in rat renal arterioles. Am J Physiol 1996;270:F69–F81.

Hebert SC. An ATP-regulated, inwardly rectifying potassium channel from rat kidney (ROMK). Kidney Int 1995;48:1010–1016.

Hebert SC, Andreoli TE. Control of NaCl transport in the thick ascending limb. Am J Physiol (Renal Fluid Electroltye Physiol) 1984;247–36:F745–F756.

Hille B. Ionic Channels of Excitable Membranes, 2nd ed. Sunderland, MA: Sinauer, 1992.

Ho K, Nichols CG, Lederer WJ, et al. Cloning and expression of an inwardly rectifying ATP-regulated potassium channel. Nature 1993;362:31–38.

Inagaki N, Gonoi T, Clemant JP, et al. Reconstitution of IK_{ATP}: An inward rectifier subunit plus the sulfonylurea receptor. Nature 1995; 270:1166–1170.

International Collaborative Study Group for Bartter-Like Syndromes. Mutations in the gene encoding the inwardly-rectifying renal potassium channel, ROMK, cause the antenatal variant of Bartter syndrome: evidence for genetic heterogeneity. Hum Mol Genet 1997;6:17–26.

Kawahara K, Anzai N. Potassium transport and potassium channels in the kidney tubules. Jpn J Physiol 1997;47:1–10.

Ketchum KA, Joiner WJ, Sellers AJ, Kaczmarek LK, Goldstein SAN. A new family of outwardly rectifying potassium channel proteins with two pore domains in tandem. Nature 1995;376:690–695.

Krapivinsky G, Gordon EA, Wickman K, Vellmirovic B, Krapivinsky L, Clapham DE. The G-protein-gated atrial K^+ channel I_{KACh} is a heteromultimer of two inwardly rectifying K^+-channel protein. Nature 1995;374:135–141.

Kubokawa M, Wang W, McNicholas CM, Giebisch G. Role of Ca^{2+}/CaMK II in Ca^{2+}-induced K^+ channel inhibition in rat CCD principal cell. Am J Physiol (Renal Fluid Electrolyte Physiol) 1995;268: F211–F219.

Lee WS, Hebert SC. The ROMK inwardly rectifying ATP-sensitive K^+ channel. I. Expression in rat distal nephron segments. Am J Physiol (Renal Fluid Electrolyte Physiol) 1995;268:F1124–F1131.

McNicholas CM, Yang Y, Giebisch G, Hebert SC. Molecular site for nucleotide binding on an ATP-sensitive renal K+ channel (ROMK2). Am J Physiol 1996;271:F275–F285.

Misler S, Giebisch G. ATP-sensitive potassium channels in physiology, pathphysiology, and pharmacology. Current Opinion in Nephrology and Hypertension 1992;1:21–33.

Rossier BC, Canessa CM, Schild L, Horisberger JD. Epithelial sodium channels. Current Opinion in Nephrology and Hypertension 1994; 3:487–496.

Simon DB, Karet FE, Rodriquez-Soriano J, et al. Genetic heterogeneity of Bartter's syndrome revealed by mutations in the K^+ channel, ROMK. Nat Genet 1996;14:152–156.

Suprenant A, North RA. P_{2X} receptors bring new structure to ligand-gated channels. TINS 1995;18:224–229.

Wang W. Two types of K^+ channel in TAL of rat kidney. Am J Physiol (Renal Fluid Electrolyte Physiol) 1994;267–36:F599–F605.

Wang W, Cassola A, Giebisch G. Arachidonic acid inhibits the secretory K^+ channel of cortical collecting duct of rat kidney. Am J Physiol (Renal Fluid Electrolyte Physiol) 1992;262–31:F554–F559.

Wang W, Cassola A, Giebisch G. Involvement of actin cytoskeleton in modulation of apical K channel activity in rat collecting duct. Am J Physiol (Renal Fluid Electrolyte Physiol) 1994;267–36:F592–F598.

Wang W, Giebisch G. Dual effect of adenosine triphosphate on the apical small conductance K^+ channel of the rat cortical collecting duct. J Gen Physiol 1991;98:35–61.

Wang W, Hebert SC, Giebisch G. Renal K^+ channels: structure and function. Annu Rev Physiol 1997;59:413–436.

Xu ZC, Yang Y, Hebert SC. Phosphorylation of the ATP-sensitive, inwardly rectifying K^+ channel, ROMK, by cyclic AMP-dependent protein kinase. J Biol Chem 1996;271:9313–9319.

68 Alport Syndrome

KARL TRYGGVASON AND PIRKKO HEIKKILÄ

BACKGROUND

Alport syndome, also termed hereditary nephritis, was initially described in 1927 by AC Alport as an inherited kidney disease characterized by hematuria and sensorineural deafness. Later, ocular lesions were also associated with the syndrome and, with the introduction of the electron microscope, irregularities and disruptions in the glomerular basement membrane (GBM) were shown to be typical for this disorder as well. The disease is progressive, usually leading to renal failure during adolescence or before middle age.

Alport syndrome is primarily inherited as an X-chromosome-linked dominant trait with an estimated gene frequency of 1:5000, but autosomal forms also exist. The defective gene in X-linked Alport syndrome was located in 1988 and 1989 to the long arm of the X chromosome. In 1990, a gene encoding a novel basement membrane (type IV) collagen α5 chain was discovered and localized to the Alport gene region on chromosome X, and this was soon followed by identification of mutations in this gene in Alport patients. More recently, mutations have also been reported in the genes for the α3 and α4 type IV collagen chains in the rarer autosomal forms of Alport syndrome. Presently, well over 100 different mutations are now identified in type IV collagen genes in Alport patients. These mutations can be considered responsible for abnormalities in the structural framework of the GBM, resulting in kidney manifestations. In this chapter we review clinical features of the disease, the molecular properties of the GBM and type IV collagen, which are the prime targets of the disease, as well as recent advances in the molecular genetics and therapy.

CLINICAL FEATURES AND DIAGNOSIS

Characteristically, Alport patients have recurrent microscopic or gross hematuria in childhood, earlier in males than in females. It usually leads to end-stage renal disease in affected males and in rare cases also in females. The hearing loss is sensorineural and primarily affects high tones. Electron microscopy usually reveals thinning and thickening of the GBM with longitudinal splits into thin layers with a basket-weave pattern (Fig. 68-1). These changes are most evident in male patients, except in boys of very young age. Lenticonus, a peculiar change of lens shape, is also frequently observed in Alport patients. Recurrent corneal erosion has also been reported. The disease is inherited and family history is present in 85% of cases. The remaining 15% may represent new mutations. Recent work has revealed a large proportion of patients with renal failure and mutations in type IV collagen without hearing loss or eye lesions. Thus, the classical clinical definition for the Alport syndrome, i.e., hereditary nephritis with hearing loss, does not apply to all patients with type IV collagen defects. Clinicians should, therefore, consider Alport syndrome as a possible diagnosis for patients with hematuria and/or renal failure, even though they lack symptoms such as hearing loss, ocular lesions or family history.

From: *Principles of Molecular Medicine* (J. L. Jameson, ed.), ©1998 Humana Press Inc., Totowa, NJ.

STRUCTURE AND MOLECULAR BIOLOGY OF THE GLOMERULAR FILTRATION BARRIER

FILTRATION BARRIER The glomerulus is a specialized vascular organ that functions as the filtration unit of plasma. Glomerular filtration is distinguished from transcapillary exchange in other organs by two characteristics: First, the glomerulus almost completely excludes plasma proteins of the size of albumin (mol wt approximately 70,000, radius 3.6 nm) and larger from the filtrate. Second, the glomerulus exhibits an extraordinary high permeability to water and small solutes. The filtration effect across the glomerulus depends on the size of the molecules; radius, which is called a size-dependent permeability barrier in the glomerulus. The filtration decreases with increasing effective molecular radius. In addition to the size, the glomerulus discriminates between molecules according to their charge, allowing greater penetration of neutral and cationic molecules than of anionic molecules of the same size.

The actual filtration barrier consists of the fenestrated capillary endothelium, the GBM of 300–350 nm in thickness, and the epithelial podocytes that are separated by the slit and connected by a thin diaphragm. Similar to basement membranes elsewhere in the body, the GBM consists of type IV collagen, laminin, proteoglycan, and nidogen/entactin. Type IV collagen forms the structural framework of the GBM together with laminin, which also plays a role in cell adhesion. Nidogen interconnects the type IV collagen and laminin networks, and proteoglycans are believed to serve as an anionic filtration barrier.

TYPE IV COLLAGEN Type IV collagen is a basement membrane specific protein that belongs to the large family of collagens that are the main extracellular structural proteins in all multicellular organisms. Collagen molecule is composed of three α chains, characterized by the repeating Gly-X-Y sequence, where X and Y can be any amino acid. The glycine residue, as every third amino acid enables the assembly of three chains into a triple-helical struc-

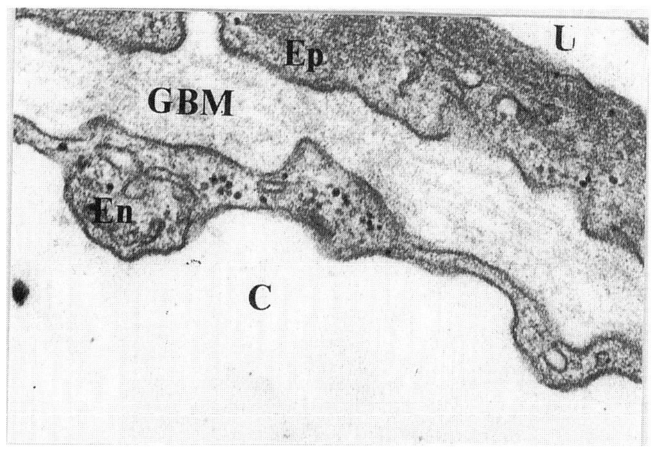

Figure 68-1 Electron micrograph of the glomerular filtration barrier in an 8-year-old Alport syndrome patient. The figure displays typical findings for the disease with irregular thinning and thickening, as well as lamellation of the GBM. C, capillary lumen; En, endothelial cell; GBM, glomerular basement membrane; Ep, epithelial cell; U, urinary space. (Courtesy of Dr. Helena Autio-Harmainen, University Hospital of Oulu, Finland.)

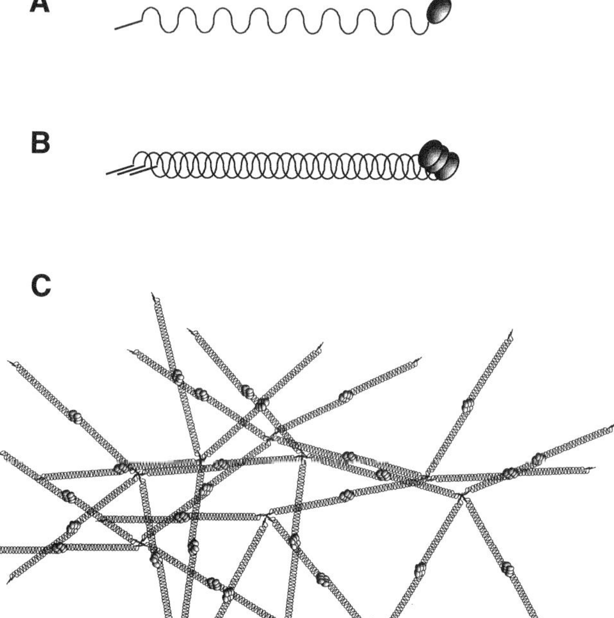

Figure 68-2 Schematic illustration of the structure and extracellular assembly of type IV collagen. **(A)** Each a chain has a 400-nm-long collagenous domain characterized by a frequently interrupted G-X-Y-repeat sequence. The interruptions, which are not shown in the figure give flexibility to the molecule and the type IV collagen network. **(B)** Three α chains form a triple-helical molecule. **(C)** Individual molecules assemble by end-to-end associations into a network-like structure into which other basement membrane proteins are bound in a largely unknown fashion. In reality, the type IV collagen network structure also contains more complex laterally aligned molecules.

ture. All collagens consist of three α chains that form the triple-helical molecule inside the cell. Once secreted from the cells, the triple-helical molecules assemble by end-to-end aggregation and lateral alignment into a tightly crosslinked network structure (Fig. 68-2). Presently, six genetically distinct type IV collagen

Table 68-1
Diseases with Linkage to Type IV Collagen Chains

Disease	*Type IV collagen α chain involved*
Genetic	
X-linked Alport syndrome	α5
X-linked Alport syndrome associated with diffuse esophageal lyomyomatosis	α5 + α6
Autosomal Alport syndrome	α3 and/or α4
Acquired	
Goodpasture syndrome	α3

α chains are known. Of those, the α1 and α2 chains are ubiquitous and can be found in all basement membranes. In contrast, the α3, α4, α5, and α6 chains are minor component chains with a more restricted tissue distribution and thus probably specialized functions. For example, molecules containing α3, α4, and α5 chains are particularly abundant in the GBM. Basement membranes containing these chains are believed to be stronger as a result of the presence of a high content of cysteine residues and, thus, disulfide crosslinks. The strength of the structural network is considered to be particularly important in basement membranes, such as those of renal glomeruli and the lens capsule, which do not have supportive collagen fibers. Molecules containing the α3–α6 chains have been shown to be involved in the pathogenesis of diseases such as Goodpasture syndrome, Alport syndrome, and/or diffuse esophageal leiomyomatosis (Table 68-1). Isoform switching (α4, α5) of type IV collagen is developmentally arrested in Alport syndrome, leading to increased susceptibility of renal basement membranes to endoproteolysis.

TYPE IV COLLAGEN GENES The mammalian type IV collagen genes are located pairwise in an unique head-to-head fashion on three different chromosomes: chromosomes 13, 2, and X (Fig. 68-3). This implies that the six genes have evolved through duplication and inversion of an ancestral gene. Subsequently, the duplicated genes have undergone two further rounds of duplication, resulting in the three head-to-head located gene pairs on different chromosomes. The type IV collagen genes are large, over 100 kb, and complex, containing 46–52 exons. The genes are termed COL4A1, COL4A2, COL4A3, COL4A4, COL4A5, and COL4A6, respectively, for the type IV collagen α1, α2, α3, α4, α5, and α6 chains.

MOLECULAR PATHOLOGY OF THE DISEASE

Mutations have been described in the COL4A5 gene in more than 100 cases of X-linked Alport syndrome. Furthermore, mutations have been identified in the COL4A3 and COL4A4 genes in autosomal recessive forms of the disease. Almost all of the mutations identified to date differ among familial groups. This, together with the complexity of the collagen genes, makes DNA-based diagnosis of Alport syndrome particularly difficult. About 15% of the mutations are large gene rearrangements, such as deletions, insertions, inversions, or duplications. The rest are small mutations, mainly large proportion of single base changes, in addition to small deletions, insertions, or duplications. The mutations can result in a complete absence of the protein (α chain) in question, a truncated protein, or a malfunctional protein. A loss of the carboxyterminal noncollagenous domain would prohibit the formation of heterotrimers. Several mutations in Alport syndrome involve replacement of a glycine residue in the collagenous domain

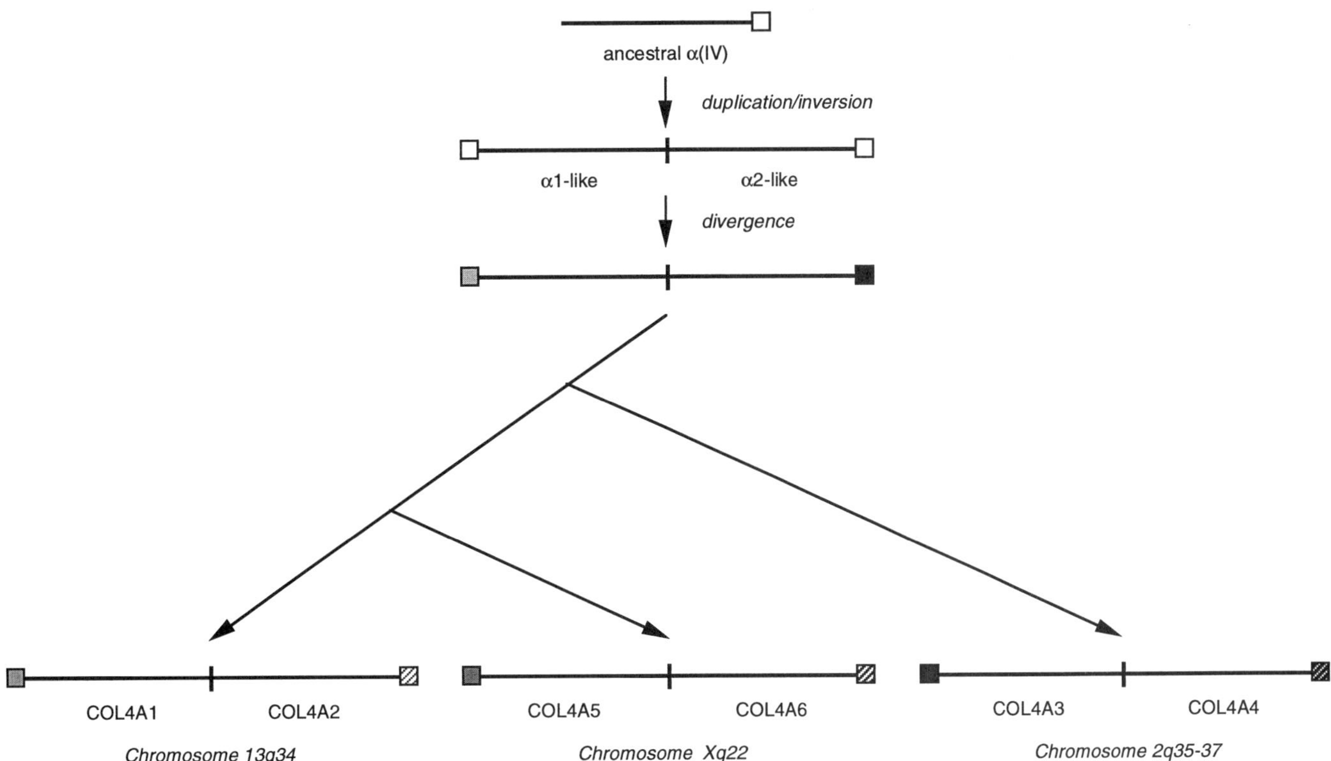

Figure 68-3 Evolution of type IV collagen genes. Analysis of the gene and protein sequences indicate that an ancestor type IV collagen α chain gene was first duplicated and inversed, followed by divergence of the genes to α1- and α2-like genes. This gene pair was later duplicated to two other chromosomes so that the α3(IV) and α4(IV) genes were formed prior to those of α5(IV) and α6(IV).

by another amino acid. Glycines at every third position are required for the formation of collagen triple helices, since this amino acid is the only amino acid small enough to fit into the interior of the tightly wound triple helix. Glycine mutations are also frequently the cause of other collagen disorders such as osteogenesis imperfecta. Based on the knowledge obtained from studies on osteogenesis imperfecta, it has been suggested that the abnormally folded triple helices are very susceptible to degradative enzymes, leading to the partial or total absence of all the α3, α4, and α5 chains. As a result, the structural framework of the GBM, which requires type IV molecules containing these polypeptide chains, becomes structurally weak and disrupted. The use of monoclonal antibodies against the α3, α4, or α5 chains in immunofluorescense microscopy of kidney biopsies may become a method to confirm the diagnosis of Alport syndrome in some cases, as an absence of these antigens can sometimes be seen in the skin basement membrane. A mouse model for the autosomal form of Alport syndrome has been produced by a collagen COL4A3 knockout. The mice develop progressive glomerulonephritis.

An interesting fact is that a clear correlation cannot be found between the nature of a mutation and the respective phenotype. A small single amino acid substitution can cause as severe symptoms as a large deletion of almost the entire collagen gene.

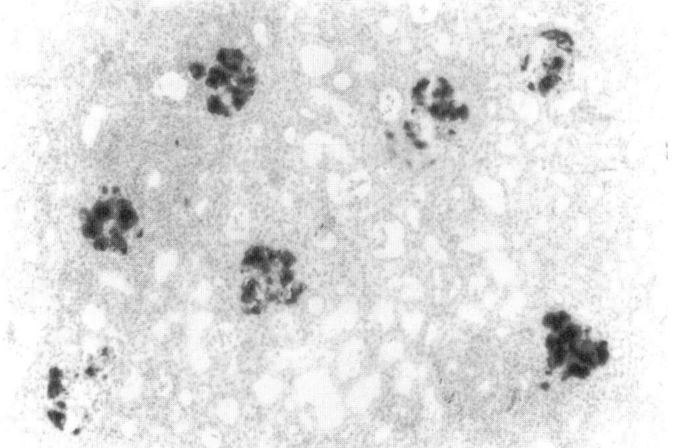

Figure 68-4 Expression of β-galactosidase in porcine kidneys following in vivo perfusion with an adenovirus containing the β-galactosidase reporter gene under the cytomegalovirus promoter. Intense expression (dark color) can be observed in almost all glomeruli, whereas little, if any, is observed in the tubular cells. (*See* color insert following p. 684.)

THERAPY

GENERAL Although the onset of hematuria occurs during early childhood, the disease usually progresses slowly. A large number of male patients enter terminal renal failure during adolescence (juvenile form), but the onset also occurs beyond 25 years of age (adult type). Usually affected males and homozygous females develop end-stage renal disease before the fifth decade of life, while heterozygous females rarely develop renal failure. There is no satisfactory and curative conservative treatment available. Patients developing end-stage renal disease are treated by hemodialysis and also by kidney transplantation whenever possible. About 5% of transplanted patients develop anti-GBM nephritis and reject the allografted kidneys.

PROSPECTS FOR GENE THERAPY As a result of this advances in molecular genetics and biology research, gene therapy may be developing into a real possibility for the treatment of hereditary diseases in the future. Although gene therapy has not yet come of age as a real therapeutic alternative, extensive research efforts are being made in that direction. Hereditary kidney diseases such as Alport syndrome, primarily affecting the renal glomeruli, could potentially be treated by somatic gene therapy, which involves the introduction of normal cDNAs or complete genes for the α3, α4, or α5 chains into glomerular cells. Recent work has already shown it to be possible to transfer foreign genes into over 85% of the glomeruli in vivo (Fig. 68-4). Thus, the stage has been set for actual gene therapy experiments in animal models of Alport syndrome. There are, however, many obstacles to overcome before we can expect the disease to be cured in humans by gene therapy. But if gene therapy is going to become a viable alternative for the treatment of genetic diseases in general, it is likely to become an option for Alport syndrome.

SELECTED REFERENCES

Adler SG, Cohen AH, and Glassock RJ. Secondary glomerular diseases. In: Brenner BM, ed. The Kidney, 5th ed. Philadelphia, PA: W.B. Saunders, 1996; pp. 1555–1558.

Alport AC. Hereditary familial congenital haemorrhagic nephritis. Br Med J 1927;1:504–506.

Atkin CL, Gregory MC, Border WA. Alport syndrome. In: Schrier WW, Gottschalk, CW, eds. Diseases of Kidney. Boston: Little, Brown, 1988; pp. 617–641.

Atkin CL, Hasstedt SJ, Menlove L, et al. Mapping of Alport syndrome to the long arm of the X-chromosome. Am J Hum Genet 1988;42: 249–255.

Barker DF, Hostikka SL, Zhou J, et al. Identification of mutations in the COL4A5 collagen gene in Alport syndrome. Science 1990;248: 1224–1227.

Brunner H, Schroder C, van Bennekom C. Localization of the gene for X-linked Alport's syndrome. Kidney Int 1988;34:507–510.

Cosgrove D, Meehan DT, Grunkemeyer JA, et al. Collagen COL4A3 knockout: a mouse model for autosoma Alport syndrome. Genes Dev 1996;10:2981–2992.

Ding J, Stitzel J, Berry P, Hawkins E, Kashtan CE. Autosomal recessive Alport syndrome: mutation in the COL4A3 gene in a woman with Alport syndrome and posttransplant antiglomerular basement membrane nephritis. J Am Soc Nephrol 1995;5:1714–1717.

Flinter FA, Abbs S, Bobrow M. Localization of the gene for classic Alport syndrome. Genomics 1989;4:335–338.

Heikkilä P, Parpala T, Lukkarinen O, Weber M, Tryggvason K. Adenovirus-mediated gene transfer into kidney glomeruli using an *ex vivo* and *in vivo* kidney perfusion system—First steps towards gene therapy of Alport syndrome. Gene Therapy 1996;3:21–27.

Heiskari N, Zhang X, Zhou J, et al. Identification of 17 mutations in ten exons in the COL4A5 collagen gene, but no mutations found in four exons in COL4A6: a study of 250 patients with hematuria and suspected of having Alport syndrome. J Am Soc Nephrol 1996;7:702–709.

Hostikka SL, Eddy RL, Byers MG, et al. Identification of a distinct type of IV collagen α chain with restricted kidney distribution and assignment of its gene to the locus of X chromosome-linked Alport syndrome. Proc Natl Acad Sci USA 1990;87:1606–1610.

Hudson BG, Reeders ST, and Tryggvason K. Type IV collagen: structure, gene organization, and role in human diseases: molecular basis of Goodpasture and Alport syndromes and diffuse leiomyomatosis. Minireview J Biol Chem 1993;268:26,033–26,036.

Kalluri R, Shield CF, Todd P, Hudson BG, Neilson EG. Isoform switching of type IV collagen is developmentally arrested in X-linked Alport syndrome leading to increased susceptibility of renal basement membranes to endoproteolysis. J Clin Invest 1997;99:2470–2478.

Knebelmann B, Breillat C, Forestier L, et al. Spectrum of mutations in the COL4A5 collagen gene in X-linked Alport syndrome. Am J Hum Genet 1996;59:1221–1232.

Lemmink HH, Mochizuki T, van den Heuvel LPWJ, et al. Mutations in the type IV α3 (COL4A3) gene in autosomal recessive Alport syndrome. Hum Molec Genet 1994;3:1269–1273.

Lemmick HH, Schroder CH, Monnens LA, Smeets HJ. The clinical spectrum of type IV collagen mutations. Hum Mutat 1997;9:477–499.

Miner JH, Sanes JR. Molecular and functional defects in kidneys of mice lacking collagen alpha 3(IV): implications for Alport syndrome. J Cell Biol 1996;135:1403–1413.

Mochizuki T, Lemmink HH, Mariyama M, et al. Identification of mutations in the α3(IV) α4(IIV) collagen genes in autosomal recessive Alport syndrome. Nature Genet 1994;8:77–82.

Renieri A, Bruttini M, Galli L, et al. X-linked Alport syndrome: an SSCP-based mutation surve over all 51 exons of the COL4A5 gene. Am J Hum Genet 1996;58:1192–1204.

Rhys C, Snyers B, Pirson Y. Recurrent corneal erosion associated with Alport's syndrome. Rapid Communication. Kidney Int 1997;52:208–211.

Saito A, Yamazaki H, Nakagawa Y, Arakawa M. Molecular genetics of renal diseases. Intern Med 1997;36:81–86.

Tryggvason K. Mutations in type IV collagen genes and Alport phenotypes. In: Tryggvason K, ed. Molecular Pathology and Genetics of Alport Syndrome, vol 117. Basel: Karger, 1996, pp. 154–171.

Tryggvason K, Zhou J, Hostikka SL, Shows T. Molecular genetics of Alport syndrome. Kidney Int 1993;43:38–44.

Yurchenco PD. Assembly of basement membranes. In: Fleischmajer R, Olsen BR, Kühn, K, eds. Structure, Molecular Biology and Pathology of Collagen, vol. 580. Ann New York Acad Sci, 1990; pp. 195–213.

69 Nephrogenic Diabetes Insipidus

DENNIS BROWN AND DENNIS A. AUSIELLO

INTRODUCTION

The neurohypophyseal antidiuretic hormone, arginine vasopressin (AVP), stimulates urinary concentration in mammals by increasing the water permeability of renal collecting ducts and by stimulating NaCl reabsorption by thick ascending limbs of Henle into the medullary interstitium. In the collecting duct, AVP binds to specific V2 receptors (V2R) on the basolateral plasma membrane of principal cells and stimulates adenylyl cyclase, which increases cytosolic cAMP levels. The increase in cAMP activates protein kinase A (PKA) and protein phosphorylation ensues. While the nature and role of the PKA substrates remains generally obscure, one phosphorylated protein is the vasopressin-sensitive water channel, aquaporin 2 (AQP2), which relocates from a pool of intracellular vesicles to the apical plasma membrane of principal cells upon vasopressin stimulation. This exocytotic insertion of water channels, illustrated in Fig. 69-1, greatly increases the water permeability of the principal cell apical membrane. Because the basolateral membrane of principal cells has a constitutively high water permeability because of the presence of two other water channels, AQP3 and AQP4, this vasopressin-induced apical exocytotic process is the rate-limiting step for increasing collecting duct epithelial cell water permeability. The urine in the tubule lumen equilibrates osmotically with the hypertonic interstitium by the bulk flow of water across the collecting duct principal cells, and the urine is concentrated.

Defective urinary concentration has long been recognized in man and in animal models such as the Brattleboro DI rat and the nephrogenic diabetes insipidus (NDI) mouse. The molecular basis for many of these related disorders has been examined and elucidated, thanks to the cloning and sequencing of two of the key proteins involved, the V2R and the vasopressin-sensitive collecting duct water channel, AQP2. This brief review will discuss cell and molecular biological evidence showing that mutations resulting in defective targeting and/or function of the V2R and the AQP2 water channel can both lead to distinct forms of NDI. Type I congenital nephrogenic DI (CNDI), the more frequent X-linked form, is caused by mutations in the vasopressin receptor, whereas type II CNDI is an autosomal recessive disease resulting from mutations in the AQP2 water channel.

From: *Principles of Molecular Medicine* (J. L. Jameson, ed.), ©1998 Humana Press Inc., Totowa, NJ.

CONGENITAL NDI—LOCATION OF THE VASOPRESSIN V2 RECEPTOR (V2R) GENE

CNDI was first described over 50 years ago, and genetic linkage studies in several families established that it is an X-linked trait. In CNDI, arginine vasopressin production is normal, but the target cells in the kidney do not respond to the presence of circulating hormone. Thus, the transepithelial water permeability of the collecting duct remains in its low basal state, and a large volume of hypotonic urine is produced. Clinically, this condition is recognizable soon after birth and if not corrected can result in severe dehydration, hypernatremia, and damage to the central nervous system. Linkage studies showed that the gene responsible is located in the subtelomeric region of the long arm of the X chromosome in region 28 (Xq28), where the V2R gene is also located.

STRUCTURE OF THE V2R

The V2R is a 371-amino acid protein that is a member of the family of seven membrane-spanning domain receptors that couple to heterotrimeric G proteins. Other members of this large family include rhodopsin and the β_2-adrenergic receptor. Homologs of the V2R have been cloned from human, pig, and rat, and the receptor sequences are more than 90% identical. The membrane topology of the receptor, as well as several functionally important features, are illustrated in Fig.69-2. These include: (1) an extracellular N-terminus with a consensus site for N-linked glycosylation; (2) a cytoplasmic carboxy-terminus and large intracellular loop that contain several sites for serine and threonine kinase phosphorylation, and which probably play a role in receptor internalization and sequestration; (3) conserved sites for fatty acylation, which may serve as an additional membrane anchor in the C-terminal tail; and (4) two highly conserved cysteine residues in the second and third extracellular loops, which may form a disulfide bridge that is important for correct folding of the molecule and stabilization of the ligand-binding site.

CNDI AND MUTATIONS IN THE V2R

A series of reports have now identified mutations in the coding sequence of the V2R gene that can account for the production of a nonfunctional receptor by target cells in the kidney. A vast array of missense, nonsense, and frameshift mutations in various domains of the receptor coding sequence have been reviewed in detail previously, and some are illustrated in Fig. 69-3. Some result in the appearance of premature stop codons, which produce an effective null mutation by causing early truncation of the growing

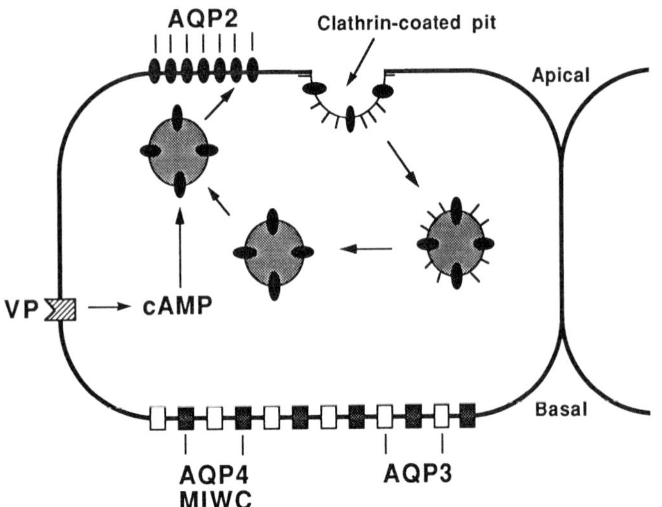

Figure 69-1 Proposed pathway of AQP2 recycling in collecting duct principal cells. AQP2 is located on intracellular vesicles that move to and fuse with the apical plasma membrane following vasopressin stimulation and a subsequent rise in intracellular cAMP levels. The water channel is then internalized via clathrin-coated pits and eventually recycles back to the apical membrane in a complex trafficking pathway that has not yet been fully elucidated. In the same cell type, two other aquaporins, AQP3 and AQP4 (also referred to as the mercurial insensitive water channel [MIWC]), are located on the basolateral plasma membrane. The membrane localization of these two proteins is not regulated by vasopressin. They are constitutively present in this membrane domain, and they are assumed to be responsible for its permanently high water permeability.

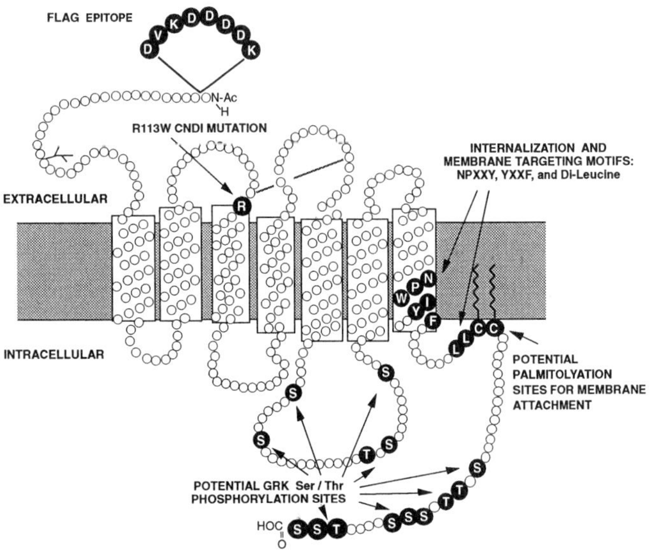

Figure 69-2 Membrane topology of the vasopressin receptor (V2R) molecule. The 371-amino acid protein has seven membrane-spanning domains, an extracellular N-terminus, and a cytoplasmic C-terminus. Several features of the molecule are illustrated, with some key residues and potential phosphorylation sites shown in black. One mutation (R113W), close to the disulfide bridge, is shown. In work from our laboratory, a FLAG epitope added to the N-terminus allows efficient immunolocalization studies to be performed and was used to demonstrate retention of the R113W mutation in the RER.

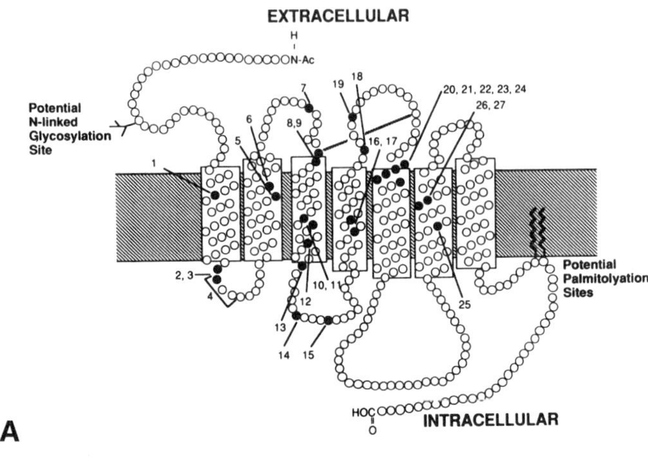

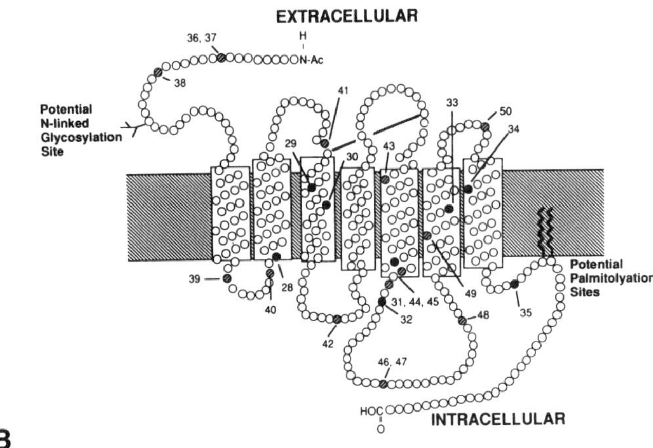

Figure 69-3 Reported mutations in the V2R, showing the diversity of affected sites and types of mutations. **(A)** Missense mutations. **(B)** Nonsense and frameshift mutations. (Taken from Holtzman et al.)

polypeptide chain. Others are single-point mutations that cause a single amino acid replacement at a functionally critical site in the receptor molecule. One such example is an arginine (R) 113 to tryptophan (W) mutation caused by a C -> T base transition. This point mutation at the end of the first extracellular loop is one amino acid toward the carboxyl-terminus from a critical cysteine residue and may interfere with the formation of an important disulfide bond within the vasopressin receptor. Interestingly, an analysis of other G-protein coupled receptors has shown that tryptophan is never found at position 113 in any functional receptor, indicating that its presence is incompatible with normal receptor function.

Mutations in the V2R sequence that still allow the production of a full-length or near full-length protein could result in CNDI by interfering with different aspects of the receptor-ligand signal transduction cascade. For example: (1) the receptor could be expressed normally at the plasma membrane, but fail to bind vasopressin; (2) the receptor could be expressed normally at the membrane, bind its ligand normally, but fail to couple to its stimulatory GTP-binding protein, so that adenylyl cyclase is not activated;(3) the mutated receptor may be incorrectly folded and might be retained for degradation in the rough endoplasmic reticulum (RER), and may never reach the cell surface; (4) changes in the ability of the receptor to be phosphorylated may affect several aspects of function, including trafficking and desensitization. So far, functional analyses of the potential cell biological mechanisms that result in CNDI have lagged behind the rapid rate at which various V2R mutants have been identified at the molecular level.

THE R133W MUTATION MODIFIES INTRACELLULAR TRAFFICKING OF THE V2R

The experiment in nature provided by the R113W V2R mutation has provided a model for the study of structural elements within receptors that permit proper folding and/or movement through the intracellular biosynthetic pathway. It has been repeatedly shown that misfolded proteins are triaged by a rigorous quality-control mechanism within the RER, and in most cases abnormally folded or assembled proteins are targeted for intracellular degradation without leaving the RER. When expressed at normal levels in vivo, the R113W V2R probably never reaches the plasma membrane in detectable amounts. Experimental overexpression of the R113W V2R in transfected LLC-PK1 cells appears to "saturate" the quality-control process, allowing at least some mutated V2R to escape degradation and reach the cell surface. Once at the cell surface, the R113W V2R can bind vasopressin, albeit at lower affinity than the wild type receptor, and can stimulate intracellular cAMP accumulation. However, even in transfected cells, the bulk of the mutated receptor is located within the RER by immunocytochemistry (Ausiello et al., unpublished results). An R337V2R mutation provides another example of receptor dysfunction because of arrested maturation and degradation before expression on the cell surface.

Thus, this particular mutation disables the V2R and the urinary concentrating mechanism, not by preventing receptor-ligand binding (although there is a shift in binding affinity), but by modifying the intracellular trafficking of the abnormal protein, such that it never reaches the plasma membrane and never comes into contact with its stimulatory ligand. A similar situation occurs in cystic fibrosis. The most common mutation in the CFTR gene product is the so-called ΔF508 mutation, again a single-point mutation. This mutation also leads to the trapping of a misfolded CFTR protein in the RER and prevents its delivery to the cell surface where it normally functions as a PKA-regulated chloride channel. Under experimental conditions that allow delivery of the ΔF508 CFTR to the cell surface, it functions normally and is regulated normally by PKA. Functional rescue of mutant V2 receptors has been demonstrated in transfected COS-7 cells by coexpression of the normal receptor sequences. Thus, it may be possible to devise therapeutic strategies that result in the correct delivery of misfolded, but otherwise functionally active, proteins to their correct location at the cell surface in vivo.

AUTOSOMAL RECESSIVE NDI—MUTATIONS IN AQUAPORIN 2

Some cases of NDI are not of the typical X-linked type, but are autosomal-recessive in nature. Alterations in the vasopressin receptor have not been found in these individuals, but instead, the defect lies within the vasopressin-regulated water channel, aquaporin 2 (AQP2). Based on two decades of studies, it was postulated that vasopressin exerts its antidiuretic effect by causing the exocytotic insertion of water channels into the apical plasma membrane of collecting duct principal cells (Fig. 69-1). The resulting increase in membrane water permeability allows osmotic equilibration to occur between the luminal fluid (urine) and the hypertonic medullary interstitium of the inner medulla.

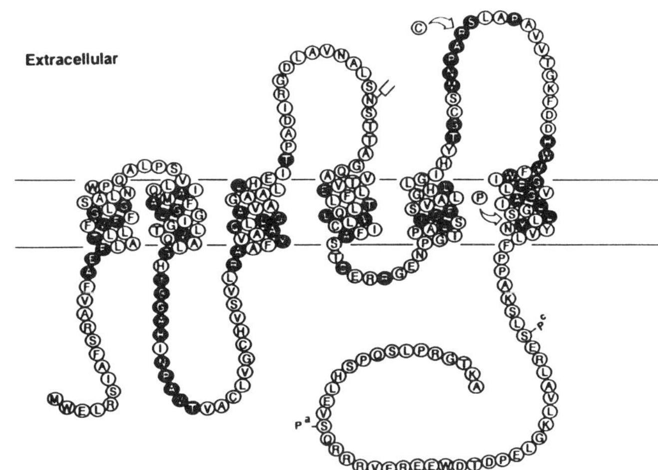

Figure 69-4 Membrane topology of the aquaporin 2 (AQP2) water channel. This 271-amino acid protein spans the lipid bilayer six times. Both N- and C-termini are in the cytoplasm. There is a consensus site for N-glycosylation in the second extracellular loop, and phosphorylation sites for PKC (Pc) and PKA (Pa) are located in the C-terminal tail. Two point mutations (R187C and S216P) that were found in NDI patients are indicated with arrows. (Taken from Deen et al.)

AQP2 was cloned and sequenced based on its homology to AQP1, and a series of studies showed that AQP2 is the vasopressin-sensitive water channel in collecting duct principal cells. In collecting duct principal cells, the membrane localization of AQP2 is tightly regulated by the antidiuretic hormone, vasopressin. In Brattleboro homozygous rats, which lack vasopressin and which have hypothalamic diabetes insipidus, AQP2 is located primarily on intracellular vesicles but is delivered to the apical plasma membrane by exocytosis following vasopressin treatment in vivo. A similar translocation was seen in isolated perfused tubules from normal rat. More recently, translocation of AQP2 from intracellular vesicles to the plasma membrane has been demonstrated in transfected renal epithelial cells in culture. This latter result shows that the AQP2 protein contains sorting information that allows it to be incorporated into a regulated pathway of exocytosis. Together, these data directly support the shuttle hypothesis of vasopressin action, which invokes a cycle of exo- and endocytosis of water channels to explain the stimulatory effect of vasopressin on collecting duct water permeability.

In contrast, the proximal tubule and thin limb water channel, AQP1, is delivered to the plasma membrane in a constitutive, nonregulated pathway that results in a permanently high membrane water permeability in these renal epithelial cells. When expressed in epithelial cells in culture, AQP1 is also delivered to the cell surface without the need for hormonal stimulation. Thus, AQP1 and AQP2 contain distinct targeting motifs that direct them to different and physiologically important intracellular transport pathways. These distinct pathways can be maintained in vitro in transfected epithelial cells, providing powerful new model systems for the investigation of aquaporin cell biology.

Important data on the role of AQP2 in non–X-linked NDI was obtained by examining the AQP2 molecule in human disease. A few examples of AQP2 mutations have now been described (Fig. 69-4), but in most cases the cause of the AQP2 inactivity is not clear. In the first patient studied, two distinct point mutations were found that resulted in a substitution of Cys for Arg^{187}, and Pro for Ser[216]. The R187C mutation occurs in a region of the third extracellular loop that is strongly conserved in members of the aquaporin family. The S216P mutation is located in the last transmembrane domain of AQP2. When mRNAs coding for these mutated proteins (which had the predicted size of 29 kDa) were expressed in Xenopus oocytes, no increase in membrane osmotic water permeability was detected above that seen in water-injected controls. However, whether the mutated proteins actually reached the cell surface of oocytes is unknown.

Mutations in the AQP2 gene that result in production of a full-length protein could have at least two consequences that would result in a loss of principal cell vasopressin-sensitivity: (1) the production of an AQP2 channel that is still vasopressin-sensitive, and is inserted into the plasma membrane after vasopressin action, but which has lost the capacity to function as a water channel; (2) the production of a water channel that is still functional, but that is no longer targeted to the plasma membrane after vasopressin action.

Other mutations could, of course, be null mutations that result in an absent or severely truncated protein. In support of the second possibility, oocyte expression studies have shown that the missense mutations R187C and S216P are impaired in their delivery to the cell surface. The trapped form of these AQP2 mutants is a 32-kDa high mannose form, indicating that the protein is blocked in the RER, in much the same way as the ΔF508 CFTR mutation is trapped inside the RER. However, it could not be determined whether these mutants were also functionally inactive water channels. That the water permeability of AQP2 can be modified by mutagenesis was shown by recent data indicating that some point mutations, including mutations in asparagine residue 123, significantly affect channel water permeability. The plasma membrane expression of this mutation was only slightly decreased from that shown by the wild type protein in oocytes.

ACQUIRED NDI

Several pathological conditions or drugs result in the syndrome of acquired NDI. Among these are lithium-induced NDI and hypokalemia (which occurs in 40% of all patients receiving lithium, polyuria in up to 35%, and NDI in 12–20%). Many studies have shown that a major cellular effect of lithium is an impairment of cAMP production that would, in principal cells, normally occur after vasopressin stimulation. While the basis for this inhibition is likely to be complex, acute lithium loading in renal epithelial cells directly inhibits adenylyl cyclase activation by competing for activation of the stimulatory GTP-binding protein subunit, Gs. The effect appears to be at the magnesium-sensitive rate limiting step in the generation of dissociated and GTP-activated Gαs-subunit, which normally activates adenylyl cyclase.

How might this modify collecting duct water permeability? Acutely, the effect would be to inhibit vasopressin-induced insertion of the AQP2 water channel into the plasma membrane of principal cells, which is a cAMP-dependent process. However, lithium also has chronic effects, and it has recently been shown that the cellular content of AQP2 protein is decreased in lithium-treated rats. This effect probably results from decreased transcription of the AQP2 gene, which is known to have a cAMP-responsive element in its 5' flanking region. Other studies have shown that dehydration of normal rats, or AVP treatment of Brattleboro rats, increases cellular AQP2 levels, implying that increased cellular cAMP "switches on" AQP2 production in principal cells. In lithium intoxication, the cellular cAMP levels would be chronically reduced, thus lowering AQP2 production at the transcriptional level.

Hypokalemia also results in NDI, and experimental hypokalemia in rats also reduces the cellular content of AQP2. Again, the precise cause is unknown, but hypokalemia causes cellular resistance to AVP, as well as directly stimulating thirst. At the cell biological level, it is known that lowering cellular potassium inhibits clathrin-mediated endocytosis and thus may interfere with the exo- and endocytosis of key proteins involved in the antidiuretic response. In particular, AQP2 is probably internalized and recycled by a process involving clathrin-coated pits, and most receptors, including the vasopressin receptor, is also dependent on clathrin-mediated endocytosis as part of its recycling pathway. Thus, interference with the correct recycling of either or both of these proteins could result in an NDI-like syndrome. Studies on tissues from potassium-depleted animals have shown a significant reduction in AVP-induced cAMP generation, which would, as in the case of lithium toxicity, result in lower transcription on the AQP2 gene and lower AQP2 levels in principal cells.

SUMMARY

With the cloning and sequencing of key proteins that are involved in the renal medullary concentrating mechanism, cell biological explanations for nephrogenic diabetes insipidus are now emerging. In congenital X-linked NDI, many mutations in the vasopressin receptor result in varying degrees of receptor inactivation, either by altering the function of the receptor itself or by preventing its proper targeting and trafficking to the plasma membrane of principal cells in the collecting duct. The rarer cases of non–X-linked NDI can, in some cases, be attributed to defects in the AQP2 water channel. Again, it is likely that functional as well as trafficking mutations will explain the NDI phenotype in cases where vasopressin-receptor activation and cAMP generation are normal. Finally, two examples of acquired NDI were presented, and potential causes of the defect based on the cellular actions of lithium and hypokalemia on AQP2 production and trafficking have been proposed.

SELECTED REFERENCES

Ausiello DA, Holtzman EJ, Gronich GH, Ercolani L. Cell signalling. In: Seldin DW, Giebisch G, eds. The Kidney: Physiology and Pathophysiology. New York: Raven, 1992; pp. 645–692.

Bai L, Fushimi K, Sasaki S, Marumo FG. Structure of aquaporin-2 vasopressin water channel. J Biol Chem 1996;271:5171–5176.

Bichet DG. X-linked nephrogenic diabetes insipidus mutations in North America and the Hopewell hypothesis. J Clin Invest 1992;92: 1262–1268.

Bichet DG, Cameron S, Davison AM. Nephrogenic diabetes insipidus. In: Graunfeld JP, Kerr D, Ritz E, eds. Oxford Textbook of Clinical Nephrology. New York: Oxford Medical, 1992; pp. 789–800.

Birnbaumer M, Seibold A, Gilbert S. Molecular cloning of the receptor for human antidiuretic hormone. Nature 1992;357:333–335.

Bonifacio JS, Suzuki CK, Klausner RD. A peptide sequence confers retention and rapid degradation in the endoplasmic reticulum. Science 1990;247:79–82.

Brown D, Orci L. Vasopressin stimulates the formation of coated pits in rat kidney collecting ducts. Nature 1983;302:253–255.

Brown D, Shields GI, Valtin H, Morris JF, Orci L. Lack of intramembranous particle clusters in collecting ducts of mice with nephrogenic diabetes insipidus. Am J Physiol 1985;249:F582–F589.

Brown D, Stow JL. Protein trafficking and polarity in kidney epithelium: from cell biology to physiology. Physiol Rev 1996;76:245–297.

Brown D, Weyer P, Orci L. Vasopressin stimulates endocytosis in kidney collecting duct epithelial cells. Eur J Cell Biol 1988;46:336–340.

Cheng S, Gregory DR, Marshall J, et al. Defective intracellular transport and processing of CFTR is the molecular basis of most cystic fibrosis. Cell 1990;63:827–834.

Cheong HI, Park HW, Ha IS, et al. Six novel mutations in the vasopressin V2 receptor gene causing nephrogenic diabetes insipidus. Nephron 1997;75:431–437.

Deen PM, Verdijk MA, Knoers NV, et al. Requirement of human renal water channel aquaporin-2 for vasopressin-dependent concentration of urine. Science 1994;264:92–95.

Deen PMT, Croes H, van Aubel RAMH, Ginsel LA, van Os CH. Water channels encoded by mutant aquaporin-2 genes in nephrogenic diabetes insipidus are impaired in their cellular routing. J Clin Invest 1995;95:2291–2296.

Dohlman HG, Thorner J, Caron MG, Lefkowitz RJ. Model systems for the study of seven-transmembrane-segment receptors. Annu Rev Biochem 1991;60:653–688.

Ecelbarger CA, Terris J, Frindt G, et al. Aquaporin-3 water channel localization and regulation in rat kidney. Am J Physiol 1995;269:F663–F672.

Echevarria M, Windhager EE, Tate SS, Frindt G. Cloning and expression of AQP3, a water channel from the medullary collecting duct of rat kidney. Proc Natl Acad Sci USA 1994;91:10,997–11,001.

Forssmann H. On hereditary diabetes insipidus. Acat Med Scand 1994;121 (Suppl. 159):9–46.

Frigeri A, Gropper MA, Kawashima M, Brown D, Verkman AS. Localization of MIWC and GLIP water channel homologs in neuromuscular, epithelial and glandular tissues. J Cell Sci 1995;108:2993–3002.

Fushimi K, Uchida S, Hara Y, Hirata Y, Marumo F, Sasaki S. Cloning and expression of apical membrane water channel of rat kidney collecting tubule. Nature 1993;361:549–552.

Hayashi M, Sasaki S, Tsuganezawa H, et al. Expression and distribution of aquaporin of collecting duct are regulated by vasopressin V2 receptor in rat kidney. J Clin Invest 1994;94:1778–1783.

Hochberg Z, Van Lieburg A, Even L, et al. Autosomal recessive nephrogenic diabetes insipidus caused by an aquaporin-2 mutation. J Clin Endocrinol Metab 1997;82:686–689.

Holtzman EJ, Ausiello DA. A molecular defect in the vasopressin V2-receptor gene causing nephrogenic diabetes insipidus. N Engl J Med 1993;328:1534–1537.

Holtzman EJ, Kolakowski LF, Ausiello DA. The molecular biology of congenital nephrogenic diabetes insipidus. In: Schlondorff D, Bonventre JV, eds. Molecular Nephrology. New York: Marcel Dekker, 1995; pp. 887–910.

Hozawa S, Holtzman EJ, Ausiello DA. cAMP motifs regulatingtranscription of the aquaporin 2 gene. Am J Physiol 1996;270:C1695–C1702.

Ishibashi K, Sasaki S, Fushimi K, et al. Molecular cloning and expression of a member of the aquaporin family with permeability to glycerol and urea in addition to water expressed at the basolateral membrane of kidney collecting duct cells. Proc Natl Acad Sci USA 1994;91:6269–6273.

Katsura T, Verbavatz JM, Farinas J, et al. Constitutive and regulated membrane expression of aquaporin-CHIP (AQP1) and aquaporin 2 water channels in stably transfected LLC-PK1 epithelial cells. Proc Natl Acad Sci USA 1995;92:7212–7216.

Lolait SJ, O'Carroll AM, Konig M, Morel A, Brownstein MJ. Cloning and characterization of a vasopressin V2 receptor and possible link to nephrogenic diabetes insipidus. Nature 1992;357:336–339.

Marples D, Christensen S, Christensen EI, Ottosen PD, Nielsen S. Lithium-induced downregulation of aquaporin-2 water channel expression in rat kidney medulla. J Clin Invest 1995;95:1838–1845.

Marples D, Frokiaer J, Dorup J, Knepper MA, Nielsen S. Hypokalemia-induced downregulation of aquaporin-2 water channel expression in rat kidney medulla and cortex. J Clin Invest 1996;97:1960–1968.

Marples D, Knepper MA, Christensen EI, Nielsen S. Redistribution of aquaporin-2 water channels induced by vasopressin in rat kidney inner medullary collecting duct. Am J Physiol 1995;269:C655–C664.

Mulders SM, Knoers NV, Van Lieburg AF, et al. New mutations in the AQP2 gene in nephrogenic diabetes insipidus resulting in functional but misrouted water channels. J Am Soc Nephrol 1997;8:242–248.

Nielsen S, Chou CL, Marples D, Christensen EI, Kishore BK, Knepper MA. Vasopressin increases water permeability of kidney collecting duct by inducing translocation of aquaporin-CD water channels to plasma membrane. Proc Soc Natl Acad Sci USA 1995;92:1013–1017.

Nielsen S, DiGiovanni SR, Christensen EI, Knepper MA, Harris HW. Cellular and subcellular immunolocalization of vasopressin-regulated water channel in rat kidney. Proc Natl Acad Sci USA 1993;90: 11,663–11,667.

Nielsen S, Smith BL, Christensen EI, Knepper MA, Agre P. CHIP28 water channels are localized in constitutively water-permeable segments of the nephron. J Cell Biol 1993;120:371–383.

Pang Y, Metzenberg A, Das S, Jing B, Gitschier J. Mutations in the V2 vasopressin receptor gene are associated with X-linked diabetes insipidus. Nat Genet 1992;2:103–106.

Robinson MG, Kaplan SA. Inheritance of vasopressin-resistant nephrogenic diabetes insipidus. Am J Dis Child 1960;99:164–174.

Rosenthal W, Seibold A, Antaramian A, et al. Molecular identification of the gene responsible for congenital nephrogenic diabetes insipidus. Nature 1992;359:233–235.

Sabolic I, Katsura T, Verbavatz JM, Brown D. The AQP2 water channel: effect of vasopressin treatment, microtubule disruption, and distribution in neonatal rats. J Memb Biol 1995;143:165–175.

Sabolic I, Valenti G, Verbavatz J, et al. Localization of the CHIP28 water channel in rat kidney. Am J Physiol 1992;263:C1225–C1233.

Sadeghi HM, Innamorati G, Birnbaumer M. An X-linked NDI mutation reveals a requirement for cell surface V2R expression. Mol Endocrinol 1997;11:706–713.

Schoneberg T, Yun J, Wenkert D, Wess J. Functional rescue of mutant V2 vasopression receptors causing nephrogenic diabetes insipidus by a co-expressed receptor polypeptide. EMBO J 1996;15:1283–1291.

Skorecki KL, Brown D, Ercolani L, Ausiello DA. Molecular mechanisms of vasopressin action in the kidney. In: Windhanger EE, ed. Handbook of Physiology: Section 8, Renal Physiology. New York: Oxford University Press, 1992; pp. 1185–1218.

Strange K, Willingham MC, Handler JC, Harris HW Jr. Apical membrane endocytosis via coated pits is stimulated by removal of antidiuretic hormone from isolated, perfused rabbit cortical collecting tubule. J Membr Biol 1988;103:17–28.

Terris J, Ecelbarger CA, Marples D, Knepper MA, Nielsen S. Distribution of aquaporin-4 water channel expression within rat kidney. Am J Physiol 1995;269:F775–F785.

Valtin H. The discovery of the Brattleboro rat, recommended nomenclature, and the question of proper controls. Ann NY Acad Sci 1982; 394:1–9.

van den Ouweland AMW, Dressen JCFM, Verdijk M, et al. Mutations in the vasopressin type 2 receptor gene (AVPR2) associated with nephrogenic diabetes insipidus. Nat Genet 1992;2:99–102.

van Lieburg AF, Verdijk MA, Knoers VV, et al. Patients with autosomal nephrogenic diabetes insipidus homozygous for mutations in the aquaporin 2 water-channel gene. Am J Hum Genet 1994;55:648–652.

Wade JB, Stetson DL, Lewis SA. ADH action: evidence for a membrane shuttle mechanism. Ann NY Acad Sci 1981;372:106–117.

Wenkert D, Schoneberg T, Merendino JJ Jr, et al. Functional characterization of five V2 vasopressin receptor gene mutations. Mol Cell Endocrinol 1996;124:43–50.

Williams RH, Henry C. Nephrogenic diabetes insipidus transmitted by females and appearing during infancy in males. Ann Int Med 1947;27:84–95.

Yamamoto T, Sasaki S, Fushimi K, et al. Localization and expression of a collecting duct water channel, aquaporin, in hydrated and dehydrated rats. Exp Nephrol 1995;3:193–201.

70 Polycystic Kidney Disease

GREGORY G. GERMINO AND LUIZ F. ONUCHIC

BACKGROUND

Renal cysts are common clinical findings, often incidentally discovered in the course of evaluating other problems. They may be either acquired or seen in association with a number of inherited and congenital disorders. The most common disorder, autosomal dominant polycystic kidney disease (ADPKD), is an important cause of end-stage renal disease (ESRD), accounting for 5–8% of the entire ESRD population. At the time of Dalgaard's sentinel description of polycystic kidney disease (PKD), death from renal failure was a frequent outcome for affected individuals. While transplantation and dialysis have improved the prognosis for those suffering from PKD, no therapies have yet been discovered that prevent or inhibit cystogenesis. Hindering their development has been an incomplete knowledge of the pathogenesis of this process. Although most types of renal cysts share some common features (cell proliferation, basement membrane abnormalities, fluid secretion), the broad range of disorders associated with renal cysts suggests that defects in multiple, possibly intersecting, pathways are responsible for cyst formation and expansion. Recent molecular genetic studies have yielded important breakthroughs that are likely to lead to the unraveling of this mystery. In this chapter, we will review these data and how they have improved our understanding of renal cystic disease.

CLINICAL FEATURES

The hallmark of this group of disorders is the replacement of normal renal parenchyma by cysts in a process that frequently results in renal impairment. The cysts vary greatly in number and size, ranging from microscopic lesions of several millimeters in diameter to very large, macroscopic structures >10 cm in width. In general, larger cysts are seen in ADPKD, tuberous sclerosis (TS), and von Hippel Lindau disease (VHL), whereas smaller cysts are more often associated with autosomal recessive polycystic kidney disease (ARPKD) and medullary cystic disease/nephronophthisis (MCDNP). The cysts increase in both number and volume in most of the disorders as the individual ages. Table 70-1 summarizes the features associated with each disorder.

The nephron segment from which cysts are derived varies among the disorders and can, on occasion, be used to help establish a diagnosis. In ARPKD, the principal renal histopathologic abnormality is cystic expansion of all generations of the collecting ducts.

From: *Principles of Molecular Medicine* (J. L. Jameson, ed.), ©1998 Humana Press Inc., Totowa, NJ.

In the neonatal form of the disease, up to 90% of the collecting ducts are involved with cysts found in both the cortex and medulla. The kidneys tend to be massively but symmetrically enlarged and are usually palpable on exam. Ultrasonography typically reveals increased echogenicity with loss of corticomedullary differentiation. The cysts often are not detectable using radiologic imaging techniques. These severely affected children typically die within the first year of life. Children affected with a less severe form have a 10–60% involvement of their collecting ducts. Their kidneys are usually less enlarged and may develop macroscropic cysts. Hypertension, progressive renal insufficiency, and liver disease (portal tract fibrosis) are the primary manifestations of the disease in this older group.

The cysts in MCDNP arise from the distal convoluted tubules and are found in the medulla and the cortico-medullary junction. Tubulo-interstitial inflammation and fibrosis are universal features and may be present even in the absence of renal cysts. The kidneys typically are small and hyperechoic on ultrasound. The cysts, which are small and heterogeneous in size, may be difficult to visualize without spécial methods that maximize resolution of the abdominal ultrasound or CT scan. Affected individuals often present with polyuria, polydypsia, and hyposthenuria, and develop progressive renal impairment. Autosomal recessive forms of the disease present in childhood and are important causes of ESRD in this age group. Rare families have been reported with a later onset of disease and an autosomal dominant pattern of inheritance.

Renal cysts develop from all nephron segments in ADPKD. The cysts begin to form *in utero* and slowly increase in size and number during the lifetime of the individual. In early stages of the disorder, the kidney may be either normal in size or slightly enlarged. Progressive cystic disease typically distorts the structure of the kidney and results in chronic renal insufficiency in approximately 50% of affected individuals. Hypertension is a common problem and is associated with a greater likelihood of developing ESRD. There is considerable intra- and interfamilial variation in the severity of disease, with a number of families displaying progressive severity in successive generations. ADPKD occasionally presents with severe manifestations in childhood. These cases tend to have inherited the disease from an affected mother and often cluster within families.

It is important to note that most of the diseases discussed above have associated extrarenal manifestations that may be major causes of morbidity or premature death (Table 70-1). Congenital hepatic fibrosis is an important cause of morbidity in children with ARPKD

Table 70-1
Genetic Renal Cystic Disorders—Clinical Features

Disease	*Inheritance*	*Kidney pathology*	*Renal manifestations*	*Extrarenal manifestations*	*Clinical onset*	*Clinical course*
ADPKD	AD	All nephron segments cyst size variable, often >1 cm	Recurrent infections, hematuria, nephrolithiasis, renal failure	Liver cysts (40%), occasional cysts in other organs (pancreas, spleen), intracranial aneurysms, aortic aneurysms, cardiac valvular abnormalities, (mitral valve) prolapse) colonic diverticiculi	3rd and 4th decades (occasionally earlier)	50% evolve to ESRD by age 60
ARPKD	AR	All portions of the collecting duct 90% involvement, infantile form 10–60% involvement, later forms cysts usually <0.5 cm	Abdominal mass, hematuria, concentrating defect renal failure	Hepatic fibrosis, portal hypertension, hypertension, pulmonary hypoplasia	Infants and children (occasionally in early adulthood)	~20% die of respiratory failure within 1st month; ESRD, hypertension, portal hypertension, infection
Bardet-Biedl Syndrome	AR	Calyceal cysts Tubulointerstial nephritis cysts usually < 0.5 cm	Polyuria, isothenuria, renal failure	Mental retardation, pigmentary retinopathy, polydactyly, obesity, hypogonadism, polydipsia	Infancy	ESRD in childhood
MCDNP	AR	Corticomedullary cysts, tubulointerstial nephritis cysts usually <0.5 cm	Polyuria, isothenuria renal failure	Growth retardation	1st and 2nd decades	ESRD common in childhood
Senior-Loken	AR	Same	Same	Pigmentary retinopathy	Same	Same
	AD	Same	Same	Normal	3rd and 4th decade	ESRD in 4th decade
Tuberous sclerosis	AD	All nephron segments, cysts range from microscopic to >1 cm	Renal tumors, occasional massive cystic disease that mimics ADPKD, occasional renal impairment	Cortical tubers, retinal hamartoma, angiofibroma, astrocytomas, cardiac rhabdomyoma, renal angiomyolipoma, renal cell carcinoma	Childhood and adulthood	Neurological complications predominate but complications of renal disease are 2nd most common cause of death
Von Hippel-Lindau Syndrome	AD	Cortical predominance cysts range from 0.5 to 3 cm	Renal carcinoma, occasional ESRD	Hemangioblastoma, cystadenocarcinoma, pheocromocytoma, occasional cysts in other organs (liver, pancreas)	3rd and 4th decades	Neurological complications and cancers are important causes of morbidity and death, renal failure uncommon

Table 70-2
Genetic Renal Cystic Disorders — Chromosome Localization

Disorder	*Prevalence*	*MIM no.*	*Chromosomal assignment*	*Protein product*
ARPKD	1/1000			
PKD1	85–95%	173900	16p13.3	Polycystin
PKD2	5–15%	173910	4q21-q23	Polycystin 2
PKD3	Rare	600666	?	?
ARPKD	1/6000–1/40,000	263200	6p21.1-p12	?
Bardet-Biedl syndrome	Rare			
BB1		209901	11q13	?
BB2		209900	16q21	?
BB3		600151	3q13	?
BB4		600374	15q22.3	?
MCDNP				
Autosomal recessive				
NPH1	85%	256100	2q13	NPHP1
NPH2	15%	?	?	?
Senior-Loken	Rare	266900	?	?
Autosomal dominant	Rare	174000	?	?
Tuberous sclerosis	1/10,000			
TSC1	~50%	191100	9q34	Hamartin
TSC2	~50%	191092	16p13.3	Tuberin
TSC/PKD	Rare	600273	16p13.3	Tuberin and polycystin
TSC3	Rare	191091	12q23-q24 (unconfirmed)	?
TSC4	Rare	191090	11q22-q23 (unconfirmed)	?
Von Hippel-Lindau Syndrome	1/40,000–1/100,000	193300	3p25-p26	G7 (elongin A homolog)

who have milder forms of renal disease, for example. These features may be helpful in establishing a specific diagnosis.

DIAGNOSIS

The diagnosis of renal cystic disease is usually established by imaging studies such as ultrasound, CT scan, or MRI. Renal size, the number and location of cysts, and the age of the individual are important parameters that help establish a diagnosis. Multiple macroscopic renal cysts are the most common presentation of ADPKD, but renal enlargement without visible cysts is more typical of ARPKD and early stages of ADPKD. Distinguishing the disorders on the basis of their radiologic appearance is not always possible, so other clinical features are usually important in establishing a specific diagnosis. The pattern of inheritance of the disease within a family is one very helpful diagnostic criterion. Massive renal enlargement in an infant whose parents do not have renal cystic disease is most likely to have ARPKD, whereas an identical presentation in a child whose parent has renal cysts almost certainly has an autosomal dominant form of PKD. Other clinical features, such as congenital hepatic fibrosis, angiomyolipomas, or cerebellar and spinal hemangioblastomas suggest ARPKD, tuberous sclerosis, VLH disease, respectively. There is considerable overlap in the clinical presentation of the various disorders, however, and an exact diagnosis based solely on clinical findings is not always possible. Genetic studies may be required to distinguish the subgroups.

GENETIC BASIS OF DISEASE

Linkage studies have yielded a number of surprising results. Many of the disorders that had been previously thought to be genetically homogeneous were found linked to more than one gene, whereas ARPKD, which had been thought to have up to four genetically distinct forms, is associated with only one locus (Table 70-2). Studies of ARPKD families with both noninfantile and severe perinatal presentations found linkage to identical markers on chromosome 6p21-cen. These studies suggest that ARPKD is genetically homogeneous and have important implications for genetic counselors. Prenatal DNA testing can now be offered to families who have previously had an affected child, if DNA material from the affected individual is available for analysis (blood, parafin-embedded specimens, and so on). Although the gene for ARPKD has not yet been isolated, it has been localized to a YAC contig of less than <3.1 Mb.

Recessive MCDNP, when present without significant extrarenal abnormalities, is a clinically homogenous disorder, yet genetic linkage studies have recently determined that it actually is comprised of at least two genetically distinct diseases. The major locus, NPH1, which accounts for ~85% of recessive MCDNP, has been mapped to chromosome 2q13. Cloning the interval in a yeast artificial chromosome contig revealed that several markers mapped to more than one locus within the NPH1 region. Further analysis determined that large-scale rearrangements were present in 80% of individuals from multiplex families and 65% of the sporadic cases. Sequence-tagged sites mapping into the interval were found to be absent in the DNA of affected individuals. Most of the individuals had large, homozygous deletions of approximately 250 kb involving a 100-kb inverted duplication. These data suggest that large rearrangements of a gene(s) at 2q13 is a common mechanism of disease in this disorder, making it the highest frequency of large rearrangements reported for any autosomal recessive trait. The recent discovery of the *NPHP1* gene will allow direct gene testing as a diagnostic test in the future. *NPHP1* was discovered to encode a 4.5-kb mRNA that is predicted to produce a novel protein of 732 amino acids whose function is presently unknown. Its only recognizable feature is a single SH3 domain. A curious and unanticipated feature is the gene's unusual pattern of expression. There is barely detectable expression in any adult organ other than muscle.

These findings are of immediate clinical use, as they permit the diagnosis of NPH1 in the majority of sporadic cases without the need for renal biopsy.

The chromosome location of NPH2 is presently unknown. It is perhaps not surprising that the clinically heterogeneous group of recessive forms of MCDNP that present with extrarenal manifestations is also genetically heterogeneous. Senior-Loken syndrome (MCDNP with retinitis pigmentosa) is not linked to chromosome 2 markers and is likely to represent yet another genetically distinct disorder. Bardet-Biedl syndrome, a group of disorders that has renal pathology similar to that of MCDNP but with mental retardation, obesity, retinitis pigmentosa, polydactyly and/or syndactyly, and hypogonadism maps to at least four loci, none of which are on chromosome 2 (Table 70-2). The chromosomal location of the gene for the autosomal dominant form of MCDNP has not yet been determined.

ADPKD has been found to be a genetically heterogenous disorder with at least three unique loci implicated in its pathogenesis. PKD1 is the most common, accounting for 85–95% of all ADPKD, and maps to chromosome 16p13.3. PKD2 is responsible for 5–15% of all ADPKD, and maps to chromosome 4. This form of ADPKD presents with an identical profile of extrarenal manifestations (liver cysts, aneurysms, and so on) but is thought to be less severe. It has recently been discovered that non-PKD1 patients live longer than PKD1 patients (median survival 71.5 vs 56.0 years), have a lower risk of progressing to renal failure, are less likely to have hypertension, tend to be diagnosed at an older age (median 69.1 vs 44.8 years), and have fewer renal cysts at the time of diagnosis. A small number of families have been discovered in which the disease does not segregate with either chromosome 16 or chromosome 4 markers (PKD3). The number of families is very small but apparently the disease is equal in severity to that seen in PKD1. This form of ADPKD has not yet been mapped, and it is possible that this subgroup also is genetically heterogeneous.

The 10-year search for *PKD1* illustrates both the challenges and opportunities offered by positional cloning. While a combination of molecular and genetic techniques rapidly localized the gene to a 500-kb gene-rich segment on 16p13.3, the large number of potential candidate genes greatly complicated the search. Two clues ultimately led to its identification. The first was the discovery that a major form of tuberous sclerosis (TSC2) mapped to the *PKD1* region. The other major "breakthrough" was provided by a family that had a child with tuberous sclerosis and renal cystic disease, whose mother and sibling only had ADPKD. Cytogenetic analysis revealed that the mother and sibling with ADPKD had balanced translocations between chromosome 16 and 22 [46XX t(16;22)(p13.3;q11.21)], whereas the child with TSC2 had an unbalanced karyotype [45XY/-16-22+der(16)(16qter-16p13.3::22q11.21-22qter)]. Since other studies had previously found loss of heterozygosity for 16p13.3 markers in TSC-associated lesions, TSC2 was hypothesized to lie within the deleted telomeric segment whereas *PKD1* was likely to be bisected by the translocation.

Further study proved both hypotheses to be true. A group of individuals with TSC2 were found to have an overlapping set of DNA deletions disrupting a gene that mapped just distal to the breakpoint (Fig. 70-1). The gene has been called tuberin and has a region of homology to a GTPase activating protein. The PKD1-associated translocation was found to bisect the adjacent gene, which encoded a 14-kb transcript. Affected individuals in the family with the translocation were discovered to have a novel mRNA of 9-kb. A small number of intragenic mutations (deletions, splice site disruption) were subsequently identified in other pedigrees that had PKD1, proving that the gene disrupted by the translocation was indeed *PKD1*.

The *PKD2* gene was discovered much more quickly. The predicted protein product of a candidate gene isolated from the minimal genetic interval on 4q22 was found to have modest homology to PKD1. A subsequent search for mutations uncovered a handful of pathogenic variants which are likely to truncate the normal protein.

MOLECULAR PATHOPHYSIOLOGY OF DISEASE

Another gene (PKD2) structurally similar to PKD1 is located on chromosome 4q22 and also causes ADPKD. This chapter will focus primarily on PKD1, including its role in the pathogenesis of cyst formation.

PKD1 GENE STRUCTURE Several features of *PKD1* and it gene product, polycystin, make it one of the most complicated disease genes yet discovered:

Size The gene encodes a 14-kb mRNA that is derived from 46 exons that extend over ~53 kb of genomic DNA. Its protein product, polycystin, is 4302 amino acids in length and likely to be a membrane-associated glycoprotein with multiple membrane-spanning segments. Both the size of the *PKD1* mRNA and its gene product are among the largest reported to date.

Unusual DNA Sequence Repeats An intron within the middle of the gene contains a ~2.5-kb segment that is 96% composed of polypyrimidines on its coding strand. Similar but much shorter elements discovered in other genes have been reported to form triple helical structures that can regulate DNA replication and RNA transcription and processing. The extreme length of this element in *PKD1* may play a role in the pathogenesis of PKD1.

Family of Homologous Sequences Greatly complicating the isolation and characterization of the gene was the discovery that ~70% of the gene was replicated in at least three copies clustered together on 16p13.1. The other loci, which also are transcribed, differ from *PKD1* by less than 5% in their shared segments. Only the last ~3.9 kb of the *PKD1* mRNA is unique and can be used to distinguish *PKD1* from its homologs. PKD2 encodes a protien called polycystin. The PKD2 gene is expressed ubiquitously, including the kidney.

POLYCYSTIN, THE PKD1 GENE PRODUCT The peptide sequence of polycystin suggests that it is likely to be a membrane glycoprotein that mediates cell–cell and/or cell–matrix interaction with a carboxy-terminal portion communicating with intracellular signaling pathways (Fig. 70-2 and 70-3). It is a novel protein with multiple domains that have homology to those of other known proteins. It is predicted to have between 7 and 11 transmembrane domains that follow its extracellular N-terminal segment of either 2500 or 3000 amino acids. Most models of the protein structure place its amino- and carboxy-terminal segments on opposite sides of the cell membrane, with the latter positioned within the cytoplasm.

The amino end of the predicted protein begins with an amino-terminal hydrophic signal sequence, which is soon followed by a pair of leucine-rich repeats (LRR). Flanking the LRRs on their amino and carboxy ends are distinctive cysteine-rich segments that are similarly found in a number of other LRR-containing proteins. The combination of both an amino and carboxy cluster with the LRRs has been previously reported for only three other protein

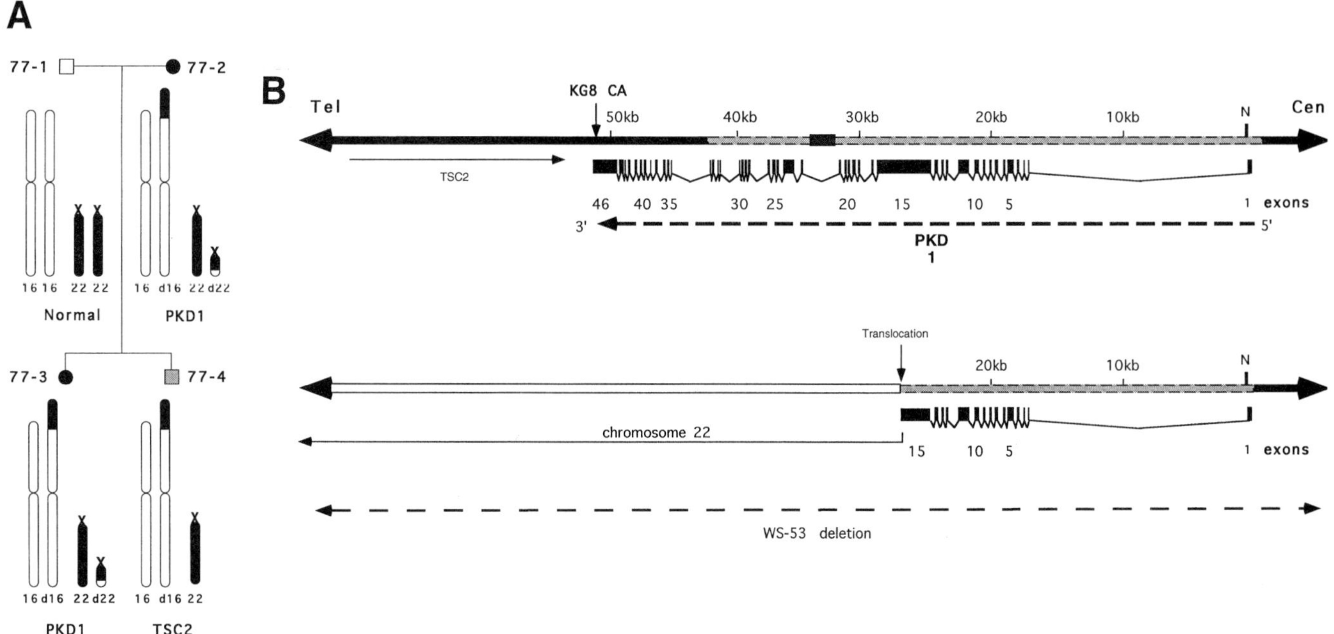

Figure 70-1 (**A**) The PKD1 Breakthrough: a pedigree with chromosomal abnormalities segregating with ADPKD and tuberous sclerosis. Unfilled box is the unaffected father (77-1). Filled symbols identify individuals affected with ADPKD (77-2, 77-3). The shaded box (77-4) identifies an individual with tuberous sclerosis and cystic disease of the kidney. The homologous pairs of chromosome 16 and 22 for each individual are schematically illustrated beneath each symbol. Individuals 77-2 and 77-3 have ADPKD and a balanced translocation [t(16;22)(p13.3;q11.21)] whereas individual 77-4 has an unbalanced translocation with loss of der22 [-16-22+der(16)(16qter→16p13.3:22q11.21 →22qter)]. *16* and *22* identify normal chromosomes whereas *d16* and *d22* define the derivative chromosomes. (**B**) Genomic structure of *PKD1*. The top line represents the chromosome segment with its orientation as listed (tel, telomere; cen, centromere). The segment is marked in kilobases (kb). *N* identifies a *Not*I restriction site that maps to the 5' end of the gene. The location of an intragenic, polymorphic microsatellite (KG8 CA) is shown. The shaded portion of the chromosome indicates the segment of the gene found replicated elsewhere on chromosome 16. The darkly stippled box within the replicated region indicates the position of the polypyrmidine tract described in the text. The numbered, linked vertical bars and boxes beneath the chromosome represent *PKD1* exons. The direction of transcription for *PKD1* and *TSC2* is indicated by the arrow above each gene name. The segment immediately below the normal chromosome illustrates the impact of the [t(16;22)(p13.3;q11.21)] translocation on the *PKD1* gene structure. The dashed line at the bottom indicates the approximate extent of a deletion that was discovered in individuals with tuberous sclerosis and severe polycystic kidney disease at any early age. (Adapted with permission from Watnick T, Germino GG. Genetic mechanisms of renal disease. Diseases of the Kidney, Schrier and Gottschalk eds. Boston: Little Brown, 1996.)

families: the trk proto-oncogenes and two developmental proteins, slit and Toll. These elements are located in the extracellular portion of each protein and are thought to mediate protein–protein interactions in cell–cell and cell–matrix recognition. The domains also may form part of the ligand-binding region of the receptors.

Another important feature of the protein sequence is a peptide module ~80 amino acids in length that is replicated 16 times. The first repeat is positioned between the LRRs and a C-lectin domain with the rest tandemly grouped after LDL-A module (Fig. 70-2). The basic unit is similar in structure to the I set of immunoglobulin (Ig) domains, being comprised of a b strand followed by a turn that links the modules but lacks the consensus cysteines. The Ig-like cluster is followed by an ~700-amino acid segment that has significant homology to the receptor for egg-jelly (REJ) in the sperm of the sea urchin. The receptor binds to matrix surrounding sea urchin eggs, and the interaction results in ion-channel activation and initiation of the fertilization process. The recent discovery that PKD2 has high homology to a family of voltage-activated ion channels has prompted some to speculate that the sea urchin sperm–egg matrix interaction may serve as a model of PKD1-PKD2 function. Finally, the short cytoplasmic tail of polycystin has an α-helical coiled-coil structure made of five heptad repeats that has been shown to interact with the cytoplasmic C-terminus of PKD2. Both naturally occuring and engineered mutations of either gene have been shown to disrupt this interaction. These data suggest that the gene products of *PKD1* and *PKD2* may function as partners in a common signaling cascade involved in tubular morphogenesis. The data also suggest that an important role of PKD1 may be to regulate the activity of PKD2.

It is interesting to note that the possible functions of polycystin as predicted by its sequence are consistent with many of the earlier hypotheses regarding the pathogenesis of ADPKD. Coordinated cell growth and morphogenesis are regulated in part by cell–matrix and cell–cell interactions. The abnormalities in extracellular matrix, regulation of tubular cell growth, epithelial cell polarity, expression profile of developmental genes, and the vectorial transport of tubular fluid observed in ADPKD cysts may be downstream effects of mutations that disrupt the function of polycystin.

MUTATION STUDIES Mutation analyses have been greatly hindered by the high sequence similarity of *PKD1* to its homologs. It has been estimated that 80–90% of all pathogenic mutations are located within the replicated portion of the gene. Only a small number of mutations have been discovered, and most have been clustered in the 3' locus-specific segment (Fig. 70-3; Table 70-3). Nonetheless, a few patterns appear to be emerging. Most of the mutations have been unique. Most of the mutant alleles have been

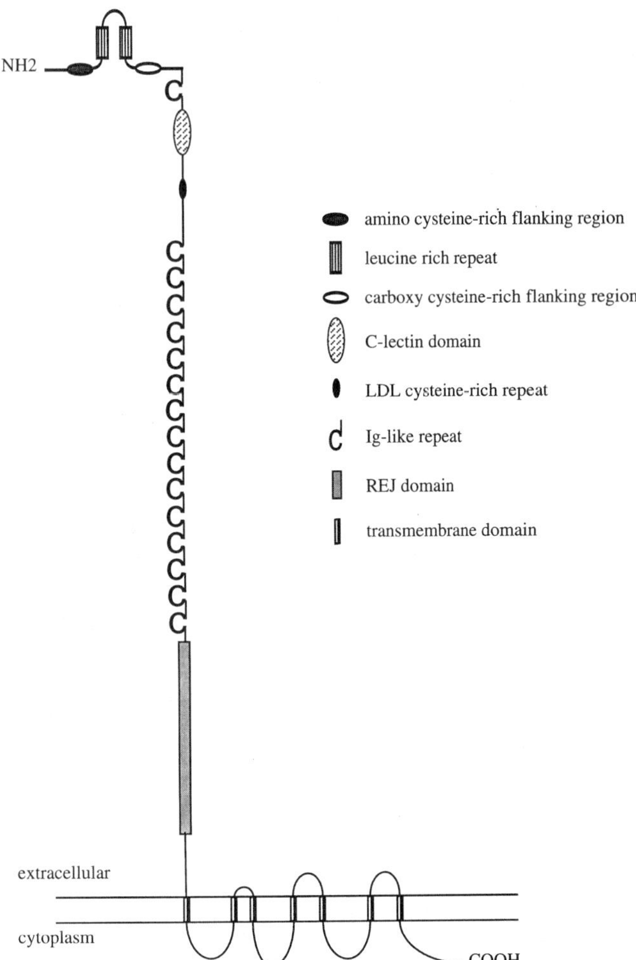

Figure 70-2 Predicted structure of polycystin, the *PKD1* gene product. Different computer analyses identify variable numbers of transmembrane (TM) spanning segments, but most models predict a final product with multiple TM elements and amino- and carboxy-termini located on opposite ends of the cell membrane. (Adapted from Burn TJ et al: Hum Mol Genet 1995;4:575–582; Hughes J et al: Nat Genet 1995;10:151–160; International Polycystic Kidney Disease Consortium. Cell 1995;81:289–298. Reprinted with permission from Watnick T, Germino GG. Molecular mechanism of renal disease. Diseases of the Kidney, Schrier and Gottschalk, eds. Boston: Little Brown, 1996.)

expressed and thought likely to produce mutant proteins lacking the final membrane-spanning regions and/or the cytoplasmic component of the protein. The model of the protein structure predicts that such abnormalities would affect membrane localization of the gene product, disrupt intracellular signaling pathways, or result in a secreted form of the protein. The mutant proteins might be able to bind their extracellular partners (some of which may be other polycystin molecules) but be unable to transmit this information across the membrane. Finally, one recent study suggests that gene conversion events between *PKD1* and its homologs may be an important mechanism causing mutations to occur.

One important goal of performing genotype/phenotype correlations is to determine genetic variants that predict more severe disease. This information can be clinically very useful as well as provide important clues to a protein's function. In the case of *PKD1*, only one pattern has been discovered that reproducibly correlates with disease severity. A small group of children has been described that is affected with a severe form of polycystic kidney disease and tuberous sclerosis (TS). They have been discovered to have deletions which remove the entire *PKD1* gene and disrupt the adjacent *TSC2* gene.

It is important to note that the children with TS and massive cystic disease had *de novo* mutations and were not members of families with documented ADPKD. Similar deletions have not been found in severely affected children born into families with classic ADPKD. In the only report of a child with early onset ADPKD in which the defect has been defined, the variant was a nonsense mutation that changed Tyr3818 to a stop codon. It is not presently known whether there is a subset of mutations associated with any of the extrarenal manifestations of ADPKD.

PKD1 GENE AND PROTEIN EXPRESSION Studies of *PKD1* gene expression have determined that it is widely expressed in both fetal and adult organs, though at variable levels (*see* Chapter 64). The highest level of gene expression appears to be in the brain. Fetal kidney and liver and cystic kidney and liver have higher levels of expression than their normal adult counterparts. The level of expression in normal adult kidney is variable, most likely reflecting differences in regional expression within the kidney.

Conflicting reports have been published describing the tissue and developmental profile of polycystin expression. Reports have differed with respect to which nephron segments have significant levels of expression, when expression is highest, and which extraepithelial cell types express polycystin. For example, one study reports that polycystin is present in the smooth muscle cells lining vessels while several other studies explicitly note its absence in these structures. There is a broad consensus, however, on several points. First, it appears likely that polycystin is widely expressed in adult tissues, though often at very low levels. For example, most investigators have detected polycystin in normal pancreatic and biliary ductules, two other cell types subject to cystic change. Second, most investigators agree that the protein is present in fetal kidney and in lesser amounts in adult kidney. One study of murine polycystin expression determined that it is highest in latc fctal and carly nconatal lifc, and drops 20-fold by thc third postnatal week. These data have been cited as evidence that PKD1 plays an important role in kidney tubule differentiation and maturation. Third, most investigators agree that the protein is membrane-associated, with the majority favoring a reporting basolateral localization. Finally, all investigators agree that the protein appears to be more abundant in cystic kidney.

The biologic significance of the transcripts encoded by the homologous loci remains unknown. It has not yet been determined whether the 21-kb, 17-kb, or 8.5-kb mRNA encoded by these loci are translated into proteins or are derived from nonfunctional pseudogenes. If the mRNA of the PKD1 homologs are translated, their protein products would include most of the important functional domains contained in the 5' end of *PKD1* and could be involved in modulating disease severity.

PKD2 GENE The gene for the second most common form of ADPKD, *PKD2*, is located on chromosome 4 and encodes a 5.4-kb mRNA. Analysis of the translated sequence predicts an integral membrane protein of ~110 kDa with 6 TM domains nested between amino- and carboxyl-termini that are likely to be intracellular. The cytoplasmic C-terminus contains an EF-Hand motif that has been shown in vitro to bind calcium. The protein sequence of PKD2 has significant homology to the voltage-activated Ca^{2+} channel a_{1E} protein and part of polycystin. An ion-channel activity

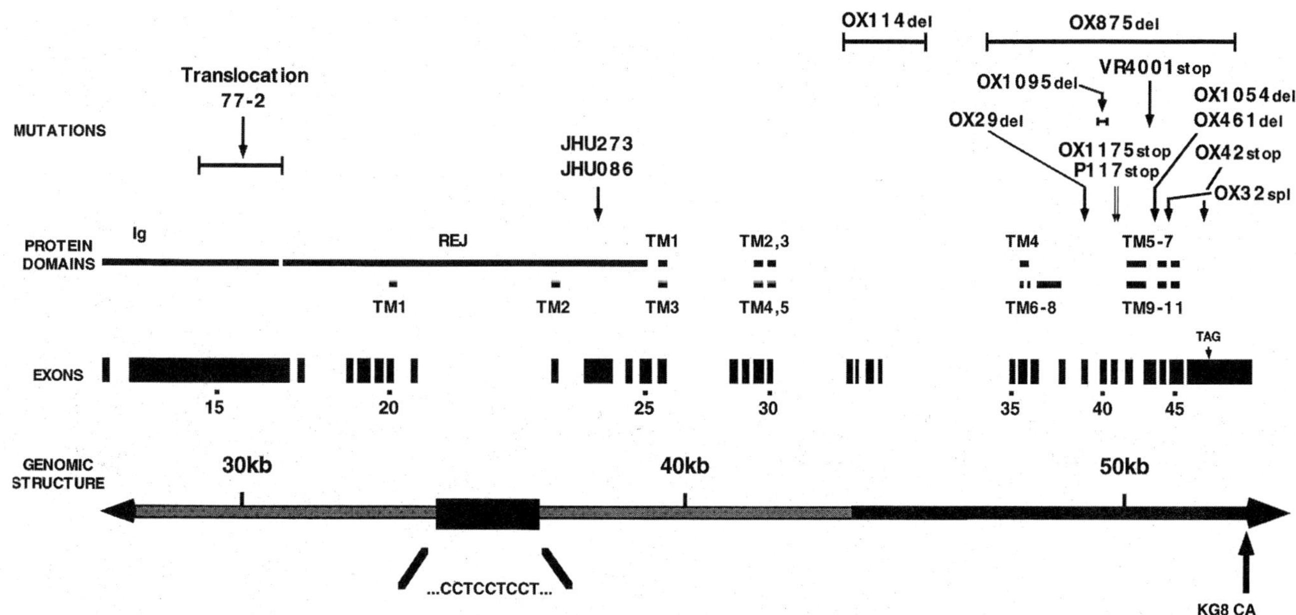

Figure 70-3 PKD1 mutations. This figure illustrates the relative location of *PKD1* exons, protein domains, and mutations. Most of the mutations reported to date have been clustered in the *PKD1*-specific portion of the gene (solid bar). The table below the figure lists the position of each mutation and describes its likely impact on the final gene product. Ig, immunoglobulin-like repeat; REJ, receptor for egg-jelly domain; TM, transmembrane segment.

Table 70-3
PKD1 Mutations

Variant name	*Type of mutation*	*Position*	*Predicted effect on protein*
77-2	Translocation	Exon 15	Truncation
JHU 273	Transversion, T→G	Exon 23	No change
	Transition, T→C	Exon 23	Missense, Met2760Thr
	Transversion, G→C	Exon 23	Missense, Arg2761Pro
	Transition, T→C	Exon 23	Missense, Met2764Thr
	Transition, T→C	Exon 23	Missense, Ileu2826Thr
JHU 086	Transversion, T→G	Exon 23	No change
	Transition, T→C	Exon 23	Missense, Met2760Thr
	Transversion, G→C	Exon 23	Missense, Arg2761Pro
	Transversion, C→G	Exon 23	Missense, Leu2763Val
	Transition, T→C	Exon 23	Missense, Met2764Thr
OX 114	Deletion, 2 kb	Intron 30–Intron 34	Frameshift deletion, 446 bp
OX 875	Deletion, 5.5 kb	Intron 34–Exon 46	Truncation
OX 29 (P35)	Deletion, 15 bp	Exon 39	In-frame deletion, 5 aa
OX 1095 (P167)	Deletion, 72 bp	Intron 39–Exon 40	In-frame deletion, 17 aa
III 2 (P117)	Transversion, C→A	Exon 41	Nonsense, Tyr3818Stop
OX 1175 (P198)	Transition, C→T	Exon 41	Nonsense, Glu3037Stop
OX 1054	Deletion, 20 bp	Intron 43	Splicing defect + intron, causes frameshift – intron, causes in-frame deletion, 22 aa
OX 461	Deletion, 18 bp	Intron 43	Splicing defect + intron causes in-frame insertion, 19 aa – intron causes in-frame deletion, 22 aa
OX 32	Transition, G→C	Intron 44	Splicing defect: in-frame deletion of exon 44
VR 4001	Transition, C→T	Exon 44	Nonsense, Gln4041Stop
OX 42	Transition, C→T	Exon 46	Nonsense, Arg4227Stop

has been proposed, though not yet demonstrated, for the *PKD2* gene product. The results of Northern blot analysis suggest that the mRNA is expressed ubiquitously. Preliminary studies have reported that the protein is likely to be membrane-associated and widely expressed in both fetal and adult tissues. In the kidney, it appears to be present in the renal tubule epithelia at the basolateral membrane. Because the protein is predicted to have only six TM-spanning regions, one model proposes that it forms either homo- or heteromultimers to create a functional channel or pore. In vitro studies, which have shown that the protein can self-associate, support this hypothesis. Whether PKD1-PKD2 heteromultimers may also be components of a functional channel remains to be determined.

ADPKD CLINICAL VARIABILITY One of the interesting features of this disease is the variability with which it presents in related members of a family. It is easy to understand how the disease may differ in severity in different pedigrees, where the mutation may differ. It is less clear why the same mutation causes different clinical presentations in genetically related individuals. The child with early onset PKD1 described above had a fraternal twin who had inherited the same *PKD1* mutation but was clinically unaffected in childhood. Variants of other modifying genes could account for some of the difference. Modifying genes have been shown to have significant effects on the clinical expression of cystic disease in murine models of PKD, for example. However, other factors are also likely to significantly alter the course of disease. The strongest evidence in support of this claim is provided by pathologic examination of human PKD kidneys. One is struck by the focality of disease—not all nephrons undergo cystic change despite all cells in each nephron sharing the same mutation of *PKD1*. Why, if every tubular cell within an affected individual's kidney or biliary tract inherits the same germline mutation and the same genetic modifiers, do only a small fraction become cystic? These observations suggest that a second, possibly rate-limiting, step must be required for cysts fo form.

Recent studies have provided a partial answer to this question for PKD1. Using a novel method for isolating DNA from the epithelial cells lining single renal cysts, it has been shown that renal cysts in ADPKD are monoclonal. Moreover, a significant fraction of cysts was found to have loss of heterozygosity (LOH) for two closely linked, polymorphic markers located within *PKD1*. Genetic analysis determined that is was the normal haplotype that was lost or mutated in cyst-lining epithelia.

An obvious challenge is reconciling the results of immunolocalization studies which suggest increased abundance of polycystin in cyst-wall lining cells with the results of the LOH study. Some have suggested that the latter phenomenon may be a consequence of the cystic state rather than an important step in its pathogenesis. While more data will be required to resolve the matter, several lines of evidence support the "two-hit" genetic model for PKD1. First, a similar process has also been recently described for hepatic cysts in ADPKD. Second, small single or oligo-basepair insertions, deletions or nonsense mutations can be detected in many cysts lacking LOH. Finally, the results of gene targeting studies in mice suggest that loss of function of both alleles is necessary for cyst formation. A *PKD1* mutation that mimics one found in human ADPKD was introduced into mice by homologous recombination. Heterozygotes had no discernible phenotype, whereas homozygotes died during the perinatal period with massively enlarged cystic kidneys, pancreatic ductal cysts, and pulmonary hypoplasia.

An important consideration is the extraordinary number of somatic mutations that must apparently occur to account for the number of cysts observed (10^2–10^4). The data suggest that *PKD1* is likely to be highly mutable. Unique genomic structural features, including unusual polypyrimidine tracts within introns 21 and 22 of the gene, might be responsible for both the high frequency of the disease within the population as well as the large number of "second hits" observed in cystic epithelia. The indistinguishable clinical presentation of all forms of ADPKD suggests that a similar two-step process occurs in each. The pattern of mutations described for PKD2 is consistent with a loss-of-function model. However, in contrast to PKD1, the relative infrequency of PKD2 and PKD3 in the population suggests that their respective genes are not highly mutable. How then, can one account for the number of second hits that must occur to account for the extraordinary number of cyts that are observed? Two models have been proposed: (1) the second hit rates of *PKD1*, *PKD2*, and *PKD3* reflect the average rate of somatic mutation in the genome rather than an unusually high rate of somatic mutation resulting from a locally mutable structure within each gene; or (2) somatic inactivation of *PKD1* may be the second step that leads to clonal expansion in the other forms of ADPKD. The second model predicts that the relative frequency of the respective forms of the disease in the population is determined by the rate of germline mutation at each genetic locus while the frequency with which cysts form is determined by the rate of somatic mutation of *PKD1*. Further study is required to determine whether either model is correct.

Regardless of whether somatic mutation of PKD1 is necessary for all forms of ADPKD, the data suggest that functional inactivation of PKD gene products is an essential step in cyst formation. These findings have important implications for investigators seeking to define polycystin's function. For example, the two-hit model suggests that PKD1 mutations are likely to result in gene products with decreased function. While one may easily imagine how mutations that result in truncated proteins with loss of essential domains impair activity, the impact of missense mutations is often more difficult to predict. The model challenges investigators to explain how these changes result in compromise of the protein's function. One must determine whether missense changes disrupt critical domains or affect the way the protein is processed and sorted through the cell (e.g., Δ508 and CFTR). The two-hit model also has important implications for investigators seeking to create suitable model systems and to develop effective therapies. Approaches that result in inactivation of the gene may be necessary to reproduce the disease state, while strategies directed at replacement of PKD gene function may reverse it.

TREATMENT/FUTURE DIRECTIONS

There presently is no cure (except for transplantation) for any of the forms of PKD, and all currently available therapies are directly available therapies are limited to managing complications associated with the diseases (hypertension, infection, pain, and so on). ADPKD offers unique opportunities for intervention, since the most severe complications of the disease typically do not develop until the fifth or sixth decade. It also poses significant challenges, however, since the therapy must be very safe. For example, we do not want to offer a treatment now to a child, with the hope of preventing ESRD in 50 years, and instead give him/her a higher likelihood of developing a cancer at age 30. Moreover, not everyone who inherits the same mutation will go on to suffer the most severe complications. One must understand the mechanism of disease if we are to offer safe and effective therapies (e.g., definition of the intersecting pathways that result in renal cystic disease may allow investigators to detour around possible blocks in signaling pathways). Alternatively, a gene product (e.g., polycystin) may function as a receptor, and competitive agonists or antagonists may be effective. One must have suitable models for testing possible therapeutic compounds or other interventions. Human cell culture systems are easily manipulated and useful for characterizing a number of aspects (transport, signaling pathways, proliferation, and so on) but have significant limitations. Genetically faithful animal models of human disease can be extremely useful when available. An exciting consequence of discovering human disease genes is that one can now use molecular genetic techniques (e.g., gene targeting) to create mice that develop human forms of PKD. These are likely to offer many new opportunities for better understanding the pathophysiology of the disease and testing therapeutic interventions.

In the short run, the discovery of genes for the various forms of PKD will have the greatest impact on our diagnostic capabilities. DNA testing can be used to evaluate relatives of an affected individual as possible donors for living related transplants in ADPKD. Genetic testing may soon be able to establish a diagnosis when individuals present with atypical features (kidneys not enlarged and only a few cysts) or an overlap syndrome (early severe cystic disease in a child, parents unaffected; ?VHL or TS). Studies correlating genotype with phenotype may identify those who would benefit most from interventions and close observation (severe early childhood forms, massive cystic disease, subarachnoid aneurysms, and so on). DNA testing may preclude renal biopsy as a diagnostic test for children with clinical features suggestive of NPH1.

An additional benefit resulting from the identification of one of the major "cystogenes" is that it is very likely to aid the discovery of others. The three types of ADPKD are virtually indistinguishable and are likely to develop as a consequence of defects in interactive factors involved in a common pathway. The protein-binding partners of polycystin are obvious candidates for PKD2 and PKD3 (and so on). Identification and characterization of the interacting proteins by means of biochemical (purification) or genetic (yeast two hybrid) techniques will likely help to define the pathways that regulate tubular morphogenesis. Finally, discovery of the *NPHP1* gene is likely to improve our understanding of the pathogenesis of another important clinical problem, chronic interstitial nephritis.

SELECTED REFERENCES

Brasier JL, Henske EP. Loss of the polycystic kidney disease (PKD1) region of chromosome 16p13 in renal cyst cells supports a loss-of-function model for cyst pathogenesis. J Clin Invest 1997;99:194–199.

Brook-Carter PT, Peral B, Ward CJ, et al. Deletion of the *TSC2* and *PKD1* genes associated with severe infantile polycystic kidney disease—a contiguous gene syndrome. Nat Genet 1994;8:328–332.

Bruford EA, Riise R, Teague PW, et al. Linkage mapping in 29 Bardet-Biedl syndrome families confirms loci in chromosomal regions 11q13, 15q22.3-q23, and 16q21. Genomics 1997;41:93–99.

Burn TJ, Connors TD, Dackowski WR, et al. The autosomal dominant polycystic kidney disease (PKD1) gene product contains a leucine-rich repeat. Hum Mol Genet 1995;4:575–582.

Carmi R, Elbedour K, Stone E M, Sheffield V C. Phenotypic differences among patients with Bardet-Biedl syndrome linked to three different chromosome loci. Am J Med Genet 1995;59:199–203.

Dalgaard OZ. Bilateral polycystic disease of the kidneys: a follow-up of two hundred and eighty-four patients and their families. Acta Med Scand 1996;Suppl 328:1–251.

Daoust MC, Reynolds DM, Bischt DG, et al. Evidence for a third genetic locus for autosomal dominant polycystic kidney disease. Genomics 1995;25:733–736.

Duan DR, Pause A, Wilson HB, et al. Inhibition of transcription elongation by the VHL tumor suppressor protein. Science 1995;269:1402–1406.

European Chromosome 16 Tuberous Sclerosis Consortium. Identification and characterization of the tuberous sclerosis gene on chromosome 16. Cell 1993;75:1305–1315.

European Polycystic Kidney Disease Consortium. The polycystic kidney disease 1 gene encodes a 14 kb transcript and lies within a duplicated region on chromosome 16. Cell 1994;77:881–894.

Geng L, Segal Y, Peissel B, et al. Identification and localization of polycystin, the PKD1 gene product. J Clin Invest 1996;98:2674–2682.

Guay-Woodford LM, Muecher G, Hopkins SD, et al. The severe perinatal form of autosomal recessive polycystic kidney disease maps to chromosome 6p21.1-p12: implications for genetic counseling. Am J Hum Genet 1995;56:1101–1107.

Hildebrandt F, Otto E, Rensing C, et al. A novel gene encoding an SH3 domain protein is mutated in nephronophthisis type 1. Nat Genet 1997;17:149–153.

Hughes J, Ward CJ, Peral B, et al. The polycystic kidney disease 1 (PKD1) gene encodes a novel protein with multiple cell recognition domains. Nat Genet 1995;10:151–160.

Ibrahgimov-Beskrovnaya O, Dackowski WR, Foggensteiner L, et al. Polycystin: in vitro synthesis, in vivo tissue expression, and subcellular localization identifies a large membrane-associated protein. Proc Natl Acad Sci USA 1997;94:6397–6402.

Konrad M, Saunier S, Heidt L, et al. Large homozygous deletions of the 2q13 region are a major cause of juvenile nephronophthisis. Hum Mol Genet 1996;5:367–371.

Latif F, Tory K, Gnarra J, et al. Identification of the von Hipple-Lindau disease tumor suppressor gene. Science 1993;260:1317–1320.

Lu W, Peissel B, Babakhanlou H, et al. Perinatal lethality with kidney and pancreas defects in mice with a targetted Pkd1 mutation. Nat Genet 1997;17:179–181.

Martinez JR, Grantham JJ. Polycystic kidney disease: etiology, pathogenesis, and treatment. [Review]. Dis Mon 1995;41:693–765.

Mochizuki T, Wu G, Hayashi T, et al. PKD2, a gene for polycystic kidney disease that encodes an integral membrane protein. Science 1996;272:1339–1342.

Palsson R, Sharma CP, Kim K, McLaughlin M, Brown D, Arnaout MA. Characterization and cell distribution of polycystin, the product of autosomal dominant polycystic kidney disease gene 1. Mol Med 1996;2:702–711.

Peral B, Ong ACM, Can Millan JL, Gamble V, Rees L, Harris PC. A stable, nonsense mutation associated with a case of infantile onset polycystic kidney disease 1 (PKD1). Hum Mol Genet 1996;5: 539–542.

Peral B, Sanmillan JL, Ong ACM, et al. Screening the 3' region of the polycystic kidney disease 1 (PKD1) gene reveals six novel mutations. Am J Hum Genet 1996;58:86–96.

Qian F, Germinao FJ, Cai Y, Zhang X, Somlo S, Germino GG. PKD1 interacts with PKD2 through a probable coiled-coil domain. Nat Genet 1997;16:179–183.

Qian F, Watnick TJ, Onuchic LF, Germino GG. The molecular basis of focal cyst formation in human autosomal dominant polycystic kidney disease type I. Cell 1996;87:979–987.

Ravine D, Walker RG, Gibson RN, et al. Phenotype and genotype heterogeneity in autosomal dominant polycystic kidney disease. Lancet 1992;340:1330–1333.

Sampson JR, Maheshwar MM, Aspinwall R, et al. Renal cystic disease in tuberous sclerosis: role of the polycystic kidney disease 1 gene. Am J Hum Genet 1997;61:843–851.

Tsiokas L, Kim E, Arnould T, Sukhatme VP, Walz G. Homo- and heterodimeric interactions between the gene products of PKD1 and PKD2. Proc Natl Acad Sci USA 1997;94:6965–6970.

Ward CJ, Turley H, Ong ACM, et al. Polycystin, the polycystic kidney disease 1 protein, is expressed by epithelial cells in fetal, adult, and polycystic kidney. Proc Natl Acad Sci USA 1996;93:1524–1528.

Watnick TJ, Piontek KB, Cordal TM, et al. An unusual pattern of mutation in the duplicated portion of PKD1 is revealed by use of a novel strategy for mutation detection. Hum Mol Genet 1997;6:1473–1481.

Zerres K, Mucher G, Bachner L, et al. Mapping of the gene for autosomal recessive polycystic kidney disease (ARPKD) to chromosome 6q21-cem. Nat Genet 1994;7:429–432.

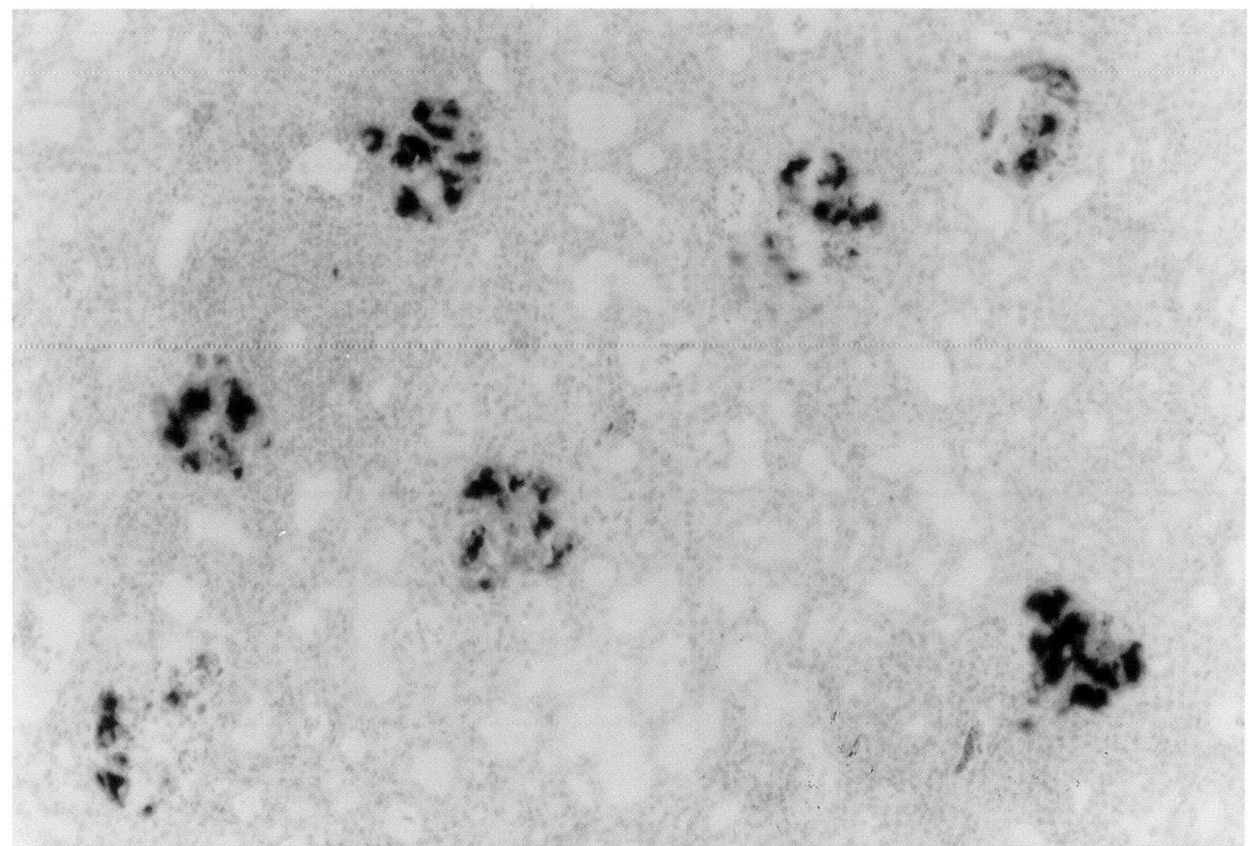

Plate 1 (Fig. 4; *see* full caption on p. 667 and discussion in Chapter 68).

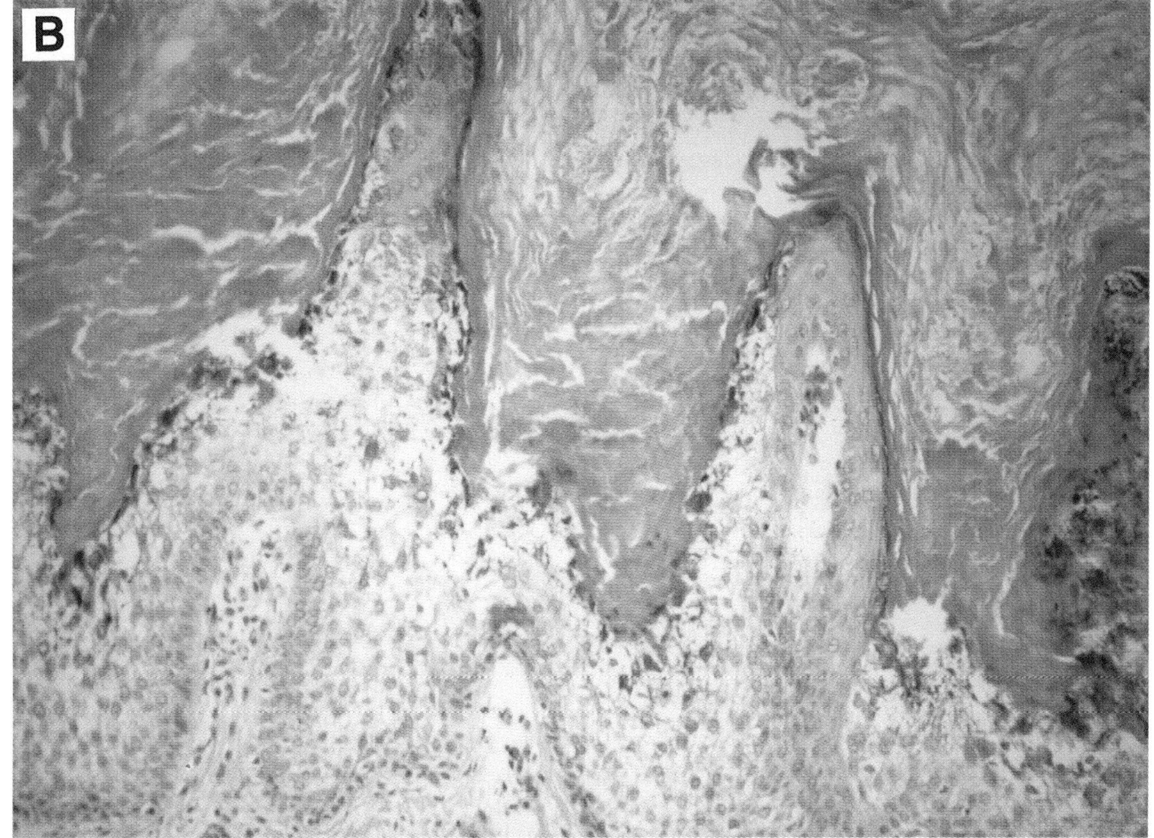

Plate 2 (Fig. 2; *see* full caption on p. 715 and discussion in Chapter 75).

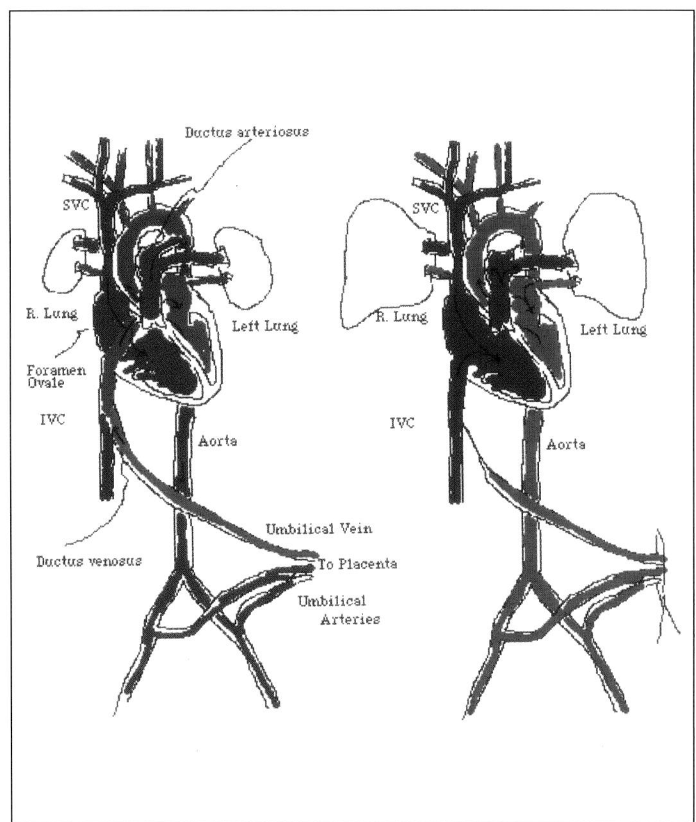

Plate 3 (Fig. 1; *see* full caption on p. 121 and discussion in Chapter 12).

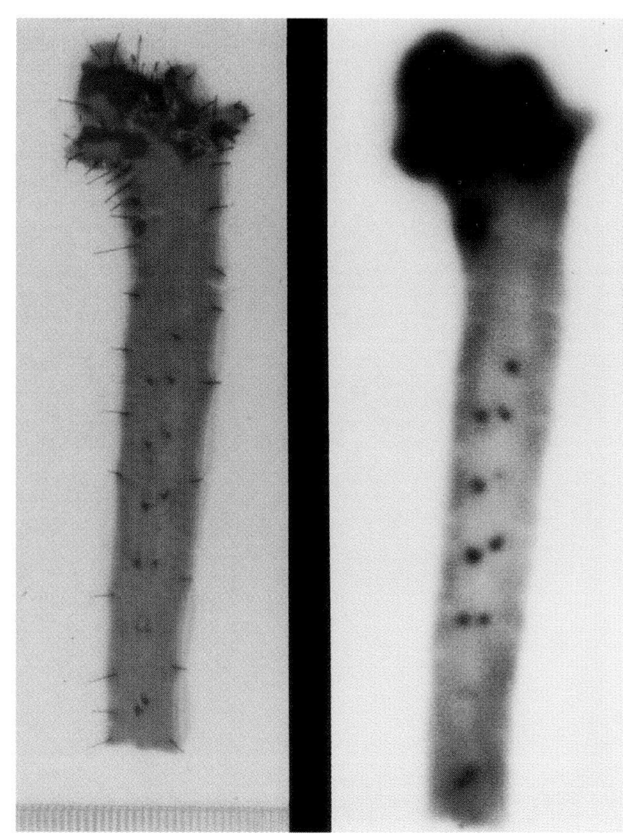

Plate 4 (Fig. 3; *see* full caption on p. 138 and discussion in Chapter 14).

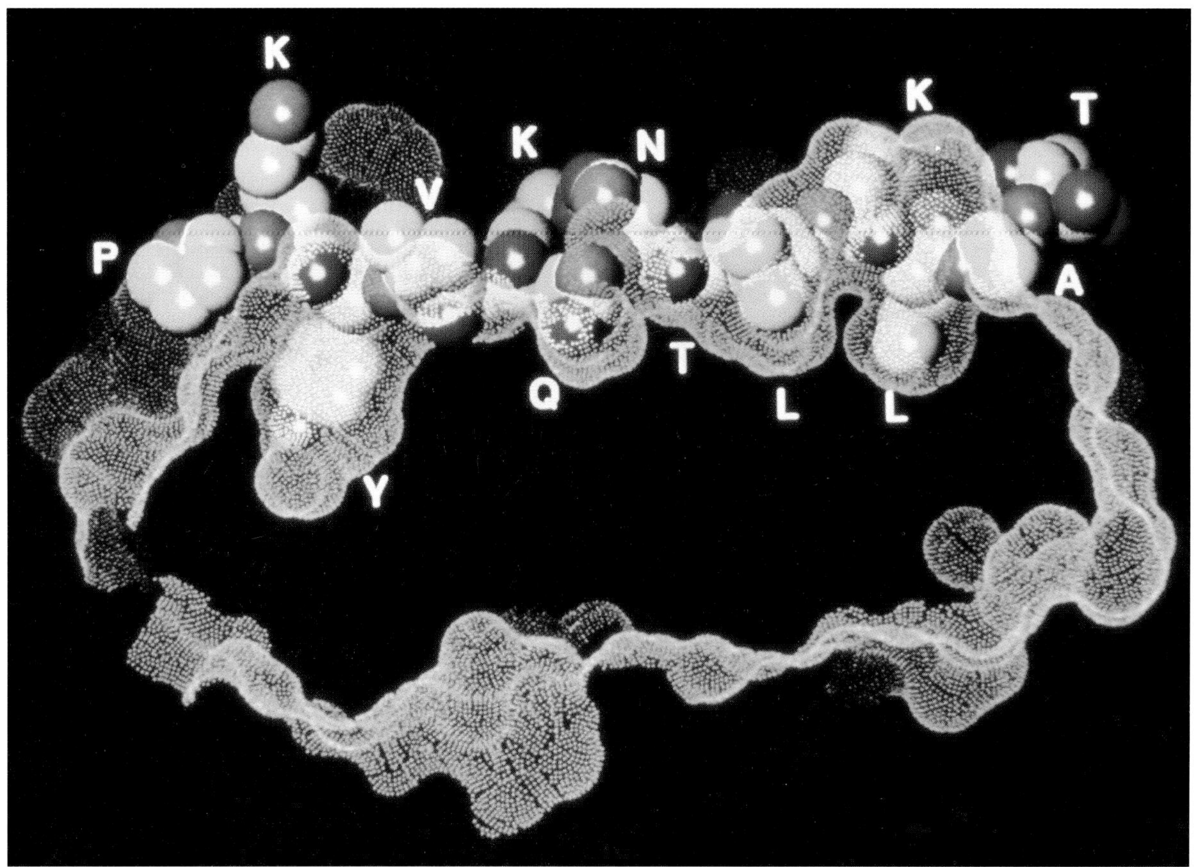

Plate 5 (Fig. 2; *see* full caption on p. 261 and discussion in Chapter 29).

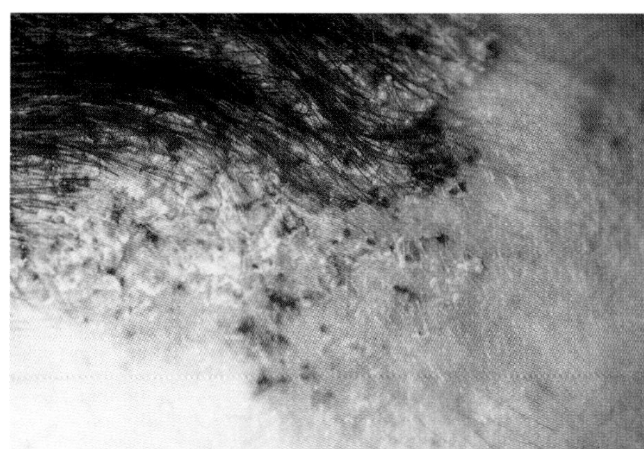

Plate 6 (Fig. 1-4; *see* full caption on p. 720-721 and discussion in Chapter 76).

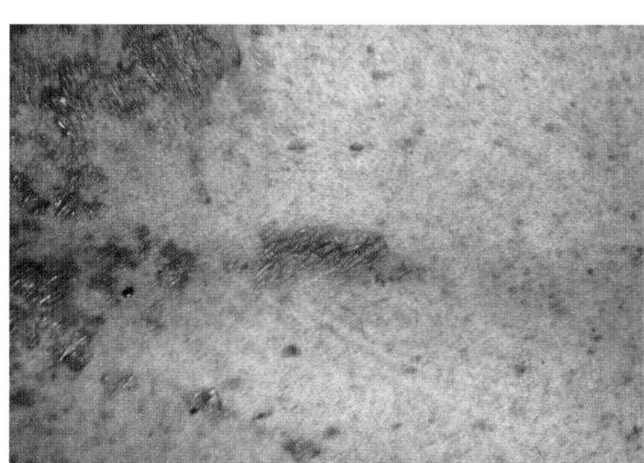

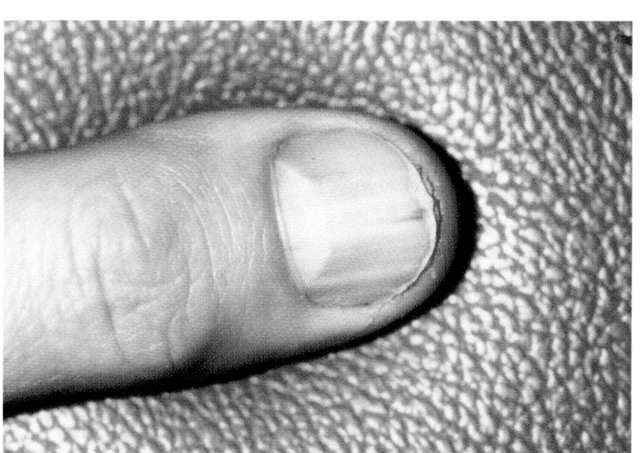

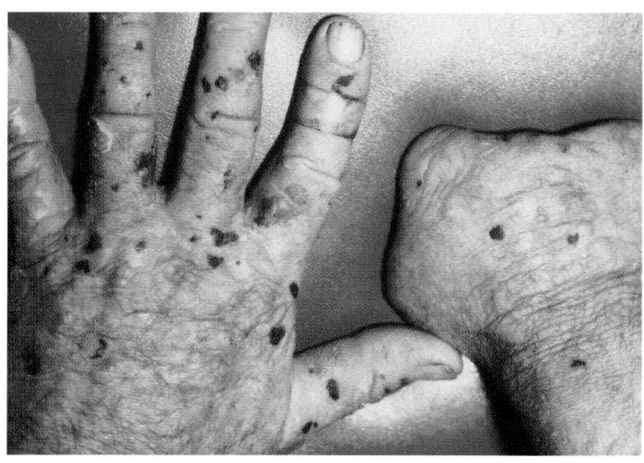

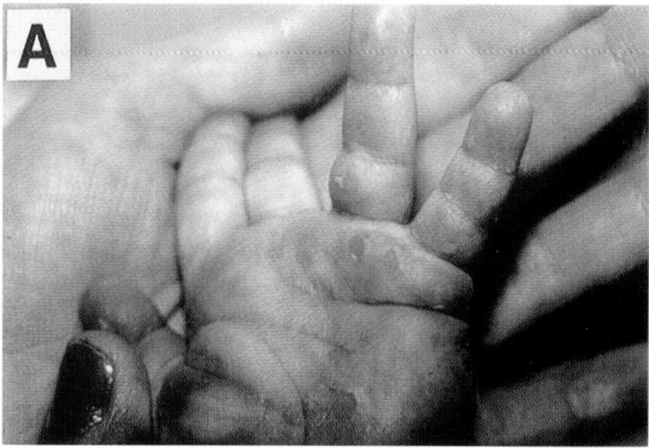

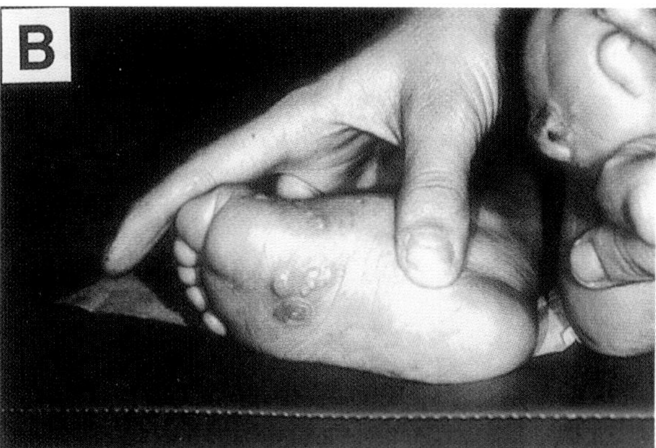

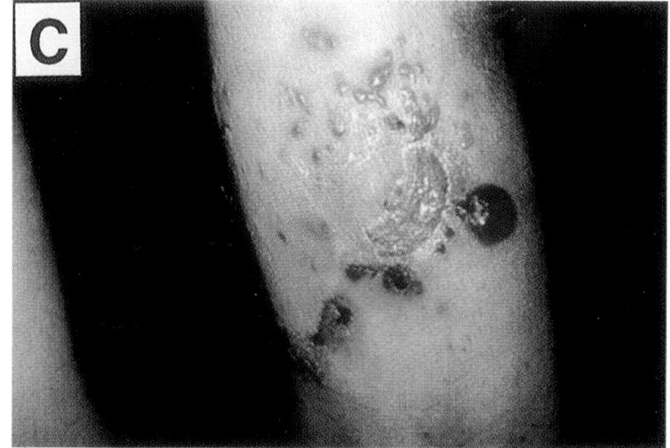

Plate 7 (Fig. 1; *see* full caption on p. 700 and discussion in Chapter 73).

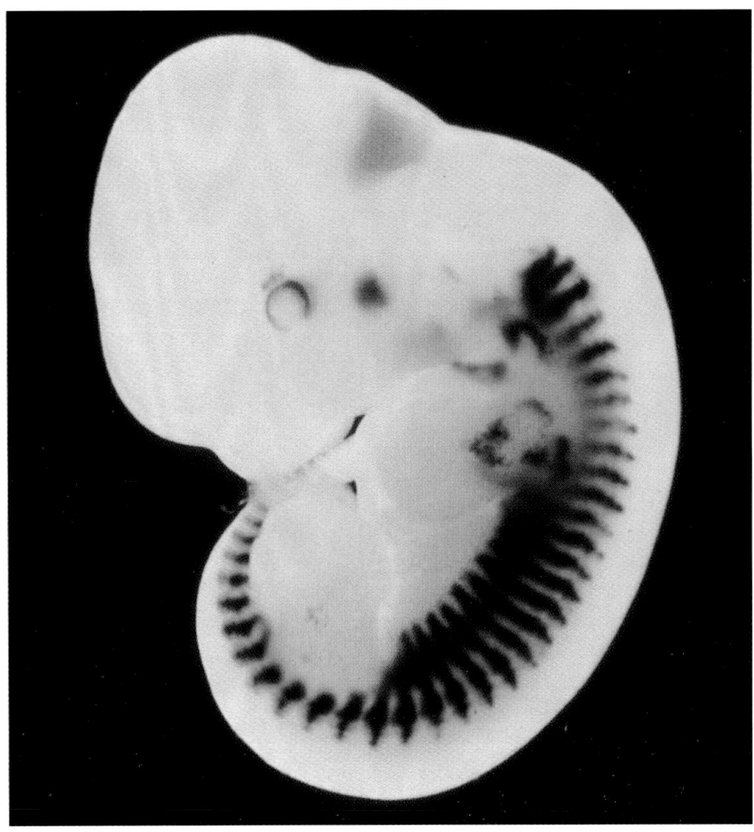

Plate 8 (Fig. 7; *see* full caption on p. 846 and discussion in Chapter 92).

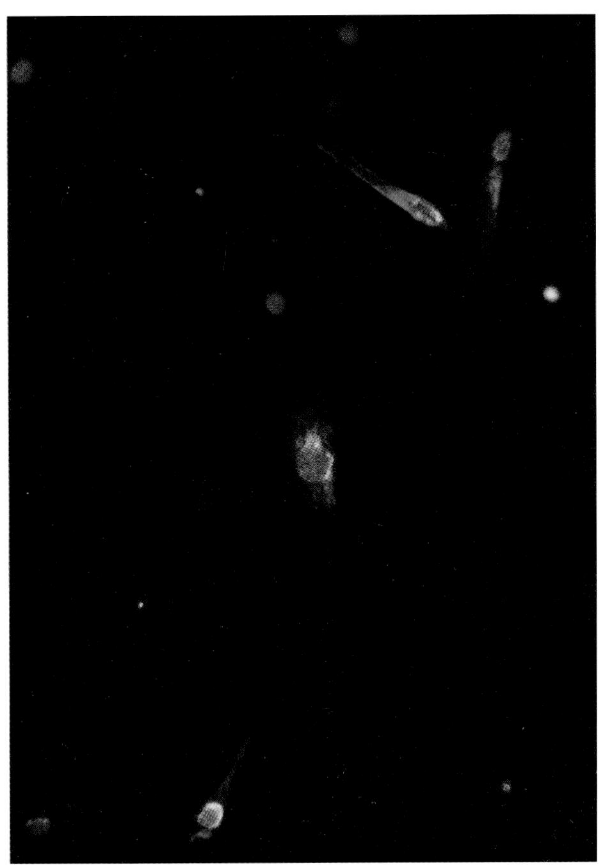

Plate 9 (Fig. 2; *see* full caption on p. 842 and discussion in Chapter 92).

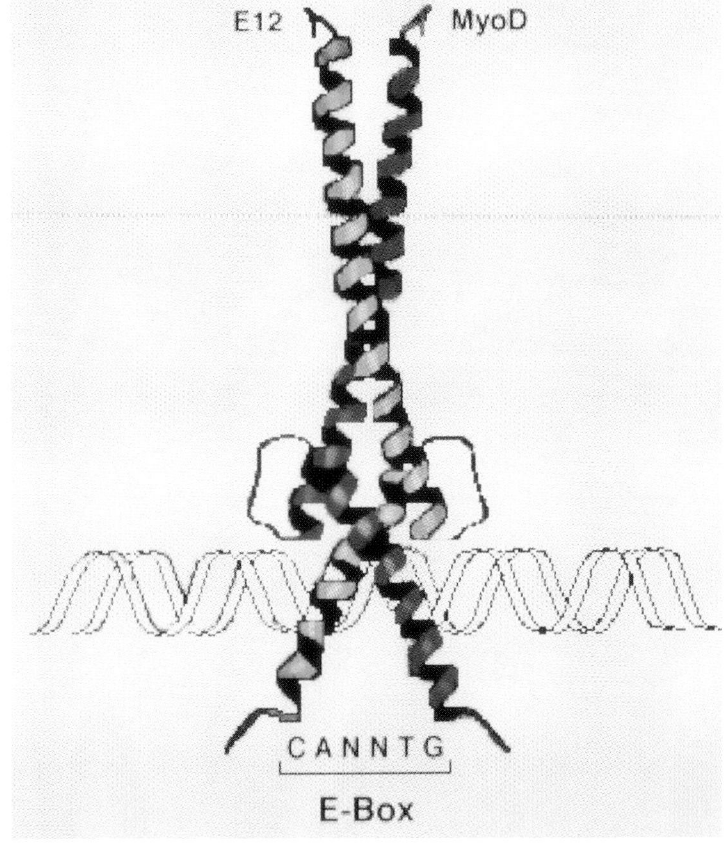

Plate 10 (Fig. 3; *see* full caption on p. 843 and discussion in Chapter 92).

71 Renal Neoplasms

Wilms' Tumor and Renal-Cell Carcinoma

KIM E. NICHOLS AND DANIEL A. HABER

INTRODUCTION

Identification of disease-related genes has been greatly facilitated by the use of positional cloning strategies. These molecular approaches, based on genetic localization rather than biologic function, have led to the isolation of genes responsible for the development of several human cancers. Among these are *WT-1*, a tumor suppressor gene implicated in the pediatric kidney cancer Wilms' tumor, and *VHL*, the gene for the Von Hippel Lindau syndrome, a disease associated with the development of renal cysts and renal-cell carcinoma. The identification of specific genes involved in the development of renal tumors may lead to a better understanding of both normal kidney development and tumor formation. For instance, *WT-1* has been shown to be required for normal formation of the kidney and gonads. Its role in the survival of renal blastemal cells and the formation of glomeruli is under active investigation. Additional insight into kidney development may follow the identification of other Wilms' tumor genes and the further characterization of the *VHL* gene.

WILMS' TUMOR

Wilms' tumor or nephroblastoma is the most common abdominal solid tumor of childhood, accounting for 5–6% of all pediatric cancers and affecting 1 in 10,000 children. The tumor was first characterized in 1899 by the surgeon Max Wilms', after whom it was named. Wilms' tumors are thought to arise from primitive renal stem cells (blastemal cells) that maintain a limited capacity to differentiate. Classical Wilms' tumors are characterized by their "triphasic" histology consisting of varying degrees of blastemal, epithelial, and stromal components. However, elements of neural or skeletal muscle differentiation may also be present. This complex histologic pattern suggests a recapitulation of early events in kidney development, consistent with the malignant transformation of a pluripotent renal stem cell.

THE KNUDSON "TWO-HIT" MODEL OF TUMORIGENESIS Although the majority of Wilms' tumors are unilateral, approximately 10% are bilateral. Bilateral cases occur at a younger age than unilateral tumors (on average 2 years earlier) and may be associated with a positive family history. These observations, analogous to those made in two other pediatric tumors, retinoblastoma and neuroblastoma, led to the "two-hit" model of tumorigenesis proposed by Knudson and Strong in the early 1970s. Based on statistical analysis of the age of incidence of unilateral versus bilateral tumors, Knudson predicted that two "rate-limiting hits" are required to initiate tumor formation. Most unilateral tumors represent sporadic cases in which these two rare genetic events have arisen in the same cell. However, children who already harbor one genetic lesion in their germline, either inherited from a parent or occuring *de novo*, require only one additional "hit" in somatic cells. The high probability of sustaining a single genetic event explains the early onset of tumors in these children and their frequent multifocal or bilateral incidence. The Knudson model has been confirmed by the demonstration of allelic losses in tumor specimens involving specific chromosomal loci and eventually by the identification of individual genes targeted by the mutational events. The two rate-limiting hits that were predicted are now understood to represent the inactivation of both alleles of a tumor suppressor gene.

While isolation of the *RB* gene involved in retinoblastoma has fulfilled all of the predictions of the Knudson model, Wilms' tumor has proved more genetically heterogeneous. Only 1% of Wilms' tumor cases show evidence of familial transmission, indicating that most bilateral tumors result from *de novo* germline mutations. This may reflect reduced fertility in individuals who carry a mutation in one allele of a gene that is involved in genito-urinary development *(see below)*. In addition, multiple genetic loci have been implicated in Wilms' tumor. *WT1*, the Wilms' tumor gene residing at the chromosome 11p13 locus, has been identified, and its properties are the subject of intensive study. Studies are currently underway to isolate the second Wilms' tumor gene localized to the chromosome 11p15 locus and a potential third Wilms' tumor gene implicated in rare familial cases.

ISOLATION OF THE WT1 TUMOR SUPPRESOR GENE AT 11p13 The development of Wilms' tumor may be associated with congenital malformation syndromes, whose characterization has proved critical to the definition of the different genetic loci contributing to Wilms' tumorigenesis. In 1964, Miller and associates described an association between the incidence of Wilms' tumor and aniridia, a malformation of the iris. The incidence of aniridia is 1 in 70 among children with Wilms' tumor, an approximately 1000-fold increase over that in the general population. Conversely, one-third of children with aniridia eventually develop Wilms' tumor. In 1978, Riccardi and coworkers discovered that children affected with the rare Wilms' tumor, aniridia, genito-

From: *Principles of Molecular Medicine* (J. L. Jameson, ed.), ©1998 Humana Press Inc., Totowa, NJ.

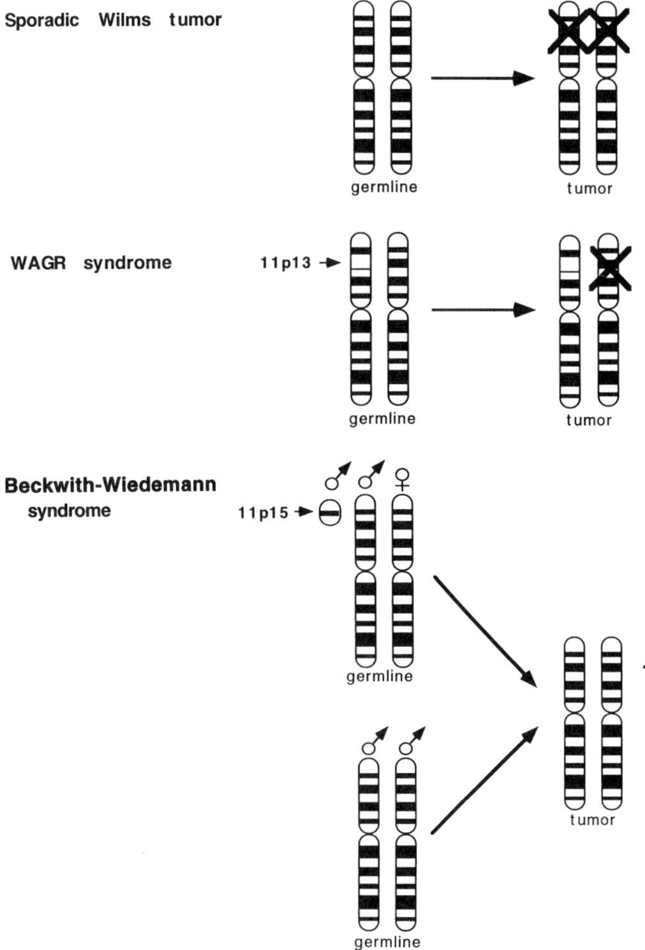

Figure 71-1 Genetic mechanisms underlying predisposition to Wilms' tumor. As predicted by the Knudson model, sporadic tumors are initiated by two rare genetic events, leading to the inactivation of both alleles of a tumor suppressor gene in a renal precursor cell. In WAGR Syndrome, genetic predisposition results from the presence of an interstitial deletion at chromosome 11p13, resulting in the loss of one *WT-1* allele in the germline. Only one subsequent genetic event in somatic cells is required for complete inactivation of *WT-1*. In Beckwith-Wiedemann Syndrome, predisposition to Wilms' tumor and other embryonic cancers is derived from the presence of an additional copy of the paternally derived chromosome 11p15 locus. This may result from partial trisomy at 11p15 or from inheritance of two chromosomes 11 from the father and none from the mother (uniparental isodisomy). These unusual genetic events presumably result in overexpression of an imprinted gene, expressed only from the paternally derived allele. The additional events leading to tumorigenesis have not been well-defined.

urinary malformations, and mental retardation (WAGR) syndrome had a constitutional deletion in one copy of chromosome 11, at band p13 (Fig. 71-1). This finding, supported by the presence of allelic losses in sporadic Wilms' tumor specimens, led to the identification of the first genetic locus involved in etiology of Wilms' tumor.

The *WT-1* gene, mapping to the smallest region of overlap between naturally-occuring deletions at chromosome 11p13, was isolated by two groups in 1990. The presence of point mutations within the gene, both in sporadic Wilms' tumor specimens and in the germline of children with genetic predisposition, confirmed its identity as the Wilms' tumor suppressor gene at the 11p13 chromosomal locus. *WT-1* encodes a transcription factor with a critical role in kidney development *(see below)*. Genito-urinary defects that are observed in children with WAGR syndrome have therefore been attributed to the reduced expression of *WT-1* during development, resulting from the loss of one germline WT1 allele (Table 71-1). Another 11p13 gene contributing to the WAGR phenotype has also been identified: the *Pax 6* gene is contiguous with *WT-1*, and constitutional loss of one germline allele results in aniridia. *Pax 6* has recently been shown to be the master gene responsible for eye development in *Drosophila*. The genetic cause of the other major defect in WAGR syndrome, mental retardation, has not been explained.

The *WT-1* gene is encoded by 10 exons, spanning 50 kb of genomic DNA. WT-1 protein migrates with a size of ~55 kDa on SDS-PAGE and contains two apparent functional domains: the carboxy-terminus (exons 7–10) contains four zinc fingers of the cysteine-histidine type, mediating specific DNA binding, while the amino-terminus contains a glutamine and proline-rich domain involved in the regulation of transcription (so-called transactivation) (Fig. 71-2). *WT-1* therefore encodes a transcription factor, predicted to regulate the expression of other genes that are important for kidney and urogenital development. WT-1 protein exists as four isoforms resulting from the presence or absence of two alternative splices in the mRNA transcript. Alternative splice I results from the insertion of 17 amino acids (exon 5) between the transactivation and DNA binding domains, and its exact function has not been determined. Alternative splice II results from the use of an alternative splice donor site in exon 9, leading to the insertion of three amino acids (lysine, threonine, serine or "KTS") between zinc fingers 3 and 4. Presence of this KTS insertion greatly reduces the DNA binding affinity of *WT-1* and has recently been shown to alter its subnuclear localization to structures that may be associated with the mRNA splicing machinery. The four isoforms are present in constant proportion in all WT-1 expressing tissues and, while WT-1 has recently been shown to dimerize in vivo, the functional consequences of the interaction between these isoforms remains unknown.

WT-1 MEDIATED TRANSCRIPTIONAL REGULATION AND GROWTH SUPPRESSION The mechanism of action of *WT-1* is not well-understood. WT-1 zinc fingers 2–4 have extensive amino acid homology to the three zinc fingers of the early growth response gene *EGR1* (also known as *NGF1-A*, *Krox 24*, and *Zif 268*), a gene induced by mitogenic stimuli and implicated in signaling pathways involved in cell proliferation. In DNA binding assays, the four zinc fingers of WT-1 bind to the GC-rich consensus sequence (5'-GCGGGGGCG-3') recognized by EGR1, although with much reduced affinity. However, other potential WT-1 DNA-binding sites have recently been proposed, including a higher affinity GC-rich site (5'-GAGTGCGTGG GAGTAGAA-3') identified from genomic DNA fragments and a TC-repeat sequence (5'-TCCTCCTCC-3') present in WT-1 responsive promoters. Definition of the optimal WT-1 DNA target site awaits a better characterization of promoter sequences that are physiologically regulated by WT-1.

Binding of WT-1 to target promoter sequences generally results in repression of transcription. WT-1 has thus been defined as a transcriptional repressor, although it is also capable of activating transcription, depending on the nature of the target promoter sequence, the presence of potential cofactors such as p53 *(see*

Table 71-1
Genetic and Phenotypic Characteristics of Congenital Syndromes Associated with Wilms' Tumor and Adult Renal-Cell Carcinoma

Locus	*Gene*	*Syndrome*	*Tumor*	*Phenotype*	*Mechanism*
Embryonal renal cancers					
11p13	WT1	WAGR	Wilms'	GU anomolies	Reduced gene dosage
11p13	WT1	Denys-Drash	Wilms' gonadoblastoma	Mesangial sclerosis pseudohermaphroditism	Gain of function (dominant negative)
11p15	?	Beckwith-Wiedemann	Wilms' hepatoblastoma adrenocortical ca	Organomegaly	Increased gene dosage
?	?	Familial cancer	Wilms'	—	—
Adult renal cancers					
3p13-14	?	Familial cancer	Renal cell ca	—	—
3p25-26	VHL	Von Hippel Lindau	Renal cell ca	Multiple cysts hemangiomas	?reduced gene dosage
7q31.1-34	Met	Familial cancer	Renal cell ca	Papillary	Tyrosine kinase activation

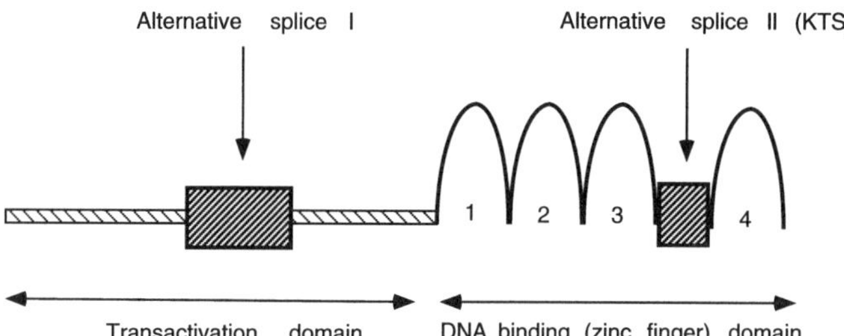

Figure 71-2 Functional domains of the *WT-1* tumor suppressor gene. WT-1 encodes a transcription factor divided into two functional domains. The carboxy-terminus comprises 4 zinc finger domains that mediate binding to specific DNA sequences, while the amino-terminus contains a transactivation domain that represses transcription from target promoters. The presence or absence of two alternative splices in the *WT-1* transcript results in four different isoforms with potentially distinct functions.

below), and mutations within *WT-1* itself. In transfection assays, *WT-1* has been shown to repress transcription from a large number of promoters containing a GC-rich sequence, including those of EGR1, insulin-like growth factor 2 (IGF-2), platelet-derived growth factor α chain (PDGF-α), Pax 2, colony stimulating factor 1, insulin-like growth factor 1 receptor (IGF1-R), transforming growth factor-β (TGF-β), epidermal growth factor receptor (EGFR), and WT-1 itself, among others. This has led to the model that *WT-1* may be a negative regulator of growth-inducing genes. However, regulation of promoter constructs by *WT-1* has proved to be a poor predictor of its effect on endogenous genes. The development of cell lines expressing *WT-1* under the control of a tightly regulated inducible promoter has shown that most of these potential *WT-1* target genes are unaffected by induction of *WT-1*. However, expression of one of these genes, EGFR, is repressed following induction of *WT-1* expression in vivo. WT-1-mediated apoptosis is preceeded by induction of the cyclin-dependent kinase inhibitor, p21. The increase in p21 occurs in a p53-independent manner.

One of the critical properties of tumor suppressor genes is their ability to arrest the growth of malignant cells or repress their tumorigenic phenotype. The retinoblastoma susceptibility gene, *RB*, mediates cell-cycle arrest in G1, while p53 can either induce a G1 block or trigger programmed cell death (apoptosis), depending on the cellular context. Reintroduction of wild-type *WT-1* into a Wilms' tumor cell line, expressing an aberrant endogenous *WT-1* transcript, results in suppression of colony formation in vitro. The few cells that emerge, expressing low levels of wild-type *WT-1*, demonstrate reduced clonogenicity in soft agar and delayed tumorigenicity in nude mice. In a model osteosarcoma cell line expressing an inducible *WT-1* gene, WT-1 isoforms lacking the KTS alternative splice trigger programmed cell death. The onset of apoptosis in these cells follows the suppression of EGFR synthesis and is prevented by constitutive expression of this growth factor receptor. *WT-1*–induced cell death in these cells may therefore result from the withdrawal of growth-factor-mediated signals required for cell survival. Although these observations have interesting implications for a role of *WT-1* in growth factor/cell death pathways in vivo, the exact function of *WT-1* during kidney development and tumorigenesis remain uncertain.

ROLE OF WT-1 IN KIDNEY AND UROGENITAL DEVELOPMENT The developmental role of *WT-1* has been closely linked with its expression pattern. By RNA *in situ* hybridization, *WT-1* transcript is detectable in cells of the developing kidney (condensed mesenchyme, renal vesicle, and glomerular epithelium), Sertoli cells of the testis, granulosa cells of the ovary, and mesothelial cells comprising the pericardial, pleural, and peritoneal surfaces. WT1 expression is also seen in stromal cells of the spleen and in the capsule of the thymus. Although normal hematopoietic cells expressing WT-1 have not been identified, high levels of mRNA expression have been found in a subset of lymphoid and myeloid leukemias. In contrast to other *WT-1* expressing tissues, presence of the *WT-1* transcript in the developing kidney is transient and associated with specific developmental structures. In the mouse, peak *WT-1* expression occurs around the time of birth, with minimal levels detected in the adult kidney. Histological analysis shows low levels of expression in the primitive blastemal stem cells, and high levels as these cells differentiate into the podocytes of glomeruli.

The critical role of *WT-1* in genito-urinary development is best demonstrated by the generation of WT1-null mice. These mice, lacking both *WT-1* alleles, fail to develop either kidneys or gonads; their vestigial renal buds lack blastemal cells and fail to differentiate following inductive stimuli. Homozygous deletion of *WT-1* in the mouse is lethal during embryonic development, possibly resulting from cardiac and diaphragmatic malformations that might be caused by the absence of *WT-1* expression in the mesothelial cells lining these organs. However, in contrast to the human WAGR syndrome, mice lacking one *WT-1* allele have no evidence of genito-urinary malformation and do not develop renal tumors.

The role of *WT-1* in genito-urinary development has also been demonstrated in humans, most prominently in Denys-Drash Syndrome (DDS). While children who have a deletion of one *WT-1* germline allele (e.g., WAGR syndrome) may have genito-urinary defects of varying severity, those with DDS display renal mesangial sclerosis progressing to renal failure and intersex disorders characterized by pseudohermaphroditism and streak gonads (Table 71-1). Virtually all patients with DDS harbor a point mutation in one *WT-1* germline allele, most commonly affecting zinc finger 3 or 4. The severe developmental defects observed in children expressing a WT-1 protein with a disrupted DNA binding domain, in contrast to those with a deleted allele, suggest that specific *WT-1* mutations may encode a dysfunctional protein. Although functionally inactive, such mutants would act in a dominant or "gain of function" manner, presumably disrupting the properties of the wild-type protein. Potential mechanisms for these so-called "dominant negative" *WT-1* mutations are discussed below.

INACTIVATION OF WT-1 IN RENAL AND MESOTHELIAL TUMORS Gross deletions affecting *WT-1* are rare, but approximately 10% of sporadic Wilms' tumors contain point mutations within the coding region, including missense, nonsense, and frameshift mutations. Missense mutations or small deletions within the zinc finger domain have been shown to disrupt DNA binding activity, whereas mutations within the amino terminus result in altered transactivational properties. Unlike other tumor suppressor genes in which both alleles must be inactivated to initiate tumor formation, a significant fraction of *WT-1* mutations observed in Wilms' tumors are heterozygous. This observation suggests that some mutations encode dysfunctional or dominant negative WT-1 proteins *(see above)*, capable of disrupting *WT-1* function despite the expression of the residual wild-type allele. One such mutant, encoding a disrupted zinc finger domain with reduced DNA binding affinity, demonstrates oncogenic effects on primary kidney cultures, consistent with a dominant transforming effect. A potential mechanism for dominant-negative *WT-1* mutations has recently been proposed, based on the observation that the amino-terminus mediates dimerization of WT-1 as well as its localization to distinct subnuclear structures. Co-expression of wild-type *WT-1* and a mutant with a disrupted DNA-binding domain results in the relocation of the wild-type protein within subnuclear structures. Dominant-negative *WT-1* mutants may therefore exert their effect by sequestering and functionally inactivating wild-type *WT-1*.

In addition to mutations disrupting *WT-1* function, other mechanisms have been reported to alter the properties of this tumor suppressor gene. RNA editing, the insertion of a nucleotide in the mRNA transcript that differs from that present within the gene itself, has been observed in rodent *WT-1*, resulting in subtle alterations in the functional properties of the encoded protein. Aberrant mRNA splicing appears to be a relatively frequent occurrence in Wilms' tumor specimens, with approximately 10% of tumors expressing a transcript with an in-frame deletion of *WT-1* exon 2. This truncated protein, which is not detected in normal *WT-1* expressing tissues, appears to result from altered splicing, rather than from a mutation within the *WT-1* gene itself. The encoded protein lacks a critical portion of the *WT-1* transactivational domain, resulting in potent activation, rather than repression, of transcription from target promoters.

The potential consequences of transcriptional activation by *WT-1* variants, in contrast to transcriptional repression by wild-type *WT-1*, are best demonstrated in desmoplastic small round cell tumor (DSRT), a rare mesothelial cell-derived pediatric malignancy. DSRT exhibits a characteristic chromosomal abnormality, consisting of a translocation between chromosomes 11p13 and 22q12. Molecular characterization of this tumor has revealed a chimeric fusion of one *WT-1* allele with the Ewing's sarcoma gene *EWS*. The translocation, analogous to that between *EWS* and other transcription factors in Ewings sarcoma and related tumors, results in the expression of a chimeric protein, containing the potent transactivation domain of EWS and zinc fingers 2–4 of WT-1. The initial genetic lesion underlying DSRT may therefore result in transcriptional activation of a subset of *WT-1* target genes.

NEPHROGENIC RESTS AND THE TIMING OF WT-1 INACTIVATION Nephrogenic rests, also termed "nephroblastomatosis" or "nodular renal blastema," represent persistent foci of primitive but nonneoplastic blastemal cells, within the otherwise normal renal tissue. Nephrogenic rests are usually microscopic, although they may measure up to several centimeters, and are not normally seen in the kidneys of children over 1 year of age. However, 30–40% of kidneys from children with unilateral Wilms' tumor, and virtually all kidneys from children with genetic predisposition, contain one or more nephrogenic rests. Untreated, nephrogenic rests may either regress spontaneously, persist, or evolve into Wilms' tumor. A potential link between the distinct histological subtypes of nephrogenic rests and the different Wilms' tumor genetic loci has been suggested: "intralobar rests," arising within the kidney lobule, are typically found in patients with aniridia and genetic abnormalities at 11p13, whereas "perilobar rests," present at the periphery of the kidney lobule, are associated with Beckwith-Wiedemann syndrome (BWS), a Wilms' tumor-associated syndrome linked to chromosome 11p15 *(see below)*. However, this correlation between histologic features and genetic loci remains to be confirmed by molecular studies.

Mutational analysis of nephrogenic rests arising within the normal kidney of sporadic Wilms' tumor cases has demonstrated that these lesions are clonally related to the associated Wilms' tumor. In two cases in which a sporadic Wilms' tumor contained a point mutation within *WT-1*, nephrogenic rests present within the uninvolved portion of the affected kidney demonstrated the identical *WT-1* mutation. Thus, nephrogenic rests may arise from renal precursor cells harboring a *WT-1* mutation, in effect constituting genetic precursors of Wilms' tumors. Inactivation of *WT-1* is therefore an early genetic event, potentially leading to the immortalization of blastemal cells and increasing the target cell population susceptible to additional genetic hits, leading to the development of Wilms' tumor.

INTERACTION BETWEEN WT-1 AND p53 In contrast to most human malignancies, p53 mutations are extremely rare in Wilms' tumor, observed in <1% of cases. Mutations in p53 appear to be specifically associated with the anaplastic variant of Wilms' tumor, a rare subtype characterized by gross chromosomal instability, resistance to chemotherapeutic agents, and having a poor clinical prognosis. The majority of p53 mutations observed in human tumors lead to amino acid substitutions that disrupt protein function while enhancing its stability, resulting in elevated levels of expression. However, most Wilms' tumors express high levels of p53 protein, despite the absence of p53 mutations. Recent observations have shown that WT-1 protein is capable of binding and stabilizing p53. In a series of eight primary Wilms' tumors, in which both *WT-1* and p53 were wild-type, the level of p53 protein was well correlated with that of WT-1. In cultured cells, binding of WT-1 to p53 alters the properties of p53, specifically blocking its ability to induce apoptosis. Thus, *WT-1* may have properties in addition to those of a classical tumor suppressor gene. In the 90% of sporadic Wilms' tumors that express low levels of wild-type *WT-1*, it may effectively disrupt p53 function, obviating the need to inactivate p53 by mutational mechanisms.

WT-1 also interacts with par-4 (prostate apoptosis response). Par-4 appears to augment WT-1-mediated repression and blocks activation by WT-1.

THE SECOND WILMS' TUMOR LOCUS: CHROMOSOME 11p15 A second genetic locus on chromosome 11, at band 11p15, has been implicated in the development of Wilms' tumor. Like 11p13, this locus has been identified both by germline abnormalities in children with genetic predisposition and by somatic allelic losses in Wilms' tumor specimens. BWS, an overgrowth syndrome characterized by visceromegaly, hemihypertrophy, macroglossia, umbilical hernia, and hypoglycemia, is notable for the increased incidence of embryonal malignancies, including adrenal carcinoma, hepatoblastoma, and Wilms' tumor (Table 71-1). In BWS cases that show familial transmission, linkage has been established to chromosome 11p15. Further, in children presenting with *de novo* BWS, striking karyotype abnormalities have been observed affecting 11p15. In contrast to the chromosomal deletions seen in WAGR syndrome, BWS has been associated with chromosomal duplication events. Partial trisomy at 11p15 has been observed, with the duplicated 11p15 locus invariably derived from the paternally inherited allele (Fig. 71-1). In BWS children without gross karyotype abnormalities at chromosome 11p15, molecular studies have revealed uniparental isodisomy, i.e., inheritance of two paternally derived chromosomes 11 and absence of any maternally derived chromosome 11.

The chromosome duplication events and the unequal parental inheritance are consistent with genomic imprinting, the differential expression of genes between maternally and paternally inherited chromosomes. Thus, an imprinted gene, whose maternal allele is silent and whose paternal allele is expressed, would be overexpressed in a child carrying two copies of the paternally inherited chromosome 11p15. Such a dosage effect would be consistent with the overgrowth features that are characteristic of BWS. One candidate gene for BWS is insulin-like growth factor 2 (*IGF-2*), a growth-inducing gene localized to 11p15 known to undergo genomic imprinting, with expression restricted to the paternal allele. Although no direct evidence has proven that overexpression of *IGF-2* is responsible for BWS, loss or "relaxation" of *IGF-2* imprinting, resulting in expression of *IGF-2* by both maternal and paternal alleles, has been observed in the germline of children with this syndrome. In addition, Wilms' tumors frequently show loss of imprinting and increased *IGF-2* expression, suggesting that this gene may contribute to tumor growth, possibly through direct activation of this growth factor receptor pathway. However, an alternative possibility has been proposed, based on the observation that *IGF-2* expression is associated with reduced expression of a contiguous putative tumor suppressor gene *H19*. *H19* is imprinted in the opposite direction to *IGF-2*, with expression restricted to the maternally derived allele. Since *H19* encodes an untranslated RNA species capable of suppressing tumorigenicity in cultured cell lines, loss of *H19* expression, with or without overexpression of *IGF-2*, may contribute to Wilms' tumorigenesis.

IGF-2 and *H19* may contribute to the etiology of BWS and potentially to the growth properties of Wilms' tumors. However, molecular mapping studies have defined a genetic locus that is distinct from these genes, and that is the specific target of allelic losses in Wilms' tumor specimens. This locus, WT2, has properties that are more characteristic of a classical tumor suppressor gene and may prove to be inactivated by point mutations and deletions, rather than by alterations in genomic imprinting. A number of other tumors, including breast cancer, cervical cancer, and leukemias, demonstrate loss of heterozygosity at 11p15, suggesting that this new tumor suppressor gene may prove to be involved in a number of different malignancies.

FAMILIAL WILMS' TUMOR AND OTHER GENETIC LOCI Although familial transmission of susceptibility to Wilms' tumor is rare, three large pedigrees have been reported, with cancer predisposition showing an autosomal dominant inheritance pattern. Linkage studies in all three families have excluded either of the chromosome 11 loci in transmission of disease susceptibility. The chromosomal location of this familial Wilms' tumor gene is currently unknown. In addition to the major genetic loci capable of initiating Wilms' tumorigenesis, other loci have been implicated in tumor progression. The contribution of the p53 gene to the anaplastic phenotype has been discussed above. In addition, 10–20% of Wilms' tumors show loss of heterozygosity at chromosomes 16q or 1p, which may be associated with a somewhat worse clinical prognosis. Finally, even the primary Wilms' tumor genetic loci on chromosome 11 may act in concert to promote tumor growth, as demonstrated by a number of tumors showing both mutations within *WT-1* and allelic losses affecting the 11p15 locus. Thus, the genetic etiology of Wilms' tumor is complex, involving potential contributions from several genes, which may play different roles during normal kidney development and tumor formation.

RENAL-CELL CARCINOMA

THE 3p13-14 RCC LOCUS Renal-cell carcinoma (RCC) is the most common malignancy of the adult kidney. In contrast to Wilms' tumor, the malignant cells are thought to originate from the tubular epithelium of the kidney, rather than from glomerular precursors, and RCC does not share the embryonic histological features of nephroblastoma. Whereas the great majority of RCCs are sporadic, they can occur in the setting of familial predisposition, demonstrating an autosomal dominant inheritance pattern. Like Wilms' tumor, RCCs arising in genetically predisposed individuals develop at an earlier age and show bilateral or multifocal involvement, although genetic susceptibility to RCC does not appear to be associated with defects in genito-urinary development. The chromosome 3p13-14 locus has been implicated in the formation of RCC, by the presence of allelic losses in tumor specimens, as well as by the transmission of translocated chromosomes involving 3p13-14 in rare familial cases. Efforts to isolate the 3p13-14 RCC gene by positional cloning techniques have been complicated by genetic events involving the von Hippel Lindau gene (*VHL*), located at a neighboring locus, 3p25-26.

VON HIPPEL LINDAU SYNDROME Hereditary RCC may occur in the setting of von Hippel Lindau (VHL) syndrome. VHL carriers develop multiple renal cysts that have the potential for malignant degeneration, tumors of the adrenal glands and pancreas, and hemangiomas of the retina and central nervous system. Cytogenetic and molecular analyses of kidney tumors from patients with VHL have demonstrated allelic losses affecting chromosome 3p25-26, culminating in the recent identification of the *VHL* gene by positional cloning techniques. Unlike WT-1, the absence of clear amino acid homology between VHL and other known proteins has made it difficult to predict the function of this potential tumor suppressor gene. *VHL* encodes a 30-kDa cytoplasmic protein, whose amino terminus contains eight copies of an acidic tandemly repeated pentamer (Gly-X-Glu-Glu-X) of uncertain significance. VHL protein has recently been found to associate with transcriptional elongation factors known as elongins, suggesting that this tumor suppressor gene may be directly involved in mRNA processing. *VHL* mRNA is expressed in a broad range of tissues, including adult brain, kidney, adrenal gland, prostate, and lung. Alternative splicing has also been observed in the *VHL* transcript, reflecting presence or absence of exon 2. While the splicing variant encoding exon 2 is the more prevalent in most normal tissues, an inverted ratio has been observed in some RCCs, suggesting a functional significance.

MUTATIONS IN THE VHL TUMOR SUPPRESSOR GENE Of patients with VHL syndrome, 39–75% have germline mutations in one *VHL* allele, with their renal cell cancers showing loss of the remaining wild-type allele. However, *VHL* mutations are not limited to RCC arising within this familial syndrome: 30–60% of sporadic nonpapillary renal-cell carcinomas contain mutations in the *VHL* gene and 80–90% show loss of heterozygosity at the VHL locus. Thus, *VHL* appears to play a major role in the development of adult renal cancers. Mutations are evenly spaced over the three exons of the gene and include insertions, deletions, splice-site abnormalities (primarily affecting exon 2), and missense and nonsense mutations. While deletions affecting the short arm of chromosome 3 have been reported in many different cancers, including sporadic pheochromocytoma, small-cell lung cancer, mesothelioma, and cancers of the breast, ovaries, colon, thyroid, prostate, and bladder, no mutations in the *VHL* gene have been identified in these tumors. Chromosome 3p may therefore contain a number of important tumor suppressor genes, with *VHL* playing a specific role in kidney tumorigenesis. The relationship between *VHL* and the familial *RCC* gene at 3p14-15 remains unclear. Like the two Wilms' tumor genes on the short arm of chromosome 11, the presence of two adult kidney cancer loci at chromosome 3p has complicated molecular and cytogenetic analyses. Sporadic RCCs may show loss of the entire chromosome region from 3p13 to the telomere, resulting in deletion of both of these loci. Rare patients with familial RCC have been reported to have both a germline translocation affecting the RCC locus at chromosome 3p13-14, as well as a mutation in the *VHL* gene in their renal cancers. These observations suggest potential functional interactions between the two chromosome 3p tumor suppressor genes involved in renal cell carcinoma.

Hereditary papillary renal carcinoma (HPRC) is histologically and genetically distinct from VHL. The HPRC gene has been localized to 7q31.1-34. Mutations have been identified in the tyrosine kinase domain of the *met* gene in HPRC families. These mutations may cause constitutive activation of the MET protein.

CONCLUSIONS

The application of molecular genetics to the study of pediatric and adult renal tumors has led to the definition of genetic loci that play critical roles in the initiation of tumorigenesis. Positional cloning strategies have led to the identification of specific tumor suppressor genes, *WT-1* and *VHL*, and may yield additional genes in the near future. Identification of these disease genes is only the first step; biochemical and functional characterization of the gene products will provide a better understanding of the abnormalities in growth and developmental pathways that result in tumor formation. *WT-1* has proved to be a paradigm for studying the critical steps in early kidney development, involving transcriptional regulation of growth inducing genes, induction of programmed cell death, and a potential role in the survival of renal blastema and the differentiation of glomeruli. The isolation of other Wilms' tumor genes that may contribute to nephroblast development and studies of *VHL* and the genetic loci involved in adult renal cancers will undoubtedly enhance our understanding of the genetic lesions that lead to cancer of the kidney.

SELECTED REFERENCES

Call K, Glaser T, Ito C, et al. Isolation and characterization of a zinc finger polypeptide gene at the human chromosome 11 Wilms' tumor locus. Cell 1990;60:509–520.

Englert C, Hou X, Maheswaran S, et al. WT1 suppresses synthesis of the epidermal growth factor receptor and induces apoptosis. Embo J. 1995;14:4662–4675.

Englert C, Maheswaran S, Garvin AJ, Kreidberg J, Haber DA. Induction of p21 by the Wilms' tumor suppressor gene WT1. Cancer Res 1997;57:1429–1434.

Fleming S. Genetics of renal tumours. Cancer Metastasis Rev 1997; 16:127–140.

Gessler M, Poustka A, Cavenee W, Neve R, Orkin S, Bruns G. Homozygous deletion in Wilms' tumours of a zinc-finger gene identified by chromosome jumping. Nature 1990;343:774–778.

Haber D, Buckler A, Glaser T, et al. An internal deletion within an 11p13 zinc finger gene contributes to the development of Wilms' tumor. Cell 1990;61:1257–1269.

Haber D, Park S, Maheswaran S, et al. WT1-mediated growth suppression of Wilms' tumor cells expressing a WT1 splicing variant. Science 1993;262:2057–2059.

Halder G, Callaerts P, and Gehring W. Induction of ectopic eyes by targeted expression of the eyeless gene in Drosophila. Science 1995; 267:1788–1792.

Henry I, Bonaiti-Pellie C, Chehensse V, et al. Uniparental paternal disomy in a genetic cancer-predisposing syndrome. Nature 1991; 351:665–667.

Hewitt SM, Fraizer GC, Wu YJ, Rauscher FJ 3rd, Saunders GF. Differential function of Wilms' tumor gene WT1 splice isoforms in transcriptional regulation. J Biol Chem 1996;271:8588–8592.

Johnstone RW, See RH, Sells SF, et al. A novel repressor, par-4, modulates transcription and growth suppression functions of the Wilms' tumor suppressor WT1. Mol Cell Biol 1996;16:6945–6956.

Knudson A, Strong L. Mutation and cancer: a model for Wilms' tumor of the kidney. J Natl Cancer Inst 1972;48:313–324.

Kreidberg J, Sariola H, Loring J, et al. WT1 is required for early kidney development. Cell 1993;74:679–691.

Ladanyi M, Gerald W. Fusion of the EWS and WT1 genes in the desmoplastic small round cell tumor. Cancer Res 1994;54:2837–2840.

Latif, F, Tory K, Gnarra J, et al. Identification of the von Hippel-Lindau disease tumor suppressor gene. Science 1993;260:1317–1320.

Little M, Wells C. A clinical overview of WT1 gene mutations. Hum Mutat 1997;9:209–225.

Maheswaran S, Englert C, Bennett P, Heinrich G, Haber D. The WT1 gene product stabilizes p53 and inhibits p53-mediated apoptosis. Genes Dev 1995;9:2143–2156.

Ogawa O, Becroft D, Morison I, et al. Constitutional relaxation of insulin-like growth factor II gene imprinting associated with Wilms' tumour and gigantism. Nat Genet 1993;5:408–412.

Okamoto K, Morison IM, Taniguchi T, Reeve AE. Epigenetic changes at the insulin-like growth factor II/H19 locus in developing kidney is an early event in Wilms' tumorigenesis. Proc Natl Acad Sci USA 1997;94:5367–5371.

Park S, Bernard A, Bove K, et al. Inactivation of WT1 in nephrogenic rests, genetic precursors to Wilms' tumour. Nat Genet 1993;5: 363–367.

Pelletier J, Bruening W, Kashtan C, et al. Germline mutations in the Wilms' tumor suppressor gene are associated with abnormal urogenital development in Denys-Drash syndrome. Cell 1991;67: 437–447.

Pritchard-Jones K, Fleming S, Davidson D, et al. The candidate Wilms' tumour gene is involved in genitourinary development. Nature 1990;346:194–197.

Pritchard-Jones K, Hawkins MM. Biology of Wilms' tumour. Lancet 1997;349:663–664.

Rauscher F, Morris J, Tournay O, Cook D, Curran T. Binding of the Wilms' tumor locus zinc finger protein to the EGR-1 consensus sequence. Science 1990;250:1259–1262.

Schmidt L, Duh FM, Chen F, et al. Germline and somatic mutations in the tyrosine kinase domain of the MET proto-oncogene in papillary renal carcinomas. Nat Genet 1997;16:68–73.

Xu YQ, Grundy P, Polychronoako C. Aberrant imprinting of the insulin-like growth factor II receptor gene in Wilms' tumor. Oncogene 1997;14:1041–1046.

DERMATOLOGY IX

SECTION EDITOR:
THOMAS S. KUPPER

CONGENITAL DISEASES OF CUTANEOUS TISSUES

PART A: SELECTED EPIDERMAL GENE MUTATIONS

72 Introduction to Selected Epidermal Gene Mutations

ANGELA M. CHRISTIANO, DANIEL B. DUBIN, AND THOMAS S. KUPPER

INTRODUCTION

Genodermatoses, or genetic disorders that primarily involve the skin, have been the subject of many monographs and reviews, and an exhaustive review of these is well beyond the scope of this section. The accessibility of skin, and the ease with which it can be observed, has allowed for the identification of well over a hundred diseases that qualify as genodermatoses, and the mode inheritance of many has been well-documented. Many of these diseases have a clear pattern of inheritance with complete penetrance (e.g., epidermolysis bullosa dystrophica), while others can arise spontaneously and are incompletely penetrant (e.g., tuberous sclerosis). More recently, an explosion of novel molecular genetic approaches and techniques have led to a series of important breakthroughs in the identification of specific gene defects underlying certain of these diseases (Table 72-1). The rate at which this is occurring ensures that any treatise that attempts to be exhaustive and current is doomed to failure. Rather than being encyclopedic and all-inclusive, we have tried to focus on several selected genodermatoses for which there has been significant experimental work performed around identifying the genetic defect. Even this is not inclusive; for example, we have not discussed in details the very elegant work that has been done by Deitz and colleagues in the identification of fibrillin as the defective gene in Marfan's syndrome, and by Hohl's group on the identification of transglutaminase as the defective enzyme in lamellar ichthyosis. The reader is referred to the primary references for more information, and several representative texts and reviews are listed below.

Most of the genodermatoses for which the gene and its protein product have been identified are listed in Table 72-2, and several are discussed at some length in the ensuing chapters. When possible, diseases in which (1) the gene has been identified, and (2) a plausible mechanism has been advanced by which the defective genotype results in the observed phenotype, have been selected for expanded discussion.

SELECTED REFERENCES

Alper JC. Genetic Disorders of the Skin. St. Louis: Mosby-Year Book, 1991.

Mallory SB, Leal-Khouri S. An Illustrated Dictionary of Dermatologic Syndromes. New York: Parthenon, 1994.

McKusick VA, Mendelian Inheritance in Man. Baltimore: Johns Hopkins University Press, 1992; 10th ed.

Novice FM, Collison DW, Burgdorf WHC, Esterly NB. Handbook of Genetic Skin Disorders. Philadelphia: WB Saunders, 1994.

Spitz, J. Genodermatoses: A Full-color Clinical Guide to Genetic Skin Disorders. Baltimore: Williams & Wilkins, 1995.

Williams ML, Elias PM. Genetically transmitted generalized disorders of cornification. Dermatol Clin 1987;5:155–178.

From: *Principles of Molecular Medicine* (J. L. Jameson, ed.), ©1998 Humana Press Inc., Totowa, NJ.

Table 72-1
Gene Mutations and Genodermatoses

Disease	*Chromosomal location*	*Gene*	*Protein*
Blistering disorders			
Epidermal			
Epidermolysis	12q13	KRT5	Keratin 5
Bullosa simplex	17q21	KRT14	Keratin 14
EB simplex with mottled pigmentation	12q13	KRT5	Keratin 5
Junctional			
EB with muscular dystrophy	8q24	PLECI	Plectin
Herlitz type	18q11.2	LAMA3	laminin 5, $\alpha 3$ chain
	1q32	LAMA3	laminin 5, $\beta 3$ chain
	1q25–31	LAMC2	laminin 5, $\gamma 2$ chain
Generalized atrophic	10q24.3	COLI7A1/BPAG2	Bullous pemphigoid
Benign EB			anitgen 2 (BPAG2)
	1q32	LAMB3	laminin 5, $\beta 3$ chain
Junctional EB with pyloric atresia	17q11-qter	ITGB4	$\beta 4$ integrin
Dystrophic			
Recessive, dominant			
Dystrophic EB's	3p21	COL7A1	Type VII Collagen
Disorders of cornification			
Epidermolytic	12q13	KRT1	Keratin 1
Hyperkeratosis	17q21	KRT10	Keratin10
Ichthyosis bullosa of Siemens	12q13	KRT2e	Keratin 2e
Lamellar ichthyosis	14q11	TGM1	Transglutaminase 1
Sjogren-Larsson	17p11.2	FAD	Fatty aldehyde dehyrogenase
Vorner's palmoplantar			
Keratoderma	17q21	KRT9	Keratin 9
Vohwinkel's syndrome	1q21	LOR	Loricrin
Other ectodermal disorders			
Pachyonychia congenita			
PC1 without cysts	12q13	KRT6a	Keratin 6a/16
	17q21	KRT16	
PC2 with Steatocystoma multiplex	17q21	KRT17	Keratin 17
White sponge nevus	12q13/17q21	KRT4/KRT13	Keratin4/13
Dyshidrotic ectodermal dysplasia	Xq12–13.1	EDA gene	EDA protein
Disorders of dermis			
Ehlers-Danlos syndrome			
Type II	9q34.2–.3	COL5A1	Type V Collegen ($\alpha 1$)
	2q31	COL5A2	Type V Collagen ($\alpha 2$)
Type IV	2q31	COL3A1	Type III Collagen ($\alpha 1$)
Type VI	1p36.2–36.3	LOH	Lysyl hydroxylase
Type VIIA	17q21–22	COL1A1	Type I Collagen ($\alpha 1$)
Type VIIB	7q21-22	COL1A2	Type 1 Collagen ($\alpha 2$)
Osteogenesis imperfecta	17q21–22	COL1A1	Type I Collagen ($\alpha 1$)
	7q21–22	COL1A2	Type 1 Collagen ($\alpha 2$)
Marfan syndrome			
MFS 1	15q21.1	FBN1	Fibrillin
Cutis laxa			
X-linked	Xq13.3	MNK	Mc-1 copper transporting ATPase
Autosomal dominant	7q11.2	ELN	Elastin
Multiple tumor syndromes			
Neurofibromatosis 1	17q	NF1	Neurofibromin
Neurofibromatosis 2	22q12.2	NF2	Schwannomin
Tuberous sclerosis			
TSC I	9q34.1	TSC1	Unknown
TSC II	16q13	TSC2	Tuberin
Basal Cell nevus syndrome	9q22.3	PTC	Patched gene product Sonic Hedgehog ligand(?)
Photosensitivity disorders			
Bloom's syndrome	15q26.1	BLM	RecQ helicase
Xeroderma pigmentosum			
XP-A	9q34.1	XPA	DNA binding protein for repair and transcription
XP-B	2q21	ERCC3/XPB	DNA helicase (unwinding to initiate repair)
XP-D	19q13.2–.3	ERCC2/XPD	DNA helicase (unwinding to initiate repair)

Table 72-1 *(continued)*

Disease	*Chromosomal location*	*Gene*	*Protein*
XP-C	3p25	XPC	DNA excision repair
XP-F	16p13.1–.2	ERCC4/XPF	DNA excision repair
XP-G	13q33	ERCC5/XPG	DNA excision repair
Cockayne Syndrome			
CSB	10q11	ERCC6	DNA excision repair (?)
CSA	5	CKN1	
Oculocutaneous albinism			
Type 1A, B, C	11q	TYR	Tyrosinase
Type II (Angelman, Prader Willi)	15q11–13	P	?, tyrosine transport (?)
Type IV	9q	TRP-1	Tyrosine-related protein
Type V	?	?	unknown
Type VIA (Hermansky-Pudlak)	10?	?	unknown
Type VIA (Chediak-Higashi)	1q43	LYST	Cell fusion protein?
Porphyrias			
Congenital erythropoietic	10q25.3–26.3	UROS	Urophorphyrinogen Synthase
Erythropoietic protoporphyria	18q21.3	FC	Ferrochetalase
Hepatoerythropoietic porphyria	1p34	UROD	Uroporphyrin oxygen decarboxylase
Porphyria Cutanea Tarda	1p34	UROD	Uroporphyrin oxygen decarboxylase
Coproporphyria	3q12	CPO	Coproporphyrinogen oxidase
Variegate porphyria	1q22	PPO	Protoporphyrin Oxidase
Selected immunodeficiency disorders			
Ataxia-telangiectasia	11q23	ATM	Cell cycle checkpoint control
Wiskott-Aldrich syndrome	Xp11.22–23	WASP	Regulates T-Cell cytoskeleton function
X-linked agammaglobulinemia	Xq21.2–22	BTK	Bruton Tyrosine kinase (B-cell development)
Chronic granulomatous disorder			
X-linked	Xp21.1	CYBB	NADPH oxidase systern, gp91 cytochrome-*b*, heavy chain
Recessive	16q24	CYBA	Cytochrome-*b*, p22phos (light chain)
	7q11.23	NCF1	47-kDa cytosolic factor
	1q25	NCF2	67-kDa cytosolic factor
Hyper-IgM syndrome	Xq26	CD40LG	Ligand for CD40, T cell mediates B-cell activation
Miscellaneous			
Menke's syndrome	Xq13.3	MCI	Mc-1copper transporter ATPase
Beare-Stevenson cutis gyrata	10q26	FGFR2	Fibroblast growth factor receptor 2
William's Syndrome	7q11.1	EL	Elastin
Werner's syndrome (progeria)	8p11.1–21.1	WRN	DNA helicase
Prolidase deficiency	19cen q13.11	PEPD	Prolidase
Homocystinuria	21q22.3	CBS	Cystathione β-synthase

Table 72-2
Genodermatoses That Predispose to Cancer

Disease	*Associated cancers*
Neurofibromatosis (*see* Chapter 106)	
NF-1	Glioma, astrocytoma, Schwannoma, sarcomas, Leukemia, retinoblastoma
NF-2	Acoustic neuromas, meningioma, glioma
Gardner's syndrome Peutz-Jeugers	Colon carcinoma
Cowden's syndrome	Breast, thyroid, uterine carcinoma and adenoma
Oculocutaneous Albinism and related disorders (*see* Chapter 79)	Melanoma, squamous, and basal cell carcinoma
Xeroderma pigmentosa and related disorders (*see* Chapter 81)	Melanoma, squamous, and basal cell carcinoma
Basal cell nevus syndrome (*see* Chapter 84)	Basal cell carcinoma
Basex syndrome	Basal cell carcinoma
Familial Melanoma/multiple mole syndrome (*see* Chapter 85)	Melanoma, pancreatic carcinoma?

73 Epidermolysis Bullosa Simplex

YIU-MO CHAN AND ELAINE FUCHS

BACKGROUND

The term "epidermolysis bullosa" (EB) was first introduced by Koebner in the late 19th century to describe a nonscarring, blistering skin disease. The name was subsequently adopted for a group of heterogenous congenital disorders that are all characterized by trauma-induced blistering of skin. The blisters may be formed intraepidermally, junctionally, or intradermally. When the blisters are formed within the basal epidermal layer of the skin, it is given the name "simplex." Today, epidermolysis bullosa simplex (EBS) constitutes a group of autosomal-dominant genetic skin diseases affecting 1 in 40,000 in the population. It is further divided into different subtypes according to the clinical severity. The penetrance in families with EBS is high, and in its most severe form, the disorder is apparent at birth.

We begin this chapter by describing the clinical and ultrastructural features of EBS and the common criteria for diagnosis. We then present the lines of evidence that led to the discovery that EBS is frequently, if not always, a result of a mutation in either of two keratin genes whose products form an extensive cytoskeletal array of 10-nm filaments in basal epidermal cells. After exploring the structural implications for the mutant keratins and their effects on keratin-filament assembly, we discuss the functional significance of the keratin network in the epidermis. Finally, we consider the impact on management and treatment of the disease.

CLINICAL FEATURES AND DIAGNOSIS

There are three major types of EBS: Dowling-Meara (D-M), Koebner (K), and Weber-Cockayne (W-C) (Table 73-1). D-M EBS is the most severe form in which blistering occurs over the entire body (Fig. 73-1). The nails may be lost, but usually regrow without dystrophy. K-EBS is intermediate in severity. Although blistering still remains generalized, it is considerably less severe and less painful. Like D-M EBS, the nails may shed and regrow without dystrophy. W-C EBS is the least severe form in which blistering is very mild and restricted mostly to the hands and feet. Unlike the other two generalized forms of EBS, symptoms in W-C EBS can be so mild that in some patients, it is not manifested until adult life, where it is detected as a result of unusually stressful exercise. Other, less-common subtypes of EBS, which are often associated with extra features such as mottled pigmentation or serous blistering and bruising, have also been reported. In all cases, blistering in EBS arises from mild mechanical trauma. In a number of cases, high temperatures seem to exacerbate the symptoms. Since blister cleavage is within the epidermis, the patient generally heals without scarring. Although blistering in some EBS cases can be very severe, the disease is rarely a threat to life. The primary complication of the disease appears to be secondary infection because of localized loss of the skin-barrier function. Ultrastructural studies show that the physical stress-induced intraepidermal blistering is caused by cytolysis within the basal layer of epidermis. Except in the most severe cases of D-M EBS, the suprabasal layers typically appear normal. In addition, as revealed by both light and electron microscopy, the basal cells from the more severe cases of EBS show marked abnormalities in basal keratin filaments (Fig. 73-2). In the basal layer of D-M EBS skin, there are usually clumps of amorphous keratin or large aggregates of keratin filaments. In contrast, the perturbations in keratin-filament networks of W-C EBS can sometimes be very small, and indeed are often barely detectable. All other cell organelles seem to be normal and intact, although aberrations in the organization of mitochondria and/or irregularities in nuclear shape have been noted.

For a proper diagnosis of EBS, a skin biopsy is necessary. Ultrastructural analysis of the skin biopsy allows the correct determination of the cleavage site in the skin, thereby differentiating EBS from other types of EB. It also allows further distinction of other blistering skin disorders, such as epidermolytic hyperkeratosis (EH), which is similar to EBS in pathology, but which affects the suprabasal layers rather than the basal layer of the epidermis.

GENETIC BASIS OF EBS

For many years, the genetic basis of EBS remained elusive, although it had long been recognized as an autosomal-dominant Mendelian trait. Despite the ultrastructural data suggesting that keratin-filament disorganization preceded cytolysis, it was often postulated that EBS might be a disease of cytolytic enzymes or that it involved transcriptional or translational alterations in keratins. Our increased knowledge about the basal epidermal keratins, K5 and K14, led to the postulate that most cases of a human genetic disease involving K5 or K14 mutations would be autosomal dominant, since most of the keratin mutations behaved in a dominant-negative fashion when introduced into cultured basal epidermal cells or when assembled with its wild-type partner in vitro. Then, when Vassar et al. introduced a mutant K14 gene into the germline of transgenic mice and discovered that the mice developed phenotypic characteristics of D-M EBS, it became clear that EBS could be generated by a mutation in one of the two basal-keratin genes. This finding explained why cultured D-M EBS

From: *Principles of Molecular Medicine* (J. L. Jameson, ed.), ©1998 Humana Press Inc., Totowa, NJ.

Table 73-1
Characteristics of the Three Major Types of Epidermolysis Bullosa Simplex

	Dowling-Meara	*Koeber*	*Weber-Cockayne*
Inheritance	Autosomal-dominant	Autosomal-dominant	Autosomal-dominant
Blistering	Body	Body	Hands/feet
Basal cell cytolysis	+	+	+
Keratin filament disorganization	+	+	+/–
Keratin clumps in basal cells	+	–	–
Abnormalities in suprabasal cells	None	None	None

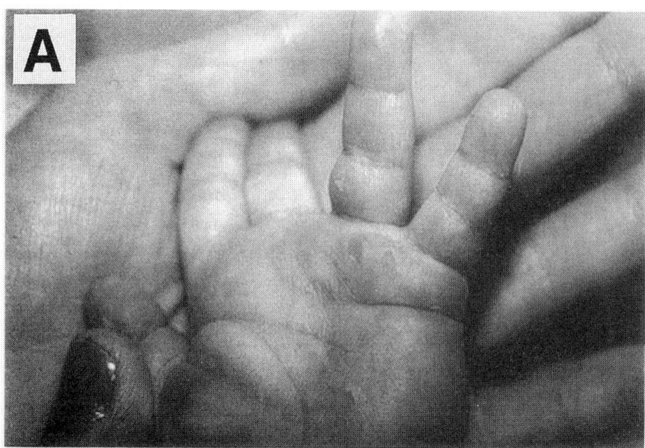

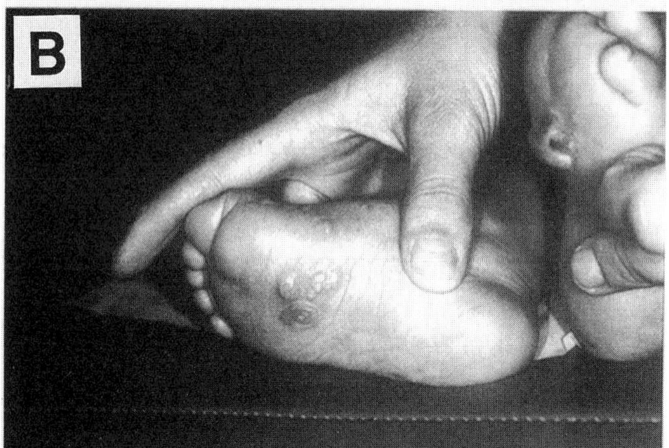

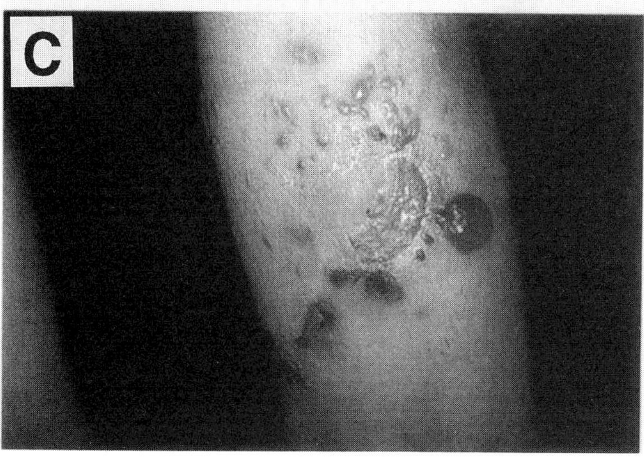

keratinocytes resembled those of normal keratinocytes transfected with a mutant K14 keratin gene.

Subsequent analyses of K5 and K14 genes of EBS patients led to the discovery of keratin mutations in all three major subtypes. Functional studies suggest that these mutations are responsible for the disorders. Additionally, whereas earlier linkage studies erroneously mapped the EBS disease to chromosome 1, more recent studies with higher lod scores map the disorder to either chromosome 12q11-q13 or 17q12-q21, the two locations where keratin K5 and K14 reside, respectively. Taken together, these lines of evidence demonstrate unequivocally that EBS can be caused by defects in the basal-specific keratin genes. Today, most EBS cases examined thus far have been found to carry point mutations in the coding region of either one of the two basal keratin genes. However, it is still possible that in some cases of EBS, the genetic defect may reside outside the K5 or K14 genes. This said, there is no convincing evidence at this time that demonstrates heterogeneity in the basic EBS disease. It has recently been shown that EBS with muscular dystrophy is a rare genetic disorder involving mutations in plectin, a keratin filament-associated protein.

Because of the relatively small size of the basal-keratin genes and their transcripts (1.8–2.1 kbp), screening for keratin mutations in EBS patients has still been conducted largely by DNA sequencing. This is particularly so when a skin biopsy is available, allowing keratinocyte culture and mRNA extraction. In one case, an antibody was used in diagnosis and analysis, and the generation of a battery of antibodies to critical regions of the keratin polypeptides may facilitate diagnoses in the future. In addition, with the introduction of methods such as conformation-sensitive gel electrophoresis (CSGE), which allow for rapid detection of single-base changes in DNA, screening for mutations in keratin genes may now become more straightforward. This method is extremely useful when a large number of patient samples are involved. It also eliminates the need to sequence the entire gene or transcript.

MOLECULAR PATHOPHYSIOLOGY OF DISEASE

The location of keratin mutations and their clinical relation is summarized in Fig. 73-3. A surprising finding emerging from the catalog of keratin mutations in different EBS subtypes is that mutations tend to be clustered, and sometimes the exact same residue is mutated in unrelated families with these diseases.

Figure 73-1 *(opposite)* Clinical pictures of EBS patients. **(A,B)** Patient with mild skin blistering on his hands and feet, typical of the mildest form of EBS, Weber-Cockayne. **(C)** Severe skin blistering of a patient who has the severe form of EBS, Dowling-Meara. (Courtesy of Amy S. Paller, Children's Hospital, Northwestern Medical School.) (*See* color insert following p. 684.)

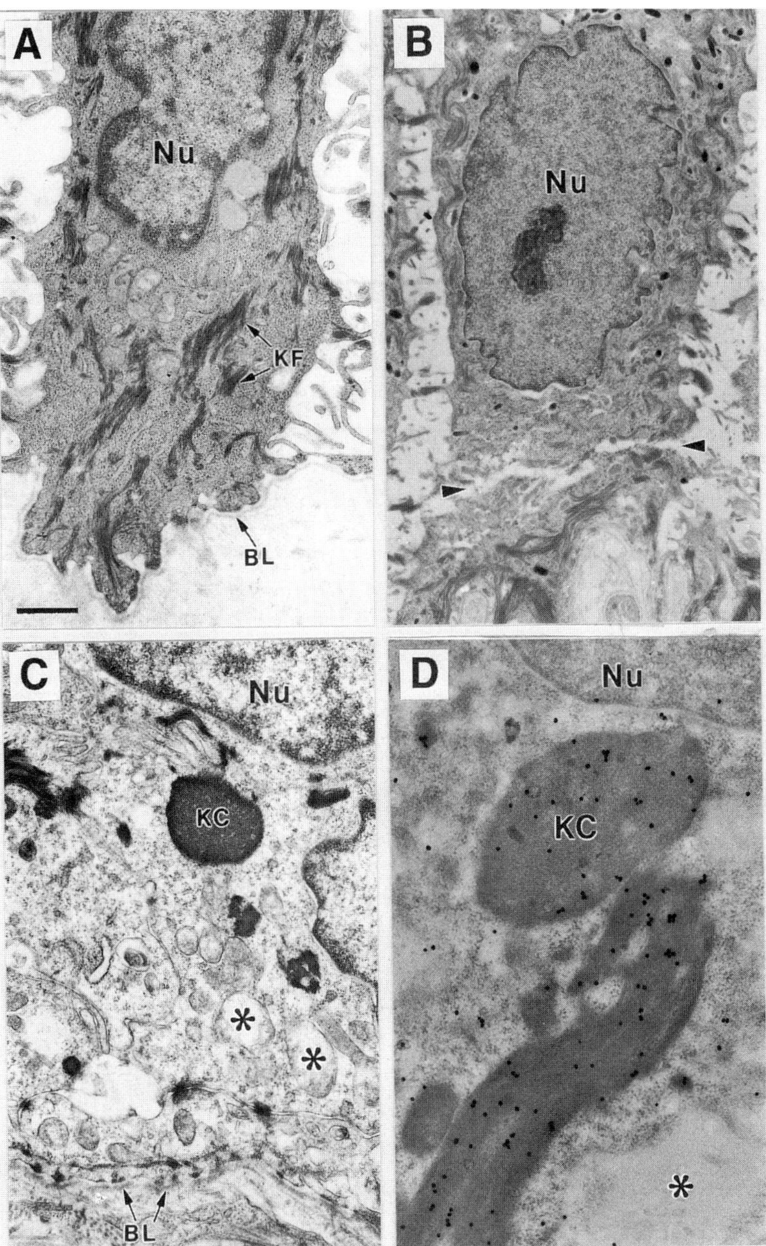

Figure 73-2 Ultrastructure of epidermis from EBS patients showing abnormalities in keratin architecture. Punch biopsies from control and EBS skins of patient volunteers were fixed and processed for conventional or immunoelectron microscopy. Shown are representative examples of epidermal cells from the basal layer of: **(A)** control skin; **(B)** patient with Weber-Cockayne EBS; **(C,D)** patient with Dowling-Meara EBS. (D) Immunogold antikeratin 14 labeling of keratin clumps and filament aggregates, typical of D-M EBS. Abbreviations: Nu, nucleus; KF, keratin filaments; BL, basal lamina; KC, keratin clump. Arrowhead in B denotes intraepidermal split beneath the nucleus, a typical feature of W-C EBS. Asterisks in C and D denote cytolysis, typical of D-M EBS basal cells. (A) Bar = 1 μm. (B) Bar = 2 μm. (C) Bar = 0.7 μm. (D) Bar = 4 μm. (Courtesy of Qian-Chun Yu, The University of Chicago.)

Approximately 60% of all sequenced D-M EBS mutations are Arg to His/Cys substitutions at codon 125 of the K14 gene. In addition, there is a strong correlation between the location of mutation within the keratin polypeptide and disease severity of EBS. Thus, whereas many of the D-M EBS keratin mutations reside in the amino (1A) or carboxy (2B) ends of the central coiled-coil rod domain of the polypeptides, Koebner mutations tend to be more centrally located within the rod segment, and W-C mutations often reside either in a nonhelical linker (L12) segment within the rod, or in the head domain of K5. In order to appreciate the significance of these findings, it is first necessary to review what is known about the overall structure of keratin filaments.

Keratins belong to the superfamily of 10-nm intermediate filaments (IFs), which, along with 6-nm actin microfilaments and 20-nm microtubules, constitute the basic features of the higher eukaryotic cytoskeleton. Keratins are encoded by multiple genes that are differentially expressed in nearly all epithelial tissues. They can be subdivided into two distinct groups, type I and type II, based on their protein sequence. Keratins assemble into obligatory heterodimers of the two subtypes. The mechanism for

K5 Mutation

No.	Subtype	Mutation	Domain
1.	M-P EBS	P23L	nonhelical head
2.	W-C EBS	I161S	nonhelical head
2.	W-C EBS	I161N	nonhelical head
3.	K-EBS	K173N	nonhelical head
4.	D-M EBS	L175F	1A conserved rod end
5.	D-M EBS	F179S	1A conserved rod end
6.	D-M EBS	Δ30deletion	1A conserved rod end
7.	W-C EBS	N193K	1A helical rod
8.	W-C EBS	M327T	L1-2 nonhelical linker
9.	W-C EBS	D328V	L1-2 nonhelical linker
10.	W-C EBS	N329K	L1-2 nonhelical linker
11.	W-C EBS	R331C	L1-2 nonhelical linker
12.	K-EBS	L463P	2B helical rod
13.	D-M EBS	I467T	2B conserved rod end
14.	D-M EBS	E475G	2B conserved rod end
15.	D-M EBS	E477K	2B conserved rod end

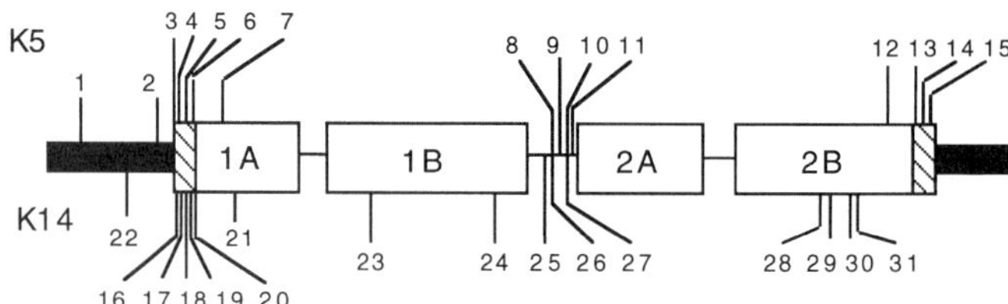

K14 Mutation

No.	Subtype	Mutation	Domain
16.	D-M EBS	M119I	1A conserved rod end
17.	D-M EBS	Q120R	1A conserved rod end
18.	D-M EBS	L122F	1A conserved rod end
19.	D-M EBS	R125C	1A conserved rod end
19.	D-M EBS	R125H	1A conserved rod end
19.	D-M EBS	R125S	1A conserved rod end
20.	D-M EBS	Y129D	1A conserved rod end
21.	EBS-rec	E144A	1A helical rod
22.	K-EBS	G107stop	nonhelical head
23.	K-EBS	Y204stop	1B helical rod
24.	K-EBS	A247D	1B helical rod
25.	W-C EBS	V270M	L1-2 nonhelical linker
26.	K-EBS	M272R	L1-2 nonhelical linker
27.	W-C EBS	A274D	L1-2 nonhelical linker
28.	K-EBS	ΔE375	2B helical rod
29.	K-EBS	I377N	2B helical rod
30.	K-EBS	L384P	2B helical rod
31.	K-EBS	R388C	2B helical rod

Figure 73-3 Summary of mutations found in patients with EBS and correlation between the location of mutation within the keratin polypeptide and disease severity of EBS. Stick figure depicts secondary structure of human keratins. Large boxes encompass the central α-helical rod domain. Hatched boxes denote the highly conserved end domains of the rod. Lines denote the nonhelical linker segments. Solid bars denote the nonhelical head and tail domains, often conserved only for a single IF type. Note D-M EBS mutations are all clustered within the highly conserved ends, whereas K-EBS mutations are more internal. In contrast, W-C EBS mutations are mostly found in the nonhelical region of keratin. Patients with EBS and Mottled Pigmentation (EBS-MP) have a mutation near the N-terminus of K5. EBS-rec is a rare recessive case.

dimerization is based on the ability of keratins to form a coiled-coil. Based on secondary-structure predictions, each keratin has a conserved central-rod domain of about 310 amino acids, which is largely α-helical. The rod domain contains a repeating heptad motif $(a\text{-}b\text{-}c\text{-}d\text{-}e\text{-}f\text{-}g)_n$ in which the a and d residues are often hydrophobic. This heptad repeat presents a hydrophobic seal on the helical surface, enabling two IF molecules, aligned in parallel, to intertwine in a coiled-coil fashion.

The α-helical rod domain can be further subdivided into four smaller regions (helix 1A, 1B, 2A, 2B), which are separated by three short stretches (approximately 12–20 residues) of nonhelical linker regions (L1, L1–2, L2) that interrupt both the heptad repeat and the helix continuity. The rod is also flanked by nonhelical head (amino-end) and tail (carboxyl-end) domains that vary in size and amino acid composition. The structure of these head and tail domains still remains unknown, although these domains are likely to protrude along the filament surface. Keratins can assemble into 10-nm filaments in vitro without auxiliary factors, indicating that this information is contained within the primary sequence of the IF polypeptide. Chemical crosslinking studies have suggested that, in the filament, linear arrays of parallel keratin heterodimers are linked in a head-to-tail fashion, with a slight overlap in their rod ends. These studies also indicate that the chains of keratin dimers are arranged antiparallelly and half-staggered relative to each other. Scanning-transmission electron microscopy studies have indicated that the width of a keratin IF can accommodate 32 keratin polypeptides, or 16 linear arrays. Structural studies on other IFs have provided similar findings. So far, most of the known EBS mutations have been found in regions that by deletion or point-mutation analyses, had already been shown to be important for IF structure and 10-nm filament assembly. Most of the known K14 and K5 point mutations of D-M EBS and K-EBS reside in the α-helical rod domains involved in coiled-coil heterodimerization (Fig. 73-3). Most of the D-M EBS mutations are clustered within the α-helical rod ends, which, in addition to being highly evolutionarily conserved, are also important for filament elongation in vivo and in vitro. Further verification that D-M EBS mutations tend to affect filament elongation stems from the engineering and testing of the precise D-M EBS mutations found in patients. This notion is particularly underscored by the recombinant DNA testing of a Y129D mutation found in a patient with an unusually severe case of D-M EBS. It is worth noting that chemically induced crosslinks have been detected between the beginning of helix 1A and the end of helix 2B, lending strong biochemical support to the notion that these segments play a critical role in the filament-elongation process. According to alignment models arising from cross-linking studies, a 1.6-nm (10–11 residue) overlap is predicted between the conserved rod ends of two head-to-tail oriented dimers. This is in good agreement with the fact that most of the D-M EBS mutations reside within the first or second heptads of helix 1A. Such associations may involve ionic associations, given that the beginning of helix 1A and the end of helix 2B are highly basic and acidic, respectively. This slight overlap between rod ends also explains why, in rotary shadowed IFs, the axial pitch is only 21–22 nm, rather than an exact half (23 nm) of the rod length. Thus, a knowledge of the severe EBS mutations has led to further experimentation and refinement of 10-nm filament structure. In contrast to the D-M EBS mutations, most of the K-EBS mutations are more internal, although still within the α-helical segments. It is interesting that Koebner mutations sometimes involve substitutions to proline residues, since it had already been shown by gene transfection and filament assembly studies that proline substitutions more centrally in the rod domain are less deleterious to those at the rod ends. On the other hand, most of the W-C EBS mutations are localized in the nonhelical domains, such as the nonhelical head of K5 and in particular, the L1-2 linker region of K5 and K14.

The majority of the L1-2 mutations reside within the carboxy end of the linker. Interestingly, in a model of linear arrays of dimers, where the helix 1A ends of one dimer have been postulated to overlap with the helix 2B ends of the next dimer in line, the carboxy ends of the L1-2 linker segments within one chain of dimers might be nearly opposite to the end-overlap segments within an adjacent row of dimers. If this model is correct, then this portion of the L1-2 linker is in a position to play a role in promoting appropriate staggered lateral associations between the linear arrays of alternating dimer chains. This segment could also participate in further stabilizing the end-overlap interaction (Fig. 73-4). The fact that mutations in the carboxyl end of the linker L1-2 region cause unraveling of filaments assembled in vitro is in agreement with this notion.

Taken together, it appears that keratin mutations giving rise to greater clinical severity cause perturbations in filament elongation, whereas mutations causing milder phenotypes often affect lateral associations within the filament (Fig. 73-5). Whereas the future may yet provide us with additional and important refinements to this trend, a knowledge of keratin structure has given us a better understanding of how the genetic defects give rise to the clinical manifestations of the disease.

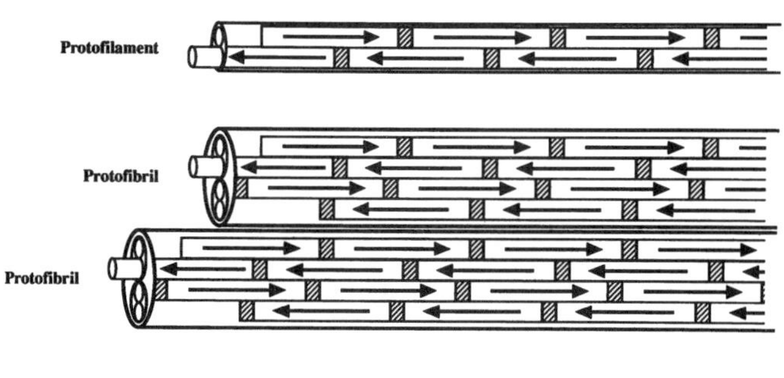

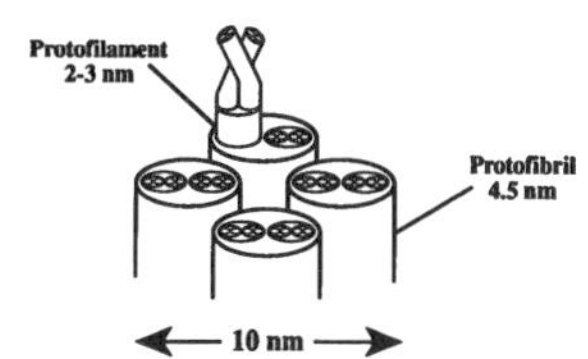

Figure 73-4 Putative alignments of subunits in IF. Box denotes rod segments of the dimer; arrows indicate orientation of polypeptides, from base (N-terminus) to tip (C-terminus). Hatched boxes denote regions of putative rod overlap between the conserved rod ends of helix 1A and 2B. In the model, near, half-staggered antiparallel dimers occur at the level of protofilament, whereas unstaggered antiparallel alignments of dimers occur at the level of interprotofibril associations.

FUNCTION OF KERATIN NETWORK

It is now known that, in mice and humans, dominant-negative keratin mutations lead to cell fragility; it therefore seems likely that keratins function by imparting mechanical integrity to cells. This said, based on dominant-negative, i.e., autosomal-dominant, mutations, it is also possible that keratin aggregates alter the cellular physiology in a gain-of-function, rather than a loss-of-function manner. This notion was ruled out by: (1) two independent discoveries of EBS patients who have rare, homozygous premature stop codon mutations in their K14 alleles; and (2) a K14 null mutant mouse, generated by gene targeting. In all cases, the basal-epidermal-keratin network is largely missing, presumably since in the absence of its partner keratin, K5 is unstable and is rapidly turned over in the keratinocytes. These data lend strong support to the hypothesis that the major function of the basal keratins is to confer physical resilience to basal cells. Additionally, these knockouts revealed the presence of a residual network of keratin filaments that had a wispy appearance, which was quite distinct from the normal K14–K5 keratin network. Further exploration uncovered the presence of a second type I keratin, K15 in basal cells. Might some EBS cases have defects in K15? Although possible, it seems unlikely based on the fact that K15 has a different distribution than K14, being more highly expressed in internal stratified-squamous epithelia than in skin. K15 knockout studies may help to resolve this new issue.

Now that we know that the function of the keratin network is to provide mechanical stability to epidermal cells, it is understandable that keratin mutations that are more disruptive on IF structure have a greater effect on the mechanical stability of the cells. Thus, whereas D-M EBS mutations cause severe cytolysis in response to mild physical trauma, W-C EBS mutations result in mild cytolysis in response to more severe mechanical stress. Since blisters in EBS are trauma-induced, only areas of the body that are constantly

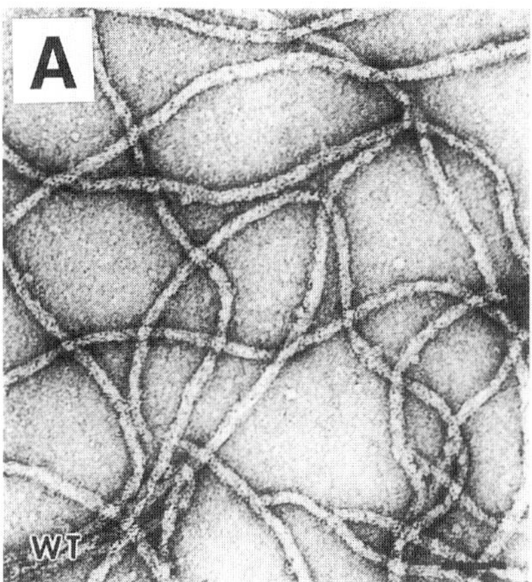

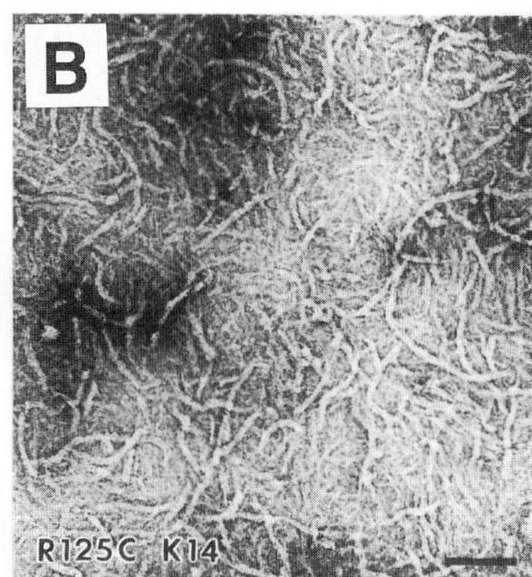

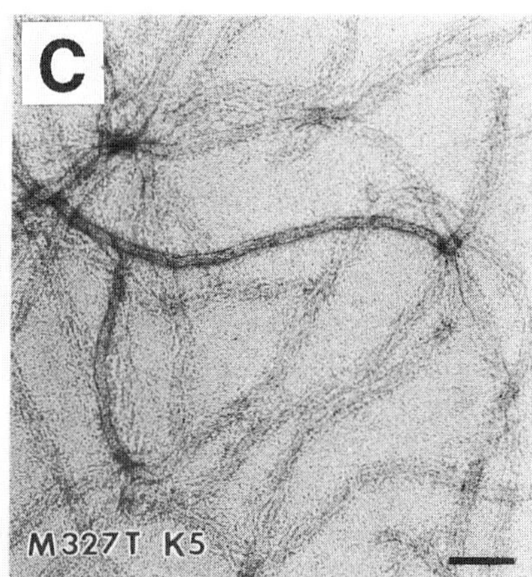

Figure 73-5 In vitro filament assembly studies of D-M EBS and W-C EBS mutants. Human K5 and K14 were expressed in bacteria, purified by FPLC, and assembled into filaments in vitro. (**A**) Filaments formed from normal K5 and K14. (**B**) Filaments formed from normal K5 and D-M EBS mutant (K14 R125C) giving rise to severely disrupted filaments. (**C**) Filament formed from normal K14 and W-C EBS mutant (K5 M327T) showing minor perturbation on IF structure, mostly unraveling of the filaments. Bar = 100 nm.

under mechanical stress, mostly the hands and feet, are subjected to blister formation in W-C EBS.

DIAGNOSIS, MANAGEMENT, AND TREATMENT

Diagnosis of EBS by ultrastructural analysis has long been a reliable method used by many physicians. In a few instances, this method has also been used for prenatal diagnosis. Understanding the genetic basis of EBS now allows for the possibility of prenatal genetic counseling for EBS, which can be done at an earlier stage in pregnancy and involves less risk to the fetus than skin biopsies.

Although the genetic basis of EBS has been elucidated, there is still no effective treatment available. The most useful treatment for EBS patients remains extensive counseling and prevention. Some patients find it useful to stay in a cool environment, as high temperature seems to worsen the condition. Since EBS has its onset at birth or early infancy and is largely trauma-induced, it is crucial for patients to learn to take good care of their health at an early age, such as avoiding activities that cause trauma. In addition, the tendency for blistering may diminish significantly over time to the point that blisters may be absent for months at a time, suggesting the disease may regress over time. Although the underlying reason for this age-dependent phenomenon remains unknown, it could be that the epidermis is naturally under less mechanical tension as it develops fully and as patients approach their adult size.

Another potential treatment is gene therapy, which is currently under extensive investigation in a number of recessive genetic disorders, such as cystic fibrosis and muscular dystrophy. Modern technology now makes it possible to introduce a missing healthy gene into the appropriate cells of the patient. The fact that EBS is inherited in an autosomal-dominant fashion makes gene therapy much more difficult, since expression of the mutant allele must be silenced. At present, the only obvious method to do this is to remove the patient's defective allele by homologous recombination technology. Whereas this should be feasible in basal keratinocytes cultured from a biopsy of the patient's skin, the frequency of homologous recombination is extremely low. Thus, even though mechanisms are already in place for grafting cultured keratinocytes back onto the patient's skin, engineering out the bad gene is likely to be very inefficient. This said, since the keratin defect is expressed in the layer of epidermis where cells can move laterally, and because the healthy keratinocyte should have a tremendous selective advantage over a cytolysing one, it is possible that a small graft of healthy keratinocytes could expand to a larger region when grafted in an area of EBS skin. If technological advances continue to be made, as they certainly have in the past, there may be hope for this type of treatment in the future.

ADDITIONAL DISORDERS OF KERATIN AND OTHER INTERMEDIATE-FILAMENT DISEASES

EBS was the first disorder of keratin to be discovered. This knowledge set the paradigm for an intermediate-filament disease. A severe filament-disrupting defect in an IF gene would be predicted to cause mechanical stress-induced degeneration in the cells in which the gene is expressed, and, ultrastructurally, there should be aggregates or clumps of IFs in these cells. It is relevant that there are more than 60 different IF genes in the human genome. These genes are differentially expressed, and at least one IF gene is expressed in nearly all cells at nearly all stages of differentiation and development. Therefore, from the time when transgenic mouse studies predicted that EBS would be a keratin disorder, it seemed likely that there are additional disorders of IF genes.

Indeed, the field has moved rapidly since the discovery of EBS. Once the paradigm was set, other potential disorders of keratin were immediately and correctly predicted. Based on the known pattern of keratin expression, and the abnormalities in the keratin networks within cells that also undergo degeneration, it was quickly determined that the following diseases are disorders of particular keratins: (1) epidermolytic hyperkeratosis (EH), a disorder of keratins K1 and K10, that results in keratin clumping and generalized cytolysis in the suprabasal layers of the epidermis; (2) a milder form of EH caused by defects in K2, a keratin expressed in the upper living layers of the epidermis; (3) epidermolytic palmar plantar keratoderma (EPPK), arising from defects in K9, a keratin that is expressed only in the suprabasal layers of palmar and plantar skin; (4) pachyonychia congenita (PC), a hair and nail degenerative disorder involving mutations in K6, K16, and K17, known to be expressed in these cells; (5) white sponge nevus, an esophageal degenerative disorder of K4 and K13, known to be expressed in the esophagus; (6) Meesman's corneal dystrophy, a corneal disorder of keratins K3 and K12; and (7) moni lethrix, a hair keratin disorder. Finally, it has recently been shown that some patients with amyotrophic lateral sclerosis (ALS), a degenerative disorder of the motor neurons, not only have abnormalities in neurofilament networks, but in addition, have point mutations in neurofilament genes. Although functional and chromosomal linkage analysis have yet to link ALS to neurofilament gene defects, it seems possible that some cases of this heterogeneous disease will have as their underlying basis neurofilament gene mutations. Another candidate disorder of IFs includes those forms of cardiomyopathies that are typified by not only cell degeneration, but also aberrations in their desmin IF networks. In the future, as more studies are conducted on degenerative cytoskeletal disorders and on the functions of intermediate filaments and their associated proteins, the list of human genetic diseases whose pathology is based on defects in IF networks will continue to grow.

ACKNOWLEDGMENTS

We would like to extend special thanks to members of the Fuchs laboratory, who over the years have contributed to many of the different findings regarding K5 and K14 and their relation to Epidermolysis Bullosa Simplex. We thank Qian Chun Yu and Amy S. Paller for some of the electron microscopy and clinical photographs used in this review.

SELECTED REFERENCES

Albers K, Fuchs E. The expression of mutant epidermal keratin cDNAs transfected in simple epithelial and squamous cell carcinoma lines. J Cell Biol 1987;105:791–806.

Albers K, Fuchs E. Expression of mutant keratin cDNAs in epithelial cells reveals possible mechanisms for initiation and assembly of intermediate filaments. J Cell Biol 1989;108:1477–1493.

Anton-Lamprecht I. Ultrastructural identification of basic abnormalities as clues to genetic disorders of the epidermis. J Invest Dermatol 1994;103:65–125.

Anton-Lamprecht I, Schnyder UW. Epidermolysis bullosa herpetiformis Dowling-Meara: report of a case and pathogenesis. Dermatologica 1982;164:221–235.

Bonifas JM, Rothman AL, Epstein EH. Epidermolysis bullosa simplex: evidence in two families for keratin gene abnormalities. Science 1991;254:1202–1205.

Bowden PE, Haley JL, Kansky A, Rothnagel JA, Jones DO, Turner RJ. Mutation of a type II keratin gene (K6a) in pachyonychia congenita. Nat Genet 1995;10:363–365.

Chan YM, Yu QC, Fine JD, Fuchs E. The genetic basis of Webercockayne epidermolysis bullosa simplex. Proc Natl Acad Sci USA 1993;90: 7414–7418.

Chan YM, Yu QC, Christiano A, et al. Mutations in the non-helical linker segment L1-2 of keratin 5 in patients with Weber-Cockayne Epidermolysis Bullosa Simplex. J Cell Sci 1994;107:765–774.

Chan YM, Anton-Lamprecht I, Yu QC, et al. A human keratin 14 "knockout": the absence of K14 leads to severe epidermolysis bullosa simplex and a function for an intermediate filament protein. Genes Devel 1994;8:2574–2587.

Chan YM, Cheng J, Gedde-Dahl T, Niemi KM, Fuchs E. Genetic analysis of a severe case of dowling-meara epidermolysis bullosa simplex. J Invest Dermatol 1996;106:327–334.

Chen H, Bonifas JM, Matsumura K, Ikeda S, Leyden WA, Epstein EH Jr. Keratin 14 gene mutations in patients with epidermolysis bullosa simplex. J Invest Dermatol 1995;105:629–632.

Cheng J, Syder AJ, Yu QC, Letai A, Paller AS, Fuchs E. The genetic basis of epidermolytic hyperkeratosis: a disorder of differentiation-specific epidermal keratin genes. Cell 1992;70:811–819.

Chipev CC, Korge BP, Markova N, et al. A leucine->proline mutation in the H1 subdomain of keratin 1 causes epidermolytic hyperkeratosis. Cell 1992;70:821–828.

Coulombe PA, Hutton ME, Letai A, Hebert A, Paller AS, Fuchs E. Point mutations in human keratin 14 genes of epidermolysis bullosa simplex patients: genetic and functional analyses. Cell 1991;166:1301–1311.

Coulombe P, Fuchs E. Elucidating the early stages of keratin filament assembly. J Cell Biol 1990;111:153–169.

Coulombe P, Chan YM, Albers K, Fuchs E. Deletions in epidermal keratins leading to alterations in filament organization in vivo and in intermediate filament assembly in vitro. J Cell Biol 1990;111: 3049–3064.

Dong W, Ryynanen M, Uitto J. Identification of a leucine to proline mutation in the keratin 5 gene in a family with the generalized Koebner type of epidermolysis bullosa simplex. Hum Mutat 1993;2:94–102.

Engel A, Eichner R, Aebi U. Polymorphism of reconstituted human epidermal keratin filaments: determination of their mass-per-length and width by scanning transmission electron microscopy (STEM). J Ultrastruc Res 1985;90:323–335.

Ehrlich P, Sybert VP, Spencer A, Stephens K. A common keratin 5 gene mutation in epidermolysis bullosa simplex—Weber-Cockayne. J Invest Dermatol 1995;104:877–879.

Figlewicz DA, Krizus A, Martinoli MG, et al. Variants of the heavy neurofilament subunit are associated with the development of amyotrophic lateral sclerosis. Human Genet. 1994;3:1757–1761.

Fine JD, Bauer EA, Briggaman RA, et al. Revised clinical and laboratory criteria for subtypes of inherited epidermolysis bullosa. J Am Acad Dermatol 1991;24:119–135.

Fine JD, Griffith RD. A specific defect in glycosylation of epidermal cell membranes: definition in skin from patients with epidermolysis bullosa simplex. Arch Dermatol 1985;121:1292–1296.

Fischer T, Gedde-Dahl T. Epidermolysis bullosa simplex and mottled pigmentation: a new dominant syndrome. Clin Genet 1979;115: 228–238.

Fuchs E. The cytoskeleton and disease: genetic disorders of intermediate filaments. Annu Rev Genet 1996;30:197–231.

Fuchs E, Coulombe PA. Of mice and men: genetic skin diseases of keratin. Cell 1992;69:899–902.

Fuchs E, Coppock S, Green H, Cleveland D. Two distinct classes of keratin genes and their evolutionary significance. Cell 1981;27:75–84.

Fuchs E, Green H. Changes in keratin gene expression during terminal differentiation of the keratinocyte. Cell 1980;19:1033–1042.

Fuchs E, Weber K. Intermediate filaments: structure, dynamics, function, and disease. Ann Rev Biochem 1994;63:345–382.

Gedde-Dahl TJ. Epidermolysis bullosa implex (intraepidermal epidermolysis bullosa) and allied conditions. In: Management of Blistering Diseases. London: Chapman and Hall Medical, 1990; pp. 189–211.

Green H. Cultured cells for the treatment of disease. Sci Am 1991;265:96–102.

Hatzfeld M, Weber K. The coiled coil of in vitro assembled keratin filaments is a heterodimer of type I and II keratins: use of site-specific mutagenesis and recombinant protein expression. J Cell Biol 1990; 110:1199–1210.

Hovnanian A, Pollack E, Hilal L, et al. A missense mutation in the rod domain of keratin 14 associated with recessive epidermolysis bullosa simplex. Nat Genet 1993;3:327–332.

Humphries MM, Sheils DM, Farrar GJ, et al. A mutation (Met to Arg) in the type I keratin (K14) gene responsible for autosomal dominant epidermolysis bullosa simplex. Human Mutation 1993;2:37–42.

Ito M, Okuda C, Shimizu N, Tazawa T, Sato Y. Epidermolysis bullosa simplex (Koebner) is a keratin disorder. Arch Dermatol 1991; 127:367–372.

Kremer H, Zeeuwen P, McLean WH, et al. Ichthyosis bullosa of Siemens is caused by mutations in the keratin 2e gene. J Invest Dermatol 1994;103:286–289.

Lane EB, Rugg EL, Navsaria H, et al. A mutation in the conserved helix termination peptide of keratin 5 in hereditary skin blistering. Nature 1992;356:244–246.

Letai A, Coulombe PA, McCormick MB, Yu QC, Hutton E, Fuchs E. Disease severity correlates with position of keratin point mutations in patients with epidermolysis bullosa simplex. Proc Natl Acad Sci USA 1993;90:3197–3201.

Letai A, Coulombe P, Fuchs E. Do the ends justify the mean? Proline mutations at the ends of the keratin coiled-coil rod segment are more disruptive than internal mutations. J Cell Biol 1992;116:1181–1195.

McLean WHI, Rygg EL, Lunny DP, Morley SM, Lane EB. Keratin 16 and keratin 17 mutations cause pachyonychia congenita. Nat Genet 1995;9:273–278.

Reis A, Hennies HC, Langbein L, et al. Keratin 9 gene mutations in epidermolytic palmoplantar keratoderma (EPPK). Nat Genet 1994; 6:174–179.

Richard G, DeLaurenzi V, Didona B, Bale SJ, Compton JG. Keratin 13 point mutation underlies the hereditary mucosal epithelia disorder white sponge nevus. Nat Genet 1995;11:453–455.

Rothnagel JA, Dominey AM, Dempsey LD, et al. Mutations in the rod domains of keratins 1 and 10 in epidermolytic hyperkeratosis. Science 1992;257:1128–1130.

Rugg EL, Morley SM, Smith FJD, et al. Missing links: Weber-cockayne keratin mutations implicate the L12 linker domain in effective cytoskeleton function. Nat Genet 1993;5:294–300.

Rugg EL, McLean WHI, Allison WE, et al. A mutation in the mucosal keratin K4 is associated with oral white sponge nevus. Nat Genet 1995;11:450–452.

Rugg EL, McLean WHI, Lane EB, et al. A functional "knockout" of human keratin 14. Genes Devel 1994;8:2563–2573.

Savolainen ER, Kero M, Pihlajeniemi T, Kivirikko KI. Deficiency of galactosylhydroxylysyl glucosyltransferase, and enzyme of collagen synthesis, in a family with dominant epidermolysis bullosa simplex. N Engl J Med 1981;304:197–204.

Steinert PM. The two-chain coiled-coil molecular of native epidermal keratin intermediate filaments is a type 1-type II heterodimer. J Biol Chem 1990;265:8766–8774.

Steinert PM, Parry DAD. The conserved Hl domain of the type II keratin 1 chain plays an essential role in the alignment of nearest neighbor molecules in mouse and human keratin 1/keratin 10 intermediate filaments at the two-to four-molecule level of structure. J Biol Chem 1993;268:2878–2887.

Steinert PM, Marekov LN, Fraser RDB, Parry DAD. Keratin intermediate filament structure: crosslinking studies yield quantitative information on molecular dimensions and mechanisms of assembly. J Mol Biol 1993;230:436–452.

Stephens K, Sybert VP, Wijsman EM, Ehrlich P, Spencer A. A keratin 14 mutational hot spot for epidermolysis bullosa simplex, dowling-meara: implications for diagnosis. J Invest Dermatol 1993;101: 240–243.

Sun TT, Eichner R, Schermer A, Cooper D, Nelson WG, Weiss RA. The transformed phenotype. In: Levine A, Topp W, van de Woude G, Watson JD, eds. The Cancer Cell, vol. 1. Cold Spring Harbor, New York: Cold Spring Harbor Laboratory, 1984; pp. 169–176.

Torchard D, Blanchet-Bardon C, Serova O, et al. Epidermolytic palmoplantar keratoderma cosegregates with a keratin 9 mutation in a pedigree with breast and ovarian cancer. Nat Genet 1994;6: 106–109.

Uttam J, Hutton E, Coulombe PA, et al. The genetic basis of epidermolysis bullosa simplex with mottled pigmentation. Proc Natl Acad Sci USA 1996;93:9079–9084.

Vassar R, Coulombe PA, Degenstein L, Albers K, Fuchs E. Mutant keratin expression in transgenic mice causes marked abnormalities resembling a human genetic skin disease. Cell 1991;64:365–380.

Yamanishi K, Matsuki M, Konishi K, Yasuno H. A novel mutation of Leu122 to Phe at a highly conserved hydrophobic residue in the helix initiation motif of keratin 14 in epidermolysis bullosa simplex. Human Mol Genet 1994;3:1171,1172.

74 Epidermolytic Hyperkeratosis

John J. DiGiovanna, Sherri J. Bale, and Peter M. Steinert

BACKGROUND

In 1902 Brocq described bullous ichthyotic erythroderma and distinguished the blistering type from the nonblistering type of congenital ichthyotic erythroderma. Whereas the original description included three unrelated patients whose clinical manifestations varied, this was probably the first description of epidermolytic hyperkeratosis (EHK). The best-recognized presentation of this rare disease is the severe, hystrix (porcupine-like) hyperkeratosis seen in adults with EHK. This appearance led to some patients' participation in traveling shows under the guise of "porcupine men." Today, the disease is named for histopathologic findings of keratinocyte lysis and associated hyperkeratosis. EHK is also known as bullous congenital ichthyosiform erythroderma, an earlier descriptive name signifying the blistering, neonatal presentation, scaling, and redness.

Information derived from a variety of approaches, including histology, ultrastructure, and molecular genetic studies in mice, and clinical, genetic, and molecular studies in humans have led to a greater understanding of EHK. The keratin intermediate-filament (KIF) network is responsible for the structural integrity of differentiated keratinocytes. Both clinical features (blistering and erosions) and morphologic studies (showing cell lysis and KIF clumps) suggested that EHK was caused by an aberration in the KIF network. This chapter will review the clinical, histologic, and ultrastructural features of EHK and the strategies used to identify the underlying defects.

CLINICAL FEATURES

The disease usually presents at birth with blistering, redness, and peeling. A generalized hyperkeratosis may develop over time either with or without erythroderma (Fig. 74-1). However, there is a striking clinical heterogeneity between EHK families. This includes differences in extent of body-surface involvement, quality of scale, presence of erythroderma, and palmar/plantar involvement. In some families, there is severe palmar-plantar involvement, whereas in others the palms and soles are normal (Fig. 74-1).

CLINICAL HETEROGENEITY IN EHK

DiGiovanna and Bale examined 52 patients with histologically confirmed EHK from 21 families and characterized specific clinical features and heterogeneity of this disorder. Patients were evaluated and graded for involvement of the palms and soles, scalp, extensor vs flexor areas, erythema, infection, and blisters. Within this group of patients, six clinical subtypes were distinguished. Several features were useful for separating patients into clinical subtypes (Table 74-1). The most distinctive characteristic was presence vs absence of severe palmar/plantar hyperkeratosis. Twenty-nine patients in six families had this finding. These patients were grouped into the PS (palm/sole hyperkeratosis) types. The remaining 15 families (23 patients) were classified as NPS (no palm/sole hyperkeratosis) types. On the basis of additional clinical characteristics, three PS types and three NPS types were identified, distinguished by presence/absence of erythroderma, quality of scale, extent of involvement, presence of digital contractures, and gait abnormality (Table 74-1).

DIAGNOSIS

In contrast to most other ichthyoses, the histopathologic picture of EHK is distinctive. There is a tremendously thickened stratum corneum and vacuolar degeneration of the upper epidermis, leading to the histologic term "epidermolytic hyperkeratosis" (Fig. 74-2). Granular cells exhibit dense, enlarged, irregularly shaped masses that were thought to be keratohyalin granules. On electron microscopic examination, clumping of filaments is observed to begin in the first suprabasal layer. These aggregated filaments have been demonstrated to be clumps of KIF that contain the terminal differentiation specific keratins 1 and 10.

GENETIC BASIS OF DISEASE

EHK is an autosomal dominant ichthyosis that occurs in approximately 1:200,000–300,000 people. However, as many as one-half of the cases have no family history and represent new mutational events.

EHK IS A KERATIN DISEASE Light and electron microscopic studies suggested that a defect in a terminal differentiation-specific epidermal-gene product might underlie EHK, causing KIF disorganization, increased numbers of keratohyalin granules, and vacuolated granular cells. Another clue came from the similarity observed in the filament clumping in EHK and epidermolysis bullosa simplex (EBS). The discovery that EBS is caused by a defect in either of the basal cell specific keratins keratin 5 or keratin 14, suggested that the keratins expressed suprabasally, keratins 1 or 10, were particularly good candidates for EHK. Compton et al. studied a large family with EHK primarily affecting the palms and soles, that segregated through three living generations. They tested for genetic linkage of the gene causing EHK to several candidate loci, including transglutaminase 1 (chromosome 14q),

From: *Principles of Molecular Medicine* (J. L. Jameson, ed.), ©1998 Humana Press Inc., Totowa, NJ.

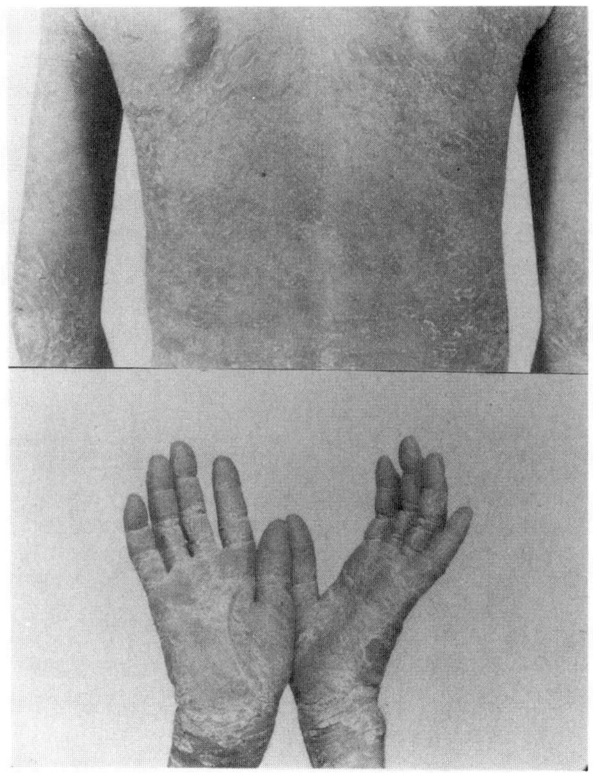

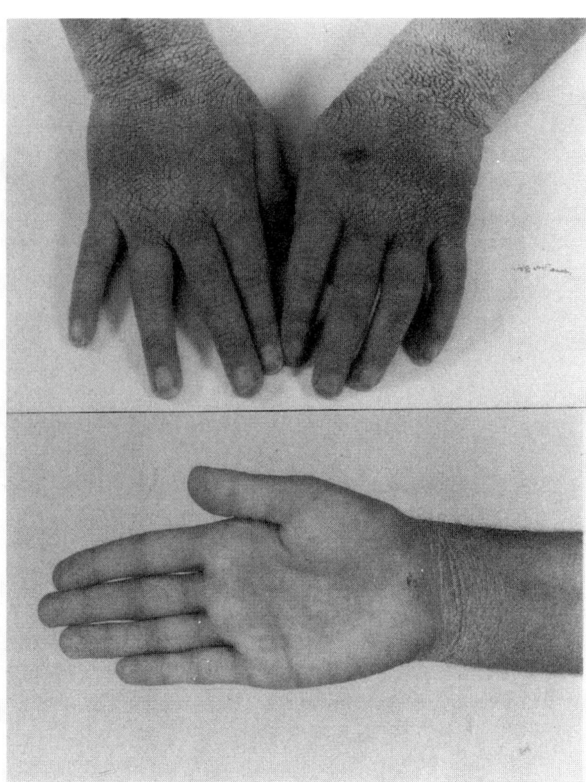

Figure 74-1 Clinical heterogeneity in EHK. Left panels: Patients with PS type (PS2) showing fine, white scale (generalized erythroderma can not be appreciated in the black and white photograph) and extensive palmar hyperkeratosis, that limits full extension of digits. Right panels: patients with NPS type (NPS1) demonstrating hystrix-type scale on the dorsum of hands and complete sparing of palmar surface (*see* DiGiovanna et al.).

Table 74-1
Characteristics of Epidermolytic Hyperkeratosis[a]

	NPS-1	*NPS-2*	*NPS-3*	*PS-1*	*PS-2*	*PS-3*
Palm/sole hyperkeratosis	–	–	–	+	+	+
Palm/sole surface	Normal	Normal	Hyperlinear, minimal scale	Smooth	Smooth	Cerebriform
Digital contractures	–	–	–	–	+	–
Scale	Hystrix	Brown	Fine, white	Mild	White scale to peel	Tan
Distribution	Generalized	Generalized	Generalized	Localized	Generalized	Generalized
Erythroderma	–	–	+	–	+	–
Blistering	+	+	+	Localized	+	Neonatal

[a]NPS indicates types without severe palm/sole hyperkeratosis; PS, types with sever palm/sole hyperkeratosis; –, absent; +, present.

loricrin and profilaggrin (both chromosome 1q), and keratin 10 (chromosome 17q). Each of these candidates could be excluded as the disease-causing gene. The locus of type II neutral-basic keratins on chromosome 12q, which includes keratin 1, was also studied. Use of several anonymous DNA markers mapped near the type II keratin locus confirmed linkage to this region, and multilocus linkage analysis further supported this location. The data strongly implicated keratin 1 as the site of the molecular defect causing EHK in this family.

Fourteen affected individuals from three other EHK families were studied by Bonifas et al. and provided some evidence for linkage to markers on chromosome 12q, whereas linkage to markers on chromosome 17q, in the region including the keratin 10 gene, were strongly excluded.

Using a fundamentally different approach, Fuchs et al. arrived at a similar conclusion that mutations in the terminal differentiation specific keratin genes underlie the pathology of EHK. They inserted a severely truncated form of the keratin 10 gene in the germline of transgenic mice. This created a dominant negative effect in the epidermis of the animals that showed clumping of KIF and other phenotypic features reminiscent of EHK.

IDENTIFICATION OF KERATIN MUTATIONS Chipev et al. sequenced the coding regions of both keratin 1 alleles of one patient in the family reported by Compton et al. A single basepair change in one allele was identified that causes a nonconservative amino acid substitution in codon 160 from leucine to proline in the H1 subdomain of the keratin 1 gene. One keratin allele of every affected member in this family had the proline substitution, whereas all unaffected members had two unsubstituted (normal) alleles. To confirm that the proline substitution was not merely a sequence polymorphism that, by chance, was segregating with EHK in this family, a further 100 alleles (from 50 normal control individuals of similar ethnic genetic background) were tested. None were found to have the mutant allele.

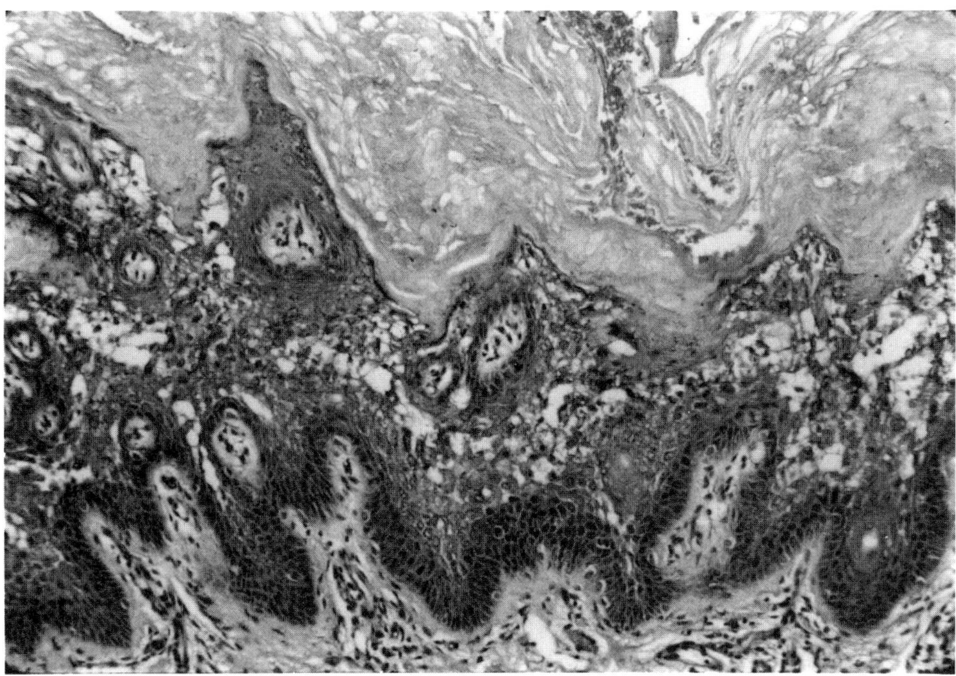

Figure 74-2 Histopathology in EHK. Tissue fixed in formalin, embedded in paraffin, and stained with hematoxylin and eosin shows epidermolysis and vacuolization of cells in the suprabasal layers of the epidermis. Extensive orthokeratotic hyperkeratosis is seen.

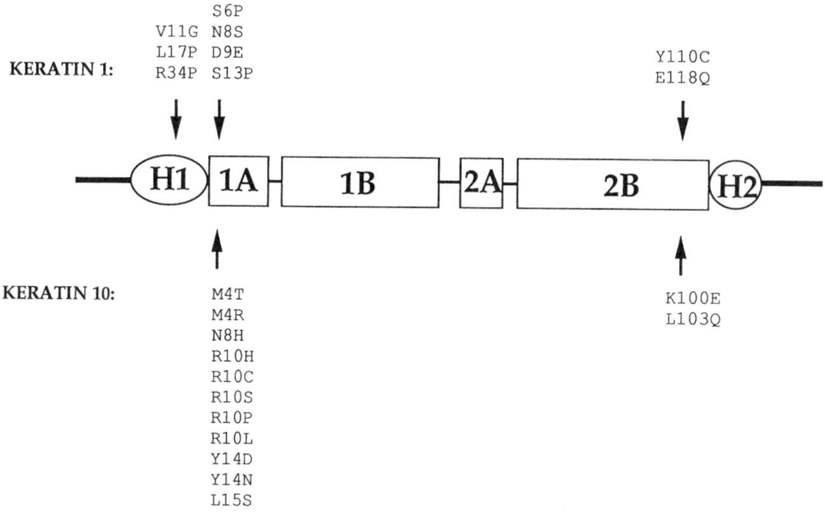

Figure 74-3 Known mutations in epidermolytic hyperkeratosis. In the center is a drawing of an idealized model of a keratin chain, displaying the four rod-domain segments, flanked by end-domain segments on either side. (Only the keratin 1 chain possesses well-defined H1 and H2 subdomains.) The locations of known amino acid substitutions, arising from point mutations, on the keratin 1 (upper) and keratin 10 (lower) chains are displayed with arrows. Notably, all substitutions occur within or immediately adjacent to the regions of the chains involved in molecular overlaps. We propose that these inappropriate substitutions destabilize the KIF so that they can no longer participate in their normal dynamic structural role in epidermal cells, ultimately leading to the pathogenesis of EHK.

Direct sequence analyses of both the keratin 1 and 10 genes has been used now to identify mutations in EHK.

From the existing catalog of EHK mutations, it is now clear that mutations in either the keratin 1 or 10 gene may cause EHK. In addition, most mutations are tightly clustered in exons 1 or 6 which encode the regions of the keratin chains forming the beginning and end of the rod domain. In particular, position 10 of the 1A rod domain segment of keratin 10 constitutes a "hot spot" for mutations (Fig. 74-3).

GENOTYPE/PHENOTYPE CORRELATION In an effort to correlate the clinical disease subtypes with specific mutations, DiGiovanna and Bale closely examined 11 families in which mutations had been found. All families with severe palmoplantar hyperkeratosis had abnormalities in keratin 1, whereas those without had abnormalities in keratin 10. Furthermore, the same mutation in keratin 10, R10H of the 1A rod domain segment, led to a wide range of NPS clinical presentations, including all three NPS subtypes.

MOLECULAR PATHOPHYSIOLOGY OF EHK

KIF STRUCTURE What is the molecular basis of these findings? Studies have recently shown that KIF are built in an hierarchical manner from individual keratin chains. First, a type I chain and a type II chain, in this case keratin 10 and keratin 1 respectively, form a heterodimer molecule by entwining their α-helical rod-domain segments. Then, pairs of molecules align in three very precise ways to form antiparallel protofilaments. This alignment may be determined in part by the H1 and H2 subdomains, which immediately flank the rod-domain segments. In addition, molecules align in parallel in rows by overlapping approximately the last 10 amino acids of the 2B segment of one molecule with the first 10 amino adds of the 1A segment of the next molecule in the row. Finally, these protofilaments align to form a KIF in groups of 12–24 in ways that are not yet known. In addition, cell-biological experiments have shown that KIF are highly dynamic structures in living cells, continuously exchanging protofilamentous units along the entire length of the KIF from soluble pools. This process is believed to be under the control of phosphorylation (which favors disassembly) and dephosphorylation (which favors reassembly). The KIF form an elaborate network throughout the epidermal cell, and interconnect with those of neighboring cells through specialized desmosomal junctions. In this way, the KIF provide three-dimensional mechanical integrity to the entire epidermis. Most of the mutations that have been observed in EHK (Fig. 74-3), and more recently in other keratin diseases, reside in the regions of the molecular overlaps.

A FUNCTIONAL ASSAY FOR KERATIN MUTATIONS Based on these structural concepts, it was shown that synthetic peptides corresponding to the molecular overlap regions encompassing the H1, 1A, and 2B rod domain segments, can be used in vitro as specific probes of the structural integrity of KIF. When added to either preformed KIF or in KIF-assembly reactions, the peptides interfere with KIF structure, leading to disassembly or failure of assembly even in 1:1 molar ratios. Presumably the peptides compete with the same sequences on the intact chains, causing destabilization, leading to disassembly. On the other hand, synthetic peptides bearing amino acid substitutions seen in the disease cases had greatly reduced capacities to disassemble KIF in vitro. From this it is concluded that the structure of the mutant keratins is seriously compromised and no longer can participate efficiently in normal dynamic behavior in the epidermal cell.

A MODEL FOR EHK PATHOGENESIS One of the hallmarks of EHK (and other keratin diseases) is the clumping of KIF. These clumps are likely caused by accumulations of the mutant keratin chain perhaps because the altered structure of the mutant keratin does not allow it to participate in the normal KIF. This accumulation of nonfunctional protein thus has secondary effects. First, there is thereby insufficient normal KIF to provide the necessary structural integrity of the cell. This may explain the cytolysis and vacuolization of cells and subsequent blistering of the suprabasal epidermal layers. In addition, the abnormal protein may interfere with the normal processes of terminal differentiation in the epidermis that involve the orderly expression and use of many other gene products, under the control of cytokines and various regulatory factors. This may explain the hyperkeratosis and erythema of some cases.

Further correlation of the clinical disease subtypes with the specific mutations should lead to a better understanding of the relationship between keratin structure and function in normal and diseased epidermis.

MANAGEMENT/TREATMENT

The management of EHK has acute and chronic aspects and varies with the clinical subtype. In the more severe, generalized types, there is usually erythema and blistering at birth. Because there is a high frequency of new mutations, the disease may not be expected and the diagnosis may not be immediately considered. Staphylococcal scalded-skin syndrome may be suspected and the infant treated with antibiotics. The newborn may require intensive care with fluid and electrolyte monitoring. Specialized skin care can minimize blistering and enhance healing of erosions. This could include lubrication to decrease friction and mechanical trauma, protective padding, specialized wound dressing, and so on. Both newborn and adult EHK skin is prone to infection, and rigorous monitoring and specific treatment of infection is essential. Over time, the skin usually thickens because of the development of hyperkeratosis. Areas of thick, hard, hyperkeratosis, which are not pliable are prone to mechanical trauma. Topical agents such as lubricants and keratolytics can reduce the thickened, rough areas and help to minimize blistering and erosion. Some patients have recurrent bouts of skin infections requiring topical or systemic antibiotics. In patients with extensive involvement, treatment with oral retinoid (isotretinoin, etretinate, acitretin) can be helpful in decreasing the hyperkeratosis and frequency of infections. However, since these drugs can enhance blistering, they must be administered carefully and used at the lowest effective doses.

SCREENING FOR MUTATIONS IN EPIDERMOLYTIC HYPERKERATOSIS Genetic screening for keratin mutations in patients diagnosed with EHK is now feasible in the clinical setting. In families in which multiple family members are affected, linkage analysis can sometimes first be used to determine if the type I or type II keratin cluster is involved. Based on these results, the focus of screening would be directed to either the keratin 10 or 1 gene, respectively. Initially, it is most productive to use an allele-specific mutation detection assay to look for the most frequently reported mutations that occur in exons 1 or 6. If this screening is negative, complete genomic DNA sequencing of all exons should be accomplished.

Many cases of EHK are caused by new mutations, and therefore linkage analysis is not feasible in these families. In screening for mutations in these sporadic EHK patients, much work in the laboratory may be eliminated if a careful clinical assessment of the patient is first made. If the patient can be categorized as having PS type, it is likely that a mutation in the keratin 1 gene is responsible for the disorder. However, if the palms and soles are uninvolved (i.e., an NPS type), a mutation in the keratin 10 gene is more likely. Screening of the appropriate gene, as outlined above, can than proceed.

In the past, prenatal diagnosis of EHK has been accomplished by obtaining skin from a fetus by ultrasound-guided biopsy. This procedure was performed between 16 and 22 weeks of fetal gestation. Although fetal skin biopsy can be used with reasonably high levels of safety and confidence, the procedure cannot be performed before the middle of the second trimester of pregnancy because of the lack of differentiation of the epidermis before that time. Alternatively, amniotic fluid cells, obtained early in the second trimester, have been shown in one study to contain aggregates of keratin filaments, allowing prenatal diagnosis of EHK. However, both of these procedures are suboptimal, forcing the parents of a fetus diagnosed with EHK to make a decision about continuation vs termination at a late stage in the pregnancy.

Prenatal diagnosis of EHK using molecular methods avoids several of the problems of fetal-skin biopsy and structural analysis of amniotic cells. Chorionic villus sampling (CVS), performed as early as 8 weeks of fetal gestation, is a relatively noninvasive technique. CVS is a procedure whereby placental trophoblast tissue is obtained via transcervical aspiration. DNA from cells obtained by CVS can be analyzed directly for keratin mutations using PCR-based methods. Results of mutation analysis can be available for the parents of the fetus before the end of the first trimester. Should the parents choose to terminate a pregnancy based on the results, the termination procedure is much simpler from a clinical standpoint, and often easier for the parents to deal with psychologically. To date, prenatal diagnosis of EHK using direct gene sequencing has been reported in a pair of twins at risk to inherit the disease from an affected father.

One caveat for DNA-based prenatal diagnosis is that the affected carrier parent should have had his or her mutation defined at a molecular level prior to the fetus being tested. Failure to do so results in a delay in providing the parents the information about the disease status of the fetus, as the parent's mutation must first be identified before the fetus can be tested. Therefore, physicians who are caring for individuals with EHK should encourage the patient to have mutation analysis accomplished prior to any pregnancy.

In some cases, although linkage analysis will have established which of the two keratin clusters is involved (i.e., type I [chromosome 17] or type II [chromosome 12]) in EHK in a particular family, that family's mutation may have not yet been identified. In these cases, indirect prenatal diagnosis can be accomplished by analysis of the fetal DNA to determine which of the two parental chromosomes the fetus has inherited from the parent with EHK (the chromosome carrying the normal keratin gene or the chromosome carrying the mutated keratin gene). However, there can be some degree of statistical uncertainty using this technique.

Until there is curative treatment for EHK, the ability to screen for the disease in at-risk fetuses leaves families with only the choice to continue or terminate the pregnancy. Many parents would be pleased if they could be assured that pregnancy with an affected fetus would never occur, rather than having to make difficult choices once the pregnancy is established. To this end, a new technology in the field of assisted reproduction, preimplantation blastomere analysis, may prove to be one answer. This technique first requires in vitro fertilization. When the cultured embryo reaches the eight-cell stage of cleavage, one cell of the blastocyst is removed and analyzed by PCR. If the analysis shows that the blastocyst carries the keratin mutation causing EHK, it would be discarded. If the tested cell does not carry the mutation, the blastocyst would be implanted into the mother's uterus so that pregnancy may be established. To date, this approach has not been used for hereditary skin disease, although it is being offered clinically for cystic fibrosis and Huntington disease.

FUTURE DIRECTIONS

The immediate prospect for the cure of EHK is not optimistic. Effective treatment will probably involve the removal of the defective keratin chain. This implies shutting off the expression of the defective allele. Several ideas for gene therapy are in progress and include, for example, the use of gene replacement by homologous recombination, and methods to specifically correct the defective allele by use of antisense oligonucleotides, ribozymes, and so on. However, at this point in time, there are a number of technical problems. A major problem is that current gene therapy procedures usually only offer a temporary correction of the gene defect: in this case corrected epidermal cells will differentiate and are then lost by desquamation. Thus, in order to avoid frequent repeated treatments, it will be necessary to identify and selectively target gene therapy to the epidermal stem cells that serve as the progenitors of the keratinocytes. Strategies should first be tested with experimental animal or cell culture model systems. Once the technical problems can be satisfactorily resolved in model systems, then in principle, a corrective regimen could proceed as follows: (1) Identification of the causative mutation in the affected individual or family; (2) isolation and in vitro culturing of epidermal keratinocytes from the patient; (3) gene therapy of the cells, isolation of corrected cell clones, and then growth into large epidermal rafts; and (4) surgical replacement of the patient's epidermis using techniques established for treatment of burn patients. Therefore, exploring novel approaches to the treatment of EHK remains an exciting challenge for the future.

SELECTED REFERENCES

Anton-Lamprecht IJ. Genetically induced abnormalities of epidermal differentiation and ultrastructure in ichthyoses and epidermolyses: pathogenesis, heterogeneity, fetal manifestation, and prenatal diagnosis. J Invest Dermatol 1983;81:149–156.

Artz AA, Compton JG, DiGiovanna JG, et al. Unpublished observations, 1994.

Bale SJ, DiGiovanna JJ. Genetic approaches to understanding the keratinopathies. Adv Dermatol 1997;12:99–113.

Bonifas JM, Bare JW, Chen MA, et al. Linkage of the epidermolytic hyperkeratosis phenotype to the region of the type II keratin gene cluster on chromosome 12. J Invest Dermatol 1992;99:524–527.

Bonifas MJ, Rothman AL, Epstein EH. Epidermolysis bullosa simplex: evidence in two families for keratin gene abnormalities. Science 1991;254:1202–1205.

Brocq L. Erythrodermie congenitale ichthyosiforme avec hyperepidermotrophie. Ann Dermatol Syph (Paris) 1902; ser 4, 4:1–31.

Cheng J, Syder AJ, Yu Q-C, et al. The genetic basis of epidermolytic hyperkeratosis, a disorder of differentiation-specific keratin genes. Cell 1992;70:811–819.

Chipev CC, Korge BP, Markova, et al. A leucine to profine mutation in the H1 subdomain of keratin 1 causes epidermolytic hyperkeratosis. Cell 1992;70:821–828.

Chipev CC, Steinert PM, Woodworth CD. An in vitro model of epidermolytic hyperkeratosis. J Invest Dermatol 1996;106:385–390.

Chipev CC, Yang J-M, DiGiovanna JJ, et al. Preferential sites in keratin 10 that are mutated in epidermolytic hyperkeratosis. Am J Hum Genet 1994;54:179–190.

Compton JG, DiGiovanna JJ, Santucci SK, et al. Epidermolytic hyperkeratosis completely segregates with the type II keratin gene cluster on chromosome 12q. Nat Genet 1992;1:301–305.

Coulombe PA, Hutton ME, Vassar R, et al. Point mutations in human keratin 14 genes of epidermolysis bullosa simplex patients: genetic and functional analyses. Cell 1991;66:365–380.

DiGiovanna JJ, Bale SJ. Clinical heterogeneity in epidermolytic hyperkeratosis. Arch Dermatol 130:1026–1035.

Epstein EH. Molecular genetics of epidermolysis bullosa. Science 1992;256:799–804.

Fuchs E, Esteves RA, Coulombe PA. Transgenic mice expressing a mutant keratin10 gene reveal the likely genetic basis for epidermolytic hyperkeratosis. Proc Natl Acad Sci USA 1992;89:6906–6910.

Golbus MS, Sagebiel RW, Filly RA, et al. Prenatal diagnosis of congenital bullous ichthyosiform erythroderma (epidermolytic hyperkeratosis) by fetal skin biopsy. N Engl J Med 1980;302:93–95.

Goldman RD, Zackroff RV, Steinert PM. Intermediate filaments: An Overview. In: Goldman RD, Steinert PM, eds. Cellular and Molecular Biology of Intermediate Filaments. New York: Plenum, 1990; pp. 3–17.

Goldsmith LA. The ichthyoses. Prog Med Genet 1976;1:185–240.

Holbrook KA, Dale BA, Sybert VP, Sagebiel RW. Epidermolytic hyperkeratosis: ultrastructure and biochemistry of skin and amniotic fluid cells from two affected fetuses and a newborn infant. J Invest Dermatol 1983;80:222–227.

Holbrook KA, Smith LT, Elias S. Prenatal diagnosis of genetic skin disease using fetal skin biopsy samples. Arch Dermatol 1993;129:1437–1454.

Ishida-Yamamoto A, Leigh IM, Lane EB, et al. Selective involvement of keratins K1 and K10 in the cytoskeletal abnormality of epidermolytic hyperkeratosis (bullous congenital ichthyosiform erythroderma). J Invest Dermatol 1992;99:19–26.

Lessin SR, Huebner K, Isobe M, et al. Chromosomal mapping of human keratin genes: evidence for nonlinkage. J Invest Dermatol 1988;91: 572–578.

Lu B, Federoff HJ, Wang Y, Goldsmith LA, Scott G. Topical application of viral vectors for epidermal gene transfer. J Invest Dermatol 1997;108:803–808.

McLean WHI, Lane EB. Intermediate filaments in disease. Curr Opin Cell Biol 1995;7:118–125.

McLean WM, Eady RAJ, Dopping-Hepenstal PJC, et al. Mutations in the 1A rod domain of keratins 1 and 10 in bullous congenital ichthyosiform erythroderma (BCIE). J Invest Dermatol 1994;102:24–30.

Miller RK, Khoun S, Goldman RD. Dynamics of keratin assembly: exogenous type I keratin rapidly associates with type II keratin in vivo. J Cell Biol 1993;122:123–135.

Paramio JM, Casanova ML, Alonso A, Jorcano JL. Keratin intermediate filament dynamics in cell heterkaryons reveals diverse behaviour of different keratins. J Cell Sci 1997;110:1099–1111.

Paller AS, Syder AJ, Chan Y-M, et al. The genetic basis of epidermal nevus, epidermolytic hyperkeratosis type. J Invest Dermatol 1994;102:576.

Parry DAD, Steinert PM. Intermediate Filament Structure. Molecular Biology Intelligence Unit, R.G. Landis Company, Austin TX, 1995.

Romano V, Bosco P, Rocchi M, et al. Chromosomal assignments of human type I and type II cytokeratin genes to different chromosomes. Cytogenet Cell Genet 1988;48:148–151.

Rosenberg M, RayChaudhury A, Shows TB, et al. A group of type I keratin genes on human chromosome 17: characterization and expression. Mol Cell Biol 1988;8:722–736.

Rothnagel JA, Dominey AM, Dempsey LD, et al. Mutations in the rod domains of keratins 1 and 10 in epidermolytic hyperkeratosis. Science 1992;257:1128–1130.

Rothnagel JA, Fisher MP, Axtell SM, et al. A mutational hot spot in keratin 10 (KRT 10) in patients with epidermolytic hyperkeratosis. Hum Mol Genet 1993;2:2147–2150.

Rothnagel JA, Longley MA, Holder RA, et al. Prenatal diagnosis of epidermolytic hyperkeratosis by direct gene sequencing. J Invest Dermatol 1994;102:13–16.

Steinert PM. Structure, function and dynamics of keratin intermediate filaments. J Invest Dermatol 1993;100:729–734.

Steinert PM, Bale SJ. How mutations in keratins cause epidermal blistering diseases. Trends Genet 1993;9:280–284.

Steinert PM, Marekov LN, Fraser RDB, et al. Keratin intermediate filament structure: crosslinking studies yield quantitative information on molecular dimensions and mechanism of assembly. J Mol Biol 1993;230:436–452.

Steinert PM, Marekov LN, Parry DAD. Conservation of the structure of keratin intermediate filaments: molecular mechanism by which different keratin molecules integrate into pre-existing keratin intermediate filaments during differentiation. Biochemistry 1993;32: 10,046–10,056.

Steinert PM, Parry DAD. The conserved Hl subdomain of type II keratin 1 chain plays an essential role in the alignment of nearest-neighbor molecules in mouse and human keratin 1/keratin 10 intermediate filaments at the two-to-four molecule level of structure. J Biol Chem 1993;268:2878–2887.

Steinert PM, Yang J-M, Bale SJ, et al. Concurrence between the molecular overlap regions in keratin intermediate filaments and the location of keratin mutations in genodermatoses. Biochem Biophys Res Commun 1993;197:840–848.

Syder AJ, Yu Q-C, Paller AS, et al. Genetic mutations in the K1 and K10 genes in patients with epidermolytic hyperkeratosis: correlation between location and disease severity. J Clin Invest 1993;93: 1533–1542.

Takahashi K, Coulombe PA. A transgenic mouse model with an inducible skin blistering disease phenotype. Proc Natl Acad Sci USA 1996;93: 14,776–14,781.

Traupe H. The epidermolytic (acanthokeratolytic) ichthyoses. In: The Ichthyoses: A Guide to Clinical Diagnosis, Genetic Counseling, and Therapy. New York: Springer-Verlag, 1989, pp. 139–153.

Verlinsky Y, Kuliev AM. Preimplantation Diagnosis of Genetic Disease: A New Technique in Assisted Reproduction. Wiley-Liss, New York, 1993.

Yang J-M, Chipev CC, DiGiovanna JJ, et al. Mutations in the H1 and 1A domains in the keratin 1 gene in epidermolytic hyperkeratosis. J Invest Dermatol 1994;102:17–23.

Yang J-M, Nam K, Park KB, et al. A novel H1 mutation in the keratin 1 chain in epidermolytic hyperkeratosis. J Invest Dermatol 1996;107: 439–441.

75 Mosaicism and Epidermal Nevi

AMY S. PALLER

BACKGROUND

Genetic mosaicism occurs when an organism contains two or more genetically different populations of cells that derive from a genetically homogeneous zygote. When mosaicism affects the skin, the resultant cutaneous patterning may follow several forms as classified by Happle: narrow or broad bands that follow Blaschko's lines; a checkerboard pattern; a phylloid pattern; or a patchy pattern without midline separation. Of these, the most common and best understood pattern follows the lines of Blaschko (Fig. 75-1), a nonrandom developmental pattern that differs from other skin-line patterns, such as dermatomes and Langer's lines of cleavage. Although never formally tested, these mosaic alterations in cutaneous morphology have been attributed to clonal proliferation of two genetically different cell populations during embryogenesis. Lesions along Blaschko's lines track linearly on extremities; the lines follow an arched S-shaped course on the sides of the trunk and abdomen, and form a striking V-shape over the dorsal midline caused by a marked caudal dip. The deviation of these designs from the expected transverse proliferation of embryonic cells has been explained by the concurrent longitudinal growth and flexion of the embryo.

The lines of Blaschko become visible in patients with various X-linked dominant genetic disorders, such as focal dermal hypoplasia, Conradi-Hünermann syndrome and incontinentia pigmenti, and in females who are carriers for certain X-linked recessive disorders, such as hypohidrotic ectodermal dysplasia. The lack of expression of the genetic mutation in all cells is thought to reflect the nonrandom inactivation of one of the X chromosomes (lyonization). These observations demonstrate a causal relationship between lyonization and lines of Blaschko, and further suggest that the lines serve as a marker of human development.

Several sporadic disorders also have cutaneous features that follow the lines of Blaschko. One of these sporadic disorders is the McCune-Albright syndrome, a disorder involving skin, bones and endocrine organs, in which hyperpigmented patches on the skin are symmetrically distributed, often along Blaschko's lines. A genetic mutation in the α-subunit of G protein that causes constitutive activation of adenylyl cyclase has been identified in patients with McCune-Albright syndrome, although a clear correlation between clinical and genetic mosaicism has not been demonstrated. This mutation is likely to be lethal, with survival possible only in the mosaic state with sufficient numbers of normal cells.

From: *Principles of Molecular Medicine* (J. L. Jameson, ed.), ©1998 Humana Press Inc., Totowa, NJ.

CLINICAL FEATURES

Epidermal nevi are organoid nevi that arise from the pleuripotential germinative cells in the basal layer of the embryonic epidermis. Lesions may not be present at birth, but tend to develop during the first few years of life. The clinical appearance of epidermal nevi varies, particularly in extent of body involvement, degree of epidermal thickening, and associated inflammation. These nevi have been classified by their major component into five major subsets: verrucous epidermal nevi and inflammatory linear verrucous epidermal nevi (keratinocyte origin); nevus comedonicus (hair follicle); nevus sebaceus (sebaceous gland); eccrine nevi (eccrine glands); and nevus syringocystadenosus papilliferus (apocrine gland). Although most patients with an epidermal nevus have no associated abnormalities, patients with the "epidermal nevus syndrome" have involvement of other organs, particularly involving the nervous system, eyes, or bones.

Epidermal nevi are almost always sporadic conditions, although rare examples of familial epidermal nevi have been described. In all forms of epidermal nevi, skin lesions tend to follow Blaschko's lines, suggesting the possibility of genetic mosaicism resulting from a postzygotic mutation.

GENETIC BASIS OF DISEASE

A subset of epidermal nevi that is clinically indistinguishable from verrucous epidermal nevi displays the typical histopathologic features of skin biopsies of patients with a rare autosomal dominant disorder, epidermolytic hyperkeratosis (EH) (Fig. 75-2A,B) (*see* Chapter 74). This type of nevus, even when extensively distributed, is not associated with other organ involvement. Epidermal nevi of the EH histologic phenotype also demonstrate ultrastructural changes similar to those of EH, with perinuclear clumping of keratin tonofilaments and epidermolysis in suprabasal layers. Epidermolytic hyperkeratosis, sometimes referred to as bullous congenital ichthyosiform erythroderma, is characterized by generalized epidermal thickening, superficial blistering, and variable-associated inflammation. A relationship between epidermal nevi of the EH type and generalized EH is further suggested by patients with generalized EH who have a parent with epidermal nevi, EH type.

The genetic basis for EH has been shown by several investigators to be mutations in the suprabasal, i.e., differentiation-specific keratins, K1 and K10 (*see* Chapter 74). These observations suggested that spontaneous somatic mutations in K1 and K10 may result in some forms of epidermal nevi. Paller et al. examined these keratin genes in three different cell types of patients with

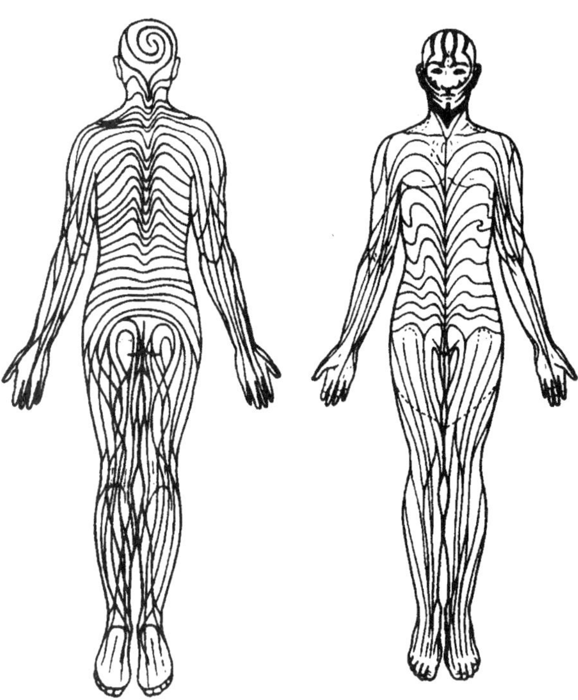

Figure 75-1 Schematic representation of the surface lines of Blaschko. Several skin diseases display epidermal patterns of clinical mosaicism that follow these lines. The lines do not follow any known underlying vascular, neural, or dermal structures, but rather are thought to arise from genetic mosaicism as a consequence of postzygotic mutation.

epidermal nevi and of their offspring with EH, and demonstrated that genetic mosaicism is the underlying cause of the clinical mosaicism of epidermal nevi of the EH type. Sequence analysis and restriction-enzyme digests of CDNA from cultured skin keratinocytes revealed defects in up to 50% of the K10 alleles in lesional skin, but not in nonlesional areas of patients with epidermal nevi (Fig. 75-3A,B). In contrast, the mutation was either absent or underrepresented in their blood and fibroblast DNA. EH offspring displayed the same mutations detected in 50% of the K10 alleles from blood DNA. K10 mutation have subsequently been shown to cause epidermal nevi of the EH type in several other patients.

MOLECULAR PATHOPHYSIOLOGY

The embryologic alterations that lead to the somatic mosaicism are poorly understood. Presumably, an earlier postzygotic mutational event would lead to more extensive cutaneous involvement and a greater likelihood of gene alteration in multiple cell types. In the studies by Paller et al., K10 mutations could be detected by restriction enzyme digests in fibroblast DNA from all three different epidermal nevi patients, in blood DNA from two of these cases and, as judged by analyses of their offspring, in germline cells of all three cases. The epidermal nevi in these patients were multiple streaks. These findings are consistent with the notion that the mosaicism in these patients with epidermal nevi was established early.

The distinctly different program of epidermal and dermal development rules out the possibility that genetic diagnosis of epidermal nevus can be made reliably from any tissue other than lesional epidermis. The presence of a keratin mutation in many different cell types of an epidermal nevus patient increases the likelihood of germline transmission, and may warrant genetic screening at early stages of pregnancy to assess whether the keratin mutation has been transmitted to the unborn offspring. Prenatal diagnosis has been performed for 15-week gestational age twins with EH by molecular analysis, born to a father affected by generalized EH. A similar approach is feasible for a parent with an extensive epidermal nevus of the EH type.

Given the parallels between EH and epidermolysis bullosa simplex (EBS), an autosomal-dominant blistering disorder caused by mutations in keratins 5 and 14, it is interesting that no mosaic disorder analogous to epidermal nevi is known for EBS (*see* Chapter 73). One explanation could be that a mutation expressed in the proliferative basal cell layer of skin, as in EBS, imparts a selective disadvantage in a mosaic state, so that the healthy basal cells would preferentially replace the cells with the expressed mutation. In contrast to basal cells, suprabasal cells terminally differentiate in upward columns of cells. Hence, as in EH, when cytolysis occurs in suprabasal cells, no compensation by lateral migration is possible, and clinical mosaicism is observed.

MANAGEMENT/TREATMENT

The current management of epidermal nevi is primarily surgical. Topical keratolytic agents are often not successful in ameliorating the cosmetic disfigurement that may result from epidermal nevi. Full-thickness excision is often difficult because of the orientation of the nevi, and is most commonly performed to completely remove nevus sebaceus, a premalignant lesion associated with a high risk of transformation to basal cell and adnexal carcinomas after puberty. Dermabrasion and the ultrapulse carbon-dioxide laser are the preferred treatments, although the pulsed-dye laser has been used successfully for patients with inflammatory linear verrucous epidermal nevi.

FUTURE DIRECTIONS

The underlying genetic basis for other types of epidermal nevi has not yet been elucidated. Interestingly, the lesions of nevus

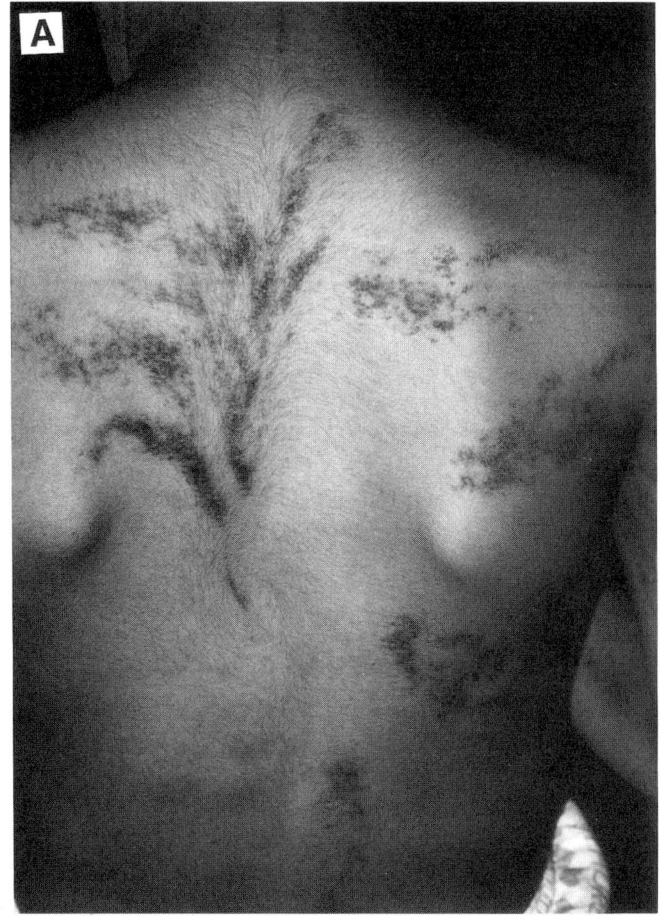

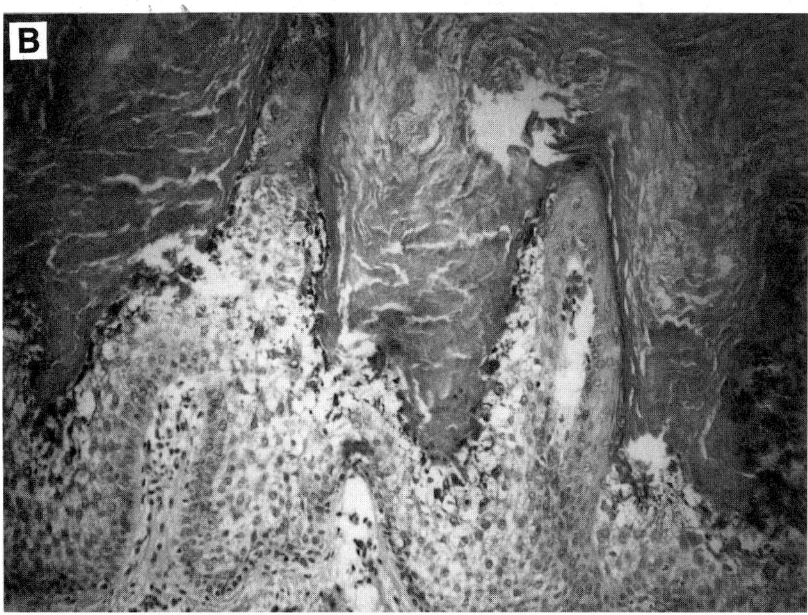

Figure 75-2 (**A**) Verrucous epidermal nevus of the EH type along the lines of Blaschko. Immediately adjacent areas of skin are clinically normal. (**B**) Lesional skin from the epidermal nevus shows normal basal cells, but hyperkeratosis and cytolysis in suprabasal cells. (*See* color insert following p. 684.)

comedonicus may show histologic evidence of epidermolytic hyperkeratosis ("nevoid follicular EH"). Generalized EH has been described in a child of a parent with nevus comedonicus at more than one site, suggesting a common mutation. Epidermal nevi are also a feature of Proteus syndrome, a multisystemic sporadic mosaic condition that is presumed to be lethal in a generalized form. DNA fingerprinting has shown single-band differences in a pair of monozygotic twins discordant for Proteus syndrome and also differences between normal and affected areas of another patient with Proteus syndrome. A *de novo* mosaic chromosome

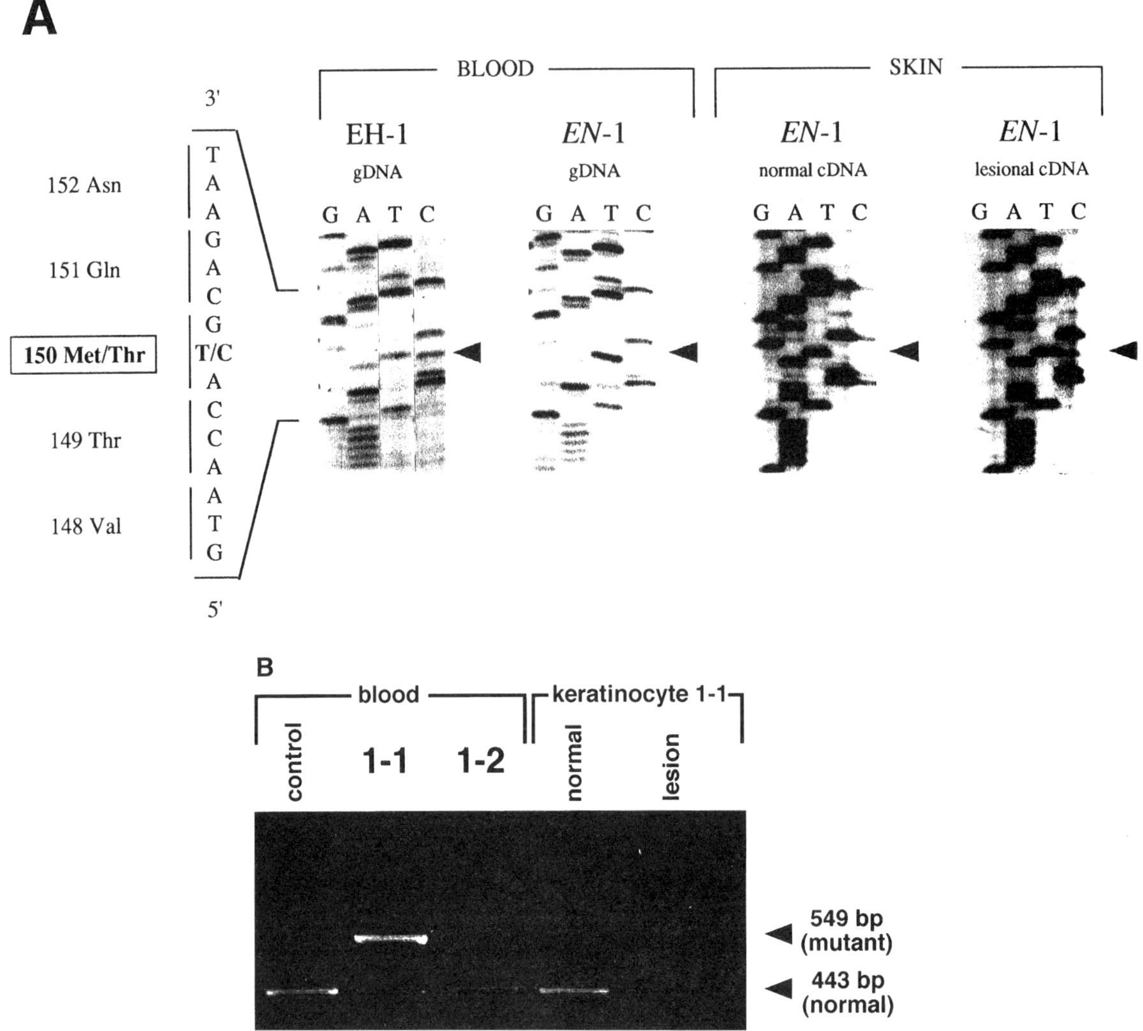

Figure 75-3 (**A**) Sequence analyses of K10 alleles from a family with epidermal nevus and EH show the mutation in lesional but not normal tissue. PCR-amplified fragments of K10-coding sequence were generated from keratinocyte cDNA or blood genomic DNA from the epidermolytic hyperkeratosis offspring and epidermal nevus parent. Note that the thymidine base is mutated to cytosine in up to 50% of the alleles in lesional skin, the same mutation that occurs in 50% of the K10 alleles of the offspring with EH, resulting in a methionine to threonine switch at amino acid 150. (**B**) Obliteration of a restriction endonuclease site in one of two K10 alleles in the epidermal nevus patient (1-1; EN-1) and offspring with EH (1-2; EH-1) shown in (A). DNA fragments with the K10 150Met→Thr mutation were amplified and digested with the restriction endonuclease Nla III. Samples were resolved by electrophoresis through agarose gels, and bands were visualized by staining with ethidium bromide. Bands characteristic of a normal and mutant K10 allele are indicated. Note that an Nla III cleavage site is lost as a consequence of the Met→Thr mutation, leading to the presence of uncleaved DNA (upper band). (Reproduced with permission from Paller AS, Syder AJ, Chan Y-M, et al. Genetic and clinical mosaicism in a type of epidermal nevus. N Engl J Med 1994;313:1408–1415.)

abnormality has been noted in still another patient with Proteus syndrome, suggesting the gene abnormality to reside within the lqll to lq25 region. Chromosomal breaks have also been demonstrated in cultured cells from epidermal nevi of the verrucous type without epidermolysis or Proteus syndrome in two patients at chromosome 1q21-25. This chromosomal localization, the site of a cluster of genes that code for several proteins specifically expressed during epidermal differentiation, including loricrin, trichohyalin, profilaggrin, involucrin, calpactin I, calcyclin, and cellular retinoic acid binding protein CRABP-II, suggests that verrucous nevi without epidermolysis may result from mosaicism of a gene mutation for one of these epidermal proteins.

At this time, localized gene therapy, either through ex vivo gene replacement and keratinocyte transplantation or by in vivo introduction, e.g., by gene-gun approach, injection of naked DNA, or liposomes, is not theoretically feasible for correction of epidermal nevi of the EH type because of the dominant-negative nature of mutations of keratin genes. With the increasing knowledge of genes that cause the clinical mosaicism of epidermal nevi, it may be feasible to correct the defect by in vivo or ex vivo deletion of the mutated gene.

SELECTED REFERENCES

Blaschko, A. Die Nervenverteilung in der Haut in ihrer Beziehung zu den Erkrankungen der Haut. In: Beilage zu den Verhandlungen der Deutschen Dermatologischen Gesellschaft: VII. Congress zu Breslau. Wilhelm Braumüller, Vienna, Austria, 1901.

Bolognia JL, Orlow SJ, Glick SA. Lines of Blaschko. J Am Acad Dermatol 1994;31:157–190.

Cohen MM Jr. Proteus syndrome: clinical evidence for somatic mosaicism and selective review. Am J Med Genet 1993;47:645–652.

Fuchs E. Intermediate filaments and disease: mutations that cripple cell strength. J Cell Biol 1994;125:511–516.

Goldman K, Don PC. Adult onset of inflammatory linear a verrucous epidermal nevus in a mother and her daughter. Dermatol 1994;189: 170–172.

Hamm H, Happle R. Inflammatory linear verrucous epidermal nevus (ILVEN) in a mother and her daughter. Am J Med Genet 1986;24:685–690.

Happle R. Akanthokeratolytischer epidermaler nävus:Vererbbar ist die akanthokeratolyse, nicht der nädvus. Hautartz 1990;40:117,118.

Happle R. Epidermal nevus syndromes. Semin Dermatol 1995;14:111–121.

Happle, R. Lyonization and the lines of Blaschko. Hum Genet 1985;70: 200–206.

Happle, R. Mosaicism in human skin: understanding the patterns and mechanisms. Arch Dermatol 1993;129:1460–1470.

Happle R. The McCune-Albright syndrome: a lethal gene surviving by mosaicism. Clin Genet 1986;29:321–324.

Lookingbill DP, Ladda RL, Cohen C. Generalized epidermolytic hyperkeratosis in the child of a parent with nevus comedonicus. Arch Dermatol 1984;223–226.

Meschia JF, Junkins E, Hofman KJ. Familial systematized epidermal nevus syndrome. Am J Med Genet 1992;44:664–667.

Moss C, Jones DO, Blight A, Bowden PE. Birthmark due to cutaneous mosaicism for keratin 10 mutation. Lancet 1995;345,596.

Nazzaro V, Ermacora E, Santucci E, Caputo R. Epidermolytic hyperkeratosis: generalized form in children from parents with systematized linear form. Br J Dermatol 1990;122:417–433.

Paller AS, Syder AJ, Chan Y-M, et al. Genetic and clinical mosaicism in a type of epidermal nevus. N Engl J Med 1994;331:1408–1415.

Rieger E, Kofler R, Borkenstein M, Schwingshandl J, Soyer HP, Kerl H. Melanotic macules following Blaschko's lines in McCune-Albright syndrome. Br J Dermatol 1994;30:215–220.

Rogers M, McCrossin I, Commens C. Epidermal nevi and 12 the epidermal nevus syndrome. A review of 131 cases. J Am Acad Dermatol 1989;20:476–488.

Rothnagel JA, Longley MA, Holder RA, Küster W, Roop DR. Prenatal diagnosis of epidermolytic hyperkeratosis by direct gene sequencing. J Invest Dermatol 1994;102:13–16.

Say B, Carpenter NJ. Report of a case resembling the Proteus syndrome with a chromosome abnormality. Am J Med Genet 1988;31:987–989.

Schwartz CE, Brown AM, Der Kaloustian VM, McGill CC, Saul RA. DNA fingerprinting: the utilization of minisatellite probes to detect a somatic mutation in the Proteus syndrome. In: Burke T, Dolf G, Jeffreys Ai, Wolff R, eds. DNA Fingerprinting: Approaches and Applications. Basel, Switzerland: Birkhauser Verlag, 1991; pp. 95–105.

Schwindinger WF, Francomano CA, Levine MA. Identification of a mutation in the gene encoding the a subunit of the stimulatory C protein of adenylyl cyclase in McCune-Albright syndrome. Proc Natl Acad Sci USA 1992;89:5152–5156.

Stosiek N, Ulmer R, von den Driesch P, Claussen U, Hornstein OP, Rott HD. Chromosomal mosaicism in two patients with epidermal verrucous nevus. Demonstration 14 of chromosomal reappoint . J Am Acad Dermatol 1994;30:622–625.

Volz A, Korge BP, Compton JG, Ziegler A, Steinert PM, Mischke D. Physical mapping of a functional cluster of epidermal differentiation genes on chromosome 1q21. Genomics 1993;18:92–99.

76 Darier's Disease and Hailey-Hailey Disease

LOWELL A. GOLDSMITH AND ERVIN EPSTEIN, JR.

INTRODUCTION

These diseases are often discussed together because of some similarities in their histopathology. They map to different chromosomal locations and the clinical differences seem much more than the similarities. They will be discussed, in turn, in this chapter.

DARIER'S DISEASE

BACKGROUND Darier's disease (DD) is an autosomal-dominant disorder characterized by altered keratinization clinically limited to the epidermis, nails, and mucous membranes. The first American patient was described by White in 1889. That patient was well until he entered the Northern army in 1862, at the age of 22, and his skin disease appeared under his knapsack after a long march. In all families studied by positional cloning with microsatellite CA repeats, the gene defective in DD maps to a site on the long arm of chromosome 12-12q23-24.1. The mapping studies exclude keratins, desmosomal proteins, integrins, and retinoic acid receptors.

CLINICAL FEATURES DD usually begins in the first or second decade but is not present at birth. Multiple discrete, scaling, rough, crusted, pruritic, frequently malodorous, and disfiguring skin papules characterize DD (Fig. 76-1). Lesions rarely are bullous or hemorrhagic (Fig. 76-2). Characteristic sites of predilection are the face, forehead, scalp, chest, and back. Although these sites have many sebaceous glands, lesions also occur commonly in sites without sebaceous glands such as the palms and soles, as well as in nonkeratinizing epithelia. Males and females are affected equally. The nails are frequently abnormal and can be a clue for early diagnosis (Fig. 76-3). They characteristically are thin and fragile (with distal cracking and notching) and have distinctive red and white bands parallel to the long axis. The hair is normal, although the scalp frequently is covered with thick greasy scales and crusts.

DD frequently is worse in the summer and often is exacerbated by ultraviolet B (UVB) light (290–320 nm) and by mechanical trauma. Lesions have been precipitated by oral lithium, phenol, or ethyl chloride spray. Common complications of DD lesions are bacterial infection and infection with herpes simplex virus, but there are no consistent immunological abnormalities. The disease does not seem to predispose to cutaneous malignancies, although basal cell carcinomas and one rare sweat-gland tumor have been reported. One family of two siblings with DD and retinitis pigmentosum is reported. Other associations reported in the literature include usually asymptomatic bone cysts. In a family with DD, one individual had concurrent renal and testicular agenesis and autoimmune thyroid disease. Epilepsy and affective disorders often have been associated with DD.

DIAGNOSIS The clinical features are associated with a distinctive histopathology that shows premature and abnormal keratinization and eosinophilic dyskeratotic cells in the spinous layer (corps ronds) and in the stratum comeum (grains). Suprabasal clefts (lacunae) are seen frequently and are interpreted as altered adhesion within the epidermis. Papillary overgrowth of the epidermis and hyperkeratosis are common.

GENETIC BASIS OF DISEASE DD is inherited as an autosomal dominant trait. The incidence of DD is at least 1:100,000 in Denmark and has been estimated to be 1:36,000 in northeast England. Cases caused by new mutations are frequent. The penetrance of the DD gene is high, at least 0.95; there is no skipping of generations in multiple pedigrees in the literature. No unique phenotype for the homozygote for the gene has been described, and there is no evidence for X-linked or autosomal-recessive forms of the disorder. There is no history of anticipation.

MOLECULAR PATHOPHYSIOLOGY OF DISEASE Several groups using positional cloning with CA microsatellite repeats have reported the localization of DD to 12q23-24.1. This is the region of the DD trait in over two dozen reported kindreds. The most recently published studies limit the DD gene to a 1- to 2-cM region between the markers D 12S234 and D12S129. This location excluded the known keratin and cytoskeletal genes, retinoid receptors, desmosomal proteins, and other cell adhesion molecules.

The basic defect is not known and it is premature to discuss details of the molecular pathophysiology, but it is worthwhile to discuss some features of the general pathophysiology.

Electron microscopic studies show basal-cell vacuolization, decreased numbers of desmosomes on the lateral borders of basal cells, separation of tonofilaments from their insertions on the cell membrane, and tonofilaments in large aggregates around the nucleus. The corps ronds have many of the characteristics of apoptotic cells. Burge et al. found no abnormality of desmosomal structure by electron microscopy or of individual desmosomal proteins by immunofluorescent studies in uninvolved DD skin.

The identical tissue histopathology seen in the genetic forms of DD rarely has been described in epidermal nevi, warty dyskeratoma (a solitary scalp or oral lesion), actinic keratoses, Grover's disease (transient acantholytic disease), and some other

From: *Principles of Molecular Medicine* (J. L. Jameson, ed.), ©1998 Humana Press Inc., Totowa, NJ.

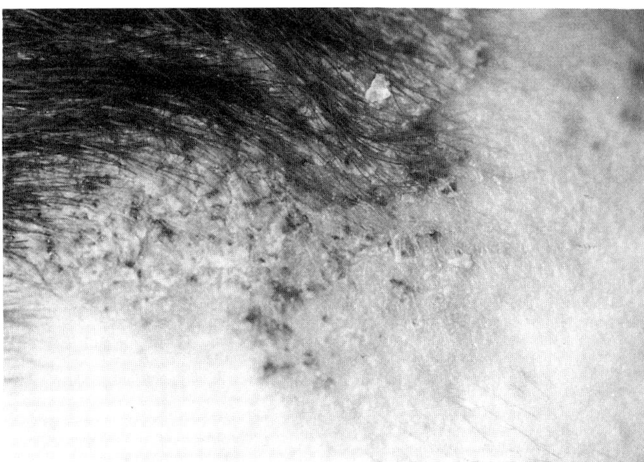

Figure 76-1 Hyperkeratotic irregular papules in Darier's disease are often on sun-exposed sites, trunk, and prominent in the hairline. (*See* color insert following p. 684.)

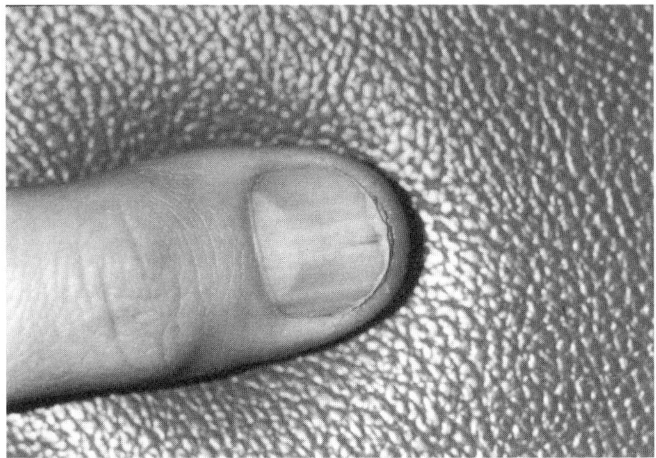

Figure 76-3 Red and white linear longitudinal bands occur in the nails of patients with Darier's disease. They are persistent and may represent clonal sites altered keratinization. (*See* color insert following p. 684.)

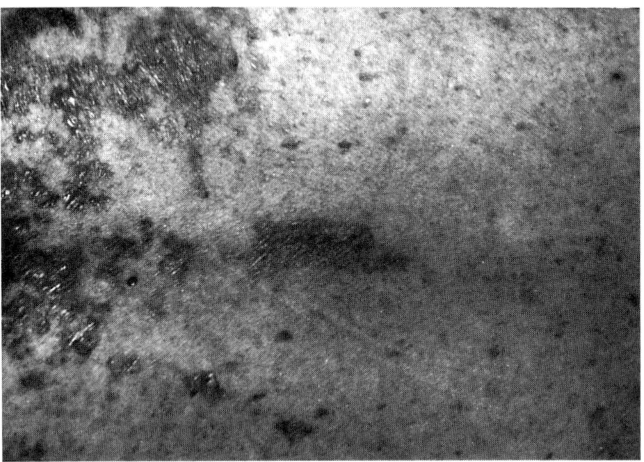

Figure 76-2 Hemorrhagic vesicle-papules occur in some kindreds with Darier's disease. This allele maps to the same 12q23-24.1 location as the common form of Darier's disease. (*See* color insert following p. 684.)

skin lesions. Hyperkeratotic papules on the dorsal surface of the hands of DD patients have a specific histopathology with a disordered acanthotic epidermis with angular, raised, church-spire-like epidermal changes. The pathology is consistent with acrokeratosis of Hopf. These lesions are almost always associated with DD, although there are rare families reported with only acrokeratosis of Hopf.

Hailey-Hailey disease is a disorder of the epidermis whose lesions have acantholysis but usually lack the extensive dyskeratotic changes seen in DD. Transient acantholytic disease (Grover's disease) occurs in middle-aged or elderly adults, usually men, has no familial incidence, and often begins after sun exposure. Individuals develop small pruritic skin lesions that are of variable duration and have the histopathology of DD. Similar lesions can be reproduced by the systemic injection of IL-4.

Chronic proliferative dermatitis is an autosomal-recessive mouse disorder that has frequent dyskeratosis and may be a model for some of the altered physiology in DD, but does not seem to be the mouse homolog of DD.

Cultured DD cells are able to induce the separation of cocultured normal keratinocytes. These data are intriguing and suggest the need for studies of DD cells in skin equivalents to determine the effect of proteolytic enzymes in the production of lesions, and especially the potential therapeutic role of protease inhibitors (and the stimulators of protease inhibitors such as transforming growth factor-β) in preventing skin lesions.

MANAGEMENT/TREATMENT As with several other genetic disorders affecting the epidermis, the disease is improved by therapy with systemic retinoids. UVB blockers are useful during the sunny portion of the year. Some patients are so sun-sensitive that systemic retinoids can be discontinued in the winter. All of the precautions relevant to systemic retinoids must be followed.

HAILEY-HAILEY DISEASE

BACKGROUND Eponymic credit for the description of "their" disease clearly belongs to the (dermatologic) brothers Hailey who in 1939 described two sets of (patient) brothers, all four of whom were affected by a clinically similar chronic skin problem.

CLINICAL FEATURES The primary lesions of Hailey-Hailey disease are small, grouped, clear vesicles that tend to spread peripherally with crusting and central clearing, leaving chronic plaques sometimes misdiagnosed as eczema or as dermatophyte or bacterial infection (Fig. 76-4). Lesions may be tender and malodorous. The usual location of lesions are the body folds—the groin and perineum, axillae, intra-, and inframammary areas—and the sides of the neck. The shoulders and upper back also frequently are affected. However, lesions unusually have been reported in a more generalized distribution on the skin and even on the mucosal surface including the vagina, buccal mucosa, and esophagus. Longitudinal white bands on the fingernails have been observed. Because of the presence of tender eroded patches, patients may find it difficult to engage in the physical activity necessary for gainful employment.

Onset is usually in the third or fourth decade but is after age 40 in approximately 12% of patients. Most patients find that their lesions are made worse by friction, heat, and sweating—with exacerbations in the summer and waning in the winter. Hailey-Hailey disease is diagnosed uncommonly, but the true incidence may well be considerably higher, for it is easy to misdiagnose lesions as a nonspecific intertrigo. Also, the common localization

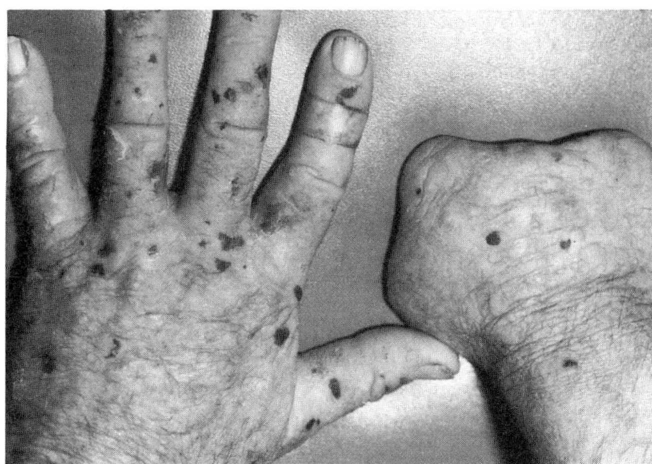

Figure 76-4 Papules and erosions characterize Hailey-Hailey disease. (*See* color insert following p. 684.)

of disease to covered sites and some reticence to discuss afflictions in those areas means that even patients' families frequently do not know of the disease and therefore are not able to enhance their physician's diagnostic suspicion.

DIAGNOSIS The diagnosis generally can be made readily by skin biopsy. Pathognomonic changes are a floating apart of suprabasal epidermal keratinocytes. Typically, the split is just above an intact basal layer, and the cells of the roof appear to be falling down into the cleft, giving an appearance that has been described as that of "a dilapidated brick wall." Lateral connections between basal cells also may be tenuous, so that the basal cells resemble a "row of tombstones."

Although biopsies usually are taken from affected sites, similar changes may be found on biopsy of skin removed for incidental purposes, e.g., for pathologic examination of a worrisome nevus, and the acantholysis related to the physical trauma to the epidermis of the biopsy procedure. Occasionally, such Hailey-Hailey–like acanthoysis is found in patients without clinically manifest Hailey-Hailey disease, but no series has been published in which such patients were carefully examined and followed for the subsequent appearance of Hailey-Hailey lesions.

Acantholysis also is characteristic of several other diseases, but generally they can be distinguished from Hailey-Hailey disease without trouble. In addition to the autoimmune types of pemphigus discussed in Chapters 88 and 89, acantholytic blisters occasionally are found in idiosyncratic reactions to several drugs, e.g., penicillamine, captopril, and norfloxacin. No antiepithelial antibodies have been found in Hailey-Hailey disease.

GENETIC BASIS Analyses of multiple published kindreds all are consistent with an autosomal-dominant inheritance. Penetrance has been reported to be incomplete but the thoroughness of examination of apparent "skipped" individuals has not always been documented. By patient history, 16% of 58 patients in one series knew of no affected relative and therefore may represent new mutations.

Linkage analysis has localized the disease gene to an approximately 5-Mb region at chromosome 3q21. This is an area lacking in genes that encode proteins known to be involved in interkeratinocyte adhesion; e.g., none of the known desmosomal protein genes map to this site. Since inheritance of disease in at least a dozen kindreds has been reported to map to this region and since no family lacking linkage to this site has been reported, it appears likely that mutations at a single genetic locus cause all cases of Hailey-Hailey disease.

MOLECULAR PATHOPHYSIOLOGY Since the gene whose mutations cause Hailey-Hailey disease has been localized but not yet identified, it is not yet possible to describe pathophysiology. Once the gene has been cloned, it will be important to explain how mutations cause several somewhat puzzling phenotypic characteristics.

These include the relatively late, noncongenital onset, the exacerbation in the summer, the usual localization to characteristic body sites despite the ability to induce blisters experimentally (e.g., by suction) at other sites and in vitro abnormalities of keratinocytes cultured from unaffected sites, the clear (albeit inconsistent) response to therapy—both to antibiotics and corticosteroids and to resurfacing *(see below)*.

MANAGEMENT/TREATMENT Standard therapy for Hailey-Hailey disease includes antibiotics—both systemic and local—and topical steroids. Responses are inconsistent, but frequent enough to warrant their use. Stronger topical steroids often are needed, and their use in the body folds may produce striae.

Since the lesions often are localized, surgical ablation has been used. Success has been reported not only with full-thickness excision (including adnexae) but also with more superficial destruction by electrodesiccation, carbon dioxide laser vaporization, dermabrasion, or liquid nitrogen freezing. This suggests that removal merely of the interfollicular epidermis may be sufficient to render the new epithelium less abnormal. This is puzzling, since experimental data indicate that the cellular abnormality is generalized including, presumably, the resurfaced epithelium.

SELECTED REFERENCES

Burge SM, Wilkinson JD. Darier-White disease: a review of the clinical features in 163 patients. J Am Acad Derm 1992;40–50.

Beck Jr. AL, Finocchio AF. Darier's disease: a kindred with a large number. Br J Derm 1977;97:335–339.

Burge SM, Wilkinson JD, Miller AJ, Ryan TJ. The efficacy of an aromatic retinoid, Tigason (etretinate), in the treatment of inflammatory and noninflammatory dermatoses. Br J Dermatol 1981;104:675–679.

Burge SM, Garrod DR. An immunohistological study of desmosomes in Darier's disease and Hailey-Hailey disease. Br J Denn 1991;124:242–251.

Burge SM, Millard PR, et al. Hailey-Hailey disease: a widespread abnormality of cell adhesion. Brit J Derm 1991;124: 329–332.

Burge SM. Hailey-Hailey disease: the clinical features, response to treatment and prognosis. Br J Derm 1992;126:275–282.

Burge SM, Schomberg KH. Adhesion molecules and related proteins in Darier's disease and Hailey-Hailey disease. Br J Derm 1992;127: 335–343.

Caulfield JB, Wilgram GF. An electron-microscope study of dyskeratosis and acantholysis in Darier's disease. J Invest Dermatol 1979;41:57–65.

Crisp AJ, Payne Rowland CME, Adams J, et al. The prevalence of bone cysts in Darier's disease: a survey of 31 cases. Clin Experiment Derm 1984;9:78–83.

Craddock N, Owen M, Burge S, Kurian B, Thomas P, McGuffin P. Familial cosegreation of major affective-disorder and Darier's disease (keratosis follicularis). Br J Psych 1994;164:355–358.

Demetree JW, Lang PG, St. Clair JT. Unilateral, linear, zosteriform epidermal nevus with acantholytic dyskeratosis. Arch Derm 1979;115: 875–877.

Dicken CH, Bauer EA, Hazen PG, et al. Isotretinoin treatment of Darier's disease. J Am Acad Dermatol 1982;6:721–726.

Foresman PL, Goldsmith LA, Ginn L, Beck AL. Hemorrhagic Darier's Disease. Arch Derm 1993;129:511,512.

Grover RW. Transient acantholytic dermatosis. Arch Dermatol 1970;101: 426–434.

Haake AR, Bartlett R, Polakowska R, Worobec S, Goldsmith LA. Is Darier's disease a defect of the cell death pathway? J Invest Derm 1994;102:596.

Hailey H, Hailey H. Familial benign chronic pemphigus. Arch Derm Syphil 1939;39:679–685.

Hedblad MA, Nakatani T, Beitner H. Ultrastructural changes in Darier's disease induced by ultraviolet irradiation. Acta Derm Venereol 1991;71:108–112.

HogenEsch H, Gijbels MJJ, Offerman E, van Hooft J, van Bekkum DW, Zurcher C. A spontaneous mutation characterized by chronic proliferative dermatitis in C57BL mice. Am J Path 1993;143:972–982.

Ikeda S, Welsh EA et al. Localization of the gene whose mutations underlie HaileyHailey disease to chromosome 3q. Hum Molec Genet 1994;3:1147–1150.

Kirtschig G, Gieler U, et al. Treatment of Hailey-Hailey disease by dermabrasion. J Amer Acad Derm 1993;28:784–786.

Matsuoka LY, Wortsman J, McConnachie P. Renal and testicular agenesis in a patient with Darier's disease. Am J Med 1985;78:873–877.

Munro CS. The phenotype of Darier's disease: penetrance and expressivity in adults and children. Br J Dermatol 1992;127:126–130.

Peluso AM, Bonifas JM, et al. Narrowing of the Hailey-Hailey disease gene region on chromosome 3q and identification of one kindred with a deletion in this region. Genomics 1995;30:77–80.

Penrod JN, Everett MA, McCreight WG. Observations on keratosis follicularis. Arch Derm 1960;82:367–370.

Wakem P, Ikeda S, Haake A, et al. Further sublocalization of the Darier disease gene on chromosome 12q and exclusion of NOS1 as a candidate gene. J Invest Derm; 1996;106:365–367.

77 Junctional Forms of Epidermolysis Bullosa

ANGELA M. CHRISTIANO AND JOUNI UITTO

INTRODUCTION

The group of heritable genodermatoses known as epidermolysis bullosa (EB) are characterized by blistering and skin and mucous membrane fragility in response to mechanical trauma. EB is divided into three major categories based on the level of tissue separation, as determined by transmission electron microscopy. Mutations in different genes encoding proteins expressed within the layers of the dermal–epidermal adhesion zone provide the molecular basis for the wide variation in clinical phenotypes of the different subtypes of EB. In the simplex forms of EB, the tissue separation occurs within the basal keratinocytes, as a result of mutations in two genes expressed in the basal keratinocytes, *KRT5* and *KRT14*. The genetics of EB simplex are covered in detail in Chapter 73. In the dystrophic forms of EB (DEB), the tissue separation occurs below the lamina densa at the level of anchoring fibrils, attachment structures extending from the lamina densa to the upper papillary dermis. In all cases of both dominantly and recessively inherited dystrophic EB studied thus far, mutations in one gene, the type VII collagen gene *(COL7A1)*, have been shown to be pathogenetic. The molecular basis of the dystrophic forms of EB is described in depth in Chapter 78.

In contrast to the genetic homogeneity observed in EB simplex and dystrophic EB, the junctional forms of EB display a remarkable degree of genetic heterogeneity, with at least six different genes implicated in pathogenesis thus far. In junctional EB (JEB), tissue cleavage occurs within the dermal–epidermal basement membrane at the level of the lamina lucida or the overlying hemidesmosomes, and, ultrastructurally, abnormalities in the region of the hemidesmosome-anchoring filament complexes are observed. In a large number of patients with both the lethal and nonlethal forms of JEB, specific mutations have been identified in the three genes encoding the constitutive polypeptides, α3, β3, and γ2, of the anchoring filament protein, laminin 5, and, recently, mutations in the genes encoding other hemidesmosomal components have also been detected in certain subtypes of JEB. For example, mutations in the gene encoding the β4 subunit of the epithelial-cell–specific integrin, α6β4, have been detected in a patient with JEB and pyloric atresia, and mutations in the gene encoding the 180-kDa bullous pemphigoid antigen (BPAG2; also known as type XVII collagen) have been demonstrated in patients with generalized atrophic benign EB, a relatively mild variant of junctional EB. Our current understanding of the molecular basis of junctional EB, emphasizes the molecular complexity of the hemidesmosome-anchoring filament complex and its role in disease.

From: *Principles of Molecular Medicine* (J. L. Jameson, ed.), ©1998 Humana Press Inc., Totowa, NJ.

THE HEMIDESMOSOME-ANCHORING FILAMENT COMPLEX

The architecture of the entire cutaneous basement membrane zone is described in detail in Chapter 78; therefore, the focus of this discussion is restricted to the hemidesmosome-anchoring filament (HD-AF) complex. The hemidesmosomes extend from the intracellular compartment of the basal keratinocytes to the lamina lucida in the upper portion of the dermal–epidermal basement membrane. Within the lamina lucida, the hemidesmosomes complex with anchoring filaments, thread-like structures that tend to concentrate below the hemidesmosomes. Biochemical studies using isolated HDs have identified five major components of the HD, consisting of polypeptides with molecular masses of 500, 230, 200, 180, and 120 kDa, and named HD1–HD5, respectively. HD2 and HD4 are now known to be identical to the 230-kDa bullous pemphigoid antigen (BPAG1) and the 180-kDa bullous pemphigoid antigen (BPAG2/COL17A1), respectively. HD3 and HD5 correspond to the β4 and α6 integrins, respectively. HD1 has been extensively studied at the protein level and may be identical to the protein plectin, yet remains to be cloned and characterized. HD1 has been shown to localize to the cytoplasmic side of the HD, in a distribution slightly above, yet almost indistinguishable from BPAG1, at the level of the cytoplasmic periphery of the HD inner plaque. The intracellular hemidesmosomal plaque comprises the 230-kDa bullous pemphigoid antigen (BPAG1), a noncollagenous protein that serves as an autoantigen in an acquired autoimmune disease, bullous pemphigoid. The 180-kDa bullous pemphigoid antigen (BPAG2), a transmembrane collagen also known as type XVII collagen (COL17A1) extends from the intracellular compartment to the extracellular space. Associated with the hemidesmosomal proteins is the basal keratinocyte-specific integrin, α6β4, which contributes to the anchoring of basal keratinocytes to the underlying basement membrane. The anchoring filaments that traverse the lamina lucida, have been shown to consist of laminin 5, a distinct member of the laminin family of proteins. Laminin 5 consists of three constitutive subunit polypeptides, the α3, β3, and γ2 chains, which form the characteristic cross-shaped trimeric structure. Clearly, mutations resulting in abnormalities in any protein component of the HD-AF network could underlie the different forms of junctional epidermolysis bullosa.

MOLECULAR HETEROGENEITY OF JUNCTIONAL EB

The junctional forms of EB display considerable phenotypic heterogeneity, and on the basis of clinical severity, the disease can be divided into the classic, Herlitz (lethal) type, and non-Herlitz (nonlethal) forms. Within the nonlethal forms, several subtypes have been described based on the associated extracutaneous manifestations and the extent and severity of the blistering tendency. This clinical heterogeneity apparently reflects the repertoire of underlying genetic lesions demonstrated thus far in at least five different genes. More precisely, mutations in different forms of JEB have now been identified in the genes encoding the macromolecular components of the hemidesmosome-anchoring filament complex.

MOLECULAR BASIS OF HERLITZ JEB: PREMATURE TERMINATION CODON MUTATIONS IN THE LAMININ 5 GENES

Early electron-microscopic data on JEB indicated ultrastructural abnormalities in the hemidesmosome-anchoring filament complexes, in which the hemidesmosomes were rudimentary and poorly formed. In the most severe, clinically devastating Herlitz type of junctional EB (Fig. 77-1), initial immunofluorescence staining for laminin 5 epitopes suggested the absence of this protein. Subsequent to the cloning of genes encoding the three constitutive polypeptides of laminin 5, mutation-detection strategies have revealed genetic lesions in each of the three genes, (*LAMA3*, *LAMB3*, and *LAMC2*), encoding the α3, β3, and γ2 chains, respectively. The majority of these mutations have been disclosed in the *LAMB3* gene, apparently reflecting the presence of two mutational hotspots leading to recurrent mutations, R42X and R635X. Also, it should be noted that, in the lethal, Herlitz form of JEB, all mutations disclosed thus far result in premature termination codons, leading to markedly reduced levels of the corresponding mRNA transcript through a nonsense-mediated mRNA decay mechanism.

MOLECULAR BASIS OF NON-HERLITZ JEB: COMPOUND HETEROZYGOUS MUTATIONS IN THE LAMININ 5 GENES

Within the nonlethal forms of JEB, laminin 5 gene mutations have been disclosed as well. In some cases, one of the mutations is a premature termination codon in one of the laminin 5 genes. However, the other genetic lesion consists of a missense mutation or an in-frame exon-skip mutation, in cases in which mutations in both alleles have been disclosed. These observations suggest that essentially full-length polypeptides with an intact carboxy-terminal end are able to assemble into trimer molecules, which serve a partial function in the anchoring filaments. This interpretation is consistent with the observation that immunofluorescence staining with an antilaminin 5 antibody, such as GB3, is positive, although frequently attenuated, in these nonlethal JEB patients.

MOLECULAR BASIS OF THE HEMIDESMOSOMAL SUBTYPES OF JEB

Whereas the molecular basis of many of the classic forms of Herlitz and non-Herlitz JEB are now well-understood on the basis of laminin 5 mutations, there is a group of patients in whom blisters form in and around the hemidesmosome (HD), and whose ultrastructural classification and clinical severity have been referred to as "pseudojunctional." The major components of the HD, consisting of polypeptides named HD1–HD5, respectively, are likely candidates for these forms of JEB. Although there may be additional structural components of the HD, these proteins are likely candidates for mutations in some of the unusual forms of EB in which cleavage occurs at the level of the HD. Ultrastructural classification of EB has identified at least three groups of patients with EB whose blisters form at the level of the HD, and whose clinical phenotype is unlike any of the classic forms of EB. These include generalized atrophic benign epidermolysis bullosa (GABEB), epidermolysis bullosa with pyloric atresia (PA-JEB), and epidermolysis bullosa with muscular dystrophy (EB/MD). Mutations have recently been identified in three HD-associated structural proteins in patients with these forms of EB, using ultrastructural and immunofluorescence data to identify candidate genes.

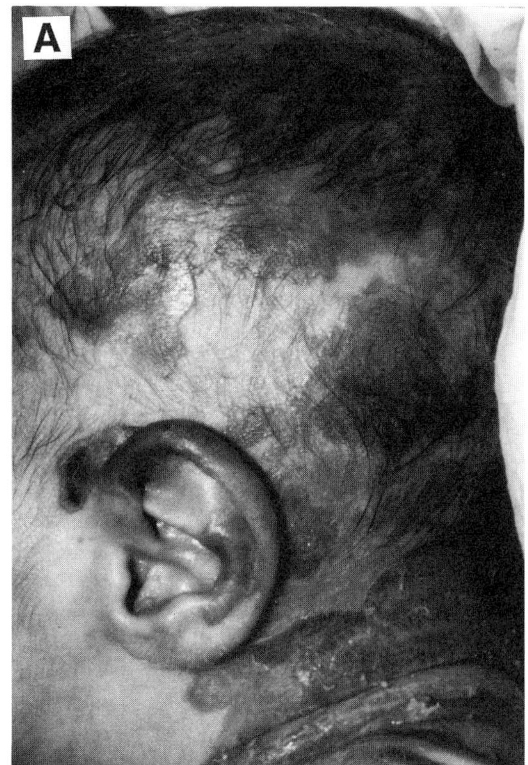

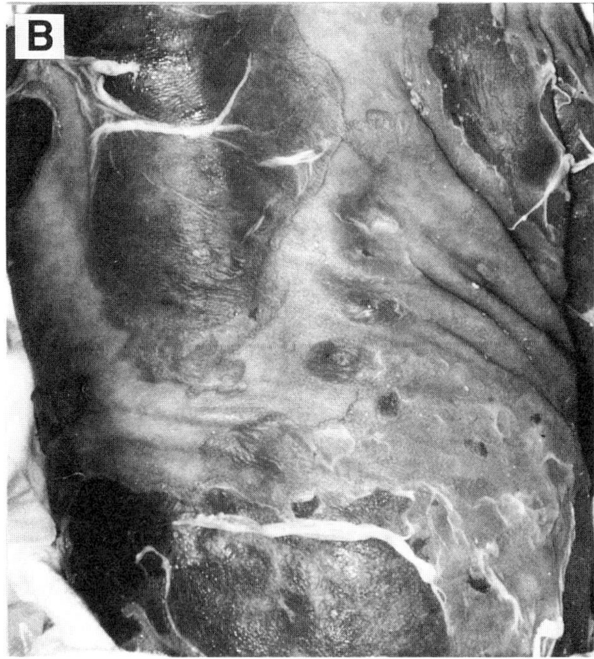

Figure 77-1 Clinical presentation of a newborn with Herlitz junctional epidermolysis bullosa. Note the widespread blistering and erosions over the neck and ears (**A**) and the back (**B**) of this affected infant.

MUTATIONS IN BPAG2 IN GENERALIZED ATROPHIC BENIGN EB

Attesting to the molecular heterogeneity of the junctional forms of EB are our recent demonstrations of specific mutations in other genes encoding structural components of the hemidesmosome-anchoring filament complex. Specifically, we have recently identified mutations in the *BPAG2* gene in a specific subset of nonlethal JEB, known as generalized atrophic benign EB. Clinically these patients demonstrate a moderately severe blistering tendency, associated with characteristic extracutaneous involvement, including dystrophy of the fingernails, focal scarring alopecia of the scalp, loss of eyelashes, dental abnormalities, and patchy macular hyperpigmentation. The first patient demonstrating genetic abnormalities in *BPAG2* had two different mutations, R1226X and 4150insG, both resulting in premature termination codons of translation; subsequently, the mutation in the original GABEB family described by Hintner and Wolff has been reported to be a premature termination codon transmitted through many branches of a large geographically inbred family. More recently, a dominantly inherited glycine substitution in *BPAG2* was identified in a GABEB family, in which the proband had inherited a premature termination codon on the second allele, whereas all carriers of the glycine substitution alone had markedly abnormal dentition and enamel pitting. Clearly, the impact of a glycine-substitution mutation in *BPAG2* also impacts upon the basement membrane of the developing tooth, a previously undisclosed function for this transmembrane collagen.

IDENTIFICATION OF β4 INTEGRIN MUTATIONS IN JEB

Yet another subtype of nonlethal JEB, a rare disorder characterized by pyloric stenosis and blistering of the skin as primary manifestations, has genetic alterations in another gene. We recently demonstrated distinct mutations in the β4 integrin gene *(ITGB4)* in a patient with this combination of clinical manifestations. The paternal mutation consisted of a 1-bp deletion causing a shift in the reading frame and premature termination codon, whereas the maternal mutation affected the donor splice site of an intron and resulted in in-frame exon skipping involving the cytoplasmic domain of the polypeptide. The phenotypic manifestation of pyloric atresia from mutations in the *ITGB4* gene suggest a tissue-specific role for this integrin both in the skin and the gastrointestinal tract.

EB AND MUSCULAR DYSTROPHY

To determine which of the candidate proteins of the HD (β4 integrin, *BPAG1*, or HD-1) is responsible for making the connection between the HD and the keratinocyte intermediate-filament network, Guo and colleagues recently reported a knockout mouse in which they targeted the ablation of *BPAG1*. Whereas the HDs in these mice were largely normal, they lacked the inner plate and demonstrated a complete severance of the connection between the HD with the intermediate-filament network. The zone of mechanical fragility of the basal keratinocytes was restricted to the region of the HD, quite distinct from the ultrastructural findings in classic EB simplex, yet strikingly similar to the cleavage plane reported in pseudojunctional EB. Unexpectedly, the *BPAG1* knockout mice also developed late-onset muscular dystonia and neurodegeneration, similar to a naturally occurring mouse, dystonia musculorum (dt). This constellation of phenotypic features together with the ultrastructural findings is remarkably consistent with the pathogenesis of EB with muscular dystrophy. On the basis of the striking similarities in the clinical phenotype of EB with muscular dystrophy and the *BPAG1* knockout mouse, it appeared likely that one of the two components of the hemidesmosomal inner plaque, *BPAG1* or HD-1, would be involved in the pathogenesis of this disorder.

HD-1 was first described as a ~500-kDa component of the hemidesmosome, and, at about the same time, an exceptionally large intermediate filament-binding protein, called plectin, was cloned from rat glioma cells. The plectin sequence has similarities to both desmoplakin and bullous pemphigoid antigen, is highly conserved between rat and human, and has a wide tissue distribution, including the central nervous system and muscle. Plectin has a remarkable number of versatile binding affinities for other proteins, including vimentin, glial fibrillary acidic protein, the neurofilament protein triplet, keratins 10 and 11, and lamin B. Although plectin is expressed in nearly all cell types, its precise cytoplasmic localization depends on the specific cell type, and it can appear diffused throughout the cell as a cytomatrix component, or in a restricted distribution as a focal adhesion protein.

Several independent lines of biochemical evidence suggest that plectin and HD-1 are the same protein, a notion confirmed by the recent cloning of human plectin. The biochemical and synthetic properties of cultured keratinocytes from patients with EB/MD using antibodies against HD-1 were studied, and plectin was found to be completely absent in the cells of several EB/MD patients. These findings strongly suggested a molecular defect in plectin/HD-1 in the pathogenesis of EB/MD, and implicated plectin/HD-1 as a novel candidate gene in the HD-AF complex. The recent definition of mutations in the plectin gene in patients with EB/MD will provide further insights into the relationship between the skin and the nervous system initially revealed by the knockout mouse, and the role of cytoskeletal and associated proteins in neurodegenerative disorders, both areas of research still in their infancy, yet of great potential scientific impact.

In summary, the junctional forms of EB reflect mutations in at least six different genes disclosed to date, and the specific clinical constellations apparently result from the combination of different types of mutations within the mutated genes (Table 77-1). Whereas the mechanism of action of these mutations has been explored at the mRNA and protein levels in many of the studies cited, the functional role of these components in HD assembly is also becoming increasingly clear through recent studies of protein–protein interactions. In the past year alone, an interaction between the 180-kDa bullous pemphigoid antigen and α6 integrin was described, the disruption of HD assembly by a tail-less β4 integrin subunit was reported, and a role for β4 integrin in signal transduction was defined. Whereas these components clearly represent functionally interdependent structural macromolecules in the dermal–epidermal adhesion zone, recent studies suggest a functionally dynamic and interactive role of some of these proteins in cell-matrix communication. Finally, it is worth noting that an extensive survey of the six genes demonstrated as candidate genes in the junctional forms of EB have thus far been negative in several families, suggesting additional, as yet undisclosed, candidate genes and uncharacterized protein components for this heterogeneous group of disorders.

APPLICATIONS OF MUTATION ANALYSIS IN PRENATAL DIAGNOSIS OF JUNCTIONAL EB

The precise understanding of the underlying mutations in junctional EB has several translational implications in terms of genetic counseling, DNA-based prenatal diagnosis, and gene therapy.

Table 77-1
Mutations in Junctional EB

Herlitz (lethal) JEB	*Consequence*	*Source*
LAMA3		
R650X/R650X	PTC/PTC	St. John's, London
R650X/R650X	PTC/PTC	St. John's, London
R650X/R650X	PTC/PTC	St. John's, London
300delG/300delG	PTC/PTC	INSERM, Nice
LAMB3		
R635X/R635X	PTC/PTC	Mayo Clinic
R635X/R635X	PTC/PTC	Seattle NEBR
R635X/R635X	PTC/PTC	St. Louis, MO
R635X/R635X	PTC/PTC	Oslo, Norway
1760delC/1760delC	PTC/PTC	INSERM, Nice
957ins77/957ins77	PTC/PTC	St. John's, London
685-1G→C/685-1G→C	PTC/PTC	Chicago, IL
Q243X/R569X	PTC/PTC	Ann Arbor, MI
R144X/R635X	PTC/PTC	Munich, Germany
1077ins77/R660X	PTC/PTC	Annandale, VA
29insC/R635X	PTC/PTC	Chicago, IL
R42X/28+2insT	PTC/PTC	Atlanta, GA
R42X/R635X	PTC/PTC	Jefferson, Philadelphia
R42X/R635X	PTC/PTC	Ann Arbor, MI
Q243X/R635X	PTC/PTC	INSERM, Nice
R635X/R635X	PTC/PTC	INSERM, Nice
R635X/R635X	PTC/PTC	INSERM, Nice
R635X/C290X	PTC/PTC	INSERM, Nice
R635X/29insC	PTC/PTC	INSERM, Nice
R635X/2910-1G→A	PTC/PTC	INSERM, Nice
R635X/R972X	PTC/PTC	INSERM, Nice
562-2A-to-G/R635X	PTC/PTC	INSERM, Nice
R635X/R635X	PTC/PTC	INSERM, Nice
Q1083X/Q1083X	PTC/PTC	INSERM, Nice
28+2insT/562-2A→G	PTC/PTC	Georgetown, Texas
R635X/R635X	PTC/PTC	Chicago, IL
Q243X/Q243X	PTC/PTC	Detroit, Michigan
R635X/R635X	PTC/PTC	St. John's, London
R42X/R42X	PTC/PTC	St. John's, London
R635X/462insT	PTC/PTC	St. John's, London
R635X/978delC	PTC/PTC	St. John's, London
R635X	PTC/?	St. John's, London
LAMC2		
Y394X/Y394X	PTC/PTC	INSERM, Nice
1070G→T/1070G→T	PTC/PTC	INSERM, Nice
R95X/R95X	PTC/PTC	INSERM, Nice
1154delT/2986+1G→A	PTC/PTC	INSERM, Nice
Nonlethal JEB	*Consequences*	*Source*
LAMB3		
R42X/E210K	PTC/Mis	St. John's London
R108X/?	PTC/?	Rockefeller NEBR
R635X/T350P	PTC/Mis	St. John's London
1367delAC	PTC/?	Chicago, Illinois
LAMC2		
2336del20→G	PTC/?	Rockefeller NEBR
1184-1G→A/1184-1G→A	Homozygous inframe exon skip	Rockefeller NEBR
BPAG2		
R1226X/4150insG	PTC/PTC	Philadelphia, PA
4003delTC/4003delTC	PTC/PTC	Salzburg, Austria
3514ins25/G627V	PTC/Mis	St. John's, London
4003 delTC/G803X	PTC/Mis	Salzburg, Austria
4003 delTC/Q1403X	PTC/PTC	Salzburg, Austria
JEB-Pyloric Atresia	*Consequence*	*Source*
β4 Integrin		
1150delC/3801+2insT	PTC/ in frame exon skip	INSERM, Nice

Most immediately relevant to patient care is the development of DNA-based prenatal diagnosis, which can be performed as early as the 10th week of gestation through chorionic villus sampling, or at the 12–15th week of gestation through amniocentesis. Because of the extensive underlying genetic heterogeneity in the junctional forms of EB, prenatal diagnosis must be based on direct demonstration of the presence or absence of both mutations, since at least seven different genes can harbor the genetic lesion in different forms of JEB, and *de novo* hotspot mutations have been observed. These approaches have been applied to DNA-based prenatal diagnosis in a number of families at risk for recurrence of Herlitz JEB. The genetic information also provides the basis for development of preimplantation diagnosis through blastomere analysis, a technological advance that would obviate the necessity of termination of the pregnancy in case of an affected fetus, if elected.

GENE THERAPY APPROACHES FOR JUNCTIONAL EB

Precise understanding of the underlying mutations, and subsequent demonstration of the functional consequences of such mutations at the mRNA and protein levels, are prerequisites for the development of gene therapy approaches for this group of devastating skin diseases. Whereas the lethal Herlitz form of JEB may represent an ensemble of unrealistic clinical challenges, we believe that several forms of JEB are realistic targets for genetic therapies, including the nonlethal forms of junctional EB, such as GABEB. Introduction of the relatively small wild-type cDNAs for BPAG2 and ITGB4 into patient keratinocytes, by *ex vivo* and in vivo methods, is more likely to be successful than for larger mRNAs, when these techniques become the standard of care for JEB in the future. Whereas the genetic basis of junctional EB is still a work in progress, and we still have much to learn about the HD-AF complex, the immediate benefits of this work have provided prenatal diagnosis for families at risk for recurrence, and, importantly, the foundation for development of gene therapy approaches to counteract JEB at the level of the molecular defect.

ACKNOWLEDGMENTS

We gratefully acknowledge the participation of the many clinicians and scientists who contributed to the original studies summarized in this review, especially John A. McGrath, Leena Pulkkinen, WH Irwin McLean, and Sirpa Kivirikko. The original studies by the authors were supported by USPHS, NIH grants PO1-AR38923 and T32-AR07561 (JU), and R29-AR43602, and the March of Dimes Birth Defects Foundation (AMC). Angela M. Christiano was the recipient of The Society for Investigative Dermatology Research Career Development Award from the Dermatology Foundation.

SELECTED REFERENCES

Aberdam D, Galliano MF, Vailly J, et al. Herlitz's junctional epidermolysis bullosa is linked to mutations in the gene (LAMC2) for the γ2 subunit of nicein/kalinin (laminin-5). Nature Genet 1994;6:299–304.

Baudoin C, Miquel C, Gagnoux-Palacois L, et al. A novel homozygous nonsense mutation in the LAMC2 gene in patients with the Herlitz junctional epidermolysis bullosa. Hum Mol Genet 1994;3:1909,1910.

Baudoin C, Miquel C, Blanchet-Bardon C, Gambini C, Meneguzzi G, Ortonne J-P. Herlitz junctional epidermolysis bullosa keratinocytes display heterogeneous defects of nicein/kalinin gene expression. J Clin Invest 1994;93:862–869.

Brown A, Copeland NG, Gilbert DJ, Jenkins NA, Rossant J, Kothary R. The genomic structure of an insertional mutation in the *dystonia musculorum* locus. Genomics 1994;20:371–376.

Brown A, Bernier G, Mathieu M, Rossant J, Kothary R. The mouse *dystonia musculorum* gene is a neural isoform of bullous pemphigoid antigen 1. Nature Genet 1995;10:301–306.

Burgeson RE, Chiquet M, Deutzmann R, et al. A new nomenclature for laminins. Matrix Biol 1994;14:209–211.

Carter WG, Kaur P, Gil SG, Gahr PJ, Wayner EA. Distinct functions for integrins α3β1 in focal adhesions and α6β4/bullous pemphigoid antigen in a new stable anchoring contact (SAC) of keratinocytes: relation to hemidesmosomes. J Cell Biol 1990;111:3141–3154.

Chavanas S, Gache Y, Tadini G, et al. A homozygous in-frame deletion in the collagenous domain of bullous pemphigoid antigen BP180 (type XVII collagen) causes generalized atrophic benign epidermolysis bullosa. J Invest Dermatol 1977;109:74–78.

Christiano AM, Uitto J. Molecular genetic diagnosis of blistering skin diseases: impact on dystrophic epidermolysis bullosa. Curr Opin in Derm 1996;3:225–232.

Christiano AM, Uitto J. Molecular diagnosis of inherited skin disorders: the paradigm of dystrophic epidermolysis bullosa. Advances in Dermatol 1996;11:199–214.

Christiano AM, Uitto J. Molecular complexity of the cutaneous basement membrane zone: revelations from the paradigms of epidermolysis bullosa. Exp Dermatol 1996;5:1–11.

Christiano AM, Pulkkinen L, McGrath JA, Uitto J. Mutation-based prenatal diagnosis of Herlitz junctional epidermolysis bullosa. Prenat Diagn 1997;17:343–354.

Christiano AM, Uitto J. Prenatal and preimplantation diagnosis of genetic skin diseases. Arch Derm 1993;129:1455–1459.

Diaz L, Ratrie H III, Saunders W, et al. Isolation of a human epidermal cDNA corresponding to the 180-kD autoantigen recognized by bullous pemphigoid and herpes gestationis sera: immunolocalization of this protein to the hemidesmosome. J Clin Invest 1990;86:1088–1094.

Eady RAJ, McGrath JA, McMillan J. Ultrastructural clues to genetic disorders of skin: the dermal-epidermal junction. J Invest Dermatol 1994;03:13S–18S.

Eady RAJ, Leigh IM, McMillan JR, et al. Epidermolysis bullosa simplex with muscular dystrophy: loss of plectin expression in skin and muscle. J Invest Dermatol 1996;106:842.

Epstein Jr EH. Molecular genetics of epidermolysis bullosa. Science 1992;256:799–803.

Fenjves ES. Approaches to gene transfer in keratinocytes. J Invest Dermatol 1994;103:70S–75S.

Fine JD, Stenn J, Johnson L, Wright T, Bock HGO, Horiguchi, Y. Autosomal recessive epidermolysis bullosa simplex: generalized phenotypic features suggestive of junctional or dystrophic epidermolysis bullosa, and association with neuromuscular diseases. Arch Dermatol 1989;125:931–938.

Fine J-D, Bauer EA, Briggman RA, et al. Revised clinical and laboratory criteria for subtypes of inherited epidermolysis bullosa: a consensus report by the subcommittee on diagnosis and classification of the national epidermolysis bullosa registry. J Am Acad Dermatol 1991;24:119–135.

Fuchs E. Genetic skin disorders of keratin. J Invest Dermatol 1992;99: 671–674.

Gache Y, Chavanas S, Lacour JP, et al. Defective expression of plectin in epidermolysis bullosa simplex with muscular dystrophy. J Invest Dermatol 1996;106:842.

Garrod, DR. Desmosomes and hemidesmosomes. Curr Opin Cell Biol 1993;5:30–40.

Giudice GJ, Emery DJ, Diaz LA. Cloning and primary structural analysis of the bullous pemphigoid autoantigen BP180. J Invest Dermatol 1992;99:243–250.

Goldman JE, Yen SH. Cytoskeletal protein abnormalities in neurodegenerative diseases. Ann Neurol 1986;19: 209–223.

Guo L, Degenstein L, Dowling J, et al. Gene targeting of BPAG1: abnormalities in mechanical strength and cell migration in stratified epithelia and neurologic degeneration. Cell 1995;81:233–243.

Hieda Y, Nishizawa Y, Uematsu J, Owaribe K. Identification of a new hemidesmosomal protein, HD1: a major, high molecular mass component of isolated hemidesmosomes. J Cell Biol 1992;116:1497–1506.

Hintner H, Wolff K. Generalized atrophic benign epidermolysis bullosa. Arch Dermatol 1982;118:375–384.

Hopkinson SB, Baker SE, Jones JCR. Molecular genetic studies of a human epidermal autoantigen (the 180-kD bullous pemphigoid antigen/BP180): identification of functionally important sequences within the BP180 molecule and evidence for an interaction between BP180 and alpha 6 integrin. J Cell Biol 1995;130:117–125.

Hynes RO. Integrins: versality, modulation, and signaling in cell adhesion. Cell 1992;69:11–25.

Jones JCR, Asmuth J, Baker SE, Langhofer M, Roth SI, Hopkinson SB. Hemidesmosomes: extracellular matrix/intermediate filament connectors. Exp Cell Res 1994;213:1–11.

Kivirikko S, McGrath JA, Baudoin C, et al. A homozygous nonsense mutation in the α3 chain gene of laminin 5 (LAMA3) in lethal (Herlitz) junctional epidermolysis bullosa. Hum Mol Genet 1995;4:959–962.

Kivirikko S, McGrath JA, Pulkkinen L, Uitto J, Christiano A. Mutational hotspots in the LAMB3 gene in the lethal (Herlitz) type of junctional epidermolysis bullosa. Hum Mol Genet 1996;2:231–237.

Li K, Tamai K, Tan EML, Uitto J. Cloning of type XVII collagen: complementary and genomic DNA sequences of mouse 180-kilodalton bullous pemphigoid antigen (BPAG2) predict an interrupted collagenous domain, a transmembrane segment, and unusual features in the 5'-end of the gene and the 3'-untranslated region of the mRNA. J Biol Chem 1993;268:8825–8834.

Li K, Giudice GJ, Tamai K, et al. Cloning of partial cDNA for mouse 180-kDa bullous pemphigoid antigen (BPAG2), a highly conserved collagenous protein of the cutaneous basement membrane zone. J Invest Dermatol 1992;99:258–263.

Lin AN, Carter DM, eds. Epidermolysis Bullosa. Basic and Clinical Aspects. New York: Springer-Verlag, 1992.

Mainiero F, Pepe A, Wary KK, et al. Signal transduction by the α6β4 integrin: distinct β4 subunit sites mediate recruitment of Shc/Grb2 and association with the cytoskeleton of hemidesmosomes. EMBO 1995;14:4470–4481.

Masunaga T, Shimizu H, Yee C, et al. The extracellular domain of BPAG2 localizes to anchoring filaments and its carboxyl terminus extends to the lamina densa of normal human epidermal basement membrane. J Invest Dermatol 1997;109:200–206.

McLean WHI, Smith FJD, Rugg EL, et al. Cloning and sequencing of the human plectin gene. J Invest Dermatol 1996;106:843.

McGrath JA, Gatalica B, Christiano AM, et al. Mutations in the 180-kD bullous pemphigoid antigen (BPAG2), a hemidesmosomal transmembrane collagen (COL17A1), in generalized atrophic benign epidermolysis bullosa. Nature Genet 1995;11:83–86.

McGrath JA, Christiano AM, Pulkkinen L, Eady RAJ, Uitto J. Compound heterozygosity for nonsense and missense mutations in the LAMB3 gene in non-lethal junctional epidermolysis bullosa. J Invest Dermatol 1996;106:775–777.

McGrath JA, Darling, T, Gatalica B, et al. A homozygous deletion mutation in the 180kD bullous pemphigoid antigen gene (BPAG2) in a family with generalized atrophic benign epidermolysis bullosa. J Invest Dermatol 1996;106:771–774.

McGrath JA, Gatalica B, Li K, et al. Compound heterozygosity for a dominant glycine substitution and a recessive internal duplication mutation in the type XVII collagen gene results in junctional epidermolysis bullosa and abnormal dentition. Am J Path 1996;148: 1787–1796.

McGrath J, McMillan J, Dunhill MGS, et al. Genetic basis of lethal junctional epidermolysis bullosa in an affected fetus: Implications for prenatal diagnosis in one family. Prenat Diag 1995;15:647–654.

McGrath JA, Ishida-Yamamoto A, O'Grady A, Leigh IM, Eady RAJ. Structural variations in anchoring fibrils in dystrophic epidermolysis bullosa: correlation with type VII collagen expression. J Invest Dermatol 1993;100:366–372.

McGrath JA, Pulkkinen L, Christiano AM, Leigh IM, Eady RAJ, Uitto J. Altered laminin 5 expression due to mutations in the gene encoding the β3 chain (LAMB3) in generalized atrophic benign epidermolysis bullosa. J Invest Dermatol 1995;104:467–474.

Meneguzzi G, Marinkovich MP, Aberdam D, Pisani A, Burgeson R, Ortonne J-P. Kalinin is abnormally expressed in epithelial basement membranes of Herlitz's junctional epidermolysis bullosa patients. Exp Derm 1992;1:221–229.

Messer A, Strominger NL. An allele of the mouse mutant dystonia musculorum exhibits lesions in red nucleus and striatum. Neuroscience 1980;5:543–549.

Niemi K-M, Sommer H, Kero M, Kanerva L, Haltia M. Epidermolysis bullosa simplex associated with muscular dystrophy with recessive inheritance. Arch Dermatol 1988;124:551–554.

Pulkkinen L, Christiano AM, Airenne T, Haakana H, Tryggvason K, Uitto J. Mutations in the γ2 chain gene (LAMC2) of kalinin/laminin 5 in the junctional forms of epidermolysis bullosa. Nature Genet 1994;6:293–298.

Pulkkinen L, Christiano AM, Gerecke D, et al. A homozygous nonsense mutation in the β3 chain gene of laminin 5 (LAMB3) in Herlitz junctional epidermolysis bullosa. Genomics 1994;24:357–360.

Pulkkinen L, Meneguzzi G, McGrath JA, et al. Predominance of the recurrent mutation R635 X in the LAMB3 gene in European patients with Herlitz junctional epidermolysis bullosa has implications for mutation detection strategy. J Invest Dermatol 1977;109:232–237.

Rousselle P, Lunstrum GP, Keene DR, Burgeson RE. Kalinin: an epithelium-specific basement membrane adhesion molecule that is a component of anchoring filaments. J Cell Biol 1991;114:567–576.

Sawamura D, Li K, Chu M-L, Uitto J. Human bullous pemphigoid antigen (BPAG1): amino acid sequences deduced from cloned cDNAs predict biologically important peptide segments and protein domains. J Biol Chem 1991;266:17,784–17,790.

Smith LT. Ultrastructural findings in epidermolysis bullosa. Arch Dermatol 1993;129:1578–1584.

Sotelo C, Guenet JL. Pathologic changes in the CNS of *dystonia musculorum* mutant mouse: an animal model for human spinocerebellar ataxia. Neuroscience 1988;27:403–424.

Spinardi L, Einheber T, Cullen T, Milner TA, Giancotti FG. A recombinant tail-less integrin β4 subunit disrupts hemidesmosomes, but does not suppress α6β4-mediated cell adhesion to laminins. J Cell Biol 1995;129:473–487.

Stanley JR, Hawley-Nelson P, Yuspa SH, Shevach EM, Katz SI. Characterization of bullous pemphigoid antigen: a unique basement membrane protein of stratified squamous epithelia. Cell 1981;24:897–903.

Stepp MA, Spurr-Michaud S, Tisdale A, Elwell J, Gipson IK. α6β4 integrin heterodimer is a component of hemidesmosomes. Proc Natl Acad Sci USA 1990;87:8970–8974.

Timpl R, Brown J. The laminins. Matrix Biol 1994;14:275–281.

Uitto J, Pulkkinen L, Smith FJ, McLean WHI. Plectin and human genetic disorders of the skin and muscle. The paradigm of epidermolysis bullosa with muscular dystrophy. Exp Dermatol 1996;5:237–246.

Uitto J, Amano S, McGrath JA, et al. Absent expression of the hemidesmosomal inner plaque protein HD-1 and its cell biological consequences in epidermolysis bullosa with muscular dystrophy. J Invest Dermatol 1996;106:842.

Vailly J, Pulkkinen L, Christiano AM, et al. Identification of a homozygous exon-skipping mutation in the LAMC2 gene in a patient with Herlitz's junctional epidermolysis bullosa. J Invest Dermatol 1995; 104:434–437.

Vailly J, Pulkkinen L, Miquel C, et al. Identification of a homozygous one basepair deletion in exon 14 of the LAMB3 gene in a patient with Herlitz junctional epidermolysis bullosa and prenatal diagnosis in a family at risk for recurrence. J Invest Dermatol 1995;104:462–466.

Verrando P, Blanchet-Bardon C, Pisani A, et al. Monoclonal antibody GB3 defines a widespread defect of several basement membranes and keratinocyte dysfunction in patients with lethal junctional epidermolysis bullosa. Lab Invest 1991;64:85–92.

Verrando P, Schofield O, Ishida-Yamamoto A, et al. Nicein (BM-600) in junctional epidermolysis bullosa: Polyclonal antibodies provide new clues for pathogenic role. J Invest Dermatol 1993;101:738–743.

Weiss DJ, Fried GW. Epidermolysis bullosa simplex associated with spinal muscular atrophy. Int J Dermatol 1993;32:589–593.

Wiche G, Becker B, Luber K, et al. Cloning and sequence of rat plectin indicates a 466-kD polypeptide chain with a three-domain structure based on a central alpha-helical coiled coil. J Cell Biol 1991;114:83–99.

Yerlinsky Y, Kuliev AM. Preimplantation Diagnosis of Genetic Diseases. A New Technique in Assisted Reproduction. New York: Wiley-Liss, 1993; pp. 1–144.

78 The Dystrophic Forms of Epidermolysis Bullosa

JOUNI UITTO AND ANGELA M. CHRISTIANO

INTRODUCTION

Significant progress has recently been made in understanding the structural features of the epidermis and dermal–epidermal junction, largely through molecular cloning of genes that encode proteins critical for the structural integrity of the cutaneous layers. Disturbances in the expression of the genes within the stratified layers of the dermal–epidermal adhesion zone provide the basis for different forms of heritable blistering skin diseases with divergent clinical presentation (Fig. 78-1).

MOLECULAR COMPLEXITY OF THE CUTANEOUS BASEMENT MEMBRANE ZONE

Electron-microscopic examination of the cutaneous basement-membrane zone (BMZ) reveals the presence of several attachment structures, critical for integrity of the stable association of epidermis and dermis (Fig. 78-1). These include hemidesmosomes that extend from the intracellular compartment of the basal keratinocytes to the lamina lucida in the upper portion of the dermal–epidermal basement membrane. Within the lamina lucida, the hemidesmosomes complex with anchoring filaments, thread-like structures that tend to concentrate below the hemidesmosomes. At the lower portion of the dermal–epidermal attachment zone, fibrillar structures known as anchoring fibrils extend from the lamina densa of the basement membrane to the papillary dermis, where they associate with basement-membrane-like structures known as anchoring plaques.

Recent molecular cloning of the cutaneous BMZ components has allowed elucidation of the structural features of the macromolecules, which constitute these dermal–epidermal attachment structures. Specifically, hemidesmosomes have been shown to consist of at least four distinct proteins. The intracellular hemidesmosomal inner plaque comprises at least two proteins, the 230-kDa bullous pemphigoid antigen (BPAG1), a noncollagenous protein that serves as an autoantigen in an acquired autoimmune disease, bullous pemphigoid; and HD1, a ~500-kDa protein belonging to the plectin family of adhesion molecules. Extending from the intracellular compartment to the extracellular space is the 180-kDa bullous pemphigoid antigen (BPAG2), a transmembrane collagenous protein, also known as type XVII collagen (COL17A1). Associated with these hemidesmosomal proteins is the basal keratinocyte-specific integrin, $\alpha 6\beta 4$, which contributes to the anchoring of basal keratinocytes to the underlying basement membrane.

The anchoring filaments, which traverse the lamina lucida, have been shown to consist of laminin 5, a distinct member of the laminin family of proteins. Laminin 5 consists of three constitutive subunit polypeptides, the $\alpha 3$, $\beta 3$, and $\gamma 2$ chains, which form the characteristic cross-shaped trimeric structure.

Early biochemical data at the protein level suggested that type VII collagen is the major, if not the exclusive, component of anchoring fibrils. Recently, type VII collagen primary structure has been elucidated through cDNA cloning, and the intron–exon organization of the entire gene has been determined.

Collectively, the data summarized above indicate that the cutaneous basement-membrane zone is a complex continuum of macromolecules that form a network providing the stable association of the epidermis to the underlying dermis. Thus, genetic lesions resulting in abnormalities in any component of this network could result in a blistering skin disease, such as the different forms of epidermolysis bullosa.

MOLECULAR BASIS OF DIFFERENT FORMS OF EPIDERMOLYSIS BULLOSA

The prototype of the diseases affecting the cutaneous BMZ is epidermolysis bullosa (EB), a group of heritable mechanobullous disorders, that manifest with considerable variability in clinical severity. Also, genetic heterogeneity is evident, and both autosomal dominant and autosomal recessive forms of EB can be recognized. Epidermolysis bullosa can be divided into three major categories based on the level of tissue separation as established by diagnostic transmission electron microscopy. In the simplex forms of EB, the tissue separation occurs within the basal keratinocytes, as a result of mutations in the basal keratin genes, *KRT5* and *KRT14*. In the junctional forms of EB, the tissue cleavage occurs within the dermal–epidermal basement membrane at the level of the lamina lucida, and ultrastructurally, the junctional forms demonstrate abnormalities in the hemidesmosome-anchoring filament complexes. In patients with the junctional forms of EB, specific mutations have been identified in the three genes encoding the constitutive polypeptides, $\alpha 3$, $\beta 3$, and $\gamma 2$, of the anchoring-filament protein, laminin 5. In addition, mutations in the genes encod-

From: *Principles of Molecular Medicine* (J. L. Jameson, ed.), ©1998 Humana Press Inc., Totowa, NJ.

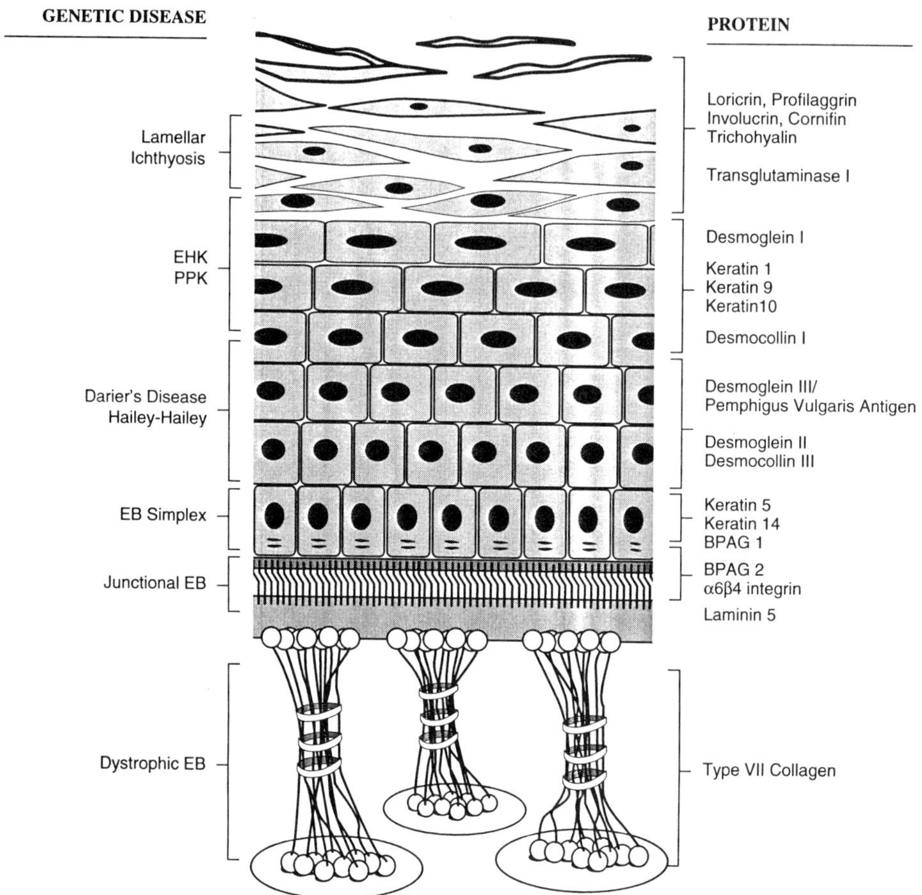

Figure 78-1 Schematic representation of the epidermis and the underlying cutaneous basement membrane zone at the dermal–epidermal junction. The skin layers affected in genetic skin diseases are indicated on the left, and the specific gene products are listed on the right. Note that tissue separation in the dystrophic forms of epidermolysis bullosa (EB) occurs below the basement membrane within the upper papillary dermis, at the level of anchoring fibrils, which consist of type VII collagen. EHK, epidermolytic hyperkeratosis; PPK, palmoplantar keratoderma; BPAG, bullous pemphigoid antigen. (Modified from Christiano AM, Uitto J. Molecular diagnosis of inherited skin disorders: the paradigm of dystrophic epidermolysis bullosa. Advances Derm 1996;11:199–213.)

ing the hemidesmosomal components have also been detected in certain subtypes of junctional EB, including mutations in the gene encoding the β4 subunit of the α6β4 integrin, and the gene encoding the 180-kDa bullous pemphigoid antigen, BPAG2, also known as type XVII collagen. (For details on the junctional forms of EB, *see* Chapter 77.)

In the dystrophic forms of EB (DEB), the tissue separation occurs below the lamina densa at the level of anchoring fibrils, critical attachment structures extending from the lamina densa to the upper papillary dermis. This chapter will illustrate the power of molecular diagnosis of blistering skin diseases by reviewing recent revelations into the molecular basis of the dystrophic forms of EB.

THE DYSTROPHIC FORMS OF EB: SPECTRUM OF CLINICAL SEVERITY

The dystrophic forms of EB (DEB), which can be inherited in either an autosomal-dominant or autosomal-recessive pattern, demonstrate extensive variability in the clinical spectrum of severity. The less severe forms, such as dominantly inherited dystrophic EB (DDEB) or the mitis type of recessively inherited DEB (RDEB), are characterized by a significant blistering tendency, but they lack the extensive mutilating scarring that is the hallmark of the severe, generalized, Hallopeau-Siemens (HS-RDEB) type of recessive dystrophic EB. In addition to cutaneous manifestations, the dystrophic forms, particularly HS-RDEB, are associated with scarring of the esophagus and corneal erosions. The combination of cutaneous and extracutaneous manifestations is associated with considerable morbidity and mortality in the most severely affected patients.

MOLECULAR GENETICS OF DYSTROPHIC EB

Several lines of evidence initially suggested that the type VII collagen gene (*COL7A1*) is the candidate gene for mutations in the dystrophic forms of EB. First, the ultrastructural diagnostic hallmark of the dystrophic forms of EB is abnormalities in anchoring fibrils, attachment structures that are composed predominantly, if not exclusively, of type VII collagen. The anchoring fibrils can be shown by transmission electron microscopy to be morphologically abnormal, reduced in number, or even completely absent. Secondly, these ultrastructural observations are reflected by changes in the immunofluorescence pattern when anti–type VII antibodies are used for staining of the skin. In normal individuals, type VII collagen epitopes are readily evident in a linear pattern at the dermal–epidermal junction, whereas in generalized HS-RDEB patients, the immunostaining is entirely negative. In dominantly

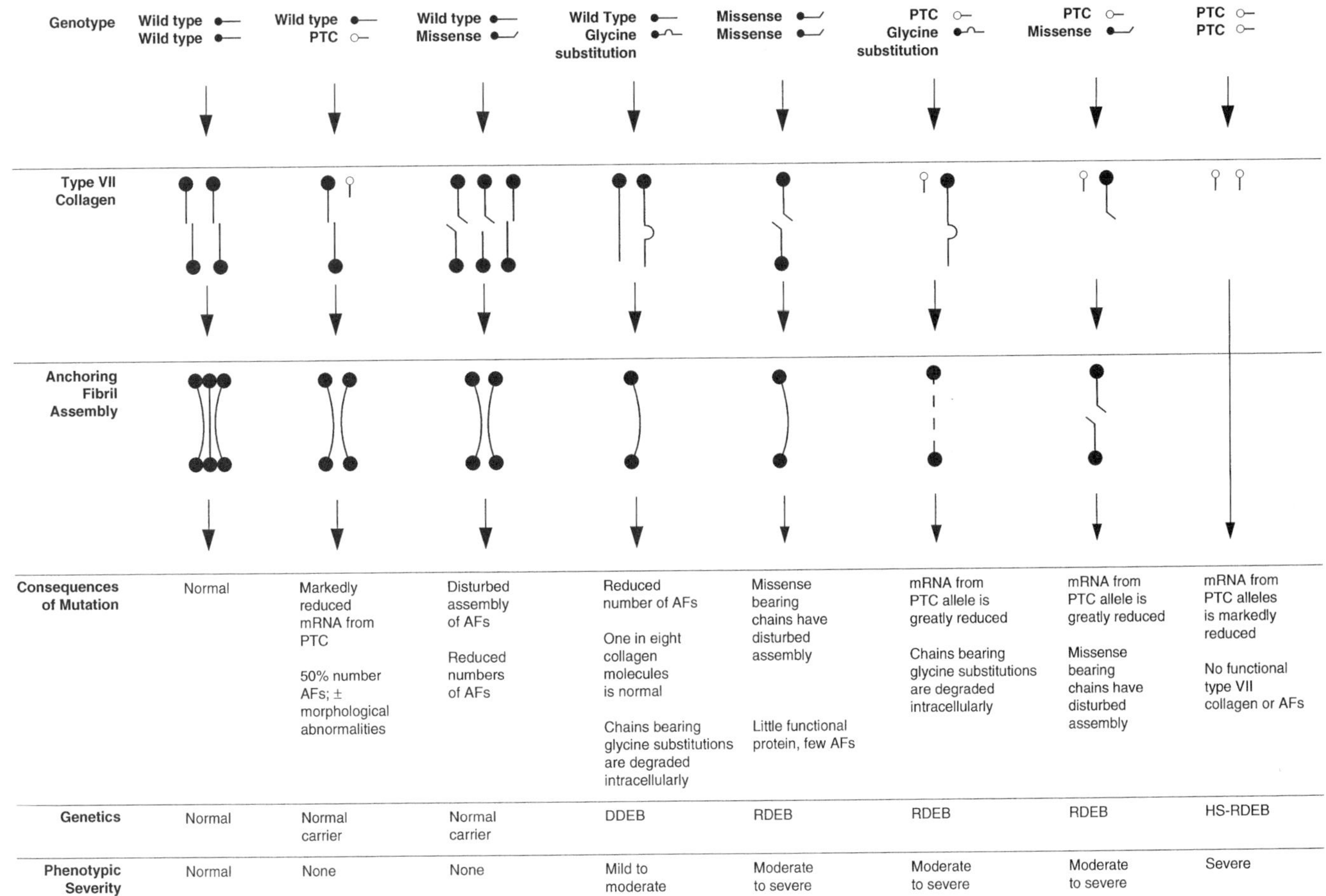

Genotype
Wild type Wild type
Wild type PTC
Wild type Missense
Wild Type Glycine substitution
Missense Missense
PTC Glycine substitution
PTC Missense
PTC PTC
Type VII Collagen
Anchoring Fibril Assembly
Consequences of Mutation
Normal
Markedly reduced mRNA from PTC
50% number AFs; ± morphological abnormalities
Disturbed assembly of AFs
Reduced numbers of AFs
Reduced number of AFs
One in eight collagen molecules is normal
Chains bearing glycine substitutions are degraded intracellularly
Missense bearing chains have disturbed assembly
Little functional protein, few AFs
mRNA from PTC allele is greatly reduced
Chains bearing glycine substitutions are degraded intracellularly
mRNA from PTC allele is greatly reduced
Missense bearing chains have disturbed assembly
mRNA from PTC alleles is markedly reduced
No functional type VII collagen or AFs
Genetics
Normal
Normal carrier
Normal carrier
DDEB
RDEB
RDEB
RDEB
HS-RDEB
Phenotypic Severity
Normal
None
None
Mild to moderate
Moderate to severe
Moderate to severe
Moderate to severe
Severe

Figure 78-2 Schematic representation of genotype-phenotype correlations based on delineation of mutations in the type VII collagen gene in different subtypes of dystrophic epidermolysis bullosa. (Modified from Christiano AM, Uitto J. Molecular diagnosis of inherited skin disorders: the paradigm of dystrophic epidermolysis bullosa. Advances Derm 1996;11:199–213.)

inherited DEB, the immunostaining reveals a near-normal pattern, whereas in the mitis forms of RDEB, the intensity of the staining can be attenuated, although clearly positive. These ultrastructural and immunofluorescent findings suggested that type VII collagen was a candidate gene for mutations in the dystrophic forms of EB. This suggestion was subsequently strengthened by demonstration of genetic linkage between the *COL7A1* locus on chromosome 3p21, and both the dominantly and recessively inherited forms of DEB.

Recent cloning of the human type VII collagen cDNA sequences has allowed us to deduce the normal structure of type VII collagen polypeptides. Cloning and elucidation of the intron–exon organization of the entire human type VII collagen gene has revealed that the gene is highly complex, consisting of a total of 118 exons, the largest number of exons in any gene reported thus far. However, *COL7A1* is relatively compact, and the exons are contained within ~32 kbp of genomic DNA. The elucidation of the intron–exon organization of *COL7A1* has provided necessary information to undertake mutation analysis of this gene in families with DEB. In fact, specific mutations have now been disclosed in over 100 kindreds with different forms of DEB.

GENOTYPE/PHENOTYPE CORRELATIONS IN DEB

The wealth of information on specific mutations in different forms of DEB allows us to begin to establish genotype–phenotype relationships. In normal skin, type VII collagen molecules form antiparallel dimers that associate through their overlapping carboxy-terminal ends. This association is stabilized by interchain disulfide bonds, and such stable type VII collagen molecules laterally aggregate to form anchoring fibrils. Thus, following the synthesis of type VII collagen, several critical steps are required for proper assembly of anchoring fibrils. Consequently, mutations affecting the synthesis of type VII collagen at the transcriptional or translational level, or those interfering with its supramolecular assembly to anchoring fibrils can result in DEB phenotype (Fig. 78-2).

SEVERE, MUTILATING HS-RDEB: PREMATURE TERMINATION CODON MUTATIONS IN COL7A1

In a number of HS-RDEB patients in whom both mutations have been disclosed thus far, the consistent genetic lesion is a premature termination codon (PTC) in both alleles of the affected individual. The major effect of a PTC mutation is reduction in mRNA abundance as a result of nonsense-mediated mRNA decay. This phenomenon appears to be coupled to the splicing process itself, since the levels of unspliced, heteronuclear RNA (hnRNA) are equivalent for both the mutant and wild-type alleles, and the decay is evident only upon comparison of processed mRNA. The PTCs result in perturbations in synthesis of type VII collagen mRNAs at the transcriptional level, which are then unable to provide templates for translation of functional polypeptides. Even if the mutant allele containing a PTC is expressed at reduced levels, the translated protein is truncated at its carboxy-terminus and is unable to assemble into anchoring fibrils. These interpretations are consistent with the ultrastructural demonstration of complete absence of the anchoring fibrils in HS-RDEB, which explains the extreme fragility of the skin, so characteristic of this phenotype (Fig. 78-2).

MILD RDEB: MISSENSE AND INFRAME DELETION MUTATIONS

In the mitis forms of RDEB, at least one, and possibly both, alleles encode for a full-length type VII collagen polypeptide. However, this allele usually contains a missense mutation that can change the conformation of the protein in a manner that anchoring-fibril assembly is perturbed. In some cases, one allele contains a missense mutation or in-frame deletion, whereas the second allele contains a PTC. The net result of the latter combination of mutations is a reduction in mutant RNA from the PTC allele at the transcriptional level, together with a mutation on the second allele, which is transcribed and presumably translated normally, yet is likely to impact on nucleation and assembly of anchoring fibrils. As a result of these more subtle mutations combined with a PTC on the other allele, mutant full-length type VII collagen molecules may be able to assemble into anchoring fibrils, which are, however, unlikely to be stabilized by disulfide bonding (Fig. 78-2). Thus, these attachment structures, although present, are weakened, resulting in moderately severe fragility of the skin, as observed in the mitis forms of RDEB.

DOMINANT DYSTROPHIC EB: GLYCINE SUBSTITUTION MUTATIONS

In the dominantly inherited forms of EB, the recurrent mutation detected thus far is the substitution of a glycine residue that occurs within the collagenous domain of the molecule characterized by the repeating Gly-X-Y amino acid sequence. Some of these nonfunctional molecules are able to associate with type VII collagen synthesized from the normal allele, through a mechanism known as dominant-negative interference. The glycine substitutions destabilize the collagen triple helix, interfere with the secretion of the molecules, and render them susceptible to intracellular degradation, thus exerting their effect at the posttranslational level. Since type VII collagen is a homotrimer consisting of three identical α1(VII) polypeptides, one out of eight triple-helical molecules (12.5%) is entirely normal, assuming equal expression of the mutant and wild-type alleles. As a result, some normal anchoring fibrils can be formed, consistent with ultrastructural demonstration of thin anchoring fibrils and the relatively mild clinical phenotype in DDEB. In addition to the classical forms of DDEB, we have recently demonstrated glycine substitution mutations in two clinical variants, known as pretibial DEB and Bart's syndrome, proving that these subtypes are indeed allelic to DDEB with mutations in COL7A1.

Collectively, the type and combination of mutations are able to predict, in general terms, the clinical severity and natural history of the disease. Since clinical severity represents a continuum in the spectrum of manifestations, the precise nature of the genetic lesions, their positions along the type VII collagen gene, and the dynamic interplay of the two mutant alleles on the individual's genetic background will determine the precise phenotype of the patient.

REVISIONS IN GENETIC COUNSELING IN DYSTROPHIC EB

As indicated above, the dystrophic forms of EB can be inherited either in an autosomal-dominant or autosomal-recessive fashion. The diagnosis of classic HS-RDEB in a patient with severe, mutilating scarring, with clinically unaffected parents, is usually made without difficulty. Similarly, inheritance of a blistering tendency and a relatively mild scarring phenotype in a vertical pattern, with multiple affected family members in several generations, allows unequivocal diagnosis of dominantly inherited DEB.

The difficulties arise during the diagnosis and ascertainment of the inheritance pattern in patients with a relatively mild phenotype and clinically normal parents. By ultrastructural analyses, these patients often demonstrate the presence, but a reduced number, of anchoring fibrils. Consequently, these cases are often diagnosed as dominant DEB, presumed to be caused by a new dominant mutation or parental germline mosaicism. This diagnosis obviously has serious implications in terms of genetic counseling of the affected individuals. If their disease is truly a new dominant mutation, the risk of their offspring being affected is one in two. In contrast, in case of a recessively inherited disease, the risk of their offspring being affected is approximately as low as in the general population, with the exception of consanguineous matings.

Careful determination of the genotype and mutation analysis of several patients with relatively mild disease and ultrastructurally detectable anchoring fibrils with positive immunofluorescence staining for type VII collagen, has demonstrated that many of them are compound heterozygotes or have homozygous missense mutations inherited in a recessive manner. For example, the first demonstration of type VII collagen mutations in the mitis type of DEB revealed the presence of a homozygous missense mutation, a methionine-to-lysine substitution (M2798K) at the carboxy-terminal end of the molecule. Similarly, in other cases, a missense mutation in one allele, including a glycine substitution in the collagenous domain, together with a premature termination codon mutation on the other allele, can result in mitis RDEB. Finally, our survey of a cohort of over 100 families, in which we have identified distinct COL7A1 mutations, only a few cases appear to be *de novo* dominant mutations at least one of them being derived from the maternal germline.

Based on these considerations, for genetic counseling purposes, it appears appropriate to consider each "new" case as a recessively inherited condition, unless proven to be a dominant mutation by molecular genetic analysis. Reclassification of DEB on the basis of the underlying mutations clearly impacts on the likelihood of the affected individual of having an affected offspring.

APPLICATIONS OF MUTATION ANALYSIS IN PRENATAL DIAGNOSIS OF EB

Precise understanding of the underlying mutations in different forms of DEB has several translational implications in terms of genetic counseling, DNA-based prenatal diagnosis, and gene therapy. Most immediately relevant to the patient care is the development of DNA-based prenatal diagnosis, which can be performed as early as the 10th week of gestation through chorionic villus sampling, or at the 12–15th week of gestation through amniocentesis. In the severe dystrophic forms of EB, such analyses can be performed either by direct mutation analyses or by genetic-linkage approaches, recognizing the fact that no evidence for genetic heterogeneity has been disclosed thus far. These approaches have already been applied to DNA-based prenatal diagnosis in over 30 families at risk for recurrence of the severe, mutilating form of RDEB. The genetic information also provides the basis for development of preimplantation diagnosis through blastomere analysis, a technological advance that would obviate the necessity of termination of the pregnancy in case of an affected fetus, if elected.

GENE THERAPY APPROACHES FOR EB

Precise understanding of the underlying mutations, and subsequent demonstration of the functional consequences of such mutations at the mRNA and protein levels, are obligatory prerequisites for the development of gene therapy approaches for this group of devastating skin diseases. It is conceivable that several forms of EB are realistic targets for genetic therapies, including RDEB. However, because of the large size of the mRNA for type VII collagen (~9.2 kbp), conventional techniques of introduction of the wild-type cDNA by viral transduction of patient keratinocytes are unlikely to be successful. For this reason, we and others have begun to explore alternative technologies, including direct introduction of genetic material into the skin cells by biolistic particle bombardment, use of ribozyme-mediated repair of mutant mRNAs by targeted *trans*-splicing, and application of chimeric RNA/DNA oligonucleotides for targeted gene correction. Thus, establishing the genetic basis of different forms of EB has provided the necessary foundation for development of gene therapy approaches to counteract these devastating skin diseases in the future.

ACKNOWLEDGMENTS

We gratefully acknowledge the participation of the many clinicians and scientists who contributed to the original studies summarized in this overview. The original studies by the authors were supported by USPHS, NIH grants PO1-AR38923 and T32-AR07561 (JU), and R29-AR43602, and by the March of Dimes Birth Defects Foundation (AMC).

SELECTED REFERENCES

Bruckner-Tuderman L. Collagens of the dermo-epidermal junction: role in bullous disorders. Eur J Dermatol 1991;1:89–100.

Burgeson RE. Type VII collagen, anchoring fibrils and epidermolysis bullosa. J Invest Dermatol 1993;101:252–255.

Christiano AM, Anton-Lamprecht I, Amano S, Ebschner U, Burgeson RE, Uitto J. Compound heterozygosity for COL7A1 mutations in twins with dystrophic epidermolysis bullosa: a recessive paternal deletion/insertion mutation and a dominant negative maternal glycine substitution result in a severe phenotype. Am J Hum Genet 1997;58:682–693.

Christiano AM, Bart BJ, Epstein EH, Uitto J. Genetic basis of Bart's syndrome: a glycine substitution in the type VII collagen gene. J Invest Dermatol 1996;106:778–780.

Christiano AM, Greenspan DS, Hoffman GG, et al. A missense mutation in the human type VII collagen gene in two siblings with recessive dystrophic epidermolysis bullosa. Nat Genet 1993;4:62–66.

Christiano AM, Greenspan DS, Lee S, Uitto J. Cloning of human type VII collagen: complete primary sequence of the α1(VII) chain and identification of intragenic polymorphisms. J Biol Chem 1994;269:20,256–20,262.

Christiano AM, Hoffman GG, Chung-Honet LC, et al. Structural organization of the human type VII collagen gene (COL7A1), composed of more exons than any previously characterized gene. Genomics 1994;21:169–179.

Christiano AM, LaForgia S, Paller AS, McGuire J, Shimizu H, Uitto J. DNA-based prenatal diagnosis of recessive dystrophic epidermolysis bullosa in ten families by mutation and haplotype analysis in the type VII collagen gene (COL7A1). Mol Med 1996;2:59–76.

Christiano AM, Lee JY-Y, Chen WJ, LaForgia S, Uitto J. Pretibial epidermolysis bullosa: genetic linkage to COL7A1 and identification of a glycine-to-cysteine substitution in the triple-helical domain of type VII collagen. Hum Mol Genet 1995;4:1579–1583.

Christiano AM, McGrath JA, Tan KC, Uitto J. Glycine substitutions in the triple-helical region of type VII collagen result in a spectrum of dystrophic epidermolysis bullosa phenotypes and patterns of inheritance. Am J Hum Genet 1996;58:671–681.

Christiano AM, McGrath JA, Uitto J. Influence of the second COL7A1 mutation in determining the phenotypic severity of recessive dystrophic epidermolysis bullosa. J Invest Dermatol 1996;106:766–770.

Christiano AM, Uitto J. Molecular genetic diagnosis of blistering skin diseases: impact on dystrophic epidermolysis bullosa. Curr Opin Derm 1996;32:225–232.

Christiano AM, Uitto J. Molecular diagnosis of inherited skin disorders: the paradigm of dystrophic epidermolysis bullosa. Advances Derm 1996;11:199–213.

Christiano AM, Uitto J. Molecular complexity of the cutaneous basement membrane zone. Revelations from the paradigms of epidermolysis bullosa. Exp Derm 1996;5:1–11.

Christiano AM, Uitto J. Prenatal and preimplantation diagnosis of genetic skin diseases. Arch Derm 1993;129:1455–1459.

Dunnill MG, McGrath JA, Richards AJ, et al. Clinicopathological correlations of compound heterozygous COL7A1 mutations in recessive dystrophic epidermolysis bullosa. J Invest Dermatol 1996;107:171–177.

Epstein EH Jr. Molecular genetics of epidermolysis bullosa. Science 1992;256:799–803.

Fine J-D, Bauer EA, Briggaman RA, et al. Revised clinical and laboratory criteria for subtypes of inherited epidermolysis bullosa: a consensus report by the subcommittee on diagnosis and classification of the National Epidermolysis Bullosa Registry. J Am Acad Dermatol 1991;24:119–135.

Fuchs E. Genetic skin disorders of keratin. J Invest Dermatol 1992;99: 671–674.

Gardella R, Belletti L, Zoppi N, Marini D, Barlati S, Colombi M. Identification of two splicing mutations in the collagen type VII gene (COL7A1) of a patient affected by the localisata variant of recessive dystrophic epidermolysis bullosa. Am J Hum Genet 1996;59: 292–300.

Hovnanian A, Hilal L, Blanchet-Bardon C, et al. Prenatal diagnosis of the Hallopeau Siemens form of recessive dystrophic epidermolysis bullosa by type VII collagen gene analysis in six pregnancies at risk for recurrence. J Invest Dermatol 1995;104:456–461.

Kon A, McGrath JA, Pulkkinen L, et al. Glycine substitution mutations in the type VII collagen gene (COL7A1) in dystrophic epidermolysis bullosa: implications for genetic counseling. J Invest Dermatol 1997;108:224–228.

Lee JY, Pulkkinen L, Liu HS, Chen YF, Uitto J. A glycine-to-arginine substitution in the triple-helical domain of type VII collagen in a family with dominant dystrophic epidermolysis bullosa pruriginosa. J Invest Dermatol 1977;108:947–949.

Lin AN, Carter DM. Epidermolysis Bullosa. Basic and Clinical Aspects. New York: Springer-Verlag, 1992.

McGrath JA, Gatalica B, Christiano AM, et al. Mutations in the 180-kD bullous pemphigoid antigen (BPAG2), a hemidesmosomal transmembrane collagen (COL17A1), in generalized atrophic benign epidermolysis bullosa. Nat Genet 1995;11:83–86.

McGrath JA, Ishida-Yamamoto A, O'Grady A, Leigh IM, Eady RAJ. Structural variations in anchoring fibrils in dystrophic epidermolysis bullosa: correlation with type VII collagen expression. J Invest Dermatol 1993;100:366–372.

Mellerio JE, Dunnill MG, Allison W, et al. Recurrent mutations in the type VII collagen gene (COL7A1) in patients with recessive dystrophic epidermolysis bullosa. J Invest Dermatol 1977;109:246–249.

Shimizu H, McGrath JA, Christiano AM, Nishikawa T, Uitto, J. Molecular basis of recessive dystrophic epidermolysis bullosa: genotype/phenotype correlation in a case of moderate clinical severity. J Invest Dermatol 1996;106:119–124.

Smith LT. Ultrastructural findings in epidermolysis bullosa. Arch Dermatol 1993;129:1578–1584.

Sullenger BA, Cech TR. Ribozyme-mediated repair of defective mRNA by targeted trans-splicing. Nature 1994;371:619–622.

Tamai K, Ishida-Yamamoto A, Matsuo S, et al. Compound heterozygosity for a nonsense mutation and a splice site mutation in the type VII collagen gene (COL7A1) in recessive dystrophic epidermolysis bullosa. Lab Invest 1997;76:209–217.

Uitto J, Christiano AM. Molecular basis of the dystrophic forms of epidermolysis bullosa: mutations in the type VII collagen gene. Arch Derm Res 1994;287:16–22.

Uitto J, Pulkkinen L, Christiano AM. Molecular basis of the dystrophic and junctional forms of epidermolysis bullosa: mutations in the type VII collagen and kalinin (laminin 5) genes. J Invest Dermatol 1994;103:39S–46S.

Uitto J, Christiano AM. Molecular genetics of the cutaneous basement membrane zone. Perspectives on epidermolysis bullosa. J Clin Invest 1992;90:687–692.

Vidal F, Aberdam D, Miquel C, et al. Integrin β4 mutations associated with junctional epidermolysis bullosa with pyloric atresia. Nat Genet 1995;10:229–234.

Vogel JC, Walker PS, Hengge UR. Gene therapy for skin diseases. Advances Derm 1996;11:383–398.

Winberg JO, Hammami-Hauasli N, Nilssen O, et al. Modulation of disease severity of dystrophic epidermolysis bullosa by a splice site mutation in combination with a missense mutation in the COL7A1 gene. Hum Mol Genet 1997;6:1125–1135.

Yerlinsky Y, Kuliev AM. Preimplantation Diagnosis of Genetic Diseases. A New Technique in Assisted Reproduction. New York: Wiley-Liss, 1993; pp. 1–144.

Yoon K, Cole-Strauss A, Kmiec EB. Targeted gene correction of episomal DNA in mammalian cells mediated by a chimeric RNA/DNA oligonucleotide. Proc Natl Acad Sci USA 1996;93:2071–2076.

Congenital Diseases of Cutaneous Tissues

Part B: Genetic Mutations That Predispose to Cancer

79 Oculocutaneous Albinism

JEAN L. BOLOGNIA

BACKGROUND

In the premolecular biology era, there were two major clinical forms of oculocutaneous albinism (OCA): tyrosinase-negative (ty-neg) and tyrosinase-positive (ty-pos). Tyrosinase is the key enzyme in the melanin biosynthetic pathway (Fig. 79-1), catalyzing three steps in the formation of melanin: (1) tyrosine to dopa (dihydroxyphenylalanine); (2) dopa to dopaquinone; and (3) 5,6-dihydroxyindole to indole-5,6-quinone. This categorization of patients was based primarily upon their clinical appearance with ty-neg patients having the most severe phenotype, i.e., white hair, gray-blue eyes, and pink skin at birth as well as throughout life. An additional diagnostic test was the incubation of anagen hair follicles with tyrosine to determine the presence (ty-pos) or absence (ty-neg) of melanin deposition.

It is now possible to go beyond the clinical findings and determine if patients have type I OCA (mutations in the tyrosinase gene) or type II OCA (mutations in the *P* gene). However, many questions still remain unanswered including the molecular bases of Hermansky-Pudlak syndrome (OCA plus platelet-storage-granule deficiency) and Chédiak Higashi syndrome (OCA plus abnormal lysosomes)* as well as the role of both melanosomal matrix proteins and tyrosinase-related proteins in the regulation of human melanogenesis.

CLINICAL FEATURES

TYPE I OCA In this autosomal-recessive disorder, the clinical features are a reflection of the amount of pigment produced in the eyes, hair, and skin. When there is a complete lack of tyrosinase activity caused by loss of function mutations in both copies of the tyrosinase gene (type IA OCA), the individuals have pink skin, white hair, and gray-blue eyes at birth and throughout life (Fig. 79-2). These are the patients who were previously referred to as having ty-neg OCA and, even with increasing age, they fail to produce any pheo- or eumelanin (Fig. 79-1). Of all the patients with OCA, this group is the one that is most susceptible to the development of cutaneous neoplasms, primarily squamous-cell carcinomas.

*Since submission of this chapter, a gene for Chédiak Higashi syndrome has been cloned, the protein product of which is similar to the yeast vacuolar sorting protein, VPS15.

From: *Principles of Molecular Medicine* (J. L. Jameson, ed.), ©1998 Humana Press Inc., Totowa, NJ.

Because of the total lack of melanin in the retinal pigmented epithelium (RPE) and in particular the fovea (Fig. 79-3), patients with type IA OCA also have very poor visual activity (20/200 to 20/400+) and many are legally blind. In addition, they exhibit marked nystagmus, photophobia, and strabismus. The photophobia is because of the discomfort associated with excess light scatter in a hypopigmented fundus, whereas the nystagmus is more difficult to explain and is perhaps related to misdirected oculomotor reflexes.

As would be expected, some mutations in the tyrosinase gene do not lead to a complete lack of enzyme activity, but rather a decrease in function (type IB OCA). At birth, children with type IB OCA are similar in appearance to those with type IA OCA, i.e., they have white skin and their hair is usually white in color. However, as patients with type IB OCA age, they acquire more pigmentation so that, depending on their racial background, their hair can develop a yellow (pheomelanin)-to-brown (eumelanin) color, pigmented nevi can appear, and a tan can even develop in sun-exposed skin. As with type II OCA *(see below)*, some patients may not have a striking albino phenotype, but they will have the ocular abnormalities characteristic of OCA, e.g., nystagmus and decreased fundal pigment. However, the ocular findings are less severe than in type IA OCA.

Type IB OCA includes those patients who were previously referred to as "yellow mutant" albinos and, for this reason, type IB OCA is sometimes referred to as ym OCA. Yellow mutant OCA was first described in an Amish family in which affected members had hair that was white at birth but became yellow over time. Even before molecular analysis of the tyrosinase gene was done, it was known that ym OCA was allelic to ty-neg (IA) OCA.

The third subgroup of type I OCA has been referred to as temperature-sensitive OCA (type I, ts). This form was first described by King et al. who noted that a patient with OCA had lightly colored hair in warm areas of the body such as the axilla, but darkly pigmented hair in cooler parts of the body such as the leg. This phenotype was analogous to that of the Himalayan mouse or the Siamese cat in which darkly pigmented hairs on the ears, paws, and nose are the reflection of a tyrosinase enzyme that has minimal activity at 37°C, but some activity at 35°C. Because the majority of patients with type I OCA are compound heterozygotes (different maternal and paternal alleles), there are a number of potential combinations (Table 79-1) such that the boundaries between type IB OCA and type I ts OCA have become blurred.

TYPE II OCA Two observations led to the hypothesis that there was at least one other gene involved in the regulation of

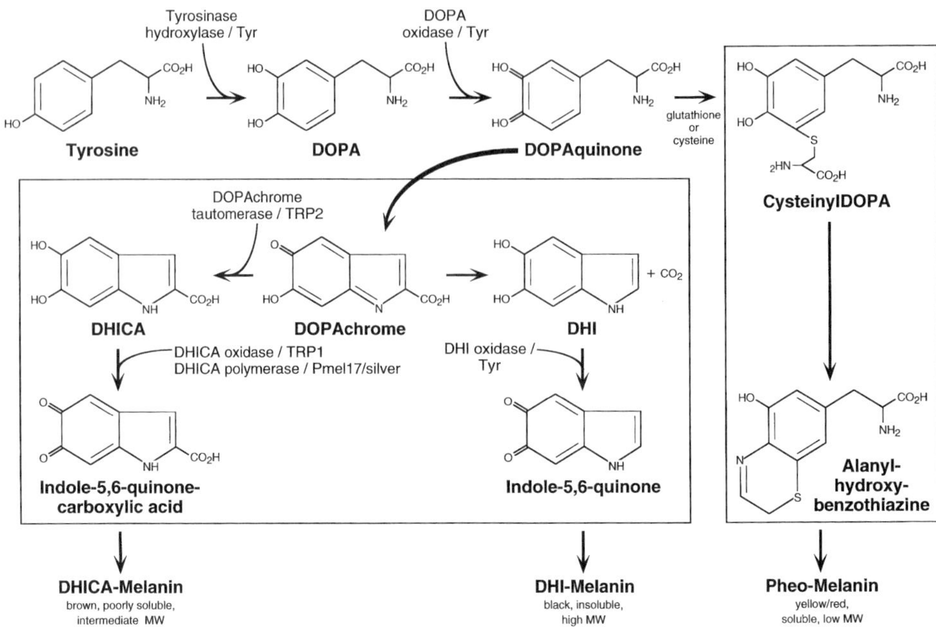

Figure 79-1 An updated version of the melanin biosynthetic pathway that incorporates observations from the 1980s and 1990s. Tyr, tyrosinase; DOPA, dihydroxyphenylalanine; DHICA, 5,6-dihydroxyindole-2-carboxylic acid; TRP1, tyrosinase related protein 1; TRP2, tyrosinase related protein 2; DHI, dihydroxyindole. (Courtesy of Vincent Hearing.)

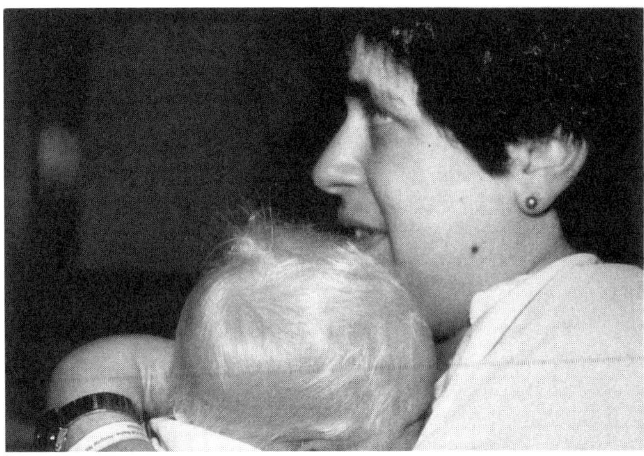

Figure 79-2 Newborn with type IA OCA who has white hair and pink skin. The pigmentary dilution is obvious when compared to her mother. (Courtesy, Yale Residents' Slide Collection.)

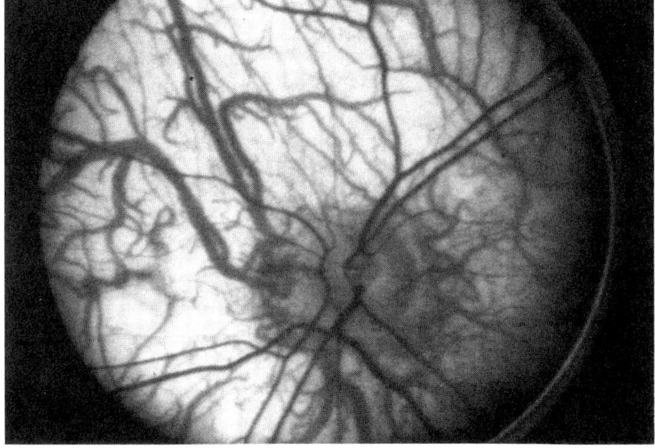

Figure 79-3 Hypopigmented fundus in a patient with type IA OCA. The vasculature is quite prominent because of the lack of pigment production in the RPE.

melanogenesis: (1) localization of the tyrosinase gene to human chromosome 11q and (2) the pigmentary dilution seen in some of the patients with Angelman and Prader-Willi syndromes (Fig. 79-4), both of which can be associated with deletions of chromosome 15q11-q13 (the two syndromes are discussed in detail in Chapter 117). Because type II OCA is an autosomal-recessive disorder, patients with type II OCA have mutations in both copies of the *P* gene located on chromosome 15q, but they have no mutations in their tyrosinase genes.

In general, type II OCA is a less severe form of pigmentary dilution as compared to type IA, although there can be an occasional patient with a fairly severe phenotype. As with type IB OCA, the skin, eyes, and hair become darker as the patient ages; however, in contrast to type IB OCA, the hair is usually not white at birth. The eventual level of pigmentation depends on the racial background of the patient and individuals, especially adults, may go undiagnosed unless compared to first-degree family members. One clinical finding, which can be rather striking when it is present, is the development of multiple solar lentigines, ranging in size from 5 mm to 2 cm.

In Caucasians living in the United States, the incidence of type II OCA is similar to that of type I OCA, approximately 1 in 36,000. However, type II OCA is more common among African Americans with an incidence approaching 1 in 10,000 and, in certain tribes in Africa, the frequency can be as high as 1 in 1100.

TYPES IV, V, AND VI OCA The designation OCA3 was given recently to an African-American child with "brown" albinism who had no detectable tyrosinase-related protein 1 (TRP-1),

Table 79-1
Relationship Between Genotype and Type I OCA Phenotype

Allele	T^+	t^-	*ym*	*ts*
T^+	Normal (T^+/T^+)	Normal (T^+/t^-)	Normal (T^+/ym)	Normal (T^+/ts)
t^-	Normal (t^-/T^+)	IA (t^-/t^-)	IB (t^-/ym)	I, ts (t^-/ts)
y	Normal (ym/T^+)	IB (ym/t^-)	IB (ym/ym)	IB (ym/ts)[a]
ts	Normal (ts/T^+)	I, ts (ts/t^-)	IB (ts/ym)[a]	I, ts (ts/ts)[a]

[a]No patient with the indicated genotype has yet been detected. ym, yellow mutant; ts, temperature-sensitive.
Adapted from Tomita, Y. J Invest Dermatol 1993;100:186S-190S.

Table 79-2
Tyrosinase and Tyrosinase-Related Proteins (TRP)

	Locus		*Chromosome*	
	Human	*Mouse*	*Human*	*Mouse*
Tyrosinase	TYR	*c*	11	7
TRP-1 (gp75)	CAS2	*b*	9	4
TRP-2 (DC tautomerase)	TRP2/DC	*slaty*	13	14

DC, dopachrome.

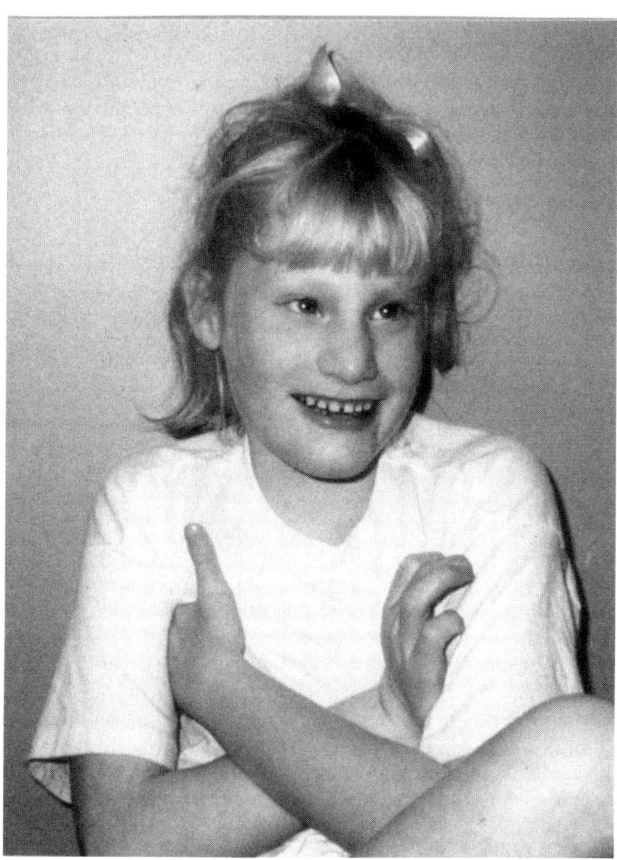

Figure 79-4 A 7-year-old girl with both type II OCA and Angelman's syndrome. (With permission from Fryburg JS, Berg WR, Lindgren V. Diagnosis of Angelman syndrome in infants. Am J Med Genet 1991;38:58-64.)

the product of a gene on chromosome 9p, which is the human homolog of the *brown* locus in the mouse (Table 79-2). This TRP family was discovered during the search for the human tyrosinase gene (Fig. 79-5). Compared to his fraternal twin, this child had diffuse pigmentary dilution characterized by light brown skin and hair. Of note, brown albinism was originally described in Africans and has also been referred to as type IV OCA.

There is a second report of two children with marked hypopigmentation of the skin and hair in association with the 9p– syndrome. The latter is characterized by craniosynostosis, midfacial hypoplasia, abdominal wall defects, and mental retardation. However, an explanation for the associated hypopigmentation was not obvious given that only one copy of the TRP-1 gene was deleted in these individuals. Type V (rufous) OCA is characterized by mahogany-red to deep-red skin, reddish-brown hair, and red-brown to brown eyes. This form of albinism has been described primarily in New Guineans and Africans.

Type VIA OCA is better known as the Hermansky-Pudlak syndrome (HPS) and type VIB OCA represents the Chédiak-Higashi syndrome (CHS). In the former, ty-pos OCA is associated with a bleeding diathesis that is caused by a defect in platelet-storage granules. Additional clinical manifestations include restrictive lung disease and granulomatous colitis secondary to deposits of ceroid-like material in these organs. This autosomal-recessive disorder is seen primarily in individuals from the Arecibo region of Puerto Rico and Holland. In the Chédiak-Higashi syndrome, the patients often have silvery-blonde hair in addition to dysfunction of neutrophils and natural killer cells that results in recurrent infections. Abnormally large melanosomes and lysosomal granules are seen in melanocytes and granulocytes, respectively. Unless bone marrow transplantation is performed, patients usually enter an "accelerated phase" characterized by pancytopenia and rarely live beyond the age of 10.

DIAGNOSIS

The diagnosis of type IA OCA can be made on the basis of clinical findings in a child or adult and then confirmed by molecular analysis of the tyrosinase gene. However, the latter is not necessary unless it provides information required for future prenatal screening or genetic counseling of family members. In patients in whom there is some pigment production, albeit reduced, clinical clues (e.g., color of hair at birth) can help to distinguish type IB from type II OCA, but molecular analysis of the tyrosinase gene and the *P* gene is the most exact method for confirming the clinical diagnosis. Of note, in type I OCA, mutations will not be identified in approximately 15% of obligate mutant alleles (personal communication, Richard King).

If there is a clinical suspicion of OCA, but the patient has a rather subtle form of the disease, i.e., one that is associated with a significant level of pigment production, it is important to examine the first-degree relatives and to have an ophthalmologist perform a complete eye examination. In addition, a complete history should be taken in patients with ty-pos OCA with special attention paid to recurrent infections or a bleeding tendency suggestive of either the CHS or HPS. Simple screening laboratory tests for these syndromes include examination of a peripheral blood smear for abnormal lysosomes within leukocytes and performance of a bleeding time.

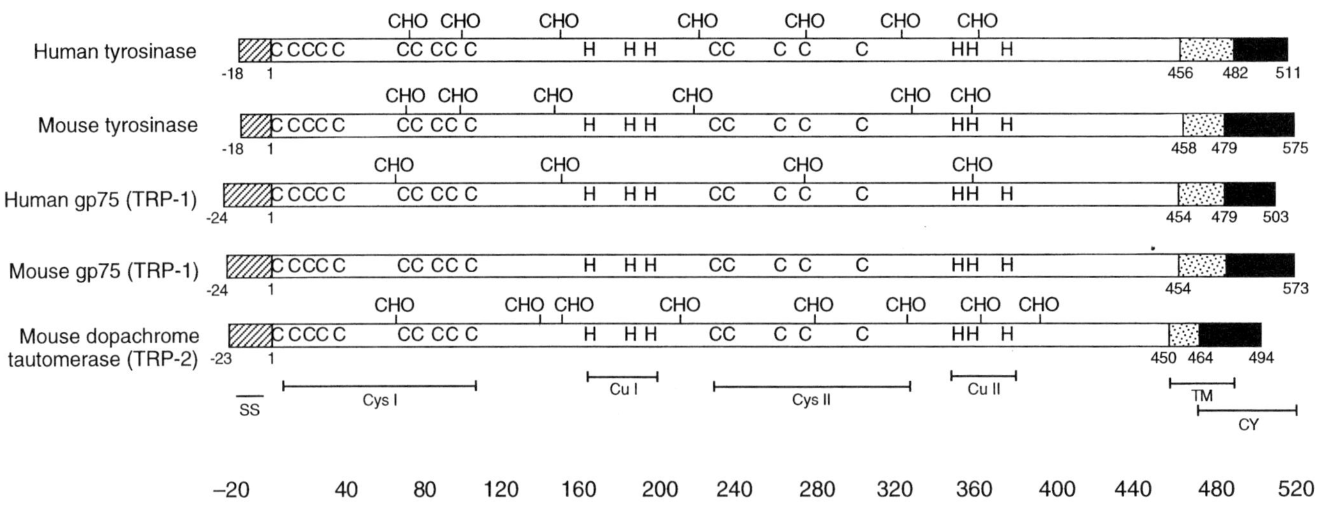

Figure 79-5 Comparison of the primary structures of the members of the tyrosinase family. The putative signal sequence (▧, SS), positions of cysteine residues (C), positions of histidine residues (H), possible N-linked glycosylation sites (CHO), putative transmembrane region (▩, TM), and potential cytoplasmic domain (CY) are indicated. Cys I and Cys II are the two cysteine-rich regions of the peptides. Cu I and Cu II are the putative copper-binding sites. The numbers indicate the positions of amino acids in the putative mature proteins. The negative numbers indicate the signal sequences. (With permission from Kwon BS. Pigmentation genes: the tyrosinase gene family and the pmel 17 gene family. J Invest Dermatol 1993;100:134S–140S.)

Other causes of diffuse pigmentary dilution of the skin, hair, and occasionally eyes should be considered and then excluded by lack of associated findings; they include Angelman, Prader-Willi (*see* Chapter 117) and Apert syndromes, phenylketonuria, histidinemia, and homocystinuria. Pigmentary dilution limited to the skin and hair is seen in Menkes' kinky hair syndrome, copper or selenium deficiency, kwashiorkor, and the EEC (ectrodactyly, ectodermal dysplasia, and clefting) syndrome.

Another entity that overlaps clinically with OCA is ocular albinism (OA), a disorder that is inherited in an X-linked fashion in the majority of patients. The gene responsible for the most common form of X-linked OA (OA1; Nettleship-Falls) has been cloned, but its function has yet to be determined. Classically, individuals with OA were said to have the eye, but not the cutaneous, findings of albinism. However, some of the patients were noted to have hypomelanotic macules or a mild generalized pigmentary dilution when compared to unaffected siblings. It is important to note that mutations in the tyrosinase gene and the *P* gene have been described in the smaller group of patients with autosomal-recessive ocular albinism.

Prenatal screening for type IA OCA has been performed successfully following molecular analysis of the tyrosinase genes in amniotic cells; obviously, such an analysis is aided by predetermination of the responsible mutations. In the past, scalp biopsies were performed between weeks 17 to 20 of gestation, and the diagnosis was based on the presence or absence of melanized melanosomes. There are no published reports to date of molecular prenatal screening for other forms of type I OCA or type II OCA.

GENETIC BASIS OF DISEASE

TYPE I Patients with type I OCA have mutations in both copies of the tyrosinase gene located on chromosome 11q. There are five exons in the tyrosinase gene and the entire gene spans more than 65 kbp of genomic DNA. Translation of tyrosinase mRNA results in a 529-amino acid polypeptide, but this includes an 18-amino acid leader peptide that is later cleaved. At least 70 different mutations have been described in patients with type I OCA and the associated phenotype depends on whether the mutations lead to a lack of enzyme activity vs a decreased level of enzyme activity. Patients with type IA OCA (the most severe phenotype) have no residual tyrosinase activity, whereas patients with types IB and I, ts have decreased or altered tyrosinase activity (*see above*). The vast majority of patients with type I OCA are compound heterozygotes, that is, the maternal allele and the paternal allele are different; unfortunately, there is no predominant mutant allele in the general Caucasian population.

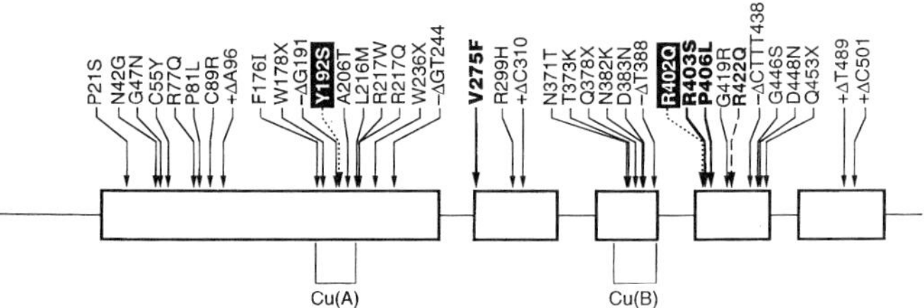

Figure 79-6 Locations of mutations in the tyrosinase gene; the five boxes represent its five exons. Mutations associated with type IA OCA are represented by solid arrows and numbers; mutations associated with type IB OCA are represented by **bold** solid lines and numbers; the mutation associated with type I, ts OCA is represented by a broken line and bold number; and sites of polymorphism are represented by dotted lines and numbers outlined in black. Cu(A) and Cu(B) are the putative copper-binding sites. (With permission from Oetting WS, King RA. Molecular basis of type I [tyrosinase-related] oculocutaneous albinism: mutations and polymorphisms of the human tyrosinase gene. Hum Mutation 1993;2:1–6.)

Several types of mutations in the tyrosinase gene have been described including missense, nonsense, and splice consensus mutations. In addition, some of the patients have had frameshift mutations, but deletions are rare. There are two dimorphic sites that are fairly common in Caucasians, at codon 192 and codon 402 (Fig. 79-6). When the sites of mutations are mapped, there is an

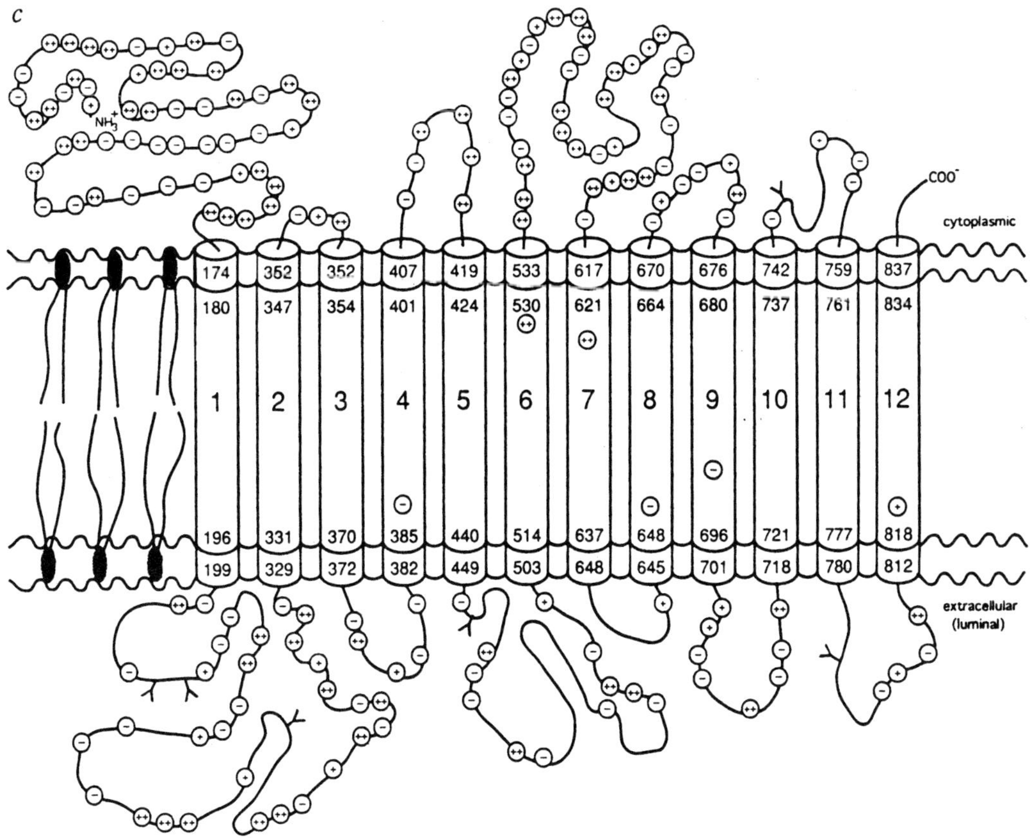

Figure 79-7 A model for the arrangement of the P polypeptide within the membrane of the melanosome; note the 12 transmembrane domains. (With permission from Rinchik EM, Bultman SJ, Horsthemke B, et al. A gene for the mouse pink-eyed dilution locus and for human type II oculocutaneous albinism. Nature 1993;361:72–76.)

obvious clustering near the amino-terminal end as well as the two putative copper-binding sites (Fig. 79-6). Although it seems logical that a mutation near one of the putative copper-binding sites would result in type IA OCA, there is limited supporting experimental evidence. For example, Spritz reported that the only amino acid substitution that involved one of the putative copper-binding histidines was associated with a mild phenotype. Also, an explanation for why amino acid substitutions at other sites result in a total lack of enzyme activity remains theoretical (*see* Type II section, *below*).

Murine tyrosinase cDNA also has been sequenced and mapped to the albino or *c* locus located on mouse chromosome 7. Pigment production has been observed in albino mice following the introduction of a minigene that contained mouse tyrosinase cDNA plus the genomic 5' noncoding flanking region.

TYPE II Type II OCA is caused by mutations in both copies of the *P* gene, which spans 250–600 kbp in chromosome segment 15q11-13 and contains 25 exons. The *P* gene is the human homolog of the pink-eyed dilution *(p)* gene on chromosome 7 in the mouse, and its protein product of 838 amino acids has 12 membrane-spanning domains (Fig. 79-7). The *P* protein was reported to have an approximately 20% homology with a tyrosine-specific transport protein from *E. coli* and given the observation that the *P* protein localizes to the melanosomal membrane, an initial hypothesis was that it was involved in the transport of tyrosine into the melanosome (Fig. 79-8). However, the exact function of the *P* protein remains unknown *(see below)*.

As with type I OCA, the majority of patients are compound heterozygotes. The types of mutations described to date include missense, splice junction, in-frame deletions, and frameshifts. An intragenic deletion of the *P* gene involving exon 7 is a commonly observed mutant allele in Africans with type II OCA. In contrast to the tyrosinase gene, the *P* gene has over 25 nonpathologic DNA sequence polymorphisms. When Caucasians with ty-pos OCA are evaluated, approximately one-third actually have type IB OCA and in 50% of the remaining patients, *P* gene mutations have been found. On the other hand, *P* gene mutations have been observed in at least 95% of Africans and African Americans with type II OCA.

In patients with either sporadic Angelman or Prader-Willi syndrome plus OCA II, one may find a deletion in either the maternal (Angelman) or paternal (Prader-Willi) copy of chromosome 15 in addition to a mutation in the second copy of the *P* gene. Uniparental disomy can also result in this constellation of findings but it is observed less commonly.

TYPE IV (BROWN) OCA (OCA3) The designation OCA3 was given to a patient who was homozygous for a single basepair deletion in the TRP-1 gene located on chromosome 9p. TRP-1 is the most abundant protein in melanocytes and is also known as gp75 (Table 79-2). Until recently, the function of TRP-1 was unknown. However, in 1994, Kobayashi et al. provided evidence that one of its functions is oxidation of dihydroxyindole-2-carboxylic acid (DHICA; Figs. 79-1 and 79-8), thus explaining the associated decrease in pigment production.

TYPE VIA The gene for HPS has been cloned recently. It encodes a transmembrane protein that may be a component of cytoplasmic organelles. Given the number of loci in the mouse

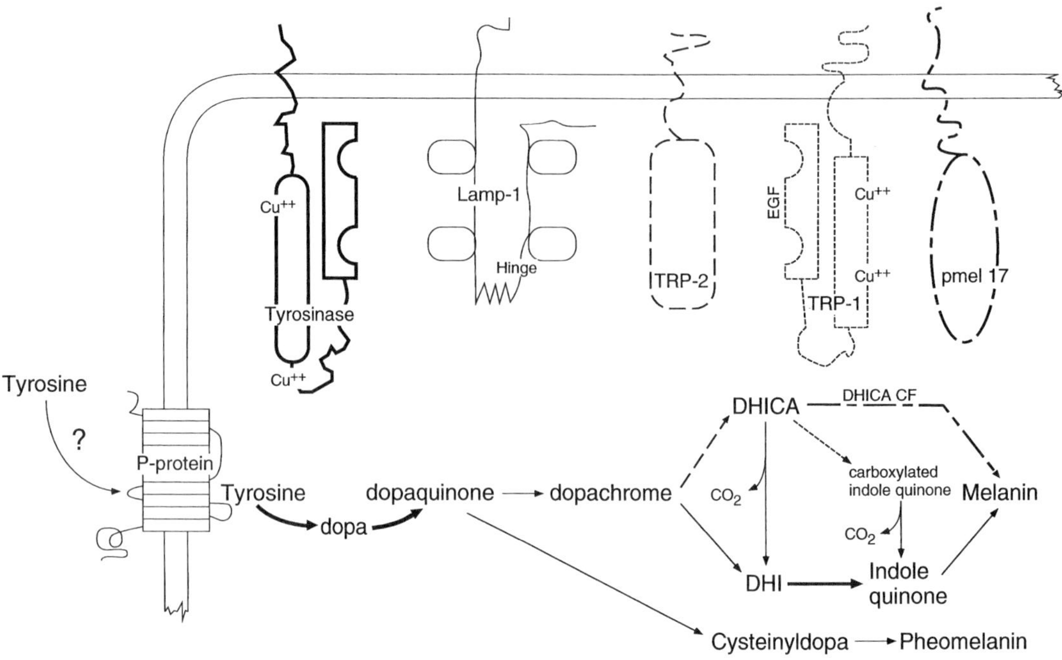

Figure 79-8 Hypothetical model of protein interactions on the melanosomal membrane. TRP-1, tyrosinase related protein 1; TRP-2, tyrosinase related protein 2; dopa, dihydroxyphenylalanine; DHICA, 5,6-dihydroxyindole-2-carboxylic acid; DHI, dihydroxyindole. (Adapted with permission from Jimbow K, Luo D, Chen H, et al. Coordinated mRNA and protein expression of human LAMP-1 in induction of melanogenesis after UV-B exposure and co-transfection of human tyrosinase and TRP-1 cDNAs. Pigment Cell Res 1994;7:311–319.)

that, when mutated, give rise to both decreased pigmentation and platelet-granule dysfunction, the possibility exists that more than one locus is responsible for HPS.

MOLECULAR PATHOPHYSIOLOGY OF DISEASE

Tyrosinase is a member of a family of copper-binding enzymes that includes hemocyanins, which explains why a pigmentary dilution is also seen in patients with Menkes' kinky-hair syndrome in which there are mutations in a copper-transporting ATPase. In patients with type IA OCA, there is a clustering of mutations in the tyrosinase gene near the two putative copper-binding sites (Fig. 79-6). Although this would seem to explain the associated phenotype, proof that amino-acid substitutions in these two regions affect copper binding is lacking *(see above)*. A total absence of enzyme activity can result from nonsense as well as frameshift mutations, but an explanation for why several of the known amino acid substitutions lead to loss of function remains theoretical. Based upon the three-dimensional structure of tyrosinase, one group of investigators proposed that the 5' end (amino-terminus) and the domain 3' of the copper B binding site (Fig. 79-6) are involved in substrate and/or cofactor binding as well as enzyme stabilization.

Several observations led to the proposal that the *P* protein might function as a tyrosine transporter including: (1) incubation of anagen hairbulbs from patients with type II OCA in the presence of excess tyrosine results in pigment production; and (2) the structural arrangement of the *P* protein (multiple transmembrane domains) is characteristic of several prokaryotic transporter proteins and significant sequence homology has been observed. Many of the *P* missense mutations that are within regions of homology occur at conserved residues, whereas mutations that result in a milder phenotype occur at less well-conserved residues. However, attempts to demonstrate abnormalities in melanosomal tyrosine transport in pink-eyed dilution murine melanocytes have been unsuccessful.

MANAGEMENT/TREATMENT

The earlier in life the diagnosis of OCA is established, the sooner interventions that have an impact on development can be instituted. It is important to assess visual acuity in each child and to provide corrective eyewear as well as access to products that are specially designed for a visually impaired person. An example of the latter is large-print materials and an excellent source for a list of such products is the American Foundation for the Blind. In addition, it is important to identify any eye abnormality such as strabismus that can be corrected either medically or surgically.

Because of the increased risk for the development of cutaneous carcinomas, a sun-protection program needs to be instituted early in life. It has been estimated that, by the age of 18 years, a person has received a majority of his or her cumulative lifetime sun exposure, emphasizing the need for early intervention. Effective measures include avoidance of midday sun, application of sunscreens, and the use of hats and clothing made of tightly woven material. The closer a patient lives to the equator, the more important this aspect of clinical care becomes. For example, in a study of albinos from Tanzania, advanced (>4 cm) cutaneous squamous-cell carcinomas were common among patients in their late 20s and early 30s and less than 10% survived beyond 30 years.

Lastly, genetic counseling should be made available to all families. Prenatal diagnosis of type IA OCA can be performed as outlined above. Because there is currently no treatment that will reverse the major forms of this genetic disorder, both patients and their parents can receive valuable information and support by joining NOAH, the National Organization for Albinism and Hypopigmentation (1530 Locust Street #29, Philadelphia, PA

19102-4415). Allogeneic bone marrow transplantation has been used successfully in patients with CHS and 1-desamino-8D-arginine (DDAVP) has been reported as a potential treatment for the bleeding diathesis associated with HPS.

FUTURE DIRECTIONS

Just as genetic studies in albino mice and pink-eyed dilution mice shed a great deal of light on the molecular pathophysiology of type IA OCA and type II OCA, respectively, so will the studies of brown and beige mice provide insights into types IV and VIB OCA. Given the dysfunction of several organelles including melanosomes, platelet-storage granules, and lysosomes in patients with HPS and CHS, it is anticipated that the protein products of the genes responsible for these disorders will play an important role in the formation and/or function of intracytoplasmic organelles. The genetic mutation in the silver mouse leads to an abnormal melanosomal matrix protein as well as altered pigmentation, and it is possible that a similar situation will exist in humans. Lastly, the slaty mouse has been shown to have a mutation in the TRP-2 gene, whose protein product is dopachrome tautomerase (Table 79-2), an enzyme involved in the melanin biosynthetic pathway that converts dopachrome to DHICA (Figs. 79-1 and 79-8). The human TRP-2 gene has been cloned and is located on chromosome 13. Although the albino phenotype has been rescued in transgenic mice *(see above)*, gene therapy for humans with type IA OCA represents futuristic thinking, especially since the majority of pigment production in the eye occurs prior to birth.

SELECTED REFERENCES

Bailin T, Oh J, Feng GH, Fukai K, Spritz RA. Organization and nucleotide sequence of the human Hermansky-Pudlak syndrome (HPS) gene. J Invest Dermatol 1997;108:923–927.

Barbosa MDFS, Nguyen QA, Tchernev VT, et al. Identification of the homologous beige and Chediak-Higashi syndrome genes. Nature 1996;382:262–265.

Barrat FJ, Auloge L, Pastural E, et al. Genetic and physical mapping of the Chekiak-Higashi syndrome on chromosome 1q42-43. Am J Hum Genet 1996;59:625–632.

Bassi MT, Schiaffino MV, Renieri A, et al. Cloning of the gene for ocular albinism type I from the distal short arm of the X chromosome. Nature Genet 1995;10:13–19.

Boissy RE, Zhao H, Oetting WS, et al. Mutation in and lack of expression of tyrosinase-related protein-1 (TRP-1) in melanocytes from an individual with brown oculocutaneous albinism: a new subtype of albinism classified as "OCA3". Am J Hum Genet 1996;58:1145–1156.

Bolognia JL, Shapiro PE. Albinism and other disorders of hypopigmentation. In: Arndt KA, LeBoit PE, Robinson JK, Wintrobe BU, eds. Cutaneous Medicine and Surgery: An Integrated Program in Dermatology. Philadelphia: Saunders, 1995; pp. 1219–1232.

del Marmol V, Beermann F. Tyrosinase and related proteins in mammalian pigmentation. FEBS 1996;381:165–168.

Durham-Pierre D, Gardner JM, Nakatsu Y, et al. African origin of an intragenic deletion of the human P gene in tyrosinase positive oculocutaneous albinism. Nature Genet 1994;7:176–179.

Falik-Borenstein TC, Holmes SA, Borochowitz Z, Levin A, Rosenmann A, Spritz RA. DNA-based carrier detection and prenatal diagnosis of tyrosinase-negative oculocutaneous albinism (OCA1A). Prenatal Diagnosis 1995;15:345–349.

Feng GH, Bailin T, Oh J, Spritz RA. Mouse pale ear (ep) is homologous to human Hermansky-Pudlak syndrome and contains a rare 'AT-AC' intron. Hum Mol Genet 1997;6:793–797.

Fukai K, Holmes SA, Lucchese NJ, et al. Autosomal recessive ocular albinism associated with a functionally significant tyrosinase gene polymorphism. Nature Genet 1995;9:92–95.

Fukai K, Oh J, Karim MA, et al. Homozygosity mapping of the gene for Cheiak-Higashi syndrome to chromosome 1q42-q44 in a segment of conserved synteny that includes the mouse beige locus (bg). Am J Hum Genet 1996;59:620–624.

Gahl WA, Pottere B, Durham-Pierre, Brilliant MH, Hearing VJ. Melanosomal tyrosine transport in normal and pink-eyed dilution murine melanocytes. Pigment Cell Res 1995;8:229–233.

Giebel LB, Spritz RA. The molecular basis of type I (tyrosinase-deficient) human oculocutaneous albinism. Pig Cell Res 1992;2(Suppl): 101–106.

Giebel LB, Tripathi RK, King RA, Spritz RA. A tyrosinase gene missense mutation in temperature-sensitive type I oculocutaneous albinism. J Clin Invest 1991;87:1119–1121.

King RA, Townsend D, Oetting W, et al. Temperature-sensitive tyrosinase associated with peripheral pigmentation in oculocutaneous albinism. J Clin Invest 1991;87:1046–1053.

Kobayashi T, Urabe K, Winder A, et al. DHICA oxidase activity of TRP1 and interactions with other melanogenic enzymes. Pigment Cell Res 1994;7:227–234.

Körner A, Pawelek J. Mammalian tyrosinase catalyzes three reactions in the biosynthesis of melanin. Science 1982;217:1163–1165.

Kwon BS. Pigmentation genes: the tyrosinase gene family and pmel 17 gene family. J Invest Dermatol 1993;100:134S–140S.

Lee S-T, RD Nicholls, S. Bundey, Laxova R, Musarella M, Spritz RA. Mutations of the *P* gene in oculocutaneous albinism, ocular albinism, and Prader-Willi syndrome plus albinism. N Engl J Med 1994; 330:529–534.

Lee S-T, Nicholls RD, Jong MTC, Fukai K, Spritz RA. Organization and sequence of the human *P* gene and identification of a new family of transport proteins. Genomics 1995;26:354–363.

Luande J, Henschke CI, Mohammed N. The Tanzanian human albino skin. Natural history. Cancer 1985;55:1823–1828.

Nagle DL, Karim MA, Woolf EA, et al. Identification and mutation analysis of the complete gene for Chediak-Higashi syndrome. Nature Genet 1996;14:307–311.

Oetting WS, King RA. Molecular basis of type I (tyrosinase-related) oculocutaneous albinism: mutations and polymorphisms of the human tyrosinase gene. Hum Mutation 1993;2:1–6.

Oetting WS, King RA. Analysis of tyrosinase mutations associated with tyrosinase-related oculocutaneous albinism (OCA1). Pig Cell Res 1994;7:285–290.

Oh J, Bailin T, Fukai K, et al. Positional cloning of a gene for Hermansky-Pudlak syndrome, a disorder of cytoplasmic organelles. Nat Genet 1996;14:300–306.

Rinchik EM, Bultman SJ, Horsthemke B, et al. A gene for the mouse pink-eyed dilution locus and for human type II oculocutaneous albinism. Nature 1993;361:72–76.

Rosemblatt S, Durham-Pierre D, Gardner JM, Nakatsu Y, Brilliant MH, Orlow SJ. Identification of a melanosomal membrane protein encoded by the pink-eyed dilution (type II oculocutaneous albinism) gene. Proc Natl Acad Sci USA 1994;91:12,071–20,075.

Shimizu H, Niizeki H, Suzumori K, et al. Prenatal diagnosis of oculocutaneous albinism by analysis of the fetal tyrosinase gene. J Invest Dermatol 1994;103:104–106.

Spritz RA. Molecular genetics of oculocutaneous albinism. Hum Mol Genet 1994;3:1469–1475.

Spritz RA, Bailin T, Nicholls RD, et al. Hypopigmentation in the Prader-Willi syndrome correlates with P gene deletion but not with haplotype of the hemizygous P allele. Am J Med Genet 1997;71:57–62.

Spritz RA, Fukai K, Holmes SA, Luande J. Frequent intragenic deletion of the P gene in Tanzanian patients with type II oculocutaneous albinism (OCA2). Am J Hum Genet 1995;56:1320–1323.

Stevens G, Ramsay JM, Jenkins T. Oculocutaneous albinism (OCA2) in sub-Saharan Africa: distribution of the common 2.7-kb P gene deletion mutation. Hum Genet 1997;99:523–527.

Wagstaff J, Hemann M. A familial "balanced" 3;9 translocation with cryptic 8q insertion leading to deletion and duplication of 9p23 loci in siblings. Am J Hum Genet 1995;56:302–309.

80 Basal Cell Nevus Syndrome

ERVIN EPSTEIN, JR.

BACKGROUND

The basal cell nevus syndrome (BCNS) (nevoid basal-cell carcinoma syndrome, Gorlin syndrome, McKusick MIM 109400) is a rare, multisystem, heritable disorder. Evidence exists for its presence in Egyptian mummies, and cases were described initially a century ago. The association of multiple basal-cell carcinomas with jaw cysts and skeletal abnormalities was well-described by midcentury, and subsequent descriptions have produced an extensive list of phenotypic abnormalities. Case reports by Howell and Caro in 1959 and by Gorlin and Goltz in 1960 focused much more widespread attention on the condition, and more recently the interest of several groups in molecular analysis of the syndrome has stimulated the collection of larger groups of patients and consequent better clinical characterization. Two recent estimates of disease frequency are 1:56,000 and 1:164,000 or greater.

CLINICAL FEATURES

Phenotypic abnormalities affect many organ systems. Individual patients have varying combinations of abnormalities, and intrafamilial variation is prominent. A listing of some of the abnormalities is given in Table 80-1.

SKIN The most notable skin abnormalities are basal-cell carcinomas (BCCs). These are the commonest human tumor—perhaps a half million are treated each year in the United States, and in sunny areas their incidence plus that of cutaneous squamous-cell carcinomas may exceed the combined incidence of all other cancers. Although the dose–reponse relationship is not straightforward, it is clear that skin damage by sunlight predisposes to BCCs. Thus, they occur frequently on sun-exposed areas and much less frequently on covered sites; they occur more commonly in sunnier areas of the world; they occur commonly in individuals with white skin and seldom in patients with darker skin (although albinos of African or Asian descent are susceptible to their development); and they occur in high numbers in patients who have defective repair of ultraviolet radiation-induced DNA damage (i.e., patients with xeroderma pigmentosum). Typically, BCCs occur in individuals of middle-to-later ages and are one to several in number.

Some individual BCCs in patients with BCNS may have the pearly, translucent, telangectactic, papular appearance of BCCs in sporadic cases but others may appear as tiny tag-like papules that may be so widespread that they are dismissed unless the examination is quite careful. Histologically they are indistinguishable from BCCs in nonfamilial cases. The role of sunlight in producing BCCs in BCNS patients, like that in sporadic cases, is not straightforward. An active role of sunlight is suggested by the reported earlier age of appearance of the first BCCs in BCNS patients in Australia than in the North West of England (47 vs 4% by age 20), the small numbers of BCCs in black-skinned BCNS patients, and the predominant localization of BCCs on sun-exposed skin sites of patients with BCNS. However, the latter localization is less strict than in patients without BCNS, for the percentage of BCCs occurring in normally covered areas (i.e., not the face and arms) is higher in BCNS patients than in sporadic patients—42 vs 13%. BCCs in BCNS patients have metastasized to the lungs and heart, as in sporadic cases, such occurrences are quite rare. Uncontrollable local invasion is less rare but still very uncommon—4 of 70 patients in one series suffered facial mutilation such as loss of an eye or an ear.

The other very common skin abnormality in BCNS patients is the presence of pits of the palms and soles (Fig. 80-1). These typically appear during the second decade, are 1–2 mm in diameter, and may be made more prominent by soaking the skin in tapwater for 15 min, thus causing swelling of the surrounding normal stratum corneum. The pits are formed by local absence of the stratum corneum. Generally, the epidermis underlying the pits is unremarkable, but BCCs have arisen from them. BCNS patients also have a higher than normal incidence of epidermal inclusion cysts—perhaps 50%. Usually these are histologically unremarkable.

JAW The most diagnostic extracutaneous abnormality is the presence of one or more cysts in the jaws. These cysts are lined by a stratified-squamous epithelium that produces parakeratotic keratinous debris and may have satellite epithelial cysts and/or islands resembling BCCs. They may be clinically silent and detected only by X-ray examination or may cause localized swelling or pain of the jaw. Their histology closely overlaps that of the odontogenic keratocysts of sporadic cases. Recurrences postoperatively are common—10/16 in one series—and loss or displacement of teeth because of local invasion of bone can occur. Malignant changes (development of squamous-cell carcinoma) in the lining are very rare. These keratocysts can develop at any age but they appear most commonly in the later part of the first decade through the second and third decade, and they are more common in the mandible than the maxilla.

SKELETAL Calcification of the falx is present commonly in patients—in one report in 100% of patients 20 years of age and older as compared to a percentage that increases with age in nor-

From: *Principles of Molecular Medicine* (J. L. Jameson, ed.), ©1998 Humana Press Inc., Totowa, NJ.

Table 80-1
Diagnostic Findings in Adults with BCNS

50% or greater frequency
Enlarged occipitofrontal circumference (macrocephaly, frontoparietal bossing, in index cases only?)
Multiple basal-cell carcinomas
Odontogenic keratocysts of jaws
Epidermal cysts of skin
High-arched palate
Palmar or plantar pits
Rib anomalies (e.g., splayed, fused, partially missing, bifid)
Spina bifida occulta of cervical or thoracic vertebrae
Calcified falx cerebri
Calcified diaphragma sellae (bridged sella, fused clinoids)
Hyperpneumatization of paranasal sinuses
49 to 15% frequency
Calcification of tentorium cerebelli and petroclinoid ligament
Calcified ovarian fibromas
Short fourth metacarpals
Kyphoscoliosis or other vertebral anomalies
Lumbarization of sacrum
Narrow sloping shoulders
Prognathism
Pectus excavatum or carinatum
Pseudocystic lytic lesion of bones (hamartomas)
Strabismus (exotropia)
14% or less, but not random
Medulloblastoma
Inguinal hernia (?)
True ocular hypertelorism
Meningioma
Lymphomesenteric cyst
Cardiac fibroma
Fetal rhabdomyoma
Ovarian fibrosarcoma
Marfanoid build
Anosmia
Agenesis of corpus callosum
Cyst of septum pellucidum
Cleft lip and/or palate
Low-pitched female voice
Polydactyly, postaxial in hands or feet
Sprengel deformity of scapula
Syndactyly
Congenital cataract, glaucoma, coloboma of iris, retina, optic nerve, medullated retinal nerve fibers
Subcutaneous calcifications of skin (possibly underestimated frequency)
Minor kidney malformations
Hypogonadism in male subjects
Mental Retardation

Reprinted with permission from Gorlin, R.J. Nevoid basal cell carcinoma syndrome. Dermatologic Clinics 1995;13:113–125.

mal individuals from 10 to 50% between ages 20 and 70. Calcification is more dense, even exuberant, in BCNS patients and is described as lamellar. Other intracranial membranes also may be calcified.

Dysmorphic changes also are reported frequently. One of the most common is an increased head size, but one recent study found increased head size only in index cases and not in their affected relatives. Large supraorbital ridges and wide-set eyes also are reported frequently as part of a characteristic facies. Ribs commonly are abnormal—bifid, flared, fused, hypoplastic, or missing—and rib abnormalities and/or spina bifida occulta of the cervical or thoracic spine occur in approximately 50% of patients. The sternum may be concave or convex, and numerous other malformations have been cataloged. Some patients have a marfanoid habitus, and many adult patients are considerably bulkier than their parents. Phalangeal lucencies were common in one series in which hand X-rays were studied, and sclerotic bone changes resembling those of metastases have been reported.

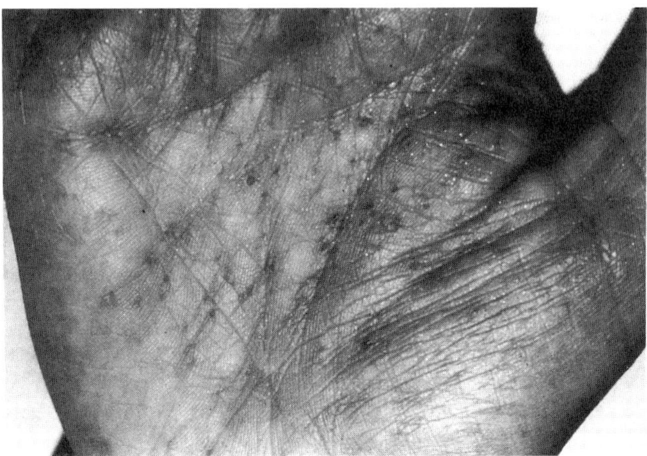

Figure 80-1 Right palm of patient with BCNS. The typical, distinctive, 2-mm in diameter pits in the stratum corneum are visible as darker spots.

VISCERAL TUMORS Medulloblastomas are the most serious extracutaneous tumors present in clearly higher frequency in BCNS patients. Like BCCs, they tend to arise at a younger age in BCNS patients than in sporadic cases (most before age 5 and half before age 2, at which age sporadic medulloblastomas are unusual). In larger series of BCNS patients, medulloblastomas have been found in 1–5% of patients, and the incidence of BCNS in patients with medulloblastomas is also 1–5%. BCNS patients with meningiomas have been reported but less commonly than those with medulloblastomas.

By contrast, ovarian fibromas are common, and these tumors frequently are calcified. They usually are asymptomatic and do not interfere with ovarian function. Cysts of the mesentery may be present, sometimes with calcification leading to notable radiological abnormalities. Several BCNS patients have had cardiac fibromas, some with onset in infancy, and in one instance a fibrous histiocytoma became so large as to necessitate cardiac transplantation.

DIAGNOSIS

Diagnosis of the classical case is straightforward, but the phenotypic variability of affected patients and the fact that all of the abnormalities may be seen, albeit less frequently, in otherwise normal individuals may make it difficult to be certain of the diagnosis, even in relatives of patients whose own diagnosis is indubitable. Both of two recent larger series proposed four major diagnostic criteria—BCCs, odontogenic keratocysts, palmoplantar pits, and lamellar calcification of the falx—and minor criteria including rib anomalies, medulloblastomas, cardiac or ovarian fibromas, and several of the other abnormalities listed in Table 80-1. For diagnosis, two major or one major plus two minor criteria are required. Without an inexpensive and sensitive screening for the underlying molecule defect, phenotype-based diagnosis is likely to continue to be difficult for many patients with less than classical findings.

GENETIC BASIS OF DISEASE

BCNS is inherited as an autosomal-dominant trait. New mutations are common (14–81% in one large series, this wide range reflecting the difficulty of being certain that unexamined parents lack all phenotypic abnormalities of the syndrome). The lack of obvious differences in phenotype according to whether disease has been inherited from the mother or the father suggests that imprinting does not underlie the phenotypic variability.

The autosomal-dominant inheritance and the cardinal manifestation of the development of BCCs in higher number and at an earlier age than in sporadic cases suggested to several observers more than a decade ago the possibility that the gene whose mutations underlie the BCNS might be a tumor-suppressor gene and that, like retinoblastomas, BCCs might require two "hits" for their development. Since one frequent mechanism of tumor-suppressor gene inactivation is allelic deletion, A. Bale and colleagues assessed BCCs arising in sporadic cases for such deletions. Indeed, they found a high incidence of loss of heterozygosity at chromosome 9q and then found significant linkage of the inheritance of BCNS to the inheritance of 9q22.3–9q31. This was confirmed rapidly by other groups. Further studies of loss of heterozygosity have confirmed an approximately 50% incidence of loss of this region with relatively little loss at other loci except at chromosome 1q. In patients with BCNS, the copy of chromosome 9q22.3–9q31 lost in BCCs is that predicted by linkage to contain the normal allele. Thus, these tumors are left with a single copy of this region, and that copy is predicted to harbor a nonfunctional allele.

No BCNS kindred has been reported in which the mutant gene fails to map to the same site on chromosome 9q, suggesting that there is a single locus whose mutations underlie all BCNS patients. Subsequent genetic mapping narrowed the region to an estimated 1.8–3.6 cM; YAC-BAC-cosmid contigs spanning the genetically delimited region were assembled; and several groups embarked on a search for isolating genes in this region. This search was capped in 1996 by the simultaneous reports by two groups of mapping of the human homolog of the *Drosophila patched* gene to the genetically defined BCNS region and of mutations of this gene in DNA both from leukocytes of BCNS patients and also from sporadic basal-cell carcinomas. Thus, it appears that this gene functions, at least in the skin, as a tumor-suppressor gene, that patients with the BCNS inherit one defective copy, and that somatic mutations that inactivate in keratinocytes the one functional allele in BCNS patients or both normal alleles in sporadic cases are a crucial step underlying the development of basal-cell carcinomas that arise sporadically. The nature of the mutations described in the skin tumors is consistent with some of them having been caused by ultraviolet radiation, as expected.

The fly *patched* gene has been studied extensively since its identification in 1989. It is a membrane-bound member of a signaling pathway that is critical in development. It acts to suppress expression of several genes, including cubitus interruptus, a member of the GLI gene family (so named because of the identification of GLI as an oncogene in human glioblastomas); *wingless*, a member of the WNT oncogene family; *decapentaplegic*, a member of the TGF-β gene family; as well as *patched* itself. It is opposed in these functions by the secreted product of the *hedgehog* gene. This pathway helps control segmentation and wing development in flies and appears to play analogous roles in vertebrates.

Mutations also have been described in BCCs in the genes encoding sonic hedgehog and smoothened, the other two members of this pathway that interact with the patched protein at the cell surface. The mutant proteins appear to act dominantly as the products of activated oncogenes, and this identification provides evidence that it is activation of the signaling pathway that determines the abnormal behavior of keratinocytes.

Thus it seems reasonable now to consider the phenotypic abnormalities in BCNS patients in two categories—developmental (e.g., rib and spine abnormalities and generalized overgrowth) and tumors (e.g., BCCs, medulloblastomas, fibromas, cysts) and to consider that the *PATCHED* gene functions in humans embryologically to direct development and postnatally to control proliferation and/or differentiation, i.e., as a tumor suppressor.

Many questions are raised by this gene identification, and the role of the hedgehog/patched signaling pathway in humans is likely to be a subject of intense investigation during the next several years.

TREATMENT

Individual BCCs in BCNS patients can be treated by the surgical approaches used for BCCs in sporadic cases. The often high number of tumors may make their excision impractical, and, e.g., cryotherapy with liquid nitrogen may be helpful for the many small lesions, especially those that are well-removed from the eye, ear, and other sites where BCCs may be particularly destructive. X-irradiation should be used with extreme caution because BCNS patients clearly are susceptible to X-ray carcinogenesis. Thus, patients successfully irradiated for medulloblastomas typically develop large numbers of BCCs in the overlying skin within a half decade. Also, instances of squamous-cell carcinomas and of fibrosarcomas with metastases have occurred soon after therapeutic irradiation of BCCs.

Several reports have documented significant reduction in the appearance of new BCCs during systemic treatment with 13-*cis*-retinoic acid but typically the side effects at the doses required to inhibit BCC growth eventually become intolerable. Topical retinoic acid and topical 5-fluorouracil may slow the growth of tumors.

SELECTED REFERENCES

Bale SJ, Amos CI, Parry DM, Bale AE. Relationship between head circumference and height in normal adults and in the nevoid basal cell carcinoma syndrome and neurofibromatosis type I. Am J Med Gen 1991;40:206–210.

Binkley GW, Johnson HHJ. Epithelioma adenoides cysticum: basal cell nevi, agenesis of the corpus callosum and dental cysts. Arch Dermat Syph 1951;63:73–84.

Bonifas JM, Bare JW, Kerschmann RL, Master SP, Epstein EH Jr. Parental origin of chromosome 9q22.3-q31 lost in basal cell carcinomas from basal cell nevus syndrome patients. Hum Mol Genet 1994;3: 447,448.

Chenevix-Trench G, Wicking C, Berkman J, et al. Further localization of the gene for nevoid basal cell carcinoma syndrome (NBCCS) in 15 Australasian families: linkage and loss of heterozygosity. Am J Hum Genet 1993;53:760–767.

Compton JG, Goldstein AM, Turner M, et al. Fine mapping of the locus for nevoid basal cell carcinoma syndrome on chromosome 9q. J Invest Dermatol 1994;103:178–181.

Dunnick NR, Head GL, Peck GL, Yoder FW. Nevoid basal cell carcinoma syndrome: radiographic manifestations including cystlike lesions of the phalanges. Radiology 1978;127:331–334.

Evans DGR, Farndon PA, Burnell LD, Gattamaneni HR, Birch JM. The incidence of Gorlin syndrome in 173 consecutive cases of medulloblastoma. Br J Cancer 1991;64:959–961.

Evans DGR, Ladusans EJ, Rimmer S, Burnell LD, Thakker N, Farndon PA. Complications of the naevoid basal cell carcinoma syndrome: results of a population based study. J Med Genet 1993;30: 460–464.

Farndon PA, Morris DJ, Hardy C, et al. Analysis of 133 meioses places the genes for nevoid basal cell carcinoma (Gorlin) syndrome and Fanconi anemia group C in a 2.6-cM interval and contributes to the fine map of 9q22.3. Genomics 1994;23:486–489.

Forssell K, Forssell H, Kahnberg K-E. Recurrence of keratocysts: a long-term follow-up study. Int J Oral Maxillofacial Surg 1988;17:25–28.

Gailani MR, Bale SJ, Leffell DJ, et al. Developmental defects in Gorlin syndrome related to a putative tumor suppressor gene on chromosome 9. Cell 1992;69:111–117.

Goldstein AM, Bale SJ, Peck GL, DiGiovanna JJ. Sun exposure and basal cell carcinomas in the nevoid basal cell carcinoma syndrome. J Am Acad Dermat 1993;29:34–41.

Goldstein AM, Pastakia B, DiGiovanna JJ, et al. Clinical findings in two African-American families with the nevoid basal cell carcinoma syndrome (NBCC). Am J Med Genet 1994;50:272–281.

Goldstein AM, Stewart C, Bale AE, Bale SJ, Dean M. Localization of the gene for the nevoid basal cell carcinoma syndrome. Am J Hum Genet 1994;54:765–773.

Golitz LE, Norris DA, Luekens CA Jr, Charles DM. Nevoid basal cell carcinoma syndrome: multiple basal cell carcinomas of the palms after radiation therapy. Arch Dermat 1980;116:1159–1163.

Goodrich LV, Milenkovic L, Higgins KM, Scott MP. Altered neural cell fates and medulloblastoma in mouse patched mutants. Science 1997;277:1109–1113.

Gorlin RJ. Nevoid basal cell carcinoma syndrome. Dermat Clinics 1995;13:113–125.

Gorlin R.J. Nevoid Basal-Cell Carcinoma syndrome. Medicine 1987; 66:98–113.

Gorlin RJ, Goltz RW. Multiple nevoid basal-cell epithelioma, jaw cysts and bifid ribs: a syndrome. N Engl J Med 1960;262:908–912.

Hahn H, Wicking C, Zaphiropoulous PG, et al. Mutations of the human homologue of Drosophila patched in the nevoid basal cell carcinoma syndrome. Cell 1996;85:841–851.

Herman TE, Siegel MJ, McAlister WH. Cardiac tumor in Gorlin syndrome. Pediatric Radiol 1991;21:234,235.

Howell JB. Nevoid basal cell carcinoma syndrome: profile of genetic and environmental factors in oncogenesis. J Am Acad Dermat 1984;11:98–104.

Howell JB, Caro MR. Basal cell nevus: its relationship to multiple cutaneous cancers and associated anomalies of development. Arch of Dermat 1959;79:67–80.

Johnson AD, Hebert AA, Esterly NB. Nevoid basal cell carcinoma syndrome: bilateral ovarian fibromas in a 3 1/2-year-old girl. J Am Acad Dermat 1986;14:371 374.

Johnson RL, Rothman AL, Xie J, et al. Human homolog of patched, a candidate gene for the basal cell nevus syndrome. Science 1996;272:1668–1671.

Leppard BJ. Skin cysts in the basal cell naevus syndrome. Clin Exp Dermat 1983;8:603–612.

Morris DJ, Reis A. A YAC contig spanning the nevoid basal cell carcinoma syndrome, Fanconi anaemia group C, and xeroderma pigmentosum group A loci on chromosome 9q. Genomics 1994;23:23–29.

Oro AE, Higgins KM, Hu Z, Bonifas JM, Epstein EH Jr, Scott MP. Basal cell carcinomas in mice overexpressing sonic hedgehog. Science 1997;276:817–821.

Peck GL, DiGiovanna JJ, Sarnoff DS, et al. Treatment and prevention of basal cell carcinoma with oral isotretinoin. J Am Acad Dermat 1988;19:176–185.

Ratcliffe JF, Shanley S, Chenevix-Trench G. The prevalence of cervical and thoracic congenital skeletal abnormalities in basal cell naevus syndrome; a review of cervical and chest radiographs in 80 patients with BCNS. Br J Radiol 1995;68:596–599.

Ratcliffe JF, Shanley S, Ferguson J, Chenevix-Trench G. The diagnostic implication of falcine calcification on plain skull radiographs of patients with basal cell naevus syndrome and the incidence of falcine calcification in their relatives and two control groups. Br J Radiol 1995;68:361–368.

Shanley S, Ratcliffe J, Hockey A. Nevoid basal cell carcinoma syndrome: review of 118 affected individuals. Amer J Med Genet 1994;50: 282–290.

Southwick, GJ, Schwartz RA. The basal cell nevus syndrome: disasters occurring among a series of 36 patients. Cancer 1979;44:2294–2305.

Strange PR, Lang PG. Long-term management of basal cell nevus syndrome with topical tretinoin and 5-fluorouracil. J Am Acad Dermat 1992;27:842–845.

Vorechovsky I, Tingby O, Hartman M, et al. Somatic mutations in the human homologue of Drosophila patched in primitive neuroectodermal tumours. Oncogene 1997;15:361–366.

Wicking C, Berkman J, Wainwright B, Chenevix-Trench G. Fine genetic mapping of the gene for nevoid basal cell carcinoma syndrome. Genomics 1994;22:505–511.

Wicking C, Shanley S, Smyth I, et al. Most germ-line mutations in the nevoid basal cell carcinoma syndrome lead to a premature termination of the PATCHED protein, and no genotype-phenotype correlations are evident. Am J Hum Genet 1997;60:21–26.

Wolter M, Reifenberger J, Sommer C, Ruzicka T, Reifenberger G. Mutations in the human homologue of the Drosophila segment polarity gene patched (PTCH) in sporadic basal cell carcinomas of the skin and primitive neuroectodermal tumors of the central nervous system. Cancer Res 1997;57:2581–2585.

Xie J, Johnson RL, Zhang X, et al. Mutations of the PATCHED gene in several types of sporadic extracutaneous tumors. Cancer Res 1997; 57:2369–2372.

Xie J, Quinn A, Zhang X, et al. Physical mapping of the 5 Mb D9S196-D9S180 interval harboring the basal cell nevus syndrome gene and localization of six genes in this region. Genes Chromosomes Cancer 1997;18:305–309.

Xie J. Nature 1998, in press.

81 Xeroderma Pigmentosum and Related Disorders

W. CLARK LAMBERT, HON-REEN KUO, AND MURIEL W. LAMBERT

INTRODUCTION

Inherited diseases with cutaneous manifestations currently believed to be associated with defective DNA repair and/or chromosomal instability, of which xeroderma pigmentosum is the prototype, are all very rare. The more important of these, discussed here, are listed in Table 81-1. Diseases above the open space are all (mainly) autosomal recessive disorders; those below it, autosomal dominant. Of the recessive diseases, there are four major entities: (1) xeroderma pigmentosum, which may occur together with a distinctive autosomal recessive disorder, Cockayne disease, and the cells of which may show some very similar changes, with failure of complementation, with those of cells from some cases with yet a third disorder, trichothiodystrophy; (2) Fanconi anemia, an important variant of which, lacking only the congenital anomalies characteristic of Fanconi anemia, is the Diamond-Blackfan syndrome (also known as the Estren-Dameshek variant of Fanconi anemia); (3) Ataxia-Telangiectasia, which shares distinctive cell culture but not clinical characteristics with two other disorders, the Nijmegen breakage syndrome and the Berlin breakage syndrome, which complement each other in complementation assays but are otherwise identical; and (4) Bloom syndrome. There is also less-well-documented evidence for defective DNA repair and/or chromosomal instability in a number of other disorders, such as progeria of various subtypes and dyskeratosis congenita.

It is likely that the genetics of some of these rare recessive diseases is much more complex than the simple phrase "autosomal recessive" would imply. A number of cell lines from different ones of these disorders test positive in at least one assay, in which chromosome abnormalities are scored following irradiation in the G2 phase of the cell cycle. This implies that these diseases are indeed related to each other. There is convincing evidence for both intragenic and intergenic genetic heterogeneity within several of these entities. Thus, different involved loci or combinations of involved loci may produce different genetic subtypes of the same disease, or even subtypes of different diseases occurring together. It is possible that the extremely complex nature of chromatin structure, with different proteins often playing more than one role, interacting with each other and possibly partially compensating for any loss or deficiency of one another, may result in specific diseases being traced only to very severe—or combined—deficiencies in these proteins. Many of the nuclear proteins identified to date as defective in one or more of these diseases are involved not only in DNA repair and maintenance of chromatin stability but also in such other cellular processes as initiation of transcription, DNA replication, and cell-cycle checkpoint controls. This may provide an explanation for some of the pleiotropic features of these disorders. A number of much more common diseases may also be related etiopathologically to less extreme defects in chromatin proteins and nuclear enzymes, but this is yet to be conclusively proved.

XERODERMA PIGMENTOSUM

BACKGROUND Xeroderma pigmentosum is a rare, [usually] autosomal recessively transmitted disease characterized by variable but usually extreme sun sensitivity associated with a marked tendency to develop precancerous lesions and, subsequently, skin cancers at a [usually] very early age in sun-exposed areas of the skin, lips, conjunctivae, and, sometimes, anterior tongue. These changes are absolutely dependent on sun exposure; sun-protected areas do not develop these changes. A subset of patients develop a progressive neurodegenerative disease, not related to sun exposure. The disease is genetically heterogeneous, with eight complementation groups known, labeled A, B, C, D, E, F, G, and V *(see below)*. Individuals in groups A, B, and G are the most sun-sensitive, whereas those in groups A and D are most prone to develop neurological disease. The first description of the disease, under the name "xeroderma" was in 1870 by Moritz Kaposi in a textbook edited by his father-in-law, Ferdinand von Hebra, professor of dermatology at the University of Vienna. Twelve years later he described additional patients and added the term "pigmentosum" to the name of the disease. The first case with neurological signs was described by Dr. Albert Neisser, better known for his work on the *Neisseria* species of bacteria named for him. In 1932, De Sanctis and Cacchione described a severely neurodegenerate case with microcephaly and mental retardation. The term "De-Sanctis-Cacchione syndrome" has subsequently been used to designate cases of xeroderma pigmentosum with a neurologic component. However, we believe that this term should only be applied in cases of severe neurologic deficiency, such as described by De Sanctis and Cacchione, with the remainder simply known as xeroderma pigmentosum with a neurological defect or component.

From: *Principles of Molecular Medicine* (J. L. Jameson, ed.), ©1998 Humana Press Inc., Totowa, NJ.

Table 81-1
Skin Disorders Associated with Defective DNA Repair and/or Chromosomal Instability

Xeroderma pigmentosum
Cockayne syndrome
Some trichothiodystrophies
Fanconi anemia
Diamond-Blackfan syndrome (Estren-Dameshek variant of Fanconi anemia)
Ataxia-telangiectasia (Louis-Barr syndrome)
Nijmegen breakage syndrome
Berlin breakage syndrome
Ataxia-telangiectasia Fresno
Bloom syndrome
Gardner syndrome (variant of Familial adenomatous polyposis [FAP] syndrome)
Turcot syndrome (variant of familial adenomatous polyposis [PAP] syndrome)
Muir-Torre syndrome (variant of the Human nonpolyposis colon carcinoma [HNPCC] syndrome)
Other diseases are also known with less well characterized DNA repair defects and/a chromosomal instabilities

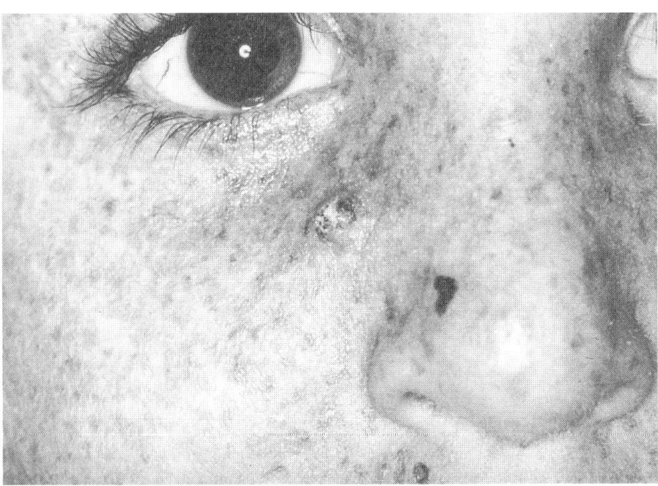

Figure 81-1 Face of a 22-month-old white male with severely sun-sensitive xeroderma pigmentosum. Note early changes, as well as a neoplasm (keratoacomthoma) on the cheek and a dysplastic melanocytic lesion on his nose. (Reproduced with permission from Lambert et al., 1998.)

The study of xeroderma pigmentosum at the cellular/biochemical level has generated many justified "firsts" in the study of human genetic diseases. In 1968, James Cleaver reported that fibroblasts derived from a patient with xeroderma pigmentosum were unable to perform the nucleotide excision type of DNA repair following exposure to short wavelength ultraviolet C light emitted by a germicidal lamp. This finding was confirmed shortly afterwards by Richard Setlow and his coworkers in cultured fibroblasts, and by John Epstein and his collaborators in an in vivo assay carried out in the skin of a xeroderma pigmentosum patient. This was the first indication of a DNA repair defect associated with a human disease. In 1972, Dirk Bootsma and his laboratory modified the autoradiography assay, which had been used to detect defective DNA repair in fibroblasts, to develop a complementation assay, which demonstrated genetic heterogeneity within xeroderma pigmentosum. This was the first such cellular/biochemical assay developed for examination of genetic heterogeneity in a human genetic disease. Rufus Day and his coworkers modified a host-cell reactivation viral assay developed in bacteria and Michael Sideman and Kenneth Kraemer and their colleagues used a further modification of this assay, the shuttle vector assay, to examine DNA repair and mutagenesis in normal and xeroderma pigmentosum cells in culture. In 1982 our laboratory, and in 1988 Richard Wood and his colleagues developed cell-free assay systems for nucleotide excision repair and used them to demonstrate defective DNA repair in xeroderma pigmentosum cell extracts in cell-free systems. The former assay has been used to show defective interaction of xeroderma pigmentosum chromatin protein complexes involved in DNA repair with nucleosomal DNA (i.e., addition of histones to damaged DNA, so as to reconstitute the DNA into nucleosomal DNA, creates a substrate on which normal chromatin DNA repair protein complexes show enhanced activity, whereas the corresponding xeroderma pigmentosum protein complexes show decreased activity on this nucleosomal DNA). The latter system has been used extensively to examine the roles of different proteins and protein complexes involved in several cellular processes, particularly initiation of transcription, and DNA repair, and to determine which of them are defective in different complementation groups of xeroderma pigmentosum. In 1992, Tanaka and his colleagues cloned a gene defective in patients in group A of xeroderma pigmentosum; five other xeroderma pigmentosum "correcting" genes have subsequently been cloned. Many other "firsts" related to cellular/biochemical studies of xeroderma pigmentosum are beyond the scope of this review.

CLINICAL FINDINGS Xeroderma pigmentosum has a worldwide distribution and has been reported in all major racial groups, including Blacks. In the United States and Europe, and probably most parts of the world, the incidence is approximately 2–4 per 10^6 live births, but it is significantly more common in certain areas, especially Japan, North Africa, and the Middle East. It has also been reported to be especially common among the Bantus of Africa. In Japan, the incidence has been estimated to be about one in 40,000 live births.

Xeroderma pigmentosum typically presents in infancy or early childhood with a sunburn following sun exposure. Less commonly, the child may cry when exposed to sunlight to the extent that this is called to the attention of a physician. Sometimes the initial sunburn may be so severe that the parents are suspected of some sort of child abuse. Depending on the sensitivity of the patient to sunlight and the extent of prior cumulative sun exposure, physical examination shows variable changes consisting of dryness (xerosis), induration, and dyspigmentation consisting of irregularly mottled freckling. The changes are absolutely limited to sun-exposed areas, and a sharp line of demarcation between involved and uninvolved skin is consistently present. As this process progresses, the freckles become larger, very irregular in shape, and some of them become darker. (Fig. 81-1). Areas of hypopigmentation and/or atrophy or scarring as well as telangiectasias also appear. These changes resemble those seen in the photoaging observed in older persons with light-complexioned skin who have undergone chronic sun exposure. They are often accompanied by eye lesions, such as extropion and entropion. A conspicuously absent feature, seen in these people but not in patients with xeroderma pigmentosum, however, is elastosis of dermal collagen.

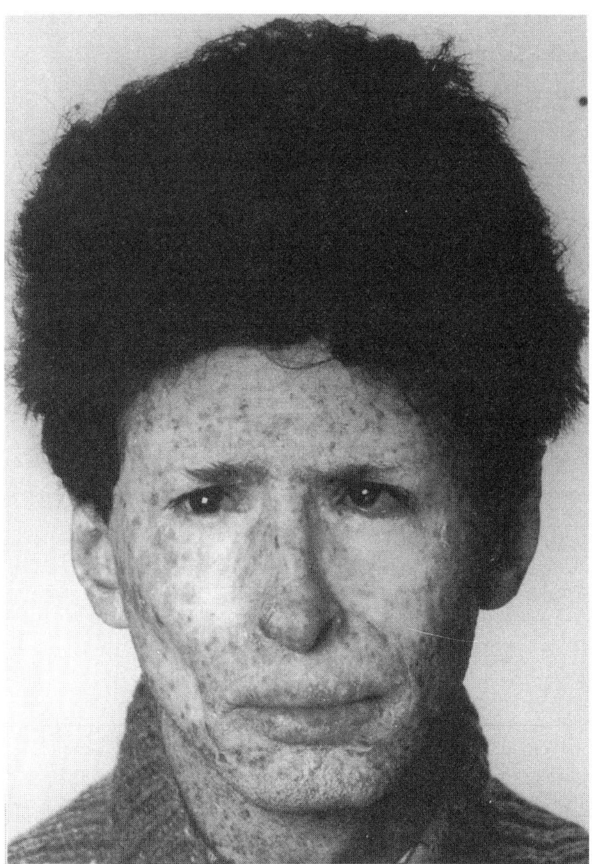

Figure 81-2 Face of a 29-year-old man with xeroderma pigmentation. Note progression of changes (compared to Fig. 81-1).

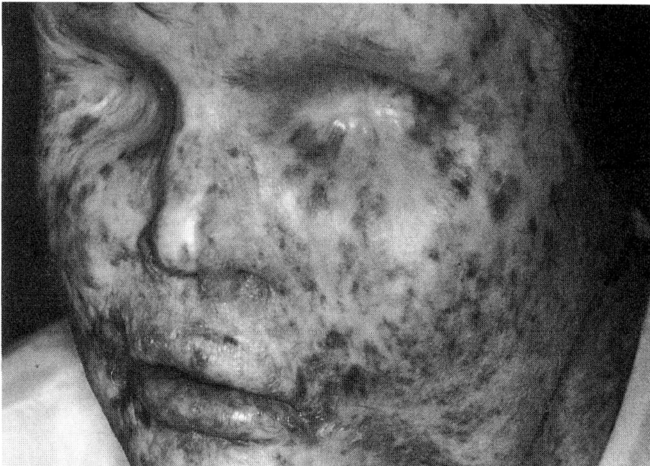

Figure 81-3 Face of a 47-year-old woman with xeroderma pigmentosum. Hundreds of neoplasms have been removed, as have both eyes.

As these changes continue to progress, premalignant and, subsequently, malignant skin lesions begin to appear (Fig. 81-1). Solar keratoses and keratoacanthomas usually appear first, followed by basal and squamous cell carcinomas and, sooner or later, melanomas (Fig. 81-2). The melanomas may arise in progressively larger and more irregularly shaped freckles; since there may be hundreds to thousands of these freckles, early detection of melanomas is often difficult. Long survival of severely sun-sensitive cases is uncommon; patients who reach middle age often show numerous neoplasms as well as extensive scarring and loss of tissue due to numerous surgical procedures carried out over the years on limited areas of skin (Fig. 81-3).

A recent review of data obtained by the Xeroderma Pigmentosum Registry has provided the first reliable information regarding the distribution of melanoma and nonmelanoma skin cancers in patients with xeroderma pigmentosum. In both normal subjects and in patients with xeroderma pigmentosum, nonmelanoma skin cancers appear over areas of greatest cumulative sun exposure (Fig. 81-4). In contrast, melanomas appear at sites of intermittent sun exposure, closely correlating to areas exposed to the sun during sunbathing (upper body in men and upper body [sparing the breasts] and legs in women) (Fig. 81-5). These data, which for Xeroderma Pigmentosum Registry patients contrast sharply with those obtained from perusal of multiple case reports of xeroderma pigmentosum in the literature, are consistent with the hypothesis that xeroderma pigmentosum is a valid model for skin cancer in the general population. There are, however, some interesting differences. Some patients with xeroderma pigmentosum develop multiple carcinomas and only a few melanomas, but others develop numerous melanomas and few or no carcinomas. At least two patients have developed numerous melanomas, which, unaccountably, have failed to metastasize, and another has shown a dramatic response of melanomas to injection with interferon-α. Computerized morphometry has found that the nuclei of melanomas arising in xeroderma pigmentosum patients are smaller and less pleomorphic than those arising in otherwise normal subjects, and in many cases these melanomas arise from solar lentigos, whereas this is rarely the case in melanomas that arise in the general population. Despite these discrepancies, however, these data indicate at least one major difference in the pathogenesis of nonmelanoma vs melanoma skin cancers in both normal subjects and in patients with xeroderma pigmentosum, even though they appear to share the same etiology, ultraviolet light damage due to sunlight.

Skin cancers of all types are about 1000 or more times more frequent in patients with xeroderma pigmentosum and arise about 40 years earlier than in the general population. If patients survive to adulthood they may have had hundreds to thousands removed, with extensive morbidity due to both the lesions, themselves, and the surgery necessary to remove them. Often, enucleation of the eyes is necessary (Fig. 81-3). In addition to skin cancers, premalignant and malignant conjunctival lesions often develop, as well as premalignant and malignant lesions of the lips and anterior tongue (Fig. 81-6). Sooner or later, patients with xeroderma pigmentosum usually die from complications due to these cancers, either from metastatic disease in developed countries or, in more primitive countries where it is impossible to treat so many tumors, from sepsis due to the tumors.

Xeroderma pigmentosum is an extremely heterogeneous disease, both clinically and genetically *(see below)*. Despite the fact that the typical patient shows extensive changes early in life, there are others with much milder disease that develops much more slowly. These patients often present much later in life, and are more difficult to diagnose, than their more typical counterparts.

In sharp contrast to the above skin, ocular, and oral stigmata, which are absolutely related to cumulative exposure to ultraviolet

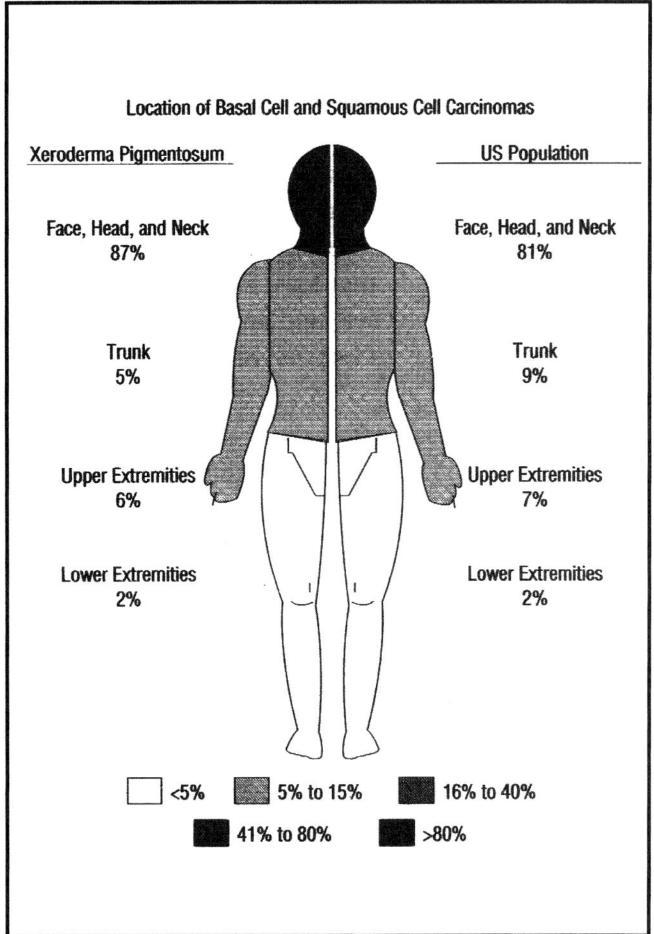

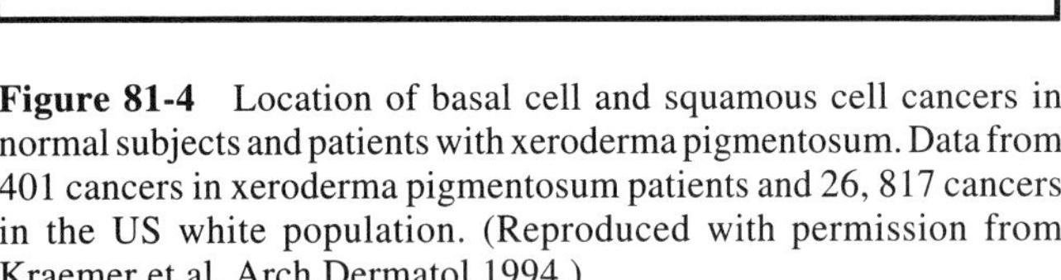

Figure 81-4 Location of basal cell and squamous cell cancers in normal subjects and patients with xeroderma pigmentosum. Data from 401 cancers in xeroderma pigmentosum patients and 26, 817 cancers in the US white population. (Reproduced with permission from Kraemer et al. Arch Dermatol 1994.)

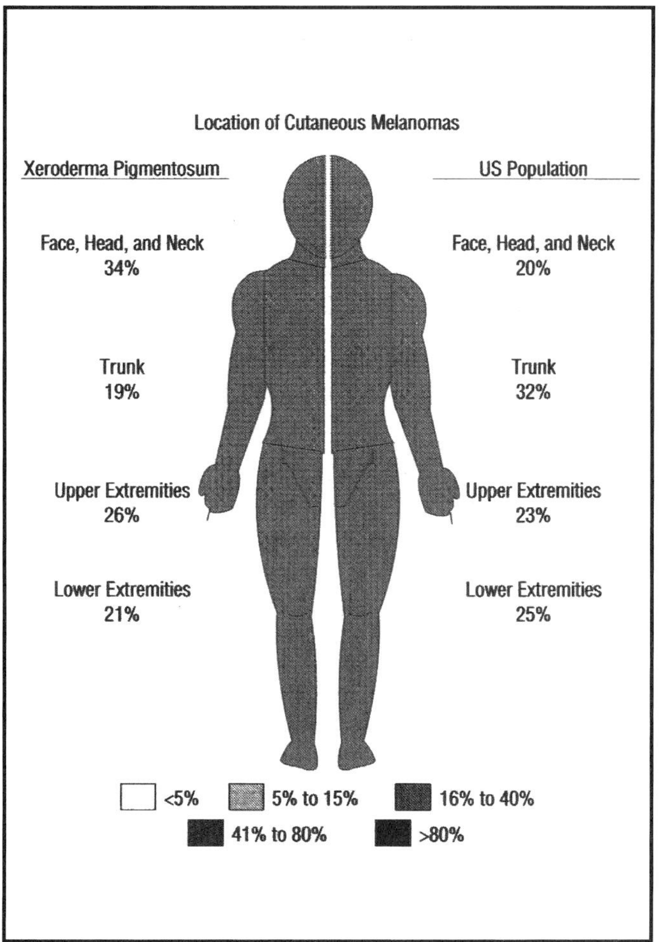

Figure 81-5 Location of melanomas in normal subjects and in patients with xeroderma pigmentosum. Data from 58 cutaneous melanomas in xeroderma pigmentosum patients and 5844 cutaneous melanomas in the general US population. (Reproduced with permission from Kraemer et al. Arch Dermatol 1994.)

radiation, neurologic abnormalities in patients with xeroderma pigmentosum occur independent of any known environmental influence. These changes affect only a minority of patients; most show either no abnormalities or subclinical abnormalities detectable only using special methods. When they do occur, these changes are progressive. The most common abnormality is loss of high-frequency hearing. Also, an abnormality in REM sleep has been reported. In most cases, however, these changes, although progressive, are mild, and the worst that most patients can expect is a need to use a hearing aid. A very small subset of patients with xeroderma pigmentosum shows severe neurologic abnormalities, as well as microcephaly, present at birth. As noted *above*, we believe that the term "De Sanctis-Cacchione syndrome" should be reserved for these unfortunate patients. Severe mental retardation is usually present. A few patients with xeroderma pigmentosum also have evidence of a second inherited disease with neurologic signs, Cockayne syndrome, as discussed *below*.

The most important diagnostic assay, for xeroderma pigmentosum, the unscheduled DNA synthesis (UDS) test, is often not done, simply because it is expensive and not really necessary for the diagnosis in many cases. Even when the test is done, further tests, using fused cells, are needed to establish the complementation group; and since these tests are also expensive, they are often not performed. Sometimes an assignment of "complementation group" is made based on clinical characteristics and the degree of depression of UDS following ultraviolet light exposure, rather than on tests using fused cells, so that the complementation group assignment is not as definitive as it should be. Nevertheless, despite these limitations, it is possible to state some significant general clinical facts about xeroderma pigmentosum complementation groups, as follows:

Complementation Group A Patients in this group are severely sun-sensitive, and some but not all of them develop, prior to age 21 years, neurodegenerative disease, which is often severe. Group A is a relatively common complementation group of xeroderma pigmentosum, and is the most common group in Japan.

Complementation Group B Only three patients in this group, one American and two in the same family in Europe, have been reported. The American patient was severely sun-sensitive, the European patients much less so. All three patients also had Cockayne syndrome.

Complementation Group C Patients in this group are moderately to severely sun-sensitive but do not usually have neurological disease, although special testing reveals a subclinical hearing loss of high frequency sounds. Group C is probably the

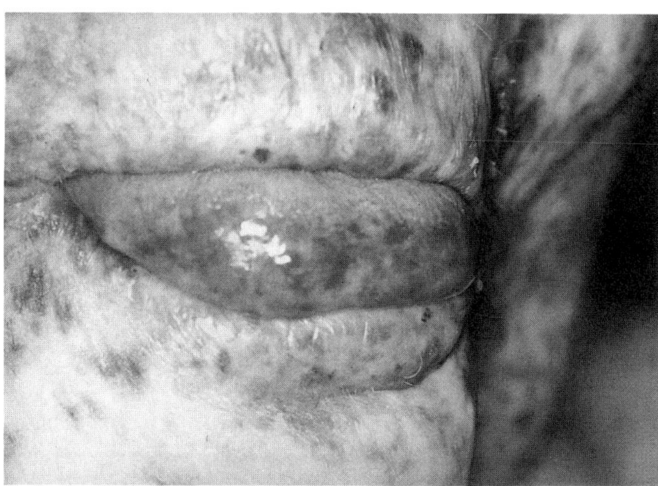

Figure 81-6 Lip and anterior tongue lesions in late xeroderma pigmentosum (same patient as in Fig. 81-3). (Reproduced with permission from Lambert et al., 1998.)

most common group worldwide, and is the most common group found in the United States, Europe, and the middle East. Two patients in this group have shown typical skin changes of xeroderma pigmentosum but have developed only melanomas that have not metastasized, and no other skin cancers.

Complementation Group D Patients in this complementation group have mild-to-moderate sun-sensitivity and typically develop neurodegeneration that is mild and of late onset. It consists mainly of deafness. It is moderately common, comprising about 20% of cases of xeroderma pigmentosum worldwide. A few patients in group D have also had unequivocal stigmata of Cockayne disease. Some patients with an entirely different disease, trichothiodystrophy, have also tested positive for the XP-D trait in the complementation assay *(see below)*.

Complementation Group E Patients in this complementation group have only mild sun sensitivity and are not usually neurologically abnormal or are minimally so. Only a few cases have been reported.

Complementation Group F Most group F patients have been moderately sun-sensitive, with development of only a few skin tumors and no neurologic abnormalities. However, one patient has been markedly sun-sensitive with severe neurological disease. Only a handful of patients have been reported, most of them Japanese.

Complementation Group G Group G patients are severely sun-sensitive. Only five patients have been reported, two of which also had unequivocal stigmata of Cockayne disease. The remaining three did not show clinically evident neurologic defects.

Complementation Group V (Variant group) Group V patients' cells test normal in the UDS assay following exposure to ultraviolet light but can be induced to show low UDS by treatment with caffeine. These patients are moderately sun-sensitive and usually are not neurologically defective. This is a relatively common group, comprising about one-third of xeroderma pigmentosum patients worldwide. It is especially common in Japan.

Dominantly Inherited Cases Two documented families—one Scottish, the other Australian—have shown an autosomal dominant pedigree for a mild type of xeroderma pigmentosum. Complementation studies have not been carried out on these patients' cells.

DIAGNOSIS In children in whom skin tumors have begun to develop, the diagnosis of xeroderma piqmentosum can usually be made with confidence purely on clinical grounds (dry, oddly pigmented, often slightly scaly skin sharply limited to sun-exposed areas, along with the tumors). In younger children, in whom tumors have not yet developed, or in older patients with milder forms of the disease, however, diagnosis may be more difficult. Children with xeroderma pigmentosum can be differentiated from those with other light-sensitive disorders by the usual tests for those disorders. For example, porphyrias can be eliminated by testing for porphyrins in the blood, urine, and feces. Although Gorlin (nevoid basal-cell carcinoma) syndrome may show multiple basal-cell cancers at an early age, the other stigmata of Gorlin syndrome (palmer pits, jaw cysts seen on X-ray) are usually easily recognizable. The dysplastic nevus syndrome may be associated with development of melanoma at a relatively young age, but the numerous dysplastic nevi usually make diagnosis relatively straightforward.

Although, ideally, one would like to perform the UDS assay *(see below)* as well as complementation group analysis on all patients with xeroderma pigmentosum, these tests are expensive, and probably need only be done when the diagnosis is in doubt. A positive UDS test is a highly specific, although not absolutely specific, indication that the patient has xeroderma pigmentosum.

The UDS test is currently performed at the following laboratories:

c/o Dr. David Bush
Department of Environmental and Toxologic Pathology Armed Forces Institute of Pathology 14th Street N.W. and Alaska Avenue
Washington, DC 20306-6000
Tel: 202-576-0222
Fax: 202-576-2164

c/o Dr. James E. Cleaver (by special arrangement only)
Laboratory of Radiobiology
University of California at San Francisco Room LR 102
3rd and Parmassus Avenue
San Francisco, CA 94143-0750
Tel: 415-476-4563
Fax: 415-476-0721

XP patients should contact, for information and support group activity:

Xerderma Pigmentation Society, Inc.
c/o Ms. Caren Mahar
PO Box 4759
Poughkeepsie, NY 12601
Tel/Fax: 914-473-9735

Physicians with patients with Xeroderma patients should contact:

Xeroderma Pigmentosum Registry
c/o W. Clark lambert, MD
Rm C-520 Medical Science Building
UMDNJ-New Jersey Medical School
185 South Orange Avenue
Newark, NJ 07103-2714
Fax: 973-972-7293

GENETIC BASIS OF DISEASE With the exception of a few families—one Scottish and one Australian family on which published data are available, a third family in North Carolina, and a possible fourth family in Ohio—in which xeroderma pigmentosum has been transmitted as an autosomal dominant trait, and one pedi-

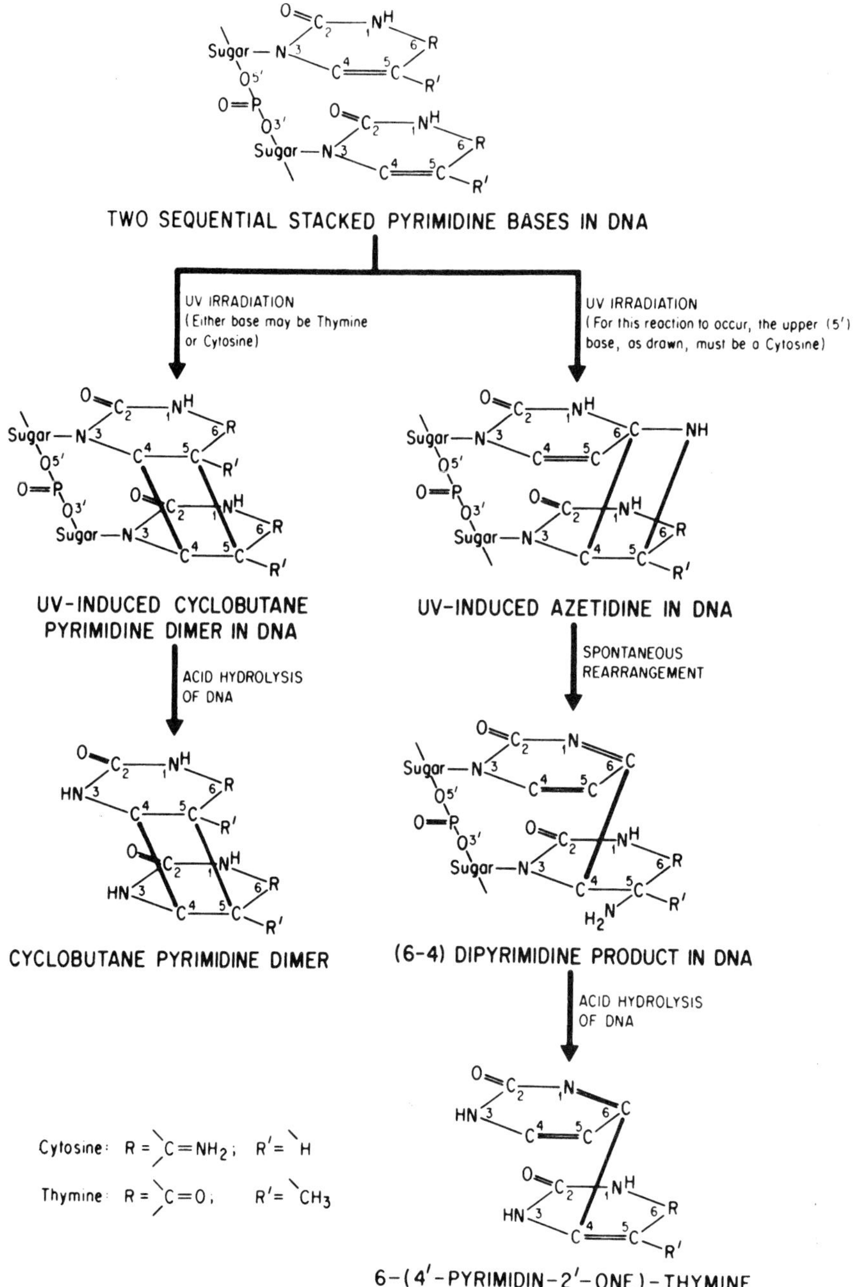

Figure 81-7 Formation of cyclobutane pyrimidine dimers and (6-4) photoproducts in cellular DNA by ultraviolet light. (From Lambert WC, Andrews AD, German J, et al. Xeroderma pigmentosum. In Thiers BH, Dobson RL, eds. Pathogenesis of Skin Disease. New York: Churchill Livingstone, 1986; pp. 576–599; with permission.)

gree in Italy in which the disease may have been sex-linked, xeroderma pigmentosum has been found to arise in pedigrees consistent with an autosomal recessive condition. The autosomal-dominant cases have all been of mild degree; none have been confirmed by UDS studies or analyzed for complementation group to date. The sex-linked cases were found to complement in xeroderma pigmentosum group A.

It has been known for many years that "classical" cases of xeroderma pigmentosum, those in complementation groups A–F, but not V, are defective in the initial, damage recognition and incision step in the nucleotide incision repair (NER) pathway of adducts introduced into cellular DNA by ultraviolet light. These adducts consist mainly of cyclobutane pyrimidine dimers and 6-4 pyrimidine-pyrimidone linkages, both of which occur between successive pyrimidines on the same strand of the duplex DNA molecule (Fig. 81-7). The dimers have outnumbered the 6-4 photoproducts by a ratio of at least two to one in most studies, but the 6-4 photoproduct causes a much greater degree of distortion in cellular DNA. Cells derived from patients with xeroderma pigmentosum have been found to be defective in repair of both adducts, but not in repair of other adducts due to reactive oxygen species generated by ultraviolet light, such as thymidine glycols, repaired by the base excision repair (BER) pathway.

Figure 81-8 outlines the base and nucleotide excision repair pathways in both mammalian cells and in cells of many other species, including yeast and *Escherichia coli*. On the left a mecha-

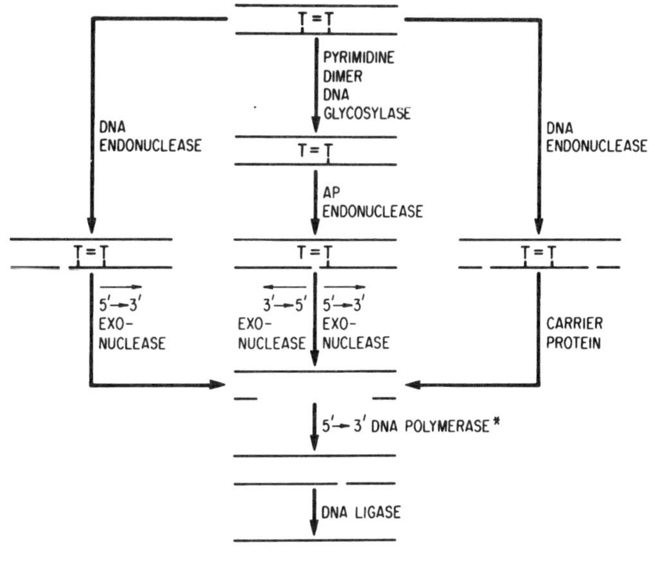

Figure 81-8 Alternate excision repair pathways proposed for both prokaryotes and eukaryotes. (From Lambert WC, Andrews AD, German J, et al. Xeroderma pigmentosum. In: Thiers BH, Dobson RL, eds. Pathogenesis of Skin Disease. New York: Churchill Livingstone, 1986; pp. 576–599; with permission.)

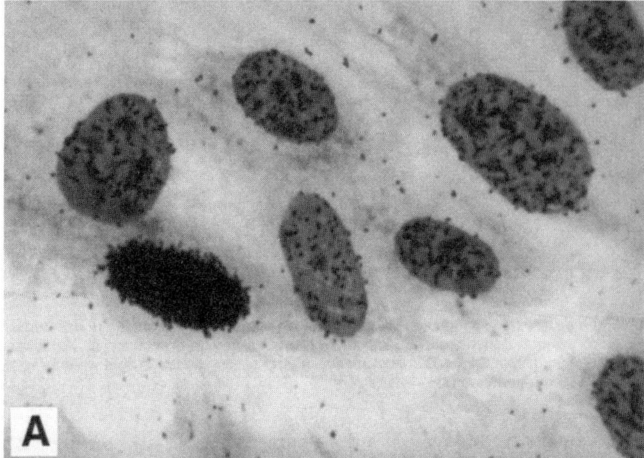

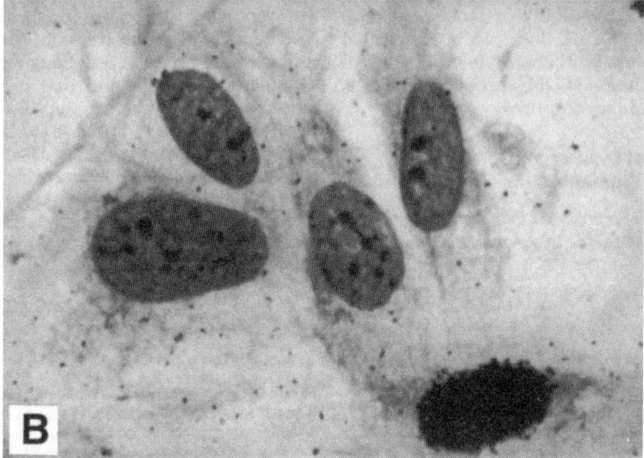

Figure 81-9 Autoradiograms of normal **(A)** and xeroderma pigmentosum, complementation group A **(B)** fibroblasts following irradiation with UV-C (254 nm) light and treatment with ^{3}H-thymidine. S-phase cells show large numbers of grains (A, lower left, and B, lower right, one cell in each), whereas cells undergoing unscheduled DNA synthesis show moderate numbers of grains (seven cells in A). Xeroderma pigmentosum, complementation group A cells show few or no grains (four cells in B). (From Lambert WC, Lambert MW. Diseases associated with DNA and chromosomal instability. In: Alper JC, ed. Genetic Disease of the Skin. St. Louis, Mosby-Year Book, 1991; pp. 320–358; with permission.)

nism is depicted in which a nick is created by an endonuclease on one side of the adduct, followed by digestion of the part of the same strand containing the adduct by an exonuclease, creating a single strand gap in the DNA. This was once thought to be the way in which mammalian NER proceeded, but is now known to be incorrect. The correct mechanism for NER in both mammalian cells and bacteria is shown on the right of the figure. A nick is made endonucleolytically on both sides of the adduct and the portion of the strand containing the adduct is removed, not necessarily by an exodonuclease. In bacteria this is mediated by the products of the *UvrABC* and *D* genes (called the UvrABC system) and the term "exinnuclease" has been used to describe the resulting combinations of enzyme activities. In mammalian cells and in yeast, these steps are mediated by protein complexes, more about which we shall explore below. The end result is again a single-stranded gap in the double-stranded DNA molecule (Fig. 81-8). In the center of Fig. 81-8 is depicted the base excision repair (BER) pathway in which an adduct, usually a simpler single-base alteration, is removed first by the action of a glycosylase, which removes the adduct so as to create an apurinic/apyrimidinic (AP) site, followed by the action of an AP endonuclease, which cuts the phosphodiester bond at the AP site. The two activities are often present in the same enzyme molecule. This eventuates, again, in the creation of a single-stranded gap in the double-stranded DNA molecule, although it is believed to be a shorter gap than that created by the NER pathway.

Whatever the mechanism, the single-stranded gap that results is then filled in by a DNA polymerase and then sealed by a DNA ligase. This affords a way to assay the process in intact cells in culture, since a small amount of DNA synthesis must occur. Replicative DNA synthesis occurs in a discrete phase of the cell cycle known as S phase, with phases both before and after it, called respectively G_1 and G_2 phases, in which no DNA synthesis occurs. However, when NER or BER are active, a small amount of DNA synthesis, called unscheduled DNA synthesis (UDS) occurs in G_1 and G_2 as well. This can be measured in UV-irradiated cells using a ^{3}H thymidine pulse followed by autoradiography, thus providing a measure of repair related DNA synthesis.

The UDS assay has become the gold standard for establishing a diagnosis of xeroderma pigmentosum in cases where the clinical diagnosis is uncertain. In this assay, a patient's cells are irradiated in culture with ultraviolet (UVB or C) light, pulsed with tritiated thymidine (an exclusive DNA precursor), and subjected to autoradiography. High-grain-count cells are discounted (as S phase cells) and low-grain-count nuclei scored as cells undergoing a limited amount of non–S-phase unscheduled DNA synthesis (UDS). Figure 81-9 shows an example of a normal and abnormal UDS test in fibroblasts; and Fig. 81-10 shows this test in lymphblastoid cells. Recently our laboratory has applied a new computerized image analysis system to these autoradiograms, which has allowed a vast improvement in the results obtained. Figure 81-11 shows a

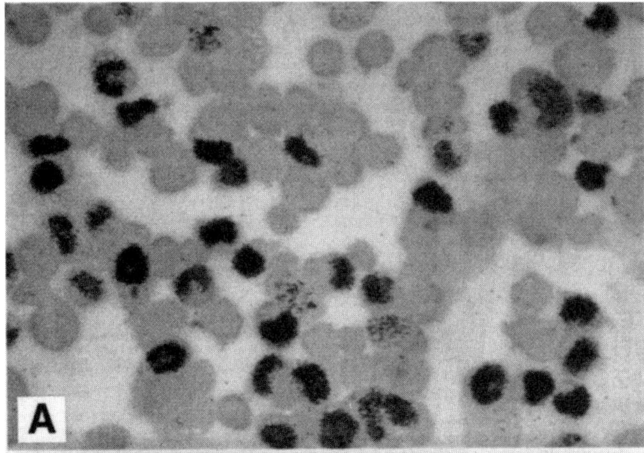

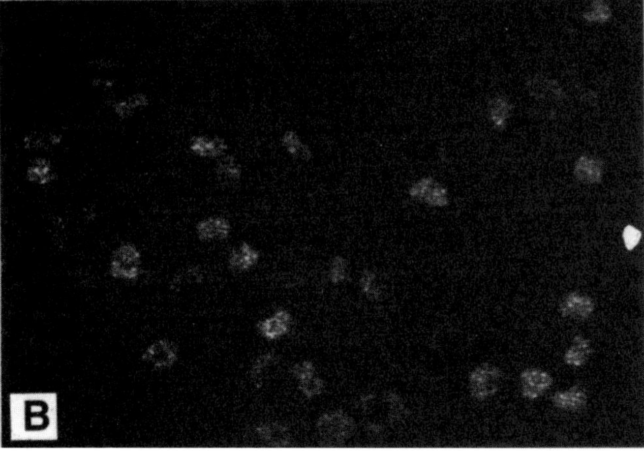

Figure 81-10 (**A** and **B**) Autoradiogram of human lymphoblastoid cells in culture following 1-h exposure to 1 m*M* methyl methanesulfonate, a DNA-damaging agent, and labeling with ^{3}H-thymidine. Cells show both scheduled (heavily labeled) and unscheduled (lightly labeled) DNA synthesis. This test, with ultraviolet radiation (UVR) or UVR-mimetic chemicals, is frequently employed in lymphoblasts or fibroblasts to confirm a clinical suspicion of xeroderma pigmentosum. This autoradiogram was examined by direct (transmission) microscopy in which the silver grains appear dark (A) and also by incident polarized light fluorescence microscopy in which the sliver grains appear bright (B), and the two images integrated by electronic image analysis (*see* Figs. 81-11 and 81-12). This eliminates most nonspecific background.

computer-generated image of a UDS assay; Fig. 81-12 shows the results generated from the assay. This system greatly facilitates and improves the accuracy of these assays. The UDS assay is, however, not completely specific; at least one normal person and one individual with hydroa vacciniforme have been found to have very low UDS levels, and, as noted above, a number of patients with trichothiodystrophy have also had low UDS results. Thus the UDS assay must be evaluated in the proper clinical context to be meaningful.

The UDS assay has also been used as the basis for the complementation assay in xeroderma pigmentosum, the first such assay to be developed in human genetics. In this assay, cells from different patients are fused and the UDS assay performed. In cells from different complementation groups, both nuclei show normal or near-normal UDS, which is not seen in cells from either patient fused with themselves (Fig. 81-13). This is interpreted as evidence for genetic heterogeneity. Nuclei of fused cells from patients in the same complementation group fail to show this phenomenon: UDS remains low.

MOLECULAR PATHOPHYSIOLOGY OF DISEASE The correlation between decreased nucleotide excision repair capability and development of skin lesions, especially skin cancer, following ultraviolet light exposure has been demonstrated in several ways. Sun protection leads to avoidance of these cutaneous lesions, which also occur in sun-exposed areas *(see above)*. Within the cutaneous lesions, mutation analysis shows that critical cancer-related genes, such as p53, are mutated with a markedly increased incidence in xeroderma pigmentosum patients. Moreover, these mutations can be traced to the types of adducts produced (and not repaired properly in xeroderma pigmentosum patients) by ultraviolet light. The roles of various products of xeroderma pigmentosum genes in the nucleotide excision repair pathway have recently become elucidated. This has been made possible by several recent developments.

The first development is the successful cloning of several xeroderma pigmentosum "correcting" genes. Successful cloning of the *XPA* gene by Tanaka et al. has been alluded to above. Some other human genes have been identified based on their ability to restore mutant, ultraviolet-sensitive rodent cells to normal following their introduction by artificial means. These genes were first termed ERCC (Excision Repair Cross-Complementing), followed by the number of the rodent cell complementation group (the rodent groups are labeled 1–11) that the human gene can complement. A number of these genes have now been cloned and found to also function to correct ultraviolet light response of cells in a xeroderma pigmentosum complementation group, at which point, by convention, they are renamed *XP* (complementation group) C genes, as *XPAC*, *XPBC*, and so on. Recently the final "C" has been deleted, so that *XPAC* is now *XPA*, and so on (Table 81-2).

The second development has been the improvement of in vitro cell-free systems for examination of nucleotide excision repair. The first of these systems, developed in our laboratory in 1983, has been most useful in elucidating the role of chromatin proteins in enhancing the repair process. The second major system, developed by Richard Wood and Tomas Lindahl in 1988, has been used to examine the role of individual proteins in nucleotide excision repair (NER). Using this system, it has been found that NER in bacteria requires 6 proteins, in mammalian cells at least 30 proteins.

The third major development has been the realization that a major protein complex serving as a regulator of initiation of human RNA polymerase II, called TFIIH, is required for NER, and that NER progresses much more rapidly in the transcribed strand of actively transcribed genes than in other DNA. TFIIH contains the products of the xeroderma pigmentosum-correcting genes *XPB*, *XPD*, and *XPG*. This fact may help to explain why some or all patients in these complementation groups have also had Cockayne syndrome, and why those Cockayne syndrome patients have been of short stature. Furthermore, those patients with trichothiodystrophy who have tested positive in the UDS assay have fallen into complementation group D (most patients) or B of xeroderma pigmentosum.

A scheme for the current concept of how these genes interact in NER has been proposed by Alan Lehmann, as follows (Table 81-2): First, the XPA gene product recognizes and binds to the damaged site in DNA via a zinc-finger domain on the XPA molecule. A

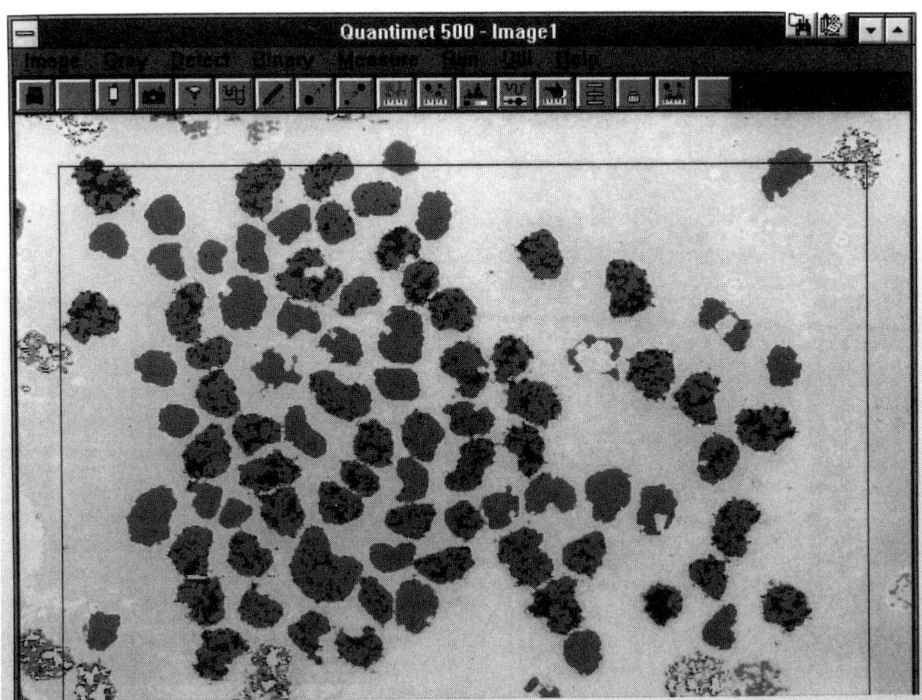

Figure 81-11 Computer-generated image generated from analysis of Figs. 81-9 and 81-10. Virtually all background has been eliminated and accurate counts of 0 to several hundred grains per nucleus may be obtained.

different domain on this same XPA protein molecule also binds to the single-stranded DNA binding protein, RPA (also known as SSB). Second, the XPA and RPA proteins act together to recruit the large TFIIH protein complex, which contains both the XPB and the XPD proteins. These latter proteins are helicases with opposite polarity, which unwind the double-helial DNA molecule, respectively, 5' and 3' to the adduct, creating a loop or "bubble" in the DNA molecule. Third, two different DNA endonucleases, one consisting of a complex of two proteins, XPF and ERCC 1, and the other consisting of the XPG protein, cut the strand of the DNA molecule containing the adduct on its 5' and 3' sides, respectively. Fourth, DNA polymerase epsilon and accessory proteins, replication factor C (RPC) and proliferating cell nuclear antigen (PNCA), fill in the resulting gap in the damaged DNA molecule. This is the step that produces the UDS phenomenon. Finally, the newly synthesized DNA is joined at its 3' end to the DNA beyond the repair gap by a DNA ligase.

This pattern of activities for the xeroderma pigmentosum gene products is, however, almost certainly quite simplistic, and should be regarded as only a first approximation of the events that occur in NER. Our laboratory, for example, has produced evidence that complementation group A cells are lacking a different product, which functions not in adduct recognition but rather in interaction of the repair proteins with chromatin. Indeed, it appears likely that, for xeroderma pigmentosum and/or some of these other disorders of DNA and chromatin instability *(see below)*, more than one biochemical defect may be necessary to produce the clinical disease. We have proposed a model, corecessive inheritance, which accounts for many of the discrepancies found in these diseases, such as, for example, the finding of a single genetic defect, in the *ATM* gene, in several different complementation groups of ataxia-telangiectasia *(see below)*. This model proposes an overlap in the function of some of these DNA repair/surveillance genes, so that the product of one can take effect where another may fail. Thus, to clinically have the disease, one must be homozygous for defective alleles (or hemizygous, should a sex-linked gene be involved) at two or more loci simultaneously. This model, should it or something like it prove correct, has profound implications for human biology. For example, it predicts extremely high carrier frequencies for these defective alleles in the general population (Fig. 81-14), so that the genes responsible for these very rare diseases may also play important roles in the etiopathogenesis of common disorders, such as cancer, ageing, and even age-related neurodegenerations. This model is by no means accepted as proven or even probable, however. It may, for example, be argued that the existence of XP "knockout" (KO) mice mitigates against it. On the other hand, KO mice are generated in inbred strains that have lost nearly half the genetic material present in the wild type, and the phenotypes of these KO mice are incomplete.

MANAGEMENT/TREATMENT Avoidance of sun exposure and vigilant surgical removal of tumors in xeroderma patients are the mainstays of treatment. It is important that surgery be performed with as little loss or destruction of normal tissue as possible, noting a high likelihood that surgery may have to be performed in the same site again and again, as malignancies continue to arise.

Particularly in severely affected small children, there is usually an interval in which skin damage due to sun exposure is evident in xeroderma pigmentosum patients, yet skin cancers have either not yet appeared or have just begun to appear. Parents at this time are hopeful that this situation may persist, but it rarely does. At this time they are loath to believe the dire prognosis their physicians present to them, and are extremely vulnerable to proponents of "alternate medicine," further compounding their problems and often draining their pocketbooks. Moreover, even if sufficient sun protection is afforded to prevent acute discomfort, this may be

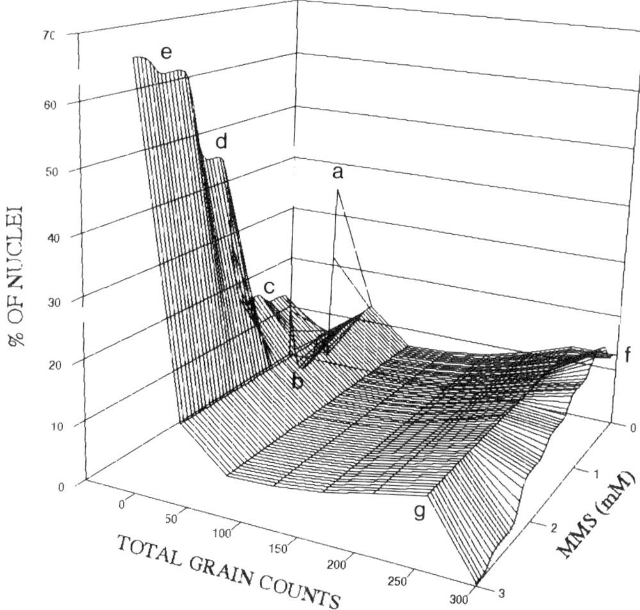

Figure 81-12 Unscheduled and scheduled (S phase) DNA synthesis in a lymphoblastoid cell line, derived from a normal individual, treated with progressively increasing doses of the DNA-damaging agent and mutagen, methyl methansulfonate (MMS). This plot was computer-generated based on grain counts and cell morphology analysis of autoradiograms of cells incubated for two hours in ^{3}H-thymidine following a 1-h exposure to MMS, performed in our laboratory using data generated by the Leitz Quantimet 500 Plus Image Analysis System (Leica, Cambridge, UK). The back plane corresponds to untreated cells; the front plane to cells treated with 3 m*M* MMS. On the far left, the proportion of cells with 0–25 grains, indicating little or no DNA synthesis, is seen. On the right, a ridge, indicative of the population of cells in S phase, each showing multiple grains, is seen. Between them is a trough in which there is overlap between low-labeled S-phase cells (mostly cells entering and leaving S phase during the radiolabeled thymidine pulse) and cells undergoing UDS. (For this reason, in this experiment, UDS was measured as loss of cells from the unlabeled population on the far left.) In untreated cells, approximately 35% of the cells showed little or no DNA synthesis (a). With progressively higher doses of MMS, this proportion fell to near zero as non–S-phase, intephase cells underwent UDS, making a modest amount of new DNA (b). At still higher doses of MMS, cells lost viability and were unable to synthesize DNA by either mechanism (c, d, and e). At the same time, cells in S phase, making large amounts of DNA progressively diminished their rate of replicative DNA synthesis (f in untreated cells to g in cells treated with 3 m*M* MMS). Determinations were made at 0.0, 0.1, 0.5, 1.0, 1.5, 2.0, 2.5, and 3.0 mM MMS with over 2500 cells counted. (Reprinted with permission from Lambert et al., 1995.)

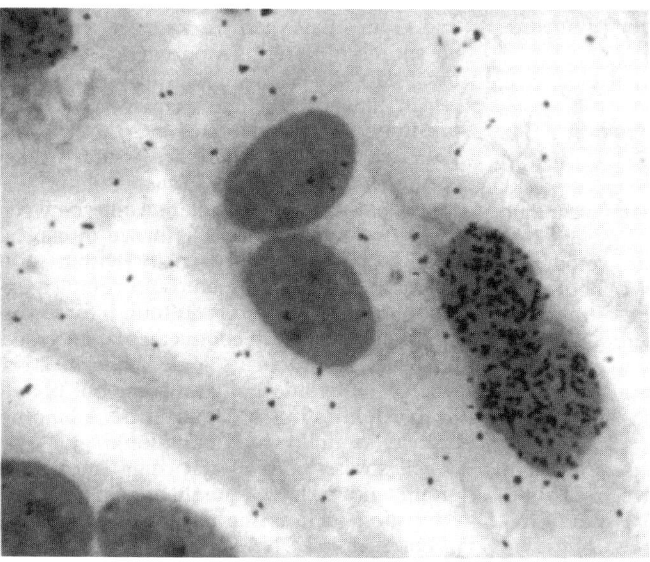

Figure 81-13 Complementation assay (UDS, fibroblasts) showing a heterokaryon (fusion product of one cell from each patient) with normal UDS and a homokaryon (fusion product of two cells from one patient) with depressed UDS. (Courtesy Dr. H. Takebe.)

insufficient to prevent the appearance of tumors later. Conversely, parents with limited resources and/or other healthy children may elect to limit the special care that they afford the child with xeroderma pigmentosum. These are difficult choices that only the family can make, and there is usually no correct or incorrect solution.

Several other modes of treatment are emerging, but they remain experimental at present. High-dose retinoids have been shown to retard rates of tumor growth. They also produce a "phasing" effect, allowing multiple tumors to be removed at one time. These high doses, however, are not without side effects, especially bone abnormalities. Application of bacterial DNA repair enzymes via topically applied microcoeles, which allow penetration of the superficial cornified layer of the skin, are also a promising approach. Dermabrasion of the skin has also been recently applied, with some success. Finally, surgical replacement of severely damaged skin by undamaged skin has been done in selected cases with some success (Fig. 81-15). Even though the replaced skin is still sun-sensitive, the accumulated mutagenic damage has not occurred, and new tumor growth is very much diminished.

In families with an affected child, prenatal diagnosis should be done whenever possible, and acceptable to the parents.

FUTURE DEVELOPMENTS Improved prenatal diagnosis of xeroderma pigmentosum using cloned genes or even in vitro selection of nonaffected embryos may become possible in the near future. Effective gene therapy, possibly using cutaneous application of corrective genes in vehicles such as microcoeles, may make it possible for patients with this disease to live nearly normal lives. If these genes play important roles in the etiopathogenesis of more common diseases, screening of the normal population for these defective alleles may allow earlier diagnosis of some of these diseases to be made. In any case, further studies on xeroderma pigmentosum are certain to provide additional information regarding human DNA repair processes and chromatin biology.

ATAXIA-TELANGIECTASIA (LOUIS-BARR SYNDROME)

BACKAROUND Ataxia-telangiectasia is an uncommon disorder characterized by development of large telangiectatic lesions on the conjunctivae and face, progressive cerebellar ataxia and other neurological deficiencies, immunological defects, and marked hypersensitivity to ionizing radiation. Although the first report of this disease is attributed to Madame Louise Barr in 1931, it may have been described earlier.

Peripheral blood lymphocytes of these patients show somatic translocations, primarily involving chromosomes 7 and 14. Cultivated cells derived from these individuals show a tendency for chromosomes to fuse at their telomeres and defective cell cycle checkpoint controls, especially following exposure to ionizing radiation.

Table 81-2
Human DNA Repair Genes and Their Nonhuman Homologs

		Homologous nonhuman genes			
Disease complementation group/gene	*Human chromosome*	*Rodent*	*Yeast S. cerevisiae*	*S. pomp*	*Putative function*
XP-A	9Q34		RAD14		Damage-specific
XP-A	8				DNA-binding protein
XP-B/CS[a]	2q21	ERCC3	(ERCC3sc)	(ERCC3sp)	DNA helicase; DNA-dependent
ATPase					
XP-C	5		RAD14		DNA endonuclease; DNA-dependent ATPase
XP-D	19q13.2	ERCC2	RAD3	rad14	DNA helicase; transcription factor
XP-E					Damage-specific DNA-binding protein; photolyase
XP-F	15	[b]			
XP-G	13q32-38	ERCC5	RAD2	rad13	DNA helicase; transcription factor
XP-V					
CS-A					
CS-B	10q11	ERCC6			
Bloom syndrome	15				
FA (FA-A-D)	9				Damage-specific DNA-binding protein (FAOA)
–	19q13	ERCC1	RAD10	swi10	RAD1-RAD10 complex: double-stranded DNA endonuclease
			RAD1	rad16	
HHR6A			RAD6		Ubiquitin-conjugating enzyme
HHR6B			RAD6		

[a]XP-B/CS is also homologous to the haywire gene in drosophila.
[b]ERCC1 and ERCC11 are candidates based on recent studies in cell-free systems.
From Lambert WC, Lambert MW. DNA repair deficiency and skin cancer in xeroderma pigmentosum. In: Mukhtar H, ed. Skin Cancer, Mechanisms and Human Releance. Boca Raton: CRC, 1994, with permission.

The disease is transmitted as an autosomal recessive disorder with four complementation groups, A, C, D, and E, currently recognized, although a number of others have also been proposed. In 1995, an international consortium identified a single gene, known as the *ATM* (Ataxia-Telangiectasia Mutated) gene, which, surprisingly, is mutated in patients in all of these complementation groups as well as some other patients with ataxia-telangiectasia not assigned to a specific group.

Heterozygotes for the *ATM* gene are believed to be at increased (two - to threefold) risk to develop certain types of cancer, particularly breast cancer in women. The breast cancer risk in these women has been proposed to be four to five times that of women in the general population, and it has been estimated that the *ATM* gene is responsible for approximately 8% of human breast cancer. However, some studies have shown lower associations between ATM gene carrier state and breast cancer, and the subject is controversial.

Three related diseases—The Nijmegen breakage syndrome, the Berlin breakage syndrome, and ataxia-telangiectasia Fresno—have clinical or cellular features closely related to those of ataxia-telangiectasia.

CLINICAL FEATURES Ataxia-telangiectasia is by far the most common entity among those discussed in this chapter, affecting approximately one individual per 30,000 live births. The pedigrees of these cases have been consistent with an autosomal recessive mode of inheritance. The Nijmegen breakage syndrome and the Berlin breakage syndrome are both characterized by microcephaly and mental retardation, but by none of the other clinical features of ataxia-telangiectasia. Ataxia-telangiectasia Fresno has clinical features of all of these diseases. If microcephaly, mental retardation, or both are present, this essentially rules out a diagnosis of ataxia-telangiectasia. However, a patient with ataxia-telangiectasia may appear to be retarded when in reality he or she is only socially repressed.

The first sign of the disease is invariably ataxia, which typically begins at about the time the child learns to walk and is progressive, so that by the age of 10 years the patient usually requires a wheelchair. The ataxia is truncal and of cerebellar type. It initially affects gait but later is of intention type as well.

A second, also very characteristic clinical finding in ataxia telangiectasia is ocular apraxia. When a patient is asked to follow an object moved across the visual fields with his or her eyes, the head is turned to follow the object, the eyes following afterward.

The characteristic telangiectatic oculocutaneous stigmata of ataxia-telangiectasia often appear years later than the neurologic signs, but by the age of 10 years almost all patients have markedly dilated, thin-walled blood vessels visible over the bulbar conjunctivae. These large vessels contrast sharply with the finely telangiectatic rash seen over the face of patients with Bloom syndrome, and do not show blistering, ulceration, or any association with sunlight. These dilated vessels are often also present on the eyelids, the bridge of the nose, on the pinnae of the external ears, and, less commonly, over the antecubital and popliteal fossae.

In addition to these stigmata, very young patients may also, occasionally, show a few gray hairs and hypertrichosis, the latter especially over the forearms.

Ataxia-telangiectasia patients are markedly prone to develop malignancies involving the lymphoid system. About 75% of these are lymphomas, most commonly B-cell lymphomas. These often occur in young patients; of the approximately one-fourth of these malignancies that arise later, most are leukemias, usually of the T-cell chronic lymphatic type. Often the malignant cells show

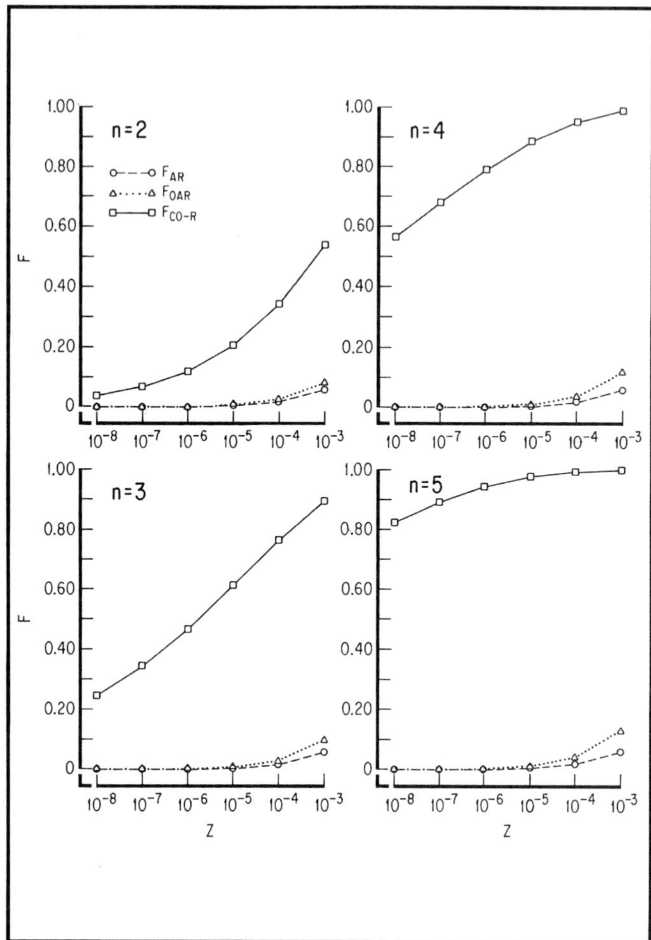

Figure 81-14 Carrier frequencies in the general population for defective alleles for DNA repair and chromosomal stability genes associated with xeroderma pigmentosum and related disorders predicted by the classical autosomal recessive (AR) and corecessive inheritance (C-RI) models. n, number of genes. (For C-RI: number of equally prevalent autosomal recessive genes which must be homozygously defective for the disease to be observed.) Z, proportion of live births in which the disease is present; F, frequency (1.00 is 100% for the population) who are carriers; F_{AR}, for AR; F_{OAR}, for oligogenic AR (i.e., AR with complementation groups); $F_{C\text{-}RI}$, for C-RI. (Reproduced with permission from Lambert and Lambert, 1992.)

inversions or translocations involving chromosome 14. Nonlymphoid malignancies, when they occur, almost always are found in older patients with ataxia-telangiectasia.

These patients are extremely radiosensitive, and may even develop an erythematous rash or other symptoms after diagnostic X-ray examination. Occasionally a patient develops a leukemia or lymphoma prior to being diagnosed with ataxia-telangiectasia. This may lead to administration of a dose of X-irradiation or of one or more chemotherapeutic agents that are contraindicated in ataxia-telangiectasia. The results are usually dramatic and tragic. It is imperative that the diagnosis of ataxia-telangiectasia be considered, and appropriate diagnostic steps taken, if necessary, prior to treating a very young patient for cancer.

Although some type of immunodeficiency is present in most patients with ataxia-telangiectasia, there is great heterogeneity in both type and degree of this between patients and often even

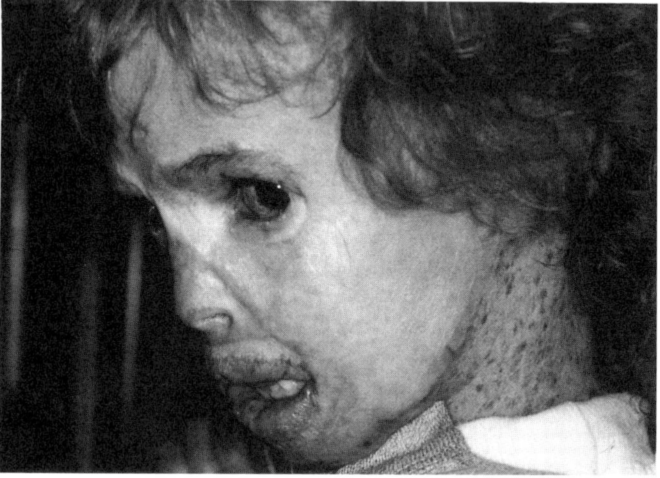

Figure 81-15 Total Facial skin replacement by surgical graft in a 7-year-old girl with severe xeroderma pigmentosa.

between siblings. Four-fifths of patients have decreased serum levels of IgG2, IgE, or IgA. Although blood T-cell counts are often normal, T-cell responsiveness to mitogens or allogenic cells is often low. At autopsy, the thymus is typically rudimentary.

About 95% of patients with ataxia-telangiectasia have elevated levels of α-fetoprotein in their sera. The 5% of patients who do not have this abnormality do not appear to differ from those that do in any other respect. In 5–10% of peripheral blood lymphocytes of most patients with ataxia-telangiectasia, there is a translocation involving chromosomes 7 and 14. Skin fibroblasts do not show these characteristic translocations.

DIAGNOSIS If early onset cerebellar ataxia, ocular apraxia and the characteristic telangiectasia of the bulbar conjunctive are all recognized, the diagnosis of ataxia-telangiectasia may be considered to be virtually established. In these cases laboratory tests are simply confirmatory. In cases in which not all of these signs are present, however, the laboratory plays a more important role. This is rather frequently the case in young children, since the telangiectatic eruption often arises years later than the ataxia and ocular apraxia. The indicated tests are serum α-fetoprotein and immunoglobulin determinations, and karyotyping and radiosensitivity assays on mitogen-stimulated peripheral blood lymphocytes and/or cultured cells. Tests for radiation-resistant DNA synthesis may also be done, but are usually a research procedure. The recent cloning of the *ATM* gene *(see below)* may soon provide molecular assay for this disease, but this is not yet available.

α-Fetoprotein levels are elevated in about 95% and serum IgE, IgG2, or IgA levels are depressed in about 80% of patients with ataxia-telangiectasia. As for most clinical laboratory tests, these studies should be done at least twice.

Cytogenetics assays of mitogen-stimulated peripheral blood lymphocytes may be complicated by the fact that ataxia-telangiectasia lymphocytes do not show an optimal mitogenic response to phytohemagglutinin. Thus a cytogenetics laboratory may return a report of "no metaphases observed." To avoid this, the laboratory should be advised to use at least one additional (higher) dose of phytohemagglutinin in separate cultures and also to harvest some of the lymphocyte cultures at 72 h rather than 48 h. This will allow metaphases to be visualized in most cases of ataxia-telangiectasia.

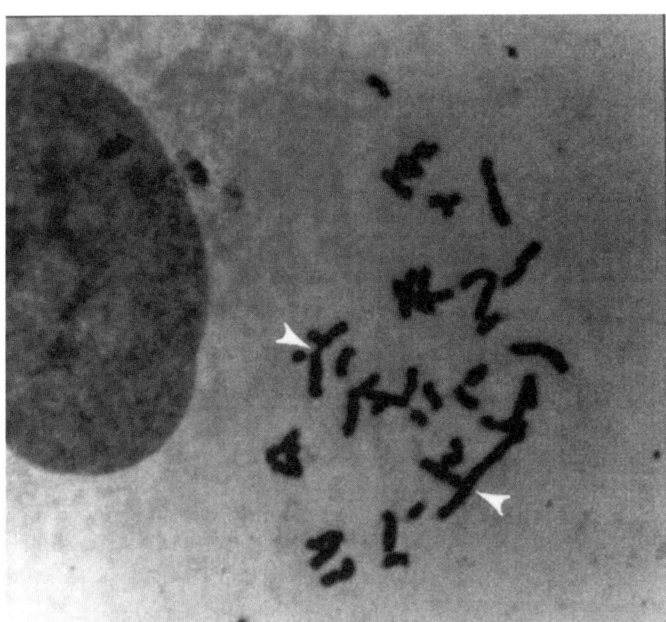

Figure 81-16 Chromosome preparation of a metaphase cell from a patient with ataxia-telangiectasia. Note fusion of telomeres (arrows).

Karyotypes of ataxia-telangiectasia cells show abnormalities, especially telomere–telomere linkages (Fig. 81-16). Most ataxia-telangiectasia patients' peripheral blood lymphocyte karyotypes show translocations between chromosomes 7 and 14 in 5–10% of metaphases examined.

Survival studies of cells derived from patients suspected of having ataxia-telangiectasia following radiation or other treatments are not routine procedures in most centers, but can provide valuable information when available. Colony-forming ability (CFA), colony survival assay (CSA), and cloning efficiency (CE) assays of peripheral blood lymphocytes irradiated with 1 Gy of X-irradiation typically show CFA values in ataxia-telangiectasia cells that are less than 20% of control levels and also less than 20% of levels of ataxia-telangiectasia heterozygotes. In some assays, heterozygote cells may show levels of activity intermediate between those of normal and those of homozygote cells.

Prenatal diagnosis is an extremely important aspect of diagnosis in a family in which a child with ataxia-telangiectasia has been identified. Until very recently the standard technique has been based on haplotype analysis of chromosome band 1 lq.22.3 in both parents and the affected child, to determine which is associated with the defective ataxia-telangiectasia gene, and then testing the DNA of the fetus, obtained either from amniocytes or from chorionic villus cells, to identify which of the parents' haplotypes have been inherited. This is then compared to the haplotypes of the affected sibling. An estimate of the likelihood of the fetus being affected is then computed. This procedure has provided extremely accurate prenatal diagnosis, due to the fact that the gene has been very well localized. Now that the *ATM* gene has been identified and cloned *(see below)*, prenatal diagnosis should become simpler and even more accurate.

GENETIC BASIS OF DISEASE Pedigrees of individual families of patients with ataxia-telangiectasia have consistently shown an autosomal recessive pattern of inheritance. However, an extensive epidemiologic study of incidence of ataxia-telangiectasia in a defined region of central-north England produced data that could not be well-fitted by any inheritance model. Subsequent examination of those reported data by two of us (WCL and MWL) indicate that they may be fitted by the corecessive inheritance model *(see above)*. However, there may be other explanations for these findings.

Cells in culture derived from patients with ataxia-telangiectasia—as well as those from patients with the Nijmegen breakage syndrome, Berlin breakage syndrome, and ataxia-telangiectasia Fresno—show a number of distinctive features: Peripheral blood lymphocytes, but not skin fibroblasts, show inversions and recombinations in chromosomes 7 and 14 in 5–10% of metaphases. All cell types tend to show chromosome breaks and a tendency of chromosomes to fuse at their telomeres (Fig. 81-16). All cells are radiosensitive and, in some but not all assays, cells derived from ataxia-telangiectasia heterozygotes show an intermediate level of radiosensitivity between that of normal cells and ataxia-telangiectasia cells. The increase in stability of p53 seen in normal cells after irradiation is significantly delayed in ataxia-telangiectasia cells and fails to reach normal levels. Ataxia-telangiectasia cells show additional breaks and other abnormalities in their metaphase chromosomes following irradiation, in excess of those seen in normal cells. Unlike normal cells, ataxia-telangiectasia cells fail to slow their rate of DNA synthesis following X-irradiation, a distinctive phenomenon termed by Painter and his colleagues "radiation-resistant DNA synthesis" (RRDR); several cell-cycle checkpoint controls, including G_1 and G_2 checkpoint controls, are defective. This phenomenon (RRDS) has been used, in fused cells, to identify complementation groups in ataxia-telangiectasia. Nuclei of cells fused from different individuals with ataxia-telangiectasia, which separately show RRDR, show normal responses to X-irradiation when the patients are in different complementation groups, but show RRDS when they are in the same group. On this basis, four complementation groups of ataxia-telangiectasia have been proposed; A, C, D, and E. What was formerly group B has been incorporated into group A. Not all of the cellular studies have produced unequivocal results, however, and additional groups have been proposed. In addition to these groups, cells from patients with the Nijmegen breakage syndrome and the Berlin breakage syndrome have been found to show similar changes in culture to those of ataxia-telangiectasia cells, but complement both each other and all ataxia-telangiectasia cell lines tested in the RRDS complementation assay. Therefore cells derived from patients with the Nijmegen breakage syndrome and the Berlin breakage syndrome are said to be in ataxia telangiectasia complementation groups V1 and V2, respectively. The complementation group analysis is essentially the only criterion that separates these latter two disorders, which are otherwise very similar in both clinical and cell culture characteristics, although different in the former from ataxia-telangiectasia.

In 1995, a large, international consortium of coinvestigators isolated and cloned a gene, which they termed the *ATM* (Ataxia-Telangiectasia Mutated) gene, which was found to be defective in each of a large group of ataxia-telangiectasia cell lines examined. Surprisingly, the *ATM* gene was defective in cells derived from patients in each of the four well-characterized complementation groups. They attributed this result to intragenic complementation, but the issue has not been resolved. They did not, in fact, explore this issue in any sort of detail, and consequently did not consider that defective alleles at one or more other genetic loci, in

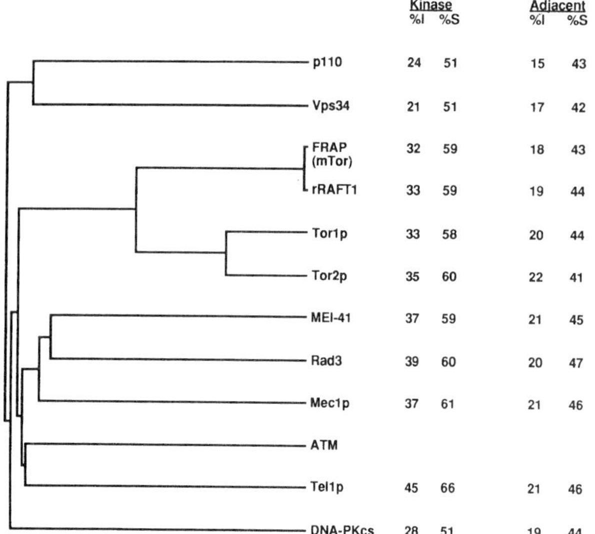

Kinase
%I %S
Adjacent
%I %S
p110 24 51 15 43
Vps34 21 51 17 42
FRAP (mTor) 32 59 18 43
rRAFT1 33 59 19 44
Tor1p 33 58 20 44
Tor2p 35 60 22 41
MEI-41 37 59 21 45
Rad3 39 60 20 47
Mec1p 37 61 21 46
ATM
Tel1p 45 66 21 46
DNA-PKcs 28 51 19 44

Figure 81-17 Sequence homology of the COOH-terminal region of the human *ATM* gene with other members of the PI3K family. At the right the % identity (I) and similarity (S) of both the kinase domains and the adjacent 10^3 amino acids is given. (Reproduced with permission from Zakian VA. Cell 1995;82:685–687.)

addition to the *ATM* gene, might be necessary to produce clinical ataxia-telangiectasia.

Based on linkage studies performed to date, the *ATM* gene is unlikely to be associated with either the Nijmegen breakage syndrome on the Berlin breakage syndrome. The *ATM* gene is on chromosome band 1 lq22-23 and has a transcript of 12 kb. Following discovery, it was quickly found to be homologous to a number of other known eukaryotic and prokaryotic genes *(see below)* and was immediately recognized as having a gene product similar to phosphatidylinositol-3-kinase.

MOLECULAR PATHOPHYSIOLOGY OF DISEASE The *ATM* gene product, predicted from its cDNA, was found to have, in the approximately 400 amino acids composing its carboxyl (-COOH) end (believed to have seroninc/threonine protein kinase activity), strong homology to a group of proteins in humans and other species known as phosphatidylinistol-3-kinases (PI3Ks). PI3Ks phosphorylate both lipids and—in proteins, serines, and threonines—play a central role in a number of signal transduction pathways, including those that regulate certain cell-cycle checkpoints and such other cellular processes as transport of certain substances across membranes.

Figure 81-17 shows the degree of sequence homology between the predicted *ATM* gene product and a number of products of other genes in the PI3K gene superfamily in various species. As is immediately apparent, the protein products of certain genes, particularly the *Drosophila melanogaster* (fruit fly) gene *MEI41*, the *Saccromyces cerevisiae* (yeast) genes *TEl 1* and *Esr 1/Mec 1*, the *S. pombe* (yeast) gene Rad 3, and the human gene *ATM* share significantly more sequence homology with each other than they do with the other gene products listed. There is also close homology with the products of the *S. cerevisiae* genes *Tor 1* and *Tor 2* and with those of their mammalian homologs, *FRAP(mTor)* and *rRAFT 1*. Slightly less homologous to all of these is the catalytic subunit (cs) of human DNA-protein kinase (DNA-PK), an important DNA repair enzyme *(see below)*. Least homologous to the other gene products within this group are those of the most homologous PI3Ks known, p110 (bovine) and Vps 34 *(S. cerevisiae)*.

Table 81-3 lists some of the properties of ataxia-telangiectasia cells along with those of cells mutant in the most homologous of these genes, *Tel 1*, *Esr 1/Mec 1*, *Rad 3* and *D. melanogaster MEI41*. Phenotypes of *S. pombe Rad 3*- and *D. melanogaster MEI41*-mutant cells clearly resemble those of ataxia-telangiectasia cells, as do those of *S. cerevisiae* cells mutant in both *Tel 1* and *Esr 1/Mec 1*. All of them are hypersensitive to several DNA damaging agents, including X-irradiation, and all show defective cell-cycle checkpoint controls, particularly following X-irradiation. Interestingly, yeast cells with a truncated mutant form of *Esr 1/Mec 1* but normal *Tel 1* show partial resistance to the lethal effects of X-irradiation when they have one or two extra normal copies of *Tel 1*. Cell lines for which this information is available also show chromosomal abnormalities, particularly defective telomere stability, and these defects are exacerbated by X-irradiation. Human ataxia-telangiectasia cells are hypersensitive to treatment with bleomycin or streptonigrin, hypersensitivities to which are present in *S. cerevisiae* cells only if mutant in both *Tel 1* and *Esr 1/Mec 1*, further reinforcing the idea that both genes together function rather like the *ATM* gene in man. The degree of overlap in these phenotypic characteristics is not perfect, however. For example, all of these nonhuman mutated cell lines are hypersensitive to ultraviolet radiation, whereas most ataxia-telangiectasia cell lines show normal sensitivity to this agent. *Esr 1/Mec 1* apparently has some function in yeast which it lacks in humans, since *Esr 1/Mec 1* mutants are lethal.

The yeast *TOR 1* and *TOR 2* gene products, working together, and their mammalian homologs, FRAP and rRAFT, working together, are required for the G_1 and S phase cell cycle progression in their respective species. DNA-PKcs, when bound to the remaining subunits of DNA-PK, kDa 70 and kDa 80, which together comprise the Ku nuclear antigen important in certain autoimmune diseases, forms an active DNA-protein kinase (DNA-PK). However this binding is in turn dependent on recognition and binding of the Ku subunits to DNA double strand (ds) breaks. Such DNA ds breaks are an important consequence of X-irradiation. DNA-PK is a serine/threonine protein kinase which activates a number of different proteins, including those that modulate certain cell-cycle checkpoints, so as to arrest the cell cycle, and the nuclear protein, p 43, which leads to stabilization of p 53, a tumor suppressor gene product the stabilization of which, following X-irradiation, is delayed in ataxia-telangiectasia cells. Activity of DNA-PK is also important in B and T lymphocytes undergoing V(D)J gene recombination. Thus a defective *ATM* gene, related to the DNA-PK gene, may be responsible for the immunodeficiency seen in ataxia-telangiectasia. Human and mouse *SCID* (Severe Combined Immuno-Deficiency) mutant cells with deficient DNA-PK activity are hypersensitive to X-irradiation, show DNA repair defects, and are unable to support V(D)J recombination. Interestingly, *S. cerevisiae* telomeres also interact with DNA double strand breaks, resulting in cell cycle arrest at the G_2 to M checkpoint.

Notably, DNA-PK does not phosphorylate lipids (such as phosphatidylinositol). It is likely that many or all of the above gene products, except the PI3Ks (p 110 and VPS-34), exert part of their effects by phosphorylation of proteins but not lipids. This further distinguishes them from PI3Ks.

Thus the *ATM* gene is a reasonable candidate to play a role in the pathophysiology of numerous cellular and clinical features of ataxia-telangiectasia. However, much needs to be done to delin-

Table 81-3
Properties of Ataxia-Telangiectasis Cells and of Cells with Mutant Genes with Product Homology to the ATM Gene

Cell type	*Lethal*	*Cell-cycle checkpoint defects*	*Chromosomal abnormalities*	*Hypersensitivities*			
				UV[a]	*X-Rays*[b]	*Chem.*[c]	*B and S*[d]
Human							
Ataxia-telangiectasia	No	Yes	Yes, with impaired telomere function	No	Yes	No	Yes
S. cerevisiae							
Mecl⁺ Tell⁺	No	No	Yes, with short telomeres	No	No	No	No
Mecl⁻ Tell⁺	Yes	Yes	—	Yes	Yes	Yes	No
Mecl⁻ Tell⁺	Yes	Yes	—	Yes	Yes	Yes	Yes
S. pombe							
Rad3⁻	No	Yes	—	Yes	Yes	Yes	—
D. melanogaster							
Mei-41⁻	No	Yes	Yes	Yes	Yes	Yes	—

[a]ultraviolet C irradiation (254 nm).
[b]X-irridation.
[c]Chemical alkylating agents (e.g., methylmethansulfonate).
[d]Bleomyein and Streptonigrin.

eate this. It is notable that the amino (-NH_3) end of all of the gene products discussed above are very different, often with little or no homology present. The presence of the same mutated gene in at least four different complementation groups of ataxia-telangiectasia is also yet to be explained.

TREATMENT/MANAGEMENT Because the ataxia and ocular apraxia usually occur in the first few years of life, whereas the characteristic oculocutaneous telangiectasias often appear much later, at about 6 or 8 years of age, the diagnosis of ataxia-telangiectasia may be suspected as one of several possible causes of the neurologic signs, but not confirmed as the cause, for an interval of as long as several years during childhood. This may complicate management as well as genetic counseling to the family. As soon as possible appropriate cytogenetic studies should be carried out. Once the diagnosis has been made, the patient should be carefully followed during childhood for evidence of development of a lymphoma, especially a B-cell lymphoma in early childhood and a T-cell leukemia later. Older patients should be screened for development of other types of cancer as well. Infections should be treated promptly and aggressively because of the immune dysfunction often present in these patients.

X-ray exposure must be carefully limited, especially therapeutic X-irradiation, as well as chemotherapeutic drugs used to treat lymphomas, which these patients are prone to develop. These modalities are often valuable and useful in ataxia-telangiectasia patients, but at carefully controlled, lower doses.

An underlying ataxia-telangiectasia should be considered in all young patients with lymphoma or leukemia prior to administration of therapeutic X-irradiation or chemotherapy. Obligate heterozygotes and other family members should be advised that the risk of developing cancer in an ataxia-telangiectasia heterozygote may be two to three times that of age-matched normal persons. This risk in female heterozygotes may be as high as five times normal for breast cancer. However, how large this increased risk is, and even whether it is present, are subjects of controversy in the current literature, and patients should be advised of the uncertainty due to this as well.

Since the prime mode of early detection of mammary cancer at present is the mammogram, which uses X-rays (which are also carcinogenic), and since ataxia-telangiectasia heterozygote cells are hypersensitive to X-rays in some (although not all) assays, this may pose a dilemma for female ataxia-telangiectasia heterozygotes. However, since the energy level of the X-rays used in mammograms is extremely low, it would seem prudent for these women to obtain regular mammograms, as well as to practice frequent periodic self-examination of their breasts.

FUTURE DIRECTIONS Many more studies of the *ATM* gene need to be, and soon will be, done. Why is it defective in all complementation groups of ataxia-telangiectasia? Are other genes involved in the etiopathogenesis of this disease as well? What is the phenotype of *ATM* knockout mice? The answers to these and other questions should be forthcoming.

Perhaps even more important than its use in elucidating the pathophysiology of ataxia-telangiectasia is the role the cloned *ATM* gene is expected to play in delineating the significance of the carrier state for this gene. What proportion of patients who are carriers develop cancer, and what kinds of cancer do they develop? Do the cancers that arise in these patients have a different course, prognosis, or biologic behavior? Is the carrier state associated with an increased sensitivity to X-irradiation or chemotherapy, and, if so, can the effectiveness of radiotherapy and chemotherapy in all patients be improved by culling these patients out and designing different dose regimens for them, with other patients able to receive higher (and thus more effective) doses?

NIJMEGEN BREAKAGE SYNDROME/ BERLIN BREAKAGE SYNDROME/ ATAXIA-TELANGIECTASIA FRESNO

These three disorders all show the same cellular abnormalities seen in ataxia-telangiectasia. However, the first two (the breakage syndromes) have different clinical manifestations (microcephaly and mental retardation, without the neurologic changes or the telangiectatic eye and skin changes seen in ataxia-telangiectasia), whereas ataxia-telangiectasia Fresno shows the clinical manifestations of all three diseases. Presumably all of these entities are associated with a predisposition to develop lymphomas and cancer, but the case numbers reported have been so small that the data base is inadequate.

The term "breakage" in the first two disorders refers to chromosome breakage in their karotypes. They are clinically very similar, and are separated on the basis of ability of their cells to complement each other in the complementation assay discussed above for ataxia-telangiectasia. Since cells from both breakage syndromes can complement those from all complementation groups of ataxia-telangiectasia they have been assigned their own complementation groups V1, for the Nijmegen breakage syndrome, and V2, for the Berlin breakage syndrome, respectively. Linkage studies indicate that neither breakage syndrome is defective at the *ATM* locus; this should (and presumably will) become elucidated by molecular studies using the cloned *ATM* gene.

BLOOM SYNDROME

BACKGROUND Bloom syndrome is a rare, autosomal recessive disorder characterized by small body size, one or both of two distinctive types of cutaneous lesions, characteristic cytogenetic abnormalities in cultured cells, and a marked predisposition to develop cancer at a young age. The cutaneous eruptions consist of a telangiectatic rash over sun exposed areas appearing in early childhood and more variable hyper- and hypopigmented areas appearing primarily on the trunk. The cancers appear in multiple organs and tissues. Bloom syndrome was first described by Dr. David Bloom, a New York City dermatologist, in 1954.

Of the multiple abnormalities present in cultured cells derived from Bloom syndrome patients (discussed below), the most characteristic are a high rate (about 10 or more times normal) of sister chromatid exchanges and multiple quadriradial figures representing abnormal linkages between two homologous chromosomes seen in cultured cells treated with bromo-deoxy-uridine. In 1995, Dr. James German and his colleagues identified and cloned the gene responsible for these and other anomalies in Bloom syndrome, which they named the *BLM* gene. This was achieved using a new cloning method, somatic crossover point mapping (SCPM) based on the *BLM* gene itself. SCPM should allow extremely rapid and precise localization of a recessive gene responsible for virtually any phenotype identifiable in cultured cells. It thus should be applicable to the study of many other recessively inherited diseases. Therefore, in addition to being of interest in the etiopathogenesis of Bloom syndrome, the *BLM* gene is likely to become an important tool in the study of inherited diseases generally, and to provide a rapid means for gene localization and cloning.

CLINICAL FEATURES Bloom syndrome is extremely rare. As of August 1993, fewer than 170 patients had been entered into the Bloom Syndrome Registry maintained by Dr. James German at the New York Blood Center in New York City.

Small, but proportionate, body size is the most characteristic and consistent sign of Bloom syndrome. Only four of 82 males and three of 53 females in the Bloom Syndrome Registry for whom this information was available as of 1995 had birth weights within two standard deviations of the normal mean. This small size persists throughout life.

Almost as characteristic as small body size is the marked tendency of Bloom syndrome patients to develop cancer at a moderately early age. These cancers are of virtually all types, with 41 carcinomas, 21 leukemias, and 4 sarcomas reported in the 165 individuals in the Bloom Syndrome Registry as of August 1993.

A telangiectatic cutaneous eruption, varying from severe to mild to undetectable, occurs over sun exposed areas, especially of the face where it tends to involve the cheeks and nose in a strikingly "butterfly" distribution (Figs. 81-18 and 81-19). Less commonly, a similar, but milder, eruption is present on the dorsa of the hands and forearms. When the facial rash is severe, it may also involve the ears, neck, and suprasternal area. In these cases, the shoulders and chest may show a mild telangiectatic eruption as well. This telangiectatic eruption does not involve other areas, however, and a telangiectatic rash on the legs, upper arms, trunk or buttocks essentially rules out Bloom syndrome as a diagnosis. This eruption is not congenital, as once thought, but rather usually appears in the first two years of life. When it is severe, loss of inferior eyelids and blistering of the inferior lip are common. Younger affected siblings often show less severe skin changes, due to being better protected by the parents. The eruption tends to be more severe in boys, possibly accounting for the fact that slightly more boys than girls have been reported to the Bloom Syndrome Registry (94 vs 71 cases). In marked contrast to the sun-damaged skin seen in xeroderma pigmentosum and to the other eruption characteristic of Bloom syndrome *(see below)*, there is no dyspigmentation associated with this eruption. Regardless of whether the eruption is present, Bloom syndrome patients tend to be hypersensitive to sunlight, in areas exposed to sun in infancy, throughout their lives (Fig. 81-20). In other areas, however, they are not particularly sun-sensitive.

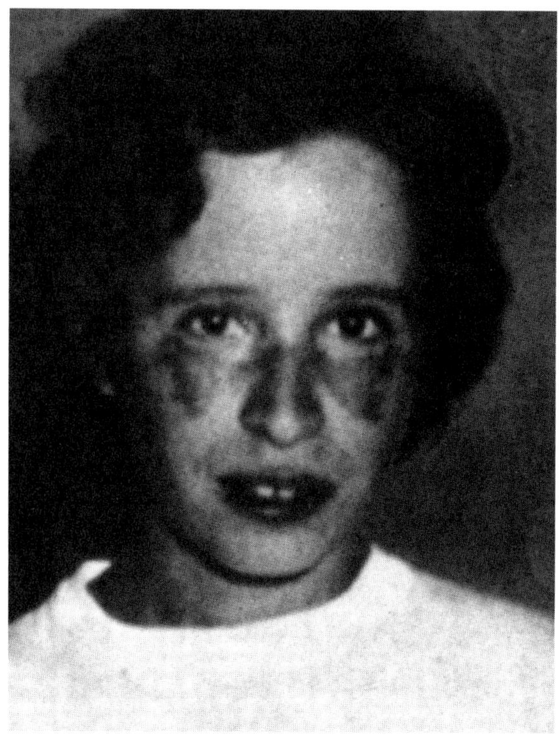

Figure 81-18 Young mother with Bloom's syndrome, demonstrating the typical telangiectatic eruption in a butterfly distribution over the malar eminences and nasal bridge. (From Friedberg EC. DNA Repair. New York: WH Freeman, 1985, with permission; and courtesy of Dr. James German.)

The second characteristic cutaneous stigma seen in many cases of Bloom syndrome consists of well-circumscribed areas of (usually) coffee-colored, *cafe au fait* type hyperpigmentation, with or without areas of hypopigmentation, located mainly over the trunk but which can occur anywhere. These areas vary widely in size and shape. The hypopigmented areas are most easily visualized using a Wood's lamp. These changes are more easily detected in dark complexioned and Black patients, and are most often noted in early childhood, rather than in infancy.

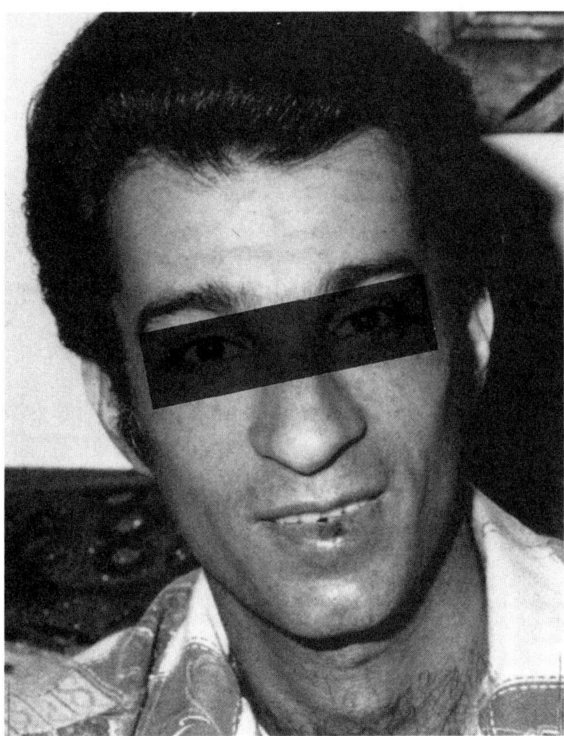

Figure 81-19 Young man with Bloom's syndrome. With much less severe "butterfly rash" but present some related lip lesion. (Courtesy of Dr. James German.)

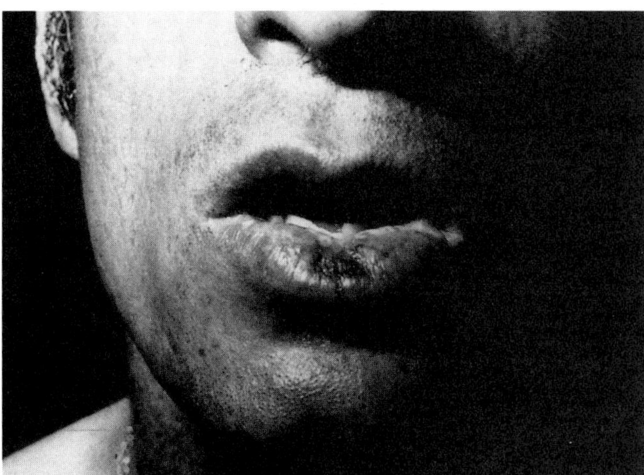

Figure 81-20 Lip of patient in Fig. 81-19. (Courtesy of Dr. James German.)

Immunodeficiency, which is generalized and very variable, is characteristic of Bloom syndrome. Most patients experience at least one severe bacterial pulmonary infection during infancy or childhood, which, if inadequately treated, may lead to severe chronic lung disease. After cancer, this has been the most common cause of death in Bloom syndrome patients. A variable degree of vomiting and diarrhea also occurs during infancy; whether it is related to an immunodeficiency is unknown. This can rapidly produce life-threatening dehydration.

Other, less constant characteristics of Bloom syndrome include a high-pitched voice, a tendency to develop diabetes mellitus, a tendency to have minor anatomic anomalies, mildly restricted intellectual ability, and, in men, small testes and a total failure of spermatogenesis; in women, reduced fertility and a short menstrual life.

DIAGNOSIS The diagnosis of Bloom syndrome usually depends on recognition of the small but proportionate stature in combination with the characteristic telangiectatic facial rash. It is unusual for the diagnosis to be made if these two features are not recognized. The small stature can be detected as in utero growth deficiency. Conversely, if the birth weight is within the normal range and the postnatal height is in the third percentile or greater, it is very unlikely that the patient has Bloom syndrome.

The diagnosis of Bloom syndrome can be confirmed cytogenetically using the Sister Chromatid Exchange (SCE) assay *(see below)*. Because the characteristic telangiectatic cutaneous eruption is not always recognizable, Dr. James German has recommended that cells obtained from the following groups of patients with abnormally small, but proportionate, stature also be examined with this assay:

1. Those with excessive numbers (i.e., more than five) *cafe au lait* macules, especially if hypopigmented macules are also present.
2. Those with unexplained immunodeficiency.
3. Those with an unexplained restriction in intelligence.
4. Those in whom diabetes mellitus develops later than the usual age of onset for Type I and earlier than this age for Type II diabetes mellitus.
5. Infertile men with abnormally small testes for which no explanation can be found.
6. Women with early onset of menopause.
7. Those patients who develop any type of cancer, especially if this occurs at a relatively young age for the type of cancer in question.

Not surprisingly, Bloom syndrome is often misdiagnosed as another type of dwarfism. Of these, it is perhaps most commonly confused with Russel-Silver dwarfism.

GENETIC BASIS OF DISEASE Bloom syndrome is transmitted by autosomal recessive inheritance with no evidence of genetic heterogeneity. This distinguishes it from most of the other major entities (xeroderma pigmentosum, ataxia telangiectasia, and Fanconi Anemia) discussed in this chapter, all of which are genetically heterogeneous.

Cultured cells derived from patients with Bloom syndrome show a number of distinctive features. Some of these are also detected in circulating lymphocytes in Bloom syndrome patients. These abnormalities include chromosome breaks, gaps, translocations, and an increased frequency of intra- and inter-chromosomal strand exchanges. The latter are detected in the Sister Chromatid Exchange assay. The results of an SCE assay on cells derived from a patient with Bloom syndrome are shown in Fig. 81-21. Note the presence of numerous sister chromatic exchanges (SCEs) as well as a balanced (i.e., symmetrical) quadriradial figure, indicative of a recombination event between two homologous chromosomes. These recombinations between homologous chromosomes are responsible for "crossovers" which occur in Bloom syndrome cells, similar to the crossovers between portions of homologous chromosomes that otherwise occur mainly in meiosis. These crossovers are exploited in a novel gene localization technique, Somatic Crossover Point Mapping (SCPM), which has recently allowed identification and cloning of the gene responsible for Bloom syndrome, the *BLM* gene *(see below)*.

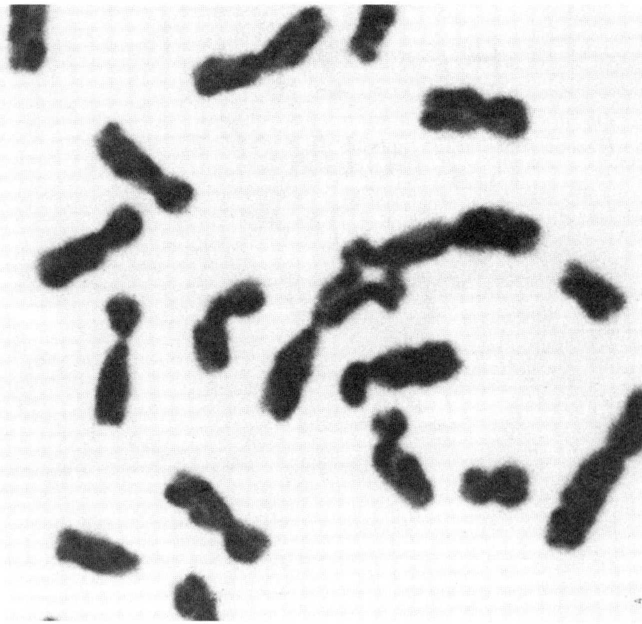

Figure 81-21 Chromosome preparation of a metaphase cell from a patient with Bloom syndrome, processed through two cell cycles so as to reveal sister chromatic exchanges. Note the presence of numerous exchanges per chromosome (identified as exchanges between dark and light strands) as well as a homologous chromosome exchange (quadriradial figure) between the long arms of chromosome 1. (Reproduced with permission from Cell cover image, V.83, #4, Nov. 17, 1995.)

Bloom syndrome cells in culture have accumulated markedly elevated numbers of mutations, compared to normal cells, in all loci in which this has been examined. These loci have included both coding sequences for actively transcribed genes and noncoding repetitive DNA.

Bloom syndrome cells in culture show a prolonged generation time and in particular a long DNA synthetic (S) phase. The rate of nascent DNA chain elongation is retarded and the distribution of DNA replication intermediates is abnormal. Bloom syndrome cells also show increased sensitivity to DNA damaging agents, including ultraviolet light, mitomycin C, ethyl methanesulfonate and *N*-nitroso-*N*-ethylurea. However, not all Bloom syndrome cells show these hypersensitivities and they do not show up in some standard assays. Moreover, no defect in a DNA repair pathway has been found in Bloom syndrome cells.

A number of enzymes associated with DNA replication and/or repair have been reported to have abnormal activities in Bloom syndrome cells. These include DNA ligase I, topoisomerase II, thymidylate synthetase, uracil-DNA glycosylase, *N*-methylpurine DNA glycosylase, 0^6-methylguanine methyltransferase, and superoxide dismutase. Interestingly, some but not all Bloom syndrome cell lines have shown these defects, and the nature of abnormalities observed has been very variable. For example, both increased and decreased activities of DNA ligase I have been reported in different cell lines by different authors, and studies on a purified uracil glycosylase from Bloom syndrome cells showed that a number of properties of the enzyme, itself, are markedly abnormal.

In 1994 James German and his colleagues noted that, in Bloom syndrome patients who are the product of nonconsanguineous matings, a proportion of peripheral blood lymphocytes are phenotypically normal. Based on this observation they developed a new technique, which they termed "Somatic Crossover Point Mapping" (SCPM). In this system, peripheral blood lymphocytes of Bloom syndrome patients are analyzed very much like progeny meiotic cells, using crossovers to obtain extremely precise mapping information. It allowed rapid localization and then cloning of the *BLM* gene, which is mutated in Bloom syndrome cells. The normal phenotype is produced by a crossover event within this gene between the parental mutations. Previously, conventional methods had already localized the *BLM* gene to chromosome band 15q26.1. The BLM gene encodes a 4437 bp cDNA encoding a 1417 amino acid peptide with homology to the RecQ helicases of *E. coli*.

The SCM technique is extremely interesting because it offers a way to exploit the BLM gene to study other inherited diseases in which the cells show associated phenotypic abnormalities.

MOLECULAR PATHOPHYSIOLOGY OF DISEASE Whether the defective *BLM* gene can account for all of the clinical, cellular, and biochemical abnormalities present in Bloom syndrome is at present unknown; however it would appear to be an excellent candidate for many of them. The *BLM* gene is homologous to the RecQ helicases in *E. coli*; these helicases are a subfamily of DExH box-containing DNA and RNA helicases. Although no universal function for the RecQ helicases has been postulated to date, a number of genes in the DExH family have been implicated in DNA repair processes. The *BLM* gene product may also have homologous functions to those of the yeast *SGS 1* gene. *SGS 1* mutants show slow growth, poor sporulation, chromosomal nondisjunction in mitosis, missegregation in meiosis, and elevated recombination frequencies. Also, an interaction between the *BLM* protein and topoisomerase II has been suggested.

MANAGEMENT/TREATMENT Upon establishing a diagnosis of Bloom syndrome, the physician should immediately notify the Bloom Syndrome Registry (even though the Registry was officially closed several years ago). The Registry (c/o Dr. James German, The New York Blood Center, 213 East 31st St., New York, NY 10023) is a very valuable source of information and support.

Patients with Bloom syndrome should avoid sunlight, although the importance of this is not nearly as great as in xeroderma pigmentosum. The clinician should be constantly on the alert for development of cancer in these patients, paying special attention to such signs as hoarseness or throat pain, mild dysphagia, hematochezia or melena, a breast lump, a positive Papanicolaou smear, abdominal discomfort or pain, intussusception, or convulsions, which might otherwise be given less notice, especially in a young patient. Unless or until the prognosis of leukemia is shown to be better if the disease is diagnosed and treated before symptoms develop, however, periodic hematologic surveillance of children with Bloom syndrome is unnecessary and may be inappropriate.

Since children with Bloom syndrome are of small stature, and also tend to be poor eaters; they should be encouraged but never coerced to eat well, and a vitamin supplement provided each day. Gastric intubation is currently being tried in a few patients, but no long-term benefit has yet been demonstrated.

Growth hormone levels in Bloom syndrome patients have been found to be normal to low normal. Exogenous administration of growth hormone has resulted, in a few cases, in development of cancer, both in Bloom syndrome patients and in other patients. This has tempered enthusiasm for administration of growth hormones to these patients.

Table 81-4
Clinical and Molecular Characteristics of Fanconi Anemia

Complementation group	*Relative frequency*	*Chromosome location of gene*	*Characteristics of gene product*
A	66.0	16q24.3	163 h Dalton protein Primary nuclear localization
B	4.3	Unknown	Unknown
C	12.7	9q22.3	63-kDa protein Primary cytoplasmic localization
D	4.3	3q22-26	Unknown
E	12.7	Unknown	Unknown

Several additional coplementation groups likely.

Counseling of patients and their families, carefully advising them of the nature of the disease, is probably the most important service the physician can provide. It is important that parents of a Bloom syndrome child be advised of the risk of having another affected child should they conceive again.

FUTURE DIRECTIONS More precise methods for diagnosing Bloom syndrome using the *BLM* gene in molecular assays will now be developed. Also the precise etiopathogenesis of this disease can now be examined in greater detail in molecular studies using this gene.

By inactivating the *BLM* gene in other types of mutant cells in culture, perhaps by using incisional mutagenesis or antisense DNA or RNA, the SCPM method should be applicable to rapid precise mapping of many other genes unrelated to the *BLM* gene.

FANCONI ANEMIA

BACKGROUND Fanconi anemia is a rare, autosomal recessive disorder characterized by diverse congenital anomalies, a predisposition to develop aplastic anemia, and an increased risk to develop cancer, particularly acute myelogenous leukemia. The clinical features of the disease are quite variable, making a diagnosis on basis of clinical findings quite difficult. This clinical heterogeneity is both interfamilial and intrafamilial. Cases in which no congenital anomaly is recognized, but who nonetheless have cell culture abnormalities and develop bone marrow changes characteristic of Fanconi anemia, are said to have the Diamond-Blackfan syndrome, also known as the Estren-Dameshek variant of Fanconi anemia.

Cells in culture derived from patients with Fanconi anemia show several distinctive characteristics, among which are an increased number, compared to cells derived from normal individuals or first-degree relatives of Fanconi anemia patients, of chromosome breaks in untreated cultures, as well as hypersensitivity to both the cytotoxic and clastogenic effects of DNA crosslinking agents such as mitomycin C, psoralen plus UVA light, and diepoxybutane. The latter property has formed the basis for development of a diagnostic test for the disease in cultured cells, known as the DEB, or diepoxybutane, test. Because the clinical manifestations of the disease are so variable, the definitive diagnosis of Fanconi anemia is currently made based on this test. Five genetic complementation groups, A, B, C, D, and E, have been defined (Table 81-4). It is very likely that several others will be found.

Fanconi anemia was first described in three brothers with congenital anomalies, anemia, and a fatty aplastic bone marrow by Guido Fanconi in 1927. The diepoxybutane test for diagnosis of Fanconi anemia was developed by Arleen Auerbach and her colleagues in 1977. Androgen therapy, one of the clinical mainstays for treatment of hypoplastic anemia short of bone marrow transplantation or gene therapy, was introduced by Nasrollah Shahidi, previously a junior associate of Fanconi. In 1992 one of the genes responsible for Fanconi anemia, the Fanconi anemia [group] C gene, was cloned by Manuel Buchwald and his associates. In 1996 two groups simultaneously reported cloning of the FAA gene. Quite recently, Lin and Walsh and their associates at the National Institutes of Health (US) Clinical Center in Bethesda, MD, performed the first successful gene therapy for Fanconi anemia using the FAC gene.

It has been proposed that Fanconi anemia heterozygotes comprise at least 0.5% of the general population. It has also been proposed that many cases of aplastic anemia without Fanconi anemia may be etiopathogenically related to this carrier state.

CLINICAL FEATURES The incidence of Fanconi anemia is thought to be similar to that of xeroderma pigmentosum, approximately 2–4 per million live births. The true incidence may be significantly higher, however, with many cases not being diagnosed. The disease appears to occur worldwide in all ethnic groups. It is much more common among Ashkenazi Jews. A recent study showed that over 1% of normal Jewish individuals of Ashkenazi ancestry are carriers of a gene for Fanconi anemia, complementation group C. This would indicate (Hardy-Weinberg law) that matings within this group would produce affected individuals in over 1/40,000 births.

Clinical features seen in some but not all patients with Fanconi anemia include the following: (1) short stature, with over 50% of patients below the fifth percentile in height, sometimes associated with low birth weight or "failure to thrive"; (2) congenital anomalies of the thumb and radius (Fig. 81-22); (3) other congenital musculoskeletal anomalies, including hip, spinal and rib malformations, and scoliosis; (4) congenital structural renal malformations, including agenesis of a kidney, fused kidneys, and misshapen kidneys; (5) hyperpigmented areas on the skin, sometimes resembling coffee colored *cafe au fait* macules. These are often large and irregular in shape (Fig. 81-23); (6) microcephaly; (7) microphthalmia; (8) congenital gastrointestinal malformations, with many patients with no observable internal defects also experiencing digestive problems; (9) hypogonadism; (10) congenital cardiac defects, especially involving the atrial or ventricular septum; and (11) mental retardation, sometimes manifested only as a learning disability without other evidence of mental deficiency. Expression of these features is extremely variable, even between affected siblings; some patients who develop aplastic anemia or acute

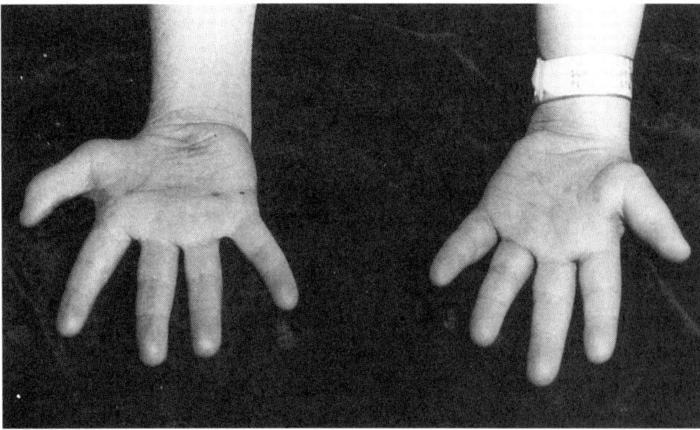

Figure 81-22 Hands and arms of patient with Fanconi anemia showing radial deformities. Such deformities are heterogeneous and not present in every patient (courtesy of Dr. N. Shahidi, University of Wisconsin, Madison, WI).

myelogenous leukemia and who have a positive DEB test show none of these features.

Viruses, including those commonly encountered in childhood, particularly the herpes varicella/zoster virus, may elicit abnormal responses in patients with Fanconi anemia, particularly thrombocytopenia and hypoplastic anemia. These viruses include, besides herpes varicella/zoster, parvovirus B 19 (the cause of fifth disease), hepatitis viruses, the Epstein-Barr virus, and cytomegalovirus. Not uncommonly the disease is first suspected and diagnosed based on a child's response to infection with one of these, particularly the former. Since most children are immunized against a number of other viruses, including rubella (German measles), rubeola (measles), mumps, and influenza A, it is unknown whether these viruses might also induce thrombocytopenia or hypoplastic anemia in Fanconi anemia patients. Bacterial infections may also induce thrombocytopenia or aplastic anemia in patients with Fanconi anemia.

In some cases, the diagnosis of Fanconi anemia is only suspected after development of aplastic anemia or, less commonly, myelodysplastic syndrome or even acute myelogenous leukemia. Anemia in Fanconi anemia patients is characteristically macrocytic, often with elevated fetal hemoglobin levels.

Patients with Fanconi anemia should be expected, sometime during childhood or early adulthood, to develop bone marrow failure and/or leukemia. Moreover, especially in patients who survive childhood, there is an increased risk of development of cancer not involving the bone marrow. These, as far as is known, may occur anywhere and may be of any type; especially common are squamous-cell carcinomas of the oral cavity, esophagus, vagina, and cervix uteri.

A more controversial issue is whether patients with Fanconi anemia have an increased susceptibility to oxygen free radicals in their cells and tissues. Hypersensitivity to agents which produce oxygen free radicals has been demonstrated convincingly in Fanconi anemia patients' cells in tissue culture (discussed below), but this hypersensitivity is lost in some of these cell lines after undergoing transformation (immortalization) in tissue culture. These transformed cells continue to test positive in other assays for Fanconi anemia. It has been proposed that patients with Fanconi anemia also show clinical evidence of this hypersensitivity, such as defective responses to bacterial infections, which induce oxygen free radical formation by neutrophils and other inflammatory cells, but this evidence can also be explained by other defects in Fanconi anemia cells, as noted above.

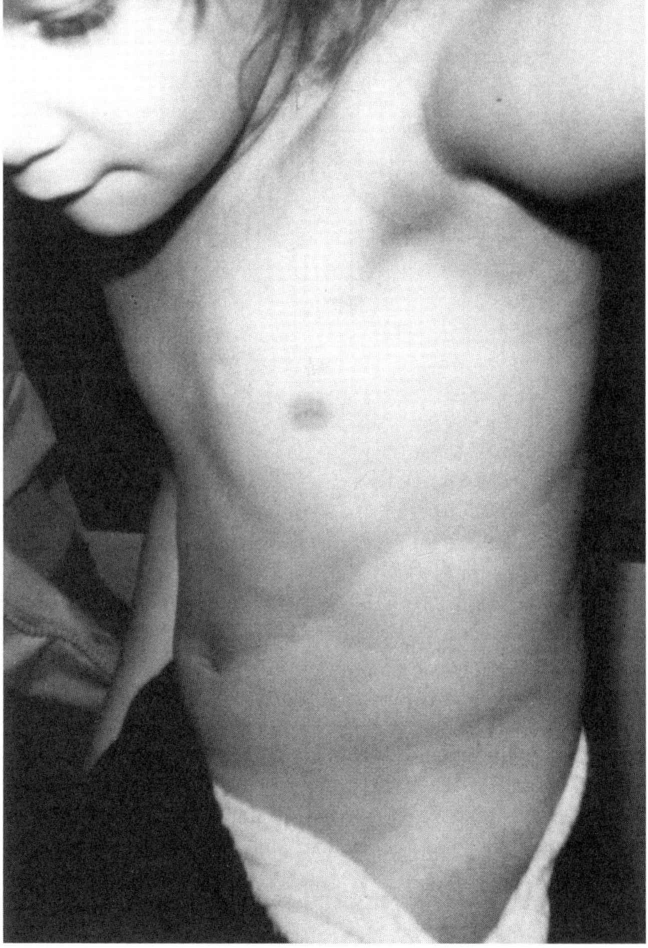

Figure 81-23 Large pigmented macule in chest of boy with Fanconi anemia (courtesy of Dr. N Shahidi).

Patients with Fanconi anemia eventually require therapy for their disease, and thus develop side effects of this therapy. Most patients receive blood transfusions, leading to a risk of iron overload. Those who receive androgen therapy develop the usual side effects of this therapy, including virilization in females and a risk of hepatotoxicity in both sexes. Increased susceptibility to infection and graft vs host disease are important potential complications of bone marrow transplantation.

DIAGNOSIS Every author of a report of a large series of cases of Fanconi anemia has emphasized the enormous clinical heterogeneity of the disease, even among siblings and, in one report, even between monozygotic twins. It is thus very difficult to make specific recommendations as to when a diepoxybutane (DEP) test should be obtained. Certainly a patient with congenital anomalies affecting the thumb or radius should be suspected of having the disease, as should a small patient with thrombocytopenia or hypoplastic, macrocytic anemia not due to folate or vitamin B 12 deficiency. Beyond this it is difficult to make a specific recommendation. The DEB test is the gold standard for the diagnosis of Fanconi anemia, and should be carried out whenever the diagnosis is seriously entertained. This test is performed by the following laboratory:

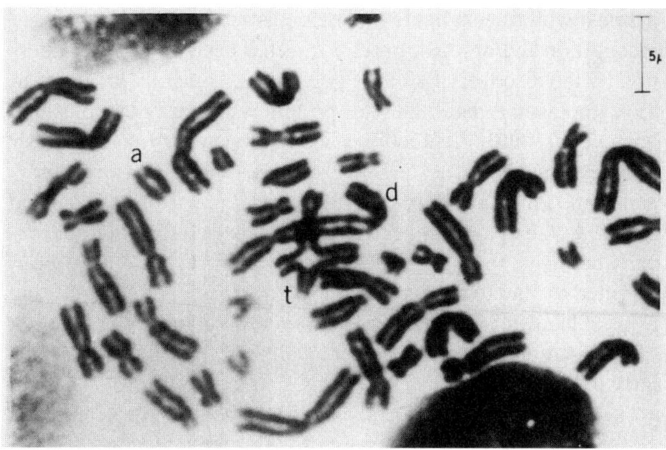

Figure 81-24 Chromosome preparation of a metaphase cell from a patient with Fanconi anemia. Note acentric (a), dicentric (d), and quadriradial (q) chromosomes (courtesy of Dr. N. Shahidi, University of Wisconsin).

c/o Dr. Arleen Auerbach
The Rockefeller University 1230 York Avenue
New York, NY 10021
212-327-7533

It is strongly recommended that the physician telephone in advance regarding optimal ways to submit samples, which must be live (never fixed) cells.

A more challenging problem is what to do with patients who test negative in the DEB assay but who have other manifestations of Fanconi anemia. Despite the great helpfulness of this test, we do not know for certain that it is 100% sensitive in detecting cases of Fanconi anemia, or 100% specific in excluding patients with other disorders.

The DEB test has been used very successfully to identify affected fetuses in prenatal diagnostic examinations of amniocytes or chorionic villi cells, and should be carried out in all cases where the parents are known heterozygotes. A more specific test, based on a known mutation in the Fanconi anemia C gene, has been used successfully in Ashkenazi Jews to identify heterozygotes *(see below)*.

GENETIC BASIS OF DISEASE Pedigrees of families of patients with Fanconi anemia have been consistent with autosomal recessive inheritance. We are unaware of any reported case in this is untrue or in doubt.

Cultured cells derived from patients with Fanconi anemia are both hypersensitive to killing by agents that produce interstrand crosslinks in cellular DNA and show markedly increased numbers of breaks and other abnormalities in metaphase chromosomes following exposure to such agents. This latter characteristic has formed the basis for the most definitive test for this disease yet available, the diepoxybutane (DEB) assay, in which cells derived from a patient suspected of having Fanconi anemia are exposed to the DNA crosslinking agent, diepoxybutane, and subsequent metaphases arrested and analyzed cytogenetically. Fanconi anemia cells show increased numbers of acentric and dicentric, as well as quadriradial, chromosomes, which result from chromosome breaks, compared to normal cells, both with and without drug treatment, although the increased frequency of abnormalities is much easier to detect in treated cultures (Fig. 81-24). In up to 30% of cases, cells derived from circulating lymphocytes fail to show these abnormalities, which are then detected in cells derived from skin fibroblasts. This is thought to be due to recombination events in the precoursers of the former cell type. If the patient is a compound heterozygote, such recomination could produce phenotypically normal cells doubly mutated or one allele and wild type on the others. With a selective growth advantage, these cells would then become predominant among circulating lymphocytes. Interestingly, the Fanconi anemia cells show a wide range in their numbers of chromosomal abnormalities, although these are consistently outside of the range of numbers seen in normal cells. Despite this variability, the diepoxybutane (DEB) test remains the gold standard on which the diagnosis of Fanconi anemia is made, due to the very variable clinical presentation of the disease, which virtually precludes use of clinical criteria to make the diagnosis in most cases.

In addition to diepoxybutane, Fanconi anemia cells are hypersensitive to other DNA crosslinking agents, including mitomycin C, nitrogen mustard (mechlorethamine), cyclophosphamide, cisplatin, and psoralen plus ultraviolet A (long wavelength) radiation. Elegant cell cycle studies have shown that this hypersensitivity is associated with prolongation of, or arrest in, the G2 phase of the cell cycle. Not only the first G2 phase but also subsequent G2 phases are prolonged after exposure to these agents.

In addition to its use in establishing the diagnosis of Fanconi anemia, the diepoxybutane test is also the basis for a complementation assay in patients known to have Fanconi anemia. Fused cells (heterokaryons) from patients in different complementation groups show numbers of metaphase chromosome abnormalities, following treatment with diepoxybutane or other DNA crosslinking agents, similar to those of similarly treated normal cells, whereas fused cells from patients in the same complementation group continue to show increased levels of chromosome abnormalities following this treatment. In this way five complementation groups, A, B, C, D, and E, of Fanconi anemia patients have now been identified. Initially, Fanconi anemia cell lines were assigned to complementation groups strictly on the basis of whether or not they complemented, in this assay, within group A. Unfortunately, all other cell lines were initially classified as "group B," regardless of whether or not they complemented each other in this assay. In consequence, some of these cell lines, once classified as in "complementation group B," are now in different complementation groups. One example is cell line HSC 62 (GM 13023), once classified as in group B, now in group D. This has led to some confusion in the literature. In reviewing the research literature on Fanconi anemia cell lines, it is important to determine precisely which cell line was examined in each study, and to corelate this information with the current complementation group classification of each cell line. Such a classification is to be found in Liu, et al., Table 1. Since only a rather small number of cell lines have been analyzed by complementation group analysis to date, it is likely that additional ones exist, beyond the five already identified, in Fanconi anemia.

A gene that corrects hypersensitivity to crosslinking agents in Fanconi anemia group C, and therefore named *FACC* now *FAC*, was isolated and portions of it cloned by Manuel Buchwald and his colleagues in 1992, who used this property as a selection method, which hastened the progress of their work. Unfortunately, this has not proved a successful strategy, to date, for isolation and cloning of other Fanconi anemia genes. The *FAC* gene does not complement Fanconi anemia cells in other complementation groups. The cDNA codes for a protein of 63 kDa, with alternative 5' and 3' untranslated sequences. Examination of available data banks has failed to identify any different human or nonhuman protein with significant amino acid sequence homology. The gene itself appears to be larger than 100 kb and has 14 exons. By *in situ* hybridization it has been mapped to chromosome band 9q22.3. The gene product localizes primarily in the cytoplasm.

A number of specific mutations have now been identified in Fanconi anemia, complementation group C, patients. These include a splice mutation in intron 4 (IVS4+4A to T), which is the predominant mutation in Ashkenazi Jews, and mutations 322delG, Q13X, R185X, and D19SV. Among the Ashkenazi, the IVS4 mutation is associated with much more severe disease than is the 322delG mutation. Alterations introduced into the gene product by site-directed mutagenesis, along with the locations of the Fanconi anemia mutations discovered to date, indicate that the carboxy (-COOH)-terminal portion of the protein is essential for activity. There is no known homolog to the human FAC gene product. The mouse *FAC* gene, found using probes based on the human sequence, is 68% homologous to it. The mouse FAC protein is identical at 65% and similar at 78% of its amino acid residues to the human FAC protein; where examined, it has a similar number of exons.

The FAA gene cDNA codes for a protein of 163 kDa with two overlapping bipartite nuclear localization signals and a partial leucine zipper consensus region. It localizes primarily in the nucleus. Again, examination of available data banks has failed to identify any different human or nonhuman protein with significant amino acid homology. The gene localizes to chromosome 16q24.3.

MOLECULAR PATHOPHYSIOLOGY OF DISEASE The molecular basis for the increased numbers of chromosome breaks and for the hypersensitivity of Fanconi anemia cells in culture to DNA crosslinking agents remains incompletely understood. It has been suggested that both defects may be due to inappropriate activation of the gene rearrangement mechanism, which normally is functional only in T and B cells undergoing final differentiation. Our laboratory has identified two endonuclease complexes in the chromatin of normal cells, pI 4.6 and pI 7.6, which cleave psoralen plus ultraviolet A light induced monoadducts as well as interstrand crosslinks. The complex, pI 7.6, acts primarily on the former type of adduct; the complex, pI 4.6, acts primarily on the latter. Using a molecularly defined substrate DNA in which the adducts were precisely localized, the exact sites of cleavage of these adducted DNAs were determined. The endonuclease complex pI 4.6, from Fanconi anemia group A cells was deficient in ability to incise DNA containing intrastrand crosslinks activity, whereas the complex, pI 7.6, was able to incise DNA containing the monoadducts. This correlates with a higher degree of sensitivity of these cells to DNA interstrand crosslinking agents. Moreover, when normal endonuclease complexes were introduced into these cells by electroporation, repair function, as measured by a computerized UDS assay based on autoradiography, was restored to normal. Fanconi anemia group A cells are also deficient in a DNA binding protein; how this relates to the endonuclease defect is under investigation.

Other laboratories have also identified DNA repair deficiencies in Fanconi anemia cell lines, but results have been inconsistent, perhaps because well-defined systems were not used. At present, the function of the FAC gene product remains unknown. While it would seem likely that it, too, is active in a DNA damage recognition and/or repair process, this has been thrown into question by the discovery that the FAC protein is mainly localized to the cytoplasm. Even if the FAC protein is primarily cytoplasmic, however, it could still function as a DNA repair enzyme. A number of other proteins that act on DNA, such as some hormone receptors and some enzymes active on DNA, are known to be localized mainly in the cytoplasm, entering the nucleus only when specifically activated to do so. Alternatively, the FAC protein has been reported to bind to the cyclin-dependent kinase, cdc2, suggesting a possible role of this protein in cell-cycle regulation. The function of the FAA gene product, which localizes to the nucleus, is similarly unknown.

In addition to increased sensitivity to both the cytotoxic and clastogenic effects of DNA crosslinking agents, Fanconi anemia cells in culture show at least three additional general features: (1) prolongation, compared to normal cells, of the G_2 phase of the cell cycle (this is in addition to the additional prolongation of G_2 following treatment with DNA crosslinking agents; (2) hypersensitivity to oxygen; and (3) overproduction of tumor necrosis factor (TNF-α). In addition to these features, X-irradiation of Fanconi anemia cells in G_2 also produces increased numbers of chromatic aberrations seen in the following metaphase, a feature Fanconi anemia cells share with a number of other genetic diseases reviewed in this chapter, as discussed above.

Fanconi anemia cells in culture grow very poorly at ambient oxygen levels (atmospheric 20%) but well at reduced oxygen tensions (atmospheric 5%). Cell-cycle/flow cytometric studies indicate that this oxygen sensitivity is associated with the elongation of the G_2 phase also seen in these cells; the G_2 phase becomes shortened at lower oxygen tensions. Even in normal cells, treatment with oxygen or reactive oxygen radicals produces elongation of the G_2 phase. It has been suggested that this effect may be due to interference of oxygen with the function of one or more DNA topoisomerases.

The hypersensitivity of Fanconi anemia cells to oxygen and to reactive oxygen species might be due to one or more of three mechanisms: (1) overproduction of reactive oxygen species in Fanconi anemia cells due to malfunction of the very complex cellular system that controls this rate of production; (2) deficient antioxidant defense mechanisms; or (3) an intrinsic inability of Fanconi anemia cells to tolerate oxygen-induced damage. Data have been reported (from a number of different laboratories) that are consistent with all three mechanisms at work in Fanconi anemia cells. However, not all cell types in Fanconi anemia patients show these deficiencies, or show them to the same extent or in the same way. In erythrocytes and leukocytes of these patients, activities of superoxide dismutase (SOD) are decreased; but in their fibroblasts, activity of at least one SOD, magnesium-SOD, is paradoxically increased. Also, transformation of Fanconi anemia fibroblasts in culture with the SV40 large T-antigenic protein has been reported to cause them to lose their hypersensitivity to oxygen. For these reasons, Liu et al. have argued that oxygen hypersensitivity is a secondary, rather than a primary, effect of mutations in Fanconi anemia genes.

Whether primary or secondary, the hypersensitivity of Fanconi anemia cells in culture to oxygen, and the associated abnormalities in these cells in antioxidant defense mechanisms, has prompted clinical use of antioxidants in Fanconi anemia patients. Following a report that treatment of Fanconi anemia fibroblasts so as to increase their activity of copper-zinc superoxide dismutase (CuZn-SOD)—an important antioxidant that reduces the oxygen species, superoxide anion (O_2)—decreased the cytotoxic effect of mitomycin C, pilot clinical trials using CuZn-SOD were initiated. These produced results suggesting that, indeed, chromosome breakage, at least, is reduced in Fanconi anemia patients receiving this treatment. These findings have also prompted Shahidi to recommend high daily doses of dietary antioxidants for Fanconi anemia patients.

It appears likely that the prolongation of the G_2 phase of the cell cycle, increased numbers of G_2 irradiation induced chromatic anomalies, and even TNF-α overproduction by Fanconi anemia cells in culture are also secondary events. The G_2-to-M cell-cycle transition is genetically controlled to proceed only if DNA damage has been repaired. Thus excess DNA damage, or inadequate DNA repair, might be responsible for G_2 prolongation, rather than a primary cell-cycle disturbance. Also, TNF-α acts preferentially during G_2 and is known to be able to prolong it. Thus TNF hypersecretion by these cells may be due to an autocrine stimulatory loop. We thus agree with Liu et al. that "A defective response (recognition or processing) to DNA lesions is likely to be a key feature of Fanconi anemia."

TREATMENT/MANAGEMENT Once a diagnosis of Fanconi anemia has been established by the diepoxybutane (DEB) test, the patient should be entered into the International Fanconi Anemia Registry (IFAR). If the DEB test is done at the Rockefeller University, this is virtually automatic, since the IFAR is in the same location. An excellent manual for patients and physicians (Frohnmayer and Frohumayer: *Fanconi Anemia. A Handbook for Families and their Physicians*) is published by the Fanconi Anemia Research Fund, Inc., 1902 Jefferson Street, Eugene, OR 97405 (tel: 503-687-4658; fax: 503-687-0548). This is also an excellent support group with which families of patients should interact.

Management of patients with Fanconi anemia has, until very recently, consisted largely of monitoring the blood and bone marrow for appearance of a premalignant or malignant clone or for development of aplastic anemia, treatment with androgens where appropriate to delay the latter, and bone marrow transplantation when one or the other of the above events seems to have progressed to the point to warrant this high-risk procedure. This entails some challenging decisions. For example, bone marrow transplants are less likely to succeed after long androgen therapy; however, androgen therapy also becomes less effective after long-term application. When, then, does one decide to discontinue androgens and opt for bone marrow transplantation? The introduction of gene therapy, for patients in complementation group C and in the future for other Fanconi anemia patients, promises to brighten this picture. Using an adenovirus vector, Liu, Walsh, and their associates have recently successfully repopulated group C patients' bone marrows with their own bone marrow cells with a corrected FACC gene introduced via an adenovirus vector into $CD34^+$ bone marrow stem cells.

At present, bone marrows of Fanconi anemia patients are examined yearly, unless a clone has been identified, in which case they are examined every 3 months. At each examination, chromosome analysis is carried out. The diepoxybutane test, already done to establish the diagnosis, should be extended to determine the complementation group. This is especially important now that it appears that it may soon become possible to offer group C patients the possibility of gene therapy. HLA typing, in anticipation of finding a bone marrow donor, is, of course, necessary.

In addition to these considerations, it is important to examine the status of other organ systems that may be affected by Fanconi anemia or its treatment. Ultrasound examination of the kidneys and urinary tract should be done. Periodic developmental assessments of children should be carried out, as well as formal hearing testing, and in all patients, blood chemistry studies, that include those for liver and kidney functions as well as iron status.

Patients should probably avoid noxious fumes, such as in automobile exhaust, gasoline, formaldehyde, herbicides, pesticides, organic solvents, and tobacco smoke. Supplementation of the diet with antioxidants, such as vitamins C and E, is also probably a wise step, even though it is uncertain whether oxygen hypersensitivity is really significant in this disease *(see above)*. Even if it is only a secondary problem, it may be well worth treating.

In addition to treating patients with Fanconi anemia, it is important that patients at risk be screened as well. The DEB test should be done on parents and siblings of patients. Also, the cloning of the FAC gene and identification of specific mutations among Ashkenazi Jews have made it possible to do molecular screening of large numbers of individuals to determine carrier status. This is now being done. This has proved to be more difficult in the FAA gene because of great heterogeneity in the mutations found.

FUTURE DIRECTIONS Since the most important problems that arise in Fanconi anemia patients are in their bone marrow cells, and since adenovirus vectored gene therapy of hematogenous stem cells has already been shown to be effective in some Fanconi anemia group C patients, it is possible that identification and cloning of other Fanconi anemia genes will lead to effective gene therapy for patients in other Fanconi anemia complementation groups. However, in some patients with Fanconi anemia, intragenic recombination, or some other event, has produced phenotypically normal clones of cells in their blood, yet they still have the disease. This indicates that gene therapy for this disease may be less effective than currently hoped. Alternatively, it is now possible to imagine that this disease may be "cured" within a decade. The term "cured" is in quotes because these patients will still have other problems, including increased tendency to develop carcinomas and whatever consequences they may have from their congenital structural abnormalities. As they come to live much longer, other problems, presently unanticipated, may also arise.

SELECTED REFERENCES

Aboussekhra A, Biggerstaff M, Shiuji MKK, et al. Mammalian DNA nucleotide excision repair reconstituted in purified protein components. Cell 1995;80:859–868.

Alter BP. Fanconi's anemia and its variability. Br J Haematol 1993;85:9–19.

Andrews AD, Halosy CL, Poh-Fitzpatrick MB. Abnormally low UV-induced unscheduled DNA synthesis in cells from a patient with hydroa vacciniforme. Photodermatology 1985;2:315–318.

Auerbach AD. Fanconi's anemia. Dermatol Clin 1985;13:41–49.

Auerbach AD, Rogatko A, Schroeder-Kurth TM. International Fanconi Anemia registry: relation of clinical symptoms to diepoxybutane sensitivity. Blood 1989;73:391–397.

Barlow C, Hirotsune JS, Paylor R, et al. ATM-deficient mice: a paradigm of ataxia telangiectasia. Cell 1996;86:159–171.

Baskaran R, Wood LD, Whitaker LL, et al. Ataxia telangiectasia mutant protein activates c-Abl tyrosine kinase in response to ionizing radiation. Nature 1997;387:516–519.

Bootsma D. The genetic defect in DNA repair deficiency syndromes. Eur J Cancer 1993;29A:1482–1488.

Brookman KW, Lamerdin JE, Thelen MP, et al. ERCC4 (XPF) encodes a human nucleotide excision repair protein with eukaryotic recombination homologs. Mol Cell Biol 1996;16:6553–6562.

Broughton BC, Thompson AF, Harcourt SA, et al. Molecular and cellular analysis of the DNA repair defect in a patient in xeroderma pigmentosum complementation group D who has the clinical features of xeroderma pigmentosum and Cockayne syndrome. Am J Hum Genet 1995;56:167–174.

Brzoska PM, Chen H, Zhu Y, et al. The product of the ataxia-telangiectasia group D complementing gene, *ATDC*, interacts with a protein kinase C substrate and inhibitor. Proc Natl Acad Sci USA 1995; 92:7824–7828.

Butturini A, Gale RP, Verlander PC, Adler-Brecher B, Gillio AP, Auerbach AD. Hematologic abnormalities in Fanconi Anemia: an International Fanconi Anemia Registry study. Blood 1994;84: 1650–1660.

Cleaver JE, Kraemer KH. Xeroderma pigmentosum. In: McKusick VE, ed. Mendelian inheritance in man, 11th ed. Baltimore: Johns Hopkins University Press, 1994;1560:2275–2281.

Cleaver JE, Volpe JP, Charles WC, Thomas GH. Prenatal diagnosis of xeroderma pigmentosum and Cockayne syndrome. Prenatal Diagn 1994;14:921–928.

Cooper PK, Nouspikel T, Clarkson SG, Leadon SA. Defective transcription-coupled repair of oxidative base damage in Cockayne syndrome patients from XP group G. Science 1997;275:990–993.

D'Andrea AD. Fanconi anaemia forges a novel pathway. Nature Genet 1996;14:240–242.

de Vries A, van Oostrom CT, Hofhuis FM, et al. Increased susceptibility to ultraviolet-B and carcinogens of mice lacking the excision DNA repair gene XPA. Nature 1995;337:169–173.

Ellis NA, Groden J, Ye T-Z, et al. The Bloom's syndrome gene product is homologous to RecQ helicases. Cell 1995;83:655–666.

Ellis NA, Lennon DJ, Proytcheva M, Alhadeff B, Henderson EE, German J. Somatic intragenic recombination within the mutated locus BLM can correct the high SCE phenotype of Bloom syndrome cells. Am J Hum Genet 1995;57:1019–1027.

Elson A, Wang Y, Daugherty CJ. et al. Pleiotropic defects in ataxia-telangiectasia protein-deficient mice. Proc Natl Acad Sci USA 1996;93:13,084–13,089.

Evens E, Bourre F, Qulliet X, et al. Different removal of ultraviolet photoproducts in genetically related xeroderma pigmentosum and trichodystrophy diseases. Cancer Res 1995;55:4325–4332.

Fanconi anaemia/Breast cancer consortium (35 authors). Positional cloning of the Fanconi anaemia group A gene. Nature Genet 1996; 14:324–328.

Fazaa B, Pierard-Franchimont C, Zghal M, Kamoun MR, Pierard GE. Nuclear morphometry in xeroderma pigmentosum-associated malignant melanomas. Am J Dermatopathol 1994;16:611–614.

Fitzgerald MG, Bean JM, Hegde SR, et al. Heterozygous ATM mutations do not contribute to early onset of breast cancer. Nat Genet 1997; 15:307–310.

Freidberg EC. DNA Repair, 2nd ed. New York, 1994; 317-365, 633–655.

Fritz E, Elsea SH, Patel PI, Meyn MS. Overexpression of a truncated human topoisomerase III partially corrects multiple aspects of the ataxia-telangiectasia phenotype. Proc Natl Acad Sci USA 1997; 94:4538–4542.

German J. Bloom's syndrome. Dermatol Clin 1995;13:7–18.

German J. Bloom's syndrome. XX. The first 100 cancers. Cancer Genet Cytogenet 1997;93:100–106.

Gillio AP, Verlander PC, Batish SC, Giampietro PF, Auerbach AD. Phenotypic consequences of mutations in the Fanconi anemia FAC gene: an International Fanconi Anemia Registry study. Blood 1997;90:105–110.

Gotti RA. Ataxia-telangiectasia. Dermatol Clin 1995;13:1–6.

Greenwell PW, Kronmal SL, Porter SE, Gassenhuber J, Obermaier B, Petes T. Tel 1: a gene involved in controlling telomere length in S. Cerevisiae, is homologous to the human ataxia-telangiectasia gene. Cell 1995;82:823–840.

Hanawalt PC. Transcription-coupled repair and human disease. Science 1994;266:1957,1958.

Hang B, Yeung AT, Lambert MW. A damage-recognition protein which binds to DNA containing interstrand cross-links is absent or defective in Fanconi Anemia complementation group A, cells. Nucleic Acids Res 1993;21:4187–4192.

Hari KL, Santerre A, Sekelsky JJ, McKim KS, Boyd JB, Hawley RS. The met-41 gene of D. melanogaster is a structural and functional homolog of the human ataxia-telangiectasia gene. Cell 1995;82:815–821.

Hartley KO, Gell D, Smith GCM, et al. DNA-dependent protein kinase catalytic subunit: a relative of phosphatidylinositol 3-kinase and the ataxia-telangiectasia gene product. Cell 1995;82:849–856.

Hoeijmakers JHJ. Nucleotide excision repair II: from yeast to mammals. Trends Genet 1993;9:211–217.

Huo YK, Wang Z, Hong JH, et al. Radiosensitivity of ataxia-telangictasia, X-linked agammaglobulinemia and related syndromes using a modified colony survival assay. Cancer Res 1994;54:2544–2560.

Jaspers NGJ, Bootsma D. Genetic heterogeneity in ataxia-telangiectasia: studies by cell fusion. Proc Natl Acad Sci USA 1982;79:2641–2646.

Jaspers NGJ, Gatti RA, Boan C, et al. Genetic complementation analysis of ataxia-telangiectasia and Nijmegen breakage syndrome: a survey of 50 patients. Cytogenet Cell Genet 1988;49:259–269.

Joenje H, Lo Ten Foe JR, Oostra AB, et al. Classification of Fanconi Anemia patients by complementation analysis: evidence for a fifth genetic subtype. Blood 1995;86:2156–2163.

Jorgensen TJ, Russell PS, Mc Ray DA. Radioresistant DNA synthesis in SV-40-immortalized ataxia-telangiectasia fibroblasts. Radiat Res 1995;143:219–223.

Kasten M. Ataxia-telangiectasia: broad implications for a rare disorder. N Engl J Med 1995;333:662,663.

Kleijer WJ, van der Kraan M, Los FJ, Jaspers NG. Prenatal diagnosis of ataxia-telangiectasia and Nijmegen breakage syndrome by the assay of radioresistant DNA synthesis. Int J Radiat Biol 1994;66:S 167–S 174.

Kohyama J, Shimohira M, Kondo S, et al. Motor disturbance during REM sleep in group A xeroderma pigmentosum. Acta Neurol Scand 1995;92:91–95.

Kraemer KH, Lee MM, Andrews AD, Lambert WC. The role of sunlight and DNA repair in melanoma and nonmelanoma skin cancer. Arch Dermatol 1994;130:1018–1021.

Kraemer KH, Lee MM, Scotto J. Xeroderma pigmentosum: cutaneous ocular and neurologic abnormalities in 830 published cases. Arch Dermatol 1987;123:241–250.

Kraemer KH, Levy DD, Parris CN, et al. Xeroderma pigmentosum and related disorders: examining the linkage between defective DNA repair and cancer. Invest Dermatol 1994;103(5 Suppl):96S–101S.

Kumaresan KR, Hang B, Lambert MW. Human endonucleolytic incision of DNA 3' and 5' to a site-directed psoralen monoadduct and interstrand cross-links. J Biol Chem 1995;270:30,709–30,716.

Kupfer GM, Yamashita T, Naf D, Suliman A, Asano S, D'Andrea AD. The Fanconi anemia polypeptide, FAC, binds to the cyclin-dependent kinase, cdc2. Blood 1997;90:1047–1054.

Lambert MW, Tsongalis GJ, Lambert WC, Hang B, Parrish DD. Defective DNA endonuclease activities in Fanconi's Anemia cells, complementation Groups A and B [now reclassified as group D]. Mutat Res 1992;273:57–71.

Lambert WC, Kuo H-R, Lambert MW. Xeroderma pigmentosum. Clinics Dermatol 1995;13:169–209.

Lambert WC, Lambert MW. Co-recessive inheritance: a model for DNA repair and other surveillance genes in higher eukaryotes. Mutat Res 1992;273:179–192.

Lambert WC, Lambert MW. DNA repair deficiency and skin cancer in xeroderma pigmentosum. In: Mukhtar H, ed. Skin cancer: Mechanisms and Human Relevance. Boca Raton: CRC, 1994; pp. 39–70.

Lambert WC, Schwartz RA. The Muir-Torre syndrome. In: Demis DJ, ed. Clinical Dermatology. Philadelphia: JB Lippincott, in press.

Lehmann AR. Nucleotide Excision repair and the link with transcription. Trends Biochem Science 1995;20:402–405.

Lehman AR, Arlett CF, Broughton BC, et al. Trichothiodystrophy: a human DNA repair disorder with heterogeneity in the cellular response to ultraviolet light. Cancer Res 1988;48:6090–6096.

Lehmann AR, Carr AM. The ataxia-telangiectasia gene: a link between checkpoint controls, neurodegeneration and cancer. Trends Genet 1995;11:375–377.

Lehmann AR, Thompson AF, Harcourt SA, Stefanini M, Norris PG. Cockayne's syndrome: correlation of clinical features with cellular sensitivity of RNA synthesis to ultraviolet radiation. J Med Genet 1993;30:679–682.

Liu JM, Buchwald M, Walsh CE, Young NS. Fanconi anemia and novel strategies for therapy. Blood 1994;84:3995–4007.

Lo Ten Foe JR, Kwee ML, Rooimans MA, et al. Somatic mosaicism in Fanconi anemia: Molecular bases and clinical significance. Eur J Hum Genet 1997;5:137–148.

Lo Ten Foe JR, Rooimans MA, Bosnoyan-Collins L, et al. Expression cloning of a cDNA for the major Fanconi anaemia gene. *FAA* Nature Genet 1996;14:320–323.

Matsumura Y, Sato M, Nishigori C, et al. High prevalence of mutations in the p53 gene in poorly differentiated squamous cell carcinomas in xeroderma pigmentosum. J Invest Dermatol 1995;105:399–401.

Morrow DM, Tagle DA, Shilow Y, Collins FS, Heiter P. Tel 1, an S. cerevisiae homolog of the human gene, mutated in ataxia-telangiectasia, is functionally related to the yeast checkpoint gene MEC 1. Cell 1995;82:831–840.

Nakane H, Takeuchi S, Yuba S, et al. High incidence of ultraviolet-B or chemical carcinogen induced skin tumors in mice lacking the xeroderma pigmentosum group A gene. Nature 1995;337:165–168.

Nelson BR, Fader DJ, Gillard M, Baker SR, Johnson TM. The role of dermabrasion and chemical peels in the treatment of patients with xeroderma pigmentosum. J Amer Acad Dermatol 1995;32: 623–626.

Nishigori C, Moriwaki S, Takebe H, Imamura S. Gene alterations and clinical characteristics of xeroderma pigmentosum group A patients in japan. Arch Dermatol 1995;130:191–197.

Nouspikel T, Lalle P, Leadon SA, Cooper PK, Clarkson SG. A common mutational pattern in Cockayne syndrome patients from xeroderma pigmentosum group G: implications for a second XPG function. Proc Natl Acad Sci USA 1997;94:3116–3121.

Pandita TK, Pathak S, Geord CR. Chromosome end associations, telomeres and telomerase activity in ataxia-telangiectasia cells. Cytogenet Cell Genet 1995;71:86–93.

Parshad R, Tarone RE, Price EM, Sanford KK. Cytogenetic evidence for differences in DNA incision activity in xerodermal pigmentosum group A, C and D cells after X-irradiation during G_2 phase. Mut Res 1993;294: 149–155.

Paulovich AG, Hartwell LH. A checkpoint regulates the rate of progression through S phase in S. cerevisiae in response to DNA damage. Cell 1995;82:841–847.

Randal J. ATM gene discovery may quiet cancer risk debate. J Natl Cancer Inst 1995;87:1350,1351.

Reardon JT, Bessho T, Kung HC, Bolton PH, Sancar A. In vitro repair of oxidative DNA damage by human nucleotide excision repair system: Possible explanation for neurodegeneration in xeroderma pigmentosum patients. Proc Natl Acad Sci USA 1997;94:9463–9468.

Robbins JH, Brumback RA, Moshell AN. Clinically asymptomatic xeroderma pigmentosum neurological disease in an adult: evidence for a neurodegeneration in later life caused by defective DNA repair. Eur Neurol 1993;33:188–190.

Robert C, Sarasin A. Xeroderma pigmentosum: what may be expected from biological studies? Ann Dermatol Venereol 1995;121:434–439.

Sancar A. Mechanisms of excision repair in mammalian cells. Science 1994;266:1954–1956.

Sands AT, Abuin A, Sanchwz A, Conti CJ, Bradley A. High susceptibility to ultraviolet-induced carcinogenesis in mice lacking XPC. Nature 1995;337:162–165.

Savitsky K, Bar-Shira A, Gilad S, et al. A single ataxia-telangiectasia gene with a product similar to PI-3 kinase. Science 1995;268: 1749–1753.

Seal G, Tallarida RJ, Sirover MA. Purification and properties of the uracil DNA glycosylase from Bloom's syndrome. Biochem Biophys Acta 1991;1097:299–308.

Stern JB, Peck GL, Haupt HM, Hollingsworth HC, Beckerman T. Malignant melanoma in xeroderma pigmentosum: search for a precursor lesion. J Am Acad Dermatol 1993;28:591–594.

Strathdee CA, Duncan AMV, Buchwald M. Evidence for at least four Fanconi anemia genes Including FACC on chromosome 9. Nature Genet 1992;1:196–198.

Strathdee CA, Garrish H, Shannon WR, Buchwald M. Cloning of cDNAs for Fanconi's anemia by functional complementation. Nature 1992; 356:763–766.

Stumm M, Gatti RA, Reis A, et al. The ataxia-telangiectasia variant genes 1 and 2 are distinct from the ataxia-telangiectasia gene on chromosome llq23.1. Am J Hum Genet 1995;57:960–962.

Swift M. Ionizing radiation, breast cancer, and ataxia-telangiectasia. J Natl Cancer Inst 1994;86:1571,1572.

Swift M, Chase CL, Morrell D. Cancer predisposition of ataxia-telangiectasia. N Engl J Med 1990;46:21–27.

Swift M, Morrell D, Massey RB, Chase CL. Incidence of cancer in 161 families affected by ataxia-telangiectasia. N Engl J of Med 1991; 325:1833–1836.

Swift M, Reitnauer PJ, Morrell D, et al. Breast and other cancers in families with ataxia-telangiectasia. N Engl J Med 1987;316:1289–1291.

Tanaka K, Miura N, Satokata I, et al. Analysis of a human DNA excision repair gene involved in group A xeroderma pigmentosum and containing a zinc-finger domain. Nature 1990;348:73–76.

Taylor AM, Boyd PJ, Mc Conville CM, Thacker S. Genetic and cellular features of ataxia-telangiectasia. Int J Rad Biol 1994;65:65–70.

Taylor EM, Broughton BC, Botta E. et al. Xeroderma pigmentosum and trichothyodystrophy are associated with different mutations in the XPD (ERCC2) repair/transcription gene. Proc Natl Acad Sci USA 1997;94:8658–8663.

Tu Y, Bates S, Pfeifer GP. Sequence-specific and domain-specific DNA repair in xeroderma pigmentosum and Cockayne syndrome cells. J Biol Chem 1997;272:20,747–20,755.

Turner ML, Moshell AN, Corbett DW, et al. Clearing of melanoma in situ with intralesional interferon alfa in a patient with xeroderma pigmentosum. Arch Dermatol 1995;130:1491–1494.

Walsh CE, Nienhuis AW, Samulski RJ, et al. Phenotypic correction of Fanconi anemia in human hematopoietic cells with a recombinant adeno-associated virus vector. J Clin Invest 1994;94:1440–1448.

Weemaes CMR, Hustinx TWJ, Scheres JMIC, et al. A new chromosomal instability disorder: the Nijmegen breakage syndrome. Acta Paediatr Scand 1981;70:557.

Wegner R-D, Metzger M, Hanefeld F, et al. A new chromosomal instability disorder confirmed by complementation studies. Clin Genet 1988;33:20–23.

Weyl Ben Arush M, Rosenthal J, Dale J, et al. Ataxia-telangiectasia and lymphoma: an indication for individualized chemotherapy dosing: Report of treatment in a highly inbred Arab family. Pediatr Hematol Oncol 1995;12:163–169.

Young BR, Painter RB. Radioresistant DNA synthesis and human genetic diseases. Hum Genet 1989;82:113–120.

Youssoufian H. Localization of Fanconi anemia C protein to the cytoplasm of mammalian cells. Proc Natl Acad Sci USA 1994;91:7975–7979.

Zakian VA. ATM-related genes: what do they tell us about functions of the human gene? Cell 1995;82:685–687.

Zhang N, Chen P, Khanna KK, et al. Isolation of full-length ATM cDNA and correction of the ataxia-telangiectasia cellular phenotype. Proc Natl Acad Sci USA 1997;94:8021–8026.

82 The Skin as a Vehicle for Gene Therapy

SOOSAN GHAZIZADEH, TADEUSZ M. KOLODKA, AND LORNE B. TAICHMAN

INTRODUCTION: DNA AS A NEW FORM OF DRUG THERAPY

Gene therapy involves the introduction and expression of new genetic material in a subset of somatic cells for therapeutic purposes and links the capacity for identifying and cloning new genes together with the ability to introduce and express these recombinant constructs in specific cell types. Gene therapy is a fast-moving, but young, enterprise. For the moment, much of the effort is concentrated on developing effective methods for gene transfer and gene expression. Clinical trials are underway covering a broad range of target cells and disorders, but in almost all instances the goal is to establish safety not efficacy. None of the current trials involves gene transfer to epidermal cells. The purpose of this chapter is to review the current state of knowledge for gene therapy, particularly as it applies to epidermal keratinocytes and dermal fibroblasts. Gene transfer to melanocytes and Langerhans cells is outside the scope of this review.

Gene therapy has features that offer a new approach to the treatment of disease (Table 82-1). Unlike previous pharmacological agents, DNA has the potential to become a permanent part of the cell and the cell's descendants by integrating into the chromosome and replicating along with the host chromosome. In this way, the newly introduced DNA is inherited by all descendant cells and therefore is a potential permanent therapy. If the gene or its expression is restricted to a specific subset of cells and if the gene product remains intracellular, unwanted toxic effects on nontargeted cells, commonly encountered with classical drug therapy, will not be seen. Gene therapy also enjoys another more subtle feature that simplifies development of new applications. For more classical drug-based therapies, each new drug has its own unique half-life, mode of action, distribution, and so on. In gene-based therapies, the same "drug" is used throughout, namely a polynucleotide. What differs is the sequence of nucleotides and the information encoded therein. This simplifies commercial manufacturing and implies that once the hurdles of safety and efficacy are overcome, new applications will be forthcoming at a very rapid rate.

FEATURES OF CUTANEOUS BIOLOGY RELEVANT TO GENE THERAPY

RENEWAL In epidermis, loss of surface cells is balanced by mitotic replication of a progenitor population located primarily in the basal compartment (Figure 82-1). This progenitor population consists of two types of replicating cells: a stem cell, the true progenitor; and amplifying cells, which undergo a limited number of rounds of replication followed by terminal differentiation and migration out of the basal compartment. As seen in Figure 82-1, the only cell that remains in the epidermis is the stem cell. Amplifying cells and terminally differentiated cells are eventually lost. If the goal of gene therapy is to provide a new gene product for prolonged periods, the target of gene insertion must be the stem cell. Putative stem cells have been localized both to the bulge region of the hair follicle by virtue of their prolonged cell cycle and to regions of interfollicular epidermis by virtue of intense staining with antibodies to β1 integrins.

CULTURE MODELS Cutaneous biology is fortunate to have several culture models that permit in-depth analysis of gene transfer and gene expression under controlled conditions and allow for accurate preclinical testing prior to human clinical trials. These models range from the relatively simple submerged cultures in which keratinocyte growth is favored but differentiation is poor, to the more complex organotypic culture in which the in vivo architecture is approximated. In addition, these cultures have been used for autologous grafting in severe thermal injuries, suggesting that stem cells are present in culture.

BARRIER A primary function of skin is to act as a barrier. Attempts, therefore, to introduce new genetic information into cells within the skin will encounter a permeability barrier and an interconnected, multilayered epidermis, making access to the progenitor population of keratinocytes problematic.

IN VIVO AND EX VIVO GENE THERAPY

There are two basic approaches to gene therapy (Table 82-2). In vivo transfer involves insertion of the new gene directly into the tissue, whereas ex vivo transfer involves gene transfer to cells while in culture, followed by transplantation to the donor. Accessibility of epidermis makes the in vivo approach attractive, but the barrier property and the multilayered nature of the tissue prevent easy access to the basal or progenitor population. Ex vivo gene therapy is more complex, requiring additional cultivation and grafting steps. But the ex vivo approach does offer two advantages: first, gene transfer methods generally work more effectively in culture than in vivo; second, with ex vivo therapy, the performance of genetically altered keratinocytes can be assessed prior to transplantation. One drawback with ex vivo therapy is the requirement for grafting, especially for keratinocytes. Autologous grafting of cultured epithelial sheets has been established for burn

From: *Principles of Molecular Medicine* (J. L. Jameson, ed.), ©1998 Humana Press Inc., Totowa, NJ.

Table 82-1
How Gene Therapy Differs from Classical Pharmacological Therapy

DNA can become a permanent part of the cell and be inherited by its descendants.
If gene transfer or gene expression is restricted to a particular cell type, unwanted side effects on other cell types are reduced or eliminated.
In gene therapy, the "drug" is a polynucleotide, for all applications.

Table 82-2
Comparison of Ex Vivo and In Vivo Gene Therapy

In vivo	*Ex vivo*
Direct transfer to tissue	Involves gene transfer to cells in culture followed by transplantation
Preclinical testing not possible	Allows preclinical testing of gene altered cells in advance of therapy
Gene transfer usually less efficient	Gene transfer techniques work optimally in culture

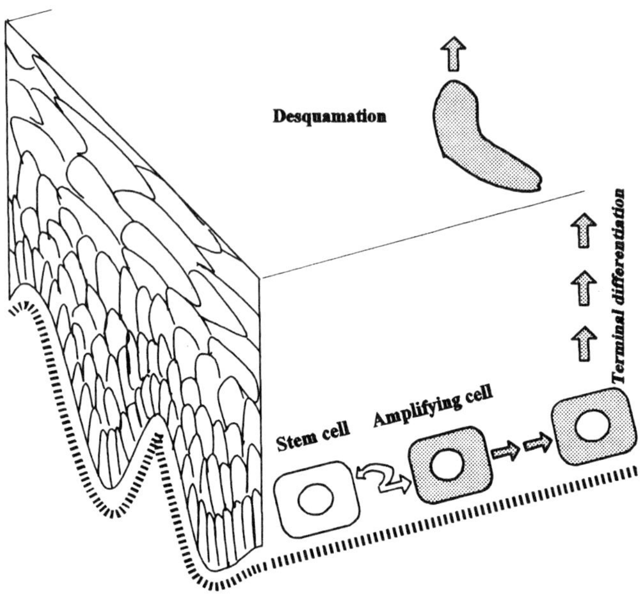

Figure 82-1 Keratinocyte renewal in a stratified squamous epithelium. The progenitor population of cells in epidermis consist of stem cells, the true progenitor cell, and amplifying cells that undergo a limited number of cycles of replication followed by terminal differentiation. Amplifying and terminal differentiating cells are eventually lost from the tissue by desquamation. Only the stem cell remains as a permanent resident of the epidermis. For long-term gene therapy, the stem cell must be the target of gene transfer.

therapy, but these techniques require full-thickness excision at the recipient graft site, a procedure that usually leads to scarring and contracture. Ex vivo gene therapy with fibroblasts may be more acceptable as autologous gene-altered fibroblasts can be implanted without having to excise normal tissue at the graft site.

GENE TRANSFER

GENE TRANSFER BY TRANSFECTION Transfection involves gene transfer with purified DNA in a plasmid vector. There are several methods for transfection in vitro, each designed to facilitate DNA delivery to the interior of the target cell. For example, in calcium phosphate-mediated transfection, formation of a calcium phosphate precipitate entrains DNA and facilitates accessibility to the cell surface and endocytic uptake. In liposome- or lipid-mediated transfection, transport of the DNA through cell membranes is facilitated by membrane fusion. Electroporation works by creating temporary holes in the cell membrane through which DNA may enter. Transfer of DNA in vivo has been achieved by use of the "gene gun," which accelerates microscopic gold particles coated with DNA and forces the projectiles into the cell interior. Recently, intradermal injection of purified DNA into mouse or pig skin has been shown to result in expression of the encoded gene product in dermal fibroblasts as well as overlying epidermal keratinocytes. The mechanism of DNA uptake by any transfection method is unclear.

Transfection methods are simple to use and can achieve transfer of relatively large molecules (>8 kbp). However, transfection in most cell types is inefficient, achieving gene transfer in a small percentage (usually 1–10%) of the target population. Transfected DNA does not ordinarily integrate into the chromosome of the target cell and, as a result, is diluted out by repeated cycles of cell replication. Expression, therefore, is transient, reaching peak levels in 2–3 days and abating after 5–10 days. However, expression can persist for much longer periods if the cell does not ordinarily cycle, such as mature muscle cells.

GENE TRANSFER BY VIRAL TRANSDUCTION The use of viral vectors to transduce cells for gene therapy capitalizes on the capacity of viruses to insert and express their own genetic material in a cell with high efficiency. To harness the transducing powers of a viral vector, an infectious, but crippled virus is constructed in which viral genes required *in trans* for viral replication are replaced by a gene(s) of interest. The infectious property of the virus is maintained, but deletion of essential viral genes renders the vector replication incompetent, unable to complete its life cycle in the target cell. The end result is a system for efficiently introducing and expressing new genetic information in a cell without the risk of reinfection and viral spread. Assembly of viral vectors is carried out in packaging cell lines that are designed to constitutively express *in trans* the deleted viral genes.

Three types of viruses have been approved for use in human gene therapy trials: adenovirus, retrovirus, and adeno-associated virus (*see* Table 82-3). Adenovirus vectors are noted for high titers and their ability to transduce nonreplicating cells, a feature that allows transduction of tissues with a low mitotic index. Adenoviral vectors have been used to transduce keratinocytes in vivo. As the vector does not have a mechanism for integration or self renewal, it does not persist and expression is lost within several days. Adenovirus vectors can be toxic at high multiplicities of infection and development of an immunological response limits duration of expression and prevents reinoculation. Attempts to reduce the immunological rejection by reducing the antigenicity of the vector or suppressing the immunoresponsiveness of the host have met with some success.

Retrovirus vectors are currently the most widely used agents for gene transfer in clinical trials. These RNA vectors are derived from the Moloney murine leukemia virus and require cell replication for successful infection, as there is no mechanism to transport the viral replication complex into the nucleus. A reverse-tran-

Table 82-3
Viral Vectors for Gene Therapy

	Retrovirus	*Adenovirus*	*AAV*
Virus structure	RNA	Linear, duplex DNA	Linear, single-stranded DNA
Titer (CFU/mL)	10^6–10^7	10^{11}–10^{12}	10^3–10^6
Insert size	7–8 kbp	~10 kbp	5.2 kbp
Target cell	Replicating cells	Replicating and nonreplicating cells	Replicating and nonreplicating cells
Integration	At random sites	No integration	Wild-type integrates at chromosome 19q13
In vivo transfer	Not reported in skin	Very effective in variety of tissues	Bronchial airway epithelial cells
Safety concerns	Insertional mutagenesis	Toxicity at high input	Without known pathology

scribed, double-stranded DNA copy of the viral genome integrates at high efficiency in the host-cell genome at random sites. Integration provides a mechanism for ensuring persistence of vector sequences in descendant cells. Retrovirus vectors are therefore quite suitable for transducing stem cells, if these cells can be induced to replicate. Recent advances in retrovirus vector design include: (1) high-titer stocks by encapsidating the viral genome in the capsid protein of vesicular stomatis virus, thereby enabling concentration to titers $\geq 10^9$ colony forming units per mL (CFU/mL) and expanding its host range; (2) lentivirus vectors capable of transducing nondividing cells; (3) receptor-binding sequences allowing targeting to a specific cell type; and (4) vectors with inactivated 5' promoter sequences that may allow unfettered expression of an internal promoter. A concern with retrovectors is the potential for mutagenesis at the site of integration. However, the likelihood of disrupting a vital gene is remote and no untoward effects of retroviral transduction have been reported to date in human trials.

Cultured keratinocytes are highly transducible with recombinant retroviruses. At titers above 5×10^6 CFU/mL, all clonogenic keratinocytes in the culture are transduced. In culture, putative stem cells are successfully transduced with no apparent loss of growth potential. No one has yet succeeded in using retrovirus vectors for direct gene transfer to epidermis or dermis, either for short-term or prolonged expression.

Wild-type adenoassociated virus has several features that make it an attractive vector system including the lack of any known pathology associated with infection, its ability to infect nonreplicating cells, and its potential for integrating at a specific site in the chromosome. However, the size of the transgene it can transfer is limited and site-specific integration is likely to require the presence of the viral *rep* gene, further limiting the size of the transgene.

Papillomaviruses induce benign warts and condyloma in stratified squamous epithelia. Papillomaviruses have not received much attention as a vector but two factors make these viruses particularly attractive for keratinocyte gene therapy. First, they have a natural tropism for keratinocytes of stratified squamous epithelium; second, their circular DNA genome replicates as a stable, multicopy episome. Three viral genes are required for episomal replication: an origin of replication, the E1 and E2 genes. The E5, E6, and E7 genes, which encode products with oncogenic potential, can be removed without loss of episomal replication. No packaging cell line for papillomavirus is available. However, infectious, but empty viral capsids have been produced by expressing viral-capsid genes at high levels. It may be possible to develop this system further to produce infectious, replication-incompetent papillomavirus.

Table 82-4
Potential Applications for Cutaneous Gene Transfer

Treatment of a cutaneous disorder (inherited or acquired)
Vaccination
Systemic delivery of gene product
Creation of an enzyme reservoir for processing of circulating metabolites

EXPRESSION OF THE THERAPEUTIC GENE

For gene therapy to succeed, the therapeutic gene must not only be inserted in the target cell it must also be expressed at a level sufficient to achieve a therapeutic effect. Some gene products may need to be regulated to achieve a suitable response. Promoters from Moloney murine leukemia virus, SV40, and cytomegalovirus have been widely used and provide high level activity in a variety of cell types including keratinocytes. For reasons that remain unclear, activity from these viral promoters remains stable while the host cell is maintained in culture, but drops precipitously when the same cells are transplanted to an animal host. The mechanism behind this tissue-induced inactivation is unknown but may be related to methylation of cytosine residues in the viral promoter. Experiments with fibroblasts, myoblasts, and hepatocytes suggest that tissue-specific promoters normally active in the particular cell type are not subject to this inactivation. The use of keratinocyte-specific promoters to overcome this inactivation has not been reported.

GENE THERAPY FOR INHERITED AND ACQUIRED CUTANEOUS DISORDERS

INHERITED DISORDERS An inherited cutaneous disorder in which the mutant gene has been identified and the normal allele cloned is a candidate for gene therapy (Table 82-4). However, there is a key difference between dominant and recessive disorders in terms of their suitability for gene therapy (Fig. 82-2). In a dominant disorder, the mutant phenotype is induced by a single copy of the mutant allele. The presence of the normal allele in the same cell has no sparing effect. Expressing an additional copy of the normal allele is therefore not likely to alter this situation. For example, epidermolysis bullosa simplex (*see* Chapter 73) and epidermolytic hyperkeratosis (*see* Chapter 74) are two dominantly inherited skin diseases in which mutation in keratin structural genes cause collapse of the intermediate filament network and cytolysis. Insertion of an additional normal allele is not likely to offset the disruptive effects of the mutant protein on the filament network. A more effective therapy is likely to require selective inactivation of the mutant gene by homologous recombination or by an antisense or ribozyme strategy.

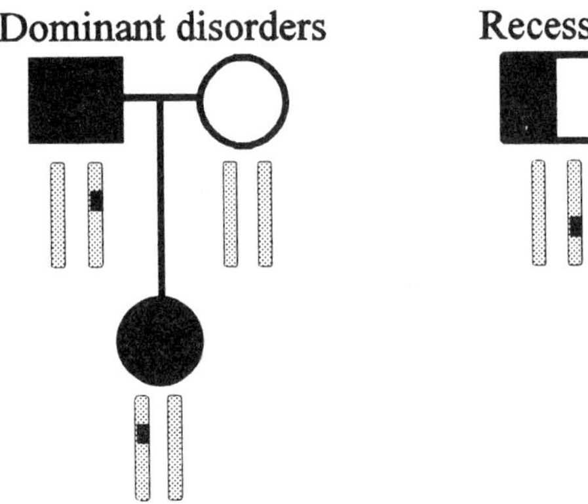

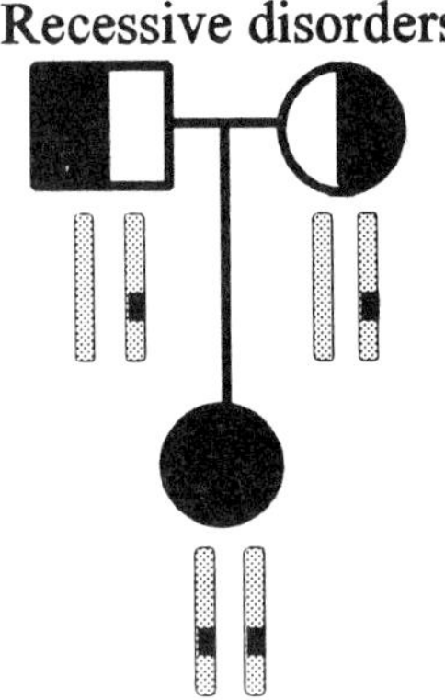

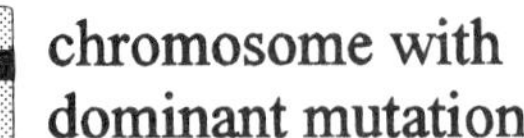

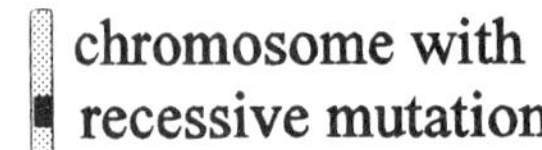

Figure 82-2 Gene therapy for dominant and recessive disorders. In a dominant disorder, a single mutation in one of the two alleles causes the mutant phenotype, whereas, in a recessive disorder, both alleles must be mutated for the mutant phenotype to be present. In carriers of a recessive disorder, the presence of one normal allele spares the cell from the mutant phenotype. Insertion and expression of a normal allele in a recessive disorder is therefore likely to result in reversion to the normal phenotype, whereas such a strategy is not likely to succeed for a dominant disorder.

Recently, a new methodology has been described that may allow targeted correction of a known dominant point mutation. A chimeric DNA/RNA oligonucleotide homologous to a specific host sequence in all but one nucleotide is introduced into a cell, and by a mechanism possibly involving DNA mismatch repair, the host sequence is altered to correspond with that of the oligonucleotide. In this way, the point mutation in the hemoglobin β allele was corrected. The use of chimeric DNA/RNA oligonucleotides has not been described in cutaneous cells.

In a recessive disorder, the mutant phenotype appears when both alleles in a cell are mutant (Fig. 82-2). Inserting a normal allele into cells from such an individual is likely to recreate conditions resembling the carrier state in which there is a single copy of the mutant and the normal allele. Lamellar ichthyosis *(LI)* is a case in point. LI is a recessive disorder associated with mutations in keratinocyte transglutaminase I (TGaseI) and results in abnormal epidermal differentiation and defective barrier function. By inserting a copy of the normal TGaseI allele into LI-keratinocytes, a more normal phenotype is evident when these gene-altered cells are grafted to athymic mice. Among the changes seen in the genetically modified epithelium were reduced hyperkeratosis, a more normal distribution of filaggrin and a reduction in transepidermal water loss. Although gene therapy is not possible over the entire epidermis, it may be possible to treat selective areas of skin. If the gene-corrected cells possess a selective growth or attachment advantage, they may be capable of replacing the defective epithelium.

ACQUIRED DISORDERS It is not clear at this time what acquired cutaneous disorders might be approached with gene therapy. Several factors are responsible for this lack of clarity. First, because of the untried nature of keratinocyte gene therapy, clinical trials are likely to be approved only for cutaneous disorders in which all current therapies have proven to be unsatisfactory. Second, because of limitations on the size of the transferred gene, only a single gene can be effectively transferred. Therefore, the disease in question must be one that can be treated with a single gene product. Third, with current methods of in vivo gene transfer, expression is transient, thereby limiting applications to conditions such as wound healing.

Table 82-5
Examples of Systemic Uptake of a Gene Product Released by Cells Located in Skin

Cell	*Protein*
Keratinocyte	α1-antitrypsin
	apo E
	Factor IX
	Growth hormone
	IL-6
Fibroblast	Growth hormone
	Erythropoietin
	Factor VIII
	Transferrin

CUTANEOUS GENE TRANSFER FOR SYSTEMIC DISORDERS

Expressing new genetic information in skin may be used to induce effects that have systemic implications. Three types of systemic applications are described:

VACCINATION Uptake and expression of naked plasmid DNA by epidermal and dermal cells can be followed by development of long-lasting humoral and cellular immune responses to the encoded protein, suggesting that intradermal gene vaccination may constitute an alternative to traditional immunization. For example, when mice receive an intradermal injection of a plasmid encoding the influenza nucleoprotein, antinucleoprotein antibodies and cytotoxic T lymphocytes developed and the mice gain resistance to challenge with a heterologous strain of influenza virus. The mechanism of immunization is not well-understood. Immunogenicity of plasmid DNA is not based on the level of protein expression, but rather the presence of short immunostimulatory DNA sequences in the plasmid backbone that elicits production of proinflammatory cytokines by keratinocytes and antigen-presenting cells. The induction of immune responses may also involve transfection of skin-derived dendritic cells that localize to the draining lymph node.

SYSTEMIC DELIVERY Systemic delivery from epidermis was first demonstrated in the case of apolipoprotein E (apo E), a 34-kDa protein naturally secreted by keratinocytes. Insertion of a recombinant tagged apo E gene under the control of a viral promoter into keratinocytes with subsequent grafting to athymic mice resulted in the presence of both the endogenous and the tagged apo E in the animal's bloodstream. Systemic delivery of apo E may be useful for the treatment of familial hypercholesterolemia III. Other gene products that have been induced in keratinocytes and delivered systemically include human growth hormone, factor IX, and α1 antitrypsin (Table 82-5).

METABOLIC PROCESSING OF A CIRCULATING SUBSTRATE In inherited metabolic disorders with a nonfunctional enzyme and toxic accumulation of its substrate, one therapy has been to replace the missing enzyme by injection. Gene-transfer techniques may allow creation of a permanent intracellular enzyme reservoir to metabolize circulating substrate. A case in point is severe-combined immunodeficiency caused by mutation in adenosine deaminase (ADA). ADA normally deaminates deoxyadenosine (dAdo) to produce deoxyinosine. In ADA deficiency, dAdo accumulates in the bloodstream and is toxic to T- and B-cell development. Classical therapy for this disease has been to furnish ADA enzyme either by injection or by transfusion of red-blood cells. Recently, human gene therapy trials have successfully introduced the ADA gene into peripheral lymphocytes and hematopoietic stem cells. Dermal fibroblasts transduced with an ADA-retrovirus vector have been shown to express high levels of the enzyme and deaminate significant quantities of the dAdo substrate and the suggestion has been made to employ these cells to create a cutaneous enzyme reservoir.

CONCLUSION

If gene therapy is an infant science, cutaneous gene therapy is at an earlier, embryonic stage. To date no clinical trials have been initiated or approved using skin as the target organ. The first clinical trials are likely to entail genetic vaccination as this application does not require sustained expression of the gene product and methods are in place for gene transfer and expression. For applications that require long-term expression of a gene product, two hurdles must be overcome: If ex vivo gene transfer is to be attempted, then methods for autologous transplantation of the genetically modified cells must be developed that are not destructive to tissues at the recipient site; if in vivo gene transfer is to be used, then vectors must be available that efficiently integrate into the host genome or undergo autonomous episomal replication. Cutaneous gene therapy will undoubtedly bring a new dimension to the treatment of cutaneous as well as systemic disorders.

SELECTED REFERENCES

Blaese RM, Culver KW, Miller DA, Carter CS, Fleisher T, Clerici M. T lymphocyte-directed gene therapy for ADA-SCID: initial trial results after 4 years. Science 1995;270:475–480.

Choate KA, Medalie DA, Morgan JR, Khavari PA. Corrective gene transfer in the human skin disorder lamellar ichthyosis. Nature 1996;2:1263–1267.

Cole-Strauss A, Yoon K, Xiang Y, et al. Correction of the mutation responsible for sickle cell anemia by an RNA-DNA oligonucleotide. Science 1996;273:1386–1389.

Fenjves ES. Approaches to gene transfer in keratinocytes. J Invest Dermatol 1994;103:70S–75S.

Fenjves ES, Smith J, Zaradic S, Taichman LB. Systemic delivery of secreted protein by grafts of epidermal keratinocytes: prospects for keratinocyte gene therapy. Hum Gene Ther 1994;5:1241–1248.

Freiberg RA, Choate KA, Deng H, Alperin ES, Shapiro LJ, Khavari PA. A model of corrective gene transfer in X-linked ichthyosis. Hum Mol Genet 1997;6:927–933.

Garlick JA, Katz AB, Fenjves ES, Taichman LB. Retrovirus-mediated transduction of cultured epidermal keratinocytes. J Invest Dermatol 1991;97:824–829.

Greenhalgh DA, Rothnagel JA, Roop DR. Epidermis: an attractive target tissue for gene therapy. J Invest Dermatol 1994;103:63S–69S.

Khavari PA, Krueger GG. Cutaneous gene therapy. Dermatol Clin 1997;15:27–35.

Krueger GG, Morgan JR, Jorgensen CM, et al. Genetically modified skin to treat disease: potential and limitations. J Invest Dermatol 1994;103: 76S–84S.

Mathor MB, Ferrari G, Dellambra E, et al. Clonal analysis of stably transduced human epidermal stem cells in culture. Proc Natl Acad Sci USA 1996;93:10,371–10,376.

Mulligan RC. The basic science of gene therapy. Science 1993;260:926–932.

Muzyczka N. Use of adeno-associated virus as a general transduction vector for mammalian cells. Curr Topics Microbiol Immunol 1992;158:98–129.

Raz E, Carson DA, Parker SE, et al. Intradermal gene immunization: the possible role of DNA uptake in the induction of cellular immunity to viruses. Proc Natl Acad Sci USA 1994;91:9519–9523.

Vogel JC, Walker PS, Hengge UR. Gene therapy for skin diseases. Adv Dermatol 1996;11:383–398.

Wilson JM. Adenoviruses as gene-delivery vehicles. N Engl J Med 1996;334:1185–1187.

Acquired Diseases of Cutaneous Tissues

83 Acquired Diseases of Cutaneous Tissues

Introduction

THOMAS S. KUPPER

INTRODUCTION

Over 2000 skin diseases have been described to date, and the majority of these are not genodermatoses, but rather are acquired over the course of the individual's lifetime. Many of these are likely to have a genetic component that is presently undefined. In addition, the skin can be an important indicator of systemic disease, including metabolic, oncologic, and infectious disorders. A careful and encyclopedic description of all acquired skin diseases, and skin signs of systemic disease, is well beyond the scope of this section and is further precluded by considerations of space. The reader is referred to several excellent comprehensive textbooks of Dermatology (listed below). In compiling this section, we elected not to simply list a large number of skin diseases (for which the etiopathogenesis is often completely obscure); rather, we decided to focus on several selected important skin diseases for which the molecular genetic basis is currently being rigorously explored.

Cutaneous oncology is a particularly important area in modern dermatology; much of what we know about the mechanism of carcinogenesis in animal models and humans stems from the study of murine models of cutaneous carcinogenesis. The molecular genetics of the most common skin cancers are discussed, including squamous-cell carcinoma, basal-cell carcinoma, and melanoma. These cancers all share, at least to some extent, an etiopathogenesis based on ultraviolet B (UVB)-radiation-mediated DNA damage. Genodermatoses associated with excessive sensitivity to UVB irradiation with respect to cutaneous carcinogenesis are discussed in Chapter 81. Less-common skin cancers, including cutaneous T-cell lymphoma (CTCL), are not discussed in detail here. This interesting non-Hodgkins lymphoma, which, in its most common form (mycosis fungoides), represents a malignancy of mature ($CD7^-$), memory (CD45RO), skin homing (CLA^+), or helper ($CD4^+$) T cells, often presents initially as an inflammatory skin disease. A comprehensive review of these lymphomas was recently published *(see below)*. Merkel-cell carcinomas and fibrosarcomas are beyond the scope of this section.

Psoriasis and atopic dermatitis (Chapters 86 and 87) are, collectively, the most common inflammatory skin diseases that appear also to have a genetic basis, and significant evidence has emerged implicating T cells and the immune system in their etiopathogenesis. Moreover, the type of T cell involved (CLA+, CD45RO, or CD3+ T cells) in the initiation of lesions of psoriasis and atopic dermatitis shares many cell-surface markers with the transformed skin-homing T cell of CTCL *(see above)*. Whereas T cells, antigen-presenting cells, and cytokines are important in the pathogenesis of psoriasis and atopic dermatitis, there is evidence that a more complex polygenic pattern of inheritance underlies these diseases. Although certain major histocompatibility complex (MHC) associations appear to be solid, other of these candidate genes are likely to not be directly related to the immune system. However, it is important to recall that immunosuppression mediated by drugs such as cyclosporin and FK506 can clinically suppress these diseases. Bullous diseases, discussed in Chapters 88 and 89, often involve an immune-mediated assault on structural elements of the skin. The relevant antigen in pemphigus vulgaris was recently found to be a cadherin-like adhesion molecule. The gene defect in a form of junctional epidermolysis bullosa involves the deficiency of a molecule first described in the context of the blistering disease bullous pemphigoid (the BPAG1) as an antigen. Finally, Chapters 90 and 91 describe two classes of disease long considered to have an autoimmune etiology: lupus erythematosis and scleroderma. It has been extremely difficult to dissect the pathogenesis of these complex diseases, and physicians have had to attempt to classify and treat these disorders in the absence of a clearly defined etiologic mechanism. These chapters review the current state of knowledge about these diseases, and suggest future directions for clinical investigation.

It is important for internists and other physicians to appreciate that there are many important skin signs of systemic diseases, and it is unreasonable to expect nondermatologists to be conversant in these. In addition, as our pharmacologic armamentarium grows and new powerful systemic therapies emerge, the already large number of drug reactions involving skin will grow. Excellent texts exist that include photographs and descriptions of these disorders, and the reader more than casually interested is encouraged to seek these out. Unfortunately, the molecular bases for most of these skin manifestations of systemic disease or drug reactions remain completely unknown. As our understanding of the molecular basis of skin disease grows, it is anticipated that this state of affairs will change. Space precludes an exhaustive discussion of other acquired skin diseases in this section.

SELECTED REFERENCES

Champion RH, Burton JL, Ebling FJG. Rook's Textbook of Dermatology, 5th ed. London: Blackwell Scientific, 1992.

Fitzpatrick TB, Eisen AE, Wolff K, Freedberg IM, Austen, KF. Dermatology in General Medicine, 4th ed. New York: McGraw Hill, 1993.

Frank MM, Austen KF, Clamen HN, Unanue ER. Samter's Immunologic Diseases, 5th ed. Boston: Little Brown, 1994.

Koh H, Foss. Cutaneous T Cell Lymphoma. St. Louis: Mosby-Year Book, 1996.

From: *Principles of Molecular Medicine* (J. L. Jameson, ed.), ©1998 Humana Press Inc., Totowa, NJ.

84 Basal- and Squamous-Cell Carcinomas

PAUL NGHIEM AND THOMAS S. KUPPER

EPIDEMIOLOGY

In 1996, nearly one million skin cancers were diagnosed in the United States alone. This number approaches the sum of all other types of cancer combined. Malignant transformation can occur in each of the three major call types of the epidermis: the basal cells, the squamous cells, or the pigment-producing melanocytes. Cancer of the melanocytes, or malignant melanoma, is the most lethal and, fortunately, least common type of skin cancer. Of approximately 38,000 cases in 1996, there were approximately 7000 deaths. (Melanoma will be covered in Chapter 85.) The nonmelanoma skin cancers, basal-cell carcinoma (BCC) and squamous-cell carcinoma (SCC), together comprise more than 95% of skin cancers, but cause few deaths as they rarely metastasize. Early diagnosis and excision is highly effective in treating all three forms of skin cancer, including melanoma.

It is now well-established that ultraviolet (UV) radiation, especially in the UVB range from approximately 280–320 nanometers, is responsible for most skin cancers. However, the complex pathway from sun exposure encountered in youth to skin cancers developing years later is only beginning to be unraveled.

RISK FACTORS FOR NONMELANOMA SKIN CANCER

ULTRAVIOLET LIGHT Australia has served as an inadvertent experiment on the effects of sunlight on minimally pigmented skin following the colonization of this sunny land with Caucasians from the British Isles. Whites in Australia have the highest rates of skin cancer of any people in the world, much higher than their British relatives who remained in the north or the Australian Aborigines who are protected by darker skin. Similar trends exist in the United States where southerners have higher rates of all three types of skin cancer than their less-exposed northern relatives.

At the molecular level, sunlight has also left telltale signs of its association with skin cancer. One of several types of mutations that can be induced by UV radiation involves adjacent cytosines on the same strand of DNA and is essentially unique to this mutagen. Specifically, light induces the formation of aberrant chemical bonds between adjacent cytosines. These so-called cyclobutane-pyrimidine dimers are then misread by DNA polymerase, causing them to be paired with adenine instead of guanine. When the next strand is copied, the adenines are paired with thymines instead of the original cytosines resulting in a so-called C-to-T mutation in the original strand of DNA. C-to-T mutations occurring in adjacent pyrimidines are highly suggestive of UV radiation as no other mutagen routinely causes this change. A high percentage of DNA mutations detected in skin cancer involve such signature mutations. Interestingly, the vast majority of these mutations occur in the nontranscribed strand of DNA, as the transcriptional machinery has significant DNA repair capacity and typically corrects mutations in the transcribed strand prior to replication.

INHERITED CANCER SYNDROMES Basal-cell nevus syndrome (BCNS) and xeroderma pigmentosum are examples of familial skin cancer syndromes. Both of these diseases have contributed to our understanding of the etiology of sporadic skin cancers and are covered in detail in separate chapters in this text. In basal-cell nevus syndrome, hundreds or thousands of basal-cell carcinomas (BCCs) develop in sun-exposed areas. In this autosomal dominant disorder, one copy of the human homolog of drosophila *patched*, a tumor-suppressor gene, is mutated, leading to multiple developmental abnormalities in addition to these tumors. The molecular pathway involving this tumor suppressor will be discussed below as it is relevant in sporadic BCCs as well.

In xeroderma pigmentosum, defective DNA repair enzymes allow rapid accumulation of UV-induced mutations. Xeroderma pigmentosum patients suffer from profound sun damage after trivial UV-light exposures and develop all three types of skin cancer within the first decades of life.

IMMUNE SUPPRESSION Through an important but poorly understood mechanism, the immune system plays a significant role in controlling skin cancers. This hypothesis is derived from the observation that organ transplant patients on prolonged immunosuppression with agents such as cyclosporine, prednisone, and azathioprine have markedly increased risks of developing basal- and especially squamous-cell carcinomas. By 20 years after kidney transplantation and beginning immunosuppression, approximately 40% of patients have developed SCCs and/or BCCs as compared with 6% for the age-matched normal population. The rates are even higher following heart transplantation, as these patients require more intensive immunosuppression and undergo transplantation later in life when precancers are presumably more advanced.

In addition to elevated rates of occurrence, SCCs especially tend to be highly aggressive when they develop in the setting of immune compromise, with a much higher rate of metastasis and lack of response to therapy, especially if immunosuppression is continued. Whereas these epidemiologic studies support the concept of tumor surveillance, we do not know the critical mecha-

From: *Principles of Molecular Medicine* (J. L. Jameson, ed.), ©1998 Humana Press Inc., Totowa, NJ.

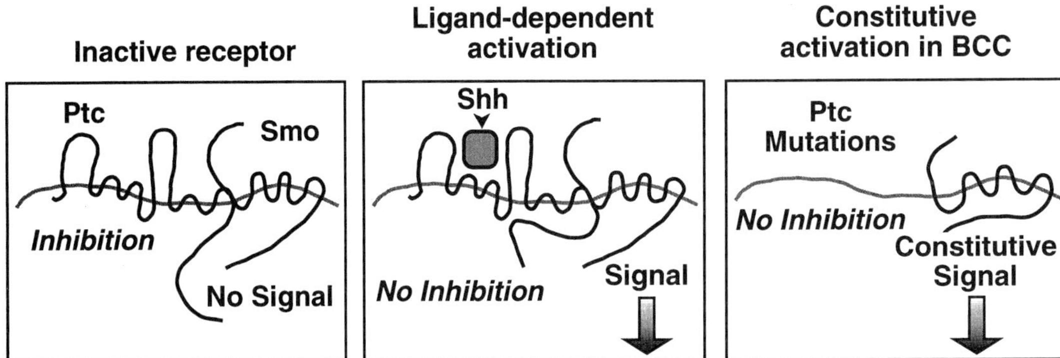

Figure 84-1 Proposed model of *Sonic Hedgehog* (Shh) signaling pathway in vertebrates, relevant in development and BCC. Shh is a diffusible signaling molecule that binds the 12 transmembrane-spanning receptor *patched* (Ptc), which is mutated in both BCNS and in many sporadic BCCs. The binding of Shh to wild-type Ptc causes disinhibition of the pathway, allowing the seven transmembrane-spanning receptor *Smoothened* (Smo) to transmit an intracellular signal affecting cellular differentiation. The critical nature of this pathway in vertebrate development is demonstrated by transgenic mice deficient in either Shh or Smo which have a phenotype of multiple skeletal and neurological defects and die before birth. Mutation or loss of Ptc (and its normal inhibitory action on Smo) causes constitutive signaling by this pathway, and leads to the development of BCCs. (Adapted from Stone DM, et al. Nature 1996;384:133.)

nisms by which the immune system recognizes most nascent skin cancers yet fails to detect others (the ones that progress). Are the products of mutant cancer-associated genes expressed as novel antigens? Does immunosuppression induced by UV light (which is potent enough to block immune-related diseases such as psoriasis for example) play a clinically relevant role in allowing tumor progression? Do tumors actively suppress the immune system by engaging the lymphocyte Fas apoptotic pathway or elaborating diffusible factors? Answers to these questions have biological and potential therapeutic implications.

HUMAN PAPILLOMA VIRUS The E6 protein product of human papilloma virus (HPV) types 16 and 18 has been shown to induce ubiquitin-mediated degradation of the p53 tumor-suppressor protein. This mechanism is believed to be central in the strong association of these particular subtypes of HPV with SCC. Genital warts caused by HPV, the most common sexually transmitted disease, is also relevant in cervical carcinoma (HPV types 6, 11, 16, and 18). SCCs are also associated with some cases of immunocompromised patients with disseminated HPV lesions.

MOLECULAR ETIOLOGY OF NONMELANOMA SKIN CANCER

BASAL-CELL CARCINOMA Two lines of investigation, genetic-disease linkage analysis and drosophila developmental biology, converged in 1996 to shed some light on the molecular basis of BCCs by identifying the affected gene in the BCNS. The developmental role of this gene product is suggested by the constellation of findings in this syndrome: jaw cysts, rib, vertebral, and shoulder abnormalities; characteristic pitting of the palms; and numerous BCCs. The affected gene, *Patched*, is 67% identical between human and fly at the nucleotide level and functions in the hedgehog (drosophila) or sonic hedgehog (vertebrate) signaling pathway. In vertebrates, sonic hedgehog (Shh) is involved in the development of motor, serotonergic, dopaminergic, and forebrain neurons, vertebrae, hindgut mesoderm, and distal limb structures. As depicted in Fig. 84-1, this pathway involves the diffusible signal protein, Shh, as well as *Patched* (Ptc) and *Smoothened* (Smo), both of which are transmembrane receptors. The normal function of Ptc appears to be the inhibition of intracellular signaling by Smo except in the presence of Shh. Loss of signaling in this pathway through the targeted disruption of either the diffusible activator protein, Shh, or the intracellular signaling molecule, Smo, leads to numerous developmental defects and embryonic lethality in transgenic mice. Conversely, loss of Ptc is associated with constitutive signaling through this pathway and the development of BCCs.

In BCNS, patients have lost a single copy of the *Patched* gene, which is encoded on chromosome 9. In a classic pattern analogous to that described for retinoblastoma and other tumor suppressor genes, this leads to a disease that is autosomal dominant at the level of the individual but autosomal recessive at the cellular level. The loss in all cells of the body of one functional copy of the tumor suppressor gene leaves only a single copy as a target of mutagens or possible errors in DNA replication. In a normal individual, a sporadic mutation of a given tumor suppressor in a somatic cell would have a minimal effect as the second copy would remain functional, but in an affected individual, a single sporadic mutation would leave the cell without function of that tumor suppressor, leading to cancer in that cell's progeny.

Although it appears that, in BCNS, loss of *Patched* function underlies development of BCCs, what is the mechanism in the much more common sporadic BCCs? Several early studies suggest that *Patched* is also mutated in a significant number of sporadic BCCs. In these cases, typically one copy is deleted by allelic loss of the 9q22 chromosomal region which encodes *Patched*, whereas the other is the target of an inactivating mutation in its sequence often as a result of a characteristic CC-to-TT mutation from UV light. Studies of *Patched* mutations in sporadic BCCs are difficult because of its large size (4330 bp) and the fact that virtually all tumors characterized thus far have distinct mutations. Recent data suggest that, although many mutations in sporadic BCCs occur in the *Patched* gene, mutation of other target proteins can also induce these tumors. Specifically, mutations have been found in the *Smoothened* gene in several sporadic BCCs as well. Indeed, when an activating mutant version of the *Smoothened* gene was overexpressed in the skin of transgenic mice, they developed BCC-like lesions. This mutation thus activated the *Smoothened* protein to generate its signal even in the absence of *Sonic hedgehog*. The nature of the signal from *Smoothened* has also recently been elucidated. A critical target of *Smoothened* signaling is a zinc finger transcription factor called Gli1. As one would predict for a target of this pathway, overexpression of Shh and loss of *Patched* both cause an upregulation of Gli1. Moreover, Gli1 is upregulated in sporadic BCCs (46 of 47 cases) but not in SCCs (0 of 10 cases). Thus, this pathway can be disrupted at several sites, all of which appear to cause an upregulation of the Gli1 transcription factor, which mediates the effects of *Sonic hedgehog*.

SQUAMOUS-CELL CARCINOMA The 1980s brought exciting progress in understanding the molecular basis of carcinomas arising in a classic model of multistage carcinogenesis in mouse skin. The experimental design involves shaving an area of mouse skin, applying a single dose of an "initiator" chemical such as DMBA (dimethylbenzanthracene), followed by twice-weekly applications of a "promoter" such as TPA (tetradecanoyl-phorbol-acetate). This treatment leads to benign skin tumors called papillomas, a small percentage of which eventually become invasive carcinomas. Elegant experiments led to the discovery that the initiator causes mutations in the *ras* gene most often in the 12th, 13th, or 61st codons. When the normal cellular form of the Harvey *ras* (H-*ras*) gene is mutated in such a manner it loses its ability to act as a GTPase-activating protein (hence becoming unable to turn off G protein-mediated signaling) and is referred to as an activating H-*ras* mutant. Whereas activated H-*ras* is adequate to transform the immortalized mouse NIH-3T3 cell line, it is incapable of transforming primary cell lines. Presumably, H-*ras* is complementing pre-existing mutations in the immortalized 3T3-cell line not present in normal cells. For example, the combination of H-*ras* with an oncogenic version of *fos* is capable of transforming normal epidermal cells. In the mouse multistage paradigm, H-*ras* mutation by an initiator must be followed by weeks of promotion, involving (among other things) repeated activation of protein kinase C, known to alter the differentiation state of cells. Unfortunately, the critical targets of this second stage of mutagenesis, promotion, remain unknown in this model of chemically induced SCCs.

A further limitation in this model system is that the vast majority of human SCCs are induced by UV light rather than chemicals. What is the relevance of *ras* mutations in typical human SCCs arising in sun-exposed areas? *Ras* mutations are present in a minority (13% in one study) of human SCCs, and evidence exists that this mutation favors an increased growth rate and diminished ability of keratinocytes to differentiate, both features that may be relevant at least to the early stages of tumorigenesis. On the other hand, a larger proportion (30%) of benign and self-regressing skin tumors called keratoacanthomas displayed *ras* mutations, arguing that activating *ras* mutations are neither capable of causing a malignant transformation nor adequate in maintaining growth of benign tumors.

More recently, mutations have been discovered in the p53 gene which are likely to be relevant as they are present in a large fraction (between 60 and 90%) of human SCCs and bear the hallmark of UV-induced damage, the C-to T substitution. p53 is a tumor suppressor that functions in at least two important ways: (1) It halts the cell cycle following DNA damage allowing repair to occur prior to DNA synthesis; and (2) it induces programmed cell death in cells in which DNA damage is too extensive for reliable repair. The loss of p53 function would thus favor tumorigenesis as DNA mutations could accumulate in cells much more rapidly. Indeed, at least one copy of p53 may be lost at a surprisingly early stage in the UV induction of cancer as p53 mutations are detectable in more than 70% of "normal" skin samples from sun-exposed sites on patients who had developed skin cancers elsewhere. No p53 mutations were detected in skin from sun-protected sites on control individuals without skin cancer. High rates of p53 mutations were also noted in the common premalignant lesions known as actinic keratoses.

p53 mutant cells typically display nuclear accumulation of p53-immunoreactivity that represents nonfunctional p53 protein. Clones of cells displaying such immunoreactivity were present in sun-exposed skin at 10 times the rate of sun-protected skin. Interestingly, sun-exposed skin was five times more likely to have large clones than was sun-protected skin, arguing that sunlight was acting both to induce the mutations and to promote their subsequent growth.

Whereas p53 mutations are likely to be relevant, there is ample evidence to suggest that they are not sufficient in keratinocyte carcinogenesis. In p53-knockout mice challenged with chemical carcinogens, both initiation and promotion steps were required, although carcinomas did develop more rapidly than in wild-type mice. Importantly, mutant *ras*, even in the setting of homozygous p53 loss, was not adequate to induce carcinoma in this model, which required promotion with TPA, an activator of protein kinase C. The relevant targets of TPA in this system remain unknown. Similar arguments about the insufficiency of p53 mutations in the induction of SCCs are derived from humans with Li-Fraumeni syndrome, in which one copy of p53 is lost in the germline. Patients with Li-Fraumeni syndrome suffer from extremely high rates of leukemia, breast carcinoma, and soft-tissue sarcoma, yet not of sun-induced skin cancers.

SUMMARY

A series of molecular events is required to generate a true cutaneous carcinoma and, within the past few years, some of the critical steps have been identified. In the case of basal-cell carcinomas, the discovery of *Patched* is a development that will further our understanding of these most common cancers. Major questions include: Is *Patched* necessary for the development of BCCs or do other molecular pathways exist for generating these cancers? Is its homozygous loss in a cell sufficient for malignant transformation? What is the nature of the signal generated in the Sonic hedgehog pathway by Smoothened? Can it be pharmacologically inhibited in order to revert tumor cells to their normal phenotype?

The puzzling observation that sunlight exposure in youth participates in carcinogenesis decades later may be partially explained by the following: (1) p53 mutations are detectable very early on in life following UV exposure and even when present on only one chromosome seem to lead to a modest growth advantage likely as a result of decreased apoptosis of these cells following UV. (2) Homozygous p53 mutations and, to a lesser degree, certain heterozygous mutations favor the accumulation of genetic mutations because of loss of function of this critical guardian-of-the-genome protein. (3) Estimates as to the number *(n)* of genetic mutations required for malignant transformation to carcinoma vary from 2 to 7, whereas the probability that a given cell has acquired mutations in all *n* genes needed to generate a cancer increases as the *n*th power of age. Taken together, these observations argue that youthful UV exposure may damage cells, allowing subsequent UV exposure to more effectively accumulate the mutations required to generate a cancer.

For squamous-cell carcinoma, although p53 and activated H-*ras* appear relevant, ample evidence suggests that more steps are required for complete malignant transformation, as mutant H-*ras*, even in the setting of doubly p53-negative keratinocytes is inadequate for carcinogenesis. In squamous-cell carcinoma, a series of genetic hits, the accumulation of which is favored by the loss of p53 function, is likely to be the route to malignancy. It would appear that some of these critical hits by sunlight are directed against target proteins that have not yet been identified.

SELECTED REFERENCES

Alcedo J, Ayzenzon M, Von Ohlen T, Noll M, Hooper JE. The *Drosophila smoothened* gene encodes a seven-pass membrane protein, a putative receptor for the hedgehog signal. Cell 1996;86:221–232.

Chen Y, Struhl G. Dual roles for *patched* in sequestering and transducing Hedgehog. Cell 1996;87:553–563.

Corominas M, Kamino H, Leon J, Pellicer A. Oncogene activation in human benign tumor of the skin (keratoacanthomas): is *HRAS* involved in differentiation as well as proliferation? Proc Natl Acad Sci USA 1990;86:6372–6376.

Dahmane N, Lee J, Robins P, Heller P, Ruiz i Altaba A. Activation of the transcription factor Gli1 and the Sonic hedgehog signalling pathway in skin tumors. Nature 1997;389:876–881.

Fan H, Oro AE, Scott MP, Khavari PA. Induction of basal cell carcinoma features in transgenic human skin expressing Sonic Hedgehog. Nat Med 1997;3:788–792.

Hahn H, Wicking C, Zaphiropolous PG, et al. Mutations of the human homolog of drosophila *patched* in the nevoid basal cell carcinoma syndrome. Cell 1996;85:841–851.

Jonasen AS, Kunala S, Price GJ, et al. Frequent clones of p53-mutated keratinocytes in normal human skin. Proc Natl Acad Sci USA 1996;93:14,025–14,029.

Leffell DJ, Brash DE. Sunlight and skin cancer. Sci Am 1996;275: 52–59.

Stone DM, Hynes M, Armanini M, et al. The tumor-suppressor gene *patched* encodes a candidate receptor for Sonic hedgehog. Nature 1996;384:129–134.

Unden AB, Zaphiropoulos PG, Bruce K, Toftgard R, Stahle-Backdahl M. Human *patched* (PTCH) mRNA is overexpressed consistently in tumor cells of both familial and sporadic basal cell carcinoma. Cancer Res 1997;57:2336–2340.

van den Heuvel, Ingham PW. *smoothened* encodes a receptor-like serpentine protein required for hedgehog signalling. Nature 1996;382: 547–551.

Xie J, Murone M, Luoh S, Ryan A, Gu Q, Zhang C, Bonifas J, Lam C, Hynes M, Goddard A, Rosenthal A, Epstein E, de Sauvage F. Activating *Smoothened* mutations in sporadic basal-cell carcinoma. Nature 1998;391:90–92.

85 Melanoma Genetics

Daniel B. Dubin and Saumyen Sarkar

INTRODUCTION

Cancer is currently being viewed as the cellular accumulation of activated oncogenes and inactivated tumor suppressor genes (*see* Chapter 7). Detailed studies on the genetics of adenocarcinoma of the colon have provided the empirical framework for the stepwise genetic progression of benign proliferations to frank malignancy. Similar to adenocarcinoma of the colon, melanoma has a putative precursor lesion, the dysplastic nevus, and may arise sporadically or in clusters within predisposed families.

Recently, germline mutations have been identified in several hereditary cancer syndromes, including Gardner's syndrome (APC), familial breast and ovarian cancer (BRCA1/2), and basal-cell nevus syndrome (BCNS) (PATCHED). Mutations in these cancer-predisposing genes are intriguing as they have been found in both sporadic and inherited malignancies. Identification of these genes has already resulted in the commercialization of a genetic-screening test (BRCA1/2) for familial breast and ovarian cancer. The discovery of veritable "melanoma-susceptibility genes" would facilitate the development of not only screening and diagnostic tests, but also gene-reconstitution treatment strategies.

The increasing incidence of melanoma and the dismal prognosis for advanced-stage disease have spurred investigation for genetic alterations responsible for sporadic and inherited forms of melanoma. Linkage analysis in melanoma-prone kindreds and karyotyping of melanomas and their derived cell lines have implicated nonrandom abnormalities of chromosomes 1, 6, 7, 9, and 10 in the pathogenesis of melanoma. Several candidate melanoma-predisposing genes and loci have been reported; however, controversy regarding the identity of veritable "melanoma-susceptibility genes" abounds.

CHROMOSOME 1

Investigators have identified alterations of chromosome 1 in primary melanomas and melanoma cell lines. The majority of these mutations have represented deletions or translocations involving 1p22–36. However, one group has reported t (1:19) translocations involving 1q in 3 cases of advanced stage melanoma. Another study identified 4/30 melanoma cell lines with transforming *N-ras* mutations that map to 1p22; however, given their relative infrequency, there is concern that such *N-ras* mutations may represent an epiphenomenon of transformation. The beta chain of NGF maps to the 1p22 region, but no alterations in this gene have been found in melanoma.

Using restriction-fragment-length polymorphism analysis, one group demonstrated loss of heterozygosity (LOH) for 1p in 15/35 melanomas and 11/21 melanoma cell lines, thus suggesting the residence of a melanoma suppressor gene in this region. Certain genetic studies have linked alterations in the 1p32-36 region, which contains the Rh gene, to melanoma and the dysplastic nevus syndrome in distinct families; however, this association has been questioned by other studies.

CHROMOSOME 6

Deletions in the 6q1 2–27 region are the most common chromosome 6 alterations that have been found in melanoma. Although the proto-oncogenes c-*ros* and c-*myb* have been mapped to the long arm of chromosome 6, mutations of these genes in melanoma are not common. Reported LOH of the 6q22–23 and 6q24–27 regions in melanoma implies that melanoma suppressor gene(s) may reside in these loci. Microcell melanoma cell hybrids into which a normal chromosome 6 has been introduced lose their capacity to form tumors in nude mice. The loss of the normal chromosome 6 from these melanoma-cell hybrids results in a restoration of their tumorigenicity in nude mice.

CHROMOSOME 7

Duplication of all or part of chromosome 7 has been reported in 36/58 advanced stage melanomas in a recent study. Similar duplications of chromosome 7 have been found in glioblastoma cell lines in which overexpression of c-*erbB*, a component of the epidermal growth factor receptor (EGF) occurs. The notion that overexpression of c-*erbB* could contribute to tumorigenesis in melanoma is intriguing but not proven.

CHROMOSOME 9

By genetic-linkage analysis, a locus responsible for melanoma predisposition has been mapped to a 2-cM interval in the chromosomal region 9p21. This locus could function to act as a somatically recessive tumor suppressor gene in the manner proposed by Knudson. Consistent with this notion, the 9p21 locus is the site of frequent somatic chromosomal deletions and/or translocations in melanoma tumor cells and cell lines. Linkage data and mutational analysis have suggested that the cyclin-dependent kinase inhibitors (CDKI), p16 and p15, both of which map to the 9p21–22 region, represent the mts-1 and mts-2 genes, respectively. In fact, p16 and/or p15 deletions and/or mutations

From: *Principles of Molecular Medicine* (J. L. Jameson, ed.), ©1998 Humana Press Inc., Totowa, NJ.

have been detected in tumors such as pancreatic adenocarcinoma, esophageal adenocarcinoma, non–small-cell lung carcinoma, leukemia, lymphomas, osteosarcomas, bladder carcinomas, glioblastoma, and mesothelioma.

Mechanistically, the CDKIs p15, p16, and possibly p18, the protein product generated from the alternative reading frames of the INK4a gene, represent attractive tumor-suppressor gene candidates (*see* Chapter 6). The CDKIs act to reinforce the START checkpoint that regulates G1 to S phase transition. By inhibiting cyclin-dependent kinases (CDKs), CDKIs prevent phosphorylation of Rb. Therefore, Rb continues to bind tightly and inactivate the transcription factor E2F, which is essential for driving the G1 to S phase transition. Both p15 and p16, when transfected into transformed mammalian-cell lines can diminish their proliferative capacity. Furthermore, p15 is upregulated by TGF-β, a cytokine which inhibits cellular proliferation in vivo. Therefore, it is an attractive hypothesis to consider that loss of p15 results in a loss of TGF-β–maintained restraint of proliferation.

Since p15, p16 deletions/mutations are more common in either tumor-derived cell lines or tumor explants than in the primary tumors, there is concern that loss of p15/p16 function may represent an epiphenomenon of transformation. In fact, a recent report that cites in vitro upregulation of p16 as a key event in the terminal stage of growth arrest in senescence could explain why p16 but not p15 is commonly inactivated in established melanoma cell lines. However, the detection of p15/p16 mutations in some primary tumors has preserved hope that these genes do represent mts-1 and mts-2.

Although p16 gene mutations in melanoma cell lines are well documented, linkage studies in kindreds with familial melanoma syndrome linked to 9p21–22 have been inconclusive. One study identified six relevant mutations of p16 in 9/18 kindreds. A second study found a single common p16 mutation in 13/15 families. Recently, germline mutations of p16, one of which has been independently tightly linked to two Australian melanoma pedigrees, have been reposted in 5/33 (18%) of patients with a family history of melanoma. On the other hand, in an analysis of 38 melanoma-prone families, 13 of which segregate 9p linkage, only two relevant mutations of p16 were detected. Furthermore, p16/19 knockout mice demonstrated a greater than expected spontaneous development of lymphomas and sarcomas. The knockout data and the mixed-linkage studies raise doubt as to whether or not p16 represents the authentic MLM gene.

Could p15 be MLM? Kamb et al. did not find relevant p15 (mts-2) mutations or deletions in their analysis of melanoma-cell lines and germline DNA derived from melanoma prone kindreds. However, we (SS) have found homozygous p15 deletions of exon 2 in 6/10 human melanoma cell lines; by contrast, no homozygous p16 deletions of exon 2 were detected in these same cell lines. Two of the cell lines in which p15 deletions were detected were primary tumor-cell cultures. In cell lines without homozygous deletion of p15, several mutations of both p15 and p16 were noted. The final word on p15's role in melanoma is pending further study.

CHROMOSOME 10

Translocations and deletions of chromosome 10 have been described in a dysplastic nevus, early-stage melanoma, and late-stage melanomas. No specific genes on chromosome 10 have been implicated. One group found both chromosome 10 deletion and chromosome 7 duplication in 10/58 of advanced-stage melanomas. This association may actually be greater since LOH of regions of chromosome 10 may occur without gross cytogenetic loss. Nowell has hypothesized that chromosome 10 may contain a trans-acting suppressor of c-*erbB*. In theory, the combination of loss of expression of the erbB suppressor and gain of an extra copy of c-*erbB* would provide a proliferative advantage.

OTHER RELEVANT GENES

Two studies have found *ras* mutations in 5–25% of melanoma tumors. However, Gerhard et al. analyzed 58 patients with sporadic melanoma and concluded that the distribution of *ras* mutations did not differ from that in a normal population.

Recently, a specific germline cyclin-dependent kinase 4 (CDK4) mutation that renders it resistant to CDKI inhibition has been detected in two melanoma pedigrees with an inheritance not linked to a locus on 9p21. This CDK4 mutation may subvert the delicate START checkpoint that is maintained in part by CDKIs such as p16 and p15 and, thus, confer a proliferative advantage to cells with such a mutation.

Several lines of evidence have implicated p53 and Rb mutations, two guardians of the START checkpoint, as pathogenic in the development of melanoma. In one study, mutations of p53 were found in 85% of primary and metastatic melanoma. Additionally, patients with Li-Fraumeni syndrome (-/p53) as well as up to 7% of survivors of hereditary retinoblastoma (-/Rb) have been reported to develop melanoma. Further evidence that p53 and Rb alterations may be important in the pathogenesis of melanoma can be gleaned from a transgenic mouse line whose melanocytes express large T antigen, a putative inactivator of p53 and Rb function. These transgenic mice develop ocular and cutaneous melanomas.

CONCLUSIONS

The literature is flush with circumstantial evidence implicating alterations of various genes and chromosomal regions in the pathogenesis of melanoma. Given the lessons of colon adenocarcinoma progression, manifestation of the melanoma phenotype likely requires the accumulation of several genetic hits, but not necessarily in any particular order. Furthermore, the array of genetic alterations necessary and sufficient for melanoma development in any one tumor may represent only a small subset of the genetic mutations that could potentially combine to cause melanoma. Cytogenetics and molecular analysis have defined several chromosomal regions in which putative melanoma suppressor genes may lie. However, the identification of true "melanoma susceptibility genes" will likely require further linkage analysis in melanoma-prone kindreds, functional studies, and more detailed sequencing of candidate chromosomal regions.

SELECTED REFERENCES

Cannon-Albright L, Goldgar D, Meyer L. Assignment of a locus for familial melanoma, MLM to chromosome 9p13-p22. Science 1992; 258:1148–1152.

Cannon-Albright LA, Kamb A, Skolnick M. A review of inherited predisposition to melanoma. Semin Oncol 1996;23:667–672.

Dracopoli N, Harnett S, Bale B, et al. Loss of alleles from the distal short arm of chromosome 1 occurs late in melanoma tumor progression. Proc Natl Acad Sci USA 1989;86:4614–4618.

Fitzgerald M, Harkin D, Silva-Arrieta S. Prevalance of germ-line mutations in p16, p19 ARF and CDK4 in familial melanoma: analysis of a clinic base population. Proc Natl Acad Sci USA 1996;93:8541–8545.

Greene MH. Genetics of cutaneous melanoma and nevi. Mayo Clin Proc 1997;72:467–474.

Hannon G, Beach D. p15 INK4B is a potential effector of TGF-β-induced cell cycle arrest. Nature 1994;371:257–261.

Hunter T, Pines J. Cyclins and cancer II: cyclin D and CDK inhibitors come of age. Cell 1994;79:573–582.

Hussussian C, Strvewing J, Goldstein A. Germline p16 mutations in familial melanoma. Nat Genet 1994;8:15–21.

Kamb A, Liu Q, Hhapshaman K, et al. Rates of p16 (MTS1) mutations in primary tumors with 9p21 loss. Science 1994;265:416,417.

Kamb A, Shattuck-Eidens D, Eeles R. Analysis of the p16 gene (CDKN2) as a candidate for the chromosome 9p melanoma susceptibility locus. Nat Genet 1994;8:22–26.

Mintz B, Silvers W. Transgenic mouse model of malignant skin melanoma. Proc Natl Acad Sci USA 1993;90:8817–8821.

Parmiter A, Nowell P. Cytogenetics of melanocytic tumors. J Invest Dermatol 1993;100:2545–2585.

Sarkar S, Kupper T. The putative 9p21 tumor suppressor gene for sporadic malignant melanoma: p15INK4b may be more important than p16INK4a (Abstract). J Invest Dermatol 1995;104:568.

Serrano M, Hannon G, Beach D. A new regulatory motif in cell-cycle control causing specific inhibition of cyclin D/CDK4. Nature 1993;366:704–707.

Wolfel T, Hauer M, Schneider J, et al. A $p16^{INK4a}$-insensitive CDK4 mutant targeted by cytolytic T lymphocytes in a human melanoma. 1995;269:1281–1284.

Zuo L, Weger J, Yang B, et al. Germlinc mutations in the $p16^{INK4a}$ binding domain of CDK4 in familial melanoma. Nat Genet 1996;12:97–99.

86 Psoriasis

JAMES T. ELDER AND JOHN J. VOORHEES

BACKGROUND

HISTORICAL PERSPECTIVES Psoriasis was first clearly described by Celsus (25 BC–45 AD), and conditions resembling psoriasis are present in the works of Hippocrates. In 1809 Robert Willan was the first to accurately describe the various forms of psoriasis, which were finally recognized as one entity and distinguished from leprosy by von Hebra in 1841. The association of psoriasis with a distinctive form of arthritis was first recognized by Alibert in 1818. Careful histopathologic studies of psoriasis were first carried out by Auspitz, Unna, and Munro in the late 1800s.

DISEASE DEFINITION Psoriasis is a chronic, inflammatory, hyperproliferative disease of the skin, scalp, nails, and joints, affecting 1–2% of the United States population at an estimated annual cost of $1.6 billion in 1985. Psoriasis is found worldwide, although its frequency varies widely among different ethnic groups. It has a variety of clinical presentations, most of which eventuate into erythematous, scaly plaques with or without nail disease, and arthritis. Susceptibility to psoriasis is unmistakably heritable, but environmental factors, notably trauma, stress, and infections, are also important determinants of disease onset and severity. At the cellular level, psoriasis is characterized by: (1) markedly increased epidermal proliferation and incomplete differentiation; (2) elongation, dilatation, and "leakiness" of the superficial plexus of dermal capillaries; and (3) a mixed inflammatory and immune-cell infiltrate of the epidermis and papillary dermis. A multitude of plausible pathomechanisms can be envisaged for psoriasis. However, true molecular insight into the cause of psoriasis is lacking. As stated by Lomholt over 30 years ago:

> *Question upon question may be asked—the disease is capricious and refuses to part with its innermost secret.*

SCOPE In this chapter, we will review what has been accomplished to solve the long-standing riddle of psoriasis, particularly in the areas of immunology and genetics. In addition, we will attempt to summarize its protean clinical manifestations, and review its diagnosis, differential diagnosis, and management.

CLINICAL FEATURES

SKIN Several types of psoriatic skin lesions are recognized, including chronic plaque, guttate, pustular, inverse, palmoplantar, and generalized (Fig. 86-1). Of these, chronic plaque lesions are by far the most common, and over time, most other forms eventuate into chronic plaque disease. The typical chronic plaque is a well-demarcated, erythematous lesion with loose, silvery scales that can vary from a few millimeters to many centimeters in diameter. The scale can be lifted off the surface of lesions, revealing a shiny base and microscopic points of bleeding (Auspitz sign). Lesions are typically located over the extensor surfaces of the extremities, and often display striking symmetry. Other areas of predilection include the scalp, umbilicus, intergluteal cleft, and genitalia. Plaques may assume a variety of shapes, described as annular, circinate, gyrate, and serpiginous. Scalp lesions can be particularly thick and refractory to therapy, and often show a sharp cutoff at the hairline. With the exception of childhood cases, the face is usually spared. Eruptive, or guttate psoriasis (Latin *gutta*, "drop") appears rapidly as tens to hundreds of 5- to 10-mm papules on the trunk and proximal extremities, usually in young patients following a streptococcal or other upper respiratory-tract infection. Generalized pustular psoriasis presents as waves of sterile pustules 2–3 mm in diameter that appear on erythematous skin, usually accompanied by fever. This is the form of psoriasis most likely to evolve into erythroderma, defined as total-body skin involvement. Inverse psoriasis presents as red plaques with moist scaling, typically located in the inframammary or inguinal folds, umbilicus, intergluteal cleft, axillae, or under the prepuce. Sebopsoriasis lesions feature a more yellowish, greasy scale in the scalp, facial, presternal, and upper back—a distribution reminiscent of seborrheic dermatitis. Localized pustular psoriasis of the palms and soles and geographic tounge are unusual forms, probably distinct from psoriasis.

NAILS Psoriasis produces three distinctive nail changes, at least one of which can be found in approximately 50% of psoriasis patients (Fig. 86-2). These include pitting, onychodystrophy, (destruction of the nail plate), and "oil drop" spotting. Pits are typically well-demarcated, randomly distributed, 1- to 2-mm depressions in the surface of the nail plate, produced by defective terminal differentiation of keratinocytes in the nail matrix. Onychodystrophic changes arise from disease of the nail bed and range from separation of the nail plate (onycholysis) to thick, yellowish, crumbly nails, to complete loss of the nail, especially in pustular cases. Oil-drop spots are orangish-to-brown discolorations underneath the nail, resulting from the leakage of serum proteins through the nail-bed capillaries.

JOINTS Essentially the only systemic manifestation of psoriasis, psoriatic arthritis typically presents between the ages of 35 and 45, usually but not always after onset of skin disease (Fig. 86-3).

From: *Principles of Molecular Medicine* (J. L. Jameson, ed.), ©1998 Humana Press Inc., Totowa, NJ.

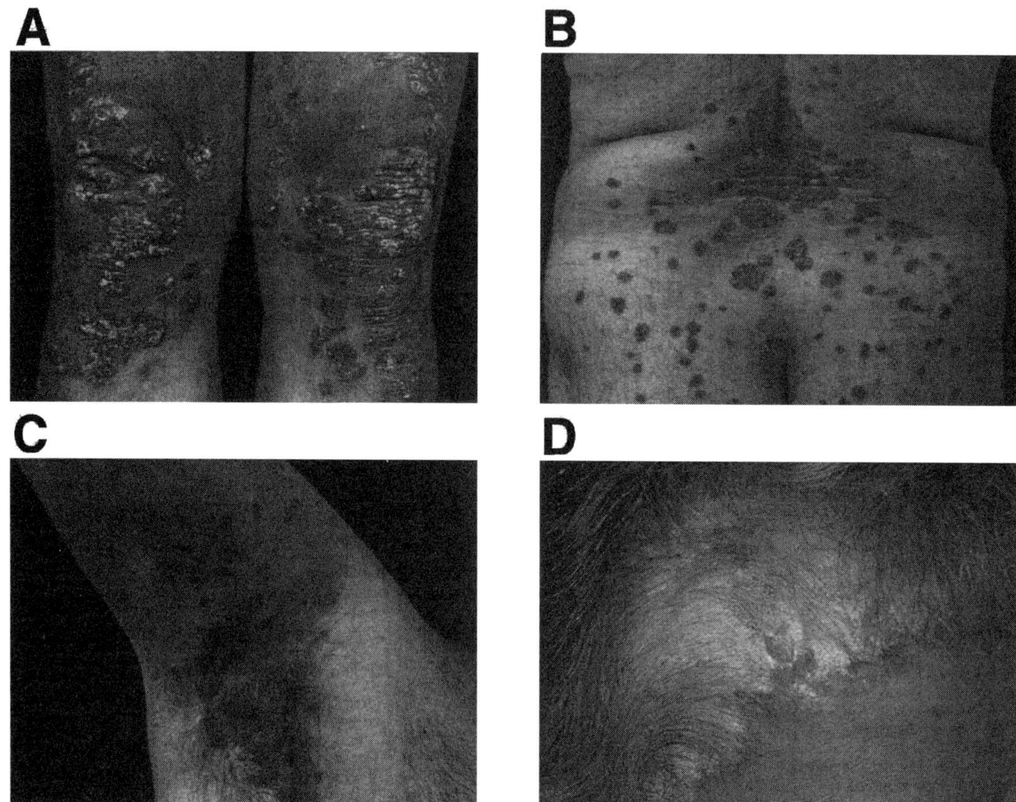

Figure 86-1 Morphology of psoriasis skin lesions. **(A)** Chronic plaque lesions of the knees. Note silvery scale that reveals a shiny base when removed. **(B)** Guttate and chronic plaque lesions of the lower back. **(C)** Inverse (intertriginous) psoriasis of the axilla. **(D)** Scalp psoriasis. Note thick, adherent scale and relatively sharp cutoff at the hairline. (Photos courtesy of Harrold Carter and James Rasmussen.)

The incidence of arthritis in psoriatics is unclear, but is at least three times that of the general population. Disease is oligoarticular and asymmetrical in over 80% of patients, and is most severe in the small joints of the hands and feet and the large joints of the legs. Involvement of the distal interphalangeal joints distinguishes psoriatic from rheumatoid arthritis, which tends to be more proximal and symmetrical. Fortunately, only approximately 5–8% of psoriatic arthritis patients develop highly severe, deforming joint disease (arthritis mutilans). Enthesopathy is the result of mononuclear cell accumulation at tendon or ligament insertions, and can progress to involve the entire digit (dactylitis, "sausage digit").

COURSE The natural history of psoriasis is highly unpredictable. Onset is usually in childhood to the early 20s, with a median age of 15–20 years and over 75% of cases presenting by the age of 40 *(see below)*. Typically, lesions wax and wane, and may reappear in the same or in different locations. Approximately 25% of patients experience a complete remission at some point in their lives, which may last from 1 to 50 years. The Köebner phenomenon, also known as the isomorphic response, refers to the tendency of psoriasis to arise at sites of cutaneous injury. The phenomenon is reported by 25% of patients, requires epidermal and possibly high dermal injury, and is usually seen in the setting of flaring rather than stable or regressing disease.

DIAGNOSIS

CLINICAL EVALUATION Based on the foregoing clinical features, the diagnosis of psoriasis is generally straightforward. The Auspitz sign is well-known but is neither sensitive nor specific for psoriasis. Fungal infection, seborrheic dermatitis, chronic eczema, candidiasis, cutaneous T-cell lymphoma, drug eruptions, syphilis, pityriasis rosea, lichen planus, and lupus erythematosus can present an occasional diagnostic challenge. Skin biopsy can be very useful in these cases.

HISTOPATHOLOGY The histopathologic features of psoriasis are variable yet distinctive (Fig. 86-4). These include: (1) epidermal edema and hyperplasia; (2) loss of the granular layer with retention of keratinocyte nuclei (parakeratosis) with or without collections of neutrophils in the stratum corneum; (3) dilatation and tortuosity of the superficial dermal capillaries; and (4) a moderate mononuclear cell infiltrate of the epidermis and dermis *(see below)*.

LABORATORY Several serologic, hematologic, and metabolic abnormalities may be present. However, they have no value as diagnostic tests because of lack of sensitivity and specificity. Whereas antistreptolysin O titers suggestive of recent infection are found in 30–40% of psoriasis patients, specific *Streptococci* can often be recovered from intertriginous sites, and *Staphylococcus aureus* colonization is increased in frequency, the diagnostic value of cultures and examination of skin scrapings is limited to ruling in other entities, rather than ruling out psoriasis. Mild anemia with folate and iron deficiency is common, and negative nitrogen balance is occasionally seen, because of loss of these nutrients in scale. Acute-phase reactants including C-reactive protein and α-2 macroglobulin correlate with elevated erythrocyte-sedimentation rate and disease severity. Serum uric acid levels are also increased in about one third of patients, although frank gout is rare. Psoriasis displays very strong HLA associations that correlate with age of onset and disease severity *(see below)*; however, HLA typing is only a research tool at this time.

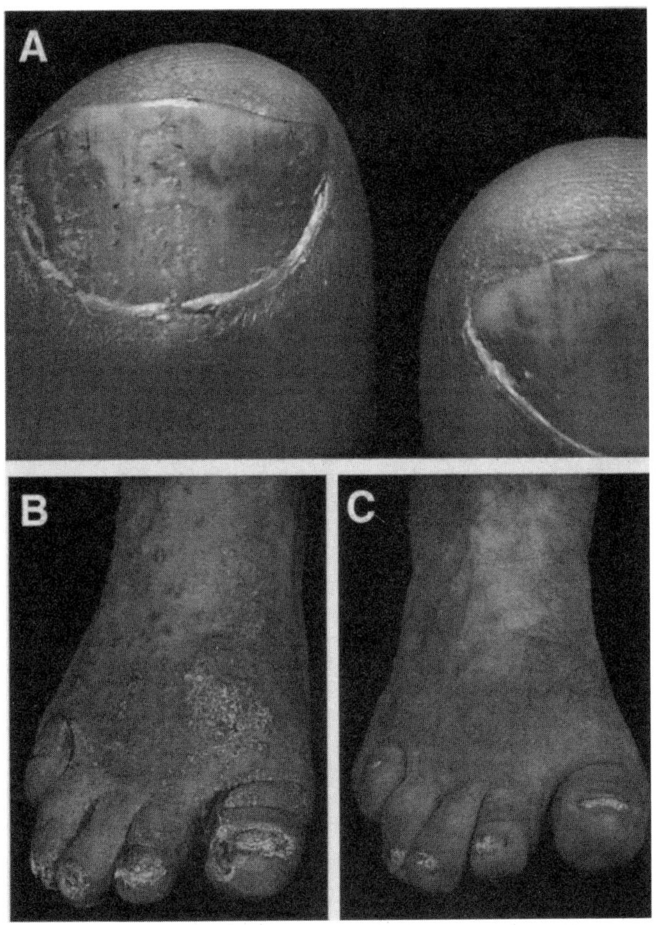

Figure 86-2 Psoriasis of the nails. **(A)** Fingernail involvement. Note presence of pits, onycholysis, and oil-drop spotting. **(B,C)** Toenail involvement, before (B) and after (C) 4 months of CsA therapy. (B) Note thickening and yellowish discoloration as well as periungual involvement. (C) Note that nail and skin involvement improve markedly after CsA treatment. (Photos courtesy of Harrold Carter and James Rasmussen.)

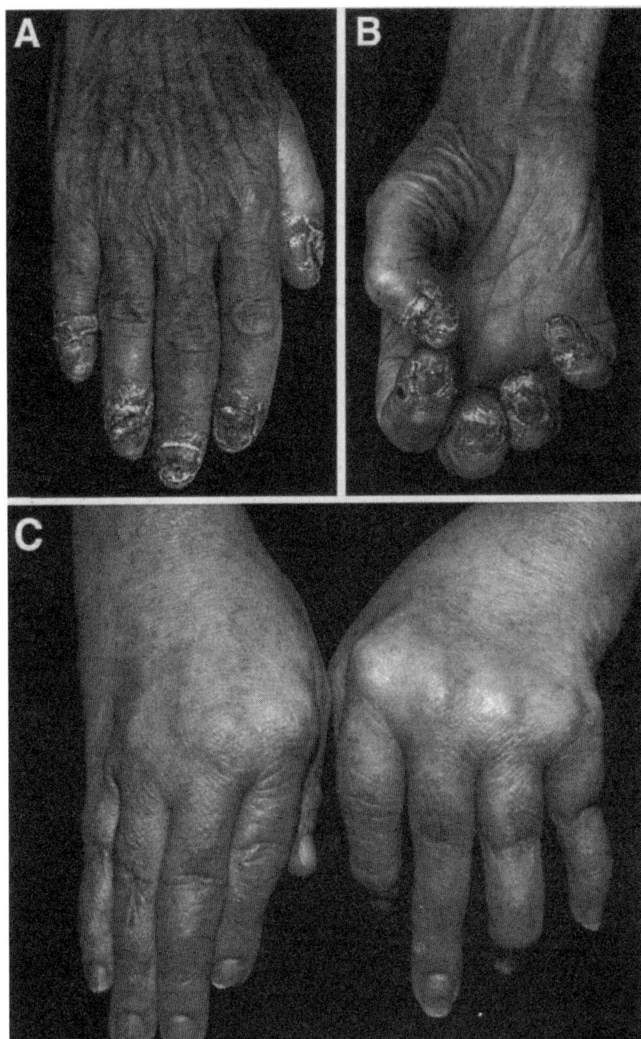

Figure 86-3 Psoriatic arthritis. **(A)** Note fusiform swelling of the middle digit (enthesopathy), accentuation of DIP involvement in association with severe nail disease. **(B)** Same patient as (A); note limited range of motion. **(C)** Arthritis mutilans. Note progressively more severe distal involvement. (Photos courtesy of Harrold Carter and James Rasmussen.)

GENETIC BASIS OF DISEASE

GENETIC EPIDEMIOLOGY Although the inheritance patterns found in certain psoriasis kindreds seem to suggest autosomal-dominant inheritance with reduced penetrance (Fig. 86-5), the weight of evidence from population-based studies indicates that susceptibility to psoriasis is determined by multiple genes as well as environmental stimuli (multifactorial inheritance). Two parameters are often used for estimating the genetic component of multifactorial diseases: heritability (h^2), that portion of the variability in the manifestation of psoriasis ascribable to genetic factors; and risk ratio (λ_R), the risk of psoriasis in relatives of degree R relative to the general population. Psoriasis displays one of the highest h^2 values known in the multifactorial diseases (0.8–0.9). Although identical-twin concordance rates were much lower in Australia than in Scandinavia, h^2 (which depends on the ratio of concordance rates in identical vs fraternal twins) was very similar in both locations. Given the therapeutic effects of ultraviolet (UV) light *(see below)*, it is possible that sun exposure may be an important environmental factor in psoriasis. At present, it is not clear how many genes are involved in psoriasis; however, the parameter λ_R can be used to infer that the number must be greater than 1. λ_R is also a useful measure of the practicability of identifying genes in multifactorial diseases. For specific genes to be identifiable by genetic-linkage methods, λ_R for siblings (termed λ_S) should exceed a value of 3. In psoriasis, estimates of λ_S vary from 4 to 10.

JUVENILE-ONSET PSORIASIS Two types of psoriasis have been distinguished, largely on the basis of age of onset. The onset of psoriasis peaks between 15 and 25 years, with onset before the age of 40 in 75–90% of patients. A second, much smaller, peak is detectable at 65–70 years of age. Psoriatics who are under 40 years old at onset are much more likely to have affected first degree relatives (Fig. 86-6A), to express known HLA susceptibility alleles, and to experience severe and recurrent disease. As adult-onset psoriatics display a different HLA profile, this population may actually have a different disease, more closely related to the spondyloarthropathies.

HLA ASSOCIATIONS AND THE EFFECT OF LINKAGE DISEQUILIBRIUM There can be no doubt that one or more genes in the HLA locus strongly influence psoriasis susceptibility.

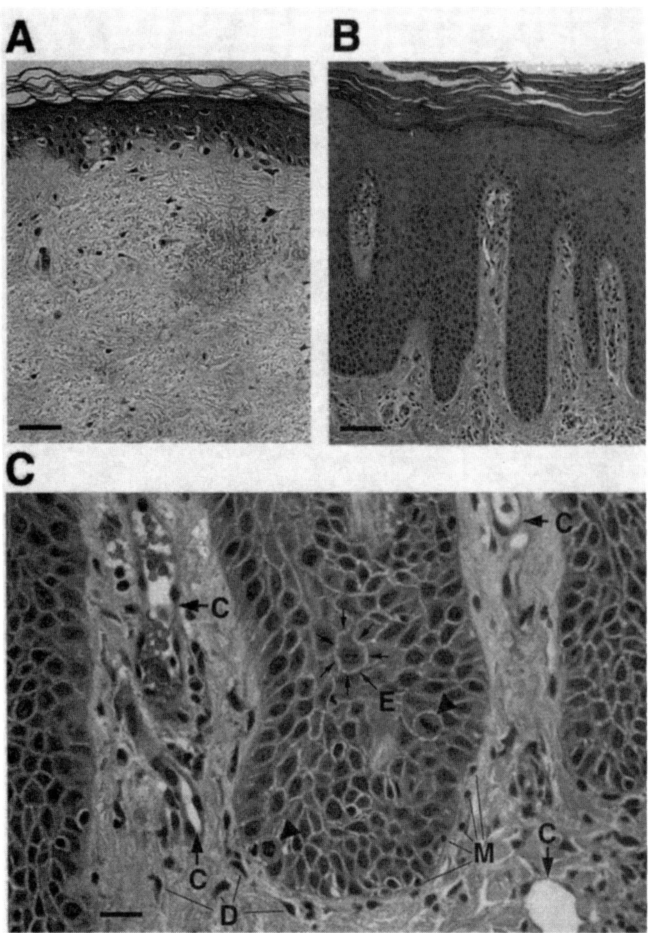

Figure 86-4 Histopathology of psoriasis. **(A)** Normal skin (scale bar = 60 μ). **(B)** Chronic plaque psoriasis (scale bar = 150 μ). Compared to normal skin, note striking regularity of epidermal downgrowth (acanthosis), loss of the granular layer, and retention of nuclei in the stratum corneum (parakeratosis). **(C)** Psoriasis lesion, high-power view (scale bar = 30 μ). Note prominent capillary dilatation (C), dermal dendritic cells, identifiable by their plump nuclei (D), mononuclear cell infiltrate in the dermo-epidermal junctional zone (M), widening of the extracellular spaces (E), and mitotic keratinocytes (arrowheads). (Photomicrographs courtesy of Harrold Carter, James Varani, and John Headington.)

HLA-B13, -B17, -B39, -B57, -Cw6, and -Cw7 (Class I), as well as HLA-DR4 and -DR7 (Class II), all show highly significant positive associations, especially in juvenile-onset disease (Fig. 86-6B). Whereas HLA-Cw6 has consistently produced the strongest associations with psoriasis worldwide, the frequencies of Cw6 and DR7 are approximately the same in psoriatic patients. The tendency of Cw6 and DR7 to be found together is not confined to psoriatics, but is also observed in the general population (allelic association). Population and family studies have revealed the basis of this allelic association: Cw6 and DR7 are linked together on the same chromosome much more often than would be predicted by chance in both affected and unaffected individuals (linkage disequilibrium).

Linkage disequilibrium in HLA is not confined to Cw6 and DR7, but involves multiple alleles at *HLA-A*, *-B*, and *-C* in the Class I region, several loci in the Class III region, and *HLA-DRA*, *-DRB*, *-DQA*, and *-DQB* in the Class II region (Fig. 86-7). (Curiously, disequilibrium does not appear to extend to *HLA-DP*.) Through the use of family studies, these allele combinations can be shown to be caused by cosegregation on the same haploid chromosome, and are therefore referred to as haplotypes. Certain haplotypes are particularly prevalent in one or more world populations, and appear to be of ancient origin. It is estimated that all HLA haplotypes found worldwide today represent one of approximately 50 of these so-called ancestral haplotypes or their recombinants.

The ancestral HLA haplotype 57.1, which carries HLA-B57 in addition to HLA-Cw6 and -DR7, is 15 times more common in German psoriatics than in the German population. However, this haplotype is neither necessary nor sufficient for disease, as only about 35% of German psoriatics carry 57.1, and only 20–25% of the German 57.1^+ population develops psoriasis. Studies of those rare individuals carrying only the Class I or Class II "ends" of this haplotype strongly suggest that the major susceptibility determinant resides on its Class I end, in the vicinity of *HLA-C*. However, several lines of evidence indicate the susceptibility determinant is not HLA-Cw6 itself, but rather an allele at one of at least 10 other genes in the centromeric HLA Class I region. At this writing, the HLA-linked susceptibility gene remains to be identified.

NON-HLA GENES Several laboratories are conducting genome-wide searches for psoriasis susceptibility genes, using both recombination-based and affected sibling pair (ASP) methods of linkage analysis (*see* Chapter 4 for a discussion of genetic analysis methods). In insulin-dependent diabetes mellitus, at least six such non-HLA loci have been confirmed using these methods (*see* Chapter 57). Two large-scale genome-wide scans for psoriasis susceptibility loci have recently been published (Trembath et al., 1997; Nair et al., 1997). Both of these studies confirmed HLA involvement and identified a candidate region on the short arm of chromosome 20. One study (Nair et al.) confirmed an earlier report of a non-HLA locus on the distal long arm of chromosome 17 (Tomfohrde et al., 1994), and identified a region of linkage on the long arm of chromosome 16. Interestingly, this region coincides with a confirmed region of linkage to Crohn's disease. Psoriasis is seven times more common in Crohn's disease patients than in the general population. It is attractive to speculate that a proinflammatory genetic mutation or polymorphism common to both diseases may reside in this chromosomal region.

MOLECULAR PATHOPHYSIOLOGY OF DISEASE

EVOLUTION OF LESIONS Early lesions of psoriasis display mast-cell degranulation, capillary dilatation, papillary dermal edema, and the appearance of a mononuclear infiltrate. However, the exact sequence of events in emerging lesions has been a subject of debate since the late 19th century. Most studies agree that as mononuclear cells begin to invade the epidermis, intercellular edema (spongiosis) of basal keratinocytes appears, followed by focal vacuolization, and patchy loss of granular layer keratinocytes and the appearance of parakeratotic cells with or without neutrophilic infiltration of the stratum corneum. During this transition, the time required for keratinocyte transit from the basal layer to the granular layer decreases from 2 weeks to 2 days, the keratinocyte mitotic rate increases approximately 10-fold, and a characteristic pattern of altered keratin synthesis ensues, with a transition in suprabasal keratins from keratins 1 and 10 to keratins 6 and 16. More chronic lesions continue to be markedly hyperplastic, resulting in a regular pattern of epidermal thickening (acanthosis) with greatly elongated and edematous rete ridges, dilation, and tortuosity of superficial capillaries, and a complete loss of granular cells with diffuse parakeratosis.

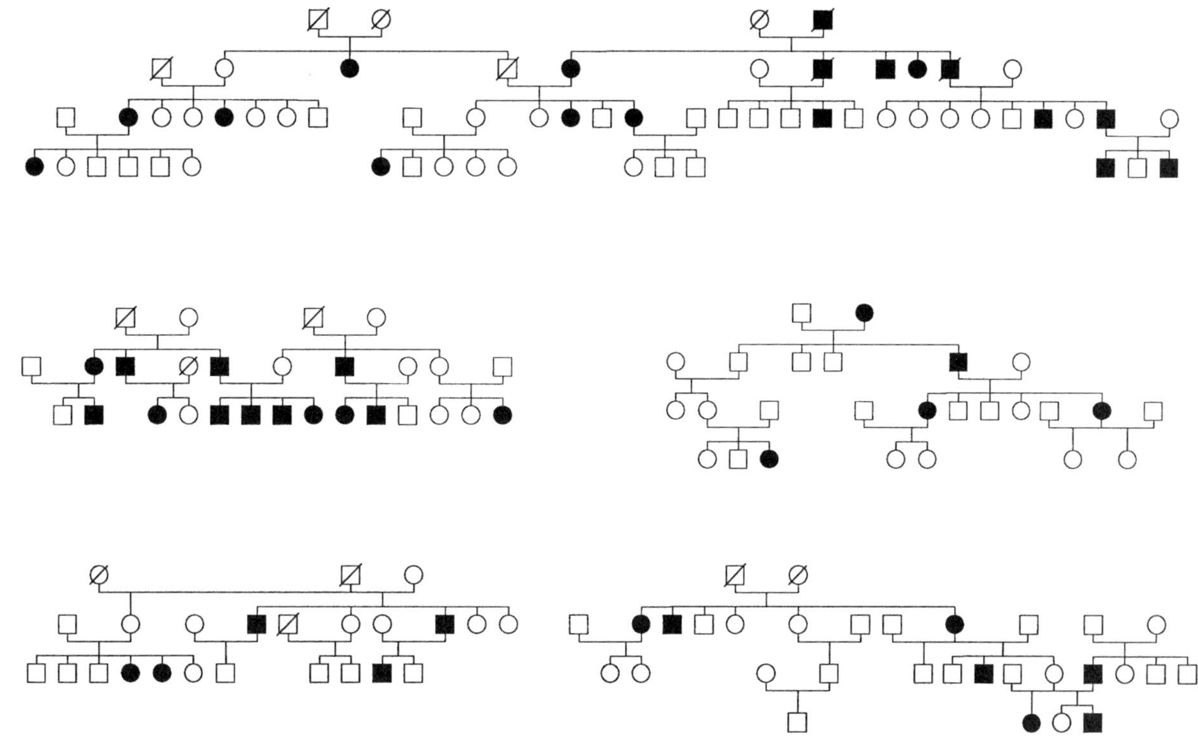

Figure 86-5 Examples of multiplex psoriasis pedigrees. Note generation-to-generation and male-to-male transmission, suggestive of autosomal dominant inheritance with reduced penetrance. (Modified from Nair et al., Human Heredity 1995;45:219–230.)

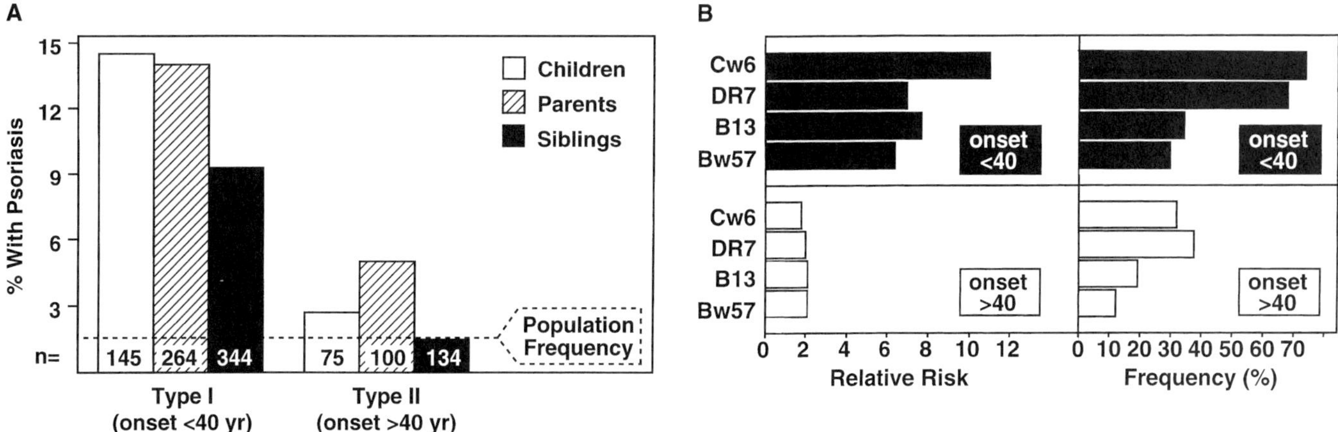

Figure 86-6 (A) Increased heritability of juvenile-onset (type I) psoriasis. (B) HLA associations in Type I vs Type II psoriasis. (From Elder et al., Arch Dermatol 1994;130:216–224.)

THE CASE FOR T-CELL INVOLVEMENT Given its known specificity for T cells, the marked efficacy of the immunosuppressant cyclosporine A (CsA) in psoriasis has provided important functional evidence of T-cell involvement. Besides cyclosporine, other T-cell–specific immunosuppressants including FK506, peptide T, anti-CD3 and -CD4 monoclonal antibodies (MAb), and diptheria toxin-coupled interleukin-2 (IL-2) have all proven efficacious in limited studies, albeit not without side effects. Additional evidence for T-cell involvement comes from reports of disease exacerbation after IL-2 and interferon-γ (IFN-γ) therapy, and after bone marrow transplantation from a psoriatic donor. Conversely, complete clearing of severe psoriasis has been reported after transplantation from a nonpsoriatic donor.

In recent years, it has become increasingly clear that psoriatic lesions contain substantial numbers of dendritic antigen-presenting cells (APCs) in addition to T cells. Most of the T cells present are not naive, but rather memory T cells capable of binding to skin-specific homing receptors on superficial dermal capillary endothelial cells. In addition, accessory factors required for efficient T-cell activation are present in the lesion, including costimulatory APC surface ligands such as B7-1 and B7-2, and a rich cytokine milleu produced by surrounding keratinocytes, mast cells, and mononuclear cells. Several lines of evidence argue for ongoing T-cell activation by antigen in the lesion itself. These include: (1) the presence of actively dividing memory T cells in contact with APCs in the dermis and epidermis of psoriatic lesions; (2)

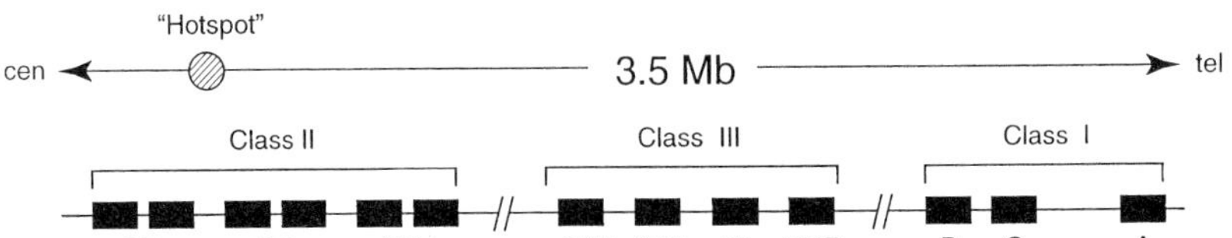

"Hotspot"

cen ← 3.5 Mb → tel

Class II — Class III — Class I

Ancestral Haplotype:	Race	DP	DQ	DR	C4B	C4A	Bf	TNF	B	C	A
57.1	C,M,N		9	7	1	6	S	L	57	w6	1
13.1	C,M		2	7	1	3	S	?	13	w6	30
7.1	C		6	15	1	3	S	L	7	w7	3
8.1	C		2	3	1	0	S	S	8	w7	1
18.2	C		2	3	0	3	F1	L	18	w5	30
46.1	M		9	9	2	4	S	S	46	w1	2
65.1	C		5	1	1+2	2	S	L	65	w8	?

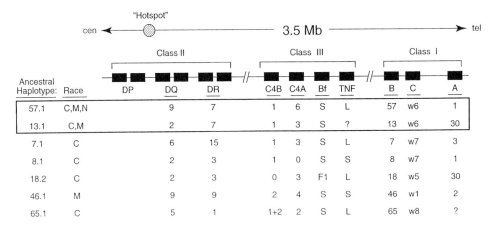

Figure 86-7 HLA region map, showing ancestral haplotypes. Psoriasis-associated ancestral haplotypes are boxed. Depiction of HLA loci are incomplete and not to scale. cen, centromere; tel, telomere; Mb, megabases; C, Caucasoid; M, Mongoloid; N, Negroid. "Hotspot" indicates approximate region of loss of linkage disequilibrium described in the text. (Data from Degli-Epsoti et al., Immunogenetics 1992;36:345–356, Hum Immunol 1992;34:242–252, and Wu et al., Hum Immunol 1992;33,89–97.)

oligoclonal usage of TCR Vβ chains in the $CD8^+$ subset of lesional T cells; and (3) maintenance of the psoriatic phenotype after transplantation of lymph node-free, split-thickness skin to globally immunodeficient (SCID) mice. Thus, psoriatic lesions appear to feature all components of the classical "ternary complex" required for T-cell activation: MHC, antigen, and the responding T-cell receptor. It is attractive to speculate that preferential Vβ subset usage reflects an important role for superantigen as the initial stimulus for T-cell activation, followed by further activation by nominal antigen; however, this concept remains to be confirmed.

Both helper ($CD4^+$) and suppressor ($CD8^+$) T cells are present in lesions, with most $CD8^+$ cells being found in the epidermis and most $CD4^+$ cells in the dermis. A case has been made for greater importance of $CD8^+$ T cells, based on: (1) the strength of MHC class I associations in psoriasis; (2) the principle that Class I molecules usually present antigens to $CD8^+$ T cells; (3) the evidence for oligoclonal expansion of $CD8^+$ T-cells; and (4) the selective depletion of $CD8^+$ by UVB light treatment. Whereas this is an attractive hypothesis, it does not explain why IL-2, IFN-γ, and IL-12 strongly predominate over IL-4, -5, and -10 in psoriatic lesions, fitting the so-called Th1 lymphokine profile usually considered characteristic of $CD4^+$ helper T cells. However, it must be remembered that both $CD4^+$ and $CD8^+$ cells can contribute to the Th1 lymphokine profile. Adding to the complexity, we have already discussed the confounding effects of linkage disequilibrium on the interpretation of Class I vs Class II associations in psoriasis, and there is evidence that anti-CD4 MAbs can clear psoriasis. Therefore, until more is known, it seems prudent to acknowledge the potential roles of both $CD4^+$ and $CD8^+$ T cells in lesion development.

Recently, T cells cloned from psoriatic lesions have been used to prepare lymphokine-rich conditioned media. Interestingly, these media stimulated the proliferation of short-term keratinocyte cultures from uninvolved skin of psoriasis patients, but not cells cultured from normal epidermis. Neutralization studies showed that IFN-γ was a major mitogen in the context of other as-yet-unidentified lymphokines in the conditioned medium, whereas it is growth inhibitory when used alone. In the long-term, however, keratinocyte proliferation in psoriasis appears to be maintained by autocrine stimulation of the EGF receptor via one of at least three EGF-like growth factors: TGF-α, amphiregulin, and HB-EGF.

Based on the foregoing observations, the following working model for maintenance of psoriatic lesions can be envisaged (Fig. 86-8): Memory T cells enter the skin, having been directed to the skin by upregulated adhesion molecules on activated endothelial cells. Once present in epidermis and dermis, these T cells may encounter bacterial and/or viral superantigens, leading to an expansion of a subset of cells with restricted utilization of TCR Vβ chains. These superantigen-activated cells will also encounter foreign or host-derived standard antigens on the surfaces of dendritic antigen-presenting cells, to which a limited number of the superantigen-activated T cells will respond by further expansion in the presence of appropriate costimulatory signals. T-cell activation causes release of IFN-γ, which may in turn stimulate keratinocyte proliferation, whereas IL-2 and other lymphokines may promote further activation of T cells, APCs, endothelial cells, and/or keratinocytes via a cytokine cascade. Alternatively, T cells may exert sublethal damage to keratinocytes, which respond by entering a wound-healing pathway of epidermal differentiation. Whether the psoriatic keratinocyte is genetically more susceptible to growth stimulation by lymphokines from these T cells requires further study.

MANAGEMENT/TREATMENT

In view of its genetic basis, lifelong duration, and low mortality, avoidance of toxicity is a cornerstone of psoriasis therapy. Nevertheless, effective treatment of moderate to severe psoriasis can entail substantial toxicity and demands careful management.

Because of incomplete terminal differentiation, the stratum corneum of the psoriatic plaque is fragile and presents a defective barrier to epidermal water loss. Recent research has shown that loss of epidermal barrier function is a trigger for keratinocyte production of various pro-inflammatory cytokines and adhesion molecules including IL-8, TNF-α, and ICAM-1. Emollients have long played an important role in psoriasis therapy, presumably by improving barrier function. Although the density of the bacterial flora in psoriasis lesions is double that of normal skin, antibiotic treatment is only occasionally helpful.

CORTICOSTEROIDS/RETINOIDS/VITAMIN D Whereas the antipsoriatic efficacy of topical and systemic steroids has been known since the 1950s, their cellular target remains unclear. Irrespective of their site of action, it is now clear that steroids

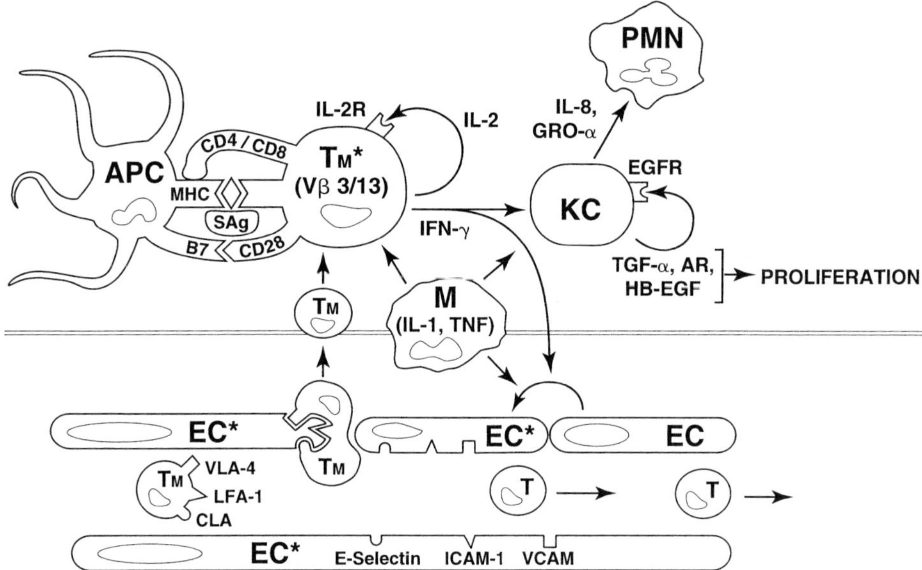

Figure 86-8 Model for T-cell pathogenesis of psoriasis. APC, dendritic antigan presenting cell; MHC, HLA Class I or Class II molecules; SAg, superantigen; T, T cell; Tm, memory T cell; Tm*, superantigen-activated memory T cell; M, monocyte/macrophage; KC, keratinocyte; PMN, polymorphonuclear leukocyte; EC, endothelial cell; EC*, activated endothelial cell expressing E-selectin (receptor for CLA), ICAM-1 (receptor for LFA-1), and VCAM (receptor for VLA-4). (*See text* for details.)

exert their beneficial effects via binding to specific nuclear receptors, which serve as ligand-dependent transcription factors. These nuclear receptors are encoded by a superfamily of related genes that encompasses the receptors for not only corticosteroids, but also other effective antipsoriatic agents including vitamin D derivatives and retinoids. At present, the full spectrum of steroid-responsive genes is unknown; however, steroids are known to inhibit the transcription of major immunomodulatory genes such as IL-2 by interfering with the binding of other activating transcription factors such as AP-1. Systemic steroids were initially highly popular but are now little used because of their well-known complications as well as "rebound" flaring of disease upon their withdrawal. In their stead, many different topical corticosteroid preparations of varying potency and vehicle formulations have appeared. Systemic side effects and local effects such as atrophy and hypopigmentation are a concern for only the most potent of these compounds, generally fluorinated derivatives.

Retinoids and vitamin D3 derivatives constitute the other two "legs" of the "therapeutic triad" of nuclear receptor ligands with antipsoriatic effects. The synthetic retinoid etretinate has been used for nearly 20 years, especially in pustular and guttate flares alone or in combination with ultraviolet light. Recently, a topical retinoid has been found to be effective; this compound may interfere with AP-1 activity in addition to activating retinoic acid receptors. Topical vitamin D3 derivatives have also emerged as useful compounds in the 1990s. At present, the major vitamin D3-related compound is calcipotriol, a short-lived structural analog of 1,25 dihydroxy vitamin D3, which lacks most of the hypercalcemic side effects of vitamin D3 itself. As with the corticosteroids, the cellular and molecular targets of retinoid and vitamin D3 action remain unclear. Both classes of compounds have profound effects upon keratinocyte differentiation, and must be used with care in psoriasis, as they produce their own characteristic patterns of skin irritation.

ULTRAVIOLET LIGHT Psoriasis therapy with combinations of high-energy ultraviolet B (UVB) light (290–320 nm) with crude coal tar was introduced in 1925, and the combination of psoralens with lower-energy UVA light (320–400 nm) followed in 1974. Initially, both regimens were thought to act directly on keratinocyte proliferation. However, it is now recognized that both therapies induce immunosuppression in addition to a complex pattern of keratinocyte effects, including immunosuppressive cytokine production and induction of apoptosis.

CYCLOSPORINE A As discussed earlier, CsA exerts potent antipsoriatic effects, with nearly immediate clearing of psoriasis when used at transplantation dose of 14 mg/kg/d. The drug remains highly effective at less nephrotoxic doses as low as 3 mg/kg/d. Its mechanism of action is thought to involve binding to the protein cyclophilin, with subsequent inhibition of the calmodulin-dependent protein phosphatase regulatory subunit calcineurin B and subsequent inability to translocate a component of the transcription factor NF-AT from the cytoplasm to the nucleus of the T cell.

METHOTREXATE As in the case of UV therapy, methotrexate was initially thought to exert its effects via inhibition of keratinocyte proliferation. However, it is effective under doses and schedules of administration that fail to inhibit keratinocyte proliferation in vitro. It now appears that this drug exerts profound antiinflammatory effects by promoting the extracellular accumulation of adenosine.

OTHER AGENTS Anthralin is a strong reducing agent long used topically in psoriasis, either alone or in combination with UVB light. Although quite effective, its use is limited by skin staining and irritation. Its mechanism of action is likely to be multifactorial. Sulfasalazine is a systemic drug that is effective in a subset of psoriasis patients, with only limited toxicity and the advantage of low cost. Its mechanism of action is also unknown, but is thought to be anti-inflammatory and/or immunosuppressive.

FUTURE DIRECTIONS

As can be appreciated from the previous sections, it appears that the actions of nearly all antipsoriatic drugs can be understood in terms of immunosuppressive and/or antiinflammatory effects, with T-cell activation as a likely primary target via the ternary complex of APC, antigen, and T-cell receptor in the context of appropriate accessory signals. Thus it is not surprising that a variety of novel molecular approaches to blocking this activation event are currently under development. These include vaccination against specific peptides of the TCR Vβ families characteristic of oligoclonal and presumably pathogenic T cells; administration of soluble CTLA-4 to block the accessory signal; administration of IL-10 to shift the lymphokine phenotype away from the disease-associated Th1 and toward the countervailing Th2 state; and additional agents that can block T-cell signal transduction with fewer side effects than CsA and FK506.

As a genodermatosis, the question remains whether psoriasis will prove to be amenable to gene therapy. The issue of direct correction of mutant gene function must await further identification of the genes involved. Assuming that defective gene function can be documented in bone-marrow-derived cells, it will not be unreasonable to expect to reintroduce the normal version of the gene via autologous transplantation of genetically engineered stem cells or long-lasting hematopoietic precursors of appropriate lineage. Moreover, inasmuch as simple approaches to introduction of DNA into the skin by direct injection or even topical application are proving to be feasible, it is also reasonable to consider the introduction of various immunomodulators at the level of the gene, rather than the cognate protein. Under either scenario, the future prospects of gene therapy for psoriasis deserve serious consideration.

SELECTED REFERENCES

Barker JN, Griffiths CE. Progress in psoriasis. Psoriasis: from gene to clinic. London, UK, 5-7 December 1996. Mol Med Today 1997;3:193,194.

Bata-Csorgo Z, Hammerberg C, Voorhees JJ, Cooper KD. Kinetics and regulation of human keratinocyte stem cell growth in short-term primary ex vivo culture. Cooperative growth factors from psoriatic lesional T lymphocytes stimulate proliferation among psoriatic uninvolved, but not normal, stem keratinocytes. J Clin Invest 1995;95:317–327.

Chang JC, Smith LR, Froning KJ, et al. CD8+ T cells in psoriatic lesions preferentially use T-cell receptor V beta 3 and/or V beta 13.1 genes. Proc Natl Acad Sci USA 1994;91:9282–9286.

Christophers E, Sterry W. Psoriasis. In: Fitzpatrick TB, Eisen AZ, Wolff K, Freedberg IM, Austen KF, eds. Dermatology in General Medicine. New York: McGraw-Hill, 1993; pp. 489–514.

Cronstein BN, Naime D, Ostad E. The antiinflammatory effects of methotrexate are mediated by adenosine. Adv Exp Med Biol 1994;370:411–416.

Degli-Esposti MA, Leaver AL, Christiansen FT, Witt CS, Abraham LJ, Dawkins RL. Ancestral haplotypes: conserved population MHC haplotypes. Hum Immunol 1992;34:242–252.

Elder J. Transforming growth factor-alpha and related growth factors. In: Luger T, Schwarz T, eds. Epidermal Growth Factors and Cytokines. New York: Marcel Dekker, 1994; pp. 205–240.

Elder J. Cytokine and genetic regulation of psoriasis. In: Dahl M, ed. Advances in Dermatology. St. Louis: Mosby-Year Book, 1995; pp. 99–134.

Elder JT, Nair RP, Guo SW, Henseler T, Christophers E, Voorhees JJ. The genetics of psoriasis. Arch Dermatol 1994;130:216–224.

Fry L. Psoriasis. Br J Dermatol 1988;119:445–461.

Greaves MW, Weinstein GD. Treatment of psoriasis [see comments]. N Engl J Med 1995;332:581–588.

Henseler T. The genetics of psoriasis. J Am Acad Dermatol 1997; 37:S1–S11.

Henseler T, Christophers E. Psoriasis of early and late onset: characterization of two types of psoriasis vulgaris. J Am Acad Dermatol 1985;13:450–456.

Krueger JG, Wolfe JT, Nabeya RT, et al. Successful ultraviolet B treatment of psoriasis is accompanied by a reversal of keratinocyte pathology and by selective depletion of intraepidermal T cells. J Exp Med 1995;182:2057–2068.

Lander ES, Schork NJ. Genetic dissection of complex traits. Science 1994;265:2037–2048.

Mangelsdorf DJ, Evans RM. The RXR heterodimers and orphan receptors. Cell 1995;83:841–850.

Modlin RL. Th1-Th2 paradigm: insights from leprosy. J Invest Dermatol 1994;102:828–832.

Morganroth GS, Chan LS, Weinstein GD, Voorhees JJ, Cooper KD. Proliferating cells in psoriatic dermis are comprised primarily of T cells, endothelial cells, and factor XIIIa+ perivascular dendritic cells. J Invest Dermatol 1991;96:333–340.

Moss P, Charmley P, Mulvihill E, et al. The repertoire of T cell antigen receptor beta-chain variable regions associated with psoriasis vulgaris. J Invest Dermatol 1997;109:14–19.

Nair RP, Henseler T, Jenisch S, et al. Evidence for two psoriasis susceptibility loci (HLA and 17q) and two novel candidate regions (16q and 20q) by genome-wide scan. Hum Mol Genet 1997;6:1349–1356.

Nickoloff BJ, Kunkel SL, Burdick M, Strieter RM. Severe combined immunodeficiency mouse and human psoriatic skin chimeras. Validation of a new animal model. Am J Pathol 1995;146:580–588.

Nickoloff BJ, Naidu Y. Perturbation of epidermal barrier function correlates with initiation of cytokine cascade in human skin. J Am Acad Dermatol 1994;30:535–546.

Northrop JP, Crabtree GR, Mattila PS. Negative regulation of interleukin 2 transcription by the glucocorticoid receptor. J Exp Med 1992;175: 1235–1245.

Stem RS. Psoriasis. Lancet 1997;350:349–353.

Tomfohrde J, Silverman A, Barnes R, et al. Gene for familial psoriasis susceptibility mapped to the distal end of human chromosome 17q. Science 1994;264:1141–1145.

Trembath RC, Clough RL, Rosbothem JL, et al. Identification of a major susceptibility locus on chromosome 6p and evidence for further disease loci revealed by a two stage genome-wide search in psoriasis. Hum Mol Genet 1997;6:813–820.

Vallat VP, Gilleaudeau P, Battat L, et al. PUVA bath therapy strongly suppresses immunological and epidermal activation in psoriasis: a possible cellular basis for remittive therapy. J Exp Med 1994;180: 283–296.

Winchester R. Psoriatic arthritis. In: Fitzpatrick TB, Eisen AZ, Wolff K, Freedberg IM, Austen KF, eds. Dermatology in General Medicine. New York: McGraw-Hill, 1993; pp. 515–527.

Wong RL, Winslow CM, Cooper KD. The mechanisms of action of cyclosporin A in the treatment of psoriasis. Immunol Today 1993; 14:69–74.

87 Atopic Dermatitis and Atopy

DONALD Y. M. LEUNG AND LARRY BORISH

BACKGROUND

Atopic dermatitis (AD) is a chronic inflammatory skin disease frequently seen in patients with a personal or family history of asthma and allergic rhinitis. The term atopic dermatitis was first introduced in 1933 by Hill and Sulzberger in recognition of this close association between AD and respiratory allergy. During the past 10 years, there have been extraordinary strides made in our understanding of the immunopathogenesis of allergic diseases. In particular, this constellation of inherited illnesses have now been demonstrated to be associated with activation of a specific group of cytokine genes encompassing interleukin (IL)-3, IL-4, IL-5, IL-13, and granulocyte-macrophage colony-stimulating factor (GM-CSF). The molecular basis for selective activation of this cytokine gene cluster and their immunologic consequences are now actively being pursued by many laboratories. However, it is clear that allergic diseases result from a polygenic inheritance pattern that not only involves cytokine-gene activation but other less-well-defined gene products as well. In addition, the clinical expression of allergic diseases is highly dependent on a complex interaction between the host and its environment, e.g., allergen exposure. This chapter will review some of these recent developments and their clinical implications.

DIAGNOSTIC AND CLINICAL FEATURES OF AD

The diagnosis of AD is based on the constellation of clinical features in Table 87-1. Approximately 50% of patients develop AD by the first year of life, and an additional 30% between age 1 and 5 years. Nearly 80% of patients with AD eventually develop allergic rhinitis or asthma later in childhood. Many of these patients outgrow their skin disease as they are developing respiratory allergy. This observation is consistent with the concept that the clinical expression of allergic disease is determined in part from local tissue allergen sensitization and compartmentalization of the immune response in the skin vs the respiratory mucosa.

SKIN REACTION PATTERNS IN AD Intense pruritus and cutaneous reactivity are the hallmarks of AD. Scratching may be intermittent throughout the day but is usually worse in the early evening and night. Patients with AD also have a reduced threshold for pruritus. Clinically, this is supported by the observation that allergens, reduced humidity, excessive sweating, and irritants— e.g., wool, acrylic, soaps, and detergents—can exacerbate pruritus and scratching.

From: *Principles of Molecular Medicine* (J. L. Jameson, ed.), ©1998 Humana Press Inc., Totowa, NJ.

Several types of inflammatory skin lesions are commonly seen in AD. Acute lesions are intensely pruritic, and characterized by erythematous papules over erythematous skin. These are associated with extensive excoriations, erosions, and serous exudate. Subacute dermatitis is characterized by erythematous, excoriated, scaling papules. Chronic dermatitis is characterized by thickened skin, accentuated skin markings (lichenification), and fibrotic papules. In chronic AD, all three stages of skin reactions usually coexist in the same individual. At all stages of AD, patients usually have dry skin. Skin distribution and reaction patterns vary according to the patient's age and disease chronicity. During infancy, the AD is generally more acute and primarily involves the face, scalp, and the extensor surfaces of the extremities. In older patients who have had long-standing skin disease, the rash is characterized by the chronic form of dermatitis with lichenification and localization to the flexural areas of the extremities.

ROLE OF ALLERGENS IN AD Serum IgE levels are elevated in 80–85% of patients with AD. Approximately 85% of patients have positive immediate skin tests or RAST for specific IgE to a variety of food and inhalant allergens. However, positive immediate skin tests to specific allergens do not always indicate clinical sensitivity and patients who outgrow AD frequently continue to have positive skin tests. Indeed, May first made a distinction between symptomatic and asymptomatic hypersensitivity based on the observation that AD patients with positive food skin tests did not always have positive challenges to the foods implicated by IgE responses. These clinical observations suggest that the relationship between IgE and clinical disease is not exclusively dependent on IgE-mediated mast-cell degranulation.

Well-controlled, double-blind, placebo-controlled food challenge studies (DBPCFC) have, however, demonstrated that food allergens can exacerbate skin rashes in at least a subset of patients particular young children with AD. Importantly, elimination of putative food allergens in such patients results in significant improvement of their skin disease. As patients grow older, they outgrow their food allergy, but a majority of them become sensitized to inhalant allergens. Whereas sensitization to inhalant allergens in most cases reflects the development of coexisting respiratory allergy—e.g., asthma or allergic rhinitis—a number of clinical studies suggest that inhalation or contact with aeroallergen may play a role in the exacerbation of AD.

CUTANEOUS INFECTIONS Patients with AD have an increased tendency to develop viral, fungal, and bacterial skin infections. These infections are generally localized to the skin. Deep-seated infections suggest the possibility of hyperimmunoglobulinemia E

Table 87-1
Diagnostic Features of Atopic Dermatitis[a]

Major features
Pruritus
Typical appearance and distribution of skin lesions
Facial and extensor involvement in infancy and early childhood
Flexural involvement and lichenification by adolescence
Chronic or frequently relapsing course (duration >6 weeks)
Personal or family history of either AD or respiratory allergy
Minor features
Increased susceptibility to skin infections, particularly *S. aureus*
Xerosis (dryness of the skin)
Early age of onset
Multiple positive immediate prick skin tests
Elevated serum IgE levels
Ichthyosis; keratosis pilaris; hyperlinearity of palms
Nonspecific hand/foot dermatitis
Scalp dermatitis, e.g., cradle cap

[a]Modified from Hanifin and Rajka.

syndrome or another immunodeficiency syndrome. Viral infections include herpes simplex, vaccinia, warts, molluscum contagiosum, and papilloma virus. The most common viral infection is herpes simplex, which tends to spread locally or can become generalized. Superficial fungal infections also appear to occur more frequently in atopic individuals. The potential importance of these dermatophyte infections is suggested by the reduction of AD skin severity following treatment with antifungal agents such as ketoconazole.

Considerable attention has focused on the contribution of *Staphylococcus aureus* colonization and infection to the severity of AD. *S. aureus* is found in over 90% of AD skin lesions. Honey-colored crusting, extensive serous weeping, folliculitis, and pyoderma indicate bacterial infection usually secondary to *S. aureus* in patients with AD. The importance of *S. aureus* in AD is supported by the observation that not only patients with impetiginized AD, but also AD patients without superinfection show clinical response to combined treatment with antistaphylococcal antibiotics and topical corticosteroids.

Recent studies suggest that *S. aureus* exacerbates or maintains skin inflammation in AD by secreting a group of toxins known to act as superantigens that stimulate marked activation of T cells and macrophages. Since staphylococcal enterotoxins (SEs) are globular proteins of 24–30 kDa, the possibility that they could act as allergens has also been studied. In this regard, it has been found that nearly half of AD patients produce IgE directed to staphylococcal toxins, particularly SEA, SEB, and toxic shock syndrome toxin-1 (TSST-1). This is of interest because staphylococci isolated from AD skin lesions predominantly secrete one of these three exotoxins. These findings suggest the possibility that local production of SEs at the skin surface could cause IgE-mediated histamine release and thereby trigger the itch–scratch cycle that can exacerbate AD.

IMMUNOLOGIC FINDINGS IN ATOPIC DERMATITIS

A number of observations suggest an underlying immunoregulatory abnormality in AD (Table 87-2). Studies of T-cell clones support the concept that activation of a subpopulation of helper cells leads to the release of cytokines important in the pathogenesis of AD. In mice, two types of $CD4^+$ T-cell clones have been

Table 87-2
Immunologic Features of Atopic Dermatitis

Increased IgE production
Immediate skin-test reactivity to multiple allergens
Increased basophil spontaneous histamine release
Decreased CD8 suppressor/cytotoxic number and function
Increased expression of CD23 on mononuclear cells
Chronic macrophage activation with increased secretion of GM-CSF, PGE_2, and IL-10
Expansion of IL-4–, IL-5–, and IL-13–secreting Th2-like cells
Decreased numbers of IFN-γ–secreting Th1-like cells

described, based on their pattern of cytokine secretion. T-helper type 1 (Th1) cells secrete IL-2 and interferon (IFN)-γ, but not IL-4 or IL-5. In contrast, Th2 cells produce IL-4, IL-5, and IL-13, but not IFN-γ. IL-4 and IL-13 act as IgE isotype-specific switch factors, and induce the expression of VCAM-1, an adhesion molecule involved in the migration of mononuclear cells and eosinophils into sites of tissue inflammation. IL-5 promotes the differentiation, vascular endothelial adhesion, and survival of eosinophils and also enhances histamine release from basophils. In contrast, IFN-γ inhibits IgE synthesis as well as the proliferation of Th2 cells.

The lack of IFN-γ production, as well as the concomitant activation of IL-4, IL-5, and IL-13 is thought to play a critical role in the pathogenesis of AD (Fig. 87-1). In support of the concept that this profile of cytokines arises from the selective activation of Th2, as compared to Th1, cells are a number of studies demonstrating increased frequency of allergen-specific T-cells producing increased IL-4 and IL-5, but little IFN-γ in the peripheral blood and skin lesions of patients with AD. IL-4 inhibits IFN-γ production and downregulates the differentiation of Th1 cells. In addition, atopic monocytes have been found to have elevated cAMP phosphodiesterase and secrete increased levels of IL-10 and prostaglandin E_2. Both IL-10 and PGE_2 inhibit IFN-γ production and may therefore contribute to the decreased IFN-γ production by AD PBMC.

IMMUNOHISTOLOGY OF ATOPIC DERMATITIS

IMMUNOHISTOLOGIC FINDINGS The histologic features of AD depend on the acuity and therefore the duration of the skin lesion. Uninvolved or clinically normal skin of AD patients is histologically abnormal and demonstrates mild hyperkeratosis, epidermal hyperplasia, and a sparse dermal cellular infiltrate consisting primarily of T lymphocytes. Acute lesions are characterized by marked intercellular edema (spongiosis) of the epidermis, and intracellular edema noted as ballooning of the keratinocytes. A sparse epidermal infiltrate consisting primarily of T lymphocytes is frequently observed. In the dermis, there is a marked perivenular inflammatory-cell infiltrate consisting predominantly of lymphocytes, and occasional monocyte-macrophages. Eosinophils, basophils, and neutrophils are rarely present in the acute lesion. In chronic lichenified lesions, the epidermis is hyperplastic with elongation of the rete ridges, prominent hyperkeratosis, and minimal spongiosis. Increased numbers of Langerhans cells are present in the epidermis, and macrophages dominate the dermal mononuclear cell infiltrate. The number of mast cells are increased in number but are generally fully granulated. Endothelial cells of the superficial venular plexus and deep venules are hypertrophied with enlarged nuclei and prominent nucleoli.

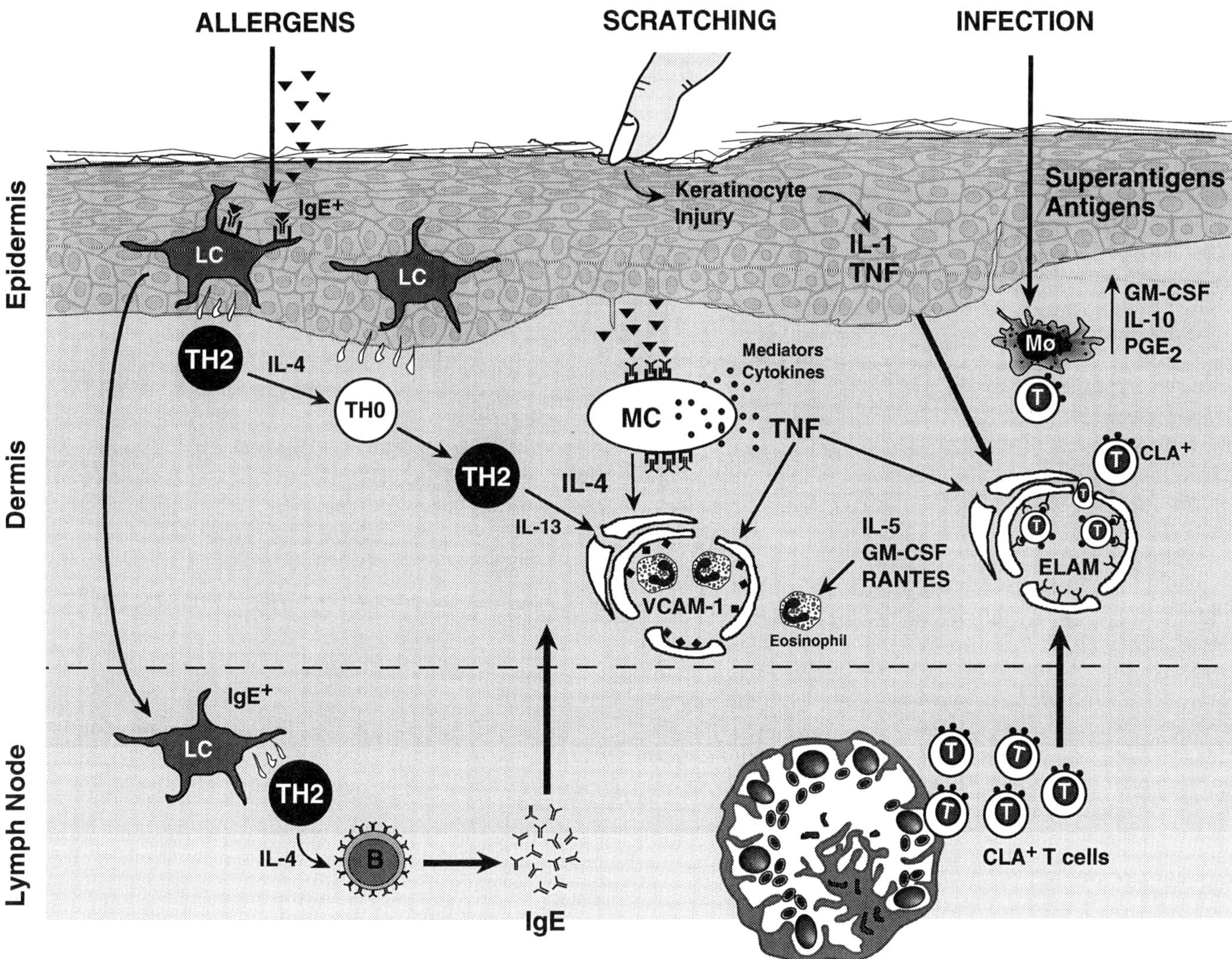

Figure 87-1 Cellular and cytokine interactions involved in the pathogenesis of atopic dermatitis. (Reproduced with permission from Leung et al. J Allergy Clin Immunol 1995;96:302–319.)

PATTERNS OF CYTOKINE EXPRESSION IN AD SKIN LESIONS The pattern of cytokines expressed locally play a critical role in modulating the nature of tissue inflammation. Therefore, an analysis of cytokine expression in AD is critically dependent on the acuity or duration of the skin lesion. The *in situ* hybridization (ISH) technique has been used to investigate the expression of IL-4, IL-5, and IFN-γ messenger RNA (mRNA) in skin biopsies from clinically normal (uninvolved), acute (erythematous AD lesions of <3 days' duration), and chronic (>2 weeks' duration) skin lesions of patients with AD. As compared with normal control skin, uninvolved skin of patients with AD had a significant increase in number of cells expressing IL-4, but not IL-5 or IFN-γ, mRNA. Acute and chronic skin lesions, when compared to normal skin or uninvolved skin of AD patients, had significantly greater numbers of cells that were positive for mRNA for IL-4 and IL-5. However, neither acute AD or uninvolved AD skin contained significant numbers of IFN-γ mRNA-expressing cells.

As compared with acute AD, chronic AD skin lesions had significantly fewer IL-4 mRNA-expressing cells, but significantly greater IL-5 mRNA-expressing cells. T-cells constituted the majority of IL-5–expressing cells in acute and chronic AD lesions. Chronic lesions also expressed significantly greater numbers of activated IL-5 mRNA-expressing eosinophils than acute lesions. These data indicate that although cells in acute and chronic AD lesions are associated with increased activation of IL-4 and IL-5 genes, acute skin inflammation in AD is associated with a predominance of IL-4 expression, whereas maintenance of chronic inflammation is predominantly associated with increased IL-5 expression and eosinophil infiltration. In addition, chronic AD lesions are associated with overexpression of GM-CSF and IL-10 expression.

MULTIFUNCTIONAL ROLE OF IgE IN AD SKIN INFLAMMATION

Although the histologic features of AD closely resembles a type IV delayed-type hypersensitivity (DTH) reaction, several lines of evidence indicate that AD is not a conventional DTH reaction, and furthermore that IgE-mediated mechanisms play a role in the pathogenesis of AD. T cells that infiltrate into conventional DTH skin reactions (e.g., tuberculin skin reactions) secrete IFN-γ and therefore induce the expression of HLA-DR on skin keratinocytes. In contrast, keratinocytes in the AD skin lesion do not express HLA-DR. More direct evidence that the T cells in skin lesions of AD differ from the Th1 cells in conventional DTH has come from studies demonstrating increased IL-4 and IL-5, but not IFN-γ, mRNA expression in acute AD skin lesions. Furthermore, Th2 cells have been found to be just as effective in inducing skin inflammation as Th1 cells. However, the mediation of skin inflammation by Th2 cells is IL-4, but not IFN-γ, dependent. Taken together, these data suggest that two histologically indistinguishable cutaneous DTH reactions exist: The first is mediated by IFN-γ–secreting Th1 cells found in conventional DTH reactions. The second is mediated by IL-4– and IL-5–secreting Th2 cells and involves allergen-induced, cell-mediated reactions.

There are several mechanisms by which IgE molecules can contribute to the induction of a mononuclear cell infiltrate. In this regard, clinically significant allergen-induced reactions are associated with an IgE-dependent biphasic response. In such reactions, following exposure to allergen, mast cells bearing IgE directed to the relevant allergen release various mediators and cytokines into local tissue within 15–60 min of allergen challenge. This immediate reaction likely contributes to the acute pruritus and erythema observed after exposure of AD patients to relevant food and inhalant allergens.

Several hours after this immediate reaction begins to subside, there is onset of an IgE-dependent late-phase reaction (LPR) characterized initially by expression of leukocyte adhesion molecules on postcapillary venular endothelium, followed by the infiltration of eosinophils, neutrophils and mononuclear cells into the inflamed area. Granulocytes reach their maximum cell accumulation at 6–8 h, and by 24–48 h after onset of the reaction, the cellular infiltrate consists predominantly of mononuclear cells. Using ISH, Kay and coworkers have reported that the cellular infiltrate in allergen-induced late-phase skin reactions express increased mRNA for IL-3, IL-4, IL-5, and granulocyte-macrophage colony-stimulating factor but no mRNA for IFN-γ. These results suggest that the T cells infiltrating into the allergen-induced LPR, similar to allergen-specific T cells grown from AD skin lesions, are Th2-like cells.

Langerhans cells and macrophages infiltrating into the AD skin lesion bear IgE antibody. Binding of IgE to Langerhans cells occurs via both high-affinity and low-affinity IgE (CD23) receptors. Macrophages can express CD23 in response to IL-4. Allergens have been demonstrated to activate IgE-bearing macrophages in an IgE-dependent manner with the formation of leukotrienes, PAF, IL-1, and TNF. The activation of IgE-bearing Langerhans cells and macrophages by allergens could thus contribute to the skin inflammation associated with AD.

There is also mounting evidence that IgE-bearing Langerhans cells in AD skin play an important role in cutaneous allergen presentation to Th2 cells. Of note, IgE-bearing Langerhans cells from AD skin lesions, but not Langerhans cells that lack surface IgE, are capable of presenting house-dust-mite allergen to T cells. These results suggest that cell-bound IgE on Langerhans cells facilitate binding of allergens to Langerhans cells prior to their processing and antigen presentation.

Although allergen challenges and experimental models suggest the participation of specific mechanisms of inflammation, it should be emphasized that an analysis of the AD skin lesion does not allow simple classification discretely into an IgE-mediated LPR or a T-cell–mediated immune reaction. Thus, in all likelihood, the mononuclear cell infiltrate in the AD skin lesion reflects a combination of both IgE-dependent mast cell/basophil degranulation and Th2-cell–mediated responses elicited during acute exposures to allergen and other antigens or superantigens.

Finally, although the release of a variety of mediators, e.g., histamine and proteases into the skin following challenge by allergens trigger acute pruritus in AD, clinical studies suggest that the actual development of eczematoid skin rashes is dependent on the skin trauma inflicted by scratching. Once the itch–scratch cycle is triggered, the mechanisms by which scratching promotes inflammation of the skin is suggested by a number of recent observations demonstrating the keratinocyte is an important epidermal source of cytokines including IL-1, IL-6, IL-8, GM-CSF, and TNF-α. In this regard, any injury including mechanical trauma to the keratinocyte will result in the release of cytokines that can induce inflammation through a number of actions. This includes the release of IL-1, TNF-α, and IL-4, which are critical cytokines in the induction of adhesion molecules, such as ELAM-1, ICAM-1, and VCAM-1 that attract lymphocytes, macrophages, and eosinophils into cutaneous sites of inflammation. At this stage, a wide variety of resident and infiltrating cells are then capable of secreting cytokines and mediators that sustain the inflammation. AD therefore results from a combination of specific and nonspecific cellular mechanisms that serve to trigger and maintain skin inflammation.

TARGETING OF Th2-LIKE CELL RESPONSE IN ATOPIC SKIN

Taken together, AD and asthma are both associated with the local infiltration of Th2-like cells, allergen sensitization, the development of chronic local tissue inflammation and the presence of organ-specific (cutaneous vs bronchial) hyperreactivity that may be caused by underlying tissue inflammation. The potential mechanisms that determine tissue specificity of Th2 cell responses in different allergic diseases are therefore of interest. In this regard, studies in experimental animal models have demonstrated heterogeneity in the ability of memory T cells to migrate to mucosal vs nonmucosal tissues. This tissue-selective homing is regulated in large part at the level of T-lymphocyte recognition of vascular endothelial cells (EC) via the interaction of differentially expressed T-lymphocyte homing receptors (HR) and their EC ligands. In humans, lymphocyte/EC adhesion molecule pairs thought to participate in tissue-selective lymphocyte homing include the skin-selective HR, cutaneous lymphoid antigen (CLA), and peripheral lymph node HR, L-selectin.

It has been found that T cells migrating into the skin are highly enriched for the CLA-expressing memory T-cell subset, whereas memory T cells isolated from the airways of asthmatics are predominantly CLA negative. Thus, the propensity of a given individual to develop AD as opposed to asthma may depend on differences in the skin- vs lung-seeking behavior of their memory/effector T cells. Children with food-induced AD provide an opportunity for determining whether there is a relationship between the tissue specificity of a clinical reaction to an allergen and the expression of HR on T cells activated in vitro by the relevant allergen. In this regard, a recent study assessed the expression of CLA and L-selectin on peripheral blood T cells from patients with AD and milk-induced eczema, and compared their HR expression, following stimulation with casein to T cells collected from patients with allergic eosinophilic gastroenteritis, milk-induced enterocolitis, or nonatopic healthy controls. The casein-reactive T cells from patients with milk-induced eczema displayed significantly higher levels of CLA than *Candida albicans*-reactive T cells from the same patients, and either casein- or *C. albicans*-reactive T cells from nonatopic controls or noneczematous atopic patients.

Further evidence for the relationship between CLA and cutaneous T-cell responses in AD has been provided by Babi et al. These investigators analyzed the CLA phenotype of circulating memory T cells in AD vs asthmatic patients who were sensitized with house dust mite. When peripheral blood $CLA^+CD3^+CD45RO^+$ T cells were separated from $CLA^-CD3^+CD45RO^+$ T cells, the mite-specific T-cell proliferation response in patients with AD sensitized to dust mite was localized to CLA^+ T cells. In contrast, mite-sensitive asthmatics had strong mite-dependent proliferation responses in their CLA^- T-cell subset. The link between CLA expression and skin disease-associated T-cell effector function in AD was demonstrated by the observation that freshly isolated circulating CLA^+ T cells in AD patients, but not normal controls, selectively demonstrated spontaneous production of IL-4, but not IFN-γ. These observations strongly support the concept that, in human allergic diseases, immunologic mechanisms exist to target memory Th2 cells to specific organs.

GENETICS OF ATOPIC DERMATITIS AND ATOPY

When the classic studies of Cooke and Van der Veer in 1916 first introduced the concept of allergic sensitization, familial predisposition was considered an important component of these conditions. However, atopy and allergic disorders such as AD are complex genetic diseases that do not follow simple Mendelian inheritance patterns. For atopy and AD, the challenges involved in understanding their genetics include the difficulty of dissecting out the roles of many genes, each with variable degrees of involvement in any given individual. Genetic studies have been difficult because identification of atopic individuals is also confounded by the role of environmental influences. In this regard, atopic, genetically at-risk individuals do not necessarily develop an allergic disease nor are people with allergic disease always carriers of any given disease gene. Nevertheless, there has been considerable progress made in identifying potential genes involved in the inheritance of atopy.

GENETIC STUDIES OF ATOPIC DERMATITIS A familial predisposition to AD as a manifestation of atopy is well-established. Among subjects with AD, 50–67% have a history of either one or both parents having an atopic disorder and the risk of a child developing AD is 25–30% with a history of a single parent with atopy and 50–75% with a dual history. In addition to an inherited predisposition to AD mediated through atopy, additional genetic factors may specifically predispose to the development of dermatitis. An extensive study of allergy in families in Switzerland confirmed that bronchial asthma, allergic rhinitis, and AD were genetically linked. However, the history of respiratory atopic diseases in relatives of probands with AD was significantly lower than that observed for probands with asthma or allergic rhinitis.

Twin studies are a useful means to assess the presence of a genetic contribution in complex genetic diseases in which there are contributions from both genetic and environmental influences. Twins, whether monozygotic (MZ) or dizygotic (DZ), if raised in the same household, share much of the same environmental influences. However, whereas MZ twins have identical genomes, DZ twins on average have only half their chromosomes in common. Thus a higher concordance rate of a given condition in MZ twins provides evidence for the presence of genetic influences. These data provide the information to produce a heritability estimate, an estimate of the relative contributions to a given condition provided by genetic as opposed to environmental factors. The most extensive investigation of twins for AD was the Swedish Twin Study, which identified a concordance rate of AD of 15% in MZ and 5% for DZ twin pairs. Studies of AD in Danish twins found much higher concordance rates for AD but also confirmed a higher rate in MZ (77%) than DZ twins (15%). These authors concluded that genetic factors play a decisive role in the development of AD.

GENETICS OF IgE Genetic studies of AD have been problematic because of variable diagnostic criteria among different studies. The identification of IgE and establishment of its role as the basis for allergic sensitization has provided an improved basis for performing genetic studies of atopy. Both the ability to accurately quantify total IgE and to identify the presence of specific IgE toward a given allergen by either skin testing or serum immunoassays have become objective means for phenotyping atopic subjects.

Twin studies of elevated serum IgE performed by Hopp and Townley in 61 monozygotic twin pairs and 46 dizygotic pairs revealed a heritability estimate of 0.61. Several additional studies have placed the heritability index of serum IgE in at 0.60–0.70. These twin studies unambiguously establish a genetic component to the inheritance of elevated serum IgE. Several additional studies have used segregational analysis to attempt to identify the mechanism for this inheritance. Cookson and Hopkin studied the familial occurrence of elevated IgE in 239 members of 43 families recruited by the presence of an asthmatic proband. Ninety percent of the atopic children had one or more atopic parents. These authors concluded that the high IgE phenotype appeared to be inherited as an autosomal-dominant trait with a variable clinical expression. In contrast, Meyers and Marsh studied the inheritance pattern of total serum IgE and concluded that there was evidence for a major IgE-regulating gene that is inherited via an autosomal-recessive model, but confounded with other familial and polygenetic factors. Their studies demonstrated evidence of this major IgE-regulating gene effect only in some families. Parks et al. studied serum IgE levels from 42 families based on an asthmatic proband and determined that a polygenic heritability model best explained the data. These conflicting results are consistent with either an autosomal recessive gene acting in combination with a polygenic component or, alternatively, the presence of a single major gene that is only operative in some families or ethnic groups, but not in others. Thus, even though it provides a more objective basis for phenotyping subjects, the use of total IgE data in segregational analyses has failed to produce unambiguous conclusions regarding its mechanism of inheritance. This confusion results primarily from the impossibility of controlling for environmental factors that influence serum IgE levels.

LESSONS FROM THE GENETICS OF ASTHMA AND BRONCHIAL HYPERREACTIVITY Similar to the results observed with AD and IgE, genetic studies of asthma have produced conflicting results. As with AD, this also reflects variable diagnostic criteria and the lack of a definitive biochemical or laboratory marker. Edfors-Lubs reviewed nearly 7000 twins in the Swedish Twin Study and reported a diagnosis of asthma in 3.8% of the study population. The concordance rate for asthma was 19% in monozygotic twins and only 4% in dizygotic twins. Most investigators have found higher concordance rates for asthma in twins. Falliers et al. reviewed the literature and reported 30–80% concordance rates for asthma in monozygotic twins and 4–45% in dizygotic twins. As with the IgE studies, these data support a hereditary component in the development of asthma.

More importantly, several studies have now addressed the question of whether asthma is inherited in part separately from atopy. Sibbald recruited asthmatic individuals and investigated the presence of asthma and positive skin tests in the nuclear family. They reported that asthma was more frequent in parents (13%), offspring (9%), and siblings (8%) of the asthmatic probands and there were no significant differences whether or not the subjects were allergic (extrinsic) asthmatics or nonallergic (intrinsic) asthmatics. As would be expected, the prevalence of atopic disorders in general (asthma, allergic rhinitis, or atopic eczema) were higher in the relatives of extrinsic than intrinsic asthmatics. They concluded that asthma and atopy are inherited independently and that the presence of atopy enhances the likelihood of asthma being expressed.

Other studies have investigated the genetics of bronchial hyperreactivity (BHR). Longo et al. performed familial analyses of BHR and documented increased occurrence of BHR in the parents of asthmatic probands. Konig and Godfrey studied exercise challenge and skin-test responses in the nuclear families of 12 children with asthma. A positive exercise challenge developed in 43% of family members and 45% of subjects with at least one positive skin test responded positively. Townley and coworkers found increased BHR in 47 nuclear families of patients with asthma when compared with 26 families with no asthma or family history. Subjects without a personal history of asthma, but from families with a history of asthma, showed bimodal distributions in their BHR, whereas control subjects from families without a history of asthma or allergy had a single uniform distribution. A bimodal distribution was also found in the nonasthmatic parents of asthmatic children. All of these observations supported an inherited component to BHR unrelated to atopy. The segregational analyses of Townley's group supported a genetic component of BHR, but not by a single gene. The consensus of these investigations, however, suggests that in addition to a general susceptibility to the atopic diseases, there may also be a separate inherited tendency to develop asthma. Unfortunately, easily reproductive objective measures of cutaneous hyperreactivity do not exist, but given the parallels between asthma and AD the possibility that cutaneous hyperreactivity may be genetically transmitted in AD must be considered as well.

POSITIONAL CLONING STUDIES OF ATOPIC DISORDERS With diseases such as the atopic disorders for which the responsible gene is unknown, the approach to identifying disease-causing genes frequently utilizes positional cloning. This technique is based on the presence of highly polymorphic markers whose location on the human genome have been mapped. Markers located close to the disease-causing gene will link to the disease when multiple kindreds are analyzed. The frequency of crossover events permits estimation of the distance between the genome marker and the disease gene. Identification of a closely linked marker is followed by "chromosomal walking" until the mutant gene is identified. In the atopic disorders with their variable expression, polygenic inheritance, and the challenges of unambiguously phenotyping subjects, such an approach will be particularly challenging. In addition to all of these previously discussed difficulties that will confound attempts at positional-based cloning, a final challenge is derived from the high frequency of these disorders. This results in the incumbent danger that even though one parent may not be atopic or have an atopic disorder they could still be the carrier of the relevant disease gene.

Despite these difficulties, investigators have utilized positional cloning technology to define the genetic basis for atopy. Cookson and colleagues defined atopic individuals through the presence of either having allergen-specific IgE or a high total serum IgE. Their initial studies of 40 nuclear and 3 extended families was consistent with an autosomal dominant inheritance. Segregational analysis of 7 extended families showed a linkage to the chromosome 11q marker D11S97 and produced a maximal lod score of 5.58. Subsequently, additional studies of 64 families and sib-pair analysis on 743 subjects confirmed this linkage. Analysis of 11q demonstrated that this marker mapped close to the gene for the β chain of the high-affinity IgE receptor. These investigators were able to link atopy to 3 specific amino acid substitutions within the fourth transmembrane hydrophic domain of the β chain. The function of the β chain remains unclear insofar as the α and γ chains are sufficient for transducing activating signals and it is not obvious how the three conservative amino acid substitutions they describe may alter signal transduction. However, it is possible that hydrophobic interactions between transmembrane domains may be critical for proper assembly of the IgE receptor and that, although not necessary for triggering histamine release, the β chain may modulate different signaling pathways. Modulation of cytokine production by a base substitution would be consisting with the biological activity of an asthma gene. Unfortunately, several reports have been unable to confirm these data, although two other groups have confirmed a linkage to this locus The basis for these conflicting results is unclear, except to argue that the development of atopy is a complex genetic process with possibly many genes and pathways leading to the development of the clinical phenotype.

CANDIDATE ATOPIC GENES Because of the difficulties inherent in positional-based cloning strategies, many investigators have opted for an approach based on performing linkage analysis with several specific candidate genes. The basis for this approach is to argue that the genes that cause the atopic disorders are, in fact, known. Specifically, certain proteins may be either abnormally regulated or otherwise function inappropriately to produce atopy and the allergic diseases. These candidate genes include cytokine genes such as *IFN-*γ and *IL-12*, cytokine-receptor genes, the ε heavy-chain gene, the low-affinity receptor for *IgE (FceRII)*, *CD40* and its ligand, and numerous other genes. Additional genes, such as those responsible for increased PGE_2 production and *cyclic AMP-phosphodiesterase* activities are candidate genes more specific for AD. Similarly both the *IL-10* gene and gene(s) controlling its expression may contribute to the diminished cellular immune responses characteristic of this disorder. However, this review will focus on studies of the major histocompatibility complex (MHC) and the cytokine gene complex on chromosome 5.

Linkages have been proposed between MHC class I and class II antigens and both the presence of atopic disease and the specificity of allergen responses. MHC class II alleles are responsible for mediating the genetic component of immune responsiveness to specific antigenic epitopes. Whereas specific MHC alleles have been proposed to link to atopic phenotype, such a linkage has not been well-established. With what is known about the function of the MHC molecules, there is no obvious biochemical basis for the MHC to regulate development of either atopy or an atopic disease. Linkages to MHC are at best likely only to explain a heritable basis for the specific immune response to a given allergenic epitope. Linkages of immune responsiveness to Amb a V and the ryegrass antigens Lol p I and II have been linked to specific *MHC* loci. However, a clinically important role for *MHC* loci in regulating even specific immune responses to allergens is unlikely given the degeneracy of the binding of allergenic epitopes to class II antigens. Thus, both clinical observations and twin studies on the presence of IgE to specific allergens are more consistent with environmental influences (i.e., presence and concentration of antigen) than by genetic factors.

Several other genes have proved to be better candidates for inducing atopy and allergic diseases. These include numerous genes that regulate IgE production, eosinophilia, and mast-cell proliferation. A surprising number of these genes are clustered on the long arm of chromosome 5, between 5q22 and 5q31. This cluster includes the genes for *ILs-3, -4, -5, -9, -13,* and *GM-CSF*. *IL-4* and *IL-13* are responsible for initiation of ε germline transcription, which in combination with signals generated by CD40 acting through the CD40 ligand leads to the IgE isotype switch. IL-5 is an eosinophilopoietin and is an activating factor for mature eosinophils. Additional factors contributing to eosinophil activation and survival are GM-CSF and IL-3. Proliferation and increased releasability of mast cells is a characteristic feature of atopic diseases and represents a T-cell–dependent process. Within this cluster, both IL-3 and IL-9 function as mast cell growth and differentiating factors, whereas IL-3 also enhances histamine release. Of these genes *IL-4, IL-13,* and *IL-5*, as well as *IL-3* and *GM-CSF* are particularly tightly linked, separated by only approximately 300 kbp.

To some extent, these genes are under shared regulatory control. Thus, GM-CSF, IL-3, IL-4, and IL-5 have all been identified at the sites of allergic reactions. The transcriptional dysregulation of these cytokines may be the basis for the atopic state. Thus, when T-lymphocyte clones are generated towards the dust mite allergen, the clones from atopic donors are characterized by the transcriptional activation of IL-4, whereas those obtained from nonatopic donors are characterized by IFN-γ and IL-2, but not IL4. That genes in close proximity may be coregulated has been observed for several other gene clusters such as has been described for the IL-1 gene cluster (*IL-1a, IL-1b,* and *IL-1ra*) and the *MHC complex*. Such coregulation does not preclude the possibility that under appropriate conditions one or more genes may be transcribed nonsynchronously.

It has therefore been proposed that regulatory elements associated with these genes may be responsible for inducing the atopic state, that these elements may be linked to specific chromosomal markers, and, therefore, that the genetic predisposition to atopy can be identified by the presence of these markers. Two groups have now reported their results utilizing linkage analyses of polymorphisms present on chromosome 5q to asthma or elevated serum IgE. Marsh et al. analyzed 170 individuals from 11 extended Amish families by sib-pair analysis. Utilizing a series of markers within the region 5q31.1 these authors found evidence for genetic linkages to high IgE phenotype for five markers within a narrow region (1.4 cM) of 5q31.1. No linkage was found to specific IgE. Similar results were obtained by Bleeckers' group in a study of 92 nuclear families from northern Holland. Via sib-pair analyses these investigators demonstrated highly significant linkages to both total IgE and to bronchial hyperreactivity with three markers within the chromosome 5q31.1 cytokine gene cluster. In summary, although much work remains to elucidate the genetics of atopic diseases such as AD and asthma, several potential genes have been identified and this is likely to be an exciting area of investigation in the future.

MANAGEMENT OF AD

Current treatment of AD is directed at symptom relief and reduction of cutaneous inflammation and the reduction of exacerbating factors are critical for effective management. Factors that must be considered and eliminated include irritants, allergens, and emotional stresses. Systemic antimicrobial therapy, particular antistaphylococcal antibiotics, is often necessary because AD skin has enhanced binding properties for *S. aureus* and, because of the frequent scratching, becomes secondarily infected. Maintenance of daily skin care with hydration of the skin and appropriate use of topical steroids to reduce skin inflammation is critical. Therapy must be individualized and is dependent on whether the patient is experiencing an acute flare or dealing with the management of chronic AD.

For patients who are poorly controlled on conventional therapy, alternative therapies should be considered. Ultraviolet light therapy may be a useful adjunctive therapeutic modality. Under professional supervision, UVB can be effective and has been found to have antiinflammatory effects in part because of its ability to inhibit lymphocyte trafficking and antigen-processing. Photochemotherapy with oral psoralen therapy followed by UVA (PUVA) may also be helpful in patients with severe disease. However, PUVA is reserved for patients with more recalcitrant disease because of the expense, and the potential increased risk of skin cancer.

Since patients with AD manifest abnormalities in immune regulation, therapy directed toward correction of their immune dysfunction represents an alternative approach. In this regard, therapeutic trials using several experimental immunomodulators or immunosuppressive agents have been reported. IFN-γ, a cytokine that downregulates Th2-cell function, has been found in placebo-controlled trials to reduce clinical severity associated with AD and decrease total circulating eosinophil counts. Cyclosporine, a drug that downregulates cytokine production, has also been reported in double-blind, placebo-controlled trials to cause a significant improvement in AD. Cyclosporine therapy did, however, lead to mild renal and liver toxicity. Thus, the side effects associated with prolonged systemic cyclosporine therapy make it an unlikely candidate for chronic treatment of AD. Of note, FK506, an analog of cyclosporine, has recently been used topically in clinical trials and found to be efficacious with no significant side effects. In addition, the new high-potency phosphodiesterase inhibitors may be useful in targeting the increased PDE activity in atopic monocytes and have demonstrated promising preliminary clinical results.

FUTURE DIRECTIONS

The current review has attempted to highlight several important advances in our understanding of the immunopathogenesis of AD. These include the observation that IgE has a multifunctional role in the pathogenesis of allergic inflammation. Aside from its involvement in IgE-mediated degranulation of mast cells/basophils, it is also involved in the activation of macrophage/monocytes and the stimulation of Th2 cells. Many of the critical cytokines involved in the pathogenesis of AD and the potentially important mechanisms by which inflammation occurs at the sites of allergic responses have now been identified. These important new advances will allow scientists in the future to target certain candidate genes to determine whether their abnormal regulation or altered function contributes to the molecular basis of atopy. Elucidation of the key genes involved in atopy is likely to provide new methods for classifying atopic diseases, particularly with respect to diagnosis, disease severity, and possibly response to therapy. Considering the complexity of multiple genes involved in atopy it is difficult to envision the use of gene therapy in the foreseeable future.

Novel immunologic therapies for chronic allergic diseases are likely to include the modulation of Th2 cells and their cytokines targeting specific organs. Recent studies with experimental immunomodulatory and immunosuppressive agents are promising and serve as proof of the concept that therapies that downregulate T-cell function and cytokine secretion are effective in reducing the clinical severity of AD. As our understanding of the immunopathogenesis of allergic responses continues to grow, manipulation of the immune response in AD and other allergic diseases is likely to become an exciting new direction in the treatment of this fascinating group of illnesses.

ACKNOWLEDGMENTS

The author would like to thank Maureen Sandoval for her assistance in the preparation of this manuscript. Supported in part by NIH grants AR 41256, RR00051, and HL36577.

SELECTED REFERENCES

Abernathy-Carver KJ, Sampson HA, Picker LJ, Leung DYM. Milk-induced eczema is associated with the expansion of T cells expressing cutaneous lymphocyte antigen. J Clin Invest 1995;95:913–918.

Babi LFS, Picker LJ, Soler MTP. Circulating allergen-reactive T cells from patients with atopic dermatitis and allergic contact dermatitis express the skin-selective homing receptor the cutaneous lymphocyte-associated antigen (CLA). J Exp Med 1995;181:1935–1940.

Bieber T, de la Salle H, Wollenberg A, et al. Human epidermal Langerhans cells express the high affinity receptor for immunoglobulin E (FcεRI). J Exp Med 1992;175:1285–1290.

Blumenthal M, Mendell N and Yunis E. Immunogenetics of atopic diseases. J Allergy Clin Immunol 1980;65:403–405.

Bochner BS, Klunk DA, Sterbinsky SA, Coffman RL, Schleimer RP. IL-13 selectively induces vascular cell adhesion molecule-1 expression in human endothelial cells. J Immunol 1995;154:799–803.

Chan SC, Hanifin JM. Immunopharmacologic aspects of atopic dermatitis. Clin Rev Allergy 1993;11:523–542.

Chandrasekharappa SC, Rebelsky MS, Firak TA, LeBeau MM, Westbrook CA. A long-range restriction map of the interleukin-4 and interleukin-5 linkage group on chromosome 5. Genomics 1990;6:94–99.

Collee JM, de Vries HG, Gerritsen J. Allele sharing on chromosome 11q13 in sibs with asthma. Lancet 1993;ii:936.

Cooke RA, van der Veer A. Human sensitization. J Immunol 1916;1:201–305.

Cookson WOCM, Hopkin JM. Dominant inheritance of atopic immunoglobulin E responsiveness. Lancet 1988;1:86–88.

Cookson W, Sharp PA, Faux JA, Hopkin JM. Linkage between immunoglobulin E responses underlying asthma and rhinitis and chromosome 11q. Lancet: 1989;1:1292–1295.

Cooper KD. New therapeutic approaches in atopic dermatitis. Clin Rev Allergy 1993;11:543–560.

Edfors-Lubs MI. Allergy in 7000 twin pairs. Acta Allergol (Kbh) 1971;26:207–219.

Falliers CI, de A Cardoso RR, Bane HN, et al. Discordant allergic manifestations in monozygotic twins: genetic identify versus clinical, physiologic, and biochemical differences. Allergy 1971;47:207–219.

Hamid Q, Boguniewicz M, Leung DYM. Differential *in situ* cytokine gene expression in acute vs. chronic atopic dermatitis. J Clin Invest 1994;94:870–876.

Hanifin JM, Rajka G. Diagnostic features of atopic dermatitis. Acta Derm Venereol 1980;92:44–47.

Hill LW, Sulzberger MB. Yearbook of Dermatology and Syphilology. Chicago: Year Book Medical Publisher, 1933; pp. 1–70.

Hopp RJ, Bewtra AK, Watt GD, Nair NM, Townley RG. Genetic analysis of allergic disease in twins. J Allergy Clin Immunol 1984;73:265–270.

Jones SM, Sampson HA. The role of allergens in atopic dermatitis. Clin Rev Allergy 1993;11:471–490.

Kay AM, Ying S, Varney V, et al. Messenger RNA expression of cytokine gene cluster, interleukin 3 (IL-3), IL-5, and granulocyte/macrophage colony-stimulating factor, in allergen-induced late-phase cutaneous reactions in atopic subjects. J Exp Med 1991;173:775–778.

Konig P, Godfrey S. Prevalence of exercise-induced bronchial liability in families of children with asthma. Arch Dis Child 1973;48:513–518.

Lacour M, Hauser C. The role of microorganisms in atopic dermatitis. Clin Rev Allergy 1993;11:491–522.

Lee SK, Metrakos JD, Tanaka KR, Heiner DC. Genetic influence on serum IgE levels. Pediatr Res 1980;14:60–63.

Leung DYM, Geha RS. Clinical and immunologic aspects of the hyper IgE syndrome. In: Hematology Oncology Clinics of North America. Philadelphia: Saunders, 1988; pp. 81–100.

Leung DYM, Travers JB, Norris DA. Superantigens in skin disease. J Invest Dermatol 1995;105:37S–42S.

Leung DYM, Harbeck R, Bina P, Hanifin JM, Reiser RF, Sampson HA. Presence of IgE antibodies to staphylococcal exotoxins on the skin of patients with atopic dermatitis: evidence for a new group of allergens. J Clin Invest 1993;92:1374–1380.

Leung DYM. Atopic dermatitis: the skin as a window into the pathogenesis of chronic allergic diseases. J Allergy Clin Immunol 1995;96:302–319.

Leung DYM, Rhodes AR, Geha RS, Schneider L, Ring J. Atopic dermatitis. In: Fitzpatrick TB, Eisen AZ, Wolff K, Freeberg IM, Austen KF, eds. Dermatology in General Medicine. New York: McGraw-Hill, 1993; pp. 1543–1564.

Longo G, Strinati R, Puli F, Fumi F. Genetic factors in nonspecific bronchial hyperreactivity. Am J Dis Child 1987;141:331–334.

Lympany P, Welsh K, MacCochrane G, Kemeny DM, Lee TH. Genetic analysis using DNA polymorphism of the linkage between chromosome 11q13 and atopy and bronchial hyperresponsiveness to methacholine. J Allergy Clin Immunol 1992;89:619–628.

Marsh D, Hsu SH, Roebber M, et al. HLA-Dw2—a genetic marker for human immune response to short ragweed allergen RAS: I. Response resulting primarily from natural antigenic exposure. J Exp Med 1982;155:1439–1451.

Marsh DG, Neely JD, Breazeale DR, et al. Linkage analysis of IL-4 and other chromosome 5q31.1 markers and total serum immunoglobulin E concentrations. Science 1994;264:1152–1156.

May CE. Objective clinical laboratory studies of immediate hypersensitivity reactions to foods in asthmatic children. J Allergy Clin Immunol 1976;58:500–515.

Meyers D, Marsh D. Report on a national institute of allergy and infectious diseases sponsored workshop on the genetics of total immunoglobulin E levels in humans. J Allergy Clin Immunol 1981;67: 167–170.

Moffatt MF, Sharp PA, Faux JA, Young RP, Cookson WOCM, Hopkin JM. Factors confounding genetic linkage between atopy and chromosome 11q. Clin Exp Allergy 1992;22:1046–1051.

Mosmann TR, Cherwinski H, Bond MW, Giedlin MH, Coffman R. Two types of murine helper T cell clones. I. Definition according to profiles of lymphokine activities and secretory proteins. J Immunol 1986;136: 2348–2357.

Mudde GC, Van Reijsen FC, Boland GJ, DeGast GC, Bruijnzeel PLB, Bruijnzeel-Koomen CAFM. Allergen presentation by epidermal Langerhans cells from patients with atopic dermatitis is mediated by IgE. Immunology 1990;69:335–341.

Parks T, Felix K, Rice T, Subbarao PV, Marimuthu KM, Rao DC. A genetic study of immunoglobulin E and atopic disease based on families ascertained through asthmatic children. Hum Hered 1990;40:69–76.

Patore S, Fanales-Belasio E, Albanesi C, Chinni LM, Giannetti A, Girolomoni G. Granulocyte macrophage colony-stimulating factor is overproduced by keratinocytes in atopic dermatitis. Implications for sustained dendritic cell activation in the skin. J Clin Invest 1997;99: 3009–3017.

Postma DS, Bleecker ER, Amelung PJ, et al. Genetic susceptibility to asthma- bronchial hyperresponsiveness coinherited with a major gene for atopy. N Engl J Med 1995;333:894–900.

Rich SS, Roitman-Johnson B, Greenberg B, Roberts S, Blumenthal MN. Genetic analysis of atopy in three large kindreds; no evidence of linkage to D11S97. Clin Exp Allergy 1992;22:1070–1076.

Schnyder UW. Neurodermititis—Asthma—Rhintis. Eine genetisch-allergologisch studie. Acta Genet Stat Med 1960;10(Suppl 18):1–106.

Schultz Larsen F, Holm NV, Henningsen K. Atopic dermatitis. A genetic-epidemiologic study in a population-based twin sample. J Am Acad Dermatol 1986;15:487–494.

Shirakawa TS, Li A, Dubowitz M, et al. Association between atopy and variants of the β-subunit of the high affinity Immunoglobulin E receptor. Nat Genet 1994;7:124–129.

Shirakawa TS, Morimoto K, Hashimoto T, Furuyama J. Linkage between severe atopy and chromosome 11q in Japanese families. Clin Genet 1994;46:228–232.

Sibbald B. Extrinsic and intrinsic asthma: influence of classification on family history of asthma and allergic disease. Clin Allergy 1980;10: 313–318.

Sistonen P, Johnsson V, Koskenvuo M, Aho K. Serum IgE levels in twins. Hum Hered 1980;30:155–158.

Townley RG, Bewtra AK, Nair NM, Brodkey FD, Watt GD, Burke KM. Methacholine inhalation challenge studies. J Allergy Clin Immunol 1979;64:569–574.

Tsicopoulous A, Hamid Q, Varney V, et al. Preferential messenger RNA expression of Th1-type cells (IFN-γ+, IL-2+) in classical delayed-type (tuberculin) hypersensitivity reactions in human skin. J Immunol 1992;148:2058–2061.

Vercelli D, Geha RS. Regulation of IgE synthesis: from membrane to the genes. Springer Semin Immunopathol 1993;15:5–16.

Vercelli D, Jabara HH, Lee B, Woodland N, Geha RS, Leung DYM. Human recombinant interleukin-4 induces FcεR$_2$/CD23 on normal human monocytes. J Exp Med 1988;167:1406–1416.

88 Pemphigus Foliaceus and Pemphigus Vulgaris

JANET A. FAIRLEY, XIANG DING, GEORGE J. GIUDICE, AND LUIS A. DIAZ

BACKGROUND

Pemphigus is a group of autoimmune disorders characterized by spontaneous intraepidermal blisters and epidermal-specific autoantibodies. Blister formation occurs by the histologically distinctive loss of epidermal cell–cell adhesion, termed acantholysis. The two major forms of the disease are pemphigus vulgaris (PV) and pemphigus foliaceus (PF). In PV, the epidermal-cell separation occurs just above the basal layer of the epidermis, whereas, in PF, the cell separation occurs at the more superficial level of the granular-cell layer of the epidermis. Although PV and PF are diseases described all over the world, there is an endemic form of PF that has been observed in Brazil since the turn of the century and recently in Colombia. This endemic form of PF is also known as "fogo selvagem" (FS; wild fire). Prior to the advent of immunosuppressive therapy, the mortality caused by these disorders was extremely high.

The histological hallmark of PV and PF, epidermal-cell detachment, has been known since the early 1940s. However it was not until the mid-1960s that a new insight into the pathogenesis of these disorders was gained with the discovery of PV and PF antiepidermal autoantibodies. The following years confirmed the diagnostic value of these autoantibodies and also brought convincing experimental data linking the epidermal-cell detachment seen in these patients with binding of antiepidermal autoantibodies to their target antigens. The true autoimmune nature of PV and PF was tested experimentally, addressing both the autoantibody side as well as the autoantigen side of the reaction. The autoantibody titers in patients were found to correlate well with disease activity and currently are used to follow the therapeutic response of these patients. It was also documented that neonates born to PV mothers presented a blistering disease probably caused by transplacental passage of maternal autoantibodies. These clinical observations suggested a pathogenic role for PV autoantibodies. Experimentally, it was found that the IgG fractions from PV and PF sera promoted cell detachment in primary epidermal-cell cultures and in organ cultures of human skin. In the early 1980s, other studies convincingly demonstrated that PV and PF autoantibodies were indeed pathogenic. In these experiments intraperitoneal injections of the IgG fraction of PV and PF sera were shown to induce intraepidermal blisters in neonatal mice. The injected animals duplicated the key clinical and histological features of the human diseases.

From: *Principles of Molecular Medicine* (J. L. Jameson, ed.), ©1998 Humana Press Inc., Totowa, NJ.

The search for epidermal antigens recognized by PV and PF autoantibodies lead to the characterization of those molecules as components of the desmosome. It had previously been established that desmosomes contain transmembrane glycoproteins and plaque proteins. The desmosomal glycoproteins were characterized as desmoglein 1 (Dsg1, 165 kDa), desmoglein 2 (identified in colonic epithelium), desmoglein 3 (Dsg3, 130 kDa mol wt), and the desmocollins. Furthermore, it is currently accepted that these glycoproteins are members of the cadherin family of cell adhesion molecules. PV and PF autoantibodies recognized calcium-dependent conformational epitopes on the extracellular domain of Dsg3 and Dsg1, respectively (Fig. 88-1).

Finally, PF, and less commonly PV, may also be triggered by medications, most commonly penicillamine. However, captopril, penicillin, ampicillin, and rifampin have also been associated with pemphigus-like eruptions. A paraneoplastic form of pemphigus has been recently reported associated in a great number of cases with underlying lymphoproliferative disorders. The autoantibody response in these patients is complex and directed against desmosomal and hemidesmosomal antigens.

CLINICAL FEATURES

PV is the most common form of pemphigus in the United States and is characterized by the spontaneous development of blisters arising on normal appearing skin (Fig. 88-2A). The lesions are typically flaccid bullae that rupture easily, producing denuded areas of skin and erosions that are slow to heal. The disease usually begins in the oral mucosa, where, because of the fragility of the blisters, the predominant lesions are erosions. Though the oral mucosa is the most common site of involvement, the disease may affect other squamous epithelium including the esophagus, conjunctiva, larynx, vagina, urethra, cervix, and rectum. The disease may remain localized to the mucosae, but generally progresses over a period of months to involve the glabrous skin. The onset of disease is most commonly between the fourth and sixth decade of life, however any age group may be affected.

PF has a different clinical appearance than PV, exhibiting superficial vesicles that rupture easily, producing erosions and crusting (Fig. 88-3A). The skin lesions in PF appear most commonly on the head and neck regions. In chronic cases, these excori-

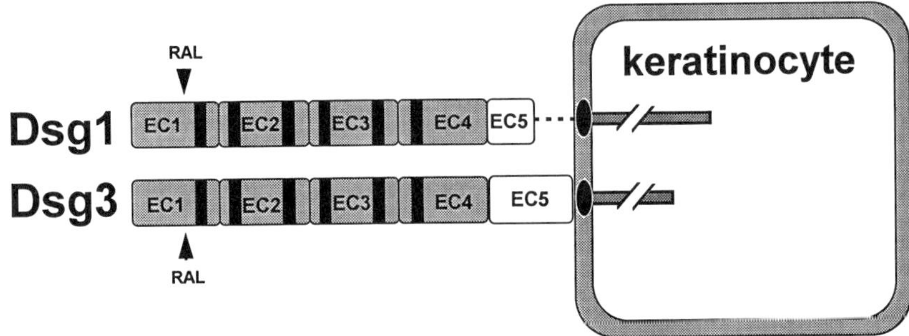

Figure 88-1 Schematic of Dsg1 and Dsg3. Dsg1 and Dsg3 are both transmembrane proteins with an intracellular, extracellular domain, and a single transmembrane domain. The extracellular domains of both Dsg1 and Dsg3 contain four cadherins repeats (EC1-4). Within the cadherin repeats, the black bars represent calcium-binding sites, and the RAL is the putative cell–cell recognition site.

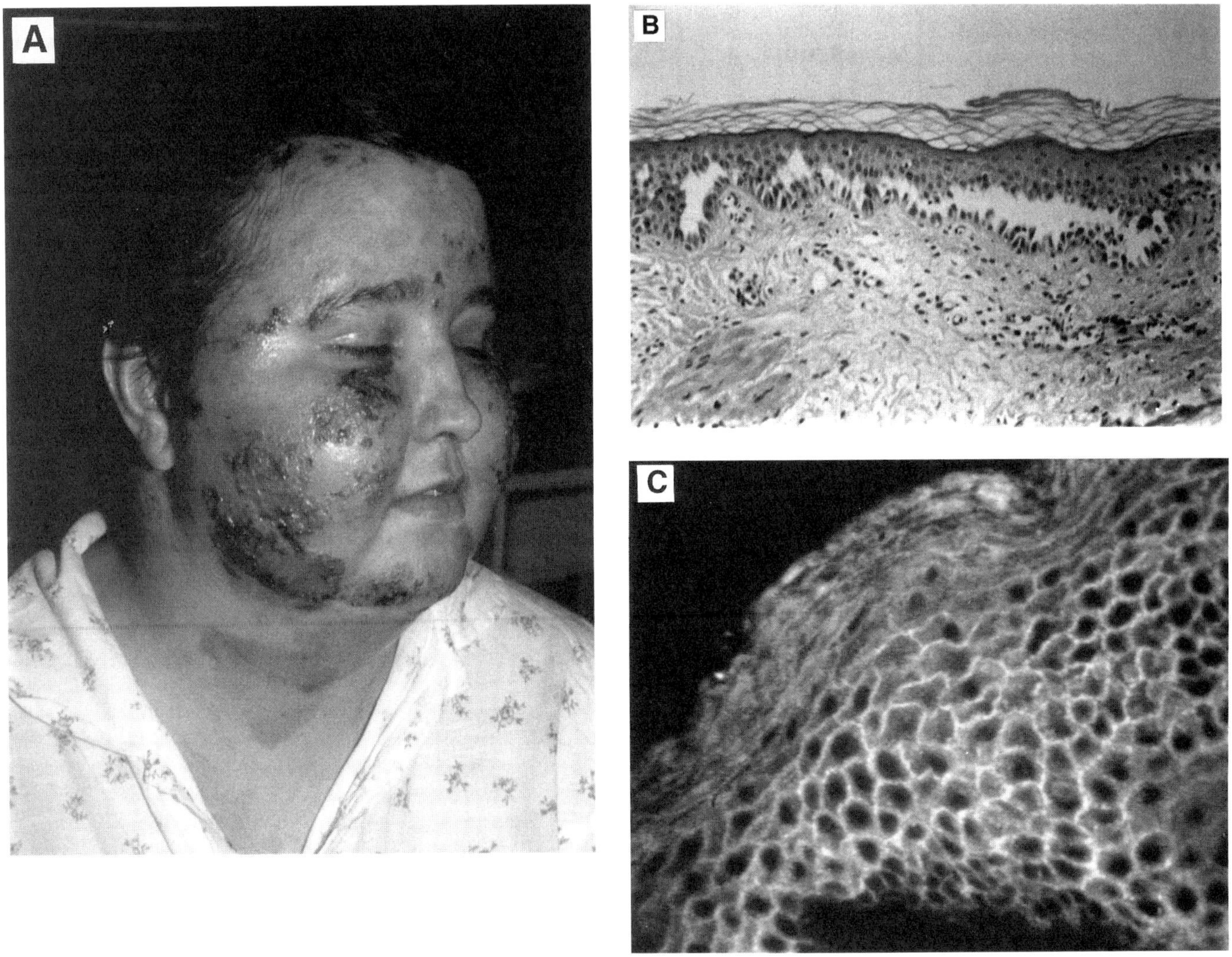

Figure 88-2 Clinical, histologic, and immunologic features of PV. PV patients typically have flaccid blisters and erosions that can become widespread **(A)**. Histologically, biopsies of PV show suprabasilar acantholysis, with the retention of the basal cells on the dermis **(B)**. Patients have both tissues-bound and circulating autoantibodies directed against the cell surface of the keratinocyte. **(C)** The results of indirect IF performed with PV serum using monkey esophagus as a substrate.

ated lesions may become more hyperkeratotic, verrucous, or vegetating plaques. In other cases, the disease may progress to an exfoliative erythroderm. In contrast to PV, the mucous membranes are spared. The clinical, immunological and histologic features of endemic PF are identical to sporadic nonendemic PF.

DIAGNOSIS

The diagnosis of pemphigus is based on clinical, histologic, and immunologic criteria. Biopsies from the lesional skin of patients with PV reveals intraepidermal vesicles occurring just above the basal-cell layer. Basal keratinocytes remain attached to

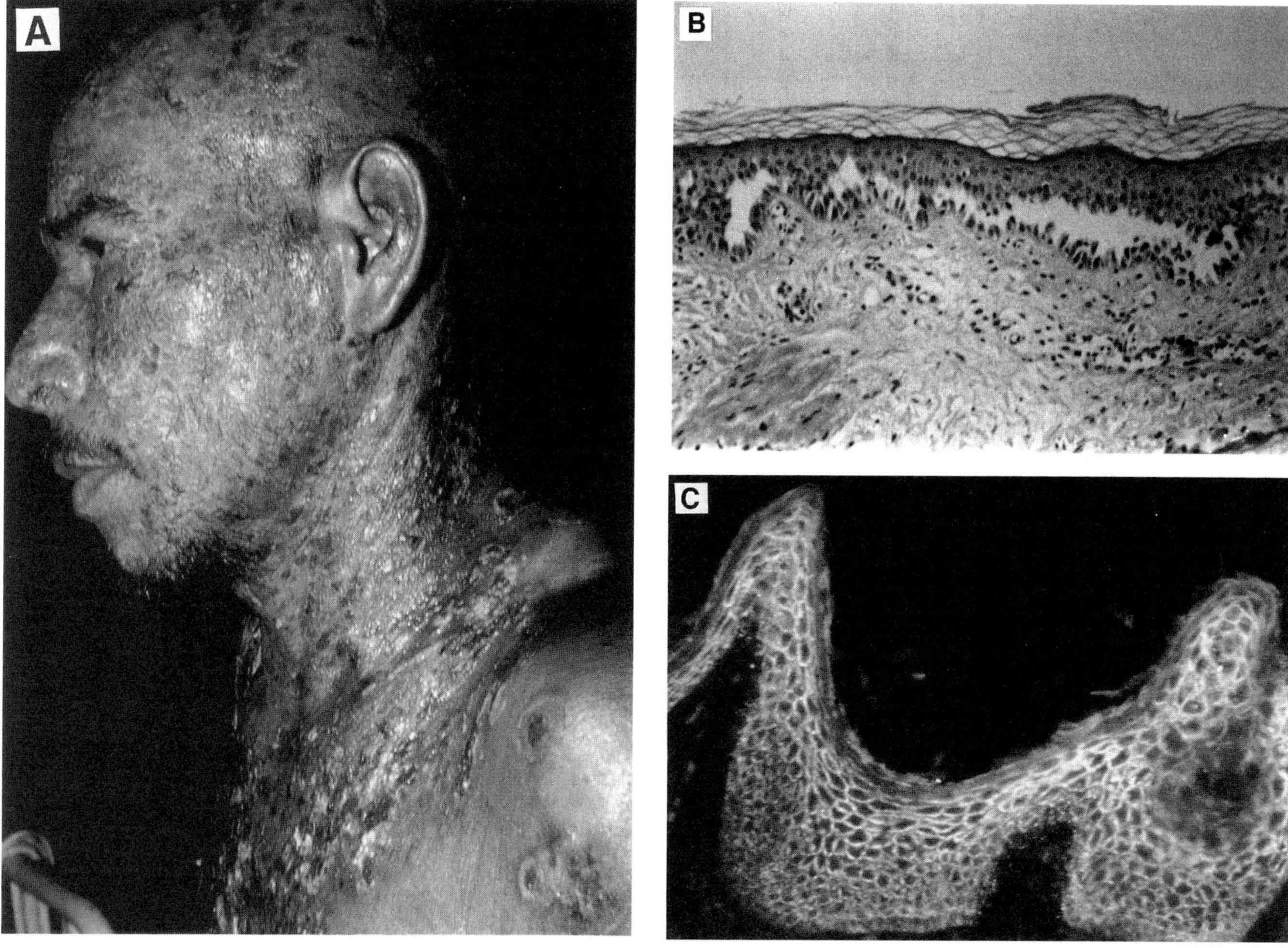

Figure 88-3 Clinical, histologic, and immunologic features of PF. This patient with endemic PF has widespread erosions and crusting on the head and neck (**A**). A skin biopsy specimen shows an intraepidermal vesicle occurring in the granular-cell layer (**B**). Indirect IF of this patient's serum shows ICS staining, using human skin as a substrate (**C**).

the dermis, producing the histological "tombstone" sign (Fig. 88-2B). The dermis may show edema and inflammation with the presence of eosinophils in early lesions, and plasma cells in older lesions. The histology of PF also shows intraepidermal vesicles, but occurring high in the epidermis, within or just below the granular-cell layer (Fig. 88-3B). Older lesions of PF may also show hyperkeratosis and thickening of the epidermis.

Immunofluorescence (IF) studies are extremely helpful in confirming the diagnosis of pemphigus. Direct IF, performed on perilesional biopsies shows typical deposition of IgG and/or C3 in the epidermal intercellular spaces (ICS) in 100% of patients with active disease. Indirect IF studies of patients' sera demonstrate circulating autoantibodies that produce an ICS staining pattern on stratified squamous epithelial substrates. Indirect IF tests yield positive results in 80–90% of patients with active disease. Though occasionally PF autoantibodies may bind preferentially to the upper layers of the epidermis, and PV autoantibodies more suprabasilarly, in general the two disorders cannot be differentiated on the basis of indirect or direct IF (Figs. 88-2C and 88-3C). In the majority of patients, the serum autoantibody titers correlate well with extent and disease activity.

Recent advances in the characterization of the antigens recognized by PV and PF autoantibodies have led to the application of other techniques to precisely diagnose these disorders. Immunoblotting and immunoprecipitation have defined the PV antigen as Dsg3, a glycoprotein of 130 kDa and the PF antigen as a 160-kDa glycoprotein, Dsg1. Specialized laboratories can perform immunoblotting and immunoprecipitation (or ELISA) techniques to test patients' sera. A positive result by immunoprecipitation is seen only in PF and PV sera if assayed with recombinant antigens (Dsg3 or Dsg1).

GENETIC BASIS OF DISEASE

Like many other human autoimmune diseases, PV and PF have been associated with certain HLA specificities. Since there is a high frequency of PV cases in the Ashkenazi Jewish background population, the HLA associations have been examined in two groups: Jewish and non-Jewish PV patients. The Jewish group shares the (HLA-B38, SC21, DR4, DQw8) and (HLA-B35, SC31, DR4, Dqw8) extended haplotype, whereas the non-Jewish group share the (HLA Bw55, Drw6, SB45, Dqw5) extended haplotype. These susceptibility alleles are thought to be inherited as a dominant trait in the Jewish group of PV patients. HLA studies have demonstrated that FS is associated with a high frequency of HLA DR1 and/or HLA D4 genes. Moreover, FS patients appear to possess the DRB1*0102 gene as a susceptibility factor (relative risk

[RR] = 7.3, $p = 0.002$) and DQB1*0201 as a gene that confers resistance to FS (RR = 0.04, $p = 0.006$). Recently it has been shown that these alleles are not present in Brazilian Indians affected by FS. Instead, 6 out of 10 Indians of the Xavante tribe with FS shared the HLA DRB1*0404 gene that was present in only 5 out of 74 of the Xavante controls, conferring a RR of 9.6 ($p = 0.002$). These findings have been confirmed recently in other Brazilian Indian tribes. It is interesting to note that the amino acid sequence of residues 67–74 of the third hypervariable region of the DRB1 gene, i.e., LLEQRRAA, is shared by DRB1*0102 (susceptibility gene of non-Indian FS patients) and DRB1*0404, DRB1*1402, and/or DRB1*1406 found with increased frequency in FS patients occurring in Brazilian Indians.

MOLECULAR PATHOPHYSIOLOGY OF DISEASE

Following the experimental demonstration that PV and PF autoantibodies are pathogenic in the mouse model system (Figs. 88-4 and 88-5), efforts were concentrated in dissecting the molecular mechanisms leading to acantholysis. It has been well-established that PV and PF autoantibodies induce epidermal-cell detachment in the mouse model independent of complement activation, i.e., C5-deficient strains of mice and neonatal mice depleted of complement by cobra-venom treatment continue to develop extensive blistering disease when passively transfused with PF or PV IgG fractions. Furthermore, in a series of studies we have demonstrated that F(ab')2 and Fab fragments from PF and PV IgG are also pathogenic, suggesting that these autoantibodies may trigger cell detachment by simple binding to their target epitopes on the ectodomain of Dsg1 and Dsg3, respectively. This binding may impair the adhesive function of these molecules. Other potential mechanisms involved in pemphigus acantholysis have been suggested. For example, it has been reported that activation of keratinocyte plasminogen activator (PA) by PV and PF autoantibodies may trigger epidermal-cell detachment. This hypothesis was reinforced by detecting elevated values of PA in epidermal-cell cultures treated with PV or PF IgG. This elevation was abolished by previous treatment of the cultures with dexamethasone, which also abolishes the pathogenic effect of these antibodies. However, this finding could not be reproduced in vivo using the mouse model system. Recently other hypotheses have been put forward, i.e., that PV and PF autoantibodies may bind the keratinocyte surface domain of Dsg1 or Dsg3 and trigger intracellular responses leading to collapse of the cytoskeleton and impairment of cell adhesiveness. These theories need further experimental testing.

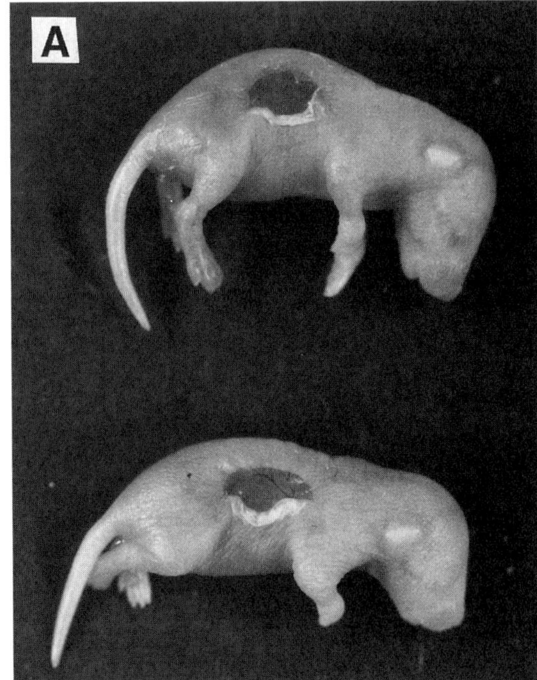

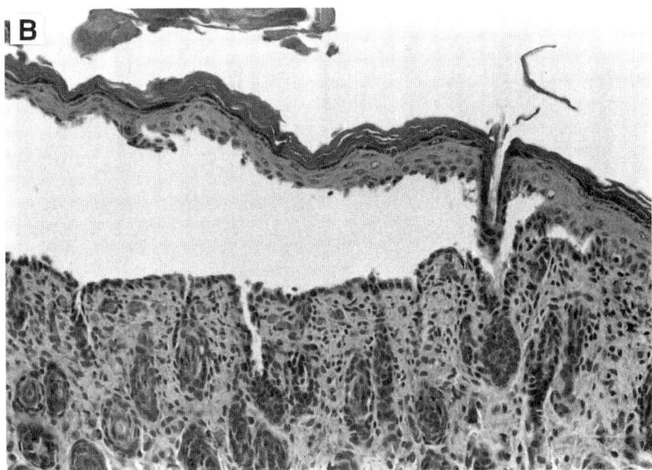

Figure 88-4 Passive-transfer mouse model of PV. Neonatal BALB/c mice injected with purified IgG from PV patient's sera reproduced the clinical (**A**), histologic (**B**), and immunologic features of the disease.

Mapping the epitopes recognized by pathogenic PV and PF autoantibodies on Dsg3 and Dsg1 has been hampered by the conformational nature of these regions of the molecules. Furthermore, it appears that the calcium-binding domains of the extracellular regions of Dsg1 and Dsg3 also modulate the optimal recognition and binding of autoantibodies. However the availability of the cDNAs of both desmogleins have opened new approaches to further analyze these conformational epitopes. For example, in recent studies the cDNAs of Dsg1 and Dsg3 have been expressed in the baculovirus system as soluble glycoproteins that are highly immunoreactive with patients' sera. Autoantibodies to Dsg3 have been purified by affinity chromatography from patients' sera utilizing full-length recombinant Dsg3 and shown to be pathogenic in the mouse system. Moreover, preadsorption of patients' sera with recombinant Dsg3 will abrogate the pathogenic effect in the passive-transfer experiments. These studies prove convincingly that anti-Dsg3 autoantibodies in PV sera are indeed pathogenic and responsible for inducing the lesions in PV patients. Similarly, Dsg1 recombinant protein produced in the baculovirus system has been used to immunoadsorb PF autoantibodies. Like in the PV cases, it has been demonstrated that anti-Dsg1 autoantibodies are pathogenic and responsible for inducing the disease in patients.

Both Dsg1 and Dsg3 share common features with the cadherin family of cell adhesion molecules. Dsg1 and Dsg3 are both transmembrane proteins that have an N-terminal extracellular domain and an intracellular C-terminal domain. The extracellular region contains a series of five repeat domains, termed EC1 to EC5 (Fig. 88-1). The first four of these domains are homologous cadherin repeats. A series of three pairs of calcium-binding sites are also located within these first four extracellular domains. These calcium-binding sites have been hypothesized to be crucial in cell–cell adhesion, and also appear to be important in autoantibody

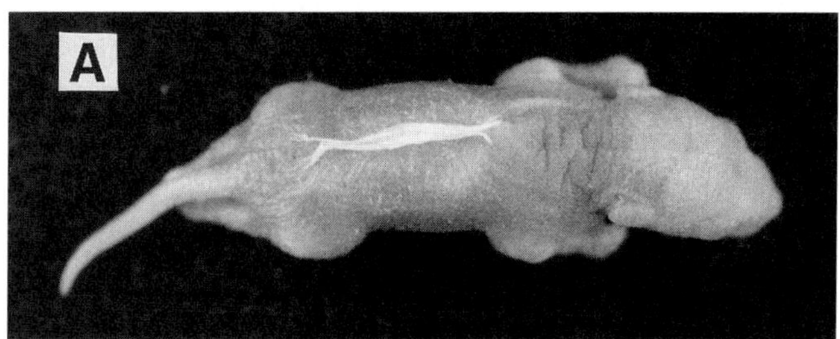

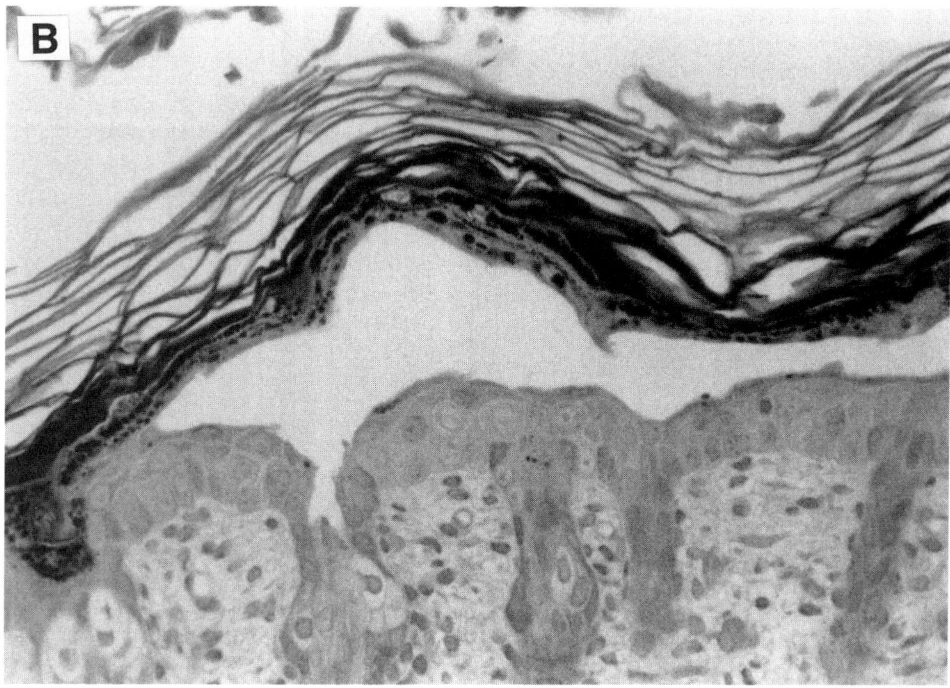

Figure 88-5 Passive-transfer mouse model of PF. Injection of purified IgG from the serum of a PF patient produces superficial erosions in neonatal BALB/c mice (**A**). A biopsy shows acantholysis in the granular-cell layer of the epidermis (**B**).

recognition. A three-amino acid sequence near the amino terminus (RAL) is the putative cell–cell recognition site. The region just outside the transmembrane domain (EC5) shows the greatest divergence between Dsg1 and Dsg3, as a portion of this region is deleted in Dsg1. The importance of the intracellular domain is its function in integrating the desmosomal proteins with the cytoskeleton. Within desmosomes, the 93-kDa desmosomal plaque protein, plakoglobin, is believed to be crucial in linking desmosomes with the cytoskeleton. Plakoglobin is part of both the PV and PF complex, and is believed to directly bind to both Dsg1 and Dsg3.

The genes for both Dsg1 and Dsg3 are located on chromosome 18. *In situ* hybridization and immunofluorescence have been used to localize Dsg1 and Dsg3 in the epidermis. Dsg3 is expressed more strongly in the basal and lower spinous layers of the epidermis, whereas Dsg1 was expressed throughout the epidermis, but appeared to gradually increase during differentiation. This difference in the site of expression of Dsg1 and Dsg3 in the epidermis may help to explain the level at which blistering occurs in PF in comparison to PV.

MANAGEMENT/TREATMENT

Despite the tremendous advances in understanding the molecular pathogenesis of PV and PF, the mainstay of treatment remains corticosteroids and immunosuppressive agents. Prior to immunosuppressive therapy, the 5-year mortality of PV approached 100%. The prognosis in PF was slightly better, with a 40–60% mortality rate. In recent years, despite the effective steroid and immunosuppressive therapy, the 5-year mortality remains between 5 and 15%. In mild cases, ultrapotent topical or intralesional steroids may be of value; however, the vast majority of cases will require systemic glucocorticoids. Prednisone is the most commonly used steroid, with an initial dose of approximately 1 mg/kg/d. If no response is seen, this may be increased to 1.5–2 mg/kg/d, not to exceed 100–120 mg/d in our experience. A slow tapering is required to prevent relapse of the disease. Cytotoxic agents, including azathioprine, cyclophosphamide, and methotrexate may be used as the sole therapeutic agents in patients in whom steroids are contraindicated, but more commonly are used in conjunction with prednisone as steroid-sparing agents. The dose of azathioprine and cyclophosphamide is 1–2 mg/kg/d, and 5–15 mg/wk for methotrexate.

Plasmapheresis may be used as a adjunct therapy in patients with refractory disease to cause an acute drop in circulating antibody titers. However, a rebound rise in autoantibody titers will occur if the patient in not concurrently on adequate immunosuppressive therapy. Parenteral gold has been successfully used in the therapy of PV, but because of the incidence of side effects over long-term therapy (dermatitis, nephrotoxicity, blood dyscrasias), its use has been limited. Other drugs occasionally reported to be effective in pemphigus include cyclosporine, etretinate, and dapsone. Extracorporeal photopheresis has also been recently reported as an alternative therapy for pemphigus, although the results are too preliminary to currently recommend it as a treatment.

Patients undergoing steroid and immunosuppressive therapy must be monitored with a variety of laboratory tests including CBC, liver enzymes, creatinine, urinalysis, and X-rays looking for toxicity, underlying infections, or evidence of osteoporosis. In addition, indirect IF studies of the patient's serum every 6–8 weeks may provide valuable information in monitoring the effectiveness of the patient's therapy.

FUTURE DIRECTIONS

The past 10 years have shown remarkable progress in understanding the pathogenicity of the autoantibodies in PF and PV. Furthermore, the advances in desmosomal biology have furthered our understanding in how antidesmosomal autoantibodies may induce cell detachment in these patients. Furthermore, the availability of full-length recombinant protein for Dsg1 and Dsg3 will allow the dissection of epitopes recognized on these molecules not only by pathogenic autoantibodies by also by T cells from patients. It is expected that within the next few years the cellular mechanisms of autoantibody production in PV and PF will be disclosed. These relevant pathogenic epitopes on Dsg3 and Dsg1 should pave the way for more specific therapies, including induction of immunological tolerance to these molecules. Newer drugs may also be available to modulate the immunopathological events happening at the level of the target cells. Finally the endemic form of PF seen in Brazil might offer the unique opportunity of identifying the etiological agent of PF. This finding could have a major impact in understanding human autoimmunity.

ACKNOWLEDGMENTS

This work was supported in part by grants R37 AR32081, R01 AR32599, R01 AR40410, and T32 AR07577 from the National Institutes of Health and by the Department of Veterans Affairs.

SELECTED REFERENCES

Amagai M, Klaus-Kovtun V, Stanley JR. Autoantibodies against a novel epithelial cadherin in pemphigus vulgaris, a disease of cell adhesion. Cell 1991;67:869–877.

Amagai M, Hashimoto T, Green KJ, Shimizu S, Nishikawa T. Antigen-specific immunoabsorption of pathogenic autoantibodies in pemphigus foliaceous. J Invest Dermatol 1995;104:895–901.

Amagai M, Hashimoto T, Shimizu N, Nishikawa T. Absorption of pathogenic autoantibodies by the extracellular domain of pemphigus vulgaris antigen (Dsg3) produced by baculovirus. J Clin Invest 1994;94:59–67.

Ahmed AR, Yunis EY, Khatri K, et al. Major histocompatibility complex haplotypes studies in Ashkenazi Jewish patients with pemphigus vulgaris. Proc Natl Acad Sci USA 1990;87:7658–7662.

Anhalt GJ, Labib R, Voorhees JJ, et al. Induction of pemphigus in neonatal mice by passive transfer of IgG from patients with the disease. N Engl J Med 1982;306:1189–1196.

Anhalt GJ, Kim SC, Stanley JR, et al. Paraneoplastic pemphigus: an autoimmune mucocutaneous disease associated with neoplasia. N Engl J Med 1990;323:1729–1735.

Beutner EH, Jordon RE. Demonstration of skin antibodies in the sera of pemphigus vulgaris patients by indirect immunofluorescent staining. Proc Soc Exp Bio Med 1964;117:505–510.

Cerna M, Fernandez-Vina M, Friedman H, et al. Genetic markers for susceptibility to endemic Brazilian pemphigus foliaceus (fogo selvagem) in Xavante Indians. Tissue Antigens 1993;42:138–140.

Diaz LA, Sampaio SAP, Rivitti EA, et al. Endemic pemphigus foliaceous (fogo selvagem): II. Current and historical epidemiological studies. J Invest Dermatol 1989;92:4–12.

Fine J-D. Drug therapy: management of acquired bullous skin disease. N Engl J Med 1995;333:1475–1484.

Koch PJ, Mahoney MG, Ishikawa H, et al. Targeted disruption of the pemphigus vulgaris antigen (desmoglein 3) gene in mice causes loss of keratinocyte cell adhesion with a phenotype similar to pemphigus vulgaris. J Cell Biol 1997;137:1091–1102.

Korman NJ, Eyre RW, Klaus-Kovtun V, et al. Demonstration of an adhering-junction molecule (Plakoglobin) in the autoantigens of pemphigus foliaceus and pemphigus vulgaris. N Engl JMed 1989;321. 631–635.

Lever WF. Pemphigus vulgaris. In: Lever WF, ed. Pemphigus and Pemphigoid. Springfield, IL: Charles C. Thomas, 1965; pp. 15–72.

Lin MS, Mascaro JM Jr, Liu Z, Espana A, Diaz LA. The desmosome and hemidesmosome in cutaneous autoimmunity. Clin Exp Immunol 1997;107:9–15.

Moraes JR, Moraes ME, Fernandez-Vina M, et al. HLA antigen and the risk for the development off pemphigus foliaceus (fogo selvagem) in endemic areas of Brazil. Immunogenetics 1991;33:388–391.

Morioka S, Lazarus G, Jensen P. Involvement of urokinase-type plasminogen activator in acantholysis induced by pemphigus IgG. J Invest Dermatol 1987;89:474–477.

Rock B, Labib RS, Diaz LA. Monovalent Fab' immunoglobulin fragments from endemic pemphigus foliaceus autoantibodies are pathogenic to BALB/c mice by passive transfer. J Clin Invest 1990; 85:296–299.

Roscoe JT, Diaz LA, Sampaio SAP, et al. Brazilian pemphigus foliaceus autoantibodies are pathogenic to BALB/c mice by passive transfer. J Invest Dermatol 1985;85:538–541.

Takiechi M. Cadherins: a molecular family essential for selective cell-cell adhesion and animal morphogenesis. Trends Genet 1987; 3:213–217.

Zhou S, Ferguson DJ, Allen J, Wojnarowska F. The location of binding sites of pemphigus vulgaris and pemphigus foliaceus autoantibodies: a post-embedding immunoelectron microscopic study. Br J Dermatol 1997;136:878–883.

89 Bullous Pemphigoid, Cicatricial Pemphigoid, and Pemphigoid Gestationis

GRANT J. ANHALT AND DIYA F. MUTASIM

BACKGROUND

The term "pemphigoid" applies to several different clinical disorders that share the clinical appearance of blisters, the histologic finding of subepidermal blister, and circulating and skin-bound IgG antibodies against a component of the basement membrane zone (BMZ) (Table 89-1). Extensive skin involvement in the elderly population occasionally leads to significant morbidity. In addition, therapy with systemic corticosteroids and immunosuppressive agents may be associated with significant adverse effects.

CLINICAL FEATURES

The exact incidence of pemphigoid is not known, but it is estimated to be twice that of pemphigus vulgaris (PV). Its incidence in Great Britain is estimated at 1 per 100,000 per year in 1985 and 7.63 per million in France in 1995. There are three closely related pemphigoid diseases, namely bullous pemphigoid (BP), cicatricial (mucosal) pemphigoid (CP), and pemphigoid (herpes) gestationis (HG).

BULLOUS PEMPHIGOID This disease appears to be a phenomenon of the aging immune system, with peak incidence very late in life (Figs. 89-1 and 89-2). There is no known HLA Class II gene that confers susceptibility for the disease. However, in herpes gestationis, there appears to be an HLA Class II-linked susceptibility. Approximately 60–85% of HG patients are HLA-DR3 positive. More strikingly, approximately 45% of women affected with the disease are heterozygote HLA-DR3/DR4.

The disease tends to be generalized with predilection for the lower abdomen, inner thighs, groin, and axillae. The characteristic blisters are pruritic and appear on either normal-appearing or erythematous, urticarial base. When blisters rupture, denuded areas may become crusted and occasionally invaded by bacterial pathogens.

The course and prognosis of BP varies. Most treated patients go into a clinical remission within several months without need for further treatment.

CICATRICIAL PEMPHIGOID This is a relatively rare condition characterized by chronic blistering and scarring of mucosal surfaces covered by stratified squamous epithelium. Involved organs include the ocular conjunctiva, nasal pharynx, oral pharynx, larynx, upper esophagus, and anogenital mucosa. The marked tendency for scarring in this disorder leads to high morbidity secondary to loss of vision, esophageal strictures, and fibrotic scarring of other mucous membranes.

PEMPHIGOID GESTATIONIS Also known as herpes gestationis (HG), this is a relatively rare disease seen during pregnancy. The disorder often begins in the second or third trimester of pregnancy. It tends to recur in subsequent pregnancies and may be elicited by challenge with oral contraceptives. Lesions tend to involve the abdomen and then spread peripherally. The clinical appearance of the lesions is similar to that of BP.

DIAGNOSIS

HISTOPATHOLOGY Histopathologic examination of an early intact blister reveals a subepidermal blister with a mixed inflammatory infiltrate that is rich in eosinophils. The blister cavity contains serum, fibrin, and inflammatory cells.

DIRECT IMMUNOFLUORESCENCE The ideal substrate for this test is a biopsy of normal-appearing skin adjacent to a lesion (Fig. 89-3). A properly performed test from such a specimen is positive in 100% of BP patients. There is continuous linear deposition of C3 and IgG along the epidermal BMZ. Direct IF in HG and CP is similar to that of BP.

INDIRECT IMMUNOFLUORESCENCE The most commonly used substrate for this test is monkey esophagus. Other stratified squamous epithelia including normal human skin may also be used. Most patients with BP have circulating IgG autoantibodies against the BMZ. These antibodies bind to basement membrane molecules of stratified squamous epithelia.

Indirect IF is usually negative in most patients with HG by the standard methods. The anti-BMZ antibodies can, however, be detected by complement-fixation amplification (HG factor assay) or Western blotting. Approximately 25% of patients with CP have circulating anti-BMZ antibodies as detected by standard indirect IF.

IMMUNOELECTROMICROSCOPY (IEM) Direct IEM reveals the in vivo bound immune deposits (C3 and IgG) to be within the lamina lucida of the BMZ as well as basal-cell hemidesmosomes. Indirect IEM reveals that the circulating BP antibodies are directed against both the basal-cell hemidesmosomes as well as the lamina lucida. The findings in HG and CP are similar.

From: *Principles of Molecular Medicine* (J. L. Jameson, ed.), ©1998 Humana Press Inc., Totowa, NJ.

Table 89-1
The Pemphigoid Disorders

Disorder	*Bullous pemphigoid*	*Cicatricial pemphigoid*	*Pemphigoid gestationis*
Distribution of lesions	Flexures, neck, abdomen	Oral, ocular, anogenital	Abdomen, extremities
Tendency for scarring	–	+	–
Subepithelial blister	+	+	+
IgG and C3 at the BMZ	+	+	+
IgA at the BMZ	Rare	Occasional	–
Serum anti-BMZ antibodies detected by:			
Indirect Immunofluorescence	70%	25%	20%
Complement fixation	80%	?	50%
Western blotting or immunoprecipitation	95%	80%	80%
Target antigen in BMZ			
Location	Hemidesmosome and lamina lucida	Hemidesmosome, lamina lucida and lamina densa	Hemidesmosome and lamina lucida
Molecule	BP 180, BP 230	BP 180, BP 230, laminin 5, other	BP 180, rare BP 230

BMZ, basement membrane zone; BP 180, bullous pemphigoid antigen, mol wt 180 kDa; BP 230, bullous pemphigoid antigen, mol wt 230 kDa.

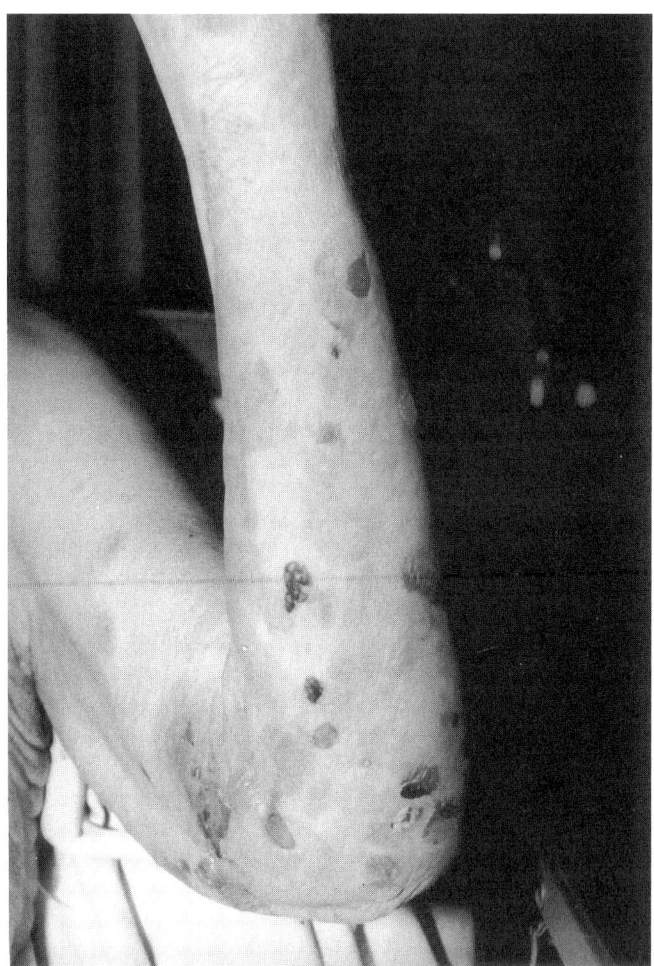

Figure 89-1 This is an elderly individual with generalized bullous pemphigoid.

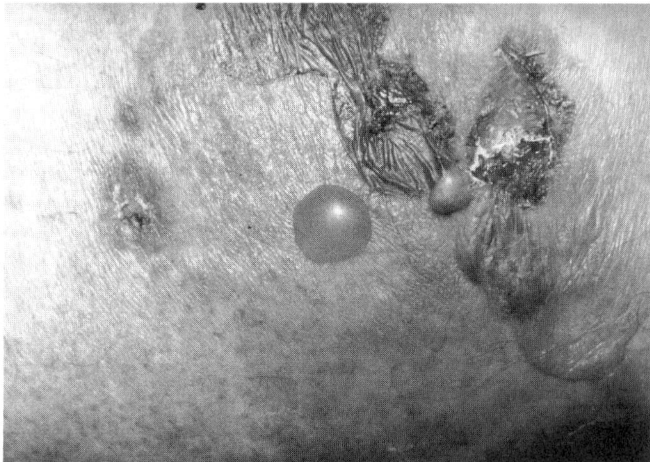

Figure 89-2 This is a close-up of the lesions revealing urticarial plaques and bullae.

PATHOPHYSIOLOGY

THE BULLOUS PEMPHIGOID ANTIGENS It is established that there are two protein antigens recognized by autoantibodies in bullous pemphigoid. Recently it has also been established by use of a passive-transfer animal model that that interaction of these autoantibodies with one of these proteins in vivo is directly responsible for blister formation.

The first pemphigoid antigen to be cloned and sequenced has been called either the BPAg1 or the BP230 antigen, and has an estimated molecular weight of 230 kDa in sodium dodecyl sulfate-polyacrylamide gel electrophoresis (SDS-PAGE). The hemidesmosome is an organelle that mediates a stable interaction between the keratin intermediate filament proteins of the basilar pole of the keratinocyte and transmembrane adhesion molecules that anchor the basal cell to the underlying lamina densa of the basement membrane. The BPAg1 is the major protein of the cytoplasmic plaque of the hemidesmosome, and its presumed (but not proven) function is to mediate this interaction. It is notable that the BPAg1 has approximately 30% sequence homology with desmoplakin I, the major plaque protein of the desmosome—an organelle that serves a similar function in mediation of cell—cell adhesion. BPAg1 has been mapped to chromosome 6 (6p12-p11) in the human and to the proximal region of chromosome 1 in the mouse.

The second pemphigoid antigen to be characterized is called the BPAg2 or the BP180 antigen, and has an estimated molecular

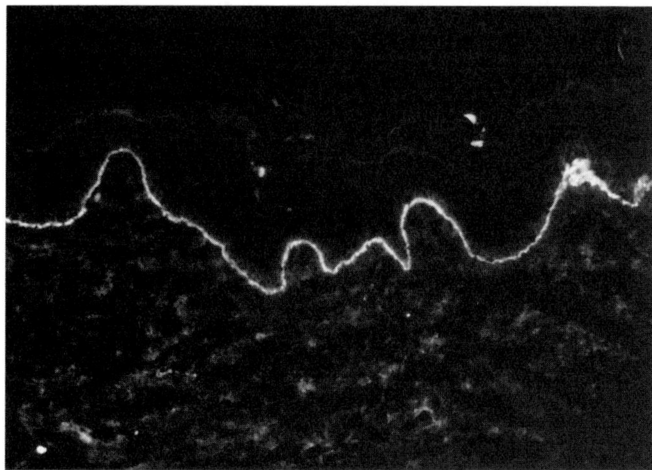

Figure 89-3 Direct immunofluorescence of perilesional skin of patient with bullous pemphigoid. Note the continuous linear deposition of complement (C3) along the epidermal basement membrane.

weight of 180 kDa in SDS-PAGE. The BPAg2 has been mapped to chromosome 10 (10q24.3) in the human and to the distal end of chromosome 19 in the mouse. It is a unique molecule, with many important structural features. It is a transmembrane molecule with a type 2 orientation, the carboxy-terminus being in the extracellular space and the amino-terminus being intracellular. The extracellular domain has lengthy collagenous domains, characterized by the presence of Gly-X-Y repeats, and this finding has led to an additional proposed name for the molecule, collagen type XVII. This portion of the molecule is presumed to interact with adhesion molecules of the lower lamina lucida/lamina densa to anchor the basal cell in place. The hypothesis that this molecule is important in normal epithelial adhesion is supported by the recent observation of kindreds in which a mutation of the BP180 gene results in a nonlethal, but generalized form of congenital epidermolysis bullosa. Immediately adjacent to the transmembrane domain of the BPAg2 there is a noncollagenous domain that contains the immunodominant epitope of the protein. Giudice and Diaz identified a polypeptide of 14 amino acids from this epitope that is recognized by the majority of human sera in bullous pemphigoid and herpes gestationis. Subsequently, they identified the corresponding region of the murine BPAg1 and found no significant homology between the human and murine epitope. This was a critical observation that allowed these investigators to subsequently develop a passive-transfer model in the mouse to define the immunopathologic events that lead to blister formation in vivo.

MECHANISMS OF BLISTER FORMATION For many years, it had been assumed that the sequence of events leading to blister formation in the human disease had been as follows: (1) Loss of tolerance to the BP antigens leads to autoantibody production and binding to the hemidesmosome. (2) Tissue-bound autoantibody activates the complement cascade. (3) Generation of chemotactic fragments of complement such as C3a and C5a recruit neutrophils and eosinophils to the site of bound autoantibody. (4) Release of proteolytic enzymes from the polymorphs degrades the BP antigens or other important adhesion molecules at the site. (5) Subepidermal blister formation ensues. This hypothesized sequence of events has now been confirmed and clearly defined in vivo by the use of an animal model. In this model, the 14-amino acid polypeptide, encoding the immunodominant epitope of the murine BPAg2 was synthesized, and antibodies against it were raised in rabbits. These antibodies were then transfused into neonatal mice, and within 24 h, cutaneous inflammation and blister formation was apparent. The induced blisters showed subepidermal separation, deposition of rabbit IgG and murine C3 along the basement membrane zone, and infiltration of the base of the blister with polymorphonuclear leukocytes. Blister formation was not observed if the model was manipulated to inhibit complement activation by bound anti-BPAg2 antibody. This was demonstrated by transfusing the antibody into C5 deficient strains of mice, into Balb/c mice depleted of complement by pretreatment with cobra venom factor, or by the infusion of F(ab')2 fragments of the rabbit anti-BPAg2 antibodies into newborn mice. If the mice were depleted of circulating polymorphonuclear cells prior to antibody infusion, blister formation was also not observed. In related studies, the role of proteases released from eosinophils in the degradation of the BPAg2 was defined. Abundant message for a 92-kDa gelatinase was found in eosinophils at the base of blisters in humans with lesions of BP. In vitro studies confirmed that the eosinophil-derived gelatinase degraded the BPAg2 in the extracellular collagenous domains. In total, these studies provide compelling evidence for the proposed immunopathogenesis of lesions in BP.

It is not clear what role, if any, antibodies specific for the BPAg1 play in the development of lesions. Passive transfer of human antibodies against the BPAg1 do not produce any inflammation in the skin of mice. Rabbits that are immunized to the antigen and have circulating anti-BPAg2 antibodies do not develop any cutaneous lesions. These animals do exhibit an unusual inflammatory reaction to ultraviolet radiation. In this circumstance, erythematous doses of ultraviolet light produce marked epidermal inflammation and keratinocyte necrosis. This suggests that antibodies against the BPAg1 may cause some secondary inflammatory events in vivo, but it appears that antibodies against the BPAg2 are really of primary pathogenic importance. It is not clear why patients should simultaneously make autoantibodies against two completely unrelated protein antigens, although a similar phenomenon is observed in autoimmune thyroiditis, where autoantibodies develop against discrete but unrelated antigens that are related to each other only by close physical proximity.

MANAGEMENT

Pemphigoid is a disorder that results from an abnormal immune response and that has prominent inflammatory features. Therapy for pemphigoid should suppress inflammation and/or the immune response. If therapy fails, the elderly patient with extensive erosions may develop complications such as fluid loss, electrolyte imbalance, bacterial colonization with potential sepsis, scarring, and decubitus ulcers.

Most patients with generalized BP require systemic therapy. The most commonly used systemic agents are the corticosteroids. Immunosuppressive drug therapy with chemotherapeutic agents should be considered for patients who require high maintenance doses of corticosteroids, patients who develop corticosteroid side effects, and patients whose disease does not respond completely to corticosteroid therapy. The most commonly used immunosuppressive agents are azathioprine, cyclophosphamide, methotrexate, and cyclosporine. Treatment of CP and HG follows the same principles as that of BP.

FUTURE DIRECTIONS

In the past decade, extensive information has been derived about the molecular structure of BP antigens. A recent animal model confirmed the pathogenic role of BP antibodies in the induction of skin lesions. Future research should be directed toward understanding the mechanisms for the immune response that results in the production of BP antibodies.

SELECTED REFERENCES

Anhalt GJ, Bahn CF, Labib RS, et al. Pathogenic effects of bullous pemphigoid autoantibodies on rabbit corneal epithelium. J Clin Invest 1981;68:1097–1101.

Anhalt GJ, Jampel HD, Patel HP, et al. Bullous pemphigoid autoantibodies are markers of corneal epithelial hemidesmosomes. Invest Ophthalmol Vis Sci 1987;28:903–907.

Bedane C, McMillan JR, Balding SD, et al. Bullous pemphigoid and cicatricial pemphigoid autoantibodies react with ultrastructurally separable epitopes on the BP180 ectodomain: evidence that BP180 spans the lamina lucida. J Invest Dermatol 1997;108:901–907.

Giudice GJ, Emery DJ, Diaz LA. Cloning and primary structural analysis of the bullous pemphigoid autoantigen BP 180. J Invest Dermatol 1992;99:243–250.

Giudice GJ, Emery DJ, Zelickson BD, Anhalt GJ, Liu Z, Diaz LA. Bullous pemphigoid and herpes gestationis autoantibodies recognize a common non-collagenous site on the BP180 ectodomain. J Immunol 1993;151:5742–5750.

Jonkman MF, deJong MC, Heeres K, et al. 180-kD bullous pemphigoid antigen (BP180) is deficient in generalized atrophic benign epidermolysis bullosa. J Clin Invest 1995;95:1345–1352.

Jordon RE, Kawana S, Fritz KA. Immunopathologic mechanisms in pemphigus and bullous pemphigoid. J Invest Dermatol 1985;85:72s–78s.

Katz SI, Hertz KC, Yaoita H. Herpes gestationis: immunopathology and characterization of the HG factor. J Clin Invest 1976;57:1434–1441.

Li KH, Sawamura D, Giudice GJ, et al. Genomic organization of collagenous domains and chromosomal assignment of human 180-kDa bullous pempigoid antigen-2, a novel collagen of stratified squamous epithelium. J Biol Chem 1991;266:24,064–20,469.

Liu Z, Diaz LA, Troy JT, et al. A passive transfer model for the organ-specific autoimmune disease, bullous pemphigoid, using antibodies generated against the hemidesmosomal antigen, BP180. J Clin Invest 1993;92:2480–2486.

Liu Z, Giudice GJ, Swartz SJ, et al. The role of complement in experimental bullous pemphigoid. J Clin Invest 1995;95:1539–1544.

Liu Z, Roopenian DC, Zhou X, et al. beta2-microglobulin-deficient mice are resistant to bullous pemphigoid. J Exp Med 1997;186:777–783.

Mutasim DF, Diaz LA. The relevance of immunohistochemical techniques in the differentiation of subepidermal bullous diseases. Amer J Dermatopath 1991;13:77–83.

Mutasim DF, Morrison LH, Takahashi Y, et al. Definition of bullous pemphigoid antibody binding to intracellular and extracellular antigen associated with hemidesmosomes. J Invest Dermatol 1989;92: 225–230.

Stahle-Backdahl M, Inoue M, Giudice GJ, Parks WC. 92-kD gelatinase is produced by eosinophils at the site of blister formation in bullous pemphigoid and cleaves the extracellular domain of recombinant 180-kD bullous pemphigoid autoantigen. J Clin Invest 1994;93: 2022–2030.

Stanley JR, Hawley-Nelson P, Yuspa SH, et al. Characterization of bullous pemphigoid antigen: a unique basement membrane protein of stratified squamous epithelia. Cell 1981;24:897–903.

90 Cutaneous Lupus Erythematosus

RICHARD D. SONTHEIMER

BACKGROUND

Lupus erythematosus (LE) is an extremely heterogenous autoimmune disease process that has the potential to involve every major organ system within the body. Involvement of internal organs is designated as systemic LE (SLE), whereas involvement of the skin is referred to as cutaneous LE. Some LE patients have only SLE and others only cutaneous LE, however, most will have features of both SLE and cutaneous LE. Polyclonal B-cell activation with resultant production of autoantibodies to a number of nuclear and cytoplasmic antigens is a hallmark of LE. Multiple genetic and environmental factors are thought to conspire to produce the mosaic of clinical and laboratory features that constitutes the LE disease process.

The skin is a major target in LE—cutaneous disease is the second most common overall clinical disease manifestation, and skin disease is the second most frequent way that this autoimmune disorder first presents itself. Unfortunately, the molecular basis of most forms of skin involvement in LE is poorly understood owing in large part to the absence of reliable in vitro or in vivo models of this pattern of cutaneous inflammation. Thus, a discussion of this subject must be allowed some degree of freedom concerning the extrapolations that naturally flow from an analysis of a diverse set of isolated clinical, pathological, and immunopathological observations as has been reported for LE. This overview will focus especially on the immunological effector mechanisms that might be responsible for the characteristic pattern of cutaneous inflammation that is seen in this disorder.

This chapter will review our current understanding of the etiology and pathogenesis of LE-specific skin disease (LESSD), the type of cutaneous involvement that is histopathologically unique to individuals having LE. Cutaneous vasculitis, a form of LE-nonspecific skin disease, can be seen in LE patients but also is seen in a number of other disease processes other than LE. Space does not allow discussion of the causal mechanisms of LE non specific skin disease. In its strictest sense, the term "cutaneous LE" might be used to refer to all forms of skin lesions that occur as the result of the underlying LE autoimmune process; however, in practice most use this term synonymously with LESSD.

CLINICAL FEATURES

The classification system popularized by James N. Gilliam divided LESSD (cutaneous LE) into three subgroups—acute cutaneous LE (ACLE), subacute cutaneous LE (SCLE), and chronic cutaneous LE (CCLE) (a comprehensive color atlas illustrating the many ways that LE can be expressed in the skin can be found in Sontheimer RD et al.). Similarities and differences exist in the clinical and laboratory features associated with these three forms of cutaneous LE (Table 90-1). LESSD lesions can exist as an isolated event (e.g., localized classical discoid LE [DLE], which is the most commonly encountered variety of CCLE) or can accompany underlying SLE disease activity (e.g., ACLE). However, LESSD lesions that occur in the context of SLE are indistinguishable clinically and pathologically from those that occur as an isolated event. Although it is possible that each of these three major forms of LESSD has a unique etiopathogenesis, it is much more likely that each represents a variation on a common underlying theme with host factors such as genetic differences and environmental stimuli such as exposure to ultraviolet (UV) light accounting for the differences in phenotypic expression.

Several clinical observations concerning LESSD can serve as clues to the underlying pathogenesis of this pattern of cutaneous inflammation. When nonlesional skin of an LE patient is injured in any way, LESSD can be precipitated at the site of injury (i.e., the Köebner phenomenon). Autografting experiments have revealed LESSD to be recipient site dominant, i.e., grafts of nonlesional autologous skin transplanted into an area of LESSD inflammation assume the clinical and pathological features of the recipient site. In some patients, LESSD, especially SCLE, can be induced by exposure to certain drugs including hydrochlorothiazide, procainamide, D-penicillamine, sulfonylureas, oxyprenolol, griseofulvin, piroxicam, naproxen, PUVA, spironolactone, and diltiazem.

Photosensitivity is a clinical hallmark of LE occurring in as many as 80–90% of certain cutaneous LE subsets such as SCLE. In addition to precipitating or exacerbating cutaneous LE activity, exposure to UV light is also capable of aggravating the underlying systemic autoimmune abnormalities. The abnormal cutaneous response to UV light in LE patients is delayed in time, usually taking days to weeks to become fully apparent. The degree of abnormal sensitivity to sunlight and artificial sources of UV light can wax and wane over an individual patient's disease course. As previously mentioned, certain photosensitizing drugs such a hydrochlorothiazide and griseofulvin are capable of inducing some forms of LESSD such as SCLE. Some studies have indicated that circulating humoral factors may predispose to the development of cutaneous LE photosensitivity.

Most LE patients respond normally to minimal erythema dose testing, however, some reports have suggested decreased minimal

From: *Principles of Molecular Medicine* (J. L. Jameson, ed.), ©1998 Humana Press Inc., Totowa, NJ.

Table 90-1
Comparison of the Major Forms of LE-Specific Skin Disease[a]

Disease features	*ACLE*	*SCLE*	*Classical DLE*
Clinical features of skin lesions			
Induration	0	0	+++
Scarring	0	0	+++
Pigment changes	+	++	+++
Follicular plugging	0	0	+++
Hyperkeratosis	+	++	+++
Photosensitivity	+++	+++	+
Distribution of lesions			
Face	+++	+	+++
Scalp	+	+	+++
Ears	+	+	+++
Extensor arms, forearms	++	+++	++
V-area of neck	++	+++	++
Histopathology			
Thickened basement membrane	0	+	+++
Intensity of lichenoid infiltrate	+	++	+++
Periappendageal inflammation	+	+	+++
Lupus band			
Lesional	++	++	+++
Nonlesional	++	+	0
Antinuclear antibodies	+++	++	+
Ro/SS-A antibodies			
By immunodiffusion	+	+++	0
By ELISA	++	+++	+
Antinative DNA antibodies	+++	+	0
Hypocomplementemia	+++	+	+
Risk for developing SLE	+++	++	+

+++, strongly associated; ++, moderately associated; +, weakly associated; 0, negative, no association.
[a](Adapted with permission from Table 1.4 of Sontheimer RD, et al.)

erythema doses in some individuals. In the classical phototesting studies, the action spectrum of LESSD appeared to be restricted to the ultraviolet B (UVB) spectrum; however, more recent studies have suggested that ultraviolet A (UVA) radiation can contribute to the photosensitive states experienced by some subsets of LE, especially SCLE. Single- and repeated-dose exposure of nonlesional skin to UV light can result in the production of typical cutaneous LE lesions. These UV light-induced lesions have identical histopathological features to idiopathic LE skin lesions. The earliest histopathological change in a UV light-induced skin lesion is perivascular accumulation of mononuclear cells—these changes clearly predate the appearance of immunoglobulin and complement deposits at the dermal–epidermal junction. Some photochallenge studies have suggested that UVB exposure preferentially induces the epidermal changes of LESSD, whereas UVA predominantly produces the dermal changes.

DIAGNOSIS

The diagnosis of LESSD is certain when the expected histopathological changes are seen in a skin lesion that is clinically consistent with a form of cutaneous LE. Dermatomyositis skin lesions can at times be difficult to distinguish from some forms of LESSD on routine histopathology alone. Whereas qualitative differences exist between ACLE, the pattern of pathological change in each of these forms of LESSD is that of a lichenoid tissue reaction. Experimental evidence suggests that other examples of the lichenoid tissue reaction such as lichen planus and graft-vs-host skin disease are the result of T-lymphocyte–mediated autoimmune injury within the skin.

PATHOLOGY

EPIDERMAL CHANGES Epidermal keratinocyte hyperproliferation in cutaneous LE lesions is associated with normal early differentiation and premature terminal differentiation. In addition, epidermal Langerhans cells are decreased in density and display a perturbed morphology.

However, the primary focus of change within the epidermis is at the basal cell layer with hydropic or liquefactive degeneration of basal keratinocytes being the most prominent change. Activated lymphocytes and macrophages can be seen admixed with these degenerating basal keratinocytes. The intimate association of activated lymphocytes with the degenerating epidermal basal cells has led to the speculation that autoantigen-specific lymphocytes might mediate keratinocyte cytotoxicity in LESSD. The presence of elevated serum levels of soluble interleukin (IL)-2 receptors in certain cutaneous LE subsets also indirectly supports a role for activated T cells in the pathogenesis of this form of LESSD. Epidermal keratinocytes in LESSD lesions express HLA class II antigen, ICAM-1, and the B7-3 costimulatory ligand. In addition, preliminary in vitro studies have suggested the existence of phenotypic variation in tumor necrosis factor (TNF)-α–induced ICAM-1 expression by epidermal keratinocytes from cutaneous LE patients.

DERMAL–EPIDERMAL JUNCTION CHANGES There is thickening of the epidermal basement-membrane zone in chronic

LESSD lesions such as DLE. This appears to result from basal lamina reduplication that occurs as a result of the hyperproliferation and premature death that occurs within the epidermal basal-cell compartment.

DERMAL CHANGES Mononuclear-cell infiltration around blood vessels and dermal appendages is a constant feature of LESSD. CD4 T lymphocytes that express class II histocompatibility antigens comprise the majority of this infiltrate. These cells express other T-cell–activation markers such as the IL-2 receptor and thymidine incorporation to only variable degree. Monocytes and macrophages are seen to a lesser extent and B cells are quite rare. The infiltrating T cells are predominately of the helper-inducer, memory phenotype ($CD4^+$, $CD45RA^-$, $CD45RO^+$) and express CD28/CTLA-4. There do not appear to be significant qualitative differences in the inflammatory infiltrate seen in DLE and SCLE lesions. Some workers have reported that γ/δ T-cell receptor-positive T cells are virtually nonexistent in the epidermis and dermis of CCLE lesions, whereas others have suggested that T cells having a specific γ/δ receptor phenotype (V-γ2/V-δ2) are preferentially expanded within the epidermal and dermal T-cell infiltrates of CCLE lesions. The presence of γ/δ T cells would suggest the possibility of an antigen-specific response to stress proteins induced within the epidermis by environmental stimuli such as UV light.

The dermal microvasculature is a major focus of cellular inflammation within the dermis. Several studies have suggested that HLA-DR antigens are expressed at lower levels on dermal microvascular endothelial cells than is normal in DLE and SLE skin lesions. Dermal mucin deposition can be a prominent feature of LESSD lesions. Recent studies have suggested the possibility that circulating factors in LE patients that parallel SLE disease activity can stimulate exaggerated production of glycosaminoglycans by dermal fibroblasts.

SUBCUTANEOUS CHANGES Subcutaneous inflammation is relatively rare in LE; however, lupus panniculitis (profundus) can at times be the dominant cutaneous change. The histologic pattern is a lobular lymphocytic panniculitis. Perivascular infiltration with lymphocytes, plasma cells, and histiocytes in the deep dermis and subcutaneous fat is usually seen; this can extend to the point of lymphoid nodule formation. Vessel-wall thickening and invasion by mononuclear cells ("lymphocytic vasculitis") can also be observed. There is a distinct absence of polymorphonuclear leukocytes. Hyaline fat necrosis can be seen as well as prominent fibrinoid degeneration of collagen. Mucinous degeneration and calcification in established lesions occurs over time.

IMMUNOPATHOLOGY

Immunoglobulin (IgG, IgA, IgM) and complement (C3, C4, membrane-attack complex) components can be found in a band-like array along the dermal–epidermal junction of both lesional and nonlesional skin of LE patients. Elution of such immunoreactants from the skin of SLE patients has suggested that they contain antinuclear and anti–basement membrane zone reactivity. Ultrastructural studies have localized these deposits to structures below the lamina densa that are associated with type VII collagen (autoantibodies to type VII collagen are produced by some patients with SLE who develop vesiculobullous skin lesions ["vesiculobullous SLE"]). These deposits have been shown to follow the appearance of the perivascular mononuclear-cell infiltrate in UV-induced LE skin lesions by 4–6 weeks and thus are probably not causally involved as a primary factor in the pathogenesis of LESSD. Experimental studies in mice have shown that deposition of immunoglobulin at the dermal–epidermal junction can result from charge interaction alone when cationized antibody or immune complexes are present.

A pattern of IgG deposition different from the LE band has been observed to occur in SCLE patients. This dust-like array of IgG deposition is seen most prominently over the epidermal basal cells and has been suggested to correlate with the presence of circulating Ro/SS-A autoantibodies. The ability to detect this subtle immunofluorescence finding appears to vary somewhat between laboratories, suggesting that technical issues might be important to its detection.

In LE panniculitis/profundus, immunoglobulin and complement deposits are usually found in blood vessel walls of the deep dermis and subcutis by direct immunofluorescence.

ULTRASTRUCTURAL CHANGES

Early electron microscopic studies identified paramyxovirus-like structures within lesions of DLE; however, similar tubuloreticular structures have also been found in other settings such as dermatomyositis and Sjögren's syndrome. Considerable evidence now suggests that these "lupus inclusions" are not directly related to viral infection since they can be reproduced in cells in vitro as a result of excessive stimulation with interferon (IFN)-α or -β.

GENETIC BASIS OF DISEASE

HLA associations have been reported for several forms of LESSD. SCLE has been associated most strongly with HLA-B8, DR3, DRW6, DRW52, and DQW1/DQW2. This the HLA haplotype that is even more strongly associated with Ro/SS-A autoantibody production, the serological marker for SCLE. Nucleotide sequence analysis of DQW1/DQW2 alleles in patients who produce Ro/SS-A antibody have demonstrated that 100% have a glutamine residue at position 34 of the outermost domain in the DQA1 chain and a leucine at position 26 of the DQB1 chain. Partial or complete genetic deficiency of C2 and C4 is also associated with SCLE. CCLE (DLE) has been a found to correlate with the presence of HLA-B7, B8, Cw7, DR2, DR3, DQW1, and DQA1*0102. Like SCLE, DLE has been associated with genetic deficiency of C2, C4, and C5. There is no specific autoantibody marker for CCLE. No specific HLA associations have been reported for ACLE; however, ACLE lesions usually occur in the context of SLE and SLE has been most closely associated with HLA-DR2 and DR3.

Non-HLA genetic associations have also been reported for CCLE. DLE has been observed to be present at increased frequency in female carriers of X-linked chronic granulomatous disease, which is now known to result from genetic deficiency of reduced nicotinamide dinucleotide phosphatase (NADPH). In addition, IL-1 receptor antagonist and TNF-α gene polymorphisms have been associated with SLE; however, the role that this plays in the expression of cutaneous LE has not been fully determined. Preliminary evidence has argued against an association between SCLE and TNF-α polymorphism.

MOLECULAR PATHOPHYSIOLOGY OF DISEASE

The foregoing clinical and laboratory observations suggest that LESSD is the result of a genetically determined autoimmune

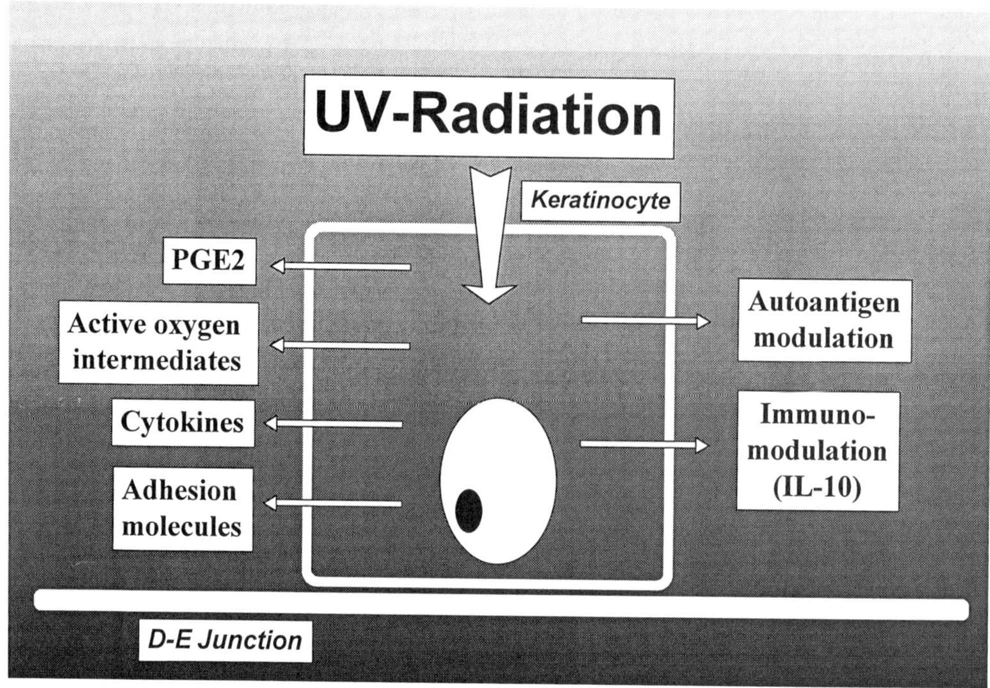

Figure 90-1 Modulation of Ro/SS-A autoantigen in epidermal keratinocytes following exposure to UVB irradiation. Lefeber, Norris, and coworkers first reported that UVB irradiation of human epidermal keratinocytes in culture resulted in the translocation of normally intracellular Ro/SS-A autoantigen to the surface of viable. Ro/SS-A antibody from the circulation would then be able to bind to these surface-expressed autoantigens, targeting the cells for injury through immune effector mechanisms such as antibody-dependent cell-mediated cytotoxicity. Golan et al. first presented data suggesting that greater degrees of Ro/SS-A autoantibody binding could be observed on the surface of cultured epidermal keratinocytes of LE patients following UVB compared to keratinocytes from normal individuals.

response to cutaneous autoantigens that is mediated by autoantibodies, immune complexes composed of autoantibodies and autoantigens, or autoantigen-specific T cells. The tempo and extent of this form of autoimmune inflammation can be impacted by various environmental stimuli foremost among which is exposure to UV light.

The photoreceptor for cutaneous LE has not been identified; however, some have argued that it might be DNA. Earlier work attempting to explain the molecular basis of photosensitivity in LE patients suggested that the pathologic immune response might be directed against neoantigens generated in the skin by the action of UV light on DNA. A murine model of some of the histopathological and immunopathological changes associated with cutaneous LE was produced by exposing the skin of mice that had been immunized to thymidine dimers to UV light. In addition, several investigators have argued that LE patients have abnormal UV light-altered DNA-repair capacity. However, the role played by UV-induced DNA injury and repair in the pathogenesis of human LESSD remains to be determined.

Most attention over the past decade has been directed to the idea that some forms of Ro/SS-A autoantibody-associated, photosensitive cutaneous LE such as SCLE and neonatal LE might result from the interaction of Ro/SS-A antibody from the circulation with Ro/SS-A antigen that has been transported to the surface of epidermal keratinocytes as a result of exposure to UVB (Fig. 90-1). The following observations support this hypothesis. Ro/SS-A autoantibodies are extremely prevalent in SCLE and there is a strong correlation between Ro/SS-A antibody levels and skin disease activity in neonatal LE. The dust-like pattern of IgG deposition seen in human SCLE lesions has been experimentally reproduced in nude mice bearing human skin explants by the passive transfer of Ro/SS-A autoantibody derived from LE patient sera.

UVB-induced Ro/SS-A antigen modulation in keratinocytes has now been confirmed by several groups, and it has been suggested that this phenomenon might be enhanced in keratinocytes from LE patients compared to those from normal individuals. It has not yet been determined whether differential UVB-induced expression of the molecular constituents of Ro/SS-A ribonucleoprotein particles (Ro60, Ro52, La/SS-B, calreticulin) might occur in the epidermal keratinocytes of LE patients compared to normal individuals. UVB-induced apoptosis might be responsible for the translocation of Ro/SS-A autoantigen to the cell surface. Autoantibody binding to the exposed antigens on the surface of keratinocytes could result in tissue injury through complement-mediated lysis or antibody-dependent cell-mediated cytotoxicity. Infection by alphaviruses such as sindbis also appears to be capable of inducing cell-surface expression of Ro/SS-A antigens as a result of virus-induced apoptosis. It is also possible that UV light might cause the expression of stress-related autoantigens in keratinocytes of LE patients that could then become the target of a pathological immune response.

Although quite attractive, the hypothesis that UVB-induced Ro/SS-A antigen modulation is a causative factor in photosensitive LESSD still remains unproven. Several arguments can be made against this hypothesis. Most Ro/SS-A antibody-positive Sjögren's syndrome patients do not develop SCLE or deliver infants with neonatal LE skin lesions, even though they have equally high levels of Ro/SS-A autoantibody (most studies have

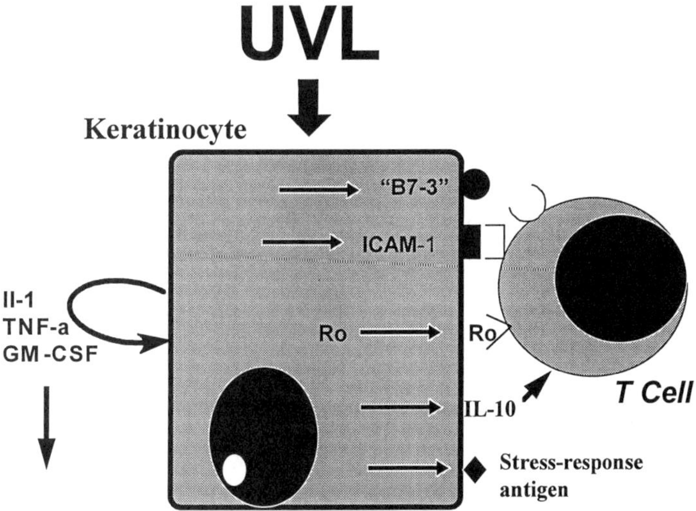

Figure 90-2 Possible mechanisms of T-cell interaction with epidermal keratinocytes of an LE patient following exposure to UVB irradiation.

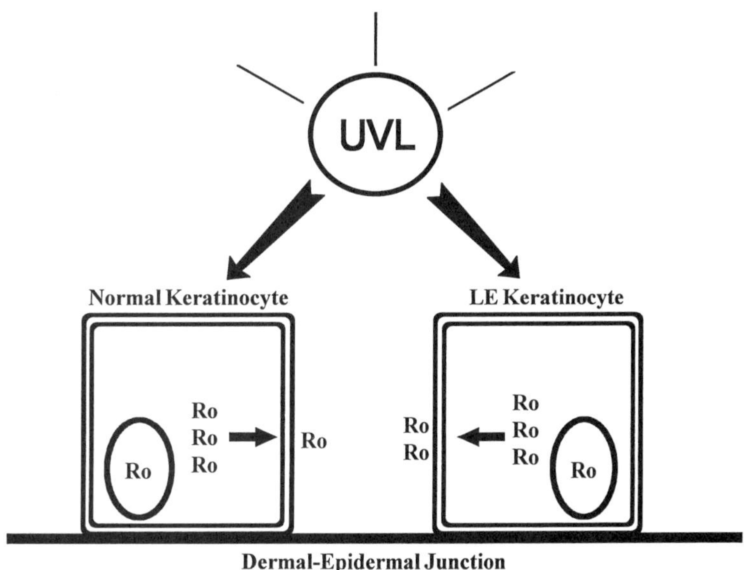

Figure 90-3 Events occurring in epidermal keratinocytes following exposure to UVB that could be relevant to the pathogenesis of LE-specific skin disease.

not found distinctive differences in the Ro/SS-A polypeptide specificities of the autoantibodies found in SCLE and Sjögren's syndrome). In addition, from the preliminary data that is available, there does not appear to be a positive correlation between Ro/SS-A antibody levels and disease activity in adults with SCLE. Also only a very small percentage of newborns exposed to maternal Ro/SS-A autoantibody production *in utero* develop either neonatal LE or congenital heart block. To date, no in vitro or in vivo experimental system involving UVB-induced Ro/SS-A autoantigen modulation in epidermal keratinocytes has reproduced the pattern of histopathological change that is typical of LESSD.

It is conceivable that Ro/SS-A antibodies in photosensitive cutaneous LE patients represent only a marker for Ro/SS-A antigen-specific T cells and that such autoreactive T cells may represent the primary immunological effector mechanism for photosensitive LESSD (Fig. 90-2). Increasing evidence suggests that many of the autoantibodies seen in LE are antigen driven and preliminary studies have identified ribonucleoprotein autoantigen-specific T cells from LE patients, including 52-kDa Ro/SS-A-specific T cells. As previously mentioned, the pathology of LESSD shares many features with other T-cell–mediated skin disorders such as lichen planus and graft-vs-host skin disease. However, to date, Ro/SS-A antigen-specific T cells have not been identified in LESSD lesions. If such cells exist they might be expected to be increased in density in LESSD lesions compared to the peripheral blood.

In addition to modulating intracellular ribonucleoprotein autoantigens, UV light also has a number of other proinflammatory effects on epidermal keratinocytes (Fig. 90-3). UV light can upregulate proinflammatory molecules such as IL-1α, TNF-α, GM-CSF, IL-6, IL-10, IL-12, MIP-1 and 2, prostaglandin E, proteases, oxygen free radicals, and histamine. It is conceivable that genetically determined enhanced expression or defective metabolic turnover of one or more of these products might occur in LE patients; however, there is currently little data that directly addresses this possibility. As previously mentioned, TNF-α polymorphism has been associated with SLE, and IL-1-receptor antagonist gene polymorphism has been implicated as a genetic factor in cutaneous LE.

UVB irradiation of murine and human skin can result in the generation of immunological tolerance to antigens applied to the skin at the site of irradiation. Increasing evidence suggests that UVB-induction of IL-10 by epidermal keratinocytes or recruited dermal macrophages might play an important role in the generation of this state of active tolerance. Since T-suppressor cell function has often been observed to be defective in SLE patients and murine models of SLE, one could question whether UVB induction of normal amounts of IL-10 within the epidermis of an LE patient might fail to produce an adequate state of physiological tolerance to epidermal autoantigens that are modulated by UVB exposure or epidermal neoantigens that are generated by UVB. Alternatively, genetically determined aberrations in IL-10 expression following UVB might also result in inadequate generation of tolerance signals leading to autoimmune responses to cutaneous autoantigens. At the moment there is no direct data to either support either of these speculations.

MANAGEMENT/TREATMENT

Effective treatment of LESSD usually requires systemic therapy with anti-inflammatory or immunosuppressive agents. Approximately 80% of patients respond to one or a combination of the aminoquinoline antimalarials such as hydroxychloroquine (Plaquenil), chloroquine (Aralen), or quinacrine. When antimalarial therapy is not successful in fully suppressing disease activity, alternative therapy with other anti-inflammatory drugs including dapsone, isotretinoin/etretinate, gold, clofazamine, and thalidomide can be beneficial. Long-term systemic corticosteroids and antimetabolite/cytotoxic immunosuppressives such as methotrexate, azathioprine, and cyclophosphamide are reserved for potentially disabling forms of cutaneous disease.

Aminoquinoline antimalarials have been associated with a diverse set of actions on cell physiology and pathways of inflammation. Which of their many molecular effects is most important to their value in LESSD is not at all certain. One of the few common actions shared by the aminoquinoline antimalarials and the rather diverse group of other drugs that are of value in cutaneous LE (e.g., dapsone, retinoids, auranofin) is their ability to scavenge oxygen free radicals, perhaps yielding a clue to an important mechanisms of cellular inflammation in LESSD. Thalidomide is another drug that can have a profoundly beneficial effect on LESSD. Recent studies have determined that thalidomide powerfully inhibits the production of TNF-α, a UVB-inducible epidermal cytokine that has been implicated in the pathogenesis of cutaneous LE.

FUTURE DIRECTIONS

The absence of a working in vivo or in vitro model of LESSD has greatly hindered our understanding of the molecular and genetic basis of this distinctive form of cutaneous inflammation. Whereas there are murine models of some of the clinical and immunological features of SLE, such animals, even when challenged with UV light do not reproducibly develop clinical skin lesions or develop the typical histopathological changes associated with LESSD. One exception is the MRL mouse. These mice, under some conditions, spontaneously develop patchy hair loss that is associated with very mild pathological and immunopathological changes typical of LESSD. It would be quite interesting to determine whether MRL mice that are crossed with transgenic mice that overexpress UVB-inducible proinflammatory cytokines such as IL-1α, TNF-α, or MIP in epidermal basal cells might more reliably express an LESSD pathology and thus provide a better model for cutaneous LE inflammation.

Much could also be done with the tools of modern molecular biology to determine whether variant expression of UVB-inducible proinflammatory cytokines might occur in the epidermal cells of LE patients compared to normal individuals. For example, RT-PCR and Northern blot analysis might be used to examine sequential suction blister-derived epidermal biopsies from UV light-challenged nonlesional skin of LE patients to determine whether the kinetics of UV light-induced cytokine production might be different in LE patients compared to normal individuals.

Systematic studies to detect evidence of oligoclonal T-cell-receptor gene rearrangement are also needed to determine whether T-cell expansion of the type associated with antigen-driven T-cell stimulation might be present in LESSD lesions. Efforts to clone Ro/SS-A autoantigen-specific T cells from SCLE skin lesions could also prove rewarding.

SUMMARY AND CONCLUSIONS

David Norris has proposed a four-step model for the pathogenesis of LESSD: (1) exposure to UV light induces the release of proinflammatory epidermal and dermal mediators such as IL-1 and TNF-α; (2) these mediators induce changes in epidermal and dermal cells including the induction of adhesion molecules and promotion of the translocation of normally intracellular autoantigen such as Ro/SS-A to the surface of epidermal cells; (3) autoantibody from the circulation binds to autoantigens such as Ro/SS-A that have been translocated to the surface of epidermal keratinocytes; and (4) keratinocyte cytotoxicity ensues as the result of lymphoid cells that have been recruited from the circulation, recognizing and responding to the Fc domains of autoantibody molecules bound to autoantigen expressed on the surface of keratinocytes (i.e., antibody-dependent cell-mediated cytotoxicity). Although this remains among the most attractive hypotheses for the explanation of Ro/SS-A antibody-associated forms of LESSD such as SCLE and neonatal LE, it does not address the pathogenesis of other forms of LESSD such as DLE that are not associated with Ro/SS-A antibody or other known autoantibody specificity. Better in vitro and in vivo experimental models will be required to more fully understand the molecular basis of all forms of LESSD.

ACKNOWLEDGMENTS

This work was supported by NIH grant AR19101 and the resources of the University of Texas Southwestern Skin Disease Research Core Center (AR41940).

SELECTED REFERENCES

Boumpas DT, Fessler BJ, Austin HA III, Balow JE, Klippel JH, Lockshin MD. Systemic lupus erythematosus: emerging concepts. Part 2: Dermatologic and joint disease, the antiphospholipid antibody syndrome, pregnancy and hormonal therapy, morbidity and mortality, and pathogenesis. Ann Inter Med 1995;123:42–53.

Casciola-Rosen LA, Anhalt G, Rosen A. Autoantigens targeted in systemic lupus erythematosus are clustered in two populations of surface structures on apoptotic keratinocytes. J Exp Med 1994;179:1317–1330.

Furukawa F. Animal models of cutaneous lupus erythematosus and lupus erythematosus photosensitivity. Lupus 1997: 6:193–202.

Golan TD, Elkon KB, Gharavi AE, Krueger JG. Enhanced membrane binding of autoantigens to cultured keratinocytes of systemic lupus erythematosus patients after ultraviolet B/ultraviolet A irradiation. J Clin Invest 1992;90:1067–1076.

Kawashima T, Zappi EG, Lieu TS, Sontheimer RD. Impact of ultraviolet radiation on the cellular expression of Ro/SS-A-autoantigenic polypeptides. Dermatology 1994;189:6–10.

Lee LA. Neonatal lupus erythematosus. J Invest Dermatol 1993;100:9S–13S.

Norris DA. Pathomechanisms of photosensitive lupus erythematosus. J Invest Dermatol 1993;100:58S–68S.

Rosen A, Casciola-Rosen L, Ahearn J. Novel packages of viral and self-antigens are generated during apoptosis. J Exp Med 1995;181: 1557–1561.

Sontheimer RD, Provost TT. Lupus erythematosus. In: Sontheimer RD, Provost TT, eds. Cutaneous Manifestations of Rheumatic Diseases, 1st ed. Baltimore: Williams & Wilkins, 1996; pp. 1–71.

91 Scleroderma (Systemic Sclerosis) and Morphea

EDWIN A. SMITH AND E. CARWILE LEROY

BACKGROUND

The term "scleroderma," referring to dermal fibrosis, has been applied to two distinct illnesses. One of these, systemic sclerosis, is a generalized vascular and fibrotic autoimmune disease affecting multiple organs, including the lungs, gastrointestinal tract, heart, and kidneys. In contrast, localized scleroderma is limited to the skin. Because there is little evidence that localized scleroderma can become systemic sclerosis and with the likelihood that these represent different etiologies and pathogeneses, systemic sclerosis and localized scleroderma will be treated separately.

SYSTEMIC SCLEROSIS (SSc)

HISTORY Notwithstanding a suggestive case report of scleroderma by Curzio of Naples in 1753, the earliest definitive clinical and pathological reports of scleroderma date from the mid-19th century, the same era in which Raynaud described the phenomenon bearing his name (1862) and associated it with scleroderma. That cardiac fibrosis can be of clinical significance was documented by Weiss in 1943, and the association of renal failure and scleroderma was made by Moore and Sheehan in 1952. Recent emphasis has been on understanding the pathophysiology of the disease with a hope that knowledge of the immunologic features as well as the causes of both the fibrosis and the vascular disease will lead to prevention or better treatment.

EPIDEMIOLOGY The incidence of systemic sclerosis is estimated at between 4 and 20 per million per year, a broad range because of the likelihood of unrecognized and misclassified cases. Estimates of the prevalence of disease meeting the ACR (American College of Rheumatology) preliminary criteria (*see* Table 91-1) range from 50,000 to 300,000 in the United States. It has been estimated, using more liberal criteria (Raynaud's phenomenon, abnormal nailfold capillaries, and positive tests for antinuclear antibodies) to identify persons suffering from "scleroderma spectrum disorders," that the population prevalence ranges from 67 to 265 per 100,000.

Systemic sclerosis is unusual in children, but has its onset throughout adult years. There is a suggestion that African Americans are at a moderately increased risk, but the illness is found in all racial groups and in all locales. Females are affected about three times more often than are males, and this difference is even more striking in young adult years. Associations have been made between the occurrence of systemic sclerosis and particular occupational exposures, including silica (gold and coal miners), vinyl chloride (industrial plastics workers), and organic solvents. Studies vary widely on the association of systemic sclerosis with HLA haplotypes, but several reports have found an association with HLA-DR5. Among selected scleroderma patients, the occurrence of certain autoantibody types has been associated with certain HLA class II alleles *(see below)*.

CLINICAL FEATURES Systemic sclerosis has been divided into two distinct types, differing in clinical course, types of organ involvement, and autoantibody profiles (Table 91-2). These two types, diffuse cutaneous systemic sclerosis (dcSSc) and limited cutaneous systemic sclerosis (lcSSc), differ in the extent of maximal skin involvement. In lcSSc, the skin thickening is limited to the face and areas distal to the elbows and knees, whereas, in dcSSc, the sclerosis is proximal as well as distal, and frequently involves the trunk. The clinical differences between limited and diffuse cutaneous systemic sclerosis are outlined in Table 91-3.

LcSSc is the more insidious of the two forms of the disease with mild symptoms which may go unreported to a physician for years or decades. Raynaud's phenomenon in the typical lcSSc patient has often been occurring since teenage or young adult years with symptoms of esophageal reflux or dysphagia occurring at a later date. It is often only with the occurrence of digital ulcers, telangiectases, or symptoms of pulmonary hypertension and right-sided heart failure that the diagnosis is made. Anticentromere antibodies are associated with lcSSc in Caucasian patients and their occurrence in a patient whose only symptom is Raynaud's phenomenon suggests that this illness is likely to develop. However, these antibodies are found in only approximately 40% of patients with lcSSc and can occur in other diseases than SSc.

Early dcSSc is very different from lcSSc, with a much more abrupt onset of symptoms. Although Raynaud's phenomenon is also common in this form of the disease, it may follow other symptoms. The earliest skin manifestation is edema of the extremities followed over a period of months by progressive induration of the dermis. This induration usually proceeds from distal to proximal

From: *Principles of Molecular Medicine* (J. L. Jameson, ed.), ©1998 Humana Press Inc., Totowa, NJ.

Table 91-1
Preliminary Criteria for Classification of Systemic Sclerosis (Scleroderma)

For the purposes of classifying patients in clinical trials, in population surveys, and for other studies, a person shall be said to have systemic sclerosis (scleroderma) if the one major or two or more minor criteria listed below are present. Localized forms of scleroderma, eosinophilic fascitis, and the various forms of pseudoscleroderma are excluded from these criteria.

A. Major criterion
   1. Proximal scleroderma: Symmetric thickening, tightening, and induration of the skin of the fingers and the skin proximal to the metacarpophalangeal or metatarsophalangeal joints. The changes may affect the entire extremity, face, neck, and trunk (thorax and abdomen).

B. Minor criteria
   1. Sclerodactyly: above-indicated skin changes limited to the fingers.
   2. Digital pitting scars or loss of substance from the finger pad: depressed areas at tips of fingers or loss of digital pad tissue as a result of ischemia.
   3. Bibasilar pulmonary fibrosis: bilateral reticular pattern or lineonodular densities most pronounced in basilar portions of the lungs on standard chest roentgenogram; may assume appearance of diffuse mottling of "honeycomb lung." These changes should not be attributable to other primary lung disease.

Table 91-2
Clinical Features of Systemic Sclerosis

Musculoskeletal
- Digital flexion contractures
- Tendon friction rubs
- Muscle weakness (when myositis present)
- Calcinosis
- Arthritis

Gastrointestinal involvement
- Esophageal reflux
- Dysphagia (diminished peristalsis or stricture)
- Delayed gastric emptying
- Malabsorption
- Alternating diarrhea and constipation

Pulmonary
- Interstitial fibrosis
- Pulmonary hypertension

Cardiac
- Pericarditis
- Myocardial fibrosis
- Tachyarrhythmias
- Conduction blockade
- Heart failure

Renal
- Hypertensive renal failure

Neurologic
- Entrapment neuropathies (including trigeminal neuralgia)

Table 91-3
Comparison of Clinical Features of Limited and Diffuse Cutaneous Systemic Sclerosis

	lcSSc	*dcSSc*
Onset	Insidious	Abrupt
Initial symptom	Raynaud	Raynaud or swelling
Skin involvement	Distal	Distal and proximal
Lung involvement	Pulmonary hypertension	Fibrosing alveolitis
Heart involvement	Secondary to pulmonary hypertension	Myocardial fibrosis
Renal involvement	Very unusual	Hypertensive renal crisis
ANA profile	Anticentromere	Anti-Scl-70 (antitopoisomerase I) Anti RNA polymerase

on the extremities and often involves the trunk. These dcSSc patients are more likely than the lcSSc patients to develop the more severe manifestations of SSc, including pulmonary fibrosis, hypertensive renal crisis, and heart failure or arrhythmias. Antibodies to topoisomerase I (30–50% of dcSSc patients) or to RNA polymerases I, II, and III (10–40%) are associated with dcSSc.

Vascular Manifestations The vascular lesion in systemic sclerosis, luminal narrowing of small arteries and arterioles as a result of intimal proliferation, is widespread and similar in all involved organs. Microvascular involvement is seen in the form of dermal telangiectases and loss of capillaries in all vascular beds. This capillary loss can be demonstrated by in vivo widefield nailfold microscopic examination of the capillaries just proximal to the cuticle. The characteristic changes of systemic sclerosis seen by this technique are capillary loop dilatation and areas of avascularity. Because these changes are not seen in primary Raynaud's phenomenon, they are very useful from a prognostic point of view in evaluating persons who have recently developed symptoms. The vascular lesions are directly associated with several distinct clinical problems, including Raynaud's phenomenon, pulmonary hypertension, and renal insufficiency.

Raynaud's Phenomenon The nearly universal occurrence of Raynaud's phenomenon (a reversible decrease in digital blood flow on exposure to cold with subsequent postischemic vasodilatation) underscores the vascular nature of systemic sclerosis. Although this is a common complaint among otherwise healthy persons (occurring in approximately 5% of the general population), it is also the most frequent initial symptom of systemic sclerosis. Patients complain of color changes (blanching or cyanosis), numbness, and/or pain in response to a cold stimulus and there is often a reactive hyperemia with rewarming. Raynaud's phenomenon in systemic sclerosis results from the superimposition of physiologic cold-induced vasoconstriction on the already pathologically reduced luminal diameter.

The ischemia resulting from the digital vascular lesions can result in irreversible changes, including tapering of the palmar fingertip pad, ulcerations of the fingertips and over the proximal interphalangeal joints, and infarction of digital tips.

Renal Involvement The characteristic kidney involvement seen in systemic sclerosis is much more likely to occur in dcSSc than lcSSc, and usually occurs early in the illness when the skin is undergoing rapid fibrosis. A sudden onset of severe hypertension is followed by progressive azotemia. This "scleroderma renal crisis" results from secretion of large quantities of renin by the juxtaglomerular apparatus in response to the decreased blood flow caused by the arteriolar luminal narrowing. The resulting formation of angiotensin causes further vasoconstriction and reduction of renal blood flow, leading to severe hypertension and diminished glomerular filtration. Shearing of erythrocytes within the altered renal vasculature can result in a microangiopathic hemolytic anemia. Until the invention of angiotensin-converting enzyme inhibitors (*see* Management section, *below*), renal crisis led invariably to renal failure or death.

Pulmonary Hypertension Pulmonary hypertension in systemic sclerosis can be the result of either of two pathologic processes. Fibrosing alveolitis *(see below)* resulting in restrictive pulmonary mechanics can result in chronic hypoxemia with secondary pulmonary hypertension. However, an increase in pulmonary vascular resistance can occur without fibrotic parenchymal lung disease as a result of the intimal lesion in the pulmonary arterioles. This isolated pulmonary hypertension is seen almost exclusively in lcSSc, where it often remains silent for decades after the occurrence of the initial manifestations of the disease. The earliest clinical manifestation is usually exertional dyspnea with overt right-sided heart failure developing later in the course.

Telangiectasia The development of dilated cutaneous blood vessels in the skin is usually a later-developing manifestation of systemic sclerosis. These telangiectases are most common on the face, palms, fingers, and lips.

Fibrotic Manifestations ***Dermal Fibrosis*** The early edematous phase of skin changes is followed by progressive thickening and tightening of the skin as a result of deposition of extracellular matrix (primarily collagen) in the dermis. This usually proceeds from distal to proximal locations on the extremities. The skin becomes indurated, difficult to pinch into a fold, and tight over bony prominences. The patient may complain of itching or burning sensations. Involvement of underlying structures such as tendons and muscles gives rise to flexion contractures of the fingers and a diminished maximal oral aperture. The maximal extent of skin fibrosis is usually reached in the first 2 or 3 years of disease, followed by progressive atrophy that is perceived as improvement by the patient and clinical examiners. However, this improvement generally does not result in diminished digital contractures. This spontaneous regression of dermal sclerosis has led to many therapies being heralded as beneficial to the course of SSc, only to be later discounted in more rigorous trials.

Pulmonary Fibrosis The development of restrictive lung disease as a result of interstitial pulmonary fibrosis has become the most common factor accounting for increased mortality in systemic sclerosis. As stated above, it is much more common in patients with dcSSc than in limited disease. Symptoms (dyspnea on exertion, nonproductive cough) are often delayed until the disease is far advanced. Chest roentgenograms are insensitive to the detection of early lung disease, but show interstitial fibrosis when the disease has progressed. Less-advanced cases of restrictive lung disease may be established by pulmonary function testing in which decreases in vital capacity and gas diffusion are found. Computerized tomographic scanning of the pulmonary parenchyma by high-resolution techniques can identify both early fibrosis and the presence of alveolitis which gives a "ground glass" appearance to the areas of inflammation. This alveolitis presumably represents the prefibrotic stage of the illness.

Pulmonary fibrosis results in dyspnea, first on exertion and then at rest. The development of pulmonary hypertension followed by right heart failure frequently precedes death.

Cardiac Involvement Several types of heart involvement occur in SSc. Symptomatic pericarditis is less common than is an echocardiographic finding of increased pericardial fluid. Reversible myocardial ischemia as a result of the vascular disease in small vessels results in contraction band necrosis, followed by patchy myocardial fibrosis. Clinical manifestations include varying degrees of heart block, arrhythmias, and congestive heart failure. Left ventricular pressure overload may result from the systemic hypertension associated with renal crisis, and right ventricular hypertrophy followed by failure often results from pulmonary hypertension.

Digestive System Involvement Involvement of the gastrointestinal system in SSc follows only Raynaud's phenomenon as a common clinical manifestation. Diminished smooth muscle motor activity of the distal two-thirds of the esophagus is the most frequent problem and results in dysphagia and esophageal reflux. With chronic reflux esophagitis, stricture can develop. Diminished peristalsis also occurs throughout the remainder of the GI tract. Delayed gastric emptying may worsen esophageal reflux. Small-bowel involvement resulting in malabsorption with weight loss is uncommon, but may be severe in the individual patient. More frequently, stasis results in bacterial overgrowth within the small intestine with deconjugation of bile salts and subsequent development of diarrhea. Colonic involvement results in stasis and constipation. Thinning of the colonic mucosa results in wide mouth diverticuli, which are usually asymptomatic.

DIAGNOSIS The diagnosis of SSc rests on clinical grounds according to the preliminary classification criteria established by the American College of Rheumatology (ACR) (Table 91-1). Many persons have illnesses that do not fulfill these intentionally insensitive, but specific, criteria, yet clearly have either early or incomplete forms of SSc.

GENETIC BASIS OF SSc As for all autoimmune diseases, the pathogenesis of SSc is felt to involve interacting genetic and environmental factors, although the precise nature of neither is completely understood. Whereas SSc is not inherited in the classical Mendelian sense, some reproducible serological manifestations are regulated by immune-response genes. DNA methods of typing HLA alleles have demonstrated close associations with disease-specific autoimmune manifestations. This link of the immunogenetic profile is much closer to the autoantibody profile than it is to the subset of SSc (lcSSc or dcSSc) or to any specific clinical or outcome parameter. The genetic hypothesis of SSc has been bolstered by rare reports of familial occurrence and by the fact that the autosomal-dominant animal model, the Tsk/+ mouse, expresses disease-specific autoantibodies (anti-topo I and anti-RNAP I) in addition to dermal fibrosis.

Whereas understanding of direct links between immune events and the vascular, cutaneous, or visceral fibrosis of SSc remains elusive, the presence of distinct autoimmune features in Ssc permits hypotheses similar to those for other autoimmune disorders. These hypotheses include: (1) an altered T-cell repertoire that fails to discriminate certain antigens as "self;" (2) one or more key immune events initiated by these self antigens and involving the trimolecular complex (MHC, TCR, antigen) that leads to the expansion and activation of self-reactive T cells; and (3) the elaboration of cytokines to provide help for B cells that express surface Ig molecules that recognize specific autoantigens such as centromere proteins, topoisomerase I, or RNA polymerase. In the specific case of SSc, these elaborated cytokines are also hypothesized to activate fibroblasts and cause endothelial cell damage and proliferation. When fully understood, many specifics of this general autoimmune paradigm should provide the basis for therapeutic immune intervention.

Antigen-presenting cells employ HLA molecules to present MHC-restricted epitopes to the heteromultimeric T-cell receptor (TCR). The expression of both the HLA and TCR are under genetic control. TCR genes utilize combinatorial mechanisms (V-J-D) to express a remarkable diversity. Most epitopes are recognized by T cells containing α/β chains in their TCRs. To date, no clonal selection of α/β T cells has been observed in either the blood or target organs (gut or lung) of SSc patients. A less prevalent subset of T-cells expresses only γ/δ chains in their TCRs. These cells seem to favor intestinal subepithelial sites and can be clonally expanded by either antigens or superantigens, the latter being microbial products that activate and expand T cells by ligating TCRs outside the cleft in which they receive MHC-restricted antigens. Normally, individuals express 10–20 different types of delta chains on their γ/δ TCRs. In groups of Ssc patients, however, γ/δ TCRs from blood, lungs, or gut biopsies display five or fewer junctional region sequences, indicating oligoclonal expansion. These studies by White et al. show expanded Vd1 ⊕ γ/δ T cells and lead to the hypothesis that the gut serves as a reservoir of γ/δ T cells where they are exposed to external influences (e.g., toxic oil, conjugated tryptophan, trichloroethylene in drinking water, possibly viruses) in response to which they expand, perhaps migrate, and potentially respond to similar influences in inhaled air. The function of this oligoclonal expansion of γ/δ T cells, including cytokine secretion and B-cell help, is poorly understood in general, and particularly, in SSc. Because T lymphocytes respond to short peptides, precise epitope mapping of these Vd ⊕, γ/δ TCRs might be a fruitful future area of study to design peptides that engage this particular T cell but block its expansion.

Both afferent (i.e., related to antigen processing or recognition) and effector (e.g., null complement haplotypes or differences in other immune-inflammatory mediators) immune-response genes have been shown to be associated with SSc to a statistically, but perhaps not clinically, significant degree. No conclusive link between class I HLA types and SSc has been demonstrated. Several class II associations have been made with different results, depending on ethnic origin of the population being studied. Positive associations with DR 3 and 5 (now 11) and negative associations with DR 2 (now 15), 7, and 9 have been made. Logistic-regression analysis has identified the primary class II HLA association to be with DQA1*0501, with the DR associations being explainable by linkage dysequilibrium. Ethnic differences between Europeans, Japanese, African Americans, and Native American Indians are substantial, but generally mirror autoimmune disease associations in those populations.

When HLA molecules and autoantibody types are examined in groups of SSc patients regardless of clinical pattern (lcSSc or dcSS), impressive associations between serology and HLA alleles can be demonstrated. For example, in one study of 42 SSc patients with anticentromere antibodies, 100% were either heterozygous or homozygous for Gly or Tyr (polar residues) rather than leucine (a nonpolar residue) at position 26 of the DQB1 molecule (a position in the peptide-binding groove of the HLA-DQ molecule). However, that 71% of the healthy population and 69% of SSc patients without anticentromere antibodies also have either one or two alleles containing such a polar residue at position 26 makes the likelihood of having anticentromere antibodies if one has such an allele very low. This indicates a major environmental influence. In the case of SSc patients expressing antitopoisomerase I autoantibodies, the polar residue in DQB1 conferring "susceptibility" is at position 30. These intriguing observations both indirectly strengthen the case that the autoimmune serology may be playing a pathogenetic role in the disease and raise the possibility of ultimately immunizing the highly susceptible individual to a blocking peptide. It should be noted that these susceptibility residues reside in the second hypervariable region of the DQB1 chain in contrast to the situation in rheumatoid arthritis or type I diabetes mellitus in which "shared epitopes" reside in the third hypervariable region of the DRB1, highlighting the lack of present understanding of functional differences between DQ and DR HLA molecules in antigen presentation. These class II HLA-autoantibody associations are strong, even if at present they are poorly understood.

Class III HLA molecules, which influence effector functions such as complement activation and tumor necrosis factor (TNF)-α cytokine secretion, are encoded by genes located between those of classes I and II on chromosome 6. A null genotype for one of the isoforms of the fourth component of complement, C4A (tightly linked to the general autoimmune haplotype [B8, DR3]) is characterized by a large gene deletion in the class III region, and is associated with several autoimmune disorders, particularly lupus and SSc. In English patients with SSc, C4A null alleles are present in 50% of patients studied. The functional implications of this gene deletion are unknown but nonetheless intriguing.

MOLECULAR PATHOPHYSIOLOGY OF DISEASE The pathophysiology of systemic sclerosis is incompletely understood, and the primary etiology(ies) remains completely obscure. Because evidence of the vascular lesion is seen so early in the course of the illness, theoretical constructs that attempt to explain all features of the illness as being secondary to the vascular lesion have been made. However, it is possible that both the vascular and fibrotic features of the illness result from some other cause, possibly immunologic or toxic. That the immunologic and microvascular lesions are already evident when the first clinical manifestations occur makes understanding the seminal event very difficult.

The Vascular Lesion The marked abnormalities seen in the blood vessels prompted searches for the cause of the endothelial-cell damage and proliferation. It is not clear whether alterations in platelet function (elevated plasma β-thromboglobulin levels and increased circulating platelet aggregates) are a cause or result of the vascular disease. Injury to or activation of the endothelium is supported by the elevated circulating levels of von Willebrand factor and endothelin (both synthesized and released by endothelial cells) and loss of endothelial reserve by diminished levels of angiotensin-converting enzyme. It has been proposed that the T lymphocytes found infiltrating the perivascular areas in early dermal lesions are the cause of the endothelial injury. Clearly, these interstitial lymphocytes leave the circulation by way of the endothelial cells. Increased expression of intercellular adhesion molecule 1 (ICAM-1) on endothelial cells of active dermal lesions

Table 91-4
Antinuclear Antibodies in Systemic Sclerosis

Antigen recognized	*Incidence (all SSc)*	*SSc Type (incidence)*
Centromere	10–20%	lcSSc 40%
Topoisomerase I (Scl-70)	15–25%	dcSSc 25–50%
RNA polymerase I, II, III	10–25%	dcSSc 20–45%
U3RNP (fibrillarin)	5–45%	dcSSc 5%
Th	5%	lcSSc
U1RNP	5–35%	lcSSc

and the demonstration that infiltrating lymphocytes bear cell surface leukocyte adhesion factor 1 (LFA-1), the ligand for ICAM-1, indicate a mechanism for the presence of T cells in the perivascular infiltrates. The endothelial cells also express increased amounts of endothelial leukocyte adhesion molecule 1 (ELAM-1 or E-selectin). That T cells may be important in causing endothelial injury is supported by the finding of elevated levels of granzyme-1 and antibodies to granzyme-1 in sera of SSc patients. This enzyme is able to lyse endothelial cells possibly in association with perforin and via a programmed cell death (apoptosis) pathway.

Immunologic Aspects Integral immunologic features of SSc include the presence of specific autoantibodies (*see* Table 91-4), infiltration of the skin by lymphocytes and macrophages, and the demonstration of abnormal amounts of certain cytokines in the blood, lungs, and dermis. Nests of lymphocytes (primarily T cells) and macrophages are found in the dermis, particularly in the deeper reticular area, where fibrosis is most intense. Subset analysis shows these infiltrating lymphocytes to be $CD4^+$ cells bearing α/β T-cell receptors.

The occurrence of antinuclear antibodies in the sera of patients with systemic sclerosis approaches 100%. All types of staining patterns may be seen, but nucleolar patterns are more specific. Associations have been made between the presence of antibodies to certain purified nuclear antigens and clinical manifestations of SSc. Antibodies to centromeres (kinetochore plates) occur in approximately 40% of patients with lcSSc, but in only 2–5% of patients with dcSSc. On the other hand antibodies to topoisomerase I (also known as Scl-70) are present much more frequently in dcSSc (30–40%). The presence of these latter antibodies is therefore also associated with rapid skin thickening, pulmonary interstitial fibrosis, and renal crisis.

Antibodies to RNA polymerase types I, II, and III are also seen frequently in dcSSc, and account for the frequent occurrence of antinucleolar ANA staining. There are marked racial differences in the occurrence of the various autoantibodies in the clinical subsets of SSc, making the regulation of expression of these specific antibodies of interest. Linkage of certain autoantibody types with specific HLA loci has been demonstrated *(see above)*.

Inflammatory Aspects SSc, with only moderate elevations of circulating acute-phase reactants, is not an overwhelmingly inflammatory condition. The only area in which polymorphonuclear leukocytes have been demonstrated to be present in increased numbers is in pulmonary lesions. When alveolar cells are obtained for analysis by bronchoalveolar lavage, increased numbers of PMNs, eosinophils, and macrophages are seen. These macrophages are activated, as evidenced by increased production of fibronectin in cell culture. Analysis of the fluid obtained by BAL has demonstrated increased levels of several cytokines. The PMN chemoattractant IL-8 is present in increased quantities in such fluid. Cytokines that increase fibroblast proliferation (platelet-derived growth factor, PDGF) and matrix synthesis (transforming growth factor type 1, TGF-1) are also present in increased concentrations.

Systemic Sclerosis (SSc) and the Extracellular Matrix (ECM) Many abnormalities of the ECM have been documented in SSc, and it is likely that many more will be forthcoming. Recent awareness that cells derive informational signals directly from ECM via integrins as well as from cytokines and growth factors bound to ECM has both substantially increased the momentum to define ECM components and placed ECM modular motifs in a central position in the study of cell behavior in fibrosis (Fig. 91-1). As an example, skin fibroblasts behave quite differently with regard to collagen secretion and metalloproteinase production when cultured on three-dimensional collagen lattices in contrast to monolayer tissue-culture plastic.

A detailed review of the components of the ECM is beyond the scope of this discussion. Suffice it to say that there are 19 collagens composed of 33 genes, 8 laminins, 5 thrombospondins, alternatively spliced fibronectins and cytotactins, and wide variations in the charge and size of a family of proteoglycans that have recently been completely renamed. That collagens are the most diverse of the modular protein families thus far characterized can be appreciated visually from Fig. 91-1. The common structural characteristic of collagens is the primary structure Gly-X-Y, which, by virtue of the absence of a side chain on glycine in peptide linkage, folds into a tight and strong α helix. When this helix is uninterrupted for 1000 or more residues, collagen fibrils with impressive tensile strength are formed, characteristic of skin, bone, tendon, and blood vessels. Collagens with interrupted helices and specialized globular modules may participate in other ways in ECM function. Collagens, fibronectins, and proteoglycans may interact with cells in adhesive ways, cytotactins and thrombospondins may function in antiadhesive ways. Cell–matrix interactions via a large number of integrin surface cell membrane receptors trigger signaling cascades and, via reorganization and clustering of intracellular cytoskeletal elements, can direct cell shape, movement, division, and secretion. The cell–matrix interactions of fibroblasts and endothelial cells are under intense study presently and understandings of direct relevance to SSc can be anticipated.

The SSc lesional skin fibroblast has been known since 1972 to differ from normal fibroblasts, with overproduction of collagen being the first abnormality described. Whereas its in vitro proliferative response to PDGF is less than that of control fibroblasts, it proliferates in response to TGF-β1, whereas control cells do not, and it does not see bFGF as a mitogen, whereas control cells do. When control cells are exposed to TGF-β1, they express some of the phenotypic traits of the activated SSc fibroblast, including the heightened expression of the PDGF receptors α and β.

In vivo healthy skin fibroblasts rarely express collagen α1(I) mRNA but, in SSc lesions, fibroblasts in the vicinity of mononuclear-cell perivascular inflammatory infiltrates express this message. Immunolocalization studies of this same microenvironment can identify TGF-β1 and PDGF AA. It is also the site of microvascular endothelial-cell abnormalities and presumably of perivascular fibrosis as well. Using a combination of in vitro and in vivo techniques, the matrix molecules shown to be overexpressed in the Ssc microlesion are collagens type I, III, V, VI, and VII,

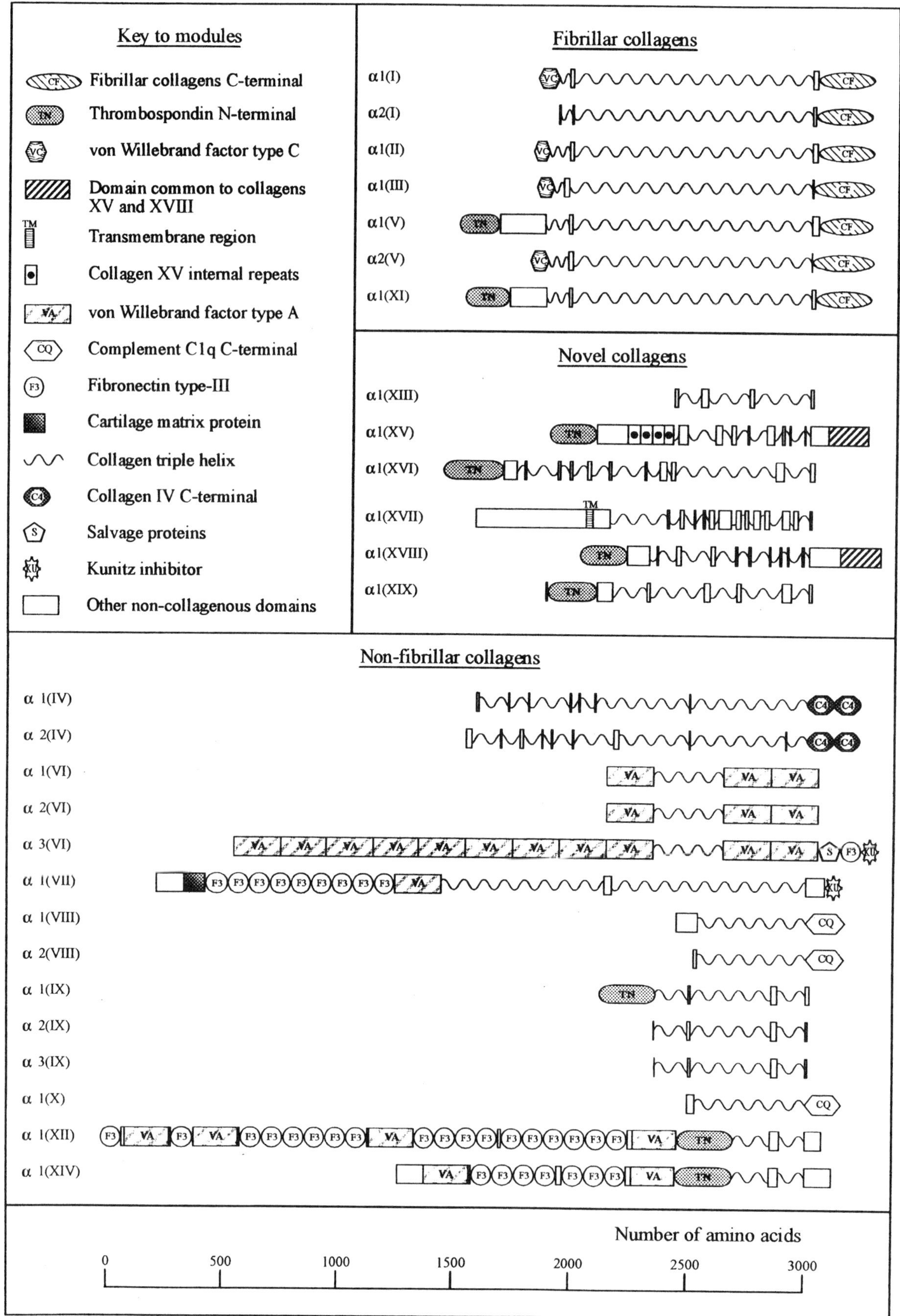

Figure 91-1 A graphic presentation of the diversity of collagens. (Reproduced with permission from Karger S, Basel AG. The collagen superfamily. Int Arch Allergy Immunol 1995;107:484–490.)

Table 91-5
Cytokines Possibly Involved in the Pathogenesis of Systemic Sclerosis

Monocyte/macrophage derived	
	IL-1, IL-6, IL-8, TGF-β, PDGF, fibronectin
Lymphocyte derived	
	IL-2,
Platelet derived	
	TGF-β, PDGF
Endothelial	
	Endothelin
Fibroblast	
	Fibronectin, IL-6, VEGF (vascular endothelial growth factor)

fibronectin, and cytotactin (tenascin). Fibroblast exposure to TGF-β1 upregulates these same matrix molecules in a prolonged fashion. The data to-date suggest that the molecular site of upregulation of these matrix molecules is pretranslational in that there is an increased level of steady-state mRNA present. Evidence also exists that suggests both an increased rate of mRNA synthesis and a decreased rate of mRNA decay, in the case of the best-studied collagen, type I. Regarding mRNA synthesis, directed by 5' promoter elements, at least 4 *cis*-acting DNA response elements can be shown to bind at least three distinct protein-transcription factors, including a collagen-binding factor (CBF) binding a CCAAT motif, the ubiquitous Sp1 binding a series of G-C–rich boxes, and a c-Krox factor binding several G rich motifs. How these interactions combine to initiate transcription and which ones are critical to the fibrosis of Ssc remains to be elucidated. Nonetheless, the area of the transcriptional control of ECM synthesis, the interruption of the widespread and prolonged stimulation by TGF-β1, and ultimately the modulation of ECM production in SSc remains a potentially important area for therapeutic intervention.

Cytokines Several cytokines have been implicated in the pathogenesis of systemic sclerosis (Table 91-5). Elevations of IL-2, IL-4, IL-6, and IL-8 have been demonstrated in the sera of patients. Both IL-2 and IL-2-receptor levels seem to mirror the activity of fibrosis that is occurring and therefore indicate involvement of the immune system. IL-2 has no direct effects on fibroblasts, but has been reported to increase TGF-β release by macrophages. Cytokines that directly affect fibroblast proliferation and matrix synthesis are involved in fibrotic lesion.

Platelet-Derived Growth Factor (PDGF) PDGF, which exists as either homo- or heterodimers of A and B chains, is a potent mitogen for fibroblasts. Rich sources of this protein include platelet α granules and macrophages, both cell types known to be activated in SSc. PDGF α receptors, which recognize all PDGF isoforms, are increased by TGF-β in scleroderma fibroblasts but not in normal dermal fibroblasts. That PDGF AA, which signals only via α receptors, is found in scleroderma lesions makes it likely that this cytokine is important in fibroblast proliferation in systemic sclerosis. Both PDGF AA and BB are found in increased concentration in fluid removed from the lungs of systemic sclerosis patients by bronchoalveolar lavage.

Transforming-Growth Factor β (TGF-β) TGF-β has quite contrasting effects on cells depending on cell type and on their state at the time of study. Interest in TGF-β in SSc stems from the fact that this is the most potent stimulator of fibroblast synthesis of extracellular matrix known. TGF-β is produced by megakaryocytes, macrophages, and T cells, particularly TH-2 type. Whereas no increases in blood levels of TGF-β are seen in systemic sclerosis patients, other evidence implicates this cytokine in the areas of occurring lesions. *In situ* expression of TGF-β mRNA in dermal lesions has been demonstrated. As mentioned above, TGF-β causes dermal fibroblasts of scleroderma lesions to proliferate via increased expression of PDGF α receptors and response to PDGF A ligand. In the lung lesion, increases in TGF-β type 1, but not type 2, have been measured in bronchoalveolar lavage fluid and increases in TGF-β mRNA are seen in mononuclear cells obtained by this means.

Interleukin-6 IL-6, a product of macrophages and fibroblasts, has been shown to be produced in vitro by scleroderma fibroblasts at levels up to 30 times that of normal fibroblasts. Although IL-6 is a stimulator of collagen synthesis only at very high concentrations, it inhibits fibroblast synthesis of tissue inhibitor of metalloproteases (TIMP). Produced locally, IL-6 may therefore promote fibrosis by inhibiting collagenase activity.

Basic Fibroblast Growth Factor (bFGF) bFGF, a stimulator of fibroblast proliferation, has been found in dermal lesions. Fibroblasts themselves produce bFGF and it may thus be involved in an autocrine role in fibroblast proliferation in systemic sclerosis.

Interferon-γ A product of T cells, interferon (IFN)-γ actively suppresses fibroblast collagen synthesis. Serum levels of IFN-γ have been found to be depressed in systemic sclerosis and in vitro stimulation of peripheral blood T cells fails to elicit the increase in interferon gamma production seen in normal T cells. Therefore, a defect in T cells of systemic sclerosis patients resulting in an inability to suppress fibrosis may exist.

Interleukin-1 IL-1, primarily a product of macrophages, is able to stimulate fibroblast extracellular-matrix synthesis. Increased sensitivity of systemic sclerosis fibroblasts in culture to stimulatory effects of IL-1β has been demonstrated. There has been recent evidence that systemic sclerosis fibroblasts from clinically involved dermis are able to produce IL-1α and that this cytokine is responsible for increases in PDGF-A and IL-6 production by these cells. This intriguing possibility would link several of the abnormal cytokine productions seen in systemic sclerosis together into a pathogenetically meaningful cytokine "cascade."

Endothelin Endothelin is the potent smooth muscle contracting peptide derived from endothelial cells. Increased blood levels of endothelin have been described in both primary Raynaud phenomenon and in SSc, and some evidence indicates that levels are further increased with exposure to cold. Elevated levels are found in patients with pulmonary hypertension and also fibrotic lung involvement. There is evidence indicating that endothelin can increase fibroblast collagen-synthetic rates, a finding that links the vascular and fibrotic lesions seen in SSc.

MANAGEMENT Because the etiology of SSc remains so obscure, treatment is directed to each of the clinical problems presented by the disease. It is hoped that with better understanding, treatment directed at the underlying disease processes can be developed.

Skin Involvement Because spontaneous skin softening almost always occurs with time, uncontrolled trials are difficult to interpret, and enthusiasm over proposed therapies must be tempered. There are many reports of dramatic improvements, but these therapies have often failed when studied in a prospective and randomized fashion.

D-Penicillamine is widely used to treat the dermal thickening, based on its inhibition of collagen crosslinking and facilitation of collagen degradation. Several uncontrolled studies have demonstrated improvement in the extent of skin thickening. A multicenter, randomized trial comparing high-dose and low-dose D-penicillamine is currently underway, and not until its results are known can one assuredly state that D-penicillamine is an effective therapy for SSc. If therapy with D-penicillamine is undertaken, the dose should be gradually increased to 1–1.5 g/d, a dose that must be maintained for 6 months to a year to see any clinically important improvements. Many patients experience side effects with gastrointestinal symptoms being the most common. Renal (hematuria, proteinuria) and hematological (leukopenia, thrombocytopenia) adverse reactions are of greater concern and close monitoring is required.

Immunosuppression with glucocorticoids and/or cytotoxic chemotherapy is not effective in changing the skin disease. Chlorambucil and 5-fluorouracil has been shown to be ineffective. IFN-γ, which decreases fibroblast collagen synthesis, has been reported to decrease skin thickening in patients with SSc in uncontrolled trials, but has been associated with some exacerbation of vascular problems.

Raynaud's Phenomenon (RP) Modifications of both behavior and environment are necessary to avoid cool temperatures. β-blockers may worsen RP by allowing unopposed α-adrenergic stimulation. Behavioral therapy with biofeedback may reduce the frequency or severity of attacks, although the evidence suggests that this is more effective in primary than in secondary Raynaud's phenomenon.

Calcium-channel blockers are the most commonly used pharmacologic therapies, but there is no definitive proof of their efficacy in SSc. The sustained release form of nifedipine is prescribed most commonly. Calcium-channel blockade causes inhibition of gut smooth muscle contraction and may therefore increase esophageal reflux or delay peristalsis in the stomach or gut. Prazosin (an α-adrenergic blocker) can be used instead of, or in addition to, calcium-channel blockers. Platelet inhibitors (low-dose aspirin and dipyridamole) are used, although there is no definitive proof of their efficacy. Nitroglycerin paste can be applied at the bases of the most affected digits to promote arterial dilatation.

Stellate ganglion blockade to bring about temporary sympathectomy may greatly alleviate pain and induce vasodilatation. Infection of a digital ulcer requires local cleansing, and application of an antibacterial ointment may be helpful. Occasionally infection is so rapidly progressive or advanced to the point of osteomyelitis that therapy with parenteral antibiotics is indicated. Surgical therapy has been used to treat severe RP. Whereas cervical sympathectomy may reduce attack frequency and severity for a short time, symptoms usually recur and it is, therefore, not recommended. Digital sympathectomy has been promoted as more selective and having longer-lasting effects than cervical sympathectomy, but this procedure is still investigational. Amputation of a phalanx or digit may quickly relieve pain, and is sometimes the most effective means of dealing with infection.

Renal Involvement The development of hypertensive renal disease in a SSc patient is a medical emergency because irreversible loss of renal function may result. The discovery of angiotensin-converting enzyme (ACE) inhibitors has changed the natural history of SSc. Any elevation in blood pressure should be taken quite seriously, and when persons who have had low-to-normal pressures develop elevations that are still within the normal range of < 140/90 mmHg, they should be evaluated for renal disease. During the early stages of treatment, captopril rather than other ACE inhibitors is recommended because its shorter half-life allows greater flexibility in dosing. For those who remain hypertensive, captopril should be maintained and other hypotensive agents added using whatever combination of drugs allows normal blood pressures to be obtained. Antihypertensive therapy should be continued, even if renal failure ensues, since there are reports of return of sustained renal function even after dialysis.

Pulmonary Disease No controlled, prospective trial has shown any drug to alter the course of SSc interstitial lung disease. All patients should be vaccinated for *Streptococcus pneumoniae* and influenza. Patients with severe fibrosis may benefit symptomatically from oxygen. Because fibrotic interstitial lung disease is associated with alveolar inflammation, therapy to reduce this inflammation has been undertaken in uncontrolled trials. Daily oral cyclophosphamide (100 mg/d) significantly increased the forced vital capacity (FVC) of patients with alveolitis. This treatment must be undertaken advisedly, however, as no controlled trial has been undertaken. Pulmonary hypertension remains a difficult problem in the management of SSc, and is often involved in the demise of these patients.

Pulmonary hypertension may occur either as a complication of interstitial fibrosis or as isolated pulmonary hypertension in the absence of interstitial lung disease. This latter form of severe pulmonary hypertension occurs almost exclusively in patients with limited cutaneous SSc. Echocardiography with Doppler allows estimation of peak systolic pulmonary artery pressure by a noninvasive means. Results of treatment studies of pulmonary hypertension complicating SSc have been quite variable. The long duration of pulmonary vascular disease before it becomes symptomatic leads to fixed vascular lesions that may not be amenable to vasodilation. Calcium-channel blockers may lower pulmonary artery resistance, but their effect on survival is unknown.

Cardiac Disease Pericarditis usually responds to nonsteroidal antiinflammatory drugs or to low-dose corticosteroids. Treatment of left-ventricular dysfunction involves the use of digoxin, diuretics, and afterload-reducing agents. Long-term therapy with captopril has been shown to improve systolic and diastolic function in some patients. Nifedipine has been shown to improve myocardial perfusion and cold-induced myocardial ischemia, but no information is available on long-term clinical effects. Antiarrhythmic drugs are used to treat symptomatic ventricular arrhythmias.

Gastrointestinal Manifestations Antireflux measures (small, frequent meals; avoiding recumbency after eating; elevation of the head of the bed) are recommended for all SSc patients because of the universal occurrence of esophageal reflux. Damage to the esophageal mucosa from acid reflux can be reduced by use of acid lowering drugs such as H_2-blockers or proton-pump inhibitors. Cisapride, which increases gastrointestinal motility by enhancing acetylcholine release at the myenteric interface, has improved upper gastrointestinal symptoms in clinical trials. Esophageal strictures are sought by barium studies and respond to dilation.

Malabsorption with diarrhea, weight loss and malnutrition, bloating, distention, and abdominal pain may result from hypoperistalsis of the small bowel. A 2-week treatment with antibiotics—e.g., tetracycline, amoxicillin, or metronidazole—may help by diminishing bacterial overgrowth and relieve symptoms of recurrent diarrhea. The occurrence of pseudoobstruction is associated with vomiting and radiographic evidence of dilated bowel. Any precipitating causes (opioid narcotics, electrolyte abnormalities) should be corrected. Surgical exploration should be avoided as the outcome is usually very poor.

LOCALIZED SCLERODERMA (MORPHEA)

EPIDEMIOLOGY The incidence and prevalence of localized scleroderma are unknown, but minor types are quite common and may not come to medical attention. It occurs primarily in young adults and children, with a slight predominance in females. All races are affected. There is no known occupational or exposure risk.

CLINICAL FEATURES There are several varieties of morphea, including guttate, plaque, generalized, and linear. These can occur either singly or as several types in the same patient. Guttate morphea are small (few millimeter), oval lesions occurring on the neck and chest. Plaque morphea are a few centimeters to a few inches in diameter and can become generalized with widespread involvement. Initially lesions are erythematous or violaceous lesions that evolve into waxy, ivory-colored skin thickening with a surrounding violaceous border. If these lesions become generalized, the appearance can resemble that of systemic sclerosis, but there is no sclerodactyly, Raynaud's phenomenon, or internal organ involvement. Linear scleroderma occurs most commonly in children and appears as band-like areas of induration along a particular myotome. There is atrophy of the skin, underlying subcutaneous tissue, muscle, and even osseous involvement. When involving the face (*en coup de sabre* lesion), facial hemiatrophy may result. This lesion is similar to (or may be the same as) the Parry-Romberg syndrome. Linear scleroderma, when involving a limb, often results in shortening, severe contractures, and considerable disability.

Histologically, morphea does not differ from the findings in systemic sclerosis, with a chronic inflammatory cell infiltrate in the inflammatory border, and monotonous increase in dermal collagen.

The clinical course of most morphea is to spontaneously soften, but to leave areas of atrophy and depigmentation. Occasionally there can be complete resolution. Progression to systemic sclerosis has been reported, but is so extraordinarily rare as to be reportable. Morphea is not associated with Raynaud's phenomenon, esophageal dysmotility, interstitial lung disease, or renal involvement.

Various nonspecific immunological abnormalities have been reported in morphea, including hypergammaglobulinemia, antinuclear antibodies, anti–single-stranded DNA antibodies, antihistone antibodies, and rheumatoid factor. Systemic sclerosis specific antibodies (antitopoisomerase, anticentromere, anti-RNA polymerase) are not found in patients with linear scleroderma. Although there was initial enthusiasm, when many patients with morphea were found to have antibodies to *Borrelia burgdorferi*, that this signified the cause of morphea, later studies using PCR to search for this organism's DNA in morphea lesions have been unsuccessful. It is now felt that *Borrelia* infection plays no role in causing morphea.

GENETIC BASIS OF DISEASE The occurrence of multiple family members with localized scleroderma is very unusual. No predisposing genetic lesion or HLA type has been associated with the occurrence of lesions.

MOLECULAR PATHOGENESIS The increases in dermal collagen are of the same types seen in systemic sclerosis—I and III. Immunohistochemically determined increases in TGF-β have been described in the active margins of the lesion in close association with fibroblasts shown to be secreting procollagen. Very few other details concerning the molecules involved in pathogenesis have been described.

TREATMENT No treatment has been demonstrated to alter the course of localized scleroderma. Often morphea lesions are self-limiting, running a course from initiation to disappearance in several years. D-penicillamine has been applied to more progressive lesions, and in those individuals who may go on to generalized morphea. No controlled study regarding use of this medication has been completed. Deforming linear scleroderma may require plastic surgery. When a limb has become so deformed as to inhibit function, amputation with prosthetic replacement should be considered.

SELECTED REFERENCES

Briggs D, Black CM, Welsh K. Genetic factors in scleroderma. Rheum Dis Clin NA 1990;16:31–51.

Briggs DC, Stephens C, Vaughan R, Welsh K, Black CM. A molecular and serologic analysis of the major histocompatibility complex and complement component C4 in systemic sclerosis. Arthritis Rheum 1993;36:943–954.

Brown JC, Timpl R. The collagen superfamily. Int Arch Allergy Immunol 1995;107:484–490.

Cannon PJ, Hassar M, Case DB, Casarella WJ, Sommers SC, LeRoy EC. The relationship of hypertension and renal failure in scleroderma (progressive systemic sclerosis) to structural and functional abnormalities of the renal cortical circulation. Medicine 1974;53:1–46.

Donoghue JF. Scleroderma and the kidney. Kidney Int 1992;41:462–477.

Feghali CA, Bost KL, Boulware DW, Levy. Mechanisms of pathogenesis in scleroderma: I. Overproduction of Interleukin 6 by fibroblasts cultured from affected skin of patients with scleroderma. J Rheumatol 1992;19:1202–1211.

Fleischmajer R. Localized and systemic scleroderma. In: Lapiere CM, Krieg T, eds. Connective Tissue Diseases of the Skin. New York: Marcel Dekker, 1993; pp. 295–314.

Hirakata M, Okano Y, Pati U, et al. Identification of autoantibodies to RNA polymerase II: occurrence in systemic sclerosis and association with autoantibodies to RNA polymerases I and III. J Clin Invest 1993;91:2665–2672.

Legerton CW III, Smith EA, Silver RM. Systemic sclerosis (scleroderma): clinical management of its major complications. Rheum Dis Clin NA 1995;21:203–216.

Ludwicka A, Ohba T, Trojanowska M, et al. Elevated levels of platelet derived growth factor and transforming growth factor-β1 in bronchoalveolar lavage fluid from patients with scleroderma. J Rheum 1995;22:1876–1883.

Masi AT, Rodnan GP, Medsger TA Jr, et al. Preliminary criteria for the classification of systemic sclerosis (scleroderma). Arthritis Rheum 1980;23:581–590.

Medsger TA Jr. Systemic sclerosis (Scleroderma), localized forms of scleroderma, and calcinosis. In: McCarty DJ, Koopman WJ, eds. Arthritis and Allied Conditions. Philadelphia: Lea and Febiger, 1993; pp. 1253–1292.

Okano Y, Steen VD, Medsger TA. Autoantibody reactive with RNA polymerase III in systemic sclerosis. Ann Int Med 1993;119: 1005–1013.

Reveille JD, Durban E, MacLeod-St. Clair MJ, et al. Association of amino acid sequences in the HLA-DQB1 first domain with the antitopoisomerase I autoantibody response in scleroderma (progressive systemic sclerosis). J Clin Invest 1992;90:973–980.

Reveille JD, Owerbach D, Goldstein R, Moreda R, Isern RA, Arnett FC. Association of polar amino acids at position 26 of the HLA-DQB1 first domain with the anticentromere autoantibody response in systemic sclerosis (scleroderma). J Clin Invest 1992;89: 1208–1213.

Seibold JR, Furst DE, Clements PJ. Why everything (or nothing) seems to work in the treatment of scleroderma. J Rheum 1992;19: 673–676.

Seibold JR. Connective tissue diseases characterized by fibrosis. In: Kelley WN, Harris ED Jr, Ruddy S, Sledge CB, eds. Textbook of Rheumatology. Philadelphia: Saunders, 1993; pp. 1113–1143.

Sollberg S, Peltonen J, Uitto J, Jimenez SA. Elevated expression of β1 and β2 integrins, intercellular adhesion molecule 1, and endothelial leukocyte adhesion molecule 1 in the skin of patients with systemic sclerosis of recent onset. Arthritis Rheum 1992;35:290–298.

Uziel Y, Krafchik BR, Silverman ED, Thorner PS, Laxer RM. Localized scleroderma in childhood: a report of 30 cases. Sem Arthritis Rheum 1994;23:328–340.

Yamakage A, Kikuchi K, Smith EA, LeRoy EC, Trojanowska M. Selective upregulation of platelet-derived growth factor a receptors by transforming growth factor β in scleroderma fibroblasts. J Exp Med 1995;175:1227–1234.

MUSCULOSKELETAL X

SECTION EDITOR:
LAURENCE KEDES

92 Muscle Development and Differentiation

ERIC N. OLSON

INTRODUCTION

Vertebrate species contain dozens of different skeletal muscles, each with unique positions, sizes, shapes, contractile properties, and patterns of innervation. In recent years, dramatic progress has been made toward understanding the genetic pathways that control the formation and patterning of skeletal muscle during embryogenesis. The discovery of several families of genes that act at different steps in the developmental pathway leading to skeletal muscle formation has provided a framework for understanding the complexity of this tissue and will undoubtedly yield insight into the causes of several neuromuscular disorders, as well as provide the potential for therapeutic intervention into such diseases.

REGULATION OF MUSCLE DIFFERENTIATION IN VITRO

Much of the progress in understanding muscle development can be attributed to the fact that many of the events associated with muscle differentiation in vivo can be recapitulated in tissue culture. Immortalized muscle cell lines or skeletal myoblasts isolated from embryos proliferate in vitro in the presence of fetal bovine serum and other mitogens such as fibroblast growth factor (FGF). Myoblasts are committed to the myogenic lineage, but they do not express muscle structural genes until they are forced to exit the cell cycle. Myoblast differentiation is accompanied by irreversible withdrawal from the cell cycle, fusion to form multinucleate myotubes, and expression of a large array of muscle-specific genes whose products are required for the specialized contractile, excitable, and metabolic properties of the differentiated muscle fiber.

Several early studies suggested the existence of myogenic regulatory factors with the potential to activate muscle gene expression. Experiments in which heterokaryons were formed between skeletal muscle cells and various nonmuscle cells demonstrated that muscle genes became activated in nonmuscle cell nuclei and suggested the existence of *trans*-acting factors in muscle cells that could activate muscle gene expression. Genetic evidence for such myogenic factors was provided by experiments in which the fibroblast cell line 10T1/2 was shown to form skeletal muscle following treatment with the demethylating agent 5'-azacytidine. The frequency of conversion of 10T1/2 cells to muscle (up to 50%) suggested that one gene was responsible for establishing the myogenic phenotype following its activation by demethylation. This hypothesis was confirmed by DNA transfection experiments in which genomic DNA from myoblasts or 5'-azacytidine-treated 10T1/2 cells was shown to convert 10T1/2 cells to myoblasts with a frequency consistent with a single regulatory gene.

From: *Principles of Molecular Medicine* (J. L. Jameson, ed.), ©1998 Humana Press Inc., Totowa, NJ.

THE MyoD FAMILY OF MUSCLE-SPECIFIC TRANSCRIPTION FACTORS

The first myogenic regulatory gene to be cloned was *myoD*, which was isolated by cloning mRNAs that were expressed in myoblasts, but not 10T1/2 fibroblasts. When a cDNA clone encoding MyoD was expressed ectopically in fibroblasts, it was found to activate skeletal muscle gene expression (Fig. 92-1). Subsequently, three related genes, myogenin, Myf5, and MRF4 (also called Myf6 and herculin) were discovered. These genes, which are referred to as the MyoD family, are expressed exclusively in skeletal muscle; there is no detectable expression in cardiac or smooth muscle, despite the fact that these three muscle cell types express many of the same muscle-specific genes.

Members of the MyoD family exhibit distinct expression patterns during differentiation of muscle cells in culture. Most established muscle cell lines express either MyoD or Myf5 when they are proliferating as undifferentiated myoblasts. When induced to differentiate by exposure to growth factor-deficient medium, myogenin is rapidly upregulated immediately prior to activation of muscle structural genes. MyoD and Myf5 also continue to be expressed in differentiated myotubes. MRF4 is not expressed until late in the differentiation program.

Members of the MyoD family can induce skeletal muscle gene expression when they are introduced into a wide variety of cell types including fibroblasts, melanoblasts, chondroblasts, smooth and cardiac muscle cells, and osteoblasts. In some cell types, these factors activate the entire myogenic program, resulting in formation of multinucleate myotubes and expression of the full array of muscle-specific genes, whereas in other cell types, only a subset of muscle genes is expressed. There are other cell types, such as adipocytes, in which forced expression of the myogenic factors represses the endogenous program of cell-specific gene expression, while in other cell types the skeletal muscle program is coexpressed with the endogenous program. There are also cell types, such as hepatocytes and several types of transformed cells, in which the myogenic factors are unable to activate muscle gene expression. The failure of the myogenic factors to activate muscle gene expression in these cell types suggests either that they lack certain cofactors required by the myogenic factors or they contain inhibitors of muscle gene expression or both.

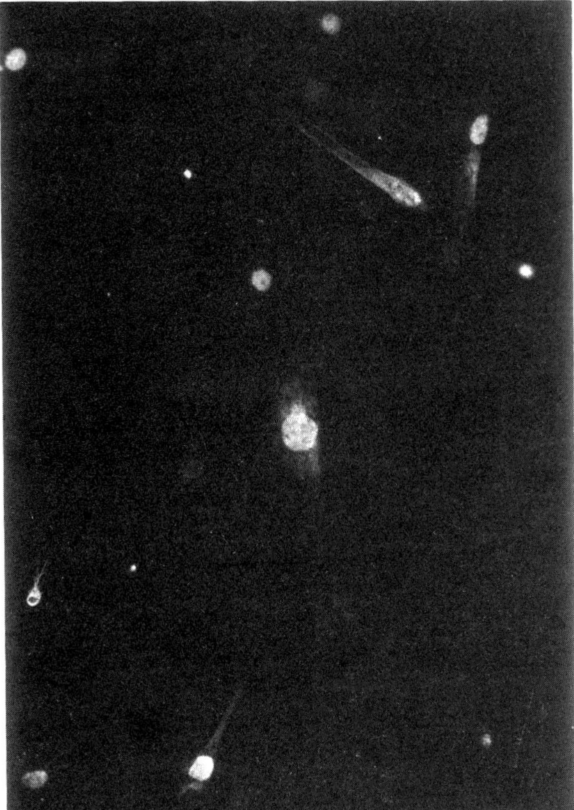

Figure 92-1 Activation of MHC expression in fibroblasts expressing exogenous MyoD. 10T1/2 fibroblasts were transfected with a MyoD expression vector. Cells were then stained using antibodies specific for MyoD (red) and myosin heavy chain (green). MyoD can been seen within the nuclei of transfected cells and myosin is expressed only in the cells that express MyoD. Figure provided by S. Tapscott, Fred Hutchinson Cancer Research Center. (*See* color insert following p. 684.)

In addition to activating the expression of muscle structural genes, members of the MyoD family regulate one anothers expression. For example, if MyoD is introduced into fibroblasts, it activates the endogenous MyoD gene as well as the myogenin and MRF4 genes. These autoregulatory interactions have been proposed as a mechanism whereby these factors amplify and maintain their expression and thereby commit cells to a myogenic fate.

THE BASIC HELIX-LOOP-HELIX FAMILY OF TRANSCRIPTION FACTORS

Members of the MyoD family share about 80% amino acid identity within a 70-amino acid segment that encompasses a region rich in basic amino acids, followed by a region postulated to adopt a helix-loop-helix (HLH) conformation in which two amphipathic α-helices are separated by an intervening loop (Fig. 92-2). Related, but more divergent, basic-HLH (bHLH) motifs are found in members of a superfamily of proteins that regulate cell proliferation and differentiation in species ranging from yeast to humans. Among these are members of the c-myc family of oncoproteins and the products of several *Drosophila* genes that regulate embryonic cell fates, including the *achaete-scute* gene products, which regulate neurogenesis, and twist, which regulates mesoderm formation.

The HLH motif mediates protein dimerization and brings together the basic regions of bHLH proteins to form a bipartite DNA binding domain that recognizes the consensus sequence CANNTG (N = any nucleotide), known as an E-box (Fig. 92-3). This DNA sequence motif is found in the control regions of numerous muscle-specific genes, where it binds the myogenic factors and mediates transcriptional activation.

The myogenic bHLH factors homodimerize inefficiently, but they readily form heterodimers with members of a family of ubiquitous bHLH proteins, known as E-proteins. There are also HLH proteins that lack basic regions and inhibit the activity of bHLH proteins by forming heterodimers incapable of binding DNA. Among this class of HLH proteins are members of the Id family.

Mutagenesis studies have revealed several functional domains in the myogenic bHLH proteins (Fig. 92-4). These factors contain transcription activation domains in their amino- and carboxyl-termini that are important for efficient activation of muscle-specific transcription. The basic regions of the myogenic factors play a dual role in the control of muscle gene expression by mediating DNA binding and by conferring muscle specificity to transcriptional activation. Fine mapping of individual amino acids in the DNA-binding domains of the myogenic factors has shown that two clusters of basic amino acids are required for binding to the E-box consensus sequence (Fig. 92-4). In addition, two adjacent amino acids, alanine-threonine, in the center of the DNA binding domains, are required for activation of muscle gene expression. These residues are conserved in the basic regions of all known myogenic bHLH proteins in species ranging from *Drosophila* and sea urchins to humans and they are absent from the basic regions of the more than 40 other bHLH proteins described to date. The specificity and conservation of these residues suggest that they represent part of an ancient mechanism for activation of muscle gene expression.

If the alanine-threonine residues in the basic region of a myogenic bHLH protein are replaced with the amino acids found at that position in the basic regions of E proteins, the resulting mutant protein will bind DNA normally, but is unable to activate muscle gene expression. Conversely, if these residues along with a third amino acid between the basic region and helix-1 of the myogenic factors are introduced in the corresponding positions in E proteins, they confer on the E proteins the ability to activate muscle gene expression.

The exact mechanism whereby amino acids in the basic region direct muscle-specific transcription is unclear. However, one possibility is that these amino acids induce an allosteric change in the myogenic factors following DNA binding, which might expose a protein interface that can interact with accessory factors required for the activation of muscle gene expression. In this regard, the crystal structure of a MyoD homodimer binding to an E-box DNA sequence has been deduced. The structure of the complex confirms that the basic region and first helix of the HLH region form a continuous α-helix. Alanine-threonine in the MyoD basic region lie within the major groove of the DNA binding site and are therefore inaccessible to other proteins. However, the interaction of these residues with the DNA appears to induce a conformational change in the protein, which may influence the proteins with which it can interact.

GROWTH FACTOR CONTROL OF MYOGENESIS

As in many cell types, differentiation of myoblasts is coupled to withdrawal from the cell cycle. Whereas many cell types can reenter the cell cycle when stimulated with mitogens, skeletal muscle cells lose the ability to reinitiate DNA synthesis when they differentiate and therefore become irreversibly committed to the postmitotic state. Because myoblasts express MyoD or Myf5

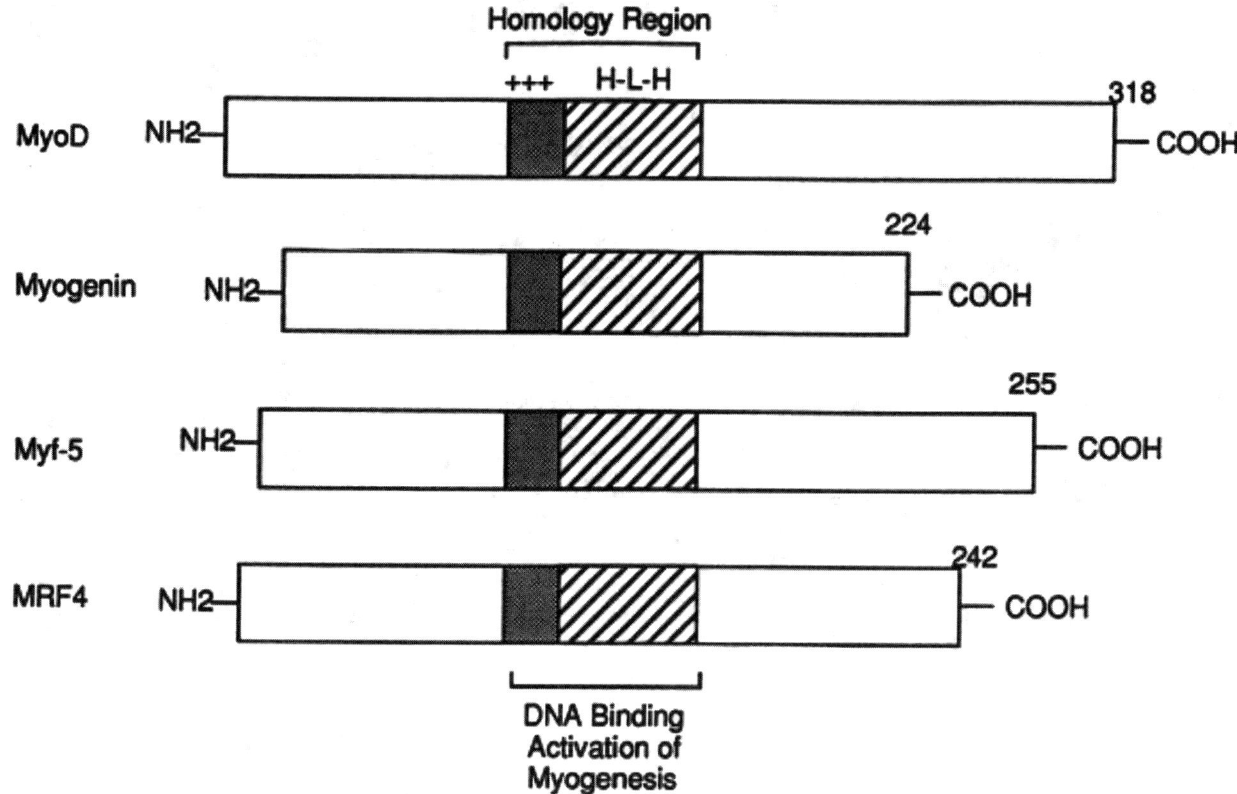

Figure 92-2 Diagramatic representation of the four myogenic bHLH proteins. A linear representation of each myogenic regulatory factor is shown. The basic (+++) and HLH regions are indicated. The number of amino acids in each protein is shown at the end of each box.

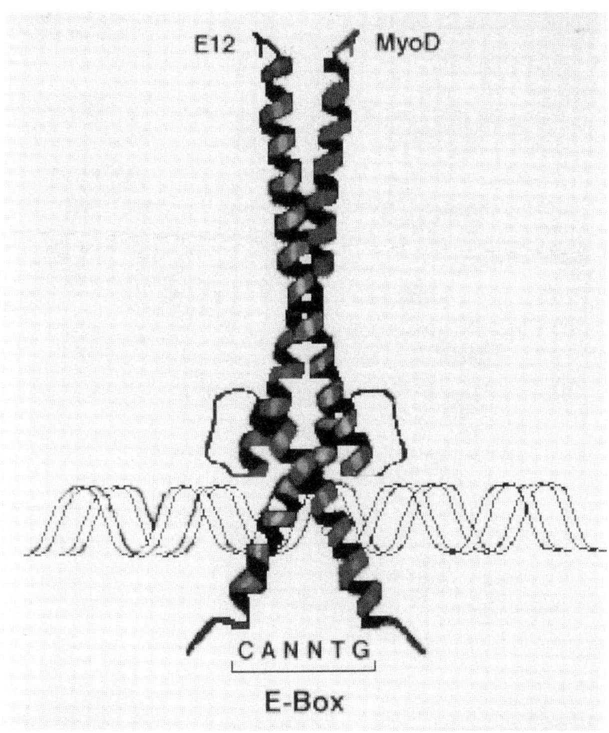

Figure 92-3 A Schematic representation of a MyoD/E12 heterodimer is shown. The basic region and helix-1 form a contiguous α-helix separated from helix-2 by an intervening loop. Each basic region recognizes half of the palindromic sequence CANNTG. E12 is represented in blue and MyoD in red. (*See* color insert following p. 684.)

(these factors are unable to induce muscle gene expression when cells are exposed to growth factors, however), there must be post-translational mechanisms that inhibit their activities. There appear to be multiple mechanisms whereby growth factors prevent myogenic bHLH proteins from activating muscle-specific genes. For example, Id proteins are expressed at high levels in proliferating undifferentiated myoblasts and are downregulated when myoblasts are induced to differentiate. Because Id proteins dimerize preferentially with E proteins, they sequester the dimerization partners for myogenic bHLH proteins in myoblasts. The downregulation of Id has been proposed to release E proteins so that they can dimerize with myogenic bHLH proteins and activate muscle-specific genes. Consistent with this model, forced expression of Id from an expression plasmid is sufficient to prevent myoblast differentiation under conditions that would normally promote differentiation. In the embryo, Id expression is also downregulated in regions of skeletal muscle differentiation.

The nuclear oncogene products Fos and Jun, which are upregulated by mitogens, can also block muscle differentiation by interfering with the activities of myogenic bHLH proteins. The inhibitory activities of Fos and Jun appear to be mediated by competition with the myogenic factors for interaction with a common cofactor required for myogenesis and by direct interactions with the myogenic factors.

Members of the MyoD family have also been shown to be targets for several protein kinases. Protein kinase C, which is activated by growth factors, can substitute for growth factors and block myoblast differentiation. The threonine residue in the center of the DNA-binding domains of the myogenic factors, which mediates muscle-specific gene activation, has been shown to be efficiently

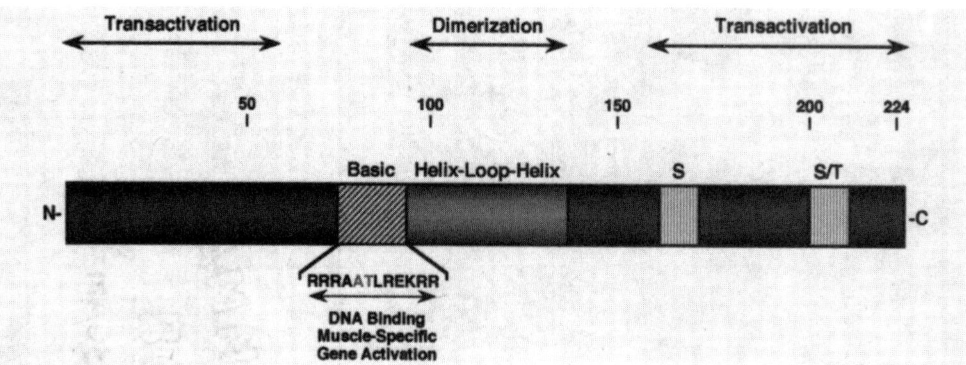

Figure 92-4 Schematic representation of the myogenin protein. Myogenin is a 224-amino acid protein with the bHLH motif near the center. The 12 amino acids within the basic region are required for sequence-specific DNA binding in conjunction with bHLH motif. The alanine-threonine in the center of the basic region are conserved in and specific to all members of the MyoD family and are important for activation of muscle-specific transcription. This threonine is also a protein kinase C phosphorylation site, which inhibits DNA binding when phosphorylated. S, S/T, serine- and serine/threonine-rich regions, respectively.

phosphorylated by PKC in vitro and in vivo. In the case of myogenin, this phosphorylation prevents DNA binding, presumably because it introduces a negative charge into the center of the DNA-binding domain, resulting in electrostatic repulsion from the DNA. FGF can induce phosphorylation of this threonine in cultured cells, resulting in repression of myogenin's ability to activate muscle gene expression. The ability of this threonine to serve as a target for growth factor-dependent phosphorylation pathways that block myogenesis demonstrates that this single amino acid plays a dual role in the control of muscle development; it is structurally important for transcriptional activation, and it serves as a target for growth factor signal transduction pathways under control of PKC.

Type-β transforming growth factor (TGF-β) also inhibits muscle differentiation by blocking the activities of the myogenic factors. In myoblasts exposed to TGF-β, myogenic bHLH proteins are expressed, and they can bind to their target DNA sequences associated with muscle-specific genes but are unable to activate expression of those genes. It has been proposed that TGF-β interferes with the expression or activity of a cofactor required by the myogenic factors to activate myogenesis.

The linkage of muscle differentiation to cell cycle withdrawal suggests that the cell cycle machinery interfaces with the mechanism for muscle gene activation. The retinoblastoma protein (Rb) has been shown to be an important regulator of cell cycle progression. Rb is a nuclear phosphoprotein that is phosphorylated in a cell cycle-dependent manner. In cycling cells, Rb is phosphorylated in a specific domain known as the "pocket," whereas in growth-arrested cells Rb is dephosphorylated. When quiescent cells are stimulated to reenter S phase, Rb becomes phosphorylated during the G1/S phase transition prior to initiation of DNA synthesis. The pocket of Rb interacts with a variety of nuclear proteins to control cell cycle progression. Among these is the transcription factor E2F, which activates the expression of several genes involved in cell proliferation. Binding of E2F to dephosphorylated Rb inactivates E2F and results in a block to proliferation (Fig. 92-5). Conversely, phosphorylation of Rb releases E2F so that it can activate cell growth. The oncoproteins encoded by several DNA tumor viruses, such as SV40 large T antigen and adenovirus E1A, also bind to the pocket of Rb, which prevents interaction between Rb and E2F, resulting in uncontrolled proliferation. These oncogenes are potent inhibitors of myogenesis and when expressed in terminally differentiated myotubes can lead to reinitiation of DNA synthesis.

MyoD has also been shown to bind to the pocket of dephosphorylated Rb. This interaction requires the basic region and first helix of MyoD and is dependent on the alanine-threonine residues in the basic region that are required for activation of muscle gene expression. Because MyoD and E2F bind the same region of Rb, they must interact with separate molecules of Rb. Exactly how MyoD binds DNA and Rb simultaneously is unclear. The role of Rb in the MyoD-DNA complex also remains to be determined.

Rb is upregulated during myogenesis and is required for irreversible exit of muscle cells from the cell cycle. Myoblasts lacking Rb are able to form myotubes and express muscle-specific genes, but they do not irreversibly exit the cell cycle and can resynthesize DNA in response to mitogenic stimulation.

The pocket of Rb is phosphorylated by cyclin-dependent protein kinases (CDKs). The CDKs are expressed constitutively throughout the cell cycle but are activated by association with regulatory proteins called cyclins. Cyclin D1 is induced during the G1 to S phase transition and activates CDK4, resulting in phosphorylation of Rb. Forced expression of cyclin D prevents activation of muscle gene expression by MyoD, presumably because it leads to inactivation of Rb, although a more direct role of the cyclin D1/CDK4 complex in phosphorylating MyoD has not been ruled out.

There is also a family of CDK inhibitors (CKIs) that act as inhibitors of cell growth by blocking CDK activity. One of these CKIs, called p21/WAF1/CIP1, is upregulated during myogenesis and is likely to play a role in locking cells out of the cell cycle. When CKI is expressed in proliferating myoblasts, it can inhibit growth and induce muscle differentiation even in the presence of high concentrations of mitogens (Fig. 92-5); p21 is also expressed in differentiating muscle cells during embryogenesis. Upregulation of p21 expression is also observed in several differentiated cell types in the embryo, suggesting it may be part of a common mechanism linking cell cycle withdrawal to activation of cell differentiation.

EMBRYONIC ORIGINS OF SKELETAL MUSCLE

The formation of skeletal muscle during embryogenesis involves the commitment of mesodermal stem cells to the skeletal muscle lineage and the subsequent differentiation of myoblasts to form multinucleate myotubes, which mature into skeletal muscle fibers. Skeletal muscle is derived from the somites, which form in a rostral-to-caudal gradient by segmentation of the paraxial mesoderm along the neural tube (Fig. 92-6). Newly formed somites

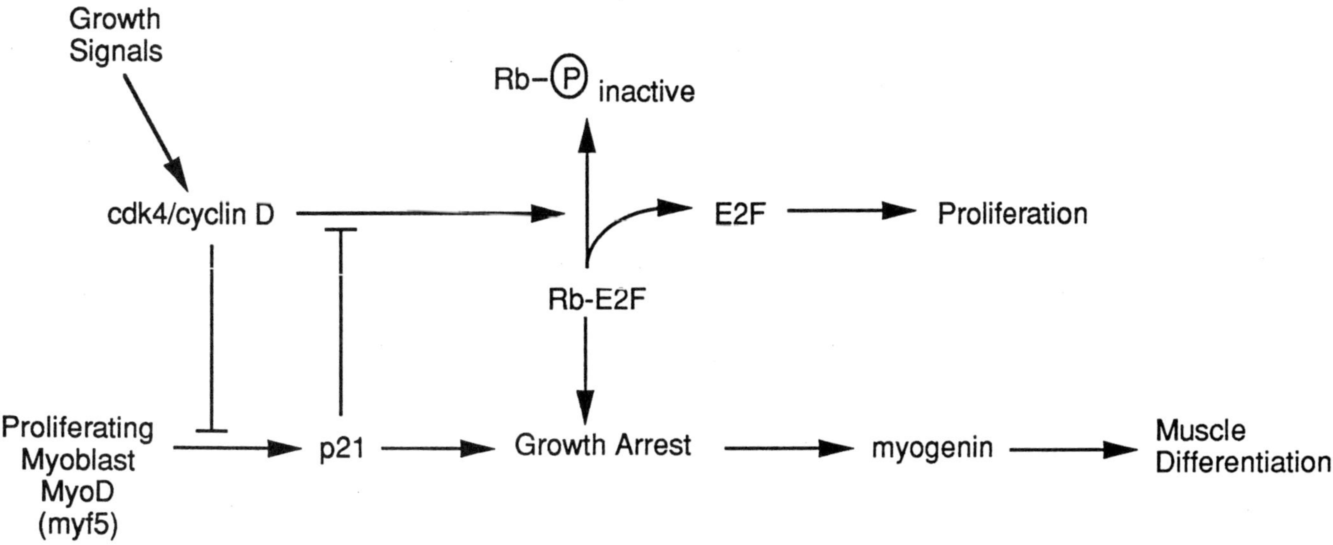

Figure 92-5 Model depicting the interaction between the cell cycle machinery and the myogenic regulatory pathway. MyoD or Myf5 are expressed in myoblasts and induce the expression of the CDK inhibitor p21 in the absence of growth factors. p21 induces growth arrest, which results in myogenin expression. Myogenin in turn activates muscle differentiation. Growth factor signals induce cyclin D1, which activates CDK4, resulting in phosphorylation of the Rb pocket, as well as inhibition of MyoD function. Phosphorylated Rb is unable to bind E2F and is therefore inactive as a growth suppressor. In the absence of growth factor signals, Rb is dephosphorylated and binds to E2F. E2F normally activates expression of genes required for cell proliferation, but it is inactivated when bound to Rb.

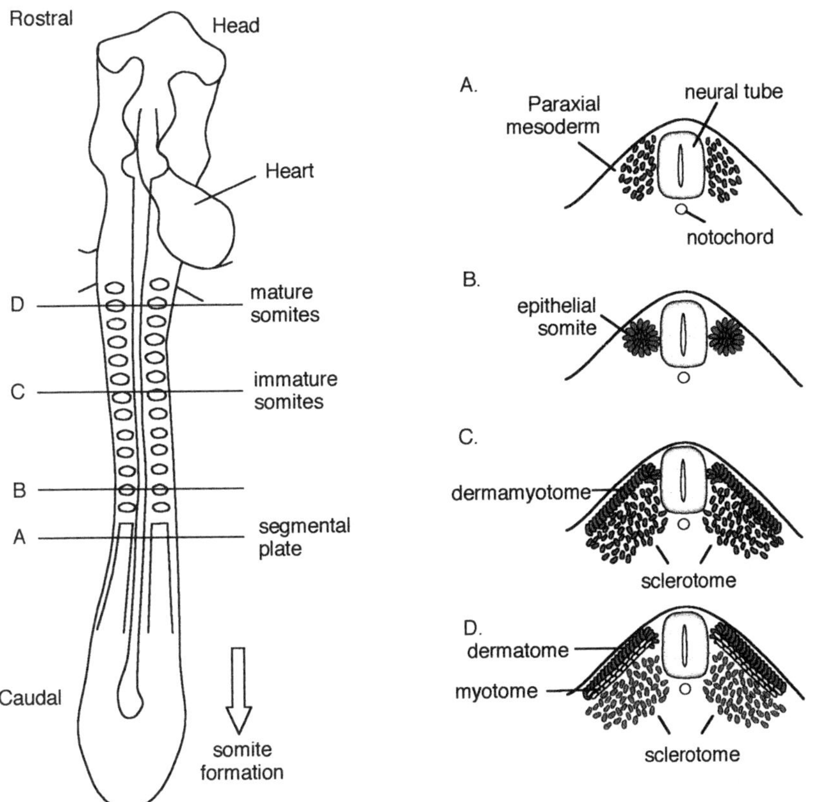

Figure 92-6 Diagrammatic representation of somite maturation. Schematic representation of an early chick embryo is shown on the left. Somites form in a rostral-to-caudal progression by segmentation of the segmental plate mesoderm. Right: cross-sections of the embryo at the indicated level. **(A)** Paraxial mesodermal cells in the segmental plates have not yet formed somites. **(B)** Newly formed somites appear as epithelial spheres. **(C)** Immature somites have become compartmentalized to form the dermamyotome and sclerotome. **(D)** Mature somites have formed the dermatome, myotome, and sclerotome.

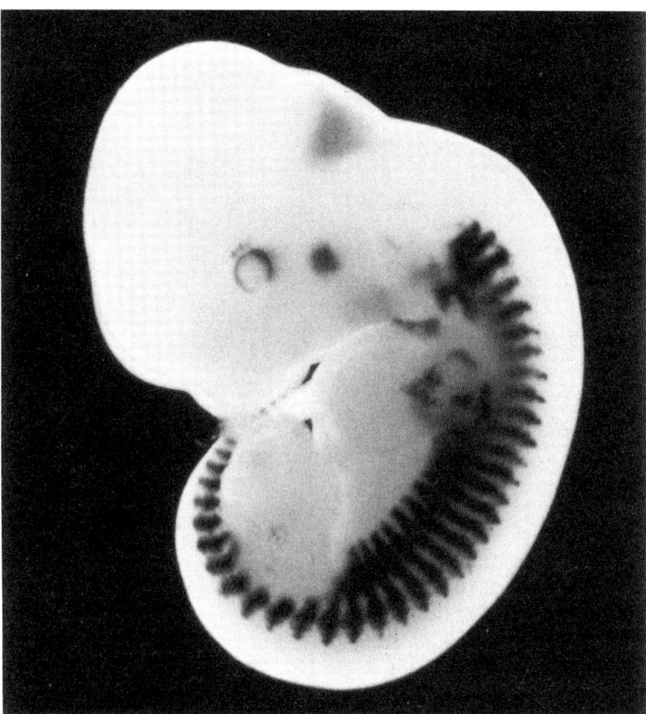

Figure 92-7 Expression pattern of a *myogenin-lacZ* transgene in an 11.5-day mouse embryo. The *myogenin* promoter was linked to a β-galactosidase reporter gene and introduced into transgenic mice. The expression of β-galactosidase activity was detected by a colorimetric assay and is shown in blue. The expression pattern of the transgene is identical to that of the endogenous gene. (*See* color insert following p. 684.)

appear as an epithelial sphere, which subsequently becomes compartmentalized to form the dermamyotome and the sclerotome. The sclerotome gives rise to the ribs and vertebrae. The dermamyotome gives rise to the myotome and dermatome, which form axial muscles of the back and the dermis, respectively. Myf5 is the first member of the MyoD family to be expressed during mouse embryogenesis, appearing in the somite at embryonic day 8 (E8). Myogenin transcripts appear in the myotome by E8.5 and MRF4 and MyoD are expressed at E9 and E10.5, respectively.

Muscle cells in the limbs arise from cells that emigrate from the ventrolateral edge of the dermamyotome. These migrating cells are committed to the myogenic lineage, but they do not express the myogenic bHLH factors until they reach the limbs. The homeobox gene *Pax3* is expressed in the migrating myogenic precursor cells. Evidence that Pax3 is involved in migration or commitment of these cells to the myogenic lineage has been provided by analysis of a mouse mutant called *Splotch*. The *splotch* mutation maps to the *Pax3* gene and results in the absence of limb muscles. Pax3 may mediate activation of MyoD and Myf5 in response to muscle-inducing signals from overlaying ectoderm. Interestingly, a chromosomal translocation resulting in structural rearrangement of the human *Pax3* gene has been associated with alveolar rhabdomyosarcoma, a malignant tumor of skeletal muscle (*see* Chapter 3).

Whereas limb muscles are derived from myogenic precursor cells that migrate from the ventrolateral edge of the dermamyotome, the axial muscles of the back are derived from the myotomal compartment of the somites. The neural tube and notochord have been shown to play important roles in somite maturation by serving as a source for signaling molecules that induce patterning of the somites. In the absence of neural tube, the myotome fails to form. In contrast, the formation of limb muscles is independent of the neural tube or notochord.

Several of the myogenic bHLH genes have been analyzed for *cis*-acting DNA sequences that direct expression in the early somites and subsequently during skeletal muscle formation. The best characterized of these genes is *myogenin*, which is controlled by DNA sequences in the proximal promoter region. When these sequences are linked to the β-galactosidase gene as a marker and are introduced into transgenic mice, they direct the expression of β-galactosidase in the exact pattern as the endogenous *myogenin* gene (Fig. 92-7). Within the *myogenin* gene control region is an E-box that binds the myogenic bHLH proteins with high affinity and a binding site for the myocyte enhancer binding factor-2 (MEF2) family of transcription factors. Together, these two families of regulators control the expression of myogenin in the somites and limb buds.

A GENETIC PATHWAY FOR2 MUSCLE DEVELOPMENT REVEALED BY GENE TARGETING IN TRANSGENIC MICE

To determine the specific roles of the myogenic bHLH genes in muscle development in vivo, these genes have been deleted from the genome of transgenic mice by homologous recombination. Remarkably, mice lacking MyoD are fully viable and show no obvious muscle abnormalities. The only apparent consequence of *MyoD* inactivation is a twofold increase in expression of Myf5. Paradoxically, mice homozygous for a null mutation of *Myf5* also develop normal skeletal muscle, but die at birth because of the absence of ribs, which results in an inability to breathe. It is unclear why Myf5, which is expressed exclusively in skeletal muscle cells, affects the formation of ribs, which are derived from the somite. One possibility is that Myf5 controls the expression of growth factors or extracellular matrix molecules by muscle cells, which are involved in regulating the behavior of adjacent rib precursor cells in the somite. When both *MyoD* and *Myf5* are inactivated in the same animal, there is a complete absence of skeletal muscle and there are no detectable myoblasts. These findings suggest that MyoD and Myf5 play overlapping roles in the generation of myoblasts. This type of genetic redundancy could occur if MyoD and Myf5 were expressed in the same cells or if they were expressed in separate cells, either of which could support normal muscle development if the other cell population were eliminated. When lacZ expression is driven by the Myf5 locus in Myf5 null embryos, muscle progenitor cells migrate aberrantly. Thus, Myf5 protein appears to be necessary for cells to respond correctly to positional cues and to adopt a myogenic fate. The phenotype of mice lacking myogenin suggests that myogenin acts in a genetic pathway downstream of MyoD and Myf5. In myogenin-null mice, myoblasts are normally specified and positioned, but there is a near-complete absence of differentiated skeletal muscle fibers. The undifferentiated myoblasts that populate the presumptive muscle forming regions of myogenin-null mice express MyoD and Myf5, indicating that these myogenic factors do not require myogenin for their expression and suggesting that they cannot direct the formation of normal skeletal muscle in the absence of myogenin.

During normal muscle development, myogenin is downregulated at birth as MRF4 becomes upregulated to high levels. MRF4 is not expressed above background levels in myogenin-null mice, which suggests that it lies downstream of myogenin in the

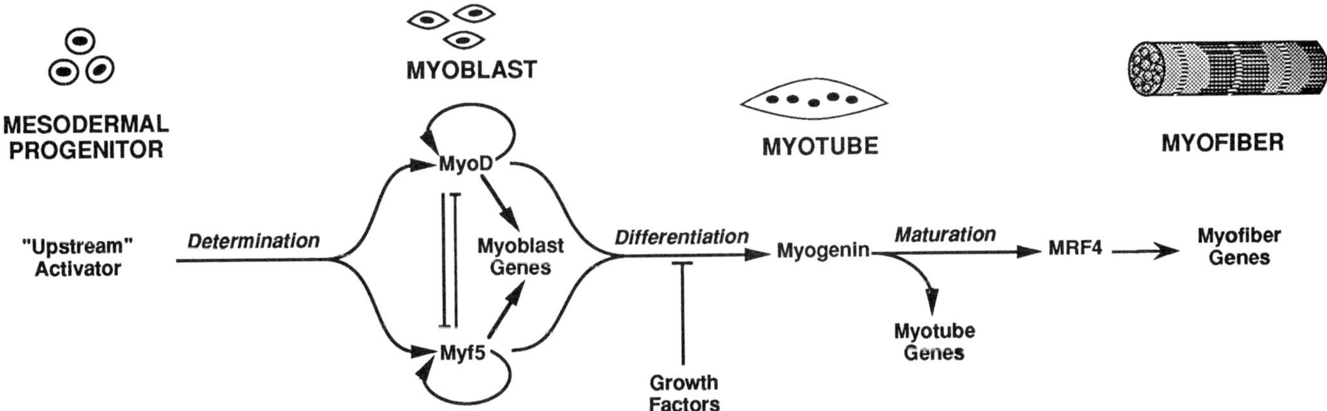

Figure 92-8 The genetic pathway for skeletal muscle development. According to this model, either MyoD or Myf5 become expressed when mesodermal precursor cells from the somite become committed to the myogenic lineage. Myoblast-specific genes are regulated by MyoD and Myf5. When the extracellular concentration of growth factors is reduced, MyoD or Myf5 activate the expression of myogenin, which in turn activates myotube-specific genes. Myogenin is normally downregulated when MRF4 is upregulated after birth. In MRF4-null mice, myogenin continues to be expressed at a high level, suggesting that MRF4 is normally required for its downregulation.

myogenic pathway. MRF4-null mice have normal skeletal muscle and are fully viable. However, myogenin is overexpressed in these mice, which suggests that it may compensate for the lack of MRF4. This upregulation of myogenin in the absence of MRF4 also suggests that MRF4 is required for the downregulation of myogenin that normally occurs in postnatal skeletal muscle.

Together, the results of gene knockout experiments suggest that muscle cell determination and differentiation are controlled by the type of genetic cascade shown in Fig. 92-8.

MEF2 FACTORS AND MYOGENESIS

The majority of skeletal muscle genes contain E-boxes in their control regions and are therefore probably directly activated by the myogenic bHLH factors. However, there are also skeletal muscle genes that lack E-boxes. Many of these genes are controlled by the myogenic bHLH factors through a cascade of events in which the myogenic factors induce the expression of intermediate regulators, which in turn activate muscle-specific genes. MEF2 proteins are among these intermediate regulators. MEF2 factors are unable to activate muscle gene expression alone, but they potentiate the transcriptional activity of bHLH proteins. This potentiation appears to be mediated by direct interactions between the DNA-binding domain of these different types of transcription factors. The MEF2 factors belong to the MADS box family of transcription factors, named for MCM1, which regulates mating type-specific genes in yeast, Agamous and Deficiens, which act as homeotic genes to control flower development in plants, and Serum Response Factor (SRF), which controls several serum-inducible and muscle-specific genes. There are four MEF2 genes in vertebrates: MEF2A,-B,-C, and -D (Fig. 92-9). The proteins encoded by these genes are nearly identical within the MADS domain, which is located at their amino-termini. The MADS domain mediates homo- and heterodimerization and DNA binding to the sequence CTA(A/T)$_4$TAG, which is found in the control regions of nearly every skeletal as well as cardiac muscle gene. Immediately adjacent to the MADS domain is a region known as the MEF2 domain, in which the MEF2 factors also share extensive homology. The function of the MEF2 domain has not yet been determined. The carboxyl-termini of the MEF2 factors are required for transcriptional activation and are subject to complex patterns of alternative splicing, which generates enormous complexity of this family.

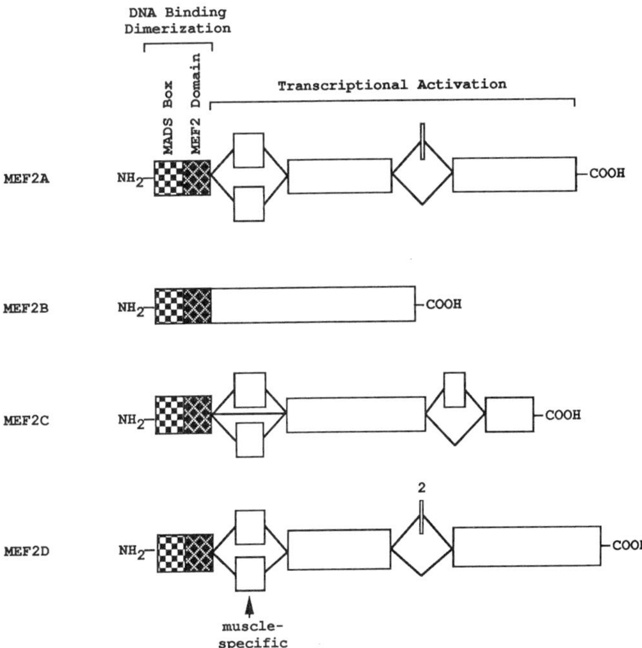

Figure 92-9 Diagrammatic representation of the proteins encoded by the four MEF2 genes. A linear representation of each MEF2 factor is shown. The MADS and MEF2 domains are indicated and alternative exons are shown.

In addition to regulating muscle structural genes, MEF2 factors have been shown to regulate the myogenic bHLH genes. The promoters of the myogenin, MyoD, and MRF4 genes have been shown to contain MEF2 sites that are essential for transcription of these genes in vivo and in vitro. During mouse embryogenesis, the MEF2 factors are expressed in the somite myotome after Myf5 and myogenin, which suggests that they do not play a role in the initial activation of these genes, but they are likely to be required for amplification and maintenance of the expression of these genes once their expression has been initiated.

MEF2 expression can be induced in nonmuscle cells by forced expression of myogenic bHLH proteins, which suggests that the

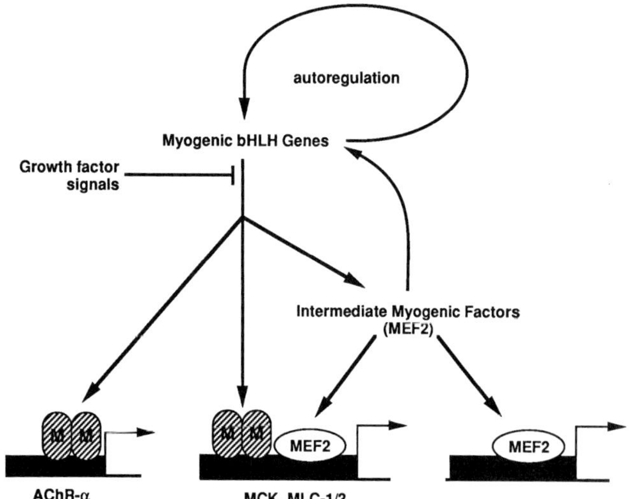

Figure 92-10 Activation of muscle gene expression by myogenic bHLH and MEF2 factors. Members of the MyoD family positively autoregulate their own expression and directly activate transcription of muscle-specific genes containing E-boxes in their control regions. MEF2 factors are induced in response to myogenic bHLH proteins and can in turn activate the expression of muscle-specific genes that lack E-boxes in their control regions. MEF2 proteins also bind the control regions of several myogenic bHLH genes and therefore participate in a positive feedback loop that amplifies and maintains the myogenic program. Myogenic bHLH proteins are shown in black, designated M.

Mef2 genes lie in a genetic pathway downstream of the myogenic bHLH genes. However, forced expression of MEF2 in fibroblasts has been shown to induce the expression of the myogenic bHLH genes and to activate muscle differentiation. This suggests that MEF2 factors and myogenic bHLH proteins function within a complex regulatory network in which members from either family of factors can autoregulate one another and crossregulate the other family members (Fig. 92-10). In this way, these two families of regulators reinforce one another's expression and drive cells toward differentiation.

The four *Mef2* genes are also expressed at the earliest stages of heart development, as well as in smooth muscle cells, suggesting that MEF2 factors may regulate muscle gene expression in multiple muscle cell types. The functions of MEF2 have been analyzed genetically in *Drosophila*, which contains only a single *Mef2* gene, called *D-mef2*, which encodes a protein that is virtually identical to the vertebrate MEF2 proteins in the MADS and MEF2 domains. The *Drosophila* MEF2 protein also binds the same DNA sequence as the mammalian factors and can activate transcription through the MEF2 site in mammalian cells. Like its vertebrate relatives, D-MEF2 is expressed specifically in myogenic precursors and their descendants during embryogenesis. *Drosophila* embryos lacking *D-mef2* contain myoblasts that are normally specified and positioned, but these cells are unable to differentiate. The severe muscle defect in these mutant flies suggests that *Mef2* provides a function required for activation of muscle gene expression in multiple muscle cell types and suggests that the genetic functions of *Mef2* have been conserved since flies and humans evolved from a common ancestor over 600 million years ago.

RELATIONSHIP OF SKELETAL MUSCLE TO OTHER TISSUES

There are several reasons to expect that networks of cell type-specific bHLH proteins may control cell determination and differentiation in cell types other than skeletal muscle. The presence of E-boxes in the control regions of numerous tissue-specific genes suggests that these genes are controlled by specific bHLH proteins. The ubiquitous expression of E-proteins also suggests the existence of cell type-specific dimerization partners for these proteins. Id proteins are also expressed in many types of undifferentiated cells. Indeed, in recent years, several cell type-specific bHLH proteins have been identified in *Drosophila* and vertebrate species. Further investigations into their mechanisms of action seems likely to reveal fundamental mechanisms for the control of tissue-specific gene expression during development.

SELECTED REFERENCES

Benezra R, Davis RL, Lockshon D, Turner DL, Weintraub H. The protein Id: a negative regulator of helix-loop-helix DNA binding proteins. Cell 1990;61:49–59.

Bengal E, Ransone L, Scharfmann R, et al. Functional antagonism between c-Jun and MyoD proteins: a direct physical association. Cell 1992;68:507–519.

Bour BA, O'Brien MA, Lockwood WL, et al. Drosophila MEF2, a transcription factor that is essential for myogenesis. Genes Dev 1995; 9:730–741.

Braun T, Rudnicki MA, Arnold HH, Jaenisch R. Targeted inactivation of the muscle regulatory gene Myf-5 results in abnormal rib development and perinatal death. Cell 1992;71:369–382.

Brennan TJ, Chakraborty T, Olson EN. Mutagenesis of the myogenin basic region identifies an ancient protein motif critical for activation of myogenesis. Proc Natl Acad Sci USA 1991;88:5675–5679.

Cheng T-C, Wallace M, Merlie JP, Olson EN. Separable regulatory elements govern myogenin transcription in embryonic somites and limb buds. Science 1993;261:215–218.

Cserjesi P, Olson EN. Myogenin induces muscle-specific enhancer binding factor MEF-2 independently of other muscle-specific gene products. Mol Cell Biol 1991;11:4854–4862.

Davis RL, Cheng P-F, Lassar AB, Weintraub H. The MyoD DNA-binding domain contains a recognition code for muscle-specific gene activation. Cell 1990;60:733–746.

Davis RL, Weintraub H. Acquisition of myogenic specificity by replacement of three amino acid residues from MyoD into E12. Science 1992;256:1027–1030.

Davis RL, Weintraub H, Lassar AB. Expression of a single transfected cDNA converts fibroblasts to myoblasts. Cell 1987;51:987–1000.

Emerson CP. Skeletal myogenesis: genetics and embryology to the fore. Curr Opin Genet Dev 1993;3:265–274.

Gu W, Schneider JW, Condorelli G, Kaushal S, Mahdavi VJ, Nadal-Ginard B. Interaction of myogenic factors and the retinoblastinoma protein mediates muscle cell commitment and differentiation. Cell 1993;72:309–324.

Halevy O, Novitch BG, Spicer DB, et al. Correlation of terminal cell cycle arrest of skeletal muscle with induction of p21 by MyoD. Science 1995;267:1018–1021.

Hasty P, Bradley A, Morris JH, et al. Muscle deficiency and neonatal death in mice with a targeted mutation in the myogenin gene. Nature 1993;364:501–506.

Kaushal S, Schneider JW, Nadal-Ginard B, Mahdavi V. Activation of the myogenic lineage by MEF2A, a factor that induces and cooperates with MyoD. Science 1994;266:1236–1240.

Konieczny SF, Emerson CP, Jr. 5-azacytidine induction of stable mesodermal stem cell lineages from 10T1/2 cells: evidence for regulatory genes controlling determination. Cell 1984;38:791–800.

Kothary FT, Surani MA, Halata Z, Grim M. The splotch mutation interferes with muscle development in the limbs. Anat Embryol 1993; 187:153–160.

Lassar AB, Paterson BM, Weintraub H. Transfection of DNA locus that mediates the conversion of 10T1/2 fibroblasts to myoblasts. Cell 1986;47:649–656.

Li L, Chambard J-C, Karin M, Olson EN. Fos and Jun repress transcriptional activation by myogenin and MyoD: the amino terminus of Jun can mediate repression. Genes Dev 1992;6:676–689.

Li L, Zhou J, James G, Heller-Harrison R, Czech M, Olson EN. FGF inactivates myogenic helix-loop-helix proteins through phosphorylation of a conserved protein kinase C site in their DNA binding domains. Cell 1992;71:1181–1194.

Lilly B, Galewsky S, Firulli AB, Schulz RA, Olson EN. D-MEF2: A MADS box transcription factor expressed in differentiating mesoderm and muscle cell lineages during *Drosophila* embryogenesis. Proc Natl Acad Sci USA 1994;91:5662–5666.

Lilly B, Zhao B, Ranganayakulu G, Paterson BM, Schulz RA, Olson EN. Requirement of MADS domain transcription factor D-MEF2 for muscle formation in Drosophila. Science 1995;267:688–693.

Ma PCM, Rould MA, Weintraub H, Pabo CO. Crystal structure of MyoD bHLH domain-DNA complex: Perspectives on DNA recognition and implications for transcriptional activation. Cell 1994;77:451–459.

Maroto M, Reshef R, Munsterberg AE, Koester S, Goulding M, Lassar AB. Ectopic Pax-3 activates MyoD and Myf-5 expression in embryonic mesoderm and neural tissue. Cell 1997;89:139–148.

Martin JF, Miano JM, Hustad CM, Copeland NG, Jenkins NA, Olson EN. A Mef2 gene that generates a muscle-specific isoform via alternative mRNA splicing. Mol Cell Biol 1994;14:1647–1656.

Molkentin JD, Olson EN. Combinatorial control of muscle development by basic helix-loop-helix and MADS-box transcription factors. Proc Natl Acad Sci USA 1996;93:9366–9373.

Morgan DO. Principles of CDK regulation. Nature 1995;374:131–134.

Murre C, McCaw PS, Baltimore D. A new DNA binding and dimerization motif in immunoglobulin enhancer binding, daughterless, MyoD, and myc proteins. Cell 1989;56:777–783.

Murre C, McCaw PS, Vaessin H, et al. Interactions between heterologous helix-loop-helix proteins generate complexes that bind specifically to a common DNA sequence. Cell 1989;58:537–544.

Nabeshima Y, Hanaoka L, Hayasaka M, et al. Myogenin gene disruption results in perinatal lethality because of severe muscle defect. Nature 1993;364:532–535.

Nevins JR. E2F: a link between the Rb tumor suppressor protein and viral oncoproteins. Science 1992;258:424–429.

Olson EN. The MyoD family, a paradigm for development? Genes Dev 1990;4:1454–1461.

Olson EN, Klein WH. bHLH factors in muscle development: dead lines and commitments, what to leave in and what to leave out. Genes Dev 1994;8:1–8.

Parker S, Eichele G, Zhang P, et al. p53-independent expression of $p21^{Cip1}$ in muscle and other terminally differentiating cells. Science 1995; 267:1024–1027.

Pollock R, Treisman R. Human SRF-related proteins: DNA-binding properties and potential regulatory targets. Genes Dev 1991;5:2327–2341.

Rao SS, Chu C, Kohtz DS. Ectopic expression of cyclin D1 prevents activation of gene transcription by myogenic basic helix-loop-helix regulators. Mol Cell Biol 1994;14:5259–5267.

Rudnicki MA, Braun T, Hinuma S, Jaenisch R. Inactivation of MyoD in mice leads to upregulation of the myogenic HLH gene Myf-5 and results in apparently normal muscle development. Cell 1992;71:383–390.

Rudnicki MA, Schnegelsberg PNJ, Stead RH, Braun T, Arnold HH, Jaenisch R. MyoD or Myf-5 is required for the formation of skeletal muscle. Cell 1993;75:1351–1359.

Schneider JW, Gu W, Zhu L, Mahdavi V, Nadal-Ginard B. Reversal of terminal differentiation mediated by p107 in Rb-/-muscle cells. Science 1994;264:1467–1471.

Shapiro DN, Sublett JE, Li B, Downing JR, Naeve CW. Fusion of PAX3 to a member of the forkhead family of transcription factors in human alveolar rhabdomyosarcoma. Cancer Res 1993;53:5108–5112.

Tajbakhsh S, Rocancourt D, Buckingham M. Muscle progenitor cells failing to respond to positional cues adopt non-myogenic fates in myf-5 null mice. Nature 1996;384:266–270.

Tapscott SJ, Davis RL, Thayer MJ, Cheng P-F, Weintraub H, Lassar AB. MyoD1: A nuclear phosphoprotein required in a myc homology region to convert fibroblasts to myoblasts. Science 1988;242:405–411.

Wachtler F, Crist B. The basic embryology of skeletal muscle formation in vertebrates: the avian model. Semin Dev Biol 1992;3:217–227.

Weintraub H. The MyoD family and myogenesis: redundancy, networks and thresholds. Cell 1993;75:1241–1244.

Weintraub H, Tapscott SJ, Davis RL, et al. Activation of muscle specific genes in pigment, nerve, fat, liver and fibroblast cell lines by forced expression of MyoD. Proc Natl Acad Sci USA 1989;86:5434–5438.

Williams BA, Ordahl CP. Pax-3 expression in segmental mesoderm marks early stages in myogenic cell specification. Development 1994; 120:785–796.

Zhang W, Behringer RR, Olson EN. Inactivation of the myogenic bHLH gene MRF4 results in upregulation of myogenin and rib anomalies. Genes Dev 1995;9:1388–1399.

93 Skeletal Muscle Structure and Function

HENRY F. EPSTEIN

INTRODUCTION

Skeletal muscle provides unparalleled examples of the interrelationships between structure and function in a biological tissue. Moreover, recent advances in molecular genetics of both humans and experimental organisms have provided models of the perturbation of structure and function in inherited disease. Three distinct systems of molecular machinery are organized to interact with one another to produce a normally contracting muscle:

1. The sarcomere with its interdigitating arrays of protein filaments that actually generate tension and perform work.
2. The sarcoplasmic reticulum and transverse-tubule system with their specialized membranes that couple the electrical signals arising from neuronal excitation with the contraction of the sarcomeres.
3. The membrane-cytoskeleton system that anchors the other two systems to the plasma membrane and to the extracellular protein matrix.

Remarkably, each of these systems is not only important for understanding muscle physiology but contains molecules whose genetic alteration is responsible for at least one specific human disease.

MYOFIBRIL STRUCTURE AND ASSEMBLY

THE SARCOMERE Skeletal muscle is composed of long fibers that were formed by the fusion of committed cells during differentiation. Each multinucleated fiber contains many microfibers or myofibrils that may be considered the units for muscle contraction. Each myofibril contains repeating assemblies of myosin and actin filaments called sarcomeres (Fig. 93-1). The sarcomeres are the physical basis of the alternating dark and light bands seen in polarized light microscopy that give striated muscle its name.

The Myosin Filament Myosin is the principal protein of the thick or myosin filaments of skeletal muscle. The sarcomeric myosin molecule of approximately 500,000 mol wt was the first multifunctional protein to be recognized, consisting of two globular head regions of about 115,000 mol wt each and a long rod-like tail region comprising the rest of the molecule. Each myosin molecule contains three pairs of distinctly encoded polypeptide chains: two heavy chains, two regulatory light chains, and two essential light chains. One of each kind of light chain and the globular portion of each heavy chain constitute each myosin head. The myosin rod contains the α-helical regions of both heavy chains supercoiled about each other.

About 300 myosin molecules assemble to form each myosin filament. The assembly has several interesting structural features. The filament is bipolar, divided in half along its long axis by a twofold axis of symmetry. In the central region, rods of myosin molecules from each half pack with another in an antiparallel manner. These interactions may represent the first steps in the assembly of the filaments. On each side of this zone, successive myosin molecules pack in parallel, staggered by about 14.5 nm, to form a right-handed helix. Myosin assembly continues until an exact filament length, 1550 nm, is reached, and then stops abruptly. This precise regulation of myosin assembly is not well understood either in molecular or physical–chemical terms.

Several additional proteins are capable of complexing with myosin and become associated with the myosin filaments. The proteins C protein and titin are among the best studied examples. The 140-kDa C protein binds to seven sites in each half-filament. These sites are separated by approximately 44 nm, skipping two myosin repeats. This observation implies that different myosins must be in nonequivalent environments within the filament. Titin is a very large (3000-kDa) protein that creates its own filament which serves as a bridge between the myosin filament and the Z line. Titin shares many structural features with C protein, including myosin binding sites, and contains a protein kinase domain with potential specificity toward myosin light chains. Other titin domains appear to form elastic springs and interact with the Z structures. Myosin filaments are separately anchored by M structures (*see below*).

The Actin Filament Actin is the principal protein of the thin or actin filaments of skeletal muscle. The actin polypeptide is 42 kDa, but it can reversibly polymerize to form long right-handed double helical filaments approximately 1.0 nm long. The assembly is coupled to the hydrolysis of ATP. The three-dimensional structure of the actin monomer has been determined, and it is a bilobed structure of 7 nm long, oriented in the direction of the polar filament axis (Fig. 93-2). The pitch of the filament axis is 36 nm with seven actin monomers per turn in each strand.

Two additional proteins are major components of actin filaments, tropomyosin and troponin. Tropomyosin is a dimer of 35-kDa polypeptides that may be identical or closely similar isoforms. The two polypeptides are highly α-helical and supercoil about one another in a very similar manner to the coils of myosin rods. Tropomyosin dimers bind to the deep groove on either side

From: *Principles of Molecular Medicine* (J. L. Jameson, ed.), ©1998 Humana Press Inc., Totowa, NJ.

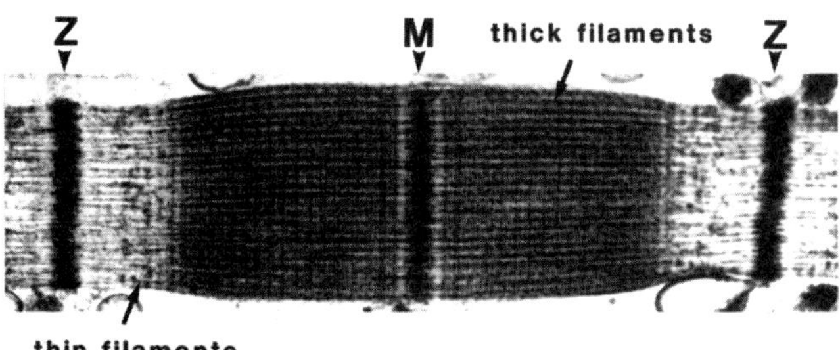

Figure 93-1 Sarcomere of skeletal muscle. Note the thick filaments that are crosslinked at the M line and thin filaments that are crosslinked at the Z line. The M and Z lines are anchored by the cytoskeleton. The vertical lines visible on the thick filaments represent the positions of myosin heads (fine lines) and of myosin-associated C-type proteins (heavier lines at every third fine line). (Courtesy of Professor Hugh E. Huxley.)

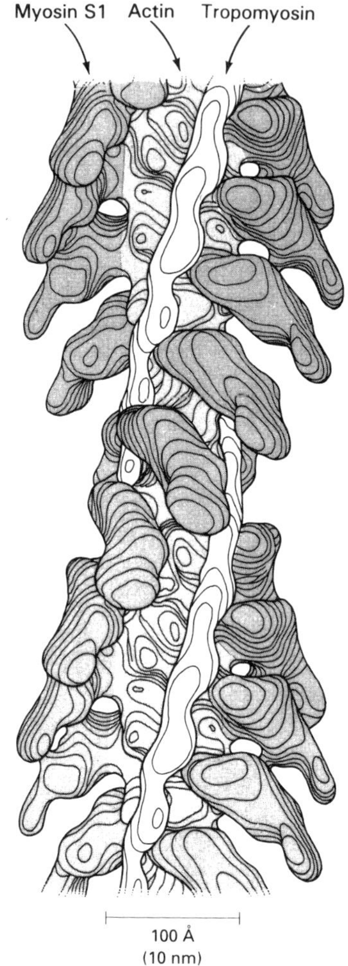

Figure 93-2 Structure of a thin filament with actin and tropomyosin present that has been saturated with myosin heads (S1 fragments). Note the helical arrangements of the proteins (From Stryer L. Biochemistry, 4th ed., New York: W H Freeman, after drawing by Drs. Ronald Milligan and Paula Flicker, with permission.)

of the actin helix. Troponin is a complex of three distinct polypeptides: troponin-T, troponin-I, and troponin-C. Troponin-T, 37 kDa, is elongated and interacts with tropomyosin. Troponin-C, 18 kDa, binds to calcium and is highly similar in three-dimensional structure to other small calcium-binding proteins, including calmodulin, parvalbumin, and the regulatory myosin light chains. Troponin-I, 24 kDa, is necessary for the formation of a functional complex with troponins T and C.

The M and Z Structures Each sarcomere contains multiple myosin and actin filaments, each kind aligned in a regular array. Within each array, the filaments are in register without any stagger and are parallel to one another. The myosin filament array is central and is flanked on each side by actin filament arrays. The symmetry of the sarcomere is similar to that of the bipolar myosin filament.

The precise alignments of these arrays require additional structures to crosslink the filaments. The myosin filaments are crosslinked in their central zones by M structures. Myomesin, a homolog of C protein and titin, is part of the M structure and is a 165-kDa myosin-binding protein. The actin filaments are crosslinked by Z structures at their distal ends. Alpha-actinin, a dimer of 100-kDa polypeptides, is an actin-binding protein, which can crosslink filaments and is a major component of the Z structure. Cap Z protein is also found in the Z structures and interacts with actin.

It is likely that more proteins will be discovered in the sarcomere that function in the assembly or alignment of the myosin and actin filaments.

THE SARCOPLASMIC RETICULUM AND TRANSVERSE TUBULE SYSTEM Because skeletal muscle fibers are large multinucleated syncytia up to 100 μM in diameter and millimeters to centimeters in length, a specialized membrane system, the transverse tubules and sarcoplasmic reticulum, couples the depolarizing signal originating from motor neurons to each of the myofibrils, even those deep within the fibers. For each of the myofibrils within the fibers and for each sarcomere unit of the myofibrils, there is a sleeve of membrane, the sarcoplasmic reticulum, which is connected via the transverse tubules to the outer plasma membrane of each fiber.

The Calcium Pump The calcium pump molecule, a 115-kDa protein, is the principal protein of the sarcoplasmic reticulum (SR). This molecular pump translocates calcium from the myofibril to the lumen of the SR. Two calcium ions are translocated per ATP hydrolyzed by the pump. The active intermediate of the pump molecule is phosphorylated. The functioning of the pump is determined by the myofibrillar calcium concentration, the availability of ATP, and the sequestering capacity of the SR. This latter function relies on the 55-kDa protein calsequestrin, which binds 40–50 calcium ions at the relatively low affinity of 1 mM.

The Calcium-Release Channel The calcium-release channel, also known as the ryanodine receptor, because the binding of that drug was critical to the original identification, is a giant oligmeric molecule composed of four 565-kDa subunits (Fig. 93-3). These channel complexes have multiple transmembrane domains that span the junctional sarcoplasmic reticulum membranes and foot domains that extend into the lumen between the transverse tubules and the sarcoplasmic reticulum. Additional proteins, including a 95-kDa junctional protein, may be important for the interaction of the calcium release channels and the voltage-sensitive channels of the transverse tubules.

Voltage-Sensitive Channel The voltage-sensitive channel of the transverse tubules is a multisubunit protein that was isolated through its interaction with the drug dihydropyridine. It was originally termed the dihydropyridine receptor and is also called the voltage sensor. The α1-subunit has a mass of 212 kDa and may be

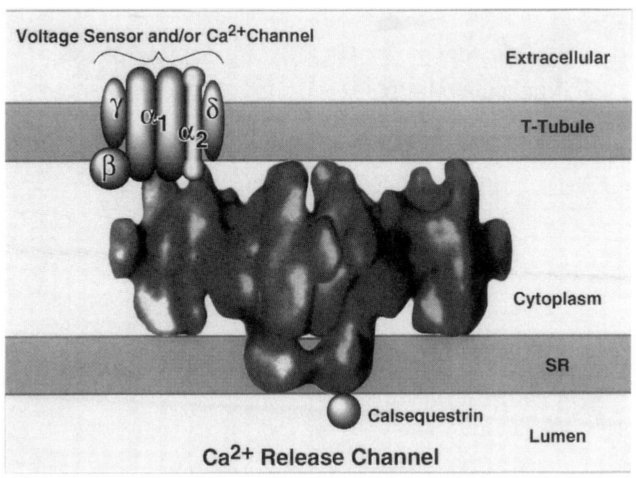

Figure 93-3 Interaction of the calcium release and voltage sensitive channels. The voltage-sensitive or sensor channel with its multiple subunits spans the transverse tubule (t-tubule) membranes and may interact with both the extracellular and cytoplasmic compartments. The calcium-release channel with its four giant subunits spans the sarcoplasmic reticulum (SR) membranes and may interact with the cytoplasm and the lumen of the SR. The voltage sensor and calcium-release channels are shown physically in the SR lumen. (Courtesy of Professors Susan L. Hamilton and Wah Chiu.)

proteolytically cleared to a 175-kDa form. The higher molecular weight form is activated by phosphorylation, whereas the smaller form has lost three phosphorylation sites and the related activation. Additional 15-kDa α2, 55-kDa β, 30-kDa γ, and 27-kDa ε subunits complex with the α1 protein. The γ-subunits are glycoproteins. A 95-kDa junctional triadic protein may be necessary for functional interactions between the tubular voltage-sensitive channel and the reticular calcium release channel (Fig. 93-3).

An interesting property of the tubular channel is that it permits calcium influx from extracellular fluids. It must be emphasized that this calcium is not directly involved in the release of calcium from the sarcoplasmic reticulum nor the subsequent activation of contraction.

THE MEMBRANE CYTOSKELETON SYSTEM The regular organization of myofibrils, sarcoplasmic reticulum, and transverse tubules in skeletal muscles suggest the existence of an underlying framework. Furthermore, the contractile action of the myofibrils necessitates their anchoring to specific sites on the plasma membranes of their muscle fibers so that the force that they produce is transmitted to the tendons and then to bone. Both of these requirements may be met by the network of protein assemblies called the membrane cytoskeleton system. The importance of this system to muscle function is emphasized by the fact that there are at least three independent membrane associated systems that anchor the actin cytoskeleton of muscle. These systems, named after the first of their constituent proteins to be identified, include the dystrophin, spectrin, and integrin-based systems.

The Dystrophin System The dystrophin system was discovered by its alteration in Duchenne-Becker muscular dystrophy. Dystrophin is actually a family of protein isoforms that are produced by alternative splicing of the transcript or alternative starts of transcription of the Duchenne genetic locus. The 427-kDa isoform functions as an integral part of a membrane-cytoskeleton system in skeletal muscle.

Muscle dystrophin is actually a member of a larger superfamily of proteins that includes α actinin and the spectrins. These proteins share an actin-binding domain near their amino terminals and a long coiled-coil rod domain. Nearer the carboxyl terminal, dystrophin has a special cysteine-rich domain and then a separate carboxyl-terminal domain.

The cysteine-rich domain is responsible for anchoring dystrophin to a complex of transmembrane glycoproteins including the 25-kDa dystrophin-associated protein, the 35- and 43-kDa dystrophin-associated glycoproteins, the 50-kDa glycoprotein adhalin, and the 43-kDa β-dystroglycan (Fig. 93-4). This complex in turn binds the extracellular 156-kDa glycoprotein α-dystroglycan, which in turn binds the 40-kDa muscle-specific laminin isoform merosin. As other laminins, merosin is a component of the extracellular basal lamina and binds to lung fibrillar protein assemblies of the extracellular matrix.

The carboxyl-terminal domain interacts with a complex of 50- to 60-kDa cytosolic proteins: α, β1, and β2 syntrophins. The syntrophins also bind to utrophin, a dystrophin homolog that may take part in a fourth membrane-cytoskeletal system and may functionally link the two systems.

The Spectrin System The earliest membrane-cytoskeletal system to be discovered was the spectrin-based complex, originally in red blood cell membranes washed free of hemoglobin or ghosts (hence spectrin-ghost protein). Spectrin exists as a dimer of an ubiquitous 284-kDa α spectrin isoform and a 270-kDa β spectrin. The β spectrin amino-terminal domain, homologous to those of α actinin and dystrophin, binds actin filaments. Both spectrin subunits contain the characteristic, long, coiled-coil rod domain, and β spectrin contains a specific domain in the rod near the carboxyl terminal that binds the 215-kDa transmembrane protein ankyrin. A muscle-specific isoform is produced by alternative splicing in the carboxyl-terminal domain. Spectrin, ankyrin, and various cytoskeletal proteins are located at specific sites on the plasma membrane including costameres which are aligned with the myofibrils, and triadic junctions (and thus appear striated) and adhesion sites near muscle-tendon junctions.

The Integrin System The integrins are a large family of protein isoforms that form tissue-specific complexes. They are transmembrane proteins that bind a variety of extracellular matrix proteins including various collagen isoforms. The integrins do not directly interact with the actin cytoskeleton, but are functionally linked to the protein vinculin and the cytoskeletal α-actinin isoform that binds actin filaments.

In the experimental organisms, *Caenorhabditis elegans* and *Drosophila*, muscle-specific β integrin isoforms are localized near the sites of apposition of Z-band-like structures and the plasma membrane. Null or "knockout" mutations of this β integrin produces a lethal disruption of membrane and myofibril organization and even of filament assembly in either organism. In *C. elegans*, nulls for vinculin have the same deleterious effect. Thus, the integrin-based system may be even more fundamental to the organization of muscle structures, especially early in development, then either the dystrophin or spectrin-based systems. Recently developed "knockout" mutations in mice cannot even form mesoderm.

CONTRACTILE FUNCTION AND REGULATION

FUNCTION

The Sliding Filament Model Contraction in skeletal muscles occurs by the sliding of actin filaments past myosin filaments (Fig. 93-5). Since myosin filaments are bipolar, the heads on each half are oriented 180° from the other half. Therefore, in contraction, the myosin heads bind and pull the polar actin filaments toward their

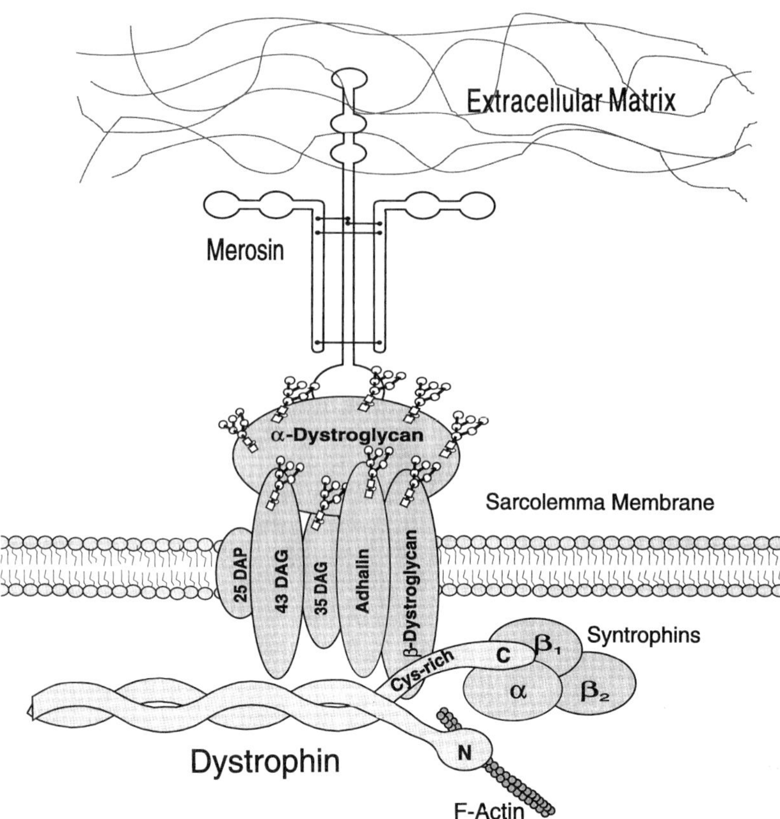

Figure 93-4 The dystrophin membrane cytoskeleton system. Dystrophin is shown interacting with the actin cytoskeleton, a complex of membrane-spanning proteins, and a complex of cytoplasmic proteins. Indirectly, dystrophin interacts with extracellular proteins and structures. This complex set of interactions is necessary for normal muscle development and function. (From Campbell KP. Cell 1995;80:675–679, with permission.)

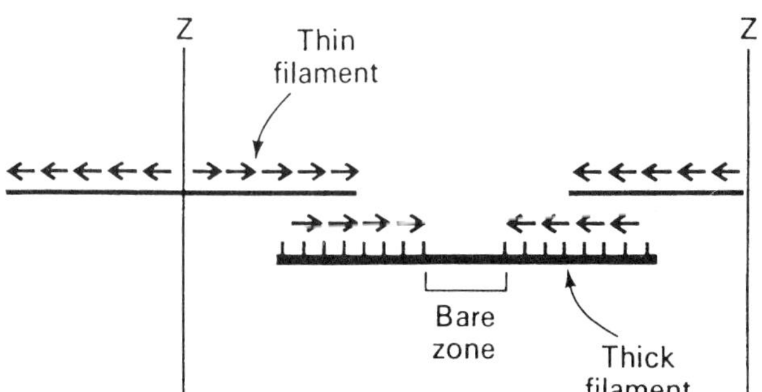

Figure 93-5 Sliding of filaments. Note changes in polarity at the Z line and in each half of the sarcomere (From Stryer L. Biochemistry, 4th ed. New York: WH Freeman, with permission.)

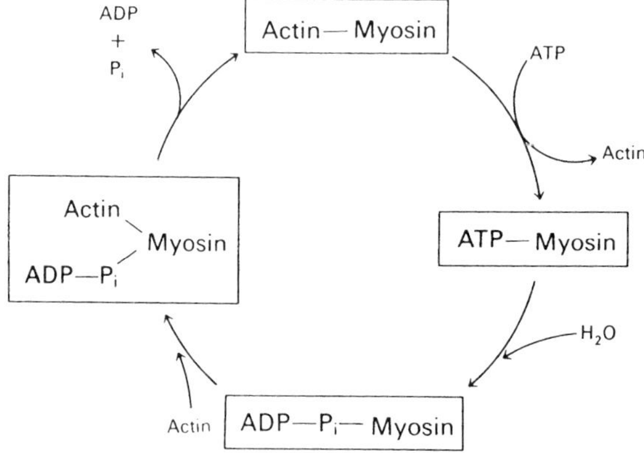

Figure 93-6 The actomyosin-ATP cycle. An outline of the main biochemical events underlying muscle contraction. (From Stryer L. Biochemistry, 4th ed. New York: WH Freeman, with permission.)

center and that of the sarcomere at the M line. In relaxation, the actin filaments move away from the sarcomere center.

In this model, the backbones of the myosin and actin filaments do not undergo significant structural changes during contraction. That is, the filaments themselves do not shrink or expand sufficiently to explain contraction and relaxation. The critical interactions and structural changes involve the association of the myosin heads and actin filaments.

The Actomyosin ATP Cycle The interactions of myosin heads with actin and ATP are the critical molecular events in muscle contraction. Actin activates myosin to bind ATP and hydrolyze it to ADP and phosphate. This activation occurs by a cycle (Fig. 93-6). Since the binding of actin, ATP, and ADP to myosin are mutually exclusive, the myosin must be placed into a special high-energy conformation (Fig. 93-7) with a finite lifetime following ATP hydrolysis. The highly transient complex of this special myosin state with actin is believed to be when actual force is generated by myosin upon actin. The cycle is completed when ADP dissociates from the actomyosin complex.

The actual muscle, the 600 heads on each myosin filament, interact with 12 neighboring actin filaments. Each actin filament can interact with three myosin filaments. With this arrangement, the probability of myosin and actin finding each other is markedly enhanced over a random distribution. At any time during

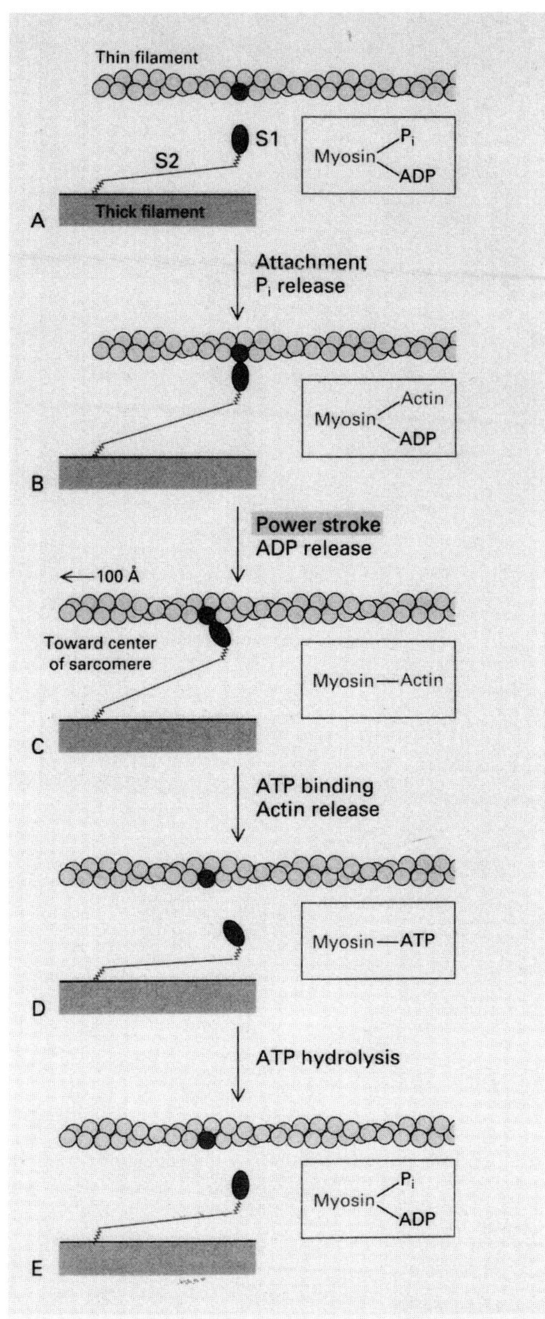

Figure 93-7 Mechanism of force generation. The biochemical events are matched to molecular structure and the power stroke of muscle contraction in this more detailed version of the actomyosin-ATP cycle. Note that movement occurs. (From Stryer L. Biochemistry, 4th ed. New York: WH Freeman, with permission.)

active contraction, every actin and myosin filament in the sarcomere is very likely to be participating in multiple actomyosin interactions.

The Myosin Head as a Protein Motor In order to accomplish the sliding of filaments and the actomyosin-ATP cycle, the myosin head must be a very specifically designed protein motor. In fact, the heads tethered artificially without their rod domains and filament organization can induce motility and tension on free actin filaments. The myosin heads are truly the business ends of thick filaments.

The three-dimensional structure of myosin heads has been determined by X-ray diffraction of protein crystals (Fig. 93-8). The head itself is a 15-nm long structure. At one end, the head has two sides, each of which contains a special site. One site binds actin in a large cleft and the opposite site binds and hydrolyzes ATP. The sites are separated by 3–4 nm. Therefore, a structural change in the region between the sites must occur in order for the binding of ATP and actin to affect one another. The opening and closing of the actin binding cleft may be part of this mechanism (Fig. 93-9).

The actual distance that a myosin head may move an actin filament has been measured. It can be as large as 10 nm. Where does this distance arise? The carboxyl terminal region of the heavy chain in the myosin head is a long α helix to which the myosin light chains attach (Fig. 93-8). This complex may serve as a lever arm where the fulcrum is either of the rod domain of the myosin molecule assembled into the backbone of a thick filament or an equivalent tether (Fig. 93-7). Evolutionarily, the myosin light chains had regulatory or modulatory functions with respect to motor functions.

REGULATION The key steps in the regulation of muscle contraction are the coupling of the excitation of muscle to the release of calcium from the sarcoplasmic reticulum and the action of calcium on the interaction of myosin and actin filaments. The uptake of calcium from the myofibril into the sarcoplasmic reticulum is the mechanism directly controlling relaxation in skeletal muscle.

Calcium Release and Uptake The contraction and relaxation of skeletal muscle ultimately is controlled by the action of motor neurons. Their release of acetylcholine presynaptically and the depolarization of the skeletal muscle plasma membrane following the binding of acetylcholine to specific receptors within specialized membrane sites postsynaptically induce muscle contraction. The absence of motor neuron input and the repolarization of the skeletal muscle plasma membrane are associated with muscle relaxation.

The depolarization of the plasma membrane directly affects the voltage-sensitive channels of the transverse tubules. Direct molecular interaction between these channels and the foot domains of the calcium-release channels of the sarcoplasmic reticulum occurs in the junctional region (Fig. 93-3). Allosteric changes in this interaction as a result of transverse tubule membrane depolarization induces a change in conformation of the calcium-release channel. This channel switches from its closed to open state, and calcium is released from the sarcoplasmic reticulum into the myofibrils.

A potential source of controversy or confusion, depending on one's viewpoint, is that both the voltage-sensitive channel of the transverse tubules and the calcium-release channel of the sarcoplasmic reticulum are themselves activated by calcium. Theoretically, calcium ions could trigger calcium-release by their action on these two molecules. However, these effects are considered to be secondary to the allosteric mechanism discussed because extracellular and junctional calcium can be eliminated without inhibition.

The allosteric interaction between the two channels is modulated by the action of other proteins. For example, activation of the voltage sensitive channels are markedly enhanced by phosphorylation of the major α1-subunits. Junctional proteins such as 95-kDa protein and other proteins of both the tubules and the reticulum may also influence the interactions of the two major channel proteins.

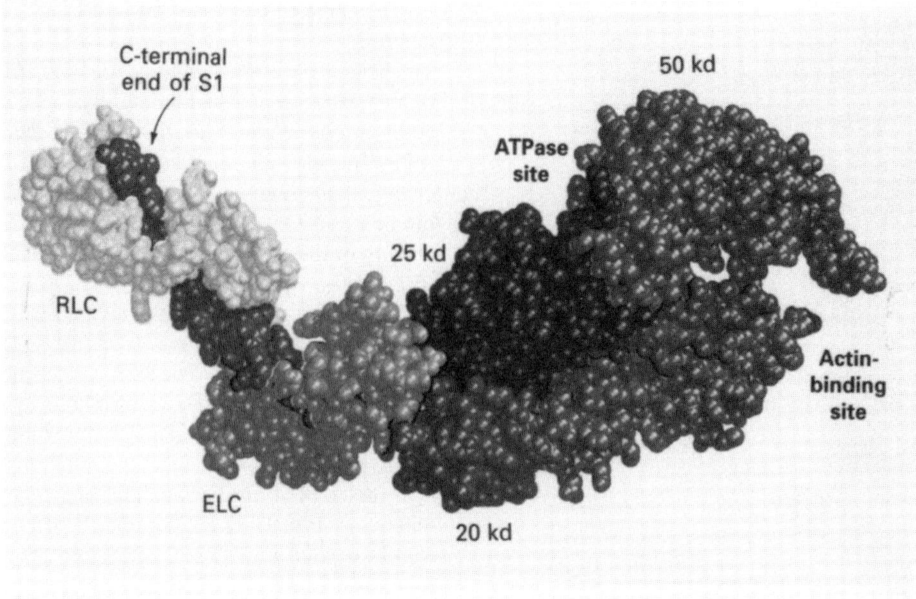

Figure 93-8 Three-dimensional structure of myosin head. Note that the balls represent individual atoms derived from X-ray diffraction of crystals of proteolytically derived S1 or myosin head. RLC is the regulatory light chain; ELC is essential light chain. (From Stryer L. Biochemistry, 4th ed. New York: WH Freeman, adapted from Ivan Rayment, with permission.)

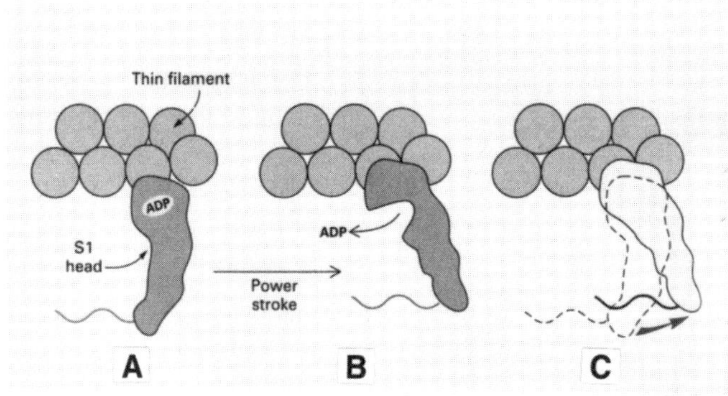

Figure 93-9 Detail of myosin head interacting with actin or thin filament. Note structural changes within myosin head and between myosin and actin. (From Stryer L. Biochemistry, 4th ed. New York: WH Freeman, after Rayment I, Holden HM, Whittaker M, Yohn CB, Lorenz M, Holmes KC, and Milligan RA, Science 1993;261:58–65, with permission.)

The uptake of calcium is controlled primarily by the calcium pump molecules of the sarcoplasmic reticulum. These molecules act as classical transport pumps; ATP is hydrolyzed by the pump in order to transport calcium ions into the reticulum lumen against an electro-chemical gradient. Secondarily, the binding of the transported calcium ions by the lumenal protein calsequestrin aids in the uptake. Essentially these processes are continuous; they are overwhelmed by the activated calcium release processes and predominate when release is deactivated.

Regulation by Calcium of Actin and Myosin Interaction The release of calcium from the sarcoplasmic reticulum into the myofibrillar space activates the cycle of actomyosin-ATP interactions (Figs. 93-6 and 93-7) and the subsequent sliding of actin filaments past myosin filaments (Fig. 93-5). The key interaction of calcium is with the troponin complexes of the actin filaments. Each actin filament with its full complement of tropomyosin and troponin may be considered as a single allosteric unit (Fig. 93-2). The binding of calcium to troponin anywhere on the actin filament changes the potential interactions of all the actin monomers.

This remarkable effect of calcium binding by troponin is mediated by two levels of conformational change. First, calcium induces a change in the troponix complex: tropomyosin interaction. Second, the activated tropomyosins rotate about each actin strand. This rotation is propagated along both strands of actin up and down the filament. The net effect of these conformational changes is the opening of sites on actin subunits for interaction with myosin heads.

The allosteric interactions of the actin filaments may also be sensitive to the binding of myosin heads.

The uptake of calcium into the sarcoplasmic reticulum leads to reversal of actomyosin activation and the conformational changes in the actin filaments.

THE MYOFIBRIL IN HEALTH AND DISEASE

Three areas of muscle biology are medically significant. First, the actin and myosin filaments of skeletal muscles represent the body's largest store of amino acids that may be mobilized for metabolic needs. Skeletal muscle, therefore, plays a necessary role in nutrition and metabolism. Second, hormones and neuronal action control the metabolic functions of muscle. Skeletal muscle is a critical tissue in the effects of diabetes. Injury or dysfunction of motor neurons leads to skeletal muscle atrophy. Third, an increasing number of inherited diseases have been traced to specific proteins of the myofibril. Many of these disorders affect both heart and skeletal muscle, consistent with the sharing of both proteins and their functions between these tissues.

MUSCLE PROTEINS AND NUTRITION Myosin and actin are the principal proteins of skeletal muscles. Although relatively stable, these proteins are continuously being degraded and synthesized. Since virtually all myosin and actin are assembled into filaments in muscle, the filaments must also be continuously assembled and disassembled. Skeletal muscle can degrade these proteins to free amino acids and, in certain cases, can oxidize the amino acids in order to synthesize ATP.

The amino acids may be reutilized by muscle or may be secreted. Nearly every tissue of the body may take up amino acids and utilize them for protein synthesis. The liver takes up alanine and can utilize it for gluconeogenesis. The glucose may be used by the liver itself or be secreted and used by other tissues. A potential cycle exists between liver and muscle. Amino acids from myofibrillar protein breakdown are secreted by skeletal muscle, taken up by liver, and used in synthesizing glucose. The glucose is secreted, taken up by muscle, and used for contraction or stored as glycogen.

Lactate from anaerobic muscle contraction may also be used by the liver for gluconeogenesis (Cori cycle). In addition to amino acids and carbohydrates, skeletal muscle oxidizes fatty acids to produce ATP.

Well-nourished persons will use fatty acid oxidation for aerobic contraction and glycolysis/glycogenolysis for anaerobic work. The utilization of protein amino acid stores becomes significant under conditions of fasting or in uncontrolled diabetic states in which glucose and fat utilization are both impaired. Prolonged starvation shuts off protein degradation, and oxidation of ketone bodies derived from prior lipid oxidation predominates.

HORMONAL AND NEURONAL CONTROL

Insulin and Diabetes The major hormone that regulates both energetics and synthetic metabolism in skeletal muscle is insulin. Insulin stimulates uptake of glucose, amino acids, and fatty acids into skeletal muscle. The synthesis of glycogen and of myofibrillar proteins is markedly increased. In diabetes mellitus of either primary β-cell pancreatic origin or a result of insulin resistance, all of these positive effects of insulin can be decreased. In severe diabetic states, they are markedly reduced. Free fatty acids are mobilized to produce ketone bodies, and the oxidation of ketone bodies becomes a major contributor to energetics in muscle and other tissues that ordinarily require insulin.

Neuronal Control Skeletal muscles require functional interactions with both motor neurons and specialized proprioceptive neurons of muscle spindles, not only for proper contractile function but also in the development and maintenance of myofibrillar proteins and structures. Muscle fibers are of two major types. Type I fibers are slow twitch, and their contraction is dependent on aerobic metabolism. Type II fibers are fast twitch, and the contraction is primarily dependent on glycogenolytic (anaerobic) metabolism. There are multiple differences in gene expression between the two fiber types, including metabolic enzymes, membrane channel protein isoforms, and myofibrillar protein isoforms. Most skeletal muscles in humans contain mixtures of the two fiber types. Some fibers show intermediate properties and represent minor subtypes.

The differentiation of and maintenance of Type I and II muscle fibers are dependent on the appropriate innervation by "slow" and "fast" motor neurons, respectively. Functional, pathological, or physical deinnervation of either type of muscle fiber leads to atrophy. Reinnervation will lead to development of a fiber of type specificity dependent upon the type of motor neuron.

The mechanism of this dependence of skeletal muscle on nerve is not fully understood. In part, skeletal muscle may respond developmentally and metabolically to its own functioning. On the other hand, neurons actively secrete various protein factors and peptides in addition to neurotransmitters such as acetylcholine. Such factors include agrin, an extracellular protein that organizes acetylcholine receptors into special membrane sites and ciliary neurotrophic factor that may stimulate skeletal muscle development and growth more generally.

Inherited Muscle Diseases Chapter 94 will discuss much of the exciting new research in inherited diseases of skeletal muscle. Also, inherited diseases of the heart may affect proteins shared with skeletal muscle. It is important to note here that there are genetic alterations of specific proteins of the myofibril, sarcoplasmic reticulum/transverse tubules, and membrane cytoskeleton that lead to alterations of skeletal muscle structure and function.

Central core disease in which the myofibrillar compartment becomes selectively depleted in affected skeletal muscle fibers can be associated with specific mutations of the β-cardiac myosin heavy-chain isoform that is shared by slow skeletal muscle fibers. The responsible genetic locus is on human chromosome 14q. The skeletal muscle defects may be associated with or independent of the development of hypertrophic cardiomyopathy in these patients.

Malignant hyperthermia in which volatile anesthetics produce uncontrollable muscular contraction and generation of heat during surgery is a result of mutations of sarcoplasmic reticulum calcium release channel. The responsible genetic locus for this disorder is on human chromosome 19q.

Duchenne and Becker muscular dystrophies are produced by a variety of mutations in the dystrophin 427-kDa isoform (Fig. 93-4). These disorders affect males primarily because the responsible genetic locus is on human chromosome Xp2.1. As discussed, dystrophin participates in one of several protein systems that anchor cytoskeletal actin filaments to the membrane and the extracellular matrix in skeletal muscle. Although primarily thought of as skeletal muscle diseases, Duchenne-Becker dystrophy patients and even female carriers may have significant cardiomyopathies because of the shared expression of dystrophin.

SELECTED REFERENCES

Alberts B, Bray D, Lewis J, Raff M, Roberts K, Watson JD. (Chapter 16 and Glossary). The Cytoskeleton. In: Molecular Biology of the Cell, 3rd ed. New York: Garland, 1994; p. 1294.

Campbell KP. Membrane organization of the dystrophin-glycoprotein complex. Cell 1995;80:675–675.

Catterall WA. Excitation-contraction coupling invertebrate skeletal muscle: a tale of two calcium channels. Cell 1991;64:871–874.

Fleischer S, Inui M. Biochemistry and biophysics of excitation-contraction coupling. Ann Rev Biophys Chem 1989;18:333–364.

Rayment I, Holden HM, Whittaker M, Yohn CB, Lorenz M, Holmes KC et al. Structure of the actin-myosin complex and its implications for muscle contraction. Science 1993;261:58–65.

Stryer L. (*Chapter 15*). Molecular Motors. In: Biochemistry, 4th ed. New York: WH Freeman, 1995; p. 1064.

94 Muscular Dystrophies

Eric P. Hoffman

OVERVIEW

Mutations of nine different genes have been shown to be causative of specific types of muscular dystrophy, and linkage studies have shown the existence of approximately six additional genes. The most common cause of muscular dystrophy is mutations of the dystrophin gene on the X chromosome: absent dystrophin results in Duchenne muscular dystrophy in males (>95% of childhood onset lethal dystrophy in males), present but abnormal dystrophin in Becker muscular dystrophy (50% adult ambulatory dystrophy in males), and 10% of isolated female dystrophy patients show symptoms as a consequence of carrier status and skewed X-chromosome inactivation. The pathophysiology of dystrophin abnormalities involves an instability of the plasma membrane of myofibers with a chronic deterioration of the muscle leading to weakness. Myotonic dystrophy is the next most frequent dystrophy, and is extremely variable, showing presentations ranging from neonatal lethality, to childhood mental retardation, adult distal weakness with myotonia, or early onset cataracts. It is dominantly inherited, with considerable variation in phenotype within families. This disease is caused by an increase in size of a trinucleotide repeat (CTG) in the 3' untranslated region of a protein kinase. The size of the expansion generally correlates with disease severity. The mechanism by which the expansion mutation causes the observed multisystemic and variable clinical features is not well-understood. Very recently, mutations of six additional genes have been identified. Mutations of calpain III, a muscle-specific membrane-bound protease, may be a relatively common cause of dystrophy in patients with normal dystrophin. Four different genes encoding specific "sarcoglycans" (transmembrane proteins that are components of the dystrophin-based membrane cytoskeleton) have recently been shown to cause relatively rare cases of Duchenne/Becker-like muscular dystrophy. Approximately 40% of neonatal onset disease, congenital muscular dystrophy, has been shown to be a result of deficiency of α2 laminin (merosin), a protein involved in attachment of myofibers to the extracellular matrix (basal lamina). In addition to profound weakness at birth, these patients show marked abnormalities of white matter by MRI studies, yet are intellectually normal. Finally, a rare X-linked recessive muscular dystrophy distinguished clinically from Duchenne/Becker muscular dystrophy by early prominent contractures and cardiac conduction defects has recently been found to be caused by mutations of a gene of unknown function in Xq28 (emerin). Additional dystrophies for which genes have been genetically mapped but not yet identified include dominantly inherited limb-girdle muscular dystrophy (chromosome 2p), fascioscapulohumeral dystrophy (4q), and oculopharyngeal muscular dystrophy (15p).

From: *Principles of Molecular Medicine* (J. L. Jameson, ed.), ©1998 Humana Press Inc., Totowa, NJ.

INTRODUCTION

Of the nine genes for which mutations have been shown to cause subtypes of muscular dystrophy, six result from abnormalities of the plasma membrane and adjacent basal lamina. Myofibers undoubtedly have a very stringent requirement for a durable and resilient plasma membrane based on two features of its normal physiology and function. First, each contraction of the myofibrils leads to a rapid and dramatic redistribution of the cytoplasm, resulting in changes of the shape of the myofiber. These shape changes would be expected to impart considerable stresses on the plasma membrane. Second, the force generated by the myofibrils must be transduced to the extracellular matrix so that the muscle group can contract and generate force as a single coordinated unit. Thus, this force transduction must be transmitted through the plasma membrane, which must be strongly reinforced to withstand these sheer forces. The study of human disease has been critical in both identifying components of the myofiber membrane cytoskeleton and in determining the relative functions of many of the components. To date, six distinct human inherited muscular dystrophies have been identified that are caused by deficiencies of the membrane cytoskeleton: one intracellular component (dystrophin; Duchenne muscular dystrophy), four transmembrane components (α, β, γ, and δ-sarcoglycans), and one extracellular component (α2 laminin). The muscular dystrophies caused by deficiency of dystrophin or any of the four sarcoglycans are quite similar histologically and clinically. This observation suggests that the progressive muscle diseases caused by these proteins may all share a similar pathogenesis, namely chronic membrane instability leading to progressive dysfunction of the muscle, and that all of the sarcoglycans and dystrophin are required for membrane stability. The deficiency of the extracellular component, α2 laminin, results in a more complicated and severe phenotype (congenital muscular dystrophy), with apparent involvement of the immune system in tissue pathology, and also abnormalities of myofiber regeneration.

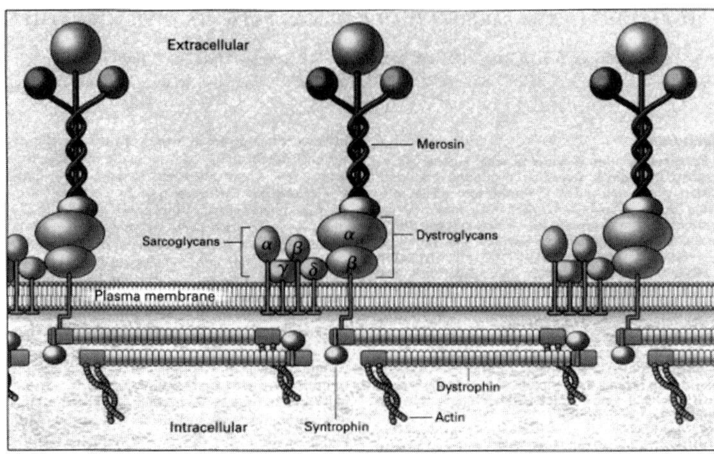

Figure 94-1 Schematic of proteins involved in muscular dystrophies. Shown is a segment of a myofiber plasma membrane, with the intracellular dystrophin-based membrane cytoskeleton, transmembrane sarcoglycans and dystroglycans, and extracellular basal lamina with laminin 2. Male Duchenne/Becker muscular dystrophy and isolated female dystrophinopathy patients are the result of abnormalities of the dystrophin protein, a common X-linked recessive disease. Rare autosomal recessive childhood-onset dystrophies are caused by mutations in any one of the sarcoglycan proteins (α sarcoglycan [adhalin], β sarcoglycan, γ sarcoglycan, and δ sarcoglycan). Many cases of neonatal onset severe congenital muscular dystrophy are caused by deficiency of α2 laminin (merosin), which is the large subunit of laminin in the myofiber basal lamina. (Reprinted with permission from Duggan et al. NEJM, 1997).

DISORDERS OF THE MEMBRANE CYTOSKELETON: DEFICIENCY OF DYSTROPHIN OR THE SARCOGLYCANS

Duchenne muscular dystrophy is one of the most common inherited disorders of humans and is the most frequent muscle disease (1/3500 live born males). Its high frequency in all world populations is a result of the high mutation rate of the gene, which in turn is largely a consequence of the enormous size of the gene (2.5 million bp). Affected children are predominantly male, because of the X-linked recessive inheritance pattern, and appear normal until about 4 or 5 years of age, when muscle weakness becomes obvious. Thereafter, there is a relentless progression of weakness and muscle wasting, leading to confinement to a wheelchair by age 14 years, and death due to respiratory failure by age 20 years (unless the patient is mechanically ventilated).

The biochemical deficiency causing the disorder remained obscure until 1987, when the Duchenne muscular dystrophy gene was identified by positional cloning techniques. The gene, which has remained 10 times larger than the next largest gene, encodes a 427-kDa protein dubbed "dystrophin," and dystrophin-deficiency is recognized to define Duchenne muscular dystrophy at the biochemical level. Mutations of the gene are deletions (55%), duplications (5%), and point mutations (40%). Partial dystrophin-deficiency, often the result of in-frame deletion mutations compatible with production of dystrophin that lacks segments of amino acids, is diagnostic of the milder and more variable Becker muscular dystrophy. Presentations of Becker dystrophy include proximal weakness, myoglobinuria, myalgias, hyperCKemia, and cardiac failure, and some patients may remain asymptomatic at advanced ages.

Female homozygotes do not exist because of the relative rarity of the disorder; females generally act as heterozygous gene carriers. However, approximately 10% of isolated female dystrophy patients express their symptoms as a consequence of heterozygosity for a dystrophinopathy. Most of these females show preferential inactivation of the X chromosome containing the normal dystrophin gene (skewed X inactivation). Presentations of isolated female carriers are as variable as in Becker muscular dystrophy in males, although the progression is often mitigated in the female patients.

Molecular diagnosis, genetic counseling, and prenatal diagnosis are well established in the dystrophinopathies. Dystrophin protein analysis of muscle biopsy, gene deletion mutation analysis, and gene linkage analysis are all routinely used. The large size of the gene complicates molecular genetic counseling and prenatal diagnosis: There is 10% recombination within the gene, and the high mutation rate leads to many "new mutations," which may effect a single egg or sperm or may cause the gonads of a parent to be a carrier but not the parent him/herself (gonadal mosaicism).

The identification of dystrophin as a major component of the membrane cytoskeleton of muscle fibers permitted use of the dystrophin protein as a probe to isolate and characterize other components. Recent research has identified three complexes of proteins that interact with dystrophin near the plasma membrane and appear to provide one type of connection between the intracellular contractile myofibrils and the extracellular matrix (Fig. 94-1). Rare childhood-onset muscular dystrophies with autosomal recessive inheritance patterns have been shown to be caused by mutations of four of the sarcoglycan proteins (Table 94-1; Fig. 94-1). No disorders have been associated with the primary defects in any of the syntrophins or dystroglycan components.

The clinical and histopathological consequences of primary disorders of dystrophin and the sarcoglycans are quite similar, and it can be safely assumed that they share a common molecular pathogenesis. Current models suggest that deficiencies of these proteins lead to membrane instability, which initiates both acute responses (hyperCKemia, myofiber necrosis) and chronic responses (progressive fibrosis, failure of myofiber regeneration, and muscle wasting/weakness). The immune system may play a role in both the acute and chronic responses, and immune suppressants such as prednisone have shown some effect in slowing the progression of

Table 94-1
Molecular Basis of the Muscular Dystrophies

Protein defect	*Disease*	*Onset of symptoms*	*Frequency*	*Characteristic clinical features*	*Gene mutations*	*Molecular diagnosis*
Dystrophin-deficiency	Duchenne muscular dystrophy	Childhood	1/3500 males (>90% of childhood-onset dystrophy)	Proximal weakness, calf hypertrophy, cardiomyopathy, 30% MR	55% deletions	Mutation, linkage analysis, protein analysis of muscle biopsy
Abnormal dystrophin	Becker muscular dystrophy	Childhood-adult	1/20,000 males (50–70% of male teen/adult-onset dystrophy)	Proximal weakness, high CK, cardiomyopathy	70% deletions	Mutation, linkage, protein of biopsy
Dystrophin mosaicism	Isolated female dystrophinopathy	Childhood-adult	1/100,000 females (10% of female dystrophy)	Proximal weakness, high CK, cardiomyopathy	60% deletions (heteroxgote)	Protein, X inactivation, mutation, linkage
α Sarcoglycan (adhalin)	SCARMD/LGMD[a]	Childhood	<1/200,000	Proximal weakness, high CK	Missense	Protein followed by mutations[b]
β Sarcoglycan	SCARMD/LGMD[a]	Childhood	<1/200,000	Proximal weakness, high CK	Missense	Protein followed by mutations[b]
δ sarcoglycan	SCARMD/LGMD[a]	Childhood	<1/200,000	Proximal weakness, high CK	Missense	Protein followed by mutations[b]
β Sarcoglycan	SCARMID/LGMD	Childhood	<1/200,000	Proximal weakness, hyperCKemia	Nonsense	Protein followed by mutations
α2-Laminin (merosin)	Congenital muscular dystrophy	Neonatal	<1/200,000	Floppiness, high CK, white matter changes by MRI	Deletion[c], nonsense	Protein, prenatal of chorionic villi
Calpain III[d]	LGMD	Childhood-adult	1/50,000?	Proximal weakness	Missense	Mutation
Emerin	Emery-Dreifuss muscular dystrophy	Childhood	<1/200,000	Contractures, proximal weakness, cardiac conduction defects	Missense	Mutation
DM kinase[e]	Myotonic dystrophy	Extremely variable	1/8,000	Neonatal floppiness, childhood MR, adult distal wasting, cataracts, frontal balding	Expansion of a CTG trinucleotide repeats	Mutation

[a]Severe childhood-onset autosomal recessive muscular dystrophy (SCARMD) and limb-girdle muscular dystrophy (LGMD) are generic descriptive diagnoses often used to describe these patients.

[b]Many muscular dystrophy patients show secondary deficiencies of sarcoglycan proteins. Thus, biochemical detection of a deficiency of a sarcoglycan protein most often does not reflect a primary deficiency (mutations) of that protein. For this reason, mutation analysis is suggested for a definitive diagnosis.

[c]Only a few mutations of the very large merosin gene have been identified to date.

[d]The clinical and molecular features of dystrophy associated with Calpain III mutations have not yet been well-defined. A multiple gene (digenic) inheritance has been proposed.

[e]The molecular pathogenesis of myotonic dystrophy is not well-understood. The disease is clearly caused by the expansion mutation in the 3' UTR of the kinase gene; however, it is not clear what genes, RNAs, or proteins are altered by this expansion.

the disease. Efforts at gene therapy are underway, although the refractory nature of mature myofibers to viral delivery systems, and the unique nature and large amount of the target muscle tissue, are hurdles currently facing this approach.

α2 LAMININ (MEROSIN) DEFICIENCY

In 1994, Tome and colleagues identified a subset of congenital muscular dystrophy patients that showed complete lack of immunostaining for the α2-laminin chain in their muscle biopsy. The α2-laminin gene (LAMA2) has been mapped to chromosome 6q22-23, and mutations have been identified in affected patients. Merosin-deficient patients are relatively uniform in clinical presentation and progression: patients are floppy at birth, with the infant unable to raise limbs against gravity. Serum creatine kinase are elevated to 2000–10,000 IU/l (normal <200 IU/l). The muscle biopsy shows a dystrophic process, with degeneration of myofibers, and a marked increase in endomysial and perimysial connective tissue with fatty infiltration. Importantly, one recent study found that 3 of 10 merosin-deficient patients studied were initially given the diagnosis of infantile polymyositis because of the presence of significant populations of inflammatory cells. This study documented focal inflammatory reaction in a young patients muscle, with concentrations of B and T cells resembling primary follicles, generally seen in spleen. These results suggested that earlier reports of the diagnosis of infantile polymyositis, with a presumed autoimmune etiology, could in fact represent a possible histological finding in inherited α2-laminin deficiency. Both $CD4^+$ and $CD8^+$ cells are seen in large numbers, both distributed throughout the biopsy and in focal aggregates.

α2 laminin is one of the three components of the heterotrimeric muscle laminin molecule (Fig. 94-1). The α2-subunit is present in muscle, the central nervous system (CNS), and schwann cells, and replaces the more ubiquitous α1 chain during the development of muscle tissue. The other two components, laminin β1 and γ1, are not tissue-specific. Laminin is a major constituent of basal lamina of most cells, where it complexes with collagen IV and other proteins to anchor cells in their tissue environment. α2 laminin is involved in neurite outgrowth in the peripheral and central nervous system. Interestingly, patients with α2 laminin deficiency show dramatic white-matter changes by MRI, although there is no overt CNS dysfunction or intellectual impairment. There is a mouse model for merosin deficiency, *dy/dy*, and the mutation in the milder of two alleles has been identified. These mice show a phenotype similar to the human disease.

Another congenital muscular dystrophy for which linkage data exist is Fukuyama congenital muscular dystrophy. This congenital muscular dystrophy is most frequently seen in Japan and shows very high serum creatine kinase levels at birth and atrophic brain. Japanese families with have been used for gene linkage studies, which have localized the gene to chromosome 9q31-33. No specific gene or gene mutations have been identified to date.

CALPAIN III DEFICIENCY A recent study has shown mutations in a gene corresponding to a muscle-specific protease, calpain III, associated with a relatively large number of childhood-adult onset muscular dystrophy inherited in an autosomal recessive pattern. The pathogenesis of the disease is not clear, and there are features of the genetics that are enigmatic and require further explanation before a strict relationship between calpain III mutations and muscular dystrophy can be assumed.

EMERY-DREIFUSS MUSCULAR DYSTROPHY A rare X-linked recessive disorder, Emery-Dreifuss muscular dystrophy, is clinically distinct from the dystrophinopathies as a result of the early presence of contractures and cardiac conduction defects requiring placement of a pacemaker. Linkage studies had shown the responsible gene to be located in Xq28, and the gene was recently identified. The novel protein (emerin) encoded by this gene shares features with other proteins involved in vesicular transport. It is localized to the nuclear membrane of skeletal and cardiac muscle cells. The molecular pathogenesis of the disorder is not clear.

MYOTONIC DYSTROPHY Myotonic dystrophy is the term used to describe one of the most common, and certainly the most variable, of the myopathic disorders. The moniker is more historical than descriptive: Only a subset of patients show myotonia or muscular dystrophy. Patients with this dominantly inherited disorder can present in the neonatal period (congenital myotonic dystrophy) with floppiness often requiring ventilatory support, in childhood with mental retardation and characteristic facies (hatchet jaw, lowset ears), in adolescence with distal weakness and wasting, or in older age with cataracts and frontal balding. The disease and corresponding severity have been strongly associated with an unstable trinucleotide repeat on the short arm of chromosome 19: Repeats of many thousands of basepairs are associated with early onset severe disease and shorter repeats associated with later onset milder disease. The repeat length changes between parent and offspring (meiotic instability), as well as within a patient (mitotic or somatic instability), such that muscle tissue has longer repeats than are present in other tissues.

The (CTG) repeat expansion is in the 3' untranslated region of a novel cAMP kinase gene (DM kinase), and an obvious assumption is that the repeat alters the expression of the kinase protein, leading to expression of disease. However, the dominant inheritance (patients are heterogotes, with a normal kinase gene in addition to the one containing the expansion mutation) and lack of sequence alterations in protein expressed by the mutant gene seem inconsistent with the dramatic variability of the clinical disease. The molecular pathogenesis is not resolved; however, three models are currently being tested: the expansion may have long-range effects on adjacent genes in the chromatin; RNA molecules containing the expansion may cause abnormalities of RNA metabolism; or the disorder may result from haploinsufficiency of the kinase or a second neighboring homeobox gene. These three mechanisms may not be mutually exclusive.

GENETICALLY DEFINED DOMINANTLY INHERITED DYSTROPHIES Three dominantly inherited, late-onset muscular dystrophies have been mapped to specific chromosome locations: limb-girdle muscular dystrophy (chromosome 2p), fascioscapulohumeral dystrophy (4q), and oculopharyngeal muscular dystrophy (15p). Fascioscapulohumeral muscular dystrophy is one of the more common dominantly inherited muscular dystrophies and shows preferential involvement of facial and upper-girdle muscles. The disorder is variable in severity, although most patients present in late teenage or adult years. The disease is strongly associated with alterations of the telomore of the long arm of chromosome 4. However, no specific gene has been implicated in the disease pathogenesis. Most patients carrying the descriptive diagnosis of limb-girdle muscular dystrophy have a recessively inherited disease, although rare families with late-onset dominant inheritance have been described. Oculopharyngeal dystrophy shows onset in later decades of life and shows progressive weakness of ocular and pharyngeal musculature. The disease is most common in French-Canadian populations.

SELECTED REFERENCES

Bione S, Maestrini E, Rivella S, et al. Identification of a novel X-linked gene responsible for Emery-Dreifuss muscular dystrophy. Nat Genet 1994;8:323–327.

Bonnemann CG, Modi R, Noguchi S, et al. Mutations in the dystrophin-associated glycoprotein β-sarcoglycan (A3b) cause autosomal recessive muscular dystrophy with disintegration of the sarcoglycan complex. Nat Genet 1995;11:266–270.

Brooke MH, Fenichel GM, Griggs RC, et al. Duchenne muscular dystrophy: Patterns of clinical progression and effects of supportive therapy. Neurology 1989;39:475–481.

Buxton, J. et al. Detection of an unstable fragment of DNA specific to individuals with myotonic dystrophy. Nature 1992;355:547,548.

Campbell KP, Crosbie RH. Muscular dystrophy. Utrophin to the rescue. Nature 1996;384:308,309.

Duggan DJ, Gorospe JR, Fanin M, Hoffman EP, Angelini C. Mutations in the sarcoglycan genes in patients with myopathy. N Engl J Med 1997;336:618–624.

Hamshere MG, Newman EE, Alwazzan M, Athwal BS, Brook JD. Transcriptional abnormality in myotonic dystrophy affects DMPK but not neighboring genes. Proc Natl Acad Sci USA 1997;94:7394–7399.

Helbling-Leclerc A, Zhang X, Topaloglu H, Cruaud C, Tesson F, Weissenbach J, et al. Mutations in the laminin alpha 2-chain gene (LAMA2) cause merosin-deficient congenital muscular dystrophy. Nat Genet 1995;11:216–218.

Hoffman EP, Brown RH, Kunkel LM. Dystrophin: the protein product of the Duchenne muscular dystrophy locus. Cell 1987;51:919–928.

Hoffman EP, Arahata K, Minetti C, et al. Dystrophinopathy in isolated cases of myopathy in females. Neurology 1992;42:967–975.

Koenig M, Hoffman EP, Bertelson CJ, Monaco AP, Feener C, Kunkel LM. Complete cloning of the Duchenne muscular dystrophy (DMD) cDNA and preliminary genomic organization of the DMD gene in normal and affected individuals. Cell 1987;50:509–517.

Ljunggren A, Duggan D, McNally E, et al. Primary adhalin deficiency as a cause of muscular dystrophy in patients with normal dystrophin. Ann Neurol 1995;38:367–372.

Miller RG, Hoffman EP. Molecular diagnosis and modern management of muscular dystrophy. Neurol Clin 1994;12:699–725.

Nagano A, Koga R, Ogawa M, et al. Emerin deficiency at the nuclear membrane in patients with Emery-Dreifuss muscular dystrophy. Nat Genet 1996;12:254–259.

Noguchi S, McNally EM, Ben Othmane K, et al. Mutations in the dystrophin-associated protein gamma-sarcoglycan in chromosome 13 muscular dystrophy. Science 1995;270:819–822.

Ozawa E, Yoshida M, Hagiwara Y, Suzuki A, Mizuno Y, Noguchi S. Dystrophin-associated proteins in muscular dystrophy. Hum Mol Genet 1995;4:1711–1716.

Pegoraro E, Mancias P, Swerdlow SH, et al. Congenital muscular dystrophy with primary laminin α2 (merosin) deficiency presenting as inflammatory myopathy. Ann Neurol 1996;40:782–791.

Pegoraro E, Schimke RN, Garcia C, et al. Genetic and biochemical normalization in female carriers of Duchenne muscular dystrophy: evidence for failure of dystrophin production in dystrophin competent myonuclei. Neurology 1995;45:677–690.

Piccolo F, Roberds SL, Jeanpierre M, et al. Primary adhalinopathy: a common cause of autosomal recessive muscular dystrophy of variable severity. Nat Genet 1995;10:243–245.

Richard I, Broux O, Allamand V, et al. Mutations in the proteolytic enzyme calpain 3 cause limb-girdle muscular dystrophy type 2A. Cell 1995;81:27–40.

Sewry C, Philpot J, Mahony D, Wilson LA, Muntoni F, Dubowitz V. Expression of laminin subunits in congenital muscular dystrophy. Neuromus Dis 1995;5:307–316.

Small K, Iber J, Warren ST. Emerin deletion reveals a common X-chromosome inversion mediated by inverted repeats. Nat Genet 1997;16:96–99.

Tinsley JM, Potter AC, Phelps SR, Fisher R, Trickett JI, Davies KE. Amelioration of the dystrophic phenotype of mdx mice using a truncated utrophin transgene. Nature 1996;384:349–353.

Toda, T, et al. Localization of a gene for Fukuyama type congenital muscular dystrophy to chromosome 9q31-q33. Nat Genet 1993;5:283–286.

Tome FM, Evangelista T, Leclerc A, et al. Congenital muscular dystrophy with merosin deficiency. Comptes Rendus Acad Sci 1994;317:351–357.

Wang JZ, Pegoraro E, Menegazzo E, et al. Myotonic dystrophy: evidence for a possible dominant-negative RNA mutation. Human Mol Genet 1995;4:599–606.

Xu H, Wu XR, Wewer UM, and Engvall E. Murine muscular dystrophy caused by a mutation in the laminin α2 (Lama2) gene. Nat Genet 1994;8:297–302.

95 Rhabdomyosarcomas

STEPHEN J. TAPSCOTT

BACKGROUND

Rhabdomyosarcomas are the most common of the soft tissue sarcomas in childhood, yet they are still a relatively rare tumor, with an incidence in the United States of 1.3–4.5 per million children per year. The histologic classification of rhabdomyosarcoma has historically relied on the expression of genes associated with skeletal muscle in some of the tumor cells, giving a subset of cells the appearance of skeletal muscle cells or myoblasts. Several histologic subcategories of rhabdomyosarcomas have also been recognized. Embryonal rhabdomyosarcomas are characterized by round or spindle-shaped cells, mixed with a variable number of eosinophilic myoblasts, sometimes showing cross-striations. Embryonal rhabdomyosarcomas occur most frequently during the first three years after birth and account for about 50–60% of rhabdomyosarcomas. Additional distinctions can be made within the group of embryonal rhabdomyosarcomas; for example, there are the botyroid and spindle-cell variants. Alveolar rhabdomyosarcomas are distinguished from embryonal rhabdomyosarcomas histologically by characteristic open spaces in pathology sections, reminiscent of alveoli in the lungs. Alveolar rhabdomyosarcomas account for approximately 20% of rhabdomyosarcomas and have a bimodal incidence distribution with peaks at approximately ages 3 and 15. A third group of pleomorphic or primitive rhabdomyosarcomas is not easily distinguished from other small round-cell tumors of childhood, such as neuroblastoma, Ewing's sarcoma, primitive neuroectodermal tumors, and non-Hodgkin's lymphoma, based on standard histology. For these primitive tumors, classification as rhabdomyosarcomas can be confirmed using antibodies or other molecular probes to genes characteristically expressed in skeletal muscle, such as desmin, myosin, or muscle creatine kinase.

RHABDOMYOSARCOMAS EXPRESS MyoD OR RELATED MYOGENIC FACTORS

Expression of the myogenic regulatory protein, MyoD, or one of the related members of this group of myogenic basic-helix-loop-helix (bHLH) proteins, which consists of MyoD, Myf5, Myogenin, and MRF4, can be used to categorize less differentiated tumors as rhabdomyosarcomas, since almost all rhabdomyosarcomas express one or more of this group of proteins. The myogenic bHLH proteins are transcription factors that orchestrate the expression of the genes that characterize skeletal muscle. Gene knockout experiments demonstrate that these genes are necessary for skeletal myogenesis, and the ability to convert nonmyogenic cells to skeletal muscle by expressing one of the myogenic bHLH proteins indicates that in many cell types, they are sufficient to mediate differentiation. In addition to activating expression of muscle structural genes, MyoD has been shown to mediate withdrawal from the cell cycle and induction of p21 expression. The role of these proteins in normal development is discussed (Chapter 92).

Given the ability of the myogenic bHLH proteins to activate transcription of skeletal muscle genes, the expression of MyoD in rhabdomyosarcomas can account for the low level of muscle differentiation seen in the tumor. In the tumors that have been analyzed, however, most of the cells in the tumor express MyoD, but very few cells express muscle structural genes and withdraw from the cell cycle, indicating that the activity of the myogenic bHLH proteins has been partially blocked. Analysis of the myogenic bHLH proteins in several tumors has demonstrated that they are not mutant, yet they are inefficient activators of muscle genes. Therefore, in the generation of rhabdomyosarcomas, the tumor cells have acquired mechanisms of preventing the normal activity of the myogenic bHLH proteins, thereby escaping cell differentiation and cell-cycle withdrawal.

Several molecular mechanisms have been identified that can prevent MyoD and related myogenic bHLH genes from activating transcription:

1. Heterodimerization with a member of the E-protein subfamily of bHLH genes (E12, E47, E2-5, E2-2) is a requirement for high-affinity DNA binding, since MyoD has a low affinity for DNA binding as a homodimer. Therefore, limiting amounts of E protein or high levels of the HLH protein Id, which competes with MyoD for heterodimerization with E proteins, could limit heterodimer formation and DNA binding.
2. A threonine residue in the DNA binding region of the MyoD protein, as well as in Myogenin, is subject to a PKC-dependent phosphorylation that can be induced by fibroblast growth factor (FGF). Phosphorylation prevents DNA binding and transcriptional activity.
3. TGF-β also blocks transcriptional activity of the myogenic bHLH proteins but does not prevent heterodimer formation or DNA binding based on in vitro binding assays.
4. Sequences adjacent to the MyoD binding sites can negatively regulate MyoD activity, possibly through interaction with other factors that can inhibit MyoD activity.

From: *Principles of Molecular Medicine* (J. L. Jameson, ed.), ©1998 Humana Press Inc., Totowa, NJ.

5. Oncogenes have been demonstrated to inhibit MyoD transcriptional activity, which could represent a direct interaction, such as with c-jun, or be mediated by other factors, such as increasing Cyclin D1 which then inhibits MyoD activity. In rhabdomyosarcomas, amplification of MDM@ has been shown to inhibit MyoD activity.

These examples represent several different basic mechanisms of preventing myogenesis mediated by MyoD and related myogenic bHLH proteins, and it remains to be determined which, if any or all, of these mechanisms play a role in the inhibition of myogenesis in rhabdomyosarcomas.

MOLECULAR GENETICS OF ALVEOLAR RHABDOMYOSARCOMAS

Cytogenetic studies identified multiple abnormalities in cells from rhabdomyosarcomas; however, alveolar rhabdomyosarcomas had a characteristic translocation between chromosome 2 and 13, t(2;13)(q35;q14). Fine mapping of the breakpoint identified *PAX3* as a candidate gene on chromosome 2, leading to the demonstration that the rearrangement occurred within the *PAX3* gene and ultimately identifying a novel chimeric transcript encoding the amino-terminal portion of the PAX3 protein from chromosome 2 and the carboxyterminal portion of a gene on chromosome 13, with homology to the fork head family of genes.

PAX3 is a transcription factor that is expressed in the neural tube, neural crest derivatives, and in the muscle precursor cells that migrate from the somites into the limb bud. Dominant, or semidominant, mutations of *PAX3* in mice, the *splotch* mutant, and humans, the Waartenberg syndrome, are noted for defects in neural crest and neural tube development. Embryos homozygous for some alleles of *splotch* have deficient limb muscle formation that can be attributed to the inadequate generation or migration of limb muscle precursor cells. This may partly be the basis for limb deformities in human variations of the Waartenberg syndrome that are homozygous for *PAX3* mutations.

The t(2;13) in alveolar rhabdomyosarcomas creates a novel gene with the transcription start site and 5-prime coding region of the *PAX3* gene and the 3' region of a gene called *FKHR* (fork head homolog rhabdomyosarcoma), a member of the fork head family of transcription factors, so-called because the prototype gene of the family was described as a mutation in Drosophila melanogaster that produced two spiked head structures (*see* Chapter 3). Additional vertebrate members of the fork head family include the hepatocyte nuclear factors (BNF-3α, BNF-3β, BNF-3γ) and brain factor-1 (BF-1). The fusion protein includes the two DNA binding domains in the carboxy-terminal half of the PAX3 protein, a paired box DNA-binding domain and a homeodomain, but disrupts the DNA-binding region of the FKHR protein. The carboxy-terminal portion of FKHR maintained in the fusion protein is rich in prolines and acidic amino acids, attributes consistent with an acidic activation domain, and transfection experiments demonstrate that the fusion protein is more potent than PAX3 as transcriptional activator of reporter constructs driven by PAX3 binding sites. Further, DNA-binding studies show that the fusion protein binds to PAX3 binding sites, but that it has a mildly altered DNA-binding affinity compared to PAX3. Therefore, the PAX3-FKHR fusion protein may have oncogenic activity based on enhanced activation of genes regulated by PAX3 or through altered binding affinity to specific DNA sequences.

While PAX3 is apparently expressed in the early migrating muscle progenitor cells, its role in development is only beginning to be understood. PAX3 expression inhibits myogenesis in cultured muscle cell lines and inhibits the ability of MyoD to activate the myogenic program in fibroblasts. The PAX3-FKHR fusion protein is a more potent inhibitor of myogenesis and MyoD activity in this system. Based on these observations and the developmental expression of PAX3 in the migrating muscle precursor cells, but not in skeletal muscle, it is possible that the normal function of PAX3 is to prevent myogenic differentiation during precursor cell migration and the fusion protein either enhances this activity or loses an element necessary to suppress this activity.

Although much less frequent than t(2;13), a t(1;13)(p36;q14) translocation has been described in some alveolar rhabdomyosarcomas. This translocation creates a fusion protein between PAX7 on chromosome 1 with the FKHR gene that is structurally very similar to the PAX3-FKHR fusion protein. PAX7 is also expressed in muscle precursor cells and is capable of binding to PAX3 sites either as a homodimer or as a heterodimer with PAX3. Therefore, each fusion protein, PAX3-FKHR and PAX7-FKHR, is expressed in myogenic precursor cells and has shared gene targets.

MOLECULAR GENETICS OF EMBRYONAL RHABDOMYOSARCOMAS

Most rhabdomyosarcomas are sporadic; however, the appearance of rhabdomyosarcomas in families with the Li-Fraumeni syndrome or the Beckwith-Wiedemann syndrome have provided valuable insights into the genetics of this tumor (*see* Chapter 7). Beckwith-Wiedemann syndrome (*see* Chapter 116) is associated with growth excess and a high incidence of tumors, including Wilms' tumor, hepatoblastoma, adrenal carcinoma, and rhabdomyosarcoma. Because of the association of Wilm's tumor with a locus on chromosome 11p13, this region was analyzed for loss of heterozygosity (LOH) in both rhabdomyosarcomas and in the Beckwith-Wiedemann syndrome. LOH of chromosome 11 was detected in a large portion of rhabdomyosarcomas, but the common region of LOH mapped to 11p15.5, similar to the mapping of the region of LOH for the Beckwith-Wiedemann syndrome. A preferential retention of the paternal allele in both embryonal rhabdomyosarcomas and in the Beckwith-Wiedemann syndrome has led to the suggestion that LOH alters the level of gene expression maintained by an imprinted allele, either decreasing expression of a tumor suppressor gene by loss of the nonimprinted allele or increasing expression of a growth-promoting gene by duplication of the nonimprinted allele.

The presence of a tumor growth suppressor gene at 11p15 has been supported by transfer of subchromosomal fragments to rhabdomyosarcoma cells. Fragments of chromosome 11 that contain 11p15 suppress growth and xenograft tumor formation in embryonal rhabdomyosarcomas, although similar experiments have not been performed in alveolar rhabdomyosarcomas, nor has parental origin of the suppressing allele been analyzed.

The gene relevant to rhabdomyosarcoma formation at 11p15 has not been clearly identified, although some candidates have been studied. Insulin-like growth factor II (IGF-2) is a maternally imprinted gene that maps to 11p15, transcriptionally silent on the maternal allele and expressed from the paternal allele. Elevated levels of IGF-2 resulting from paternal disomy associated with LOH may give a growth advantage to cells and has been postulated as the cause of the somatic hypertrophy in the Beckwith-

Wiedemann syndrome. IGF-2 has been shown to act as an autocrine growth factor in some rhabdomyosarcomas and loss of imprinting (LOI), i.e., expression of IGF-2 from both alleles has been demonstrated in alveolar rhabdomyosarcomas and embryonal rhabdomyosarcomas that do not have LOH at 11p15. The growth-promoting activity of increased IGF-2 levels may play a critical role in the generation of rhabdomyosarcomas; however, this model would not explain the somatic cell genetic experiments that implicate a tumor suppressor gene at 11p15.

A second, somewhat unusual, candidate gene that maps to 11p15 is *H19*, unusual because the *H19* transcript does not contain a conserved open reading frame and may function as a regulatory polyadenylated RNA. *H19* is imprinted in the opposite manner to *IGF2*, expressed from the maternal allele and silent on the paternal allele; therefore, loss of the maternal allele decreases *H19* expression. Transfection of *H19* into rhabdomyosarcoma cell lines suppresses both growth and tumorigenicity, making it a candidate for the 11p15 tumor suppressor gene.

Implicating imprinting as a critical factor in the LOH at 11p15 means that the transcription of numerous genes in the region might contribute to the transformed phentoype, and both *H19* and *IGF2* may contribute to the generation of rhabdomyosarcomas. Many additional genes have been mapped to the 11p15.5 region, including the cyclin-dependent kinase inhibitor $p57^{KIP2}$, the nucleosome assembly protein *hNAP2*, and the retinoblastoma-associated protein *RbAp48*. Mutations of the *p57* gene have been reported in Beckwith-Wiedemann syndrome and cause developmental abnormalities in mice that are similar to the Beckwith-Widemann syndrome, indicating that *p57* has a critical role in this syndrome. It remains to be determined whether altered expression of *p57* or other genes in this region contribute to the generation of rhabdomyosarcomas.

Rb, p53, AND ONCOGENES

Just as the association of rhabdomyosarcomas with the Beckwith-Wiedemann syndrome focused attention on 11p15, the appearance of rhabdomyosarcomas in families with Li-Fraumeni syndrome suggested that *p53* inactivation may be important for tumor formation. Analysis of *p53* abnormalities, without respect to alveolar or embryonal histologic types, indicated that approximately half of the tumors had abrogated normal *p53* function. When histologic subtype is considered, then it appears that the frequency of *p53* mutations is higher in the embryonal rhabdomyosarcomas. Differences between embryonal and alveolar rhabdomyosarcomas are further suggested by a higher frequency of *N-myc* amplification in alveolar rhabdomyosarcomas, whereas mutations in *N-ras* or *K-ras* appear to be more frequent in embryonal rhabdomyosarcomas. In contrast to *p53*, mutations in the *Rb* gene are rare in rhabdomyosarcomas.

ORIGIN OF RHABDOMYOSARCOMAS

While it is commonly believed that rhabdomyosarcomas originate from transformed muscle precursor cells, the appearance of rhabdomyosarcomas in regions that contain few muscle progenitors suggests that another mechanism may also contribute to their generation. A defining molecular feature of rhabdomyosarcomas is the expression of *MyoD* or another member of the myogenic bHLH group. *MyoD* transcription is actively suppressed in nonmuscle cells, an attribute that may be general to genes such as *MyoD* that positively autoregulate their transcription and commit a cell to a specific fate. Therefore, a cell that loses suppression of *MyoD* transcription may activate the positive feedback circuits and commit to the muscle lineage. If this happens in a nascent tumor cell, then the sufficiency of MyoD to activate terminal differentiation might eliminate that cell from the replicating population. In this regard, the loss of the suppression of *MyoD* transcription could be thought of as a protection against growth. However, if the activity of MyoD was prevented by the expression of an oncogene, such as *PAX3-FKHR*, or by the loss of other factors necessary for myogenesis, then tumor growth would continue and MyoD would not be able to induce terminal differentiation. While this model is speculative, it would account for mixed tumor phenotypes, such as the myomedulloblastoma or the rhabdomyomatous nephroblastoma.

TREATMENT AND FUTURE DIRECTIONS

The current approach to therapy of rhabdomyosarcomas combines chemotherapy, radiation therapy, and surgery. The most recent Intergroup Rhabdomyosarcoma Study (IRS-III) utilized a risk-based design that increased therapeutic intensity in groups with marginally poorer prognosis. In addition to tumor staging based on invasiveness, involvement of lymph nodes, metastasis and degree of surgical excision; tumor histology is a significant variable in predicting response to treatment. In IRS-II, the 5-year survival rate was 95% for the favorable category of botyroid, 67% for embryonal, and approximately 50% for alveolar and undifferentiated. IRS-III included therapy intensification for the groups with the less favorable prognosis and has achieved survival rates for alveolar tumors comparable to embryonal.

One challenge for the future is to determine if survival can be improved and therapy-related complications minimized by using the available molecular markers to further refine risk-based therapy. One clear question is whether tumors that are histologically classified as embryonal but have t(2;13) should be treated as alveolar or embryonal tumors. Further, is there an outcome distinction between those tumors with t(2;13) or t(1;13), or tumors with amplified *N-myc*, activated *ras*, or *p53* mutations that will help direct therapeutic decisions. The availability of rapid PCR methods to identify fusion transcripts or LOH should greatly facilitate these studies.

It would be very satisfying if further understanding of the molecular biology of rhabdomyosarcomas eventually led to rationally designed therapies. Perhaps the development of drugs that inhibit *PAX3* expression or increase *H19* expression, or ribozymes and antisense oligonucleotides that degrade the *PAX3-FKHR* fusion transcript, would be useful adjuvants to therapy.

SELECTED REFERENCES

Anand G, Shapiro DN, Dickman PS, Prochownik EV. Rhabdomyosarcomas do not contain mutations in the DNA binding domains of myogenic transcription factors. J Clin Invest 1994;93:5–9.

Barr FG, Galili N, Holick J, Biegel JA, Rovera G, Emanuel BS. Rearrangement of the PAX3 paired box gene in the paediatric solid tumour alveolar rhabdomyosarcoma. Nat Genet 1993;3:113–117.

Bengal E, Ransone L, Scharfmann R, et al. Functional antagonism between c-Jun and MyoD proteins: a direct physical association. Cell 1992;68:507–519.

Best LG, Hoekstra RE. Wiedemann-Beckwith syndrome: autosomal-dominant inheritance in a family. Amer J Med Genet 1981;9: 291–299.

Bober E, Franz T, Arnold HH, Gruss P, Tremblay P. Pax-3 is required for the development of limb muscles: a possible role fo the migration of dermomyotomal muscle progenitor cells. Development 1994; 120:603–612.

Brennan TJ, Edmondson DG, Li L, Olson EN. Transforming growth factor beta represses the actions of myogenin through a mechanism independent of DNA binding. Proc Natl Acad Sci USA 1991;88: 3822–3826.

Clark J, Rocques PJ, Braun T, et al. Expression of members of the myf gene family in human rhabdomyosarcomas. Brit J Cancer 1991; 64:1039–1042.

Crist W, Gehan EA, Ragab AH, et al. The third intergroup rhabdomyosarcoma study. J Clin Oncol 1995;13:610–630.

Davis RJ, D'Cruz CM, Lovell MA, Biegel JA, Barr FG. Fusion of PAX7 to FKHR by the variant t(1;13)(p36;q14) translocation in alveolar rhabdomyosarcoma. Cancer Res 1994;54:2869–2872.

De Chiara A, T'Ang A, Triche TJ. Expression of the retinoblastoma susceptibility gene in childhood rhabdomyosarcomas. J Natl Cancer Inst 1993;85:152–157.

Douglass EC, Valentine M, Etcubanas E, et al. A specific chromosomal abnormality in rhabdomyosarcomas. Cytogenet Cell Genet 1987; 45:148–155.

Driman D, Thorner PS, Greenberg ML, Chilton-MacNeill S, Squire J. MYCN gene amplification in rhabdomyosarcoma. Cancer 1994; 73:2231–2237.

El-Badry OM, Minniti C, Kohn EC, Houghton PJ, Daughaday WH, Helman LJ. Insulin-like growth factor II acts as an autocrine growth and motility factor in human rhabdomyosarcoma tumors. Cell Growth Diff 1990;1:325–331.

Epstein JA, Lam P, Jepeal L, Maas RL, Shapiro DN. Pax3 inhibits myogenic differentiation of cultured myoblast cells. J Biol Chem 1995;270:11,719–11,722.

Felix CA, Kappel CC, Mitsudomi T, et al. Frequency and diversity of p53 mutations in childhood rhabdomyosarcoma. Cancer Res 1992; 52:2243–2247.

Franz T. The Splotch (Sp1H) and Splotch-delayed (Sp^d) alleles: differential phenotypic effects on neural crest and limb musculature. Anat Embryo 1993;187:371–377.

Fredericks WJ, Galili N, Mukhopadhyay S, et al. The PAX3-FKHR fusion protein created by the t(2;13) translocation in alveolar rhabdomyosarcomas is a more potent transcriptional activator than PAX3. Mol Cell Biol 1995;15:1522–1535.

Galili N, Davis RJ, Fredericks WJ, et al. Fusion of a fork head domain gene to PAX3 in the solid tumour alveolar rhabdomyosarcoma. Nat Genet 1993;5:230–235.

Halevy O, Novitch BG, Spicer DB, et al. Correlation of terminal cell cycle arrest of skeletal muscle with induction of p21 by MyoD. Science 1995;267:1018–1021.

Hao Y, Crenshaw T, Moulton T, Newcomb E, Tycko B. Tumour-suppressor activity of H19 RNA. Nature 1993;365:764–767.

Jen Y, Weintraub H, Benezra R. Overexpression of Id protein inhibits the muscle differentiation program: in vivo association of Id with E2A proteins. Genes Dev 1992;6:1466–1479.

Koi M, Johnson LA, Kalikin LM, Little PF, Nagamura Y, Feinberg AP. Tumor cell growth arrest caused by subchromosomal transferable DNA fragments from chromosome 11. Science 1993; 260:361–364.

Koufos A, Hansen MF, Copeland NG, Jenkins NA, Lampkin BC, Cavenee WK. Loss of heterozygosity in three embryonal tumours suggests a common pathogenetic mechanism. Nature 1985;316:330–334.

Lai E, Clark KL, Burley SK, Darnell JE, Jr. Hepatocyte nuclear factor 3/fork head or "winged helix" proteins: a family of transcription factors of diverse biologic function. Proc Natl Acad Sci USA 1993;90: 10,421–10,423.

Lassar AB, Davis RL, Wright WE, et al. Functional activity of myogenic HLH proteins requires hetero-oligomerization with E12/E47-like proteins in vivo. Cell 1991;66:305–315.

Li L, Zhou J, James G, Heller-Harrison R, Czech MP, Olson EN. FGF inactivates myogenic helix-loop-helix proteins through phosphorylation of a conserved protein kinase C site in their DNA-binding domains. Cell 1992;71:1181–1194.

Loh WE, Jr., Scrable HJ, Livanos E, et al. Human chromosome 11 contains two different growth suppressor genes for embryonal rhabdomyosarcoma. Proc Natl Acad Sci USA 1992;89:1755–1759.

Martin JF, Li L, Olson EN. Repression of myogenin function by TGF-beta 1 is targeted at the basic helix-loop-helix motif and is independent of E2A products. J Biol Chem 1992;267:10,956–10,960.

Mulligan LM, Matlashewski GJ, Scrable HJ, Cavenee WK. Mechanisms of p53 loss in human sarcomas. Proc Natl Acad Sci USA 1990; 87:5863–5867.

Pappo AS, Shapiro DN, Crist WM, Maurer HM. Biology and therapy of pediatric rhabdomyosarcoma. J Clin Oncol 1995;13:2123–2139.

Raney RB, Hays DM, Tefft M, et.al. Rhabdomyosarcoma and the undifferentiated sarcomas. In: Pizzo PA, Poplack DG, eds. Principles and Practice of Pediatric Oncology. Philadelphia: Lippincott, 1993; pp. 769–794.

Rudnicki MA, Schnegelsberg PN, Stead RH, Braun T, Arnold HH, Jaenisch R. MyoD or Myf-5 is required for the formation of skeletal muscle. Cell 1993;75:1351–1359.

Schafer BW, Czerny T, Bernasconi M, Genini M, Busslinger M. Molecular cloning and characterization of a human PAX-7 cDNA expressed in normal and neoplastic myocytes. Nucleic Acids Res 1994;22: 4574–4582.

Scrable H, Cavenee W, Ghavimi F, Lovell M, Morgan K, Sapienza C. A model for embryonal rhabdomyosarcoma tumorigenesis that involves genome imprinting. Proc Natl Acad Sci USA 1989;86:7480–7484.

Scrable H, Witte D, Shimada H, et al. Molecular differential pathology of rhabdomyosarcoma. Genes Chromosomes Cancer 1989;1:23–35.

Skapek SX, Rhee J, Spicer DB, Lassar AB. Inhibition of myogenic differentiation in proliferating myoblasts by cyclin D1-dependent kinase. Science 1995;267:1022–1024.

Stratton MR, Fisher C, Gusterson BA, Cooper CS. Detection of point mutations in N-ras and K-ras genes of human embryonal rhabdomyosarcomas using oligonucleotide probes and the polymerase chain reaction. Cancer Res 1989;49:6324–6327.

Tapscott SJ, Weintraub H. MyoD and the regulation of myogenesis by helix-loop-helix proteins. J Clin Invest 1991;87:1133–1138.

Tapscott SJ, Thayer MJ, Weintraub H. Deficiency in rhabdomyosarcomas of a factor required for MyoD activity and myogenesis. Science 1993;259:1450–1453.

Thayer MJ, Weintraub H. Activation and repression of myogenesis in somatic cell hybrids: evidence for trans-negative regulation of MyoD in primary fibroblasts. Cell 1990;63:23–32.

Weintraub H, Genetta T, Kadesch T. Tissue-specific gene activation by MyoD: determination of specificity by cis-acting repression elements. Genes Dev 1994;8:2203–2211.

Weintraub H, Tapscott SJ, Davis RL, et al. Activation of muscle-specific genes in pigment, nerve, fat, liver, and fibroblast cell lines by forced expression of MyoD. Proc Natl Acad Sci USA 1989;86:5434–5438.

Zhan S, Shapiro DN, Helman LJ. Activation of an imprinted allele of the insulin-like growth factor II gene implicated in rhabdomyosarcoma. J Clin Invest 1994;94:445–448.

Zlotogora J, Lerer I, Bar-David S, Ergaz Z, Abeliovich D. Homozygosity for Waardenburg syndrome. Am J Hum Genet 1995;56:1173–1178.

NEUROLOGY XI

SECTION EDITOR:

JOSEPH B. MARTIN

96 Molecular Neurobiology

JOSEPH B. MARTIN AND FRANK M. LONGO

GENERAL APPROACHES FOR IDENTIFYING GENES RELEVANT TO NEUROLOGICAL DISORDERS

Recent advances in gene mapping and cloning strategies have led to the discovery of genes responsible for many neurological disorders. These disorders are often characterized by considerable phenotypic or biochemical complexity. Successes and failures of efforts to clone genes responsible for neurological disorders highlight the crucial role of skilled clinical assessment. Identification of disease-related genes is a critical step in the elucidation of the underlying disease mechanism, provides a basis for a more logical classification of disease entities, and, it is hoped, will lead to new therapies. The general principles for identifying disease-related genes are described in Part I of this textbook; in this chapter we will focus on approaches relevant to neurological disorders.

The power of the cloning strategies can be appreciated from a general quantitative perspective of the human genome (*see* Chapter 5). The genome consists of 3×10^9 base pairs (bp), and less than 5% of the entire genome encodes the estimated total of 60,000–100,000 expressed genes. These estimates predict an average of one gene every 30–50 kb throughout the genome. The average gene covers approximately 20 kb; a large gene such as the Duchenne muscular dystrophy (DMD) gene can extend for several hundred kilobases, whereas a relatively small gene can be encoded by less than 5 kb.

A typical search for a disease gene encompasses mapping the gene to a physical chromosomal location and then isolating clones containing fragments of DNA that encode all or part of the gene. One commonly employed cloning strategy consists of using probes genetically linked to the disease locus to screen libraries of yeast artificial chromosome (YAC) clones containing fragments of human DNA of 0.1–2.0 Mb (1 Mb = 1 million bases) in length. A 1-Mb segment of human genomic DNA may contain some 50 genes. Since DNA sequencing remains a tedious procedure in which a medium-sized laboratory may be capable of sequencing only several thousand base pairs per week, it would require several years to sequence one YAC clone. Thus, methods of selecting YAC clones are crucial, and after selection the search for a gene must be narrowed even further before direct DNA sequencing becomes productive. Several physical characteristics of genomic DNA can be used to guide the search for clones containing the disease-causing gene.

From: *Principles of Molecular Medicine* (J. L. Jameson, ed.), ©1998 Humana Press Inc., Totowa, NJ.

About 70% of the genome is unique-sequence DNA and contains both coding and noncoding regions. The remaining 30% is composed of repetitive DNA sequences. Some of these are clustered in a few locations (such as the telomeres), and some are dispersed throughout the genome amid short stretches of single-copy sequence of several kilobases or less. The association of these interspersed repeats with expressed genes has led to their use as crucial markers for cloning approaches. Minisatellite repeats contain repeat units of some 10–15 nucleotides, which are present with variable copy numbers in different individual genomes such that the length of the minisatellite varies across individuals. If DNA is cut using a restriction endonuclease and analyzed by Southern blot, a fragment that contains a minisatellite will also demonstrate size variation across individuals; this variation is termed a VNTR (variable number of tandem repeats) polymorphism.

Microsatellite repeats contain a repeat unit of only two, three, or four nucleotides, most commonly the dinucleotide (CA)n or variable-length runs of a single nucleotide. The high degree of polymorphism in microsatellite markers compared with restriction fragment length polymorphisms (RFLPs) and VNTR markers significantly increases the chances that a marker located near a disease locus will be informative in linkage studies. Variation in a microsatellite repeat number results in only a small change in the overall length of a microsatellite-containing DNA fragment and is therefore difficult to detect by Southern blot analysis. However, using the polymerase chain reaction (PCR), primers flanking the microsatellite can be used to amplify the DNA segment containing the repeats, and variations in repeat length of only two or three nucleotides can be detected by electrophoresis of the PCR product. Microsatellite alleles of different lengths (one microsatellite can have more than 10 different alleles) can easily be identified. Since microsatellites are typically flanked by unique-sequence DNA, a specific pair of PCR primers will usually identify a unique locus and therefore serve as a useful marker. The development of PCR and microsatellite markers has made available genetic markers that are more evenly distributed throughout the genome and more polymorphic than the previously used RFLP and VNTR markers. For most cloning approaches, several hundred evenly spaced microsatellite markers located at 10-Mb intervals are adequate for screening the entire human genome.

The goal of identifying and determining the location of all human genes is based on developing both physical and genetic linkage maps of the genome. Physical maps identify the position of a gene or locus in terms of chromosomal location. Giemsa staining of chromosomes reveals a banding pattern unique to each chromosome. The designation that the gene for myotonic dystrophy (DM) is at 19q13.3 indicates that the gene is on the long arm (q = long arm; p = short arm) of chromosome 19 at band 13.3. Cytogenetic analyses such as Giemsa banding provide a mapping resolution of several megabases. Linkage maps are derived from the establishment of genetic linkage between specific markers with distances expressed in units (centimorgans [cM]) that are a function of recombination frequency. On average, 1 cM is equal to approximately 1 Mb. The ongoing integration of physical and genetic linkage maps, which is the first stage of the Human Genome Project, will result in a comprehensive, high-density map of the human genome.

FUNCTIONAL CLONING Functional cloning (also known as "forward genetics") consists of identifying a defective enzyme or protein by standard biochemical methods based on knowledge of the disease phenotype. This approach has most commonly been used for isolating genes coding for defective enzymes associated with inborn errors of metabolism. Our meager understanding of the mechanisms underlying most neurological disorders has limited the number of disease-related genes isolated by functional cloning. Examples of genes derived by functional cloning include Lesch-Nyhan syndrome, metachromatic leukodystrophy, and Fabry's disease. Purification of the protein of interest allows antibody and oligonucleotide probes to be produced, which are used for screening DNA libraries. Oligonucleotide probes can be used to screen cDNA or genomic libraries by hybridization or PCR-based methods. Genomic or cDNA clones isolated by library screening can then be used to derive the full-length DNA sequence by isolating additional clones. The chromosomal location of the gene of interest can be established by using the clone as a probe for fluorescent *in situ* hybridization (FISH) to a resolution of 1–20 Mb.

POSITIONAL CLONING Positional cloning (also known as "reverse genetics") in a purely conceptional sense requires no knowledge of disease mechanism or underlying biochemical defects. Identification of the gene responsible for the disease of interest is established by its map position as determined by linkage analysis in affected families. The principal difficulty with this approach is that a genomic region defined by current high-resolution mapping with microsatellite markers can extend for several centimorgans (several megabases) and contain more than 50 genes. In many cases, cytogenetic rearrangements such as deletions, translocations, or the presence of trinucleotide repeats for diseases demonstrating anticipation (defined as the earlier appearance of a more severe phenotype in successive generations) have provided the necessary additional clues for gene localization. Neurological disorders for which the responsible gene was discovered primarily by positional cloning include DMD, neurofibromatosis types 1 and 2, DM, and tuberous sclerosis. Currently, the number of disease genes identified by positional cloning strategies in which phenotypic features, suspected biochemical deficits, or chromosomal rearrangements were not used to select likely gene candidates is less than 10. Lander and Schork pointed out that the only two human disease genes with point mutations (rather than rearrangements, deletions, or trinucleotide repeats) that had been identified solely by positional cloning were cystic fibrosis and diastrophic dysplasia. More recently, the gene responsible for a majority of early onset cases of Alzheimer's disease (AD), presenilin 1 *(S182)*, was also identified by positional cloning. The fact that few neurological disease genes have been identified to date purely by positional cloning points to the crucial role of a combination of clinical, phenotypical, and biochemical studies.

CANDIDATE GENE APPROACH In contrast to positional cloning, the candidate gene approach requires no knowledge of gene location. It can be used if knowledge of the disease phenotype suggests gene candidates. For example, accumulation of amyloid plaques in familial and sporadic AD raised the possibility that mutations in the β-amyloid precursor protein (APP) gene might cause some forms of familial Alzheimer's disease (FAD). Studies have shown that some 15–25% of FAD is associated with mutations in the APP gene and that these mutations can alter APP processing and contribute to amyloid formation. APP mutations have not been detected in sporadic AD. The discovery that the transmissible spongiform encephalopathies such as kuru and Creutzfeldt-Jakob disease involve aberrant metabolism of the prion protein raised the possibility that inherited spongiform encephalopathies might involve mutations in the prion protein gene. DNA sequencing demonstrated that various point mutations in this gene cause several inherited prion diseases including Gerstmann-Sträussler-Scheinker syndrome, Creutzfeldt-Jakob disease, and fatal familial insomnia. Significant genetic linkage between specific mutations in the prion protein gene and each phenotype further supported the role of these mutations in causing prion disease.

POSITIONAL CANDIDATE APPROACH The positional candidate approach uses mapping to define a genomic locus linked to the disease followed by selection of gene candidates from the identified region based on biological or phenotypic knowledge of the disease. For example, the Huntington's disease (HD) gene was mapped to 4p16.3, and YAC contigs (overlapping DNA clones) from this region were established which included many candidate transcripts. The phenotypic observation that anticipation occurs in HD families had raised the possibility that the HD gene might contain a trinucleotide repeat; thus, efforts were focused on a transcript (IT15) that contained cytosine-adenine-guanine (CAG) repeats. Expansion of the IT15 CAG repeats was established to be the mutation causing HD *(see below)*. The presence of anticipation also guided efforts to pinpoint genes with trinucleotide expansions in DM and spinocerebellar ataxia (SCA). A positional candidate approach also identified the Xq28 gene responsible for X-linked hereditary hydrocephalus. In this instance, the morphology suggested a disorder in neuronal migration as a possible explanation for the developmental defect. One of the many genes present in the linkage-derived 2-Mb candidate interval was *L1*, a cell surface protein with amino acid sequence motifs characteristic of cell adhesion molecules (CAMs). Sequencing of the *L1* gene in normal controls and in patients with hereditary hydrocephalus demonstrated several disease-associated mutations. Since there are numerous CAMs and other categories of proteins modulating neural morphogenesis, studies that focused on the *L1* gene sequence would have been difficult to justify without mapping studies first pointing to the *L1* region.

The discovery that specific apolipoprotein E *(APOE)* alleles are associated with early versus late onset of AD also resulted from a combination of gene mapping and biochemical studies. Late-onset FAD was found to be linked to chromosome 19q markers located in a region containing *APOE* and other candidate genes. Biochemical investigation showing that APOE bound to amyloid β-peptide led to studies focusing on the potential relationship between *APOE* alleles and AD. The number of disease genes found by the combined strategies of positional cloning and candidate genes will continue to increase as the locations of human transcripts are mapped at an increasing rate and microsatellite markers with finer mapping resolution are made available.

TYPICAL STEPS IN A POSITIONAL CANDIDATE APPROACH

1. DETERMINE CHROMOSOMAL LOCATION BY GENETIC LINKAGE ANALYSIS Genetic loci of disease-relevant genes are determined by establishing significant linkage between the disease phenotype and a particular form of a genetic marker at a known locus within one or more pedigrees. Significant linkage is formally determined by calculation of logarithm of odds (lod) scores. Three features of genetic linkage studies are especially crucial for successful gene mapping: (1) accurate clinical diagnosis, (2) the availability of large families, and (3) the use of informative genetic markers.

With respect to neurological disorders, the first point is of particular interest. The tremendous phenotypic complexity and the large number of overlapping features of many neurological and neuropsychiatric diseases limit the accuracy of many clinical classification systems. The phenotype of ataxia illustrates the problems of clinical nosology. Familial neurodegenerative diseases that cause ataxia can be associated with a plethora of other features such as dementia, retinitis pigmentosa, myelopathy, or neuropathy. Different combinations of these features have been used to create specific categories of hereditary ataxia. As Harding pointed out, purely clinical classification of hereditary ataxias can prove to be quite fallible. Members of the same family have been assigned to different disease categories, and individuals from families with mutations in different genes can have indistinguishable phenotypes. The latter point is of particular importance since misdiagnosis of only one individual within a pedigree or the inadvertent mixing of pedigrees with different diseases can invalidate lod scores. Fortunately, classification of inherited ataxias is becoming clearer as genotypes are established. It is important to note that the astonishing progress made in determining the genetic loci of neurological disorders has been possible because of the careful attention neurologists have given to the identification and classification of patients with familial neurological disorders.

2. ESTABLISH A GENETIC MAP AND NARROW THE CANDIDATE REGION WITH FLANKING MARKERS By using several microsatellite markers from one candidate region and multipoint linkage analysis, one can identify markers most closely flanking the disease gene and narrow the candidate region to 1–3 cM. However, the presence of chromosomal regions with lower- or higher-than-average rates of recombinations can result in up to a fivefold variation in distances determined by genetic versus physical methods. Fifty or more expressed genes may be present in a 1-Mb segment of genome.

3. ESTABLISH A PHYSICAL MAP OF THE CANDIDATE REGION Closely flanking microsatellite markers can be used to screen YAC libraries. By isolating overlapping contiguous YAC clones, a contig map is created that contains the loci of flanking microsatellite markers and therefore the candidate gene region. Contigs covering most of the human genome are now available. To narrow further the physical candidate region, clones with shorter fragments of human DNA can be derived either by subcloning fragments of YAC clones into smaller vectors or by screening cosmid or bacteriophage P1 libraries, which contain DNA fragments of up to 50 kb (cosmids) or 50–100 kb (P1) in length.

4. IDENTIFY CANDIDATE GENES IN THE REGION DEFINED BY THE CONTIG MAP Often, the most challenging step in the positional candidate approach is the identification of candidate genes interspersed over hundreds of kilobases of noncoding DNA. Presently, there is no accurate way to identify expressed genes merely by sequencing DNA. In order to isolate individual genes present in a YAC or P1 clone, DNA fragments derived from YAC or P1 clones can be used to screen cDNA libraries that contain DNA inserts derived only from expressed genes. Another method of gene isolation is known as exon trapping, or amplification, in which exons are selectively cloned based on their association with exon/intron splice junction sites. Sequencing of a candidate gene may result in several possible outcomes: the gene may be a previously discovered genc with known function, it may be a novel gene with significant sequence similarity to genes of known function and therefore may have a similar function, or the sequence may have no previously known motifs to offer a clue to function.

5. IDENTIFY DISEASE-ASSOCIATED ALTERATIONS IN DNA SEQUENCE OR STRUCTURE Once candidate genes are identified, several different strategies can be used to look for disease-associated mutations. In most cases, direct DNA sequencing of dozens of candidate genes derived from normal and disease DNA would not be feasible with current DNA-sequencing technology. Alternative strategies include focusing on genes with known or suspected functions that are likely to be relevant to the disease phenotype; screening for mutations by the technique of heteroduplex analysis or single-stranded conformation polymorphism (SSCP) analysis; and selecting genes with potentially relevant elements such as a trinucleotide repeat if one characteristic of the phenotype is anticipation.

6. PROVE THAT AN IDENTIFIED DNA ALTERATION IS THE CAUSE OF THE DISEASE DNA is highly polymorphic; for example, DNA sequence differs by 1–2 bp in every 1000 bp between two unrelated individuals. Thus, an altered DNA sequence in a candidate gene might constitute either a wild-type allele that does not cause disease, or a disease-causing mutant allele. It is possible that the "mutation" is a DNA polymorphism that is tightly linked to the disease locus but does not constitute the disease locus itself. DNA polymorphisms not causing altered phenotype are more likely not to affect transcription or protein structure and therefore are more likely to occur outside of transcription-relevant elements and open reading frames or in the third base of a codon. In contrast, disease-causing mutations often lead to nonconservative amino acid substitutions, open reading frame shifts, stop codons causing premature truncation of protein translation, disruption of transcription elements, or disruption of RNA splice sites.

Increasingly stringent criteria can be used to support the hypothesis that a given mutation is the cause of the disease phenotype: (1) all affected individuals, but none of the unaffected individuals, within a pedigree should have the mutation; (2) the mutation should not be present in a large series of unrelated controls; (3) in a case where the mutation has appeared *de novo*, the affected individual, but neither of the unaffected parents, should have the mutation; (4) protein expressed from DNA constructs containing the mutation should demonstrate altered function in vitro; or (5) transgenic animals expressing the mutant genotype should show some phenotypic features of the disease.

COMPLICATIONS AND LIMITATIONS OF GENETIC MAPPING

Many diseases or phenotypes, including those of the nervous system, have a hereditary component yct do not exhibit classical mendelian inheritance that can be attributed to a single genetic locus (*see* Chapter 4). These diseases or phenotypes have been referred to as "complex traits" and include susceptibilities to cancer, heart disease, hypertension, and diabetes. Complex traits manifesting in the nervous system may include dementia, migraine, Tourette-like syndromes, schizophrenia, and manic-depressive illness. Neurological diseases illustrate the point that genetic linkage approaches become more problematic with more complex phenotypes.

Many mechanisms can obscure modes of inheritance. Different mutations in the same gene can result in different phenotypes (allelic heterogeneity) and mutations occurring in different genes can result in the same phenotype (nonallelic genetic heterogeneity). Other features of genetic diseases that complicate mapping efforts include phenocopies, incomplete penetrance, variable expressivity, age-dependent onset of phenotype, polygenic inheritance, mitochondrial inheritance (Chapter 103), and dynamic mutations (trinucleotide repeats).

Characteristics of neurological diseases that may compound these uncertainties include the complexity of disease manifestations, common phenotypic overlap of different diseases, the lack of laboratory studies that confirm clinical diagnosis, and late age of onset. Some of the mechanisms that limit the use of linkage analysis for inherited disorders are listed below.

NONALLELIC GENETIC HETEROGENEITY Nonallelic genetic heterogeneity describes the phenomenon of individuals or families with similar clinical syndromes who have mutations in different genes. One important implication of this phenomenon is the effect on genetic linkage analysis. The calculation of lod scores often involves pooling of multiple families with the same phenotype because statistical significance is difficult to achieve with one family. If families with mutations at different loci are pooled, positive and negative lod scores may cancel each other out and linkage will be missed. For this reason, the most conservative linkage analyses are limited to one large family. One example of nonallelic genetic heterogeneity is the multiple axonal forms of Charcot-Marie-Tooth disease (CMT). The locus for CMT type 1A is 17p11.2, and the disease mutation is in the peripheral myelin protein *(PMP-22)* gene. CMT type 1B, which is less common but clinically similar to CMT type 1A, is associated with a mutation on chromosome 1q. Other neurological diseases in which similar or indistinguishable phenotypes are caused by mutations in different genes include FAD, with loci at 14q24.3, 1q31–42, and 21q21.3, and the phenotypically similar SCA types 1, 2, and 3, with loci at 6p23, 12q23–24.1, and 14q24.3–31, respectively. Retinitis pigmentosa can be caused by mutations in more than 10 different genes. Nonallelic genetic heterogeneity is likely to be one of several factors that have limited successful genetic linkage studies of schizophrenia and manic-depressive illness. The lack of distinguishable clinical subcategories and/or the clinical complexity of these diseases makes accurate phenotypic analysis difficult and is likely to lead to inappropriate pooling of different genotypes.

ALLELIC HETEROGENEITY Different phenotypes can result from different mutations in the same gene (allelic mutations). Unlike the process of nonallelic genetic heterogeneity, allelic heterogeneity is unlikely to complicate the calculation of lod scores. Examples of neurological diseases demonstrating phenotypic heterogeneity include Duchenne/Becker muscular dystrophy (dystrophin gene, Xp21.2), infantile/juvenile-onset spinal muscular atrophy (5q11.2–13.3), and familial Creutzfeldt-Jakob disease/fatal familial insomnia/Gerstmann-Sträussler-Scheinker disease (prion protein gene, 20pter–p12). Each of these mutations results in different aberrant protein isoforms or alterations in expression that apparently trigger distinct disease mechanisms and phenotypes.

PHENOCOPIES Individuals may have a clinical presentation that resembles a particular disease phenotype but has a nongenetic cause. Examples include vascular dementia appearing as FAD and toxin- or drug-induced chorea mimicking HD.

VARIABLE EXPRESSIVITY Variable expressivity occurs when the severity of a trait resulting from a mutant allele varies from mild to severe. Expression of the disease phenotype can be modified by other factors such as predisposing alleles of other genes, environmental agents, sex, and age. Variation in expression can also occur following somatic variations in trinucleotide repeats as occurs in myotonic dystrophy.

INCOMPLETE PENETRANCE Penetrance refers to the all-or-none expression of a mutant genotype. If a disease is expressed in less than 100% of individuals carrying the abnormal allele, it is said to have incomplete penetrance.

POLYGENIC INHERITANCE Some diseases are caused by concomitant mutations in multiple genes. Polygenic inheritance has been observed in a form of retinitis pigmentosa that results when mutations in both the RDS/peripherin and *ROM1* genes are present. Similarly, some forms of Hirschsprung's disease may be caused by simultaneous mutations located at 13q22 and 10q11.2. Polygenic inheritance complicates mapping studies because a mutation at one locus may not always produce an abnormal phenotype.

More advanced mapping approaches have recently been reviewed. In allele-sharing methods, one demonstrates by polymorphic marker analysis that identical copies of a candidate chromosomal region are present in affected relatives of a pedigree more often than expected by chance. This type of approach was used to establish linkage of late-onset AD to chromosome 19 even though conventional linkage studies resulted in equivocal results. A second alternative mapping strategy consists of association studies, which do not require the availability of disease pedigrees because they compare allotypes of a gene of interest across unrelated affected and unaffected individuals from one population. Association studies demonstrated that *APOE* gene allotype has a significant association with age of onset of AD and implicated the *APOE* in the underlying mechanism of AD.

If an allele or a marker is close enough to a disease-causing gene and most cases of the disease in the population arise from a small number of ancestral mutations, then association studies will demonstrate linkage disequilibrium between the marker and the disease-causing gene. Linkage disequilibrium studies are particularly useful for genetically isolated populations. The power of linkage disequilibrium analysis was demonstrated by Nikali et al, who identified a locus for infantile-onset SCA in an isolated Finnish population by using DNA samples from only four affected individuals.

NON–DISEASE-BASED APPROACHES FOR CLONING NERVOUS SYSTEM GENES

An important source of candidates for disease genes are those cloned in the context of studies elucidating basic neurobiological mechanisms. Common cloning approaches are described below.

FROM PROTEIN TO GENE As described above, purification of a protein responsible for a biological function of interest allows oligonucleotide or antibody probes to be made, which are used to screen genomic or cDNA libraries. The resulting clones can be used for FISH to determine the chromosomal localization of the gene. FISH analysis with multiple probes can define interprobe relationships with a resolution as precise as 40 kb or less. Hundreds of genes cloned in this manner have contributed to physical maps of cloned genes with known functions. As illustrated in the example of X-linked hydrocephalus and the *L1* cell adhesion molecule gene, the availability of physical maps with genes of identified functions can contribute significantly to genetic linkage studies in discovering disease-causing genes.

FROM FUNCTION TO GENE In some cases, low abundance or other properties of a protein with known function make its purification difficult. In other cases, nothing is known about the nature of the protein responsible for a specific well-characterized function. If an assay is available that quantitatively detects the function of the protein of interest, this assay can be used to clone the corresponding gene. In one functional approach known as expression cloning, 5 or 10 randomly divided fractions of cDNA clones made from messenger RNA derived from tissue normally expressing the protein are each injected into frog oocytes in which proteins encoded by cDNA clones are expressed. Oocyte protein derived from one of the cDNA fractions will contain the specific activity of interest; that cDNA fraction can be further divided, injected again into oocytes, and the activity assayed. This cycle can be repeated until one cDNA clone responsible for the activity of interest is identified.

Expression cloning has been used to identify several genes likely to be critical in our understanding of neurological disease mechanisms. A gene encoding a vesicular amine transporter that suppresses MPP+ toxicity was isolated by screening Chinese hamster ovary fibroblasts transfected with pools of cDNA derived from MPP+-resistant cells, for MPP+ resistance. In another expression cloning study, a gene expressing a cocaine- and antidepressant-sensitive human noradrenaline transporter was found by screening COS cells, transfected with pools of cDNA derived from neuroblastoma cells, for noradrenaline accumulation. The availability of clones expressing neurotransmitter transporters will be critical for determining whether neurotransmitter transport has a significant role in neurodegenerative disease.

Another function-based approach for cloning genes is the yeast two-hybrid system. This system can be used to screen libraries for proteins that bind with a known target protein of interest. A plasmid containing the gene encoding the target protein and plasmids containing cDNAs derived from a tissue of interest are used to transform yeast cells such that each transformant expresses the target protein and a protein encoded by one cDNA. The plasmids also encode a DNA binding site, a transcription activating domain, and a reporter protein such as β-galactosidase. If the target protein binds with a protein expressed by cDNA inserts, the DNA binding site and transcription activation domains are brought into close proximity, causing the reporter gene to be expressed and the transformed cell to turn blue. Blue cells are likely to contain a cDNA encoding a protein that binds to the target protein. PCR-based sequencing of the identified cDNA reveals whether it represents a known or novel gene. In a search for proteins regulating the cell cycle, the cyclin-dependent kinase Cdk2 was used as a target protein to identify a new protein, Rbr2, which is related to the retinoblastoma protein. The yeast two-hybrid system was also used to discover the huntingtin-associated protein 1 (HAP1). HAP1 binds to the N-terminal region of normal and mutant huntingtin, the protein expressed by the Huntington's disease gene.

CLONING ADDITIONAL MEMBERS OF GENE FAMILIES Different members of gene families often have similar functions. In order to discover additional genes coding for proteins with a desired function, several methods have been developed for cloning related family members. A cDNA probe corresponding to a previously cloned gene (the prototype family member) can be used to screen cDNA or genomic libraries under low stringency conditions, which allow identification of clones with similar as well as identical sequences. Clones with significant overall sequence similarity can then be used to express protein, and the protein can be assayed to establish if it has a function similar to the prototype protein. If two or more members of a gene family have been cloned, PCR primers corresponding to domains conserved across the known family members can be used to screen libraries for novel family members. This method has been used to discover three novel members of the neurotrophin gene family. Neurotrophins such as brain-derived neurotrophic factor (BDNF) are undergoing clinical trials for motor neuron disease and peripheral neuropathies. Homology of the presenilin 1 gene to one of several candidate genes in the 1q31 region contributed to the discovery of the presenilin 2 gene as an additional gene causing FAD.

CLONING HUMAN ANALOGS OF GENES CAUSING DISORDERS IN OTHER SPECIES The powerful methods of Drosophila genetics have led to the discovery of hundreds of mutations leading to phenotypes affecting the nervous system. In cases where the Drosophila phenotype has some resemblance to a human disease phenotype, probes based on the mutation-containing Drosophila gene can be used for low-stringency screening of human libraries to clone the human analog. A much smaller number of mutations have been found in mice, which have also been used to guide efforts for cloning human genes and identifying human mutations. For example, the discovery that the myelin-deficient trembler mouse contains point mutations in the *PMP-22* gene contributed to the hypothesis that CMT type 1A may be caused by mutations in human *PMP-22*.

GENOME SCANNING Two recently described techniques are being used to compare genomes from individuals with and without a given genetic disease with the hope of identifying chromosomal regions that do not match and therefore may be responsible for the phenotype. Methods such as genomic mismatch scanning (GMS) and representational difference analysis (RDA) may be particularly useful for multigene diseases.

RANDOM CLONING Several groups are conducting partial sequencing of randomly selected cDNA clones with the goal of having partial sequence (a minimum of one sequencing reaction or several hundred base pairs) from all expressed human genes. Partial cDNA sequences are generally specific to a given expressed gene and have been termed expressed sequence tags (ESTs). Some groups are focusing on human brain cDNA libraries, while others have targeted cDNA libraries made from cells relevant to pathologic processes to increase the chances of cloning disease-relevant genes. Partial sequence is often sufficient to assign a cDNA to a known gene family. Several thousand ESTs are being deposited in databases every week. Within the next 2 years virtually all expressed human genes are likely to be at least partially sequenced. Expanded cDNA sequence databases and integration with physical and genetic maps will contribute significantly to evaluation of candidate genes located in regions defined by mapping studies.

CLINICAL AND GENETIC CLASSIFICATION OF GENE DISORDERS

Genetic neurological disorders have traditionally been classified on the basis of clinicopathologic concepts of disease. Typical of classification schemes are those applied to hereditary ataxias, hereditary neuropathies, and myotonic dystrophies. Phenotypic classification criteria have also been used to establish subtypes of disorders such as Duchenne/Becker muscular dystrophy, neurofibromatosis types 1 and 2, and tuberous sclerosis types 1 and 2. The complexity, variability in phenotype, and overlapping features of these diseases limit the resolution of phenotype-based classification and complicate disease nosology. Accordingly, as new clinical studies have been undertaken these categories have been revised and continue to evolve. The derivation of tightly linked disease markers, identification of disease-causing mutations, and molecular genetic mechanisms responsible for these diseases have introduced new methodologies for disease categorization. For example, the phenotypic distinction between neurofibromatosis types 1 and 2 has been reinforced by the discovery that they are caused by mutations in different genes belonging to distinct gene families: GTPase-activating protein and the merlin cytoskeletal protein, respectively. In contrast, the finding that Duchenne and Becker muscular dystrophies are both caused by mutations of the dystrophin gene blurs the traditional distinction between these diseases. A comparison of the clinical categorization of the inherited ataxias with the identification of distinct genotypes has confirmed that mutations in different genes can lead to indistinguishable clinical syndromes. In other cases, diseases that would not have been viewed as related clinically have been found to be caused by mutations in the same gene. Both X-linked hereditary hydrocephalus and X-linked spastic paraparesis are caused by mutations in the *L1 CAM* gene. Perhaps the most dramatic example of a novel disease category evolving from discovery of new genes is the group of trinucleotide repeat diseases. To date, nine previously characterized and ostensibly largely unrelated disorders can now be considered in the context of the shared mechanism of unstable trinucleotide repeats (discussed *below*).

Hereditary neurological disorders with known gene localization are organized primarily by clinicopathologic phenotype in Table 96-1. In some cases, organization is influenced by genotype. The first group is the neurodegenerative disorders, which implies that deterioration and death of neurons occurs after normal development. These diseases may affect any portion of the nervous system. The second group is the epilepsy syndromes. The third group is the neuromuscular diseases, which affect the peripheral nervous system, the neuromuscular junction, or muscle. The fourth group is tumors of the central nervous system (CNS). The fifth group is abnormalities of development characterized by defects in neuronal development and migration. The availability of testing by DNA diagnostic laboratories is indicated in the far right column.

Different modes of inheritance occur in each of these categories. Neurological genetic disorders inherited in a mendelian autosomal dominant fashion include HD, FAD, amyotrophic lateral sclerosis (ALS), DM, CMT, familial hyperkalemic periodic paralysis, and tuberous sclerosis. Disorders with autosomal recessive traits include Friedreich's ataxia, Wilson's disease, Tay-Sachs disease, and other lysosomal disorders. X-linked recessive disorders include DMD, spinobulbar muscular atrophy (Kennedy's syndrome), Kallmann's syndrome, and fragile X syndrome.

The types of mutations causing neurological genetic disorders include gene deletions (the most common finding in DMD), translocations that interrupt the gene (neurofibromatosis type 1), and point mutations (e.g., in the superoxide dismutase gene in ALS). Point mutations can substitute an alternative base and thereby alter the amino acid sequence (missense mutations) or introduce stop codons leading to premature truncation of protein translation (nonsense mutations). These classical forms of DNA alterations are considered "static" mutations, because they generally remain stable during meiosis and provide the basis for classical mendelian inheritance. The discovery of unstable trinucleotide repeats has introduced the more recent concept of "dynamic" mutations, which account for some forms of non-mendelian inheritance such as the clinical phenomenon of anticipation.

THE CONTRIBUTION OF GENE CLONING TO ELUCIDATION OF NEUROLOGICAL DISEASE MECHANISMS

One of the strongest arguments for cloning disease genes and large-scale human genome projects is that the discovery of a disease gene leads to elucidation of pathogenetic mechanisms of disease and possible therapeutic approaches. It is important to note, however, that for a large number of the disorders listed in Table 96-1, cloning and sequencing of the gene responsible for the disease have not established the function of the gene product or fundamental principles regarding mechanisms of cell dysfunction or death. It is clear that identification of the disease gene and its product are just one part of the constellation of biological and clinical studies required to elucidate disease mechanisms. Highlighting this point of view is one of the most puzzling features of genetic neurological disorders including familial ALS and trinucleotide repeat diseases: in many diseases the mutant gene is widely expressed in many tissues, yet pathological manifestations are limited to subpopulations of cells. In some cases the nature of the protein encoded by the disease gene fits well into existing knowledge of the pathological process. Neurofibromatosis type 1 and tuberous sclerosis type 2 involve abnormal cell growth and are caused by mutations in GTPase-activating proteins, consistent with the fundamental role of GTPase in regulating cell growth.

One of the important outcomes of gene discovery is the development of tools such as antibody probes to launch the search for physiological function. Antibodies raised against the HD gene protein revealed that it is a cytoplasmic protein also associated with intracellular vesicles and therefore raised the possibility that abnormal vesicular function might contribute to the phenotype. Availability of clones with and without mutations can be used to express normal and aberrant forms of the protein to test hypotheses of protein function. An elegant example of this application is the demonstration of abnormal electrophysiologic properties of sodium channels containing specific and distinct mutations characteristic of hyperkalemic periodic paralysis and paramyotonia congenita respectively.

GENETICALLY INDUCED MECHANISMS OF CELL DEATH

The mechanism of cell death in genetic disorders remains unknown for most conditions. Three general mechanisms of mutation effects have been proposed: (1) loss of function, (2) dominant-negative effects, and (3) gain of function.

In loss-of-function disorders, the mutation leads to a deficiency in an enzyme or protein, resulting in cellular dysfunction. The best-defined examples are the lysosomal storage disorders, in which enzymatic deficiencies in complex lipid metabolism lead to accumulation of normal or abnormal cellular constituents. The mode of inheritance in these disorders can be autosomal recessive, X-linked (as for example in DMD), or the result of a combined germ cell and somatic mutation that affects both alleles (such as the removal of a growth suppressor effect as occurs in tumors like retinoblastoma or neurofibromatosis type 1).

In the case of a dominant-negative effect, the abnormal mutation competes with or abolishes the normal allelic function at either the DNA, RNA, or protein level. Although this mechanism has been postulated to be an important example of cellular dysfunction in yeast, its role in neurological disorders remains speculative. True dominant disorders such as HD and SCA1, in which the heterozygote genotype elicits the full spectrum of the disease phenotype, could be the result of either dominant-negative or true gain-of-function effects. In the latter case, the abnormal cellular function exerted by the mutation at one allele in some way renders the cell susceptible to toxic effects, whether or not the normal allele is expressed.

DISORDERS ASSOCIATED WITH TRINUCLEOTIDE REPEATS Nine neurological disorders are now recognized to be associated with abnormal expansions of trinucleotide repeats (Table 96-2). This section will provide an overview of trinucleotide repeat disorders; additional chapters will focus on HD and the SCA trinucleotide diseases. A convenient way of organizing repeat diseases and understanding their mechanisms can be based on the location of the repeat expansions within the gene. Expansions can occur in the 5' untranslated region (UTR), within the open reading frame (translated portion) of the gene, within the 3' UTR, or within introns.

Four fragile X sites (FRAXA, FRAXE, FRAXF, and FRA16A) are associated with expansions of CGG or CCG trinucleotide repeats located on the long arm of the X chromosome. Expansion of CGG trinucleotides is associated with hypermethylation of nearby CpG islands and chromosomal fragility. The FRAXA site is associated with the fragile X syndrome, the most common cause of inherited mental retardation syndromes. FRAXA is located in the 5' UTR of the *FMR1* gene, which encodes a protein identified as FMRP. Loss of FMRP is responsible for the fragile X phenotype. One model to account for the defect in fragile X syndrome is that expanded CGG repeats become methylated and become targets of methyl CpG-binding proteins that act to inhibit transcription. Studies showing decreased *FMR1* RNA and FMRP protein in fragile X patients support this loss-of-function model. In expansions of more than 200 repeats, inhibition of transcript translation also affects FMRP levels. Expansions at the FRAXE locus are associated with a milder form of mental retardation.

The second category of trinucleotide expansion diseases consists of five neurodegenerative disorders in which expansion of an open reading frame CAG repeat would be expected to lead to expanded polyglutamine tracts. The stretches of CAG repeats, which vary between 5 and 37 in the normal alleles of each condition, are increased by two- to fourfold in the mutation; increased severity of the neurological disorder demonstrates a striking correlation with larger numbers of repeats. Normal alleles identified to date never contain more than 38 CAG repeats. One possible disease mechanism is that the expanded polyglutamine tract causes a loss of protein function. The observations that deletions causing the loss of the HD and spinobulbar muscular atrophy (SBMA) genes do not lead to disease phenotypes and that HD patients homozygous for the disease allele have phenotypes similar to heterozygous patients argue against loss-of-function models. Instead, these observations suggest a gain-of-function model in which the gained function is toxic to neurons. For example, expanded polyglutamine tracts might lead to the gained function of excessive protein transglutamination. Expanded polyglutamine tracts could also acquire the function of "polar zippers" due to hydrogen bond formation between main-chain and side-chain amides of interacting proteins. In both models, loss of the function of a crucial protein(s), inhibited or depleted by aberrant interaction with expanded polyglutamine tracts, would lead to neuronal degeneration. Recent studies showing that apparent open reading frame CAG repeats are indeed translated into protein and that expanded polyglutamine tracts in the HD protein lead to a potentially deleterious interaction with the glycolysis enyzme glyceraldehyde-3-phosphate dehydrogenase (GAPDH) further encourage toxic gain-of-function models.

Gain-of-function mechanisms of polyglutamine tract diseases must also account for the findings that even though proteins associated with these neurodegenerative diseases are widely expressed by most neurons, each disease affects only a regionally specific, small subpopulation of neurons. One possibility is that each of these polyglutamine tract proteins interacts with proteins that are indeed cell type specific. Another potential mechanism of cell type specificity is that somatic instability of CAG repeats leads to greater expansions in specific cell populations. The relatively small variations of three to five in the number of triplet repeats in the HD gene occurring in different regions of the brain makes this explanation less likely.

A third category of trinucleotide repeat disorders consists of repeat expansion in the 3' UTR. So far, only one disease demonstrates expansion in this region. In DM, a GTC (CAG in the antisense) repeat in the 3' UTR of the DM kinase gene expands manyfold, from 5–40 repeats in normal alleles to several kilobases in severe cases. The DNA expansion is variable in different tissues, indicating that errors in DNA replication can occur during meiosis, as well as during subsequent somatic-cell mitosis. Since DNA sequence motifs in the 3' UTR of genes are thought to regulate transcript processing, expansions in this region might affect transcript levels and thereby alter DM kinase protein levels. Quantitative messenger RNA analysis of muscle biopsies demonstrated dramatic disease-specific decreases in DM kinase RNA in adult-onset myotonic dystrophy patients. Interestingly, levels of both the mutant and normal DM transcripts were decreased, suggesting a novel mechanism of a dominant-negative mutation occurring at the RNA level.

A second potential novel disease mechanism occurring in myotonic dystrophy is that expansion of the GTC repeat could also affect expression of nearby genes. The *DMR-N9* gene is located immediately upstream from the DM kinase gene and is expressed in neural tissue and testis. Interestingly, Jansen and colleagues have noted that in spite of characteristic cognitive impairment and testicular atrophy in DM patients, little or no DM kinase protein is present in these tissues. In contrast, the highest expression of *DMR-N9* is neural tissue and testis; therefore, alterations in its expression might better account for pathology at these sites. Studies showing that repeat expansion disrupts adjacent chromatin structure offer one mechanism by which expression of adjacent genes could be inhibited. The possibility that repeat expansions at one locus could affect expression of more than one gene by a *cis*-acting effect and that expansion-containing transcripts can affect levels

(continued on page 888)

Table 96-1
Classification of Inherited Neurological Disorders

	Disorder	Chromosomal localization	Principal clinical findings—phenotype	Mode of inheritance	Genotype/gene products/functions/ disease mechanisms	OMIM[a] number(s)
Neurodegenerative diseases	Alzheimer's disease, early onset	AD4: 1q31–42	Dementia, memory loss, typical Alzheimer's disease	AD	Mutations in presenilin 2 gene *(SM2)*; product is a putative membrane protein that may be involved in intracellular protein transport	600759
	Alzheimer's disease, early onset	AD3: 14q24.3	Dementia, memory loss, typical Alzheimer's disease	AD	Mutations in presenilin 1 gene *(S182)*; product is a putative membrane protein that may be involved in intracellular protein transport	104311
	Alzheimer's disease, late onset familial and sporadic	AD2: 19q13.2	Memory loss, dementia	Codominant	Apolipoprotein E4 associated with increased risk and earlier age of onset; in vitro, APOE3 promotes and apo E4 inhibits neurite outgrowth; APOE4 binds to Aβ peptide less avidly than APOE3, and may promote fibrillogenesis	104310
	Familial Alzheimer's disease with amyloid precursor protein mutation	AD1: 21q21.3–22.05	Rare cause of early-onset Alzheimer's disease	AD	Point mutation in *APP* gene	104760
	Huntington's disease[b]	4p16.3	Chorea, dementia, rigidity, epilepsy in juvenile patients	AD	CAG triplet repeats 5' end of gene that encodes a novel protein huntingtin → expanded polyglutamate tract in protein may cause partial loss of some physiologic functions and gain of other functions	143100
	Familial Creutzfeldt-Jakob disease	20pter–p12	Spongioform encephalopathy with dementia, myoclonus	AD	Prion protein gene mutation	123400
	Fatal familial insomnia	20pter–p12	Adult-onset insomnia	AD	Prion protein gene mutation	600072
	Gerstmann-Straüssler-Scheinker disease	20pter–p12	Spongioform encephalopathy with dementia, myoclonus	AD	Prion protein gene mutation	137440
Movement disorders	Ataxia telangiectasia	11q22.3	Cerebellar degeneration, choreoathetosis, ocular apraxia oculocutaneous telangiectasia, immunodeficiency, endocrinopathy	AR	Mutations in *ATM* gene, which codes for protein with domains similar to phosphatidylinositol 3' kinase, an intracellular growth and differentiation factor signal transduction mediator, and rad3, a DNA repair monitor/cell cycle checkpoint regulator protein; mutations found in the same gene in all complementation groups suggest intragenic complementation	208900
	Autosomal dominant cerebellar ataxia with pigmentary macular dystrophy (ADCAII)	3p12–21.1	Cerebellar ataxia, decreased vision, ophthalmoplegia, decreased vibration sense, increased deep tendon reflexes	AD	Unknown; mapped to within 8 cM	164500

Dentatorubropallido-luysian atrophy (DRPLA)	12p12.3-13.1	Ataxia, choreoathetosis, dementia, progressive myoclonus epilepsy (PME), psychiatric disorder	AD	CAG repeat expansions in *DRPLA* gene—unknown function; PME more common with larger expansions	125370
Episodic ataxia type 1 (EA-1)	12p13	Ataxic episodes lasting seconds to minutes, myokymia, paroxysmal kinesogenic choreoathetosis, acetazolamide and phenytoin responsive	AD	Potassium channel *(KCNA1)* gene mutations	160120
Episodic ataxia type 2 (EA-2)	19p13	Ataxic episodes lasting hours to days, down gaze nystagmus, headache, progressive cerebellar signs and atrophy, acetazolamide responsive	AD	Unknown	108500
Friedreich's ataxia	9q13–21.1	Onset during puberty; ataxia, dysarthria, absent reflexes, decreased vibration, joint position sense cardiomyopathy, diabetes mellitus	AR	Unknown	229300
Ataxia with vitamin E deficiency, Friedreich-like (AVED)	8q13	Same as Friedreich's ataxia but with severe vitamin E deficiency	AR	Mutations in α-tocopherol transfer protein gene *(αTTP)* → impaired binding of vitamin E to VLDL	277460
Hereditary progressive dystonia with marked diurnal fluctuation (HPD)	14q22.1–22.2	Distal lower extremity dystonia in first decade, spreads to other limbs over years; symptoms greatest in evening, decreased in morning; responds markedly to levodopa	AD? female predominance	Mutations in GTP cyclohydrolase I gene → biopterin deficiency → decreased tyrosine hydroxylase activity → decreased dopamine	128230
Machado-Joseph disease (MJD)	14q24.3–31	Ataxia, ophthalmoparesis, corticospinal signs, dystonia-rigidity, amyotrophy	AD	CAG repeat expansions in *MJD1* gene	109150
Spinocerebellar ataxia 1 (SCA1)	6p23	Ataxia, progressive dementia, spasticity, onset 3rd or 4th decade; anticipation in successive generations	AD	Expansion of trinucleotide repeat (CAG) in ataxin 1	164400
Spinocerebellar ataxia 2 (SCA2)	12q23–24.1	Features extensively overlap with SCA1, but more common hypotonia and ophthalmoplegia	AD	Unknown; anticipation observed suggesting possibility of trinucleotide repeat expansion	183090
Spinocerebellar ataxia 3 (SCA3)	14q24.3-31	Similar to Machado-Joseph disease	AD	Allelic at Machado-Joseph disease locus	183085
Spinocerebellar ataxia 4 (SCA4)	16qter-24	Ataxia, axonal neuropathy, corticospinal signs, normal eye movements	AD	Unknown	600223
Spinocerebellar ataxia 5 (SCA5)	11 centromeric	Ataxia, dysarthria	AD	Unknown	600224
Torsion dystonia	9q34	Early onset, generalized dystonia, occurs in both Ashkenazi Jewish (AJ) and non-Jewish pedigrees	AD	Unknown	128100

(continued)

Table 96-1 *(continued)*

	Disorder	Chromosomal localization	Principal clinical findings—phenotype	Mode of inheritance	Genotype/gene products/functions/ disease mechanisms	OMIM[a] number(s)
	Wilson's disease	13q14.3	Disorder of copper transport into liver: extrapyramidal signs, psychiatric disorders	AR	Mutations in gene *ATP7B*, encoding a putative copper transporting P-type membrane ATPase, 57% similar to that associated with Menkes' syndrome (MNK)	277900
Retinitis pigmentosa	Retinitis pigmentosa 1	3q21-q24	Night blindness, peripheral field loss, blindness, abnormal ERG	AD	Mutations in gene that encodes rhodopsin → interference in maturational processing of wild-type protein	180100
	Retinitis pigmentosa, peripherin-related	6p21.1–cen	Night blindness, peripheral visual loss leading to blindness	AD	Mutations in RDS/peripherin gene, a rod photoreceptor membrane protein	179605
Spastic paraplegia	Autosomal dominant familial spastic paraplegia (SPG3, SPG4, SPG6)	SPG3: 14q SPG4: 2p21–24 SPG6: 15q11.1	Pure spastic paraplegia	AD	Unknown	SPG3: 182600 SPG4: 182601 SPG6: 600363
	Autosomal recessive familial spastic paraplegia	8q	Pure spastic paraplegia	AR	Unknown	600146
	X-linked familial spastic paraplegia 2 (SPG2)	Xq21–22	Initial pure spastic paraplegia; involvement of entire CNS over years	X-LR	Myelin proteolipid protein gene mutation; allelic with Pelizaeus-Merzbacher	312920
Vascular diseases	Cerebral autosomal dominant arteriopathy with subcortical infarcts (CADASIL)	19p12	Multiple subcortical infarcts, dementia	AD	Unknown	125310
	Familial cerebral amyloid angiopathy (Dutch type)	21q21.3–22.05	Cerebral hemorrhage	AD	Point mutations in *APP* gene	104760
	Familial hemiplegic migraine	19p13	Onset 5–30 years, aura with unilateral paresis and other focal symptoms lasting 30–60 min; followed by headache, may have persistent cerebellar signs	AD	Unknown, may be related to episodic ataxia type 2	141500
	Hereditary cystatin C amyloid angiopathy (HCCAA) (Icelandic)	20p11.2	Cerebral hemorrhage	AD	Mutations in cystatin C gene, product is a cysteine protease inhibitor; forms amyloid, which deposits in the walls of cerebral vessels	105150
Miscellaneous	Abetalipoproteinemia (Bassen-Kornzwieg syndrome)	4q24	Vitamin E deficiency; neuropathy, ataxia, retinitis pigmentosa, acanthocytosis	AR	Mutations in gene coding large subunit of microsomal triglyceride transfer protein (MTP) → impairment of synthesis of VLDL	200100
	Adrenoleukodystrophy	Xq28	Leukodystrophy, hypoadrenalism, mild neuropathy, baldness, hypogonadism	X-LR	Mutations in ALD protein gene, a peroxisomal membrane transporter; associated with impaired β-oxidation of unbranched saturated very long chain fatty acids in peroxisomes	300100
	GM1 gangliosidosis	3p21.33	Mental retardation, seizures, blindness	AR	Mutations in gene encoding β-galactosidase, which cleaves the terminal saccharide of GM1; mutations → enzyme deficiency → cellular GM1 accumulation	230500

	Hypobetalipoproteinemia	2p24	Vitamin E deficiency; neuropathy, ataxia, retinitis pigmentosa, acanthocytosis	AR	Mutations of apolipoprotein β100 → low serum betalipoprotein → altered VLDL and chylomicron function	107730
	Menkes' syndrome (kinky hair disease, steely hair disease)	Xq13.3	Abnormal whitish kinky hair, growth and mental retardation, spastic quadriparesis, seizures	X-LR	Mutations in *ATP7A*, encoding MNK, a protein very similar to P-type cation-transporting membrane ATPases; may be involved in copper transport across membranes; mutations may lead to copper deficiency → copper dependent enzyme dysfunction	309400
	Pelizaeus-Merzbacher disease	Xq21–22	CNS dysmyelination; progressive neurologic deterioration	X-LR	30% have mutation in coding region of myelin proteolipid protein gene; allelic with X-linked familial spastic paraplegia 2	312080
	X-linked cutis laxa (occipital horn syndrome)	Xq13.3	Mild mental retardation, skin and joint laxity, skeletal deformities, bony horns projecting from occipital bone	X-LR	Allelic with MNK	304150
Epilepsy syndromes	Benign neonatal epilepsy 1 (EBN1)	20q13.2–13.3	Generalized seizures, neonatal onset, benign course, usually resolving at 6–12 mo, 10–15% have seizures later in life	AD	Mutations in the α-4 subunit of the neuronal nicotinic acetylcholine receptor gene	121200
	Benign neonatal epilepsy 2 (EBN2)	8q	Clinically indistinguishable from EBN1	AD	Unknown	121201
	Familial partial epilepsy	10q	Simple partial seizures, normal intelligence	AD, reduced penetrance	Unknown; mapped to within 10 cM	600512
	Juvenile myoclonic epilepsy (JME)	6p11–21.2	Onset in adolescence, myoclonic jerks, generalized tonic-clonic seizures	Uncertain	Gene locus named *EJM1*	254770
	Nocturnal frontal lobe epilepsy (ADNFLE)	20q13.2–13.3	Nocturnal seizures	AD	May be allelic with *EBN1*, also with a normal low-voltage electroencephalogram variant	600513
	Progressive epilepsy with mental retardation (EPMR)	8pter-p22	Normal at birth, generalized seizures onset age 5–10 years, severe mental retardation 2–5 years after seizure onset	AR	Unknown; mapped to within 7 cM	600143
	Progressive myoclonus epilepsy, Unverricht-Lundborg type (EPM1)	21q22.3	Generalized seizures, stimulus-reactive myoclonus, onset age 6–15, progressive	AR	Mutations in cystatin B gene	254800
Neuromuscular disorders Motor neuron diseases	Familial amyotrophic lateral sclerosis, adult, dominant (ALS1)	21q22.1	Weakness, muscle atrophy, spasticity, increased deep tendon reflexes; about 10% of cases are familial, indistinguishable clinically from sporadic form	AD	Point mutations in Cu,Zn-superoxide dismutase *(SOD1)* in some families (20%); heterogeneity exists → possible motor neuron injury due to defective detoxification of reactive oxygen species	105400
	Familial amyotrophic lateral sclerosis, juvenile recessive (ALS2)	2q33–35	Earlier onset and slower progression than ALS1	AR	Unknown	205100
	Familial amyotrophic lateral sclerosis, adult, dominant (ALS3)	11	Similar to ALS1	AD	Mutations in neurofilament protein heavy chain gene → disruption of neurofilament crosslinking	Not cited

(continued)

Table 96-1 *(continued)*

	Disorder	*Chromosomal localization*	*Principal clinical findings—phenotype*	*Mode of inheritance*	*Genotype/gene products/functions/ disease mechanisms*	*OMIM*[a] *number(s)*
	Spinal muscular atrophy (SMA) I–III	5q11.2–13.3	SMAI: infantile (Werdnig-Hoffman) disease—present by 3 months of hypotonia, proximal limb weakness, areflexia SMAII: childhood onset, limb/girdle weakness, areflexia, 70% never ambulate independently SMAIII: juvenile (Kugelberg-Welander) disease—onset after age 2, slowly progressive symmetric proximal muscle weakness sparing bulbar muscles	AR	Mapped to about 1-Mb region; region is unstable and highly polymorphic making reconciliation of mapping data difficult; two candidate genes have been identified: neuronal apoptosis inhibitory protein *(NAIP)* gene, with amino acid homology to baculovirus apoptosis inhibitory proteins, and survival motor neuron *(SMN)* gene, coding a novel 294-aa protein	SMAI: 253300 SMAII: 253550 SMAIII: 253400
	Spinobulbar muscular atrophy (Kennedy's syndrome)	Xq12	Muscular weakness and atrophy	X-LR	Trinucleotide repeats in androgen receptor gene → expanded polyglutamate tract in protein may cause partial loss of some physiologic functions and gain of other functions	313200
Muscle diseases	Becker myotonia (recessive myotonia congenita)	7q35	Similar to myotonia congenita	AR	Known *ClC-1* mutations present in about 16% unrelated cases	255700
	Central core disease (CCD)	19q13.1	Nonprogressive primarily proximal myopathy, onset in infancy	AD	Mutation in ryanodine receptor gene *(RYR1)*; allelic with MHS1	117000
	Congenital muscular dystrophy (merosin deficient) (CMD)	6q2	Weakness and hypotonia at birth, limb contractures at birth or later	AR	Probable mutations in merosin gene	156225
	Congenital myasthenic syndromes/slow-channel syndrome (SCS)	2q,17p	Weakness, fatigability, hypotonia, muscle atrophy	AD (?)	Mutations in genes encoding subunits of the acetylcholine receptor → altered channel kinetics	100690
	Duchenne/Becker muscular dystrophy (DMD/BMD)	Xp21.2	DMD: onset of muscular weakness early in life, progressive; BMD form is later onset, less severe	X-LR	Mutations in dystrophin gene resulting in complete absence or major deletions of dystrophin (DMD), or less severe derangements of dystrophin structure (BMD) → disruption of linkage between microfilaments and the trans-sarcolemmal glycoprotein complex mediating adhesion to the extracellular matrix protein merosin → may lead to membrane damage with contraction	310200
	Emery-Dreifuss muscular dystrophy	Xq28	Childhood onset, benign course with early contractures, progressive muscle wasting with humeral/peroneal predominance, cardiac conduction defects-arrhythmias, heart block	X-LR	Mutations in emerin gene; codes a 254-aa serine-rich protein, which may be membrane-anchored and has unknown function	310300

Facioscapulohumeral dystrophy	4q35	Weakness, atrophy; face and shoulder muscles	AD	Unknown; exhibits anticipation, which may be associated with successive deletions in a region of tandem repeats	158900
Fukuyama-type congenital muscular dystrophy (FCMD)	9q31-33	Weakness and hypotonia at birth, cerebral and cerebellar polymicrogyria and cerebellar cysts, ocular anomalies; overlaps with Walker-Warburg syndrome	AR	Unknown; proposed allelic with Walker-Warburg syndrome	253800
Hereditary myoglobinuria	1p32	Episodic myalgia, rhabdomyolysis, myoglobinuria presenting 2nd and 3rd decade	AR	Mutations in gene coding carnitine palmitoyltranserase II → diminished import of long-chain fatty acids into mitochondria → mitochondrial dysfunction	600650
Hyperkalemic periodic paralysis (HYPP)	17q23.1–25.3	Myotonia, periodic areflexic paralysis	AD	Point mutation in α-subunit, sodium channel (SCN4A) → impairment of sodium current inactivation; normokalemic variants occur (normoPP)	170500
Hypokalemic periodic paralysis (HOKPP)	1q32	Similar to HYPP, but attacks accompanied by hypokalemia, triggered by insulin and epinephrine, last longer and patients have no myotonia	AD	Loss of function mutations in α-1 subunit of the dihydropyridine (DHP) receptor gene, a slow voltage-gated L-type calcium channel → ? dominant negative disruption of channel function (decreased Ca^{2+} current); predominant expression in males may be hormone effect	170400
Limb-girdle muscular dystrophy, autosomal dominant 1A (LGMD1A)	5q22.3–31.3	Late (3rd decade) onset muscular dystrophy, sparing the face; slow progression	AD	Unknown; mapped to within 7 cM	159000
Limb-girdle muscular dystrophy, autosomal recessive 2A (LGMD2A)	15q15.1–21.1	Progressive symmetrical atrophy of proximal limb muscles, beginning in first two decades	AR	Mutations in calcium-activated neural protease 3 (CANP3), large subunit gene important, but probably requires another as yet unidentified mutation for disease expression (digenic model)	253600
Limb-girdle muscular dystrophy, autosomal recessive 2B (LGMD2B)	2p13–16	Pelvic girdle affected earliest; onset in late 2nd decade	AR	Unknown	253601
Malignant hyperthermia (MHS1)	19q13.1	Sensitivity to volatile anesthetics, muscle contraction	AD	Mutation in ryanodine receptor gene *(RYR1)* at 19q13.1 → ? disturbance of Ca^{2+} flux cells; when mild → excessive contraction; when severe (as in CCD?) → Ca^{2+}-mediated mitochondrial toxicity	145600
Malignant hyperthermia (MHS2,3,4)	MHS2: 17q11.2–24 MHS3: 7q21–22 MHS4: 3q13.1	Sensitivity to volatile anesthetics, muscle contraction	AD	Unknown	MHS2: 154275 MHS3: 154276 MHS4: 600467

(continued)

Table 96-1 *(continued)*

	Disorder	Chromosomal localization	Principal clinical findings—phenotype	Mode of inheritance	Genotype/gene products/functions/ disease mechanisms	OMIM[a] number(s)
	Myotonia congenita (dominant MC, Thomsen's disease)	7q35	Onset 1st decade, muscle stiffness/myotonia, muscle hypertrophy without weakness	AD	Known mutations in the chloride channel gene *(ClC-1)* account for about 15% of MC cases. Mutations cause loss of function and functional channel is likely homo-oligomer → "dominant negative" mechanism	160800
	Myotonic dystrophy	19q13.3	Multisystem disorder: cataracts, myotonia, weakness, frontal baldness, mental retardation	AD, anticipation	CTG repeats at 3' end of myotonin protein kinase gene—product is membrane associated and localized primarily to neuromuscular and myotendinous junctions; expression of adjacent genes may also be affected	160900
	Nemaline myopathy	1p13–q25	Most commonly congenital non- or slowly progressive myopathy; forms range from severe congenital to mild adult	AD (other forms AR)	Dominant form associated with α-tropomyosin gene *(TPM3)* mutation. Met9Arg mutation may increase tropomyosin-actin affinity → rod body formation	256030 (general); 161800 (dominant)
	Oculopharyngeal muscular dystrophy (OPMD)	14q11.2–13	Onset usually after age 50, ptosis, dysphagia	AD	Gene unknown; maps near cardiac β-myosin	164300
	Paramyotonia congenita (PC)	17q23.1–25.3	Cold-induced muscle stiffness (myotonia) and weakness, occasional periodic paralysis	AD	*SCN4A* mutations; allelic with HYPP	168300
	Potassium-aggravated myotonia (PAM)	17q23.1–25.3	Potassium sensitive muscle stiffness (myotonia) and weakness, occasional periodic paralysis	AD	*SCN4A* mutations; allelic with HYPP (other variants occur ("sodium-channel myotonias")	170500
	Severe childhood autosomal recessive muscular dystrophy (SCARMD, LGMD2C, LGMD2D)	13q12, 17q21	Similar to DMD or BMD	AR	17q21-linked form: mutations of adhalin gene; adhalin is a component of the membrane glycoprotein complex noted above 13q12-linked form: gene unknown	LGMD2C: 253700 LGMD2D: 600119
	Startle disease (hyperekplexia)	5q33–35	Exaggerated startle, neonatal hypertonia, nocturnal myoclonus	AD, AR	Mutations in the α-1 subunit of the inhibitory glycine receptor → mechanisms unknown, though Arg271 mutations seen in some human cases; causes decreased agonist sensitivity in a mouse model	149400
	X-linked myotubular myopathy	Xq28	Severe neonatal hypotonia, apnea, common perinatal death	X-LR	Unknown	310400
Peripheral neuropathies	Charcot-Marie-Tooth disease type 1A (CMT1A)	17p11.2–12	HMSNI: Variable onset, motor > sensory neuropathy, distal muscle atrophy, absent reflexes, high arches in feet, decreased nerve conduction velocities, ± nerve enlargement	AD	Mutations or 1.5-Mb duplication in peripheral myelin protein gene *(PMP-22)*, product is a component of compact myelin	118220
	Charcot-Marie-Tooth disease type 1B (CMT1B)	1q22	HMSNI	AD	Mutations in *MPZ* gene, product is a component of compact myelin	118200

	Charcot-Marie-Tooth disease type 1, X-linked (CMTX1,2,3)	CMTX1: Xq13.1 CMTX2: Xp22.2 CMTX3: Xq26	HMSNI	X-linked dominant	CMTX1: mutations in connexin32 gene coding a gap junction protein localized to uncompacted peripheral myelin at the nodes of Ranvier and Schmidt-Lanterman clefts; CMTX2,3: genes unknown	CMTX1: 302800 CMTX2: 302801 CMTX3: 302802
	Charcot-Marie-Tooth disease type 2A (CMT2A)	1p35–36	HMSNII: Later onset, sensorimotor axonal neuropathy, near normal nerve conduction velocities	AD	Unknown	118210
	Charcot-Marie-Tooth disease, type 4A (CMT4A)	8q13–21.1	HMSNI	AR	Unknown	214400
	Dejerine-Sottas disease type A (DSDA)	17p11.2–12	HMSNIII: Onset birth/infancy, slowly progressive sensorimotor deficits, high arches, scoliosis, ataxia, enlarged nerves, markedly decreased conduction velocities	AD	*PMP-22* mutations *(see above)*	601097 (PMP22); 145900 (Dejerine-Sottas)
	Dejerine-Sottas disease type B (DSDB)	1q22–23	HMSNIII	?	Mutations in *MPZ* gene coding P_o protein *(see above)*	145900 (Dejerine-Sottas); 159440 (P_o mutation)
	Familial amyloidotic polyneuropathy (FAP)	18q11.2–12.1	Sensory/autonomic peripheral neuropathy, cardiomyopathy	AD	Mutations in transthyretin gene → formation of amyloid	176300
	Hereditary neuropathy with pressure palsies type A (HNPPA)	17p11.2	Recurrent entrapment/pressure neuropathies, segmental demyelination	?AD	*PMP-22* deletions; CMT1A and HNPPA may be reciprocal products of unequal crossover	162500
Central nervous system tumors	Neurofibromatosis type 1 (Von Recklinghausen) (NF1)	17q11.2	Multiple neurofibromas, 1:3500 individuals, *café au lait* spots, malignant gliomas, Lisch nodules in iris	AD	Encodes neurofibromin, a member of the Ras-GTPase-activating protein (GAP) family	162200
	Neurofibromatosis type 2 (NF2)	22q12.2	Acoustic neuromas, bilateral meningiomas	AD	Deletions in the gene that encodes for merlin/schwannomin, a tumor suppressor protein with sequence similarity to tyrosine phosphatase and cytoskeleton linkage protein	101000
	Retinoblastoma	13q14.1–14.2	40% hereditary, 60% nonhereditary, multiple tumors in inherited form	AR	Rb gene mutations or deletions cause disease; Rb protein is 105-kDa tumor suppressor, DNA-binding protein	180200
	Von Hippel-Lindau type 1, 2 (VHL1, VHL2)	3p25–26	Type 1: retinal angiomas, CNS hemangioblastomas, pancreatic cysts in some; type 2: identical to type 1 plus pheochromocytoma	AD	Type 1: 56% microdeletions, deletions, insertions, nonsense mutations in VHL gene, a tumor suppressor of otherwise unknown function; type 2: 96% missense mutations in VHL gene	193300
Defects of neuronal migration and differentiation	Familial cavernous malformations of the brain	7q11.2–21	Seizures, headache, intracerebral hemorrhage, neurologic deficits	AD	Unknown	116860

(continued)

Table 96-1 *(continued)*

Disorder	*Chromosomal localization*	*Principal clinical findings—phenotype*	*Mode of inheritance*	*Genotype/gene products/functions/ disease mechanisms*	*OMIM[a] number(s)*
Familial dysautonomia, Riley-Day syndrome	9q31–33	Onset in infancy, autonomic dysfunction, taste, pain and temperature loss; seen in Ashkenazi Jewish populations	AR	Unknown	223900
Fragile X syndrome A (FRAXA)	Xq27.3	Mental retardation, decreased head size, large forehead, macro-orchidism	X-LR	CGG trinucleotide repeat expansions in 5' region of *FMR1* → transcriptional inhibition of gene due to overmethylation, as well as translational inhibition; *FMR1* product contains KH domains and RGG box, motifs found in RNA binding proteins	309550
Fragile X syndrome E (FRAXE)	Xq28	Mild mental retardation	X-LR	CGG/CCG repeat expansions, 600 kb distal to FRAXA site; developmentally regulated transcript recently found in region	309548
Hirschsprung's disease 1 (HSCR1)	10q11.2	Neonatal megacolon due to absence of Messner and Auerbach plexuses	AD	Mutations in *ret* proto-oncogene. Product (c-ret) is a receptor tyrosine kinase with extracellular domain similar to cadherins; thought to be involved in enteric neuronal migration or differentiation; mutations in *ret* also associated with multiple endocrine neoplasia type 2A	142623
Hirschsprung's disease 2 (HSCR2)	13q22	Very similar or identical to HSCR1	Dose-dependent expression homozygotes 74%, heterozygotes 21%	Mutations in the endothelin B receptor (EDNRB) gene; product is a G-protein-coupled receptor which mediates cellular calcium fluxes; mutations → loss of function; disease expression probably requires participation of other loci	600155
Hydrocephalus due to stenosis of the aqueduct of Sylvius (HSAS)	Xq28	Hydrocephalus with moderate to severe mental retardation, adducted hypoplastic thumbs (25% of cases), spastic paraparesis, aplasia or hypoplasia of the corticospinal tract and corpus callosum	X-LR	Mutations in *L1* gene—product is a multifunctional/multidomain cell adhesion molecule	307000
Kallmann syndrome	Xp22.3	Anosmia with hypogonadism (GnRH deficiency), syndrome due to failure of olfactory neuronal migration	X-LR	Mutations in gene *(KALIG-1)* which encodes protein with homology to neural-cell adhesion molecules (N-CAM)	308700
MASA syndrome (Gareis-Mason syndrome)	Xq28	Mental retardation, aphasia, shuffling gait (due to spastic paraparesis) and adducted thumbs (due to absent or hypoplastic extensor pollicis brevis and/or longus), may also have hydrocephalus	X-LR	*L1* mutations	303350

Miller-Dieker lissencephaly syndrome	17p13.3	Microcephaly, micrognathia, epilepsy, agyria due to failure of cortical neuronal migration	AD	Mutation in *LIS-1* gene coding the 45-kDa (regulatory) subunit of platelet-activating factor (PAF) acetylhydrolase; part of heterotrimeric enzyme, which inactivates PAF; PAF proposed to modulate neuronal differentiation or migration; effect of mutation on PAF unknown	247200
Norrie disease (ND)	Xp11.4	Retinal malformation, hearing loss, mental retardation	X-LR	Mutations in *ND*; sequence comparisons and modeling suggest similarity to transforming growth factor–β family/cysteine-knot motif growth factors	310600
Tuberous sclerosis type 1	9q34	1:10,000 births, mental retardation, seizures, adenoma sebaceum	AD	Unknown; may be a growth suppressor	191100
Tuberous sclerosis type 2	16p13.3	Hamartomas, epilepsy, mental retardation	AD	Gene encodes tuberin, which has homology to GTPase activating protein GAP3; effects of mutations on gene function unknown	191092
Waardenburg syndrome 1 (WS1)	2q35	Deafness, white forelock, dystopia canthorum, pigmentary abnormalities	AD	Mutation in paired box-containing *(PAX)*–3 gene; product is a transcription factor involved in embryonic patterning/neural crest migration; heterozygotes have WS1, homozygotes have WS3, which is more severe and includes upper limb abnormalities	193500
Waardenburg syndrome 2 (WS2)	3p12.3–14.1	Deafness, white forelock, dystopia canthorum, heterochromia irides, early greying	AD	Mutations in microphthalmia (MITF) gene encoding a putative basic helix-loop-helix-leucine-zipper transcription factor	193510
Walker-Warburg syndrome (WWS)	9q31–33	Lissencephaly, ocular anomalies, hydrocephalus, callosal hypoplasia, septal agenesis, congenital muscular dystrophy	AR	Unknown; proposed allelic with FCMD	236670
X-linked spastic paraplegia type 1 (XLSP or SPG1)	Xq28	Spastic paraplegia, ataxia, absent extensor pollicis longus	X-LR	*L1* mutations	312900

Abbreviations: AD, autosomal dominant; APP, amyloid precursor protein; AR, autosomal recessive; CNS, central nervous system; ERG, electroretinogram; GnRH, gonadotropin-releasing hormone; Rb, retinoblastoma; SCA, spinocerebellar ataxia; VLDL, very low density lipoprotein; X-LR, X-linked recessive.

[a]On-line mendelian inheritance in man.

[b]HD causes both dementia and movement disorder.

Table 2
Neurological Diseases Caused by Expansion of Trinucleotide Repeats

Disorders	*Site of repeat*	*Effect on gene expression*
Fragile X-A	CGG repeat 5' to translation initiation site; point mutation identified in some patients	Failure of expression of *FMR1*
Fragile X-E	CGG/CCG repeats; relationship to genes unknown	Unknown
Dentatorubropallidoluysian atrophy (DRPLA)	CAG repeat in open reading frame (ORF)	Normal gene expression
Huntington's disease	CAG repeat in ORF	IT15 transcript shows normal expression without cellular selectivity; expanded polyglutamine tract may alter huntingtin protein intersection with huntingtin-associated protein 1 (HAP1) or GAPDH
Kennedy's syndrome	CAG repeat in ORF of androgen receptor gene	Normal gene expression; polyglutamine tract in androgen receptor
Spinocerebellar ataxia type 1 (SCA1)	CAG repeat in ORF	Normal gene expression
Spinocerebellar ataxia type 3 (SCA3)/Machado-Joseph disease	CAG repeat in ORF	Unknown
Myotonic dystrophy	CTG repeat in 3' untranslated region of *DM-1* gene, 5' end of dystrophia myotonia-associated homeodomain protein gene; cases without repeats also described	Gene expression decreased; possible dominant-negative effect at RNA level
Friedreich's ataxia	GAA repeat in the first intron of the *X25* gene	Gene expression decreased

of transcripts derived from a separate allele by a *trans*-acting effect point to many new potential scenarios for the mechanism of DM.

A fourth category of trinucleotide repeat diseases is caused by expansion of a repeat in an intron. Friedreich's ataxia (FA) is caused by the expansion of a GAA triplet in intron 1 of the *X25* gene leading to decreased mRNA levels due to either inhibition of transcription or disrupted RNA splicing. The majority of FA patients tested thus far demonstrate homozygosity for expanded alleles, while some are heterozygous with a combination of one expanded allele and point mutations in the other allele. These genotypes are consistent with an autosomal recessive pattern of inheritance and a loss-of-function disease mechanism.

The discovery of triplet repeats and analysis of the ages of onset of affected individuals has given a molecular precision to old concepts such as anticipation (earlier onset of the disease in successive generations, which is associated with further expansion of the abnormal repeats in persons who are more severely affected) and has helped to account for variations in gene expression. Variations in trinucleotide repeats in HD (and particularly in DM) have given a molecular explanation for concepts of variable expressivity, in which variations in repeats occurring among individual members of the family can lead to earlier onset, or more severe symptoms and signs, as occurs in juvenile HD. Variations in the numbers of repeats in somatic cells resulting from further expansions of repeats in cells undergoing mitotic divisions, as in DM, can also explain differences in tissue involvement. Studies suggesting that other neurological and psychiatric disorders involve anticipation and the identification of other genes with trinucleotide repeats raise the possibility that additional trinucleotide repeat diseases will be discovered.

DNA-BASED DIAGNOSIS OF NEUROLOGICAL DISORDERS Many of the disorders listed in Table 96-1 have been mapped to specific chromosomes or chromosomal regions; however, the particular genes affected by mutations have yet to be identified. For some of these diseases, DNA diagnosis or presymptomatic testing is possible by family linkage analysis. Successful family linkage analysis requires that family relationships (such as paternity) are accurately established, that the clinical status of affected or unaffected individuals is accurate, that a sufficient number of family members can be genotyped, and that informative markers are available. For many patients, these requirements often rule out application of DNA diagnosis.

The rapid rate at which disease genes are being identified is rendering direct DNA diagnosis more widely applicable. In genetic diseases in which the pathological phenotype is caused by only one or a small number of well-defined mutations within a given gene, detection of the mutation is an extremely useful tool in clinical diagnosis. Methods of detecting DNA mutations for diagnostic purposes include direct sequencing of patient DNA, allele-specific oligonucleotide hybridization, differential restriction endonuclease patterns of PCR products, and analysis of single-stranded conformation polymorphisms (*see* Chapters 2 and 4).

The limitations of DNA testing in the context of neurological disorders should be emphasized. First, if the clinical diagnosis being considered is in error or if the phenotype overlaps with other disorders, the detection of normal alleles of the gene tested is of no diagnostic value. For example, in cases of suspected hereditary spinocerebellar ataxia, investigators have suggested concomitant analysis of multiple SCA genes.

Second, some diseases such as DM, neurofibromatosis, and hereditary amyloid polyneuropathy can be caused by dozens of different mutations within one gene (allelic heterogeneity). Most methods of DNA analysis focus on point mutations or relatively short segments of DNA; therefore, assessment of numerous loci scattered over a wide area of DNA becomes impractical for most clinical applications. Mutations are identified in only about two-thirds of DMD/Becker muscular dystrophy (BMD) and neurofibromatosis type 2 patients and in less than half of those with neurofibromatosis type 1. Recent advances in multiplex PCR and single-stranded chain polymorphism analysis have improved this yield; however, it is essential that the clinician be aware of the "sensitivity" of each DNA analysis.

It is also possible that focused DNA analysis could miss the presence of a novel mutation in the relevant gene. For these reasons, particularly for many genes involved in metabolic diseases, diagnostic methods based on protein properties or function are more effective and efficient than DNA-based tests. For example, dystrophin antibodies may show decreased expression or aberrant distribution of dystrophin expression in a muscle biopsy of a patient in which no DNA mutations were detected.

DNA testing can be performed by commercial laboratories, hospital-based laboratories set up for clinical applications, or academic laboratories studying a gene of interest in a research context. It must be emphasized that DNA testing should only be conducted in the context of comprehensive genetic counseling in which the implications of potential test results are fully understood and adequate support services are available. The practical and ethical implications of neurogenetic testing have recently been reviewed. A computerized directory of diagnostic and research DNA laboratories (known as Helix) is accessible by phone and fax at no cost to registered health care professionals. Laboratories are encouraged to list their services with Helix, also at no cost. Information on access and/or listing new laboratories may be obtained at the Helix office (tel: 206-528-2689; fax: 206-528-2687).

SELECTED REFERENCES

Adams MD, Kerlavage AR, Fields C, Venter JC. 3,400 new expressed sequence tags identify diversity of transcripts in human brain. Nat Genet 1993;4:256–267.

Banfi S, Zoghbi HY. Molecular genetics of hereditary ataxias. Baillieres Clin Neurol 1994;3:281–295.

Bates G, Lehrach H. Trinucleotide repeat expansions and human genetic disease. Bioassays 1994;16:277–284.

Bird T, Bennett R. Why do DNA testing? Practical and ethical implications of new neurogenetic tests. Ann Neurol 1995;38:141–146.

Bird TD. Are linkage studies boring? Nat Genet 1993;4:213,214.

Brown PO. Genome scanning methods. Curr Opin Genet Dev 1994;4:366–373.

Brown RH Jr. Amyotrophic lateral sclerosis: recent insights from genetics and transgenic mice. Cell 1995;80:687–692.

Campbell KP. Three muscular dystrophies: loss of cytoskeleton-extracellular matrix linkage. Cell 1995;80:675–679.

Campuzano V, Montermini L, Molto MD, et al. Friedreich's ataxia: autosomal recessive disease caused by an intronic GAA triplet repeat expansion. Science 1996;271:1423–1427.

Center CHL. A comprehensive human linkage map with centimorgan density. Science 1994;265:2049–2054.

Chance PF, Reilly M. Inherited neuropathies. Curr Opin Neurol 1994;7:372–380.

Collins FS. Positional cloning moves from perditional to traditional. Nat Genet 1995;9:347–350.

Davies K. Cloning the Menkes disease gene. Nature 1993;361:98.

Davies KE, Willard HF. Genetics of disease. Curr Opin Genet Dev 1995;5:295–297.

Edwards RH. Neural degeneration and the transport of neurotransmitters. Ann Neurol 1993;34:638–645.

Elmslie F, Gardiner M. Genetics of the epilepsies. Curr Opin Neurol 1995;8:126–129.

Fields C, Adams MD, White O, Venter JC. How many genes in the human genome? Nat Genet 1994;7:345–346.

Fields S, Sternglanz R. The two-hybrid system: an assay for protein-protein interactions. Trends Genet 1994;10:286–292.

Gardiner K. Human genome organization. Curr Opin Genet Dev 1995;5:315–322.

Green H. Human genetic diseases due to codon reiteration: relationship to an evolutionary mechanism. Cell 1993;74:955–956 (letter).

Harding A. Clinical features and classification of inherited ataxias. Adv Neurol 1993;61:1–14.

Harding AE. Inherited ataxias. Curr Opin Neurol 1995;8:306–309.

Hinds PW, Weinberg RA. Tumor suppressor genes. Curr Opin Genet Dev 1994;4:135–141.

Hoffman EP, Lehmann HF, Rudel R. Overexcited or inactive: ion channels in muscle disease. Cell 1995;80:681–686.

Huntington's Disease Collaborative Research Group. A novel gene containing a trinucleotide repeat that is expanded and unstable on Huntington's disease chromosomes. Cell 1993;72:971–983.

Junck L, Fink JK. Machado-Joseph disease and SCA3: the genotype meets the phenotypes. Neurology 1996;46:4–8.

Lander ES, Schork NJ. Genetic dissection of complex traits. Science 1994;265:2037–2048.

Lewin B. Genes for SMA: multum in parvo. Cell 1995;80:1–5 (comment).

Li SH, McInnis MG, Margolis RL, et al. Novel triplet repeat containing genes in human brain: cloning, expression, and length polymorphisms. Genomics 1993;16:572–579.

MacMillan JC, Harper PS. Clinical genetics in neurological disease. J Neurol Neurosurg Psychiatry 1994;57:7–15.

Martin JB. Molecular genetics in neurology. Ann Neurol 1993;34: 757–773.

Martin JB. CNS genetic disorders: loss of function, gain of function, or something else? Curr Opin Neurobiol 1995;5:669–673.

Miller RG, Hoffman EP. Molecular diagnosis and modern management of Duchenne muscular dystrophy. Neurol Clin 1994;12:699–725.

Nagafuchi S, Yanagisawa H, Ohsaki E, et al. Structure and expression of the gene responsible for the triplet repeat disorder, dentatorubral and pallidoluysian atrophy (DRPLA). Nat Genet 1994; 8:177–182.

Orr HT, Chung MY, Banfi S, et al. Expansion of an unstable trinucleotide CAG repeat in spinocerebellar ataxia type 1. Nat Genet 1993;4: 221–226.

Patel PI, Lupski JR. Charcot-Marie-Tooth disease: a new paradigm for the mechanism of inherited disease. Trends Genet 1994;10: 128–133.

Pennacchio LA, Lehesjoki AE, Stone NE, et al. Mutations in the gene encoding cystatin B in progressive myoclonus epilepsy (EPM1). Science 1996;271:1731–1734.

Pericak-Vance MA, Haines JL. Genetic susceptibility to Alzheimer disease. Trends Genet 1995;11:504–508.

Perutz MF, Johnson T, Suzuki M, Finch JT. Glutamine repeats as polar zippers: their possible role in inherited neurodegenerative diseases. Proc Natl Acad Sci USA 1994;91:5355–5358.

Prusiner SB. Biology and genetics of prion diseases. Annu Rev Microbiol 1994;48:655–686.

Prusiner SB, Hsiao KK. Human prion diseases. Ann Neurol 1994;35: 385–395.

Ptacek LJ, Johnson KJ, Griggs RC. Genetics and physiology of the myotonic muscle disorders. N Engl J Med 1993;328:482–489.

Rosenberg RN. Autosomal dominant cerebellar phenotypes: the genotype has settled the issue. Neurology 1995;45:1–5 (editorial).

Roses AD. Apolipoprotein E genotyping in the differential diagnosis, not prediction, of Alzheimer's disease. Ann Neurol 1995;38:6–14.

Servadio A, Koshy B, Armstrong D, et al. Expression analysis of the ataxin-1 protein in tissues from normal and spinocerebellar ataxia type 1 individuals. Nat Genet 1995;10:94–98.

Snipes GJ, Suter U, Shooter EM. The genetics of myelin. Curr Opin Neurobiol 1993;3:694–702.

Strittmatter WJ, Roses AD. Apolipoprotein E and Alzheimer disease. Proc Natl Acad Sci USA 1995;92:4725–4727.

Strittmatter WJ, Roses AD. Apolipoprotein E: emerging story in the pathogenesis of Alzheimer's disease. The Neuroscientist 1995; 1:298–306.

Sutherland GR, Richards RI. Simple tandem DNA repeats and human genetic disease. Proc Natl Acad Sci USA 1995;92:3636–3641.

Thomas GR, Forbes JR, Roberts EA, et al. The Wilson disease gene: spectrum of mutations and their consequences. Nat Genet 1995; 9:210–217.

Van Camp G, Vits L, Coucke P, et al. A duplication in the *L1CAM* gene associated with X-linked hydrocephalus. Nat Genet 1993;4:421–425.

Van Ommen G-JB, Breuning MH, Raap AK. FISH in genome research and molecular diagnosis. Curr Opin Genet Dev 1995;5:304–308.

Wang J, Pegoraro E, Menegazzo E, et al. Myotonic dystrophy: evidence for a possible dominant-negative RNA mutation. Hum Mol Genet 1995;4:599–606.

Wong EV, Kenwrick S, Willems P, Lemmon V. Mutations in the cell adhesion molecule L1 cause mental retardation. Trends Neurosci 1995;18:168–172.

Yazawa I, Nukina N, Hashida H, et al. Abnormal gene product identified in hereditary dentatorubral-pallidoluysian atrophy (DRPLA) brain. Nat Genet 1995;10:99–103.

Zhang JS, Longo FM. LAR tyrosine phosphatase receptor: alternative splicing is preferential to the nervous system, coordinated with cell growth and generates novel isoforms containing extensive CAG repeats. J Cell Biol 1995;128:415–431.

97 Huntington's Disease

MARCY E. MACDONALD

INTRODUCTION

In 1872 George Huntington reported a perplexing and fatal disease that afflicted some of his patients who were members of the same East Hampton Long Island families cared for by his physician father and grandfather in previous generations. The ailment, an unremitting, adult-onset "hereditary chorea," became known as Huntington's chorea but is now called Huntington's disease (HD) (OMIM 143100), to reflect the constellation of motor, psychiatric, and cognitive deficits that attend the disorder.

Huntington emphasized the familial nature of the disease, reporting that it was frequently transmitted by either affected mothers or fathers to their children, never skipping a generation, a pattern that was subsequently attributed to the inheritance of an autosomal dominant mendelian gene defect. He thought that the disorder must represent "an heirloom from generations away back in the dim past," a conjecture later supported by Vessie's observation that many of the Long Island families were descendants of immigrants from Bures, England, who arrived in New England in 1649.

The disorder is not restricted to Long Island, as Huntington believed, but is found worldwide, with the lowest prevalence in Blacks and Asians, and the highest, approximately 4–7 cases per 100,000, in populations of Western European ancestry. Finland, with its distinct genetic origin, has a lower disease prevalence than the rest of Europe. However, the frequency of the genetic defect, *HD*, is 2.5 to 3-fold higher, because at any given time an estimated two out of three gene carriers are too young to exhibit disease symptoms, which typically do not strike until middle age.

The unique clinical symptoms arise from a progressive and graded loss of neurons, primarily in the basal ganglia, that is triggered mysteriously by the *HD* gene defect. The biochemical basis for the cell loss remains an enigma, but HD is yielding to a molecular genetic approach; in 1983 *HD* was the first defect mapped to a chromosomal location using only genetic linkage to DNA markers, and a decade later it was found to be an elongated, unstable CAG trinucleotide repeat in a novel 4p16.3 gene. The nature of the mutation clarifies many of the puzzling genetic features of the ailment, and its discovery reveals that HD is one of a number of neurodegenerative diseases whose distinct pathologies are caused by the shared theme of an expanded triplet repeat.

From: *Principles of Molecular Medicine* (J. L. Jameson, ed.), ©1998 Humana Press Inc., Totowa, NJ.

CLINICAL FEATURES

Huntington's original report, a classic description of the manifestations of HD, remarked on the three disorders that together make HD a distinct clinical entity: progressive motor impairment, cognitive decline, and emotional deterioration. The majority of patients become symptomatic in midlife, as was the case in Huntington's families, but the disease can strike at any age, and approximately 10% of cases exhibit symptoms before the age of 20 (juvenile onset) or after the age of 55 (late onset).

The severity of the movement disorder, which involves both voluntary and involuntary systems, is variable, changing during the course of the disease and being more or less pronounced depending on the age of the patient when symptoms first begin. Typically, it starts subtly in midlife with clumsiness, motor restlessness, and slight adventitious movements, and progresses to frank chorea, sudden unintended movements of almost any part of the body. Although chorea is a prominent feature in most midlife and late onset-adult patients, it may not be seen in juvenile-onset HD, which follows a more aggressive course, featuring seizures, rigidity, myoclonus, or dystonia. At all ages, there is a progressive loss of voluntary motor function that is evident from abnormal eye saccades and an inability to perform tasks demanding fine motor control. Walking is also affected and patients usually assume a wide-gaited stance. As the disease steadily worsens over a period of 15–20 years, patients inevitably become incapacitated, unable to communicate by word or gesture, and incapable of eating and walking without assistance. Near the end most patients are bedridden, and, for many, death results from asphyxiation or infection arising from inhalation of food particles.

The cognitive and psychiatric deficits of HD often precede the onset of neurologic symptoms and manifest as dementia, memory loss, apathy, and bouts of deep depression. The most commonly reported initial symptoms are irritability and restlessness. Patients are unable to change easily from one task to another, job performance cannot be maintained, and most become periodically depressed and lose interest in family and work. The disease is also associated with an increased risk of suicide. Although the severity of the psychiatric and cognitive symptoms is variable, these aspects of the disease pose significant challenges for the care of HD patients.

HD is almost invariably present within a family and it is usually possible to establish the inherited nature of the disease by asking the patient or related family members for genealogical information (Fig. 97-1). The disease is transmitted by both males and females in an autosomal dominant manner, and both sexes have a

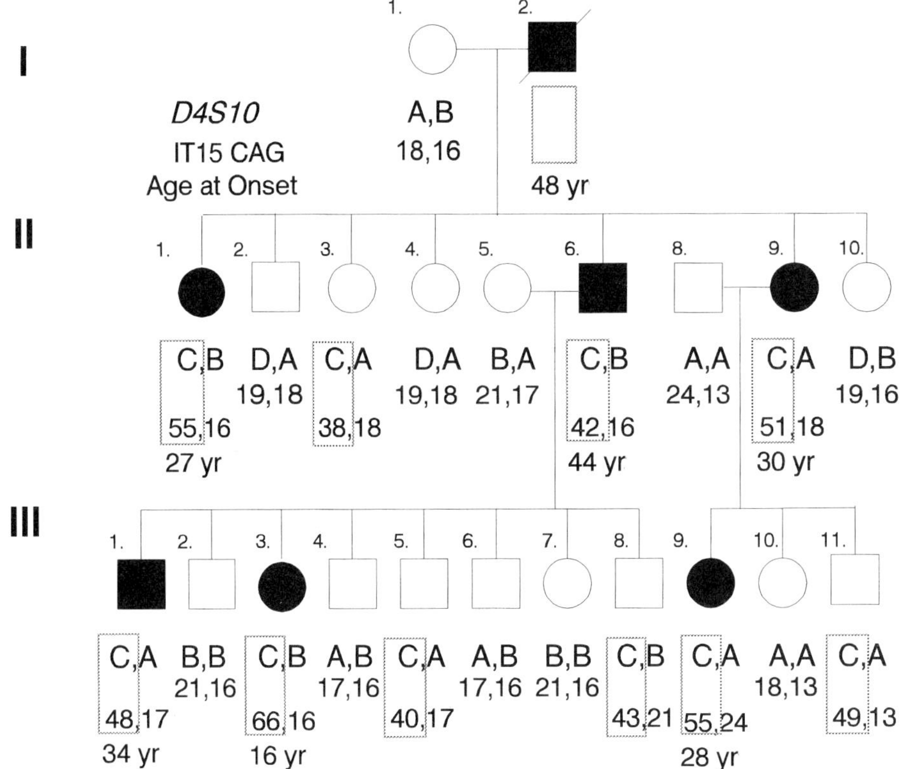

Figure 97-1 Genetic characteristics of HD. An idealized three generation **(I–III)** HD pedigree is depicted with family members—males (circles) and females (squares)—numbered sequentially. Filled symbols, clinically diagnosed members; slashed symbol, a deceased individual. Genotyping results for *D4S10* marker alleles (A,B,C,D) and the *HD* CAG repeat length measurement (IT15 CAG) at both alleles (larger shown first by convention) are shown below each symbol, with the marker alleles on the disease chromosome given within a box. The age at onset (yr) is also shown below symbols of symptomatic family members. The disease is segregating with the C allele of *D4S10*, a linked marker that exhibits 4% recombination with HD. Individuals who have inherited the C allele from their affected parent (II-1, II-3, II-6, II-9, III-1, III-3, III-5, III-8, III-9, III-11), therefore, have a 96% chance of having inherited the *HD* defect. Direct determination of the length of the *HD* CAG repeat demonstrates that all of these individuals have inherited the *HD* defect. One child (III-3) had juvenile onset due to a CAG allele of 66 repeat units but many other individuals are not yet old enough to have become symptomatic (II-3, III-5, III-8, III-11) including an elderly individual in generation II (II-3) who inherited a disease chromosome that has 38 CAG repeats.

50–50 chance of inheriting the defect, although the relatively rare juvenile form of the disease occurs most frequently as a result of transmission through the male germline. The *HD* defect is highly penetrant, and individuals who have inherited it will develop symptoms if they live a normal life span. Sadly, because HD generally strikes in middle age, the defective gene is often passed on to children before the parent is aware of his or her disorder.

PATHOLOGY

Huntington's disease-associated pathology appears to be confined to the brain. The basal ganglia, especially the striatum, is in the course of time ravaged by the disease, and the dramatic cell loss becomes evident on magnetic resonance imaging (MRI) and positron emission tomography (PET) scans. The atrophy is due to the progressive loss of one of the major striatal neuronal cell populations, the γ-aminobutyric acid (GABA)-, enkephalin-, and substance P-containing medium-sized spiny projection neurons. There is also neuronal cell loss in the globus pallidus. However, with the exception of the cortex, other brain regions are not obviously affected, and other striatal neuronal populations, such as the large acetylcholine-rich or smaller somatostatin- and neuropeptide Y-containing aspiny interneurons, are spared by the gene defect. The death of striatal neurons begins in the medial dorsal region of the caudate and progresses along posteroanterior, dorsoventral, and mediolateral axes, producing a characteristic gradient of cell loss that forms the basis of the neuropathologic evaluation of HD.

The cerebral cortex, another primary target of the gene defect, consistently exhibits a diffuse pattern of neuronal cell loss rather than the focal pathology found in the basal ganglia. Total brain weight is reduced about 20–30% in end-stage disease, a consequence of massive cell death that is especially apparent in juvenile-onset cases. Inconsistent alterations involving almost every cell population and brain region, including the thalamic and subthalamic nuclei, brain stem, and spinal cord, have been reported, but it is likely that these changes are secondary features of the disease rather than primary effects of the *HD* defect.

The obvious striatal degeneration provides an explanation for the motor and perhaps the cognitive and emotional features of HD as the basal ganglia receives inputs from cortical areas serving these functions. Loss of the striatal input to the globus pallidus probably results in the choreiform movements of HD because of increased inhibitory pallidal input to the subthalamic nucleus, a region whose destruction by other means elicits chorea. Similarly, loss of striatal input to the frontal cortex and the superior colliculus is likely to be involved in the loss of control over voluntary movements such as eye saccades.

Glutamate is the major excitatory neurotransmitter of the cortical-striatal pathway but a variety of neurotransmitters and neuropeptides are found in both regions. Indeed, these biologically active molecules appeared to be good targets for treatment schemes that are based on the idea that rectification of a neurochemical imbalance caused by the gradual loss of neuronal cells could slow or prevent the progression of disease pathology. However, a selective neurotransmitter deficit has not been found in HD, and therapeutic strategies arising from these neurochemical surveys have been ineffective.

The biochemical lesion that precipitates the apparently specific neuronal cell loss in HD remains elusive despite increasingly sophisticated cellular and neurochemical descriptions of the disease pathology. Changes in a myriad of neurotransmitters, amino acid receptors, and metabolites have been reported, and some may contribute to the clinical symptoms of HD, but these alterations are likely to be a consequence of the cell death rather than a direct effect of the disease gene. Some changes that are seen in HD, including reduced numbers of *N*-methyl-D-aspartate (NMDA) receptors, decreased glucose utilization, and elevated lactose concentration, are consistent with a currently favored hypothesis that is emerging from animal studies. This model proposes that neuronal cell death is a consequence of NMDA receptor-mediated glutamate excitotoxicity that occurs via either an acute direct mechanism or a subtle route such as a defect in energy metabolism.

CLINICAL DIAGNOSIS

Diagnosis of HD based on neurologic or psychiatric examination is relatively straightforward despite the variable age at onset and age-dependent differences in clinical presentation. In many cases the clinical diagnosis is strengthened by evidence of HD neuropathology at autopsy in a previously diagnosed family member. Because the disease almost always presents in someone with a family history of the disorder, inheritance is a commonly used diagnostic criterion, but this information may not be available when dealing with very late onset cases or adoptees, making diagnosis more difficult in these individuals.

The differential diagnosis of HD theoretically includes disorders involving voluntary and involuntary motor dysfunctions and many forms of mental illness; in practice, however, few diseases are confused with HD clinically. Some disorders with overlapping symptoms, including cortical stroke, schizophrenia, and cortical dementias, are relatively common and consequently may be initially confused with HD but are ultimately distinguished as the disease progresses. Familial diseases that exhibit HD-like symptoms, such as choreo-acanthocytosis, benign hereditary chorea, and dentatorubropallidoluysian atrophy, are very rare and also can be distinguished from HD by a variety of means including neurological examination, neuropathology, and, most recently, direct DNA testing.

GENETIC LINKAGE

In 1983 *HD* was the first gene defect mapped to a human chromosome using a genetic strategy that exploits naturally occurring DNA sequence variation (polymorphism) to search the human genome for chromosomal segments that are coinherited with the defect in disease families. Genetic linkage to polymorphic DNA markers is used first to discover the approximate chromosomal location of the defect and then to narrow progressively the amount of chromosomal DNA that must be searched to identify the mutation itself. This strategy, which does not require any knowledge of the disease gene, its function, or its mechanism of pathogenesis, is now widely used to isolate mutant genes that cause inherited human disease.

HD was an ideal candidate for pioneering this approach because it exhibits high penetrance, unique clinical manifestations, and midlife onset, which conspire to produce large, identifiable families with the disease. Genetic linkage was quickly discovered by tracing the inheritance of restriction fragment length polymorphisms (RFLPs) detected by anonymous DNA probes in HD kindred. No crossover events were observed between two *Hin*dIII RFLPs, detected by the probe G8, and the disease gene in two large pedigrees (one of American and the other of Venezuelan ancestry) producing odds of greater than 100 million to one in favor of genetic linkage between *D4S10* and *HD*. Assignment of G8 to the short arm of chromosome 4 placed *HD* close to 4p16.3, the terminal cytogenetic band of the short arm of chromosome 4.

The discovery of genetic linkage provided the means to test whether the same gene defect that resides on chromosome 4 was responsible for causing disease symptoms in all HD families. Indeed, this was proven to be the case, as all HD families genotyped exhibited linkage to *D4S10* regardless of ethnic or genetic background. The absence of nonallelic heterogeneity meant that, for the first time, an accurate predictive test could be offered to some asymptomatic individuals who are "at risk" for the disorder because a parent has the disease (*see* Fig. 97-1).

Family studies with the linked DNA markers also revealed the complete phenotypic dominance of the disorder. Rare HD homozygotes, individuals with two copies of the *HD* defect, one inherited from each affected parent, were found to be clinically indistinguishable from their affected heterozygous siblings, who have only one copy of the mutation. This surprising finding argues that the normal *HD* gene does not help delay or otherwise influence the clinical features of the disorder and demonstrates that two copies of the disease gene are not significantly more damaging than a single copy.

ISOLATION OF THE *HD* MUTATION

Genetic linkage set the stage for the isolation of the *HD* defect from the vicinity of *D4S10* (Fig. 97-2). Genotyping of a large number of HD families demonstrated that *HD* and *D4S10* displayed about 4% recombination, and linkage analysis with DNA markers located centromeric to *D4S10* revealed that the defect was located within 4p16.3 between *D4S10* and the telomere, a distance of about 6 Mb of DNA. The location cloning strategy that progressively refined the candidate region and ultimately led to the discovery of the *HD* mutation then progressed through a number of stages. Initial efforts were aimed at the generation of somatic cell and radiation hybrid mapping panels that were required for the generation of a large number of polymorphic RFLPs, variable number of tandem repeat (VNTR), and simple sequence repeat (SSR) genetic markers from 4p16.3. As new markers were cloned they were placed on the emerging genetic and physical maps of the region, and they were used for genetic linkage in HD pedigrees in an effort to find critical crossover events that would bracket the defect.

A hot spot of recombination located approximately 300 kb telomeric to *D4S10* quickly became the proximal boundary, but localization of the defect within the remaining 3.5 Mb of 4p16.3 was problematic because several crossover events within well-

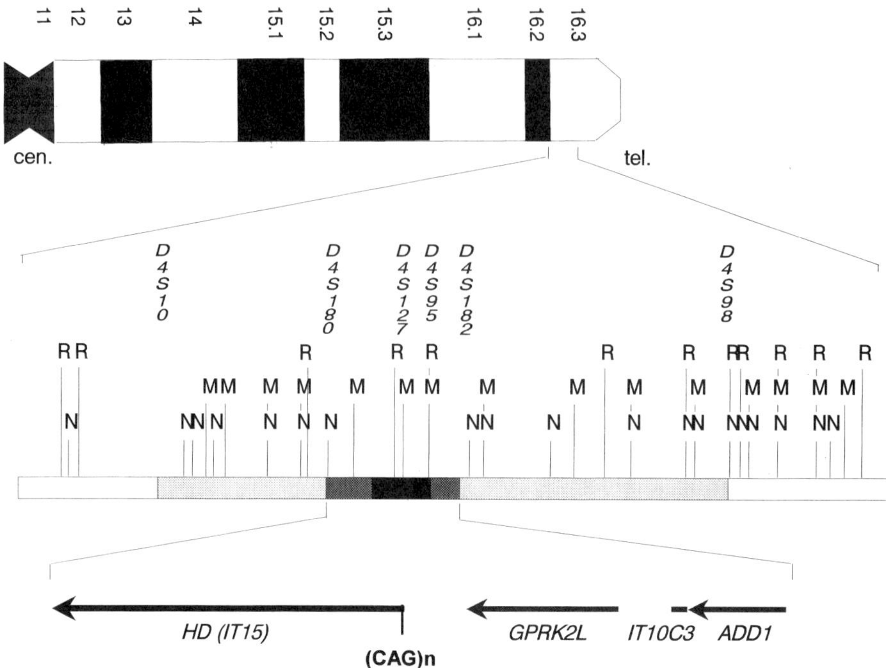

Figure 97-2 Isolation of the HD gene from 4p16.3. The long-range restriction map (R, *Nru*I site; M, *Mlu*I site; N, *Not*I site; brackets, sites that are partially cut) of about 3×10^6 bp of 4p16.3, the terminal cytogenetic band, is depicted under a schematic of the short arm of chromosome 4 (cen., centromere; tel., telomere). The unshaded region was eliminated by recombination events in HD families, placing the defect within the ~2-Mb region between *D4S10* and D4S98 (light shading). The ~500-kb region between *D4S180* and *D4S182* (darker shading) was implicated by linkage disequilibrium and initial haplotype studies, and continued haplotype analysis placed the defect within the ~150-kb region between *D4S180* and *D4S127* (darkest shading). This segment is further expanded below the restriction map to depict gene transcripts that were eliminated as candidates (ADD1, IT10C3 *GPRK2L*), thereby targeting the search to the 5' end of *IT15*, where the *HD* defect, an unstable and expanded CAG repeat, is located ([CAG]n).

characterized HD pedigrees yielded contradictory locations for the gene. A few clinically diagnosed members of HD families had inherited DNA markers from the affected parents' normal chromosome 4, suggesting that the defect must be located in the telomeric 100 kb of the chromosome. But other crossover events predicted a nonoverlapping internal location of about 2.5 Mb of DNA closer to *D4S10*. Isolation of the telomeric region as a yeast artificial chromosome (YAC) demonstrated that it was unlikely to contain the disease gene, and a few rare recombination events that favored the internal region were identified. The individuals with apparent crossover chromosomes that predicted the telomeric location were explained ultimately only by the cloning of the *HD* defect.

Linkage disequilibrium, the nonrandom association of certain marker alleles with HD chromosomes, at *D4S95* initiated a search across the entire internal candidate region with highly polymorphic VNTR and SSR markers, and highlighted a subregion that exhibited maximal linkage disequilibrium with the defect. The construction of 4p16.3 haplotypes across this relatively small segment yielded a plethora of marker haplotypes, a surprising finding that revealed for the first time that the current pool of *HD* chromosomes has arisen from more than one independent *HD* mutation or primordial chromosome. Moreover, these results suggested that the identification of a minimum collection of 4p16.3 marker alleles shared by *HD* chromosomes likely to be related by mutational ancestry might pinpoint the location of the disease gene.

A region of about 2 Mb of DNA was ultimately mapped and isolated in overlapping clone sets and candidate genes from a 500-kb segment of 4p16.3 between *D4S180* and *D4S182* were scanned for DNA sequence alterations that were unique to disease chromosomes. Several genes with sequence homology to known proteins, including the gene encoding α-adducin, *ADD1*, a novel small molecule transporter, IT10C3, a G-protein-coupled receptor kinase, *GPRK2L*, and several genes with novel DNA sequence were eliminated as *HD* gene candidates, and a rare Alu repeat insertion within an intron of *ADD1* in two affected individuals was incorrectly interpreted as being causative of HD.

Continued haplotype analysis using new polymorphic markers finally targeted a very small (150-kb) portion of the candidate region that contained the 5' end of a novel interesting transcript (IT). Cloning and sequencing of this region of the *IT15* gene revealed a polymorphic CAG trinucleotide repeat that was found to be expanded and unstable on HD chromosomes signaling the isolation of the *HD* mutation.

THE *HD* MUTATION

A plethora of studies involving individuals from HD families worldwide have confirmed the IT15 CAG repeat expansion as the universal cause of HD and serve to further delineate the characteristics of the *HD* defect. The length of the IT15 CAG repeat (Figs. 97-2 and 97-3) on normal chromosomes is variable, ranging from 6 to 35 U, and these arrays are inherited in a mendelian fashion. Immediately adjacent is a polymorphic, stably transmitted stretch of CCG codons that on normal chromosomes varies in length from 6 to 12 repeat units, while more than 90% of disease chromosomes carry 7 CCG repeats. By contrast, the CAG repeat

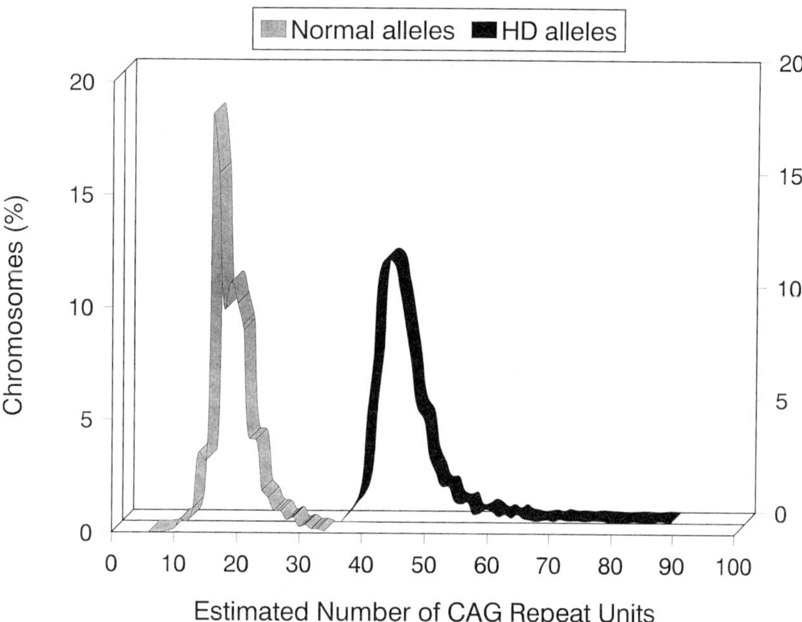

Figure 97-3 Distribution of CAG repeat lengths on HD and normal chromosomes. The frequency of CAG allele sizes reported in the literature for 2885 normal (light shading) and 3484 disease (dark shading) chromosomes, shown as a percentage of the total, is plotted against the estimated number of CAG units. These CAG repeat length determinations represent the distribution of repeat lengths at the *HD* locus in populations of disparate genetic and ethnic backgrounds from around the world. The very rare chromosomes displaying an intermediate-sized allele, overlapping with the upper end of the normal and the lower end of the disease chromosome distribution, that have been identified in families with a member who represents a new mutation to HD are not included in this data set.

on HD chromosomes ranges from 37 to more than 100 U, alleles that almost invariably change in length, increasing or decreasing in size, when transmitted from parent to offspring. In most cases, the alteration is small (<6 U), with a bias toward increases in length, but paternal transmission can result in very large increases in the number of CAG repeats. This striking intergenerational instability appears to occur during spermatogenesis, and different *HD* allele sizes among children of an *HD* gene carrier are reflected in a similar variation in sperm DNA. Moreover, identical monozygotic twins with HD develop clinical symptoms at the same time and display identical expanded CAG repeat lengths, strengthening the argument that the intergenerational instability occurs during gametogenesis rather than during embryonic development. The unstable behavior of the expanded CAG repeat during maternal transmission suggests that instability, albeit of reduced magnitude, also occurs during oogenesis. The cellular and molecular mechanisms leading to changes in CAG repeat length and the parameters that affect it, including parental age, disease status, repeat length, and a host of other biological factors, have yet to be defined.

In contrast to the evident gametic instability, the vast majority of expanded CAG repeats exhibit very limited somatic instability. Somatic variation is exhibited by some long expanded CAG repeats (>60 U), but these alterations are most evident in the cerebellum and do not correlate with the neuropathology of HD.

CLINICAL CORRELATES

Studies reporting the IT15 repeat lengths observed on the disease chromosomes of several thousand HD patients from around the world reveal that all but a few exceptional individuals have a CAG repeat in the expanded size range, confirming the universality of this mutation in diverse races, nationalities, and ethnic groups. It is apparent that rare patients with HD-like symptoms who do not have an expanded CAG allele can be explained as sample mix-ups, lab errors, or erroneous diagnoses based on atypical features. Indeed, the low rate of misdiagnosis of the disorder is also revealed by the small number of postmortem brains from patients with a clinical diagnosis of HD that do not have HD-like neuropathology.

Huntington's disease almost always occurs in individuals with a family history of the disorder, and only rarely do sporadic cases satisfy the rigorous criteria for new mutation status: living unaffected elderly parents, proof of paternity, and transmission of the disease to a child. Nonetheless, evidence that new mutation to HD does occur is provided by the identification of a few such families and the finding of a multiplicity of different 4p16.3 haplotypes on HD chromosomes, a result that was consistent with multiple origins of the mutation. Discovery of the *HD* mutation has confirmed that sporadic cases of HD are due to new mutations at the *HD* locus. These individuals, like familial HD cases, have CAG repeat lengths in the expanded disease range but their unaffected relatives with the same 4p16.3 haplotype possess a CAG repeat of intermediate size, repeats that span the gap between the normal and disease causing ranges. Indeed, many new mutations occur on the same 4p16.3 haplotype found in about one-third of unrelated HD families, suggesting that these traditional disease families share a common ancestor who was not affected by the disorder. Thus, it is likely that these intermediate allele-bearing chromosomes serve as a reservoir that can give rise to new sporadic HD cases.

The vast majority of postmortem brains assessed for HD neuropathology have an expanded CAG repeat, and the few anomalous cases (<1%) can be ascribed to atypical clinical features suggesting a distinct disorder. Because all cases of HD that have been confirmed neuropathologically display an expanded IT15

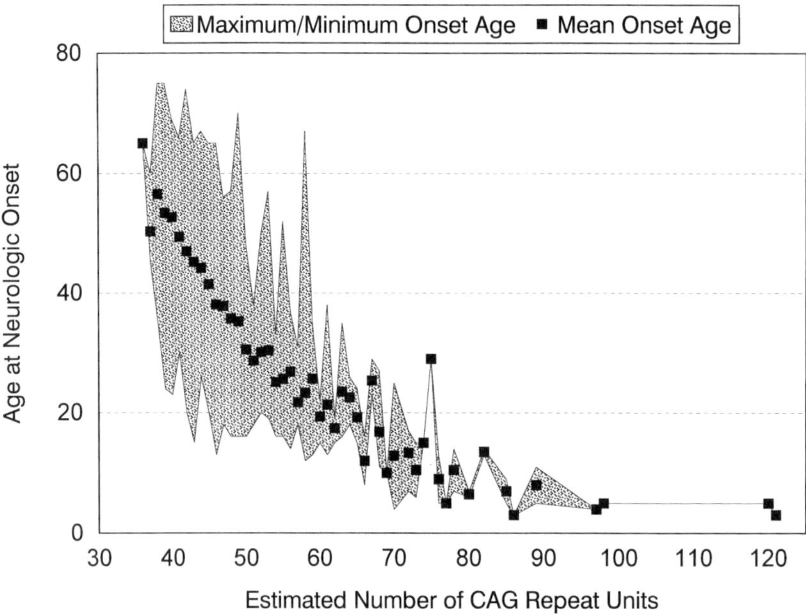

Figure 97-4 Inverse correlation between CAG repeat length and age at onset. The association of any given CAG repeat length with the age at onset of neurologic disease symptoms for 1070 HD patients reported in the literature is shown. The mean age at onset (filled squares) and the range of onset ages (shaded area) for any given CAG repeat length is depicted and the line represents the curve obtain by power regression analysis. The correlation between age at onset and CAG repeat length is highly significant across all HD allele sizes ($r = -0.87$, $p < 0.00001$), but the wide range of possible ages of onset associated with any given repeat length precludes an accurate estimate of when the disease will strike any single individual.

CAG repeat, it is unlikely that another mutation, either at the *HD* locus or elsewhere in the genome, is able to produce the constellation of clinical and neuropathological features that makes HD a unique clinical disorder.

The nature of the *HD* mutation explains much of the variation in the clinical manifestations of the disorder, including the paternal inheritance of juvenile-onset HD. The longest expanded CAG repeat lengths (>55 U) give rise to juvenile-onset HD and the shortest (35–39 U) tend not to trigger disease until very late in life (Figs. 97-1 and 97-4). CAG repeat length, therefore, is inversely correlated with age at onset of disease symptoms. Coupled with the propensity of the expanded CAG repeats occasionally to increase dramatically in length during spermatogenesis, this inverse correlation accounts for the observation that most juvenile-onset HD is inherited from fathers.

The inverse correlation between the length of the expanded IT15 CAG and age at onset of neurologic and psychiatric symptoms as well as age at death is extremely strong, even when clinical data are contributed by many different physicians. Repeat length, however, accounts for only about 50% of the variation in age at onset of clinical symptoms that is observed between individual patients with identical expanded CAG repeat lengths. Thus, it is evident that other factors, perhaps interacting genes, environmental influences, or stochastic events, are involved in determining the precise age at which the disease strikes any given individual. It has not yet been established whether the length of the CAG expansion is associated with the rate of progression of the disorder, as these studies have yielded conflicting results.

THE *HD* GENE

The polymorphic CAG repeat is located 17 amino acids from the initiator ATG codon in the first exon of a novel gene whose 67 exons span about 185 kb of 4p16.3 DNA (Fig. 97-2). The *HD* gene encodes a protein, dubbed huntington, that is more than 3140 amino acids in length including the variable segment of glutamine residues and the adjacent polyproline segment encoded by the polymorphic CAG and CCG repeats, respectively. Huntingtin's normal activity is not known, but the high degree of sequence conservation exhibited by the mouse, rat, and pufferfish *HD* homologs suggests that it performs an essential cellular function. The most divergent segment is the polyglutamine/polyproline segment at the N-terminus of the protein. The normal human gene has 12–36 glutamines, whereas the rat has 8, the mouse 7, and the pufferfish 4 consecutive polyglutamine residues at this position, strongly suggesting that the exact composition or length of the amino acid sequence of this portion of the N-terminus is not critical for huntingtin's normal activity.

Huntingtin is expressed in the cytoplasm of a wide variety of neuronal and nonneuronal tissues and cells, but its distribution does not immediately explain the distinct pattern of HD neuropathology. As a consequence of the extended N-terminal polyglutamine segment encoded by the expanded CAG repeat, the products of the normal and HD chromosomes can be distinguished in extracts of HD cells and tissues, but these two isoforms of huntingtin do not differ in their pattern of expression or intracellular location. Preliminary biochemical analysis supports the notion that both isoforms are primarily cytosolic rather than being integrally associated with particular organelles. A similar distribution of huntingtin expression is revealed by immunohistochemistry in sections of rat, monkey, and human brain tissue. Huntingtin, in both normal and HD tissue, is found in the cell bodies, dendrites, axons and terminals, but not in the nuclei, of neurons and other cell types in the brain. Thus, the primary targets of the CAG mutation, the medium-sized striatal projection neurons, are only a subset of the neuronal and nonneuronal cells that express the mutant isoform of huntingtin.

MOLECULAR MECHANISM

The means by which the expanded IT15 CAG repeat causes the pathology of HD is not evident from the sequence of the normal or mutant versions of the *HD* gene products or their apparently identical patterns of expression. Indeed, the *HD* gene is widely expressed and yet only particular populations of neuronal cells appear to be sensitive to its effects. The mutation may provoke the pathological changes by a direct action on the mature striatal neurons, it may first trigger an as yet undetected alteration within another cell type(s), or it may act during development to generate a compromised tissue that is susceptible to neuronal cell loss later in life.

At the molecular level, several modes of action can be formulated, but some of these have been eliminated by studies of the gene products. The mutation does not alter transcription of the *HD* gene, as the mRNA is expressed at comparable levels from the disease and normal alleles. It also does not prevent translation of the mRNA from the disease allele, implicating the altered structure of huntingtin, and its extended polyglutamine segment, in the pathogenesis.

The lengthened polyglutamine stretch does not cause HD by elimination of huntingtin's normal activity, because disruption of the gene does not produce disease symptoms. In humans, individuals with an *HD* gene translocation that eliminates 50% of huntingtin production do not develop HD, and mice with one copy of the *HD* gene homolog *(Hdh)* inactivated by targeted mutagenesis show no HD-like abnormality. Notably, expression of a novel truncated version of murine huntingtin's NH_2-terminus in transgenic mice appears to cause restless behavior, learning deficits, and pathology in the subthalamic nucleus, suggesting that abnormal versions of huntingtin can have neuronal and behavioral consequences. By contrast, complete inactivation of the mouse *Hdh* gene results in early embryonic death, prior to development of the nervous system, and severely reduced levels of huntingtin produce perinatal lethality and an abnormal brain phenotype, indicating that huntingtin activity is essential for normal embryonic development. Thus, the existence of HD homozygotes who make only mutant huntingtin cannot be simply explained if the mutation acts to eliminate huntington's normal activity.

The most likely hypothesis is that the expanded CAG repeat causes pathology via a gain of function mechanism in which the extended polyglutamine stretch confers a new property on huntingtin. If it increased, rather than decreased, huntingtin's normal activity, this gain of function could act through the protein's normal physiological role. Alternatively, huntingtin's inherent activity may remain intact, but the elongated polyglutamine segment may promote a new interaction of huntingtin or one of its breakdown products with a biochemical pathway unrelated to its normal physiological role. This novel interaction, the protein's gain of function, could cause either activation or inactivation of the target pathway. It has been shown that huntingtin is cleaved by a proapoptotic cysteine protease and that the rate of cleavage increases with the length of the polyglutamine tract. The role of inappropriate apoptosis in HD therefore warrants further study.

Any hypothesized mode of action of the expanded CAG repeat must explain the complete dominance of the defect, the cellular specificity, and the association of repeat length with disease severity. Dominance is expected in the gain of function model because huntingtin would probably not interfere with the new property of the HD protein, and complete dominance would be expected if a critical effective threshold for the new property was achieved with a single dose of the disease gene. The specificity could be the result of the restricted distribution of a critical interacting target protein, and the correlation with disease severity could derive from an increasing effectiveness of the interaction with lengthening of the polyglutamine stretch. Indeed, a recent study reports the cloning of a gene encoding a novel protein, HAP1, whose expression is confined to the brain and whose association with huntingtin in vitro is influenced by the length of the polyglutamine segment.

Thus, the gain of function model provides an attractive working hypothesis that emphasizes investigation of the peculiarities of the mutant isoform with its extended N-terminal polyglutamine segment. Additional protein partners for normal and HD huntingtin will emerge from a variety of biochemical and genetic studies, and the challenge will be to determine whether these candidate interactor proteins play a role in the pathogenesis of HD.

OTHER CAG REPEAT DISORDERS

Huntington's disease is one of a growing number of neurodegenerative disorders that are known to be caused by expanded and unstable trinucleotide repeats that encode extended polyglutamine segments (*see* Chapter 100). In all of these diseases, a normally polymorphic CAG repeat is expanded and unstable on disease chromosomes, and the CAG repeat is located within the coding sequence of the gene, predicting an altered protein with an extended stretch of consecutive glutamine residues.

In Kennedy's syndrome (OMIM 313200) or spinobulbar muscular atrophy (SBMA), the expanded CAG lengthens a polyglutamine segment in the androgen receptor at Xq11.2–q12, resulting, in males, in a progressive loss of anterior horn cells in the spinal cord causing progressive muscular weakness and sometimes mental retardation and mild androgen insensitivity. Reduced androgen receptor function may underlie the endocrine abnormalities, including gynecomastia and testicular atrophy that usually occurs before onset of muscle weakness, but there is no abnormal development of the genitalia. Inactivation of the androgen receptor gene, therefore, does not mimic the pathology of SBMA but rather produces testicular feminization, indicating that the expanded CAG repeat does not trigger the degeneration of the anterior horn cells by causing androgen insensitivity.

Spinocerebellar ataxia type 1 (SCA1) (OMIM 164400), a fatal progressive cerebellar ataxia characterized by muscle atrophy, decreased deep tendon reflexes, and proprioception, is caused by the loss of neurons in the cerebellum (Purkinje's cells and dentate nucleus), in the inferior olive, and in cranial nerve nuclei III, IV, IX, X, and XII. This disorder, which, like HD, is inherited as an autosomal dominant trait, is due to an expanded CAG repeat in a novel chromosome 6p gene that encodes ataxin 1, an 87-kDa protein of unknown function. Ataxin is found in the cytoplasm of nonneuronal tissues, in the nuclei of neurons from various brain regions, and in both the cytoplasm and nuclei of cerebellar Purkinje's cells. Interestingly, the *SCA1* alleles found on normal chromosomes do not encode a pure CAG stretch, as occurs at the *HD*, SBMA, and other loci; rather, the repeat is interrupted by CAT codons not found in the expanded CAG segment of the disease allele.

Machado-Joseph disease (MJD) (OMIM 109150), originally described in an Azorean Portuguese family, is one of the most frequent inherited spinocerebellar degenerative disorders. Its

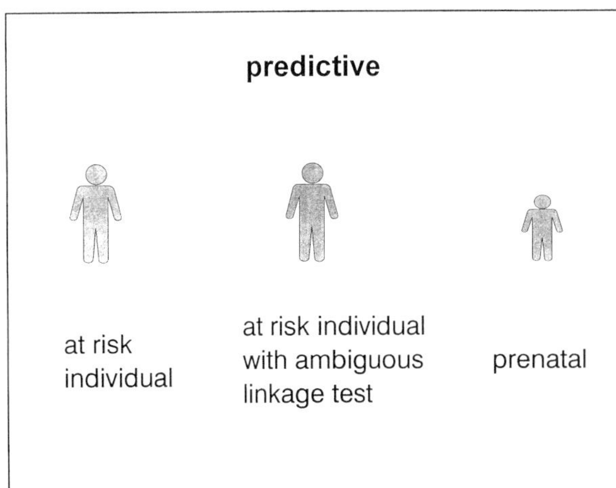

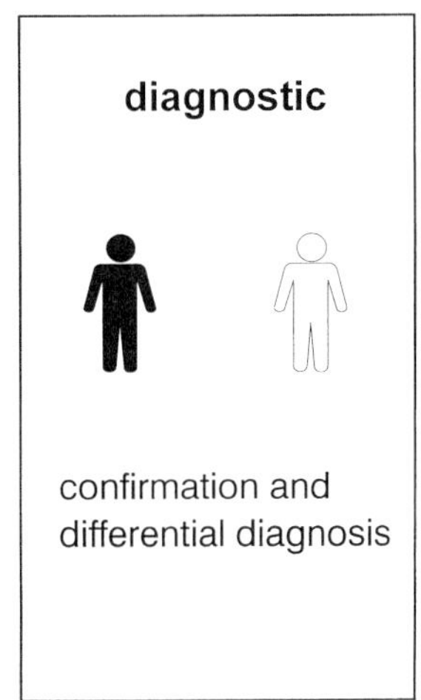

Figure 97-5 Molecular diagnosis. A diagram illustrating the uses of direct CAG repeat length measurement is shown. The direct DNA test distinguishes between normal and HD chromosomes in predictive testing of at-risk individuals, including those who have received an ambiguous result from the HD linkage test perhaps because of a crossover event between the linked markers and the disease gene and in prenatal diagnosis in at-risk pregnancies. The test is also of diagnostic value in confirming or refuting the clinical diagnosis of HD in atypical cases.

pathology involves a progressive degeneration of the spinocerebellar tracts, but the inferior olive and cerebellar cortex are not as affected, as they are in SCA1. The disorder manifests with progressive cerebellar ataxia and pyramidal and extrapyramidal signs, external opthalmoplegia, facial and lingual fasciculation, and bulging eyes. It is also autosomal dominant and is caused by an expanded CAG repeat in a novel gene encoded at 14q32.1. Spinocerebellar ataxia type 3 (SCA3), which is clinically very similar to MJD, is caused by expansion of this same CAG repeat on chromosome 14 and is therefore an allelic disorder.

Dentatorubropallidoluysian atrophy (DRPLA) (125370) is a rare autosomal dominant neurodegenerative disorder involving loss of neurons in dentatofugal and pallidofugal systems. It is a progressive motor disorder whose hallmarks are ataxia, choreoathetosis, and myoclonus, associated with epilepsy and dementia. DRPLA is due to an expanded CAG repeat located in the coding sequence of a novel gene on chromosome 12p. This expansion causes the extension of a polymorphic polyglutamine stretch in a 190-kDa cytoplasmic protein of unknown function. Haw River syndrome, a DRPLA-like disorder observed in a single African-American family in North Carolina, is an allelic disorder caused by expansion of this same CAG repeat.

The range of CAG repeat sizes on both normal and disease chromosomes is similar in each of the disorders (approximately 6–34 on normal and approximately 35–100 on disease chromosomes), and in each case CAG instability is most obvious during gametogenesis, although somatic mosaicism in the expanded alleles has been observed. In all of the disorders, the length of the CAG repeat on disease chromosomes is inversely correlated with age at onset of symptoms, so that the most severe cases, juvenile onset, are due to the longest CAG repeat lengths. The inverse correlation of age at onset of symptoms and repeat length, and the observation that striking increases in the size of the expanded CAG repeat most often occur during spermatogenesis clarify the tendency for inheritance of the earliest-onset cases from fathers.

The expanded CAG repeat at each of the disease loci produces an elongated stretch of polyglutamine in the corresponding protein resulting in structurally distinct normal and abnormal proteins, providing support for the idea that the defect is operating at the level of the altered protein in each disease. Similarly, in each disease the primary pathology is progressive neurodegeneration, albeit of different neuronal populations in different brain regions, suggesting that the neuronal cell death is caused by a common mechanism. In this scenario, the pattern of neuronal cell susceptibility would be determined by the protein context with which the extended polyglutamine stretch is presented to the cell. If the expanded CAG repeat is acting via a gain of function at the protein level in all of these neurodegenerative disorders, it may be possible to develop interventions for many of these diseases by unraveling the biochemical steps between the mutation and the cellular pathology in any one of them.

PROSPECTS

In 1983 predictive testing for HD became a reality when the discovery of the linked DNA marker, G8, made it possible to offer presymptomatic or prenatal diagnostic testing to some individuals. The linkage test, however, was only applicable to at-risk individuals for whom several family members, including a clinically diagnosed affected relative, were able and willing to donate their DNA. The ability to test a currently unaffected individual for the presence of a gene defect that will eventually cause an untreatable neurologic disease raised numerous ethical dilemmas, and pilot programs began cautiously, with an emphasis on counseling both before and after delivery of the test result. Formal guidelines, sanctioned by the International Huntington Association (IHA) and by the World Federation of Neurology (WFN), have been established to ensure high ethical standards in HD predictive testing. It is hoped that this precedent will become an important guide for predictive testing programs in other untreatable late-onset neurologic diseases.

Predictive testing in HD and the other triplet repeat expansion disorders can now be performed by measurement of CAG repeat length (Fig. 97-5). This assay provides an inexpensive method that can be applied to any at-risk individual and to prenatal testing, for confirmation of a clinical diagnosis of HD and for differential diagnosis in difficult cases. This direct DNA test is more accurate and of broader applicability than the linkage test, but the information that can be imparted to the individual undergoing testing is essentially the same. Therefore, the formal guidelines, revised to take into account the peculiar features of the assay method, are still valid, and it is recommended that they be followed for the direct test that makes use of CAG repeat length measurement.

Several inherent features of the CAG repeat complicate the interpretation of the molecular DNA test in predictive testing situations. The range of repeat sizes on normal and HD chromosomes does not overlap but may differ by as few as three repeat units. In addition, chromosomes with CAG repeat lengths that span the gap between these two distributions, intermediate alleles, are found in unaffected members of rare HD new-mutation families. These alleles can also overlap with the lower end of the HD size range, and it is not clear whether these individuals are truly "normal" or will develop HD if they have a sufficiently long life-span. It is probable that a discrete border between CAG repeat lengths that cause HD and those that do not cannot be drawn but rather that other genetic, environmental, or stochastic modifying factors become of primary significance in determining the age at onset for repeat lengths at the low end of the HD range. In addition, the intergenerational stability of the intermediate repeat lengths is also not well-established, making it difficult to assess accurately the risk of transmitting to children an allele that has expanded into the disease range.

The strong inverse correlation between age at onset and the length of the expanded CAG repeat raises an additional counseling dilemma. The number of CAG repeats can be precisely measured, and an allele size that falls within the established disease range is diagnostic of the future onset of the disease. However, the broad range of ages at onset observed for any given repeat length makes the number of CAG repeat units a dubious predictor of when symptoms of the disease will begin (*see* Fig. 97-4).

The discovery of the *HD* mutation has made the molecular diagnosis of the disease more accessible to at-risk individuals, but the availability of an accurate predictive test is a mixed blessing without a cure or effective treatment for the disorder. The gain-of-function hypothesis, in which the extended polyglutamine segment bestows a new property on the huntingtin protein, suggests that development of a therapy will require modulation or elimination of the impact of mutant huntingtin's novel property rather than simply replacing or augmenting its normal activity. For example, a specific toxic breakdown product from mutant huntingtin that inhibits another cellular process may cause neuronal cell death that could perhaps be reversed by replacing the lost activity. Alternatively, if the new property was simply an augmentation of huntingtin's normal activity, producing "too much of a good thing," the protein's normal pathway would have to be targeted to eliminate neuronal cell death. These are only two of the numerous gain of function scenarios that can be imagined to explain how the expanded CAG repeat kills neuronal cells. It is also conceivable that studies on the underlying cellular mechanisms causing neuronal cell loss in the other polyglutamine expansion diseases could generate therapeutic strategies that can be effectively applied to HD. It is clear that this devastating disorder is yielding to the molecular genetic approach, and there is little doubt that therapies based on a knowledge of the actual disease mechanism will be forthcoming. The next major advance, a therapeutic intervention that will prevent or even slow the onset of HD, will refute George Huntington's contention that this devastating disease is "one of the incurables."

ACKNOWLEDGMENTS

The author is grateful to members of the laboratory for discussion. The author's work on Huntington's disease is supported by National Institutes of Health grants NS-16367 and NS-32765, and by grants from Bristol-Myers Squibb, Inc., the Hereditary Disease Foundation, the Foundation for the Care and Cure of HD, and the Huntington's Disease Society of America.

SELECTED REFERENCES

Albin RL, Reiner A, Anderson KD, et al. Preferential loss of striato-external pallidal projection neurons in presymptomatic Huntington's disease. Ann Neurol 1992;31:425–430.

Ambrose CM, Duyao MP, Barnes G, et al. Structure and expression of the Huntington's disease gene: evidence against simple inactivation due to an expanded CAG repeat. Somat Cell Mol Genet 1994;20:27–38.

Beal MF. Huntington's disease, energy, and excitoxicity. Neurobiol Aging 1994;15:275,276.

Burke JR, Wingfield MS, Lewis KE, et al. The Haw River Syndrome: dentatorubropallidoluysian atrophy (DRPLA) in a African-American family. Nat Genet 1994;7:521–524.

Duyao MP, Auerbach AB, Ryan A, et al. Homozygous inactivation of the mouse *Hdh* gene does not produce a Huntington's disease–like phenotype. Science 1995;269:407–410.

Ferrante RJ, Kowall NW, Beal MF, et al. Selective sparing of a class of striatal neurons in Huntington's disease. Science 1985;230:561–563.

Folstein S. Huntington's disease: a disorder of families. Baltimore, MD: Johns Hopkins, 1989.

Goldberg YP, Nicholson DW, Rasper DM, et al. Cleavage of huntingtin by apopain, a proapoptotic cysteine protease, is modulated by the polyglutamine tract. Nat Genet 1996;13:442–449.

Goldberg YP, Rommens JM, Andrew SE, et al. Identification of an Alu retrotransposition event in close proximity to a strong candidate gene for Huntington's disease. Nature 1993;362:370–373.

Graveland GA, Williams RS, DiFiglia M. Evidence for degenerative and regenerative changes in neostriatal spiny neurons in Huntington's disease. Science 1985;227:770–773.

Graybiel AM. Neuropeptides in the basal ganglia. In: Martin JB, Barchas J, eds. Neuropeptides in Neurologic and Psychiatric Disease. New York: Raven, 1986:135–161.

Gusella JF. DNA polymorphism and human disease. Annu Rev Biochem 1986;55:831–854.

Gusella JF. Huntington's disease. In: Harris H, Hirschhorn K, eds. Advances in Human Genetics, vol. 20. New York, Plenum, 1991:125–151.

Gusella JF, MacDonald ME. Hunting for Huntington's disease. In: Friedmann T, ed. Molecular Genetic Medicine, vol. 3. San Diego, CA: Academic, 1993, pp. 139–158.

Gusella JF, MacDonald ME. Huntington's disease. Semin Cell Biol 1995;6:21–28.

Gusella JF, MacDonald ME. Huntington's disease: CAG genetics expands neurobiology. Curr Opin Neurobiol 1995;5:656–662.

Gusella JF, Wexler NS, Conneally PM, et al. A polymorphic DNA marker genetically linked to Huntington's disease. Nature 1983;306:234–238.

Harper PS. The epidemiology of Huntington's disease. Hum Genet 1992;89:365–376.

Huntington G. On chorea. Med Surg Reporter 1872;26:317–321.

Huntington's Disease Collaborative Research Group. A novel gene containing a trinucleotide repeat that is expanded and unstable on Huntington's disease chromosomes. Cell 1993;72:971–983.

Ikeuchi T, Onodera O, Oyake M, et al. Dentatorubral-pallidoluysian atrophy (DRPLA): close correlation of CAG repeat expansions with the wide spectrum of clinical presentations and prominent anticipation. Semin Cell Biol 1995;6:37–44.

International Huntington Association and World Federation of Neurology Research Group on Huntington's Chorea. Guidelines for the molecular genetics predictive test in Huntington's disease. Neurology 1994;44:1533–1536.

Kawaguchi Y, Okamoto T, Taniwaki M, et al. CAG expansions in a novel gene for Machado-Joseph disease at chromosome 14q32.1. Nat Genet 1994;8:221–228.

LaSpada AR, Wilson EM, Lubahn DB, et al. Androgen receptor gene mutations in X-linked spinal and bulbar muscular atrophy. Nature 1991;352:77–79.

Li X-J, Li S-H, Sharp AH, et al. A huntingtin-associated protein enriched in brain with implications for pathology. Nature 1995;378:398–402.

Mangiarini L, Sathasivam K, Seller M, et al. Exon 1 of the HD gene with an expanded CAG repeat is sufficient to cause a progressive neurological phenotype in transgenic mice. Cell 1996;87:493–506.

Mangiarini L, Sathasivam K, Mahal A, et al. Instability of highly expanded CAG repeats in mice transgenic for the Hungtingtin's disease mutation. Nat Genet 1997;15:197–200.

MacDonald ME, Ambrose CM, Duyao MP, Gusella JF. Capturing a CAGey killer. In: Davies KE, Warren ST, eds. Genome Analysis, vol 7. Cold Spring Harbor, NY: Cold Spring Harbor Laboratory, 1993, pp. 25–42.

Martin JB, Gusella JF. Huntington's disease: pathogenesis and management. N Engl J Med 1986;315:1267–1276.

Nasir J, Floresco JB, O'Kusky JR, et al. Targeted disruption of the Huntington's disease gene results in embryonic lethality and behavioral and morphological changes in heterozygotes. Cell 1995;81:811–823.

Persichetti F, Ambrose CM, Ge P, et al. Normal and expanded Huntington's disease alleles produce distinguishable proteins due to translation across the CAG repeat. Mol Med 1995;1:374–383.

Schöls L, Menezes Saecker-Vieira AM, Schöls S, et al. Trinucleotide expansion within the MJD1 gene presents clinically as spinocerebellar ataxia and occurs most frequently in German SCA patients. Hum Mol Genet 1995;4:1001–1005.

Vessie PR. On the transmission of Huntington's chorea for 300 years: the Bures family group. J Nerv Ment Dis 1932;76:553–573.

Vonsattel J-P, Myers RH, Stevens TJ, et al. Neuropathological classification of Huntington's disease. J Neuropathol Exp Neurol 1985;44: 559–577.

White JK, Auerbach W, Duyao MP, et al. Huntingtin is required for neurogenesis and is not impaired the Huntington's disease CAG expansion. Nature Genet 1997;17:404–410.

World Federation of Neurology Research Group on Huntington's Disease. Ethical issues policy statement on Huntington's disease molecular genetics predictive test. J Med Genet 1990;27:34–38.

Yazawa I, Nukina N, Hashida H, et al. Abnormal gene product identified in hereditary dentorubral-pallidoluysian atrophy (DRPLA) brain. Nat Genet 1995;10:99–103.

Zeitlin S, Liu J-P, Chapman DL, et al. Increased apoptosis and early embryonic lethality in mice nullizygous for the Huntington's disease gene homologue. Nat Genet 1995;11:155–162.

Zoghbi HY, Orr HT. Spinocerebellar ataxia type 1. Semin Cell Biol 1995;6:29–35.

98 Molecular Genetics of Alzheimer's Disease

P. H. St. George–Hyslop

INTRODUCTION

Alzheimer's disease (AD) (OMIM 104300) is a common degenerative disorder of the human central nervous system. The disease is characterized clinically by the onset of a slowly progressive impairment of memory and most other higher cognitive functions during mid to late adult life. The illness, which typically follows a progressive course over 5–15 years, ultimately renders the patient bedridden, and eventually results in death from intercurrent illness such as pneumonia. The neuropathological hallmarks of AD include the widespread loss of neurons from many areas of the brain, but especially from the cerebral cortex and hippocampus. In addition, many neurons in the cerebral cortex and hippocampus show the presence of an intracellular aggregate of fibrillary proteins composed of hyperphosphorylated Tau, which at the level of electron microscopy appear as aggregates of paired helical filaments (PHF), and at the level of light microscopy appear as neurofibrillary tangles (NFTs). Some neurons also show evidence of granulovacuolar degeneration. The final conventional neuropathological hallmark of AD is widespread and often severe extracellular deposition of the amyloid β (Aβ) peptide. These deposits of Aβ peptide, which are derived from proteolytic cleavage of the full-length precursor protein known as β-amyloid precursor protein (βAPP), may occur as amorphous spherical deposits with little associated reaction in the surrounding neuropil (diffuse or pre-amyloid plaques). Alternatively, the Aβ peptide deposits may be associated with swollen dystrophic neurites containing paired helical filaments, with activated microglia and reactive astrocytes (mature or senile plaques). It is thought, but not proven, that the mature senile plaques represent a progression from earlier diffuse plaques.

The etiology of AD appears complex. Multiple epidemiological studies have repeatedly shown that the risk for acquiring AD is age-dependent and is increased in the presence of a family history of this disease. There is also evidence from some but not all epidemiological studies that risk for AD may be increased with a prior history of significant head trauma and with lower levels of education. Less clear-cut risk factors include exposure to heavy metals such as aluminium, depression, hyperthyroidism, and a family history of Down's syndrome.

The repeated observation in multiple epidemiological surveys that a positive family history is a strong risk factor for AD clearly suggests that genetic factors play a role in this disease. Attempts to dissect the nature of this genetic contribution using epidemiological techniques have been difficult to interpret for a variety of technical reasons including the fact that the disease has a late onset that allows censoring from death (by other disorders), and the absence of definitive antimortem diagnostic tools. Thus, early studies reported risks to first-degree relatives (parents, siblings, or children) that varied between 3 and 14%. More recent studies using life-table techniques suggest that the risk to first-degree relatives is much higher and varies from 24% to over 50% by age 90. Studies of twins, which are also affected by the same confounding factors, suggest concordance rates amongst monozygotic twins of 40–50% compared with a lower concordance rate in dizygotic twins (10–15%). More recently, attempts at segregation analysis using information on family members of probands with AD have also been applied. These studies suggest that pedigrees with an early age of onset cumulatively show a pattern of segregation compatible with autosomal dominant inheritance with age-dependent penetrance. Conversely, late-onset families have a more complicated pattern of inheritance, which could be compatible with one of several genetic models including a high-frequency, low-penetrance single gene disorder or a multifactorial model in which several genes and/or nongenetic factors interact. Nevertheless, despite the apparent complexity of the general model of etiologic factors causing AD derived from the epidemiological surveys, there is clear evidence that some cases of AD are inherited through families as a simple autosomal dominant trait with complete or very high age-dependent penetrance. These families, although somewhat rare, have recently been used for molecular genetics studies, which have led to the discovery of four different genes that confer inherited risk for AD.

THE β-AMYLOID PRECURSOR PROTEIN GENE

The β-amyloid precursor protein gene (βAPP) (OMIM 104760) was the first gene found to bear mutations capable of causing early-onset familial AD (FAD). The βAPP gene, which has been mapped to chromosome 21, encodes an alternatively spliced single spanning transmembrane protein. The longer isoform, which contains 770 amino acids, contains two exons, which encode a Kunitz protease inhibitor domain and a 19–amino acid sequence homologous to the *ox*-2 antigen, and is expressed in most tissues. In contrast, a shorter isoform containing 695 amino acids is predominantly expressed in brain (Fig. 98-1). Several other rare splice forms are known. The immature protein undergoes O- and N-glycosylation and phosphorylation, and a complex pattern of

From: *Principles of Molecular Medicine* (J. L. Jameson, ed.), ©1998 Humana Press Inc., Totowa, NJ.

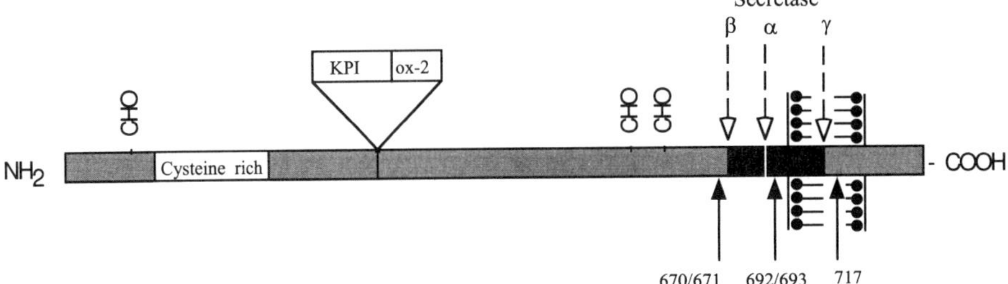

Figure 98-1 Cartoon of the functional domains of the β*APP* gene. The N-terminus is located in the extracellular domain and contains a signal peptide (not shown), a cysteine-rich region (white box), and several putative O- and N-glycosylation sites (CHO). Exons 7 and 8 of the β*APP* gene are alternatively spliced at residue 289 and encode the Kunitz protease inhibitor (KPI) and ox-2 domains, respectively. The Aβ peptide (black box) spans the end of the extracellular domain and part of the transmembrane domain. The location of the transmembrane domain is depicted by the lipid bilayer cartoon. The short C-terminal domain is intracellular. Open-headed arrows, the sites of the secretase cleavages; solid arrows, the sites of the pathogenic mutations.

Table 98-1
Missense Mutations in the βAPP Gene[a]

Codon	*Mutation*	*Phenotype*
665	Gln→Asp	Late-onset AD, no segregation
670/671	Lys-Met→Asn-Leu	FAD; increased Aβ production
673	Ala→Thr	No disease phenotype
692	Ala→Gly	FAD + cerebral hemorrhage; increased Aβ
693	Glu→Gly	Late onset AD, no segregation
	Glu→Gln	HCHWA-D
713	Ala→Val	Schizophrenia, no segregation
	Ala→Thr	AD, no segregation
717	Val→Ile	FAD; increased long Aβ isoforms
	Val→Phe	FAD
	Val→Gly	FAD

[a]Some mutations have been found in elderly asymptomatic subjects or have not been present in all affected subjects, raising the question as to whether these mutations are simple benign polymorphisms or pathogenic mutations with incomplete penetrance.

metabolism through the trans-Golgi network before passage to the cell surface *(see below)*. The Aβ peptide is a proteolytic cleavage product of the full-length protein derived from residues 672 to 711 that spans the last 28 residues of the "extracellular" domain and the first 14 residues of the transmembrane domain (encoded by exons 16 and 17). The function of the βAPP gene is unknown, although roles in cell adhesion, synaptic growth, or neural repair have been proposed. The βAPP gene may also function as a G-coupled receptor linked through an interaction in the C-terminus to $G_{0\alpha}$-protein (this putative linkage may have several levels of significance, including signal transduction and regulation of intracellular protein trafficking).

The candidacy of βAPP as the site of mutations causing AD was supported by four observations. First, a 40- to 43-amino acid proteolytic cleavage product of βAPP, termed the Aβ peptide, is a major component of the amyloid plaque of AD. Second, genetic linkage studies had implicated the existence of an FAD gene in some pedigrees in approximately the same region of chromosome 21 as the βAPP gene. Third, patients with trisomy 21, who would be expected to carry an extra copy of the βAPP gene, almost invariably develop at least the neuropathological attributes of AD by age 40. Finally, a glutamate to glutamine missense mutation at codon 693 of the βAPP gene had been discovered in subjects with a rare cerebral vascular disorder known as hereditary cerebral hemorrhage with amyloidosis (Dutch-variant) (HCHWA-D), which is characterized by severe deposition of Aβ within blood vessel walls and with modest numbers of diffuse amyloid plaques within the brain parenchyma. Subsequent analysis of the βAPP gene in some pedigrees with FAD led to the discovery of missense mutations at three other codons (Table 98-1). In addition, several other missense amino acid substitutions have been discovered, but their relationship to disease states is less clear-cut, either because they have also been observed in elderly subjects without disease or because they were not present in all AD-affected members of the kindred in which the mutation was discovered.

An examination of the position of pathogenic mutations in the βAPP gene revealed that their locations were probably nonrandom and appeared to be positioned around residues that are important in the cleavage of full-length βAPP into the 40- to 43-amino acid Aβ peptide (*see* Table 98-1). A number of studies conducted on cultured cell lines and a more limited analysis of homogenates of brain tissue suggested that βAPP is metabolized through two different routes (Fig. 98-2). The first route, known as the α-secretase pathway, involves cleavage of the full-length βAPP molecule between residues 687 and 688 (using numbering of the 770 isoform), which in effect cleaves βAPP within the residues that would form the Aβ peptide (at residues 16 and 17 of the Aβ peptide). This pathway, therefore, leads to the release of a large soluble N-terminal fragment equivalent to protease nexin II, and the retention in the membrane of a C-terminal fragment of approximately 10 kDa in size, which is then further processed by γ-secretase to render a short 20–amino acid peptide termed p3. It appears that the α-secretase (nonamyloidogenic) cleavage can occur both at the cell surface and in the secretory pathway on the way to the cell surface.

The alternate pathway for cleavage of βAPP occurs in the endosome-lysosome network either after reinternalization of surface of βAPP or during passage through the endoplasmic reticulum and trans-Golgi network. This β-secretase pathway gives rise to the Aβ peptide through N-terminal cleavage at residues 671 and 672 (770 isoform numbering) by β-secretase, and C-terminal cleavage by γ-secretase at residues that have not been clearly defined. The Aβ peptide, or rather the range of peptides with sizes varying from 40 to 43 amino acids in length, that is produced by this pathway is a normal physiologic secretory product of many cell types. However, this pathway is also thought to be the principal source of Aβ peptide forming the amyloid plaque.

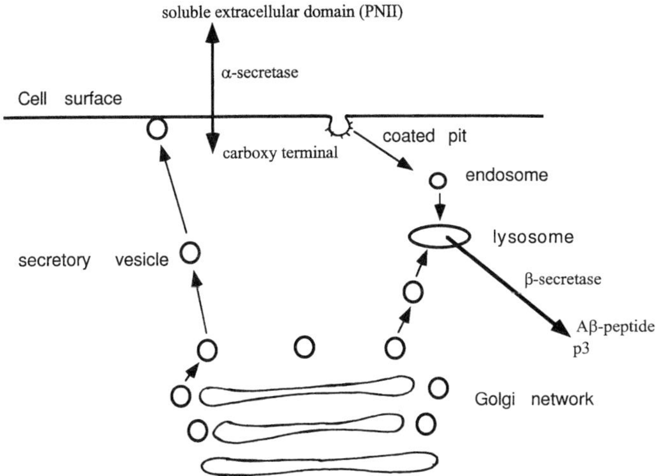

Figure 98-2 Processing pathways for βAPP. The immature βAPP protein undergoes O- and N-terminal glycosylation in the Golgi, and then either it is transported to the cell surface, where it may be cleaved within the Aβ peptide by α-secretase (nonamyloidogenic pathway) to release the soluble N-terminus while the C-terminus is cleaved by γ-secretase to generate the p3 fragment, or the mature βAPP can be cleaved in the post-Golgi endosome-lysosome pathway at the N-terminus and C-terminus of Aβ by β-secretase and γ-secretase, respectively, to liberate Aβ (amyloidogenic pathway).

While both the α-secretase and the β-secretase pathways appear to be physiological, the relative balance of the two pathways seems to be controlled by a number of events including the phosphorylation state of the cell. In addition, the pathogenic mutations in the *βAPP* gene also appear to influence the relative activities of these βAPP processing pathways. Thus, the double mutation at codon 670 and 671 which substitutes the lysine-methionine residues with asparagine-leucine (Swedish mutation) is a better substrate for β-secretase, which, as noted earlier, cleaves at the N-terminus of the Aβ peptide between residue 671 and 672 of βAPP. The Ala692Gly (Flemish) mutation and the HCHWA-D mutation at codon 692 are both located close to the putative α-secretase cleavage site between residues 687 and 688. The Ala692Gly mutation appears to inhibit normal α-secretase cleavage and therefore promotes passage through the β-secretase pathway, thus leading to a higher relative production of Aβ peptide. The Ala692Gly mutation also increases the N-terminal heterogeneity of the Aβ peptide, which may result in the production of slightly hydrophobic peptides, which could aggregate more easily into insoluble β-pleated sheet conformations.

Constitutively secreted Aβ normally terminates at residue 711 (residue 40 of the Aβ peptide). Smaller proportions of the Aβ peptide are secreted in longer isoforms with 42 or 43 amino acids ending at position 713 or 714 of βAPP. The mutations at codon 717, which are located three residues outside the C-terminus of the Aβ peptide, appear to increase the relative proportion of Aβ peptides with 42 amino acid residues. These longer isoforms are more hydrophobic and may therefore also be more prone to aggregate into β-pleated sheet conformation.

Cumulatively, the observations on the physiological processing of βAPP, and on the effects of pathogenic mutations in the *βAPP* gene have led to the thesis that the aberrant processing of full-length βAPP into the Aβ peptides is one of the central biochemical events leading to AD. One potential mechanism by which the apparent production of Aβ peptide might lead to neurodegeneration is provided by the observation that the Aβ peptide, while a physiologic product of cells, can undergo a conformational change that renders the Aβ peptide neurotoxic. As noted above, the longer isoforms (e.g., $A\beta_{1-42}$) are particularly prone to undergoing this conformational change and become neurotoxic, whereas shorter isoforms like the normally secreted $A\beta_{1-40}$ tend to be more soluble. The exact mechanisms by which cell death occurs after exposure to neurotoxic Aβ isoforms is unclear but might involve potentiation of excitotoxic injury, alterations in intracellular calcium homeostasis, and activation of apoptotic cell death pathways. Nevertheless, attempts are now being made to generate compounds that will inhibit either Aβ peptide production, Aβ peptide aggregation, or its neurotoxic effects.

APOLIPOPROTEIN E

Studies implicating the apolipoprotein (APOE) (OMIM 107741) gene as an AD susceptibility locus derived from several intersecting lines of investigation. First, genetic linkage studies conducted on a large series of late-onset AD families provided evidence suggesting the presence of genetic linkage and/or association to a region of chromosome 19q13. Second, APOE immunoreactivity had been detected in senile plaques and NFTs of patients with AD. Third, analysis of proteins in the cerebral spinal fluid that were able to bind to immobilized Aβ peptide revealed the presence of APOE. Finally, association studies revealed that inheritance of the ε4 allele (Cys112Arg) of the APOE gene is associated with 1) a copy number–dependent increase in risk of both sporadic and late-onset FAD and 2) a decrease in the age of onset for late-onset AD. Conversely, the ε2 allele confers a protective effect against late-onset AD. It also seems likely that the genotype at APOE can modify the age of symptom onset in subjects carrying certain βAPP mutations (especially Val717Ile) and perhaps the mutations in the presenilin 2 *(PS2)* gene *(see below).*

While the association between increased risk for AD with inheritance of the ε4 allele and decreased risk for AD associated with inheritance for the ε2 allele has now been confirmed in multiple studies in many different racial groups, there remains some controversy as to whether the inheritance of the ε4 allele is sufficient by itself to cause this disease. Furthermore, while the association with AD is unambiguous, some but not all studies have suggested that the ε4 allele may also be associated with a variety of other neurodegenerative diseases including Creutzfeldt-Jakob disease, Lewy body variant of AD, and multi-infarct dementia, as well as with a poorer outcome after head injury and stroke. The latter observations suggest that the apo E ε4 allele might act as a modulator of the regenerative response to selected types of neural injury. Moreover, unlike the missense mutations in the *βAPP*, *PS1*, and *PS2* genes, the predictive value of the presence of an ε4 allele in presymptomatic subjects is unclear. Nevertheless, the discovery of the presence of the ε4 allele in a subject with a clinical picture compatible with AD may have some usefulness as an ancillary diagnostic test when performed in conjunction with the usual battery of clinical tests used in the work-up of patients presenting with dementia.

The mechanism by which the inheritance of the ε4 allele of APOE increases risk for AD, and how this might be addressed therapeutically, is unclear. It has been suggested that APOE is a chaperon for Aβ and that the ε4 allele more avidly binds Aβ and either promotes assembly into pathologic fibrils or inhibits its

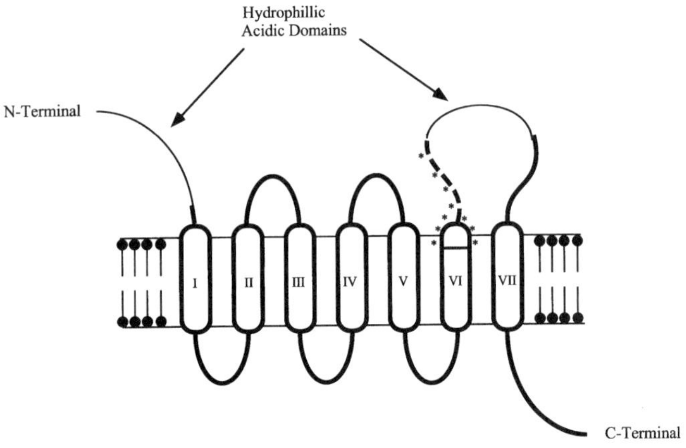

Figure 98-3 Cartoon of a putative structure of the presenilin genes. Thin lines, sequences that are poorly conserved between the presenilin 1 and presenilin 2 genes; bold lines, conserved domains. The region depicted by asterisks is alternatively spliced in some tissues.

clearance possibly through competition for the low-density lipoprotein receptor–related protein, LRP. Conversely, it has been proposed that the unphosphorylated microtubule-associated protein, Tau, which is involved in the formation of the paired helical filaments, is bound avidly by ε3 but not by ε4, thereby, in the presence ε4, more easily allowing the formation of PHF. Finally, it is possible that the different APOE alleles might exert their effects through different mechanisms of lipid recycling and/or on neural repair.

THE *PRESENILIN* GENES ON CHROMOSOME 14q24.3 AND CHROMOSOME 1

Genetic linkage studies using large numbers of pedigrees with early onset autosomal dominant FAD mapped a common locus *(AD3)* (OMIM 104311) to chromosome 14q24.3. It has been estimated that the *AD3* locus, which is associated with a particularly aggressive form of early onset AD (onset between 30 and 60 years of age), accounts for up to 50% of cases of early onset FAD. Subsequent positional cloning studies led to the isolation of a novel gene termed presenilin 1 *(PS1)* because of its association with presenile dementia of the Alzheimer type. Although the function of the *PS1* gene is unknown, the predicted amino acid sequence for the *PS1* cDNA implies that it is probably an integral membrane protein with at least seven hydrophobic membrane-spanning domains and two acidic hydrophilic domains located at the N-terminus and between transmembrane domain 6 and transmembrane domain 7 (Fig. 98-3). The amino acid sequence of the presenilin 1 protein shows strong homology to a *C. elegans* gene, sel12. Loss-of-function mutations in *sel12* suppress developmental phenotypes arising from activating mutations in the *lin12/notch* gene. While the mechanism by which *sel12* suppressed *lin12/notch* mutations is unclear, the role of notch in intercellular signaling during cell fate determination in development has suggested that the human presenilins may also have a function within signal transduction pathways. However, the amino acid sequence of presenilin 1 also shows weaker homology to that of another *C. elegans* protein, SPE-4, which is thought to be involved in membrane budding and fusion events in a membrane-bound cytoplasmic organelle derived from the Golgi network in spermatocytes of *C. elegans*. In addition, weaker amino acid sequence similarities are also present between presenilin 1 and a number of ion channels, and there is some structural similarity to G-coupled receptors, which also have seven membrane-spanning domains. Finally, studies of cDNA sequences capable of rescuing lymphocytes from apoptosis led to the isolation of a cDNA that was capable of suppressing apoptosis in T cells, and which contained the C-terminus of the *PS1* homolog called *PS2 (see below)*. As a result, three putative functions have been proposed. The first proposes a role in membrane budding and fusion events during protein trafficking in the endoplasmic reticulum or Golgi apparatus (which significantly is the site of βAPP metabolism). The second putative function is either a role in intracellular ion homeostasis (particularly calcium metabolism, which is thought to be abnormal in AD) or intracellular signaling pathways. Finally, there may be a role in modulation of cell death mechanisms. Mutational analysis of the *PS1* gene has led to the discovery of at least 12 different mutations in residues that are highly conserved in evolution (Table 98-2). Unlike the mutations in the *βAPP* gene, the *PS1* mutations have not been focused on a single domain, but are placed in the hydrophobic membrane spanning domains as well as in the hydrophilic exposed domains.

Table 98-2
Missense Mutations in the Presenilin Genes

Codon	*Location*	*Mutation*	*Phenotype*
Presenilin 1			
82	TM1	Val→Leu	FAD, onset 55 years
96	TM1	Val→Phe	FAD
115	TM1→TM2 loop	Tyr→His	FAD, onset 37 years
136	TM2	Met→Thr	FAD, onset 49 years
143	TM2	Ile→Thr	FAD, onset 35 years
146	TM2	Met→Leu	FAD, onset 45 years
163	TM3 interface	His→Arg	FAD, onset 50 years
171	TM3	Leu→Pro	FAD, onset 35 years
210	TM4 interface	Ile→Thr	FAD
231	TM5	Ala→Thr	FAD, onset 52 years
246	TM6	Ala→Glu	FAD, onset 55 years
260	TM6	Ala→Val	FAD, onset 40 years
264	TM6	Pro→Leu	FAD, onset 45 years
285	TM6→TM7 loop	Ala→Val	FAD, onset 50 years
286	TM6→TM7 loop	Leu→Val	FAD, onset 50 years
del291-319	TM6→TM7 loop	Ex10 splice defect	FAD
384	TM6→TM7 loop	Gly→Ala	FAD, onset 35 years
392	TM6→TM7 loop	Leu→Val	FAD, onset 25–40 years
410	TM7	Cys→Tyr	FAD, onset 48 years
Presenilin 2			
141	TM2	Asn→Ile	FAD (Volga German), onset 50–65 years
239	TM5	Met→Val	FAD (Florence), onset variable

Immediately following the isolation of the *PS1* gene, causing the *AD3* subtype of FAD, a second gene (termed presenilin 2) was discovered on the basis of its strong nucleotide and amino acid sequence homology to the *PS1* gene. The *PS2* gene (OMIM 600759), which is located on chromosome 1, encodes a protein of 448 amino acids and has a structural organization very similar to that of *PS1*, including at least seven transmembrane domains and two large acidic hydrophilic domains at the N-terminus and between transmembrane domain 6 and 7. The strong amino acid sequence homology (greater than 60% amino acid sequence identity) and the obvious structural similarities suggest that the *PS1* and the *PS2* genes are members of a gene family. The principal differences between these genes are in the amino acid sequence of the acidic hydrophilic domains of their respective proteins, and in the patterns of tissue specific expression. The *PS1* gene is expressed at moderate levels in most tissues, whereas the *PS2* gene is expressed at somewhat lower levels in most tissues, including brain, but is expressed at quite high levels in pancreas, skeletal muscle, and cardiac muscle. Mutational analysis of the *PS2* gene in pedigrees with FAD in which mutations in the βAPP and *PS1* genes had been excluded led to the discovery of two different mutations in the *PS2* gene; one in a pedigree of Italian origin, the other in a group of related families of Volga German ancestry. The clinical phenotype associated with mutations of the PS2 gene has a later onset than the phenotype associated with mutations in the *PS1* gene or βAPP genes (onset 50–70 years). Furthermore, it appears that the age of onset of clinical symptoms in carriers of *PS2* mutations can be dramatically modified over a range of 40 years by as yet unidentified genetic or environmental factors. A similar phenomena has been discovered with some mutations in the βAPP gene where age of onset is reduced by the presence of an APOE ε4 allele and delayed by the presence of an APOE ε2 allele, but is not observed with mutations in the *PS1* gene. A potential explanation for the differences in the clinical phenotypes associated with mutations in the different presenilin genes may arise from differences in their levels of expression or perhaps differences in their specific functions.

OTHER ALZHEIMER'S DISEASE GENES

Although four different genetic loci associated with inherited susceptibility to AD are now known, it has become clear that they do not account for all cases of FAD. Thus, while the APOE ε4 allele is a relatively common risk factor for late-onset AD, at least 40% of subjects with late onset AD (particularly those with onset after age 70 years) do not have the ε4 allele. Mutations in the presenilin 1 gene probably account for up to 70% of very early onset AD (onset before age 60). However, mutations in the βAPP and the presenilin 2 genes, which are respectively associated with onsets at 45–60 years and 50–70 years, account for only a small proportion of familial cases with ages of onset between 50 and 70 years of age. Consequently, it seems highly likely that at least one, and possibly several, other genes causing inherited susceptibility to AD must exist elsewhere in the genome. A late-onset form of AD may be caused by mutations in the mitochondrial cytochrome-c oxidase 1 and 2 genes (*see* Chapter 103). Attempts to identify these other AD susceptibility genes are currently underway using both conventional genetic linkage strategies and nonparametric association methods.

ANIMAL MODELS

In addition to providing a known starting point for biochemical studies designed to elucidate the biochemical pathophysiology of this disease, the discovery of AD susceptibility genes also provides a means to generate animal models. Such animal models would be useful both in the molecular dissection of this disease and in the preclinical testing of potential treatments. Several transgenic lines have been created using a variety of βAPP constructs, and have met with varying degrees of success. The most successful model to date has been a transgenic line in which a mutant human βAPP minigene has been placed under the control of the platelet-derived growth factor receptor β-subunit promoter. This animal model developed severe cerebral Aβ amyloidosis with abundant amyloid plaques, which showed some neuritic dystrophy and synaptic pathology. Classical NFTs, however, were not observed. The reason why this particular transgenic line was more successful in recapitulating at least part of the AD phenotype is unclear but may reflect either the strong promoter employed or a special vulnerability of the strain of mouse used. If the latter hypothesis were proven correct, mapping of other loci within the mouse genome that are capable of altering susceptibility of the mouse to AD amyloidosis could provide a rapid means to identify other human genes that would modify human susceptibility to this disease. Manipulation of the expression of these modifier genes could potentially be used therapeutically to treat human AD.

SELECTED REFERENCES

Caporaso GL, Gandy SE, Buxbaum JD, Ramabhadram TV, Greengard P. Protein phosphorylation regulates secretion of Alzheimer B/A4 amyloid precursor protein. Proc Natl Acad Sci USA 1992;89:3055–3059.

Citron M, Oltersdorf T, Haass C, et al. Mutation of the β-amyloid precursor protein in familial Alzheimer's disease increases β-protein production. Nature 1992;360:672–674.

Corder EH, Saunders AM, Risch NJ, et al. Apolipoprotein E type 2 allele decreases the risk of late-onset Alzheimer disease. Nat Genet 1994;7:180–184.

Davis RE, Miller S, Herrnstadt C, et al. Mutations in mitochondrial cytochrome c oxidase genes segregate with late-onset Alzheimer disease. Proc Natl Acad Sci USA 1997;94:4526–4531.

Farrer LA, Myers RH, Connor L, Cupples LA, Growdon JH. Segregation analysis reveals evidence of a major gene for Alzheimer disease. Am J Hum Genet 1991;48:1026–1033.

Games D, Adams D, Alessandrini A, et al. Alzheimer-type neuropathology in transgenic mice overexpressing V717F beta-amyloid precursor protein. Nature 1995;373:523–527.

Goate AM, Chartier-Harlin M-C, Mullan M, et al. Segregation of a missense mutation in the amyloid precursor protein gene with familial Alzheimer disease. Nature 1991;349:704–706.

Golde TE, Estus S, Younkin LH, Selkoe DJ, Younkin SG. Processing of the amyloid protein precursor to potentially amyloidogenic derivatives. Science 1992;255:728–730.

Goldgaber D, Lerman MI, McBride OW, et al. Characterization and chromosomal localization of a cDNA encoding brain amyloid of Alzheimer's disease. Science 1987;235:877–880.

Haass C, Koo EH, Mellon A, Hung AY, Selkoe DJ. Targetting of cell surface β-amyloid precursor protein to lysosomes: alternative processing into amyloid bearing fragments. Nature 1992;357: 500–503.

Hendricks M, van Duijn CM, Cras P, et al. Presenile dementia and cerebral hemorrhage linked to a mutation at codon 692 of the β-amyloid precursor protein gene. Nat Genet 1992;1:218–221.

Hill LR, Klauber MR, Salmon DP, et al. Functional status, education, and the diagnosis of dementia in the Shanghai survey. Neurology 1993;43:138–145.

Kang J, Lemaire HG, Unterbeck A, et al. The precursor of Alzheimer disease amyloid A4 protein resembles a cell surface receptor. Nature 1987;325:733–736.

Katzman R. Alzheimer's disease. N Engl J Med 1986;314:964–973.

Katzman R, Kawas C. The epidemiology of dementia and Alzheimer disease. In: Alzheimer disease. New York: Raven, 1994, pp. 105–122.

Kitaguchi N, Takahashi Y, Tokushima Y, Shiojiri S, Ito H. Novel precursor of Alzheimer's disease amyloid protein shows protease inhibitory activity. Nature 1988;331:530–532.

Levy E, Carman MD, Fernandez-Madrid IJ, et al. Mutation of the Alzheimer's disease amyloid gene in hereditary cerebral hemorrhage—Dutch type. Science 1990;248:1124–1126.

Mann DM, Brown A, Prinja D, et al. An analysis of the morphology of senile plaques in Down's syndrome patients of different ages using immunocytochemical and lectin histochemical techniques. Neuropathol Appl Neurobiol 1989;15:317–329.

Mullan MJ, Crawford F, Axelman K, et al. A pathogenic mutation for probable Alzheimer's disease in the APP gene at the N-terminus of β-amyloid. Nat Genet 1992;1:345–347.

Rogaev EI, Sherrington R, Rogaeva EA, et al. Familial Alzheimer's disease in kindreds with missense mutations in a novel gene on chromosome 1 related to the Alzheimer's disease type 3 gene. Nature 1995;376:775–778.

Saunders A, Strittmatter WJ, Schmechel S, et al. Association of apoliprotein E allele ε4 with the late-onset familial and sporadic Alzheimer disease. Neurology 1993;43:1467–1472.

Selkoe DJ. Normal and abnormal biology of β-amyloid precursor protein. Annu Rev Neurosci 1994;17:489–517.

Sherrington R, Rogaev E, Liang Y, et al. Cloning of a gene bearing missense mutations in early onset familial Alzheimer's disease. Nature 1995;375:754–760.

Sisodia S. Beta-amyloid precursor protein cleavage by a membrane bound protease. Proc Natl Acad Sci USA 1993;89:6075–6079.

St. George–Hyslop PH, Haines JL, Farrer LA, et al. Genetic linkage studies suggest that Alzheimer's disease is not a single homogeneous disorder. Nature 1991;347:194–197.

Strittmatter WJ, Saunders AM, Schmechel D, et al. Apolipoprotein E: high affinity binding to B/A4 amyloid and increased frequency of type 4 allele in familial Alzheimer's disease. Proc Natl Acad Sci USA 1993;90:1977–1981.

Susuki N, Cheung TT, Cai X-D, et al. An increased percentage of long amyloid β protein secreted by familial amyloid β protein precursor (BAPP717) mutants. Science 1994;264:1336–1340.

Yan SD, Chen X, Fu J, et al. RAGE and amyloid-beta peptide neurotoxicity in Alzheimer's disease. Nature 1996;382:685–691.

99 Amyotrophic Lateral Sclerosis and Related Motor Neuron Diseases

MERET E. CUDKOWICZ AND ROBERT H. BROWN, JR.

INTRODUCTION

The last decade has witnessed considerable progress in elucidating the genetic and molecular basis of inherited motor neuron diseases. Determination of specific gene defects causing motor neuron illness provides insights into the neurobiology of the motor neuron and into the pathogenesis of both inherited and sporadic forms of motor neuron disease. These insights are critical in guiding the development of treatment strategies. This chapter provides an overview of motor neuron disorders, with a particular focus on recent studies of amyotrophic lateral sclerosis.

CLINICAL FEATURES AND DIFFERENTIAL DIAGNOSIS

AMYOTROPHIC LATERAL SCLEROSIS (ALS) It is convenient to classify motor neuron diseases anatomically into three groups that involve: (1) both motor neurons in brainstem and spinal cord (lower motor neurons), and corticospinal and corticobulbar motor neurons (upper motor neurons); (2) only lower motor neurons; and (3) only upper motor neurons (Table 99-1). Amyotrophic lateral sclerosis (ALS) is a progressive neurodegenerative disease that falls into the first group. The prevalence of ALS is 4–6 cases per 100,000 with an incidence of 0.4–1.8 per 100,000. The majority of ALS cases are sporadic. However, 10–15% of cases are inherited as an autosomal dominant trait (familial ALS, autosomal dominant: FALS-AD; OMIM 105400); very rare cases have an autosomal recessive inheritance pattern. The sporadic and FALS-AD forms of ALS are clinically and pathologically identical. Age and sex are the only ALS risk factors repeatedly documented in epidemiological studies. The median age of onset is 55, and the median survival is less than five years. Ten percent of cases begin before age 40 and only rarely before age 30. There is a slight male predominance (3:2 male-to-female ratio).

The distinctive clinical and pathological features of ALS were first described in 1869 by Charcot. Clinical signs of both lower and upper motor neuron involvement are necessary for a definitive diagnosis. The former include weakness and muscle atrophy, usually beginning asymmetrically and distally in one limb, and then spreading within the neuraxis to involve contiguous groups of motor neurons. Upper motor neuron involvement is heralded by weakness with spasticity or muscle stiffness. Symptoms can begin either in bulbar or limb muscles. In this and most other motor neuron diseases, there is relative sparing of muscles of eye movement and of urinary sphincters. Respiratory failure may be an early manifestation in patients with bulbar onset. It is usually a later development in limb-onset cases and ultimately proves fatal in virtually all cases of ALS.

From: *Principles of Molecular Medicine* (J. L. Jameson, ed.), ©1998 Humana Press Inc., Totowa, NJ.

DISORDERS OF LOWER MOTOR NEURONS Several diseases are characterized by selective involvement of lower motor neurons. These are distinguished from ALS by the absence of corticospinal or corticobulbar tract involvement and, in many instances, a slower rate of progression. Multifocal motor neuropathy with conduction block (MMNCB) is a treatable lower motor neuropathy characterized by multifocal disruption of motor nerve conduction. This disease often begins asymmetrically in the upper extremities. In most instances focal onset, absence of corticospinal findings, and slow progression (several years) distinguish MMNCB from ALS. The diagnostic test for MMNCB is electromyography (EMG), which reveals focal motor conduction failure, defined by a loss of greater than 50% of the amplitude of the compound motor action potential. This disease is thought to be autoimmune, both because many affected individuals have high titers of antibodies to GM1 ganglioside and because many respond dramatically to treatment with intravenous immunoglobulin (iv Ig). Some individuals fail to respond to iv Ig but improve with high-dose cyclophosphamide therapy. Lymphoma-associated motor neuron disease is a rare disorder described in patients with both Hodgkin's and non-Hodgkin's lymphoma. Laboratory tests often reveal a monoclonal gammopathy, elevated cerebrospinal fluid (CSF) protein and the presence of oligoclonal bands in the CSF. Postpoliomyelitis muscular atrophy is a slowly progressive motor neuropathy that arises several decades after partial or complete recovery from acute, paralytic poliomyeltis. The course is slow and progressive.

Three disorders of the lower motor neuron are inherited. X-linked spinal bulbar atrophy (OMIM 313200) affects males in early adulthood and presents with slowly progressive limb weakness with prominent bulbar muscle involvement. Tendon reflexes are lost and upper motor neurons signs are absent. There are often active fasciculations about the face. Associated findings include gynecomastia, testicular atrophy, and diminished fertility. Electromyography and muscle biopsy findings show chronic denervation and reinnervation.

Table 99-1
Inherited Motor Neuron Disorders

Disease	*Defect*	*Locus*
Upper and lower motor neurons		
Amyotrophic Lateral Sclerosis		
Dominant, adult onset		
	Superoxide dismutase 1	21q
	Neurofilament heavy subunit	11
Dominant, juvenile onset		9
Recessive, juvenile onset		2q33–35
Lower motor neurons		
Spinal muscular atrophy		5q11.2–13.3
SMA I	Survival motor neuron protein	
SMA II		
SMA III		
SMA IV		
X-linked spinobulbar muscular atrophy	Androgen receptor	Xq11
GM2 gangliosidoses		
Late-onset Tay-Sachs	Hex A deficiency (α subunit)	15q23–24
Sandhoff disease	Hex A+B deficiency (β subunit)	5q11.2–13.6
AB variant	GM2 activator protein	5q
Upper motor neurons		
Familial spastic paraplegia		
Dominant		2p
		14q
		15q
Recessive		8q
X-linked	Proteolipid protein	Xq22
		Xq28

The spinal muscular atrophies (SMAs) are a group of neuromuscular disorders characterized by progressive degeneration of motor neurons in the spinal cord and brainstem. The majority of familial cases have an autosomal recessive mode of inheritance. A smaller number have an autosomal dominant or X-linked inheritance pattern. The most severe form of SMA (type I or Werdnig-Hoffmann disease; OMIM 253300) is a fulminant denervating disease of infants. With an incidence of 1 in 20,000 live births and a carrier frequency of 1:80, this is a relatively common disorder. The other forms (*see* Table 99-1) begin later in life and have a more chronic course. In type I SMA, clinical signs may be evident prenatally, as indicated by diminished fetal movements in the last two or three weeks before birth. In the neonatal period, the infants are severely weak and hypotonic. Problems with nursing and respiratory function are common. The majority of children die before age two, usually from respiratory infections and pulmonary insufficiency. Type II SMA (OMIM 253550) is a childhood form that usually appears before 18 months of age and is associated with survival of several years. Type III, or Kugelberg-Welander disease (OMIM 253400), is also a childhood form, typically beginning after 18 months of age. One may rarely encounter a late childhood or adult-onset form, which produces more pronounced distal weakness. However, it is striking that in these chronic forms, progressive, symmetric weakness is typically more proximal than distal, with leg greater than arm involvement. Indeed, before EMG studies are obtained, the severity of the proximal weakness may erroneously suggest the diagnosis of a primary muscle disease.

At least three forms of GM2 gangliosidosis (type 1, or adult-onset Tay-Sachs disease, OMIM 272800; Sandhoff disease, OMIM 268800; AB variant, OMIM 272750) may have a clinical phenotype that resembles SMA. Affected individuals usually have lifelong incoordination. In the teen or early adult years, they develop progressive proximal weakness with fasciculations, mild denervation atrophy, and EMG abnormalities indicating dysfunction of spinal motor neurons. There may be mild dysarthria and difficulty swallowing. Some patients also develop spasticity and Babinski responses attesting to corticospinal tract involvement. The primary defect in this disease is accumulation of GM2 ganglioside, a consequence of defects either in one of the two enzymes, *N*-acetyl-hexosaminidase A and B (hex A and hex B), which normally metabolize this substrate, or in the protein "GM2 activator," which normally enhances the activity of these two enzymes.

PATHOLOGY

In ALS, the pathological hallmark is selective atrophy and death of corticospinal and corticobulbar neurons in the motor cortex and motor neurons in the brainstem and spinal cord. There is an associated mild proliferation of glial cells. Affected neurons and axons often have cytoskeletal pathology with accumulations of neurofilaments and aggregates of ubiquinated proteins. There is thinning of the anterior roots of the spinal cord with preservation of the posterior sensory roots. As Charcot first noted, the lateral columns of the cord, consisting primarily of long tracts of the descending corticospinal system, may be shrunken and sclerotic. The pathological hallmark of the spinal muscular atrophies is degeneration and loss of anterior horn cells. Affected motor neurons can be strikingly chromatolytic, with swelling of the cell body, dispersion of the endoplasmic reticulum, displacement of the nucleus to an atypical, peripheral position in the soma, and nucleolar hyper-

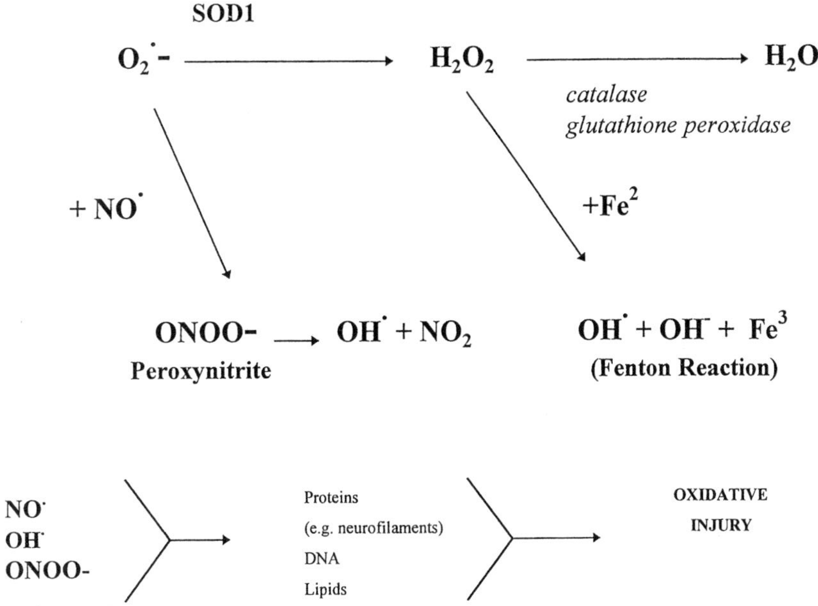

Figure 99-1 Selected normal reactions of superoxide. Top: Superoxide is normally detoxified by SOD1 to hydrogen peroxide, which is then converted to water by catalase and glutathione. Combined with nitric oxide (NO˙), superoxide can also form peroxynitrite (ONOO-), which breaks down nonenzymatically to produce hydroxyl radicals (OH˙). These may also be generated from hydrogen peroxide via Fe^{2+} (Fenton reaction). Bottom: These reactive oxygen species may oxidatively damage DNA, lipids, and proteins.

trophy. In any disease targeting spinal motor neurons, muscle biopsy may reveal evidence of both active denervation, in the form of isolated, angulated, atrophic fibers, and chronic denervation, with either successful reinnervation (fiber-type grouping) or reinnervation followed by successive denervation (atrophy of groups of fibers with identical fiber type). The major pathological abnormality in FSP is corticospinal tract degeneration, which is more pronounced caudally.

FAMILIAL SPASTIC PARAPLEGIAS Familial spastic paraplegias (FSPs) are usually transmitted as autosomal dominant traits and characterized by progressive, spastic weakness beginning in the distal legs (OMIM 182600). Recessive (OMIM 270088) and X-linked (OMIM 312900) forms are also recognized. The age of onset in FSPs varies widely. Because respiration is largely spared, most FSP patients survive several decades. Weakness of the upper extremities is distinctly unusual, as is involvement of the posterior columns and anterior horn cells. FSP may infrequently arise in "complicated" forms associated with involvement of other regions of the nervous system; for example, there may be amyotrophy, mental retardation, sensory neuropathy, and, in some infantile-onset cases, hydrocephalus.

PATHOGENESIS AND GENETICS

AMYOTROPHIC LATERAL SCLEROSIS Many causes of ALS have been proposed including atypical poliovirus infection, prion-mediated neuronal death, intoxication by exogenous metal-toxins (lead, aluminum, and other metals), autoimmune processes targeting motor neurons, and toxicity from excess excitation of the motor neuron by transmitters such as glutamate. The latter is suggested by several observations: brain levels of glutamate are reduced in ALS; glutamate transport is diminished in brains of ALS patients at autopsy; and CSF glutamate levels may be elevated. Moreover, there is growing literature documenting that glutamate is pathological for motor neurons in vitro.

In some cases of FALS, genetic studies have established that the primary defects are mutations in the gene for cytosolic, copper-zinc superoxide dismutase (SOD1). Currently, more than 50 different mutations in SOD1 have been reported exclusively in FALS. Copper-zinc superoxide dismutase is a metalloenzyme of about 153 amino acids that is expressed in all eukaryotic cells. It is one of a family of three SOD enzymes, which include manganese-dependent mitochondrial SOD (SOD2) and copper-zinc extracellular SOD (SOD3). Encoded by five exons, the SOD1 protein functions as a homodimer. Each monomer contains an active site with one ion each of copper and zinc. The primary function of the SOD1 enzyme is to detoxify the superoxide anion by conversion to hydrogen peroxide (Figure 99-1). Hydrogen peroxide is subsequently detoxified by glutathione peroxidase or catalase to form water. Hydrogen peroxide can generate free radicals by reacting with ferric ions to form the hydroxyl radical. Superoxide is potentially toxic by itself, and also can produce the more toxic hydroxyl radical either through formation of hydrogen peroxide or by reaction with nitric oxide. Superoxide interacts with nitric oxide to form the peroxynitrite anion, which may be directly toxic to cells and also generates hydroxyl radicals. An important implication of these biochemical properties of SOD1 is that FALS may arise as a consequence of abnormalities of free radical homeostasis and resulting cellular oxidative stress.

The effects of the FALS mutations on SOD1 function are not fully understood. Whether motor neurons degenerate because SOD1 activity is reduced or because the mutant protein has gained a novel, adverse function remains to be determined. In patients with these SOD1 mutations, but not in sporadic cases or in normal controls, SOD1 activity is reduced by 25–50% in red blood cell lysates, lymphoblastoid cell lines, and brain. The loss of function appears to be due to diminished stability of the mutant protein rather than a loss of intrinsic specific activity or a dominant negative interaction of mutant and wild-type protein in SOD1 heterodimers. Recently, it has been shown that in chronic, organotypic spinal cord cultures partial reduction of activity of SOD1 triggers apoptotic nerve cell death, including fulminant motor neuron death. This death process, in vitro, is reversed by agents that enhance intracellular antioxidant defenses (e.g., *N*-acetylcysteine).

These observations are somewhat enigmatic, as most diseases arising from decreased protein activity, or "loss of function," are recessive. Dominantly inherited diseases, like FALS, are thought to arise because a single mutant allele produces a mutant protein with a novel property that is in some way toxic to the cell. Three arguments indicate that the primary effect of the SOD1 mutations is gain of a toxic function. First, to date, no true null mutations have been identified in SOD1 in FALS patients. If haplo-insufficiency (50% reduction in activity from loss of the product of one allele) triggers the disease, one would anticipate some mutations that block protein expression from the mutant allele (e.g., via premature stop codons or deletions). Such null mutants are conspicuously absent. Second, in most studies, there is not a correlation between the extent of inactivation of SOD1 and any clinical measures of disease severity. The third observation, suggesting that SOD1 mutations may be cytotoxic, is that mice that overexpress high levels of mutant SOD1 protein reportedly develop a lethal, denervating, paralytic disease that resembles ALS clinically and pathologically. In these animals, dendritic processes in motor neurons show microvacuolization, resulting from defects in rough endoplasmic reticulum and mitochondria. Because the total or aggregated SOD1 activity in these animals is above normal, it is difficult to argue that the disease arises from loss of function. The possibility that the high levels of SOD1 activity in the animals triggers the neuronal degeneration is unlikely, as mice overexpressing normal SOD1 to a similar extent do not develop motor neuron disease. These findings support the hypothesis that the primary effect of the SOD1 mutations is a gain of a toxic function. The mechanisms of cytotoxicity of the mutant SOD1 molecule are unclear at this time. It is possible that: (1) the mutant enzyme precipitates to form toxic, cytoplasmic aggregates; (2) the mutant SOD1 molecule has an enhanced affinity for peroxynitrite and, consequently, produces elevated levels of nitronium ions, which catalyze nitration of tyrosines on proteins such as neurofilaments and tyrosine kinase receptors; (3) there is subnormal copper or zinc binding by the enzyme and resulting neurotoxicity from these metals; and (4) some mutant SOD1 proteins are cytotoxic because reduced detoxification of superoxide anion causes an increased level both of this anion and secondarily, peroxynitrite. The latter may nitrate protein tyrosine groups or decompose enzymatically to produce nitrogen dioxide and hydroxyl radical. Studies have also shown that certain mutations in SOD1 (A4V; G93A) catalyze oxidation by hydrogen peroxide at a higher rate than that of the wild-type enzyme, supporting the idea that oxidative reactions may be involved in the pathology of ALS.

More recently, a second genetic defect has been associated with isolated cases of ALS. Two different mutations have been identified in the heavy subunit of neurofilament in five different patients. Because these mutations were not detected in more than 300 DNA samples from normal controls, they are unlikely to be polymorphisms. It remains to be established whether these neurofilament mutations will be present in large series of either familial or sporadic ALS patients. It is pertinent, however, that transgenic mice overexpressing either normal or mutant neurofilament develop a motor neuron disease phenotype. Moreover, mice that express a point mutation in the light neurofilament subunit even more fully reproduce aspects of human ALS pathology. Further, animals intoxicated with the agent β-β-imino-diproprionitirle (IDPN) develop severe neurofibrillary pathology, particularly in the proximal axon, which disrupts axonal transport and thereby impairs motor neuron function. Together, these findings in humans and experimental animals underscore the importance of cytoskeletal protein function for motor neuron viability.

X-LINKED SPINOBULBAR MUSCULAR ATROPHY The genetic defect underlying X-linked spinobulbar muscular atrophy (SBMA) is an expansion of a normally occurring CAG trinucleotide repeat within the coding region of the gene for the androgen receptor on the X chromosome. This leads to an expanded polyglutamine tract within the receptor. The length of the repeated CAG sequence correlates with the severity of the disease. Although first identified in SBMA, this primary defect, an expanded CAG repeat domain, has now been identified in other neurodegenerative disorders including Huntington's disease (OMIM 143100), spinocerebellar ataxia (OMIM 164400), and a rare disorder known as dentatorubopallidoluysian atrophy (DRPLA) (OMIM 125370). As discussed in the chapter on Huntington's disease (Chapter 97), it remains to be established why this defect is so selectively neurotoxic, and why its pathological effect may not be evident until adult life.

FAMILIAL SPASTIC PARAPLEGIAS In the last 2 years, genetic linkage analyses have clearly documented genetic heterogeneity in FSPs. Large FSP pedigrees with dominant inheritance patterns have been linked to loci on chromosome 2p, 14q, and 15q. Other large FSP families are not linked to these loci, indicating there must be yet another locus for dominantly inherited FSP. The observation that there is genetic anticipation in some families has prompted the speculation that FSP may be a trinucleotide repeat disease. A childhood-onset form of uncomplicated FSP has recently been linked to chromosome 8q. In addition, there are both complicated and uncomplicated forms of FSP transmitted as X-linked recessive traits. Genetic studies have detected at least two loci for X-linked FSP at Xq28 and Xq22. In some families the Xq22-linked form arises from mutations in the gene for the central nervous system myelin constituent, protcolipid protein (PLP). Strikingly, different mutations in the same PLP gene cause Pelizaeus-Merzbacher disease, indicating that this disease and some forms of X-linked FSP are allelic variants.

SPINAL MUSCULAR ATROPHIES In 1990 the defect causing spinal muscular atrophies (SMA) was genetically mapped to the proximal portion of the long arm of chromosome 5 (5q11.2–13.3). Most cases of SMA are linked to this locus; it is likely that these disorders all result from mutations within the same gene (allelic heterogeneity). While the specific gene has not yet been definitively identified, two candidate genes were recently reported. Strikingly, one has homology to a viral protein known to inhibit apoptosis. This suggests that SMA might result from loss of antiapoptotic proteins normally required in critical stages of motor neuron differentiation to prevent motor neuron death. It is fortunate that, even in the absence of a definitive gene defect, prenatal testing is now available for SMA using linked polymorphisms; the accuracy of prenatal predication is 90% or greater depending on the individual family.

ANIMAL MODELS

There are currently several mouse models of hereditary motor neuron disease. These include the wobbler (wr), progressive motor neuropathy (pmn), wasted (wst), tumbler (tb) motor neuron disease 1 (mnd1), motor neuron disease 2 (mnd2), transgenic mice overexpressing mutant SOD1, and transgenic mice overexpressing light and heavy neurofilaments subunits (NF-L and NF-H). The motor neuron disease in the mnd1 and transgenic SOD1 mice are inherited as autosomal dominant and are relevant models for ALS. The NF-L and NF-H mice develop progressive weakness and muscular atrophy secondary to denervation. The spinal neurons show extensive neurofilamentous swellings that are prominent in proximal axons and within dorsal root ganglia. The remaining animal models have a lower motor neuropathy with a recessive inheritance pattern, possibly more relevant to the spinal muscular atrophies. The specific genetic defects in these animals have not yet been defined. Therapeutic trials of potential new agents for ALS are already underway in the SOD1 transgenic mice. It is hoped that this model will be a useful method to screen novel therapeutics and a tool to better understand the underlying disease process.

THERAPEUTIC OPTIONS

There is no known therapy for ALS. However, three recent therapeutic trials have been cautiously promising. Riluzole, a drug that inhibits release of glutamate at presynaptic terminals, is reported to extend survival in ALS, although there is no concomitant improvement in strength. Insulin-like growth factor 1 has been reported in preliminary communications to improve strength in ALS patients in a dose-dependent manner. It has been suggested that brain-derived neurotrophic factor (BDNF) augments respiratory function in ALS. To date, full reports of the latter two studies have not been published; it remains to be established how clinically meaningful these drugs will be in ALS. As noted above, multifocal motor neuropathy with conduction block is often effectively treated with immunosuppressive agents such as intravenous gammaglobulin or cyclophosphamide.

Currently, there are no specific treatments for X-linked SBMA, the SMAs, post-polio muscular atrophy, or the FSPs. Prevention and early treatment of respiratory infections, rehabilitation measures, bracing, and treatment of scoliosis are critical to improving and optimizing motor function.

FUTURE DIRECTIONS

Molecular biology has had a profound effect on our understanding of the motor neurons disorders—in particular, familial and sporadic ALS and the spinal muscular atrophies. The investigations of motor neuron diseases summarized here give significant insights into factors important for motor neuron viability. Exactly how important each of these factors is should hopefully become apparent in the near future. The development of several animal models of motor neuron disease should enhance our understanding of these disorders and increase our ability to screen quickly many potential therapeutic agents. One hopes that insights gained from the study of these diseases will enhance our understanding not only of motor neuron diseases but also of other neuron-selective degenerative diseases. Finally, and most importantly, one hopes that the investigation of these issues will lead to effective strategies for treating these diseases.

SELECTED REFERENCES

Bensimon G, Laomblez L, Meininger V, the ALS/Riluzole Study Group. A controlled trial of Riluzole in amyotrophic lateral sclerosis. N Engl J Med 1994;330:585–591.

Borchelt DR, Guarnieri M, Wong PC, et al. Superoxide dismutase 1 with mutations linked to familial amyotrophic lateral sclerosis do not affect wild-type subunit function. J Biol Chem 1995;270:3234–3248.

Bowling AC, Schultz JB, Brown RH Jr, Beal MF. Superoxide dismutase activity, oxidative damage and mitochondrial energy metabolism in familial and sporadic amyotrophic lateral sclerosis. J Neurochem 1993;61:2322–2325.

de Belleroche J, Orrell R, King A. Familial amyotrophiclateral sclerosis/ motor neurone disease (FALS): a review of current developments. J Med Genet 1995;32:841–847.

Deng H-X, Hentati A, Tainer JA, et al. Amyotrophic lateral sclerosis and structural defects in Cu,Zn superoxide dismutase. Science 1993; 261:1047–1051.

Gurney ME, Pu H, Chiu AY, et al. Motor neuron degeneration in mice that express a human Cu,Zn superoxide dismutase mutation. Science 1994;264:1772–1775.

LaSpada AR, Wilson EM, Lubahn DB, et al. Androgen receptor gene mutations in X-linked spinal and bulbar muscular atrophy. Nature 1991;352:77–79.

Kunst CB, Mezey E, Brownstein MJ, Patterson D. Mutations in SOD1 associated with amyotrophic lateral sclerosis cause novel protein interactions. Nat Genet 1997;15:91–94.

Lyons TJ, Liu H, Goto JJ, et al. Mutations in copper-zinc superoxide dismutase that cause amyotrophic lateral sclerosis alter the zinc binding site and the redox behavior of the protein. Proc Natl Acad Sci U S A 1996;93:12,240–12,244.

Mulder DW, Kurland LT, Offord KP, Beard CM. Familial adult motor neuron disease: amyotrophic lateral sclerosis. Neurology 1986; 36:511–517.

Price DL, Cleveland DW, Koliatsis VE. Motor neuron disease and animal models. Neurobiol Dis 1994;1:3–11.

Rosen D, Siddique T, Patterson D, et al. Mutations in Cu/Zn superoxide dismutase are associated with familial amyotrophic lateral sclerosis. Nature 1993;362:59–68.

Rothstein JD, Bristol LA, Hosler B, et al. Chronic inhibition of superoxide dismutase produces apoptotic death of spinal neurons. Proc Natl Acad Sci USA 1994;91:4155–4159.

Saugier-Veber P, Munnich A, Bonneau D, et al. X-linked spastic paraplegia and Pelizaeus-Merzbacher disease are allelic disorders at the proteolipid protein locus. Nat Genet 1994;6:257–262.

Siddique T, Deng H-X. Genetics of amyotrophic lateral sclerosis. Hum Molec Genet 1996;5:1465–1470.

Wiedam-Pazos M, Goto JJ, Rabizadeh S, Gralla EB, Roe JA, Lee MK, Valentine JS, Bresdesen DE. Altered reactivity of superoxide dismutase in familial amyotrophic lateral sclerosis. Science 1996; 271:515–518.

100 Spinocerebellar Ataxia and Other Disorders of Trinucleotide Repeats

HUDA Y. ZOGHBI

INTRODUCTION

Expansion of trinucleotide repeat sequences is now known to be the mutational mechanism in at least seven neurological disorders. These include fragile X syndrome, myotonic dystrophy (DM), spinobulbar muscular atrophy (SBMA), Huntington's disease (HD), spinocerebellar ataxia type 1 (SCA1), dentatorubropallidoluysian atrophy (DRPLA), and Machado-Joseph disease (MJD). The discovery of trinucleotide repeat expansions provides a biological explanation for "anticipation," a poorly understood clinical phenomenon frequently observed in these disorders. So far, only trinucleotide repeats with cytosine-guanine-guanine (CGG), cytosine-adenine-guanine (CAG), or cytosine-thymidine-guanine (CTG) have been associated with disease states, although other polymorphic trinucleotide repeat sequences are widespread in the human genome (please *see* Addendum).

The mechanism underlying the expansion, and occasionally the contraction, of these repeats remains unresolved. It is intriguing that the number of repeat units within the murine homologs of the genes involved in the above human disorders is relatively small, ranging from 2 to 5 repeats, and the repeats are frequently not polymorphic. This raises the question of whether dynamic mutations involving trinucleotide repeat instability are unique to humans and whether the mechanism involving pathologic expansions is influenced by the length and variability within a particular repeat.

The disorders caused by trinucleotide repeat expansions can be divided into three groups based on clinical and molecular distinctions. Five diseases have later onset and are progressively neurodegenerative. These include SBMA, HD, SCA1, DRPLA, the allelic Haw River syndrome (HRS), MJD, and the allelic spinocerebellar ataxia type 3 (SCA3). The expanding repeat in each of these disorders is $(CAG)_n$, which lies within the coding region of the respective gene, and is predicted to encode for glutamine in the protein. The number of repeats on the expanded alleles is not very large, usually about twice the number on normal chromosomes, and ranges between 37 and 121 repeats. All five diseases display a dominant inheritance pattern (modified by the effects of X inactivation in SBMA), suggesting that the phenotype cannot be simply explained by loss of the normal function of the protein after repeat expansion.

From: *Principles of Molecular Medicine* (J. L. Jameson, ed.), ©1998 Humana Press Inc., Totowa, NJ.

The clinical and molecular features of the second group of disorders include a stable nonprogressive neurologic deficit, mainly mental retardation, and large expansions (200–2000 U) of a $(CGG)_n$ repeat. The CGG repeat responsible for fragile X syndrome (FRAXA) is located in the 5' untranslated region of the *FMR1* gene and is not predicted to encode for a peptide. Expansions of the repeat in excess of 200 U result in methylation of the promoter region, shutdown of *FMR1* transcription, and absence of the FMR1 protein. FRAXE, a molecularly defined syndrome characterized by a fragile site in Xq28 and occasionally accompanied by mental retardation in some kindreds, has been shown to be caused by large expansions of a (CGG vs CCG) repeat that has not been associated with a gene thus far.

Myotonic dystrophy is in a unique category in that the mutation involves large expansions, ranging from 50 to 4000 U, of a CTG repeat that is located in the 3' untranslated portion of a gene encoding myotonin protein kinase. Myotonic dystrophy is a dominantly inherited neuromuscular disorder characterized by muscle weakness, myotonia, and several associated findings. The mechanism by which the repeat expansion leads to the phenotype in DM is unknown at this time, and it is not clear whether the repeat expansion leads to loss of normal function or to a new detrimental function in myotonin protein kinase.

Table 100-1 summarizes the salient clinical and genetic features of the various disorders caused by trinucleotide repeat expansions, and Fig. 100-1 shows the range of repeat sizes in both the normal and expanded alleles.

This chapter will focus on SCA1 and will provide a brief overview of the other trinucleotide repeat disorders.

SPINOCEREBELLAR ATAXIA TYPE 1 (SCA1)

CLINICAL FEATURES AND LABORATORY FINDINGS

The dominantly inherited SCAs are clinically and genetically a heterogeneous group of neurologic disorders characterized by variable degrees of degeneration in the cerebellum, spinal tracts, and brain stem. SCA1 (OMIM 164400) is one subtype that has been classified based on its genetic localization to the short arm of human chromosome 6.

The main clinical features in SCA1 include gait ataxia, dysarthria, and dysmetria. As the disease progresses, brain-stem involvement results in facial weakness, tongue atrophy, severe dysarthria, and dysphagia. Hyperreflexia may be detected early in the course of the disease, but in later stages the patients develop

Table 100-1
Inherited Disorders Caused by Trinucleotide Repeat Expansions

Disease	*Clinical features*	*Pathology*	*Inheritance*	*Gene locus*	*Repeat sequence and location*	*Protein*
Spinal and bulbar muscular dystrophy	Proximal muscle weakness, bulbar dysfunction, partial loss of secondary sexual characteristics	Loss of motor neurons in the spinal cord and cranial nerves	X-linked	Xq11–q12	CAG-coding	Androgen receptor
Huntington's disease	Chorea and intellectual deterioration; juvenile onset with dystonia seizures and cognitive dysfunction	Atrophy of caudate and putamen; loss of spiny neurons	AD	4p16.3	CAG-coding	Huntingtin
Spinocerebellar ataxia type 1	Ataxia, dysarthria, and brain stem dysfunction	Purkinje's cell degeneration and loss of neurons in the dentate nucleus, inferior olive, and cranial nerve nuclei	AD	6p22–p23	CAG-coding	Ataxin-1
Dentatorubro-pallidoluysian atrophy/Haw River syndrome	Progressive ataxia, myoclonus, epilepsy, chorea, and dementia	Neuronal loss in the dentate nucleus, globus pallidus, thalamus, and subthalamic nuclei	AD	12pter–p12	CAG-coding	Atrophin
Machado-Joseph disease/ spinocerebellar ataxia type 3	Ataxia, amyotrophy, bulging eyes, faciolingual fasciculations, and dystonia	Neuronal loss in the dentate nucleus, substantia nigra, and cranial nerve motor nuclei	AD	14q32.1	CAG-coding	
Fragile X syndrome (FRAXA)	Mental retardation, macrocephaly, enlarged ears, macro-orchidism, and mild skeletal anomalies	Edema and generalized increase of connective tissue in adult testes	X-linked	Xq27.3	CGG-5'UTR	FMR1
FRAXE	Possibly mental retardation	X-linked	Xq28	CGG-?		
Myotonic dystrophy	Myotonia and muscle weakness, cataracts, cardiac involvement, endocrine dysfunction, and baldness	Relative loss of type 1 muscle fibers; increased internal nuclei and degeneration of microfilaments	AD	19q13	CTG-3'UTR	Myotonin protein kinase

Abbreviations: AD, autosomal dominant; UTR, untranslated region.

muscular atrophy, hypotonia, and hyporeflexia. Other, less consistent findings observed in some patients include optic nerve atrophy, ophthalmoparesis, and loss of proprioception and vibration sense. The disease typically manifests in the third to fourth decade, progresses over 10–15 years, and results in death due to brain stem dysfunction. Earlier age of onset and increase in the severity of the phenotype in later generations, a phenomenon known as *anticipation*, has been observed in some SCA1 kindreds.

Computerized tomography and magnetic resonance imaging studies in SCA1 patients reveal atrophy of the brachia pontis and anterior lobe of the cerebellum, and enlargement of the fourth ventricle. Typical neuropathologic findings in SCA1 include cerebellar atrophy with loss of Purkinje cells and dentate nucleus neurons, presence of "torpedoes," which are swollen axons of degenerating Purkinje cells, and severe neuronal degeneration in the inferior olive and to a lesser degree in cranial nerve nuclei III, IV, IX, X, and XII. Demyelination in the restiform body, brachium conjunctivum, spinocerebellar tracts, and posterior columns is frequently noted.

The clinical and laboratory findings in SCA1 are also observed in patients with other genetically distinct hereditary SCAs, including spinocerebellar ataxia type 2 (SCA2), which maps to the long arm of chromosome 12 (12q23–24); SCA3, which maps to chromosome 14q24.3–q32; and several SCA kindreds for which the gene locus is not yet mapped.

MOLECULAR MECHANISMS CAG Repeat Expansion in SCA1 The candidate region for the SCA1 gene was determined to span approximately 1 Mb of DNA using a combination of genetic and physical mapping approaches. Genomic cosmid clones from this candidate region were screened for the presence of trinucleotide repeats given that expansion of such sequences proved to be the mutational mechanism in three other disorders that display anticipation, fragile X syndrome, DM, and HD. This approach resulted in the identification of a CAG repeat that was unstable and expanded in SCA1. Using the polymerase chain reaction (PCR),

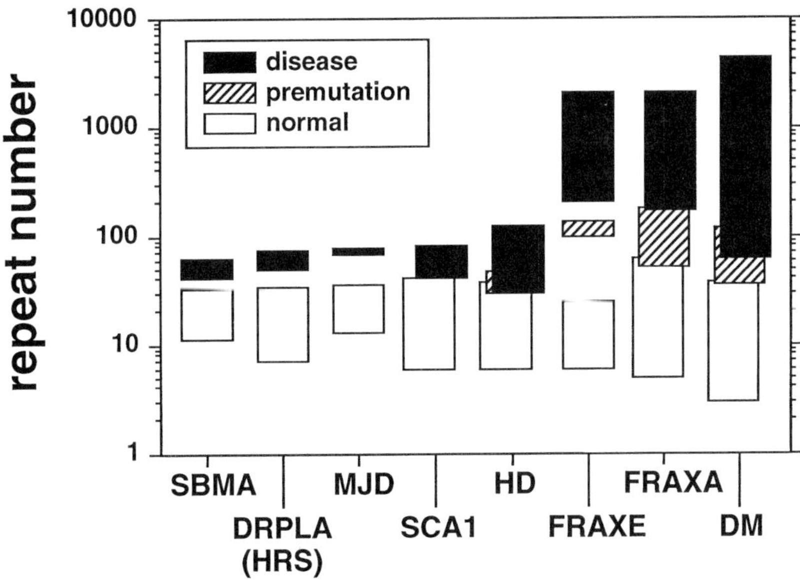

Figure 100-1 Ranges of repeat sizes in normal, premutation, and expanded alleles for eight trinucleotide repeat disorders. SBMA, spinobulbar muscular atrophy; DRPLA, dentatorubropallidoluysian atrophy; HRS, Haw River syndrome; MJD, Machado-Joseph disease; SCA1, spinocerebellar ataxia type 1; HD, Huntington's disease; FRAXE, mental retardation associated with the FRAXE chromosomal fragile site; FRAXA, fragile X syndrome; DM, myotonic dystrophy. (Figure kindly provided by Belinda J. F. Rossiter and reprinted with permission from Plenum Publishing Corporation, New York.)

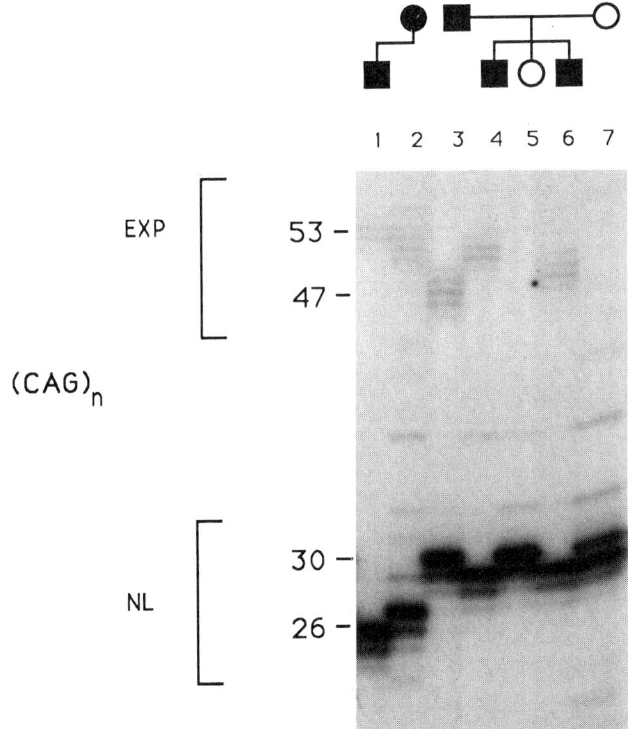

Figure 100-2 Analysis of the SCA1 CAG repeat in normal and SCA1 individuals using PCR on peripheral blood leukocyte DNA. The range for normal (NL) and expanded (EXP) CAG repeat units is indicated. (Reprinted with permission from Nature Genetics, a MacMillan Publication, Washington, DC.)

the repeat was amplified from DNAs of unaffected and affected individuals to determine the sizes of alleles. The SCA1 CAG repeat is highly polymorphic, with a heterozygosity rate of 84%. Normal individuals displayed 18 alleles, ranging from 6 to 39 repeat units, whereas individuals with SCA1 had two alleles, one within the normal range and one within a range of 40–81 CAG repeat units (Fig. 100-2). The number of trinucleotide repeat units on SCA1 chromosomes was inversely correlated with the age of onset of symptoms (Fig. 100-3). A linear correlation coefficient of –0.815 was obtained, indicating that the number of repeat units accounts for 66% of the variability in the age of onset.

Analysis of the SCA1 CAG repeat in families known to have the chromosome 6–linked form of SCA demonstrated an expanded allele cosegregating with disease in affected individuals, suggesting that expansion of this repeat is the mutational mechanism in all SCA1 families examined to date.

Features of the SCA1 CAG Repeat DNA sequence analysis of genomic and cDNA clones at the SCA1 locus revealed the following repeat configuration: $(CAG)_{12}CATCAGCAT(CAG)_{15}$. Because of the finding of CAT interruption in these clones, the configuration of the repeat on normal and SCA1 chromosomes was examined by sequence analysis and a combination of PCR and restriction analysis using *Sfa*NI, which cleaves $GCATC(N)_5$, allowing the identification of CAG tracts with CAT interruptions. These data revealed that in greater than 98% of normal chromosomes the CAG repeat is interrupted with 1, 2, or 3 CAT units. The four normal chromosomes with a contiguous CAG repeat configuration had very short repeat tracts (one with 6, one with 19, and two with 21 repeats). All SCA1 individuals examined to date, from several independent kindreds, were found to have a contiguous repeat configuration. This finding led to the hypothesis that the CAT interruptions, which break the repeat into two smaller tracts (typically less than 18 U each), may stabilize alleles with 21 or more repeats, and that the loss of the CAT interruption renders the CAG repeat unstable on SCA1 chromosomes. Studies of over 700 germline transmissions of normal alleles containing one or more CAT interspersions failed to identify instances of repeat instabil-

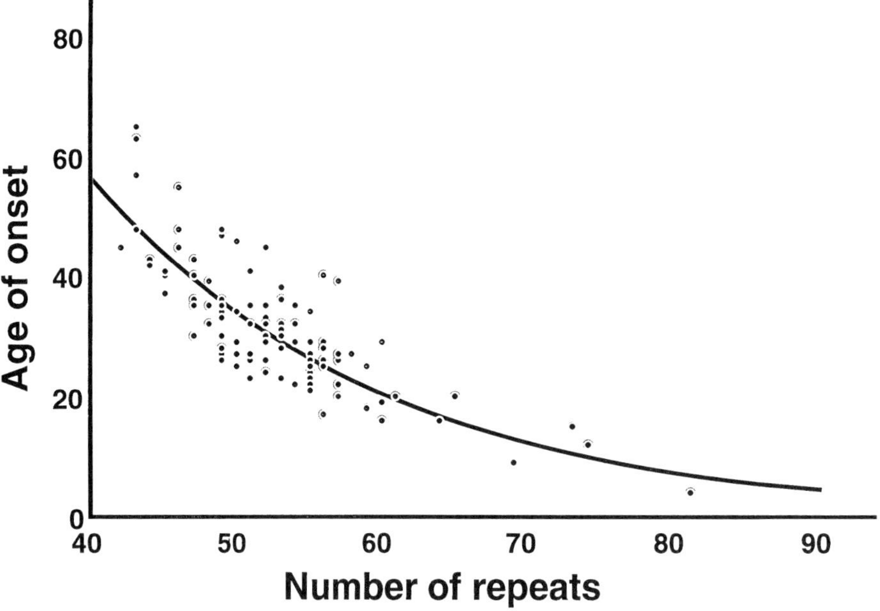

Figure 100-3 Distribution of the *SCA1* CAG repeat length versus the age of onset in year. The linear correlation coefficient is –0.8145. (Reprinted with permission from The University of Chicago Press, Chicago.)

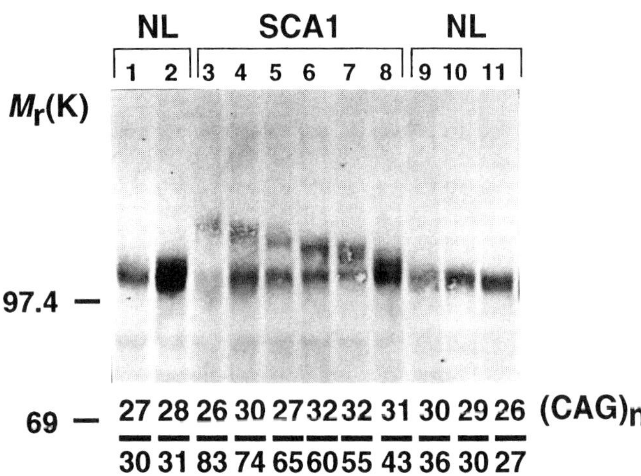

Figure 100-4 Immunoblot analysis of ataxin 1 expression in lymphoblasts from normal (NL) and SCA1 individuals. Lanes 1, 2, and 9–11, extracts from normal individuals; lanes 3–8, extracts from SCA1 patients. The number of CAG repeats on both alleles is shown. Normal and expanded alleles are translated, with the latter varying according to the number of repeat units. (Reprinted with permission from Nature Genetics, a MacMillan Publication, Washington, DC.)

ity. In contrast, expanded alleles with perfect CAG tracts are very unstable and expand or contract in 70% of transmissions. The majority of the expansions occur in paternal transmissions resulting in larger alleles and earlier age of onset, whereas contractions mostly occur in maternally transmitted alleles. Chong and colleagues demonstrated gametic and somatic heterogeneity of the expanded *SCA1* CAG repeat using single sperm and low-copy genome analysis establishing mitotic instability at this locus. Comparative low-copy genome analysis of a large interrupted normal allele (n = 39) and a small uninterrupted disease allele (n = 40) revealed somatic instability of the latter, suggesting a role of the CAT interruption in stabilizing longer repeat tracts.

Characterization of Ataxin 1, the *SCA1* Gene Product Northern blot analysis revealed that the CAG repeat is within an 11-kb transcript that is expressed in a wide variety of tissues including brain, muscle, kidney, lung, leukocytes, and placenta. Sequence analysis allowed the development of a composite sequence spanning 10,660 bp and identified a putative coding region which encodes 792–826 amino acids depending on the size of the repeat. The *SCA1* protein product, ataxin 1, appears to be a novel protein that does not share any homology with previously identified proteins. The CAG repeat is predicted to encode glutamine, and it is located 588 bp from the first methionine. The *SCA1* transcript is transcribed from both the wild-type and the expanded alleles in lymphoblasts from SCA1 patients.

The expression of ataxin 1 was evaluated in tissues from normal and SCA1 individuals using immunoblot and immunohistochemical analyses. Using ataxin 1 antiserum, lymphoblasts extracts from unaffected individuals revealed a single ataxin 1 band with an estimated molecular weight of 100 kDa (Fig. 100-4, lanes 1, 2, 9, 10, and 11). Extracts from SCA1 patients contained the 100-kDa band as well as a band showing slower electrophoretic mobility (Fig. 100-4, lanes 3–8). The size of the higher molecular-weight band in the patients varied according to the size of the expanded allele (*see* Fig. 100-4). The wild-type and expanded alleles were also translated in cerebellar tissue as well as in other brain tissues. Ataxin 1 is expressed in a variety of both neuronal and nonneuronal cells. Immunolocalization studies revealed that ataxin 1 is cytoplasmic in nonneuronal tissues and nuclear in neuronal cells, the only exception being cerebellar Purkinje cells, where it has both nuclear and cytoplasmic localization. The staining and localization of ataxin 1 was similar in regional brain tissues from SCA1 patients and controls.

PATHOGENESIS OF NEURODEGENERATION IN SCA1

SCA1 is a member of a growing family of neurodegenerative disorders caused by expansion of CAG repeats that lie within the coding portion of the involved genes and encode a glutamine tract.

A gain-of-function pathogenic mechanism has been proposed for these disorders based on numerous observations that argue against a loss-of-function mechanism. These observations include the lack of SBMA and HD phenotypes in patients with deletions of the androgen receptor and *HD* genes, respectively, and the embryonic lethal phenotype in mouse mutants lacking both copies of the murine *hd* gene. The gain-of-function model may involve cell-specific protein–protein or protein–DNA interactions, given the selective neuronal loss in face of a broad tissue expression pattern of the gene products. Alternatively, the mutated protein or its degradation products may become toxic to the cell, leading to neurodegeneration. The specificity of the degenerating neurons could be determined by the level and/or localization of the protein within those cells. The findings that the expanded alleles are translated into mutant proteins and that the sizes of the mutant proteins correlate with the number of repeats and age of onset support a gain-of-function model at the protein level. The unique expression pattern of ataxin 1 in Purkinje cells, the primary site of pathology in SCA1, may have a role in determining the specificity of the neuropathologic phenotype in this disease. To test the gain-of-function hypothesis, Burright and colleagues generated transgenic mice harboring the human *SCA1* gene with either a normal or expanded CAG tract containing 30 or 82 repeats, respectively. Expression of the transgenes was directed to the Purkinje cells using the regulatory elements of the Purkinje cell-specific gene *Pcp*-2. All transgenic mice expressing the unexpanded human *SCA1* gene were normal, whereas animals expressing the expanded *SCA1* allele developed ataxia and Purkinje cell degeneration like the human disorder. These data indicate that the expanded CAG tract within the *SCA1* gene is sufficient to produce Purkinje cell degeneration and ataxia consistent with a gain-of-function pathogenic mechanism. The availability of this mouse model will allow further studies aimed at understanding the exact molecular mechanisms leading to neurodegeneration in disorders caused by CAG repeat expansions.

It is interesting to note that both the normal and expanded repeat tracts were stable in over 125 parent to offspring transmissions. These data suggest that there may be basic differences between mice and humans with respect to DNA repair and/or replication. Alternatively, repeat instability may be affected by the chromosomal milieu and may be difficult to reproduce in the context of cDNA transgenes.

OTHER TRINUCLEOTIDE REPEAT DISORDERS

The following section will briefly review the main clinical and molecular features of the disorders caused by trinucleotide repeat expansions. Huntington's disease will not be discussed since a more detailed discussion is provided in Chapter 97.

SPINOBULBAR MUSCULAR ATROPHY Spinobulbar muscular atrophy (OMIM 313200) is an X-linked disorder characterized by proximal muscle weakness, bulbar dysfunction, and partial loss of secondary sexual characteristics. The clinical findings of lower motor neuron disease, gynecomastia, and impotence led to the hypothesis that SBMA may result from dysfunction of the androgen receptor (AR) given that this receptor is expressed in spinal and cranial motor neurons. Fischbeck and colleagues mapped the SBMA locus to the long arm of the X chromosome and subsequently determined the mutation in SBMA to be an expansion of the CAG repeat within the first exon of the AR gene. Normal alleles contain 12–30 repeats, and expanded alleles contain 40–62 repeats. The AR is a transcriptional regulatory protein, and it is proposed that the CAG repeat expansion confers a new regulatory activity that is harmful to motor neurons. Transgenic mice harboring a human AR cDNA failed to develop motor neuron disease in spite of transcription of the transgene. This lack of phenotype could be due to the low level of expression of the transgene compared with the endogenous gene, or may be due to the relatively short CAG repeat tract (45 repeats). New transgenic lines using different promoters and longer repeats are currently being generated to address these issues.

DENTATORUBROPALLIDOLUYSIAN ATROPHY Dentatorubropallidoluysian atrophy (OMIM 125370) is a rare autosomal dominant neurodegenerative disorder, characterized by progressive ataxia, myoclonus, epilepsy, chorea, athetosis, and dementia. The mutation causing DRPLA was identified using the candidate gene approach and was determined to involve an expansion of a CAG repeat within a novel gene that maps to human chromosome 12p. DRPLA patients have an expanded allele in the 54–75 repeat range in addition to the normal allele, which typically contains 7–34 repeats. The size of the expanded allele typically increases when paternally transmitted, with larger alleles causing juvenile-onset cases.

Burke and colleagues found the DRPLA mutation in an African-American family with HRS. Haw River syndrome differs from DRPLA in the absence of myoclonic epilepsy and presence of demyelination of the subcortical white matter.

The DRPLA protein is a novel protein whose function is unknown at this time; it is localized within the cytoplasm of neurons. As in SCA1, SBMA, and HD, the mutant alleles are translated into proteins of expanded length.

MACHADO-JOSEPH DISEASE AND SCA3 Machado-Joseph disease (OMIM 109150) is characterized by progressive ataxia, external ophthalmoplegia, bulging eyes, facial and lingual fasciculation, muscle atrophy, dystonia, and spasticity. Neuropathologic findings include severe neuronal loss in the striatum and substantia nigra, with moderate abnormalities in the dentate nucleus and red nucleus. The mutational mechanism in MJD involves the expansion of a CAG repeat that lies within a novel gene on chromosome 14q32.1. Normal alleles contain 14–34 repeats, whereas expanded alleles contain 61–84 repeats. SCA3 (OMIM 183085), which is clinically distinct from MJD and resembles SCA1, is also caused by CAG expansions within the *MJD* gene.

MYOTONIC DYSTROPHY Myotonic dystrophy (OMIM 160900), the most common muscular dystrophy affecting adults, is an autosomal dominant disorder with a wide range of severity from a frequently lethal form in newborns (congenital DM) to almost asymptomatic expression in adults. Clinical features include muscle weakness, myotonia, cataracts, cardiac arrhythmias, endocrine dysfunction, male-pattern baldness, and male infertility. The disease typically increases in severity and occurs earlier with successive generations, a phenomenon known as anticipation. Congenital DM, the most severe form of the disease, is characterized by severe hypotonia, respiratory insufficiency, and feeding difficulties. Congenital DM is usually transmitted from mothers, who often have mild to undetectable symptoms.

Myotonic dystrophy is caused by expansion of a CTG repeat that is located in the 3' untranslated region of a gene predicted to encode a protein kinase. The number of repeats varies from 5 to 20 in the normal population, whereas in DM families it ranges from 50 to 4000.

The DM gene product, myotonin protein kinase (Mt-Pk), was confirmed to be a serine/threonine kinase using in vitro assays of the recombinant protein. Controversy still exists as to the effects of the CTG repeat expansion on the mRNA/protein in DM. Mice lacking the myotonin protein kinase gene develop a late onset progressive myopathy, but lack other features of myotonic dystrophy, including myotonia and male infertility. Thus, the exact pathogenic mechanism of this mutation remains unclear.

FRAGILE X SYNDROME AND OTHER FRAGILE SITES Fragile X syndrome (OMIM 309550) is the most common single cause of inherited mental retardation, with an estimated incidence of 1 in 2000 live births. The main clinical feature in preadolescent males is mental retardation; in postpubescent males additional features include increased head size, enlarged ears, macroorchidism, narrow and elongated facies, and mild skeletal defects. FRAXA, which was initially mapped to Xq27.3 based on the finding of a fragile site at this location, is an X-linked disorder with unusual penetrance. Approximately 30% of female carriers have borderline IQ, and 20% of males with genetic risk for FRAXA are normal. These observations led to the "Sherman paradox," which describes increasing penetrance in successive generations. The FRAXA gene known as *FMR1* was isolated using a positional cloning approach, and the mutation was determined to be an expansion of a CGG repeat within the 5' untranslated portion of the gene. Symptomatic males have 200 or more repeat units, whereas nonpenetrant males and carrier females have 70–150 repeats, which are referred to as premutational. Females with mental retardation typically have repeats with 200 or more units, but, in general, only 30% of females with repeats over 200 have mental retardation, presumably due to the effects of X-inactivation patterns. The identification of the mutational basis of FRAXA clarified the Sherman paradox and, like other trinucleotide repeat mutations, provided a molecular basis for anticipation.

The *FMR1* CGG repeat is highly unstable in premutation alleles transmitted through a female meiosis. Females with 80 or more repeats have a virtual 100% mutation rate to a disease-causing expansion with more than 200 repeats. Sequence analysis of normal and FRAXA alleles showed that the CGG repeat is interrupted by AGG trinucleotides at regular intervals. These interruptions, which are lost in premutation alleles, may provide stability in normal alleles.

The FMR1 gene product is found in many tissues, with highest levels being observed in brain and testis. The precise function of the protein remains unknown, but it has been shown to bind RNA. The RNA-binding property of FMR1 suggests that it might be involved in regulating the expression of other genes.

The CGG expansion in FRAXA leads to methylation of the promoter region and decreased levels of the mRNA and protein. Although the majority of FRAXA cases are caused by CGG repeat expansions, a few cases have resulted from mutations that lead to the complete absence of the FMR1 protein (Fig. 100-5). A mouse mutant that is null for *Fmr1* was generated by gene targeting and was found to have learning deficits. These data clearly demonstrate that, in FRAXA, the disease results from loss of the normal function of *FMR1*.

Two additional fragile sites have been identified on the X chromosome: FRAXE (OMIM 309548) and FRAXF (OMIM 600226) in Xq28. Both of these have been associated with CGG repeat expansions. A gene (FMR2) adjacent to the FRAXE site has been cloned, and there is loss of FMR2 expression in association with CGG expansion at FRAXE. At this time there is no clinical phenotype associated with FRAXF.

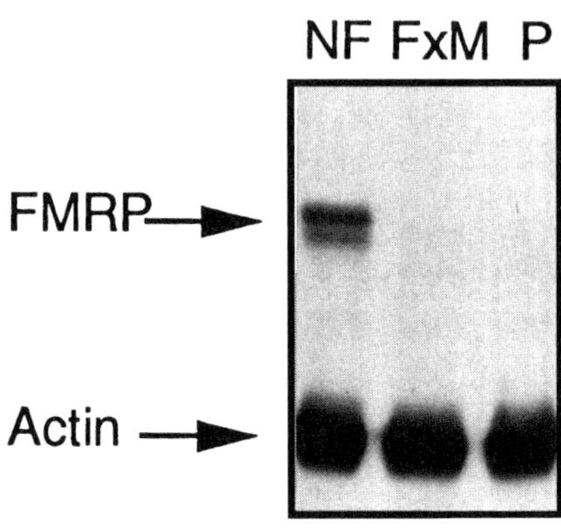

Figure 100-5 Immunoblot analysis for the FMR1 protein. NF, normal female cell line; FxM, cell line from a male with fragile X syndrome caused by a typical CGG expansion mutation; P, cell line from a patient with a nucleotide deletion in exon 5 of *FMR1* resulting in premature termination of translation; FMR1 protein cannot be detected in the cell lines from the males with mutation (P) or expansion (FxM). (Figure kindly provided by David Nelson and reprinted with permission from Nature Genetics, a MacMillan Publication, Washington, DC.)

CGG repeat expansions have been observed in two autosomal fragile sites, FRA16A (OMIM 136580) and FRA11B (OMIM 600651), on human chromosomes 16 and 11, respectively. FRA16A has not been associated with a gene yet, but the expanding CGG repeat in FRA11B is within the 5' end of the protooncogene *CBL2* and results in methylation of sequences in this region. It is interesting that FRA11B has been associated with Jacobsen syndrome (OMIM 147791), a disorder characterized by dysmorphic features, mental retardation, and deletions of 11q23–qter. This association has been observed in some families where the 11q deletion has been noted to occur on a parental chromosome carrying the expanded CGG repeat.

CLINICAL IMPLICATIONS

The finding that expansion of trinucleotide repeats is the mutational mechanism in the neurological disorders described above greatly facilitates the diagnosis of these diseases and provides options for genetic counselling. In the case of dominantly inherited ataxias, the identification of these mutations allows a rational classification of this highly heterogeneous group of diseases in addition to facilitating diagnosis. Molecular testing for trinucleotide repeat expansions should be considered as the leading diagnostic test in trying to evaluate patients with dominantly inherited ataxia, progressive degenerative disorders characterized by chorea, dementia with or without seizures, X-linked patterns of lower motor neuron disease, congenital muscle disorders and suspected DM, and mental retardation. SCA1 and MJD/SCA3 are currently estimated to account for approximately 30–40% of dominantly inherited ataxias. Thus, analysis of the CAG repeats at those two loci will provide a molecular diagnosis in a substantial number of patients. It is important to emphasize that testing for the HD, DRPLA, and SCA mutations in asymptomatic individuals who are at risk should be restricted to adults who have undergone extensive psychological and genetic counseling, given the devastating nature of these diseases. In children these tests should be limited to those already symptomatic. In the case of FRAXA, the molecular analysis of the CGG repeat is superior to the cytogenetic approach traditionally used for identifying the fragile site, owing to its sensitivity and accuracy. However, chromosomal analysis in patients with mental retardation is still extremely valuable given the relative high likelihood of identifying other cytogenetic abnormalities.

The finding that CAG repeat expansion is the mutational mechanism in several late-onset neurodegenerative disorders suggests that this will prove to be the mutational mechanism in most of them. This will facilitate the identification of the genes/mutations in several dominantly inherited ataxias and will eventually lead to understanding the pathogenesis of these diseases.

ADDENDUM

Since the submission of this chapter, several new research developments have occurred in the field of trinucleotide repeats. These mainly include the identification of new disease genes and new insight into disease pathogenesis. The following section will highlight some of the key recent developments.

The CGG repeat which expands in the fragile XE syndrome has been demonstrated to reside in the 5' UTR of a new gene termed FMR2. The expansion of an AAG repeat which resides in the first intron of a novel gene was demonstrated to be the most common mutation in Friedreich ataxia (FRDA). Normal alleles typically contain 7–32 repeats, whereas expanded alleles have more than 66 repeats. The expansion leads to lower levels of the gene product and most likely causes disease through a loss-of-function mechanism. The FRDA gene product frataxin localizes to the mitochondria and has homologs in yeast and round worm. Loss of function of the yeast frataxin homolog results in mitochondrial dysfunction and iron accumulation. These findings, together with the finding of iron deposits in heart tissue from FRDA patients, suggest that frataxin is involved in mitochondrial iron export and homeostasis.

The gene for spinocerebellar ataxia type 2 (SCA2) was identified, and the mutation involves the expansion of a translated CAG repeat within the novel protein ataxin-2. Normal alleles contain 15–29 repeats and expanded alleles contain 35–59 repeats. The SCA2 CAG repeat is interrupted by 1–3 CAA units on normal chromosomes but is a pure CAG repeat tract on expanded disease alleles. Ataxin-2 is a cytoplasmic protein of an apparent molecular weight of 150 kDa and no known homology to previously identified molecules.

Using the candidate gene approach, a small expansion in the CAG repeat located in the C-terminal portion of the α_{1A} voltage-dependent calcium channel was demonstrated to cause spinocerebellar ataxia type 6 (SCA6). The SCA6 CAG repeat contains 4–18 repeats on normal chromosomes and 21–30 repeats on disease chromosomes. It is intriguing that these small expansions, which are well within the normal range for other polymorphic CAG repeats, are pathogenic in SCA6. This finding suggests that the protein context of the CAG repeat is important and may modulate the pathogenicity of the toxic glutamine tract. Alternatively, the small expansion of the CAG repeat in the α_{1a} calcium channel may disrupt its normal function, leading to abnormal calcium homeostasis and neuronal degeneration.

Lastly, the gene for spinocerebellar ataxia type 7 (SCA7) has been identified and the mutational mechanism was demonstrated to be the expansion of a translated CAG repeat within a novel nuclear protein ataxin-7. Normal alleles contain 7–17 repeats and expanded alleles contain 38–130 repeats.

The importance of the length of the polyglutamine tract in the phenotype of each of the neurodegenerative diseases caused by CAG repeat expansion has been demonstrated by the fact that longer repeats cause earlier and typically more severe disease. New insight into the pathogenesis of neurodegenerative diseases caused by CAG repeat expansion has recently emerged from immunohistochemical studies of patient tissues and studies of transgenic mouse models.

Immunohistochemical staining of brain tissues from HD, SCA3, and SCA1 patients using the respective antisera demonstrated the presence of nuclear inclusions in affected brain regions but not in neurons spared in the disease. Transgenic mice harboring a truncated form of the huntingtin protein with an expanded polyglutamine tract, as well as SCA1 transgenic mice, had neuronal inclusions similar to those seen in patients. It is interesting that the nuclear inclusions stain positively with ubiquitin antibodies in both patient and mouse tissues. These findings point to the nucleus as the site where disease pathogenesis is mediated and raise the possibility that protein ubiquitination and the degradation pathway may be involved. Factor(s) that lead to selective neuronal loss in each of these diseases remain unknown. In the case of SCA1, the strong interaction between mutant ataxin-1 and the leucine-rich acidic nuclear protein (LANP), a protein with highest expression levels in cerebellar Purkinje cells, suggests that LANP is a candidate to be one of the factors mediating cell specificity in SCA1. Additional factors for SCA1 and other diseases could include levels of expression of the mutant proteins in the various neuronal types, as well as protein modifications that may be cell-specific.

In summary, the identification of expansion of unstable trinucleotide repeats as a mutational mechanism in human disease has proven to be one of the most exciting and clinically relevant discoveries in this decade. To date, over 12 diseases can be easily diagnosed, and families can be offered effective genetic counselling. The identification and characterization of the mutant gene products are likely to lead to better understanding of disease pathogenesis and hopefully to potential therapeutic choices in the future.

ACKNOWLEDGMENTS

The author thanks Dr. Harry T. Orr for insightful discussions throughout an exciting and productive collaborative effort. Portions of this work were supported by a grant from the National Institutes of Health (NS-27699) and by cores from the Mental Retardation Research Center and the Baylor College of Medicine Human Genome Center.

SELECTED REFERENCES

Ashley CT Jr, Wilkinson KD, Reines D, Warren ST. *FMR1* protein: conserved RNP family domains and selective RNA binding. Science 1993;262:563–566.

Babcock M, de Silva D, Oaks R, Davis-Kaplan S, Jiralerspong S, Montermini L, Pandolfo M, Kaplan, J. Regulation of mitochondrial iron accumulation by Yfh1p, a putative homolog of frataxin. Science 1997;276:1709–1712.

Bingham PM, Scott MO, Wang S, et al. Stability of an expanded trinucleotide repeat in the androgen receptor gene in transgenic mice. Nat Genet 1995;9:191–196.

Burke JR, Wingfield MS, Lewis KE, et al. The Haw River syndrome: dentatorubropallidoluysian atrophy (DRPLA) in an African-American family. Nat Genet 1994;7:521–524.

Burright EN, Clark HB, Servadio A, et al. SCA1 transgenic mice: a model for neurodegeneration caused by an expanded CAG trinucleotide repeat. Cell 1995;82:937–948.

Campuzano V, Montermini L, Molto MD, Pianese L, Cossee M, Cavalcanti F, et al. Friedreich's ataxia: autosomal recessive disease caused by an intronic GAA triplet repeat expansion. Science 1996; 271:1423–1427.

Chong SS, McCall AE, Cota J, Subramony SH, Orr HT, Zoghbi HY. Gametic and somatic tissue-specific heterogeneity of the expanded *SCA1* CAG repeat in spinocerebellar ataxia type 1. Nat Genet 1995;10:344–350.

Consortium TD-BFX. *Fmr1* knockout mice: a model to study fragile X mental retardation. Cell 1994;78:23–33.

David G, Abbas N, Stevanin G, Durr A, Yvert G, Cancel G, et al. Cloning of the SCA7 gene reveals a highly unstable CAG repeat expansion. Nature Genetics 1997;17:65–70.

Davies SW, Turmaine M, Cozens BA, DiFiglia M, Sharp AH, Ross CA, et al. Formation of neuronal intranuclear inclusions underlies the neurological dysfunction in mice transgenic for the HD mutation. Cell 1997;90:537–548.

DiFiglia M, Sapp E, Chase KO, Davies SW, Bates GP, Vonsattel JP, Aronin N. Aggregation of Huntingtin in neuronal intranuclear inclusions and dystrophic neurites in brain. Science 1997;277:1990–1993.

Dunne PW, Walch ET, Epstein HF. Phosphorylation reactions of recombinant human myotonic dystrophy protein kinase and their inhibition. Biochemistry 1994;33:10,809–10,814.

Duyao MP, Auerbach AB, Ryan A, et al. Inactivation of the mouse Huntington's disease gene homolog *Hdh*. Nature 1995;269:407–410.

Eichler EE, Holden JJA, Popovich BW, et al. Length of uninterrupted CGG repeats determines instability in the *FMR1* gene. Nat Genet 1994;8:88–94.

Gecz J, Gedeon AK, Sutherland GR, Mulley JC. Identification of the gene FMR2, associated with FRAXE mental retardation. Nat Genet 1996;13:105–108.

Gu Y, Shen Y, Gibbs RA, Nelson DL. Identification of FMR2, a novel gene associated with the FRAXE CCG repeat and CpG. Nature Genetics 1996;13:109–113.

Harper PS. Myotonic dystrophy and other autosomal muscular dystrophies. In: Scriver CR, Beandet AL, Sly WS, Valle D, et al, eds. The Metabolic and Molecular Bases of Inherited Disease, 7th ed., vol. 3. New York: McGraw-Hill, 1995; pp. 742–751.

Imbert G, Saudou F, Yvert G, Devys D, Trottier Y, Garnier J-M, Weber C, Mandel J-L. Cloning of the gene for spinocerebellar ataxia 2 reveals a locus with high sensitivity to expanded CAG/glutamine repeats and high instability. Nature Genetics 1996;14:285–291.

Jansen G, Groenen RJ, Bachner D, et al. Abnormal myotonic dystrophy protein kinase levels produce only mild myopathy in mice. Nat Genet 1996;13:316–324.

Jodice C, Malaspina P, Persichetti F, et al. Effect of trinucleotide repeat length and parental sex on phenotypic variation in spinocerebellar ataxia 1. Am J Hum Genet 1994;54:959–965.

Jones C, Penny L, Mattina T, et al. Association of a chromosome deletion syndrome with a fragile site within the proto-oncogene *CBL2*. Nature 1995;376:145–149.

Kawaguchi Y, Okamoto T, Taniwaki M, et al. CAG expansions in a novel gene for Machado-Joseph disease at chromosome 14q32.1. Nat Genet 1994;8:221–227.

Kennedy WR, Alter M, Sung JH. Progressive proximal spinal and bulbar muscular atrophy of late onset—a sex-linked recessive trait. Neurology 1968;18:671–680.

Knight SJL, Flannery AV, Hirst MC, et al. Trinucleotide repeat amplification and hypermethylation of a CpG island in FRAXE mental retardation. Cell 1993;74:127–134.

Koide R, Ikeuchi T, Onodera O, et al. Unstable expansion of CAG repeat in hereditary dentatorubral-pallidoluysian atrophy (DRPLA). Nat Genet 1994;6:9–13.

Koutnikova H, Campuzano V, Foury F, Dollé P, Cazzalini O, Koenig M. Studies of human, mouse and yeast homologues indicate a mitochondrial function for frataxin. Nature Genet 1997;16:345–351.

Kunst CB, Warren ST. Cryptic and polar variation of the fragile X repeat could result in predisposing normal alleles. Cell 1994;77:853–861.

La Spada AR, Wilson EM, Lubahn DB, Harding AE, Fischbeck H. Androgen receptor gene mutations in X-linked spinal and bulbar muscular atrophy. Nature 1991;352:77–79.

Lugenbeel KA, Peier AM, Carson NL, Chudley AE, Nelson DL. Intragenic loss of function mutations demonstrate the primary role of FMR1 in fragile X syndrome. Nat Genet 1995;10:483–485.

Maruyama H, Nakamura S, Matsuyama Z, et al. Molecular features of the CAG repeats and clinical manifestation of Machado-Joseph disease. Hum Mol Genet 1995;4:807–812.

Nagafuchi S, Yanagisawa H, Sato K, et al. Dentatorubral and pallidoluysian atrophy expansion of an unstable CAG trinucleotide on chromosome 12p. Nat Genet 1994;6:14–18.

Nancarrow JK, Kremer E, Holman K, et al. Implications of FRA16A structure for the mechanism of chromosomal fragile site genesis. Nature 1994;264:1938–1941.

Nasir J, Floresco SB, O'Kusky JR, et al. Targeted disruption of the Huntington's disease gene results in embryonic lethality and behavioral and morphological changes in heterozygotes. Cell 1995;81:811–823.

Nussbaum RL, Ledbetter DH. Fragile X syndrome. In: Scriver CR, et al. The Metabolic and Molecular Bases of Inherited Disease, 7th ed., vol, 3. New York: McGraw-Hill, 1995; pp. 795–810.

Orr H, Chung M-Y, Banfi S, et al. Expansion of an unstable trinucleotide (CAG) repeat in spinocerebellar ataxia type 1. Nat Genet 1993;4:221–226.

Paulson HL, Perez MK, Trottier Y, Trojanowsk JQ, Subramony SH, Das SS, Vig P, Mandel J-L, Fischbeck KH, Pittman RN. Intranuclear inclusions of expanded polyglutamine protein in spinocerebellar ataxia Type 3. Neuron 1997;19:333,334.

Pulst S-M, Nechiporuk A, Nechiporuk T, Gisper S, Chen X-N, Lopez-Cendes I, Pearlman S, Lunkes A, DeJong P, Rouleau GA, Auburger G, Korenberg JR, Figueroa C, Sahba S. Identification of the SCA2 gene: Moderate expansion of a normally biallelic trinucleotide repeat. Nature Genetics 1996;14:269–276.

Ranum LPW, Chung M-Y, Banfi S, et al. Molecular and clinical correlations in spinocerebellar ataxia type 1 (SCA1): evidence for familial effects on the age of onset. Am J Hum Genet 1994;55:244–252.

Reddy S, Smith DB, Rich MM, et al. Mice lacking the myotonic dystrophy protein kinase develop a late onset progressive myopathy. Nat Genet 1996;13:325–335.

Rötig A, deLonlay P, Chretien D, Foury F, Koenig M, Sidi D, Munnich A, et al. Frataxin gene expansion causes aconitase and mitochondrial iron-sulfur protein deficiency in Friedreich ataxia. Nature Genet 1997;17:In press.

Sanpei K, Takano H, Igarashi S, Sato T, Oyake M, Sasaki H, et al. Identification of the gene for spinocerebellar ataxia type 2 (SCA2) using a direct identification of repeat expansion and cloning technique (DIRECT). Nature Genetics 1996;14:277–284.

Servadio A, Koshy B, Armstrong D, Antalfy B, Orr HT, Zoghbi HY. Expression analysis of the ataxin-1 protein in tissues from normal and spinocerebellar ataxia type 1 individuals. Nat Genet 1995;10:94–98.

Siomi H, Siomi MC, Nussbaum RL, Dreyfuss G. The protein product of the fragile X gene, *FMR1*, has characteristics of an RNA-binding protein. Cell 1993;74:291–298.

Skinner PJ, Koshy B, Cummings C, Klement IA, Helin K, Servadio A, Zoghbi HY, Orr HT. Ataxin-1 with extra glutamines induces alterations in nuclear matrix-associated structures. Nature 1997;389: 971–974.

Wilson RB, Roof DM. Respiratory deficiency due to loss of mitochondrial DNA in yeast lacking the frataxin homologue. Nature Genet 1997;16:352–357.

Yazawa I, Nukina N, Hashida H, Goto J, Yamada M, Kanazawa I. Abnormal gene product identified in hereditary dentatorubral-pallidoluysian atrophy (DRPLA) brain. Nat Genet 1995;10:99–103.

Zhuchenko O, Bailey J, Bonnen P, Ashizawa T, Stockton DW, et al. Autosomal dominant cerebellar ataxia (SCA6) associated with small polyglutamine expansions in the α_{1A}-voltage-dependent calcium channel. Nature Genetics 1997;15:62–69.

Zoghbi HY. CAG Repeats in SCA6: Anticipating new clues. Neurology 1997;49:1196–1199.

Zoghbi HY. The expanding world of ataxins. Nature Genetics 1996; 14:237,238.

Zoghbi HY, Ballabio A. Spinocerebellar ataxia type 1. In: Scriver CR, et al, eds. The Metabolic and Molecular Bases of Inherited Disease, 7th ed., vol 3. New York, McGraw Hill, 1995; pp. 4559–4568.

Zoghbi HY, Caskey CT. Inherited disorders caused by trinucleotide repeat expansions. In: Harris H, Hirschorn KH, eds. Advances in Human Genetics. Eds, New York, Plenum, 1998; in press.

101 Charcot-Marie-Tooth Disease and Related Peripheral Neuropathies

JAMES R. LUPSKI

INTRODUCTION

Charcot-Marie-Tooth disease (CMT) is the most common inherited peripheral neuropathy, affecting at least 1 in 2500 individuals. Charcot-Marie-Tooth disease represents a heterogeneous collection of disorders of the peripheral nerve. It can be inherited as an autosomal dominant, autosomal recessive, or X-linked trait, and, in addition, isolated cases occur. The autosomal dominant segregation pattern is the most frequently observed, and recent molecular studies have identified an exciting novel mutational mechanism for this form—the CMT1A duplication. It is intriguing that, for one of the most common dominant disorders affecting humans, there is no mutant gene involved in the majority of cases. Instead, the disease phenotype results from having three copies of a normal non-mutated gene or a gene dosage effect secondary to an inherited or *de novo* DNA duplication. Furthermore, an intrinsic structural property of the human genome, a repeat sequence (CMT1A-REP) flanking the duplicated region, acts as a substrate for homologous recombination and an unequal crossover event. This recombination between misaligned flanking CMT1A-REP repeats appears to have a sex predilection and to occur preferentially during male gametogenesis. The identification of the CMT1A duplication has potent implications for clinical diagnosis, clinical management with respect to prognosis, counseling regarding recurrence risk, and the rational design of therapy geared at normalizing the levels of gene expression.

Hereditary neuropathy with liability to pressure palsies (HNPP) (OMIM 162500) is a less frequently diagnosed autosomal dominant peripheral neuropathy, which usually presents with a milder clinical phenotype than CMT. The patient inherits a tendency to nerve injury after mild trauma; it is likely that most affected individuals remain undiagnosed because they are either clinically asymptomatic or only minimally aware of functional disabilities. Carpal tunnel syndrome and other entrapment neuropathies are frequent manifestations of HNPP, making it difficult to distinguish from an acquired neuropathy. In the majority of cases, HNPP results from DNA deletion of the same genetic region duplicated in CMT1A. Molecular detection of the HNPP deletion secures a diagnosis suspected clinically and can be useful for distinguishing HNPP from acquired neuropathies.

From: *Principles of Molecular Medicine* (J. L. Jameson, ed.), ©1998 Humana Press Inc., Totowa, NJ.

The Dejerine-Sottas syndrome (DSS) (OMIM 145900) is a rare and severe neuropathy. Though it was initially thought to be an autosomal recessive trait, molecular studies have identified mutations in only one copy of the two homologues of the same genes that when mutated can lead to a CMT phenotype. These heterozygous mutations presumably represent dominant alleles. Thus, instead of being two completely distinct entities, DSS and CMT may more accurately represent a spectrum of related clinical findings due to allelic heterogeneity underlying the disorders; many DSS cases may result from new mutation dominant alleles.

In the past few years, molecular analyses have identified three genes: *PMP22*, *MPZ*, and *Cx32*, wherein mutations, or altered dosage of the normal gene in the case of *PMP22*, lead to inherited neuropathies. These genes provide critical reagents to study the biology of the peripheral nerves. Each gene product is important for proper structure or function of the myelin. The inherited peripheral neuropathies CMT, HNPP, and DSS thus represent "myelinopathies." Molecular genetic studies of CMT and related neuropathies have given new insights into the biology of the human peripheral nervous system and have important implications for patient care.

CLINICAL FEATURES AND PATHOGENESIS

Charcot-Marie-Tooth polyneuropathy syndrome, or the hereditary motor and sensory neuropathies (HMSN), are genetically and clinically heterogeneous disorders of the peripheral nerves characterized by an insidious onset and slowly progressive weakness of the distal muscles and mild sensory impairment. Symptoms typically appear in the first or second decade but may appear later. Children with CMT often walk on their toes, and adults consult a physician because of abnormalities of gait from a dropped foot due to dorsiflexor weakness, foot deformities such as pes cavus, or loss of balance. Cramps are a frequent complaint, are worse after long walks, and are sometimes exacerbated by cold weather. The most frequent complaint concerning hand function that may occur later in the disease is difficulty with fine finger movements. Deep tendon reflexes disappear early at the ankle and later at the patella and the upper limb.

Electrophysiologic and neuropathologic studies distinguish two major forms. Charcot-Marie-Tooth disease type 1 (CMT1) (OMIM 118200), also known as HMSNI, is a demyelinating neuropathy with moderately to severely decreased motor nerve conduction velocities (NCVs, usually <42 m/s). The conduction deficit is uniform from nerve to nerve and from nerve segment to nerve segment, suggesting a cell-autonomous defect involving the Schwann's cell. Charcot-Marie-Tooth disease type 1 is characterized by hypertrophic nerves, which may be visualized in some patients under the skin (greater auricular nerve) or palpated (ulnar and peroneal nerves).

Peripheral nerve pathology shows segmental demyelination and remyelination and frequent "onion bulb" formation, which consists of circumferentially directed Schwann cells and their processes. Charcot-Marie-Tooth disease type 1 has been characterized further with genetic linkage studies, which demonstrate the involvement of at least three loci in different families: CMT1A at 17p11.2–p12, CMT1B on 1q21.2–q23, and CMTX1 at Xq13.1. Charcot-Marie-Tooth disease type 2 (CMT2) (OMIM 118210), also called HMSNII, is characterized by normal or slightly reduced motor NCVs with decreased amplitudes and neuropathology that shows axonal loss with few if any onion bulbs. Dejerine-Sottas syndrome (HMSNIII) is a demyelinating neuropathy with clinical electrophysiologic and histopathologic features similar to, but of more severe and earlier onset than, CMT1. These classifications appear to reflect primary pathological involvement of the myelin (CMT1 and DSS) or the axon (CMT2) of the peripheral nerve.

Hereditary neuropathy with liability to pressure palsies may manifest clinically as periodic episodes of numbness, muscular weakness, atrophy, and in some cases palsies that follow relatively minor compression or trauma to the peripheral nerves. Electrophysiologic studies sometimes show mildly slowed NCV in clinically affected individuals as well as in asymptomatic "carriers." Conduction blocks can also be observed. Peripheral nerve pathology shows segmental demyelination and remyelination with tomacula or "sausage-like" focal thickenings of the myelin sheath. Ultrastructural studies reveal frequent occurrence of uncompacted myelin, particularly in the inner lamellae, due to separation of the major dense line with widened islands of cytoplasm in the Schwann cell.

MOLECULAR MECHANISMS

DNA DUPLICATION ASSOCIATED WITH CMT1A The CMT1A duplication (OMIM 118220) was identified initially in multiple US and European CMT1 families, where it was found to cosegregate with the disease in familial cases and as a new mutation in an isolated or sporadic case. The segregation of marker genotypes from within the duplicated segment in the new mutation individual suggested a mechanism of unequal crossover or nonsister chromatid exchange for the duplication. Demonstration of the CMT1A duplication in affected individuals was carried out by the following methods: detection of three alleles at a highly polymorphic dinucleotide repeat locus, dosage differences at restriction fragment length polymorphic (RFLP) alleles, detection of a duplication-specific junction fragment of 500 kb with pulsed field gel electrophoresis (PFGE) to separate large-molecular-weight fragments of *Sac*II digested genomic DNA from the affected individual, and microscopically by two-color fluorescent *in situ* hybridization (FISH) of interphase nuclei. Failure to recognize the molecular duplication can lead to misinterpretation of marker genotypes for affected individuals, identification of false recombinants, and incorrect localization of the disease locus. The CMT1A duplication was confirmed subsequently by many laboratories in patients from varied ethnic background, was shown to occur in approximately 70% of unrelated CMT1 cases, and was found in 9 out of 10 sporadic CMT1 cases. The junction fragment appeared to be identical in multiple CMT1A duplication patients of varied ethnicity, suggesting a precise recombination event to generate the duplication. Taken together, these observations suggested that the CMT1A duplication was a frequent cause of CMT that appears to have occurred *de novo* multiple and independent times in different genetic backgrounds.

Patients with the CMT1A duplication exhibit typical neuropathology of CMT1. Electrophysiologic studies in families segregating the CMT1A duplication demonstrated a clear bimodal distribution of abnormally decreased motor NCV in individuals with the CMT1A duplication, while normal NCVs appeared in those shown not to have inherited the CMT1A duplication. However, a remarkable range of motor NCV was observed in CMT1A duplication patients that was not related to age or clinical severity. Longitudinal electrophysiologic studies performed 22 years apart in one family segregating the CMT1A duplication demonstrated little change in NCV and only mild increased motor impairment. Thus, the CMT1A duplication is a good biological marker for the disease with clinical utility for diagnosis and prognosis.

Molecular studies showed that the duplication was 3 Mb in size, consisting of a tandem arrangement of a 1.5-Mb monomer unit, and that the region duplicated was flanked by an approximately 30-kb repeat called CMT1A-REP (Fig. 101-1). Physical mapping studies showed that CMT1A-REP was present in two copies on the normal chromosome as a direct repeat but in three copies on the CMT1A duplication chromosome. Probes to CMT1A-REP were shown to detect specific junction fragments in CMT1A duplication patients. These observations are consistent with a model of unequal crossover whereby misalignment between the proximal copy of CMT1A-REP and the distal copy of CMT1A-REP during meiosis and a homologous recombination event involving these misaligned repeats result in the CMT1A duplication. This model predicts a reciprocal recombination that would result in a 1.5-Mb deletion.

***PMP22* GENE DOSAGE AS A NOVEL MECHANISM FOR CMT1A** Several models were proposed to explain how the CMT1A duplication might alter the expression of a "CMT gene" to result in the disease phenotype. To investigate the gene dosage model, patients with a cytogenetically visible duplication of the short arm of chromosome 17 (17p) were subjected to electrophysiologic studies. Four patients with different cytogenetic duplications had the decreased NCV consistent with CMT1. That these patients had different breakpoints and yet, as long as they duplicated the CMT1A region, they manifested motor NCV abnormalities consistent with CMT1 lends strong support to the gene dosage model even prior to the identification of a dosage-sensitive gene that maps within the CMT1A duplication.

The identification of the dosage-sensitive gene was aided greatly by concurrent studies on the basic neurobiology of peripheral nerve regeneration and an animal model for CMT1, the *Trembler (Tr)* mouse. A subtractive hybridization strategy, using cDNA libraries constructed from crushed sciatic nerve vs noncrushed nerve to investigate genes important to nerve regeneration, identified a peripheral myelin-specific gene that was not expressed after crush injury but was expressed at a high level during nerve regeneration and maintenance. This gene mapped to mouse chromosome 11, which is syntenic to human chromosome 17p, encoded a protein of approximately 22 kDa, and was called peripheral

CMT1A Duplication

3.0 Mb
CMT1A-REP *PMP22* CMT1A-REP *PMP22* CMT1A-REP
11.1 11.2 12 13.1 13.2 13.3
17p (Duplication)
17p (Normal)
CMT1A-REP (~30kb) *PMP22* (36 kb) CMT1A-REP (~30kb)
1.5 Mb

HNPP Deletion

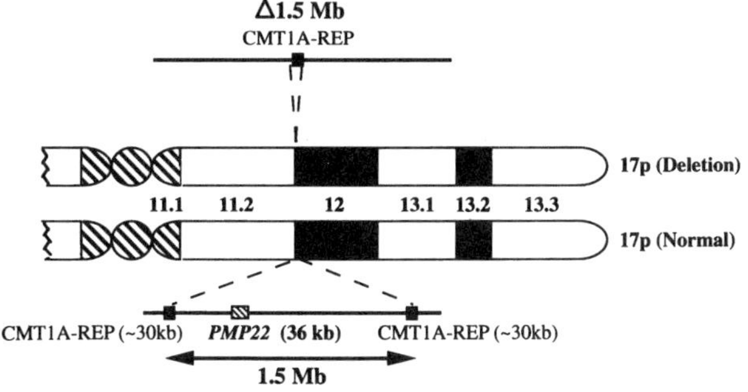

Figure 101-1 Structure of CMT1A duplication and HNPP deletion. The CMT1A duplication is a submicroscopic tandem duplication of a 1.5-Mb DNA region while the HNPP is a 1.5-Mb deletion of the same region in chromosome 17p11.2–p12. The regions on chromosome 17p are depicted, with the normal chromosome shown below and the segmentally duplicated or deleted chromosome above. Cross-hatched circles, the centromere. The normal chromosome 17p contains a 1.5-Mb region on 17p11.2–p12 flanked by homologous CMT1A-REP sequences (filled boxes in blown-up region) of approximately 30 kb in length (our unpublished observations). The *PMP22* gene (crosshatched boxes) maps within this 1.5-Mb critical region, which is duplicated in most patients with CMT and deleted in most patients with HNPP. The 1.5-Mb HNPP deletion is not detected by standard cytogenetic G-banding, and results in deletion of *PMP22* and one copy of CMT1A-REP on one chromosome. CMT1A results from three copies of *PMP22*, while HNPP results from one copy of *PMP22*. The 3.0-Mb CMT1A duplication is not detected cytogenetically, and results in two copies of *PMP22* and three copies of CMT1A-REP on the duplicated chromosome.

myelin protein–22, *Pmp*-22. *Pmp*-22 was shown to contain a mutation causing different missense amino acid substitutions in the *Tr* and allelic Tr^J mice. *Trembler* had been proposed as an animal model for CMT and for DSS based on similar electrophysiologic findings of decreased motor NCV and neuropathologic findings including onion bulb formation.

The human *PMP22* gene was isolated, shown to be expressed at a high level specifically in the peripheral nerve, and mapped within the CMT1A duplication (Fig. 101-1). Subsequently, a human *PMP22* missense mutation leading to the identical amino acid substitution identified in Tr^J mouse was found to cosegregate with the CMT1 phenotype in a nonduplication family, whose disease locus was linked to 17p11.2–p12. Similarly, a *de novo PMP22* mutation was identified in a sporadic nonduplication case of CMT1.

The identification of *de novo* and inherited *PMP22* point mutations in DSS further supports the role of *PMP22* in demyelinating peripheral neuropathies. These observations, in conjunction with the findings that rare CMT1 patients with smaller or larger duplications each include the *PMP22* gene, strongly support the hypothesis that *PMP22* is the dosage-sensitive gene in the CMT1A duplication. Further proof for the dosage hypothesis was obtained with the demonstration of elevated *PMP22* mRNA expression in biopsied peripheral nerves from CMT1A duplication patients.

A transgenic rat model of CMT1A has been created by overexpression of *PMP22*. The transgenic rats develop gait abnormalities, peripheral hypomyelination, onion bulb formation in Schwann cells, and muscle weakness. This model may facilitate the evaluation of potential treatment strategies for CMT1A

DNA DELETION ASSOCIATED WITH HNPP The HNPP deletion was identified initially in two families segregating autosomal dominant HNPP and as a *de novo* mutation in a sporadic case. The deletion was demonstrated in affected individuals by loss of RFLP alleles and by FISH. It was shown to segregate in a dominant fashion, to contain all the markers known to be duplicated in patients with the CMT1A duplication, to measure 1.5 Mb in size, and to have junctions that overlapped those of the CMT1A duplication (Fig. 101-1). Because the deletion resulted in lack of transmission of deleted alleles to affected offspring, failure to recognize the deletion could lead to erroneous exclusion of paternity or maternity. The *PMP22* gene was shown to be deleted in patients with the HNPP deletion. It was proposed as the gene whose underexpression or haploinsufficiency was responsible for HNPP. This hypothesis was substantiated by the subsequent identification of a *PMP22* frameshift mutation, leading to a nonsense codon and to a premature termination likely resulting in a null allele, in a nondeletion HNPP family.

Although some evidence exists to suggest genetic heterogeneity, the majority of patients appear to have HNPP by the deletion. The identification of similar junction fragments in multiple unrelated families suggests that a precise recombination event is involved in generating the HNPP deletion.

THE CMT1A DUPLICATION AND HNPP DELETION RESULT FROM A RECIPROCAL RECOMBINATION Physical mapping studies of the CMT1A duplication showed that CMT1A-REP was present in three copies on the duplicated chromosome. This finding led to a model for generating the duplication that predicted a reciprocal recombination product of a 1.5-Mb deletion with only one copy of CMT1A-REP remaining on the deleted chromosome. The HNPP deletion was proposed as the anticipated reciprocal recombination product. Molecular analysis in multiple patients detected three copies of CMT1A-REP on both inherited and *de novo* CMT1A duplication chromosomes, and one copy of CMT1A-REP on the deleted chromosome in both inherited and *de novo* HNPP. Furthermore, the predicted HNPP junction fragments with a CMT1A-REP probe were identified. Obviously, these two diseases cannot coexist in the same family lineage because the mutation event must cause a duplication and a deletion gamete, only one of which will appear in the fertilized egg and thus be transmitted into subsequent generations. These observations support the hypothesis that a reciprocal recombination mechanism involving CMT1A-REP is responsible for the generation of both the duplicated and deleted chromosomes. Moreover, they document the first examples in humans of mendelian syndromes resulting from the reciprocal products of unequal

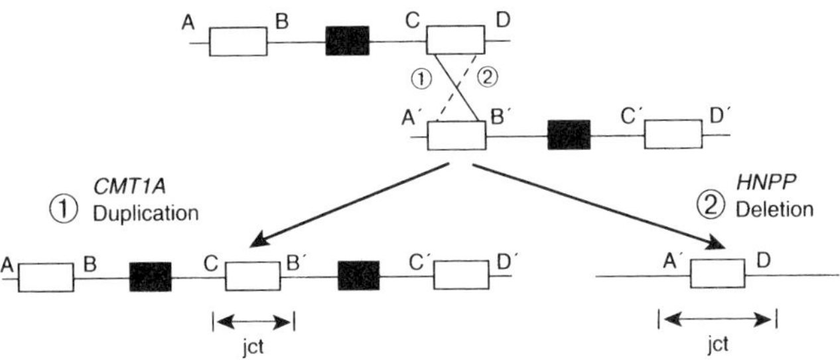

Figure 101-2 Reciprocal recombination resulting in Charcot-Marie-Tooth disease type 1A (CMT1A) or hereditary neuropathy with liability to pressure palsies (HNPP). Open boxes, CMT1A-REP; solid boxes, *PMP22*; A, B, C, and D, and A', B', C', and D', unique sequences flanking CMT1A-REP on the two chromosome homologs, respectively; circled numbers 1 and 2, the crossovers that lead to the different DNA rearrangements: CMT1A duplication or HNPP deletion; jct, specific junction fragments for the CMT1A duplication and HNPP deletion detected using a CMT1A-REP probe. (Reprinted from Lupski et al., JAMA 1993;270:2326–2330.)

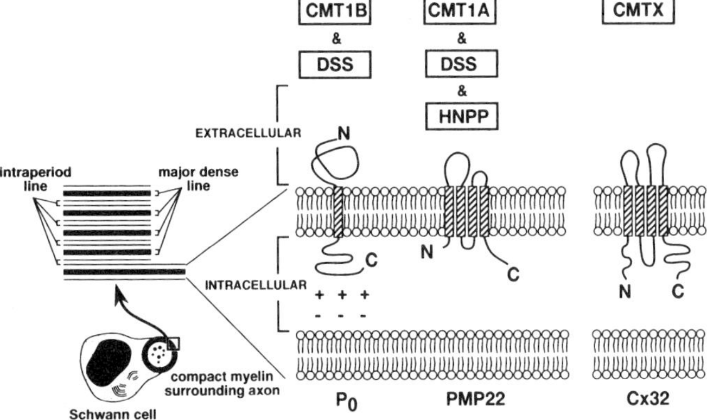

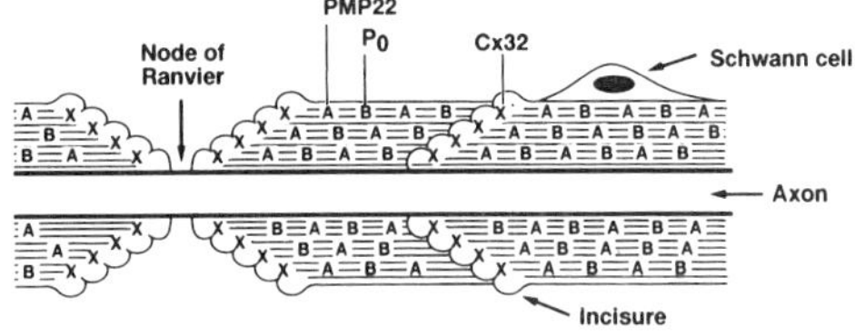

Figure 101-3 Myelin protein components and organization in the peripheral nervous system (PNS). Note that one Schwann cell myelinates a single axon in the PNS. A crosssection illustrates compact myelin organization indicating the major dense line and the intraperiod line, which are formed by apposed intracellular and extracellular membranes surfaces, respectively. The proposed structures of the major PNS myelin proteins are shown; PMP22, peripheral nerve myelin protein, 22-kDa M_r; P_0, myelin protein zero; Cx32, connexin 32. Boxes, the inherited myelin disorders associated with mutations in each myelin protein; CMT1A, Charcot-Marie-Tooth disease type 1A; HNPP, hereditary neuropathy with liability to pressure palsies; CMT1B, Charcot-Marie-Tooth disease type B; DSS, Dejerine-Sottas syndrome; CMTX, X-linked CMT. The gap in the membrane indicates the different locations of the Cx32 proteins. Bottom, the distribution as determined by immunostaining of the major PNS myelin proteins PMP22 (A), P_0 (B), and Cx32 (X) in the peripheral nerve. (Adapted from Roa and Lupski, Adv Hum Genet 1994;10:128–133.)

exchange involving large intrachromosomal segments, and provide the first example of two distinct human diseases associated with reciprocal products of the same mutational event (Fig. 101-2). Interestingly, there is a recombination hot spot within CMT1A-REP associated with the unequal crossover responsible for the CMT1A duplication and HNPP deletion, and this hot spot is located near a *mariner* insect transposon-like element.

MPZ AND _CX32_ MUTATIONS ASSOCIATED WITH MYELINOPATHIES The *MPZ* gene encodes myelin protein P_0, which is expressed uniquely by myelinating Schwann cells and is a major structural protein of peripheral myelin. P_0 is an integral myelin membrane protein with a single transmembrane domain and an extracellular domain consisting of an immunoglobulin-like structure. The latter domain is important for homophilic adhesion molecule interactions and is proposed to play a significant role in myelin compaction. Homozygous P_0 knockout mice have clinical features similar to CMT1, including hypomyelination and uncompacted myelin.

The locus for the human P_0 gene was mapped to 1q22–q23 by FISH, the same region implicated in CMT1B. Heterozygous *MPZ* mutations have been identified in CMT1B, isolated CMT1, and DSS (Fig. 101-3). Many mutations are in regions that encode the extracellular domain and may result in a perturbation of homophilic interactions necessary for myelin compaction.

The *Cx32* gene encodes the gap junction protein, connexin 32. *Cx32* mRNA is expressed at high levels in the peripheral nerve but also in the liver. Multiple *Cx32* mutations were identified in families with X-linked CMT1 (CMTX1). Immunohistochemical staining of connexin 32 at the nodes of Ranvier and at Schmidt-Lanterman incisures suggests that it may form the intracellular gap junctions that connect the folds of Schwann's cell cytoplasm (*see* Fig. 101-3). These junctions have been proposed to allow transfer of ions, nutrients, and small molecules around and across the compact myelin to the innermost myelin layers, indirectly providing sustenance to the axon as well. This could explain the combination of myelin disruption and axonal degeneration that occurs with *Cx32* mutations in CMTX1.

PATHOPHYSIOLOGY

The three genes identified to date, *PMP22*, *MPZ*, and *Cx32*, involved in the inherited myelinopathies CMT1, HNPP, and DSS, each encode highly expressed integral myelin membrane proteins. The biology of protein P_0 is perhaps the best understood, because of extensive structural studies, the analysis of the properties of adhesion molecules in cell culture systems, the availability of a P_0 knockout mouse, and the multiple *MPZ* mutations in CMT1 and DSS, which are enabling genotype/phenotype correlations. All evidence points to an important role for P_0 in the maintenance of proper myelin compaction by acting as a homophilic adhesion molecule facilitating the tight compaction of apposed extracellular membrane faces along the intraperiod line of peripheral nerve myelin.

The exact biological function of *PMP22* remains unknown. However, by analogy to *MPZ* and mutational alterations leading to CMT1 and DSS, and in combination with ultrastructural studies showing loss of myelin compaction in HNPP patients where the phenotype is now known to result from haploinsufficiency of *PMP22*, it is likely that the PMP22 protein plays a role in maintaining myelin compaction. One proposed hypothesis regarding *PMP22* function is that it may be involved in the intramembrane contact important to myelin integrity, since many of the mutations associated with inherited neuropathies occur in regions encoding the transmembrane domains. Whatever the exact function for

PMP22, it is clear that a critical amount of the protein is required, since either overexpression or underexpression by only 50% results in a disease phenotype. The studies on the role of *PMP22* inherited neuropathies delineate the concept of a "gene expression window" for a dosage-sensitive gene. This concept has potent implications for gene therapy.

The underlying pathophysiology in CMT1 and related demyelinating neuropathies may therefore be related to a disturbance of myelin compaction, resulting in the abnormal motor NCV, which then leads to the clinical manifestations. The identification of other genes wherein mutations result in a CMT1 phenotype would facilitate a better understanding of the biology of the normal peripheral nerve.

CLINICAL IMPLICATIONS

MOLECULAR DIAGNOSIS The CMT1A duplication is the causative mutation for the majority of autosomal dominant CMT1 and occurs as a new mutation in 90% of sporadic CMT1 cases. Given its high frequency, the detection of the CMT1A duplication is a useful diagnostic test in patients with inherited as well as sporadic peripheral neuropathy. In a patient with an electrophysiological diagnosis of CMT1, detection of the CMT1A duplication establishes the exact molecular form of the disease in that family. This makes it possible to diagnose or exclude with a simple blood test other family members who are at risk of developing the disease, enables prenatal diagnosis to be offered, and may provide prognostic information.

The HNPP deletion appears to be the causative mutation in the majority of autosomal dominant and sporadic HNPP cases. Hereditary neuropathy with liability to pressure palsies is a milder disease than CMT, and, because the symptoms can be episodic and transient, individuals may be less likely to seek medical attention. It can be a difficult clinical diagnosis to make and requires a high index of suspicion. Therefore, molecular testing can be very helpful. The HNPP deletion should be suspected in the following clinical situations: (1) any family showing dominantly inherited pressure palsies, (2) families with multiple members affected with carpal tunnel syndrome or other entrapment neuropathies, and (3) all patients with a recurrent demyelinating mononeuropathy or polyneuropathy of undetermined etiology, since electrophysiological studies can show evidence for conduction block. The detection of the HNPP deletion establishes a precise molecular diagnosis, enables presymptomatic diagnosis in family members at risk, can be useful for prognosis, and will promote preventive measures to avoid nerve pressure or trauma to susceptible areas such as the elbows, wrists, and at the fibular neck of the legs. Although the exact prevalence of HNPP is unknown, sporadic cases should be nearly as common as sporadic CMT1A, since the HNPP deletion and CMT1A duplication represent reciprocal recombination products.

Molecular diagnostic testing is available commercially for the detection of the CMT1A duplication and the HNPP deletion in the United States and is also performed in molecular diagnostic laboratories throughout the world. In the first 18 months of testing in the United States, the CMT1A duplication was detected in 21% of 2421 individuals with a clinical suspicion of CMT. Intriguingly, 20 suspected CMT patients were found to have the HNPP deletion even prior to launching of the molecular assay for HNPP. This emphasizes the extreme variability of clinical expression of these inherited peripheral neuropathies, the limitations of a clinical

Increasing Severity →

Dejerine-Sottas Syndrome / *PMP22, MPZ* point mutations

Severe CMT1A / homozygous duplication

CMT1A and CMT1B / *PMP22, MPZ* point mutations

X-linked CMT(♂ > ♀) / *Cx32* point mutations

CMT1A / 1.5 Mb duplication

HNPP / 1.5 Mb deletion

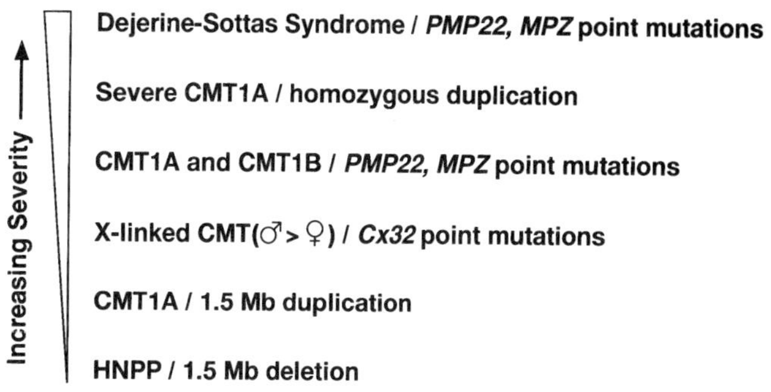

Figure 101-4 Clinical neuropathy phenotype/genotype correlations. Left, clinical phenotypes with the trend toward increasing severity listed from bottom to top; right, are shown the types of mutations found. The inherited primary demyelinating peripheral neuropathies are clinically heterogeneous with a wide variability of clinical expression and can have overlap of symptoms. However, molecular analysis enables recognition of some trends for phenotype/genotype correlations.

diagnosis when evaluating these patients, and the diagnostic value of molecular testing. During the 6 months since the launch of molecular testing for the HNPP deletion, 28% of 166 individuals suspected clinically of having HNPP have tested positive for the deletion.

Molecular diagnostic testing for *Cx32* mutations is also available commercially in the United States. Mutation in *Cx32* appears to be the most common alteration found in nonduplication CMT1. Detection of these mutations has important clinical implications for genetic counseling regarding recurrence risk, since it establishes the X-linked form of the disease in the family.

PHENOTYPE/GENOTYPE CORRELATIONS Charcot-Marie-Tooth disease is well-established as a disorder with extreme variability of clinical expression. Some of this variability may have reflected genetic heterogeneity. However, not only is there interfamilial clinical heterogeneity but there is also significant intrafamilial clinical heterogeneity. Families segregating the CMT1A duplication may have substantive variability among affected individuals; the degree of motor NCV decrease can also vary. Clinical variability can even be observed in identical twins with the CMT1A duplication. It has been proposed that this clinical variability may reflect the gene dosage phenomena underlying CMT1A. Patients with the CMT1A duplication have no abnormal gene product, but, instead, their disease reflects abnormally increased expression of *PMP22*. Altered gene expression levels may be more susceptible to modifier gene and/or environmental effects than gene mutations resulting in aberrant proteins.

There is a wide variability of clinical expression for each of the inherited demyelinating neuropathies and clinical diagnostic categories may overlap. Nevertheless, molecular analyses enable some phenotype/genotype correlations as guidelines. Patients with the HNPP deletion usually have a milder disease than those with the CMT1A duplication. The point mutations in *PMP22* and *MPZ* give missense amino acid substitutions, which result in aberrant proteins that will usually lead to a more severe clinical CMT1 or DSS phenotype than the duplication form (Fig. 101-4). The severity of the disease likely reflects the extent of the mutation's effect on the protein function in myelin compaction. Missense amino acid substitutions may be more detrimental than null mutation by having a dominant-negative effect in a multimeric structure.

CONCLUSIONS

Molecular genetic analysis of the demyelinating neuropathies CMT1 and HNPP has uncovered a novel mutational mechanism whereby a reciprocal recombination involving a misaligned flanking repeat sequence results in both the CMT1A duplication and HNPP deletion. These studies have illuminated the role that gene dosage may play in causing a disease phenotype, which has important implications for therapeutic strategies, and which may underlie the basis of the extreme clinical variability. The identification of these specific molecular lesions has resulted in the availability of molecular procedures for establishing or excluding a secure diagnosis, enabling presymptomatic and prenatal diagnosis, and providing prognostic information.

The identification of the myelin genes *PMP22*, *MPZ*, and *Cx32*, wherein structural gene alterations can result in demyelinating neuropathy phenotypes, has led to a better understanding of the molecular basis of CMT1, HNPP, and DSS, and has provided important tools to investigate further the biology of the peripheral nerve. Multidisciplinary approaches have enabled us to understand the molecular bases for and pathophysiology of CMT and other myelinopathies, and they highlight the importance of myelin compaction for proper nerve function. These findings provide a clear focus for efforts to elucidate the cascade of events beginning with a mutation in a gene or altered gene dosage leading ultimately to recognizable diseases phenotypes. This knowledge will be instrumental to the design of rational therapies for these diseases.

SELECTED REFERENCES

Bergoffen J, Scherer SS, Wang S, et al. Connexin mutations in X-linked Charcot-Marie-Tooth disease. Science 1993;262:2039–2042.

Chance PF, Abbas N, Lensch MW, et al. Two autosomal dominant neuropathies result from reciprocal DNA duplication/deletion of a region on chromosome 17. Hum Mol Genet 1994;3:223–228.

Chance PF, Alderson MK, Leppig KA, et al. DNA deletion associated with hereditary neuropathy with liability to pressure palsies. Cell 1993;72:143–151.

Chance PF, Bird TD, Matsunami N, Lensch MW, Brothman AR, Feldman GM. Trisomy 17p associated with Charcot-Marie-Tooth neuropathy type 1A phenotype: evidence for gene dosage as a mechanism in CMT1A. Neurology 1992;42:2295–2299.

Garcia CA, Malamut RI, Parry GS, Liu P, Lupski JR. Clinical variability in identical twins with the Charcot-Marie-Tooth disease type 1A duplication. Neurology 1995;45:2090–2093.

Hayasaka K, Himoro M, Sato W, et al. Charcot-Marie-Tooth neuropathy type 1B is associated with mutations of the myelin P_0 gene. Nat Genet 1993;5:31–34.

Hayasaka K, Himoro M, Sawaishi Y, et al. *De novo* mutation of the myelin P_0 gene in Dejerine-Sottas disease (hereditary motor and sensory neuropathy type III). Nat Genet 1993;5:266–268.

Hoogendijk JE, Hensels GW, Gabreels-Festen AAWM, et al. De-novo mutation in hereditary motor and sensory neuropathy type 1. Lancet 1992;339:1081–1082.

Kaku DA, Parry GJ, Malamut R, Lupski JR, Garcia CA. Nerve conduction studies in Charcot-Marie-Tooth polyneuropathy associated with a segmental duplication of chromosome 17. Neurology 1993;43: 1806–1808.

Killian JM, Tiwari PS, Jacobson S, Jackson RD, Lupski JR. Longitudinal studies of the duplication form of Charcot-Marie-Tooth polyneuropathy. Muscle Nerve 1996;19:74–78.

Kulkens T, Bolhuis PA, Wolterman RA, et al. Deletion of the serine 34 codon from the major peripheral myelin protein P_0 gene in Charcot-Marie-Tooth disease type 1B. Nat Genet 1993;5:35–39.

Lupski JR. DNA diagnostics for Charcot-Marie-Tooth disease and related peripheral neuropathies. Clin Chem 1996;42:995–998.

Lupski JR. Molecular genetics in clinical practice V. Charcot-Marie-Tooth disease: A gene dosage effect. Hospital Practice 1997;32:83–122.

Lupski JR, Chance PF, Garcia CA. Inherited primary peripheral neuropathies: molecular genetics and clinical implications of CMT1A and HNPP. JAMA 1993;270:2326–2330.

Lupski JR, Montes de Oca-Luna R, Slaugenhaupt S, et al. DNA duplication associated with Charcot-Marie-Tooth disease type 1A. Cell 1991;66:219–232.

Lupski JR, Wise CA, Kuwano A, et al. Gene dosage is a mechanism for Charcot-Marie-Tooth disease type 1A. Nat Genet 1992;1:29–33.

Nicholson GA, Valentijn LJ, Cherryson AK, et al. A frame shift mutation in the *PMP22* gene in hereditary neuropathy with liability to pressure palsies. Nat Genet 1994;6:263–266.

Palau F, Lofgren A, De Jonghe P, et al. Origin of the *de novo* duplication in Charcot-Marie-Tooth disease type 1A: unequal nonsister chromatid exchange during spermatogenesis. Hum Mol Genet 1993;2: 2031–2035.

Patel PI, Lupski JR. Charcot-Marie-Tooth disease: a new paradigm for the mechanism of inherited disease. Trends Genet 1994;10:128–133.

Patel PI, Roa BB, Welcher AA, et al. The gene for the peripheral myelin protein PMP-22 is a candidate for Charcot-Marie-tooth disease type 1A. Nat Genet 1992;1:159–165.

Pentao L, Wise CA, Chinault AC, Patel PI, Lupski JR. Charcot-Marie-Tooth type 1A duplication appears to arise from recombination at repeat sequences flanking the 1.5 Mb monomer unit. Nat Genet 1992;2:292–300.

Raeymaekers P, Timmerman V, Nelis V, et al. Duplication in chromosome 17p11.2 in Charcot-Marie-Tooth neuropathy type 1a (CTM1a). Neuromuscul Disord 1991;2:93–97.

Reiter LT, Murakami T, Koeuth T, et al. A recombination hotspot responsible for two inherited peripheral neuropathies is located near a mariner transposon-like element. Nat Genet 1996;12:288–297.

Roa BB, Ananth U, Garcia CA, Lupski JR. Molecular diagnosis of Charcot-Marie-Tooth disease type 1A and hereditary neuropathy with liability to pressure palsies. LabMedica International 1995;12:22–24.

Roa BB, Dyck PJ, Marks HG, Chance PF, Lupski JR. Dejerine-Sottas syndrome associated with point mutation in the peripheral myelin protein 22 *(PMP22)* gene. Nat Genet 1993;5:269–273.

Roa BB, Garcia CA, Suter U, et al. Charcot-Marie-Tooth disease type 1A: association with a spontaneous point mutation in the *PMP22* gene. N Engl J Med 1993;329:96–101.

Roa BB, Lupski JR. Molecular genetics of Charcot-Marie-Tooth neuropathy. Adv Hum Genet 1994;22:117–152.

Sereda M, Griffiths I, Puhlohofer A, et al. A transgenic rat model of Charcot-Marie-Tooth disease. Neuron 1996;16:1049–1060.

Shaffer LG, Kennedy GM, Spikes AS, Lupski JR. Diagnosis of CMT1A duplications by interphase FISH: Implications for testing in the cytogenetics laboratory. Am J Med Genet 1997;69:325–331.

Suter U, Moskow JJ, Welcher AA, et al. A leucine-to-proline mutation in the putative first transmembrane domain of the 22-kDa peripheral myelin protein in the trembler-J mouse. Proc Natl Acad Sci USA 1992;89:4382–4386.

Suter U, Welcher AA, Ozcelik T, et al. *Trembler* mouse carries a point mutation in a myelin gene. Nature 1992;19:241–244.

Suter U, Welcher AA, Snipes GJ. Progress in the molecular understanding of hereditary peripheral neuropathies reveals new insights into the biology of the peripheral nervous system. Trends Neurosci 1993;2:50–56.

Valentijn LJ, Baas F, Wolterman RA, et al. Identical point mutations of *PMP-22* in *Trembler-J* mouse and Charcot-Marie-Tooth disease type a. Nat Genet 1992;2:288–291.

Warner LE, Hilz MJ, Appel SH, et al. Clinical phenotypes of different MPZ (PO) mutations may include Charcot-Marie-Tooth type 1B, Dejerine-Sottas, and congenital hypomyelination. Neuron 1996; 17:451–460.

Wise CA, Garcia CA, Davis SN, et al. Molecular analyses of unrelated Charcot-Marie-Tooth (CMT) disease patients suggest a high frequency of the CMT1A duplication. Am J Hum Genet 1993;53:853–863.

Yoshikawa H, Dyck PJ. Uncompacted inner myelin lamellae in inherited tendency to pressure palsy. J Neuropathol Exp Med 1991;50:649–657.

Yoshikawa H, Nishimura T, Nakatsuji Y, et al. Elevated expression of messenger RNA for peripheral myelin protein 22 in biopsied peripheral nerves of patients with Charcot-Marie-Tooth disease type 1A. Ann Neurol 1994;35:445–450.

102 Molecular and Genetic Basis of Prion Diseases

STANLEY B. PRUSINER

INTRODUCTION

Prions cause a group of human and animal neurodegenerative diseases that are now classified together because their etiology and pathogenesis involve modification of the prion protein (PrP). Prion diseases are manifest as infectious, genetic, and sporadic disorders (Table 102-1). These diseases can be transmitted among mammals by the infectious particle designated "prion." Despite intensive searches over the past three decades, no nucleic acid has been found within prions; yet, a modified isoform of the host-encoded PrP designated PrP^{Sc} is essential for infectivity. In fact, considerable experimental data argue that prions are composed exclusively of PrP^{Sc}. Earlier terms used to describe the prion diseases include transmissible encephalopathies, spongiform encephalopathies, and slow virus diseases.

The quartet of human prion diseases are frequently referred to as kuru, Creutzfeldt-Jakob disease (CJD) (OMIM 123400), Gerstmann-Sträussler-Scheinker (GSS) (OMIM 137440) disease, and fatal familial insomnia (FFI) (OMIM 600072). Kuru (OMIM 245300) was the first of these diseases to be transmitted to experimental animals, and it is likely that kuru spread among the Fore people of Papua New Guinea by ritualistic cannibalism. The experimental and presumed human-to-human transmission of kuru led to the belief that prion diseases are infectious disorders caused by unusual viruses similar to those causing scrapie in sheep and goats. Yet, a paradox was presented by the occurrence of CJD in families; it appeared to be a genetic disease. The significance of familial CJD remained unappreciated until mutations in the protein coding region of the *PrP* gene on the short arm of chromosome 20 were discovered. The earlier finding that brain extracts from patients who had died of familial prion diseases inoculated into experimental animals often transmitted disease posed a conundrum that was resolved with the genetic linkage of these diseases to mutations of the *PrP* gene.

CJD is a rare disorder with an annual worldwide incidence of about 1 case per 10^6 people. Less than 1% of CJD cases are infectious, and most of those appear to be iatrogenic. Between 10 and 25% of prion disease cases are inherited, while the remaining cases are sporadic. Patients with CJD frequently present with dementia, but approximately 10% of patients exhibit cerebellar dysfunction initially. Kuru was once the most common cause of death among New Guinean women in the Fore region of the Highlands but has virtually disappeared with the cessation of ritualistic cannibalism. Patients with either kuru or GSS usually present with ataxia, while those with FFI manifest insomnia and autonomic dysfunction.

From: *Principles of Molecular Medicine* (J. L. Jameson, ed.), ©1998 Humana Press Inc., Totowa, NJ.

Scrapie is the most common natural prion disease of animals. One outbreak of scrapie followed the vaccination of sheep for looping ill virus with formalin-treated extracts of ovine lymphoid tissue unknowingly contaminated with scrapie prions. Two years later, more than 1500 sheep developed scrapie from this vaccine. While the transmissibility of experimental scrapie became well established, the spread of natural scrapie within and among flocks of sheep remained puzzling. Parry argued that host genes were responsible for the development of scrapie in sheep. He was convinced that natural scrapie is a genetic disease which could be eradicated by proper breeding protocols. He considered its transmission by inoculation of importance primarily for laboratory studies and communicable infection of little consequence in nature. Other investigators viewed natural scrapie as an infectious disease and argued that host genetics only modulates susceptibility to an endemic infectious agent.

The offal of scrapied sheep in Great Britain is thought to be responsible for the current epidemic of bovine spongiform encephalopathy (BSE) or mad cow disease. Prions in the offal from scrapie-infected sheep appear to have survived the rendering process that produced meat and bone meal (MBM). The MBM was fed to cattle as a nutritional supplement. After BSE was recognized, MBM produced from domestic animal offal was banned from further use. Since 1986, when BSE was first recognized, more than 150,000 cattle have died of BSE. Whether humans will develop CJD after consuming beef from cattle with BSE prions is of considerable concern.

As our knowledge of the prion diseases increases and more is learned about the molecular and genetic characteristics of prion proteins, these disorders will undoubtedly undergo modification with respect to their classification. Indeed, the discovery of PrP and the identification of pathogenic *PrP* gene mutations have already forced us to view these illnesses from perspectives not previously imagined.

THE PRION CONCEPT

Once an effective protocol was developed for preparation of partially purified fractions of scrapie agent from hamster brain, it

Table 102-1
Human Prion Diseases

Disease	*Etiology*
Kuru	Infection
Creutzfeldt-Jakob disease	
Iatrogenic	Infection
Sporadic	Unknown
Familial	*PrP* mutation
Gerstmann-Sträussler-Scheinker disease	*PrP* mutation
Fatal Familial Insomnia	*PrP* mutation

became possible to demonstrate that those procedures which modify or hydrolyze proteins produce a diminution in scrapie infectivity. At the same time, tests done in search of a scrapie-specific nucleic acid were unable to demonstrate any dependence of infectivity on a polynucleotide, in agreement with earlier studies reporting the extreme resistance of infectivity to ultraviolet irradiation at 254 nm.

Based on these findings, it seemed likely that the infectious pathogen capable of transmitting scrapie was neither a virus nor a viroid. For this reason the term prion was introduced to distinguish the proteinaceous infectious particles that cause scrapie, CJD, GSS, and kuru from both viroids and viruses. Hypotheses for the structure of the infectious prion particle included: (1) proteins surrounding a nucleic acid encoding them (a virus), (2) proteins associated with a small polynucleotide, and (3) proteins devoid of nucleic acid. Mechanisms postulated for the replication of infectious prion particles ranged from those used by viruses to the synthesis of polypeptides in the absence of nucleic acid template to posttranslational modifications of cellular proteins. Subsequent discoveries have narrowed hypotheses for both prion structure and the mechanism of replication.

Considerable evidence supporting the prion hypothesis has accumulated over the past decade. Furthermore, the replication of prions and their mode of pathogenesis also appear to be without precedent. After a decade of severe criticism and serious doubt, the prion concept is now enjoying considerable acceptance.

DISCOVERY OF THE PRION PROTEIN

Once the dependence of prion infectivity on protein was clear, the search for a scrapie-specific protein intensified. While the insolubility of scrapie infectivity made purification problematic, we took advantage of this property, along with its relative resistance to degradation by proteases, to extend the degree of purification. In subcellular fractions from hamster brain enriched for scrapie infectivity, a protease-resistant polypeptide of 27–30 kDa, later designated PrP 27–30, was identified; it was absent from controls. Radioiodination of partially purified fractions revealed a protein unique to preparations from scrapie-infected brains.

Purification of PrP 27–30 to homogeneity allowed determination of its NH_2-terminal amino acid sequence. These studies were particularly difficult because multiple signals were found in each cycle of the Edman degradation. Whether multiple proteins were present in these "purified fractions," or a single protein with a ragged NH_2 terminus was present, was resolved only after data from five different preparations were compared. When the signals in each cycle were grouped according to their intensities, of strong, intermediate, and weak, it became clear that a single protein with a ragged NH_2 terminus was being sequenced. Determination of a single, unique sequence for the NH_2 terminus of PrP 27–30 permitted the synthesis of an isocoding mixture of oligonucleotides that was subsequently used to identify incomplete PrP cDNA clones from Syrian hamster (SHa) and mouse (Mo). cDNA clones encoding the entire open reading frames (ORF) of SHa and Mo PrP were subsequently recovered.

PrP is encoded by a chromosomal gene and not by a nucleic acid within the infectious scrapie prion particle. Levels of PrP mRNA remain unchanged throughout the course of scrapie infection—an unexpected observation, which led to the identification of the normal PrP gene product, a protein of 33–35 kDa, designated PrP^C. PrP^C is protease-sensitive and soluble in nondenaturing detergents, while PrP 27–30 is the protease-resistant core of a 33- to 35-kDa disease-specific protein, designated PrP^{Sc}, which is insoluble in detergents. Progress in the study of prions was greatly accelerated by the discovery of PrP and determination of its N-terminal sequence. Indeed, all of the elegant molecular genetic studies in humans and animals as well as many highly informative transgenetic investigations have their origin in the purification of PrP 27–30 and the determination of its N-terminal sequence.

***PrP* GENE STRUCTURE AND ORGANIZATION** The entire ORF of all known mammalian and avian *PrP* genes is contained within a single exon (Fig. 102-1). This feature of the *PrP* gene eliminates the possibility that PrP^{Sc} arises from alternative RNA splicing; however, mechanisms such as RNA editing or protein splicing remain a possibility. The two exons of the *SHaPrP* gene are separated by a 10-kb intron: exon 1 encodes a portion of the 5' untranslated leader sequence, while exon 2 encodes the ORF and 3' untranslated region. The Mo and sheep *PrP* genes are comprised of three exons with exon 3 analogous to exon 2 of the hamster. The promoters of both the SHa- and *MoPrP* genes contain multiple copies of G-C-rich repeats and are devoid of TATA boxes. These G-C nonamers represent a motif that may function as a canonical binding site for the transcription factor Sp1.

Mapping *PrP* genes to the short arm of human (Hu) chromosome 20 and the homologous region of Mo chromosome 2 argues for the existence of *PrP* genes prior to the speciation of mammals. Hybridization studies demonstrated fewer than 0.002 *PrP* gene sequences per ID_{50} unit in purified prion fractions, indicating that a nucleic acid encoding PrP^{Sc} is not a component of the infectious prion particle. This is a major feature that distinguishes prions from viruses, including those retroviruses that carry cellular oncogenes and from satellite viruses that derive their coat proteins from other viruses previously infecting plant cells.

Although *PrP* mRNA is constitutively expressed in the brains of adult animals, it is highly regulated during development. In the septum, levels of *PrP* mRNA and choline acetyltransferase were found to increase in parallel during development. In other brain regions, *PrP* gene expression occurred at an earlier age. *In situ* hybridization studies show that the highest levels of PrP mRNA are found in neurons.

HUMAN PRION DISEASES

CLINICAL MANIFESTATIONS OF HUMAN PRION DISEASES The human prion diseases are manifest as infectious, inherited, and sporadic disorders, and are often referred to as kuru, CJD, GSS, and FFI, depending on the clinical and neuropathological findings (*see* Table 102-1).

Infectious forms of prion diseases result from the horizontal transmission of infectious prions, as occurs in iatrogenic CJD and

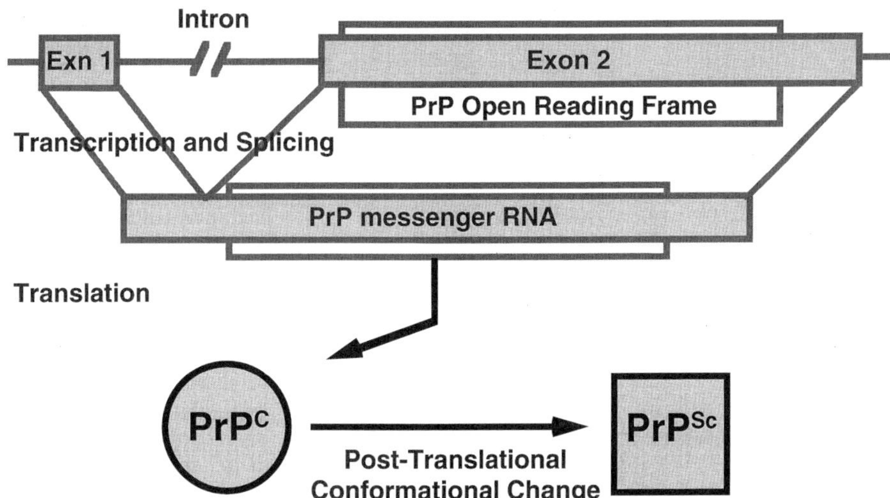

Figure 102-1 Structure and organization of the chromosomal *PrP* gene. In all mammals examined the entire ORF is contained within a single exon. The 5' untranslated region of the *PrP* mRNA is derived from either one or two additional exons. Only one *PrP* mRNA has been detected. PrP^{Sc} is thought to be derived from PrP^{C} by a posttranslational process. The amino acid sequence of PrP^{Sc} is identical to that predicted from the translated sequence of the DNA encoding the *PrP* gene, and no unique posttranslational chemical modifications have been identified that might distinguish PrP^{Sc} from PrP^{C}. Thus, it seems likely that PrP^{C} undergoes a conformational change as it is converted to PrP^{Sc}.

kuru. Inherited forms, notably GSS, familial CJD, and FFI, constitute 10–15% of all cases of prion disease. A mutation in the ORF or protein coding region of the *PrP* gene has been found in all reported kindreds with inherited human prion disease. Sporadic forms of prion disease comprise most cases of CJD and possibly some cases of GSS. How prions arise in patients with sporadic forms is unknown; hypotheses include horizontal transmission from humans or animals, somatic mutation of the *PrP* gene ORF and spontaneous conversion of PrP^{C} into PrP^{Sc}. Numerous attempts to establish an infectious link between sporadic CJD and a preexisting prion disease in animals or humans have been unrewarding.

DIAGNOSIS OF HUMAN PRION DISEASES Human prion disease should be considered in any patient who develops a progressive subacute or chronic decline in cognitive or motor function. Typically adults between 40 and 70 years of age, patients often exhibit clinical features helpful in providing a premorbid diagnosis of prion disease, particularly sporadic CJD. There is as yet no specific diagnostic test for prion disease in the cerebrospinal fluid. A definitive diagnosis of human prion disease, which is invariably fatal, can often only be made from the examination of brain tissue. Over the past decade, knowledge of the molecular genetics of prion diseases has made it possible to diagnose inherited prion disease in living patients using peripheral tissues.

A broad spectrum of neuropathological features in human prion diseases precludes a precise neuropathological definition. The classic neuropathological features of human prion disease include spongiform degeneration, gliosis, and neuronal loss in the absence of an inflammatory reaction. When present, amyloid plaques that stain with α-PrP antibodies are diagnostic.

The presence of protease-resistant PrP (PrP^{Sc} or PrP^{CJD}) in the infectious and sporadic forms and most of the inherited forms of these diseases implicates prions in their pathogenesis. The absence of PrP^{CJD} in a biopsy specimen may simply reflect regional variations in the concentration of the protein. In some patients with inherited prion disease, PrP^{Sc} is barely detectable or undetectable; this situation seems to be mimicked in transgenic (Tg) mice, which express a mutant *PrP* gene and spontaneously develop neurologic illness indistinguishable from experimental murine scrapie.

In humans and Tg mice that have no detectable protease-resistant PrP but express mutant PrP, neurodegeneration may, at least in part, be caused by abnormal metabolism of mutant PrP. Because molecular genetic analyses of PrP genes in patients with unusual dementing illnesses are readily performed, the diagnosis of inherited prion disease can often be established where there was little or no neuropathology, atypical neurodegenerative disease, or misdiagnosed neurodegenerative disease, including Alzheimer's disease.

Although horizontal transmission of neurodegeneration to experimental hosts was for a time the "gold standard" of prion disease, it can no longer be used as such. Some investigators have reported that transmission of the inherited prion diseases from humans to experimental animals is frequently negative when using rodents, despite the presence of a pathogenic mutation in the *PrP* gene, while others state that this is not the case with apes and monkeys as hosts. The discovery that Tg(MHu2M) mice are susceptible to Hu prions promises to make feasible transmission studies that were not practical in apes and monkeys.

The hallmark common to all of the prion diseases, whether sporadic, dominantly inherited, or acquired by infection, is that they involve the aberrant metabolism of the prion protein. Making a definitive diagnosis of human prion disease can be rapidly accomplished if PrP^{Sc} can be detected immunologically. Frequently, PrP^{Sc} can be detected by either the dot-blot method or Western immunoblot analysis of brain homogenates, in which samples are subjected to limited proteolysis to remove PrP^{C} prior to immunostaining. The dot-blot method exploits enhancement of PrP^{Sc} immunoreactivity following denaturation in the chaotropic salt, guanidinium chloride. Because of regional variations in PrP^{Sc} concentration, methods using homogenates prepared from small brain regions can give false-negative results. Alternatively, PrP^{Sc} may be detected *in situ* in cryostat sections bound to nitrocellulose membranes followed by limited proteolysis to remove PrP^{C} and guanidinium treatment to denature PrP^{Sc}, and thus enhance its avidity for α-PrP antibodies. Denaturation of PrP^{Sc} *in situ* prior to immunostaining has also been accomplished by autoclaving fixed tissue sections.

In the familial forms of the prion diseases, molecular genetic analyses of *PrP* can be diagnostic and can be performed on DNA extracted from blood leukocytes antemortem. Unfortunately, such testing is of little value in the diagnosis of the sporadic or infectious forms of prion disease. Although the first missense *PrP* mutation was discovered when the two *PrP* alleles of a patient with GSS were cloned from a genomic library and sequenced, all subsequent novel missense and insertional mutations have been identified in PrP ORFs amplified by the polymerase chain reaction (PCR) and sequenced. The 759 bp encoding the 253 amino acids of PrP reside in a single exon of the *PrP* gene, providing an ideal situation for the use of PCR. Amplified PrP ORFs can be screened for known mutations using one of several methods, the most reliable of which is allele-specific oligonucleotide hybridization. If known mutations are absent, novel mutations may be found when the PrP ORF is sequenced.

When PrP amyloid plaques in brain are present, they are diagnostic for prion disease as noted above. Unfortunately, they are thought to be present in only about 10% of CJD cases, and by definition all cases of GSS. The amyloid plaques in CJD are compact (kuru plaques). Those in GSS are either multicentric (diffuse) or compact. The amyloid plaques in prion diseases contain PrP. The multicentric amyloid plaques, which are pathognomonic for GSS, may be difficult to distinguish from the neuritic plaques of Alzheimer's disease except by immunohistology. In the GSS kindreds the diagnosis of Alzheimer's disease was excluded because the amyloid plaques failed to stain with β-amyloid antiserum but stained with PrP antiserum. In subsequent studies, missense mutations were found in the *PrP* genes of these kindreds.

In summary, the diagnosis of prion disease may be made in patients on the basis of (1) the presence of PrP^{Sc}, (2) mutant PrP genotype, or (3) appropriate immunohistology, and should not be excluded in patients with atypical neurodegenerative diseases until one or preferably two of these examinations have been performed.

INFECTIOUS PRION DISEASES

KURU For many decades kuru devastated the lives of the Fore Highlanders of Papua New Guinea. The high incidence of the disease among women left a society of motherless children raised by their fathers (Table 102-2). It was unusual in the Fore region to see an older woman. With the cessation of traditional warfare, older men are now found. Many of these older men have had a succession of wives, each dying of kuru after leaving several children. Because contamination during ritualistic cannibalism appears to have been the mode by which kuru spread among the Fore people, and since cannibalism had ceased by 1960 in the Fore region, the patients now developing kuru presumably were exposed to the kuru agent more than three decades ago. In many cases, histories from patients and their families of the episode in which they cannibalized the remains of a near relative who had died of kuru have been obtained, presumably providing the source of infection. That the kuru prions could remain apparently quiescent in these patients for periods of three decades and then manifest in the form of a fatal neurological disease is supported by incubation periods of over 7.5 years in some monkeys inoculated with kuru agent.

Table 102-2
Infectious Prion Diseases of Humans

Diseases	*No. of cases*
A. Kuru (1957–1982)	
1. Adult females	1739
2. Adult males	248
3. Children and adolescents	597
Total	2584
B. Iatrogenic Creutzfeldt-Jakob disease	
1. Depth electrodes	2
2. Corneal transplants	1
3. Human pituitary growth hormone	90
4. Human pituitary gonadotropin	5
5. Dura mater grafts	65
6. Neurosurgical procedures	4
Total	167

IATROGENIC CREUTZFELDT-JAKOB DISEASE Accidental transmission of CJD to humans appears to have occurred by corneal transplantation, contaminated EEG electrode implantation, and surgical operations using contaminated instruments or apparatus (*see* Table 102-2). A cornea unknowingly removed from a donor with CJD was transplanted to an apparently healthy recipient, who developed CJD after a prolonged incubation period. Corneas of animals have significant levels of prions, making this scenario seem quite probable. The same improperly decontaminated EEG electrodes that caused CJD in two young patients with intractable epilepsy were found to cause CJD in a chimpanzee 18 months after their experimental implantation.

Surgical procedures may have resulted in accidental inoculation of patients with prions during their operations, presumably because some instrument or apparatus in the operating theater became contaminated when a CJD patient underwent surgery. Although the epidemiology of these studies is highly suggestive, no proof for such episodes exists.

Since 1988, 65 cases of CJD after implantation of dura mater grafts have been recorded. All of the grafts were thought to have been acquired from a single manufacturer whose preparative procedures were inadequate to inactivate human prions. One case of CJD occurred after repair of an eardrum perforation with a pericardium graft.

Thirty cases of CJD in physicians and health care workers have been reported; however, no occupational link has been established. Whether any of these cases represent infectious prion diseases contracted during care of patients with CJD or processing specimens from these patients remains uncertain.

HUMAN GROWTH HORMONE THERAPY The possibility of transmission of CJD from contaminated human grown hormone (HGH) preparations derived from human pituitaries has been raised by the occurrence of fatal cerebellar disorders with dementia in more than 90 patients, ranging in age from 10 to 41 years (*see* Table 102-2). While one case of spontaneous CJD in a 20-year-old woman has been reported, CJD in patients under 40 years of age is very rare. These patients received injections of HGH every 2–4 days for 4–12 years. Interestingly, most of the patients presented with cerebellar syndromes which progressed over periods varying from 6 to 18 months. Some patients became demented during the terminal phases of their illnesses. This clinical course resembles kuru more than ataxic CJD in some respects. Assuming these patients developed CJD from injections of prion-contaminated HGH preparations, the possible incubation periods range from 4 to 30 years. The longest incubation periods are similar to those (20–30 years) associated with recent cases of kuru. Many patients received several common lots of HGH at various times during their prolonged therapies, but no single lot was administered to all the American patients. An aliquot of one lot of HGH has been reported to transmit CNS disease to a squirrel monkey after a prolonged incubation period. How many lots of the HGH might have been contaminated with prions is unknown.

Although CJD is a rare disease with an annual incidence of approximately 1 out of a million people, it is reasonable to assume that CJD is present with a proportional frequency among dead people. About 1% of the population dies each year, and most CJD patients die within one year of developing symptoms. Thus, we estimate that 1 in 10^4 dead people have CJD. Since 10,000 human pituitaries were typically processed in a single HGH preparation, the possibility of hormone preparations contaminated with CJD prions is not remote.

The concentration of CJD prions within infected human pituitaries is unknown; it is interesting that widespread degenerative changes have been observed in both the hypothalamus and the pituitary of sheep with scrapie. The forebrains from scrapie-infected mice have been added to human pituitary suspensions to determine if prions and HGH copurify. Bioassays in mice suggest that prions and HGH do not copurify with currently used protocols. Although these results seem reassuring, especially for patients treated with HGH over much of the last decade, the relatively low titers of the murine scrapie prions used in these studies may not have provided an adequate test. The extremely small size and charge heterogeneity exhibited by scrapie and presumably CJD prions may complicate procedures designed to separate pituitary hormones from these slow infectious pathogens. Even though additional investigations argue for the efficacy of inactivating prions in HGH fractions prepared from human pituitaries using 6 *M* urea, it seems doubtful that such protocols will be used for purifying HGH, since recombinant HGH is available.

Molecular genetic studies have shown that most patients developing iatrogenic CJD after receiving pituitary-derived HGH are homozygous for either methionine (M) or valine (V) at codon 129 of the PrP gene. Homozygosity at the codon 129 polymorphism has also been shown to predispose individuals to sporadic CJD. Interestingly, valine homozygosity seems to be overrepresented in these HGH cases compared with the general population.

Five cases of CJD have occurred in women receiving human pituitary gonadotropin.

INHERITED PRION DISEASES

FAMILIAL PRION DISEASE The recognition that approximately 10% of CJD cases are familial posed a perplexing problem once it was established that CJD is transmissible. Equally puzzling was the transmission of GSS to nonhuman primates and mice, since most cases of GSS are familial. Like sheep scrapie, the relative contributions of genetic and infectious etiologies in the human prion diseases remained a conundrum until molecular clones of the *PrP* gene became available to probe the inherited aspects of these disorders.

***PrP* MUTATIONS AND GENETIC LINKAGE** The discovery of the *PrP* gene and its linkage to scrapie incubation times in mice raised the possibility that mutation might feature in the hereditary human prion diseases. A proline (P)→leucine (L) mutation at codon 102 was shown to be linked genetically to development of GSS with a logarithm of odds (LOD) score exceeding 3 (Fig. 102-2). This mutation may be due to the deamination of a methylated CpG in a germline *PrP* gene resulting in the substitution of a thymine (T) for cytosine (C). The P102L mutation has been found in 10 different families in nine different countries, including the original GSS family. Amyloid plaques isolated from patients with GSS (P102L) were found to be composed of PrP molecules with an L at residue 102 based on protein sequencing of purified peptides. Patients with GSS who have a P→L substitution at PrP codon 105 have also been reported.

Some patients with a mutation at codon 117 have a dementing or telencephalic form of GSS, while others have an ataxic form of the disease. In both forms of GSS (A117V), PrP amyloid plaques were found as well as spongiform degeneration. The factor or factors that determine the different phenotypes of this disease are unknown.

Patients with PrP mutations at codons 198 and 217 were once thought to have familial Alzheimer's disease but are now known to have prion diseases, on the basis of PrP immunostaining of amyloid plaques and *PrP* gene mutations. A genetic linkage study of this family produced a LOD score exceeding 6. Patients with the codon 198 mutation resulting in a phenylalanine (F)→serine (S) substitution have numerous neurofibrillary tangles (NFT) that stain with antibodies to tau (τ) protein and have amyloid plaques that are composed largely of a PrP fragment extending from residues 58 to 150. Since the F198S mutation is not contained within the major PrP peptide of the amyloid plaques, patients heterozygous at codon 129 were chosen to determine whether this peptide is derived from the mutant protein. Like the results of studies with GSS (P102L) and GSS (Y145Stop), protein sequencing showed that the PrP peptides are derived exclusively from the mutant protein. Similar results were found with PrP peptides from a patient of Swedish ancestry with the codon 217 mutation resulting in a glutamine (Q)→arginine (R) substitution. The neuropathology of patients with the codon 217 mutation was similar to that of patients with the codon 198 mutation.

One patient with a prolonged neurologic illness spanning almost two decades who had PrP amyloid plaques and NFTs was found to have an amber mutation of the *PrP* gene resulting in a stop codon at residue 145. Staining of the plaques with α-PrP peptide antisera suggested that they might be composed exclusively of the truncated PrP molecules. That a PrP peptide ending at residue 145 polymerizes in amyloid filaments is to be expected since an earlier study noted above showed that the major PrP peptide in plaques from patients with the F198S mutation was an 11-kDa PrP peptide beginning at codon 58 and ending at approximately 150. A synthetic PrP peptide containing residues 90–145 was found to adopt an α-helical or β-sheet structure depending on the solvent as determined by 2D-NMR, FTIR spectroscopy, and fiber diffraction.

An insert of 144 bp at codon 53 containing six octarepeats has been described in patients with CJD from four families all residing in southern England (*see* Fig. 102-2). This mutation must have arisen through a complex series of events since the human *PrP* gene contains only five octarepeats, indicating that a single recombination event could not have created the insert. Genealogic investigations have shown that all four families are related, arguing for a single founder born more than two centuries ago. The LOD score

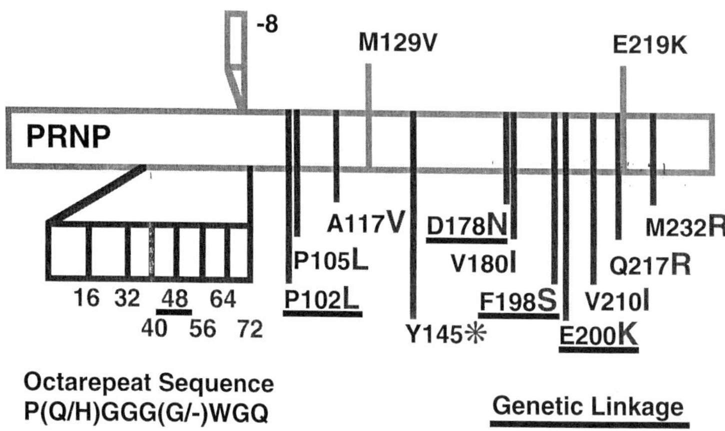

Figure 102-2 Human prion protein gene (PRNP). Large gray rectangle, the open reading frame; above the rectangle, human PRNP wild-type coding polymorphisms; below the rectangle, mutations that segregate with the inherited prion diseases. Single letter code for amino acids is as follows: A, Ala; D, Asp; E, Glu; F, Phe; I, Ile; K, Lys; L, Leu; M, Met; N, Asn; P, Pro; Q, Gln; R, Arg; S, Ser; T, Thr; V, Val; Y, Tyr.The wild-type human *PrP* gene contains five octarepeats [P(Q/H)GGG(G/-)WGQ] from codons 51 to 91. Deletion of a single octarepeat at codon 81 or 82 is not associated with prion disease; whether this deletion alters the phenotypic characteristics of a prion disease is unknown. There are common polymorphisms at codons 117 (A→A) and 129 (M→V); homozygosity for M or V at codon 129 appears to increase susceptibility to sporadic CJD. Octarepeat inserts of 16, 32, 40, 48, 56, 64, and 72 amino acids at codons 67, 75, or 83 are designated by the small rectangle below the ORF. These inserts segregate with familial CJD, and genetic linkage has been demonstrated where sufficient specimens from family members are available. Point mutations are designated by the wild-type amino acid preceding the codon number and the mutant residue follows, e.g., P102L. These point mutations segregate with the inherited prion diseases, and significant genetic linkage (underlined mutations) has been demonstrated where sufficient specimens from family members are available. Mutations at codons 102 (P→L), 117 (A→V), 198 (P→S), and 217 (G→A) are found in patients with GSS. Point mutations at codons 178 (A→A), 200 (G→L), and 210 (V→I) are found in patients with familial CJD. Point mutations at codons 198 (P→S) and 217 (G→A) are found in patients with GSS who have PrP amyloid plaques and neurofibrillary tangles. Additional point mutations at codons 145 (Y→Stop), 105 (P→L), 180 (V→I), 208 (A→H), and 232 (M→A) have been recently reported.

for this extended pedigree exceeds 11. Studies from several laboratories have demonstrated that two, four, five, six, seven, eight, or nine octarepeats in addition to the normal five are found in individuals with inherited CJD, whereas deletion of one octarepeat has been identified without the neurologic disease.

For many years the unusually high incidence of CJD among Israeli Jews of Libyan origin was thought to be due to the consumption of lightly cooked sheep brain or eyeballs. Recent studies have shown that some Libyan and Tunisian Jews in families with CJD have a *PrP* gene point mutation at codon 200 resulting in a glutamate (E)→lysine (K) substitution. One patient was homozygous for the E200K mutation, but her clinical presentation was similar to that of heterozygotes, arguing that familial prion diseases are true autosomal dominant disorders. The E200K mutation has also been found in Slovaks originating from Orava in northern Slovakia, in a cluster of familial cases in Chile, and in a large German family living in the United States. Some investigators have argued that the E200K mutation originated in a Sephardic Jew whose descendants migrated from Spain and Portugal at the time of the Inquisition. It is more likely that the E200K mutation has arisen independently multiple times by the deamidation of a methylated CpG as described above the codon 102 mutation. In support of this hypothesis are historical records of Libyan and Tunisian Jews indicating that they are descended from Jews living on the island of Jerba off the southern coast of Tunisia where Jews first settled around 500 BC and not from Sephardim. Although genetic linkage was established for the P102L mutation, some investigators continued to hold the view that an environmental cofactor was necessary and that mutant *PrP* genes render individuals susceptible to the ubiquitous "scrapie virus." This "virus" was also provided as an explanation for what was mistakenly interpreted as incomplete penetrance of the codon 200 mutation in familial CJD. From life-table analyses, we now recognize that if carriers with the codon 200 mutation live long enough they eventually develop prion disease (Fig. 102-3).

Many families with CJD have been found to have a point mutation at codon 178 resulting in an aspartate (D)→asparagine (N) substitution. In these patients as well as those with the E200K mutation, PrP amyloid plaques are rare; the neuropathologic changes generally consist of widespread spongiform degeneration. Recently, a new prion disease called fatal familial insomnia, which presents with insomnia, was described in three Italian families with the D178N mutation. The neuropathology in these patients with FFI is restricted to selected nuclei of the thalamus. It is unclear whether all patients with the D178N mutation or only a subset present with sleep disturbances. It has been proposed that the allele with the D178N mutation encodes an M at position 129 in FFI while a V is encoded at position 129 in familial CJD. The discovery that FFI is an inherited prion disease clearly widens the clinical spectrum of these disorders and raises the possibility that other degenerative diseases of unknown etiology may be caused by prions. The D178N mutation has been linked to the development of prion disease with a LOD score exceeding 5. Studies of PrP^{Sc} in FFI and familial CJD caused by the D178N mutation show that after limited proteolysis the M_r of the FFI PrP^{Sc} is about 1 kDa smaller. Whether this difference in protease resistance reflects distinct conformations of PrP^{Sc} that give rise to the different clinical and neuropathologic manifestations of these inherited prion diseases remains to be established.

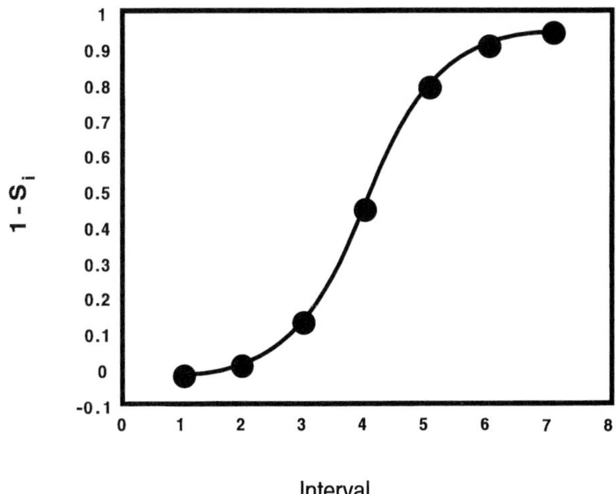

Figure 102-3 Cumulative probability of developing CJD ($1\text{-}S_i$) as a function of age in the *PrP*-E200K carriers. Intervals are the ages of the carriers in decades.

A valine (V)→isoleucine (I) mutation at PrP codon 210 produces CJD with classic symptoms and signs. The V210I mutation is thought to be incompletely penetrant, as the E200K mutation was previously thought to be. It seems likely that, if a sufficiently large number of people with the V210I mutation could be analyzed, complete penetrance that is age-dependent would be found.

Other point mutations at codons 208 and possibly 232 also segregate with inherited prion diseases. The codon 208 mutation results in the substitution of arginine (R) for histidine (H). The patient presented with a progressive dementia and widespread myoclonus was subsequently observed. The diagnosis of CJD was conformed at autopsy. Patients with the codon 232 mutation present with dementia; this mutation is particularly notable since it lies within the C-terminal signal sequence that is removed from *PrP* when the GPI anchor is attached.

PRP GENE POLYMORPHISMS

POLYMORPHISMS AT CODONS 129 AND 219 At PrP codon 129, an amino acid polymorphism for the M→V has been identified (*see* Fig. 102-2). This polymorphism appears able to influence prion disease expression, not only in inherited forms, but also in iatrogenic and sporadic forms of prion disease. A second polymorphism resulting in an amino acid substitution at codon 219 (E→K) has been reported in the Japanese population, in which the K allele occurs with a frequency of 6%.

DOES HOMOZYGOSITY AT CODON 129 PREDISPOSE TO CJD? Studies of Caucasian patients with sporadic CJD have shown that most are homozygous for M or V at codon 129. This contrasts with the general population, in which frequencies for the codon 129 polymorphism in Caucasians are 12% V/V, 37% M/M, and 51% M/V. In contrast, the frequency of the V allele in the Japanese population is much lower and heterozygosity at codon 129 (M/V) is more frequent (18%) in CJD patients than the general population, where the polymorphism frequencies are 0% V/V, 92% M/M, and 8% M/V.

While no specific mutations have been identified in the *PrP* gene of patients with sporadic CJD, homozygosity at codon 129 in sporadic CJD is consistent with the results of Tg mouse studies. The finding that homozygosity at codon 129 predisposes to CJD supports a model of prion production which favors interactions between PrP molecules that are homologous in the H1 and H2 regions. Structural prediction studies suggest that PrP has four regions of secondary structure denoted H1, H2, H3, and H4. The H1 and H2 regions are thought to undergo a conformational change when PrPC is converted into PrP^{Sc}.

CODON 129 MAY INFLUENCE IATROGENIC CJD Susceptibility to infection may be partially determined by the PrP codon 129 genotype, analogous in principle to the incubation-time alleles in mice. In 16 patients (15 Caucasian, 1 African-American) from the United Kingdom, United States, and France with iatrogenic CJD from contaminated growth hormone extracts, 8 (50%) were V/V, 5 (31%) were M/M, and 3 (19%) were M/V. Thus, a disproportionate number of patients with iatrogenic CJD were homozygous for valine at PrP codon 129, and heterozygosity at codon 129 may provide partial protection. Whether these associations are strongly significant awaits statistical analysis of larger samples. Thousands of children who received pituitary growth hormone extracts are still at risk for the development of CJD. Fortunately, the use of genetically engineered growth hormone will eliminate this form of iatrogenic CJD in the future.

Approximately 15% of patients with sporadic CJD develop ataxia as an early sign, accompanied by dementia. Most, but not all, patients with ataxia have compact "kuru" plaques in the cerebellum. Patients with ataxia and compact plaques exhibit a protracted clinical course, which may last up to 3 years. The molecular basis for the differences between CJD of shorter and longer duration have not yet been fully elucidated; however, some preliminary analyses have suggested that patients with protracted, atypical clinical courses are more likely to be heterozygous at codon 129.

CODON 129 AND INHERITED PRION DISEASES Homozygosity at codon 129 has been reported to be associated with an earlier age of onset in the inherited prion disease caused by the 6 octarepeat insert, but not by the E200K mutation, in Libyan Jews. As noted above, the FFI phenotype is found in patients with the D178N mutation who encode a Met at codon 129 on the mutant allele, while those with dementing illness (familial CJD) encode a V at 129. Homozygosity for either M or V at codon 129 is thought to be associated with an earlier age of onset for the D178N mutation.

BOVINE SPONGIFORM ENCEPHALOPATHY

EPIDEMIC OF MAD COW DISEASE Beginning in 1986, an epidemic of a previously unknown disease appeared in cattle in Great Britain. This disease was initially named bovine spongiform encephalopathy (BSE) but is frequently called "mad cow" disease. BSE was shown to be a prion disease by demonstration of protease resistant PrP in brains of ill cattle. Based mainly on epidemiologic evidence, it has been proposed that BSE represents a massive common source epidemic that has caused more than 150,000 cases to date. In Britain, cattle, particularly dairy cows, were routinely fed meat and bone meal (MBM) as a nutritional supplement. The MBM was prepared by rendering the offal of sheep and cattle using a process that involved steam treatment and hydrocarbon solvent extraction. The extraction process produced protein- and fat-rich fractions; the protein, or greaves, fraction contained about 1% fat, from which the MBM was prepared. In the late 1970s, the price of tallow prepared from the fat fraction fell, making it no longer profitable to use hydrocarbons in the rendering process. The resulting MBM contained about 14% fat, and it is postulated

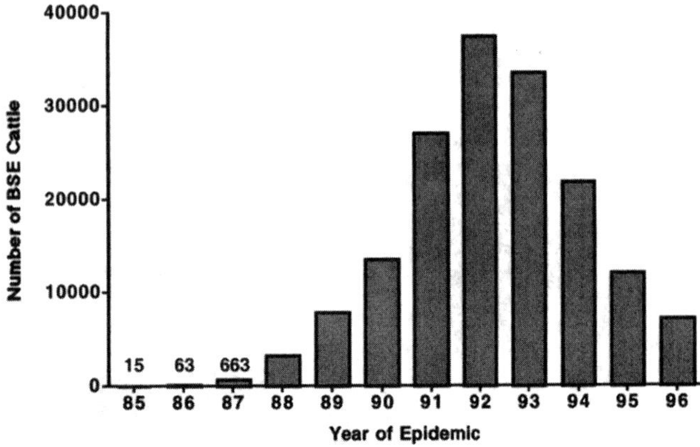

Figure 102-4 Annual incidence of bovine spongiform encephalopathy in Great Britain. All cases were confirmed clinically and neuropathologically. Statistics compiled by John Wilesmith of the Central Veterinary Laboratory at Weybridge, England.

that the high lipid content protected scrapie prions in the sheep offal from being completely inactivated by steam.

Since 1988 the practice of using dietary protein supplements for domestic animals derived from rendered sheep or cattle offal has been forbidden in the United Kingdom. By 1992 the BSE epidemic seems to have reached a peak, with over 35,000 cattle afflicted (Fig. 102-4). In 1993 less than 32,000 cattle were diagnosed with BSE, and in 1994 the number was approximately 22,000. The recent statistics argue that the epidemic is now under control as a result of the 1988 food ban.

CROSSING A SPECIES BARRIER Assuming the above postulate is correct, then only sheep prions were present initially in the contaminated MBM. Since the species barrier depends, at least in part, on the amino acid sequences of PrP in the donor host and recipient, the similarity between bovine and sheep PrP was probably an important factor in initiating the BSE epidemic. Bovine PrP differs from sheep PrP at seven or eight residues depending on the breed of sheep. As the BSE epidemic expanded, infected bovine offal began to be rendered into MBM which contained bovine prions.

TRANSMISSION OF BSE TO EXPERIMENTAL ANIMALS Brain extracts from BSE cattle have transmitted disease to mice, cattle, sheep, and pigs after intracerebral inoculation. Transmissions to mice and sheep suggest that cattle preferentially propagate a single "strain" of prions. Seven BSE brains all produced similar incubation times as measured in each of three strains of inbred mice.

Of particular importance to the BSE epidemic is the recent transmission of BSE to the nonhuman primate marmoset after intracerebral inoculation followed by a prolonged incubation period. The potential parallels with kuru of humans, confined to the Fore region of New Guinea, are worthy of consideration. While it seems likely that kuru was transmitted orally, as proposed for BSE among cattle, some investigators argue that other than oral routes were important since oral transmission of kuru prions to apes and monkeys has been difficult to demonstrate.

There is no example of zoonotic transmission of prions from animals to humans based on many epidemiological studies that have attempted to implicate scrapie prions from sheep as a cause of CJD. Whether BSE poses any risk to humans is unknown, but four farmers with BSE-afflicted cattle have died of CJD during the past 2 years.

PRION PROPAGATION

The concept of the species barrier for prion transmission was introduced three decades ago based on transmission studies of experimental scrapie in sheep, goats, and rodents. The initial molecular studies of the prion species barrier were performed using Tg(*SHaPrP*) mice. The *SHaPrP* transgene rendered mice susceptible to SHa prions, implying that the species barrier between Syrian hamsters and mice is due to one or more of the 16 amino acid substitutions that distinguish *SHa* from *MoPrP*. Like SHa prions, Hu prions inoculated into non-Tg mice produced disease infrequently after a prolonged incubation period. Based on our experience with Tg(*SHaPrP*) mice, we produced Tg(*HuPrP*) mice, but surprisingly they remained refractory to Hu prions. When the Tg(*HuPrP*) were crossed with Prnp$^{0/0}$ mice in which the MoPrP was disrupted, the resulting Tg(*HuPrP*)Prnp$^{0/0}$ mice became susceptible to infection with Hu prions (Table 102-3). This indicates that MoPrP^{C} inhibited the conversion of HuPrP^{C} into HuPrP^{Sc}. These findings and others described here make it likely that, besides PrP^{C} and PrP^{Sc}, a third component participates in the formation of nascent PrP^{Sc}. We presume that this third component is a macromolecule and that it is a protein; though it remains as yet unidentified, we have provisionally designated this third component "protein X."

The site at which PrP^{C} binds to protein X must be within the Mo-encoded residues of chimeric PrP^{C}, since Tg(*MHu2M*) mice were found to be susceptible to Hu prions irrespective of the presence of endogenous MoPrP^{C} (Table 102-4). We interpret these results to mean that the Mo sequences in chimeric PrP^{C} enable it to compete effectively with MoPrP^{C} for binding to protein X.

We envision that, during the propagation of prions, a complex of homotypic PrP^{Sc} and PrP^{C} binds to protein X. This pairwise interaction of PrP^{Sc} with PrP^{C} and the stoichiometry of the conversion reaction make it doubtful that PrP^{Sc} itself is protein X. Although the function of protein X in the formation of PrP^{Sc} is unknown, it seems likely that protein X acts in some manner to facilitate the formation of nascent PrP^{Sc}.

PrP^{Sc} FORMATION The formation of nascent PrP^{Sc} is a posttranslational process that seems to occur after PrP^{C} reaches the cell surface. Transgenetic studies argue that PrP^{C} and PrP^{Sc} form a complex during the conversion of PrP^{C} into nascent PrP^{Sc}. Although SHa transgenes provided considerable information about some of the features of PrP^{Sc} formation, use of the more divergent *HuPrP* transgene has greatly extended our understanding. Tg(*MHu2M*)Prnp$^{0/0}$ mice that express only chimeric PrP^{C} were resistant to Mo prions; whereas Tg(*MHu2M*)FVB mice expressing both chimeric and MoPrP^{C} were susceptible to Mo prions but the incubation time was prolonged. In contrast, Tg(*MHu2M*)Prnp$^{0/0}$ mice inoculated with either Hu or chimeric MHu2M prions exhibited similar incubation times (*see* Table 102-4).

To assess the specificity of PrP^{C} binding to PrP^{Sc} in the central domain delimited by codons 96 to 167, we studied the influence of pathologic mutations and a polymorphism. Tg(*MHu2M*) mice were resistant to Hu prions from a patient with GSS who carried the P102L mutation but were susceptible to prions from patients with familial CJD who harbor the E200K mutation (*see* Table 102-4C). Engineering the P102L mutation into the chimeric transgene rendered the Tg(*MHu2M*-P101L) mice susceptible to the GSS prions from the brain of a patient who died of GSS and carried the P102L mutation (Fig. 102-5). Studies of Tg(*HuPrP*)Prnp$^{0/0}$ mice expressing M or V at the polymorphic codon 129 demonstrated the

Table 102-3
Transmission of Hu Prions to Tg(*HuPrP*)/Prnp$^{0/0}$ Mice

Recipient mouse line	*Inoculum*[a]	*Incubation time (mean d ± SEM)*	*(n/n$_0$)*
A. Tg(*HuPrP*)FVB mice			
Tg(*HuPrP*)152/FVB	sCJD(RG)	721	(1/10)[b]
Non-Tg152/FVB	sCJD(RG)	701	(1/10)[b]
Tg(*HuPrP*)152/FVB	sCJD(RG,purified rods)	677	(1/10)[b]
Non-Tg152/FVB	sCJD(RG,purified rods)	643 ± 42	(3/10)[b]
B. Tg(*HuPrP*)Prnp$^{0/0}$ mice			
Tg(HuPrP)152/Prnp$^{0/0}$	sCJD(RG)	263 ± 2	(6/6)
Tg(*HuPrP*)152/Prnp$^{0/0}$	sCJD(EC)	254 ± 6	(9/9)
Tg(*HuPrP*)152/Prnp$^{0/0}$	iCJD(364)	262 ± 8	(6/6)
Tg(*HuPrP*)440/Prnp$^{0/0}$	iCJD(364)	164 ± 2	(7/7)
C. Tg(*HuPrP*)Prnp$^{+/0}$ mice			
Tg(*HuPrP*)152/Prnp$^{+/0}$	sCJD(RG)	>370	(0/2)
Tg(*HuPrP*)152/Prnp$^{+/0}$	iCJD(364)	>400	(0/4)

[a]All samples were 10% (w/v) brain homogenates, unless otherwise noted, that were diluted 1:10 prior to inoculation. Patient's initials referring to inocula are given in parentheses. sCJD, sporadic CJD; iCJD, iatrogenic CJD; n/n$_0$, number of animals/number of inoculated animals.

[b]Extended observations of transmissions previously reported.

Table 102-4
Transmission of Hu Prions to Tg(MHu2MPrP) Mice

Inoculum[a]	*Incubation time (mean d ± SEM)*	*(n/n$_0$)*
A. Tg(*MHu2M*)FVB mice inoculated with sporadic or infectious CJD		
sCJD(RG)	238 ± 3	(8/8)[b]
sCJD(EC)	218 ± 5	(7/7)[b]
iCJD(364)	232 ± 3	(9/9)[b]
iCJD(364)[c]	231 ± 6	(9/9)
sCJD(MA)	222 ± 1	(4/4)
B. Tg(*MHu2M*)Prnp$^{0/0}$ mice inoculated with sporadic or infectious CJD		
sCJD(RC)	207 ± 4	(8/10)
sCJD(RG)	191 ± 3	(10/10)
iCJD(364)	192 ± 6	(8/8)
iCJD(364)[c]	211 ± 5	(8/9)
sCJD(MA)	180 ± 5	(8/8)
sCJD(RO)	217 ± 2	(9/9)
C. Tg(*MHu2M*)Prnp$^{0/0}$ mice inoculated with inherited GSS or CJD		
GSS(JJ,P102L)	>310	(0/10)
fCJD(LJ1,E200K)	170 ± 2	(10/10)
fCJD(CA,E200K)	180 ± 9	(9/9)
fCJD(FH,E200K)	>290	(0/7)

[a]All samples were 10% (w/v) brain homogenates unless otherwise noted that were diluted 1:10 prior to inoculation. Patient's initials referring to inocula are given in parentheses. If the *PrP* gene of the patient carried a mutation, then the mutation is noted after the patients initials. sCJD, sporadic CJD; iCJD, iatrogenic CJD; GSS, Gerstmann-Sträusssler-Scheinker disease with the codon 102 mutation; fCJD, familial CJD with the codon 200 mutation.

[b]Transmissions previously reported.

[c]This is a second inoculum prepared from a different brain region of iatrogenic CJD patient 364.

influence of this residue within the central domain on prion propagation (Fig. 102-6). When the 129 residue within the central domain was the same in PrP^{Sc} of the inoculum and PrP^{C} of the recipient mouse, incubation times were substantially shortened. These findings demonstrate that single amino acid mismatches at codon 102 or 129 prolong the incubation time; whereas, a mismatch at codon 200 does not. Although the results reported here argue that prion propagation is facilitated by homology within the central domains of HuPrP^{C} and HuPrP^{Sc}, other investigations with *SHa/MoPrP* transgenes demonstrate that the requirements for sequence similarity may vary with different species and strains of prions.

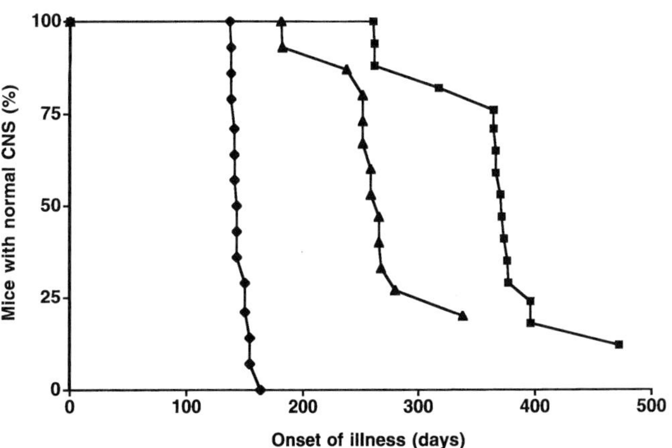

Figure 102-5 Spontaneous and transmissible neurodegeneration in Tg(*MHu2M*-P102L)69/Prnp$^{0/0}$ mice. Uninoculated Tg(*MHu2M*-P102L)69/Prnp$^{0/0}$ mice were observed for the spontaneous development of neurologic disease (squares). At ~70 days of age, Tg(*MHu2M*-P102L)69/Prnp$^{0/0}$ mice were inoculated intracerebrally with brain homogenate prepared from either a patient with GSS who carried the P102L mutation (diamonds) or another patient who died of sporadic CJD (triangles).

Since MoPrP^{C} can inhibit the formation of HuPrP^{Sc} in the presence of a substantial excess of HuPrP^{C}, this contends that Mo protein X has a higher affinity for MoPrP^{C} than it does for HuPrP^{C} (*see* Table 102-3B,C). MoPrP^{C} prevented HuPrP^{Sc} formation whether the inoculum contained amorphous aggregates of PrP^{Sc} or ordered arrays of prion rods composed of PrP 27–30 molecules

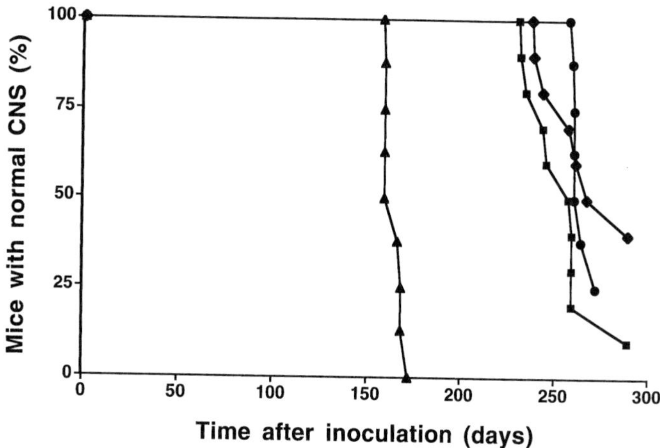

Figure 102-6 Amino acid mismatches at the codon 129 polymorphism prolong the incubation times of Tg(*HuPrP*)/Prnp$^{0/0}$ mice. Tg(*HuPrP*-M129)440/Prnp$^{0/0}$ mice were inoculated intracerebrally with a case of iatrogenic CJD (364A, triangles). Tg(*HuPrP*-V129)152/Prnp$^{0/0}$ mice were inoculated with iatrogenic CJD (364A, diamonds) and sporadic CJD (EC, squares; RG, circles). All the CJD cases were from individuals homozygous for M/M at codon 129.

(*see* Table 102-3A). If MoPrP^{C} had been more inhibitory when the prion rods were inoculated, then we would suppose that a single MoPrP^{C} molecule could bind to multiple HuPrP^{Sc} molecules and prevent the formation of nascent HuPrP^{Sc}, but this is not the case.

We assume that the stoichiometry of PrP^{C} and PrP^{Sc} that form a complex is approximately 1:1. Whether this complex is composed of two or more PrP molecules is uncertain. Although some investigators have argued that the formation of nascent PrP^{Sc} involves the formation of PrP amyloid fibrils, there is much evidence to the contrary. Purified preparations of PrP^{Sc} from brain possess an amorphous ultrastructure and do not form amyloid polymers except when PrP^{Sc} undergoes partial proteolysis to produce PrP 27–30 in the presence of a nondenaturing detergent. Isolated PrP amyloid plaques contain primarily fragments of PrP, and several synthetic PrP peptides spontaneously polymerize into amyloids when dispersed in water. In vitro conversion of PrP^{C} into a protease resistant form that is presumed to be equivalent to PrP^{Sc} by mixing a greater than 50-fold excess of PrP^{Sc} with labeled PrP^{C} has been reported. Interestingly, the binding of PrP^{C} to PrP^{Sc} was found to be dependent on the same residues that render Tg(*MH2M*) mice susceptible to SHa prions, and it seems to be strain dependent. Whether PrP^{C} actually undergoes a conformational change that is characteristic of PrP^{Sc} or the binding of PrP^{C} to PrP^{Sc} renders it protease resistant without actually undergoing this conformational transition remains to be established.

EVIDENCE FOR PROTEIN X BINDING TO THE C-TERMINUS OF PrP^{C} Since truncation experiments show that the N-terminal 67 residues of mature PrP are dispensable, it seems likely that the site at which PrP^{C} binds to protein X is at the C-terminal end of PrP^{C}. A comparison of predicted amino acid sequences shows sufficient variation from codon 167 to 231 between Hu and Mo as well as similarity between SHa and Mo to account for our results. The location of residue 215 is particularly interesting; in HuPrP, it is an I, while in MoPrP it is a V and in SHaPrP a T.

In contrast to SHaPrP, HuPrP differs from MoPrP at four additional amino acids that lie C-terminal to residue 215. Any or all of these substitutions besides residue 215 could explain the difference in susceptibility between Tg(*HuPrP*)FVB and Tg(*SHaPrP*)FVB mice to Hu and SHa prions, respectively. Two of the four additional residues that distinguish HuPrP from MoPrP lie at positions 219 and 220. While these residues might participate in the binding of PrP^{C} to protein X, it seems unlikely that residues at 228 or 230 are involved in the binding to protein X since they are adjacent to the GPI anchor which is attached to an S residue at 231. The proposed model is consistent with our findings that chimeric MHu2MPrP^{C} but not HuPrP^{C} is converted into PrP^{Sc} in the presence of MoPrP^{C}, and HuPrP^{C} is converted into PrP^{Sc} in the absence of MoPrP^{C} (*see* Table 102-3).

DOES PROTEIN X FUNCTION AS A MOLECULAR CHAPERONE? How PrP^{C} unfolds and refolds into PrP^{Sc} is unknown, but the profound change in protein structure that occurs during this process is likely to be associated with a large activation barrier. Whether protein X functions as a molecular chaperon that lowers this barrier remains to be established; consistent with such a role for protein X is the apparent lack of PrP^{Sc} binding. Changes in the inducibility of heat shock proteins (Hsp) as well as their subcellular distribution, some of which function as molecular chaperones, have been found in scrapie-infected cells and raise the possibility that protein X might be an Hsp. Alternative possibilities for protein X include scaffolding or assembly proteins that provide a milieu for the PrP isoforms to interact as well as the *bcl-2* protein, which was found with the yeast two-hybrid system to bind PrP. Another possibility is that protein X features in the transient or as yet undetected chemical modification of PrP^{C} that facilitates its refolding into PrP^{Sc}.

MODELING OF GSS IN TRANSGENIC MICE

The codon 102 point mutation found in GSS patients was introduced into the *MoPrP* gene and Tg(*MoPrP*-P101L)H mice were created expressing high (H) levels of the mutant transgene product. The two lines of Tg(*MoPrP*-P101L)H mice designated 174 and 87 spontaneously developed CNS degeneration, characterized by clinical signs indistinguishable from experimental murine scrapie and neuropathology consisting of widespread spongiform morphology and astrocytic gliosis and PrP amyloid plaques (Fig. 102-7). By inference, these results contend that *PrP* gene mutations cause GSS, familial CJD, and FFI.

Brain extracts prepared from spontaneously ill Tg(*MoPrP*-P101L)H mice transmitted CNS degeneration to Tg196 mice and some Syrian hamsters. The Tg196 mice express low levels of the mutant transgene product and do not develop spontaneous disease. Many Tg196 mice and some Syrian hamsters developed CNS degeneration between 200 and 700 days after inoculation, while inoculated CD-1 Swiss mice remained well. Serial transmission of CNS degeneration in Tg196 mice required about 1 year, while serial transmission in Syrian hamsters occurred after about 75 days. Crossing the Tg196 mice with Prnp$^{0/0}$ mice produced recipient Tg196/Prnp$^{0/0}$ mice that developed CNS degeneration in more than 95% of the inoculated animals in approximately 190 days. Serial transmission of CNS degeneration in Tg196/Prnp$^{0/0}$ mice required about 220 days, while serial transmission in Syrian hamsters occurred after approximately 75 days. These findings and those from other studies suggest that mutant and wtPrP interact, perhaps through protein X, to modify the pathogenesis of the dominantly inherited prion diseases.

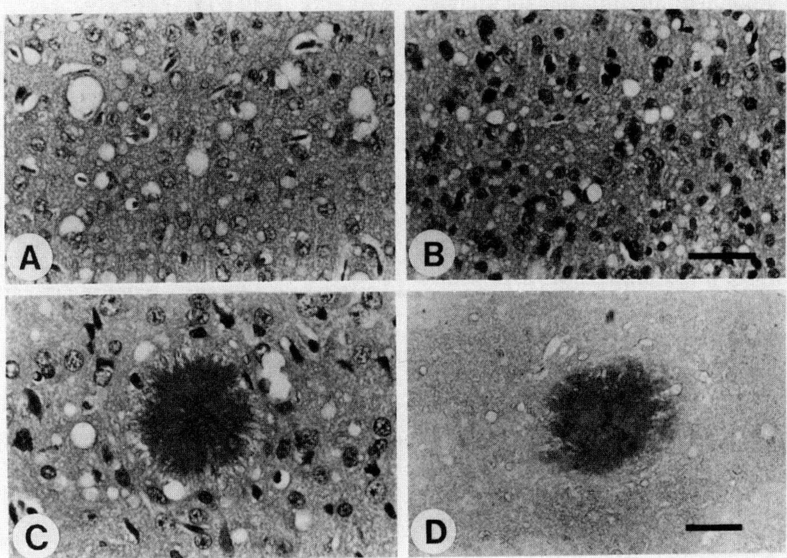

Figure 102-7 Neuropathology of Tg(*MoPrP*-P101L) mice developing neurodegeneration spontaneously. The mice harbor transgenes carrying the PrP point mutation found in GSS(P102L) of humans. **(A)** Vacuolation in cerebral cortex of a Swiss CD-1 mouse that exhibited signs of neurologic dysfunction at 138 days after intracerebral inoculation with ~10^6 ID_{50} units of RML scrapie prions. **(B)** Vacuolation in cerebral cortex of a Tg(*MoPrP*-P101L) mouse that exhibited signs of neurologic dysfunction at 252 days of age. **(C)** Kuru-type PrP amyloid plaque stained with periodic acid Schiff in the caudate nucleus of a Tg(*MoPrP*-P101L) mouse that exhibited signs of neurologic dysfunction. **(D)** PrP amyloid plaques stained with α-PrP antiserum (RO73) in the caudate nucleus of a Tg(*MoPrP*-P101L) mouse that exhibited signs of neurologic dysfunction. Bars: in B (also applies to A) = 50 μm; in D (also applies to C) = 25 μm.

THERAPEUTIC APPROACHES TO PRION DISEASES

There is no known effective therapy for treating or preventing CJD. There are no well-documented cases of patients with CJD showing recovery either spontaneously or after therapy, with one possible exception. Since people at risk for inherited prion diseases can now be identified decades before neurologic dysfunction is evident, the development of an effective therapy is imperative.

PRENATAL SCREENING FOR PrP MUTATIONS The inherited prion diseases can be prevented by genetic counseling coupled with prenatal DNA screening, but such testing presents ethical problems. For example, during the childbearing years, the parents are generally symptom-free and may not want to know their own genotype.

GENE THERAPY AND ANTISENSE OLIGONUCLEOTIDES Unexpectedly, ablation of the *PrP* gene in Tg($Prnp^{0/0}$) mice has not affected the development of these animals, and they remain healthy at almost two years of age. Since $Prnp^{0/0}$ mice are resistant to prions and do not propagate scrapie infectivity, gene therapy or antisense oligonucleotides might ultimately provide an effective therapeutic approach. Mice heterozygous ($Prnp^{0/+}$) for ablation of the *PrP* gene had prolonged incubation times when inoculated with mouse prions. This finding is in accord with studies on Tg(*SHaPrP*) mice in which increased SHaPrP expression was accompanied by diminished incubation times.

INHIBITORS OF β-SHEET FORMATION Because the absence of PrP^C expression does not provoke disease, it seems reasonable to conclude that scrapie and other prion diseases are a consequence of PrP^{Sc} accumulation rather than an inhibition of PrP^C function. The function of PrP^C remains unknown to date. These findings suggest that perhaps the most effective therapy may evolve from the development of drugs that block the conversion of PrP^C into PrP^{Sc}. Since the fundamental event in both the formation of PrP^{Sc} and the propagation of prions seems to be the unfolding of α helices and their refolding into β sheets, drugs targeting this structural transformation would seem likely to be efficacious.

Whether dyes like Congo red that bind to PrP amyloid will be effective in vivo in preventing the formation of PrP^{Sc} remains to be established. Congo red has been reported to inhibit the formation of PrP^{Sc} in cultured scrapie-infected mouse neuroblastoma cells, but the mechanism by which this occurs is unknown.

Dextran sulfates have been used to delay the onset of scrapie in laboratory animals; however, these compounds are only effective when given before or concurrently with the prion inoculum. The inhibitory effect of dextrans on prion propagation has been most pronounced in animals inoculated intraperitoneally. The mechanism by which the sulphated sugar polymers inhibit PrP^{Sc} formation in cultured cells and animals is unknown.

Injection of corticosteroids into mice at the time of intraperitoneal inoculation of prions resulted in the prolongation of the incubation time. These results suggested that the immune system played a role in the initial phase of scrapie infection as did studies with spleenless mice. Studies with nude mice and more recently SCID mice showed that incubation times were unaltered compared with controls after intracerebral inoculation; in contrast, SCID mice were not susceptible to prions inoculated intraperitoneally. Studies of lymphoid tissues after intraperitoneal inoculation of prions showed that the follicular dendritic cells that are thought to function in the presentation of antigens selectively accumulated PrP^{Sc}. In SCID mice no focal accumulations of PrP^{Sc} in lymphoid tissues have been found.

Chronic treatment with the antifungal drug amphotericin started at the time of intracerebral inoculation prolonged incubation periods in mice and hamsters. Administration of amphotericin to humans with CJD had no therapeutic effect; likewise, the antiviral drug amantidine was also ineffective. HPA-23 is an inhibitor of viral glycoprotein synthesis. When given to scrapie-infected animals around the time of inoculation, but not later, it profoundly extends the length of the incubation period. The effects in human CJD are uncertain. Interferon was used in experimental scrapie of rodents, but the incubation times were unaltered.

Although antibodies have been raised against the scrapie prion protein and these crossreact with prion proteins in CJD human brains, passive immunization or even vaccination would seem to be of little value. CJD and scrapie both progress in the absence of any immune response to the offending prions; however, neutralization of scrapie prion infectivity was accomplished when the infectious particles were dispersed into detergent–lipid–protein complexes.

RESISTANT BREEDS OF SHEEP With the discovery that QQ homozygosity at codon 171 appears to render Suffolk sheep susceptible to scrapie while QR and RR sheep are resistant, the notion of breeding scrapie-resistant sheep as Parry proposed seems quite reasonable. The screening procedures for identifying QQ sheep are simple and could be applied in an agricultural setting with ease.

CONCLUDING REMARKS

PRIONS ARE NOT VIRUSES The study of prions has taken several unexpected directions over the past few years. The discovery that prion diseases in humans are uniquely both genetic and infectious has greatly strengthened and extended the prion concept. To date, 19 different mutations in the human *PrP* gene all resulting in nonconservative substitutions have been found either to be linked genetically to or to segregate with the inherited prion diseases (*see* Fig. 102-2). Yet, the transmissible prion particle is composed largely, if not entirely, of an abnormal isoform of the prion protein designated PrP^{Sc}. These findings argue that prion diseases should be considered pseudoinfections, since the particles transmitting disease appear to be devoid of a foreign nucleic acid and thus differ from all known microorganisms as well as viruses and viroids. Because much information, especially about scrapie of rodents, has been derived using experimental protocols adapted from virology, we continue to use terms such as infection, incubation period, transmissibility, and end-point titration in studies of prion diseases.

PRION BIOLOGY If, as recently suggested, several yeast proteins induce alternative metabolic states through a prion-like mechanism, then perhaps PrP^C also exists in more than one physiologic state. The transformation of PrP^C to an alternative metabolic isoform might be facilitated by protein X. Interestingly, one prion-like protein in yeast (Sup 35) seems to require intermediate levels of the molecular chaperone (Hsp 104) to undergo transformation to [PSI^+]. In the filamentous fungus *Podospora anserina*, the *het-s* locus controls the vegetative incompatibility; conversion from the S^s to the s state seems to be a posttranslational, autocatalytic process.

Might protein X function as a chaperone that mediates a conformational change in PrP^C that alters its cellular function in the absence of PrP^{Sc} or a pathologic *PrP* gene mutation? In the presence of PrP^{Sc}, protein X might catalyze the conversion of PrP^C into PrP^{Sc}. Whatever the mechanism of PrP^{Sc} formation, this process seems to be unprecedented in biology, and its elucidation promises to have implications far beyond the prion diseases.

ACKNOWLEDGMENTS

I thank M Baldwin, D Borchelt, G Carlson, F Cohen, C Cooper, S DeArmond, R Fletterick, M Gasset, R Gabizon, D Groth, R Koehler, L Hood, K Hsiao, Z Huang, V Lingappa, K-M Pan, D Riesner, M Scott, A Serban, N Stahl, A Taraboulos, M Torchia, and D Westaway for their help in these studies. This work was supported by grants from the National Institutes of Health (NS-14069, AG-08967, AG-02132, NS-22786, and AG-10770) and the American Health Assistance Foundation, as well as by gifts from Sherman Fairchild Foundation and Bernard Osher Foundation.

SELECTED REFERENCES

Alper T, Cramp WA, Haig DA, Clarke MC. Does the agent of scrapie replicate without nucleic acid? Nature 1967;214:764–766.

Basler K, Oesch B, Scott M, et al. Scrapie and cellular PrP isoforms are encoded by the same chromosomal gene. Cell 1986;46:417–428.

Bockman JM, Kingsbury DT, McKinley MP, Bendheim PE, Prusiner SB. Creutzfeldt-Jakob disease prion proteins in human brains. N Engl J Med 1985;312:73–78.

Brown P, Preece MA, Will RG. "Friendly fire" in medicine: hormones, homografts, and Creutzfeldt-Jakob disease. Lancet 1992;340:24–27.

Büeler H, Fischer M, Lang Y, et al. Normal development and behaviour of mice lacking the neuronal cell-surface PrP protein. Nature 1992;356:577–582.

Chapman J, Ben-Israel J, Goldhammer Y, Korczyn AD. The risk of developing Creutzfeldt-Jakob disease in subjects with the PRNP gene codon 200 point mutation. Neurology 1994;44:1683–1686.

Chernoff YO, Lindquist SL, Ono B, Inge-Vechtomov SG, Liebman SW. Role of the chaperone protein Hsp104 in propagation of the yeast prion-like factor [psi+]. Science 1995;268:880–884.

Collinge J, Sidle KC, Meads J, Ironside J, Hill AF. Molecular analysis of prion strain variation and the aetiology of 'non variant' CJD. Nature 1996;383:685–690.

Fradkin JE, Schonberger LB, Mills JL, et al. Creutzfeldt-Jakob disease in pituitary growth hormone recipients in the United States. JAMA 1991;265:880–884.

Gajdusek DC. Unconventional viruses and the origin and disappearance of kuru. Science 1977;197:943–960.

Gajdusek DC. Genetic control of nucleation and polymerization of host precursors to infectious amyloids in the transmissible amyloidoses of brain. Br Med Bull 1993;49:913–931.

Gajdusek DC, Gibbs CJ, Jr, Alpers M. Experimental transmission of a kuru-like syndrome to chimpanzees. Nature 1966;209:794–796.

Goldfarb LG, Petersen RB, Tabaton M, et al. Fatal familial insomnia and familial Creutzfeldt-Jakob disease: disease phenotype determined by a DNA polymorphism. Science 1992;258:806–808.

Goldfarb L, Korczyn A, Brown P, Chapman J, Gajdusek DC. Mutation in codon 200 of scrapie amyloid precursor gene linked to Creutzfeldt-Jakob disease in Sephardic Jews of Libyan and non-Libyan origin. Lancet 1990;336:637–638.

Hsiao K, Baker HF, Crow TJ, et al. Linkage of a prion protein missense variant to Gerstmann-Sträussler syndrome. Nature 1989;338:342–345.

Hsiao K, Dlouhy S, Farlow MR, et al. Mutant prion proteins in Gerstmann-Sträussler-Scheinker disease with neurofibrillary tangles. Nat Genet 1992;1:68–71.

Huang Z, Gabriel J-M, Baldwin MA, Fletterick RJ, Prusiner SB, Cohen FE. Proposed three-dimensional structure for the cellular prion protein. Proc Natl Acad Sci USA 1994;91:7139–7143.

Kahana E, Milton A, Braham J, Sofer D. Creutzfeldt-Jakob disease: focus among Libyan Jews in Israel. Science 1974;183:90,91.

Kaneko K, Peretz D, Pan K-M, et al. Prion protein (PrP) synthetic peptides induce cellular PrP to acquire properties of the scrapie isoform. Proc Natl Acad Sci USA 1995;92:11,160–11,164.

Kitamoto T, Tateishi J. Human prion diseases with variant prion protein. Philos Trans R Soc Lond. B Biol Sci 1994;343:391–398.

Kocisko DA, Come JH, Priola SA, et al. Cell-free formation of protease-resistant prion protein. Nature 1994;370:471–474.

Masters CL, Gajdusek DC, Gibbs CJ Jr. Creutzfeldt-Jakob disease virus isolations from the Gerstmann-Sträussler syndrome. Brain 1981;104:559–588.
Medori R, Tritschler H-J, LeBlanc A, et al. Fatal familial insomnia, a prion disease with a mutation at codon 178 of the prion protein gene. N Engl J Med 1992;326:444–449.
Palmer MS, Dryden AJ, Hughes JT, Collinge J. Homozygous prion protein genotype predisposes to sporadic Creutzfeldt-Jakob disease. Nature 1991;352:340–342.
Pan K-M, Baldwin M, Nguyen J, et al. Conversion of α-helices into β-sheets features in the formation of the scrapie prion proteins. Proc Natl Acad Sci USA 1993;90:10,962–10,966.
Parry HB. Scrapie disease in sheep. Oppenheimer, D. R. ed. New York: Academic, 1983.
Petersen RB, Tabaton M, Chen SG, et al. Familial progressive subcortical gliosis: presence of prions and linkage to chromosome 17. Neurology 1995;45:1062–1067.
Poulter M, Baker HF, Frith CD, et al. Inherited prion disease with 144 base pair gene insertion. 1. Genealogical and molecular studies. Brain 1992;115:675–685.
Prusiner SB. Novel proteinaceous infectious particles cause scrapie. Science 1982;216:136–144.
Prusiner SB. Molecular biology of prion diseases. Science 1991; 252:1515–1522.
Prusiner SB. The prion diseases. Sci Am 1995;272:48–57.
Prusiner SB. Prion diseases and the BSE crisis. Science 1997;278: 245–251.
Prusiner SB, Groth DF, Bolton DC, Kent SB, Hood LE. Purification and structural studies of a major scrapie prion protein. Cell 1984;38: 127–134.
Prusiner SB, Scott M, Foster D, et al. Transgenetic studies implicate interactions between homologous PrP isoforms in scrapie prion replication. Cell 1990;63:673–686.
Spudich S, Mastrianni JA, Wrensch M, et al. Complete penetrance of Creutzfeldt-Jakob disease in Libyan Jews carrying the E200K mutation in the prion protein gene. Mol Med 1995;1:607–613.
Stahl N, Baldwin MA, Teplow DB, et al. Structural analysis of the scrapie prion protein using mass spectrometry and amino acid sequencing. Biochemistry 1993;32:1991–2002.
Telling GC, Parchi P, DeArmond SJ, et al. Evidence for conformation of the pathologic isoform of the prion protein enciphering and propagating prion diversity. Science 1996;274:2079–2082.
Telling GC, Scott M, Hsiao KK, et al. Transmission of Creutzfeldt-Jakob disease from humans to transgenic mice expressing chimeric human-mouse prion protein. Proc Natl Acad Sci USA 1994;91: 9936–9940.
Telling GC, Scott M, Mastrianni J, et al. Prion propagation in mice expressing human and chimeric PrP transgenes implicates the interaction of cellular PrP with another protein. Cell 1995;83:79–90.
Wells GAH, Scott AC, Johnson CT, et al. A novel progressive spongiform encephalopathy in cattle. Vet Rec 1987;121:419,420.
Westaway D, Goodman PA, Mirenda CA, McKinley MP, Carlson GA, Prusiner SB. Distinct prion proteins in short and long scrapie incubation period mice. Cell 1987;51:651–662.
Wickner RB. [URE3] as an altered URE2 protein: evidence for a prion analog in Saccharomyces cerevisiae. Science 1994;264:566–569.
Wilesmith JW, Hoinville LJ, Ryan JBM, Sayers AR. Bovine spongiform encephalopathy: aspects of the clinical picture and analyses of possible changes 1986–1990. Vet Rec 1992;130:197–201.

103 Genetic Basis of Mitochondrial Disease

DONALD R. JOHNS

INTRODUCTION

Structural, biochemical, or genetic derangement of mitochondria is the common feature of the mitochondrial encephalomyopathies. This diverse group of disorders has a wide spectrum of clinical manifestations (Tables 103-1 and 103-2) that affect the eye, central nervous system, peripheral nervous system, and the somatic organs. The differential dependence of nearly all organ systems on oxidative metabolism is reflected in the variable, protean clinical manifestations of mitochondrial disorders. There is also a wide array of ages and modes of onset, course, and progression, ranging from severe infantile diseases to chronic neurodegenerative diseases of the elderly.

Establishment of the molecular genetic basis of many of the mitochondrial diseases has occurred at a rapid pace since the first human mitochondrial DNA (mtDNA) mutations were discovered in 1988. A number of different types of pathogenetic mtDNA mutations have been associated with a variety of clinical phenotypes, and the roster of mtDNA mutations and phenotypes continues to grow. The potential role of mtDNA mutations is also being investigated in the pathogenesis of more prevalent diseases, in addition to the traditional mitochondrial diseases.

Our emphasis will be on the molecular genetic basis and clinical features of mitochondrial encephalomyopathies with known pathogenetic mtDNA mutations.

STRUCTURE AND FUNCTION OF MITOCHONDRIA AND MITOCHONDRIAL DNA

Mitochondria contain a complex array of biochemical pathways that are involved in intermediary metabolism. The inner mitochondrial membrane encompasses the matrix space, which is the site of the tricarboxylic acid cycle and fatty acid oxidation. The five polypeptide complexes of the respiratory chain and ATP synthase are assembled in the inner mitochondrial membrane. The oxidation of a variety of substrates produces reducing equivalents that are sequentially transferred via the electron transport chain to reduce molecular oxygen to water. An electrochemical gradient is produced by the coupled translocation of protons and the redox potential is used by ATP synthase to produce ATP. The mitochondrial production of ATP for energy requiring cellular processes by this process is known as oxidative phosphorylation.

From: *Principles of Molecular Medicine* (J. L. Jameson, ed.), ©1998 Humana Press Inc., Totowa, NJ.

Mitochondria are the only animal cellular organelles that contain their own extrachromosomal DNA, distinct from the overwhelming majority of cellular DNA found in the nucleus. Human mtDNA is a small (16,569-nucleotide) double-stranded, circular molecule that encodes 13 protein subunits of four different biochemical complexes of oxidative phosphorylation. MtDNA also encodes the 24 structural RNAs (2 ribosomal RNAs and 22 transfer RNAs) required for the intramitochondrial translation of these subunits. The mtDNA-encoded tRNAs are also involved in the cleavage of the polycistronic transcript into individual messenger RNAs and tRNAs, and the $tRNA^{Leu(UUR)}$ has a unique role in transcription termination. The noncoding D (displacement)-loop is the site of regulatory regions that control transcription and replication. MtDNA mutations are found in each type of mitochondrially encoded gene (Fig. 103-1).

Mitochondria probably evolved from independent organisms that became endosymbiotically incorporated into the cell. Consequently, they replicate, transcribe, and translate their DNA independently of nuclear DNA. However, cellular and mitochondrial function are interdependent. The nuclear DNA-encoded proteins that are subunits of oxidative phosphorylation and all of the other myriad macromolecular compounds required for mitochondrial structure and function (e.g., mitochondrial DNA replication, transcription, and translation) must be imported from the cytoplasm into the correct position within the mitochondria.

Several unique features of mtDNA help explain its role in the pathogenesis of disease. mtDNA has no introns (so that a random mutation will usually strike a coding DNA sequence), has no protective histones, has no effective DNA repair system, is exposed to oxygen free radicals generated by oxidative phosphorylation, and mutates more than 10 times more rapidly than nuclear DNA. mtDNA is strictly maternally inherited and does not recombine; thus, mitochondrial DNA mutations sequentially accumulate along maternal lineages. This property has made mtDNA sequence variation an invaluable tool for evolutionary biologists and forensic scientists, and has provided important normative data to help determine the pathogenetic significance of newly discovered mutations.

A number of other mtDNA characteristics are central to understanding mitochondrial disease. Each mitochondrion contains 2–10 mtDNA molecules, and each cell contains multiple mitochondria (polyplasmy). Thus, normal and mutant mtDNA can coexist within the same cell, a condition known as heteroplasmy, which allows an otherwise lethal mutation to persist. The presence of either completely normal or completely mutant mitochondrial DNA is known as homoplasmy. During cell division, mitochondria are unevenly

Table 103-1
Neurological Manifestations of Mitochondrial Diseases

Ophthalmoplegia	Sensorineural hearing loss
Stroke-like episodes	Ataxia
Seizures	Dementia
Myoclonus	Peripheral neuropathy
Optic neuropathy	Vascular headache
Myopathy	Myelopathy

Table 103-2
Systemic Manifestations of Mitochondrial Diseases

Cardiac conduction defects	Fanconi proximal nephron dysfunction
Cardiomyopathy	Glomerulopathy
Diabetes mellitus	Hepatopathy
Short stature	Intestinal pseudo-obstruction
Pigmentary retinopathy	Pancytopenia
Lactic acidosis	Psychiatric disease (depression)

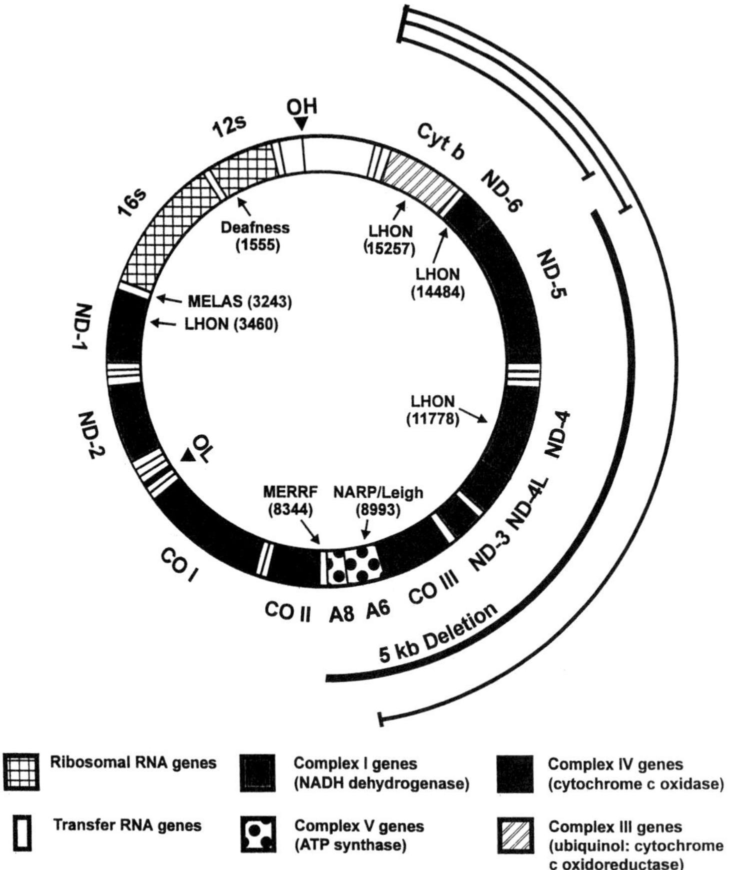

Figure 103-1 Schematic diagram of human mitochondrial DNA and the most prominent pathogenetic mutations. Inside the circle, point mutations in structural and protein-coding genes, with the clinical phenotype and the nucleotide position of the mutation; arcs outside the circle, the position of the most common single deletion, which is 5 kilobases in length, and the multiple deletions; *MERRF*, myoclonic epilepsy with ragged red fibers; MELAS, mitochondrial encephalomyopathy, lactic acidosis, and stroke-like episodes syndrome; LHON, Leber's hereditary optic neuropathy; *NARP*, neuropathy, ataxia, and retinitis pigmentosa; Leigh, maternally inherited Leigh's disease. (Reproduced with permission from NEJM 1995;333:638–644.)

partitioned into the daughter cells through the process of replicative segregation, and the proportion of mutant and normal mtDNA molecules can thereby shift. Thus, population genetics, as opposed to mendelian genetics, govern mtDNA. Selection pressures apply at the molecular, cellular, and organismal levels. The critical proportion of mutant mtDNA required for deleterious phenotypic expression is known as the threshold effect, and varies among individuals, among organ systems, and within a given tissue depending on the delicate balance of oxidative supply and demand.

The dual genetic input into the complexes of oxidative phosphorylation by both the nuclear and mitochondrial genomes, as well as complex intergenomic communication and the reactions required for import of proteins into the mitochondria, provides a wide variety of sites at which mitochondrial function can be altered.

The classic mitochondrial phenotypes described below are caused by both gross structural rearrangements (single deletions, multiple deletions, duplications) and by mtDNA point mutations. Mutations that are likely to cause a severe, lethal impairment of oxidative phosphorylation (gross structural defects, point mutations in critical regions) are only viable if they are heteroplasmic. In contrast, the majority of the milder, missense mtDNA mutations in protein-coding genes are homoplasmic. Pathogenetic mtDNA point mutations have been found in each type of mtDNA gene, but tRNA mutations predominate in mitochondrial encephalomyopathy phenotypes and protein-coding gene mutations predominate in Leber's hereditary optic neuropathy (LHON). A point mutation in the 12S ribosomal RNA gene is associated with both spontaneous and antibiotic-associated sensorineural deafness (OMIM 561000) (*see* Fig. 103-1).

CLASSIC MITOCHONDRIAL ENCEPHALOMYOPATHY PHENOTYPES

Many diseases were provisionally classified as mitochondrial disorders on the basis of abnormal mitochondrial morphology, biochemistry, or a pattern of maternal inheritance. The first direct proof that mtDNA was involved in disease pathogenesis was the finding of large deletions in the mtDNA of patients with mitochondrial myopathies and the description of a missense mutation in the mtDNA of patients with LHON. Over the next several years, the molecular genetic basis of the classic mitochondrial encephalomyopathies was elucidated. Although these disorders are relatively uncommon, they were the first molecularly defined examples of many cardinal neurological diseases, including stroke: mitochondrial encephalomyopathy, lactic acidosis, and stroke-like episodes (MELAS) syndrome; seizures: MELAS and myoclonic epilepsy with ragged red fibers (MERRF) syndrome; and optic neuropathy: LHON.

CHRONIC PROGRESSIVE EXTERNAL OPHTHALMOPLEGIA This disease (OMIM 258450) is characterized by ptosis, ophthalmoplegia, and limb myopathy. Additional clinical features (*see* Tables 103-1 and 103-2) may also occur, as may the laboratory abnormalities characteristic of mitochondrial disorders (Table 103-3). Patients with chronic progressive external ophthalmoplegia (CPEO) have abnormal skeletal muscle biopsies, with abnormal proliferating mitochondria that cause "ragged red fibers," a histological hallmark of the severe biochemical defects in oxidative phosphorylation found in many mitochondrial encephalomyopathies. The occurrence of a number of somatic and central nervous system findings with CPEO are known as the CPEO-plus syndromes. Kearns-Sayre syndrome (OMIM 530000) is a subset of CPEO-plus that begins before age 20 and is characterized by CPEO and atypical pigmentary retinopathy, with the ancillary features of elevated cerebrospinal fluid protein, ataxia, or heart block.

Most patients with CPEO have large, single deletions in mtDNA, and the presence of a pigmentary retinopathy is a strong predictor of a deletion. Almost all single mtDNA deletions occur sporadically and the mechanism of deletion formation is unknown, but recombination or slippage during replication are plausible. The junction of most deletions contains directly repeated sequences, including a 13/13 nucleotide direct repeat "hot spot" that accounts for about 25% of all deletions. Approximately half of all deletions are bounded by other direct repeats, and one-quarter have no apparent direct repeat. A few patients have partially duplicated mtDNA molecules. Many patients who lack an mtDNA deletion or duplication have a point mutation at nucleotide position 3243.

AUTOSOMALLY TRANSMITTED MULTIPLE MITOCHONDRIAL DNA DELETIONS The autosomal inheritance of multiple mtDNA deletions implies a primary defect in a nuclear DNA gene that has secondary qualitative effects on mtDNA and thus typifies a defect in intergenomic communication. Multiple mtDNA deletions have diverse manifestations, but most are variants of CPEO with specific additional features. This syndrome (OMIM 550000) is characterized by multiple deletions that differ from single deletions in their inheritance pattern, their location within the mitochondrial genome, and their molecular structure. Multiple mtDNA deletions can be transmitted in both autosomal dominant and autosomal recessive patterns. The identity of the nuclear encoded gene(s) that influences the regulation and function of normal mtDNA in a *trans*-acting manner is not known but has been linked in Finnish families to chromosome 10q23.3–24.3. Tissue-specific autosomally transmitted depletion of mtDNA, which represents a quantitative mtDNA defect caused by an intergenomic communication error, has also been described. mtDNA deletions can be detected reliably by molecular genetic methods, but require skeletal muscle as the source of DNA.

Table 103-3
Possible Laboratory Findings in Mitochondrial Diseases

"Ragged red fibers" on skeletal muscle biopsy
Elevated serum and cerebrospinal fluid lactate concentration
Myopathic potentials on electromyography
Axonal and demyelinating peripheral neuropathy on nerve conduction studies
Sensorineural hearing loss on audiogram
Cardiac conduction defects
Basal ganglia calcification or focal signal abnormalities on magnetic resonance imaging studies
Altered phosphorus magnetic resonance spectroscopy
Defects in oxidative phosphorylation on biochemical studies
Molecular genetic demonstration of mtDNA mutation

MITOCHONDRIAL ENCEPHALOMYOPATHY, LACTIC ACIDOSIS, AND STROKE-LIKE EPISODES The mitochondrial encephalomyopathy, lactic acidosis, and stroke-like episodes (MELAS) syndrome (OMIM 540000) is characterized by seizures and stroke-like events that cause subacute brain dysfunction, cerebral structural changes, and several other common clinical and laboratory features (*see* Tables 103-1 through 103-3). The maternal inheritance of the MELAS syndrome may be obscured because of mild or oligosymptomatic clinical features in relatives. In 80% of cases, a point mutation at nucleotide 3243 in the transfer $RNA^{Leu(UUR)}$ gene is the cause. Other mutations in this gene, which appears to be a common site of pathogenetic mutations, have also been found in MELAS probands. The 3243 mtDNA mutation appears to be the most pleiomorphic pathogenetic mutation and is also associated with nondeletion CPEO, myopathy, deafness, diabetes, and dystonia.

MYOCLONIC EPILEPSY WITH RAGGED RED FIBERS SYNDROME The myoclonic epilepsy with ragged red fibers (MERRF) syndrome (OMIM 545000) consists of myoclonus, seizures, cerebellar ataxia, and mitochondrial myopathy. Pathogenetic mutations have been demonstrated at nucleotide positions 8344 and 8356 in the $tRNA^{Lysine}$ gene. Neurological (*see* Table 103-1) and laboratory (*see* Table 103-3) features common to other mitochondrial encephalomyopathies are seen. Maternal relatives may be asymptomatic or may have partial clinical syndromes, including lipomas in a characteristic "horse-collar" distribution and hypertension.

NEUROPATHY, ATAXIA, AND RETINITIS PIGMENTOSA/MATERNALLY INHERITED LEIGH'S DISEASE The syndrome of neuropathy, ataxia, and retinitis pigmentosa (NARP) (OMIM 551500) is characterized by proximal weakness, sensory neuropathy, developmental delay, ataxia, seizures, dementia, and retinal

Table 103-4
Pathogenetic mtDNA Point Mutations

Nucleotide position	*mtDNA gene*	*Clinical phenotype*	*Nucleotide change*	*Amino acid substitution*
1555	12S rRNA	Deafness	A to G	NA
3243	$tRNA^{Leu(UUR)}$	MELAS	A to G	NA
			Diabetes	
3260	$tRNA^{Leu(UUR)}$	Cardiomyopathy	A to G	NA
3271	$tRNA^{Leu(UUR)}$	MELAS	T to C	NA
3303	$tRNA^{Leu(UUR)}$	Cardiomyopathy	A to G	NA
3460	ND-1	LHON 1°	G to A	Ala 52 Thr
8344	$tRNA^{Lys}$	MERRF	A to G	NA
8356	$tRNA^{Lys}$	MERRF	T to C	NA
8993	ATPase 6	NARP/Leigh's	T to G[a]	Leu 156 Arg
			T to C	Leu 156 Pro
11778	ND-4	LHON 1°	G to A	Arg 340 His
13708	ND-5	LHON 2°	G to A	Ala 458 Thr
14484	ND-6	LHON 1°	T to C	Met 64 Val
15257	Cytochrome-*b*	LHON 1°/2°	G to A	Asp 171 Asn

Note: The numeral in the amino acid substitution column refers to the position of the mutant codon in the mtDNA-encoded protein. ND-1, ND-4, ND-5, and ND-6—1st, 4th, 5th, and 6th subunits of NADH dehydrogenase; ATPase 6—6th subunit of ATP synthase; MELAS—mitochondrial encephalomyopathy, lactic acidosis, and stroke-like episodes syndrome; MERRF—myoclonic epilepsy and ragged red fibers; NARP/Leigh's—neuropathy, ataxia, and retinitis pigmentosa/maternally inherited Leigh's disease; cardiomyopathy—hypertrophic cardiomyopathy and skeletal myopathy; LHON—Leber's hereditary optic neuropathy; 1°—primary, 2°—secondary LHON-associated mtDNA mutation; NA—not applicable since mutations are in ribosomal or transfer RNAs; Ala—alanine; Thr—threonine; Leu—leucine; Arg—arginine; Pro—proline; His—histidine; Met—methionine; Val—valine; Asp—aspartic acid; Asn—asparagine.

[a]Only pathogenetic mtDNA point mutation that is a transversion mutation.

pigmentary degeneration. This maternally inherited disorder is associated with two different heteroplasmic missense mutations at nucleotide position 8993 in the ATPase 6 gene. High proportions of the same mutations are also seen in maternally inherited Leigh's disease. The point mutations associated with these and other mitochondrial disorders are readily detected by molecular genetic analysis of mtDNA extracted from muscle, blood, and urine.

LEBER'S HEREDITARY OPTIC NEUROPATHY Leber's hereditary optic neuropathy (OMIM 535000) was the first disease in humans pathogenetically linked to heritable point mutations in mtDNA, and it may serve as a paradigm for homoplasmic missense mutation-mediated mitochondrial diseases. The core clinical phenotype is painless, subacute, bilateral visual loss with central scotomas and dyschromatopsia. The mean age of onset is 23 years, and three to four times as many males are affected as females.

LHON bears little clinical resemblance to the other mitochondrial diseases but was first classified as such on the basis of its maternal inheritance pattern. The pathophysiology of visual loss appears to involve both genetic and epigenetic factors. The mtDNA mutations exhibit a great deal of genetic heterogeneity with mutations in at least eight genes that encode subunits of three biochemical complexes. Four mutations, at nucleotide positions 11778, 3460, 15257, and 14484, are thought to have primary pathogenetic importance in multiple probands (Table 103-4; *see also* Fig. 103-1).

Several other mtDNA mutations have been associated with LHON that may have secondary pathogenetic roles in LHON. The prevalence of a secondary mutation at nucleotide position 13708 in the ND-5 gene is significantly increased in association with four different primary mutations. An X-linked nuclear DNA factor has been postulated to explain the marked male predominance, but the evidence has been conflicting. The most important epigenetic factors are exposure to alcohol and tobacco.

The diversity of the primary LHON-associated mtDNA mutations is reflected in genotype-specific clinical phenotypes. The most outstanding differential feature is the prognosis for visual recovery, which varies nearly 10-fold depending on the mutation. The causative mtDNA mutations of some variants of LHON, such as LHON plus dystonia (OMIM 516006.0002) and subacute optic neuropathy and myelopathy, have also been determined.

Analysis of the pathogenetic importance of LHON-associated mtDNA mutations illustrates the issues involved in determining the pathogenicity of any mtDNA mutation. A definitive cause-and-effect relationship between an mtDNA mutation and a clinical phenotype can be difficult to establish. MtDNA is highly polymorphic, there is dissociation of genotype and phenotype, different mutations can be associated with the same phenotype, the same mutation can be associated with different phenotypes, and epigenetic factors can affect clinical manifestations.

PATHOPHYSIOLOGY OF MITOCHONDRIAL DNA MUTATIONS

There is a complex, poorly understood relationship between the various mtDNA mutations, the resulting impairment of oxidative phosphorylation, and the associated clinical phenotypes. One important experimental system that has made major contributions to the understanding of mtDNA mutations is the rho° cell line. Recipient cell lines are rendered devoid of endogenous mtDNA and are fused with donor cytoplasts that harbor the mtDNA mutation of interest. The resultant cybrid contains the nucleus of the recipient cell line and the cytoplasm (including the mitochondria and mtDNA) of the diseased cell line. This system can be used to study the mitochondrial protein synthesis and the biochemical phenotype of oxidative phosphorylation defects in cybrid cell lines with variable proportions of mutant and normal mtDNA. There are no animal models of mitochondrial disease, and there is a large gap between detailed data at the molecular and cellular level, and the complex clinical observations in patients.

All well-characterized mtDNA deletions eliminate at least one tRNA gene, and the deleted region appears to be transcribed but not translated. Indeed, there is a severe, generalized defect of translation that causes impaired mitochondrial protein synthesis and oxidative phosphorylation defects. The limited clinical expression of mtDNA deletions may reflect both heteroplasmy and differential tissue distribution. Clinically sporadic single deletions must have arisen in the oocyte or early in development, prior to the divergence of the three primary germ cell layers.

Pathogenetic tRNA mutations also impair mitochondrial messenger RNA translation and cause deficits in mitochondrial protein synthesis and in oxidative phosphorylation. The different clinical phenotypes seen in mutations in different tRNA genes imply some subtle functional differences among them, although impairment of oxidative phosphorylation must be a central feature of their pathogenicity. Age-related decline in oxidative metabolic capacity, differential tissue susceptibility, heteroplasmy, and interaction with tissue-specific nuclear DNA-encoded isozymes of oxidative phosphorylation subunits explain some of the intra- and interfamilial clinical heterogeneity, as well as the progressive course of the mitochondrial diseases.

The primary LHON-associated missense mtDNA mutations are usually homoplasmic and may occur alone or in combination with a number of secondary mutations. The LHON-associated mutations studied to date cause subtle, complex-specific impairment of oxidative phosphorylation. Many characteristic features of LHON, such as the long latency to onset, the acute nature of the vision loss, and clinical involvement confined to the optic nerve, are not explained adequately by such a mechanism. The allelic missense mutations in the ATPase 6 gene associated with NARP and Leigh's disease mutate a highly conserved leucine residue and impair ATP production via blockage of the ATPase proton channel. These mutations show a unique trait among pathogenetic mtDNA mutations in that the clinical phenotype appears to be dependent on the proportion of mutant to wild-type mtDNA.

A mouse model of mitochondrial myopathy has been created by generating a knockout of the heart/muscle isoform of the adenine nucleotide translocator (Ant 1). The null mice exhibit mitochondrial proliferation, a defect in coupled respiration, and increased serum lactate levels. Adult mice also had severe exercise intolerance.

ORGAN SYSTEM MANIFESTATIONS OF MITOCHONDRIAL DNA MUTATIONS

Virtually all tissues of the body are dependent to some extent on oxidative metabolism and thus can be affected by mtDNA mutations. The somatic manifestations listed in Table 103-2, first noted in association with the classic mitochondrial diseases, may be the dominant or initial clinical symptom and may provide the first opportunity for consideration of a mitochondrial diagnosis. These somatic manifestations may be important comorbid features.

The neurological manifestations of mitochondrial disorders, involving both the central and peripheral nervous systems, have dominated the literature and have been reviewed elsewhere. Less well known are the nonneurological manifestations of mtDNA mutations. The ophthalmological manifestations of mtDNA mutations are very prominent, with involvement of virtually the entire visual axis from lids, cornea, and extraocular muscles to the occipital cortex. The cardinal eye findings include ptosis, ophthalmoplegia, optic neuropathy, pigmentary retinopathy, and cortical visual field defects.

Cardiovascular manifestations are also common in the mitochondrial disorders and can be life-threatening, comorbid features. These manifestations include dilated and hypertrophic cardiomyopathy (OMIM 510000), conduction disease and heart block, Wolff-Parkinson-White syndrome, and most recently hypertension. Cardiomyopathy has been the dominant clinical feature in association with several tRNA mutations, particularly in the $tRNA^{Leu(UUR)}$ gene, which harbors a disproportionately large number of mutations.

Endocrine manifestations are frequent, and the prevalence of diabetes mellitus is higher than expected in the mitochondrial encephalomyopathies (*see* Chapter 47). The islet cells of the pancreas are extremely metabolically active and are susceptible to disruption of oxidative phosphorylation. The diabetes mellitus associated with mtDNA mutations is mainly due to a defect in insulin secretion. Diabetes mellitus has been linked with a heteroplasmic point mutation in the $tRNA^{Leu(UUR)}$ gene at nucleotide position 3243, usually, but not exclusively, in association with sensorineural hearing loss (OMIM 520000). Diabetes mellitus is a treatable, co-morbid feature of a number of mitochondrial diseases and can be the dominant, presenting manifestation of an mtDNA mutation. Hypoparathyroidism and symptomatic hypocalcemia have been noted in association with Kearns-Sayre syndrome.

Gastrointestinal manifestations of mtDNA mutations include colonic pseudo-obstruction, hepatopathy, chronic diarrhea, and weight loss. The most prominent renal manifestation of mtDNA mutations has been a Fanconi type of nonselective proximal nephron dysfunction, with consequent aminoaciduria, phosphaturia, and glycosuria. A glomerulopathy and the lactic acidosis associated with mitochondrial disorders may also bring these patients to the attention of the nephrologist. Pearson's syndrome (OMIM 557000) of exocrine pancreas dysfunction and a sideroblastic hypoproliferative anemia and pancytopenia occurs in association with large-scale single mtDNA deletions. Other forms of sideroblastic anemia or aplastic anemia may also be associated with acquired or inherited mtDNA mutations. Psychiatric manifestations, most notably depression, have been noted in association with multiple mtDNA deletions.

ROLE OF MITOCHONDRIAL DNA MUTATIONS IN COMMON DISEASES

The role of mtDNA mutations in common, socioeconomically significant diseases is under active investigation. The genetic basis of many prevalent diseases is complex, and does not follow simple, single-gene mendelian inheritance. The study of mitochondrial diseases such as LHON has illustrated the potential for complex pathophysiological interaction between genetic and epigenetic factors. As a result of these interactions, mtDNA mutations may be involved in subsets of common diseases, such as diabetes mellitus, in which the maternal inheritance pattern is not prominent.

The tissue-specific accumulation of somatic (noninherited) mtDNA mutations may be more relevant to late-onset degenerative disorders than are inherited mtDNA mutations or gross structural derangements that occur at the gametic level. The high mutation rate and poor repair capacity of mtDNA contributes to the buildup of mtDNA mutations in postmitotic tissues or those with a slower turnover rate. Environmental factors may also affect mtDNA; the antiretroviral drug azidothymidine depletes muscle mtDNA and causes an acquired mitochondrial myopathy.

The accumulation of mtDNA mutations and the consequent deficit in ATP production beyond a threshold level in certain critical neuronal subpopulations may contribute to the pathogenesis of neurodegenerative diseases, particularly those that become more common with age, such as Alzheimer's disease and Parkinson's disease. Mitochondrial energy deficits have been postulated to contribute to neuronal injury via an excitotoxic mechanism that implicates many of the currently identified mediators of cell injury and death. These mechanisms may also contribute to arguably the most prevalent human condition, aging (OMIM 502000) itself. Ames and colleagues have outlined an elegant scenario that incorporates a rapidly accumulating body of data about the role of mitochondria in animal and human aging. They posit that cumulative, age-dependent mitochondrial dysfunction, mediated to a significant degree by oxidative damage to mtDNA and other mitochondrial macromolecules, is a major contributor to aging at the cellular, tissue, organ-system, and whole-organism level.

FUTURE STUDIES

Data about the role of mtDNA mutations in the pathogenesis of human disease has accumulated rapidly since 1988. The availability of the complete human mtDNA sequence and a wealth of knowledge about variations in that sequence have been crucial to our nascent understanding of the pathogenetic role of mtDNA mutations. Detailed study of mitochondrial disease has also provided insight into fundamental biological processes such as oxidative phosphorylation and aging.

There are a number of fertile areas for future work on the molecular genetic basis of mitochondrial disease, based in part on our knowledge of the complex interaction of nuclear and mitochondrial genes. The majority of oxidative phosphorylation subunits are encoded by nuclear genes, and pathogenetic mutations in these genes will be discovered. There are multiple nuclear genes involved in the coordinate regulation of mtDNA, and the identification of one such defect in intergenomic communication is underway. The discovery of the nuclear gene defect underlying the mtDNA depletion phenotype, which may involve the control of mtDNA replication, is technically more difficult, because of the autosomal recessive inheritance and the small sibships. The complex pathway by which nuclear DNA-encoded proteins reach their ultimate destination in the correct intramitochondrial compartment affords a number of vulnerable points for mutations, including the chaperon proteins.

mtDNA mutations appear to be pathogenetic in an expanding array of human conditions and diseases, and the repertoire of mtDNA mutations is by no means exhausted. The phenotypic borders of the mitochondrial diseases will broaden, and novel clinical syndromes will be described, at least partially on the basis of newly discovered pathogenetic mtDNA mutations. Pathogenetic mtDNA mutations have been discovered in each type of mtDNA gene, and there does not appear to be any constraint to prevent all 37 (22 tRNAs, 13 proteins, 2 rRNAs) mtDNA genes from harboring them. The role of mtDNA mutations in more prevalent neurological diseases, such as multiple sclerosis and Parkinson's disease, will continue to be an active area of investigation. In multiple sclerosis, for instance, there may be a dominant nuclear DNA gene mutation(s) that interacts with and is modified by mtDNA mutations.

Advances in our understanding of the molecular genetic basis of mitochondrial diseases have already had a profound impact on their detection and evaluation. A set of sensitive and specific molecular genetic tests has been developed for a number of the mitochondrial encephalomyopathies. The unequivocal establishment of the diagnosis of a mitochondrial disease by such molecular genetic methods is a prerequisite for proper genetic counseling and, ultimately, treatment. To date, the advances in diagnosis of these diseases have not been paralleled by therapeutic advances, but at least we are now aware of the biochemical target for such therapy and are able to avoid ineffective or inappropriate therapy. For example, using in vitro replication run-off assays, it has been possible to selectively inhibit the replication of mutant mitochondrial DNA by using peptide nucleic acids complementary to the mutant sequence. Mitochondrial gene therapy for these disorders must overcome a number of obstacles (e.g., the unique mtDNA genetic code and the requirement for specific targeting to the correct intramitochondrial compartment) from those encountered in the search for effective nuclear gene therapy, but it is not beyond the realm of possibility in the future.

ACKNOWLEDGMENT

This work was supported by a grant from the National Eye Institute of the National Institutes of Health (RO1-EY10864).

SELECTED REFERENCES

Anderson S, Bankier AT, Barrell BG, et al. Sequence and organization of the human mitochondrial genome. Nature 1981;290:457–465.

Attardi G, Schatz G. Biogenesis of mitochondria. Annu Rev Cell Biol 1988;4:289–333.

Beal MF, Hyman BT, Koroshetz W. Do defects in mitochondrial energy metabolism underlie the pathology of neurodegenerative disease? Trends Neurosci 1993;16:125–31.

Brown MD, Wallace DC. Molecular basis of mitochondrial DNA disease. J Bioenerg Biomembr 1994;26:273–289.

Cann RL, Stoneking M, Wilson AC. Mitochondrial DNA and human evolution. Nature 1987;325:31–36.

Clayton DA. Structure and function of the mitochondrial genome. J Inherit Metab Dis 1992;15:439–447.

Cullom ME, Heher KL, Savino PJ, Miller NR, Johns DR. Leber's hereditary optic neuropathy masquerading as tobacco-alcohol amblyopia. Arch Ophthalmol 1993;111:1482–1485.

Dalakas MC, Illa I, Pezeshkpour GH, Laukaitis JP, Cohen B, Griffin JL. Mitochondrial myopathy caused by long-term zidovudine therapy. N Engl J Med 1990;322:1098–1105.

Davis RE, Miller S, Herrnstadt C, et al. Mutations in mitochondrial cytochrome c oxidase genes segregate with late-onset Alzheimer disease. Proc Natl Acad Sci USA 1997;94:4526–4531.

DiMauro S, Moraes CT. Mitochondrial encephalomyopathies. Arch Neurol 1993;50:1197–1208.

Graham BH, Waymire KG, Cottrell B, Trounce IA, MacGregor GR, Wallace DC. A mouse model for mitochondrial myopathy and cardiomyopathy resulting from a deficiency in the heart/muscle isoform of the adenine nucleotide translocator. Nat Genet 1997;16:226–234.

Holt IJ, Harding AE, Petty RKH, Morgan-Hughes JA. A new mitochondrial disease associated with mitochondrial DNA heteroplasmy. Am J Hum Genet 1990;46:428–433.

Johns DR. Therapy of mitochondrial encephalomyopathies. In: Johnson RT, Griffin JW, eds. Current therapy in neurologic disease. vol. 4. Philadelphia: B. C. Decker, 1993: pp. 329–332.

Johns DR. Genotype-specific phenotypes in Leber hereditary optic neuropathy. Clinical Neuroscience 1994;2:146–150.

Johns DR. Mitochondrial DNA mutations and eye disease. In: Wiggs JL, ed. Molecular genetics of ocular disorders. New York, Wiley-Liss, 1994: pp. 197–214.

Johns DR. Mitochondrial DNA and disease. N Engl J Med 1995;333: 638–644.

Johns DR. The other human genome: mitochondrial DNA and disease. Nat Med 1996;10:1065–1068.

Johns DR, Hurko O. Preferential amplification and molecular characterization of junction sequences of pathogenetic deletion in human mitochondrial DNA. Genomics 1989;5:623–628.

Johns DR, Rutledge SL, Stine OC, Hurko O. Directly repeated sequences associated with pathogenic mitochondrial DNA deletions. Proc Natl Acad Sci USA 1989;86:8059–8062.

Johns DR, Smith KH, Miller NR, Sulewski ME, Bias WB. Identical twins who are discordant for Leber's hereditary optic neuropathy. Arch Ophthalmol 1993;111:1491–1494.

King MP, Attardi G. Injection of mitochondria into human cell leads to a rapid replacement of the endogenous mitochondrial DNA. Cell 1988;52:811–819.

Moraes CT, Ciacci F, Silvestri G, et al. Atypical clinical presentations associated with the MELAS mutation at position 3243 of human mitochondrial DNA. Neuromuscul Disord 1993;3:43–50.

Newman NJ. Leber's hereditary optic neuropathy: new genetic considerations. Arch Neurol 1993;50:540–548.

Pfanner N, Craig EA, Meijer M. The protein import machinery of the mitochondrial inner membrane. Trends Biochem Sci 1994;19: 368–372.

Poulton J. Duplications of mitochondrial DNA: implications for pathogenesis. J Inherit Metab Dis 1992;15:487–498.

Prezant TR, Agapian JV, Bohlman MC, et al. Mitochondrial ribosomal RNA mutation associated with both antibiotic-induced and non-syndromic deafness. Nat Genet 1993;4:289–294.

Santorelli FM, Shanske S, Macaya A, DeVivo DC, DiMauro S. The mutation at nt 8993 of mitochondrial DNA is a common cause of Leigh's syndrome. Ann Neurol 1993;34:827–834.

Schon EA, Hirano M, DiMauro S. Mitochondrial encephalomyopathies: clinical and molecular analysis. J Bioenerg Biomembr 1994;26: 291–299.

Shigenaga MK, Hagen TM, Ames BN. Oxidative damage and mitochondrial decay in aging. Proc Natl Acad Sci USA 1994;91:10,771–10,778.

Shoffner JM. Maternal inheritance and the evaluation of oxidative phosphorylation diseases. Lancet 1996;348:1283–1288.

Shoffner JM, Brown MD, Torroni A, et al. Mitochondrial DNA variants observed in Alzheimer disease and Parkinson disease patients. Genomics 1993;17:171–184.

Silvestri G, Ciafaloni E, Santorelli FM, et al. Clinical features associated with the A→G transition at nucleotide 8344 of mtDNA ("MERRF mutation"). Neurology 1993;43:1200–1206.

Suomalainen A, Kaukonen J, Amati P, et al. An autosomal locus predisposing to deletions of mitochondrial DNA. Nat Genet 1995;9:146–151.

Taylor RW, Chinnery PF, Turnbull DM, Lightowlers RN. Selective inhibition of mutant human mitochondrial DNA replication in vitro by peptide nuclear acids. Nat Genet 1997;15:212–215.

Zeviani M. Nucleus-driven mutations of human mitochondrial DNA. J Inherit Metab Dis 1992;15:456–471.

104 Malignant Hyperthermia and Central Core Disease

DAVID H. MACLENNAN AND BEVERLEY A. BRITT

MALIGNANT HYPERTHERMIA

BACKGROUND The recorded history of malignant hyperthermia (MH) began in 1900, when several, often fatal, cases of unexpected fever and "convulsions" during anesthesia in the operating room were reported. It was not until Denborough and colleagues (1961) reported 10 cases in a single Australian family, however, that it was realized that MH is inherited as an autosomal dominant abnormality. In 1966 it was discovered that pigs afflicted with porcine stress syndrome also develop MH reactions that are virtually identical to human MH, providing an excellent experimental model for MH. By 1970 the site of the primary defect could be assigned to skeletal muscle rather than brain. Muscle fascicles from MH-susceptible (MHS) patients were shown to be more sensitive than normal to the contracture-inducing properties of caffeine and halothane, providing the basis for the caffeine/halothane contracture test for MH susceptibility. In a landmark paper, Harrison (1975) showed that dantrolene sodium is an effective antidote, reversing the symptoms of an MH reaction. In the early 1980s the Ca^{2+}-release channel of skeletal muscle sarcoplasmic reticulum from both humans and swine was shown to be hypersensitive to Ca^{2+}-, caffeine-, and halothane-induced channel opening. Subsequent genetic analysis has shown that abnormalities in the Ca^{2+}-release channel of skeletal muscle sarcoplasmic reticulum (the ryanodine receptor, OMIM 180901) are linked to MH in a large proportion of MH families.

CLINICAL FEATURES

Individuals susceptible to malignant hyperthermia (OMIM 145600) may respond to the administration of potent inhalational anesthetics and depolarizing skeletal muscle relaxants with a rising end tidal CO_2, skeletal muscle rigidity, tachycardia, unstable and rising blood pressure, hyperventilation, cyanosis, a falling arterial oxygen tension (PaO_2), an increasing arterial carbon dioxide tension ($PaCO_2$), lactic acidosis, and, eventually, fever. Cellular damage brings about electrolyte imbalance with an early elevation in serum of K^+, Mg^{2+}, and Ca^{2+} and a later rise in the serum and urine of muscle proteins such as creatine kinase and myoglobin. If therapy is not initiated immediately, the patient may die within minutes from ventricular fibrillation, within hours from pulmonary edema or coagulopathy, or within days from neurological damage (postanoxic cerebral edema or encephalopathy) or obstructive renal failure, the latter resulting largely from the release of muscle proteins such as myoglobin into the circulation and thence into the renal tubules. During convalescence, acute muscle soreness, and muscle edema may develop.

Central core disease (CCD) (OMIM 117000) is a rare, nonprogressive myopathy, presenting in infancy, and characterized by hypotonia, proximal muscle weakness, and susceptibility to malignant hyperthermia. Additional variable clinical features include pes cavus, kyphoscoliosis, foot deformities, congenital hip dislocation, and joint contractures. Although signs may be severe, up to 40% of patients demonstrating central cores may be clinically normal. Diagnosis is made on the basis of the lack of oxidative enzyme activity in central regions of skeletal muscle cells, observed upon histological examination of muscle biopsies. Electron microscopic analysis shows disintegration of the contractile apparatus, ranging from blurring and streaming of the Z lines to total loss of myofibrillar structure. The sarcoplasmic reticulum and transverse tubular systems are increased in content and are, in general, less well structured. NADH-tetrazolium reductase reactions reveal pale circular areas designated as central cores. Mitochondria are depleted in the cores but may be enriched around the surfaces of the cores. The disorder is inherited as an autosomal dominant trait with variable penetrance, and it is tightly linked to defects in the Ca^{2+}-release channel gene.

The King-Denborough syndrome (OMIM 145600) is characterized in children by particular congenital abnormalities such as short stature, scoliosis, pectus deformity, delay in motor development, ptosis, low-set ears, antimongolian slanted eyes, cryptorchidism, and susceptibility to malignant hyperthermia. This syndrome is inherited as an autosomal dominant trait, but it is not yet known whether it is linked to defects in the Ca^{2+}-release channel gene.

EPIDEMIOLOGY MH crises develop most commonly in individuals between the ages of 3 and 30, and the number of MH reactions declines progressively in age groups above 30. Reactions are rare before the age of 3 or after the age of 78. Males are slightly more affected, in terms of both incidence of reactions and positive biopsies, perhaps because of their larger and stronger musculature. Many individuals experiencing MH reactions have had previous uneventful general anesthetics, often of long duration and with known triggering agents.

From: *Principles of Molecular Medicine* (J. L. Jameson, ed.), ©1998 Humana Press Inc., Totowa, NJ.

INCIDENCE The incidence of MH is about 1 in 15,000 anesthetics in children and about 1 in 50,000 to 1 in 100,000 anesthetics in adults. These reported incidences are probably marked underestimates of the true incidence of MH susceptibility because of the incomplete penetrance of the gene and the difficulty in defining mild reactions, including masseter muscle spasm. The incidence of masseter muscle rigidity in children in the United States is about 1 in 100 anesthetics. The corresponding figure for masseter muscle rigidity in Canada is only about 1 in 1000 to 1 in 2000 anaesthetics, perhaps due to different protocols for anesthesia. Of those US children who have had anaesthetic-induced masseter muscle rigidity and, subsequently, had muscle biopsies, 50% were positive in the caffeine/halothane contracture test for MH susceptibility. If these frequencies were truly indicative of MH susceptibility, then the incidence of MH in the general population would be as high as 1 in 200.

DIAGNOSTIC TESTS

MH episodes may occur in individuals who have inherited muscle diseases with deleterious phenotypes such as central core disease, King-Denborough syndrome, Duchenne muscular dystrophy, myotonia fluctuans, and, possibly, other myopathies. MH susceptibility is seldom associated with ill health, although serum creatine kinase is often elevated and potential associations with chronic muscle pain, chronic fatigue, and muscle weakness are being investigated. Accordingly, one of the most important goals of MH research is to prevent MH episodes through identification of MHS individuals in advance of anesthesia. The in vitro caffeine/halothane contracture test (CHCT and IVCT) was developed as a diagnostic test for MH susceptibility on the premise that muscle fibers from MHS individuals might be more sensitive than normal to these agents, which induce contractures. The North American test protocol and the European test protocol have been standardized on this premise.

The CHCT and IVCT have been devised to be a valuable clinical test, assuring that appropriate anesthetics are administered to those patients who are MHS, while permitting those diagnosed as normal to be treated with normal anesthetic routines. Sensitivity approaching 100% is crucial to avoid false negative diagnoses, since failure to detect MH susceptibility can result in a serious or fatal outcome. Specificity should also be high to avoid false positive diagnoses, but false positive diagnosis will not result in life-threatening anesthetic reactions.

The current CHCT is carried out under strict protocols, and those who perform the tests should be experienced and highly competent. Under these conditions, the CHCT and IVCT currently achieve 97–99% sensitivity, and only 78–92% specificity (Ørding et al. 1997; Allen et al. 1998). The tests detect abnormal responses to caffeine- and halothane-induced rises in intracellular Ca^{2+}. This is a complex process, because the outcome of the contracture test depends on the interplay among a very large number of competing reactions within muscle cells, including, as a minimum, Ca^{2+} release and reuptake, and muscle contraction and relaxation. The multifactorial nature of the regulation of the contracture response could, occasionally, give a test result that is discordant with genetic evidence. While a false-positive test result does not pose any significant problem for clinicians, inaccurate diagnoses create serious difficulties for geneticists attempting to link the inheritance of MH susceptibility to inheritance of a specific allele. In any case where the CHCT has been positive, it is strongly recommended that non-triggering anesthetic routines be followed.

MOLECULAR GENETICS

LINKAGE OF THE *RYR1* GENE TO MALIGNANT HYPERTHERMIA Early studies of porcine MH established a linkage group for the porcine *HAL* gene, the glucose phosphate isomerase gene (*GPI*), and the gene for 6-phosphogluconate dehydrogenase (*PGD*), located near the centromere of pig chromosome 6. The homologous region around the human *GPI* locus was found to be on the long arm of chromosome 19, making this a candidate region for human MH. Cloning of the human skeletal muscle ryanodine receptor (*RYR1*) cDNA led to the localization of *RYR1* to human chromosome 19q13.1, in the same region as human *GPI*. Linkage studies showed cosegregation of MH in 23 meioses in nine families, leading to a lod score (the logarithm of the odds favoring linkage vs nonlinkage) of 4.2 for a recombinant fraction of 0.0. The probability of linkage of more than 10,000 to 1 identified *RYR1* as a candidate gene for MH in humans.

PORCINE MALIGNANT HYPERTHERMIA MUTATION The demonstration of linkage of *RYR1* to MH led to parallel searches in both pigs and humans for sequence differences in the *RYR1* gene between MH and normal individuals. In a comparison of the cDNA sequences of MH (Pietrain) and normal (Yorkshire) pigs, the substitution of T for C at nucleotide 1843, leading to the substitution of Cys for Arg at amino acid residue 615, was the only amino acid sequence alteration found. Tight linkage between inheritance of the mutation and inheritance of MH was established in a study of backcrosses between British Landrace heterozygous animals of the *N/n* genotype and homozygous MH animals of the *n/n* genotype. A lod score of 102, favoring linkage, was found for a recombinant fraction of 0.0 in tests of 376 animals, including 338 informative meioses.

HUMAN MALIGNANT HYPERTHERMIA MUTATIONS The demonstration of linkage between MH and a mutation in porcine *RYR1* led to a search for the corresponding mutation in human MH families. The equivalent human mutation, Cys for Arg^{614}, was first found in a single family of five members, in which it segregated with MH. This mutation has been found in about 4% of MH families worldwide. In many of these MH families, it segregated with individuals who have been diagnosed by the CHCT as MHS, but, in a few of these MH families, linkage has not been observed. If linkage cannot be demonstrated, at least three alternatives explanations must be considered: (1) the Arg^{614}-to-Cys mutation may not be causal of MH; (2) a second MH allele may be segregating in the family; or (3) the phenotypic diagnosis, based on the CHCT, may result from factors other than genetic MH.

The assignment of the Arg^{614}-to-Cys mutation as causative of human MH has a strong genetic and biochemical basis. First, the corresponding mutation is linked to porcine MH with a lod score of 102, favoring linkage for a recombinant fraction of 0.0. Second, the mutation has been found across a species barrier, between swine and humans, where it frequently segregates with MH. Third, in biochemical studies of the porcine channel, a measurable defect has been observed in the closing of the Ca^{2+}-release channel. Finally, when expressed in muscle cells, the mutant form of the ryanodine receptor has been shown to release Ca^{2+} in response to lower levels of added caffeine or halothane than the normal channel. Accordingly, explanation (1) cannot be readily accepted.

By contrast, explanations (2) and (3) can be more readily accepted as a cause of linkage discordance. The segregation of two MH mutations in a single family could lead to apparent discordance, if only one mutation were being analyzed, even though

Table 104-1
***RYR1* Mutations Associated with Human MH and CCD**

Mutation	*Exon*	*Association*	*Occurrence*
Cys35Arg	2	MH	1 Family
Arg163Cys	6	MH, CCD	2%
Gly248Arg	9	MH	2%
Gly341Arg	11	MH	6%
Ile403Met	12	MH, CCD	1 Family
Tyr522Ser	14	MH, CCD	1 Family
Arg552Trp	15	MH	1 Family
Arg614Cys	17	MH	4%
Arg614Leu	17	MH	2%
Arg2162Cys	39	MH, CCD	4%
Arg2162His	39	MH	1 Family
Val2167Met	39	MH	8% (6 Swiss)
Thr2205Met	40	MH	1 Family
Gly2434Arg	45	MH	4%
Arg2435His	45	MH, CCD	1 Family
Arg2458Cys	46	MH	4%
Arg2458His	46	MH	4%

concordance might exist for each mutation. Since the sensitivity and the specificity of the CHCT and IVCT are less than 100%, it is highly probable that the occasional discordance between the CHCT- and the DNA-based diagnoses, at least for the Arg^{614}-to-Cys mutation, arises from inaccuracy in the CHCT. The phenotype determined from the CHCT may have resulted from genetic factors not related directly to MH susceptibility and might be attributed to variation arising from the multifactorial nature of the contracture response.

Continued analysis of the DNA sequence of ryanodine receptors from probands from MH families has associated MH with 17 mutations at 14 sites present in 40% of MH families (Table 104-1). Thus, the causal MH mutations in 60% of MH families have yet to be found. The search for additional MH mutations in *RYR1* is hampered largely by the size of the gene. The coding sequence in the cDNA is over 15,000 bp long. The gene is 161,000 bp long and contains 106 exons. The MH mutations found to date have clustered in exons 2–17 and 39–46 (*see* Table 104-1). If additional mutations continue to cluster in a few exons, mutant searches will be much less onerous than might be anticipated, considering the length of the coding sequence in the gene.

CENTRAL CORE DISEASE MUTATIONS An important feature of CCD is its close association with susceptibility to malignant hyperthermia. This association has led investigators to establish linkage between CCD and markers in the long arm of chromosome 19, including markers in *RYR1*. Analysis of *RYR1* cDNA sequences in several CCD families has led to the discovery of five mutations that are linked to CCD and MH (*see* Table 104-1).

SEARCHING FOR ADDITIONAL MHS LOCI Linkage of MH to chromosome 17q (OMIM 154274) in several families has been reported, making candidates of the sodium channel α-subunit gene *(SCN4A)* and two subunits of the dihydropyridine receptor, *CACNLB1* and *CACNLG*, located on chromosome 17q11.2-q24. In subsequent studies, however, linkage of MH to chromosome 17q and to the candidate genes was ruled out in other nonchromosome 19-linked European families. Vita et al. (1995) have suggested that paramyotonia congenita and other demonstrated defects of the sodium channel α-subunit protein might have been associated with abnormal responses to succinylcholine, including muscle rigidity.

MH has also been linked to chromosome 7q (OMIM 154276), with a lod score less than 3 in a single family. The presence of the gene encoding the α2/δ subunit of the dihydropyridine receptor (CACNL2A OMIM 114204) on chromosome 7q21-22 established it as a candidate gene for MH, but sequencing of this candidate gene has not led to the identification of a causal mutation.

Several large, non-chromosome 19-linked European MH families have been included in a systematic linkage study using a set of polymorphic microsatellite markers covering the entire human genome (Robinson et al., 1997). A single family was first linked to chromosome 3q3.1 (OMIM 600467) with a lod score of 3.22, and two more candidate loci were identified. The first was chromosome 1q (OMIM 601887 1q32), the site of a candidate gene, *CACNL1A3*, encoding the α1-subunit of the DHP receptor (CACNA1S OMIM 114208); the second resides on chromosome 5p (MHS6 OMIM 601888), where no known candidate has been mapped; the third provides evidence for at least one other unspecified locus.

Analysis of the chromosome 1q-linked family led to the discovery of the mutation of G3333 to A in the *CACNL1A3* gene (OMIM 114208), leading to the mutation of Arg1086 to His in the α1-subunit of the L-type voltage-dependent calcium channel. This mutation segregated with MH in a large pedigree, yielding a two-point lod score of 4.38 at a recombination fraction of 0 (Monnier et al., 1997). This mutation is located in the loop between domains III and IV of the channel, where it is spatially separated from other mutations in the gene, previously shown to be causal of hypokalemic periodic paralysis, and which are not associated with MHS. This study suggests that there is a direct functional interaction between the III-IV loop of the α-subunit of the DHP receptor and the ryanodine receptor, which can lead to susceptibility to MH, probably through defective regulation of the Ca^{2+}-release channel. The DHP receptor mutation does not lead to any other symptoms of ion channel disease, suggesting that it does not affect L-type calcium channel function.

It is still difficult to project the proportion of MH families that will eventually be linked to causal mutations in *RYR1* and in other gene loci. At least 50% of MH families are now linked to *RYR1*. A significant number of true MH families show a high correlation with inheritance of *RYR1* markers, but are not fully concordant. Evidence that in vitro contracture tests have less than complete specificity will require re-evaluation of the role of *RYR1* in these high correlation families. Other MH loci clearly exist, but only one or a few families have been linked to each of the other MH loci identified to date, indicating that MH mutations in these loci are rare. Causal mutations in *RYR1* will most likely be found in a large proportion of families when linkage problems are worked out.

PHYSIOLOGICAL BASIS

Examination of the early and late events in the development of a halothane-induced MH reaction in swine have proven very informative. Blood chemistry studies have revealed that lactic acidosis, presumably originating in glycogenolysis and glycolysis, and the release of K^+, Mg^{2+}, and Ca^{2+} from muscle, the target tissue, occur within seconds of the time that halothane reaches the muscle. Observed rises of serum K^+ to as high as 7–8 m*M* have been considered to be sufficient to cause cardiac arrest in at least some patients. A rise in body temperature usually occurs only after 15 or 20 min, and perhaps even substantially longer. On the basis of measurements of oxygen uptake, the major source of heat production has been shown to be anaerobic, arising from the breakdown of creatine phosphate and ATP. The neutralization of bicarbonate in the blood by lactic acid and the direct production of CO_2 by the tricarboxylic acid cycle gives rise to CO_2 in the blood and expired air. The release of Ca^{2+} into the blood from the muscle was the first indication that a disturbance in Ca^{2+} homeostasis in muscle was the primary defect in MH.

Studies of the mechanisms controlling changes in muscle tension have revealed that the interaction of actin and myosin is regulated by Ca^{2+} and that Ca^{2+} regulation is mediated through the Ca^{2+}-binding protein, troponin. Muscle Ca^{2+} concentrations are regulated by the activities of Ca^{2+} pumps and channels located in the sarcoplasmic reticulum and transverse tubular systems. Ca^{2+} also plays a role in the control of glycolysis in muscle through its activation of phosphorylase kinase.

Higher rates of Ca^{2+}-induced Ca^{2+} release, particularly at low levels of inducing Ca^{2+}, were observed in membrane vesicle preparations from both human and porcine muscle and closure of single porcine MH channels at high Ca^{2+} concentrations has been shown to be inhibited. In studies of single Ca^{2+}-release channels from humans, an abnormally high caffeine sensitivity was detected in MH individuals. In sarcoplasmic reticulum from MHS swine, ryanodine binding, which is dependent on the open state of the Ca^{2+}-release channel, was enhanced. Thus, comparative biochemical and physiological studies have implicated the Ca^{2+}-release channel as a potential causal factor for MH.

The Ca^{2+}-release channel has been isolated from skeletal muscle as a huge tetrameric complex. The complex consists of a relatively small transmembrane domain and a large, multidomain, cytoplasmic segment. Single, isolated Ca^{2+}-release channel proteins, when incorporated into planar lipid bilayers, form ligand-gated channels with a conductance greater than 100 pS in 50 m*M* Ca^{2+}. Ca^{2+} release is activated by μ*M* Ca^{2+}, m*M* ATP, and m*M* caffeine, and is inhibited by m*M* Mg^{2+} and by m*M* calmodulin. In muscle cells, the primary activation of the Ca^{2+}-release channel probably occurs through its interaction with the dihydropyridine receptor.

DNAs encoding the Ca^{2+}-release channel of skeletal muscle sarcoplasmic reticulum have been cloned from rabbit and human muscle. They encode proteins containing about 5035 amino acids with masses of about 564,000 Dalton. Transmembrane sequences are located at the COOH-terminal end of the molecule. Predicted ATP, Ca^{2+}, and calmodulin-binding sites are clustered in two sites in the molecule. One lies in the proposed transmembrane domain in the COOH-terminal end of the protein, encompassing the region between amino acid residues 4253–4499, and the other lies between about residues 2400 and 3000.

It is of interest that six out of eight MH or CCD mutations lie between amino acids 163 and 614 (*see* Table 104-1), suggesting that this region of the molecule forms a third regulatory domain in the Ca^{2+}-release channel. The sequence surrounding Arg^{614} is homologous to a sequence in the inositol 1,4,5-trisphosphate (IP_3) receptor, to which IP_3 binds to activate Ca^{2+} release. MH mutations are also found in residues 2433 and 2434. The second MH regulatory domain is also homologous to a sequence in the IP_3 receptor. Another interesting feature of the known MH mutations is that 13 of the 17 involve either loss or gain of arginine. This suggests that positive changes within the two MH domains are critical to regulatory function.

A defect in the Ca^{2+}-release channel giving rise to abnormal Ca^{2+} regulation within skeletal muscle could account for all of the signs of MH. If the Ca^{2+}-release channels had longer open times in the presence of anesthetic agents, intracellular Ca^{2+} might be chronically elevated, resulting in muscle contracture and activation of the first steps in glycogenolysis through activation of phosphorylase kinase. Muscle contracture and the pumping of excessive amounts of cytoplasmic Ca^{2+} back to the lumen of the sarcoplasmic reticulum would consume large amounts of ATP, thus generating high quantities of heat. The ADP formed would stimulate glycolysis and the mitochondrial oxidation of pyruvate derived from glucose. These hypermetabolic responses would lead to depletion of ATP, glycogen, and oxygen; to the production of excess glucose, lactic acid, CO_2, and heat; and, ultimately, to the disruption of cellular integrity and to intra- and extracellular ion imbalance.

MANAGEMENT

DIAGNOSIS An acute MH episode is recognized by the presence of a number of nonspecific clinical indicators that illustrate muscle contracture, muscle breakdown, and hypermetabolism, including fever. A clinical grading scale (Larach et al. 1994) has been developed to assess the likelihood that each event represented acute MH. The CHCT is a widely used and valuable clinical test for diagnosis of MH status in families in which MH susceptibility is segregating. DNA-based diagnosis of MH susceptibility is currently possible in only about 10–15% of MH families. As more mutations are uncovered and linked to MH, DNA-based diagnosis should become the diagnostic method of choice.

ELECTIVE ANESTHESIA Anesthesiologists identify many patients at risk through case histories, which include information on their kinship to individuals who have had an MH reaction and/or a combined history of a persistently elevated creatine kinase with chronic and incapacitating muscle pain and cramps. For patients known or suspected of having malignant hyperthermia, anesthetic routines are changed to any desired combination of nontriggering anesthetics (barbiturates, tranquillizers, narcotics, propofol, ketamine, nitrous oxide, and local anesthetics). Propofol is especially advantageous, not only because of the rapid reawakening, but also because propofol appears to normalize MH muscle. For this reason, however, propofol should not be used for muscle biopsies for the diagnosis of MH.

EMERGENCY TREATMENT FOR MH REACTIONS Under present-day standard anesthetic practice, heart rate, blood pressure, end tidal CO_2 production, arterial oxygen saturation (SaO_2), and body temperature are monitored during the course of anesthesia. An increase in several of these may lead to the diagnosis of MH. When this occurs, the administration of the MH-triggering anesthetic is stopped immediately, without waiting for further confirmation of the diagnosis. The gas machine is replaced with a clean gas machine. If this is not possible, then at least the soda lime, the corrugated anesthetic tubing, and the ventilating bag are changed. The antidote, dantrolene, is administered at a dose of 1.0 mg/kg/min until muscle tone softens; fever, heart rate, and respiratory rate decline significantly toward normal; and blood gases normalize. Although internal and external cooling has been the usual practice, it no longer seems necessary, since dantrolene by itself effectively lowers body temperature. The patient is hyperventilated with 100% oxygen. Sodium bicarbonate is given for partial correction of metabolic acidosis. Regular insulin may be infused if serum potassium and blood glucose are elevated. Furosemide and mannitol are infused to prevent the onset of acute renal failure. In addition, furosemide stops the sodium overload that may develop in the face of overly large doses of sodium bicarbonate, while mannitol helps to prevent muscle and brain edema. These practices have lowered the death rate from MH episodes from over 80% to less than 7% in recent years, but neurological, muscle, and kidney damage still contribute to the morbidity resulting from MH reactions.

FUTURE DIRECTIONS

Research over the past quarter century has led to partial understanding of the physiological and genetic basis for MH, but many goals are yet to be attained. Perhaps the most important immediate goal is to define all of the genes and all of the mutations in those genes that are causal of human MH. The development of DNA-based diagnostic tests for MH susceptibility, replacing the current invasive and expensive CHCT, should then permit accurate identification of those members of MH families who are MHS. This will assure that MHS individuals will receive a regiment of "safe" anesthetics, while normal family members can utilize more conventional anesthetics.

A second goal will be to understand the functional consequences of the structural alterations in the Ca^{2+}-release channel that lead to its involvement in MH episodes. Very little is known about the structural and functional domains of the Ca^{2+}-release channel and how mutations in the domains affect channel gating. MH mutations are clustered between residues 35 and 614 in a clear regulatory domain that corresponds to the IP_3 binding and activation domain for the Ca^{2+}-release function of the IP_3 receptor. MH mutations also appear between residues 2162 and 2458 in a second predicted regulatory domain. Future structure/function analyses will lead to the understanding of important regulatory domains in the Ca^{2+}-release channel and of their response to pharmaceutical intervention.

A third goal will be to understand, at the physiological level, how MH mutations in *RYR1* and possibly other genes relate to mutation-associated abnormalities in muscle cells. The question of how morphologically abnormal central cores form in muscle, from an *RYR1* mutation that also causes MH, raises another important question, of how chronic variation in Ca^{2+} levels in a muscle cell can affect its physiology. A corollary of this question is: How do mutations in alternate genes, leading to other myopathies, also affect Ca^{2+} regulation in muscle cells resulting in anesthetic-induced malignant hyperthermia? The answers to these and other questions will arise from ongoing investigations of the genetics and physiology of these interesting abnormalities.

ACKNOWLEDGMENTS

We thank our many colleagues for advice and discussion in the preparation of this review. Research grants to DHM, supporting original work from his laboratory, were from the Medical Research Council of Canada (MRCC), the Muscular Dystrophy Association of Canada (MDAC), the Heart and Stroke Foundation of Ontario (HSFO), and the Canadian Genetic Diseases Network of Centers of Excellence.

SELECTED REFERENCES

Adeokun AM, West SP, Ellis FR, et al. The G1021A substitution in the RYR1 gene does not cosegregate with malignant-hyperthermia susceptibility in a British pedigree. Am J Hum Genet 1997;60:833–841.

Allen GC, Larach MG, Kunselman AR. The sensitivity and specificity of the caffeine halothane contracture test: a report from the North American Malignant Hyperthermia Registry. Anesthesiology, 1998; in press.

Ball SP, Johnson KJ. The genetics of malignant hyperthermia. J Med Genet 1993;30:89–93.

Berman MC, Harrison GG, Bull AB, Kench JE. Changes underlying halothane-induced malignant hyperthermia in Landrace pigs. Nature 1970;225:653–655.

Britt BA. Malignant hyperthermia: a review. In: Schonbaum E, Lomax P, eds. Thermoregulation: pathology, pharmacology and therapy. New York: Pergamon, 1991; pp. 179–292.

Britt BA, Kalow W. Hyperrigidity and hyperthermia associated with anesthesia. Ann NY Acad Sci 1968;151:947–958.

Brownell AKW. Malignant hyperthermia: relationship to other diseases. Br J Anaesth 1988;60:303–308.

Denborough MA, Forster JFA, Lovell RRH. Anaesthetic deaths in a family. Br J Anaesth 1962;34:395,396.

Dubowitz V, Pearse AGE. Oxidative enzymes and phosphorylase in central-core disease of muscle. Lancet 1960:23,24.

Elbaz A, Vale-Santos J, Jurkat-Rott K, et al. Hypokalemic periodic paralysis and the dihydropyridine receptor (CACNL1A3): genotype/phenotype correlations for two predominant mutations and evidence for the absence of a founder effect in 16 caucasian families. Am J Hum Genet 1995;56(2):374–380.

Ellis FR, Harriman DGF. A new screening test for susceptibility to malignant hyperpyrexia. Br J Anaesth 1973;45:638.

European MH Group. Malignant hyperpyrexia: a protocol for the investigation of malignant hyperthermia (MH) susceptibility. Br J Anaesth 1984;56:1267–1269.

Fleischer S, Inui M. Biochemistry and biophysics of excitation-contraction coupling. Annu Rev Biophys Biophys Chem 1989;18:333–364.

Fontaine B, Vale-Santos J, Jurkat-Rott K, et al. Mapping of the hypokalaemic periodic paralysis (HypoPP) locus to chromosome 1q31-32 in three European families. Nat Genet 1994;6(3):267–272.

Hall LW, Woolf N, Bradley JW, Jolly DW. Unusual reaction to suxamethonium chloride. Br Mol J 1966;2:1305.

Harrison GG. Control of the malignant hyperpyrexic syndrome in MHS swine by dantrolene sodium. Br J Anaesth 1975;47:62–65.

Iaizzo PA, Lehmann-Horn F. Anaesthetic complications in muscle disorders. Anesthesiology 1995;82:1093–1096.

Iles DE, Lehmann-Horn F, Scherer SW, et al. Localization of the gene encoding the $\alpha 2/\delta$-subunits of the L-type voltage-dependent calcium channel to chromosome 7q and analysis of the segregation of flanking markers in malignant hyperthermia susceptible families. Hum Mol Genet 1994;3:969–973.

Iles DE, Segers B, Sengers RC, et al. Genetic mapping of the beta 1- and gamma-subunits of the human skeletal muscle L-type voltage-dependent calcium channel on chromosome 17q and exclusion as candidate genes for malignant hyperthermia susceptibility. Human Molecular Genetics 1993;2(7):863–868.

Jurkat-Rott K, Lehmann-Horn F, Elbaz A, et al. A calcium channel mutation causing hypokalemic periodic paralysis. Hum Mol Genet 1994;3(8):1415–1419.

Kalow W, Britt BA, Terreau ME, Haist C. Metabolic error of muscle metabolism after recovery from malignant hyperthermia. Lancet 1970;ii:895–898.

Keating KE, Quane KA, Manning BM, et al. Detection of novel RYR1 mutation in four malignant hyperthermia pedigrees. Hum Mol Genet 1994;3(10):1855–1858.

King JO, Denborough MA. Anaesthetic-induced malignant hyperpyrexia in children. J Pediatr 1973;83:37–40.

Larach MG for the North American Malignant Hyperthermia Group. Standardization of the caffeine halothane muscle contracture test. Anesth Analg 1989;69:511–515.

Larach MG, Landis JR, Shirk BS, Diaz M. Prediction of malignant hyperthermia susceptibility in man: improving sensitivity of the caffeine halothane contracture test. Anaesthesiology 1992;77:A1052.

Larach MG, Localio AR, Allen GC, et al. A clinical grading scale to predict malignant hyperthermia susceptibility. Anesthesiol 1994; 80(4):771–779.

Lehmann-Horn F, Iaizzo PA. Are myotonias and periodic paralyses associated with susceptibility to malignant hyperthermia? Brit J Anaesth 1990;65(5):692–697.

Lehmann-Horn F, Sipos I, Jurkat-Rott K, et al. Altered calcium currents in human hypokalemic periodic paralysis myotubes expressing mutant L-type calcium channels. Soc Gen Physiol Ser 1995;50:101–113.

Lerman J. Controversies in paediatric anaesthesia. Can J Anaesth 1988;35:S18–S22.

Levitt RC, Olckers A, Meyers S, et al. Evidence for the localization of a malignant hyperthermia susceptibility locus (MHS2) to human chromosome 17q. Genomics 1992;14(3):562–566.

Loke JCP, MacLennan DH. Bayesian modelling of muscle biopsy contracture testing for malignant hyperthermia susceptibility. Anesthesiology 1998; in press.

MacLennan DH. Discordance between phenotype and genotype in malignant hyperthermia. Curr Opin Neurobiol 1995;8:397–401.

MacLennan DH, Otsu K, Fujii J, et al. The role of the skeletal muscle ryanodine receptor gene in malignant hyperthermia. In: Haj AE, ed. Molecular Biology of Muscle—a Symposium of the Society for Experimental Biology, vol. 46. Cambridge, UK: Company of Biologists, 1992; pp. 189–201.

MacLennan DH, Phillips MS. Malignant hyperthermia. Science 1992; 256:789–794.

McKenzie AJ, Couchman KG, Pollock N. Propofol is a "safe" anaesthetic agent in malignant hyperthermia susceptible patients. Anaesth Intensive Care 1992;20:165–168.

Monnier N, Procaccio V, Stieglitz P, Lunardi J. Malignant-hyperthermia susceptibility is associated with a mutation of the alpha 1-subunit of the human dihydropyridine-sensitive L-type voltage-dependent calcium-channel receptor in skeletal muscle. Am J Hum Genet 1997; 60:1316–1325.

Mulley JC, Kozman HM, Phillips HA, et al. Refined genetic localization for central core disease. Am J Hum Genet 1993;52:398–405.

Olckers A, Meyers DA, Meyers S, et al. Adult muscle sodium channel alpha-subunit is a gene candidate for malignant hyperthermia susceptibility. Genomics 1992;14(3):829–831.

Ørding H, Brancadoro V, Cozzolino S, et al. In vitro contracture test for diagnosis of malignant hyperthermia following the protocol of the European MH Group: results of testing patients surviving fulminant MH and unrelated low-risk subjects. The European Malignant Hyperthermia Group. Acta Anaesthesiol Scand 1997 Sep;41(8)955–966.

Ørding H, for the European Malignant Hyperthermia Group. In vitro contracture test for diagnosis of malignant hyperthermia following the protocol of the European MH group: Results of testing patients surviving fulminant MH and unrelated low-risk subjects. Acta Anaesthesiol Scand, 1997; in press.

Phillips MS, Fujii J, Khanna VK, et al. The structural organization of the human skeletal muscle ryanodine receptor (*RYR*1) gene. Genomics 1996;34:24–41.

Phillips MS, Khanna VK, De Leon S, et al. The substitution of Arg for Gly2433 in the human skeletal muscle ryanodine receptor is associated with malignant hyperthermia. Human Mol Genet 1994;3(12): 2181–2186.

Ptacek LJ, Gouw L, Kwiecinski H, et al. Sodium channel mutations in paramyotonia congenita and hyperkalemic periodic paralysis. Ann Neurol 1993;33(3):300–307.

Robinson RL, Monnier N, Wolz W, et al. A genome wide search for susceptibility loci in three European malignant hyperthermia pedigrees. Hum Mol Genet 1997;6(6):953–961.

Rosenberg H, Fletcher JE. Masseter muscle rigidity and malignant hyperthermia susceptibility. Anesth Analg 1986;65:161–164.

Shuaib A, Paasuke RT, Brownell KW. Central core disease: clinical features in 13 patients. Medicine 1987;66:389–396.

Shy GM, Magee KR. A new congenital non-progressive myopathy. Brain 1956;79:610–621.

Sipos I, Jurkat-Rott K, Harasztosi C, et al. Skeletal muscle DHP receptor mutations alter calcium currents in human hypokalaemic periodic paralysis myotubes. J Physiol (Lond) 1995;483(Pt 2):299–306.

Sudbrak R, Golla A, Hogan K, et al. Exclusion of malignant hyperthermia susceptibility (MHS) from a putative MHS2 locus on chromosome 17q and of the alpha 1, beta 1, and gamma subunits of the dihydropyridine receptor calcium channel as candidates for the molecular defect. Hum Mol Genet 1993;2(7):857–862.

Sudbrak R, Procaccio V, Klausnitzer M, et al. Mapping of a further malignant hyperthermia susceptibility locus to chromosome 3q13.1. Am J Hum Genet 1995;56:684–691.

Vita GM, Olckers A, Jedlicka AE, et al. Masseter muscle rigidity associated with glycine 1306-to-alanine mutation in the adult muscle sodium channel alpha-subunit gene. Anesthesiology 1995;82(5): 1097–1103.

Zorzato F, Fujii J, Otsu K, et al. Molecular cloning of cDNA encoding human and rabbit forms of the Ca^{2+} release channel (ryanodine receptor) of skeletal muscle sarcoplasmic reticulum. J Biol Chem 1990;265:2244–2256.

105 Retinoblastoma

A Current Review

Joan M. O'Brien

BACKGROUND AND HISTORY

Retinoblastoma (OMIM 180200) is the most common ocular tumor of childhood, occurring in 1 in 18,000 live births. In 1809 the disease was first recognized and described with careful anatomical drawings by James Wardrop, an ophthalmologist in Edinburgh. He maintained that retinoblastoma could be cured by early enucleation (removal of the eye involved with the tumor). His hypothesis was not confirmed in his own lifetime, since in that era children with this disease presented late, with widespread metastases. The advent of a cure for primary retinoblastoma coincided with the development of the ophthalmoscope. Once intraocular disease could be visualized and diagnosed, Wardrop's hypothesis was confirmed. Rudolph Virchow believed the tumor had a glial origin, and therefore, the malignancy was termed glioma retinae. Frederick Verhoeff defined retinoblastoma as an undifferentiated neuroblastic tumor of the retina, and this designation was soon adopted by the American Ophthalmological Society. Benign variants of retinoblastoma are termed retinoma and retinocytoma.

Retinoblastoma is a disease of infancy and early childhood, with the majority of cases diagnosed before the age of 4 years. In 1971 Alfred Knudsen proposed the "two-hit hypothesis," based on an epidemiological review of 48 cases of retinoblastoma. He analyzed the patient's disease with respect to unilaterality or bilaterality, age at diagnosis, sex of patient, and family history of disease. The author concluded that retinoblastoma could be caused either by a germinal mutation or a somatic mutation. Knudsen hypothesized that the number of new heritable cases decreases over time because the occurrence of a second event at a constant rate is less likely in a declining population of undifferentiated cells. David Comings elaborated upon Knudsen's hypothesis by suggesting that mutations responsible for the phenotype could occur to inactivate both alleles of a single responsible gene.

These hypotheses were confirmed by cloning of the retinoblastoma gene *(Rb)* (*see* Chapter 7). A close linkage of the tumor predisposition with the esterase-D locus was first described, placing the gene on chromosome 13q14. This was followed by Thaddeus Dryja's observation of overlapping deletions in familial cases, suggesting a more precise genetic locus. Subsequently, in collaboration with Stephen Friend and colleagues, *Rb* was cloned.

From: *Principles of Molecular Medicine* (J. L. Jameson, ed.), ©1998 Humana Press Inc., Totowa, NJ.

Shortly thereafter, using a strategy involving chromosomal walking in the region 13q14.1, Yuen Kai Fung and colleagues provided "structural evidence for the authenticity of the human retinoblastoma gene." Wen-Hwa Lee and coworkers published the gene's full sequence nearly simultaneously. Knudsen's hypothesis was specifically confirmed in the paper by Fung and colleagues; in a bilateral case a mutation at the *Rb* locus was detected not only in the tumor but also in fibroblast DNA, suggesting a germline initiating event. In a unilateral patient, both of two mutational events (a 3' deletion and a total deletion) were found in the tumor only, with the fibroblast DNA showing no deletion at the retinoblastoma locus. This suggested that the initiating event for unilateral retinoblastoma was somatic, occurring only within the transformed cells of the retina.

CLINICAL FEATURES

The clinical features of retinoblastoma are useful to predict the underlying genetic basis for the disease in individual patients. Children with germline mutations at the retinoblastoma locus generally present earlier in life, and because the initial event has occurred in every cell, the second event is a frequent one, resulting in bilateral and multifocal disease of the retina. In contrast, children with a somatic form of the disease have two mutations which occur sporadically within a single retinal cell. The likelihood of both events occurring within one retinal cell is low; therefore, these children present later with unilateral, unifocal disease.

Although such clinical observations generally correlate with genetic background, exceptions do exist. At least 15% of unilateral patients harbor germline mutations at the *Rb* locus. Any patient with a germinal mutation at this site has increased risk for the development of osteogenic sarcoma (OMIM 259500), soft tissue sarcoma, melanoma (malignant melanoma, OMIM 155600; uveal melanoma, OMIM 155720; malignant intraocular melanoma, OMIM 155700), breast carcinoma (familial, OMIM 114480; type 1, OMIM 113705), and gastrointestinal carcinoma (OMIM 175100). Additionally, 3–7% of children with bilateral disease develop primitive neuroectodermal tumors (PNETs) of midline structures of the brain. This disease entity has been described as trilateral retinoblastoma (cf., retinoblastoma, OMIM 180200), since a striking resemblance exists between the neuroblastic tumors arising bilaterally in the retina and in the brain.

Children with germline *Rb* mutations clearly have a lifelong neoplastic predisposition this requires careful surveillance.

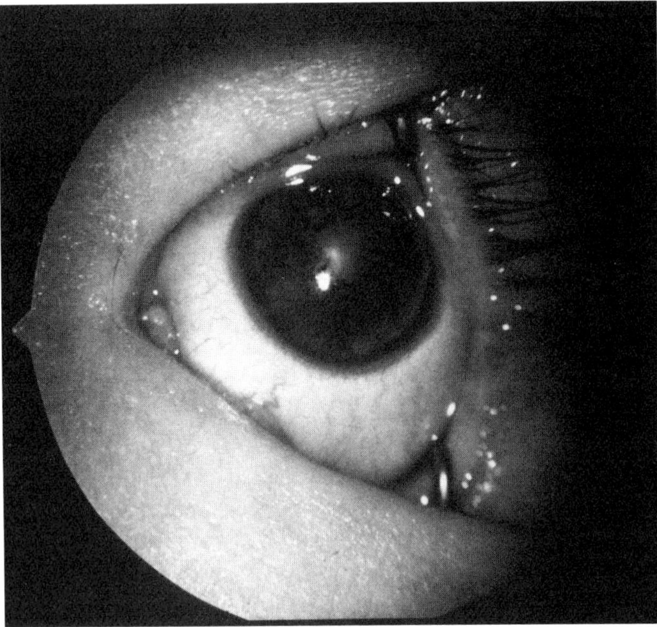

Figure 105-1 Leukocoria. In this case, the white pupil is associated with persistent hyperplastic primary vitreous, a congenital anomaly of ocular development. This entity is in the differential diagnosis of retinoblastoma, but leukocoria and retinoblastoma need not be synonymous.

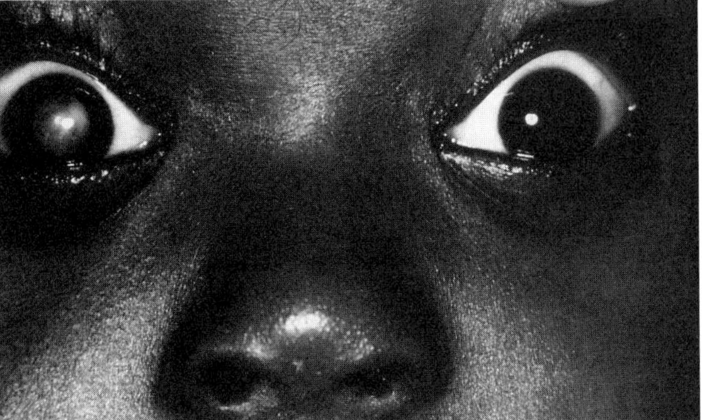

Figure 105-2 Leukocoria. In this case, the child has bilateral retinoblastoma with the larger tumor on the right producing leukocoria.

These children are also at risk for the development of multiple retinal tumors over the first 4 years of life. The major clinical challenge is to manage the recurrent primary tumors with as little risk to vision as possible, while minimizing iatrogenic inducers of second tumor development (e.g., treatment of primary tumors with external beam radiation, which has been associated with an increased rate of osteogenic sarcoma occurrence within the radiation field).

DIAGNOSIS

Children with retinoblastoma classically present with leukocoria or a white pupillary reflex (Figs. 105-1 and 105-2). However, patients with this disease may present with a wide variety of signs and symptoms and, in some cases, accurate diagnosis may be difficult. Retinoblastoma can be masked by hyphema (blood in the anterior segment of the eye, in front of the iris), a situation that is observed when the tumor has induced neovascularization of the iris. Children can present with orbital signs and symptoms that mimic preseptal cellulitis.

Retinoblastoma patients may also show signs of intraocular inflammation and may be thought to have vitritis. Coats' disease (exudative vitreoretinopathy/familial, OMIM 133780), an exudative retinopathy that can produce massive yellow white deposits, may be mistaken for retinoblastoma. Retinal dysgenesis syndromes, such as Norrie's disease (OMIM 310600), may also suggest retinoblastoma. Occasionally, the large ridges associated with retinopathy of prematurity appear mass-like, and retinoblastoma must be excluded. Myelinated nerve fibers, tuberous sclerosis with glial hamartomas of the retina and optic disc, and ocular staphylomas all may be confused with this tumor. A congenital anomaly of ocular development, persistent hyperplastic primary vitreous, also belongs in the differential diagnosis of this disease (*see* Fig. 105-1).

The diagnosis of retinoblastoma is made with retinal fundoscopy and imaging studies. Because calcification of the tumor is common, ultrasound examination to identify pathognomonic calcification is frequently helpful in the diagnosis. Most other lesions considered in the differential diagnosis do not calcify. A computed tomography (CT) scan of the brain and orbits is essential to examine the extent of ocular involvement and to detect calcification within the tumor, as well as to evaluate midline structures to exclude the presence of a concomitant PNET. Magnetic resonance imaging (MRI) is rarely necessary, although in children with orbital signs at presentation or any suggestion of optic nerve invasion by CT scan, an MRI with gadolinium contrast enhancement can be useful in planning a surgical approach to the patient.

All children should be examined at birth to confirm a bilateral red reflex, and to exclude the diagnosis of retinoblastoma or other retinal disease. Any child under 6 years of age who presents with a white pupillary reflex should be considered to have retinoblastoma until an alternative diagnosis can be confirmed. If the retina cannot be clearly visualized by an ophthalmologist—for example, because of intraocular inflammation or intraocular blood—the child should undergo an imaging study. Retinoblastoma must be excluded prior to any surgical intervention because of the risk that occult tumor may be disseminated systemically. Even fine-needle aspiration biopsy is contraindicated in children suspected of having retinoblastoma.

GENETIC BASIS OF DISEASE

Prior to the identification of the retinoblastoma susceptibility gene, many researchers believed that malignancy resulted primarily from the activation of oncogenes. Experiments in which normal cells were fused with tumor cells, with resultant suppression of neoplastic features, suggested that normal cells could also contain genetic elements capable of suppressing malignant transformation. Cloning of the retinoblastoma locus provided the first unequivocal proof of this theory and permitted identification of the gene's function as a tumor suppressor. This discovery had important implications for the study of malignancy, leading to a search for other tumor suppressor genes. Mutations or deletions of tumor suppressor genes are associated with loss of function and with deregulated growth of cells. The *Rb* gene was thought to control an important point in the pathway of regulated cellular growth. Progression toward malignancy occurs in the absence of this gene product.

Inactivation of the *Rb* locus was subsequently recognized to occur not only in retinoblastoma and osteogenic sarcoma but also

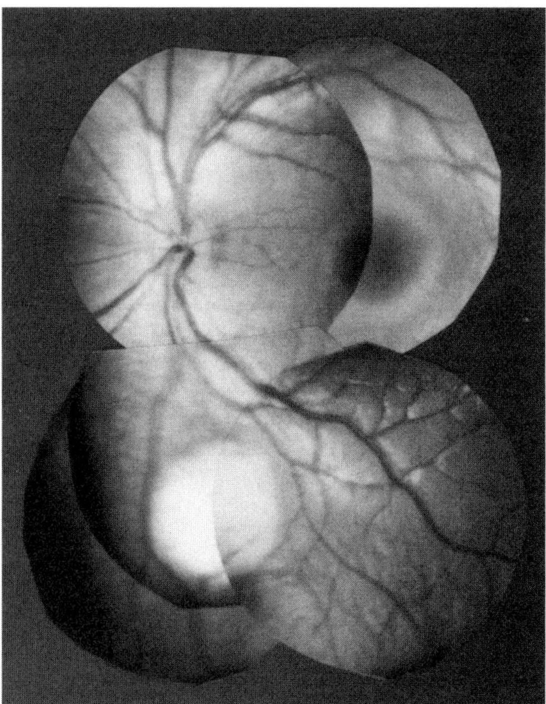

Figure 105-3 Untreated unifocal, unilateral retinoblastoma. In general, unifocal lesions are not recognized until they are considerably larger than this. With unilateral retinoblastoma, visual decrement is not appreciated by the child or the parents until the disease is advanced, since the opposite eye is unaffected and has normal vision. Most children with unilateral disease have sporadic, somatic *Rb* gene alterations, and are at low risk for second-tumor development.

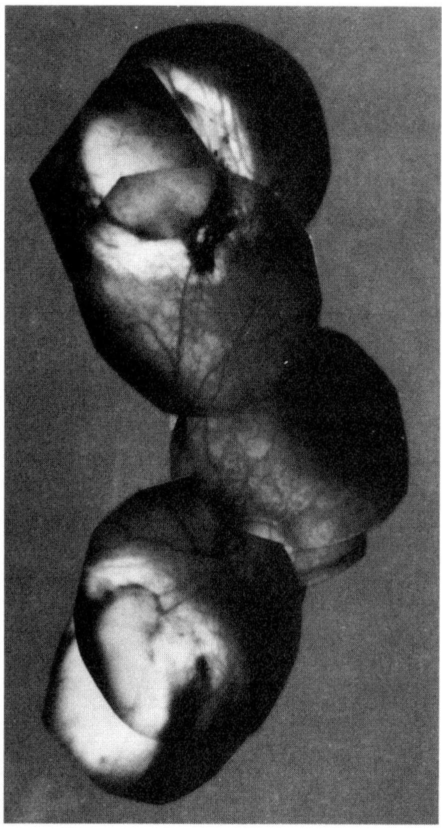

Figure 105-4 Treated multifocal, bilateral retinoblastoma associated with germline mutation at the Rb locus. The gray, diaphanous appearance of the superior lesion is associated with disease activity. The white, calcified lower lesion is treated and inactive.

in a number of other neoplastic processes, including breast carcinoma, small-cell lung carcinoma (OMIM 182280), bladder carcinoma (OMIM 109800), prostate carcinoma (OMIM 176807), and primary leukemia (OMIM 151390). It was discovered that the gene product was ubiquitously expressed in normal tissues. These observations suggested that *Rb* gene deletion or mutation could have a central role in transformation in a spectrum of histopathologically distinct malignancies.

In patients with germinal mutations at the *Rb* locus, every cell lacks one functional gene copy. The reason these children are predisposed to develop tumors of bone at an increased rate compared with tumors of other histologic origin is unclear. The risk for children with retinoblastoma to develop a second cancer of some type is approximately a 45%, 35-year risk. This risk may be increased after treatment with agents that damage DNA, such as irradiation or chemotherapy. Often, however, treatment options in children with retinoblastoma are limited. In many children, radiation therapy is required in order to retain vision and to treat the primary tumor. Figures 105-3 and 105-4 show, respectively, a unilateral and bilateral case of retinoblastoma. Treated and untreated forms are demonstrated.

MOLECULAR PATHOPHYSIOLOGY OF DISEASE

In some patients with retinoblastoma, the retinoblastoma gene is deleted in its entirety. An internal deletion of one exon or a point mutation at an important splice site may also occur, resulting in disruption of the gene product's function. The Rb protein (pRb) is known to play a key role in interacting with cell-cycle regulators (E2F and the cyclins) in the regulation of transcription, and in producing terminal differentiation of particular cell types. The protein is phosphorylated in a cell cycle-dependent manner, and the phosphorylation state regulates the activity of pRb. A number of DNA tumor virus gene products, including SV40 T antigen, adenovirus E1A, and human papilloma virus E7, bind preferentially to the underphosphorylated form of pRb, and this binding may inactivate the protein, resulting in transformation of the cell toward malignancy.

NATURE OF GENE DEFECT The retinoblastoma gene is 180 kb in length and contains 27 exons. The normal message encoded by the gene is 4.7 kb in length: 2.7 kb represent coding sequence, and 2 kb represent noncoding sequence. The resultant protein contains 928 amino acids (Fig. 105-5). The promoter of the retinoblastoma gene contains a CpG island, and it is very GC rich. The promoter also contains consensus sequences for the transcription factors E2F-1, ATF, and SP-1. The 27 exons that comprise *Rb* range in size from 31 to 1889 nucleotides in length. The largest intron is greater than 60 kb long, and the smallest intron is less than 80 bp in length. Exon 1 contains 5' untranslated sequences and the first methionine, which correspond to the 5' end of the mRNA.

A number of mutations that have been observed in the retinoblastoma gene affect one of two conserved regions, areas that are also required for Rb gene product (pRb) binding to viral oncoproteins. Mutations have also been observed in the promoter region of the retinoblastoma gene in areas corresponding to recognition sequences for the ATF and SP-1 transcription factors. The identification of mutations in SP-1 and ATF sites in retinoblastoma

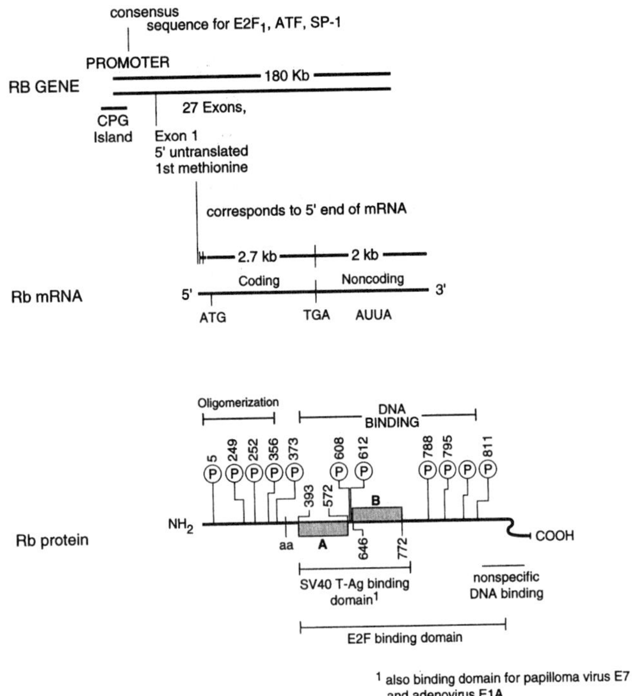

Figure 105-5 Retinoblastoma gene, mRNA, and protein structures.

families suggests that these sequences within the promoter may act as regulators of Rb gene transcription and are of phenotypic significance.

STUDIES OF mRNA AND PROTEIN The retinoblastoma protein is constitutively and ubiquitously expressed in human cells. The protein has a half-life of about 12 h. Regulation of Rb is accomplished posttranslationally (changes in expression and degradation are less important). pRb is activated and deactivated through phosphorylation events or through association with other cellular proteins. Compartmentalization within the nucleus may also play a role in the regulation of pRb.

In a number of cases where the retinoblastoma gene contains a mutation, its mRNA is truncated. The resultant protein loses function, particularly in the conserved domains where viral binding occurs, regions designated A and B. The amino acid sequence of the retinoblastoma protein suggests that it contains a number of globular domains and a hydrophilic tail. Of these, the A and B globular domains have been better defined, through mapping to the C terminus by deletion mutagenesis studies. These viral binding domains appear important to retinoblastoma protein function. Presumably, this localization of function explains why viruses have evolved to bind to this region and thereby to inactivate pRb. Activities that appear to be localized to the A-B region include suppression of growth in cell culture, adherence to nuclear components, and binding to transcription factors, as well as phosphorylation during the G1 phase of the cell cycle. Not surprisingly, these are the regions frequently observed to be deleted or to contain mutations in patients with retinoblastoma. Normal progression through the cell cycle is mediated by phosphorylation of pRb with consequent release of bound transcription factors, which act in a cascading fashion (Fig. 105-6). In cases in which the Rb gene is defective, the G1 block mediated by underphosphorylated pRb is missing, and division with cellular proliferation occurs in a less regulated fashion.

pRB: ROLE IN REGULATING TRANSCRIPTION To date, more than 30 separate cellular proteins have been identified that bind to pRb. This diverse group of proteins has been characterized to include transcription factors, regulators of growth, protein phosphatases, and protein kinases, as well as nuclear matrix proteins. Of these associated proteins, the best described is the transcription factor E2F-1. The E2F binding domain on pRb encompasses both the A and B regions involved in binding to viral oncoproteins and extends beyond these toward the carboxy-terminus. Apparently, the underphosphorylated form of pRb functions to bind and sequester members of the *E2F* family. Since E2F recognition sites are found in the promoters of a number of genes, the interaction between E2F and pRb is significant in growth regulation. The *E2F* consensus nucleotide sequence TTTCGCGC is found in the *TK* promoter, c-*myc*, b-*myb*, Cdc2, *E2F-1*, and, importantly, in the dihydrofolate reductase gene *(DHFR)*. E2F activates transcription of these downstream genes when it is released from binding to pRb. The dihydrofolate reductase gene is active in DNA synthesis which occurs during the S phase of the cell cycle. As indicated in Fig. 105-6, certain members of the E2F family bind to the Rb protein with greater affinity. Other E2F family members demonstrate greater binding affinity for p107 or p130, other members of the retinoblastoma family of genes.

In summary, when pRb is phosphorylated through the action of cyclin-Cdk complexes, E2F is released, which results in upregulation of transcription at targeted consensus sequences in the promoter regions of a variety of growth promoting genes. This includes genes such as the *DHFR* and *DNA polymerase*, which are necessary for DNA synthesis to occur in S phase. The presence of normal underphosphorylated pRb results in sequestration of E2F and its consequent inability to bind to the consensus sequence of numerous downstream genes. This binding may constitute a significant part the pRb-mediated G1 block. The Rb protein may also contain a transrepressor domain which mediates cell cycle arrest when bound to E2F.

pRB AND THE CELL CYCLE Studies investigating the role of the retinoblastoma gene in cell cycle progression have, in the majority of instances, focused on the phosphorylation status of the protein (*see* Chapter 6). Hypophosphorylated Rb protein predominates in G0 and G1, while in the S, G2, and M phases of the cell cycle the Rb protein is hyperphosphorylated. Phosphorylation events occur in at least three phases of the cell cycle: mid G1, S, and in the G2/M transition. Underphosphorylated forms of pRb mediate growth inhibition in G0 and G1 through binding of multiple transcription factors. The mid-G1 phosphorylation of pRb inactivates its tumor suppressor activity. Transcription factors and other proteins are freed to upregulate transcription and to allow the cell to progress through the cell cycle. The phosphorylation status of the retinoblastoma protein and its interactions with other gene products are demonstrated in Figs. 105-5 and 105-6. It appears that physical complex formation between cyclins D1, D2, and D3 with Cdk4, Cdk6, and cyclin E with Cdk2 results in phosphorylation of pRb. Cdks are catalytic subunits which are expressed at stable levels throughout the cell cycle; however, Cdk activity is modulated by cell cycle-dependent changes in the levels of different cyclins.

Eventually, the retinoblastoma gene product is restored to its dephosphorylated form, and this process may be mediated by protein phosphatase 1 (PP1). The catalytic subunit of PP1 binds to pRb in vitro. Other phosphatases will likely be identified that are

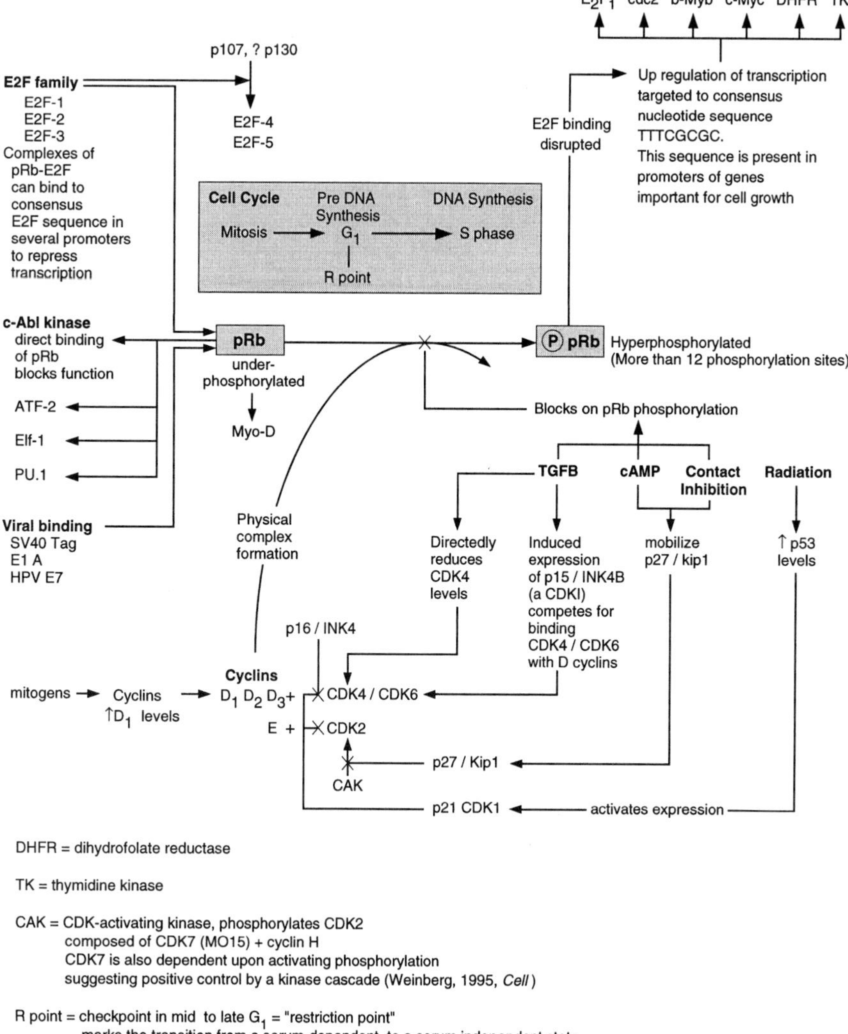

Figure 105-6 Function of the retinoblastoma gene product.

capable of dephosphorylating pRb. It is the hypophosphorylated form of pRb that binds most strongly to DNA. In addition, the hypophosphorylated form is "tethered" to nuclear structures, as demonstrated in experiments involving the extraction of cellular components through the use of salt and detergent solutions. Consistent with these findings, the hypophosphorylated form binds most specifically to other nuclear proteins. These observations suggest that the phosphorylation of pRb reduces its nuclear interactions, thereby allowing disassociation of Rb protein from the nuclear subcompartment during precise stages of the cell cycle.

In order for critical phosphorylations to occur in this complex protein, serine and threonine residues must be available for the phosphorylation event. The location of these residues is provided in Fig. 105-5. Furthermore, the protein must also contain binding sites for kinases and phosphatases. Given the complex interactions of this gene product with cell cycle proteins, it is reasonable to suggest that large deletions in the gene may have far-reaching effects upon its ability to regulate cell cycle progression.

pRB AND TERMINAL DIFFERENTIATION The role of retinoblastoma gene product in producing terminal differentiation has been carefully studied in muscle differentiation. The product of the retinoblastoma gene was found to bind directly to MyoD, a basic helix loop protein. MyoD appears to act as a muscle-specific transcription factor, capable of activating downstream structural genes in muscle, as well as mediating myogenic differentiation in different cell types. When pRb is inactivated, the progression from myoblast to myotube in culture is inhibited. Myotubes are generally felt to represent terminally differentiated structures; yet these will reenter the cell cycle in the presence of pRb inactivation. In a number of transgenic models, inactivation of the *Rb* gene appears to result in failure of terminal differentiation in neuronal tissues as well as in hematopoietic cells. These cell types are distinguished by the requirement for terminal differentiation in order to achieve full function. Interestingly, in these models muscular development is not affected.

RETINOBLASTOMA-RELATED PROTEINS The retinoblastoma gene is part of a larger family of genes that share homology. p107 and p130 inhibit E2F-mediated transcriptional activation and also appear to produce a G1 block. Whereas the retinoblastoma gene product binds preferentially to E2F-1, E2F-2, and E2F-3, p107 appears to bind preferentially to a distinct subset of the E2F family, E2F-4, and E2F-5. The sequence homology between these genes is greatest in the regions that correspond to the SV40 T antigen-binding domain in the retinoblastoma protein.

These E2F family members may exhibit a tissue-specific activity. For example, growth arrest in cervical carcinoma cells is mediated by p107 but not by pRb. If tissue specificity exists for this family, it could provide one explanation for the observation that patients with retinoblastoma gene mutations initially develop tumors of the retina, and subsequently develop bony tumors, particularly osteogenic sarcoma, at greatly increased frequency. Tissue-specific activity could suggest why children with the germline form of retinoblastoma are not more prone to tumors involving every cell that contains a retinoblastoma gene mutation. In certain tissues, other Rb family members could exert a protective function.

pRB AND CANCER Study of the retinoblastoma gene and its product must initially focus on normal pathways for cell cycle progression and normal regulatory blocks on this progression. The absence of retinoblastoma gene product has cascading effects on regulation of downstream genes. Regulation of the cell cycle is an important process, which allows time for DNA repair before DNA synthesis occurs. Since the *Rb* gene is ubiquitously expressed, the tissue specificity of tumors that occur in children with retinoblastoma gene deletions has never been adequately explained. Recognition of the retinoblastoma family of genes and the potential for these genes to be tissue-specific in their action is a line of investigation that remains to be fully explored. Clearly, the pathway involving the retinoblastoma gene product is complex and interacts with many other pathways, including those involving cyclins, Cdks, transcription factors, growth factors, and nuclear DNA. As growth regulatory pathways are seen to converge, important points of intersection may be identified where crucial elements could be modified in the treatment of cancer.

MANAGEMENT/TREATMENT

Children with retinoblastoma are difficult to manage because the disease involves an extremely important sensory system, vision, and because in many cases the disease is inherited or is heritable. When families receive this diagnosis for their infant, they almost invariably experience feelings of guilt and responsibility. Siblings and offspring of patients with bilateral retinoblastoma need to be examined by an ophthalmologist early in life, which can place additional stress on the family. The major challenge in clinical management of children with retinoblastoma is to maintain their vision, while minimizing their exposure to second tumor-inducing effects of traditional treatment modalities. Because these patients are at risk for second-tumor development, they need to be monitored closely, including routine imaging of midline brain structures to exclude the development of PNETs. With early detection and treatment, retinoblastoma is a disease that is cured in its primary form in the majority of cases. Morbidity and mortality arise mainly when second tumors develop. Families of children with retinoblastoma require strong and consistent support from physicians committed to long-term tumor surveillance.

STANDARD TREATMENT MODALITIES The treatment modality first recommended by James Wardrop, and subsequently found to be curative in many cases, is enucleation. This can be an extremely difficult treatment for patients with bilateral disease. In these cases, preservation of both eyes is attempted, if at all possible. Retinoblastoma invades the brain through the optic nerve; therefore, any tumor present at the surgical margin of the optic nerve is an undesirable clinical outcome. The surgical approach to enucleation must facilitate obtaining a long section of optic nerve. In general, when enucleation is performed in children, the eye is removed with preservation of the conjunctiva, Tenon's capsule, and extraocular muscles. An orbital implant is placed, and this implant is usually integrated with the extraocular muscles so that it will move. The implant is covered completely with layers of Tenon's capsule and conjunctiva so that it is not readily visible. A prosthesis is then fitted over the orbital implant. An unfortunate side effect of enucleation in very small children is that orbital growth may be somewhat diminished in the absence of a viable globe.

External beam radiation is an extremely effective modality for the treatment of primary retinoblastoma. This modality avoids the necessity for enucleation and can provide useful vision in cases where tumors regress away from vital visual structures such as the macula and the optic nerve. Regrettably, external beam radiation therapy does increase the risk for second tumors within the radiation field, and has the unfortunate effect of producing mid-face hypoplasia, particularly in very young patients. Children who have received external beam radiation need to be carefully followed for the development of second tumors both within and outside the field of radiation. Furthermore, endocrine deficiencies can be observed if the hypothalamus and pituitary are in the radiation field, and children should be followed presumptively for endocrine and growth deficiencies. Precise radiation-therapy planning in children with retinoblastoma is extremely important. From an ophthalmologic perspective, the retinal disease needs to be followed carefully for the first 4–5 years of the child's life, as multiple recurrences of bilateral disease typically occur during this period. Lateral radiation ports sometimes can be designed to avoid the lens, eliminating cataract formation, which precludes viewing new neoplasms as these develop. Occasionally, anterior radiation ports are required in the treatment of large tumors, particularly when this is the only option for ocular preservation. In children who receive this treatment, cataracts almost invariably develop. Tumors are then followed for growth with serial ultrasound examinations.

Laser photoablation involves the use of an indirect laser on a head-mounted indirect ophthalmoscope. Tumors of less than 4 mm in basal diameter and less than 4 mm in height are generally amenable to this treatment. The tumor is covered with small laser burns, and the retinal surround is ablated with a lower-power setting. A precise treatment, laser photoablation can be used for tumors anywhere in the eye but is particularly useful for tumors near vital structures, which can be carefully avoided with this modality.

Cryotherapy involves placing a cryoprobe (a freezing metal instrument) on the sclera external to an observed focus of new tumor development. The sclera is indented to confirm the location of the cryoprobe with respect to the tumor with visualization through an indirect ophthalmoscope. The cryoprobe, properly situated, is then activated with a foot pedal. A triple freeze–thaw cryotechnique is performed, which ablates the tumor and the surrounding retina. Cryotherapy is useful in tumors of approximately 4 mm in basal diameter and height. Tumors at the equator or more-anterior locations may be more easily approached through cryotherapy. On the other hand, cryotherapy does incite more intraocular inflammation and produces more pain in children than laser photoablation.

Trials of primary chemotherapy for the treatment of intraocular retinoblastoma have recently been initiated. Preliminary results from groups in the United States, England, France, and Canada suggest that chemotherapy, especially in combination with laser photoablation, may be useful in treating primary intraocular retinoblastoma. Chemotherapy is also useful as an adjunctive modality in children who have previously undergone external beam radiation therapy and who develop a tumor recurrence that is not amenable to any other treatment modality. Repeat radiation therapy is unlikely to result in good visual outcome, and in these cases, a course of chemotherapy may be considered.

An alternative method of delivering localized radiation directly to a tumor involves suturing a radioactive plaque on the sclera external to the region of tumor occurrence. This modality can be used to treat tumors that are larger than those amenable to laser photoablation or cryotherapy. Less localized than laser photoablation or cryotherapy, plaque therapy is effective in tumors in the far periphery of the eye, where structures vital to vision are not directly affected by the tumor or by the treatment. Complications including radiation vasculopathy and vitreous hemorrhage can occur, particularly if high doses of radiation are delivered through this modality. Furthermore, visual outcomes are not ideal if the plaque is placed posteriorly in the eye in proximity to the optic nerve or macula.

DEVELOPMENT OF NEW INTERNATIONAL CLASSIFICATION SYSTEM TO EVALUATE TREATMENT OUTCOMES The Reese Ellsworth classification system was based on the ophthalmologist's view of retinoblastoma using a direct ophthalmoscope. Since the advent of indirect ophthalmoscopy, tumors anterior to the ocular equator have been associated with better visual outcomes. Tumors at these anterior locations now can be easily visualized and are distant from important visual structures. Retinoblastoma is a rare disease, and, therefore, outcomes from a variety of centers need to be compared in order to provide useful information. At a meeting in Toronto, in July of 1994, consensus for the development of a new international classification system was achieved. Once implemented, this classification system will allow a tumor's size and location to be described uniformly among centers and across countries. This will permit more-objective evaluation of various therapeutic protocols as they emerge, as well as facilitating the assessment of combined modality therapy.

CURRENT STATUS OF GENETIC SCREENING The retinoblastoma gene is large, spanning 180,000 bp. In families where an informative polymorphism is available, restriction fragment length polymorphism (RFLP) analysis is a relatively rapid and straightforward method for genetic screening. This technique, however, is difficult to employ for the great majority of children with this disease, who do not have affected family members. Seventy percent of children with retinoblastoma do not have germline mutations but rather have sporadic somatic mutations occurring within a single retinal cell. Of the remaining 30% of children with the bilateral germinal form of retinoblastoma, only 10% have positive family histories. Genetic testing as it is currently employed with RFLP analysis requires an informative polymorphism, typically found when two or more affected family members' DNA is available for analysis. If blood and tumor DNA are available from only a single patient, the test becomes less informative. However, in these cases, if loss of heterozygosity is observed, the mutant allele often can be identified. An alternative method, sequencing the retinoblastoma gene, is time and labor intensive, and may not provide a result within the appropriate time frame for clinically relevant diagnosis. The need for a rapid test for germline mutation carriers is apparent, and this is a focus of ongoing research.

MONITORING OF CHILDREN FOR SECOND-TUMOR DEVELOPMENT For many years, children with an initial presentation of retinoblastoma were first evaluated with bone scan, lumbar puncture for cerebrospinal fluid cytology, and bone marrow aspirates and biopsies. The routine use of these tests has not yielded any earlier diagnoses of metastatic retinoblastoma, nor have serial bone scans proven to be useful in early diagnosis of osteogenic sarcoma. For this reason, a multidisciplinary clinic has been instituted at the University of California, San Francisco, in which experts with different perspectives and areas of expertise evaluate children with retinoblastoma for long-term cancer risk. In this clinic, children are monitored for endocrine deficiencies resulting from external beam radiation therapy. They are evaluated by a specialist in craniofacial plastics in order to ameliorate problems associated with mid-face hypoplasia in the setting of previous radiation. An ophthalmologist evaluates the patient's vision and retina to exclude the possibility of reactivations in the primary tumor, as well as to exclude radiation- and chemotherapy-related retinopathy and vasculopathy. In many cases, visual rehabilitation devices are recommended. An ocularist is present to refit the prosthesis over the orbital implant as the child grows. Pediatric oncologists perform complete histories and physical examinations on these children. To pinpoint any behavioral problems or learning difficulties, the children are also evaluated by school specialists and nurse specialists. Children are evaluated annually, and an attempt is made to see siblings on the same day. Having children seen in this clinic minimizes the number of physician visits required for each family and allows for discussion of patient problems from a multidisciplinary perspective.

The goal in reducing physician visits while maintaining comprehensive care is to minimize trauma to the child and to the family. This illness is lifelong, potentially familial, and requires surveillance, treatment, and genetic counseling. The emphasis, however, in a yearly clinic visit is on preventive care and on the high rate of cure. We have found that retinoblastoma families provide each other with strong support, and often families arrange to attend this clinic together so that ties established in infancy (when the children may be seen monthly for examinations under anesthesia) are maintained during childhood. Families with a new diagnosis of retinoblastoma are often best reassured by referral to this clinic, where it is apparent that older children with the same diagnosis are leading successful lives.

FUTURE DIRECTIONS

Since the cloning of the retinoblastoma gene, its complex role in regulating transcription and progression through the cell cycle has become the focus of intense research. In certain cells, the retinoblastoma gene product seems to be important in determining terminal differentiation. In many cancers, the retinoblastoma gene is altered or its pathway is deregulated, suggesting that this gene may act along one of several important pathways which should maintain the cell in a nonneoplastic state.

It is very likely that absence of functional retinoblastoma gene product results in deregulation of other downstream genes. When future treatment at the molecular level is considered, simple replacement of the retinoblastoma gene or its product may not completely reverse this cascade of downstream events. As the retinoblastoma gene pathway is clarified, however, important branch points may be identified and possibly reversed. Genetic intervention for this disease will require a more complete understanding of the role of the retinoblastoma gene in individual tissues, its normal regulation, and the multiple ways in which it can become deregulated to produce neoplasia.

Retinoblastoma, when it occurs in children, represents a highly penetrant, almost purely genetic cancer. Environmental factors that may act to increase predisposition to adult cancers play a very small role in this disease. If genetic therapy is contemplated, it may be best employed in diseases that are predominantly genetic in origin and that permit early intervention (as in children born of parents with the retinoblastoma phenotype).

Advances are required in genetic testing so that prenatal diagnosis of retinoblastoma can be routinely and reliably established. Early referral of retinoblastoma patients dramatically affects visual outcome and treatment options. When treatment is initiated, multimodality programs should minimize toxicity and second-tumor risk associated with individual modalities. Finally, evaluating treatment outcomes for this rare disease can best be accomplished through multicenter trials utilizing a uniform tumor classification system.

SELECTED REFERENCES

Bandara LR, La Thangue NB. Adenovirus E1a prevents the retinoblastoma gene product from complexing with a cellular transcription factor. Nature 1991;351:494–497.

Brehm A, Miska EA, McCance DJ, et al. Retinoblastoma protein recruits histone deacetylase to repress transcription. Nature 1998;391: 597–601.

Buchkovich K, Duffy LA, Harlow E. The retinoblastoma protein is phosphorylated during specific phases of the cell cycle. Cell 1989;58: 1097–1105.

Chellappan SP, Hiebert S, Mudryj M, Horowitz JM, Nevins JR. The E2F transcription factor is a cellular target for the RB protein. Cell 1991;65:1053–1061.

Chen PL, Scully P, Shew JY, Wang JY, Lee WH. Phosphorylation of the retinoblastoma gene product is modulated during the cell cycle and cellular differentiation. Cell 1989;58:1193–1198.

Chittenden T, Livingston DM, Kaelin WG Jr. The T/E1A-binding domain of the retinoblastoma product can interact selectively with a sequence-specific DNA-binding protein. Cell 1991;65:1073–1082.

Comings DE. A general theory of carcinogenesis. Proc Natl Acad Sci USA 1973;70:3324–3328.

Connolly MJ, Payne RH, Johnson G, et al. Familial, EsD-linked retinoblastoma with reduced penetrance and variable expressivity. Hum Genet 1983;65:122–124.

DeCaprio JA, Ludlow JW, Figge J, et al. SV40 large tumor antigen forms a specific complex with the product of the retinoblastoma susceptibility gene. Cell 1988;54:275–283.

DeCaprio JA, Ludlow JW, Lynch D, et al. The product of the retinoblastoma susceptibility gene has properties of a cell cycle regulatory element. Cell 1989;58:1085–1095.

Durfee T, Becherer K, Chen PL, et al. The retinoblastoma protein associates with the protein phosphatase type 1 catalytic subunit. Genes Dev 1993;7:555–569.

Friend SH, Bernards R, Rogelj S, et al. A human DNA segment with properties of the gene that predisposes to retinoblastoma and osteosarcoma. Nature 1986;323:643–646.

Fung YK, Murphree AL, T'Ang A, Qian J, Hinrichs SH, Benedict WF. Structural evidence for the authenticity of the human retinoblastoma gene. Science 1987;236:1657–1661.

Goodrich DW, Wang NP, Qian YW, Lee EY, Lee WH. The retinoblastoma gene product regulates progression through the G1 phase of the cell cycle. Cell 1991;67:293–302.

Gu W, Schneider JW, Condorelli G, Kaushal S, Mahdavi V, Nadal-Ginard B. Interaction of myogenic factors and the retinoblastoma protein mediates muscle cell commitment and differentiation. Cell 1993;72:309–324.

Harris H, Miller OJ, Klein G, Worst P, Tachibana T. Suppression of malignancy by cell fusion. Nature 1969;223:363–368.

Helin K, Lees JA, Vidal M, Dyson N, Harlow E, Fattaey A. A cDNA encoding a pRB-binding protein with properties of the transcription factor E2F. Cell 1992;70:337–350.

Horowitz JM, Park SH, Bogenmann E, et al. Frequent inactivation of the retinoblastoma anti-oncogene is restricted to a subset of human tumor cells. Proc Natl Acad Sci USA 1990;87:2775–2779.

Hu QJ, Dyson N, Harlow E. The regions of the retinoblastoma protein needed for binding to adenovirus E1A or SV40 large T antigen are common sites for mutations. EMBO J 1990;9:1147–1155.

Knudson AG Jr. Mutation and cancer: a statistical study of retinoblastoma. Proc Natl Acad Sci USA 1971;68:820–823.

Lee WH, Brookstein R, Hong F, Young LJ, Shew JY, Lee EY. Human retinoblastoma susceptibility gene: cloning, identification, and sequence. Science 1987;235:1394–1399.

Lee WH, Shew JY, Hong FD, et al. The retinoblastoma susceptibility gene encodes a nuclear phosphoprotein associated with DNA binding activity. Nature 1987;329:642–645.

Leone G, DeGregori J, Sears R, et al. Myc and Ras collaborate in inducing accumulation of active cyclin E/Cdk2 and E2F. Nature 1997;387: 422–426.

Li W, Fan J, Hochhauser D, et al. Lack of functional retinoblastoma protein mediates increased resistance to antimetabolites in human sarcoma cell lines. Proc Natl Acad Sci USA 1995;92:10,436–10,440.

Magraghi-Jaulin L, Groisman R, Naguibreva I, et al. Retinoblastoma protein represses transcription by recruiting a histone deacetylase. Nature 1998;391:601–605.

Mancini MA, Shan B, Nickerson JA, Penman S, Lee WH. The retinoblastoma gene product is a cell cycle–dependent nuclear matrix-associated protein. Proc Natl Acad Sci USA 1994;91:418–422.

Mittnacht S, Weinberg RA. G1/S phosphorylation of the retinoblastoma protein is associated with an altered affinity for the nuclear compartment. Cell 1991;65:381–393.

Nevins JR. E2F: a link between the Rb tumor suppressor protein and viral oncoproteins. Science 1992;258:424–429.

Rustgi AK, Dyson N, Bernards R. Amino-terminal domains of c-myc and N-myc proteins mediate binding to the retinoblastoma gene product. Nature 1991;352:541–544.

Sellers WR, Rodgers JW, Kaelin WG Jr. A potent transrepressor domain in the retinoblastoma protein induces cell cycle arrest when bound to E2F sites. Proc Natl Acad Sci USA 1995;92:11,544–11,548.

Sparkes RS, Murphree AL, Lingua RW, et al. Gene for hereditary retinoblastoma assigned to human chromosome 13 by linkage to esterase D. Science 1983;219:971–973.

Verhoeff FH, Jackson E. Minutes of proceedings, 62nd Annual Meeting. Trans Am Ophthalmol Soc 1926;24:38.

Whyte P, Buchkovich KJ, Horowitz JM, et al. Association between an oncogene and an anti-oncogene: the adenovirus E1A proteins bind to the retinoblastoma gene product. Nature 1988;334:124–129.

106 Neurofibromatosis

Type 1 and Type 2

JAIME O. CLAUDIO AND GUY A. ROULEAU

INTRODUCTION

Neurofibromatosis is a Mendelian genetic disorder that primarily affects the nervous system. It is characterized by an inherent predisposition to develop tumors of the brain and spinal cord, and a variety of neoplastic abnormalities involving tissues derived from neural crest cells or from the neural ectoderm. It consists of two major types that are genetically and phenotypically distinct: neurofibromatosis type 1 (NF1; OMIM 162200) and neurofibromatosis type 2 (NF2; OMIM 101000).

The first medical description of NF1 can be traced back in the 16th century to an Italian physician and naturalist, Ullise Aldrovandi; but the eponymous credit is ascribed to a German pathologist, Friedrich Daniel von Recklinghausen, who first described the cellular component of the tumors seen in this disease in 1882. However, von Recklinghausen made no distinction between NF1 and NF2 despite the fact that J. H. Wishart, then President of the Royal College of Surgeons of Edinburgh, reported in 1822 the first documented case of NF2; the patient, Michael Blair, suffered from tumors of the dura matter, brain, and both "auditory nerves." The genetic distinction between NF1 and NF2 became clear in 1987 when the genes responsible for these disorders were localized to separate chromosomes. The mapping of the *NF1* locus to the proximal long arm of chromosome 17 and *NF2* to the long arm of chromosome 22 established a precise classification and set the pace for the positional cloning of the *NF1* and *NF2* genes.

COMPARISONS BETWEEN NF1 AND NF2

DIAGNOSTIC CRITERIA The National Institutes of Health Consensus and Development Conference Statement in 1987 recommended the numerical classification of the neurofibromatoses and set up guidelines on diagnostic criteria for NF1 and NF2. This original set of criteria has been expanded for NF2 (Table 106-1) to accommodate diagnosis of individuals with no family history.

CLINICAL FEATURES Although NF1 and NF2 are distinct disorders, both show remarkable variable clinical expressivity. Both disorders usually present early; NF1 at about age 10 and NF2 in early teens or 20s. The major defining features of NF1 include *café au lait* spots, peripheral neurofibromas, and Lisch nodules. Additionally, an NF1 patient may suffer from orthopedic problems such as scoliosis and pseudoarthrosis, may develop plexiform neurofibromas, or may be intellectually handicapped. A fraction of NF1 cases develop myeloid leukemia (OMIM 151410). Tumors such as rhabdomyosarcomas, optic gliomas, phaeochromocytomas, and neurofibrosarcomas may occur. By contrast, the hallmark of NF2 is the occurrence of bilateral vestibular schwannomas; however, schwannomas may occur on any cranial nerve, nerve root, or peripheral nerve. Meningiomas (OMIM 156100) occur in approximately 50% of patients, and ependymomas occur rarely. Optic gliomas do not occur in NF2 but juvenile subcapsular lenticular opacities are common, often presenting before tumors arise, and so may be a useful predictive test for at risk individuals. For NF2, *café au lait* spots and peripheral nerve schwannomas are infrequent, but when present may cause misdiagnosis as NF1. The most useful distinguishing feature for differential diagnosis between the two disorders is the absence of axillary freckling and Lisch nodules, and the lower number of *café au lait* spots in NF2. Furthermore, NF1 individuals never develop bilateral vestibular schwannomas.

There are two subtypes of NF2, often referred to by eponyms: the mild Gardner subtype and the severe Wishart subtype. Gardner is generally characterized by late onset (usually >25 years) of bilateral vestibular schwannomas and few associated brain or spinal tumors. Wishart is a serious and earlier onset subtype (usually <25 years) with rapid and progressive growth of bilateral vestibular schwannomas accompanied by multiple intracranial and spinal schwannomas, meningiomas, and ependymomas.

MOLECULAR GENETICS OF THE NEUROFIBROMATOSES

The predisposition to develop NF1 or NF2 is inherited as an autosomal dominant trait, but the diseases manifest as recessive traits at the cellular level. This genetic paradox is analogous to the two-hit mechanism in retinoblastoma (OMIM 180200), in which an individual inherits a mutant copy of the gene in an autosomal dominant pattern but develops tumors only when an inactivating somatic mutation occurs in the otherwise normal homolog. This results in the recessive expression of the disease phenotype in affected cells leading to tumor formation. Thus, the *NF1* and *NF2* genes are considered as recessive tumor suppressors.

NF1 is a more common disease than NF2, with a birth incidence of 1:3000, compared to 1:37,500 for NF2 (Table 106-2). However, NF2 is a more serious disease, with a mean actuarial survival of 15 years after diagnosis, whereas NF1 does not affect life-span.

From: *Principles of Molecular Medicine* (J. L. Jameson, ed.), ©1998 Humana Press Inc., Totowa, NJ.

Table 106-1
Diagnostic Criteria for NF1 and NF2

I. Neurofibromatosis Type 1

NF1 may be diagnosed in an individual when two or more of the following are present:

1. Six or more *café au lait* macules with diameters of more than 5 mm in prepubescent patients and more than 15 mm in postpubescent patients.
2. One plexiform neurofibroma or two or more neurofibromas of any type.
3. Freckling in the axillary or inguinal region.
4. A distinctive osseous lesion as sphenoid dysplasia or thinning of long-bone cortex, with or without pseudoarthrosis.
5. Optic glioma.
6. Two or more Lisch nodules (iris hamartomas).
7. A parent, sibling or child with neurofibromatosis 1 on the basis of the above criteria.

II. Neurofibromatosis Type 2

NF2 may be diagnosed when one of the following is present:

1. Bilateral eighth cranial nerve masses seen by magnetic resonance imaging with gadolinium.
2. A parent, sibling, or child with NF2 plus:
   a. Unilateral eighth cranial nerve mass or
   b. Any one of the following:
      i. Neurofibroma.
      ii. Meningioma.
      iii. Glioma.
      iv. Schwannoma.
      v. Posterior subcapsular cataract or opacity at a young age.
3. Unilateral vestibular schwannoma plus one or more of the following:
   a. Neurofibroma.
   b. Meningioma.
   c. Glioma.
   d. Schwannoma.
   e. Posterior subcapsular cataract or opacity at a young age.
4. Multiple meningiomas (two or more) plus unilateral vestibular schwannoma.
5. Multiple meningiomas (two or more) plus:
   a. Neurofibroma.
   b. Glioma.
   c. Posterior subcapsular cataract or opacity at a young age.

Source: NIH Development Conference (1987) and Short et al. 1994.

Table 106-2
Comparisons of NF1 and NF2

Characteristic	*NF1*	*NF2*
Other names	von Recklinghausen's disease Peripheral neurofibromatosis	Bilateral acoustic neurofibromatosis Central neurofibromatosis
Chromosomal location	17q11.2	22q12.1
Inheritance	Autosomal dominant	Autosomal dominant
Expression	Recessive	Recessive
Age of onset	First decade	Second decade
Birth incidence	1:3000	1:37,500
Penetrance	Close to 100%	Close to 100%
Mutation rate	$3.0–5.0 \times 10^{-5}$	$1.0–8.0 \times 10^{-6}$

Both types share certain genetic features, such as high penetrance and high frequency of new mutations. For example, as many as 50% of cases are reported to have no family history and so represent new mutations. The penetrance for both diseases is close to 100%.

THE *NF1* AND *NF2* GENES For diseases with no known biochemical abnormality, positional cloning now offers a way to isolate the primary gene defect. The *NF1* and *NF2* genes were identified using this approach. Thus, the search for the gene responsible for each disorder began by mapping the neurofibromatosis loci to specific chromosomes, narrowing down the region, and identifying genes within the defined critical interval. For *NF1*, two translocation breakpoints within the critical region helped identify the gene, whereas big chromosome deletions (which segregated with the disease in families) provided clues for the positional cloning of the *NF2* gene.

IDENTIFICATION OF THE *NF1* GENE AND ITS PROTEIN NEUROFIBROMIN In 1987, two groups reported the localization of the *NF1* locus to the long arm of chromosome 17. Using anonymous DNA sequences and cloned genes that detect restriction fragment length polymorphisms (RFLPs), both groups independently identified genetic markers near the centromere that are linked to the *NF1* locus. Fine genetic mapping by an international collaboration established a more precise localization of the *NF1* gene (Fig. 106-1A). Subsequently, two different chromosomal translocations in two NF1 patients, t(1;17) and t(17;22), were mapped to the *NF1* region. These chromosomal abnormalities served as key reagents for the identification of the *NF1* gene and provided evidence that NF1 is caused by loss of function mutations. To search for genes within the translocation breakpoint, screening was focused on genes lying within this region. The mouse leukemia gene, *Evi-2*, maps to the distal region of mouse chromosome 11, which is syntenic to the *NF1* region on human chromosome 17. Studies on the human homolog of *Evi-2* *(EVI2A)* indicated that it mapped in between the two translocation breakpoints, which are 50 kb apart. Subsequently, two other genes, *EVI2B* and oligodendrocyte-myelin glycoprotein *(OMGP)* were discovered within the 50-kb interval. All three genes were considered good candidates for the disease; *Evi-2* is a known protooncogene involved in murine myeloid tumors, whereas OMPG is a cell adhesion molecule in myelin of the nerve sheath and expressed only in schwann cells and oligodendrocytes. However, further analyses indicated that none of the three genes were disrupted by either translocation nor was there any sequence alteration within these genes in NF1 patients. Nevertheless, this strategy allowed the cloning of genomic DNA in the region. By searching for phylogenetically conserved DNA fragments and using these to screen cDNA libraries, a gene was identified that spanned the translocation breakpoint. On further analyses, deletions and point mutations within the cDNAs confirmed the identity of the *NF1* gene. Concomitantly, another group reported the insertion of a 500-bp sequence in an NF1 patient that, in subsequent studies, was shown to be an *Alu*I repeat that altered the splicing pattern of the *NF1* gene, thereby causing exon skipping during RNA processing.

The NF1 gene spans at least 350 kb and consists of 59 exons that are processed to yield a transcript of 11–13 kb. Transcription proceeds in telomeric direction opposite to the direction of transcription of the three genes (*EVIA2*, *EVI2B*, and *OMGP*) that are embedded within an intron of the *NF1* gene (Fig. 106-1A). The *NF1* gene encodes for a protein of 2818 amino acids with an estimated molecular weight of 250–320 kDa. The NF1 protein, called neurofibromin, has a central 381-amino acid domain with sequence

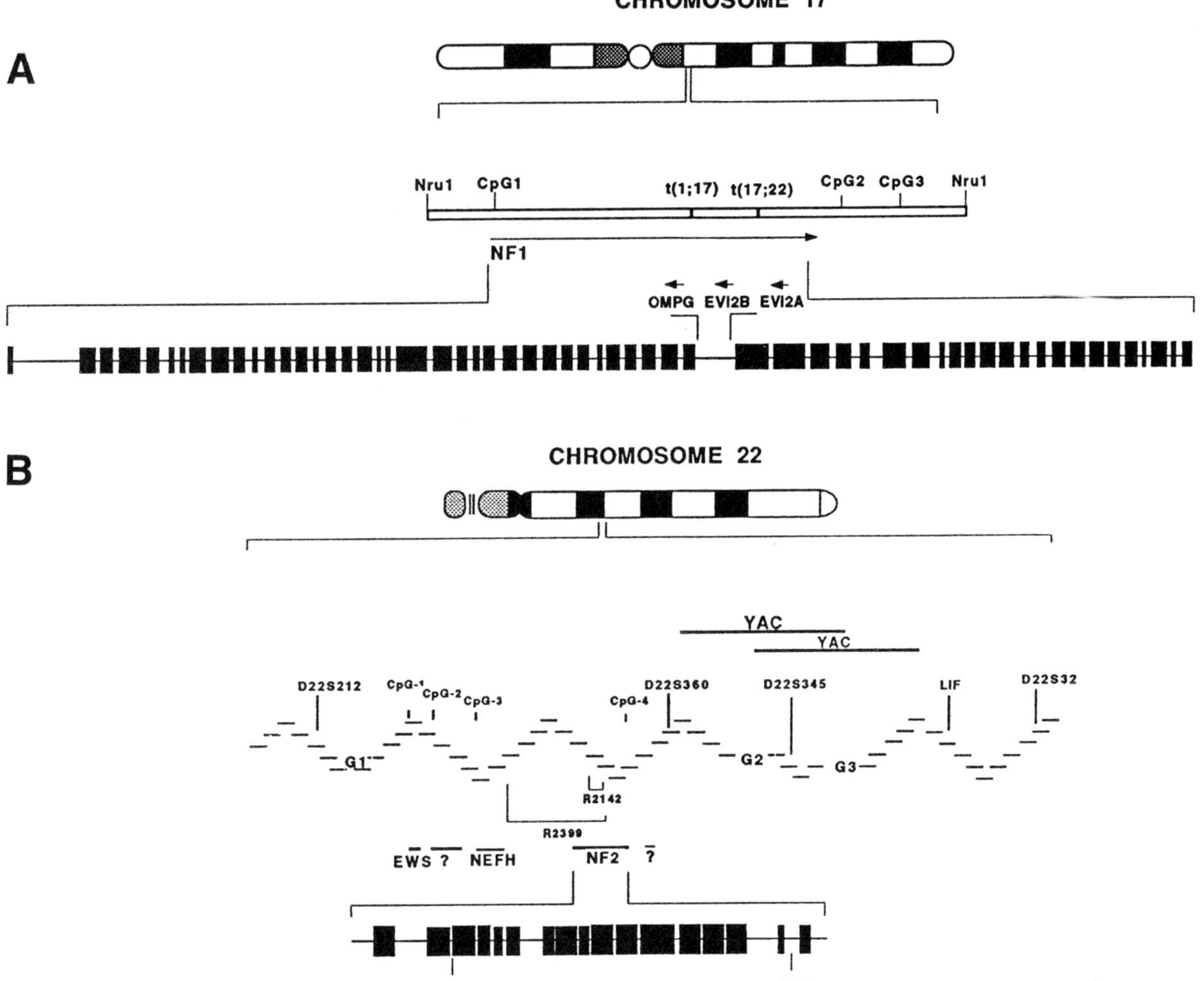

Figure 106-1 (**A**) The *NF1* locus in the pericentromeric region of chromosome 17. Fine genetic mapping by pulsed-field gel electrophoresis identified a 600-kb *Nru*I fragment within which two translocation breakpoints from two NF1 patients were identified. The translocation breakpoints, t(1;17) and t(17;22), were mapped 50 kb apart. Three CpG islands, known marker of the 5' region of a gene, are shown within the *Nru*I fragment. The organization of the 59 exons of the *NF1* gene, shown as black bars, and the three genes originally considered as good candidates (*EVI2A*, *EVI2B*, and *OMPG*) embedded in an intron of the *NF1* gene, are indicated. The three genes are transcribed in centromeric direction opposite to the direction of transcription of the *NF1* gene (**B**). Regional map of the *NF2* locus on the long arm of chromosome 22. Cosmid contig shown as overlapping horizontal lines provided the path for the chromosome walk leading to the identification of the *NF2* gene. G1, G2, and G3 are gaps within the contig; the G2 and G3 are each spanned by yeast artificial chromosome (YAC). The location of 4 CpG islands is shown in between the markers D22S212 and D22S360. The two patients who showed abnormal fragments as detected by hybridization using C13 and C16 probes are indicated as R2399 and R2142 (the extent of the deletion in each patient is shown). The relative position of EWS, NEFH, NF2, and two unidentified genes are shown. Transcription of all the identified genes proceeds in telomeric direction except for pK1.3 and BAM22 (not shown), which are transcribed in centromeric direction. The NF2 gene is shown with its 17 coding exons in black bars. The position of C13 and C16 probes are also shown (modified from Rouleau et al., 1993).

similarity to p21-*ras* GTPase-activating proteins (GAP) and to IRA1 and IRA2, known yeast inhibitory regulators of the RAS signal transduction pathway. This domain, the NF1-GAP-related domain (NF1-GRD), may be alternatively spliced generating an additional 21-amino acid residue that retains GAP activity.

MUTATION ANALYSIS OF THE *NF1* GENE Deletions, insertions, base substitutions, and splice site mutations in the *NF1* gene have been described in a number of NF1 cases. No hot spot for mutations has yet been identified; however the majority of mutations result in a truncated and presumably nonfunctional protein. Mutations in the *NF1* gene have also been reported in a variety of malignancies and tumor syndromes from non-NF1 patients, including melanomas (OMIM 155600) and neuroblastomas, colon adenocarcinomas, myelodysplastic syndrome, and anaplastic astrocytomas. NF1 patients with mosaicism for an *NF1* mutation have been reported and may explain some cases of "new" mutation in a sibship. A somatic mutation was identified in a benign neurofibroma from an individual with a known constitutional deletion of the other *NF1* allele. Homozygous inactivation of both *NF1* alleles has also been found in the leukemia cells of patients with neurofibromatosis type 1.

IDENTIFICATION OF THE *NF2* GENE AND ITS PROTEIN SCHWANNOMIN Molecular genetic studies in sporadic and NF2-associated meningiomas and schwannomas originally suggested a common pathogenic mechanism for these tumors by the loss of heterozygosity for distinct chromosome 22 loci. These results were the starting point for genetic linkage analysis in NF2 pedigrees. An anonymous RFLP marker, D22S1, frequently reduced to hemizygosity in NF2-related tumors, was used to map the *NF2* gene to the long arm of chromosome 22. A combination of multipoint linkage analysis using a large kindred and molecular analysis of NF2 tumors with either interstitial or terminal deletions of chromosome 22 resulted in the exclusion of two possible candidate genes in the region. These genes include the "breakpoint cluster region" (BCR) implicated in the t(9;22) Philadelphia chromosome characteristically seen in chronic myelogenous leukemia (OMIM 151410) and the PDGF-β, the homolog of the *sis* oncogene that encodes the platelet derived growth factor (PDGF). As more closely linked polymorphic markers were developed, it became possible to analyze families for genetic heterogeneity. Such study led to the conclusion that NF2 is a genetically homogeneous disease involving only one major gene, distinct from the *NF1* gene on chromosome 17. Further segregation studies in affected families and characterization of large germline deletions in NF2 pedigrees narrowed the localization of the *NF2* locus to the interval flanked by D22S212 and D22S32, a one million-bp region small enough to positionally clone the *NF2* gene (Figure 106-1B).

As part of the cloning strategy, unrelated NF2 individuals were screened for chromosomal rearrangement within this 1-Mb interval using pulsed-field gel electrophoresis (PFGE) and single-copy DNA probes. Yeast artificial chromosome (YAC) and cosmid contiguous sequences, known as contigs, spanning the candidate region were constructed to provide the path for the chromosome walk to identify candidate genes (Figure 106-1B). This process uncovered two major probes for the identification of the gene. One probe, C16, detected an abnormal fragment in two individuals with NF2, whereas another probe, C13, located 40 kb centromeric to C16, was deleted in both patients (Figure 106-1B). Further characterization of the C13 probe showed that it is phylogenetically conserved, suggesting that a gene may be encoded within this DNA fragment. Using C13 to screen a fetal human cDNA library, a 2-kb cDNA clone (N1.1) was isolated that mapped backed by fluorescence *in situ* hybridization to the NF2 region. When the gene isolated was screened for mutations in NF2 individuals, sequence alterations were found that segregated with the disease. Independently, by chromosome walking and a combination of exon trapping and cDNA library screening, another group identified a candidate cDNA with a sequence identical to N1.1. Together, these data provided incontrovertible evidence that the cloned cDNA encodes for the protein mutated in NF2.

The *NF2* gene spans about 100 kb of genomic sequence and consists of at least 17 exons that encodes for a 595-amino acid protein called schwannomin (alternately merlin), with an estimated molecular weight of 69–80 kDa. In human tissue Northern blots, transcripts of different sizes (7.0, 4.4, and 2.6 kb) are expressed ubiquitously. It is uncertain whether these transcripts are generated by alternate polyadenylation signal or by alternative splicing of the *NF2* gene. Indeed, there are reports of different splicing patterns of the *NF2* gene, but the biological significance of the mRNA variants has not yet been understood.

Schwannomin belongs to a gene superfamily involved in linking plasma membrane protein to the cytoskeleton. This superfamily includes erythrocyte band 4.1, talin, a group of proteins known as the ezrin, radixin, and moesin (ERM) family and a rapidly expanding family of protein tyrosine phosphatases (Figure 106-2).

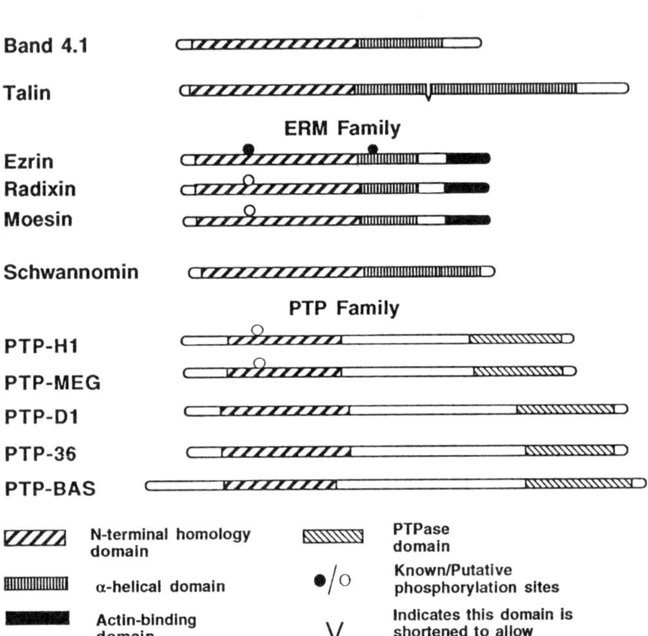

Figure 106-2 Schematic structural model of schwannomin and related proteins. Schwannomin belongs to a superfamily that includes erythrocyte band 4.1, talin, ERM family, and protein tyrosine phosphatase family. The members of this superfamily have common structural organization: a globular amino-terminal domain followed by a region rich in α-helical structure and a highly charged carboxy-terminal domain. The overall homology of schwannomin to the ERM proteins is 48% but the amino-terminal half of schwannomin is 62% identical to the same region in ERM family. Lower amino acid homology is seen between band 4.1, protein tyrosine phosphatases, and talin (~43% at the amino-terminus). The tyrosine phosphorylation sites for ezrin are conserved in the ERM family but not in schwannomin. The putative tyrosine phosphorylation sites of two of the tyrosine phosphatases are also shown. The last 32 amino acids at the carboxy-terminus of the ERM proteins are responsible for binding to actin; the amino terminal region binds to CD44. The actin-binding domain of the ERM family is not conserved in schwannomin. The amino-terminal domain of band 4.1 interacts with glycophorin C and its carboxy-terminal domain binds to the actin-spectrin complex in erythrocytes. Similarly, talin links integrins to vinculin through its amino- and carboxy-terminal domains, respectively.

MUTATION STUDIES OF THE *NF2* GENE Identification of inactivating mutations in tumors from NF2 patients, in sporadic schwannomas and meningiomas, and in other tumors not seen in NF2 provided evidence that the *NF2* gene is involved in the genesis of these tumors. Parallel mutation analyses of blood and tumor DNA had confirmed the two-hit mechanism of tumorigenesis in NF2 and proved that the *NF2* gene encodes for a recessive tumor suppressor. The observation that the *NF2* gene is mutated in the majority of sporadic meningiomas put to an end the controversy that another gene, closely linked to *NF2*, is implicated in the genesis of meningiomas. About 40% of meningiomas have no chromosome 22 abnormalities, suggesting that a yet-unidentified gene on another autosome must be involved. Evidence supporting a major role of the *NF2* gene in other tumors like melanomas, breast carcinomas, and mesotheliomas (OMIM 156240) has not been

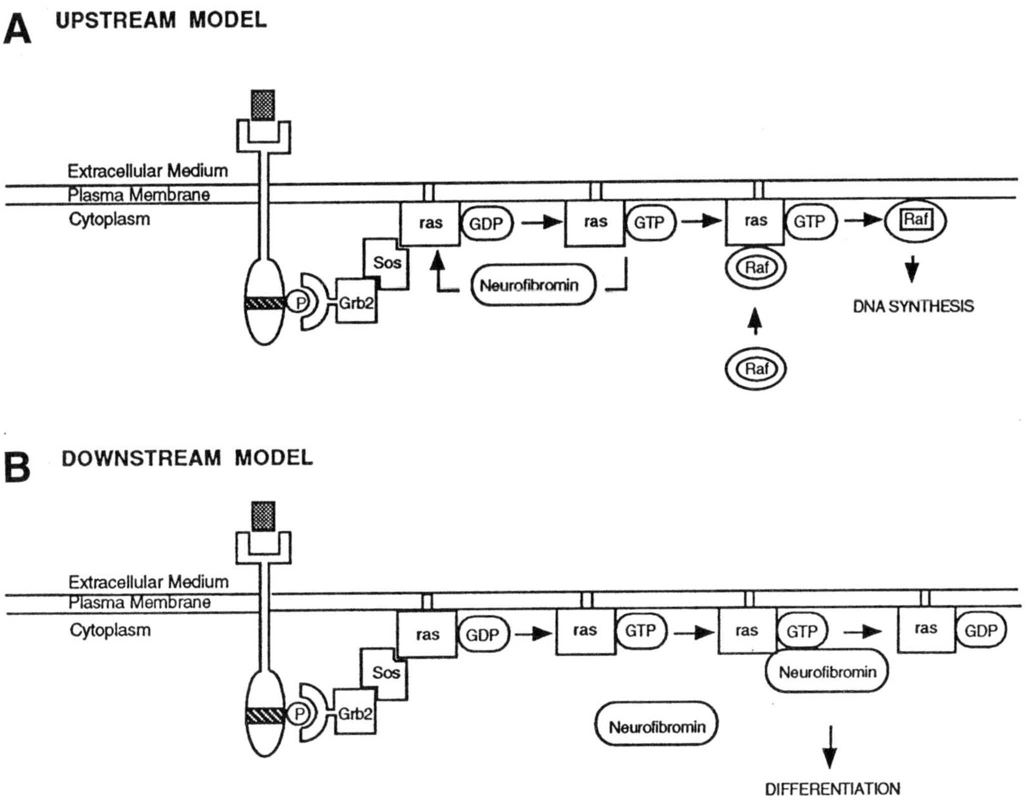

A UPSTREAM MODEL

B DOWNSTREAM MODEL

Figure 106-3 Models of neurofibromin function. **(A)** Upstream model depicting neurofibromin as downregulator of p21-*ras* activity. A growth factor interacting with its receptor initiates the signaling process through p21-*ras* protein. Binding of the growth factor results in phosphorylation of the receptor which, in turn, results in binding of Grb2/Sos to the receptor. This process activates p21-*ras* by promoting exchange of bound GDP for GTP. The level of accumulation of active p21-*ras*-GTP depends on the degree of activation by Sos and the degree of inactivation by neurofibromin, which promotes the hydrolysis of GTP. The activation of p21-*ras* leads to recruitment and activation of cytoplasmic Raf, thereby initiating a kinase cascade by a pathway that is not yet well-defined. This process results in DNA synthesis leading to cell division. **(B)** Downstream model of neurofibromin as an effector of differentiation, either alone or in complex with p21-*ras*. The binding of a growth factor to its receptor promotes phosphorylation of the receptor that, in turn, results in binding of Grb2/Sos to the receptor. The amino-terminal domain of Sos then activates p21-*ras* by exchange of GDP to GTP. The activation of p21-*ras* allows it to interact with neurofibromin; such interaction allows neurofibromin (or in complex with p21-*ras*) to act as an effector of the *ras*-mediated differentiation signal. Loss of function of neurofibromin would cause inhibition of the differentiation signal, and in effect promote cell division.

compelling, and no mutation of the *NF2* gene has been found in gliomas (OMIM 137800).

Most *NF2* gene mutations that have been identified result in truncated protein that is presumably nonfunctional. Missense mutations are rare and comprise only a minor percentage of mutations.

Germline mutation analyses correlating genotype to phenotype have not been conclusive. Three comprehensive studies have suggested that mild manifestations of the disease seem associated with mutations that preserve the C-terminus of the protein or with alterations involving missense or in-frame small deletions. Germline mutations have been identified in only about one-third of NF2 patients screened for alteration in the entire coding region of the *NF2* gene. However, because of the genetic homogeneity of *NF2*, it is unlikely that there is another gene involved. The most reasonable explanation for the unaccounted mutations is the possibility that mutations occur within the promoter and other regulatory sequences, and because large deletions affecting both intron and exons are not detected by polymerase chain reaction (PCR) screening method. No hot spot for mutation has been identified.

FUNCTIONAL ANALYSIS OF NEUROFIBROMIN AND SCHWANNOMIN

NEUROFIBROMIN A clue to the function of neurofibromin came from the sequence homology of its central domain to mammalian GAP and to yeast IRA1 and IRA2. These proteins downregulate p21-*ras* by accelerating the hydrolysis of p21-*ras*-GTP to inactive p21-*ras*-GDP. Thus, a mutant neurofibromin is thought to be unable to control the continuous mitogenic signal brought about by the unrestricted activity of p21-*ras*. The first evidence supporting this paradigm known as the "upstream model" (Fig. 106-3A) came from experiments in yeast transfected with the NF1-GRD. Expression of the NF1-GRD in yeast promoted the hydrolysis of GTP by p21-*ras* and was able to complement the heat-shock sensitive phenotype of *ira1* and *ira2* yeast mutants. However, there are observations that contradict this model. For example, active p21-*ras* does not accumulate in mutant cells whose neurofibromin has been lost by mutation, such as neuroblastoma and melanoma cell lines; activated p21-*ras* can cause cell cycle arrest in rat schwann cells, and induce differentiation and block proliferation in rat phaeochromocytoma cell line PC12; and third, other members of the *ras* superfamily, like R-*ras* p23 protein, which is regulated by neurofibromin and interacts with Bcl-2, a suppressor of programmed cell death (apoptosis), are expected to be affected by the loss of neurofibromin, thereby altering the apoptotic function of Bcl-2. These discrepancies can be explained by an alternate model known as the "downstream model," which postulates that neurofibromin receives a signal from activated p21-*ras* to promote differentiation (Fig. 106-3B). Therefore, a mutant neurofibromin would be unable to block cell proliferation because it can no longer affect cell differentiation from a p21-*ras* signal.

Further evidence supporting the model that neurofibromin may function as a negative regulator of p21-*ras* is derived from experiments on primary cell cultures of schwann cells, and neural crest- and placode-derived sensory neurons from *Nf1* (–/–) embryos. Whereas *Nf1* (–/–) neurons extend neurites and survive without neurotrophins in vitro, their wild-type counterparts die rapidly in the absence of NGF and BDNF. Schwann cells from null mutant embryos develop elaborate processes and, like the neurons from these mutant mice, have elevated levels of Ras-GTP. *Nf1* (–/–) neurons survive and acquire mature morphological characteristics in the absence of neurotrophins, just as if Ras signaling pathways were activated constitutively. Similarly, studies on hematopoietic cells from *Nf1* (–/–) mice showed that loss of the *Nf1* gene leads to an increased and prolonged rise in Ras-GTP levels in myeloid cells after granulocyte/macrophage colony stimulating factor (GM-CSF) stimulation, defining a role for neurofibromin in regulating GM-CSF signaling through Ras in hematopoietic cells.

Studies on the subcellular distribution of neurofibromin showed that it can associate with cytoplasmic microtubules. It is postulated that the interaction of neurofibromin to tubulin reduces its ability to downregulate p21-*ras*. This observation suggests that neurofibromin may suppress tumor formation in normal cells by an even more complex mechanism.

SCHWANNOMIN The homology of schwannomin to a group of proteins known to function in maintaining cellular integrity provides evidence of a novel site of action of tumorigenesis. Although there is no current working model for the molecular basis of schwannomin in suppressing tumors of the nervous system, knowledge of its function has been based primarily on studies of members of the band 4.1 superfamily (Fig. 106-2). For example, schwannomin is postulated to normally act like erythrocyte band 4.1, which links transmembrane glycoproteins to the spectrin–actin complex of the cytoskeleton; or like talin, which interacts with vinculin and integrins, thereby regulating organization of cell shape. More closely related to schwannomin are ezrin, radixin, and moesin, which act as structural linkers between cell surface glycoprotein CD44 and actin-based cytoskeleton. These proteins are found preferentially in dynamic structures; ezrin is found in actin-containing cell-surface structures, moesin is found in microspikes, blebs, retraction fibers, filopodia, and lamellipodia; radixin is found in the cell-to-cell adherens junctions. Mutation of schwannomin may thus lead to unstable cell–cell and cell–matrix interactions leading to changes in cell shape, loss of contact inhibition, and cell migration. The transient phosphorylation of ezrin on tyrosine residues following exposure to epidermal growth factor, and of radixin in response to PDGF, provide insights into possible activation of schwannomin by a receptor-specific mechanism leading to a possible downstream signaling pathway. However, although schwannomin has several putative tyrosine phosphorylation sites, no phosphorylation site involved in a putative signaling pathway has been identified by in vivo or in vitro experiments.

Studies on the expression of schwannomin in human and mouse tissues show widespread but cell type-specific expression. It is expressed in neural crest-derived cells, endothelial cells, and erythrocytes. Functional studies of schwannomin in vitro have demonstrated that it can reverse the v-Ha-*ras*-induced anchorage-independent phenotype of NIH-3T3 cells. Additionally, when NIH-3T3 fibroblasts are transfected with the full-length NF2 cDNA, a concomitant one-third reduction of growth rate, as well as phenotypic changes (such as extension of varying number of thin processes) are observed compared to controls. These data support the tumor suppressor function of the *NF2* gene.

ANIMAL MODELS

Various breeds of domestic cattle are thought to develop multiple neurofibromas and schwannomas. Similarly, neurofibromas, schwannomas, and neurofibrosarcomas are known to develop in bicolor damsel fish. These are often cited as models of NF1 although they do not completely mimic the human disease. Several attempts to use chemical mutagens to introduce mutation and consequently generate mice with the neurofibromatosis phenotype have been unsuccessful in the past. Therefore, the technology of using embryonic stem cells to introduce mutations in mice, known as the "knockout" technique, remained the best recourse to model the disease. The identification and subsequent findings of high conservation of the mouse homologs of the *NF1* and *NF2* genes made it possible to study the genetic defect in mice using this strategy. Experiments to model *NF1* and *NF2* by gene targeting have generated mice that are genetically identical to neurofibromatosis patients. For *NF1*, a heterozygous mouse mutant has been generated by disruption of the gene by homologous recombination. Homozygous mutant embryos die *in utero* at around 14.5 days postcoitum due to severe malformation of the heart and hyperplasia of neural crest-derived sympathetic ganglia. This finding, not surprising since no human homozygote has been identified, suggests that neurofibromin plays an important role in cardiac organogenesis. Heterozygous animals do not develop the clinical abnormalities characteristic of the human disease, but they have increased predisposition to develop phaeochromocytoma and myeloid leukemia, two phenotypes that are seen, albeit infrequently, in NF1. They also exhibit learning and memory deficits. Similar efforts to generate NF2 mutant mice have confirmed that embryonic lethality defines the phenotype of homozygous mice. Although the exact clinical phenotype of both disorders are hardly reproducible in mice, these heterozygous mutant mice will be useful in understanding the molecular pathogenesis of the disorder and designing efficient therapeutic approaches.

MANAGEMENT AND THERAPEUTIC OPTIONS

Neurofibromatosis is an extremely difficult disease to manage because it involves the coordination of different health care professionals such as neurosurgeons, genetic counselors, otolaryngologists, opthalmologists, educational psychologists, and dermatologists, among others. The disfiguring defect, dermal neurofibroma, and learning disabilities in children with NF1 require strong psychosocial support. Similarly, NF2 patients may need social support from teachers of communication of the deaf. As at-risk individuals have a 50% chance of transmitting the disease to their offspring, proper management of neurofibromatosis patients includes genetic counseling. Currently, multidisciplinary centers in North America and Europe and several lay organizations are working as support groups for neurofibromatosis patients. Information about the National Neurofibromatosis Foundation can be accessed through the internet at http://www.neurofibromatosis.org.

Because of the variable clinical expressivity of the disease, management and treatment vary with each patient, even within families. Surgery is still the mainstay of treatment for NF1 and NF2. Treatments for symptomatic patients with NF2 include radiotherapy, including gamma knife treatment, although surgery remains the treatment of choice. The prognosis for surgical excision is very good.

FUTURE PROSPECTS

The cloning of the genes for NF1 and NF2 has made the screening of at-risk individuals possible by molecular genetic analysis rather than by undergoing a series of neurological, ophthalmological, and audiometric tests. However, genetic testing is not yet readily available except in nonservice research laboratories studying the disease. Given the large size of both genes, especially *NF1*, direct DNA mutation screening will take a few years to become economically feasible and easily accessible. An alternative method to direct mutation screening by DNA analysis lies in the observation that the majority of mutations are predicted to result in truncated proteins. Thus a protein with altered size can be readily detected by a combination of reverse transcription-PCR and in vitro translation known as protein truncation assay. However, this method only predicts the site of mutation and thus still has to be complemented with a routine technique of DNA analysis.

The prospects of gene therapy are still uncertain. However, a better understanding of the molecular pathogenesis of the disease may provide clues in developing chemotherapeutic agents. This conventional approach may be a more practical method of providing more immediate therapeutic options for patients with neurofibromatosis.

ACKNOWLEDGMENTS

JOC is a student of the National Cancer Institute of Canada, supported with funds from the National Cancer Society. GAR is funded by the Medical Research Council of Canada, Fond de Recherche en Santé du Québec and the National Neurofibromatosis Foundation. We apologize for authors not included in the references due to space limitations.

SELECTED REFERENCES

Andersen LB, Ballester R, Marchuk DA, et al. A conserved alternative splice in the von Recklinghausen neurofibromatosis (NF1) gene produces two neurofibromin isoforms, both of which have GTPase-activating protein activity. Mol Cel Biol 1993;3:487–495.

Ballester R, Marchuk D, Boguski M, et al. The NF1 locus encodes a protein functionally related to mammalian GAP and yeast IRA proteins. Cell 1990;63:851–859.

Barker B, Wright E, Nguyen K, et al. Gene for von Recklinghausen neurofibromatosis is in the pericentromeric region of chromosome 17. Science 1987;236:1100–1102.

Boguski MS, McCormick F. Proteins regulating *ras* and its relatives. Nature 1993;366:643–654.

Bollag G, Clapp DW, Shih S, et al. Loss of *NF1* results in activation of the Ras signaling pathway and leads to aberrant growth in haematopoietic cells. Nat Genet 1996;144–148.

Brannan CI, Perkins AS, Vogel KS, et al. Targeted disruption of the neurofibromatosis type-1 gene leads to developmental abnormalities in heart and various neural crest-derived tissues. Genes Dev 1994; 8:1019–1029.

Cawthon R, Weiss R, Xu G, et al. A major segment of the neurofibromatosis type 1 gene: cDNA sequence, genomic structure, and point mutations. Cell 1990;62:193–201.

Evans DRG, Huson SM, Donnai D, et al. A genetic study of type 2 neurofibromatosis in the United Kingdom. II. Guidelines for genetic counseling. J Med Genet 1992;29:847–852.

Gutmann DH. New insights into the neurofibromatoses. Curr Opin Neurol 1994;7:166–171.

Jacks T, Shih TS, Schmitt EM, et al. Tumour predisposition in mice heterozygous for a targeted mutation in *Nf1*. Nature Genet 1994;7:353–361.

Kim HA, Rosenbaum T, Marchionni MA, et al. Schwann cells from neurofibromin deficient mice exhibit activation of p21*ras*, inhibition of cell proliferation ad morphological changes. Oncogene 1995; 11:325–335.

Largaespada DA, Brannan CI, Jenkins NA, Copeland NG. *Nf1* deficiency causes Ras-mediated granulocyte/macrophage colony stimulating factor hypersensitivity and chronic myeloid leukemia. Nat Genet 1996;12:137–143.

Li Y, O'Connell P, Breidenbach HH, et al. Genomic organization of the neurofibromatosis 1 gene (NF1). Genomics 1995;25:9–18.

Li Y, Bollag G, Clark R, et al. Somatic mutations in the neurofibromatosis gene in human tumors. Cell 1992;69:275–281.

Lutchman M, Rouleau GA. The neurofibromatosis type 2 gene product, schwannomin, suppresses growth of NIH 3T3 cells. Cancer Res 1995;55:2270–2274.

Marchuk DA, Collins FS. Molecular genetics of neurofibromatosis 1. In: Huson SM, Hughes RAC, eds. The Neurofibromatoses. London: Chapman and Hall Medical, 1994, pp. 23–49.

Maynard J, Kranczak M, Upadhyaya M. Characterization and significance of nine novel mutations in exon 16 of the neurofibromatosis type 1 (NF1) gene. Hum Genet 1997;99:647–676.

McClatchey AI, Saotome I, Ramesh V, et al. The *Nf2* tumor suppressor gene product is essential for extraembryonic development immediately prior to gastrulation. Genes Dev 1997;11:1253–1265.

McCormick F. *Ras* signaling and NF1. Curr Opin Genet Dev 1995; 5:51–55.

Mérel P, Hoang-Xuan K, Sanson M, et al. Screening for germ-line mutations in the NF2 gene. Genes Chromosome Cancer 1995;12:117–127.

Narod SA, Parry DM, Parboosingh J, et al. Neurofibromatosis type 2 appears to be a genetically homogeneous disease. Am J Hum Genet 1992;51:486–496.

O'Connell P, Cawthon RM, Viskochil D, White R. The NF1 translocation breakpoint region. Ann NY Acad Sci 1991;615:319–331.

Rouleau GA, Wertelecki W, Haines JL, et al. Genetic linkage of bilateral acoustic neurofibromatosis to a DNA marker on chromosome 22. Nature 1987;329:246–248.

Rouleau GA, Merel P, Lutchman M, et al. Alteration in a new gene encoding a putative membrane-organizing protein causes neurofibromatosis type 2. Nature 1993;363:515–521.

Ruttledge MH, Sarrazin J, Rangaratnam S, et al. Evidence for the complete inactivation of the NF2 gene in the majority of sporadic meningiomas. Nature Genet 1994;6:180–184.

Ruttledge MH, Andermann AA, Phelan CM et al. Type of mutation in the neurofibromatosis type 2 gene *(NF2)* frequently determines severity of disease. Am J Hum Genet 1996;59:531–342.

Sawada S, Floreel S, Purandare SM, Ota M, Stephens IC, Viskochil D. Identification of NF1 mutations in both alleles of a dermal neurofibroma. Nat Genet 1996;14:110–112.

Seizinger BR, Rouleau GA, Ozelius LJ, et al. Genetic linkage of von Recklinghausen neurofibromatosis to the nerve growth factor receptor gene. Cell 1987;49:589–594.

Side L, Taylor B, Cayouette M, Conner E, Thompson P, Luce M, Shannon K. Homozygous inactivation of the NF1 gene is bone marrow cells from children with neurofibromatosis type 1 and malignant myeloid disorders. N Engl J Med 1997;336:1713–1720.

Silva AJ, Frankland DN, Marowitz Z, Friedman E, Lazlo G, Cioffi D, Jack ST, Bourtchuladze R. A mouse model for the learning and memory deficits associated with neurofibromatosis type 1. Nat Genet 1997; 15:281–284.

Short PM, Martuza RL, Huson SM. Neurofibromatosis 2: clinical features, genetic counselling and management issues In: Huson SM and Hughes RAC, eds. The Neurofibromatoses: a pathogenic and clinical overview. London: Chapmann and Hall, 1994, pp. 414–444.

Tikoo A, Varga M, Ramesh V, Gusella J, Maruta H. An anti-ras function of neurofibromatosis type 2 gene product (NF2/Merlin). J Biol Chem 1994;269:23,387–23,390.

Trofatter JA, MacCollin MN, Rutter JL, et al. A novel moesin-, ezrin-, radixin-like gene is a candidate for the neurofibromatosis 2 tumor suppressor. Cell 1993;72:791–800.

Viskochil D, Buchberg A, Xu G, et al. Deletions and a translocation interrupt a cloned gene at the neurofibromatosis type 1 locus. Cell 1990;62:187–192.

Vogel KS, Brannan CI, Jenkins NA, et al. Loss of neurofibromin results in neurotrophin-independent survival of embryonic sensory and sympathetic neurons. Cell 1995;82:733–742.

Wallace M, Marchuk D, Anderson L, et al. Type 1 neurofibromatosis gene: identification of a large transcript disrupted in three NF1 patients. Science 1990;249:181–186.

White R, Viskochil D, O'Connell P. Identification and characterization of the gene for neurofibromatosis type 1. Curr Opin Neurobiol 1991; 1:462–467.

107 Brain Tumors

Mark A. Israel

INTRODUCTION

Tumors of the central nervous system (CNS) are a remarkably diverse group of neoplasms and the diversity of their origins is reflected in their biological behavior and clinical manifestations. Primary CNS tumors occur infrequently compared to other tumor types, yet approximately 15,000–20,000 Americans are afflicted each year. In contrast to the relative rarity of these tumors in adults, brain tumors are the second most common type of tumor seen during childhood occurring with an incidence of 2.2–2.5 cases per 100,000 children per year. The incidence of brain tumors wanes during early adulthood, although they again occur with increasing frequency in the fourth decade of life, after which the incidence continues to increase. The incidence of brain tumors in the elderly is rising, although the reason for this is unknown.

CLINICAL PRESENTATION

Depending on the site of occurrence and the degree to which a tumor has progressed at presentation, an individual's signs and symptoms may be focal or diffuse. Small, slow-growing tumors deep in the brain may have few, if any, clinical manifestations, while a rapidly growing tumor of the motor cortex can have profound consequences early in its course. Since specific functions reside in characteristic locations in the brain, the site of a tumor can often be predicted by deficits identified during a neurological examination. Eventually symptoms attributable to increased intracranial pressure such as morning headache, vomiting, and lethargy predominate if the flow of cerebral spinal fluid is compromised. The most common presenting symptom in all age groups is headache, and seizures are the second most common. Other more subtle symptoms include personality changes and gastrointestinal disturbance. Typically symptoms develop over a subacute or chronic course. Rarely, the onset of symptoms is acute and may be associated with compression of critical brain regions in the temporal lobe or cerebellum against the skull (herniation), requiring immediate intervention.

Tumors that occur at CNS sites other than the cerebrum, such as the base of the skull, the cerebellum, or the brain stem may have distinctive clinical characteristics. Schwannomas occurring in the acoustic nerve may cause a cerebellopontine angle syndrome including disturbances of hearing, balance, taste, and sensation on the face. Posterior fossa tumors oftentimes lead to deficits of gait, coordination, and balance, while brain-stem lesions are associated with cranial nerve dysfunction. Tumors of the spinal cord may present with local symptoms attributable to a tumor's location along the spinal column or with symptoms that occur at a site distant from the tumor due to involvement of sensory and motor neuronal tracts.

Approximately 25% of tumors occurring outside the CNS eventually metastasize to the brain, although this is more common in adults than in children. Carcinomas of the lung, breast, and colon, as well as melanoma and renal cell carcinoma, are among the most common such tumors. Their signs and symptoms mimic those of primary brain tumors occurring at similar locations. Frequently there are multiple sites of metastatic involvement when a patient presents for treatment. While primary intracranial tumors of adults rarely metastasize, brain tumors of children more frequently spread throughout the neuroaxis and to distant sites, causing otherwise unexpected symptoms.

PATHOLOGY

Approximately 60% of primary brain tumors arising in adults exhibit cytological and immunohistochemical evidence of astrocytic lineage. Oligodendrogliomas are less frequent, accounting for only about 5% of glial tumors. Mixed tumors expressing evidence of both astrocytic and oligodendroglial differentiation are rather commonly seen. Brain tumors of adults very rarely exhibit evidence of neuronal differentiation. During childhood a different spectrum of brain tumors is observed. The most common childhood brain tumors are supratentorial, low-grade astrocytomas, although astrocytomas of the cerebellum and brain stem occur almost as frequently. Medulloblastoma is the third most common brain tumor that occurs during childhood.

Several different nosologies have been proposed for the pathological classification of brain tumors, since the pioneering work of Cushing and Bailey. The World Health Organization (WHO) classification of CNS tumors, now the most widely used, incorporates three separate types of criteria based on anatomical site, histologic type, and degree of malignancy (Table 107-1). The pathology of astrocytic tumors is particularly relevant to this text because most advances in our understanding of the molecular basis for the malignant behavior of CNS tumors have been in the characterization of astrocytomas. Typically these tumors are infiltrative, and they are morphologically and cytologically heterogeneous. Various grading schema for astrocytic tumors have been proposed. These share a focus on the degree of tumor cell anaplasia.

From: *Principles of Molecular Medicine* (J. L. Jameson, ed.), ©1998 Humana Press Inc., Totowa, NJ.

Table 107-1
Pathological Classification of Central Nervous System Tumors According to the World Health Organization

Tumors of neuroepithelial tissue	**Cysts and tumor-like lesions**
Astrocytic tumors	Rathke cleft cyst
Oligodendroglial tumors	Epidermoid cyst
Ependymal tumors	Dermoid cyst
Mixed gliomas	Colloid cyst of the third ventricle
Choroid plexus tumors	Enterogenous cyst
Neuroepithelial tumors of uncertain origin	Neuroglial cyst
Neuronal and mixed neuronal-glial tumors	Granular cell tumor
Pineal parenchymal tumors	Hypothalamic neuronal hamartoma
Embryonal tumors	Nasal glial heterotopia
Tumors of cranial and spinal nerves	Plasma cell granuloma
Schwannoma	**Tumors of the sellar region**
Neurofibroma	Pituitary adenoma
Malignant peripheral nerve sheath tumor	Pituitary carcinoma
Tumors of the meninges	Craniopharyngioma
Tumors of meningothelial cells	**Local extensions from regional tumors**
Mesenchymal, nonmeningothelial tumors	Paraganglioma
Primary melanocytic lesions	Chordoma
Tumors of uncertain histogenesis	Chondroma
Lymphomas and hemopoietic neoplasma	Carcinoma
Malignant lymphomas	**Metastatic tumors**
Plasmacytoma	**Unclassified tumors**
Granulocytic sarcoma	
Others	
Germ cell tumors	
Germinoma	
Embryonal carcinoma	
Yolk sac tumor	
Choriocarcinoma	
Teratoma	
Mixed germ cell tumors	

CLINICAL EVALUATION

Patients in whom a brain tumor is suspected should undergo imaging studies. Evaluation of such patients has been greatly facilitated by the development of sensitive and specific modalities of neuroimaging. Computerized tomography (CT) and magnetic resonance imaging (MRI) both with and without contrast enhancing agents are the mainstays of diagnosis and patient evaluation. Enhancing agents are of particular usefulness in high-grade tumors, as these typically increase contrast between normal and malignant tissue.

MRI is the preferred diagnostic technique because it gives a more accurate image of tumor margins and is more sensitive than CT in identifying hydrocephalus and in evaluating tumor associated edema and hemorrhage. MRI also provides multiplanar images that assist in treatment planning. Most CNS tumors are visible on MRI scanning, although as many as 50% of some tumor types, such as low-grade gliomas, do not enhance with gadolinium. Other tests, such as visual field evaluations and electroencephalography, may contribute to the evaluation of brain tumor patients.

MOLECULAR MECHANISMS AND GENETICS

The recognition of cancer as a disorder of genes has provided impetus for the molecular analysis of brain tumors and focused attention on the possibility of identifying new agents and new modalities of treatment. Cancer arises when mutations that provide a growth advantage to cells lead to their unregulated proliferation within the CNS (Table 107-2). Tumor suppressor genes and oncogenes are two distinctive groups of genes that contribute to the development of brain tumors. Mutations in tumor suppressor genes can inactivate their ability to inhibit cell growth, whereas oncogenes contribute to cancer because inappropriate expression or expression of an altered protein stimulates cell growth. Tumor suppressor genes function recessively, and both alleles of a tumor suppressor gene must be inactivated for its phenotype to be manifest (*see* Chapter 105). Oncogenes act dominantly and mutation of one allele confers an altered phenotype on affected cells. Such a mechanism of dominant cellular activation has been found in Gds mutations in somatotropes (*see* Chapter 48).

CANCER PREDISPOSITION A predisposition for the development of brain tumors has been recognized as a part of several different complex inherited syndromes (Table 107-3). Some of these syndromes present with signs and symptoms attributable to multisystem disorders, and malignant tumors are only one of many disabling or life-threatening manifestations of the disorder. Other heritable syndromes have as their primary manifestation the development of malignant tumors. Tumor suppressor genes are responsible for some of these syndromes, a finding consistent with the model of tumorigenesis, first put forth by Knudson.

The familial occurrence of tumors is most evident when the inherited predisposition is widely expressed throughout the affected family. The Li-Fraumeni syndrome (OMIM 151623) is such a disorder that frequently results from the inheritance of a

Table 107-2
Frequently Occurring Cytogenetic and Genetic Alterations in Brain Tumors

Tumor	*Cytogenetic changes*	*Genetic alterations*
Astrocytoma	$1p^-,9p^-$,del10,$13q^-$, $17p^-,17q^-$,19q,$22p^-$,DMs[a]	*P53,RB1,NF1,EGFR,* C-*ros,met,gli,*c-*myc,ckd4,neu,ras*
Oligodendroglioma	$1p^-,9p^-,19q^-$	
Medulloblastoma	$17p^-,6q^-$,16q,DMs	
Meningioma	$22q^-$	*NF2*

[a]DMs, double minute chromosomes.

Table 107-3
Hereditary Syndromes Associated with Brain Tumors

Hereditary disorder	*OMIM no.*	*Prominently associated CNS malignancies*
Syndromes with multisystem presentations		
Neurofibromatosis Type I	162200	Glioma
Neurofibromatosis Type II	101000	Meningioma, acoustic neuroma, schwannoma, ependymoma
Tuberous sclerosis	191100	Giant cell astrocytoma
von Hippel-Lindau	193300	Hemangioblastoma
Ataxia-telangiectasia	208900	Glioma
Common variable immunodeficiency	240500	Glioma
Syndromes with cancer as primary symptoms		
Turcot syndrome	276300	Medulloblastoma
Li-Fraumeni syndrome	151623	Glioma, medulloblastoma, ependymoma, choroid plexus
Hereditary retinoblastoma	180200	Retinoblastoma, pineablastoma
Gorlin syndrome	109400	Medulloblastoma, meningioma

mutated *p53* gene (*see* Chapter 7). Members of families affected by this syndrome typically have an increased frequency of many different tumors that occur earlier in life than is expected when they occur sporadically. Gliomas tend to be among the commonly occurring brain tumors, although medulloblastomas and choroid plexus tumors also occur. *p53* germline mutations have also been identified in young patients with glioblastoma who do not have a family history of brain tumors or increased tumor incidence. Patients with multifocal astrocytomas are also more likely than other glioma patients to have germline *p53* mutations.

Another cancer predisposition syndrome in which brain tumors are a particularly prominent characteristic and the molecular basis is known is Turcot's syndrome (OMIM 276300). Affected patients, who typically have both a malignant brain tumor and multiple colorectal adenomas, can carry germ-line mutations of either the *APC* gene or a DNA mismatch-repair gene (*see* Chapter 7). A predisposition for the development of brain tumors is clearly associated with other inherited disorders in which the development of malignancy may not be the first or primary manifestation of the inherited syndrome (Table 107-3). The two most widely recognized groups of such disorders are the phacomatoses and the immunodeficiency syndromes. Neurofibromatosis occurs in patients with mutations in the *NF1* gene, which functions in a signal transduction pathway important for cell growth. *NF1* (OMIM 162200) was cloned following localization of this locus to chromosome 17q11.2 by extensive linkage analysis and the identification of two neurofibromatosis patients with chromosomal translocation breakpoints at 17q11.2 (*see* Chapter 106). Using DNA from patients with these breakpoints, the *NF1* gene was identified as being interrupted by the rearrangement and recognized to encode a guanosine triphosphatase activating protein, neurofibromin. Brain tumors are the most lethal manifestation of neurofibromatosis. Tuberous sclerosis (OMIM 191100) also predisposes to CNS malignancies, and mutations have been identified recently in the TSC1 (tuberous sclerosis complex 1) gene on chromosome 9q34.

MOLECULAR PATHOLOGY OF BRAIN TUMORS

Astrocytomas The different histologic grades of astrocytomas in adults correspond to clonal populations of malignant cells that acquire sequential genetic alterations. Each mutation provides an additional growth advantage to the tumor cell leading to that cell becoming the predominant cell type and the most likely target for the next mutation. This model is consistent with clinical experience that documents highly malignant tumors arising within low-grade tumors. Other data relevant to this model come from the evaluation of tumors of different histologic grades for a number of different oncogenetic alterations. Genetic changes observed in low-grade tumors are also found in higher grade tumors, while other alterations seem to occur only in tumors of the highest malignant grades. To date, the study of astrocytic tumors has focused on the loss of DNA from chromosomes 1p, 9p, 10, 13q, two different loci on chromosome 17p, 17q, 19q, and the telomeric portion of 22q. At some of these loci, known or putative tumor suppressor genes are located. Deletions in 9p21-9p22 probably target *CDKN2*, which encodes a known tumor suppressor gene, *P16*. *P16* is an inhibitor of cdk4, a cyclin-dependent kinase that functions to promote cell growth. Interestingly, cdk4 is sometimes amplified in glioblastomas that have a normal *P16*.

p53, located on chromosome 17p, has been found to be mutated in approximately 30–40% of gliomas. The frequency of *p53* mutation does not vary among the different histologic grades of tumor. The retinoblastoma gene, *RB1* (OMIM 180200), is a well-characterized tumor suppressor gene located on chromosome 13q14 (*see* Chapter 105). Disruption of the *RB1* locus and mutations in the *RB1* gene have been found in all grades of astrocytoma suggesting a role for *RB1* in the development of astrocytomas. The *NF1* locus at 17q is a likely candidate for being the gene altered in those tumors that show cytogenetic evidence of DNA loss in this chromosomal region, although *NF1* involvement in sporadically occurring gliomas has not been well-defined. No convincing evidence of the involvement of specific genes has yet emerged for other chromosomal sites altered in astrocytomas. Deletion of chromosome 10 occurs in up to 80% of glioblastomas and is seen rarely in low-grade astrocytomas. Loss of chromosome 10 occurs frequently, but smaller deletions suggest that different loci on 10p and 10q24 may be involved. A tumor suppressor gene *(PTEN)*, which encodes a putative protein tyrosine phosphatase gene, has been localized to chromosome 10q23. Mutations in *PTEN* have been found in one-third of glioblastoma cell lines and in 17% of primary glioblastomas.

Little is known regarding the oncogenes that may be important in the pathogenesis of astrocytic tumors. The oncogene most frequently implicated is *EGFR*, which encodes the epidermal growth factor (EGF) receptor. *EGFR* is amplified and mutated in glioblastomas. These altered forms of the molecule may contribute to unregulated growth by assuming a conformation corresponding to the activated form of the receptor. Other oncogenes activated in gliomas, albeit infrequently, include c-*ros*, *met*, and *Neu* (c-*erbB-2*), *MYC*, *HRAS*, and *NRAS*, which have all been observed to be highly-expressed in some glial tumors, although their contributions to tumorigenesis are unknown.

Pilocytic astrocytomas frequently have a rather benign clinical course, and their precise relationship to other astrocytomas is not understood. *p53* mutations are rare in pilocytic astrocytomas. Also, while the occurrence of these tumors in patients with neurofibromatosis strongly suggests that this gene will be involved in sporadic pilocytic astrocytomas, mutations in *NF1* have not yet been detected in pilocytic astrocytomas.

Oligodendrogliomas Cytogenetic studies of oligodendrogliomas have shown frequent deletions of chromosomes 1p, 9p, and 19q13.2–13.4, although in none of these locations have specific tumor suppressor genes been implicated. The *p53* locus has been examined in a number of oligodendrogliomas and mixed oligoastrocytomas, although evidence for mutations was found in less than 10% of tumors examined. *EGFR* is not amplified in oligodendrogliomas, and other oncogenes have not been implicated.

Meningiomas Most meningiomas (OMIM: 156100) arise from cells of the arachnoid membrane and are typically benign, although they have a distinct propensity to recur. These tumors occur frequently in patients with neurofibromatosis type 2 (NF2; OMIM 101000), which occurs as a result of mutations of the *NF2* gene on chromosome 22q. Since deletion of chromosome 22q is found frequently in both vestibular schwannomas and meningiomas, tumors that occur in patients with NF2, the *NF2* gene is likely to be inactivated in sporadic meningiomas, although this has not yet been documented. There is also preliminary evidence for a second tumor suppressor locus on 22q that contributes to the pathogenesis of meningiomas. No oncogenes are known to be amplified in meningiomas, and deletion or mutation of *p53* occurs infrequently. Deletions of loci on chromosomes 1p, 9q, and 17p have been observed in malignant meningiomas, which occur infrequently.

Medulloblastomas Medulloblastomas (OMIM 155255) occur most commonly in children, and are seen frequently in two inherited cancer syndromes, the Turcot syndrome and Gorlin's syndrome (OMIM 109400). In Turcot syndrome, familial adenomatosis of the colon is combined with CNS tumors, including both glioma and medulloblastoma. The APC gene is mutated in the germ line of patients with Turcot syndrome, but this gene has not been found to be altered in sporadically occurring medulloblastomas. In Gorlin's syndrome, multiple basal cell carcinomas are associated with medulloblastoma. The gene for this syndrome is on chromosome 9q22.3–31, but evidence for the loss of genetic material at these loci is infrequently found in sporadic medulloblastoma. Although chromosome 17p is a frequent site of deletion in medulloblastoma, and medulloblastoma occurs in Li-Fraumeni families, *p53* mutations have not been found in sporadically occurring medulloblastoma. Several studies, however, have suggested the presence of a second tumor suppressor gene on 17p13 distal to *p53*. Other genetic changes rarely identified in medulloblastoma are deletions of chromosome 6q and 16q.

MOLECULAR PATHOPHYSIOLOGY Mutations in genes important for the development of brain tumors manifest themselves by their effect on growth regulation and contribute to the invasive characteristics of malignant brain tumors. Probably the most important of these is the pathway mediated by the EGF receptor, which binds EGF or TGF-α and has tyrosine kinase activity when activated. The proliferation of some astrocytic tumors may occur as the result of autocrine stimulation, since some tumors that express the *EGFR* gene also synthesize and secrete EGF or TGF-α. Similarly, the platelet derived growth factor (PDGF) receptor and PDGF are sometimes found in the same tumor. Other growth factors that may contribute to glioma tumor cell proliferation include insulin-like growth factor I, basic fibroblast growth factor, and vascular endothelial cell growth factor, although the latter two seem to function primarily as angiogenic factors. Interestingly, several members of the TGF-β family of growth factors produced by some high-grade astrocytic tumors have immunosuppressant properties.

Extracellular matrix proteins and integrins, the cell surface receptors that recognize them, play key roles in mediating the production of tumor-derived proteases and the migration of tumor cells. Brain tumors produce several different types of proteases. The highest grade astrocytomas, glioblastoma multiforme (OMIM 137800), are unusual in that they contain high levels of the extracellular matrix protein vitronectin, which is not seen in the normal brain, as well as expressing the receptors for vitronectin, $\alpha_v\beta_3$ and $\alpha_v\beta_5$.

THERAPY

Therapy for malignant brain tumors is tumor-specific but typically involves surgery and radiation therapy. Neuro-oncology has been an important beneficiary of the technical advances that have characterized these two therapeutic approaches over the last several decades, and patients with localized, noninvasive tumors can frequently be cured. Radiosurgical techniques for precisely targeting tumor tissue with a very high dose of radiation are currently being evaluated. Some brain tumors, such as medulloblastoma, are sensitive to chemotherapy, which plays an important role in the management of some patients with this tumor. A role for adjuvant chemotherapy, in particular nitrosurea-based regimens, for the treatment of glial tumors is also widely recognized. Very high-dose chemotherapy utilizing combinations of drugs such as thiotepa and carboplatinum supported by autologous bone marrow transplantation or peripheral stem cell rescue are currently being evaluated.

FUTURE DIRECTIONS

The emerging description of a molecular basis for the pathogenesis of brain tumors and advances in molecular biology have led to new opportunities for improving the care of brain tumor patients. Evaluation of *EGFR* amplification or mutation of *p53* as prognostic markers may one day lead to new diagnostic and prognostic tools. Ongoing attempts to develop new anticancer drugs that target specific molecules in various growth regulatory pathways may prove useful against brain tumors, and this is especially true for tyrosine kinase inhibitors. Several different growth factor receptors implicated in the proliferation of brain tumors have tyrosine kinase activity, and drugs targeted at inhibiting this enzymatic activity will soon enter clinical trials.

Gene therapy for the treatment of brain tumors has also attracted considerable interest because of animal studies that suggest that at least two very distinct strategies are capable of curing animals with established brain tumors. One such strategy involved inoculation of rat C6 glioma cells transfected with an antisense mRNA for insulin-like growth factor 1 into nontransfected tumor. In association with an immune response, the established tumor disappeared. In other experiments the retroviral mediated transfer of the herpes simplex virus thymidine kinase gene to tumor cells has been pursued. Infected cells become sensitive to the cytotoxic effects of Ganciclovir, a guanine analog that disrupts cellular proliferation when it is phosphorylated by the viral thymidine kinase. Ongoing gene therapy trials for the treatment of brain tumor patients using such a viral prodrug strategy are currently ongoing and should provide insights important for the development of this new modality of treatment.

ACKNOWLEDGMENT

I wish to thank Dr. Jim Fick and Dr. Fred Barker for thoughtful comments and ideas in preparing this manuscript, and Ms. Lucy Avila for her editorial assistance.

SELECTED REFERENCES

Bishop JM. Molecular themes in oncogenesis. Cell 1991;64:235–248.

Black PM. Brain tumors. N Engl J Med 1991;324:1471–1476.

Fick J, Israel MA. Gene therapy for diseases of the nervous system. West J Med 1994;161:260–263.

Hamilton SR, Liu B, Parsons RE, et al. The molecular basis of Turcot's syndrome. N Engl J Med 1995;332:839–847.

James CD, Mikkelsen T, Cavenee WK, Collins VP. Molecular genetic aspects of glial tumour evolution. Cancer Surv 1990;9:631–644.

Kleihues P, Burger PC, Scheithauer BW, in collaboration with L. H. Sorbin and pathologists in 14 countries. Histological Typing of Tumours of the Central Nervous System, 2nd ed. Springer-Verlag, New York, 1993.

Knudson AG. Mutation and cancer: statistical study of retinoblastoma. Proc Natl Acad Sci USA 1971;68:820–824.

Li J, Yen C, Liaw D, et al. PTEN, a putative protein tyrosine phosphatase gene mutated in human brain, breast, and prostate cancer. Science 1997;275:1943–1947.

Malkin D, Li FP, Strong LC, et al. Germ line p53 mutations in a familial syndrome of breast cancer, sarcomas, and other neoplasms. Science 1990;250: 1233–1238.

Marchuk DA, Collins FS. Molecular genetics of neurofibromatosis 1. In: The Neurofibromatoses: A Pathogenetic and Clinical Overview. Eds. Huson SM, Hughes RAC. Chapman & Hall Medical, London, 1994, pp. 23–44.

Miller BA, Gloeckler R, Lynn A, et al. Seer Cancer Statistics Review 1973–1990. Department of Health and Human Services, Public Health Service, NIH, NCI Bethesda, MD, 1993.

van Slegtenhorst M, de Hoogt R, Hermans C, et al. Identification of the tuberous sclerosis gene TSC1 on chromosome 9q34. Science 1997;277:805–808.

Wen PY, Schiff D. Clinical evaluation of patients with astrocytomas. In: Black P McL, Schoene WC, Lampson LA, eds. Astrocytomas: Diagnosis, Treatment, and Biology. Boston: Blackwell, 1993, pp. 26–29.

Zülch KJ. Brain Tumors: Their Biology and Pathology, vol. 3. Berlin: Springer-Verlag, 1986, pp. 1–323.

PSYCHIATRY XII

SECTION EDITOR:
CHARLES B. NEMEROFF

108 Molecular Mechanisms and Regulating Behavior

PAUL M. PLOTSKY AND CHARLES B. NEMEROFF

INTRODUCTION

Elucidating the molecular genetic underpinnings of behavior represents the "Holy Grail" of neuroscience and is of particular interest to psychiatry. Despite the difficulty inherent in this ambitious goal, the past decade has witnessed promising strides toward this aim in large part because of the armamentarium of molecular, genetic, and imaging tools currently available. In studies on species ranging from aquatic snails (to worms to birds to rodents) to humans, increasing evidence indicates that there is a major heritable component to virtually every behavior in all organisms.

GENERAL CONSIDERATIONS IN GENETIC STUDIES OF BEHAVIORAL TRAITS

Several important assumptions are implicit in any genetic studies of behavior. First, although a given behavior may have a heritable component, this does not necessarily imply that a complex behavior is entirely attributable to an inherited gene or set of genes. Second, it is imperative to recognize that, even though genes probably do not code for behavior in a direct way, this does not exclude the possibility that an individual gene cannot play a critical role in the expression of a behavior. Third, it should be appreciated that most complex behaviors and behavioral dysfunctions are likely to be polygenetic and not regulated by a single gene. Fourth, the age-old nature versus nurture controversy must be replaced with the realization that the genetic/biological substrate with which an organism is born is modifiable by nongenetic factors or, put another way, the full expression of a behavioral phenotype is shaped by a complex interaction of genetic and environmental factors.

It is highly improbable that a gene encodes a single behavior. Individual genes code for specific proteins (i.e., enzymes, structural proteins, trophic factors, neurotransmitters, receptors, and so on). A given behavior is generated by neural circuits composed of multiple, interconnected neuronal elements. The development, differentiation, function, and connectivity of each neuron is dependent on the coordinated activity of a multitude of genes. The products of these genes interact with one another and their local environment, thus giving rise to coordinated neuronal activation subserving some particular behavior or set of behaviors. It follows from this reasoning that a particular gene does not explicitly code for a behavior. For instance, if a particular molecule in the signaling cascade of a behavior-related neurocircuit is absent, it is easy to envision the disruption of the behavioral component that would normally be elicited by activation of that neurocircuit. Finally, there is a growing appreciation for the complexity of the interaction between the genetic endowment and nongenetic factors. For example, an individual may inherit a defective copy of a gene coding for a catabolic liver enzyme necessary for elimination of certain heavy metal complexes. If this individual accepts employment at a battery factory where exposure to heavy metal complexes occurs, the genetic vulnerability will be expressed as sickness and/or death as a result of the accumulation of these poisons. However, if the individual avoids such exposure, the potential vulnerability may ever be realized. This concept of a preexisting genetic vulnerability requiring some nongenetic trigger for expression of the phenotype has been readily adopted by developmental psychologists and psychiatrists to explain the acquisition of "released behaviors" or the etiology of psychiatric disease and substance abuse.

From: *Principles of Molecular Medicine* (J. L. Jameson, ed.), ©1998 Humana Press Inc., Totowa, NJ.

The foregoing exposition suggests that requisite to the successful investigation of the genetic basis of behavioral traits or etiology of psychiatric illness, it is necessary to: (1) develop replicable measurement techniques and methods to accurately define the target biological and behavioral phenomena, (2) demonstrate that the biological and behavioral measures are related to the normal or pathophysiology, and (3) establish an association between the biological and behavioral measures in human or animal studies.

TOOLS OF THE TRADE

It is now generally accepted that genetic factors contribute to the expression of various behavioral and psychiatric disorders in humans. From this, it follows that there must be underlying biological differences associated with differences in behavior. Unfortunately, there are currently few replicated findings that identify the specific biological substrates necessary for normal behavior in humans or lower animals (vide infra). Indeed, it is unlikely that the study of normal behaviors will lead to the identification of the underlying genetic determinants of behavior. The classic approach in human genetics has been and continues to be the study of abnormal or unusual phenotypes using family, twin, and adoption studies to assess the epidemiology of these phenotypes. By understanding the biological/genetic mechanisms responsible for abnormal behavior, it should be possible to unravel the mechanisms involved in normal behavior. Clearly, the most convincing evidence for a genetic etiology of an illness or of a normal behavioral phenotype is the identification of a gene product that is always associated with the disorder and that can be established as necessary for expression of the phenotype.

Recent advances in molecular biology have provided geneticists with an increasing set of tools for such studies. In the past, linkage studies were not practical for humans because of the scarcity of available markers. However, in the past decade, the discovery of restriction fragment length polymorphisms (RFLPs), and the subsequent demonstration that RFLPs were inherited as simple Mendelian traits, have accelerated linkage mapping of loci responsible for many human diseases. The availability of these RFLP markers has ushered in the decade of genome mapping projects as well as making it at least theoretically possible to systematically screen families using these markers. Thus far, however, nearly all diseases mapped follow clear Mendelian, single-locus segregation patterns. In contrast, many common familial diseases such as diabetes, some forms of alcoholism, and many psychiatric diseases, such as schizophrenia and depression, are more complex; these diseases appear to be familial and clearly have a (poly)genetic component that may not display simple Mendelian transmission.

Complex behaviors and psychiatric diseases have yielded only slowly, if at all, to these approaches. This may be, in part, because of the polygenetic nature of these behavioral traits or to the important influence of nongenetic factors on the expression of these traits. Among the problems plaguing such studies are lack of sufficiently large genotypically or phenotypically pure populations, the relative inability of current diagnostic instruments to differentiate subcategories of these diseases, which probably occur on a continuum, and the lack of any convincing biochemical or anatomical marker.

In the past few years, a new class of human mutation, referred to as a trinucleotide repeat amplification, has been identified. Trinucleotide DNA repeats, which can expand to hundreds or even thousands of repeating triplets, have been found in many genetic diseases, including myotonic dystrophy, fragile X syndrome (types A and E), Kennedy's disease, Huntington's disease, and type 1 spinocerebellar ataxia. Interestingly, evidence indicates that the amplified DNA trinucleotide repeat underlies the clinical phenomenon termed genetic anticipation. Two components of genetic anticipation, greater severity and earlier age at onset in subsequent generations, are features of several psychiatric illnesses (i.e., schizophrenia and bipolar affective disorder). Furthermore, the concept of these trinucleotide repeats as regions of unstable DNA provides a compelling alternative to the traditional multifactorial polygenic theories: Many deviations from a single-gene mode of inheritance in psychiatric twin and family studies, which previously served as strong proof for more than one etiologic gene, can be easily explained by the non-Mendelian behavior of unstable DNA.

In animal studies, more interventionist strategies may be attempted to assess the relationship of a particular gene to behavior. It is now considered routine to create a series of transgenic animals. Usually, the initial studies are concerned with production of a "knockout" model, in which a particular gene or gene product is totally or partially inactivated. In some cases, an "overproduction" paradigm is created, as has been done to create a mouse model of Cushing's disease. The second stage is often the creation of a series of transgenic animals carrying target gene constructs, or promoter–reporter constructs, in which systematic mutagenesis of the promoter region has been performed. In each of these experimental paradigms, most commonly performed in fruit flies and mice, transfer of the construct into the organism is assessed, followed by biochemical, physiological, and/or behavioral testing.

NONGENETIC FACTORS

It is now abundantly clear that developmental windows exist during which the central nervous system (CNS) is extremely sensitive to environmental and emotional insults that shape how the organism will subsequently perceive and respond to its environment. This interaction between the organism's genetic endowment (e.g., genotype) and the local environment (i.e., uterine, intrinsic, extrinsic) suggests a high degree of plasticity during this critical period that may contribute to individual (phenotypic) differences, even among identical twins. It has been postulated that life experiences, especially those occurring during the pre- and neonatal periods of central nervous system development, exert a significant influence on phenotypic development at the cellular, as well as at the organismal, levels. Developing a comprehensive understanding of the nature and the mechanism(s) underlying this plasticity remains a major goal of biological psychiatry.

Communication between the genome and the environment is bidirectional. Development of the CNS proceeds along a fundamental genetic program that specifies the interrelationships among larger categories of neurons via mechanisms, including cell differentiation and chemoaffinity for the establishment of appropriate synaptic connections. As demonstrated in numerous species, the developing nervous system contains an excess number of synaptic connections, many of which will be lost during development. This process of synaptic sculpting or pruning occurs in response to the level of impulse activity along each connection and, thus, is environmentally mediated. Neuronal activity within a developing network selectively stabilizes only those emerging contacts (presynaptic) whose postsynaptic (receiving) cell is receptive to the process at a particular moment. The activation of a specific gene is not necessary for constructing a specific individual synaptic contact. Instead, the fine structuring of synaptic contacts follows a pattern determined by epigenetic factors, which build on a foundation of less finely structured neuronal networks that were specified by a basic genetic program. This high degree of flexibility leads to individual variability even among organisms sharing the same genes (i.e., identical twins). These responses to the external environment are capable of modifying gene expression within responsive cells at the microscopic level of fine structure and biochemistry as well as permanently altering the behavior of the central nervous system on a macroscopic level. The mechanistic aspects of this long-term "imprinting" by early experience remains to be fully elucidated, but is likely to involve alterations in gene expression via processes of DNA methylation or demethylation, activation of transcription factors, changes in protein phosphorylation state, as well as the participation of neurotrophic factors. It is particularly important to remember that these individual changes in neuronal circuitry may be either adaptive or maladaptive.

This preamble leads to the following questions:

1. To what degree is a particular behavioral trait or psychiatric disease determined by genetic and developmental factors?

2. To what degree is any given behavioral trait or psychiatric disease environmentally or socially determined?

We will attempt to address these questions in the remainder of this chapter through the presentation of specific examples primarily drawn from preclinical research. A comprehensive analysis of human studies of the genetic contributions to the development of major psychiatric illnesses is presented in Chapters 109–111 of this section.

OF SNAILS, FLIES, AND MICE: GENES AND BEHAVIOR

SENSITIZATION IN THE MARINE MOLLUSK Several invertebrate models have provided important insights into the effects of the genome on behavior. These invertebrate models offer the advantage of a more tractable central nervous system combined with comparatively simple, stereotyped behaviors. One such model system, which has been helpful in defining cellular and molecular events associated with simple forms of learning and memory, is the gill- and siphon-withdrawal reflex of the marine mollusk *Aplysia californica*. One simple form of nonassociative learning in this reflex is sensitization, which refers to an increase in the strength of the defensive withdrawal and the response to previously neutral stimuli after exposure to threatening stimuli. A single stimulus to the tail initiates the withdrawal and gives rise to a short-term sensitization that persists for minutes to hours. Repeated application of the stimulus results in a long-term sensitization that can persist for days to weeks. The deposition of this long-term memory is associated with the growth of synaptic connections, protein synthesis, and alterations in gene expression.

The fundamental mechanism underlying both short- and long-term sensitization is an increase in the synaptic strength of a monosynaptic connection between identified mechanoreceptor sensory neurons and effector motor neurons. An in vitro model of sensitization exists: Reconstructed synapses occurring in dissociated cell culture demonstrate the homologous phenomenon of facilitation. Biophysical studies suggest that the increase in synaptic strength observed in facilitation is secondary to an enhancement in transmitter release by the sensory neuron and an increase in postsynaptic excitability resulting from decreased potassium flux in the motor neuron.

Despite the similarity in the cellular processes of short- and long-term sensitization, the short- and long-term processes differ in important ways. The short-term change involves covalent modification of preexisting proteins and alteration of pre-existing intercellular connections. Short-term sensitization does not require *de novo* protein synthesis and is refractory to inhibition of transcription or translation. Conversely, long-term facilitation requires protein and mRNA synthesis, which must occur within a relatively narrow time window for facilitation to be manifest. Thus, the gene products required for short-term memory are pre-existing and turn over relatively slowly, whereas long-term memory requires the synthesis of new gene products. At least some of these new gene products drive structural changes in the synapse. Long-term, but not short-term sensitization, is associated with the formation of new synaptic contacts of the sensory cells onto the motor neurons.

The binding of serotonin to its receptor on the sensory neuron appears to be both necessary and sufficient to induce sensitization. Just as for physical stimuli, a single application of serotonin will produce short-term sensitization, whereas repeated or continuous application will induce long-term changes. Serotonin binding activates an adenylyl cyclase that increases the intracellular concentration of cAMP, which in turn triggers the dissociation of the regulatory and catalytic subunits of protein kinase A (PKA). Activated catalytic PKA remains in the cytoplasmic compartment, primarily in presynaptic terminals, where it phosphorylates protein substrates, which contribute to prolongation of the presynaptic action potential and the enhancement of neurotransmitter release.

In contrast, long-term facilitation induces these as well as additional changes in the neurons; some of these changes impinge on the nucleus and result in alterations of gene expression. Stimuli producing long-term facilitation also induce a translocation of active catalytic PKA subunit to the nucleus, where proteins regulating transcription from cAMP response elements (CRE) are presumed to be phosphorylated. One family of proteins thought to be phosphorylated under these conditions are the CRE-binding (CREB) proteins. The necessity of PKA-driven expression from CREs for long-term facilitation is demonstrated by the fact that interference with the CRE expression prevents the establishment of long-term facilitation.

The identity of some of the genes induced by long-term facilitation has been elucidated. These are divided into two categories: early effectors and late effectors. Early effector products include N-terminal ubiquitin hydroxylase, which appears to effect the ubiquitin-mediated proteolytic cleavage of the regulatory subunit of PKA, thus maintaining the activity of the catalytic subunit, even in the absence of cAMP, clathrin, and an NCAM-related cell adhesion molecule. These latter two proteins, as well as many late effector products, appear to be involved in the structural elaboration of the synapse that occurs with long-term facilitation.

The dependency of long-term facilitation on transcription and translation displays a remarkably narrow temporal window. Inhibition of either transcription or translation at times greater than one hour after the last training session are without effect on the development of long-term facilitation. This critical period of sensitivity to transcription and translation is referred to as the consolidation phase. The existence of the *consolidation phase* suggests that there is a rapid initial expression of genes in response to the training regimen, and that the expression of these genes ultimately results in the establishment and stable maintenance of the increased synaptic strength associated with long-term facilitation and sensitization. The fact that mere covalent modification of existing transcription factors is not sufficient for the establishment of facilitation suggests that training starts a cascade of gene activation wherein constitutively expressed transcription factors induce temporally early genes that activate later effector genes; it is these later effector genes that are ultimately responsible for the morphological and biophysical changes associated with facilitation.

Several members of both early- and late-phase gene families have been identified. An Aplysia homolog of the mammalian C/EBP transcription factor family has been identified (ApC/EBP) and is known to possess an upstream CRE and to be regulated by cAMP. ApC/EBP is known to have the properties of an immediate–early gene: Its expression is not detected in unstimulated cells but is induced in stimulated cells, even in the presence of protein synthesis inhibitors. ApC/EBP expression is necessary for the establishment of long-term facilitation as shown by experiments blocking the expression or the actions of the protein. These interventions block the establishment of long-term facilitation without affecting short-term facilitation. Thus ApC/EBP represents at least one member of the early-phase gene family.

Other investigations have identified six proteins, the expression of which are altered during the acquisition of long-term facilitation. Two of these, clathrin and tubulin, increase in expression, whereas the other four, which appear to be immunoglobulin-related cell adhesion molecules displaying sequence homology to vertebrate NCAM and Drosophila fasiculin II, decrease in expression. The decreased expression of the cell adhesion molecules, designated apCAM, is thought to lead to a removal of adhesion molecules at sites of neuronal connections, promoting defasiculation and destabilizing adhesive contacts as a prelude to the synaptic remodeling and elaboration of long-term facilitation. Increased expression of the cytoskeletal proteins contribute to both the increased intracellular protein trafficking and the more extensive synaptic architecture resulting from synaptic remodeling.

The dissection of the molecular processes associated with long-term sensitization and facilitation in this seemingly simple monosynaptic reflex of Aplysia has yielded insights into the cellular and molecular events surrounding nonassociative learning. Additionally, we have seen that environmental events can influence (alter) the expression of genes, and that this altered gene expression results in altered behavior at both the synaptic and organismal level. The following corollaries are derived from these observations:

1. The seemingly simple process of learning in this reflex arc requires the coordinated expression of several genes, suggesting that the search for one gene/one behavior linkages may be futile.
2. Genetic defects along this pathway are likely to result in deficiencies in learning and memory processes.

THE SEX LIFE OF FLIES CNS regulation of sex-specific behaviors in Drosophila has been studied with great intensity, in the context of genetic factors that influence the development of sexually differentiated aspects of this insect. These studies have been particularly useful in strengthening the "single-gene" approach to behavior resulting from the availability of numerous mutant phenotypes. Three categories of genetic variations that can disrupt reproductive behaviors have been described:

1. Mutants isolated with regard to courtship defects.
2. General behavioral and neurological variants including sensory and learning mutants, whose defects include subnormal reproductive performance.
3. Mutations of genes within the sex-determination regulatory hierarchy of Drosophila.

Overall, these studies have clearly revealed that mutagenesis of genes, seemingly far removed from the regulation of behavior, can have direct consequences on it. Such studies have also highlighted the fact that the study of the genetic basis of behavior requires the study of genomes and their functional organization, rather than of single genes alone.

Drosophila males display a highly stereotyped courtship and mating behavior including orienting, following, tapping, singing, licking, mounting, and copulating behaviors toward receptive females. Mutations of a single gene, named period (*per*), result in alterations of the fly's circadian rhythms and, therefore, disrupt behaviors based on these rhythms. Males carrying a mutant *per* gene generate a courtship song that lacks the characteristic smooth sinusoidal pattern of frequencies and, hence, is much less effective in inducing receptivity in females. This demonstrates both that a single gene can influence multiple complex behaviors and that a single gene is capable of determining a single behavior. More recent work has mapped specific behavioral motifs within the *per* gene. Two species of flies, *D. melanogaster* and *D. simulans*, show similar 24-h circadian rhythms, but perform courtship songs with differing periods. When transgenic animals are constructed between these two species, a short region in the middle of the *per* gene was shown to control song period: *D. melanogaster* carrying the mid-region from *D. simulans* will sing with the period of *D. simulans* and vice versa.

The courtship behavior of *D. melanogaster* also illustrates the importance of regional gene expression in determining behavior. Sexual development in these flies is controlled by the complement of X chromosomes in each cell. Cells harboring one X chromosome give rise to male anatomical structures and behaviors in adult flies, while cells that have two X chromosomes lead to female anatomy and behaviors. Single-X male cells and double-X female cells activate separate but overlapping sets of sex-determining genes that give rise to the phenotypic differences. The generation of genetic mosaic flies carrying mixtures of male and female cells throughout the nervous system allowed the identification of those regions that are responsible for various components of the courtship ritual. Discrete regions of the fly brain have been identified in mosaic animals as being responsible for male pattern behavior in attraction to females (antennal lobe and mushroom body), initiating courtship (trigger zone) and orienting, tapping, following and licking (dorsocaudal brain), singing (rostral thoracic ganglion), and mounting and copulating (caudal thoracic ganglion). These observations suggest that the correct expression of sex-determining genes in several discrete anatomical loci are responsible for specific components of a complex suite of behaviors.

Drosophila have also contributed to our understanding of the molecular events of learning. Male flies react to pheromones from impregnated females with a prolonged cessation of mating behavior toward all females. Calcium/calmodulin-dependent protein kinase II (CaMKII) is another intracellular protein kinase that has been implicated in induction of molecular changes associated with learning, with mechanisms similar to those discussed for PKA in the case of the Aplysia (*vide supra*). Male flies engineered to express a thermosensitive CaMKII fail to remember their rejection by impregnated female flies when their CaMKII is inactivated. CaMKII-mediated learning in Drosophila bears additional similarities to PKA-mediated learning in Aplysia. The relevant substrate for CaMKII appears to be the potassium channel protein EAG. Mutations of the EAG protein produce learning impairment similar to CaMKII inactivation, and the EAG protein is a substrate of CaMKII in vitro. The full circuit appears to involve pheromone activation of neurons in the trigger region, which increases intracellular calcium levels. The increased calcium activates CaMKII, which phosphorylates the EAG potassium channel protein. Phosphorylation increases potassium efflux and decreases neuronal firing. The reduction in firing of trigger region neurons removes the stimulus to initiate the suite of courtship behaviors.

Drosophila behavior is rich and complex. As such, and similar to the case in higher vertebrates and mammals, early experience affects behavioral development of Drosophila. Therefore, Drosophila can be used to study the developmental mechanisms by which organisms optimize their behavioral repertoires to enhance their chances of survival. Female responsiveness to courting males is modified by early experience. This type of developmental plasticity permits adjustment of intrinsically determined responses to visual targets, so that these insects can take into account the actual characteristics of the developing animal's environment. The "fine tuning" of basic genetic patterns of behavior introduces the possibility of inclusion of "cultural" and "social" elements into courtship and mate choice in insects. Conceptually, the role of developmental plasticity modification of genetic programs has broad theoretical and practical implications.

OF BIRD BRAINS AND MICE

HOW DO BIRDS SING? On any given morning, the sound of singing birds brings delight and pleasure. Birds sing to attract mates and, therefore, the development of mechanisms to produce and decode these songs is of reproductive and evolutionary importance. Several discoveries have shaped the recent study of brain substrates for birdsong. First, the failure of deaf birds to reproduce a song from memory supported the postulated existence of a song template. Attempts to test this idea led to the observation that song control is lateralized, as is language in humans. These observations stimulated the identification of brain sites of lateralization and auditory control of voice. Neurophysiological studies have shown that auditory information reaches the song control system. Lesions of the lateral magnocellular nucleus of the anterior neostriatum or area X affect song development in young birds, but not the maintenance of song in adults, which suggests this region acts as a site for song learning.

Isolation of behavioral components that contribute to the learning and production of song in birds has focused on the relationships between the vocal and respiratory systems. The temporal pattern of birdsong is primarily accomplished from the timing of activity in the bird's respiratory muscles. It appears that birds can simultaneously produce two different temporal patterns from the left and right halves of their vocal organ. The archistriatal and midbrain vocal nuclei in the brain innervate some of the respiratory centers in the medulla. Comparisons of the vocal and auditory systems between taxa indicate that different groups may use different neural circuits to achieve similar vocal–auditory behavior.

Now that the basic mechanisms of the actual control of birdsong learning and production are established, researchers will be able to perform interspecies comparisons of both the neurocircuitry and the genes involved in the generation of this complex behavior. Since this behavior is modifiable, analysis of birdsong at the genetic level may provide a model system for studies of the interaction between genetic and environmental factors.

HOW NOT TO BUILD THE BETTER MOUSE By studying a diverse set of gene mutations, important insights into the roles that the given gene product plays in the biological process may be gained. Gene mapping and gene manipulation studies in the mouse have yielded some of the most exciting findings in the genetic investigation of mammalian behavior. After years of studying various behavioral characters in the mouse using selective breeding techniques, it is clear that most are heritable and are specified by complexes of genes or quantitative trait loci (QTLs). The introduction of methods to perform highly efficient mutagenesis of the mouse germline has led to mutations that are of considerable value, including mutations of genes that have yet to be cloned or characterized. Once marked by such methods, these genes can be mapped to high resolution and then cloned. The use of primer templates based on a gene of interest that was characterized in another species has also provided a very productive method of cloning particularly important genes. Application of these approaches has resulted in the identification of the mouse gene for circadian periodicity, numerous neurotransmitter receptors, channels, and reuptake transporters. Gene mutations or knockouts can also be induced to yield animal models of human heritable diseases, as demonstrated with the partial knockout of glucocorticoid receptor function, gene knockouts of serotonin receptors, and knockout of dopamine transporters. Such disease models permit research into the etiology of the given disease and evaluation of potential therapeutic regimens. However, the difficulties inherent in constructing valid models of psychiatric diseases or addictive syndromes in lower mammals must be appreciated.

WARRIOR MICE: THE MOLECULAR GENETICS OF AGGRESSION Building on data derived from mouse lines selected for either nest-building behavior or attack latency, researchers are focusing in on the gene or genes that contribute to aggressive behavior. Several molecular genetic mouse lines have recently been created that display increased aggression. The first of these was produced by knockout of the monoamine oxidase-A (MAOA) gene. These animals were characterized by elevated brain serotonin and norepinephrine concentrations as pups, and as adults they displayed enhanced intermale aggression, attempts to mount nonreceptive females, and reduced immobility in the forced swim test. Interestingly, rats treated prenatally with an MAO inhibitor have a reduced cortical serotonergic innervation as adults and various alterations in serotonin levels during development. A deficit of central serotonin has been associated with impulsive violence, depression, suicidality and alcoholism. Mice with knockout of the gene encoding for α-calmodulin–dependent protein kinase II (CaMKII), an enzyme necessary for activation of tryptophan hydroxylase required for serotonin biosynthesis, also leads to increased defensive aggression. The next target for gene knockout was the 5-HT1B receptor, as previous studies indicated that agonists of this receptor reduced aggressive behavior. Indeed, mice lacking this receptor exhibited greatly increased intermale aggression (decreased latency to attack, increased number of attacks, increased intensity of attacks) in classical tests. These observations are consonant with neurochemical and behavioral data from studies of monkeys and humans. Somewhat surprising have been reports of increased aggression and lack of social inhibition in null mutant mice lacking the neural nitric oxide synthase gene. Overall, these observations support the thesis that there are likely to be multiple routes, both genetic and environmental, to hyperaggressive behavior.

RODENT ADDICTS Considerable effort has been directed toward identifying the genetic contributions to substance abuse behavior. Psychostimulant drugs are believed to primarily interact with monoaminergic neurons. Most research efforts in this field have focused on the analysis of those central dopaminergic circuits believed to serve as the substrate for reward, leading to the dopamine hypothesis of psychostimulant addiction. This hypothesis proposes that enhancement of dopamine neurotransmission in the mesolimbic pathway is fundamental to the reinforcing properties of many drugs of abuse.

One approach to studies of the genetic basis of substance abuse is to construct congenic animal lines with different mesotelencephalic dopamine systems, using selective breeding techniques. Then, genomic markers (QTLs) associated with sensitivity to alcohol or cocaine can be identified, thus allowing the candidate genes that demonstrate linkage to markers associated with these behaviors to be cloned by position. In addition, Southern blot hybridization techniques can be used to identify genetic polymorphisms of dopamine receptor subtype loci in mice and rats. In fact, polymorphisms of the D2, D3, and D4 dopamine receptor loci have been observed. The influence of the D2-like receptors in reward and addictive behaviors can be assessed by pharmacogenetic studies. Together, these approaches permit a molecular analysis of both known and previously unknown genes regulating various aspects (e.g., tolerance, sensitization, dependence, withdrawal) of substance abuse behavior. (An exceilent review of the current status of this research area may be found in Self and Nestler.)

A common screening technique to assess sensitivity to cocaine is to measure locomotor responses to drug administration. In this way, it has been possible to characterize the effects of cocaine on the dopamine transporter. Thus, central dopaminergic system involvement has been studied in different strains of mice that exhibit differential sensitivity to cocaine. In these studies, C57BL/6 mice were less activated than DBA/2 mice after cocaine, though both strains had equivalent brain cocaine concentrations at the times and doses tested. Interestingly, treatment with a selective dopamine uptake inhibitor produced greater locomotor activation in DBA/2 mice than in C57BL/6 mice, even though binding studies with a selective dopamine uptake ligand revealed no between-strain differences, in caudate putamen or nucleus accumbens Kd or Bmax. Specific D1 or D2 antagonists produced dose-dependent decreases in locomotor activity, again showing no between-strain differences and the D2 antagonist completely reversed cocaine-induced activation in both strains. These findings demonstrate that C57BL/6 and DBA/2 mice differ in dopamine-related behaviors and suggest that dopaminergic processes may mediate genetic differences in cocaine sensitivity. Recent work in rats has confirmed the importance of dopamine receptors in substance abuse, as priming with a D2 agonist triggered relapse of self-administration behavior, whereas treatment with a D1 agonist inhibited this drug-seeking behavior.

The dopamine transporter represents an important regulator of dopaminergic activity. Cocaine, one of the best characterized of the psychostimulant drugs, fulfills the dopamine hypothesis by blocking the dopamine transporter and, thus, by preventing reuptake of the neurotransmitter, enhancing its synaptic concentration. A good concordance exists between binding of cocaine analogs to the dopamine transporter and changes in locomotor activity. Abundant data suggest that vulnerability to both the toxic and addictive effects of cocaine may be significantly influenced by genetic differences in both humans and animals. Even within the brain, differences in the dopamine transported are apparent. This difference may arise from differences in glycosylation of the polypeptide. The observation that cocaine is commonly abused along with other drugs has given rise to the hypothesis that common biochemical pathways may mediate the reinforcing or addictive properties of drugs of abuse. Of particular interest is the recent creation of a dopamine transporter knockout mouse line. Studies of these animals clearly demonstrate the importance of the dopamine transporter to overall function of central dopmaninergic circuits. In the knockout animals, evoked dopamine remains in the region of the synaptic cleft approximately 100 times longer than in normal mice. Furthermore, the knockout mice do not respond to cocaine, supporting the postulate that the primary site of cocaine's action is at the transporter. This animal model, along with those created with partial knockouts or transporter mutants, should be quite helpful in elucidating the basis for substance abuse, as well as for testing putative therapeutic approaches.

THE HYPOTHALAMIC-PITUITARY-ADRENAL AXIS, CUSHING'S DISEASE, AND DEPRESSION IN RODENTS

Patients with a number of psychiatric disorders exhibit profound disturbances of hypothalamic-pituitary-adrenal (HPA) axis function. Patients with severe depression often show evidence of increased HPA axis activity, such as a premature escape from the cortisol suppressant action of the synthetic glucocorticoid dexamethasone, elevations of cerebrospinal fluid levels of corticotropin releasing factor (CRF), and increased adenohypophysial and adrenal volumes. It is currently unknown whether these changes are primarily the result of defective glucocorticoid feedback inhibition or inappropriate secretion of CRF and/or arginine vasopressin. However, it is clear that normalization of the hyperactive HPA system occurs during successful antidepressant pharmacotherapy of depressive illness. Both elevation of CRF and of glucocorticoids are associated with signs and symptoms resembling depression in both humans and animals, giving rise to the idea that HPA axis dysfunction may precede the onset of depressive illness.

The connection between HPA axis dysfunction and depression has been tested in numerous animal models, including chronic exposure to stress, maternal separation, a transgenic model of CRF overexpression, and a transgenic model of partial glucocorticoid receptor knockout.

The hypothalamic peptide CRF is released in response to various stressors and increases pituitary adrenocorticotropin secretion, which then drives adrenal glucocorticoid production. Extrahypothalamic CRF serves as a neurotransmitter/neuromodulator and has been shown to play an important role in behavioral responses to stress. The transgenic mouse model of CRF overproduction was developed to examine the endocrine and behavioral effects of chronic CRF excess. These transgenic mice CRF display the expected endocrine abnormalities of the HPA axis, such as elevated plasma levels of ACTH and glucocorticoids. The CRF transgenics also exhibited an increase in anxiogenic behavior, an effect known to occur following central administration of CRF in animals, which was partially reversed by administration of a CRF antagonist. Continuing studies of these animals suggests that CRF transgenics and related transgenics such as CRF promotor mutants and CRF receptor mutants may provide a valuable tool for investigating the long-term effects of dysregulation of central CRF neurocircuits.

Another interesting transgenic mouse model was created by expression of a type II glucocorticoid receptor antisense RNA in the brain that results in impairment of glucocorticoid receptor function. These mice display endocrinological characteristics similar to those seen in depression, including hyperactivity of the HPA axis and resistance to dexamethasone negative feedback. When treated with the tricyclic antidepressant desipramine, hypothalamic glucocorticoid receptor mRNA concentration and binding activity increased. At the same time, circulating levels of adrenocorticotropin hormone and corticosterone decreased. These studies suggest that antidepressants affect HPA axis activity via modulation of glucocorticoid receptor gene expression; however, such studies do prove that this is a direct effect rather than an indirect action mediated through changes in other factors (i.e., neurotransmitters, G-proteins, neurotrophic factors) that secondarily alter glucocorticoid receptor expression. Nonetheless, this animal model represents an important advance in our understanding of the interactions between the HPA axis and depression and certainly warrants further study.

DISCUSSION

Psychiatry, like much of the rest of medicine, has entered a new and exciting age demarcated by the rapid advances and the promise of molecular biology and neuroscience. This promise is presaged by the ability to generate knockout (e.g., null mutant) and overexpression transgenic organisms for the study of specific genes (*vide supra*). In addition, some success has been realized in the elucidation of molecular mechanisms underlying several brain disorders that lie at the intersection of neurology and psychiatry, including identification of mutations on chromosomes 1, 14, and 21, which appear to be associated with the early onset, dominantly inherited form of Alzheimer's Disease and a mutant gene on chromosome 4 associated with Huntington's Disease; unfortunately neither of these diseases is currently treatable.

Progress at the molecular level has furthered our understanding of phenylketonuria (PKU), a well-characterized disease that can be readily treated if identified by early screening. PKU, a classic example of success in the prevention of a genetic disease, is a genetic disorder in which an inborn error of metabolism (e.g., disruption of the hydroxylation of phenylalanine to tyrosine) leads to mental retardation if left untreated. Treatment is a relatively straightforward matter of removing phenylalanine from the diet beginning soon after birth. At least five known genes, which have been cloned, are involved in hydroxylation of phenylalanine, synthesis of tetrahybrobiopterin, and regeneration of this cofactor. More than 170 mutations of the human phenylalanine hydroxylase gene have been identified, and these account for approximately 99% of the mutations causing hyperphenylalaninemia. The aggregate PKU gene frequency is polymorphic in many human populations with the mutations highly stratified by region and population, thus reflecting a variety of mechanisms (i.e., founder effect, genetic drift, hypermutability, selection) for their occurrence and distribution. These studies have served notice that the relationship between genotype and clinical outcome is more complex than was originally suspected and is a function of multiple effects.

The enthusiasm for the promise presented by a molecular approach to understanding mechanisms of behavior and psychopathology, however, must be tempered by the recognition that the brain is an exceedingly complex organ shaped by more than the mere unfolding of a proscribed genetic program. Substantial evidence indicates that intrinsic and extrinsic environmental factors play a major role in the transition from genotype to phenotype. Perhaps the most compelling and well-documented example in neuroscience concerns the functional reorganization of the visual cortex in response to visual deprivation during development, a principle known as activity-dependent plasticity. Such activity-dependent plasticity fine tunes the basic genetically specified pattern of neuronal connectivity, thus assigning "weights" to particular neurocircuits in a process that may turn out to be either adaptive or maladaptive.

While the ability to engineer organisms that either over- or underexpress a particular gene has led to impressive advances in studies of the molecular basis of behavior and disease; these studies also highlight the remarkable adaptability of the brain to the absence of proteins that are believed to play critical roles in synaptic signaling. In the case of the null mutant paradigm, it must be appreciated that the knockout organism represents not only the absence of a single gene product, but potential compensatory alterations in a number of developmental, physiological, or even behavioral processes. These compensatory mechanisms might result in either the absence of an expected phenotypic change or the expression of phenotypic abnormalities, which then may be mistakenly attributed to the null mutation. Furthermore, these putative compensations depend, not only on the targeted gene, but also on the background genotype of the animal. Thus, studies that claim to demonstrate a linkage between a single gene mutation and a complex behavior, as recently claimed in studies suggesting that a polymorphism of the D4 dopamine receptor gene on the short arm of chromosome 11 accounted for approximately 10% of the genetic variation in the trait referred to as "novelty seeking," must be viewed with some degree of skepticism. The overall message, then, is that caution is warranted when inferring a tight relationship between a single gene and a particular behavioral phenotype or psychopathology, given the ability of the brain to compensate for deficits during development and its ability to modify synaptic connectivity as a function of experience.

Molecular forays into the basis of behavior and neural disorders is a very young field and is likely to hold many surprises. For instance, it has now been established that mutations and deletions of genes encoded in mitochondrial DNA cause heritable CNS disorders that do not follow simple Mendelian genetics. The extent to which genetic defects in mitochondrial DNA contribute to human disease is currently unknown. The mechanism of anticipation, a phenomenon in which each succeeding generation of affected individuals exhibits an earlier age of disease onset, eluded explanation for many years. This phenomenon is now attributed to the progressive expansion of trinucleotide repeats in mutant genes of successive generations.

The molecular genetic approach will undoubtedly yield important insights into the biological mechanisms underlying normal and abnormal brain function and behavior. However, it should be appreciated that the primary virtue of this approach lies in deciphering general principles of the biological organization of the brain and behavior rather than revealing the linkage between single genes and complex behaviors. Behavioral and neurobiological traits are complex, likely to be variable, and influenced by a large number of genes and environmental factors. In fact, it can be argued that the development of the CNS and emergent qualities, such as an individual organism's behavioral phenotype, are best described as complex nonlinear processes. This line of reasoning suggests that when contemplating complex functions such as behavior, we might need to look for fundamental units of organization larger than that of single genes alone. In fact, the precedent for such a paradigm shift is evident in the neuroscience where the focus has changed from the analysis of the characteristics of single neurons to neurocircuit analysis or the analysis of shifting populations of neurons when attempting to understand mechanisms underlying complex behaviors or processing tasks. The single gene, as the single neuron, represents a potentiality, the expression of which is highly dependent on its interactions with the local environment. Therefore, it would not be unreasonable to expect that groups of genes specified by some higher level of organization might represent the functionally relevant unit in determining a behavioral phenotype. In this scenario, some genes might belong to more than one functional gene group, much as a single neuron may belong to multiple neurocircuits. This sharing of "valence" genes or neurons might provide an intrinsic mechanism for integration of multimodal information. Furthermore, this type of organization, whether one is referring to neurons or to genes, implies a hierarchical organization of functional groups necessary for the generation of emergent qualities.

A number of interesting predictions may be made on the basis of such an organizational scheme. For instance, the mutation of a single gene within a functional gene group may be important as a trigger to alter expression levels of other genes within a group in a coordinated fashion. Identification of these cascades in gene expression might lead to insights into inherent features of CNS organization and of constellations of genes or gene groups that specify a complex phenotype, whether it be temperament or some other heritable aspect of behavior. As stated by Gerlai, "Genes, especially as they affect brain function, are not expressed in a vacuum but rather in the rich personal context of individual experience. Perhaps, the most important contribution of research in molecular aspects of psychiatry will be the characterization of the intrinsic vulnerabilities to psychiatric disorders so that we can, for the first time, have control over one variable in the complex simultaneous equation of Nature and Nurture that shapes brain and behavior." If the molecular genetic approach to studies of brain and behavior moves in this direction, then medicine and psychiatry are indeed headed into an exciting new age, likely to be characterized by tremendous advances leading to the reduction of needless human suffering — this represents the great promise and the beginning of a long journey.

SELECTED REFERENCES

Bailey CH, Alberini C, Ghirardi M, Kandel ER. Molecular and structural changes underlying long-term memory storage in Aplysia. Adv Second Messenger Phosphoprotein Res 1994;29:529–544.

Barinaga M. Missing Alzheimer's gene found. Nature 1995;269:917,918.

Beaulieu S, Rousse I, Gratton A, Barden N, Rochford J. Behavioral and endocrine impact of impaired type II glucocorticoid receptor function in a transgenic mouse model. Ann NY Acad Sci 1994;746:388–391.

Benjamin J, Li L, Patterson C, Greenberg BD, Murphy DL, Hamer DH. Population and familial association between the D4 dopamine receptor gene and measures of novelty seeking. Nat Genet 1996;12:81–84.

Bhatnagar S, Shanks N, Plotsky PM, Meaney MJ. Hypothalamic-pituitary-adrenal responses to stress in neonatally handled and nonhandled rats: differences in facilitatory and inhibitory neural pathways. In: McCarty R, Aguilera G, Sabban E, Kvetnansky R, eds. Stress: Molecular Genetic and Neurobiological Advances. New York: Gordon and Beach, 1996.

Black I. Trophic interactions and brain plasticity. In: Gazzaniga, MS, ed. The Cognitive Neurosciences. Cambridge, MA: MIT Press, 1995;9–17.

Cases O, Seif I, Grimsby J, et al. Aggressive behavior and altered amounts of brain serotonin and norepinephrine in mice lacking MAOA. Science 1995;268:1763–1766.

Caskey CT, Pizzuti A, Fu YH, Fenwick RG, Jr, Nelson DL. Triplet repeat mutations in human disease. Science 1992;256:784–787.

Chen D, Rainnie DG, Greene RW, Tonegawa S. Abnormal fear response and aggressive behavior in mutant mice deficient for α-calcium-calmodulin kinase II. Science 1994;266:291–294.

Ebstein RP, Novick O, Umansky R, et al. Dopamine D4 receptor (D4DR) exon III polymorphism associated with the human personality trait of Novelty Seeking. Nat Genet 1996;12:78–80.

Eichelmann B. Aggressive behavior: from laboratory to clinic quo vadit? Arch Gen Psychiatry 1992;49:488–492.

Ferrus A, Canal I. The behaving brain of a fly. Trends Neurosci 1994;17:479–486.

Gerlai R. Gene-targeting studies of mammalian behavior: Is it the mutation or the background genotype? TINS 1996;19:177–181, 188,189.

Giros B, Jaber M, Jones SR, Wightman RM, Caron MG. Hyperlocomotion and indifference to cocaine and amphetamine in mice lacking the dopamine transporter. Nature 1996;379:606–612.

Greenspan RJ. Understanding the genetic construction of behavior. Sci Am 1995;272:72–78.

Hall JC. The mating of a fly. Science 1994;264:1702–1714.

Hawkins RD, Kandel ER, Siegelbaum SA. Learning to modulate transmitter release: Themes and variations in synaptic plasticity. Ann Rev Neurosci 1993;16:625–665.

Hen R. Mean genes. Neuron 1996;16:17–21.

Hirsch HV, Tompkins L. The flexible fly: experience-dependent development of complex behaviors in Drosophila melanogaster. J Exp Biol 1994;195:1–18.

Hubel DH, Wiesel TN, LeVay S. Plasticity of ocular dominance columns in monkey striate cortex. Philos Trans Roy Soc Lond [Biol] 1977;278:377–409.

Huntington's Disease Collaborative Research Group. A novel gene containing a trinucleotide repeat that is expanded and unstable on Huntington's Disease chromosome. Cell 1993;72:971–983.

Hyman SE, Nestler EJ. The Molecular Foundations of Psychiatry. Washington: American Psychiatric, 1993; pp. 173–191, 193–224.

Konishi M. An outline of recent advances in birdsong neurobiology. Brain Behav Evol 1994b;44:279–285.

Konishi M. Pattern generation in birdsong. Curr Opin Neurobiol 1994a;4:827–331.

Kupfermann I. Genetic determinants of behavior. In: Kandel ER, Schwartz JH, Jessell TM, eds. Principles of Neural Science, 3rd ed. New York: Elsevier, 1991; pp. 987–996.

Kyriacou CP, Hall JC. Genetic and molecular analysis of Drosophila behavior. Adv Genet 1994;31:139–186.

McDonald JD. Using high-efficiency mouse germline mutagenesis to investigate complex biological phenomena: genetic diseases, behavior, and development. Proc Soc Exp Biol Med 1995;209:303–308.

McEwen BS. Stressful experience, brain, and emotions: Developmental, genetic, and hormonal influences. In: Gazzaniga MS, ed. The Cognitive Neurosciences. Cambridge, MA: MIT, 1995; 1117–1135.

McInnes LA, Freimer NB. Mapping genes for psychiatric disorders and behavioral traits. Curr Opin Genet Dev 1995;5:376–381.

Muller U, Aguet M, Babinet C, Shih JC, De Maeyer E. Aggressive behavior and altered amounts of brain serotonin and norepinephrine in mice lacking MAOA. Science 1995;268:1763–1766.

Nelson RJ, Demas GE, Huang PL, et al. Behavioral abnormalities in male mice lacking neuronal nitric oxide synthase. Nature 1995;378:383–386.

Osborne KA, Robichon A, Burgess E, et al. Natural behavior polymorphism due to a cGMP-dependent protein kinase of Drosophila. Science 1997;277:834–836.

Owens MJ, Nemeroff CB. The role of corticotropin-releasing factor in the pathophysiology of affective and anxiety disorders: laboratory and clinical studies. Ciba Found Symp 1993;172:296–308.

Pennisi E. What makes fruit flies roam? Science 1997;277:763–764.

Pepin MC, Pothier F, Barden N. Antidepressant drug action in a transgenic mouse model of the endocrine changes seen in depression. Mol Pharmacol 1992;42:991–995.

Pepin MC, Pothier F, Barden N. Impaired type II glucocorticoid-receptor function in mice bearing antisense RNA transgene. Nature 1992; 355:725–728.

Petronis A, Kennedy JL. Unstable genes—unstable mind? Am J Psychiatry 1995;152:164–172.

Phillips TJ, Crabbe JC, Metten P, Belknap JK. Localization of genes affecting alcohol drinking in mice. Alcohol Clin Exp Res 1994;18:931–941.

Plomin R. The role of inheritance in behavior. Science 1990;248:183–188.

Post RM. Molecular biology of behavior. Targets for therapeutics. Arch Gen Psychiatry 1997;54:607,608.

Ramboz S, Saudou F, Ait Amara D, et al. 5-HT1B receptor knock out-behavioral consequences. Behav Brain Res 1996;73:305–312.

Ritz MC, Kuhar MJ. Psychostimulant drugs and a dopamine hypothesis regarding addiction: update on recent research. Biochem Soc Symp 1993;59:51–64.

Saudou F, Ait Amara D, Dierich A, et al. Enhanced aggressive behavior in mice lacking 5-HT_{1B} receptor. Science 1994;265:1875–1878.

Scott AW, Griffin SA, Luedtke RR. Genetic polymorphisms at the rat and murine loci coding for dopamine D2-like receptors. Mol Brain Res 1995;29:347–357.

Scriver CR. Whatever happened to PKU? Clin Biochem 1995;28:137–144.

Self DW, Barnhart WJ, Lehman DA, Nestler EJ. Opposite modulation of cocaine-seeking behavior by D1- and D2-like dopamine receptor agonists. Science 1996;271:1586–1589.

Self DW, Nestler EJ. Molecular mechanisms of drug reinforcement and addiction. Ann Rev Neurosci 1995;18:463–495.

Sluyter F, Bult A, Lynch CB, van Oortmerssen GA, Koolhaas JM. A comparison between house mouse lines selected for attack latency or nest-building: evidence for a genetic basis of alternative behavioral strategies. Behav Genet 1995;25:247–252.

Stenzel-Poore MP, Heinrichs SC, Rivest S, Koob GF, Vale WW. Overproduction of corticotropin-releasing factor in transgenic mice: a genetic model of anxiogenic behavior. J Neurosci 1994;14:2579–2584.

Taylor BJ, Villella A, Ryner LC, Baker BS, Hall JC. Behavioral and neurobiological implications of sex-determining factors in Drosophila. Dev Genet 1994;15:275–296.

Tolliver BK, Belknap JK, Woods WE, Carney JM. Genetic analysis of sensitization and tolerance to cocaine. J Pharmacol Exp Ther 1994;270:1230–1238.

Vadasz C, Kobor G, Lajtha A. Motor activity and the mesotelencephalic dopamine function. I. High-resolution temporal and genetic analysis of open-field behavior. Behav Brain Res 1992;48:29–39.

Wallace DT, Lott MT, Shoffner JM, Ballinger S. Mitochondrial DNA mutations in epilepsy and neurological disease. Epilepsia 1994; 35:543–550.

Weiss F, Hurd YL, Ungerstedt U, Markou A, Plotsky PM, Koob GF. Neurochemical correlates of cocaine and ethanol self-administration. Ann N Y Acad Sci 1992;654:220–241.

Whitaker-Azmitia PM, Druse M, Walker P, Lauder JM. Serotonin as a developmental signal. Behav Brain Res 1996;19–29.

Willner P. Animal models of depression: validity and applications. Adv Biochem Psychopharmacol 1995;49:19–41.

Womer DE, Jones BC, Erwin VG. Characterization of dopamine transporter and locomotor effects of cocaine, GBR 12909, epidepride, and SCH 23390 in C57BL and DBA mice. Pharmacol Biochem Behav 1994;48:327–335.

109 Schizophrenia

Ming T. Tsuang and Stephen V. Faraone

INTRODUCTION

Psychiatry, with the rest of medicine, has entered the age of molecular genetics, but we are far from the stage of molecular diagnosis or treatment. Although schizophrenia researchers have produced suggestive evidence implicating specific chromosomal loci, the molecular genetic basis of the disease remains a mystery: Its mode of inheritance is unknown, and the loci that have been implicated are unlikely to account for a substantial proportion of the disease's etiology. In contrast, family, twin, and adoption studies have taught us much about the genetic epidemiology of schizophrenia. In doing so, they have provided a solid foundation for a new generation of molecular studies that promise to unravel the genetics of this complex disorder.

FAMILY STUDIES

Many of the studies from the first half of the twentieth century were completed prior to the creation of structured diagnostic criteria. These early studies showed the following risks for schizophrenia to relatives of schizophrenic probands: parents, 5.6%; siblings, 10.1%; offspring, 12.8%. Note that the risk to parents is less than the risk to siblings, yet most genetic models predict that these risks would be similar. It is relatively uncommon for schizophrenic people to marry and have children. When both parents had schizophrenia, the risk to children was much greater (36.6%). In the early studies, the risks to second-degree relatives ranged from 4.2% for half-siblings to 2.4% for uncles and aunts. First cousins had an average risk of 2.4%. Because the risk for schizophrenia in the general population was 0.8%, these familial risk figures are strongly suggestive of an important genetic component in the transmission of schizophrenia.

Compared with these early reports, more recent studies used more rigorous research methods and narrower, criterion-based definitions of schizophrenia. Overall, these studies confirm the familial nature of schizophrenia, but they report risk figures that are lower than those seen in earlier studies. For example, Tsuang, Winokur, and Crowe reported the risk of schizophrenia to first-degree relatives of schizophrenics to be 3.2%, compared with 0.6% for relatives of nonpsychiatric controls. Guze, Cloninger, Martin, and Clayton reported comparable figures of 3.6 and 0.56%, respectively. In both studies, the increased risk for schizophrenia among relatives of schizophrenics remained statistically significant despite the lower prevalence figures.

From: *Principles of Molecular Medicine* (J. L. Jameson, ed.), ©1998 Humana Press Inc., Totowa, NJ.

The reduced prevalence rates of schizophrenia in the more recent studies are probably because of differences in diagnostic procedures. For example, the figure of 3.2%, obtained when using stringent Washington University criteria, increases to 7.8% if the schizophrenia category is broadened to include atypical schizophrenics (e.g., schizoaffective disorder, psychosis not otherwise specified). Thus, the risk figures for schizophrenia based on modern criteria are similar to the figures obtained by the earlier European studies when atypical cases are included.

The exclusion of atypical schizophrenia cases from family studies may also explain why two family studies failed to find familial transmission in schizophrenia. Pope et al. found no cases of schizophrenia among first-degree relatives of their schizophrenic probands. Abrams and Taylor found the risk for schizophrenia to be only 1.6% among 128 first-degree relatives of schizophrenics. Although certain methodological problems may explain these results, it is also possible that they are because of diagnostic practices. Despite the caveats noted, contemporary figures as well as those reported in earlier studies suggest that the risk for schizophrenia in first-degree relatives exceeds the observed rate in the general population by 5–10 times. Of course, environmental factors can also cause familial transmission. Thus, twin and adoption studies must be examined to verify that genes—not the environment—underlie the familial transmission of schizophrenia.

TWIN STUDIES

After pooling the results of extant twin studies, Kendler found concordance rates of 53% for monozygotic (MZ) twin pairs and 15% for dyzygotic (DZ) twin pairs. This strongly implicates a genetic component for schizophrenia. Yet, the concordance rate for MZ twin pairs is not 100%; thus, environmental factors must play a crucial role in the etiology of schizophrenia. When concordance rates are translated into "heritabilities" (the proportion of the liability to schizophrenia resulting from genetic factors), 70% of the variance is attributed to genetic factors. Thus, there is a substantial role for environmental factors in the expression of schizophrenia. Several possibilities exist. Some forms of schizophrenia could be caused completely by environmental factors such as birth complications or viral infection. Alternatively, it may be that all cases of schizophrenia require a genetic susceptibility that is only expressed in some environmental circumstances.

A nongenetic explanation for the schizophrenia twin data is that MZ twins are exposed to more similar environmental factors than DZ twins. This hypothesis can be tested by looking at twins raised in different environments. A high concordance rate for monozygotic twin pairs reared apart would refute the theory that sharing the same predisposing environment leads to the higher concordance rate in monozygotic twin pairs. Among the 17 such monozygotic twin pairs that have been observed, 11 (65%) were concordant for schizophrenia. This strengthens the hypothesis that both genes and environment play a causal role in the development of schizophrenia.

ADOPTION STUDIES

Adoption studies can disentangle genetic and environmental sources of etiology by showing if biological or adoptive relationships explain the familial transmission of disease. Heston examined 47 children who had been separated from their biological schizophrenic mothers within 3 days of birth. These children were raised by adoptive parents with whom they had no biological relationship. He also examined a control group of 50 persons who had been separated from nonschizophrenic mothers. Both groups studied were adults at the time of examination. If genes caused schizophrenia, then the biological children of schizophrenic mothers should have a higher risk for schizophrenia, regardless of who raised them as children. In contrast, if the parenting relationship caused schizophrenia, then separating children from a schizophrenic parent should prevent them from having schizophrenia. Heston's results supported a genetic etiology of schizophrenia: Five children of schizophrenic mothers became schizophrenic; in contrast, none of the children of nonschizophrenic mothers became schizophrenic.

Kety et al. carried out adoption studies of schizophrenia in Denmark. In the Greater Copenhagen area, 5500 children had been separated from their biological families by adoption between 1923 and 1947. Of these children, 33 who later became schizophrenic were studied along with 33 nonschizophrenic adoptees. The investigators examined the biological relatives of these schizophrenic and nonschizophrenic adoptees. They diagnosed 21% of the biological relatives of schizophrenic adoptees with schizophrenia or a related disorder. In contrast, only 11% of the biological relatives of nonschizophrenics had schizophrenia. There were no differences in rates of schizophrenia between the adoptive relatives of the schizophrenic and nonschizophrenic adoptees. One component of the Kety et al.'s study was similar to Heston's study. Children born to schizophrenic families but raised by nonschizophrenic families were compared with children born to, and raised by, nonschizophrenic parents. Schizophrenia and related disorders were found in 32% of the former group but only in 18% of the latter group.

Kety et al.'s sample also included some persons who had been born of nonschizophrenic parents but raised by a schizophrenic parent. If the fact of being reared by a schizophrenic parent caused schizophrenia, then these persons should be likely to suffer from schizophrenia. However, this was not so: Being raised by a schizophrenic parent did not predict schizophrenia in children who were not genetically predisposed to the disorder (i.e., who did not have a schizophrenic biological parent).

The adoption studies show that genetic factors mediate the transmission of schizophrenia. However, these studies also have some limitations. Most importantly, although the adopted children had been separated from the mother soon after birth, they had spent 9 months in the mother's uterus. During that time, the mother could have transmitted to the fetus some nongenetic biological or psychosocial factor that might have resulted in the child's schizophrenia 15 years later.

Fortunately, the Danish researchers could examine whether or not *in utero* influences might have explained their results. Kety et al. found that 13% of paternal half siblings of schizophrenic adoptees had schizophrenia compared with only 2% of paternal half siblings of nonschizophrenic adoptees. Paternal half siblings have different mothers. Therefore, these results cannot be explained by in utero effects. Indeed, the fact that a higher rate of schizophrenia was found among these half-siblings from the father's side, than in the half-siblings of the controls, is compelling evidence for the genetic basis of schizophrenia.

QUANTITATIVE MODELS OF GENETIC TRANSMISSION

A classic Mendelian model of inheritance will not adequately describe the genetic transmission of schizophrenia. Thus, more complex models are needed to describe the genetic transmission of the disorder. Quantitative or mathematical modeling studies provide a strategy for doing so. Such studies are discussed briefly below.

Single major locus models (SMLs) propose that the pair of genes present at a single locus is responsible for the transmission of schizophrenia. Results of SML analyses have not consistently supported single-gene transmission. SML models accurately predict the general population prevalence, the prevalence in offspring of schizophrenics, and the prevalence in siblings of schizophrenics. However, segregation analyses that provide statistical tests of model adequacy reject single-gene transmission. Those that cannot rule out the model note that the rate of schizophrenia among the MZ co-twins of schizophrenic patients and the offspring of two schizophrenics are underpredicted by the SML model.

The failure to find an SML model that unequivocally accounts for the familial transmission of schizophrenia has led to the testing of polygenic models. These models assume that genes found at more than one locus are responsible for the familial pattern of the disorder. There are two types of polygenic models. Oligogenic models postulate a relatively limited number of loci (e.g., less than 10), whereas multifactorial polygenic (MFP) models propose a large, unspecified number of loci (e.g., more than 100).

Studies that compared SML and oligogenic models agree that there are no dramatic differences between their abilities to account for the familial transmission of schizophrenia. Further, the oligogenic models are similar to the SML model in predicting that the majority of individuals with the schizophrenic genotype will not develop schizophrenia. Simulation studies by Risch suggest that multilocus models including gene interactions may be needed to account for the familial pattern of illness in schizophrenia. Notably, the rate of schizophrenia among the MZ co-twins of schizophrenic patients (which is underpredicted by SML models) is correctly predicted by oligogenic models that include a small number of genes that interact with one another.

Unlike oligogenic models, MFP models do not specify the number of loci involved in schizophrenia. Instead they assume that there are many interchangeable loci; genes at these loci have small, additive effects on the individuals predisposition for schizophrenia. This model assumes that all individuals have some unobservable "liability" or predisposition to develop schizophrenia. Gottesman and Shields noted five points in favor of MFP models. First, like other MFP disorders, schizophrenia is found with varying severities. Second, the risk for schizophrenia is greater for persons with many schizophrenic relatives than for persons with few schizophrenic relatives. Third, the risk to a person increases as a function of the severity of a schizophrenic relative's illness. Fourth, nonschizophrenic individuals from the schizophrenia spectrum can be conceptualized as having a liability close to but not exceeding the threshold for schizophrenia. Finally, MFP disorders are expected to respond slowly to natural selection. Further, as discussed above, the SML model underpredicts the rate of schizophrenia among the MZ co-twins of schizophrenic patients. Thus, the twin studies of schizophrenia are consistent with the MFP model.

Overall, the MFP results are more promising than the SML results. In particular, path analytic MFP studies support the hypothesis that schizophrenia is to a large extent a disorder with a mostly genetic multifactorial etiology. Under this model, genetic factors account for 60–70% of the familial pattern of schizophrenia. Environmental factors are important to a much lesser degree. Overall, the results suggest that the MFP model deserves serious consideration. These results cannot rule out, however, the possibility of a mixed model in which an SML component and a MFP component both exist. However, attempts to fit such a mixed model have not been able to determine the mode of transmission.

THE SEARCH FOR GENES

In the 1980s, some preliminary findings implicated a gene on the short arm of chromosome 5. Interest in this area was initially motivated by the report of a single family in which two cases of schizophrenia each had a distinct abnormality of this chromosome. Subsequently, Sherrington et al. studied seven British and Icelandic families having schizophrenia in at least three generations. These investigators demonstrated genetic linkage to the part of chromosome 5 that had been previously implicated. Taken together, these two findings suggested that a schizophrenia gene would be found.

Unfortunately, other linkage studies could not replicate this linkage finding and some clearly excluded the chromosome 5 locus as being involved in schizophrenia. What can we make of these conflicting results? Some argued that, if more than one gene can cause schizophrenia, then both the positive and the negative findings can be correct. However, as more and more studies fail to find linkage to chromosome 5, it becomes more reasonable to conclude that the original positive finding may be a false result resulting from the play of chance. This now seems likely given that the group that produced the original finding of linkage found that evidence for it diminished when they extended their original sample.

Recent data implicated a pseudoautosomal locus in the etiology of schizophrenia. The pseudoautosomal region is a small portion of the Y chromosome that crosses over with the X chromosome during meiosis. If a gene from the pseudo-autosomal region causes schizophrenia, we would expect the following pattern of sex-specific transmission. Pairs of siblings with schizophrenia should be more likely to have the same sex if their father is schizophrenic but no such sex concordance is expected if the mother is schizophrenic. Since this pattern was found among schizophrenic families, the pseudoautosomal region was proposed to be the locus for a schizophrenia gene. In subsequent work, support for the pseudoautosomal hypothesis was inconsistent. Crow et al. showed that the estimated recombination fraction at the putative pseudoautosomal locus was greater for females compared with males, a fact that was not consistent with the known greater recombination fraction for males in the pseudoautosomal region. Thus, the same group suggested that a schizophrenia gene might reside in a nearby sex-specific region of the X and Y chromosomes. Their linkage analysis found some support for a dominant X-Y model of transmission in which homologous genes on X and Y contributed to the genetic susceptibility to schizophrenia.

A locus for schizophrenia on the sex chromosomes had also been suggested by cytogenetic studies. As reviewed by DeLisi et al., this work shows that schizophrenic patients have increased rates of the sex chromosome aneuploidies XXX and XXY. Other anomalies include long Y chromosomes, duplications in the heterochromatin regions of some chromosomes, inversion of a chromosome 9 region, fragile sites on chromosomes 9, 17, and 3, and trisomies of chromosomes 5 and 8. Since those reviews, Nanko et al. reported an association between schizophrenia and pericentric inversion of chromosome 9, Malaspina et al. described an association between schizophrenia and partial trisomy of chromosome 5p, and another study found a balanced 6:11 chromosomal translocation in a three-generation family with psychosis.

Although the available literature suggests that cytogenetic abnormalities cause some cases of schizophrenia, these abnormalities must account for only a small fraction of all schizophrenia. Some studies report no chromosome anomalies among patients with schizophrenia, and all positive studies report relatively low rates. For example, based on their review of ten studies that comprised 7519 patients, DeLisi et al. estimated the prevalence of sex chromosome anomalies among schizophrenic patients to be 0.5%.

A potential linkage to chromosome 22 has also generated much interest. Pulver et al. suggested the possibility of linkage to the long arm of chromosome 22, and consistent findings were reported by other investigators. However, a collaborative study reported by Pulver et al. excluded linkage to chromosome 22 loci, and another study could not find evidence of linkage. In addition, an association study to a marker at 22q12 found evidence for linkage disequilibrium with schizophrenia. Recently, Gill et al. reported a combined analysis of 11 schizophrenia linkage data sets. As a group, these data provided statistically significant evidence for linkage. However, their analyses also suggested that the putative schizophrenia gene would account for no more than 2% of the liability to develop the disorder.

The studies of chromosome 22 provide hope that the molecular genetic basis of schizophrenia will be uncovered. It seems likely that several genes in an oligogenic system may account for the genetic contribution to the disorder. In this regard, it is also notable that potential linkages have been reported to chromosomes 3p and 8p and also to the short arm of chromosome 5. Moreover, recent evidence implicated a schizophrenia gene on chromosome 6p in a series of 186 Irish schizophrenia families collected by Kendler et al. Findings consistent with their work have subsequently been reported, although not consistently.

SCHIZOPHRENIA-RELATED CONDITIONS

The available molecular genetic data suggest that multiple genes may cause schizophrenia. If so, then they might not be detectable without reducing measurement error and creating measures that more directly assess the genotype and its biological or behavioral consequences. Genetic epidemiological studies suggest that there are other disorders and conditions that are caused by the same genes that cause schizophrenia. Schizophrenia-related psychiatric disorders have been called "schizophrenia spectrum disorders" to convey the idea of a spectrum of disorders related to schizophrenia. Likewise, we use the term "neurobiologic spectrum disorders" to refer to measures of brain functioning that are not psychiatric disorders, but can be considered to be evidence of abnormal brain function related to the schizophrenia genotype. The criterion for defining a disorder as in the schizophrenia spectrum is straightforward: It must occur more frequently among the biological relatives of schizophrenic patients than the relatives of people who do not have schizophrenia. This provides some evidence that their expression is mediated by one or more of the genes that also lead to schizophrenia.

PSYCHIATRIC SPECTRUM DISORDERS Approximately 9% of the first-degree relatives of schizophrenic patients will have a psychotic disorder that does not meet criteria for either schizophrenia or a mood disorder. The most common of these are "schizoaffective disorder" and "psychosis, not otherwise specified (NOS)." Notably, schizoaffective disorder is also found among the relatives of patients with bipolar disorder. This has led some investigators to conclude that schizophrenia and bipolar disorder may have genes in common. In this view, the two disorders are at opposite ends of a "continuum of psychosis" and the schizoaffective patients lie in the middle. This idea is controversial and is now the subject of much research.

In addition to these psychotic disorders, psychiatrists have observed for many years that the relatives of schizophrenic patients had "eccentric personalities." They also noticed poor social relations, anxiety in social situations, and limited emotional responses among the family members of schizophrenics. Less frequently observed were mild forms of thought-disorder, suspiciousness, magical thinking, illusions, and perceptual aberrations.

Psychiatric genetic researchers have focused on the familial prevalence of three disorders: schizotypal, schizoid, and paranoid personality disorders. Numerous studies have documented the increased prevalence of schizotypal personality disorder (SPD) in the biological relatives of chronic schizophrenic probands. These results have demonstrated consistency across family studies, adoption studies, and twin studies. Although two studies failed to find a higher rate of SPD among relatives of schizophrenic probands, most studies suggest that the biological relatives of schizophrenics demonstrate "subthreshold" pathology in the form of schizotypal personality disorder. The prevalence of such disorders in schizophrenic families has been estimated at between 4.2 and 14.6%. If "probable" SPD is included, estimates may run as high as 26.8%.

Results for schizoid and paranoid personality disorders (PDs) have been less consistent. Baron et al. found higher rates of paranoid PD in the relatives of schizophrenic probands (7.3%) versus control probands (2.7%). However, their results have been criticized for artificially inflating estimates of paranoid PD in relatives on the grounds that the sample of research diagnostic criteria (RDC)-defined schizophrenic probands may have also included delusional disordered probands. Moreover, family studies suggest that schizophrenia and delusional disorder are not genetically related to one another. For example, Winokur found paranoid traits in relatives of delusional disorder patients, but not in the relatives of schizophrenics. Kendler et al. showed that rates of DSM-III paranoid PD were not increased in the relatives of schizophrenics, but were increased in relatives of patients with delusional disorder. Thus, there is not strong evidence favoring paranoid PD as a member of the schizophrenia spectrum.

Regarding schizoid PD, Kety et al. and the Danish adoption studies are most frequently cited as providing the evidence which potentially refutes a schizoid-schizophrenia genetic link. A more recent replication in an adoption sample indicated findings similar to Kety and coworkers' earlier report. Also, Baron et al., reported that the relatives of schizophrenics had a slightly higher rate of schizoid PD than controls (1.6 vs 0%). Also, compared to family members of controls, the family members of schizophrenics demonstrated a significantly higher rate of probable SPD (12.1 vs 6.5%). Kendler et al. found an increased prevalence of a combined "schizotypal-schizoid" PD in biological relatives of schizophrenics, but their results did not allow for a distinction between "schizotypal" and "schizoid" traits. Thus, as with paranoid PD, strong evidence has yet to be presented in establishing a link between schizophrenia and schizoid PD. Clearly, among Axis-II disorders, Schizotypal PD is the strongest candidate for a relatively mild illness which is genetically related to schizophrenia.

NEUROBIOLOGIC SPECTRUM DISORDERS It seems unlikely that there will be a one-to-one correspondence between genetically influenced processes in the brain and the clinical phenomena that define diagnostic categories. Since psychiatric signs and symptoms may be relatively remote effects of the genotype, linkage studies might be more fruitful if they focus on measures more closely tied to brain function. Moreover, a putative indicator may measure only one component of the schizophrenia genotype. This would be likely if more than one gene caused the disorder—a very reasonable hypothesis for schizophrenia. To paraphrase Matthysse, minor genes for schizophrenia might be major genes for some index of central nervous system dysfunction. If so, these neurobiologic phenotypes could help clarify the genetic etiology of the disorder.

The search for neurobiologic phenotypes has previously uncovered several excellent candidates. These include eye-tracking dysfunction, attentional impairment, allusive thinking neurologic signs, neuropsychological impairment, and characteristic auditory-evoked potentials. A comprehensive review of each of these is beyond the scope of this chapter. However, an examination of neuropsychological studies will provide a useful example.

Studies of the children of schizophrenic patients provide consistent evidence for their poorer performance on perceptual-motor speed tests. Other studies found significant deficits in perceptual-motor speed tests among the adult relatives of schizophrenics. Tests of mental control/encoding (also referred to as measures of short-term memory or selective attention) are also impaired among relatives of schizophrenics. For example, several studies reported children of schizophrenic patients to have lower Wechsler arithmetic subtest scores than controls. Also, children of schizophrenic patients do poorly on digit span tasks when these tasks include a distraction component. Sorting tests (e.g., the Wisconsin Card Sorting Test) have implicated abstraction and concept formation as deficits among relatives of schizophrenic patients. Some studies found deficits in verbal learning and memory among relatives of schizophrenic patients; in contrast, visual–spatial general ability and visual–spatial learning and memory have usually not been impaired in these subjects. Impairments in motor function have been found consistently among the children of schizophrenic patients, usually as soft neurological signs such as disturbed gait, poor balance, incoordination, and motor impersistence.

In summary, studies of neuropsychological functioning among relatives of schizophrenic patients point to deficits in sustained attention, perceptual-motor speed, concept formation and abstraction and, to a lesser extent, mental control/encoding and verbal learning and memory. The domains impaired in relatives are promising as potential indicators of the schizophrenia genotype because they are consistent with the cognitive dysfunctions thought to be central to schizophrenic patients themselves.

CLINICAL IMPLICATIONS

Psychiatric genetic research has not produced new diagnostic technologies or new therapies for schizophrenic patients. There is little doubt that, in the long run, the discovery of etiological genes will lead to treatments that are more effective, along with molecular genetic diagnostic markers that will identify high-risk individuals. Improved diagnostic technologies raise the possibility of designing primary prevention and other early intervention strategies for preschizophrenic individuals.

Although the major clinical contributions of genetic research in schizophrenia may be decades away, this line of research has led to advances in diagnosis, treatment, and genetic counseling that should be useful to the practicing clinician.

DIAGNOSIS Because schizophrenia is familial, the art of diagnosis should be extended from diagnosing patients to diagnosing entire families. Indeed, we have found that a comprehensive psychiatric family history is one of the most illuminating sources of information in a diagnostic interview. By determining what psychiatric illnesses occur in the patient's family, the clinician may be more precise in the diagnosis of the patient.

The psychiatric family history is most helpful for "atypical" patients who are not clearly schizophrenic or mood-disordered. It is also useful when little data about the patient are available. Nevertheless, such data should be routinely collected because, in all cases, it helps the clinician develop and test diagnostic hypotheses.

The use of family history data is straightforward and intuitive. For example, consider the case of a 30-year-old patient who is admitted to a hospital for the first time with the psychotic symptoms of both schizophrenia and the affective symptoms of bipolar disorder, without clearly meeting criteria for any disorder. If the patient has two schizophrenic siblings, a provisional diagnosis of schizophrenia would certainly be in order. If these siblings had bipolar disorder and/or major depression, the diagnosis of bipolar disorder would receive more consideration.

Of course, "familial diagnosis" should be used cautiously. It is an adjunct to—not a replacement for—clinical psychiatric diagnosis. Most importantly, the absence of schizophrenia among relatives should not be used to infer that the patient being diagnosed does not have schizophrenia. In fact, because of schizophrenia's complex mode of inheritance, many patients with schizophrenia will not have relatives with the disorder.

TREATMENT Knowledge of the genetics of schizophrenia should influence its therapy in three ways. First, if a patient has relatives with the disorder, their response to specific biological treatments should be considered in choosing a therapy for the patient. Although little is known about the pharmacogenetics of psychotropic drugs, clinical experience shows that, in some cases, biologically related schizophrenic patients may respond best to the same medication. However, controlled research is needed before practice guidelines can be established.

The second influence of genetic findings on treatment is in the area of medication compliance. Many schizophrenic patients refuse to take their medication; others do not actively refuse, but find it difficult to maintain their prescribed regimen. These problems can be reduced by discussing the genetic etiology of schizophrenia when teaching patients about their illness. Many still hold naive beliefs about the etiology of their disorder; they are quick to attribute it to events in the past, life circumstances, or their own psychological inadequacies. These beliefs (sometimes delusional) may make it difficult for a patient to accept the biological roots of their problems. For many psychiatric disorders, genetic data provide the quickest and most convincing means of showing patients how biology plays a role in their condition.

A third therapeutic use of genetic data relates to family therapy, especially for those that do assume that the illness was directly or indirectly caused by deviant family interaction. An educational component attempts to reduce the family's self-blame for the illness. Once families learn about the genctic and biological bases of the illness, they can discard guilty feelings and more productively cooperate in the treatment of their relative. Understanding biological bases also helps families accept the necessity of medication.

GENETIC COUNSELING Many patients, along with their relatives, are concerned about the potential recurrence of schizophrenia among family members. In the absence of knowledge of DNA markers from linkage analysis or risk figures from a known model of genetic transmission, we can use the available family study data to make predictions. For example, it is reasonable to tell a schizophrenic patient that the risk to siblings for severe psychotic illness is about 10%. The risk to an identical twin would be about 55%. Unfortunately, little is known about complicated family structures (e.g., the risk to a child who has a schizophrenic father and sibling).

When genes for schizophrenia are discovered, it will become possible to predict its onset in apparently healthy individuals. After a link has been confirmed, we can identify individuals within a pedigree who are marker-positive and disease-negative, but who have not yet passed through the period of risk for the illness. We would then predict that these individuals would later manifest the disorder. Thus, linkage analysis carries with it the promise of substantially increasing our understanding of etiology with hopes of providing leads toward primary prevention.

SELECTED REFERENCES

Barondes SH, Alberts BM, Andreasen NC, et al. Workshop on schizophrenia. Proc Natl Acad Sci USA 1997;94:1612–1614.

Crow TJ. Current status of linkage for schizophrenia: polygenes of vanishingly small effect or multiple false positives? Am J Med Genet 1997;74:99–103.

Crow TJ. Nature of the genetic contribution to psychotic illness—a continuum viewpoint. Acta Psychiatr Scand 1990;81:401–408.

Faraone SV, Tsuang MT. Methods in Psychiatric Genetics. In: Tohen M, Tsuang MT, Zahner GEP, eds. Textbook in Psychiatric Epidemiology. New York: Wiley, New York, 1994.

Faraone SV, Tsuang MT. Quantitative models of the genetic transmission of schizophrenia. Psychol Bull 1985;98:41–66.

Faraone SV, Kremen WS, Lyons MJ, Pepple JR, Seidman LJ, Tsuang MT. Diagnostic accuracy and linkage analysis: How useful are schizophrenia spectrum phenotypes? Am J Psychiatry 1995;152:1286–1290.

Gottesman II. Schizophrenia Genesis: The Origin of Madness. New York: Freeman, 1991.

Gottesman II, McGue M. Mixed and mixed-up models for the transmission of schizophrenia. In: D. Cichetti, ed. Thinking Clearly About Psychology: Essays in Honor of Paul E. Meehl. University of Minnesota Press, 1990.

Gottesman II, Shields J. Schizophrenia and Genetics: A Twin Study Vantage Point. New York: Academic, 1972.

Gottesman II, Shields J. Schizophrenia: The Epigenetic Puzzle. Cambrdige, UK: Cambridge University Press, 1982.

Guze SB, Cloninger R, Martin RL, Clayton P. A follow-up and family study of schizophrenia. Arch Gen Psych 1983;40:1273–1276.

Kendler KS. Overview: A current perspective on twin studies of schizophrenia. Am J Psychiatry 1983;140:1413–1425.

Kendler KS, Gardner CO. The risk for psychiatric disorders in relatives of schizophrenic and control probands: A comparison of three independent studies. Psychol Med 1997;27:411–419.

Kety SS, Rosenthal D, Wender PH, Schulsinger F, Jacobson B. Mental illness in the biological and adoptive families of adopted individuals who have become schizophrenic: a preliminary report based on psychiatric interviews. In: Rieve RR, Rosenthal D, Brill H, eds. Genetic research in psychiatry. Baltimore, MD: Johns Hopkins University Press, 1975.

Kremen WS, Seidman LJ, Pepple JR, Lyons MJ, Tsuang MT, Faraone SV. Neuropsychological risk indicators for schizophrenia: A review of family studies. Schiz Bull 1994;20:103–119.

Kremen WS, Tsuang MT, Faraone SV, Lyons ML. Using vulnerability indicators to compare conceptual models of genetic heterogeneity in schizophrenia. J Nerv Ment Dis 1992;180:141–152.

Portin P, Alanen YO. A critical review of genetic studies of schizophrenia. II. Molecular genetic studies. Acta Psychiatr Scand 1997;95:73–80.

Risch N. Linkage strategies for genetically complex traits. I. Multilocus models. Am J Hum Genet 1990;46:222–228.

Straub RE, MacLean CJ, O'Neill FA, Wash D, Kendler KS. Support for a possible schizophrena vulnerability locus in region 5q22-31 in Irish families. Mol Psychiatry 1997;2:148–155.

Tsuang MT, Faraone SV. Genetic heterogeneity of schizophrenia. Psychiatria Et Neurologia Japonica 1995;97:485–501.

Tsuang MT, Faraone SV. Schizophrenia. In: Winokur G, Clayton P, eds. Medical Basis of Psychiatry, 2nd ed. Philadelphia, PA: Saunders, 1994.

Tsuang MT, Faraone SV, Lyons MJ. Advances in psychiatric genetics. In: Costa e Silva JA, Nadelson CC, Andreasen NC, Sato M, eds. International Review of Psychiatry, Vol. I. Washington: American Psychiatric, 1993

Tsuang MT, Faraone SV, Lyons MJ. Identification of the phenotype in psychiatric genetics. Eur Arch Psychiatr Neurol Sci 1993; 243: 131–142.

Tsuang MT, Lyons MJ, Faraone SV. Heterogeneity of schizophrenia: conceptual models and analytic strategies. Br J Psychiat 1990; 156:17–26.

Tsuang MT, Winokur G, Crowe RR. Morbidity risks of schizophrenia and affective disorders among first-degree relatives of patients with schizophrenia, mania, depression and surgical conditions. Br J Psychiat 1980;137:497–504.

Turecki G, Rouleau GA, Joober R, Mari J, Morgan K. Schizophrenia and chromosome 6p. Am J Med Genet 1997;74:195–198.

110 Affective Disorders

FRANCIS J. MCMAHON AND J. RAYMOND DEPAULO, JR.

BACKGROUND

In this chapter, we will attempt to outline the current state of knowledge about the genetics of affective disorders. The inclusion of this subject in a textbook of molecular medicine could be viewed as premature, since an understanding of the pathophysiology of the affective disorders on the molecular level is not yet in our grasp. Nevertheless, clinical research over the last century has established a major role for genetic factors in the etiology of the affective disorders. We will describe how molecular approaches to the affective disorders follow from this knowledge. We will also outline the major challenges in the path to a molecular understanding of the affective disorders.

The top–down approach of neuroscience, which attempts to fashion theories of pathogenesis out of an understanding of the component molecules of the nervous system, has so far not succeeded in establishing the molecular basis of the affective disorders. This is not surprising in view of the enormous complexity of receptors, ligands, second messengers, and synaptic connections in the brain. However, the impressive body of work in molecular neuroscience over the past 40 years has succeeded in establishing the context against which genetic findings may ultimately be interpreted.

The bottom–up approach of modern genetics is radically different. Instead of reasoning from component parts, the genetic approach first exploits the great wealth of genetic variation in an attempt to identify a gene or genes that are tied to the phenotype of interest in a predictable manner. This is the goal of linkage and association studies, which we will discuss in depth later. Once such a gene is identified, work can proceed logically to identifying a change in the gene's sequence of nucleotides that alters the structure and function of the protein product, that is, a mutation. At that point, the genetic approach may join hands with molecular neuroscience in formulating a theory of pathogenesis based on both genetic variation and biochemistry.

Affective disorders is the term applied to a range of illnesses manifested by pathologic changes in mood, one's attitude toward self, and the sense of bodily well-being. In this chapter we will not focus on the myriad illnesses that engender affective changes as a secondary feature of some larger disease process, such as cancer; rather, we will focus on those illnesses that, to the best of our knowledge and observation, constitute a primary change in the affective realm of mental life.

From: *Principles of Molecular Medicine* (J. L. Jameson, ed.), ©1998 Humana Press Inc., Totowa, NJ.

HISTORY

The affective disorders have been recognized in some form since antiquity. Galen and Aristotle write of patients suffering from melancholia and mania, whose symptomatology would be very familiar to modern psychiatrists. Later in Anatomy of Melancholy, Burton provided a bridge between the classical authors and medieval notions of mental illness, placing what we would now call affective disorders at the heart of his complex nosology of mental disorders. But it was the work of eighteenth- and nineteenth-century physicians, such as Benjamin Rush, Wilhelm Griesinger, and especially Emil Kraepelin, that provided the basis of our modern conceptualization of affective disorders as disease entities, distinct from schizophrenia or dementia, and characterized by cyclic or periodic changes that may be depressive or manic in character.

NOSOLOGY

UNIPOLAR VS BIPOLAR DISORDER The only major nosologic advance over these pioneers was introduced by Leonhard, who in the late 1950s showed that there were marked differences in age at onset and clinical course between patients with only depressions compared to those who also experienced mania at some time in their lives. This fundamental observation has been confirmed many times over in clinical studies, but has not yet been correlated with any robust differences in laboratory findings. Nevertheless, Leonhard's unipolar/bipolar distinction has become the basis of our clinical terminology. This chapter will focus on those studies undertaken since the adoption of the unipolar/bipolar distinction, reflecting its enormous impact on the field.

OTHER APPROACHES The Diagnostic and Statistical Manual of Mental Disorders, 4th ed. (DSM-IV) recognizes six major types of affective disorder (Table 110-1). In addition, several "specifiers" are listed for most of the major types, based on such things as the presence or absence of hallucinations or delusions, a seasonal pattern of episodes, or other clinical features. Calculation of all possible unique combinations of types and specifiers yields some 2655 subtypes of affective disorder. While all specifiers meet some minimum standard of reliability, validation of even the most widely recognized subtypes remains weak at best.

The International Classification of Diseases (ICD-10) contains a classification of major affective disorder that is very similar to that in the DSM. The exceptions are bipolar II disorder, which is not included as a separate category in the ICD-10, even though hypomania is included as a subtype of manic disorder. ICD-10 also

Table 110-1
DSM-IV Classification
of Affective (Mood) Disorders, Major Subtypes

Depressive disorders
Major depressive episode
Dysthymic disorder
Depressive disorder NOS
Bipolar disorders
Bipolar I disorder
Bipolar II disorder
Cyclothymic disorder
Bipolar disorder NOS
Mood disorder NOS
Related condition listed under "Schizophrenia and other psychotic disorders":
Schizoaffective disorder

provides fewer specifiers than DSM-IV. Finally, there are differences between the ICD-10 and the DSM-IV in the types of schizoaffective disorder and their clinical definitions.

The pragmatic value of such catalogs as DSM-IV and ICD-10 notwithstanding attempts to break down the affective disorder phenotype beyond the level of the unipolar/bipolar distinction have not proven very fruitful. There do appear to be differences in prognosis and possibly treatment response for some types of depression, and patients who experience distinct mood elevations less severe than those seen in mania (hypomanias) may be distinguished by family history, longitudinal course, and comorbidity from other patients. Still, the similarities among patients with unipolar or bipolar illness seem to far outweigh the differences. Further distinctions must likely await molecular discoveries of a fundamental nature.

CLINICAL FEATURES

CLASSIC DESCRIPTIONS The German psychiatrist Emil Kraepelin is widely viewed as the father of the clinical study of manic-depressive disorder. Based on his clinical observations, he advanced one of the broader concepts of manic-depressive disorder, encompassing modern bipolar and unipolar disorder as well as milder disturbances of the affective realm. As he states in the 8th edition of his classic textbook:

> *Manic-depressive insanity encompasses, on the one hand, the whole area of the so-called periodic and cyclic forms of mental illness, on the other hand, simple mania, the majority of illnesses designated as melancholia, and also a not insignificant proportion of cases of amentia (stupor). Finally, we also must include certain mild, even trivial colorings of mood—sometimes periodic, sometimes chronic—which can either be seen as prodromes of more serious disturbances or as phenomena that blend without sharp borders into the area of personal disposition.*

Whether Kraepelin's broad concept will prove valid must await the results of genetic research. But the clarity of his approach, his sharp differentiation between schizophrenia and manic-depressive disorder, and his appreciation for all of the clinical nuances of the illness, make his writings very valuable even for the modern reader.

DESCRIPTIVE VARIABLES **Age at Onset** Depression and mania can occur in children, although affective disorders are usually first diagnosed in adolescents and adults. However, the precise definition of the time when a mood disorder actually begins is often not possible on clinical grounds alone. The onset may be manifested in by the first treatment contact, the first clear episode, the first symptoms, or by some clinically occult process that bears no obvious relationship to symptoms.

Defining even these arbitrary markers of onset can be problematic. Age at onset data is usually collected retrospectively, which introduces some biases. Further, disease onset may be precluded by death from an unrelated cause, or onset may occur after the patient is examined and thus goes unobserved. Ascertainment biases can also significantly affect age at onset observations (e.g., clinical samples often contain more severe cases with earlier onset). In addition, several epidemiologic studies have described earlier onset of unipolar or bipolar disorder among persons born after 1945. This so-called cohort effect is of mysterious origin, but may result from several environmental and cultural phenomena, as well as recall bias.

Despite these issues, there is reasonably good agreement in the literature about age at onset for the affective disorders. The first episode of mania or major depression in bipolar I disorder tends to occur around the age of 20 years. For unipolar disorder, the first major depression occurs later, toward the early thirties, on average. Studies give conflicting results as to the onset of bipolar II (BPII) disorder. Some suggest an age at onset between that of bipolar I (BPI) and recurrent unipolar disorder, while other studies have suggested an age at onset for BPII that is very close, if not identical, to that of BPI.

Several points are clear. There are no marked differences in age at onset between males and females. In both bipolar and unipolar disorders, age at onset tends to be lower when there are many affected relatives, probably because of the increased burden of both genetic and nongenetic risk factors in such families.

Attempts to define clinical subtypes of affective disorder beyond the unipolar/bipolar level based on age at onset have, in general, produced a few striking differences. There is a remarkable clinical similarity between affective disorder beginning in young and late adulthood. However, people with early-onset bipolar disorder do appear to be more likely to experience psychotic symptoms (i.e., hallucinations or delusions).

Several disease that models account for the delayed onset of affective disorders have been proposed (for a review, *see* McMahon and DePaulo, 1996). Within families, several studies have suggested that age at onset declines in successive generations. Such anticipation may point to a role for genes with expanding triplet repeat sequences in affective disorders. Ultimately, however, a full understanding of age at onset in mood disorders must await discovery of the genetic factors involved.

Drug Response Treatment of affective disorders relies on two broad classes of pharmacologic agents: antidepressants and mood stabilizers, such as lithium.

The antidepressants are often classified according to their molecular structure or the major neurotransmitter systems they affect. However, it is not at all certain whether an antidepressant's known effects on neurotransmitter systems bears any direct relationship to its therapeutic action. Similarly, while the pharmacologic and side-effect profiles of the major mood stabilizers are well known, the mechanism of their therapeutic action remains mysterious.

Several investigators have attempted to classify persons with affective disorders according to their response or nonresponse to a particular drug or class of drugs. Unfortunately, this approach has revealed little. Aside from the methodologic difficulties inherent in classifying patients as "responders" or "nonresponders," a nosology based on treatment response embodies a logical fallacy. Simply stated, if a patient responds to a treatment that has been used successfully in disease X, then the patient must have had disease X. While morphine quickly relieves the symptoms of heart failure, we do not conclude that cancer patients who feel better when treated with morphine actually have heart failure.

Still, classification by treatment response may have some value in producing more homogeneous populations of patients for genetic linkage studies. For example, several studies have shown that a family history of bipolar disorder predicts response to lithium, and others have suggested that lithium-responsive bipolar disorder may fit a Mendelian model of inheritance better than bipolar disorder as a whole.

Comorbidity The affective disorders are often complicated by other mental disorders, particularly substance abuse and anxiety disorders. That this comorbidity is more than just an understandable consequence of the impairments of depression or mania is shown by family studies. The same diagnoses that tend to co-occur with affective disorder also occur with increased frequency in the affectively well relatives of affectively ill probands. For example, Gershon et al. (1982) reported a greater lifetime risk of cyclothymic personality, generalized anxiety disorder, alcoholism, and drug abuse among first-degree relatives of probands with major affective disorder compared to unaffected control probands.

Comorbidity may also prove valuable as a means of differentiating different genetic forms of affective disorder. For example, MacKinnon et al. (1997) have shown an increased incidence of panic disorder only among the bipolar relatives of probands who suffer from both bipolar disorder and panic disorder. If particular comorbid illnesses occur in certain genetic subtypes of affective disorder, then the power and resolution of genetic linkage studies might be improved by partitioning family samples according to comorbid illnesses.

EPIDEMIOLOGY **Epidemiologic Catchment Area Study** While the high prevalence of the affective disorders has been suggested since antiquity, precise estimates of prevalence awaited the advent of modern epidemiologic methods. In 1978, the largest systematic study of the epidemiology of mental disorder in the United States was undertaken by investigators at five universities. Approximately 20,000 individuals aged 18 and older were selected for study out of a population that even included those living in institutions, such as nursing homes, psychiatric hospitals, and prisons. Face-to-face evaluations were carried out by nonclinicians using a structured interview, the Diagnostic Interview Schedule (DIS). Diagnoses were assigned based on the DSM-III. The ECA study clearly established that affective disorders, particularly major depression and dysthymia are quite prevalent in the community (Table 110-2). Females report more major depression and dysthymia than males, but similar rates of bipolar disorder, consistent with previous studies. The ECA found very little difference in prevalence between groups in different socioeconomic classes, races, or metropolitan areas. This would be expected if the prevalence of affective disorder is determined primarily by genetics. Furthermore, the ECA established the high rate of substance abuse comorbidity in affective disorder, particularly BPI, where over 60% of subjects with this illness reported abuse or dependence with alcohol and/or other drugs.

Table 110-2
Lifetime Prevalence[a] of Affective Disorder by Sex, Age, and Ethnicity: ECA and NCS Data

	Bipolar I	*Bipolar II*	*Major depression*	*Dysthymia*
ECA				
Men	1.6	NS[b]	12.7	4.8
Women	1.7	NS	21.3	8.0
Total	1.6	NS	17.1	6.4
NCS				
Men	0.7	0.4	2.6	2.2
Women	0.9	0.5	7.0	4.1
Total	0.8	0.5	4.9	3.2
18–29 years	1.1	0.7	5.0	3.0
30–44	1.4	0.6	7.5	3.8
45–64	0.3	0.2	4.0	3.6
65+	0.1	0.1	1.4	1.7
White	0.8	0.4	5.1	3.3
Black	1.0	0.6	3.1	2.5
Hispanic	0.7	0.5	4.4	4.0

[a]Per 100 persons.
[b]NS, not specified.

National Comorbidity Survey This large epidemiologic study was undertaken to complement the ECA, collecting data on prevalence, comorbidity, and risk factors for mental disorders in a national sample of approximately 8100 respondents aged 15–54 years. Evaluations were carried out by nonclinicians using a modification of the DIS. Diagnoses were assigned based on the revised version of the DSM-III (DSM-III-R). The NCS results support the high prevalence of affective disorders in the community, with lifetime prevalence estimates that actually exceed those seen in the ECA for some diagnoses (Table 110-2). Like the ECA, the NCS also found more unipolar disorder among females and only small differences in prevalence between groups in different socioeconomic classes, races, or metropolitan areas. NCS data also revealed considerable comorbidity between substance use disorders and affective disorders. Comorbidity of alcohol use disorders and major depression was particularly striking, especially between alcohol dependence and major depression in females and blacks.

DIAGNOSIS

BASICS: MOOD, SELF-ATTITUDE, VITAL SENSE Patients suffering from an affective disorder manifest a pathologic change in mood in at least two ways: in degree and responsiveness. The patient with major depression, for example, will experience a sad, low, or indifferent mood that fails to be dispelled by events that would usually be pleasurable or cheering. Similarly, the patient with mania will experience an elated, expansive, or irritable mood that does not change appropriately in response to disappointments or negative consequences of the patient's behavior. While a patient with an affective disorder will usually experience some variability of mood—for example, diurnal mood variation in major depression—this variability typically loses the close relationship to daily events and experiences characteristic of normal mood variability.

When we speak of a change in self-attitude, we mean a change in the way one views one's self in comparison to one's usual standards of personal worth. Self-attitude represents the aggregate of one's judgements about personal talents, achievements, character, and future. While sometimes difficult to examine, self-attitude is a diagnostically very important feature of affective disorder that can be helpful in distinguishing episodes of affective disorder from nonpathologic mood changes.

During an episode of affective disorder, the self-attitude typically changes in the same direction as the mood. Thus, the depressed patient will see himself as a failure, as unworthy of love, as reproachable. He may be preoccupied with guilt, past failures, or personal shortcomings. In severe cases, the future seems very bleak and thoughts of death or suicide may be present. All of these symptoms belong to the changes in self-attitude seen in affective disorder.

The vital sense is another aspect of the affective realm typically influenced by an affective disorder. The vital sense refers to one's feeling of physical well-being and bodily health. The vital sense encompasses changes in energy, stamina, sleep, and appetite, but is not restricted to these obvious bodily functions. For some patients, a change in vital sense will manifest only as a subtle change in subjective cognitive skills, such as concentration or memory. For other patients, vital sense changes will be the chief complaint at presentation, leading to the suspicion or diagnosis of a physical illness other than depression.

In major depression, vital sense is typically decreased, with feelings of exhaustion, fatigue, or achiness. Sleep may be increased or decreased, but is typically not perceived as refreshing or restful. Food may lose its appeal, leading to weight loss. All drives are decreased, with a loss of libido, appetite, and interest.

In mania, the opposite applies. Patients boast of limitless energy, strength, and stamina. The need for sleep is reduced, brief naps are perceived as completely restorative, and total sleeplessness may persist for days. All appetites are increased, which may lead to inappropriate sexual behavior or excessive use of alcohol.

In making the diagnosis of an affective disorder, it is important to examine all three aspects of the affective realm in detail. Changes may be subtle, may not be discovered unless enquired about, and may require skillful probing. Finally, it is difficult to overstate the value of longitudinal observation over time, particularly in milder cases of major depression. Longitudinal observation may also help identify rapid cycling, where patients may alternate quickly between mania and major depression, or mixed states, with simultaneous features of both mania and depression. These clinical features often call for particular treatment approaches.

CRITERION SYSTEMS Rationale Whereas the diagnosis of affective disorder is often not difficult for the skilled observer, variations in clinical practice and experience can lead to a lack of agreement among clinicians as to the correct diagnosis. For example, the US/UK diagnostic study found that, in 1972, the diagnosis of affective disorder was much less common among hospitalized patients in the United States than in the United Kingdom, raising concerns about diagnostic practices on both sides of the Atlantic. This finding added impetus to the movement to formulate and adopt standardized diagnostic criteria for the affective disorders and indeed for all mental illnesses. The Diagnostic and Statistical Manual of Mental Disorders (DSM) and its equivalent sections in the International Classification of Diseases (ICD) represent the current incarnation of this movement.

Reliability vs Validity The value of standardized diagnostic criteria lies in their ability to increase the reliability with which a diagnosis can be assigned. Reliability describes how often two different clinicians will make the same diagnosis when they examine the same patient. Thanks largely to the advent of standardized criteria, it is now safe to assume that most patients diagnosed with mania in New York would have been given the same diagnosis if they had been examined by psychiatrists in Iowa, London, or Frankfurt.

Diagnostic reliability is a necessary first step in discovering the molecular causes of any disease. Without reliability, there is no basis for assuming that any two people with the same diagnosis share any etiologic or pathogenic features in common. In this regard, the advent of reliable diagnostic criteria has been a major element in the progress toward understanding affective disorders on the molecular level. However, reliability can never be perfect, neither does perfect reliability assure validity. Until the genetic basis of the affective disorders is understood, we cannot be sure that the current diagnostic entities are valid disease entities, that is, that they bear a predictable relationship to events outside the affective realm, such as a change in the coding sequence of a gene.

Diagnostic and Statistical Manual of Mental Disorders The DSM-IV lists operational criteria for diagnosing affective disorder. These criteria, while imperfect, do allow affective disorder to be diagnosed with high reliability by experienced clinicians. As discussed above, the DSM also delineates criteria for many related conditions, some of which are commonly seen among the relatives of probands with major affective disorders. The degree to which these conditions overlap with, or are distinct from, the major affective disorders, is another question that can best be answered once the genetic causes of the major subtypes are known.

GENETIC BASIS OF DISEASE

A genetic basis for the affective disorders, while long-suspected and supported by family, twin, and adoption studies, still awaits molecular elucidation. In this section, we will review the evidence supporting a genetic basis for affective disorders. We will also discuss the results of association and linkage studies, which, while still provisional, may lead to the identification of specific genes and mutations.

FAMILY STUDIES Family studies have accomplished two important goals in the study of affective disorders. First, they have confirmed the familial nature of these illnesses—a necessary part of the genetic hypothesis. Necessary, but not sufficient: Many things, ranging from wealth to eating habits, are familial without being genetic. This is why twin and adoption studies, covered later, are also of great importance. Second, family studies have provided essential information about the range of disease phenotypes associated with the putative affective disorder genes, by revealing which types of illnesses run in the families of patients with affective disorder and which do not.

In other genetic disorders, family studies have also been a valuable tool for discerning the mode of inheritance, through segregation analysis. Segregation analyses have yielded conflicting results when applied to affective disorders, probably because the method does not readily accommodate etiologic heterogeneity, a fact of life likely to strongly affect the study of most psychiatric disorders. In addition, recent studies have suggested that transmission of bipolar affective disorder (BPAD) is influenced by the sex of the transmitting parent. Such parent-of-origin effects, which may reflect imprinting or mitochondrial inheritance, further obscure Mendelian transmission patterns.

Table 110-3
Lifetime Morbid Risks for Affective Disorders and Schizophrenia in Families

Proband (N)	*Risk (%) for first-degree relatives*[a]			*Study*
	Bipolar[b]	*Unipolar*	*Schizophrenia*	
BIPOLAR (134)	17.7	22.4	0.0	Mendlewicz and Rainer, 1974
BIPOLAR (100)	3.9	9.1	3.0	Tsuang et al., 1980
UP (225)	2.2	11.0	1.6	
UNAFF (160)	0.2	5.9	0.6	
BIPOLAR (145)	17.5	20.4	–	Baron, 1981
UP (110)	0.2	18.1	–	
BPI (96)[c]	8.6	14.0	0.2	Gershon et al., 1982
BPII (34)	7.1	17.3	0.5	
UP (30)	3.0	16.6	0.0	
UNAFF (43)	0.5	5.8	0.0	
BPI (97)	6.2	21.9	–	Endicott et al., 1985[d]
BPII (30)	11.0	17.6	–	
UP (121)	3.3	29.3	–	
BPI (151)	8.1	22.8	1.0	Andreasen et al., 1987
BPII (76)	9.3	26.2	0.4	
UP (330)	3.5	28.4	0.3	
BPI (251)	8	45	–	Winokur et al., 1995
UP (313)	1	45	–	
UNAFF (305)	1	53	–	
BIPOLAR (1114)	10.5	21.9	0.6	Mean risk across studies
UP (1129)	2.4	26.2	0.6	
UNAFF (508)	0.6	21.6	0.5	

[a]Age-corrected by various methods.
[b]For studies that specify relatives diagnoses as bipolar I or bipolar II, includes both diagnoses.
[c]BPI includes probands and relatives with bipolar I and schizoaffective-manic disorders.
[d]Rates not age-corrected.

Classic The classic family studies of affective disorders were carried out in the early part of this century, before the advent of modern methodologic approaches. Despite this limitation, many of the classic family studies yielded conclusions that modern researchers have only confirmed, albeit with greater precision.

The 1936 study of Elliot Slater is perhaps the best example. Slater studied 315 probands with recurrent, major affective disorder collected from the cardfiles of the Munich Genealogical Institute, where he studied under the pioneering psychiatric geneticist Bruno Schulz. Slater calculated the lifetime risk for various mental illnesses among the parents and children of his probands. His paper was one of the first to use age-corrected estimates of lifetime risk, such as the Strömgren method, which adjusts for the fact that relatives of different ages have passed through different proportions of the period of risk.

Slater's main finding was that the parents and children of probands with manic-depressive disorder had a lifetime risk of developing the illness themselves (morbid risk) of about 15%. Although Slater did not collect unaffected control probands for comparison, based on contemporary prevalence estimates he concluded that "manic-depression" and suicide were increased among the parents and children of the probands, while schizophrenia "criminality" and "imbecility" were not. These results forced Slater to revise his own view that there existed a relationship between the predisposition to schizophrenia and to manic-depressive disorder. He concluded instead that "...such speculations, however, appear to me now to be unjustified..." Although statistical and diagnostic approaches have changed, Slater's risk estimates are not very different from those obtained in more modern family studies, detailed below.

Modern Modern family studies are distinguished from the most of the classic studies by three methodologic advances:

1. Use of operational diagnostic criteria.
2. Use of age-corrected risk estimates.
3. Use of control procedures, such as examination of relatives by investigators who were blind to the proband's diagnosis, and use of unaffected probands, allowing more precise estimates of relative risk of illness for relatives of affected probands.

The modern studies also incorporate the unipolar/bipolar distinction when selecting probands and reporting results.

The main findings of the modern family studies are presented in Table 110-3. These studies were selected based on proband sample sizes of over 100, diagnostic assessment by direct interview, and clinical evaluations performed blind to the diagnostic status of the proband. While absolute risks vary across studies, three conclusions are clear:

1. Major affective disorder is familial: There is an increased risk for major affective disorder among the relatives of affected probands compared to the relatives of unaffected probands.

2. Bipolar and unipolar disorder are distinct, but related: There is an increased risk of both unipolar and bipolar forms of affective disorder among the relatives of probands with bipolar disorder, while among the relatives of probands with unipolar disorder, risk is increased only for the unipolar form of the illness.
3. Major affective disorder is different from other major mental illnesses: The risk for other major mental illnesses such as schizophrenia, is not increased among the relatives of probands with major affective disorder. However, affective disorders and schizophrenia may still share etiologic determinants, as suggested by some authorities.

Family studies have clearly established the distinct familiality of major affective disorder and support the validity of the unipolar/bipolar distinction. However, as noted above, family studies alone cannot establish an unambiguous etiologic role for genetic factors. For this, lacking confirmed linkage reports or identified genes, twin and adoption studies remain the best source of data.

TWIN STUDIES The rationale of twin studies is simple: Since monozygotic (MZ) (identical) twins presumably carry the same genetic endowment, if one twin falls ill with a genetic illness, the other would be expected to fall ill as well, that is, be concordant. On the other hand, dizygotic (DZ) (fraternal) twins should have a lower concordance rate, since they share, on average, only half their genes. Concordance rates are usually calculated from the number of pairs where both co-twins are affected divided by the total number of pairs studied (pairwise concordance). Tetrameric correlations, which also take into account pairs where both co-twins are unaffected, are sometimes calculated as well. In probandwise concordance rates, the proportion of affected probands with an affected co-twin is reported.

It is important that the implicit assumptions of the twin method be borne in mind. First, it is assumed that ascertainment into the study is independent of concordance. For this reason, systematic ascertainment is important; nonsystematic studies usually overestimate concordance rates. It is also assumed that MZ and DZ twins differ only in the proportion of shared genes. We now know that MZ twins are not always genetically identical, because of somatic mosaicism, and may be more likely to experience similar environmental events than DZ twins. Still, high concordance rates among MZ twins, particularly if coupled with lower concordance rates among DZ twins, strongly suggest an etiologic role for genetic factors. Some researchers have developed biometrical models that, when applied to large samples of twins, provide estimates of the relative contributions of genes and environment to the variance in the phenotype, and in some cases distinctions can be made between shared (familial) and unshared environmental influences.

Classic The classic twin study of major affective disorders was published by Rosanoff, Handy, and Plesett (1935). In a retrospective chart-review study, 90 twin pairs were evaluated, at least one of whom suffered from "manic depressive syndromes." Although their methods were crude by today's standards, the authors obtained concordance estimates that are in good agreement with those of modern studies. Rosanoff et al. estimated a MZ pairwise concordance rate of 69.6% and a DZ concordance rate of 22.9%, based on same-sex twins. He concluded correctly that genetic factors play an important etiologic role, but, in some cases at least, nonhereditary factors are also required to cause the illness.

Modern The few modern twin studies of major affective disorder are distinguished by large, systematically ascertained samples. Some also have used operational diagnostic criteria and control procedures, such as blind assessment.

The largest study of bipolar disorder (110 twin pairs) was based on the Danish Twin Registry. In this study, MZ co-twins of probands with "manic-depressive disorders" had a probandwise concordance rate of 67%, significantly greater then the 20% seen in DZ twins. These figures were 79 and 19%, respectively, for MZ and DZ co-twins of probands with more narrowly defined bipolar disorder. Monozygotic co-twins of probands with unipolar disorder had a concordance rate of 54%, compared to a 24% rate seen in dizygotic twins.

These concordance rates are approximated by most other large, systematic twin studies. The results strongly support a major role for genetic factors in bipolar disorder, but offer less support for a major genetic role in unipolar disorder. Furthermore, the less than 100% concordance rate in bipolar disorder suggests that (barring undetected mosaicism) nongenetic factors are also important in the expression of the bipolar phenotype.

The largest twin sample studied for unipolar disorder comes from the Virginia Twin Registry. This population-based registry contains over 1700 female twins, with 742 complete pairs. Kendler et al. have studied these women using repeated self-report questionnaire assessments. Estimates of heritability of major depression ranged from 33 to 70%, depending on the reliability of the case definition: The more reliable case definitions were associated with higher heritability estimates. Kendler concludes that "major depression, as assessed over the lifetime, may be a rather heritable disorder of moderate reliability rather than a moderately heritable disorder of high reliability."

Twin studies have made a major contribution to our understanding of the role of genetic factors in affective disorders. While they certainly increase our confidence in a major etiologic role for genes in these illnesses, twin studies cannot provide data as to the particular genes involved. Still, future twin studies may help contribute to the refinement of our nosologic and disease-recognition strategies, which are critical steps in the road to the identification of disease genes.

ADOPTION STUDIES While twin studies lend strong support to a major role for genetic factors in major affective disorder, these studies do not readily distinguish between shared genes and shared environment. Twins generally share the same uterine environment and, being the same age, experience the same family environment at the same developmental stages. Moreover, MZ twins, perhaps owing to their similarity in appearance and temperament, may be exposed to more environmental similarity than DZ twins.

Adoption studies offer a way out of this conundrum. There are two basic designs:

1. The affected parent design, where the risk of illness is compared for the adopted versus biological offspring of affected parents; or
2. The affected adoptee design, where the risk of illness is compared for the biological vs adoptive parents of affected adoptees.

Even the best adoption studies cannot entirely exclude the environmental contributions of affected parents. For example, adoption usually occurs in the first days or weeks after birth, so that exposure to the biological mother's intrauterine environment is not eliminated. The advent of ovum donation and gestation by surrogate mothers may eventually set the stage for an adoption study that avoids this problem.

The first adoption study in bipolar disorder was conducted by Mendlewicz and Rainer (1977), using the affected adoptee design with several different control groups. They found that the adoptive parents of affected adoptees had an observed rate of affective disorder that was not higher than that seen in the adoptive parents of unaffected adoptees or in the biological parents of children with poliomyelitis. In contrast, the biological parents of the adoptees with bipolar disorder showed a 16-fold increased rate of affective disorders. Several subsequent adoption studies of BPAD confirm these findings. Thus, while family environment probably plays a role in major affective disorders, there is little evidence that it is a major causative factor.

LINKAGE AND ASSOCIATION STUDIES While family, twin, and adoption studies all support a major role for genes in the etiology of the major affective disorders, these study designs do not indicate in any way which genes are involved. Linkage and association studies, on the other hand, are designed to locate specific genes. In linkage studies, we assess the co-inheritance within a family of the disease phenotype and particular genetic markers whose location on the chromosomes is known. These can either be phenotypic markers, such as red-green color blindness, candidate genes, or anonymous polymorphic DNA markers.

In association studies, we assess the co-occurrence within a large population of the disease phenotype and a particular form (allele), of a gene of interest. A specialized type of association study, the linkage disequilibrium study, looks for fragments of ancestral founder chromosomes defined by associated DNA markers lying very near the actual disease allele.

Linkage Results Over 50 linkage studies of BPAD have been performed to date. Although initial results were disappointing, more recent studies have yielded replicated findings that may ultimately lead to the identification of important disease genes. The major regions of interest are discussed below.

HLA Two early reports of linkage between bipolar disorder and a particular set of human leukocyte antigens have never been replicated and probably represent a false-positive result.

The X Chromosome An X-linked gene has been hypothesized to play an etiologic role in affective disorders since at least 1934, when Rosanoff hypothesized an X-linked "activating factor" to explain the higher prevalence of affective disorder among women. More direct evidence of X-linkage was suggested by Winokur, Clayton, and Reich's classic study of BPAD and protan/deutan color blindness (1968). The evidence of X-linkage seemed even stronger when two other groups reported linkage between BPAD and protan/deutan color blindness or glucose 6-dehydrogenase deficiency.

Despite these early results, X-linkage of BPAD, while not entirely disproven, has not been supported by the mass of molecular evidence. Ultimately, X-linkage was not supported in Baron's original pedigree set, when highly polymorphic DNA markers were used. The reliance on relatively uninformative phenotypic markers and large multigenerational families with few opportunities for male-to-male transmission may explain the failure to find support for X-linkage in many studies, but the early positive findings of X-linkage have never been fully explicated. While an X-chromosome locus for BPAD cannot be ruled out, if it exists, it must be a relatively "weak" locus or play a significant role in only a small minority of families.

Chromosome 11 The report of linkage of BPAD to the DNA markers HRAS and INS on chromosome 11 was greeted with great excitement. Following on the successful detection of the chromosome 4 linkage in Huntington disease, this report seemed to be further proof of the promise of polymorphic DNA markers in detecting linkages for complex neuropsychiatric disorders.

Although the initial report of chromosome 11 linkage, like that for the X chromosome, was not confirmed, the reasons for this failure were clear, and provided important lessons for the field. The linkage evidence rested on study of a large pedigree from the relatively inbred Old Order Amish. The rationale for studying the Amish in the first place was quite legitimate: It was hoped that this genetically isolated population, founded by relatively few initial settlers about three centuries ago, would be less likely to contain many different BPAD disease genes, and thus the power to detect linkage might be correspondingly greater.

Unfortunately, this same genetic isolation and in-breeding make the Amish population problematic in several ways: (1) in large, inbred kindreds, linkage evidence may rest disproportionately on data from one or a few individuals; (2) linkage evidence in large pedigrees with a few affected relatives is derived primarily from unaffected individuals, whose phenotype could change or who may carry the disease allele but not manifest the phenotype (incomplete penetrance); and (3) it is difficult or impossible to be sure that a large, inbred pedigree stems from a single ill founder, leading to genetic heterogeneity within the pedigree, decreasing the power to detect true linkage

The re-evaluation of the chromosome 11 linkage results in the Amish pedigrees indicated that each of these problems had a hand in the demise of the linkage finding. Previously missing genotype data on 10 individuals decreased the LOD score at HRAS from 4.08 to 2.36 ($\theta = 0$). The most dramatic effect on the LOD scores resulted from a phenotype change from unaffected to affected in one or two key individuals, lowering the LOD score to $-1.75 (\theta = 0)$. Although these individuals may actually be phenocopies, they cannot be ignored, since there is, as yet, no way of identifying phenocopies independent of the linkage data. Extension of the original pedigree into right and left branches further reduced the LOD score well into the exclusionary range, probably as a result of multiple ancestral sources of illness in the Amish kindred leading to different disease genes segregating in different branches.

Based in part on the experience with the Amish study, linkage analysts now recommend that for complex phenotypes like affective disorder, several special precautions should be taken in the design and analysis of linkage studies. First, linkage results—particularly in large pedigrees—should be recalculated several times, each time changing the diagnosis (or genotype) of one person in the pedigree, to be sure that the results do not depend too heavily on any one individual. Second, it is important to detect multiple ancestral sources of illness and consider this fact in the linkage model. Third, affected-only linkage methods should always be part of a linkage study of diseases with late and variable age at onset or suspected incomplete penetrance. Results that are not supported by the affected-only analyses should be viewed with appropriate suspicion.

Recent The results of the second generation of linkage studies of BPAD are beginning to appear, distinguished from the first generation by larger sample sizes, use of nonparametric (affected relative pairs) as well as parametric linkage methods, and the universal use of highly polymorphic DNA markers. A reported linkage to chromosome 18p has been independently replicated. Other reports also suggest additional loci on the long arm of chromosome 18. New reports suggesting linkage to Xq26, and to chromosomes 4p and 21q have also appeared; the latter has been replicated in an independent series of pedigrees.

Berrettini et al. reported evidence of linkage between BPAD and polymorphic DNA markers within the pericentromeric region of chromosome 18. While overall LOD scores were not significant, several individual families yielded LOD scores consistent with linkage and affected sib-pair and affected pedigree-member results were statistically significant.

Stine et al. also reported evidence of linkage between BPAD and markers on 18p, within the same region implicated by Berrettini et al. On average, a highly significant 64% of sib-pairs affected with bipolar or recurrent unipolar disorder shared alleles of a DNA marker in this region. Stine et al. also found evidence of linkage to markers on 18q. Significant excess sharing of paternally, but not maternally, transmitted alleles was observed at three neighboring 18q markers. The evidence of linkage to loci on both 18p and 18q was strongest in the families with affected or transmitting fathers. In this set of families, the peak LOD score was 3.51 on chromosome 18q; LOD scores in the families with an affected or transmitting mother were negative. Similar results were seen in affected sib-pair analyses. Such a parent-of-origin effect for BPAD had been suggested by previous studies and has also been detected in a reanalysis of the Berrettini et al. data. Three other groups have since published weakly supportive evidence for an 18q locus in BPAD, and the group reporting the original 18q linkage has found further evidence of linkage to 18q in a new set of families.

Caveats and Outlook Recent linkage reports suggest that, in contrast to earlier findings, linkage findings in BPAD, particularly on chromosomes 18 and 21, are not only detectable but replicable. Linkage methods work best when one or only a few genes underlie the phenotype of interest, while in complex phenotypes like BPAD, linkage results are more difficult to interpret, with many false positives and false negatives. The uncertainties inherent in the linkage study of BPAD mean that linkage findings, even when confirmed, are unlikely in themselves to provide fundamental insights. Such insights must await the identification of specific genes and mutations. While such an achievement is clearly visible on the horizon, very large sample sizes or the fortuitous discovery of an expanding triplet repeat, linkage disequilibrium effect, or cytogenetic abnormality will probably be necessary in order to localize linkage with the precision necessary for the commencement of gene-identification approaches.

The linkage studies of BPAD to date suggest that neither a single major locus nor a large number of genes, each of very small effect, will be found to underlie the phenotype. As has been shown for other complex phenotypes, like IDDM, it appears that a few genes of moderate effect (each conferring a relative risk of disease that is two to five times greater than that for persons not carrying the disease allele), probably acting in concert but with considerable heterogeneity in different populations, will ultimately be identified.

ASSOCIATION FINDINGS The association approach is a method that complements linkage studies, typically by focusing on candidate genes, i.e., genes, the function of which makes them plausible candidates for a pathophysiologic role in BPAD. The association approach hypothesizes that when a gene underlies a given phenotype, certain alleles of that gene should be more commonly found in patients than in unaffected controls. Association methods look for a correlation between gene and phenotype in a population, while linkage methods look for this correlation within families. In linkage disequilibrium studies, association methods are used to detect marker alleles that lie so close to a disease gene that recombination between the marker and the disease gene occurs only rarely. Association approaches are more sensitive than linkage approaches in the face of significant genetic heterogeneity. But, like linkage approaches, association approaches are subject to false-positive findings, particularly when patient and control groups are not well-matched.

Tyrosine hydroxylase is the rate-limiting enzyme in the synthesis of catecholamine. An association between alleles of the gene encoding tyrosine hydroxylase, which maps to the tip of chromosome 11p, has been suggested by some studies, but the potential of a false-positive association has not been ruled out. Similarly, a few studies point to an association between BPAD or manic behavior and the gene for MAO-A, on Xp11. A number of studies have reported and association between affective disorder and polymorphisms near the serotonin transporter gene, but these may prove to be false-positive findings arising from population differences between cases and controls (for a review, *see* Greenberg et al.). Other reported associations have either proved to be spurious or have repeatedly failed to be replicated.

To date, only one study of BPAD has used the linkage disequilibrium approach across the genome. However, searching within a linked chromosome region for alleles associated with the phenotype is becoming a standard approach to narrowing the implicated chromosome region so that gene-identification studies can be accomplished efficiently. For this approach, genetically isolated populations are particularly useful.

Caveats and Outlook Association studies have the potential to contribute significantly to the search for genes underlying BPAD. However, the selection of appropriate candidate genes is problematic. As pointed out by Crowe, all 20,000 genes expressed in the human brain are potential candidates. Even if it were possible to carry out the needed 20,000 association experiments, almost all of the positive findings would prove spurious, given the strong prior odds against any particular gene's being involved in BPAD. Narrowing candidate genes to those brain-expressed genes lying within areas of replicated linkage may offer a solution to this dilemma. Furthermore, the power of association methods to narrow linked regions via linkage disequilibrium may prove to be of great value in the identification of disease genes through physical mapping approaches. Once the first etiologic mutation is identified in BPAD, identification of the other important genes will be hastened. For example, sequence analyses have revealed that genes can be grouped into families or superfamilies, with similarities in sequence predicting similarity of function. A gene known to cause BPAD thus strongly implicates other genes in the same family as candidates.

MOLECULAR PATHOPHYSIOLOGY

HOW GENETIC DEFECTS COULD CAUSE MOOD DISORDER Genetic studies of the affective disorders promise to revolutionize our understanding of molecular pathophysiology by implicating specific mutations as causal events leading to a mood disorder. But genetic findings alone will be insufficient. As stated at the beginning of this chapter, the genetic findings will only be interpretable in the context of detailed knowledge about the structure and function of the brain.

One can speculate that genes encoding transcription factors (especially genes that regulate circadian rhythms, and the family of stress-induced immediate-early genes), neurotransmitter transporters, and second-messengers (such as G proteins) may ultimately be implicated by genetic studies of affective disorders. Data from family studies suggest that genes containing triplet-repeat sequences or genes in the mitochondrial genome are worthwhile candidates for study. Still, linkage and association methods offer the best hope for revealing which of the numerous good candidate genes actually play an etiologic role. Association methods are also the best way to identify genes that, while not themselves etiologic, play an important role in modifying the expression of the affective disorder phenotype. Indeed, when a disease is caused by many different highly pathogenic mutations, each of which is rare or uncommon, modifier loci may be the most important identifiers of those at risk for the disease. The apo E4 association with Alzheimer disease is a good example of a modifier locus that is of greater significance in the general population than any given causative disease allele.

MANAGEMENT/TREATMENT

HOW DISCOVERY OF A GENE WILL AFFECT MANAGEMENT AND TREATMENT The discovery of even one major gene underlying the affective disorders will revolutionize management and treatment. The identification of gene carriers among patients presenting for treatment will aid in accurate diagnosis using a much more valid method of disease classification—that based on the specific mutation involved—than is currently possible. It will also become possible to develop treatments that are truly rational, i.e., based on an understanding of the pathophysiology of the illness at the molecular level. Today, although currently available treatments are effective for the vast majority of patients with major affective disorders, we do not know why our treatments work when they work or why they fail when they fail. It is even possible that some of the mutations underlying major affective disorder will be amenable to gene therapy, raising the possibility of truly curative treatments for this devastating group of illnesses.

SELECTED REFERENCES

American Psychiatric Association. Diagnostic and Statistical Manual of Mental Disorders, 4th ed. Washington: American Psychiatric,1994.

Berrettini WH, Ferraro TN, Goldin LR, et al. Chromosome 18 DNA markers and manic-depressive illness: evidence for a susceptibility gene. Proc Natl Acad Sci USA 1994;91:5918–5921.

Bertelsen A, Harvald B, Hauge M. A Danish twin study of manic depressive disorders. Brit J Psychiat 1977;130:330–351.

Baron M, Freimer NF, Risch N, et al. Diminshed support for linkage between manic depressive illness and X-chromosome markers in three Isralei pedigrees. Nat Gen 1993;3:49–55.

Cavazzone P, Alda M, Turecki G, et al. Lithium-responsive affective disorders: no association with the tyrosine hydroxylase gene. Psychiatry Res 1996;64:91–96.

Crowe RR. Candidate genes in psychiatry: an epidemiological perspective. Am J Med Genet (Neuropsychiatr Genet) 1993;48:74–77.

Gershon ES, Hamovit J, Guroff JJ, Nurnberger JI, Goldin LR, Bunney WE. A family study of schizoaffective, bipolar I, bipolar II, unipolar and normal control probands. Arch Gen Psychiatry 1982;39:1157–1167.

Greenberg BD, McMahon FJ, Murphy DL. Serotonin transporter candidate gene studies in affective disorders and anxiety: promises and potential pitfalls. Mol Psychiatry, in press.

Hall JG. Genomic imprinting: review and relevance to human diseases. Am J Hum Genet 1990;46:857–873.

Kelsoe JR, Ginns EI, Egeland JA, et al. Re-evaluation of the linkage relationship between chromosome 11p loci and the gene for bipolar affective disorder in the Old Order Amish. Nature 1989;342:238–243.

Kendler KS. Twin studies of psychiatric illness: current status and future directions. Arch Gen Psychiatry 1993;50:905–915.

Kendler KS, Neale MC, Kessler RC, Heath AC, Eaves LJ. The lifetime history of major depression in women. Arch Gen Psychiatry 1993; 50:863–870.

Kessler RC, McGonagle KA, Zhao S, et al. Lifetime and 12-month prevalence of DSM-III-R psychiatric disorders in the United States:esults from the National Comorbidity Survey. Arch Gen Psychiatry 1994; 51:8–19.

Kraepelin E. Manic-Depressive Insanity and Paranoia. Edinburgh: E & S Livingstone, 1921.

Lander ES, Schork NJ. Genetic dissection of complex traits. Science 1994;265:2037–2048.

Leonhard K. Aufteilung der endogenen Psychosen. Berlin: Akademie-Verlag, 1957.

MacKinnon DF, McMahon FJ, Simpson SG, McInnis MG, DePaulo JR. Panic disorder with familial bipolar disorder. Biol Psychiatry 1997;42:90–95.

Mahieu B, Souery D, Lipp O, et al. No association between bipolar affective disorder and a serotonin receptor (5-HT2A) polymorphism. Psychiatry Res 1997;70:65–69.

McInnis MG, McMahon FJ, Chase G, Simpson SG, Ross CA, DePaulo JR. Anticipation in bipolar affective disorder. Am J Hum Genet 1993;53:385–390.

McMahon FJ, Hopkins PJ, Xu J, et al. Linkage of bipolar affective disorder to chromosome 18 markers in a new pedigree series. Am J Hum Genet 1997;61:1397–1404.

McMahon FJ, DePaulo JR. Genetics and age at onset. In: Shulman KI, Tohen M, Kutcher S, eds. Mood Disorders Throughout the Lifespan. New York: Wiley-Liss, 1996; pp. 35–48.

McMahon FJ, Stine OC, Meyers DA, Simpson SG, DePaulo JR. Patterns of maternal transmission in bipolar affective disorder. Am J Hum Genet 1995;56:1277–1286.

Mendlewicz J, Rainer JD. Adoption study supporting genetic transmission in manic-depressive illness. Nature 1977;268:327–329.

Risch N. Linkage strategies for genetically complex traits. Am J Hum Genet 1990;46:229–241.

Rosanoff, AJ, Handy LH, Plesset IR. The etiology of manic-depressive syndromes with special reference to their occurrence in twins. Am J Psychiatry 1935;91:725–740.

Rubensztein DC, Leggo J, Goodburn S, Walsh C, Jain S, Paykel ES. Genetic association between monoamine oxidase A microsatellite and RFLP alleles and bipolar affective disorder: Analysis and meta-analysis. Hum Mol Genet 1996;5:779–782.

Shields J, Gottesman II. Man, Mind, and Heredity: Selected Papers of Eliot Slater on Psychiatry and Genetics. Baltimore: Johns Hopkins, 1971.

Stine OC, Xu J, Koskela R, et al. Evidence for linkage of bipolar disorder to chromosome 18 with a parent-of-origin effect. Am J Hum Genet 1995;57:1384–1394.

Straub RE, Lehner T, Luo Y, et al. A possible vulnerability locus for bipolar affective disorder on chromosome 21q22.3. Nat Genet 1994;8:291–296.

Tsuang MT, Faraone SV. The Genetics of Mood Disorders. Baltimore: Johns Hopkins, 1990.

Weissman MM, Bruce ML, Leaf PJ, Florio LP, Holzer C. Affective Disorders. In: Robins LN, Regier DA, eds. Psychiatric Disorders in America: The Epidemiologic Catchment Area Study. New York: Free Press, 1991.

Winokur G, Clayton PJ, Reich R. Manic-Depressive Illness, St. Louis: CV Mosby, 1969.

World Health Organization. The ICD-10 classification of mental and behavioural disorders: clinical descriptions and diagnostic guidelines, 10th ed. Geneva: World Health Organization, 1992.

Young RC, Klerman GL. Mania in late life: focus on age at onset. [Review]. Am J Psychiatry 1992 Jul, 1995;149:867–876.

111 Alcoholism

Eric J. Devor and Arthur Falek

INTRODUCTION

The many biochemical, familial/genetic, and molecular studies of alcoholism carried out in recent years are representative of the state of psychiatric genetics. This is to say that, despite the fact that there have been great advances made in each of these areas, the grail still eludes us; no precise mechanism has yet been elucidated to explain the transmission of risk, though there is ample evidence that vertical risk transmission does occur. On the other hand, it is also true that the gap in the ring is closing. As with nearly every major complex disease, including the psychiatric disorders, studies of the biochemistry, genetic epidemiology, and molecular biology of alcoholism are inexorably converging on a unifying model of pathogenesis. The exact nature of the model is unknown at present, but some of its general features have been defined, even though this has occurred primarily through discovering what is not included. Naturally, at this stage all knowledge is of value, and in this context it is useful to always keep in mind the great aphorism of Sherlock Holmes that, when all else is eliminated, whatever remains, however unlikely, must be the truth! In this chapter, therefore, we will give as much weight to negative evidence as we will to positive evidence and will use both to provide the general outlines of a model of the genetics of alcoholism.

One fact may be stated at the outset: that there is a plethora of evidence of the vertical transmission of risk in alcoholism; that is to say, the disease runs in families. Indeed, the familiality of alcoholism is one of its oldest and most robust features. The notion that heredity plays a significant role in alcoholism is an old one, dating perhaps back to the origins of alcoholic beverages themselves. References to the familiality of alcoholism and to the "passing on" of the disease from generation to generation may be found in the writings of the ancient Grecks, including both Aristotle and Plutarch, as well as those of the ancient Chinese. Moreover, it is clear in those writings that such ideas came to them from even more remote times. Interestingly, it was recognized, even in the oldest surviving records, that alcoholism was not a simple disease. Rather, complex and even contradictory patterns of inheritance were described. In some works, the scope of the inheritance of alcoholism was expanded to include presumed pleiotropic effects. For example, Long, reporting on his survey of the offspring of alcoholics in 1879, noted that 21% of the "inherited diseases" observed among these offspring could be attributed to alcoholism in the parents.

From: *Principles of Molecular Medicine* (J. L. Jameson, ed.), ©1998 Humana Press Inc., Totowa, NJ.

A classic early, systematic study of alcoholism was reported by Crothers in 1909. In that study, Crothers found that 70% of the more than 4000 alcoholics he had treated over a 35-year period had relatives whose own drinking habits could be described as moderate to excessive. Since then, virtually every study of alcoholics has confirmed of Crothers' conclusion that susceptibility of alcohol abuse/alcoholism is familial, and it can be accepted that "something that runs in families" is operating to produce at least part of the observed patterns of risk. The questions that still remain are: What is this something, and how does it operate?

A NATURAL HISTORY OF ALCOHOLISM

As with most psychiatric and neuropsychiatric disorders, a consensus definition of alcoholism is difficult to come by. However, the definition of alcoholism by Keller, quoted in Goodwin and Guze, is an acceptable working definition: "The repetitive intake of alcoholic beverages to a degree that harms the drinker in health or socially or economically, with indication of inability consistently to control the occasion or amount of drinking." This reference to so-called "loss of control" is an important feature in the discussion of heterogeneity among alcoholics, a topic we will take up later on.

Generally speaking, the epidemiology of alcoholism is also not well-defined. More is known about the patterns of drinking in general than about alcoholism *per se*. However, it is known that gender, age, education, socioeconomic status (SES), and ethnicity all play a role in the lifetime risk of alcoholism. Surveys of lifetime risk from Europe and a few from the United States agree that the reasonable "ballpark" figures are from 3 to 5% among males and from 0.1 to 1% among females. Taking these numbers as an average, it has been shown that African Americans in urban settings have higher rates of alcoholism than do Caucasians, whereas Orientals in all settings have consistently lower rates. Native Americans, who were frequently branded as ubiquitously heavy drinkers, display a great range of alcoholism prevalence and, in fact, some groups are now known to have very low rates. A further complication are the observations that women tend to begin heavy drinking at a later age than do men, and that African Americans begin to drink at younger ages than do whites of comparable SES. Clearly, there are complex interactions among epidemiologic variables that tend to make it difficult to do more than just describe these general tendencies.

Regardless of the patterns of occurrence, one thing is clear: Alcoholism is a behavioral disorder, and the behavior at the root of the disease is the consumption of large quantities of alcohol on repeated occasions. The reasons for this consumption are often obscure and may be unknown. But as consumption progresses and the amounts consumed increase, there are some common behavioral sequelae. As problems related to drinking excessively become greater, the alcoholic often attempts to hide the condition by drinking alone, hiding bottles, and sneaking drinks. This behavior is almost always accompanied by feelings of guilt and remorse. Guilt and remorse, in their turn, lead to more drinking and a vicious circle is established.

Alcoholics often display symptoms of anxiety and depression. They attempt to relieve these symptoms in the short term by their drinking, but in the long term these same symptoms are exacerbated by that drinking. In addition to either inducing or enhancing low mood, irritability, anxiety, and violence, long-term alcohol consumption has the unusual capability of producing amnesia—the classic alcoholic "blackout." Beyond these behavioral effects of the prolonged use of alcohol in large amounts, there are also serious medical complications. Chief among these is, of course, cirrhosis of the liver but nearly every organ system is affected either directly or indirectly by years of heavy alcohol consumption.

One result of the years of study of end-organ damage in alcoholism is the evidence that the medical effects of alcohol consumption themselves appear to be under some genetic control. A classic alcoholic twin study in which concordance rates for alcoholism were assessed among 15,924 male twins also included data on alcoholic cirrhosis and psychosis. Concordance rates of 21.1% among monozygotic (MZ) twin pairs and 5.4% among dizygotic (DZ) twin pairs for psychosis and 14.6% among MZ twin pairs and 5.4% among DZ twin pairs for cirrhosis were reported. The authors of that study concluded that the alcoholism concordance rates among these twin pairs could not entirely account for the observed concordances of the medical and psychiatric sequelae, and that this constituted evidence that organ-specific complications themselves have an underlying genetic risk not associated with the overall alcoholism genetic risks. Other medical conditions for which some evidence of independent genetic risk is emerging include alcoholic cardiomyopathy and alcoholic pancreatitis.

THE GENETICS OF ALCOHOLISM

GENETIC EPIDEMIOLOGY We alluded early on to the evidence suggesting the vertical transmission of risk in alcoholism. Here, we will present some of this evidence in more detail because, as will become clear, the devil really is in the details.

Evidence of a genetic predisposition for any disease comes primarily from twin and adoption studies whereas the nature, or "architecture" of that genetic component comes mainly from family studies. Historically, the appeal of twin studies has been that they provide a means for assessing the relative contributions of genetic and nongenetic factors to the overall phenotype. The model twin paradigm asserts that, since MZ twins are genetically identical and DZ twins share only half of their genes on average, a greater similarity, or concordance, among MZ twins vs DZ twins for a particular trait can be taken as *de facto* evidence of a genetic component. The strength of that genetic component can thus be gaged by the degree of difference in MZ vs DZ concordance. This, of course, assumes that all other factors are equal!

Since 1960, a number of large twin studies of alcoholism, or of traits indicative of alcoholism, have been conducted. One of the most widely cited is the 1966 study of 902 male Finnish twin pairs in which three major components of drinking behavior were identified. These were frequency of drinking, amount of alcohol consumed, and loss of control over consumption. Among these three components, only loss of control failed to exhibit evidence of genetic control. The other two, frequency of drink and amount consumed, displayed modest heritabilities of 0.39 and 0.36, respectively for frequency. Subsequent studies of 11,500 Finnish twin pairs of both sexes and of 7500 Swedish twin pairs of both sexes confirmed these results by demonstrating heritability estimates for frequency of consumption and amount consumed in the range of 0.30–0.40.

One of the earliest twin studies that focused on alcohol abuse rather than upon consumption was the 1960 study of 174 Swedish male twin pairs by Kaij and colleagues. This study, along with a similarly focused examination of 850 American twin pairs, suggested that alcohol abuse itself had a heritability in the same 0.30–0.40 range as did consumption. This pattern was further supported by the classic twin study of clinically defined alcoholism conducted by Hrubek and Omenn mentioned previously. Thus, it appears clear from twin studies that overall, about one-third of the risk for consuming and abusing alcohol is a result of genetic factors.

One indication of a major advance in heritability studies in recent years is the trend toward separating risk by gender. Among the early studies of twin pairs, only one reported heritability estimates sexes separately. Those investigators noted that, based on their sample size, the difference in male-specific heritability of 0.37 and female-specific heritability of 0.25 for alcohol intake was statistically significant. In more recent studies, the evidence of heritable factors operating to differentially mediate risk of alcohol abuse and alcoholism among men and women has been compelling. Kendler and colleagues examined a sample of 1030 like-sex twin pairs using various definitions of alcoholism and found that, while all definitions provided evidence in favor of a genetic contribution to risk, only their broadest definition was conclusive in showing a concordance of 47% among MZ twins and 32% among DZ twins. Importantly, their data indicated alcoholism was under some genetic control in both sexes, though the nature of this genetic component was likely to be different among women than among men. This impression has been substantiated by the results of a large Australian twin survey. There, it was reported that proband-wise concordance rates were 57% among male MZ twin pairs vs 33% among male DZ twin pairs. These rates compared to proband-wise concordances of 29% among female MZ twin pairs vs 19% among female DZ twin pairs.

The Australian Twin Survey went further and examined concordances among opposite-sex twin pairs. It was found that the risk of alcoholism among the male co-twins of female affecteds was four times that among the female co-twins of male affecteds (60 vs 15%). In the terms of the classic formulation of the multifactorial model of disease risk, these findings suggest a substantially higher loading for risk among affected women than among affected men. That is, women have a much higher liability threshold than do men. A somewhat different conclusion was reached in an earlier study by of 114 male twin pairs and 55 female twin pairs. An observed proband-wise concordance of 76% among male MZ twin pairs compared to 53% among male DZ twin pairs and 39% among female MZ twin pairs compared to 42% among females DZ twin pairs. While these data would tend to deny the presence of a genetic contribution to risk among the female affected, they did not examine opposite-sex pairs in order to assess differential risk loads. Even so, when the details of the extant twin data are sorted out, the overall evidence points toward a complex and interactive model of the genetic control of risk in which gender appears to play a major role. This should, of course, surprise no one.

A similarly complex set of phenomena are available in the results of the numerous, excellent adoption studies of alcoholism. The theory underlying the adoption study paradigm is a sound one. If the nature of liability transmission is substantially genetic, then at-risk adoptees, in whom the nongenetic familial milieu has been changed from high risk to low risk, should still develop the disorder in question at a higher rate than controls from a low-risk setting and nearly equal to their high-risk relatives in high-risk environments. However, if this paradigm is true, one of the earliest adoption studies of alcoholism was an inauspicious start. In the early 1940s, Roe reported that there were no differences in risk among adoptees compared with low-risk controls and, therefore, no genetic factors. The series of Danish adoption studies carried out in the early 1970s have served to relegate the Roe results to a less significant status. In the Danish series, a rigorous design selected subjects who were adopted away at an early age and had no subsequent contact with their biological relatives. The excellent records obtained through the Danish registries allowed comparison of both male and female adoptees of alcoholic parents, not only with matched controls from nonalcoholic parents but with their nonadopted same-sex siblings. This three-way comparison revealed that the adopted-away sons of alcoholic parents were four times as likely to become alcoholic than were the adopted-away sons of nonalcoholics, but nearly equal to their nonadopted male siblings. As before, however, the adopted-away daughters of alcoholic parents displayed no increased risk nor did their nonadopted same sex siblings. The rate for the adopted-away daughters of alcoholic parents was around 2% compared to 3% among their nonadopted siblings and 4% among the controls! In these studies, however, was an observation that was later to prove to be a key element in a massive record-linking Swedish adoption study. Investigators observed that not only were the adopted-away sons of alcoholic parents at much higher risk for becoming alcoholic than were the controls, but their alcoholism tended to be much more severe and had an earlier age of onset.

A research team headed by Bohman, Cloninger, and Sigvardsson set out in the late 1970s to make use of the excellent adoption registry data available in Sweden and also to use the gold mine of mandatory registrations of individuals with the government-run Temperance Board. Linking these databases together enabled the classification of 862 Swedish males adopted prior to age 3 on the basis of severity of alcohol abuse, not only among the adoptees themselves, but among both their biological and adoptive parents as well. This permitted the data to be subdivided among four groups; e.g., adoptees with and without a family history of alcohol abuse in either their biological or adoptive families, by level of severity of abuse, and to use both adopted and biological controls. A significant genetic heterogeneity and gene–environment interaction was demonstrated in these samples. The study showed that adoptees having both pre- and postnatal risks were more than four times as likely to become alcoholic as were adoptees from low-risk backgrounds (27 vs 6%). Making use of the same record-linking study design, the same pattern of risk was demonstrated among female adoptees. Beyond this, the wealth of information gathered in this study, including the crucial severity classifications, revealed in detail the pattern of greater severity and earlier age of onset among some male adoptees that was hinted at in other studies.

The results of the Swedish adoption study design led to the now famous formulation of Type I and Type II alcoholism. This formulation held that there were three clinical and etiologic subtypes of alcoholism. The first, termed Type I or milieu-limited alcoholism, in which both male and female subjects developed the disorder, is marked by adult onset and a less severe course, that was receptive to treatment. The Type II, or male-limited, form was expressed primarily among males and was marked by onset in the early teens, much more severe symptoms, including criminality related to alcohol abuse and low treatment success. Among the female relatives of these Type II alcoholics, there was an increased risk of somatization disorder rather than alcohol abuse. Somatization is characterized by numerous physical and emotional complaints, including pains, gastrointestinal disturbance, anxiety, sexual and marital maladjustment, and mood disorder for which no causes can be found. Such individuals have a long and florid medical history. This condition, also called Briquet's syndrome, was found in the female relatives of another type of alcoholism found in this study, in which males displayed severe antisocial, criminal behavior, and low treatment success. Among these female relatives, however, the somatization disorder appeared at a much higher frequency and was itself more severe than that seen in the female relatives of the Type II alcoholics.

In the years since the original presentation of the Type I/Type II alcoholism formulation there have been detractors and critics of the idea, but the weight of evidence from other investigators has tended to favor the view that alcoholism is not a unitary disorder, that there are in fact clinically and etiologically distinct subtypes of alcoholism. Recently, a much-anticipated replication of this earlier study was presented. This replication again employed the large-scale record-linking study design and was composed of 577 male and 660 female adoptees from Sweden. The results confirm the Type I/Type II dichotomy and reinforce the earlier conclusion that the more severe Type II form has a substantially greater genetic component of risk. The question remains, however, as to the architecture of that genetic component, and it is here that family studies have shed some light.

Familial/genetic studies of alcoholism have been conducted by many investigators for many years and, regardless of the definitions used, the ascertainment schemes employed, and the extent of the studies, it is clear that alcoholism aggregates in families. In one investigation, hospitalized alcoholics were studied, and it was found that 34% of their male relatives and 9% of their female relatives were themselves alcoholic. Even higher recurrence rates were found elsewhere. In another series, 54% of male relatives and 17% of female relatives of probands were also alcoholic compared to 20 and 4% of the male and female relatives of controls. Overall, the recurrence risks in relatives of alcoholics have been found in family studies to be as much as seven times higher than in relatives of nonalcoholics. Of course, as much, and more, data regarding the nature of recurrence risks have been gathered from the many twin and adoption studies of alcoholism. The true power of the family study design, however, emerged along with the sophisticated analytical methods of genetic epidemiology in the 1980s.

The methods of genetic epidemiology descend both analytically and philosophically from the multifactorial model of risk in complex, common diseases. These methods permit the investigator to decompose the genetic and nongenetic components of liability and to assess the genetic architecture of the heritable component. It is further possible to use these methods to determine the relative contributions of major gene loci and of a polygenic background in shaping the heritable component. One of the earliest applications of the method of complex segregation analysis to the question of risk transmission in alcoholism was the 1987 family study by Gilligan and colleagues. Utilizing the pedigree information on a sample of 286 hospitalized alcoholics, the investigators determined that the families of male alcoholics were etiologically heterogeneous. Some of the families seemed to be like the families of the female probands. These were termed Type I-like in reference to the Cloninger typology scheme. Other families appeared to resemble Type II male-only families and were designated as Type II-like. Heritability estimates for alcoholism in the Type I-like families were in the range of 0.20. In the Type II-like families, it was found to be very high: 0.88. Segregation analyses of these families then revealed that there was significant genetic heterogeneity among male alcoholics, and that there were two distinct genetic architectures associated with the different levels of heritability. The less heritable Type I familial form was marked by a polygenic architecture, whereas the highly heritable Type II form was found to be under the control of a single dominant major gene effect. Two additional features of that study must be mentioned, however. The first is that no departures from purely Mendelian transmission were reported for the major locus but, second, in order for the major locus model to fit, the penetrances of the major gene conferring increased risk were required to be both gender-specific and quite low. Penetrance refers to the probability that an individual carrying a risk gene will actually express it in the form of the disease. An example of a completely penetrant disease gene is Huntington's chorea, wherein every person who inherits the gene eventually develops the disease if he or she lives long enough. Among males, penetrance estimates for alcoholism were less than 30% and, among females, penetrance estimates were less than 10%. The difficulty here is that these are penetrances that could look almost nongenetic in a family sample.

In a subsequent study using the same segregation analysis methods, another group reported that the genetic architecture of risk in a sample of 35 multigenerational families was indeed consistent with a major genetic effect, but that a single, major Mendelian genetic locus was not the basis of the effect. Recently, a reanalysis of these data using a more sophisticated model was reported. This third-generation technique indicated that non-Mendelian transmission of the major effect on risk was consistent with a genetic architecture involving the presence of a "few" major loci contributing to risk in a developmental progression. This newest result is completely in line with the developmental model of alcoholism risk summarized later in this chapter.

The genetic epidemiology of alcoholism has advanced our knowledge to a point where the useless notion of factors "versus" each other, whether they be genetic vs nongenetic, major gene vs polygenes, or shared vs nonshared, can be dispensed with. What has emerged is a more sophisticated view that all factors contribute to risk, and that their relative effects change over time. What remains to be done is to find these factors, especially the genetic factors, define them, and then build an understanding of how they work.

MOLECULAR AND BIOCHEMICAL GENETICS One of the legacies of the single-factor era in alcoholism research, and of psychiatric genetics research in general, has been the notion of "the" gene. Whether it was the gene for alcoholism, or the gene for schizophrenia, or the gene for depression, the search was focused on finding that one gene that by its very presence conferred increased risk to developing the disorder in question. This idea encouraged us to make hopeful-looking lists of potential candidate genes and to begin to assess their roles in "causing" our disease (*see*, for example, the impressive list of potential candidate genes for alcoholism provided by Devor and Cloninger, 1989:31). The result of this was that the single causal gene idea entered the molecular era nearly unchanged from the biochemical marker era.

An ideal example of this notion is the HLA-association study paradigm. In one investigation, Corsico and colleagues typed a sample of 30 alcoholics for 11 HLA-A antigens, 16 HLA-B antigens, and 9 HLA-DR antigens. They compared their HLA types with two different control groups with the result that significant associations for increased HLA-B40 and HLA-D3 frequencies and for decreased HLA-DR4 frequency were observed. The authors concluded from these statistical associations that alcoholism must have a significant genetic component, and that the HLA system is a major component of risk. Numerous investigators, including Gilligan and Cloninger, have noted that, for such studies, the number of markers tested and the sample sizes used can have a substantial influence on the chances of finding an association and that the statistical analyses must be corrected for the number of tests performed. This is to say, the more you look, the more chance you run of coming across a false-positive. Here, then, replication of an association would seem to be key, and it is worth noting that none of the HLA associations with alcoholism have survived this test.

In the molecular era, a scenario similar to the HLA studies has already occurred. In 1990, Blum and colleagues announced a statistically significant association between a restriction fragment-length polymorphism (RFLP) near the human D2-dopamine receptor gene (*DRD2*), on chromosome 11q22-q23 and alcoholism. An RFLP is a marker found in the DNA base sequence itself that appears to be linked to a risk gene.* The Blum et al. data showed that one of two variant DNA sequences, or alleles, of an RFLP revealed near the D2 dopamine receptor gene by the DNA restriction enzyme Taq I was present in a significantly higher number of alcoholics than controls. Their announcement of this association launched a flood of replication studies using a clone for the human *DRD2* gene that, for a time, resembled a virtual cottage industry. The field of psychiatric genetics was consumed by the debate as to whether or not *DRD2* played a role in alcoholism risk and whether or not it may act as a modifier of severity. To date, dozens of papers have been published addressing these and other questions about *DRD2*. While the arguments still continue in the psychiatric genetics literature, the importance of the *DRD2* gene in alcoholism has decreased.

Lost in the debate about the role that DRD2 may or may not play in alcoholism was an interesting aspect of the context of the initial claim of association. The clone of the *DRD2* gene was only one of nine markers selected and, among these, only three displayed polymorphisms for the enzymes used in the study. Several of the other markers had known RFLPs with other enzymes and yet these RFLPs were not screened. Thus, of the nine markers cited, only three polymorphisms were studied, but DRD2 was significant. The point of this digression is to note an interesting sociological aspect of such studies. Once the DRD2 association was reported everything else was ignored, including some odd methodology in the original paper. Over time, the weight of evidence has turned

*For many readers the RFLP may be only an historical phenomenon. A brief history and detailed description of the RFLP, its immediate successors, and their roles in the development of molecular genetic studies of disease, may be found in Devor (1992).

against an association of DRD2 with alcoholism, not in the least because no adequate functional mutation or pathophysiologic mechanism has been found to explain it. This is not to say, however, that DRD2 and the other dopamine receptors are irrelevant to the pathogenesis of psychiatric disorders. Indeed, credible evidence involving DRD2 in other forms of substance abuse is coming to light, and the D4 dopamine receptor, DRD4, has been tentatively associated with schizophrenia. Thus, research on the dopamine receptors continues and will do so for some time to come. However, the story of DRD2 and alcoholism is a perfect example of the single, causal gene paradigm.

It is interesting to note that one of the markers unsuccessfully studied in the original Blum et al. paper was monoamine oxidase (MAO). The relationship between the activity of MAO and alcoholism is one of the most replicated finding in all of psychiatric genetics. There are two isoforms of this enzyme, MAO-A and MAO-B, each having its own substrate affinities and kinetic properties. The two isoforms are encoded by separate genes located together on the X-chromosome (Xp11.3). The two genes appear to have arisen from a common ancestral form via a duplication. Interest in MAO and its role in alcoholism began with the 1977 study of Wiberg and colleagues who reported significantly lowered MAO-B activities among alcoholics when compared with controls. Since that report, the finding of decreased MAO activity among alcoholics has been replicated many times. Moreover, studies of MAO activity and the alcoholic subtypes defined by Cloninger have consistently found that the more severe and more genetically determined Type II alcoholics have the lowest activities among alcoholics and controls.

Reich proposed in 1988 that a marker of genetic susceptibility to a disease must pass three specific tests:

1. The marker itself must be highly heritable.
2. The marker must be present in as yet unaffected offspring of affecteds.
3. There must be demonstrable increase in risk among the relative of affecteds who carry the marker vs the relatives of affecteds who do not carry the marker.

The years of study of MAO would suggest that it passes all three of these tests. The activity of the enzyme has been shown to be under the influence of a single major gene. Familial studies of the sons of alcoholics showed that MAO meets the second criterion. Other family studies have demonstrated a greater risk of alcoholism and other psychopathologies among the relatives of alcoholics who have low MAO activities vs the relatives of alcoholics who have more normal enzyme activities. The weight of evidence would seem to support the conclusion that MAO activity is in fact a genetic marker of risk in alcoholism but, as has been the case for all other aspects of such research, some newer studies have cast some doubt on this conclusion. In one of these, the first molecular marker for *MAO-B*, a dinucleotide repeat located in one of the noncoding regions of the *MAO-B* gene itself was studied in a sample of 74 alcoholics and 34 nonalcoholic controls. No association of the molecular marker with alcoholism could be demonstrated in their data. Moreover, a follow-up family study has asserted that one of the findings of lowered MAO-B activities among alcoholics and alcoholic subtypes was confounded by gender differences in enzyme activities. Once these differences were accounted for, the statistical significance of the lower activity levels among the alcoholic subtypes could not be replicated. However, in that reanalysis, the investigators did find a significant difference in MAO activity, but only among males. Thus, even for an association as apparently robust as that between MAO and alcoholism, more work will be required to understand the nuances.

One marker that has also been studied among alcoholics for many years but for which the nuances do appear to be understood is the mitochondrial aldehyde dehydrogenase, *ALDH2*. A dominant mutation in the human *ALDH2* gene, located on chromosome 12q24, results in the loss of enzymatic activity in the liver. This defect reduces the conversion of acetaldehyde to acetic acid and is associated with the well-known "flushing" reaction in response to alcohol ingestion. This reaction is characterized by facial flushing, nausea, palpitations, and lightheadedness, and appears to be the consequence of slowed removal of acetaldehyde from the body. Historically, the flushing reaction has been associated with Asian populations and this correlates well with the distribution of the mutant allele ALDH2*2. Also, it is believed that the ALDH2*2 mutation represents a protective factor against alcoholism in populations in which it occurs, and this belief has been well-substantiated. In support of the allelic association, more detailed physiologic and psychologic analyses of the ALDH2*2 mutation phenotype have served to further reinforce the idea that it plays a protective role in alcoholism. Thus, ALDH2 represents the best known case of a genetic modifier of risk of alcoholism (*see* the discussion of secondary genotype/genotype interactions, *below*).

Finally, while there are many biochemical and molecular studies of alcoholism under way worldwide, few have produced potential markers of the status of MAO and ALDH2, by providing solid evidence that they do play some role in influencing risk, and none have passed the tests proposed by Reich. One that comes close is adenylate cyclase (AC). First reported by Tabakoff and colleagues, the activity of platelet AC in the presence of cesium fluoride was found to be significantly lower among alcoholics than among controls. This lowered activity was also found in lymphocytes of alcoholics. Subsequent familial/genetic studies of AC activity suggested that the phenomenon was under the primary control of a single major gene. The familial/genetic study suggested that the major gene involved in the regulation of AC activity and in the association with alcoholism was the G protein, G_s, that activates AC in response to receipt of a stimulus at a cellular receptor. This model has subsequently been verified by other investigators, and future studies of this phenomenon will finally determine the status of AC as a marker.

A DEVELOPMENTAL MODEL OF ALCOHOLISM

The information presented in this chapter forms a paradox of a sort. Given that the genetic epidemiology of alcoholism overwhelmingly supports the proposition that there is a substantial genetic component to risk, why has there not been one single gene identified as a true genetic risk locus? The answer lies in the nature of the methods used to look for risk genes and in the way that risk is understood or, better said, misunderstood. Twin studies and adoption studies are able to provide evidence that "something" is being transmitted in the families of alcoholics that burdens the relatives of affecteds with higher risk of becoming alcoholics themselves. These studies are also able to determine how much of this "something" is genetic in nature. Within this context, studies of the genetic epidemiology of alcoholics have performed brilliantly and have for once and for all time buried the utterly useless dichotomy of genetic vs environmental cause. The family studies have performed equally well in their appointed task of attempting

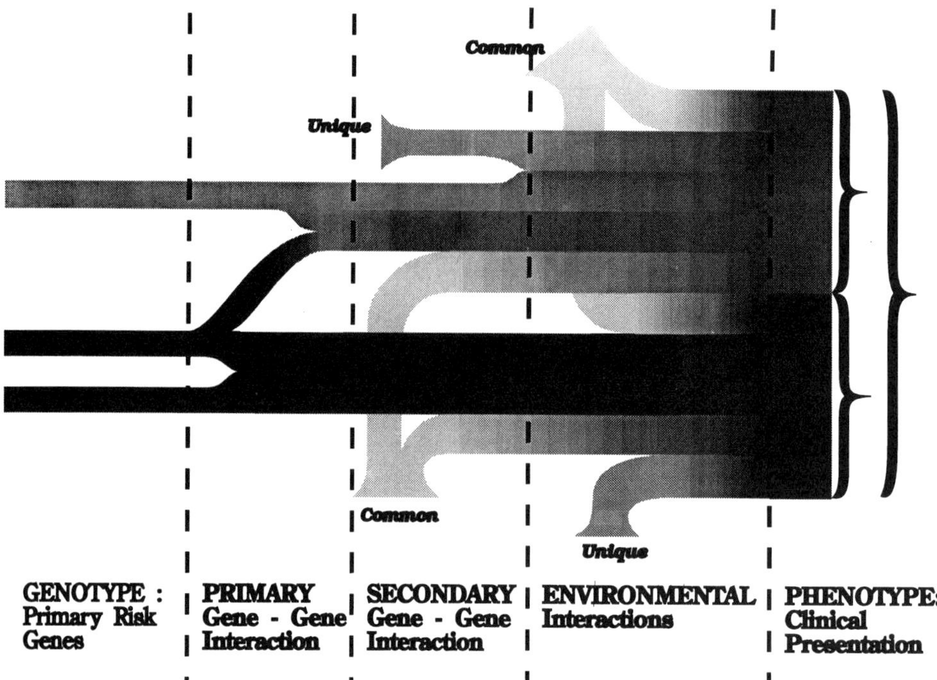

Figure 111-1 Graphic representation of a developmental genetic model of alcoholism. Part 1 indicates the existence of several primary risk genes. Part 2 demonstrates the possibility of interactions between these primary genes. Part 3 allows for other genes in the genome to interact with the primary genotype, further modifying it. Part 4 incorporates factors from the environment in the same interactive manner. Part 5 indicates that what is actually seen clinically is the end result that has been shaped by a lifelong process of interaction and modification. (Used with permission from Devor, 1993.)

to fashion a genetic architecture of the underlying risk. These studies have shown that, whatever the genetics may eventually turn out to be, the single major genetic locus with some or no multifactorial background will not be it. Accepting this interpretation of the state-of-the-field leads to an awkward question. Why is there no gene for alcoholism? The answer may be found in a cognitive dissonance that affects much of psychiatric genetics but one that is slowly abating. The field recognizes the multifactorial, oligogenetic nature of risk underlying common, complex disorders but has continued to approach it as if it were a single major gene phenomenon. The way to break out of this stalemate is simply to replace the single gene paradigm with a new one. This, obviously, is not easily accomplished, but a recent paper by Benjamin and Gershon acknowledges that this change is occurring and that thinking in psychiatric genetics has turned toward pursuit of genes of small effect that, together with the rest of the genome and the environment, both determine and influence risk.

In 1993, a dynamic developmental model of alcoholism was proposed as a heuristic device for abandoning the single gene mind-set. Later, specific implications of this model for linkage and association studies were outlined. The intellectual heritage of this developmental model can be traced to the seminal evolutionary genetics of Wright, to the concepts of canalization and epigenetics proposed by Waddington, and to the elegant multifactorial disease model formulated by Guze, Reich, and Cloninger. The philosophical impetus behind the model is eloquently summarized by Konner in *The Tangled Wing*:

> *Now that the discussion of heredity versus environment has transcended the "versus," passing beyond the question, Which? and the only slightly less useless question, How much? to the mature question, How? we must prepare ourselves to face the fact that this last is not one question at all, but thousands. For each system, for each moment in development, we may have on our hands a different balance, a different division of labor, a different integration of the functions of the genes and of the world.*

Here, then, is the mind-set that is replacing the single-gene linkage analysis search for "the" gene for complex diseases.

A developmental model of alcoholism is presented in Fig. 111-1. The model is composed of five parts. The first part represents the fundamental, pristine state present at fertilization, in which there exists a set of alcoholism-specific genes that confer "primary risk" to developing the disease. These genes are representatives of a finite pool of risk gene loci that segregate alleles more or less independently in the human population, with each allele conferring a specific increase in liability on the individuals who inherit it. For schizophrenia, a disorder in which risk among relatives falls off precipitously with decreasing degrees of relatedness, Reich postulates that the pool may be as small as two or three loci. For alcoholism, it may not be many more and, in the absence of inbreeding or phenotypic assortative mating, the presence of any of the risk alleles in any particular combination could be essentially random. However, when two or more primary risk-enhancing alleles are present in any one individual the possibility of primary gene–gene interactions exists. This is shown in the second part of the model in Fig. 111-1.

The primary gene–gene interaction effects depend on which genetic combinations are present, and these could range from simple additive risk loading (in which each gene adds to the overall risk of developing the disease without regard to which other genes are present) to true nonlinear epistatic effects (in which the increase in risk is greater than a simple sum of these effects and does depend on which other genes are present). Beyond this level of primary risk loading is a secondary level of gene–gene interactions (part 3), which recognizes the fact that the primary risk genotype exists in a developmental milieu composed of the rest of the genome. Thus, secondary gene–gene interactions may occur that involve genes that are not alcoholism-specific. Some of these secondary genes may exert a unique effect, affecting one or a few primary risk genotypes, or they may exert a common effect, affecting most or all primary risk genotypes. As was alluded to earlier in this chapter, such secondary interactions may increase the risk loading conferred by the primary genotype, or they may be protective and decrease the risk loading.

Part 4 of this model explicitly recognizes the role of nongenetic factors in modifying the entire relevant genotype. These environmental interactions may, as with secondary gene–gene interactions, be unique or specific to a small number of genotypes by acting through, for example, one particular secondary interaction pathway, or they may be ubiquitous, affecting most or all possible genic combinations. The overall effect of this interactive, developmental model is to precisely produce the types of clinical variations observed (e.g., age of onset, sex differences, response to treatment, severity, and familiality).

The practical experience with alcoholism to date does suggest that relatively few distinct alcoholic subtypes exist. This, in turn, permits us to speculate that the levels of interaction may be few, the actual number of primary risk loci and secondary modifying loci is small, or both. In this case the situation is manageable, and the search for these genes will ultimately be successful.

In closing, we refer to a sentiment written near the opening of the molecular era of alcoholism research that has proven to be prophetic, but remains true. In referring to the search for alcoholism risk genes, "the task is enormous, the pitfalls many, and the cost high, yet the payoff is staggering—a fundamental understanding of the genetics of an addiction and a realistic program of intervention based upon that understanding" Devor and Cloninger, 1989:29).

SELECTED REFERENCES

Babor TF, Hesselbrock V, Meyer RE, Shoemaker W. Types of Alcoholics: Evidence for Clinical, Experimental, and Genetic Research, vol. 708. New York: The New York Academy of Sciences, 1994.

Blum K, Nobel EP, Sheridan PJ, et al. Allelic association of human dopamine D2 receptor gene in alcoholism. JAMA 1990;263: 2055–2060.

Crothers TD. Heredity in the cause of inebriety. Brit Med J 1909;2: 659–661.

Devor EJ. Introduction: A brief history of the RFLP. In: Devor EJ, ed. Molecular Applications in Biological Anthropology. Cambridge, UK: Cambridge University Press, 1992; pp. 1–18.

Devor EJ. Why there is no gene for alcoholism. Behavior Genet 1993;23:145–151.

Devor EJ, Cloninger CR. Genetics of alcoholism. Annu Rev Genet 1989;23:19–36.

Dinwiddie SH. Genetics of alcoholism. In: Miller NS, ed. The Principles and Practice of Addictions in Psychiatry. Philadelphia: WB Saunders, 1997; pp. 26–34.

Eighth special report to the U.S. Congress on alcohol and health. U.S. Department of Health and Human Services. NIH Publication No. 94–3699, 1994.

Goodwin DW, Guze SB. Psychiatric diagnosis, 4th ed. Oxford, UK: Oxford University Press, 1989.

Gordis E. Genes and the environment in complex diseases: a focus on alcoholism. Mol Psychiatry 1997;2:282–286.

Hill SY. Vulnerability to alcoholism in women: genetic and cultural factors, vol. 12. In: Galanter M, ed. Recent Developments in Alcoholism. Women and alcoholism. New York: Plenum, 1995; pp. 9–28.

Holden C. A cautionary genetic tale: the sobering story of D2. Science 1994;264:1696–1697.

Hrubek Z, Omenn GS. Evidence of genetic predisposition to alcoholic cirrhosis and psychosis: twin concordances for alcoholism and its biologic end-points by zygosity among male veterans. Alcohol Clin Exp Res 1981;5:207–215.

Jellinek EM. Phases of alcohol addiction. Q J Stud Alcohol 1952;13:673–684.

Kidd KK, Pakstis AJ, Castiglione CM, et al. DRD2 haplotypes containing the TaqI A1 allele: implications for alcoholism research. Alcohol Clin Exp Res 1996;20:697–705.

Konner M. The Tangled Wing. New York: Holt, Rinehart, and Winston, 1982.

Long JF. Use and abuse of alcohol. Trans Med Soc North Carolina 1879;26:87–100.

Nestler EJ. Molecular mechanisms of drug addictions. J Neurosci 1992;12:2439–2450.

Palmer TN. The Molecular Pathology of Alcoholism. New York: Oxford University Press, 1991.

Parsian A, Chakrawverty S, Fisher L, Cloninger CR. No association between polymorphisms in the human dopamine D3 and D4 receptors genes and alcoholism. Am J Med Genet 1997;4:281–285.

Reich T. Biologic marker studies in alcoholism. New Engl J Med 1988;318:180–182.

Sigvardsson S, Bohman M, Cloninger CR. Replication of the Stockholm adoption study of alcoholism. Confirmatory cross-fostering analysis. Arch Gen Psychiatry 1996;53:681–687.

The Genetics of Alcoholism, Alcohol Health and Research World, vol. 19(3). US Department of Health and Human Services, NIH Publication No. 96–3466, 1995.

Watts TD, Wright R Jr. Alcoholism in minority populations. Charles C. Thomas, Springfield, 1989.

Yuan H, Marazita ML, Hill SY. Segregation analysis of alcoholism in high density families: a replication. Am J Med Genet (Neuropsych Genet) 1996;67:71–76.

Genetic Basis of Congenital Malformations

XIII

Section Editor:
Ethylin Wang Jabs

112 Waardenburg Syndrome

ANDREW P. READ

BACKGROUND

AUDITORY-PIGMENTARY SYNDROMES IN HUMANS AND OTHER ANIMALS "What can be more singular than the relation between blue eyes and deafness in cats?" asked Charles Darwin in his *Origin of the Species*. In fact, the combination of hearing loss and pigmentary abnormalities is known in many other mammals, including dogs, horses, cattle, mink, mice, and humans. Most commonly, the skin or fur is white-spotted, sometimes white all over, and one or both eyes are blue. These syndromes are quite distinct from albinism. In albinos, melanocytes are present but produce no melanin as a consequence of an enzyme defect, usually lack of tyrosinase. In contrast, auditory-pigmentary syndromes are caused by a physical absence of melanocytes; this is associated with hearing loss but not with any visual problems. (Albinos suffer from poor eyesight because of a characteristic misrouting of optic nerve fibers.) Usually the absence is patchy, with areas of normal and depigmented tissue. In the inner ear, the stria vascularis of the cochlea contains melanocytes, and an absence of melanocytes correlates with a nonfunctioning cochlea, as judged by the lack of an endocochlear potential. Melanocytes are necessary for this function, but melanin is not, because albinos have normal hearing.

MELANOCYTES AND THE NEURAL CREST Melanocytes are migratory cells, originating in the neural crest of the embryo. Thus the underlying cause of auditory-pigmentary syndromes is either a failure of neural crest differentiation, failure of melanocyte precursors to migrate correctly, or failure to differentiate and survive in their end location.

CLINICAL AND GENETIC HETEROGENEITY OF HUMAN AUDITORY-PIGMENTARY SYNDROMES Human auditory-pigmentary syndromes have been described under many names and are undoubtedly highly heterogeneous. Autosomal-dominant, autosomal-recessive, and X-linked forms have been described, with or without other syndromic features. Waardenburg syndrome (WS) is a heterogeneous entity named after the Dutch ophthalmologist and geneticist who published the first comprehensive description in 1951. In this chapter I will review the classification of WS and describe the role of the *PAX3* and *MITF* genes in its etiology. Other related genes and syndromes will be discussed more briefly.

From: *Principles of Molecular Medicine* (J. L. Jameson, ed.), ©1998 Humana Press Inc., Totowa, NJ.

CLINICAL FEATURES

The subtypes of Waardenburg syndrome are listed in Table 112-1. Other related conditions are discussed in the section on Diagnosis.

WAARDENBURG SYNDROME TYPE 1 Waardenburg's original description was of "developmental anomalies of the eyelids, eyebrows and nose root with pigmentary defects of the iris and head hair and with congenital deafness." The eyelid abnormality is dystopia canthorum *(see below)*. Other features are summarized in Table 112-2. The incidence is about 1/40,000.

WAARDENBURG SYNDROME TYPE 2 Arias pointed out that families could be divided into two types, those in which all affected people had dystopia canthorum (Type 1) and those in which dystopia was never seen (Type 2). The remaining features are similar in both types (Table 112-2). Figure 112-1 shows the contrasting facial appearances. In most studies, WS2 is one to two times as frequent as WS1.

WAARDENBURG SYNDROME TYPE 3 (KLEIN-WAARDENBURG SYNDROME) WS3 is extremely rare. The original patient described by Klein had very severe contractures and hypoplasia of her shoulders, arms, and hands, in addition to extensive depigmentation and other features of WS1. She resembled a WS1 homozygote reported by Zlotogora et al. (1995). Later reports have been of patients with WS1 plus mild contractures affecting the arms or fingers. These are probably a rare variant presentation of WS1. Some "WS3" patients have relatives with WS1; in several cases, PAX3 mutations have been described, and PAX3 is known to be expressed in the limb buds *(see below)*.

WAARDENBURG SYNDROME TYPE 4 (WAARDENBURG-SHAH SYNDROME) Shah reported a series of Indian babies with depigmentation and Hirschsprung disease, who died before their hearing could be assessed. Recently, the genetic basis of this recessive combination of WS2 and Hirschsprung disease has been unraveled *(see below)*.

DIAGNOSIS

CRITERIA FOR DIAGNOSING WAARDENBURG SYNDROME The label Waardenburg Syndrome is best confined to cases where the hearing loss is sensorineural, congenital, and nonprogressive, and where the inheritance is autosomal-dominant. Differential diagnoses include albinism (melanocytes are present but unpigmented, no hearing loss), vitiligo (postnatal onset and fluctuating course of depigmentation, no hearing loss), and piebaldism (extensive congenital depigmentation, no hearing loss, mutations in the *KIT* oncogene). Coincidental hearing loss can complicate the diagnosis.

Table 112-1
The Four Types of Waardenburg Syndrome

Type	*MIM no.*	*Inheritance*	*Features*
1	193500	AD	Dystopia canthorum
2	193510	AD	No dystopia
3 (Klein-Waardenburg)	148820	AD? (most cases sporadic)	Dystopia + limb abnormalities
4 (Waardenburg-Shah)	277580	AR	Hirschsprung disease

Table 112-2
Features of Waardenburg Syndrome Type 1 and Type 2

	Feature	*WS1, %*	*WS2, %*
Major criteria	Congenital sensorineural hearing loss >25dB	57	77
	Iris pigmentary abnormality		
	Heterochromia: eyes of different colors; or clearly demarcated segments of different colors in one eye;	20	50
	Isochromia: characteristic brilliant blue eyes	15	25
	White forelock in hair	45	25
	Dystopia canthorum	98	Absent
	Affected first-degree relative.		
Minor criteria	Several areas of congenitally hypopigmented skin	35	10
	Medial flaring of eyebrows with synophrys	65	Rare
	Broad high nasal root	75	Rare
	Hypoplasia of the alae nasi	Common	Rare
	Graying of the hair before age 30	Common	25

For Waardenburg syndrome, the Waardenburg Consortium defined an affected person as someone having two major, or one major and two minor criteria. The criteria are given in Table 112-2, along with estimated penetrances in WS1 and WS2, from the study of Liu et al. The apparently somewhat higher incidence of hearing loss and heterochromia in WS2 is probably an artefact of ascertainment: Without dystopia as a guide, patients are not diagnosed unless they show several other features of WS.

DIFFERENTIAL DIAGNOSIS OF TYPE 1 AND TYPE 2 WAARDENBURG SYNDROME Because dystopia is specific and highly penetrant, WS1 can be diagnosed with confidence and shows little or no genetic heterogeneity. The inner canthi are displaced outward so that the palpebral fissures are short, with little of the sclerae showing on the medial side of the pupil; the inferior lacrimal punctae lie in front of the cornea, and there is a broad high nasal root with synophrys (confluent eyebrows). Experience shows that dystopia canthorum needs to be assessed by measuring the inner canthal, interpupillary, and outer canthal distances (a,b,c respectively, in millimeters) with a rigid ruler held in front of the head, and then applying the formula

$$W = X + Y + a/b$$

where

$$X = (2a - 0.2119c - 3.909)/c$$

and

$$Y = (2a - 0.2479b - 3.909)/b$$

This rather abstruse measure (the numbers come from a discriminant analysis) has proved extremely effective for distinguishing WS1 ($W > 1.95$) from WS2 ($W < 1.95$). By contrast, clinical impression, even by skilled judges, has proved unreliable. The distinction is important to make because, as shown below, it holds the key to molecular diagnosis.

TYPE 2 WS AND OTHER RELATED SYNDROMES WS2 is not homogeneous. Clinical definition is arbitrary, and molecular studies show heterogeneity. About 20% of families have mutations in the *MITF* gene *(see below)*. Rare patients with Hirschsprungs disease plus features of WS2 (and thus describable as WS4) have an endothelin defect *(see below)*.

Many patients with auditory-pigmentary syndromes do not fall into any of the categories described above, and many other ill-defined auditory-pigmentary syndromes are listed in the literature, but little is known of the underlying genetics. In thinking about their clinical classification, it is useful to try to distinguish melanocyte-specific defects from more general neurocristopathies. Neurocristopathies arise early in embryonic development, whereas death of melanocytes can occur at any time. Nevertheless, this distinction is not always clear-cut. WS1 is mainly caused by dysfunction of the embryonic neural crest, but people with WS1 also often suffer premature graying of their hair 15–30 years after their neural crest completed its differentiation.

GENETIC BASIS OF WAARDENBURG SYNDROME

TYPE 1 WAARDENBURG SYNDROME Linkage to 2q35 and the Sp Mouse Model WS1 is relatively homogeneous genetically. Linkage was first demonstrated to the marker ALPP (alkaline phosphatase, placental isozyme) in 1989. ALPP maps to the distal long arm of chromosome 2. Recent collaborative studies using a microsatellite polymorphism from the *PAX3* gene suggest that all WS1 but no WS2 maps to this region. The map position was originally claimed to be 2q37, but more recent results suggest 2q35-q36. This region shows strongly conserved synteny with the proximal part of mouse chromosome 1, and a search of the corresponding mouse map suggested a likely homolog, *Splotch*. The heterozygous *Sp* mouse has no hearing loss, but nor do many

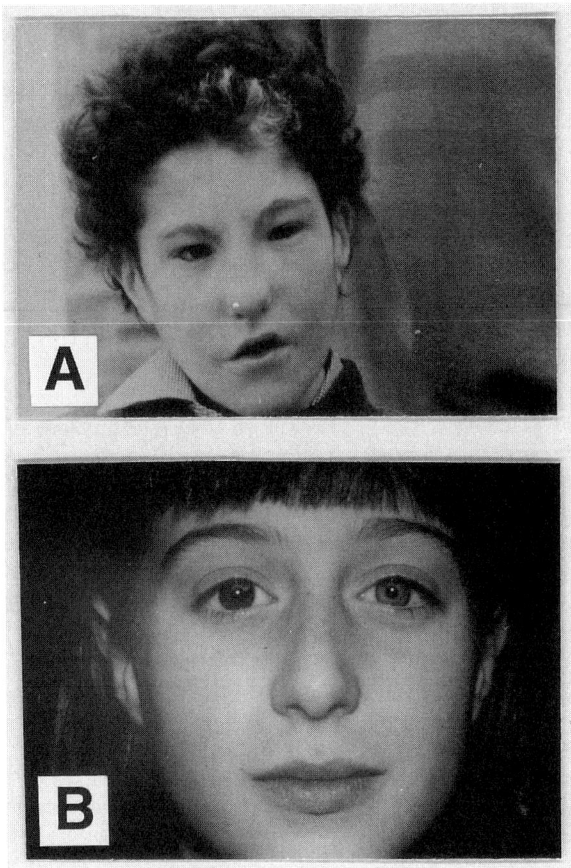

Figure 112-1 Facial appearance in (A) Type 1 and (B) Type 2 Waardenburg syndrome. Note dystopia canthorum in the patient in Panel A. This patient has a chromosomal deletion del(2)(q34q36.2) and is mentally retarded in addition to showing typical features of Type 1 WS. Neither Type 1 nor Type 2 WS is normally associated with any mental retardation.

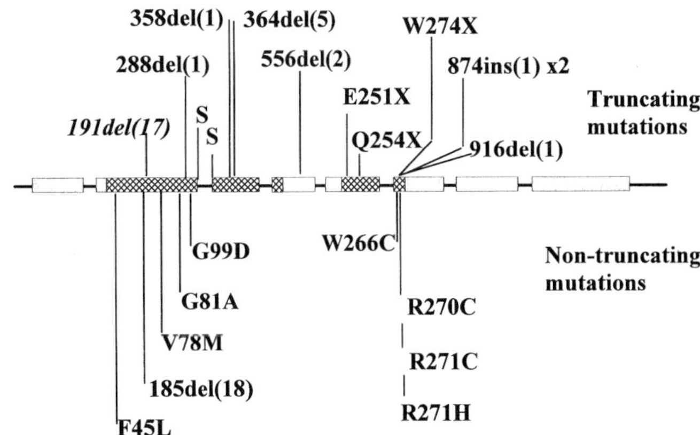

Figure 112-2 PAX3 mutations seen in Manchester patients with WS1. The eight exons of the PAX3 gene are shown, with the paired box in exons 2–4 and the homeobox in exons 5–6 shaded. Mutations expected to truncate the gene product are above the gene diagram, those expected to produce a full-length product are below. Note that, whereas truncating mutations are distributed across most of the gene, amino acid substitutions are pathogenic only when located in the 5' part of the paired box and the 3' part of the homeobox. These regions are critical for DNA binding by the PAX3 protein.

humans with WS1, and phenotypes of orthologous mouse and human mutants are often somewhat different. On some genetic backgrounds, *Sp* mice have a broad snout, probably corresponding to dystopia canthorum in man.

The PAX3/pax-3 Gene A candidate gene, *pax-3*, mapped to this region in the mouse and was expressed in the developing nervous system of the early embryo in a pattern compatible with the pathology, both of *Sp* and of WS1. The human homolog is *PAX3*, originally called *HuP2*. Searches revealed mutations in both Sp and WS1.

PAX3 is a very interesting gene. PAX genes, in both mouse and man, form a family of nine closely related genes. All share a paired box, a highly conserved 128 amino acid DNA-binding domain found in organisms from *Drosophila* to man. As well as the paired box, *PAX3*, *PAX6*, and *PAX7* have a homeobox. All the PAX genes are believed to encode transcription factors; the expression pattern of PAX3 in the early embryo is described below. *PAX3* was the first human homeobox gene shown to carry mutations causing inherited disease.

Other PAX Genes in Human Syndromes *PAX6* mutations cause aniridia and other abnormalities of the anterior chamber of the eye. Mutations in *PAX2* have been seen in a few families with combinations of eye (e.g., optic nerve coloboma) and kidney problems. The molecular pathology of all these conditions appears to involve haploinsufficiency. In each case there is a good mouse homolog, *sey* (small eye) and *krd* (kidney and retinal defects), respectively.

TYPE 2 WAARDENBURG SYNDROME In perhaps 20% of WS2 families the mutation maps to the proximal short arm of chromosome 3, and in some of these families mutations have been demonstrated in *MITF*, the human homolog of the mouse *microphthalmia* gene. The human *MITF* and mouse *mi* genes encode another transcription factor, a basic helix-loop-helix leucine zipper protein. Only about 20% of families with WS2 show evidence (by linkage or mutation screening) of involvement of *MITF*; the gene(s) responsible for 80% of WS2 have yet to be mapped or identified.

TYPE 3 WAARDENBURG SYNDROME In a few cases, *PAX3* mutations have been described. PAX3 is expressed in the developing limb muscles, and WS3 is probably a variant presentation of WS1.

TYPE 4 WAARDENBURG SYNDROME Mutations in the endothelin 3 or endothelin receptor B genes (on chromosomes 20 or 13, respectively) have recently been described in well-characterized affected patients with a combination of WS2-like pigmentary abnormalities and Hirschsprung disease.

MOLECULAR PATHOPHYSIOLOGY

EXPRESSION OF PAX3 In the mouse, *pax-3* is expressed in the developing nervous system starting at d 8–8.5 postcoitum. Expression occurs along the length of the neural tube, but only in the posterior part, including the neural crest. Expression is seen in various parts of the developing brain, and *pax-3* expressing cells migrate into the limb buds. The patterns of expression are described in more detail in the reviews cited at the end of this chapter. Preliminary studies in human embryos reveal a similar pattern. The expression pattern fits well with the observed features of WS1 and *Sp*, although as is usual in these cases, only a subset of expressing tissues is affected.

MOLECULAR PATHOLOGY OF PAX3 MUTATIONS *PAX3* mutations have been found in many families with WS1, but not in families with WS2. Figure 112-2 shows the mutations that

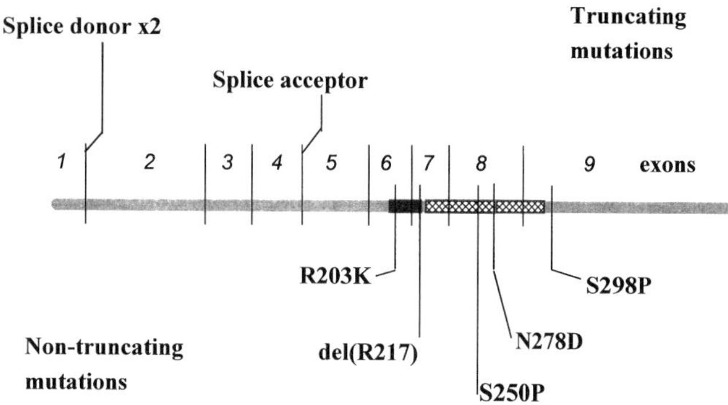

Figure 112-3 MITF mutations seen in Manchester patients with WS2. The gene has nine exons and encodes a DNA-binding basic domain (hatched in exon 6) and helix-loop-helix and leucine zipper dimerization domains (shaded, in exons 8–9). Mutations expected to truncate the gene product are above the gene diagram, those expected to produce a full-length product are below.

have been described in Manchester; similar mutations have been found by other groups within the Waardenburg Consortium. It is noteworthy that the mutations are very heterogeneous, including a complete deletion of the gene, truncating (nonsense or frameshifting) changes spread through exons 2–6, splice site mutations and amino acid substitutions. The substitutions are all of amino acids in the 5' part of the paired domain or the third (recognition) helix of the homeodomain. All of the amino acids involved are highly conserved across species and are known to take part in critical protein-DNA contacts in other PAX and homeodomain genes.

All of these changes produce the same clinical result, WS1. We conclude that WS1 is caused by a dosage effect in people heterozygous for a loss-of-function mutation.

As deaf people frequently marry, homozygotes may occur, and one case has been described. The child had severe depigmentation and limb contractures, but unexpectedly, considering the phenotype of homozygous *Splotch* mice, no neural tube defect. Nevertheless, it is likely that most *PAX3* mutations that cause WS1 in heterozygous people would be lethal in homozygotes.

Substitutions of asparagine 47 in the PAX3 paired domain may possibly produce a special phenotype. The mutation N47H was seen in the only known example of familial WS3, whereas a different substitution of the same amino acid, N47K, occurred in a family whose phenotype was described as craniofacial-deafness-hand syndrome (MIM 122880). Conceivably, these mutations represent a gain of function. Unambiguous (but somatic, not inherited) gain of function mutations of PAX3 are seen in the pediatric tumor alveolar rhabdomyosarcoma. In these tumors, a chromosomal translocation t(2;13)(q35;q14) creates a novel chimeric gene out of the 5' parts of *PAX3* and the 3' part of another transcription factor gene, *FKHR*.

MOLECULAR PATHOLOGY OF MITF MUTATIONS

Figure 112-3 shows human MITF mutations described in patients with WS2. All of these cases are dominant. In the mouse, both dominant and recessive alleles of *mi* are known. The difference can be explained by dominant negative effects of mutants that sequester the product of the normal allele in inactive dimers. Some of the human WS2 mutations would be predicted to be recessive in mice; however, maybe human homozygotes would be much more severely affected, as in mice. Transcripts and protein products of these mutant genes have not yet been studied.

MANAGEMENT AND TREATMENT OF WAARDENBURG SYNDROME

Apart from possible early graying of the hair, all features of Waardenburg syndrome are nonprogressive, and treatment is symptomatic. Early screening is important to identify hearing loss in infants.

FUTURE DIRECTIONS

For the known genes, *PAX3* and *MITF*, the major problem is the inability to predict the severity of symptoms of WS1 or WS2. Both conditions are variable even within families, so that severity must depend on the action of unidentified modifier genes. This makes genetic counseling difficult. Identifying the modifier genes and identifying the genes responsible for the bulk of WS2 are priorities. Although *PAX3* and *MITF* are known to be transcription factors, very little is known about their upstream regulators or downstream targets in the embryo. Knowing these might help identify genes for other auditory-pigmentary syndromes, as well as shedding light on an important part of embryonic development.

Gene therapy for WS seems problematic. *PAX3* and *MITF* have roles in basic pattern formation and differentiation in the embryonic neural crest. This makes them biologically interesting genes, but also makes it difficult to imagine effective postnatal gene therapy.

SELECTED REFERENCES

Asher JH, Harrison RW, Morell R, Carey ML, Friedman TB. Effects of Pax3 modifier genes on craniofacial morphology, pigmentation, and viability: a murine model of Waardenburg syndrome variation. Genomics 1996;34:285–298.

Asher JH, Sommer A, Morell R, Friedman TB. Missense mutation in the paired domain of PAX3 causes craniofacial-deafness-hand syndrome. Hum Mutat 1996;7:30–35.

Baldwin CT, Hoth CF, Amos JA, da-Silva EO, Milunsky A. An exonic mutation in the HuP2 paired domain gene causes Waardenburg's syndrome. Nature 1992;355:637–638.

Barsh GS. Pigmentation, pleiotropy and genetic pathways in humans and mice. Am J Hum Genet 1995;57:743–747.

Chakravarti A. Endothelin receptor-mediated signaling in Hirschsprung disease. Hum Mol Genet 1996;5:303–307.

Epstein DJ, Vekemans M, Gros P. Splotch (Sp2H), a mutation affecting development of the mouse neural tube, shows a deletion within the paired homeodomain of Pax-3. Cell 1991;67:767–774.

Farrer LA, Grundfast KM, Amos J, et al. Waardenburg syndrome (WS) type 1 is caused by defects at multiple loci, one of which is near ALPP on chromosome 2: first report of the WS Consortium. Am J Hum Genet 1992;50:902–913.

Foy C, Newton VE, Wellesley D, Harris R, Read AP. Assignment of WS1 locus to human 2q37 and possible homology between Waardenburg syndrome and the Splotch mouse. Am J Hum Genet 1990;46:1017–1023.

Galili N, Davis RJ, Fredericks WJ, et al. Fusion of a fork head domain gene to PAX3 in the solid tumour alveolar rhabdomyosarcoma. Nat Genet 1993;5:230–235.

Hanson I, Fletcher JM, Jordan T, et al. Mutations at the PAX6 locus are found in heterogeneous anterior segment malformations including Peters' anomaly. Nat Genet 1994;6:168–173.

Hemesath TJ, Steingrimsson E, McGill G, et al. Microphthalmia, a critical factor in melanocyte development, defines a discrete transcription factor family. Genes Dev 1994;8:2770–2780.

Hofstra RM, Osinga J, Tan-Sindhunata G, et al. A homozygous mutation in the endothelin-3 gene associated with a combined Waardenburg type 2 and Hirschsprung phenotype (Shah-Waardenburg syndrome). Nat Genet 1996;12:445–447.

Hoth CF, Milunsky A, Lipsky N, Sheffer R, Clarren SK, Baldwin CT. Mutations in the paired domain of the human PAX3 gene cause Klein-Waardenburg syndrome (WS-III) as well as Waardenburg syndrome Type 1 (WS-1). Am J Hum Genet 1993;52:455–462.

Klein D. Historical background and evidence for dominant inheritance of the Klein-Waardenburg syndrome (Type III). Am J Med Genet 1983;14:231–239.

Liu XZ, Newton VE, Read AP. Waardenburg syndrome Type 2: phenotypic findings and diagnostic criteria. Am J Med Genet 1995;55:95–100.

Nobukuni Y, Watanabe A, Takeda K, Skarka H, Tachibana M. Analyses of loss-of-function mutations of the MITF gene suggest that haploinsufficiency is a cause of Waardenburg syndrome type 2A. Am J Hum Genet 1996;59:76–83.

Pandya A, Xia XJ, Landa BL, et al. Phenotypic variation in Waardenburg syndrome: mutational heterogeneity, modifier genes or polygenic background? Hum Mol Genet 1996;5:497–502.

Puffenberger EG, Hosoda K, Washington SS, et al. A missense mutation of the endothelin-B receptor gene in multigenic Hirschsprung's disease. Cell 1994;79:1257–1266.

Sanyanusin P, Schimmenti LA, McNoe LA, et al. Mutation of the PAX2 gene in a family with optic nerve colobomas, renal anomalies and vesicoureteral reflux. Nat Genet 1995;9:358–363.

Steel KP, Barkway C. Another role for melanocytes: their importance for normal stria vascularis development in the mammalian inner ear. Development 1989;107:453–463.

Steel KP, Bock GR. Hereditary inner-ear abnormalities in animals: relationship with human abnormalities. Arch Otolaryngol 1983;109:22–29.

Steingrimsson E, Moore KJ, Lamoreux ML, et al. Molecular basis of mouse microphthalmia (mi) mutations helps explain their developmental and phenotypic consequences. Nat Genet 1994;8:256–263.

Strachan T, Read AP. PAX genes. Curr Opin Genet Dev 1994;4:427–438.

Stuart ET, Kioussi C, Gruss P. Mammalian PAX genes. Annu Rev Genet 1994;28:219–236.

Tassabehji M, Newton VE, Liu XZ, et al. The mutational spectrum in Waardenburg syndrome. Hum Mol Genet 1995;4:2131–2137.

Tassabehji M, Newton VE, Read AP. Waardenburg syndrome type 2 caused by mutations in the human microphthalmia (MITF) gene. Nat Genet 1994;8:251–255.

Tassabehji M, Read AP, Newton VE, et al. Waardenburg syndrome patients have mutations in the human homologue of the Pax-3 paired box gene. Nature 1992;355:635,636.

Waardenburg PJ. A new syndrome combining developmental anomalies of the eyelids, eyebrows and nose root with pigmentary defects of the iris and head hair and with congenital deafness. Am J Hum Genet 1951;3:195–253.

Xu W, Rould MA, Jun S, Desplan C, Pabo CO. Crystal structure of a paired domain-DNA complex at 2.5Å resolution reveals structural basis for Pax developmental mutations. Cell 1995;80:639–650.

Zlotogora J, Lerer I, Bar-David S, Ergaz Z, Abielovich D. Homozygosity for Waardenburg syndrome. Am J Hum Genet 1995;56:1173–1178.

113 Greig Cephalopolysyndactyly Syndrome and Limb Disorders

KARL-HEINZ GRZESCHIK

INTRODUCTION

In the process of dissecting the factors governing the formation of hands and feet from the limb buds, human genetic disorders in which polydactyly or syndactyly occurs can provide clues to the genes involved in separating and defining the outline of limb elements in normal development. The identification by the positional cloning strategy of a gene believed to be responsible for Greig cephylopolysyndactyly syndrome, a rare developmental disorder, characterized by craniofacial abnormalities and malformations of hands and feet, can serve as a paradigm for the value of this approach, since it drew attention to GLI3, a gene not previously expected to be involved in regulation of human development. Greig syndrome appears to result from haploinsufficiency of this gene. *GLI3* is a member of a zinc finger gene family that includes *Krüppel*, a gene that was known to regulate development in Drosophila. Nevertheless, the involvement of a zinc finger gene in mammalian development had not been demonstrated earlier.

The identification of a candidate gene involved in human limb development called for the application of the powerful methods of genetic dissection of this gene in the mouse. Such a combination of candidate gene search in human developmental malformations and gene analysis in animal model systems holds the promise to teach how genes develop the human gestalt.

CLINICAL FEATURES OF GREIG CEPHALOPOLYSYNDACTYLY SYNDROME

Greig cephalopolysyndactyly syndrome (GCPS, OMIM 175700) is a rare developmental disorder characterized by craniofacial abnormalities and postaxial polydactyly of the hands, preaxial polydactyly of the feet, and syndactyly of the fingers and toes. It shows autosomal dominant inheritance with full penetrance but with marked inter- and intrafamilial variability.

Characteristic limb and skull manifestations observed in more than 50 patients are listed in Table 113-1. Hand and foot malformations are mostly bilateral. If unilateral, a hand is more often affected than a foot. Postaxial polydactyly is common in the hands and preaxial polydactyly in the feet: The thumbs are frequently broad with a broad nail and a malformed distal phalanx, sometimes with a bifid tip. Radiographs of the hands can reveal preaxial polydactyly that is not noted on physical examination. Postaxial polydactyly of the hands usually manifests as a pedunculated postminimus, sometimes merely as a small cutaneous tag, with or without hypoplastic nail and a bony fragment as phalanx. The additional finger articulates at the ulnar side of the hand, mostly at the proximal or middle phalanx of the fifth finger; the fifth metacarpal bone is not affected (Fig. 113-1A).

In the feet, preaxial polysyndactyly is the most common malformation, including duplication of the distal phalanx of the hallux, of both phalanges, of both phalanges and metatarsus, and rarely of metatarsus alone (Fig. 113-1B). Broad halluces with broad nails are common. The fifth metatarsal bone, if not duplicated, is often broad and markedly altered in shape. Postaxial polydactyly of the feet has been observed occasionally resulting from duplication of the fifth toe (eventually only a single bony fragment is found) and broadening or duplication of the fifth metatarsal bone. Also in the feet, polydactyly sometimes was noted on radiographs only.

Syndactyly affects hands and feet as a constant feature but with some variability in its extent. It is mostly cutaneous in the feet, varying from mild webbing between the first two or three toes to complete cutaneous fusion, sometimes also with nail fusion. In the hands, bony fusion was reported on the distal phalanges of third to fourth fingers and of third to fifth fingers.

The craniofacial manifestations are variable and consist of a macrocephaly with a broad prominent forehead, a broad nasal root and brachycephaly (Fig. 113-1C). In individuals with large crania, the interpupillary distance will often be increased. The impression of hypertelorism is confirmed only rarely if canthal indices are used for correction. Prognosis for the mental and physical development of affected individuals is good. Advanced bone age seems to be a frequent finding in GCPS, suggesting an influence of the GCPS gene on bone development.

DIFFERENTIAL DIAGNOSIS

The wide variability of manifestations raised the question of whether or not other genetic entities thought to be distinct syndromes are not merely variants of the GCPS.

Acrocallosal syndrome (ACLS, OMIM 200990) is an autosomal recessive condition that shares manifestations with GCPS. However, neurological findings such as the severe mental retardation, hypotonia, and absence of corpus callosum in ACLS, are very

From: *Principles of Molecular Medicine* (J. L. Jameson, ed.), ©1998 Humana Press Inc., Totowa, NJ.

Table 113-1
Skull and Limb Manifestations in GCPS Patients[a]

Malformation	*Number observed*
Craniofacial	
Macrocephaly	23/44
High, broad forehead	25/36
Frontal bossing	21/36
Broad nasal bridge	30/38
Hands	
Preaxial polydactyly	
Clinical	4/41
Radiological	8/22
Postaxial polydactyly	
Clinical	36/46
Radiological	10/22
Broad thumbs	37/40
Syndactyly	33/40
Feet	
Preaxial polydactyly	
Clinical	40/49
Radiological	21/26
Postaxial polydactyly	
Clinical	3/39
Radiological	3/26
Broad halluces	26/29
Syndactyly	43/47

[a]Data compiled from Ausems et al. 1994, according to references described therein. When radiographs were performed after surgical treatment in patients with polydactyly, this item is scored clinically (+) and radiologically (–).

rare in GCPS. Also, the type of polydactyly differs and the syndactyly is less severe in ACLS, generally affecting only the proximal portion between the second and third toes. Since no linkage was found on chromosome 7 in patients with acrocallosal syndrome, it is very unlikely that acrocallosal syndrome and Greig syndrome are allelic disorders.

Greig syndrome can be so mild as to be indistinguishable from the normal. Therefore, preaxial polydactyly type IV, or uncomplicated polysyndactyly (OMIM 174700), a dominant trait characterized by broad duplicated thumbs that are radially deviated and duplication of the halluces or second toes, with syndactyly of the second and third toes, may be Greig syndrome. Also, *crossed polydactyly*, a condition with autosomal dominant inheritance, characterized by polydactyly of the hands and feet with discrepancy of the axes of polydactyly between hands and feet, which occasionally shows syndactyly but no associated craniofacial abnormalities might be Greig syndrome.

THE MOLECULAR GENETICS OF GCPS

IDENTIFICATION OF A GCPS CANDIDATE GENE The genetic locus of GCPS had been assigned to chromosome 7p13 by three balanced translocations associated with GCPS in different families with one chromosome breakpoint in this band. This assignment was corroborated by the detection of three sporadic cases carrying overlapping deletions in 7p13, as well as by tight linkage of GCPS to the epidermal growth factor receptor gene in 7p13–p12.

In a positional cloning effort, the translocation breakpoint region was covered with a contiguous restriction map employing arbitrary DNA fragments and the cDNA of the gene *GLI3* as hybridization probes. *GLI3* had been isolated by homology to the zinc-finger gene GLI, which is amplified in gliomas, and mapped to 7p13. It was considered a potential candidate gene for Greig syndrome, both on the basis of its map position and its homology to the *Drosophila* gene *Krüppel*, which is involved in the regulation of development. Since the GCPS translocation breakpoints were found to interrupt the genomic segment coding for the distal half of the *GLI3* gene, and since the interstitial deletions of 7p observed in three Greig patients also eliminated the *GLI3* gene region, it could be postulated that haploinsufficiency of *GLI3* might evoke the developmental malformations in at least some of the Greig syndrome patients. The size of the *GLI3* gene could be determined as at least 280 kb. The transcribed *GLI3* sequence is composed of 15 exons with the most 3' exon spanning about 2.5 kb of continuously transcribed DNA. The gene is flanked by a CpG island that lies on the 5' side and that is in close proximity to the first exon detected by the cloned *GLI3* cDNA. The presence of other genes in this region that might be affected by deletions or positional effects resulting from the translocation events, however, still cannot be excluded. Two large introns of 70 kb each in the 5' region of the *GLI3* gene would leave ample room for additional genes.

PROPERTIES OF GLI3 The *GLI3* gene belongs to the human *GLI-Krüppel* gene family. It encodes a zinc-finger protein of 1596 amino acids and an apparent molecular mass of 190 kDa. Multiple regions of sequence similarity aside from the zinc-finger region suggest that other aspects of function are shared among the members of this gene family of DNA-binding proteins. The gene is expressed in a wide variety of human adult tissues. Because of their ability to bind specific DNA sequences, zinc-finger proteins are generally considered to be transcription factors. The high similarity between the binding specificities of the members of this family suggests, however, that these genes may assume their specific function only through their developmentally regulated expression or interaction of other nonhomologous protein domains with additional cellular factors.

ANIMAL MODELS FOR GCPS

Additional evidence for the influence of *GLI3* on the embryonal development of limbs and skull is derived from the allelic mouse mutations *extra toes* (*Xt*) *anterior digit deformity* (*add*), and possibly also from the mouse mutant *Polydactyly Nagoya* (*Pdn*). The spontaneous semidominant mouse mutation extra toes affects limb development with almost complete penetrance in heterozygotes but variable expressivity (Fig. 113-2). Several *Xt* alleles have been reported since and mapped to a region on mouse chromosome 13 homologous to human chromosome band 7p13.

The *Xt* mutation in a (C3Hx101)F_2 mouse was shown to be a deletion of at least 80 kb beginning at the 5' side of the *GLi3* gene. In a second *Xt* allele, Xt^J, a more downstream deletion was detected extending from the first zinc-finger motif towards the 3' end of the gene spanning at least 30 kb. The *Xt* heterozygotes show phenotypic peculiarities similar to GCPS patients: predominantly preaxial polydactyly of the hind limbs and a postaxial nubbin on the forelimbs. They also often have an enlarged interfrontal bone and some show hydrocephaly.

Brachyphalangy (Xt^{bph}) is a radiation-induced allele that has similar effects to *Xt* but is distinguishable in both heterozygotes and homozygotes. Unlike *Xt* heterozygotes, Xt^{bph} heterozygotes usu-

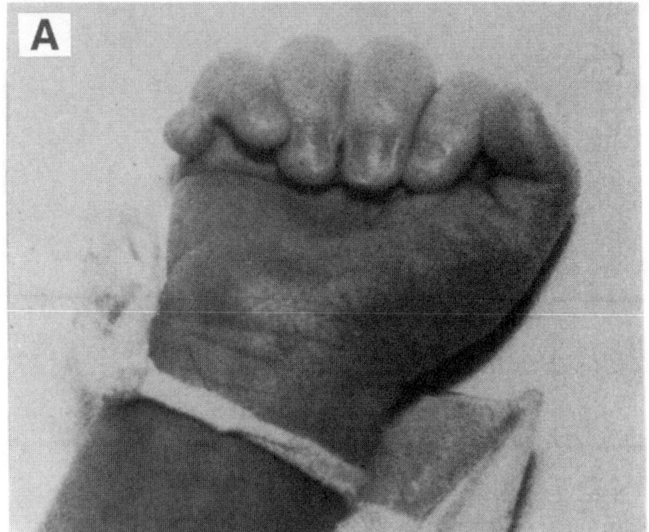

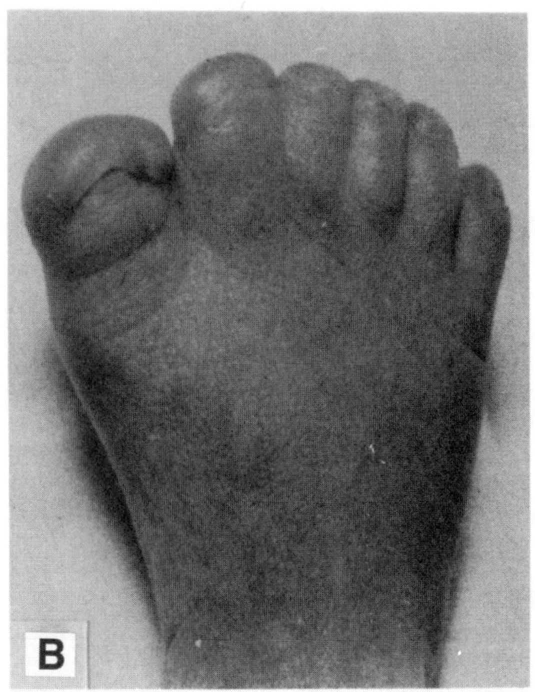

Figure 113-1 **(A)** Right hand, **(B)** foot, from patients with Greig Cephalopolysyndactyly Syndrome. (Reproduced with permission from Gollop and Fontes, Am J Med Genet 1985;22:59–68.)

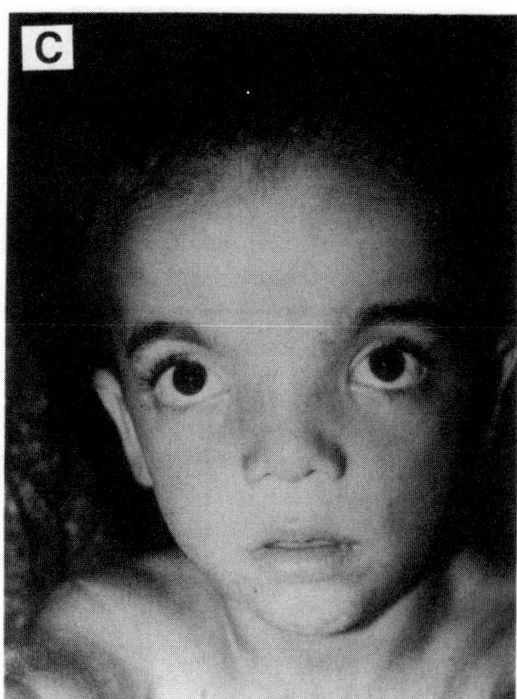

Figure 113-1 *(continued)* **(C)** Head from patient with Greig Cephalopolysyndactyly Syndrome. (Reproduced with permission from Gollop and Fontes, Am J Med Genet 1985;22:59–68.)

ally have an abnormal sternum and occasionally show syndactyly. All *Xt* alleles are homozygous lethal with more extreme limb and craniofacial defects as well as additional abnormalities of the brain, the central nervous system, and sense organs.

The *Pdn* mouse mutation is very likely to be allelic to *Xt*, but no effects on genomic structure nor expression of *GLI3* could be demonstrated yet.

The recessive mouse mutant add is an allele of the gene affected in *Xt*. This mutant was generated by insertional mutagenesis in mice. The *add* mutation originates from a transgene insertion within the segment deleted in $Xt^{(C3Hx101)F_2}$ at a maximal distance of about 44 kb from the transcription start of *Gli3*. The *add* insertion replaced only 1 bp of the wild-type sequence. Since the *GLi3* RNA expression level in homozygous *add/add* mice showed a reduction similar to that observed in heterozygous *Xt*/+ mice but no alteration of the transcript size, it can be postulated that the insertion of foreign material disturbed a region important for transcriptional control of *Gli3*.

In homozygous *add/add* mice the forelimb is disorganized. The morphology of the thumbs is always altered, and sometimes the adjacent finger has an extra phalanx. The effect of the *Xt* and *add* mutants on the phenotype of the feet is summarized in Table 113-2. The anterior digit duplications in extra-toes mutants are similar to the phenotype of homozygous ci^{w} *Drosophila* flies, which are caused by a mutation in the *Drosophila Gli* protein *cubitus interruptus* (*Ci*). This homology in function throughout the animal kingdom suggests that *Gli* proteins are part of a very basic, conserved signaling pathway.

MOLECULAR PATHOPHYSIOLOGY OF GLI3 DEFICIENCY

GLI3 AS A TRANSCRIPTIONAL REGULATOR Based on the phenotypic similarities of *Xt* heterozygotes with GCPS and the molecular evidence that homologous genes are affected in both species, it is possible to analyze the physiological role of *GLI3* and the consequences of its deficiency by comparing *GLI3* expression in normal embryonic development with the effects in *Xt* mice in organs not readily available for analysis in Greig patients.

The consequence at the molecular level of both *Xt* deletions as well as the GCPS mutations detected so far is the complete absence of *GLI3* expression from the affected locus. This haploinsufficiency results only in a small number of minor malformations. *Xt/Xt* homozygotes on the other hand, despite the complete lack of expression from both genes, generally survive until birth; however, with a number of severe malformations. These stress the

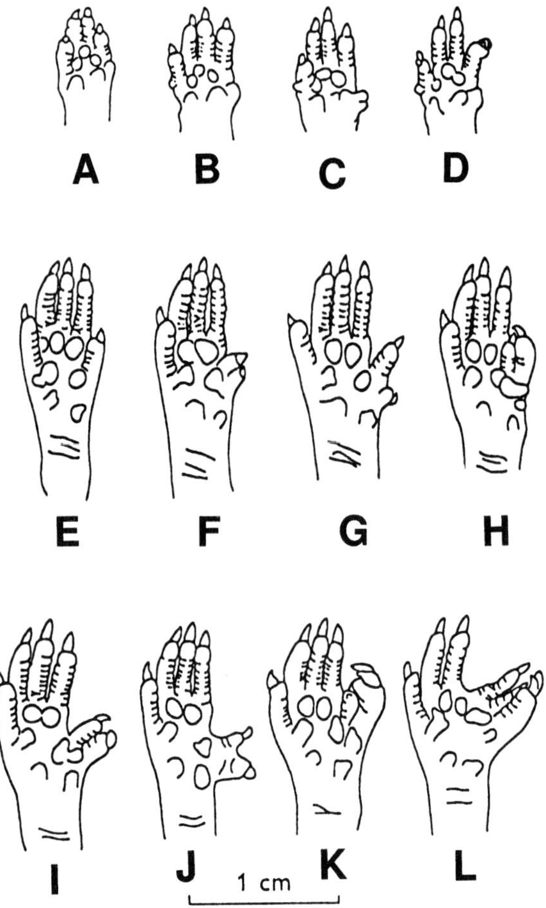

Figure 113-2 Plantar views of the feet of +/+ and *Xt*/+ mice. **(A)** +/+ right forefoot **(B–D)** *Xt*/+ right forefeet, **(E)** +/+ right hind foot, **(F–L)** Xt/+ right hind feet. Note short, broad, or bifid polluces and postaxial nubbin of tissue on forefeet and preaxial polysyndactyly of hind feet. (Reproduced with permission from Johnson et al., J Embryol Exp Morphol 1967;17:543–581.)

general importance of the *Gli3* protein as a determinator of many parts of the body plan. At the same time, it appears that most of the development can occur without any *Gli3* protein. This may reflect the presence of other very similar *Gli* genes. Lethality may result from the lack of a functioning *Gli3* gene after birth rather than from developmental defects.

The spatial and temporal pattern of high *Gli3* expression in mouse embryos correlates well with the *Xt* phenotype. The highest level of *Gli3* expression is found in limb buds, the developing craniofacial mesenchyme, and the brain, the most severely affected structures in *Xt*/*Xt* homozygous mice. In addition, *Gli3* is highly expressed in the intercerebral disk anlage and in the sternal cartilage, both in regions affected by *Xt* mutations. Thus, the proper amount of *Gli3* product appears crucial in areas where it is particularly highly expressed.

Possible mechanisms for such a dosage-sensitive regulatory system have been elucidated by the analysis of other *Krüppel*-type zinc-finger genes. In *Drosophila*, the *Krüppel* product, the prototype, can both activate and repress gene expression through interaction with a single DNA-binding site. The opposite regulatory effects of the *Krüppel* protein are concentration-dependent, and they require distinct portions of the protein such as the N-terminal region for activation and the C-terminal region for repression. The

Table 113-2
Induction of Digits According to *Gli3*[a] Alleles Present in Mice

Alleles	*Phenotype*
+/+	Normal digit number
add/+	Normal digit number
add/*add*	One thumb is changed
Xt/+	One extra toe
Xt/*add*	Two extra toes
Xt/*Xt*	Up to four extra toes

[a] *Gli3* expression inversely correlates with the number of digits formed.

Krüppel zinc-finger type transcription factor is able to form homodimers through sequences located within the C-terminus. The *Krüppel* monomer is a transcriptional activator. At higher concentration, *Krüppel* forms a homodimer and becomes a repressor that functions through the same target sequences as the activator.

Most important for the understanding of *GLI* function is the observation that during limb development in the *Drosophila Gli* protein Ci acts both as a repressor and activator of *decapentaplegic* (*dpp*) transcription in a concentration-dependent manner. The expression of *Dpp*, a homolog of the mammalian bone morphogenetic proteins (BMP), is normally repressed by low levels of *Ci*. An increase of *Ci* levels by *hedgehog protein* (*Hh*) signaling might overcome this regulation and result in *dpp* activation.

This dual function of a *Gli* protein during limb development in *Drosophila* might represent an evolutionarily conserved aspect of patterning by *Hh* family members. *Sonic Hh* plays an important role in mammalian limb development by specifying in conjunction with *BMP* pattern across the anteroposterior axis of the limb. A function for *GLI3* in the control of *SHH* signal production together with the control of *SHH* signal reception, may be consistent with the clinical observations in Greig Syndrome.

GLI3 IN LIMB DEVELOPMENT A wealth of experimental results on the regulation of limb development allows to speculate on the role that *Gli3* might play in this context. Limb formation in the vertebrate embryo is initiated by local proliferations of mesenchymal cells forming a bulge under the ectoderm, which is induced to form an apical ectodermal ridge (AER) at the anterior-to-posterior (first-to-fifth digit) rim of the limb bud by maintaining undifferentiated proliferating mesenchyme in the immediately subjacent area (Fig. 113-3). The AER also elaborates pattern along the proximal-distal axis (i.e., humerus to digits). A region in the posterior mesenchyme, the zone of polarizing activity (ZPA), controls patterning in the anterior-posterior axis. Genes involved in the induction and maintenance of this process in vertebrates are indicated in Fig. 113-3. Distal skeletal morphogenesis is a late event in limb development. Mesenchymal condensations occur in a sequence to become adult skeletal elements.

Several steps in this developmental cascade seem to be sensitive to the proper amount of *Gli3* product: In mouse embryos, *Gli3* expression in the period from day 7 to 12 of gestation at first is strong in undifferentiated mesenchyme of the developing limb. Then it becomes confined to the interdigital mesenchyme between the precartilageous rays of the future digits and the interzonal mesenchyme. Later, *Gli3* is highly expressed in the perichondrium, a mesenchymal layer of cells surrounding the developing cartilageous intermediate of the bones to be formed.

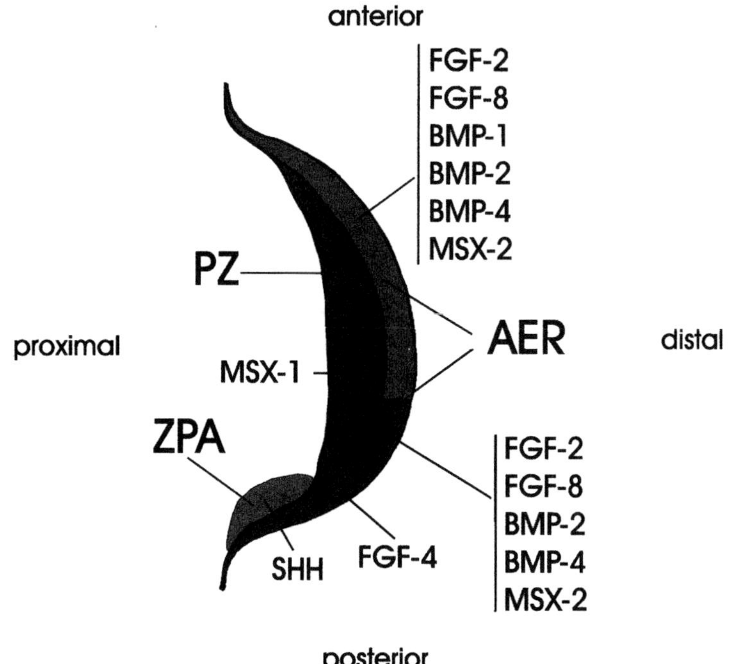

Figure 113-3 Molecules involved in pattern specification during limb bud development. Dorsal view of the limb bud. AER, apical ectodermal ridge: The ridge releases factors from signal to the underlying cells to maintain a high mitotic state and patterning activities. PZ, progress zone: Cells in the underlying mesenchyme progressively acquire more distal fates in the course of limb outgrowth. ZPA, zone of polarizing activity: Posterior mesenchyme cells express *Sonic hedgehog* (*SHH*) and exhibit polarizing activity, i.e., an active role in coordinating pattern formation at the growing tip of the limb by establishing a dynamic system of positional values in three dimensions. SHH induces FGF4 expression, and its own expression is maintained by FGF4 and a dorsalizing factor from the dorsal ectoderm, WNT7a. The full names of the factors are given in Table 113-3.

The level of *Xt* expression inversely correlates with the number of digits formed (Table 113-2). There is no indication for a polarized *Gli3* expression along the anterior-posterior axis. However, it seems that the developmental field on the anterior side of the limb mesenchyme is more affected by a reduction of gene dosage than the posterior. This reduction may directly determine the additional digits. Alternatively, lack of transcriptional control by the *Gli3* protein may initially result in an increased size of the limb and AER that would induce formation of additional digits. Various additional consequences of *Gli3* reduction, such as bones with aberrant shapes, fused or elongated bones, and syndactylies suggest that also inducing steps further downstream, such as apoptosis separating digital elements, are influenced by the level of *Gli3* product.

CANDIDATE GENES FOR HUMAN LIMB DEVELOPMENT

Each of the genes organizing size and shape of individual bones and the separation of individual fingers by apoptosis and outgrowth can be altered resulting in oligo- or polydactyly, syndactylies, or ectrodactyly. As outlined for Greig syndrome, the hint for an association of a gene with a function can originate from the study of human malformations or from candidate genes detected in animal models.

Only a few of the many human syndromes associated with malformations of hands and feet could be linked to candidate genes on specific human chromosomes. In rare cases, distinct mutations of candidate genes are known to cause malformations. The rich collection of candidate genes originating from the study of limb development in animal models awaits its exploitation for the study of human development. Table 113-3 compiles the fragmentary information from these three sources.

CONCLUSIONS

PERSPECTIVE OF MOLECULAR DIAGNOSTICS *GLI3* spans at least 280 kb of genomic DNA. Little more than the cDNA and intron–exon boundaries have been sequenced so far. The upstream gene sequences that are potentially important for gene regulation still have to be analyzed in detail. The known intron–exon structure will stimulate the search for mutations in this gene; however, a clinical routine application is not readily available.

FUTURE RESEARCH The recessive mutation in *add/add* mice seems to reduce the expression of the *Gli3* gene and thus produce less of an otherwise normal protein. This reduction induces overgrowth only in the most sensitive developmental fields, mainly the most anterior part of the forelimbs (thumb and, eventually, digits). All other mutations analyzed so far on the molecular level in Greig patients or *Xt* mice are deletions or translocations, null mutations, probably eliminating transcription completely.

Whereas the mouse system provides advantages for studies of embryonal stages, of homozygotes, and gene rescue studies in transgenic animals, analysis of human developmental mutations holds the promise for a larger variety of mutations in individual unrelated Greig patients. These studies will show if only complete loss of one gene copy results in the Greig phenotype. If not, the position of mutations in the *GLI3* gene should indicate domains essential for functionality, the analysis of which in turn might

Table 113-3
Human Chromosome Regions Potentially Governing Limb Development

Gene	*Name*	*Chromosomal location*	*Syndrome affecting limb development*
LMX1	LIM homeobox transcription factor 1	1q22–23	
INHBB	Inhibin, beta B	2cen–q13	
PAX8	Paired box homeotic gene 8	2q12–q14	
EN1	Engrailed homolog 1	2q13–q21	
HOXD	Homeo box D cluster	2q31	
HOXD13	Homeo box D13	2q31	Synpolydactyly syndrome
EVX2	Even-skipped homeo box 2	2q24.3–q31	
		2q24–q31	Split hand split foot
DLX1	Distal-less homeo box 1	2q32	
DLX2	Distal-less homeo box 2	2q32	
INHA	Inhibin, alpha	2q33–q34	
IHH	Indian hedgehog (Drosophila) homolog	2	
GLI2	GLI-*Krüppel* family member GLI 2	2	
		4p16	Adelaide type craniosynostosis
MSX1	msh (Drosophila) Homeo box homolog 1	4p16.3–p16.1	
FGFR3	Fibroblast growth factor receptor 3	4p16.3	Achondroplasia, Thanatophoric dysplasia, Hypochondroplasia
FGF2	Fibroblast growth factor 2	4q25–q27	
MSX2	msh (Drosophila) Homeo box homolog 2	5q34–q35	(Boston-type craniosynostosis)
		6q21	Split hand split foot
		7p15–21	Saethre-Chotzen syndrome
HOXA	Homeo box A cluster	7p15–p14	
EVX1	Even-skipped homeo box 1	7p15–p14	
INHBA	Iinhibin, beta A	7p15–p13	
GLI3	GLI-*Krüppel* family member GLI 3	7p13	Greig cephalopolysyndactyly syndrome
		7q11–q22	EEC syndrome
DSS1	Deleted in SHFM1	7q22.1	Split hand split foot (SHFM1)
DLX5	Distal-less homeo box 5	7q22	
DLX6	Distal-less homeo box 6	7q22	
WNT2	Wingless-type MMTV integration site 2, homolog	7q31	
PAX4	Paired box homeotic gene 4	7q32	
		7q36	Complex bilateral polysyndactyly
		7q36	Triphalangeal thumb
SHH	Sonic hedgehog (Drosophila) homolog	7q36	
EN2	Engrailed homolog 2	7q36	
BMP1	Bone morphogenetic protein 1	8p21	
FGFR1	Fibroblast growth factor receptor 1	8p12	Pfeiffer syndrome
		10q24–q25	Split hand split foot (SHFM3)
FGF8	Fibroblast growth factor 8	10q25–q26	
FGFR2	Fibroblast growth factor receptor 2	10q25.3–q26	Apert syndrome, Pfeiffer syndrome, Jackson-Weiss syndrome (Crouzon syndrome)
FGF4	Fibroblast growth factor 4	11q13.3	
WNT1	Wingless-type MMTV integration site 1, homolog	12q13	
GLI	Glioma-associated oncogene homolog	12q13	
INHBC	Inhibin, beta C	12q13.1	
BMP4	Bone morphogenetic protein 4	14	
HOXB8	Homeo box B8	17q21–q22	
WNT3	Wingless-type MMTV Integration site 3, homolog	17q21–q22	
		17q23.1–q24.2	Hunter-McAlpine craniosynostosis
SOX9	SRY (sex-determining region Y)-box 9	17q24.3–q25.1	Campomelic dysplasia
BMP2	Bone morphogenetic protein 2	20p12	
		Xq26–26.1	X-linked split hand split foot (SHFM2)
WNT7a	Wingless-type MMTV Integration site 7a, homolog	—	

help to identify other genes on which the *GLI3* product acts to regulate development and other factors cooperating with *GLI3* in this function.

The genomic sites upstream of the *Gli3* transcription start that are disturbed by the add insertion are candidates for promoter regions governing transcription of *Gli3* itself.

The variety of effects on different organ systems manifested by homozygous *Xt* mice encourages one to search systematically for mutations influencing *GLI3* expression or functionality in the multitude of human developmental defects other than the Greig syndrome.

DEVELOPMENTAL DEFECTS ASSOCIATED WITH *GLI3* MUTATIONS

The disturbance of anterior development resulting in digit duplications in *extra toes* mutants in the mouse or GCPS in humans is reflected by the disturbance of anterior wing development in mutants of the Drosophila *GLI* homolog Cubitus interruptus (*Ci*). At a low level of expression wild-type Ci protein is tethered to microtubules in the cytoplasm of anterior cells. The N-terminal segment including the zinc finger domain is proteolytically cleaved and transferred to the nucleus to repress transcription of Hedgehog (*Hh*) and other genes, thus ensuring anterior development. Hh expression in posterior cells signals to adjacent anterior cells. There, Ci is released from the microtubules and no longer cleaved proteolytically, resulting in an apparent increase of intact Ci molecules. Target genes such as Decapentaplegic (*Dpp*) are upregulated, possibly by an activating function of Ci. Sequence comparison between GLI and Ci proteins indicates that several regions, in addition to the ZFD, are conserved, suggesting that functional roles of individual domains might be similar.

In vertebrates, *GLI3* appears to be the only *GLI* family member expressed at the anterior margin of the limb bud, while the expression domains of all three GLI proteins overlap in the center of the bud. Employing Ci as a model for GLI protein action and assuming that GLI1, 2, and 3 can replace each other in the function of Hh downregulation, one can speculate that a reduction in the amount of GLI3 by a mutation results at the anterior margin of the limb bud in a GLI protein level which is insufficient to prevent *Shh* expression. Indeed, ectopic *Shh* expression at the anterior margin of the limb buds is observed in *Xt* as well as other polydactylous mice. This might mimic a second ZPA and lead to ectopic anterior mirror image induction of extra digits such as in experimentally induced anterior *Hh* expression in chick limb development.

These conclusions drawn from model organisms are corroborated by the analysis of GLI3 mutations in GCPS patients without obvious cytogenetic lesions in 7p13. The majority of point mutations observed so far resulted in transcriptional stop signals upstream of or within the zinc finger region, potentially resulting in a nonfunctional product. However, mutations affecting more downstream exons are associated with GCPS as well, indicating functional importance of the affected protein domains C-terminal of the ZFD. Recently, two other clinically distinct developmental disorders, Pallister-Hall syndrome (*PHS*) and postaxial polydactyly type A (*PAP-A*), were linked by genetic studies in families to the chromosome segment encompassing *GLI3*. Mutation analysis subsequently found stop mutations potentially resulting in truncations of the GLI protein between the ZFD and domain 3 in PHS, and C-terminal of domain 3 in PAP-A.

One might speculate that GCPS mainly is due to haploinsufficiency, a reduction in the amount of functional GLI3 resulting from various types of mutations, PHS due to a protein lacking domains C-terminal of the ZFD, and PAP-A due to the lack of domains C-terminal of the microtubular anchor. However, the low number of mutations detected in these syndromes so far prohibits a general conclusion.

These recent findings and the multitude of effects on different organ systems manifested by homozygous *Xt* mice encourage further systematic searching for mutations influencing *GLI3* expression or functionality in the multitude of human developmental defects besides the Greig syndrome.

SELECTED REFERENCES

Ausems MGEM, Ippel PF, Renardel de Lavalette PAWA. Greig cephalopolysyndactyly syndrome in a large family: a comparison of the clinical signs with those described in the literature. Clin Dysmorphol 1994;3:21–30.

Buscher D, Bosse B, Heymer J, Ruther U. Evidence for genetic control of sonic hedgehog by Gli3 in mouse limb development. Mech Dev 1997;62:175–182.

Cohn MJ, Tickle C. Limbs: a model for pattern formation within the vertebrate body plan. TIG 1996;12:253–257.

Domínguez M, Brunner M, Hafen E, Basler K. Sending and receiving the *hedgehog* signal: control by the *Drosophila* Gli protein cubitus interruptus. Science 1996;272:1621–1625.

Greig DM. Oxycephaly. Edinburgh Med J 1926;33:189–218.

Hui C-C, Joyner AL. A mouse model of Greig cephalopolysyndactyly syndrome: the *extra-toes*^{J} mutation contains an intragenic deletion of the *Gli3* gene. Nat Genet 1993;3:241–246.

Johnson DR. *EXt*ra toes: a new mutant gene causing multiple abnormalities in the mouse. J Embryol Exp Morph 1967;17:543–581.

Kang S, Graham JMJr, Haskins Olney A, Biesecker LG. *GLI3* frameshift mutations cause autosomal dominant Pallister-Hall syndrome. Nat Genet 1997;15:266–268.

Marigo V, Johnson RL, Vortkamp A, Tabin CJ. Sonic hedgehog differentially regulates expression of GLI and GLI3 during limb development. Dev Bio 1996;180:273–283.

Masuya H, Sagai T, Moriwaki K, Shiroishi T. Multigenic control of the localization of the zone of polarizing activity in limb morphogenesis on the mouse. Dev Biol 1997;182:42–51.

Mo R, Freer AM, Zinyk DL, et al. Specific and redundant functions of Gli2 and Gli3 zinc finger genes in skeletal patterning and development. Development 1997;124:113–123.

Pohl TM, Mattei M-G, Rüther U. Evidence for allelism of the recessive insertional mutation add and the dominant mouse mutation extra-toes (*Xt*). Development 1990;110:1153–1157.

Radhakrishna U, Wild A, Grzeschik K-H, Antonarakis SE. Mutation in *GLI3* in postaxial polydactyly type A. Nat Genet 1997;17:269–271.

Roberts DJ, Tabin C. The genetics of human limb development. Am J Hum Genet 1994;55:1–6.

Ruiz i Altaba A. Catching a Gli-mpse of Hedgehog. Cell 1997;90:193–196.

Ruppert JM, Vogelstein B, Arheden K, Kinzler KW. *GLI3* encodes a 190-kilodalton protein with multiple regions of *GLI* similarity. Mol Cell Biol 1990;10:5408–5415.

Schimmang T, Lemaistre M, Vortkamp A, Rüther U. Expression of the zinc finger gene *Gli3* is affected in the morphogenetic mouse mutant extra-toes (*Xt*). Development 1992;116:799–804.

Tabin C. The initiation of the limb bud: growth factors, Hox genes, and retinoids. Cell 1995;80:671–674.

Vortkamp A, Gessler M, Grzeschik K-H. *GLI3* zinc-finger gene interrupted by translocations in Greig syndrome families. Nature 1991;352:539,540.

Vortkamp A, Heid C, Gessler M, Grzeschik K-H. Isolation and characterization of a cosmid contig for the GCPS gene region. Hum Genet 1995;95:82–88.

Wild A, Kalff-Suske M, Vortkamp A, Bornholdt D, König R, Grzeschik K-H. Point mutations in human GLI3 cause Greig syndrome. Hum Mol Genet 1997;6:1979–1984.

114 Fibroblast Growth Factor Receptor-Related Skeletal Disorders

Craniosynostosis and Dwarfism Syndromes

MAXIMILIAN MUENKE, CLAIR A. FRANCOMANO, M. MICHAEL COHEN, JR., AND ETHYLIN WANG JABS

BACKGROUND

Unique mutations in three human fibroblast growth factor receptors (FGFR1, FGFR2, and FGFR3) have been identified as causing various skeletal disorders that affect the skull (craniosynostosis syndromes) and the growth of the long bones (dwarfism syndromes). Craniosynostosis is the premature fusion of one or more cranial sutures. It is relatively common, with an estimated birth prevalence of 340 per million. More than 90 syndromes are associated with craniosynostosis, and the majority are inherited in an autosomal dominant manner. The best known of these include Crouzon, Jackson-Weiss, Pfeiffer, Apert, and Saethre-Chotzen syndromes. These syndromes have in common premature synostosis of the coronal sutures of the skull, underdevelopment of the midface, some cases having variable abnormalities of the extremities and other organ systems. All are inherited as autosomal dominant traits, most with complete penetrance and variable expressivity. Although viewed clinically as distinct entities, Crouzon, Jackson-Weiss, Pfeiffer, and Apert syndromes have now been shown to be allelic, with alterations in the same gene (*FGFR2*). Other craniosynostosis syndromes also shown to be caused by *FGFR* mutations include Beare-Stevenson cutis gyrata syndrome, Crouzon syndrome with acanthosis nigricans, and a craniosynostosis syndrome associated with a unique *FGFR3* point mutation. Interestingly, the two former conditions have dermatologic findings, but the first disorder is associated with *FGFR2* mutations, whereas the second is secondary to a *FGFR3* mutation. In contrast, there are two craniosynostotic conditions with mutations in transcription factors. Craniosynostosis, Boston type, is a result of a mutation in a homeobox gene, *MSX2*, and Saethre-Chotzen syndrome has been linked to mutations in the *TWIST* gene, a basic helix-loop-helix transcription factor. It has been suggested that the FGFRs are part of the same signaling pathway as TWIST.

Three dwarfing conditions—achondroplasia, hypochondroplasia, and thanatophoric dysplasia—have long been considered a family of skeletal dysplasias because of clinical and radiographic similarities. The phenotypic spectrum ranges from neonatal lethal thanatophoric dysplasia to mild hypochondroplasia, with achondroplasia somewhere in between. Overlap with the craniosynostosis syndromes is seen in thanatophoric dysplasia, in which cloverleaf skull occurs much more frequently in Type 2 than in Type 1. Recent observations have led to the delineation of a newly recognized syndrome in this family of disorders, which is more severe than achondroplasia but less so than thanatophoric dysplasia; the condition is called severe achondroplasia with developmental delay and acanthosis nigricans (SADDAN). It is now recognized that all four of these disorders are caused by mutations in *FGFR3*.

Comparison of specific mutations in *FGFR*s and their phenotypes is providing new insights into the role of these receptors in normal and abnormal bone development. Furthermore, these mutations provide molecular signposts to complement clinical descriptions of this family of disorders. First, we will introduce the clinical features of these craniosynostosis and dwarfing syndromes and then discuss their genetic basis.

CLINICAL FEATURES

CROUZON SYNDROME Crouzon syndrome (OMIM 123500) is among the earliest described and most commonly inherited causes of craniosynostosis. In addition to premature fusion of the skull bones, this syndrome is characterized by shallow orbits, ocular proptosis, and midface hypoplasia (Fig. 114-1A). Craniosynostosis commonly involves the coronal suture leading to brachycephaly with shortening of the anteroposterior diameter of the skull. Additional findings include frontal bossing, hypertelorism, strabismus, beaked nose, mandibular prognathism, high arched palate, dental malocclusion, and conductive hearing loss. On occasion, mental deficiency has been observed. The most consistent finding is severe-to-moderate ocular proptosis because of shallow orbits. The hands and feet are not involved, in contrast to other craniosynostosis syndromes. Crouzon syndrome has a birth prevalence of 15.5 per one million newborns and accounts for approximately 4.5% of all cases of craniosynostosis. This syndrome has an autosomal dominant mode of inheritance with high penetrance and moderate variability in phenotypic expression. On occasion, families with extreme variability have been reported. New mutations represent 56% of all cases, and there is evidence of an advanced paternal age effect. Instances of two affected sibs

From: *Principles of Molecular Medicine* (J. L. Jameson, ed.), ©1998 Humana Press Inc., Totowa, NJ.

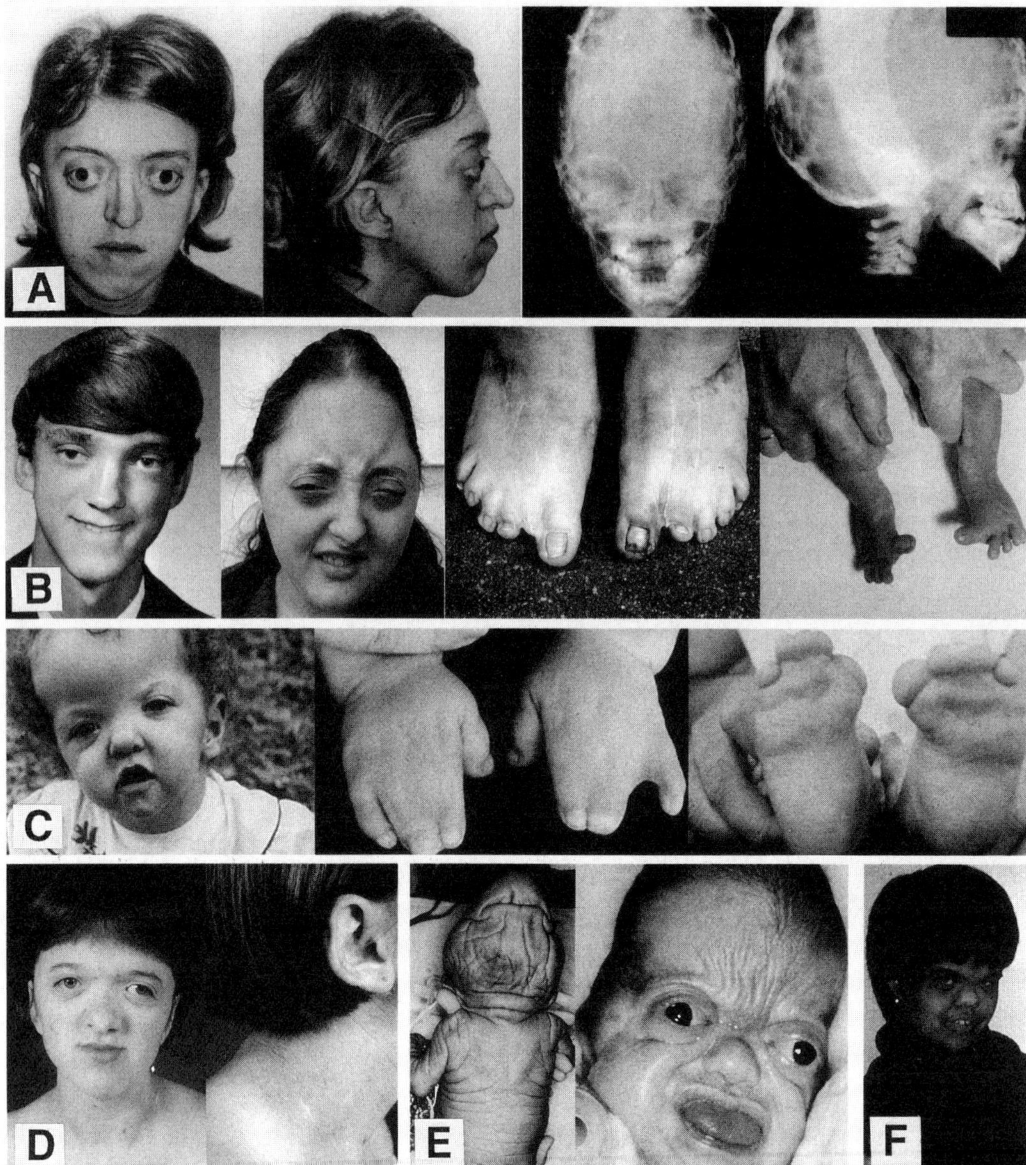

Figure 114-1 (**A**) Crouzon syndrome: Mother with ocular proptosis, divergent strabismus, hypertelorism, and midfacial hypoplasia. Note marked digital impressions on radiograms of the skull. (From Jones, Smith's Recognizable Patterns of Human Malformation, 1997, p. 421.) (**B**) Jackson-Weiss syndrome: two members of the Amish pedigree, one who is mildly affected with brachycephaly and hypertelorism and the other with turribrachycephaly. Feet anomalies of large great toes, syndactyly, and medial deviation. (From Fig. 1 of Jabs et al. Nature Genet 8:275–279,1994; Fig. 1C of Li et al. Genomics 22:418–424, 1994.) (**C**) Apert syndrome: Infant with severe brachycephaly, frontal bossing, ocular proptosis, hypertelorism, and midfacial hypoplasia. Note significant syndactyly. (From Fig. 2 of Park et al. Am J Hum Genet 57:321–328, 1995.) (**D**) Crouzon syndrome and acanthosis nigricans: female with brachycephaly, ocular proptosis, hypertelorism. Dermatologic manifestations of hyperpigmentation, hyperkeratosis, and melanocytic nevi. (**E**) Beare-Stevenson cutis gyrata syndrome: Note fine and coarse wrinkling of the skin with facial features of ocular proptosis and midface hypoplasia. (From Fig. 1 of Przylepa et al. Nature Genet 13:492–494, 1996; Fig. 12 of Hall et al. Am J Med Genet 44:82–89, 1992.) (**F**) SADDAN syndrome: Female with facial features similar to achondroplasia and hyperpigmentation.

born to unrelated parents with normal phenotypes raises the possibility of germline mosaicism.

CROUZON SYNDROME WITH ACANTHOSIS NIGRICANS A subgroup of patients with Crouzon syndrome have a dermatologic disorder—acanthosis nigricans and melanocytic nevi (Fig. 114-1D; OMIM 134934.0011). These skin findings with craniosynostosis breed true as an autosomal dominant condition. Acanthosis nigricans is characterized by verrucous hyperplasia of the skin, particularly in flexural areas. Histopathological findings include marked papillomatosis, the epidermis being thin and hyperpigmented. Acanthosis nigricans is heterogeneous, and many cases are associated with insulin resistance. This is of interest, since insulin binds to the classic insulin receptor and insulin-like growth factor receptors, which are expressed in keratinocytes. Other endocrine abnormalities (including obesity) and certain malignancies are known causes of acanthosis nigricans, and an association with certain congenital disorders, including Crouzon syndrome, is well-recognized. Acanthosis nigricans associated with Crouzon syndrome is rare and atypical in several ways. It usually occurs in females and its onset is often early, apparent in childhood

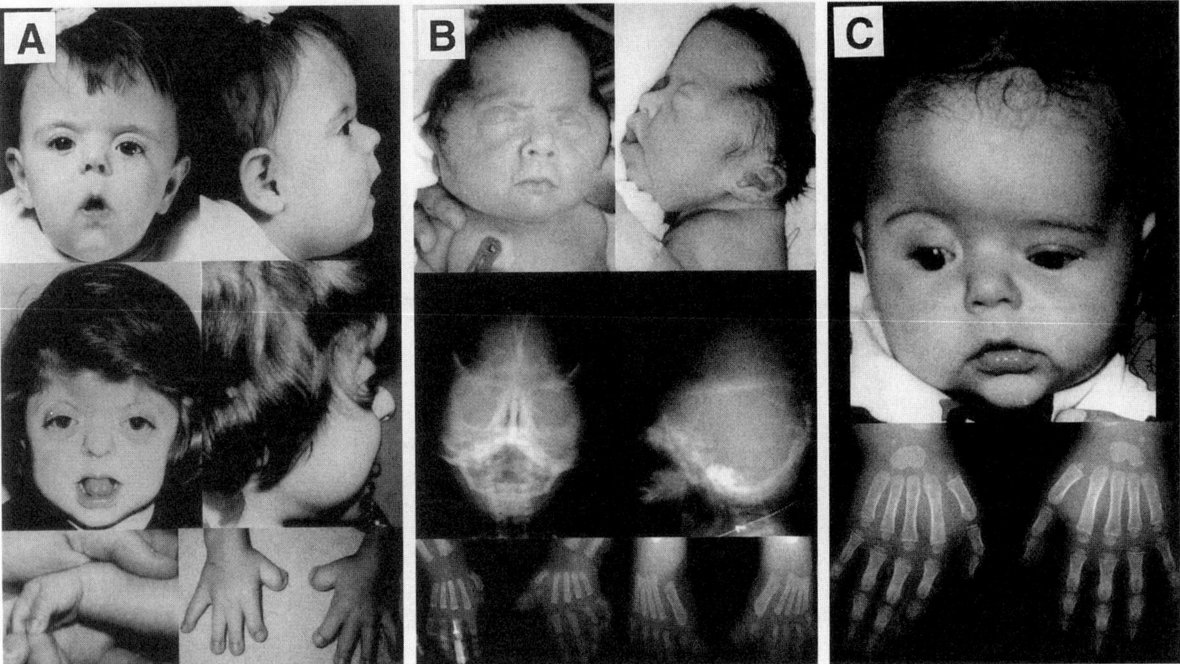

Figure 114-2 (**A**) Pfeiffer syndrome: Craniosynostosis of the coronal sutures, mild protrusion of her eyes, mildly broad thumbs, and great toes in a sporadic patient with the common *FGFR1* mutation. Craniosynostosis with more severe ocular protrusion, very broad thumbs and great toes and a splice mutation in exon 9 (IgIIIc) of *FGFR2* in a patient with familial Pfeiffer syndrome. (From Fig. 5 of Schell et al. Hum Mol Genet 4:323–328, 1995.) (**B**) Cloverleaf skull resulting from synostosis involving multiple sutures in a newborn with sporadic Pfeiffer syndrome and *FGFR2* mutation. Note the broad thumbs and broad medially deviated great toes on X-rays. (**C**) *FGFR3*-associated coronal synostosis: plagiocephaly resulting from unicoronal synostosis. Note the coned epiphyses and fused metacarpal bones on radiograms of the hands in the same patient with *FGFR3* 749C→G (Pro252Arg) mutation. (From Gripp et al., J Pediatr, in press.)

and always by puberty. It is distributed in a distinctive pattern, in the perioral, periorbital, and nasolabial areas as well as the neck, axillae, chest, breasts, and abdomen. Cementomas of the jaws have been found in a number of cases. Additional findings may include choanal atresia and hydrocephalus.

BEARE-STEVENSON CUTIS GYRATA SYNDROME Beare-Stevenson cutis gyrata syndrome (OMIM 123790) is a rare condition with only nine isolated cases reported to date. It is presumed to be autosomal dominant because of associated advanced paternal age. It is characterized by furrowed skin (cutis gyrata), acanthosis nigricans, craniosynostosis with craniofacial dysmorphism, digital anomalies, umbilical and anogenital anomalies, and early death (Fig. 114-1E). The most striking feature of this syndrome is the cutis gyrata with a corrugated appearance resembling the fine ribbing of corduroy. Large and deep folds are seen on the forehead, palms, soles, and perianal/genital regions. The craniofacial features of Beare-Stevenson syndrome are similar to the other craniosynostosis syndromes with downslanting of the palpebral fissures, ocular hypertelorism and proptosis, strabismus, dysmorphic ears, choanal atresia, and palatal anomalies. The majority have cloverleaf skull deformities with hydrocephalus, but some patients have a Crouzon-like appearance. In addition, a prominent umbilical stump, genital abnormalities (bifid scrotum, prominent scrotal raphe, rugose labia majora), and anal anomalies (anteriorly placed anus, tissue mounding of the anus) have been noted. Other unusual features include natal teeth, bifid or accessory nipples, pyloric stenosis, and a coccygeal tail.

JACKSON-WEISS SYNDROME Jackson-Weiss syndrome (OMIM 123150) is characterized by craniosynostosis and foot anomalies (Fig. 114-1B). This condition was first reported in an Amish kindred with 88 affected individuals examined and another 50 reported to be affected. The condition is inherited in an autosomal dominant pattern with high penetrance and phenotypic expression so variable that the entire spectrum of dominantly inherited craniofacial dysostoses-acrocephalosyndactylies (e.g., Saethre-Chotzen and Pfeiffer syndromes, with the exception of Apert syndrome) appeared to be represented within this kindred. The facial features include proptosis, maxillary hypoplasia, and frontal prominence.

Unlike Crouzon syndrome, the degree of craniosynostosis and shallow orbits is mild to moderate, and none of the over 130 affected individuals in the Amish family are known to have undergone surgical intervention. Another distinguishing feature is that patients with Jackson-Weiss syndrome have the consistent manifestation of abnormal clinical and/or radiographic appearance of the feet, which can occur in the absence of any craniofacial features. Affected individuals have mild cutaneous syndactyly (especially of the second and third toes), broad great toes (broad metatarsal and proximal phalanges) with medial deviation, metatarsal and tarsal fusions (calcaneus, cuboid, navicular, and cuneiform), and/or abnormally shaped metatarsal and tarsal bones. Hand abnormalities are rare. The birth prevalence of this disorder is unknown, but several familial cases have been reported in the literature.

PFEIFFER SYNDROME Pfeiffer syndrome (OMIM 101600) is characterized by craniosynostosis, broad thumbs, and broad great toes (Fig. 114-2A,B). Craniofacial features are variable and secondary to synostosis, usually involving the coronal sutures.

Findings include a turribrachycephalic skull, midfacial hypoplasia with relative mandibular prognathism, beaked nose, low nasal bridge, hypertelorism, downslanting palpebral fissures, ocular proptosis, strabismus, highly arched palate, and crowded teeth. Anomalies of the hands and feet differ from any other craniosynostosis syndrome. Characteristically, the thumbs and great toes are broad and medially deviated (varus deformity). Brachydactyly is often present, as is partial soft tissue syndactyly of the fingers and toes. Radiographic findings of the hands include malformed and fused phalanges of the thumbs, short middle phalanges (brachymesophalangy) to complete absence, symphalangism (complete osseous fusion of proximal, middle, and distal phalanges that occurs over several years), and occasional fusion of the proximal ends of the fourth and fifth metacarpals. The distal phalanx of the great toe is broad, and the proximal phalanx is malformed. Broad and short first metatarsals and fusion of carpal and tarsal bones have been described. Additional manifestations may include cloverleaf skull (Fig. 114-2B), fusions of cervical and lumbar vertebrae, cubitus valgus, synostosis of the radio-humeral and ulnar-humeral joints, shortened humerus, abnormalities of the pelvis, coxa valga, and talipes calcaneovarus. Abnormalities affecting other organ systems are of low frequency and include hearing deficit, optic nerve hypoplasia, choanal atresia, bifid uvula, supernumerary teeth, gingival hypertrophy, widely spaced nipples, anal atresia or malpositioned anus, pyloric stenosis, umbilical hernia, and bifid scrotum. Intelligence is usually normal, although mental deficiency has been observed, particularly in sporadic cases. Rare CNS anomalies include hydrocephaly, Arnold-Chiari malformation, and seizures. The birth prevalence of Pfeiffer syndrome is not known. Its inheritance pattern is autosomal dominant with complete penetrance and variable expressivity. In addition to familial occurrence, sporadic cases resulting in new mutations are well-known.

FGFR3-ASSOCIATED CORONAL SYNOSTOSIS SYNDROME This craniosynostosis syndrome has been defined in patients with a unique point mutation in *FGFR3* (OMIM 134934.0014). Clinical findings in over 70 patients from more than 30 unrelated families include bi- or unicoronal synostosis, midface hypoplasia, downslanting palpebral fissures, and ptosis (Fig. 114-2C). It is of note that some mutation carriers do not show any signs of craniosynostosis, having only macrocephaly or even normal head size. Sensorineural hearing loss is seen in some, as is developmental delay. Hand and foot anomalies are found in some, but not all, affected individuals and include brachydactyly with characteristic radiographic findings, such as thimble-like middle phalanges, coned epiphyses, and tarsal fusions. Some patients have broad halluces that are not deviated. It is of interest that this specific *FGFR3* mutation was identified in several affected individuals with unicoronal synostosis from a large prospective series, some of which were previously thought to be caused by intrauterine constraint. Height is normal, in contrast to FGFR3-associated dwarfism syndromes. The mode of inheritance is autosomal-dominant. Several previously reported families could be demonstrated to have this specific *FGFR3* mutation, one of which was called "craniosynostosis-type Adelaide." Based on results from an ongoing prospective study, it appears that the mutation associated with this syndrome may be common in sporadic or familial patients with uni- or bicoronal synostosis whose findings do not fit into any of the classic craniosynostosis syndromes.

APERT SYNDROME Apert syndrome (OMIM 101200) is characterized by craniosynostosis, midface hypoplasia, and symmetric syndactyly of the hands and feet, with a variety of other anomalies (Fig. 114-1C). Craniofacial features are characteristic for Apert syndrome and differ from those of other craniosynostosis syndromes. The cranium is disproportionately high, and the brain is megalencephalic. During infancy, a wide midline calvarial defect is present, extending from the root of the nose to the posterior fontanelle. Bony islands form and coalesce until the gap is completely covered by bone during the third year of life. Although the coronal suture is fused at birth, the anterolateral fontanelles are abnormally large, and both the lambdoid and squamosal sutures are patent. Turribrachycephaly is commonly observed with a flattened occiput and a steep forehead. The cranial base is malformed and often asymmetric. The anterior cranial fossa is very short. Additional craniofacial anomalies include hypertelorism, proptosis secondary to shallow orbits, downslanting palpebral fissures, and frequently strabismus. Hyperopia, myopia, or astigmatism can be found frequently. The nasal bridge is low, and the nose is beaked. Midfacial hypoplasia gives the impression of relative mandibular prognathism. Hearing deficit is secondary to otitis media and is related to the high frequency of cleft palate or bifid uvula. Furthermore, congenital fixation of the stapedial footplate has been reported in a number of cases. Dental anomalies include delayed and/or ectopic eruption, shovel-shaped incisors, and malocclusion. Upper-airway compromise is secondary to reduced nasopharyngeal and oropharyngeal space and poses a risk for obstructive sleep apnea, cor pulmonale, and even sudden death.

Characteristic abnormalities of the hands and feet are symmetric. The mid-digital hand mass minimally involves the second, third, and fourth fingers. The first and fifth fingers may be joined to the mid-digital hand mass or may be free. Similar patterns of syndactyly occur in the feet. Additional limb anomalies include limited mobility at the glenohumeral joint as a constant feature that progressively worsens with growth. Slight limitation of elbow extension and rotation occurs commonly, but is nonprogressive in nature. The humerus is commonly shortened to some degree. Radiographically, lack of segmentation of some joints in the hands cannot be observed at birth, but progressive ossification is found with time.

Vertebral anomalies particularly cervical fusions are common. Variable degrees of fusion may be observed involving the articular facets, the neural arch or transverse processes, or block fusion of the vertebral bodies. Ossification may not always be evident in early radiographs, although signs of impending fusion may include irregularity in vertical orientation of the vertebral bodies and narrowing of the involved intervertebral spaces. In childhood, the growth pattern in Apert syndrome consists of a slowing of linear growth so that most values fall between the 5th and 50th percentiles. From the onset of adolescence to adulthood, slowing becomes more pronounced. This two-step deceleration results in large measure from rhizomelic shortening of the lower limbs. The adolescent growth spurt takes place within the normal time frame.

Intelligence in patients with the Apert syndrome varies from normality to mental deficiency. In patients who had craniectomies performed the first year of life, no significant differences in IQ were found between retarded and nonretarded outcome. It has been speculated that the mental deficiency is secondary to CNS abnormalities, such as malformations of the corpus callosum, the limbic structures, gyral abnormalities, hypoplasia of the cerebral white matter, and heterotopic gray matter. Gyral abnormalities, megalencephaly, and distortion ventriculomegaly are very com-

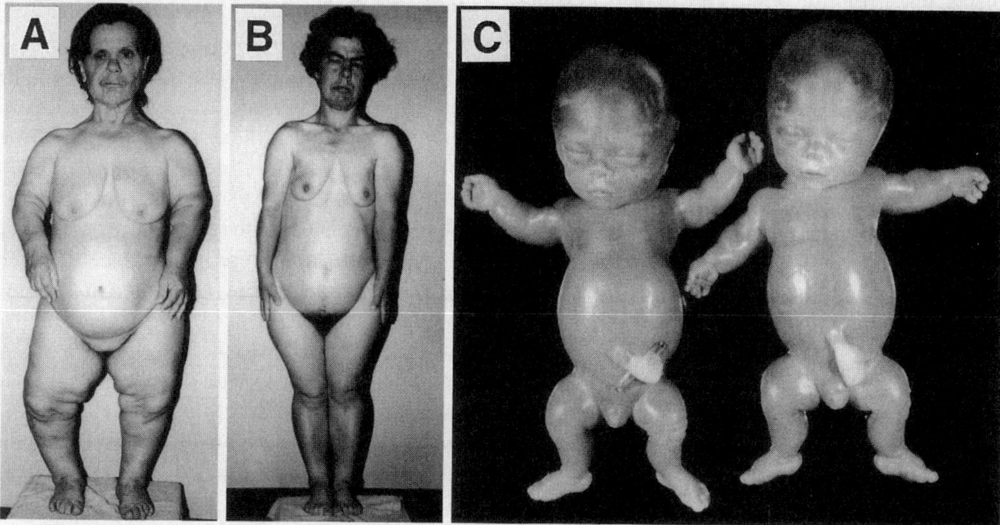

Figure 114-3 (**A**) Achondroplasia: Note macrocephaly, rhizomelic shortening, leg bowing (From Cohen MM, Jr. The Child with Multiple Birth Defects, 2nd ed., New York: Oxford University Press, 1997; p. 213). (**B**) Hypochondroplasia is associated with normal face and relatively proportional, short stature (From Cohen MM, Jr. The Child with Multiple Birth Defects, 2nd ed., New York: Oxford University Press, 1997; p. 213). (**C**) Thanatophoric dysplasia type 1 stillborn twins (Courtesy of MM Cohen, Jr.).

mon. Progressive hydrocephalus may occur on occasion but not nearly as frequently as in Pfeiffer or Crouzon syndromes or with cloverleaf skull deformities.

Cutaneous manifestations include skin dimples at the shoulders, elbows, and knuckles. Excess sweating is common. Acneiform lesions are particularly prevalent on the face, chest, and back. Additional skin findings include hyperkeratoses of the midplantar and lateral plantar surface, hypopigmentation of the skin, and paronychial infections with the feet being more commonly involved than the hands.

Apert syndrome is mostly sporadic, although over one dozen familial instances with autosomal-dominant inheritance pattern are known. Gonadal mosaicism has been postulated in a family with two affected sibs and unaffected parents. The rarity of familial cases can be explained by reduced genetic fitness of affected individuals because of the severe malformations and the presence of mental deficiency in many cases. Increased paternal age at the time of conception has been found in a large series of sporadic cases, and exclusive paternal origin of new mutations has been confirmed on a molecular level. Birth prevalence of Apert syndrome is 15.5 per one million births. The mutation rate is calculated to be 7.8×10^{-6} per gene per generation. Apert syndrome accounts for about 4.5% of all cases of craniosynostosis.

ACHONDROPLASIA Achondroplasia (OMIM 100800) is the most common cause of human dwarfism, with an estimated birth prevalence of 25–66.7 per one million live births. It is inherited as an autosomal-dominant condition, but more than 80% of cases represent new mutations. The phenotype predominantly involves the skeletal system, although manifestations are seen in other organ systems as a result of bony compression. Affected persons are short, with rhizomelic (proximal) shortening of the arms and legs and a disproportionately long trunk (Fig. 114-3A). Often the hands exhibit a "trident" configuration, with separation between the fourth and third fingers resulting in a three-pronged appearance. True megalencephaly is seen, with absolute enlargement of the head circumference in more than 75% of cases. Typical facial characteristics include frontal bossing and midface hypoplasia.

Affected infants often have a thoraco-lumbar gibbus that is usually reducible and resolves as the child begins to sit and walk independently. Frequently, the gibbus is replaced by an exaggerated lumbar lordosis in early childhood, although the gibbus may persist into adulthood and may require surgical correction. Hypotonia is frequently observed in infancy and usually becomes less pronounced with age. Although major motor milestones are usually delayed, intelligence is generally normal unless hydrocephalus or other major complications involving the central nervous system intervene. Final adult height typically ranges from 118 to 145 cm for males and 112 to 136 cm for females.

The major medical complications of achondroplasia result from bony compression of the neuroaxis and the respiratory system. A small foramen magnum is found in almost all cases, and may lead to compression of the cervico-medullary junction and result in a high cervical myelopathy and/or central respiratory complications in early childhood, if the medulla is compromised. Small airway passages may lead to airway obstruction with potentially severe obstructive apnea. Recurrent otitis media is a frequent complication in early childhood and may require placement of pressure-equalizing tubes to minimize the risk of hearing loss.

Radiographic features of achondroplasia include short limbs with short, thickened tubular bones and short phalanges and metacarpals. The ribs are short with concave ends, and the growth plates are notched with a V-shaped appearance. Proximal fibular overgrowth is a frequent observation. The sternum is thick and wide. The vertebral bodies are typically short, flat and "bullet-shaped" in infancy. There is a decrease in the interpediculate distance as one progresses to the caudal end of the spine, in contrast to the increase in this dimension seen in persons who do not have achondroplasia. The vertebrae have short pedicles, which further compromise the dimensions of the spinal canal and contribute to symptoms of spinal stenosis in adulthood. Neuroradiologic evaluation of the brain and skull typically demonstrates enlarged ventricles and marked reduction in the size of the foramen magnum.

Morphologic evaluation of the growth plate in achondroplasia demonstrates normal, well-organized endochondral ossification in many growth plates, but disruption of the growth plate in some weight-bearing joints, with short columns of chondrocytes and widening of the septa between the columns.

HYPOCHONDROPLASIA Hypochondroplasia (OMIM 146000) has many clinical similarities to achondroplasia, but is generally milder overall and typically has less craniofacial involvement. Short stature may not be recognized until the child is 2–3 years of age and is less pronounced than usually seen in achondroplasia (Fig. 114-3B). The height range may overlap with that of the general population, and the condition may be underdiagnosed. Hands and feet are broad and wide, but the trident appearance seen in achondroplasia is not usually apparent. At least one paper has reported an increased frequency of learning disabilities among this population.

The radiographic features of hypochondroplasia are also similar to, but milder than, those seen in achondroplasia. The long bones appear short and wide, with mild flaring of the metaphyseal-epiphyseal junctions. The skull is relatively normal in appearance, with only mild midface hypoplasia and frontal bossing. The interpediculate distance in the lumbar spine may stay constant or decrease as one progresses from rostral to caudal. The bone and cartilage in hypochondroplasia look relatively normal on morphologic evaluation, with minimal shortening of the chondrocytic columns and thickening of the matrix between the columns.

THANATOPHORIC DYSPLASIA Thanatophoric dysplasia (OMIM 187600) takes its name from the Greek "thanos," meaning death. Children affected with this condition almost invariably die in the perinatal period, with only a few survivors into early childhood documented in the literature. Early death is caused by severe respiratory compromise, secondary to an extremely small chest, perhaps exacerbated by medullary compression secondary to a small foramen magnum. Thanatophoric dysplasia is the most common of the neonatal lethal skeletal dysplasias. Clinical features include severe short-limbed dwarfism, curvature of the long bones, megalencephaly, and disproportionately long trunk with short ribs (Fig. 114-3C). The condition has been separated into two types, based on the presence or absence of curved tibiae and fibulae. The cloverleaf skull deformity is more often seen with straight tibiae and fibulae (Type 2). Type 1 is generally characterized by curved long bones and the absence of cloverleaf skull. Histopathology of the growth plate is typically irregular with few proliferative and hypertrophic chondrocytes. The hypertrophic zone of the growth plate is replaced by fibrous-appearing tissue, particularly at the periphery of the growth plate.

SADDAN Three patients have been recognized with a newly defined syndrome named SADDAN, for severe achondroplasia with developmental delay and acanthosis nigricans (Fig. 114-1F). All three patients were initially diagnosed as having achondroplasia, but were recognized as severe cases, with more profound dwarfism and bowing of the limbs than is typical for achondroplasia. All three cases exhibited acanthosis nigricans (an overlap with Crouzon syndrome with acanthosis nigricans and Beare-Stevenson syndrome) and had severe developmental delay, a highly unusual observation in achondroplasia. Radiographic features are intermediate between those of achondroplasia and thanatophoric dysplasia, and to date no chondro-osseous histopathology has been studied. One phenotypic case of thanatophoric dysplasia Type 1 with long-term survival and the R248C mutation associated with this diagnosis, and not SADDAN, has also been associated with acanthosis nigricans.

DIAGNOSIS

Patients with craniosynostosis syndromes are brought to medical and surgical attention because of abnormal head shape. Standard radiologic criteria are used to make the diagnosis of craniosynostosis. The three-dimensional CAT scan is the preferred tool for documentation of prematurely fused sutures and facial dysmorphism. Craniosynostosis cannot be diagnosed radiologically in adults because the sutures are normally fused. Associated increased intracranial pressure can be detected by radiological (*see* radiogram in Fig. 114-1A), ophthalmologic, and neurological examination, and CAT or MRI scan. A dysmorphology examination is required to detect the presence of associated features such as midface hypoplasia, and digital and anal anomalies. Clinical examination and dermatologic consultation with histologic examination of the skin can document such findings as acanthosis nigricans. Molecular diagnosis may involve analysis of the *FGFR1*, *FGFR2*, *FGFR3*, *MSX2*, or *TWIST* genes.

Diagnosis of dwarfism syndromes is still made predominantly on clinical and radiographic grounds. There are cases of intermediate severity between achondroplasia and hypochondroplasia, for whom molecular analysis may help to clarify the diagnosis. However, in the vast majority of cases, the diagnoses of achondroplasia, hypochondroplasia, and thanatophoric dysplasia can be made based on clinical observations and radiographic analysis. Unusual cases, such as those with acanthosis nigricans, unusually severe dwarfism, or mental deficiency, should be studied for the *FGFR3* mutation associated with SADDAN or other possible *FGFR3* mutations. The detection of the molecular basis of these disorders allows for prenatal as well as postnatal diagnosis. However, there are several problems in the application of molecular diagnostic testing, including the difficulty in predicting the severity of the phenotypic expression in affected individuals.

GENETIC BASIS OF DISEASE

The genetic bases of the craniosynostosis and short-stature syndromes described above have been elucidated very recently. The identification of the genes involved in these disorders has been a prime example of the so-called positional candidate gene approach. As an initial step toward gene identification, linkage analysis in large families aided in the mapping of the respective syndrome loci. Using microsatellite markers from throughout the genome, achondroplasia was mapped to DNA markers located in chromosome band 4p16. Both Crouzon and Jackson-Weiss syndrome were linked to chromosome 10q25–q26. Pfeiffer syndrome was shown to be heterogeneous with one locus on 8cen, a second locus on 10q25–q26. Because of the lack of large families with Apert syndrome, this disease could be excluded from 8cen markers and was shown to be consistent with linkage to 10q25–26. Similarly, a new autosomal-dominant craniosynostosis syndrome was excluded from the 8cen and 10q25–q26 regions, respectively, and was consistent with linkage to 4p16. Based on the chromosomal map position and the expression pattern, the *FGFR*s located in the same chromosomal regions were examined as candidate genes. Mutations were identified in *FGFR2* on chromosome 10q25–q26 as the cause for Crouzon, Jackson-Weiss, Pfeiffer, Apert, and Beare-Stevenson cutis gyrata syndromes. Mutations in *FGFR1* gene on 8p11.1 were identified in a subset of families with Pfeiffer syndromes. *FGFR3* on 4p16 is known to be involved in achondroplasia, hypochondroplasia, thanatophoric, and SADDAN, and was shown to cause Crouzon syndrome with acanthosis nigricans and, most recently, FGFR3-associated coronal synostosis syndrome. Thus far, no human disorder has been associated with *FGFR4*, which is located in 5q35.

FIBROBLAST GROWTH FACTOR RECEPTORS Four human FGFRs have been described, all coding for a cell-surface protein with an extracellular region with three immunoglobulin-like domains (IgI, IgII, IgIII), a transmembrane segment, and a split cytoplasmic tyrosine kinase domain (Fig. 114-4). The four FGFRs exhibit an amino acid identity of 55–72%, but differ in their ligand affinity and their tissue and temporal distribution. Structural diversity of the FGFRs is generated by alternative splicing (Fig. 114-4A), which leads to transmembrane receptors or secreted receptors consisting of one, two, or three Ig domains and different carboxyterminal halves of IgIII. IgII, the interloop region, and the N-terminus of IgIII are implicated in ligand binding. In addition, C-terminal sequences of IgIII appear to be important for ligand specificity, although they do not directly interact with their ligands, the fibroblast growth factors (FGFs). FGFs regulate cell proliferation, differentiation, and migration in many different tissues through complex signaling pathways. To date, 15 structurally related proteins of the mammalian FGF family have been identified and are associated with a wide spectrum of functions such as angiogenesis, wound healing, embryonic development, and malignant transformation. The ligand-induced activation of the FGFR kinase activity is mediated by receptor dimerization, which results in transphosphorylation of one receptor molecule by the other in the dimer. The autoactivated FGFR can then bind and phosphorylate intracellular signal transduction proteins and thus activate downstream pathways.

Xenopus, chicken, and mouse *FGFR*s encode proteins similar to human FGFR1 with a high amino acid identity of 78–98%. For the *Drosophila* (*DFR1*) and the *Xenopus* (*FGFR*) homologs, mRNA expression was shown in the mesoderm during embryogenesis. In *Xenopus*, posterior and ventral mesoderm development was blocked by a dominant-negative FGFR. Distinct spatial and temporal mRNA expression of *FGF*s and *FGFR*s, observed in the mouse, further supports roles for this group of ligands and receptors in embryogenesis. Whereas *FGFR1* and *FGFR2* mRNAs are coexpressed in prebone/precartilage structures, such as during craniofacial bone formation, *FGFR3* is expressed in the cartilage growth plates of long bones during endochondral ossification.

MUTATIONS IN *FGFR*s CAUSE CRANIOSYNOSTOSIS AND DWARFISM SYNDROMES Both linkage and mutation analysis demonstrated genetic heterogeneity in Pfeiffer syndrome. Mutations have been identified in sporadic and familial Pfeiffer syndrome in *FGFR1* and *FGFR2*. A common mutation, a C-to-G transversion in exon 5 of *FGFR1* has been detected in all affected individuals of more than 20 unrelated families with Pfeiffer syndrome. This missense mutation, 755C→G, predicts a P252R substitution in the IgII-IgIII linker region, which is highly conserved in FGFRs through evolution as well as among the four human FGFRs. In this respect, it is of great interest that the 755C→G transversion predicting a P252R substitution in the IgII-IgIII linker region of *FGFR1* causing Pfeiffer syndrome is at an identical position to the 755C→G change in *FGFR2* in Apert syndrome and the 749C→G mutation in *FGFR3*, causing FGFR3-associated coronal synostosis syndrome (Fig. 114-4B,C; *see below*).

The second gene known to be involved in Pfeiffer syndrome is *FGFR2*. Approximately 18 different mutations have been shown in familial and sporadic cases, the majority of which either (1) destroy a specific paired cysteine residue (C342) crucial for the formation of IgIII within the ligand binding region of FGFR2 or (2) introduce an additional unpaired cysteine, which likely interferes with the normal protein structure. Aberrant splicing of exon 9 (exon IIIc or exon B) in *FGFR2* was proposed to account for a subgroup of cases. The phenotypic consequences of mutations affecting exon 9 of *FGFR2* are remarkable for their pleiotropic effects resulting in three distinct craniosynostosis syndromes: Crouzon, Jackson-Weiss, and Pfeiffer syndrome (Fig. 4B; *see below*).

Molecular analyses of over 80 cases of Crouzon syndrome has revealed 30 different FGFR2 mutations. The majority of these mutations occur in IgIII, the ligand binding region of the extracellular domain. Over half of the mutations are in exon 9 (exon IIIc or exon B), which forms the second half of IgIII, with the others occurring primarily in exon 7 (exon IIIa or exon U), which forms the first half of IgIII (Fig. 114-4A,B). The mutations are missense, splicing, and small in-frame deletions and insertions. As in Pfeiffer syndrome, in the majority of cases, these mutations result in the loss or gain of the amino acid cysteine, and the most frequently mutated amino acid is C342. Mutation of this cysteine residue is predicted to affect the formation of the disulfide bond, which is critical to forming the tertiary structure of IgIII and determine its binding specificity and affinity.

FGFR2 normally undergoes alternative splicing resulting in isoforms with different spatiotemporal expression (Fig. 114-4A). The BEK or FGFR2 isoform that includes the product from exon 9 (exon IIIc or exon B) is expressed predominantly in primordial bone. The keratinocyte growth factor receptor (KGFR) isoform, which includes the product from exon 8 (exon IIIb or exon K), is expressed primarily in epithelial lined structures. *FGFR2* mutations that only affect exon 9 and the specific expression pattern of this isoform (BEK) in primordial bone are consistent with skeletal changes seen in Pfeiffer and Crouzon syndromes. In contrast, mutations in exon 7 present in both isoforms (BEK and KGFR) would be expected, not only to result in a skeletal phenotype but also in anomalies involving epithelial structures. Interestingly, there are documented cases of low imperforate anus and anorectal fistulas in Crouzon syndrome patients with exon 7 mutations. *FGFR2* mutations in both exon 7 and 9 have also been identified in Jackson-Weiss syndrome. In fact, Jackson-Weiss, Crouzon, and Pfeiffer syndromes share a common mutation, C342R. The original Amish family in the description of Jackson-Weiss syndrome had a mutation predicting an A344G substitution that was also found in Crouzon syndrome. The extensive phenotypic variability in this large kindred suggests the involvement of modifying gene(s). A number of these FGFR2 mutations, including C342R, have been demonstrated to cause constitutive activation of the receptor by aberrant intermolecular disulfide-bonding.

FGFR2 mutations were also detected in Beare-Stevenson cutis gyrata syndrome. In three sporadic cases, two novel missense mutations were identified predicting an amino acid to be replaced by a cysteine. Two patients had the identical Y375C substitution in the transmembrane domain, and one had a S372C change in the carboxyl-terminal end of the linker region between IgIII and the transmembrane domain (Fig. 114-4B,C). In two other patients, neither of these mutations as found suggesting further genetic heterogeneity. The phenotype of this syndrome is consistent with the mutations occurring in regions that would affect both the BEK (exon 9 or IIIc) and KGFR (exon 8 or IIIb) isoforms and their coexpression, because the BEK isoform is expressed normally in

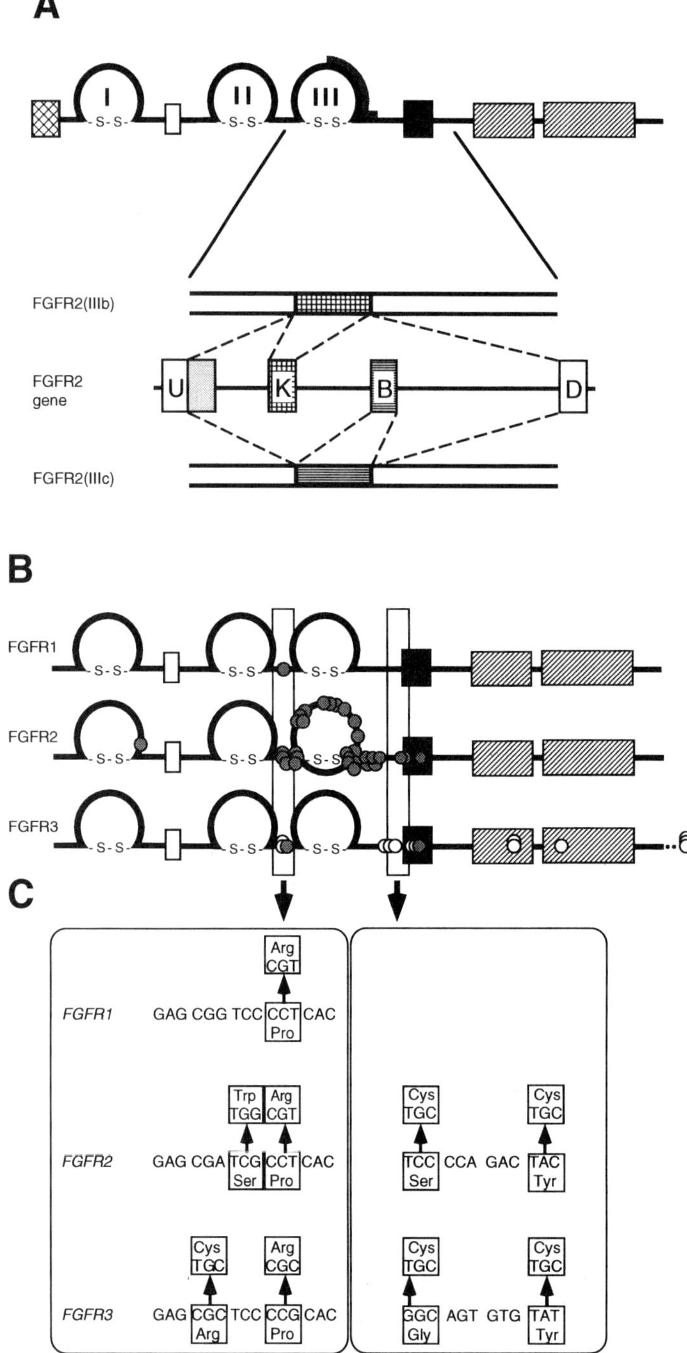

Figure 114-4 (**A**) Schematic diagram of the mammalian fibroblast growth factor receptor (FGFR) putative protein structure with signal peptide (hatched box), three immunoglobulin-like (Ig) domains (loops), and an acidic region (open box) between first and second Ig-like domain, transmembrane domain (black box) and a split tyrosine kinase domain (striped box). Alternative splicing with differential exon use, as shown for the human *FGFR2* gene, generates receptor variants that differ in the second half of their third Ig-like domain and presumably their ligand-binding properties. Exons U (upstream, exon IIIa, or 7) and D (downstream containing transmembrane domain, exon 10) flank the alternatively used exons K (KGFR, exon 8) or B (BEK, exon IIIc, or 9) in the resulting mRNA, which constitute the IgIIIb or IgIIIc isoforms, respectively (*see text* for details). (**B**) Schematic diagram of the genes encoding FGFR1, FGFR2, and FGFR3 with the positions of the mutations reported in craniosynostosis (gray circles), including Pfeiffer, Apert, Crouzon, Crouzon with acanthosis nigricans, Beare-Stevenson cutis gyrata, and Jackson-Weiss syndrome, and short-stature syndromes (white circles) including achondroplasia, hypochondroplasia, thanatophoric, and SADDAN. (**C**) Nucleotide sequence of the interloop region between IgII and IgIII with three adjacent amino acids recurrently affected by unique mutations identified in Pfeiffer syndrome (*FGFR1*), Apert syndrome (*FGFR2*), *FGFR3*-associated craniosynostosis syndrome (*FGFR3*), and thanatophoric dysplasia (*FGFR3*). It is of note that the identical C-to-G substitution in *FGFR1*, *FGFR2*, and *FGFR3* predicting a proline to arginine change causes different craniosynostosis syndromes. The analogous amino acids in FGFR2 for Beare-Stevenson cutis gyrata syndrome and FGFR3 for thanatophoric dysplasia type 1 are mutated to produce an extra cysteine residue.

skeletal structures and the KGFR is expressed in tissues involved in the development of the skin, umbilicus, and anogenital organs.

In Apert syndrome, two recurring mutations in exon U (or exon 7) of *FGFR2* account for the overwhelming majority of several hundred cases studied worldwide. These are a 934C→G transversion resulting in a S252W substitution in the linker region between IgII and IgIII in about 70% and a 937C→G change resulting in a P253R substitution in 30% (Fig. 114-4B,C). These two distinct amino acid substitutions in FGFR2, which result in Apert syndrome, are both bulky substitutions that may alter the relative orientation of IgII and IgIII, thus affecting the binding of FGF ligands or dimerization with other FGFRs.

FGFR3-associated coronal synostosis is caused by a recurrent single-point mutation (749C→G) predicting a P252R substitution in the IgII/III interlinker region of FGFR3 in over 30 unrelated families. Interestingly, this common mutation occurs precisely at the analogous position within the *FGFR3* protein as the mutations in FGFR1 (P252R) in Pfeiffer syndrome and FGFR2 (P253R) in Apert syndrome (Fig. 114-4B,C). It has been speculated that the FGFR1 Pro252Arg and FGFR3 Pro250Arg mutations influence FGFR2 signaling, thereby causing the craniosynostosis phenotype. The observation that patients with FGFR1 or FGFR3 mutations tend to have a milder phenotype than those seen with FGFR2 mutations and that Apert syndrome, the most severe phenotype in the spectrum of FGFR2 mutations, is caused by the equivalent Pro252Arg mutation in FGFR2, is consistent with this possibility.

In Crouzon syndrome with acanthosis nigricans, a recurrent mutation predicting a A391E substitution occurs in the transmembrane domain of FGFR3 (Fig. 114-4B). The phenotypes associated with FGFR3 mutations are consistent with its spatiotemporal expression. FGFR3 is expressed in primordial bone, ectoderm, epithelial-lined structures, and skin. The majority of FGFR3 mutations are reported in dwarfism conditions, achondroplasia, thanatophoric dysplasia, and hypochondroplasia (Fig. 114-4B). The association of nondwarfism and even nonskeletal phenotypes with FGFR3 mutations reveals the potential for a wide range of pleiotropic effects as well as locus heterogeneity in Crouzon syndrome. Thus, the effects of the FGFR3 mutations in Crouzon syndrome with acanthosis nigricans, FGFR3-associated coronal synostosis syndrome, and those for the different dwarfism syndromes must be functionally distinct.

More than 95% of cases of achondroplasia are caused by one of two mutations in *FGFR3* (1138G→A is most common, 1138G→C is least common), both of which result in the substitution of an arginine residue for the normal glycine at amino acid 380 in the transmembrane domain of the protein. Interestingly, this alteration is one of the most frequent mutation in the human genome, with an estimated mutation frequency between 5.5×10^{-6} and 2.8×10^{-5} per gamete generation. The transmembrane domain affected by this mutation is important, not only as a cell-membrane anchor, but also in signal transduction.

Hypochondroplasia is less genetically homogeneous, with approximately 70% caused by a K540L substitution in the first tyrosine kinase domain of the FGFR3 protein. Mutations for the rest have not yet been identified. Several linkage studies have suggested that some cases of hypochondroplasia may be caused by mutations at a locus distant and distinct from *FGFR3*, but mutations at other gene loci have not yet been recognized.

Thanatophoric dysplasia (TD) Type 1 is caused by series of mutations in the *FGFR3* gene, one of which results in R248C, located in the Ig II/II interloop region (Fig. 114-4B,C). In contrast, Type 2 (TD2; associated with straight limbs with or without cloverleaf skull) is associated with a unique recurring mutation predicting a K650N substitution in the second tyrosine kinase domain of FGFR3. The identical amino acid (K650M) is altered in three patients with SADDAN. In vitro studies have demonstrated that the G380R substitution in achondroplasia, the K540L change in hypochondroplasia, and the K650N alteration in TD2 all are associated with constitutive (ligand-independent) activation of FGFR3. The downstream effects of this constitutive activation and the mechanism whereby it is translated into the phenotypic effects of these mutations are not, as yet, understood.

MOLECULAR PATHOPHYSIOLOGY OF DISEASE

How these FGFR mutations alter the intracellular signaling pathway to cause the autosomal dominant phenotypes seen in the craniosynostosis and dwarfism syndromes is poorly understood. The abnormal phenotypes in the FGFR-related skeletal disorders are not simply caused by a deletion of one copy of the gene. This is supported by naturally occurring deletions in humans and also by gene knockout experiments in the mouse. Although individuals with a deletion of the short arm of chromosome 4 have one copy of *FGFR3* deleted, they do not have any of the characteristic findings of achondroplasia or thanatophoric dysplasia. Thus, the phenotypes in these skeletal disorders cannot be explained by the classic model of a mutation-induced haploinsufficiency. Further evidence for the unique nature of the identified *FGFR* mutations comes from knockout studies in transgenic mice. Heterozygous animals that are deleted for one copy of *Fgfr1*, *Fgfr2*, or *Fgfr3*, respectively, appear to be developmentally and anatomically normal. Recent studies provide further evidence that the abnormal phenotypes in FGFR-associated craniosynostosis and dwarfism syndromes are not a result of a loss-of-function, but rather from a gain-of-function of the mutated receptor molecule. This evidence comes from mutation-induced receptor activation and targeted *Fgfr* gene disruption experiments in the mouse. Biochemical studies have demonstrated that an *FGFR2* mutation (Cys342Tyr) found in Pfeiffer and Crouzon syndromes and *FGFR3* mutations in achondroplasia and types 1 and 2 thanatophoric dysplasia result in ligand-independent, constitutive activation of the receptor. This conclusion is supported by studies of *Fgfr3* knockout mice, which exhibit overgrowth of the long bones and axial skeleton suggesting that FGFR3 is a negative regulator of bone growth. However, individuals with FGFR3-associated coronal synostosis and Crouzon syndrome with acanthosis nigricans have normal long-bone growth. It is therefore doubtful that this mutation leads to constitutive FGFR3 activation in the same tissue distribution as the achondroplasia, TD-1, and TD-2 mutations.

MANAGEMENT AND FUTURE DIRECTIONS

Multidisciplinary team approach is required for the management of the craniofacial, audiologic, ocular, oral, dental, skeletal, hand, foot, and skin abnormalities found in these conditions. Management is symptomatic and psychosocial support is often indicated. Recommendations for follow-up and management are reviewed for chondrodysplasias by Horton and Hecht (1993) and for craniosynostosis by Cohen (1986). Further studies of development pathways, animal models, cell biologic aspects, and biochemical signal transduction components involved in the pathogenesis and in the modification of the phenotype are required. Chemical inhibitors of FGFRs have been developed. As yet, no approaches to the management of these conditions have been devised using techniques of gene therapy.

ACKNOWLEDGMENTS

This work was supported in part by NIH Grants P50 DE11131 and RO1 DE11441 (EWJ.), by NIH grants HD2873 and HD29862 (M.M.) and the Division of Intramural Research, National Human Genome Research Institute NIH (C.A.F.; M.M.).

SELECTED REFERENCES

Baker KM, Olson DS, Harding CO, Pauli RM. Long-term survival in typical Thanatophoric dysplasia type 1. Am J Med Genet 1997;70:427–436.

Bellus GA, Bamshad MJ, Przylepa KA, et al. Severe achondroplasia with developmental delay and acanthosis nigricans (SADDAN): phenotypic analysis of a new skeletal dysplasia caused by fibroblast growth factor receptor 3 Lys650Met mutation (submitted).

Bellus GA, Gaudenz K, Zackai EH, et al. Identical mutations in three different fibroblast growth factor receptor genes in autosomal dominant craniosynostosis syndromes. Nat Genet 1996;14:174–176.

Bellus GA, McIntosh I, Smith EA, et al. A recurrent mutation in the tyrosine kinase domain of fibroblast growth factor receptor 3 causes hypochondroplasia. Nat Genet 1995;10:357–359.

Cohen MM Jr. Craniosynostosis: Diagnosis, Evaluation, and Management. New York: Raven, 1986; pp. 413–590.

Cohen MM Jr, Kreiborg S. An updated pediatric perspective on the Apert syndrome. Am J Dis Child 1993;147:989–993.

Cohen MM Jr, Kreiborg S. Skeletal abnormalities in the Apert syndrome. Am J Med Genet 1993;47:624–632.

Cohen MM Jr, Kreiborg S. The hands and feet in Apert syndrome. Am J Med Genet 1995;56:82–96.

El Ghouzzi V, Le Merrer M, Perrin-Schmitt F, et al. Mutations of the TWIST gene in Saethre-Chotzen syndrome. Nat Genet 1997;15:42–46.

Gripp KW, McDonald-McGinn DM, Gaudenz K, et al. Identification of a genetic cause for isolated unilateral coronal synostotis: A unique mutation in the fibroblast growth factor receptor 3. J Pediatr 1998, in press.

Hall BD, Cadle RG, Golabi M, Morris CA, Cohen MM Jr. Beare-Stevenson cutis gyrata syndrome. Am J Med Genet 1992;44:82–89.

Horton WA, Hecht JT. The chondroplasias. In: Royce, PM; Steinmann, B, eds. Connective Tissue and its Heritable Disorders: Molecular, Genetic, and Medical Aspects. New York: Wiley-Liss, 1993; pp. 641–675.

Howard TD, Paznekas WA, Green ED, et al. Mutations in TWIST, a basic helix-loop-helix transcription factor, in Saethre-Chotzen syndrome. Nat Genet 1997;15:36–41.

Jabs EW, Muller U, Li X, et al. A mutation in the homeodomain of the human MSX2 gene in a family affected with autosomal dominant craniosynostosis. Cell 1993;75:443–450.

Jabs EW, Li X, Scott AF, et al. Jackson-Weiss and Crouzon syndromes are allelic with mutations in fibroblast growth factor receptor 2. Nat Genet 1994;8:275–279.

Lajeunie E, Ma HW, Bonaventure J, Munnich A, Le Merrer M, Renier D. FGFR2 mutations in Pfeiffer syndrome. Nat Genet 1995;9:108.

Meyers GA, Orlow SJ, Munro IR, Przylepa KA, Jabs EW. Fibroblast growth factor receptor 3 (FGFR3) transmembrane mutation in Crouzon syndrome with acanthosis nigricans. Nat Genet 1995; 11:462–464.

Moloney DM, Wall SA, Ashworth GJ, et al. Prevalence of Pro250Arg mutation of fibroblast growth factor receptor 3 in coronal craniosynostosis. Lancet 1997;349:1059–1062.

Muenke M, Gripp KW, McDonald-McGinn DM, et al. A common mutation in the fibroblast growth factor receptor 3 (FGFR3) gene defines a new craniosynostosis syndrome. Am J Hum Genet 1997;60:555–564.

Muenke M, Schell U. Fibroblast growth factor receptor mutations in human skeletal disorders. Trends Genet 1995;11:308–313.

Muenke M, Schell U, Hehr A, et al. A common mutation in the fibroblast growth factor receptor 1 gene in Pfeiffer syndrome. Nat Genet 1994;8:269–274.

Oldridge M, Lunt PW, Zackai EH, et al. Genotype-phenotype correlations for nucleotide substitutions in the IgII-IgIII linker of FGFR2. Hum Mol Genet 1997;6:137–143.

Online Mendelian Inheritance in Man (OMIM). Center for Medical Genetics, Johns Hopkins University (Baltimore, MD) and National Center for Biotechnology Information, National Library of Medicine (Bethesda, MD), 1997. World Wide Web URL: http://www3.ncbi.nih.gov/omim/

Park W-J, Bellus GA, Jabs EW. Mutations in fibroblast growth factor receptors: phenotypic consequences during eukaryotic development. Am J Hum Genet 1995;57:748–754.

Przylepa KA, Paznekas W, Zhang M, et al. Fibroblast growth factor receptor 2 mutations in Beare-Stevenson cutis gyrata syndrome. Nat Genet 1996;13;492–494.

Reardon W, Winter RM, Rutland P, Pulleyn LJ, Jones BM, Malcolm S. Mutations in the fibroblast growth factor receptor 2 gene cause Crouzon syndrome. Nat Genet 1994;8:98–103.

Rousseau F, Bonaventure J, Legeall-Mallet L, et al. Mutations in the gene encoding fibroblast growth factor receptor-3 in achondroplasia. Nature 1994;371:252–254.

Rousseau PL, Saugier P, Le Merrer M, et al. Stop codon FGFR3 mutations in thanataphoric dwarfism type 1. Nature Genet 1995;10:11,12.

Rutland P, Pulleyn LJ, Reardon W, et al. Identical mutations in the FGFR2 gene cause both Pfeiffer and Crouzon syndrome phenotypes. Nat Genet 1995;9:173–176.

Schell U, Hehr A, Feldman GJ, et al. Mutations in FGFR1 and FGFR2 cause familial and sporadic Pfeiffer syndrome. Hum Mol Genet 1995; 4:323–328.

Shiang R, Thompson LM, Zhu YZ, et al. Mutations in the transmembrane domain of FGFR-3 cause the most common genetic form of dwarfism, achondroplasia. Cell 1994;78:335–342.

Tavormina PL, Bellus GA, Webster M, et al. A novel skeletal dysplasia with developmental delay and acanthosis nigricans is caused by a Lys650Met mutation in fibroblast growth factor receptor 3. Am J Hum Genet, in press.

Tavormina PL, Shiang R, Thompson LM, et al. Thanatophoric dysplasia (types I & II) caused by distinct mutations in fibroblast growth factor receptor 3. Nat Genet 1995;9:321–328.

Wilkie AOM, Slaney SF, Oldridge M, et al. Apert syndrome results from localized mutations of FGFR2 and is allelic with Crouzon syndrome. Nat Genet 1995;9:165–172.

115 Aarskog-Scott Syndrome

JEROME L. GORSKI

INTRODUCTION

Aarskog-Scott syndrome, or Faciogenital dysplasia (FGDY, MIM 305400), is an uncommon X-linked recessive developmental disorder that primarily affects skeletal morphogenesis. The condition was first described by Aarskog and Scott in the early 1970s. Mutations in FGD1, the gene responsible for Aarskog-Scott syndrome, result in a developmental disorder affecting specific skeletal structures that include elements of the face, cervical vertebrae, and distal extremities. Genetic and biochemical analyses show that FGD1 encodes a guanine nucleotide exchange factor (GEF), or activator, for Cdc42, a member of the Rho family of Ras-like GTPases. Rho proteins comprise a family of at least eight distinct proteins that are involved in the control of a wide variety of cellular functions, including the organization of the actin cytoskeleton, the control of cellular division, and the transcriptional regulation of gene expression. Together, members of the Rho protein family and their activators regulate cell shape, adhesion, and migration, properties that are involved in tissue morphogenesis. The identification that FGD1, the gene responsible for Aarskog-Scott syndrome, is a RhoGEF and a component of the Rho signal transduction pathway suggests that other components of this signaling pathway will be found to be responsible for defects in mammalian morphogenesis.

CLINICAL FEATURES OF AARSKOG-SCOTT SYNDROME

PHYSICAL MANIFESTATIONS OF THE DISEASE The Aarskog-Scott syndrome, or Faciogenital dysplasia (FGDY), phenotype consists of a characteristic set of facial and skeletal anomalies, disproportionate short stature, and urogenital malformations. The cardinal features of this disease are summarized in Table 115-1 and illustrated in Fig. 115-1.

Facial Features The face is typically round and the forehead broad with ridging of the metopic suture. Facial features typically consist of widely-spaced eyes (hypertelorism), ptosis, down-slanting palpebral fissures, and a short up-turned (anteverted) nose (Fig. 115-1). The philtrum is commonly long and the maxilla is typically hypoplastic. A variety of external ear anomalies have been described, including low-set ears, posteriorly-rotated auricles, and thickened over-folded helixes.

From: *Principles of Molecular Medicine* (J. L. Jameson, ed.), ©1998 Humana Press Inc., Totowa, NJ.

Musculoskeletal Features Impaired growth is another major manifestation of the disease; growth retardation usually becomes apparent during the first few years of life, and affected males rarely exceed 160 cm in height. Stature is disproportionate and the distal extremities are most severely shortened (Fig. 115-1). Hands and feet are broad and short. Interphalangeal joints are typically hypermobile; however, camptodactyly and contractures of the interphalangeal joints have also been observed. The majority of affected males have a pectus excavatum and inguinal hernias. Typically, relative to affected males, the phenotype of obligate female heterozygotes is mild and limited to relative short stature and a subtler form of the characteristic craniofacial anomalies.

Radiographic Abnormalities Radiographic findings are usually limited to the cervical spine and distal extremities; these abnormalities are summarized in Table 115-1. About half of the affected males have a cervical spine abnormality such as spina bifida occulta, odontoid hypoplasia, fused cervical vertebrae, and ligamentous laxity with subluxation. Radiographic abnormalities of the hands and feet typically consist of shortened digits, hypoplasia of the terminal phalanges, clinodactyly, fusion of the middle and distal phalanges, and retarded bone maturation. Other radiographic abnormalities include maxillary hypoplasia, additional pairs of ribs and other segmentation anomalies, and calcified intervertebral disks.

Urogenital Anomalies The scrotum typically appears bifid. Scrotal folds commonly extend ventrally around the base of the penis to form what resembles a shawl. Cryptorchidism is common; penile hypospadius has also been reported.

Other Features Although mild-to-moderate mental retardation has been described in some affected males, it does not appear to be a consistent feature. Affected males have been observed to have a delayed eruption of teeth; some have congenitally missing teeth. Other anomalies occasionally occur including cleft lip and palate and congenital heart defects. Some males have a single palmar crease or distally placed axial triradii. Affected males and obligate carrier females both appear to have normal fertility.

Epidemiology Population surveys estimate that FGDY occurs with a recognized frequency of approximately 1 per one million in the general population. However, because it is likely that mildly affected individuals would not be detected, it is probable that the disease frequency is actually higher than this estimate.

EMBRYOLOGIC CORRELATIONS Mutations that result in the Aarskog-Scott syndrome alter the size and shape of a limited number of specific cartilaginous and bony elements but leave other skeletal structures unaffected. Similar abnormalities have been observed in the *short-ear* (*se*) and *brachypodism* (*bp*) mouse

Table 115-1
Primary Clinical and Radiographic Features of FGDY

Anatomical region or system	*Clinical features*
Craniofacial	Broad forehead, abnormally formed ears, hypertelorism, down-slanted palpebral fissures, ptosis, maxillary hypoplasia, anteverted nostrils, hypodontia and malocclusion (cleft lip and palate, enamel hypoplasia)[a]
Musculoskeletal	Disproportionate short stature, distally shortened limbs and brachydactyly, pectus excavatum, soft tissue syndactyly of the digits, interphalangeal joint hypermobility, camptodactyly and clinodactyly, broad feet, inguinal hernias (single palmar crease, abnormal dermatoglyphics)
Urogenital	Shawl and bifid scrotum, crytorchidism (hypospadius, renal hypoplasia)
Miscellaneous	Mild-to-moderate mental retardation, strabismus, growth hormone deficiency (congenital heart defects)
Radiographic Features	Spina bifida occulta, odontoid hypoplasia, cervical vertebral defects and ligamentous laxity, calcified intervertebral disks, additional ribs, hypoplastic phalanges, retarded bone age (osteochondritis dissecans)

[a]Items in parentheses are less commonly observed.

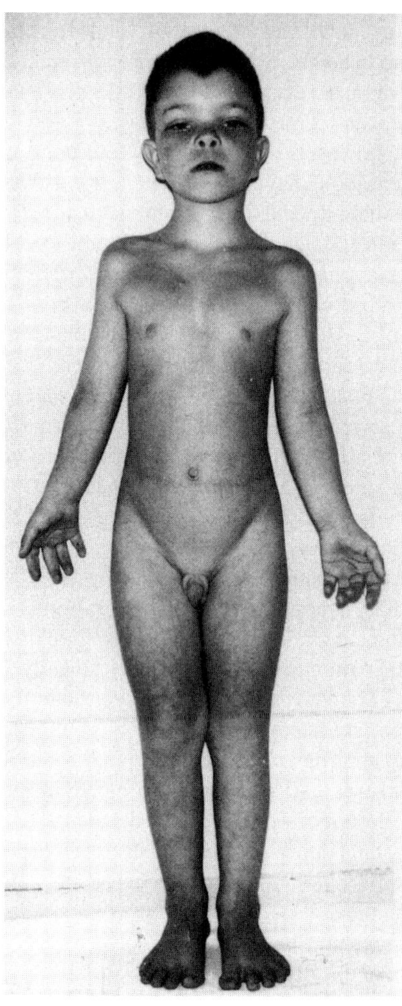

Figure 115-1 Aarskog-Scott syndrome. Facial features are characterized by a broad forehead, a widow's peak, hypertelorism, bilateral ptosis of the upper eyelids, midface hypoplasia, a depressed nasal bridge, anteverted nose, and low-set ears. Stature is short and disproportionate with shortened distal extremities; hands and feet are short and broad. Bilateral inguinal herniorrhaphy scars are present. Consequential to scrotal folds joining ventrally over the base of the penis, an abnormal penoscrotal configuration is present. (Courtesy R Gorlin, University of Minnesota.)

mutants. During development, *se* and *bp* embryos manifest abnormalities in the formation of a characteristic subset of skeletal progenitors. During mammalian embryogenesis, the first observable sign of skeletal morphogenesis is the aggregation of mesenchymal cells into regions of high cell density termed condensations; these condensations represent the initial outlines of future skeletal elements. The mesenchymal cells within these condensations later elaborate extracellular matrix and differentiate into cartilage and bone cells; final skeletal shapes result from a combination of partial cell loss (apoptosis), the fusion of adjacent condensations, and the coordinated resorption and deposition of bone by osteoclasts and osteoblasts. *Se* and *bp* embryos exhibit abnormalities in the size and shape of specific skeletal condensations, anomalies that result in the mutant phenotype. The similarity of these mutations to Aarskog-Scott syndrome suggests that, like *bp* and *se* mice, FGDY males may have an altered pattern of skeletogenesis that affects a limited number of specific skeletal progenitors. Additional analyses will be required to verify this hypothesis.

DIFFERENTIAL DIAGNOSIS Several other inherited conditions, including Noonan syndrome, Robinow syndrome, and Leopard syndrome, share clinical features with Aarskog-Scott syndrome; shared features include short stature, hypertelorism, and hypogonadism. Pseudohypoparathyroidism and hydantoin embryopathy also share several physical features with FGDY. In combination with the distinctive radiographic abnormalities, the characteristic pattern of craniofacial abnormalities, disproportionate short stature, shortening of the distal extremities, and characteristic urogenital anomalies distinguish Aarskog-Scott syndrome from these other conditions. Unlike these other conditions, FGDY is an X-linked recessive trait; therefore, a demonstrated X-linked pattern of inheritance assists in confirming the diagnosis.

MOLECULAR GENETICS OF AARSKOG-SCOTT SYNDROME

AARSKOG-SCOTT SYNDROME GENE, FGD1, MAPS TO REGION Xp11.21 Gene Localization Pedigree analyses of families segregating FGDY strongly suggested an X-linked recessive pattern of inheritance; subsequent genetic linkage studies mapped the responsible locus to the pericentric region of the X chromosome. The observation of a mother and son who both displayed all of the major features of FGDY in association with a reciprocal X;8 chromosome translocation tentatively localized the disease gene to the X-chromosomal breakpoint, region Xp11.21. The observation that, in the affected female, the translocated X chromosome was active in the majority of cells examined, suggested that the translocation breakpoint directly interrupted the disease gene. By isolating the rearranged X chromosome in a rodent somatic cell hybrid, mapping experiments sublocalized the FGDY-specific breakpoint to an estimated 350-kb region within distal Xp11.21.

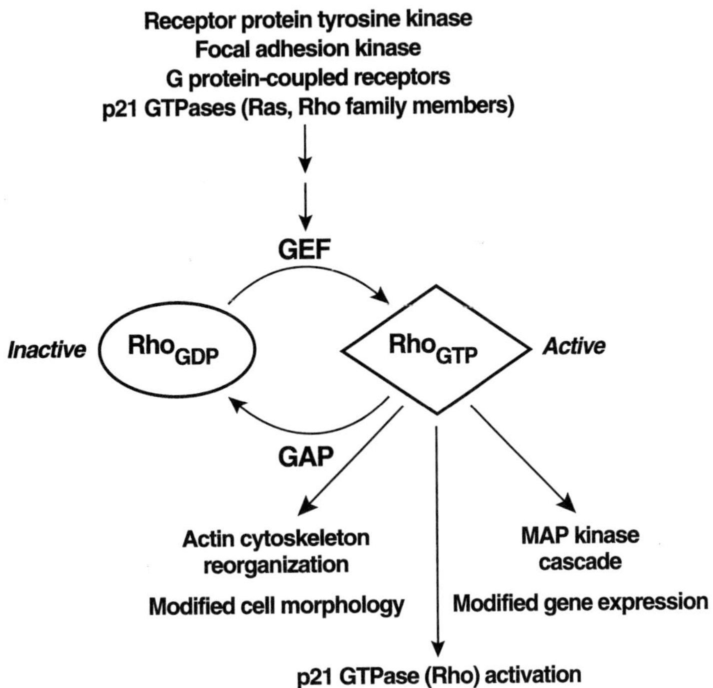

Figure 115-2 RhoGEFs activate Rho proteins by catalyzing the exchange of GDP for GTP. A variety of stimuli lead to the activation of Rho protein family members via RhoGEFs, including the p21 GTPase Ras, receptor protein tyrosine kinases, and G-protein-coupled receptors. Activated Rho leads to modified cell morphology by a reorganization of the actin cytoskeleton, a modulation of gene transcription by the activation of mitogen-activated protein (MAP) kinase cascade, and the sequential activation of other Rho family member proteins. RhoGAP facilitates the hydrolysis of GTP and the Rho protein inactivation.

Positional Cloning The FGDY-specific X;8 breakpoint was used as a molecular signpost to positionally clone the Aarskog-Scott syndrome gene. Using DNA markers flanking the disease-specific breakpoint, a YAC contig of the region was assembled; DNA clones derived from this contig were used to identify regional transcripts and identify a cDNA clone, designated FGD1, that spanned the disease-specific breakpoint. A number of lines of evidence indicated that FGD1 was the gene responsible for Aarskog-Scott syndrome:

1. FGD1 was mapped to Xp11.21, the region known to contain the Aarskog-Scott syndrome gene.
2. The FGD1 gene was directly disrupted by a disease-specific X;8 translocation breakpoint.
3. FGD1 mRNA was expressed in tissues involved in the disease phenotype including fetal craniofacial bones.

The identification of additional FGD1 mutations in affected FGDY males, including an insertional mutation predicted to result in a severely abbreviated and nonfunctional FGD1 protein, confirmed that FGD1 was the gene responsible for the Aarskog-Scott syndrome.

Genomic Organization The complete FGD1 cDNA is 4439 nucleotides in length, a result consistent with the 4.4-kb transcript detected by Northern blot analysis. The FGD1 transcript contains a 2883-nucleotide open reading frame (ORF) that encodes a protein of 961 amino acids with a predicted mass of 107 kDa. Comparative sequence analyses show that the FGD1 gene is composed of 18 exons that span 51 kb of genomic DNA. Exons range from 1210 to 31 bp in size; intron sizes range from 23 kb to 106 bp in size. RNase protection and primer extension analyses show that the FGD1 promoter belongs to a GC-rich, TATA-less class of promoters.

Mutation Analyses Genomic analyses have failed to identify a common structural rearrangement among FGDY patients. These results suggest that FGD1 mutations will be highly heterogeneous. Expression studies indicate that FGD1 is not expressed in readily biopsied tissues such as lymphocytes and fibroblasts; these results suggest that DNA-based analyses will be necessary to identify individual FGD1 mutations. A determination of the genomic structure of the FGD1 gene provides a means for designing DNA-based diagnostic analyses to detect FGD1 mutations. For example, primers designed to polymerase chain reaction amplify each of the FGD1 exons may provide a means of detecting FGD1 mutations by performing single-strand conformational polymorphism (SSCP) analysis.

FGD1 ENCODES A RHOGEF, A REGULATOR OF CDC42 SIGNAL TRANSDUCTION

Comparative Analyses Comparative sequence analysis indicated that FGD1 encoded a Rho guanine nucleotide exchange factor (RhoGEF). RhoGEFs form a family of cytoplasmic proteins that activate the GTPase Ras-like family of Rho proteins by catalyzing the exchange of bound GDP for free GTP (Fig. 115-2). The p21 GTPase superfamily and the biological roles of the family members are summarized in Table 115-2.

The RhoGEF family consists of at least 16 distinct members. Like FGD1, all members contain a 200-amino acid RhoGEF motif; in a number of RhoGEF family members, this domain has been shown to be necessary and sufficient for catalyzing the GDP/GTP exchange for Rho protein family members. In addition, all RhoGEF domains are paired with pleckstrin homology (PH) domains; PH domains are thought to be essential for the proper cellular localization of RhoGEF proteins to the cytoskeleton. In addition to the RhoGEF and PH domains, most RhoGEF proteins contain other types of functional domains that are commonly found in signaling

Table 115-2
p21 GTPase Superfamily Members

Family	*Family members*	*Biological function*
Ras	H-ras, Ki-ras, N-ras, R-ras, rap1A/B, rap2A/B, ralA/B, TC21	Regulation of cell growth Regulation of cell differentiation
Rho	RhoA, RhoB, RhoC, RhoG, Cdc42, Rac1, Rac2, TC10	Actin cytoskeleton organization Regulation of gene expression Regulation of cell growth
Rab/ARF	Rab1,...,Rab26, ARF1,...,ARF6	Vesicle transport
Ran	Ran1	Importation of nuclear proteins

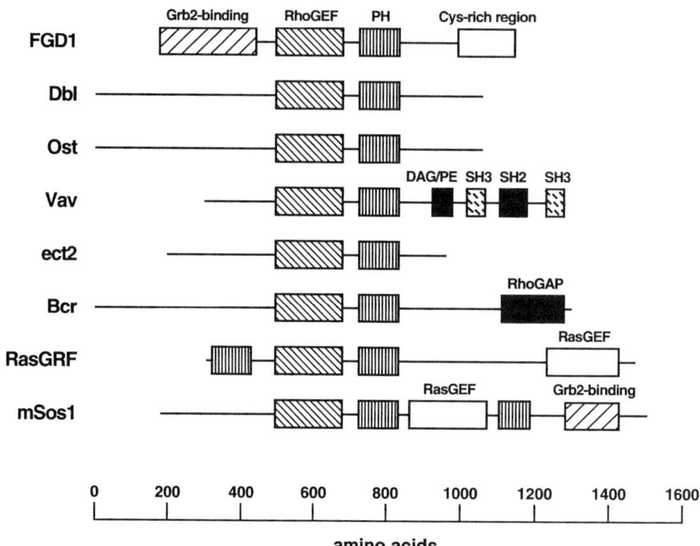

Figure 115-3 Schematic representation of the domain structure of the FGD1 protein compared to other RhoGEF proteins. Domains are drawn approximately to scale. FGD1 contains at least four distinct domains, including a RhoGEF domain and a pleckstrin homology (PH) domain, motifs common to all RhoGEF family members. FGD1 also contains a cysteine-rich zinc finger-like (Cys-rich) motif and a putative Src-homology 3-binding (Grb2-binding) region. Vav contains Src-homology 3 (SH3), Src-homology 2 (SH2), and a putative diacylglycerol/phorbol ester-binding (DAG/PE) zinc butterfly motif; Bcr contains a Rho GTPase activator protein (RhoGAP) domain. RasGRF and mSos1 contain a Ras guanine nucleotide exchange factor (RasGEF) domain.

molecules. For example, although RasGRF and mSos1 both contain RhoGEF domains, they also contain RasGEF motifs (Fig. 115-3), a result suggesting that these proteins may act as two-headed exchange factors by mediating the activation of both the Rho and Ras signaling pathways. Most of the RhoGEFs identified, including Dbl, ect2, and Ost were discovered by virtue of their transforming capability through gene transfer experiments; other RhoGEFs, including Cdc24, Bcr, mSos1, RasGRF, and Vav, were identified by their role in cell growth regulation. As shown in Fig. 115-2, the signaling cascade that couples RhoGEFs to upstream components remains elusive. The specific biological function of many of the RhoGEF family members remains to be determined.

Biochemical Studies In vivo and in vitro studies indicate that FGD1 is a RhoGEF for Cdc42, a member of the Rho protein family. When microinjected into cultured cells, the FGD1 RhoGEF domain induces fibroblasts to form filopodia, actin-associated membrane complexes generated by activated Cdc42. The FGD1 RhoGEF domain specifically binds to the Cdc42 protein, and FGD1-dependent filopodia formation is blocked by complexing Cdc42 to other Cdc42-binding proteins. In addition, in FGD1 expressing fibroblasts, stress-activated protein kinase (SAPK)/c-Jun N-terminal kinase (JNK) activity is stimulated in a manner similar to that obtained with constitutively activated Cdc42. Together, these results indicate that FGD1 is a specific RhoGEF for Cdc42.

FGD1 ENCODES ADDITIONAL STRUCTURAL DOMAINS

A Zinc Finger Motif A comparative analysis of FGD1 showed that it contained two additional conserved structural motifs (Fig. 115-3). Like the proto-oncogene RhoGEF member Vav, the 3' region encoded a 50-amino acid cysteine-rich zinc finger-like motif that was similar to, but distinct from, the diacylglycerol/phorbol ester-binding regulatory domain of protein kinase Cγ. The Vav zinc finger motif is functionally significant; mutations in the conserved cysteine residues abolish transforming activity. Similar putative regulatory domains have been identified in a variety of Ras-associated proteins, including the Raf proto-oncogene, the RhoGAP *n*-chimerin, and diacylglycerol kinase. The observation that the predicted FGD1 sequence contains a zinc finger-like domain suggests that the FGD1 protein may interact with lipid second messenger molecules. Therefore, it is possible that the FGD1 protein may interact with, or be modified by, the components of multiple signal transduction pathways.

A Putative Grb2-Binding Region An analysis of the FGD1 protein showed that the 5' region was remarkably proline-rich and that proline constituted 22% of the first 250 amino acid residues.

Table 115-3
Actin-Associated Membrane Complexes

Complex type	*Involved Rho family member*	*Biological function*	*Proteins*[a]
Focal adhesion	Rho	Cellular adhesion	Integrin, vinculin, talin, PTK, FAK, tensin, paxillin, zyxin, ERM, α-actinin
Filopodia	Cdc42	Cellular morphology	Vinculin, fimbrin, talin, PTK, α-actinin, ERM
Lamellipodia	Rac	Cellular movement	Talin, fimbrin, integrin, PTK, α-actinin, ERM
Cortical stress fibers	Rho	Cellular morphology	Fodrin-spectrin, ankyrin, PTK, adhesion molecules
Adherens junction	?	Cellular adhesion	Cadherin, catenin, vinculin, PTK, filamin, α-actinin, ERM

[a]Known to comprise an actin-associated membrane complex; PTK, protein tyrosine kinase; FAK, focal adhesion kinase; ERM, ezrin, radixin, and moesin.

Since proline-rich regions may contain Src-homology 3 (SH3) binding domains, the 5' portion of the derived FGD1 protein sequence was compared to other sequences known to contain SH3 binding sites. An analysis showed that FGD1 contained two putative SH3 binding sites that exhibited strong similarity to the functionally significant regions of several proteins with demonstrated Grb2 binding activity, including the RasGEF, mSos1. Recently, it has been shown that Grb2 selectively binds the proline-rich motifs of the mSos1 protein to form a link in a signal transduction pathway that functionally ties tyrosine kinase receptors to Ras. Among the identified Ras and RhoGEF family members, mSos1 is unique in containing an SH3 (or Grb2)-binding domain. The identification of a putative proline-rich SH3 binding domain in FGD1 implies that, like Sos, the location and/or activity of the FGD1 protein may be modified by Grb2-like proteins.

MOLECULAR PATHOPHYSIOLOGY OF AARSKOG-SCOTT SYNDROME

Identified FGD1 mutations included a frame shift mutation and a chromosomal rearrangement, mutations predicted to result in the total absence of FGD1 protein; therefore, a loss of FGD1 appears to result in the FGDY phenotype. In *S. cerevisiae*, *S. pombe*, *D. melanogaster*, and *C. elegans*, the loss of a RhoGEF activity is functionally equivalent to the loss of the target Rho protein. Although the structural and functional diversity of the RhoGEF protein family indicates that FGD1 is not the only Cdc42 RhoGEF, it is logical to expect that within expressing cells FGD1 mutations will reduce or modify Cdc42 activity. Therefore, it is likely that an examination of the molecular biology of Cdc42 and the other Rho proteins will illuminate the biological role of FGD1.

RHO PROTEINS REGULATE THE ORGANIZATION OF THE ACTIN CYTOSKELETON AND GENE EXPRESSION The mammalian Rho protein family (listed in Table 115-2) consists of at least eight distinct proteins and three subfamilies: Rho, Cdc42, and Rac. Each Rho protein has at least 50–55% homology with any of the others and 30% homology to Ras.

Regulation of the Actin Cytoskeleton Rho proteins are part of a signal transduction pathway that modulates a cell's response to external stimuli by reorganizing the actin cytoskeleton to regulate cellular morphology. Regulated changes in the actin cytoskeleton are required for cytokinesis, cell motility, and cell–cell interactions. Therefore, by regulating the actin cytoskeleton, Rho proteins and their activators regulate cell shape, adhesion, and migration, properties critical to tissue morphogenesis. Expressed in cells, Rho proteins elicit a distinctive actin-associated membrane complex; these complexes, their biological function, and the involved Rho proteins are listed in Table 115-3. In fibroblast cells, microinjection analyses show that activated Cdc42 stimulates the

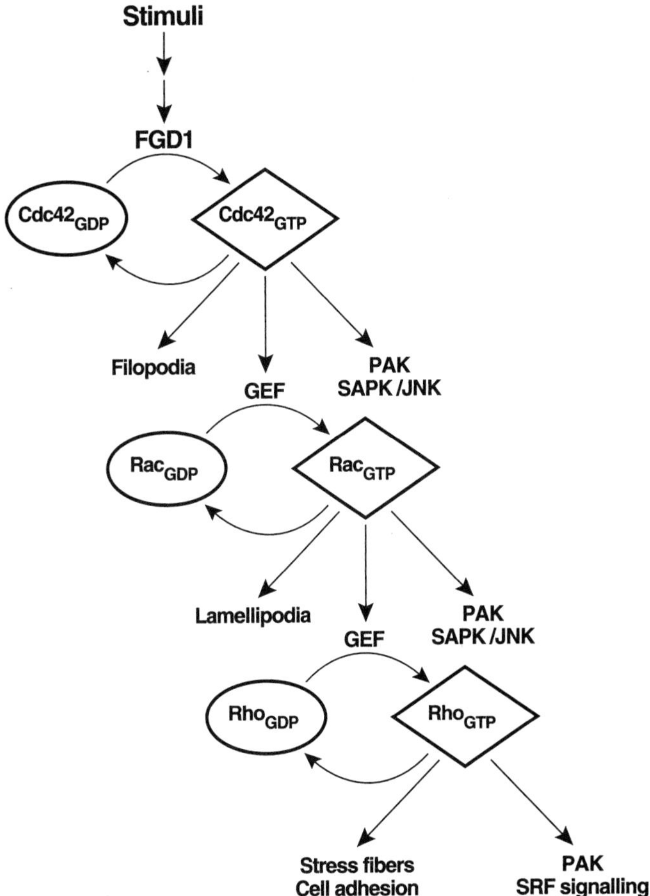

Figure 115-4 Rho protein family members are activated in a hierarchical cascade. The activation of Cdc42 by FGD1 leads to the sequential activation of Rac and Rho. Activated Cdc42 results in the formation of filopodia, whereas activated Rac leads to the formation of lamellipodia; activated Rho results in the formation of actin stress fibers and focal adhesions. Cdc42 and Rac activate the stress-activated protein kinase (SAPK)/c-Jun N-terminal kinase (JNK) mitogen-activated protein kinase (MAPK) cascade via the Ser/Thr kinase PAK; Rho is required for signaling via PAK to modulate gene transcription through the serum response factor (SRF).

formation of microspikes, or filopodia; in *S. cerevisiae*, Cdc42 is required for polarized cell growth and bud formation. Related studies show that Rac regulates the formation of lamellipodia and cell ruffles, and that Rho stimulates the formation of focal adhesions and cortical stress fibers. These same experiments show that Rho proteins are activated in a hierarchical cascade (Fig. 115-4), and that activated Cdc42 stimulates the sequential activation of Rac and Rho to sequentially elicit filopodia, lamellipodia, and stress fibers. More recently, use of cell-free assays and intact cell systems show that Rho regulates several enzymes involved in phosphoinositol metabolism, including phosphoinositide 3-kinase, phosphatidylinositol 4-phosphate 5-kinase, and phospholipase D. These results suggest that Rho may regulate the reorganization of the actin cytoskeleton through the metabolism of phospholipid metabolites. However, the exact relationship between Rho, phospholipid metabolism, and the actin cytoskeleton remains to be determined.

Mitogen-Activated Protein Kinase (MAPK) Cascade Rho proteins are also part of a signal transduction pathway that activates MAPK cascades to modulate gene transcription. Kinases belonging to the MAPK family are used throughout evolution to control cellular responses to external signals, such as growth factors, inductive signals, and nutrient status. MAPKs have received particular attention, because many of these enzymes translocate to the cell nucleus to modulate the action of transcription factors. Recent studies show that Cdc42 and Rac activate the stress-activated protein kinase (SAPK)/c-Jun N-terminal kinase (JNK) MAPK cascade via the Ser/Thr kinase PAK. In contrast, Rho is required for modulating gene transcription through the serum response factor (SRF), results that suggest the existence of a novel signaling pathway (Fig. 115-4).

Implications for Morphogenesis In addition to the identification of FGD1 as a RhoGEF, several lines of evidence indicate that Rho proteins are critical to development. In *Drosophila*, Cdc42 and Rac1 dominant-negative mutations result in specific developmental defects, including anomalies in the outgrowth of peripheral neurons and abnormal myoblast fusion, defects of cellular polarity that are consistent with the role of Rho proteins in regulating cellular morphology. Cdc42 and Rac1 mutations result in distinct phenotypes, results suggesting that different Rho proteins play specific roles during development. Transgenic mice carrying dominant-negative Rac mutations have similar developmental defects in neurogenesis. In addition, Cdc42 mutations in *S. cerevisiae* and *S. pombe* result in abnormalities in cellular morphology.

FGD1 mutations could alter morphogenesis in at least two ways. Since FGD1 stimulates Cdc42 to activate the SAPK/JNK MAPK cascade, consequential to FGD1 mutations, diminished Cdc42 activity could alter SAPK/JNK activity and critically change patterns of gene transcription. Alternatively, since FGD1 stimulates Cdc42 to form filopodia, as a result of FGD1 mutations, diminished Cdc42 activity could alter cellular morphology. Since the actin cytoskeleton regulates cell shape, adhesion, and migration, altered patterns of cellular morphology are likely to play a critical roles in skeletogenesis. Additional studies will be necessary to determine how FGD1 mutations perturb human morphogenesis.

FUTURE DIRECTIONS

With advances in the molecular understanding of disease processes, it has been appreciated that many diseases, such as the proliferative diseases of cancer, atherosclerosis, and psoriasis, result from a malfunction in signal transduction. This recognition has led to intensive research and the development of therapies based on the modification of cellular signaling in diseased cells. The identification of FGD1 as a RhoGEF and a component of Rho signal transduction suggests that other inherited abnormalities of human morphogenesis may also be the result of defects in embryonic signal transduction. Recent experiments have shown that cellular signal transduction pathways can be successfully modulated by a variety of reagents, including small molecules, antibodies, DNA encoding dominant-negative proteins, antisense RNA, and target-specific RNA ribozymes. The continued development of these reagents may provide a means for selectively correcting altered patterns of embryonic signal transduction in the future.

Several Ras-associated proteins have been found to be responsible for human genetic diseases. Neurofibromin, the protein defective in von Recklinghausen neurofibromatosis, contains a RasGAP domain homologous to the catalytic domains of p120-GAP. Tuberin, the gene responsible for the form of tuberous sclerosis mapped to chromosome 16 (TSC2), has some homology to the GAP3 protein. The gene responsible for choroderemia (CHM), a retinal degeneration syndrome, was found to be similar to a Rab geranylgeranyl transferase.

Among identified RhoGEF family members, FGD1 is the first to be directly implicated in causing an inherited human disease. However, the involvement of FGD1 in human morphogenesis implies that other components of the Rho signaling cascade may also be critical to embryonic development and responsible for related and/or unrelated inherited birth defects. An analysis of FGD1, in the context of its normal function and regulation, is likely to provide important new information regarding the roles that RhoGEF proteins and, by inference, Rho proteins play in signal transduction and mammalian development.

SELECTED REFERENCES

Aarskog D. A familial syndrome of short stature associated with facial dysplasia and genital anomalies. J Pediatr 1970;77:856–861.

Bard J. Morphogenesis: The Cellular and Developmental Processes of Developmental Anatomy. Cambridge, UK: Cambridge University Press, 1990, pp. 120–180.

Boguski MS, McCormick F. Proteins regulating Ras and its relatives. Nature 1993;366:643–653.

Bray D. Protein molecules as computational elements in living cells. Science 1995;376:307–312.

Cerione RA, Zheng Y. The Dbl family of oncogenes. Curr Opin Cell Biol 1996;8:216–222.

Chant J, Stowers L. GTPase cascades choreographing cellular behavior: movement, morphogenesis, and more. Cell 1995;81:1–4.

Erlebacher A, Filvaroff EH, Gitelman SE, Derynck R. Toward a molecular understanding of skeletal development. Cell 1995;80:371–378.

Gebbink MF, Kranenburg O, Poland M, van Horck FP, Houssa B, Moolenaar WH. Identification of a novel, putative Rho-specific exchange factor and a RhoA-binding protein: control of neuronal morphology. J Cell Biol 1997;137:1603–1613.

Gorlin RJ, Cohen MM Jr, Levin LS. Syndromes of the Head and Neck, 3rd ed. Oxford: Oxford University Press, 1990; pp. 295–297.

Hall A. Small GTP-binding proteins and the regulation of the actin cytoskeleton. Annu Rev Cell Biol 1994;10:31–54.

Hall BK, Miyake T. The membranous skeleton: the role of cell condensations in vertebrate skeletogenesis. Anat Embryol 1992;186:107–124.

Hart MJ, Eva A, Zangrill D, et al. Cellular transformation and guanine nucleotide exchange activity are catalyzed by a common domain on the Dbl oncogene product. J Biol Chem 1994;269:62–65.

Jockusch BM, Bubeck P, Giehl K, et al. The molecular architecture of focal adhesions. Annu Rev Cell Dev Biol 1995;11:379–416.

Kingsley DM. What do BMPs do in mammals? Clues from the mouse short-ear mutation. Trends Genet 1994;10:16–21.

Lemmon, MA, Furguson KM, Schlessinger J. PH domains: diverse sequences with a common fold recruit signaling molecules to the cell surface. Cell 1996;85:621–624.

Levitzki A. Targeting signal transduction for disease therapy. Curr Opin Cell Biol 1996;8:239–244.

Nobes CD, Hall A. Rho, Rac, and Cdc42 GTPases regulate the assembly of multimolecular focal complexes associated with actin stress fibers, lamellipodia, and filopodia. Cell 1995;81:53–62.

Olson MF, Pasteris NG, Gorski JL, Hall A. Faciogenital dysplasia protein (FGD1) and Vav, two related proteins required for normal embryonic development, are upstream regulators of Rho GTPases. Curr Biol 1996;6:1628–1633.

Pasteris NG, Buckler JM, Cadle A, Gorski JL. Genomic organization of the faciogenital dysplasia (FGD1, Aarskog syndrome) gene. Genomics 1997;43:390–394.

Pasteris NG, Cadle A, Logie LJ, et al. Isolation and characterization of the faciogenital dysplasia (Aarskog-Scott syndrome) gene: a putative rho/rac guanine nucleotide exchange factor. Cell 1994; 79:669–678.

Pawson T. Protein modules and signalling networks. Nature 1995;373: 573–580.

Porteous MEM, Goudie DR. Aarskog syndrome. J Med Genet 1991; 28:44–47.

Schwartz MA, Schaller MD, Ginsberg MH. Integrins: emerging paradigms of signal transduction. Annu Rev Cell Dev Biol 1995;11:549–599.

Stossel TP. On the crawling of animal cells. Science 1993;260:1086–1094.

Treisman R. Regulation of transcription by MAP kinase cascades. Curr Opin Cell Biol 1996;8:205–215.

Vojtek AB, Cooper JA. Rho family members: activators of MAP kinase cascades. Cell 1995;82:527–529.

Zheng Y, Fischer DJ, Santos MF, et al. The faciogenital dysplasia gene product FGD1 functions as a Cdc42Hs-specific guanine-nucleotide exchange factor. J Biol Chem 1996;271:33,169–33,172.

116 Beckwith-Wiedemann Syndrome

Ellen R. Elias, Michael R. DeBaun, and Andrew P. Feinberg

BACKGROUND

Beckwith-Wiedemann syndrome (BWS) is one of the most common overgrowth syndromes, with an estimated incidence of 1/14,000 births. Independently described by Beckwith in 1963 and Wiedemann in 1964, it was originally called the EMG syndrome for its three main features: exomphalos, macroglossia, and gigantism.

Patients with BWS present with a distinctive craniofacial phenotype and may have multiple congenital anomalies. Macrosomia is present at birth and accelerated growth occurs during early childhood. In addition, asymmetry of the limbs may develop over time. Patients with BWS, particularly those with clinically significant limb asymmetry, have an increased risk of developing intra-abdominal malignancies.

BWS is caused by a gene in chromosomal band 11p15.5. Autosomal-dominant transmission has been documented, though most cases are sporadic. A greater likelihood of maternal vs paternal transmission and increased penetrance when inherited from the mother have been reported, but have not been evaluated systematically in a large number of families.

CLINICAL FEATURES

BWS is a heterogeneous syndrome that can have many different presentations. All or a few of cardinal features of the syndrome can be present at birth. Thus, the diagnosis of BWS can be obvious or difficult in the neonatal period depending on the set of characteristic features observed. BWS can be suspected at birth because of macrosomia, macroglossia, and the presence of abdominal wall defects, which range in spectrum from diastasis recti or umbilical hernia in the milder cases to omphalocele in the most severe case. In addition to these cardinal features, visceromegaly or enlargement of the internal organs (liver, spleen, kidneys, pancreas, and occasionally the heart) may be identified. Adrenal cytomegaly with associated cysts, a rare pathological finding (Table 116-1), is a hallmark of BWS. The classic craniofacial features associated with BWS include facial nevus flammeus, maxillary hypoplasia with a broad nasal bridge, and a prominent occiput (Fig. 116-1). Characteristic ear lobe creases/pits are a distinctive if not pathomnemonic finding in children with other features of BWS. Microcephaly is seen in a small number of cases. Table 116-2 lists the common craniofacial features associated with BWS.

From: *Principles of Molecular Medicine* (J. L. Jameson, ed.), ©1998 Humana Press Inc., Totowa, NJ.

In addition to dysmorphic features, macroglossia, and abdominal wall defects, other congenital anomalies may be present. These include cardiac defects and, occasionally, cardiomegaly and abnormalities of the gastrointestinal tract. Genital anomalies are common, including cryptorchidism and enlargement of the labia and clitoris. Many other anomalies, such as cleft palate, supernumerary nipples, and syndactyly have been reported with variable frequencies in patients with BWS and are listed in Table 116-3.

CLINICAL COURSE

The clinical course during the neonatal period is most remarkable for hypoglycemia, often quite severe. This is felt to be caused by insulin hypersecretion from hypertrophied pancreatic islet cells. Polycythemia may also be problematic. Macrosomia is present at birth, and the growth velocity is greater than normal during the early years of life. The musculoskeletal system in children with BWS can be variably affected. Asymmetry of the musculoskeletal system may manifest as an increase in muscle bulk, bone length, or both. In addition, patients may have scoliosis or chest wall asymmetry independent of asymmetry of the long bones. Bone age is often advanced in early childhood but typically subsides by adolescence. After 4–6 years of age, growth velocity decreases, and puberty is usually achieved at the normal time. Asymmetry, seen in 13–18% of patients, may not be present at birth, but often manifests itself in infancy and early childhood.

Patients with BWS generally have intellectual function in the normal range, although no study of formal cognitive evaluations has been completed. Central nervous system damage and subsequent intellectual impairment may result from severe neonatal hypoglycemia if not adequately managed.

Patients with BWS have an increased risk of cancer. The risk is age-dependent, with most cancers occurring before 5 years of age and virtually all before 10 years. The risk of cancer appears to be higher in children with limb asymmetry, although the magnitude of asymmetry needed to confer a high risk of cancer has not been quantified. Common tumors in patients with BWS include Wilms' tumor, adrenocortical carcinoma, neuroblastoma, and hepatoblastoma. Extraabdominal malignancies are much less common in patients with BWS, but have been reported, including rhabdomyosarcoma, glioblastoma, and cardiac fibrous harmartoma.

DIAGNOSIS

The diagnosis of BWS is suspected on the basis of clinical phenotype. A constellation of abnormalities including macrosomia, macroglossia, abdominal wall defects, mid-face hypoplasia,

Table 116-1
Pathological Findings in BWS

Adrenal cytomegaly and cysts
Visceromegaly
Nephromegaly
Prominent lobulation
Persistent nephrogenesis
Medullary dysplasia/sponge kidneys
Hepatomegaly
Splenomegaly
Hyperplasia of islets of Langerhans

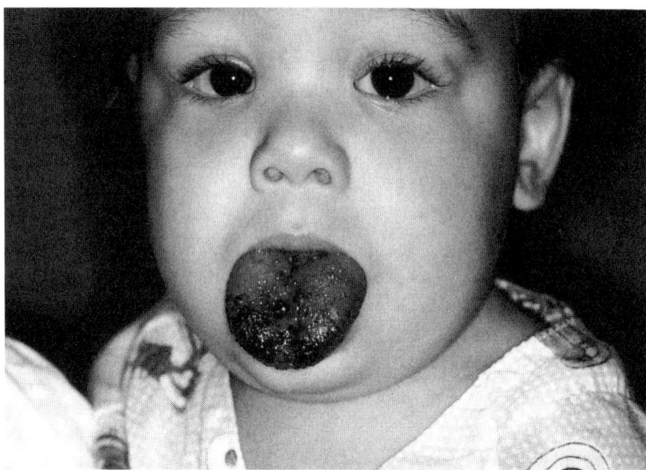

Figure 116-1 Beckwith-Wiedemann patient with maxillary hypoplasia, broad nasal bridge, telecanthus, and macroglossia.

Table 116-2
Clinical Features in BWS

Macroglossia
Macrosomia
Abdominal wall defects
Diastasis recti
Umbilical hernia
Omphalocele
Craniofacial dysmorphism
Facial nevus flammeus
Ear pit/creases
Prominent occiput
Maxillary hypoplasia
Wide and flat nasal bridge
High arched palate
Frontal ridging
Mild microcephaly

Table 116-3
Congenital Anomalies Associated with BWS

More common
Cardiac defects/cardiomegaly
Genitourinary anomalies
Gastrointestinal anomalies
Less common
Supernumerary nipples
Inguinal hernia
Skeletal anomalies
Cleft palate
Diaghragmatic defects
Chest wall deformities
Clinodactyly/polydactyly
Neural tube defect
Imperforate anus

and ear pits or creases should prompt the clinician to consider BWS. The diagnosis of BWS within the first days of life is important so that precautionary measures may be taken to prevent hypoglycemia. Hypoglycemia occurs in the majority of newborns within the first days of life and may manifest with seizures. This is in contrast to infants of diabetic mothers who may present with macrosomia but who often are hypoglycemic at birth. Infants of diabetic mothers may also have other congenital anomalies, but do not present with macroglossia, abdominal wall defects, and the typical ear creases seen in an infant with BWS. Macroglossia may also be observed in storage diseases such as Type II glycogen storage disease as well as in neurofibromatosis and hypothyroidism. Neurofibromatosis can be distinguished by its dermatological findings, and congenital hypothyroidism is usually detected on newborn screening. Most patients with storage diseases do not present with impressive macroglossia at birth.

Other rare syndromes that should be considered in the differential diagnosis include Simpson-Golabi-Behmel syndrome, Proteus syndrome, and Perlman syndrome. Simpson-Golabi-Behmel syndrome is an X-linked disorder with a phenotype similar to BWS, including macrosomia, macroglossia, and a predisposition to Wilms' tumor. Patients, in addition, may show cleft lip and/or palate, unusual alveolar grooves, and skeletal anomalies. An abnormality in glypican-3, which binds to IGF2, has recently been reported in Simpson-Golabi-Behmel patients. Proteus syndrome involves gigantism, macrocephaly, hemihypertrophy, enlargement of the limbs, and risk of malignancy, but has distinctive dermatologic manifestations. Perlman syndrome, involving prenatal overgrowth, renal hamartomas and a depressed nasal bridge, may be part of a continuum with BWS, although patients do not usually have macroglossia, midline abdominal defects, or hemihypertrophy.

Other common overgrowth syndromes include Sotos syndrome (cerebral gigantism), Weaver syndrome, and Marshall-Smith syndrome. Sotos syndrome is characterized by early overgrowth and advanced bone age, hypotonia, and mild cognitive impairment in most patients. Facial features are notable for macrocephaly, downslanting palpebral fissures, and a prominent chin. Neoplasms of the kidney and liver have been reported in Sotos syndrome patients, although this is less frequent than in BWS. Weaver syndrome patients also show accelerated growth and advanced bone age. Characteristic facies include a broad forehead, large ears, and a small chin. Patients with Marshall-Smith syndrome show accelerated skeletal growth, but often manifest failure to thrive and severe, life-threatening respiratory problems. Characteristic features include prominent eyes, low-set ears, and choanal narrowing in some individuals. Patients with Sotos syndrome, Weaver syndrome, and Marshall-Smith syndrome can be distinguished from patients with BWS by the marked differences in their physical features and clinical course.

Prenatal diagnosis of BWS is possible, made on the basis of second trimester ultrasound detection of large fetal size, polyhydramnios, and abdominal wall defects. A positive family history

Table 116-4
Clinical Issues and Management

Neonatal
Hypoglycemia
Airway/feeding problems
Surgical management of GU/GI anomalies
CT and ultrasound for baseline assessment of intra-abdominal cancer
Early childhood
Audiology exam
Musculoskeletal exam
Assessment of asymmetry of the limb
Cancer surveillance
Ultrasound of kidney/liver/adrenal every 3 months from birth until 7 years of age
α fetoprotein every 6–12 weeks of age until age 3[a]

[a]The efficacy for screening for hepatoblastoma with alphafetal protein has not been proven. However, anecdotal reports have indicated that this tumor biomarker may be of potential benefit.

is helpful in those cases of BWS acquired as a dominant trait. Chromosomal analysis in a few cases has revealed a translocation or duplication involving 11p15.5, but most patients with BWS have normal chromosomes.

MANAGEMENT/TREATMENT

The initial management of the newborn with BWS (Table 116-4) must first address the neonatal hypoglycemia, which may be prolonged and quite severe. The macroglossia may cause airway and/or feeding difficulties. Cardiac evaluation, including chest radiographs, electrocardiogram, and echocardiogram are indicated if congenital heart disease is suspected. Surgical intervention may be necessary for the abdominal wall defects and genitourinary abnormalities. Ultrasound of abdominal organs should be performed to rule out the presence of congenital tumors, which may require surgical excision and/or chemotherapy. Polycythemia is another common neonatal problem, which tends to subside without intervention.

Beyond the neonatal period, the most important aspect of management is tumor surveillance. Cancer screening has traditionally consisted of serial abdominal sonography to detect Wilms' tumor, the most common cancer in this group, from birth until 7 or 8 years of age. Other than anecdotal reports, there have been limited data to support cancer screening. Nevertheless, screening for Wilms' tumor in this high-risk cancer population appears prudent. If one plans to do such screening, then screening intervals should be less than 6 months because of the doubling time of Wilms' tumor. Despite the decreasing incidence of Wilms' tumor with age, the doubling time of this cancer does not allow for longer screening intervals. There have been no published prospective studies demonstrating the benefit of screening for the other cancers, such as hepatoblastoma with α fetoprotein or neuroblastoma with urinary catecholamines. However, hepatoblastoma is a very aggressive tumor in which early diagnosis and complete surgical resection markedly improves survival. In contrast, factors predicting survival in children with neuroblastoma are more biological and demographically determined, such as N-myc copy number or age. Thus, preliminary data suggest screening for neuroblastoma is unlikely to be effective.

Other aspects of management may include an early audiology exam to detect hearing loss, orthopedic intervention for leg length discrepancy, urologic management of complex genitourinary anomalies, and speech and language therapy for the consequences of macroglossia.

MODE OF INHERITANCE

BWS is transmitted as an autosomal-dominant trait, with increased penetrance when transmitted from a carrier mother when compared to the father. Discordant monozygotic twins have also been described. These differences in parental origin-specific penetrance are most likely explained by genomic imprinting, a differential modification of the two parental chromosomes in the gamete or zygote, leading to differential function of the two chromosomes in the offspring. Imprinting is by definition reversible, and it usually refers to monoallelic expression of a specific parental allele of a gene. Several genes in mouse and man have been shown to be imprinted. Notably, the insulin-like growth factor-II gene (IGF-2) is expressed exclusively from the paternal allele in most tissues (exceptions are the choroid plexus, leptomeninges, and adult liver). IGF-II is an autocrine growth factor in cancer and has mitogenic effect on cells mediated by signaling at the IGF-I receptor. Approximately 100 kb telomeric to IGF-2 on 11p15 is the gene H19, which acts as an untranslated RNA and is reciprocally imprinted, that is, expressed only from the maternal allele. H19 has shown growth inhibitory effects on cultured tumor cells. IGF2 and H19 are interesting with regard to BWS because of their chromosomal location and potential growth properties.

Based on parental origin-specific differential penetrance data alone, BWS could involve an imprinted gene normally expressed only from the paternal allele, which is somehow activated on the maternal allele in carrier mothers. Alternatively, BWS could represent a gene normally only expressed from the maternal allele, and thus a mutant copy is only phenotypically apparent when transmitted from the mother.

CHROMOSOMAL ALTERATIONS IN BWS

BWS was localized to 11p15 by genetic linkage analysis. While BWS predisposes to Wilms' tumor and other embryonal tumors, it is unlinked to the known Wilms' tumor gene on 11p13 (WT1). Interestingly, a wide variety of embryonal neoplasms, to which BWS patients are susceptible, including rhabdomyosarcoma, hepatoblastoma, and Wilms' tumor, show loss of allelic heterozygosity (LOH) of 11p15 in tumors. Thus, using polymorphic markers, one can demonstrate that one copy of 11p15 is lost in these tumors. Strikingly, almost all cases of LOH involve the maternal allele, again suggesting that an imprinted gene on 11p15 may be involved in the pathogenesis of BWS or cancer.

Rare patients with BWS show cytogenetic abnormalities (Table 116-5) involving chromosome 11p. These include both balanced rearrangements and unbalanced duplications. The balanced germline chromosomal rearrangements (including translocations and inversions) lie near the end of 11p (generally 11p15.4–p15.5), and they involve the maternally inherited chromosome. In contrast, the unbalanced rearrangements are of paternal origin. The unbalanced rearrangement breakpoints are distributed throughout 11p, and what seems to be important is the extra chromosomal material, which always includes 11p15. Furthermore, carriers of the unbalanced rearrangement breakpoints are themselves unaffected, suggesting that the duplications, not the breakpoints themselves, are pathogenic in the chromosome duplication patients.

Table 116-5
Genetic Abnormalities in BWS

Chromosomal rearrangements (~1%)
Balanced translocations and inversions
Involve 11p15
Maternal chromosome affected
Translocation carriers unaffected
Involves K_VLQT1 gene
Unbalanced translocations
Relative trisomy of 11p including 11p15
Paternal chromosome affected
Uniparental disomy (~10%)
Region between β globin and H-ras on 11p15
Paternal duplication with maternal loss
Occurs postzygotically (mosaic)
Loss of imprinting (~20%)
Activation of the normally silent maternal IGF-2 gene
Occurs in 70% of embryonal tumors, in both BWS and non-BWS patients
Mutation of $p57^{KIP2}$ (~5%)

The balanced chromosomal rearrangements in BWS are consistent with either mechanistic hypothesis for an imprinted gene. Thus, the rearrangements could interrupt the coding sequence of a gene normally expressed only from the maternal chromosome, or they could epigenetically activate a gene near the breakpoints on the maternal chromosome that is normally silent on that chromosome. The paternal duplications, however, would suggest that the latter model is correct, that the BWS gene is normally only expressed from the paternal chromosome. Thus, one would be affected by BWS if one had two functional copies of the gene. Normal individuals with one paternal and one maternal chromosome would have only one functional copy. Patients with a paternal duplication would have two, and patients with a balanced rearrangement of the maternal allele would somehow activate their normally silent copy of the BWS gene.

GENOMIC IMPRINTING AND BWS GENES

Strong molecular evidence for genomic imprinting in BWS derives from the observation that 10% of BWS patients have paternal uniparental disomy (UPD) of 11p15. Thus, their maternal chromosome has been replaced with a paternal chromosome over a region extending from the β-globin gene on 11p15 to the H-ras gene. UPD could be pathogenic either by causing loss of the normally expressed maternal gene or duplication of a normally expressed and imprinted paternal gene. UPD in the original reports was suggested to be associated with an increased risk of malignancy. However, other laboratories have not confirmed that finding, and it is unwise to quote a risk of malignancy based on the presence or absence of UPD. Prenatal diagnosis might be done using UPD as a marker, on single cells by PCR, as it has been performed on single circulating cells in BWS patients. The problem with that approach is that the sensitivity of the test is limited to the frequency of UPD, which is 10% or less. Furthermore, in contrast to UPD in Prader-Willi syndrome, UPD in BWS is mosaic in patients, with no more than 90% of peripheral blood lymphocytes or skin fibroblasts showing UPD. Thus, it is likely that UPD cases arise by mitotic recombination in early embryogenesis.

One feature of the BWS germline rearrangements that is inconsistent with a single-gene hypothesis for this disorder is that there are two distinct regions of BWS balanced rearrangement breakpoints, with one located approximately 250 kb centromeric to IGF-2, and a second cluster located 4 Mb centromeric to the first, on the opposite side of the β-globin gene cluster. Because it seems most unlikely that a single gene could span all of these breakpoints, it is conceivable that the breakpoints themselves could influence expression of a BWS gene at some distance, similar to mechanisms observed in both yeast and Drosophila. Furthermore, some human birth defects are caused by spreading inactivation from an X chromosome to a fused autosome in patients with X-autosome translocations.

Genomic imprinting also appears to play an important role in the tumors to which BWS patients are susceptible. Thus, approximately 70% of Wilms' tumors show loss of imprinting (LOI) affecting the IGF-2 and H19 genes. In tumors, the maternal allele of IGF-2 is abnormally activated, and the maternal allele of H19 is abnormally silenced. Other embryonal tumors also show LOI, including rhabdomyosarcoma and hepatoblastoma, and thus LOI appears to be a general feature of embryonal tumors. In addition, a "CpG island," a region rich in CG dinucleotides, appears to distinguish maternal and paternal chromosomes, with the paternal chromosome methylated and maternal chromosome unmethylated. DNA methylation is a covalent modification of cytosine that tends to mark nonexpressed genes but in this case marks the paternal chromosome. In tumors with LOI, the maternal allele is abnormally methylated. Thus, the maternal chromosome appears to undergo an epigenetic switch from a maternal to a paternal epigenotype, with activation of IGF-2, loss of expression of H19, and methylation characteristic of the paternal chromosome. Thus, LOI is the functional equivalent in a tumor of UPD in embryogenesis.

Normal tissues of BWS patients also show LOI of IGF-2; however, this affects only approximately 10% of patients. BWS patients with LOI also show the switch from an unmethylated to a methylated CpG island on the maternal chromosome, again suggesting a shift from a maternal to a paternal epigenotype. However, IGF-2 cannot be the only gene involved in BWS, because it shows abnormal imprinting in only a minority of patients.

Mutations have been described in $p57^{KIP2}$ in patients with BWS. $p57^{KIP2}$ is an inhibitor of several G1 cyclin/Cdk complexes (*see* Chapter 116-6), and it is a negative regulator of cell proliferation. The $p57^{KIP2}$ gene is imprinted and only the maternal allele is expressed. Mice lacking $p57^{KIP2}$ develop some but not all abnormalities that resemble BWS.

A third genetic change in BWS in rearrangement of the K_VLQT1 gene, a voltage-gated potassium channel formerly associated only with the cardiac conduction disorder long QT syndrome. All of the balanced germline chromosomal rearrangements in this region involve this gene. Its role in BWS is supported by the discovery that K_VLQT1 is also imprinted, with preferential expression from the maternal allele. However, imprinting is relaxed in some postnatal tissues, as well as prenatal and postnatal heart, accounting for the lack of parent of origin effect in long QT syndrome.

A model representing how several different types of genetic alterations could lead to abnormal imprinting in BWS is shown in Fig. 116-2. This model incorporates what is known about LOI of target genes, alterations in DNA methylation, and chromosomal rearrangements in BWS. The model emphasizes the importance of regarding genomic imprinting as a developmental process that may be altered at several different stages in BWS and cancer.

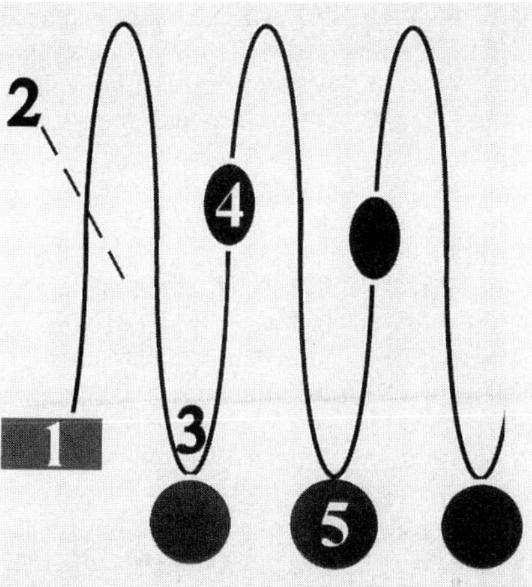

Figure 116-2 A model of genomic imprinting in Beckwith-Wiedemann syndrome. An imprint organizing center (red rectangle) exerts a long-range *cis*-acting influence on IGF-2 and other imprinted genes (blue ellipses) via alterations in chromatin structure (represented as DNA loops). This imprint-organizing center establishes the imprinting mark as maternal or paternal. This effect is propagated outward during development, similar to the organizing center on the X-chromosome. Imprinting is maintained in part by allele-specific methylation of CpG islands as well as interactions with *trans*-acting proteins (green circles). According to this model, loss of imprinting could arise by any of several mechanisms (numbered in the figure): (1) deletion or mutation in the imprint-organizing center itself, which would lead to a failure of parental origin-specific switching in the germline; (2) separation of the imprint organizing center from the imprinted target genes, as seen in BWS germline chromosomal rearrangement cases; (3) abnormal methylation of CpG islands; (4) local mutation of regulatory sequences controlling the target imprinted genes themselves; or (5) loss of or mutations in *trans*-acting proteins that maintain normal imprinting. (Figure modified from Feinberg, et al. 1994, with permission.)

DIAGNOSTIC TESTING

Karyotypic abnormalities are seen in fewer than 1% of BWS patients and generally involve the K_VLQT1 gene. LOI of IGF2 is observed in 20–60% of patients, depending on the report, although we believe the more conservative figure is correct. UPD occurs in about 10% of patients. $p57^{KIP2}$ mutations occur in only 5% of patients. Thus, there is no single diagnostic test for BWS, and the sensitivity of any given test is low. At this point, the most useful test for counseling purposes is UPD. That is because, although the frequency of UPD is low, it would indicate a zero recurrence risk when present, because UPD occurs postzygotically. In contrast, diagnosis of an imprinting mutation (LOI), or mutation of $p57^{KIP2}$ or K_VLQT1 would warrant investigation of other family members for a similar alteration. It is important to emphasize that diagnostic testing for BWS is at the research stage, and that identification of additional target genes should increase the sensitivity and specificity of such testing.

CONCLUSIONS

In summary, BWS involves several 11p15 genes that are imprinted. One of these, IGF2, is normally expressed from the paternal allele and is abnormally activated in patients with LOI. A second gene, $p57^{KIP2}$, is expressed from the maternal allele patients and is mutated in a small fraction of patients. A third gene, K_VLQT1, is expressed from the maternal allele and rearranged in most BWS patients with balanced germline chromosomal rearrangements. The phenotype may be explained in part by the variable involvement of these specific genes, as well as additional as yet unidentified imprinted genes. Of all BWS patients, 1% or fewer show rearrangements of K_VLQT1, approximately 10% show uniparental disomy of 11p15, at least 20% involve LOI of IGF2, but most are sporadically occurring and without a defined genetic abnormality. Currently, the most useful genetic test in evaluating the family of a BWS patient, as with most genetic disorders, is a good family history. It is particularly important to examine infant photographs and to obtain a neonatal history on first-degree relatives of the affected patient. If a family appears to show dominantly transmitted BWS, then the risk to future offspring is 50%.

An interesting and provocative aspect of BWS is that the phenotype appears to abate with age, as does the risk of malignancy. Given that epigenetic factors may play a role in controlling genomic imprinting, it is possible that those factors could be modified epigenetically using novel therapeutic approaches. For example, drugs such as 5-aza-2'-deoxycytidine, which cause hypomethylation of DNA, might eventually present a novel form of gene therapy for disorders of abnormal imprinting such as BWS. Such ideas are at the earliest in vitro experimental stages, but one cannot help but speculate that, because BWS involves, at least in part, epigenetic changes to the chromosome, these changes might be experimentally or therapeutically reversible.

ACKNOWLEDGMENTS

This work was supported by NIH Grant CA 65145 (APF).

SELECTED REFERENCES

Aleck KA, Hadro TA. Dominant inheritance of Wiedemann-Beckwith syndrome: further evidence for transmission of "unstable premutation" through carrier women. Am J Med Genet 1989;33:155–160.

Beckwith JB. Extreme cytomegaly of the adrenal fetal cortex, omphalocele, hyperplasia of the kidneys and pancreas and Leydig-cell hyperplasia; another syndrome? Presented at the Annual Meeting of the Western Society of Pediatric Research, Los Angeles, Nov 1963.

Bischoff FZ, Feldman GL, McCaskill C, Subramian S, Hughes MR, Shaffer LG. Single cell analysis demonstrating somatic mosaicism involving 11p in a patient with paternal isodisomy and Beckwith-Wiedemann syndrome. Hum Mol Genet 1995;4:395–399.

Feinberg AP, Kalikin LM, Johnson LA, Thompson JS. Loss of imprinting in human cancer. Cold Spring Harbor Symp Quant Biol 1994; 59:357–364.

Hao Y, Crenshaw T, Moulton T, Newcomb E, Tycko B. Tumor-suppressor activity of H19 RNA. Nature 1993;365:764–767.

Hatada I, Ohashi H, Fukushima Y, et al. An imprinted gene p57KIP2 is mutated in Beckwith-Wiedemann syndrome. Nat Genet 1996;14:171–173.

Henry I, Bonaitijk-Pellie C, Chehensse V, et al. Uniparental paternal disomy in a genetic cancer-predisposing syndrome. Nature 1991;351: 665–667.

Hoovers JMN, Kalikin LM, Johnson LA, et al. Multiple genetic loci within 11p15 defined by Beckwith-Wiedemann syndrome rearrangement breakpoints and subchromosomal transferable fragments. Proc Natl Acad Sci USA 1995;92:12,456–12,460.

Koufos A, Grundy P, Morgan K, et al. Familial Wiedemann-Beckwith syndrome and a second Wilms tumor locus both map to 11p15.5. Am J Hum Genet 1989;44:711–719.

Lee MP, Hu RJ, Johnson LA, Feinberg AP. Human K_VLQT1 gene shows tissue-specific imprinting and encompasses Beckwith-Wiedemann syndrome chromosomal rearrangements. Nat Genet 1997;15:181–185.

Lee MP, DeBaun M. Randhawa G, Reichard BA, Elledge SJ, Feinberg AP. Low frequency of p57KIP2 mutations in Beckwith-Wiedmann syndrome. Am J Hum Gen 1997; 61:304–309.

Litz CE, Taylor KA, Qiu JS, Pescovitz OH, de Martinville B. Absence of detectable chromosomal and molecular abnormalities in monozygotic twins discordant for the Wiedemann-Beckwith syndrome. Am J Med Genet 1988;30:821–833.

Lubinsky M, Herrmann J, Kosseff AL, Opitz JM. Autosomal-dominant sex-dependent transmission of the Wiedemann-Beckwith syndrome. Lancet 1974;1:932.

Mannens M, Hoovers JMN, Redeker E, et al. Parental imprinting of human chromosome region 11p15.3-pter involved in the Beckwith-Wiedemann Syndrome and various human neoplasia. Eur J Hum Genet 1994;2:3–23.

Moulton T, Crenshaw T, Hao Y, et al. Epigenetic lesions at the H19 locus in Wilms tumour patients. Nat Genet 1994;7:440–447.

Ogawa O, Eccles MR, Szeto J, et al. Relaxation of insulin-like growth factor-II gene imprinting implicated in Wilms tumour. Nature 1993;362:749–751.

Pettenati MJ, Haines JL, Higgins RR, Wappner RS, Palmer CG, Weaver DD. Wiedemann-Beckwith syndrome: presentation of clinical and cytogenetic data on 22 new cases and review of the literature. Hum Genet 1986;74:143–154.

Pilia G, Hughes-Benzie RM, MacKenzie, et al. Mutations in GPC3, a glypican gene, cause the Simpson-Golabi-Behmel overgrowth syndrome. Nat Genet 1996;12:241–247.

Ping AJ, Reeve AE, Law DJ, Young MR, Boehnke M, Feinberg AP. Genetic linkage of Beckwith-Wiedemann syndrome to 11p15. Am J Hum Genet 1989;44:720–723.

Rainier S, Dobry C, Feinberg AP. Loss of imprinting in hepatoblastoma. Cancer Res 1995;55:1836–1838.

Rainier S, Johnson LA, Dobry CJ, Ping AJ, Grundy PE, Feinberg AP. Relaxation of imprinted genes in human cancer. Nature 1993; 362:747–749.

Reik W, Maher ER. Imprinting in clusters: lessons from Beckwith-Wiedemann syndrome. Trends Gent 1997;13:330–334.

Schroeder WT, Chao L-Y, Dao DD, et al. Nonrandom loss of maternal chromosome 11 alleles in Wilms tumors. Am J Hum Genet 1987;40:413–420.

Shackney SE, McCormack GW, Cuchural GJ. Growth rate patterns of solid tumors and their relation to responsiveness to therapy. Ann Int Med 1978;89:107–121.

Sippell WJ, Partsch CJ, Wiedemann HR. Growth, bone maturation and pubertal development in children with the EMG syndrome. Clin Genet 1989;35:20–28.

Steenman MJC, Rainier S, Dobry CJ, Grundy P, Horon I, Feinberg AP. Loss of imprinting of IGF2 is linked to reduced expression and abnormal methylation of H19 in Wilms' tumor. Nat Genet 1994;7:433–439.

Treuner J, Schilling FH. Neuroblastoma mass screening: the arguments for and against. Euro J Cancer 1995;31A:565–568.

Weksberg R, Shen DR, Fei YL, Song QL, Squire J. Disruption of insulin-like growth factor 2 imprinting in Beckwith-Weidemann syndrome. Nat Genet 1993;5:143–150.

Wiedemann HR. Complex malformatif familial avec hernia, ombilicale et macroglossie—un syndrome nouveau? J Genet Hum 1964;13:223–232.

Wiedemann HR. Tumors and hemihypertrophy associated with Wiedemann Beckwith syndrome (Letter). Euro J Ped 1983;141:129.

Yan Y, Frisen J, Lee MH, Massague J, Barbacid M. Ablation of the CDK inhibitor p57Kip2 results in increased apoptosis and delayed differentiation during mouse development. Genes Dev 1997;11:973–983.

Zhan SL, Shapiro DN, Helman LJ. Activation of an imprinted allele of the insulin-like growth factor-II gene implicated in rhabdomyosarcoma. J Clin Invest 1994;94:445–448.

Zhang P, Liegeois NJ, Wong C, et al. Altered cell differentiation and proliferation in mice lacking p57KIP2 indicates a role in Beckwith-Wiedemann syndrome. Nature 1997;387:151–158.

117 Prader-Willi and Angelman Syndromes

ROBERT D. NICHOLLS

BACKGROUND

Congenital disease in a patient usually involves a mutation in a gene that obeys established rules of Mendelian inheritance. This chapter describes two genetically related syndromes that do not conform to these principles and thereby give rise to totally independent clinical disorders. Prader-Willi syndrome (PWS) was first described by three German physicians, Prader, Labhart, and Willi, in 1956, and represents the most common form of syndromic genetic obesity. PWS was originally called the HHHO syndrome for its main features of hyperphagia, hypotonia, hypogonadism, and obesity. Angelman syndrome (AS) was first described by the British pediatrician, Harry Angelman in 1965, in which he coined the term "Happy Puppet syndrome," as it described two of the cardinal features of AS, a happy disposition with unprovoked laughter and severe ataxic movements. PWS and AS each occur at a frequency of about 1/10,000 to 1/20,000 births.

PWS and AS are each caused by genetic abnormalities in chromosome 15q11–q13, which involve imprinted genes. Imprinting refers to a class of non-Mendelian inheritance, in which specific genes or chromosomal regions are "marked" differently in the male and female germline. Following fertilization, this allows a somatic cell to know which parent the "marked" gene came from, and leads to parent-of-origin specific gene expression during development. We do not yet know why imprinting occurs, though much is being learned about the complexities and role of imprinting in AS and PWS, which has important implications for not only diagnosis of these two syndromes, but also as a means of potential therapeutic intervention in the future.

CLINICAL FEATURES AND NATURAL HISTORY OF PRADER-WILLI SYNDROME

DIAGNOSTIC CRITERIA The clinical phenotype of PWS is characterized by neonatal hypotonia and developmental delay, followed by postnatal onset of hyperphagia with subsequent obesity and other features, including short stature, hypogonadism, and mild-to-moderate mental retardation (Fig. 117-1A). These features have been organized into a set of clinical diagnostic scoring criteria for infancy and early childhood or childhood-to-adult periods. However, since most of the clinical features are relatively nonspecific, and non-PWS patients with other disorders can meet the score required to ascertain PWS, these criteria are meant to suggest a possible diagnosis of PWS and the need for further molecular tests *(see below)*, not that a given patient has the syndrome.

NEONATAL HYPOTONIA AND FAILURE TO THRIVE Decreased fetal activity during the perinatal period has been associated with PWS. This is followed by severe hypotonia in the neonatal period, with feeding difficulties requiring gavage or other feeding methods. There is failure to thrive and developmental delay in the neonatal/infancy period. Physical therapy is important as a therapeutic approach to poor muscle tone and may help prevent scoliosis and improve ability to exercise in later life.

HYPERPHAGIA AND OBESITY The onset of hyperphagia in PWS is between 1 and 6 years of age, with consequent severe obesity. Obesity is perhaps the most significant clinical feature of PWS, since it is life-threatening by the third decade without dietary and behavioral intervention. Hyperphagia in PWS appears to be driven by a failure to reach satiety, thought to be hypothalamic in origin. This results in a high energy intake, which coupled with low activity levels, short stature, and a decreased caloric requirement (for fat-free mass), results in severe obesity that has potentially morbid consequences without intervention, most commonly due to cardiopulmonary failure. However, with dietary and behavior modification, including incorporation of an exercise program, significant weight losses can be achieved, with medical, psychological, and social benefits to the patient. The latter occur because severe obesity in PWS is associated with poor self-image and social acceptance. Early diagnosis and intervention is particularly critical for these aspects.

Hyperphagia is associated with food-seeking behavior, obsession with food, and behavioral problems when food is restricted *(see below)*. PWS patients also have a thick, viscous saliva and inability to vomit. There is a specific pattern of fat distribution which is predominantly truncal and involves the proximal limbs. PWS individuals tend to have 30–40% body fat even when near ideal weight for height. The role of increased adipose tissue lipoprotein lipase is unknown. Diabetes mellitus is present in 10–20% of patients.

HYPOGONADISM PWS patients have hypogonadism, secondary to hypogonadotropism. Hypogonadism is characterized by genital hypoplasia, delayed or incomplete gonadal maturation, delayed puberty, and infertility in males and females.

SHORT STATURE AND SMALL HANDS AND FEET PWS patients have short stature, a consequence of secondary growth hormone (GH) deficiency. The basis for GH deficiency is not known. Therapeutic application of GH has been shown to not only

From: *Principles of Molecular Medicine* (J. L. Jameson, ed.), ©1998 Humana Press Inc., Totowa, NJ.

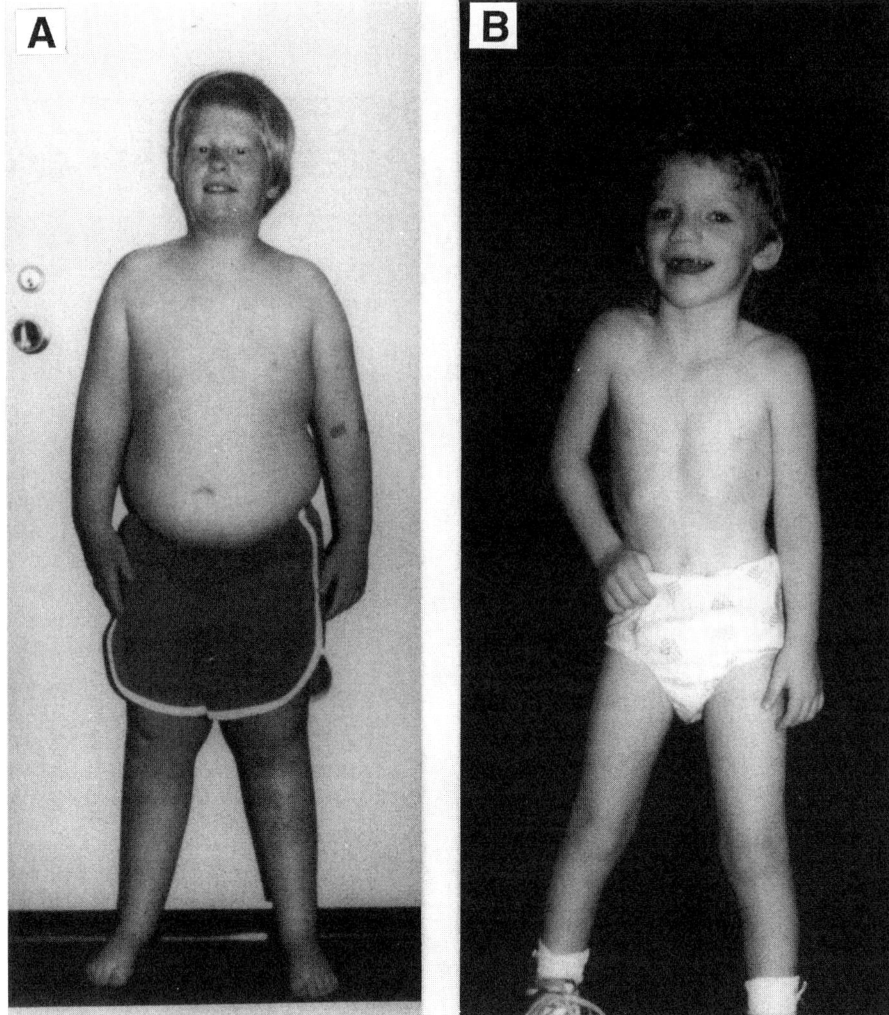

Figure 117-1 Clinical phenotype of children with **(A)** Prader-Willi syndrome or with **(B)** Angelman syndrome. Note the central obesity, short stature, small hands and feet, and almond-shaped eyes/narrow bifrontal diameter in the PWS child, and the happy disposition, wide-spaced mouth, and teeth, and broad stance of the AS child. (Reprinted with permission from Butler MG. Prader-Willi syndrome: current understanding of cause and diagnosis. Am J Med Genet 1990;35:319–332 [A]; and Williams CA, Zori RT, Stone JW, et al. Maternal origin of 15q11–13 deletions in Angelman syndrome suggests a role for genomic imprinting. Am J Med Genet 1990;35:350-353 [B]).

increase height, but also to increase the muscle mass and decrease fat mass. This results in improved muscle tone, with consequent less problems from effects of hypotonia, and decreased obesity with improvements in behavior, self-image, and social acceptance; these may lead to an increase in measurable IQ. PWS patients have small hands and feet, compared to height, particularly evident after midchildhood, suggesting delay in distal limb maturation, but the basis for this is not known.

MENTAL RETARDATION AND LEARNING AND BEHAVIORAL DISORDERS PWS patients have mild-to-moderate mental retardation (IQ in the 20–100 range, usually 40–80), but they also have learning disabilities, particularly of speech, and reading disabilities. Interestingly, PWS patients also fulfill criteria for obsessive–compulsive disorder. There are many behavioral and emotional problems, such as temper tantrums, stubbornness, rage, violence, and stealing. Many of these abnormal behaviors may be associated with hunger and food-seeking behavior. PWS patients also have other unique behavioral features, such as skill with jigsaw puzzles.

CRANIOFACIAL There is mild craniofacial dysmorphism in most PWS patients, including a narrow bifrontal diameter and almond-shaped palpebral fissures, which may be upslanting, and down-turned mouth, with thin upper lip. At least the down-turned mouth may be a consequence of hypotonia, but it is not clear if the craniofacial features represent a primary embryonic defect or secondary consequence of abnormal brain development.

OTHER FEATURES The hypopigmentation of the hair, skin, and eyes seen in one-half to two-thirds of PWS patients is associated with presence of a cytogenetic deletion and almost certainly results from deletion of the *P* gene. However, since mutations in the *P* gene cause the autosomal-recessive condition, oculocutaneous albinism type 2 (OCA2), in humans and mice, it is unclear why deletions lead to hypopigmentation in PWS (and AS) patients. PWS patients also often display skin picking, perhaps indicating a decreased pain sensitivity, and abnormal temperature control. The somnolence often seen in PWS patients appears not to be a direct consequence of the obesity in the syndrome. Therefore, it is possible that there is a specific sleep (and possibly circadian rhythm) disturbance in PWS, but this requires further research.

DIFFERENTIAL DIAGNOSIS FOR PWS Many of the syndromes that require differential diagnosis with PWS also display obesity, endocrine abnormalities (e.g., growth, hypogonadism, diabetes), and mental retardation. These include Bardet-Biedl syndrome, Borjeson-Forssman-Lehmann syndrome, Cohen syndrome, Albright hereditary osteodystrophy (including pseudohypoparathyroidism [PHP1a] and pseudo-PHP [PPHP]), Smith-Magenis syndrome, Fragile X syndrome, and other rare conditions. Congenital hypotonia in infancy can have many causes, and molecular diagnostics may be important here for PWS *(see below)*. "Acquired" PWS-like conditions also exist, arising from tumors or other insults to the brain, predominantly in the region of the hypothalamus.

CLINICAL FEATURES AND NATURAL HISTORY OF ANGELMAN SYNDROME

CLINICAL DIAGNOSTIC CRITERIA AS is associated with gait ataxia (jerky, unsteady, stiff with upheld arms), tremulousness, seizures typically beginning after 1–6 years of age, hyperactivity, severe mental retardation, absence of verbal speech, microbrachycephaly, protruding tongue and drooling, wide-spaced mouth and teeth, and a happy disposition with inappropriate laughter (Fig. 117-1B). AS patients display abnormal electroencephalograms (EEGs), with a characteristic pattern of large amplitude slow-spike wave activity (usually 2–3 Hz), which is facilitated by eye closure. The EEG abnormalities are a useful diagnostic guide for AS, although after the second decade of life, the EEG can appear normal. Mild cerebral atrophy has been seen on CT scan in about 30% of patients.

NEONATAL/INFANCY FEATURES AS children appear normal at birth, but soon suffer severe developmental delay. From early childhood, AS patients have developmental delay, with no development of speech, a smiling, happy disposition, ataxia and limb tremulousness, and microbrachycephaly. Seizures usually begin by 3–6 years of age.

MOVEMENT DISORDER Gross motor milestones are delayed, although hyperkinetic movements of the trunk and limbs may be seen in early infancy. Tremulousness may begin as early as 6 months. Most AS children are ambulatory, but there is a prancing ataxic gait with tendency to lean forward, pronounced in running, with upheld arms flexed at the elbows and wide-spaced legs. More severely affected children are very stiff, shaky, and jerky when walking, and some individuals remain nonambulatory.

SEIZURES Seizures typically begin after 1 year of age but usually before 3 years. They can be severe, episodic, of all types, but mostly major motor type or minor type, requiring anticonvulsant medication. However, no one medication has proven effective for seizures in AS and usually depends on the minor or major motor type. Seizures can be confused with the tremulousness and jerky movements seen in AS. While the abnormal EEG may be associated with seizure behavior, an abnormal EEG can persist even when seizures are controlled. Seizures may decrease in frequency or cease by the teenage years.

INAPPROPRIATE LAUGHTER An apparent happy disposition typifies the AS child. In addition, most reactions to mental or physical stimuli are accompanied by laughter or similar facial expressions. This behavior has an onset early in childhood. It does not appear to be related to the seizure disorder. Sometimes irritability and hyperactivity can also be present.

MENTAL RETARDATION AND SPEECH Developmental milestones are greatly delayed, although formal testing is difficult because of absence of formal speech, hyperactivity, motor difficulties, and attention deficit. Nevertheless, IQ scores are in the severely retarded range, although AS children perform better on receptive social skills, and it is believed that cognitive abilities are higher than thought from developmental testing. Most AS children have one to four words, at most, although a few rare cases with milder presentation *(see below)* have up to 10–20 words. Nevertheless, most AS children are able to follow and understand commands, except for cases with severe seizures and hyperactivity. In higher-functioning individuals, there may be nonverbal language, such as some degree of sign language.

CRANIOFACIAL The microcephaly present in some AS patients may be a secondary result of developmental brain abnormalities, associated with decelerated growth by 1 year of age. Many of these patients also have a flattened occiput, some with a distinct occipital groove. Brachycephaly is a common finding in AS. The mandible is normal in size but can appear large because of a forward and upward orientation, with midface hypoplasia, a thin upper lip, and deep-set eyes. A wide mouth and wide-spaced teeth are often present, and prognathia can result from excessive chewing. Facial dysmorphism is not present at birth.

OTHER FEATURES Virtually all AS individuals display features of hyperactivity, both constant movement (including running), and handling and mouthing of objects in infancy. This may improve in adults. There is attention deficit, which in severe cases prevents facial and social cues, but in others allows sufficient attention for developmental training programs. Sleep abnormalities consisting of short periods of sleep and abnormal sleep/wake cycles are characteristic of AS. The role of abnormal circadian rhythms and other features of sleep and hyperactivity remain to be assessed. The hypopigmentation of the hair, skin, and eyes seen in one-half to two-thirds of AS patients likely results from deletion of the *P* gene, as explained above for PWS. It is present only in PWS and AS patients with deletions of 15q11–q13. AS patients also share intriguing behavioral features, such as love of water, of bright, shiny objects, and of music. About 5% of AS patients show obesity.

DIFFERENTIAL DIAGNOSIS FOR AS Conditions that need to be considered in the differential diagnosis of AS include Rett syndrome, a neurodegenerative syndrome affecting girls only, distinguished by the history of regression and loss of acquired skills, the alpha-thalassemia-mental retardation syndrome, X-linked (ATRX syndrome), ataxic cerebral palsy with less severe mental retardation, and others.

CLINICAL MANAGEMENT OF THE SYNDROMES

For PWS, feeding and behavior management are critical, particularly from an early age. Appetite suppressant agents have not generally been successful in PWS. Growth hormone replacement for height, improved muscle-to-fat mass, and associated behaviors is beneficial during childhood, but is still controversial. Learning disabilities require evaluation and may require speech therapy. Early intervention with physical therapy can significantly help difficulties associated with poor muscle tone. While hormonal treatment can be applied to hypogonadism, the benefits are not clear.

For AS, the principle management issues relate to seizure control (in which no one anticonvulsant has been successful) and to hyperactivity, sleep disturbances, and education. It would also be

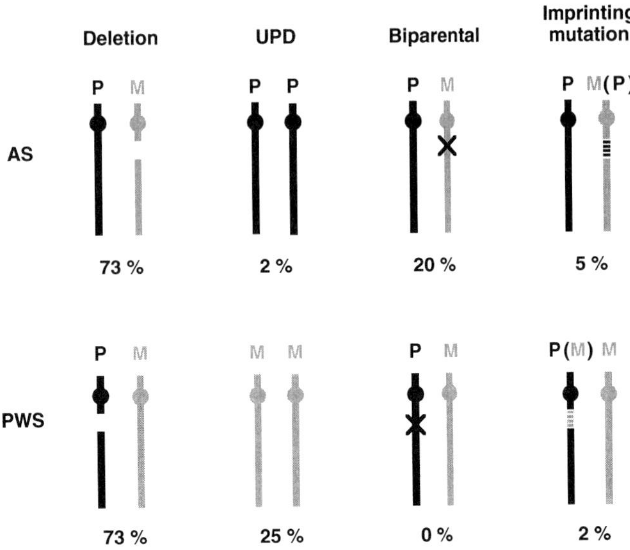

Figure 117-2 Molecular classes of Prader-Willi and Angelman syndromes. The chromosome 15 genotypes (and frequency) are shown for the major classes of AS and PWS. UPD, uniparental disomy; P, paternal (black); M, maternal (gray); M(P), maternal inheritance with paternal imprint (or epigenotype); P(M), paternal inheritance with maternal epigenotype; X, structural gene mutation. (*See text* for details.)

beneficial to treat the ataxia and tremulousness of the limbs in AS, since this may improve the ability to learn sign language, or, potentially, computer skills, both very difficult for AS individuals.

Although the biological basis of AS and PWS are unknown, both syndromes are likely to arise predominantly from failure of an aspect of neural development during embryogenesis (particularly the hypothalamus or associated structure for PWS and the cerebellum or other limbic structure in AS). However, some features of both syndromes clearly have postnatal onset, including in AS of seizures (and their resolution) and coarsening of the facial appearance during the first two decades of life, and in PWS of hyperphagia (hypotonia and poor feeding ability may prevent this in infancy and early childhood), behavioral disturbances, and small hand and foot size. No consistent abnormality has been identified in PWS or AS by biochemical, endocrine, or anatomical studies.

GENETIC BASIS OF PRADER-WILLI AND ANGELMAN SYNDROMES

CHROMOSOME 15 There are multiple molecular genetic mechanisms that can lead to PWS and AS (Fig. 117-2), but despite this complexity, each leads to a common gene deficit. Each molecular mechanism that leads to PWS and AS abolishes imprinted (parent-of-origin)-specific expression, such that paternal gene expression is abrogated in PWS (one or more genes) and maternal gene expression is silenced in AS (probably one gene). Chromosome 15q11–q13 is now known to have three subregions (Fig. 117-3):

1. A proximal region containing genes that are expressed from the paternally inherited chromosome only (hence each of these genes is a candidate to play a role in PWS).
2. A central region containing a gene, or genes, expressed from the maternally inherited chromosome only (and thus this gene is a candidate for AS).
3. A distal region containing genes that are expressed from both alleles and thus show normal Mendelian inheritance, (which includes a cluster of gamma-aminobutyric acid (GABA) class A receptor genes and the *P* gene involved in the autosomal-recessive disorder OCA2).

CYTOGENETIC DELETIONS Cytogenetically visible deletions of 15q11–q13 were first observed in PWS by Ledbetter and colleagues in 1981 and in AS by Latt and Magenis and their colleagues in 1987. Although initially thought that the deletions in PWS and AS would be adjacent, it was first shown in 1989 that the majority of the deletions in PWS and AS are in fact of a very similar size. This conclusion was supported by the cloning of a yeast artificial chromosome (YAC) contig spanning 15q11–q13, which showed that about 4 Mb of DNA was deleted in these PWS and AS patients. It is likely that specific sequences at the proximal and distal breakpoints predispose to recombination, to generate the common deletion. Although the deletion size is generally the same in PWS and AS, from the study of differently sized deletions in rare patients, it was subsequently realized that the PWS and AS genes do in fact map to adjacent chromosome regions (Fig. 117-3).

PARENTAL ORIGIN OF DELETIONS Since the majority of deletions in PWS and AS are the same size, it was initially an enigma as to how two different clinical syndromes arise. However, the use of cytogenetic and molecular polymorphisms led to the findings that all deletions in PWS are paternal in origin, and all deletions in AS are maternal in origin (Fig. 117-2). Therefore, the parental origin determines the clinical nature of the syndrome, and both parental contributions of chromosome 15q11–q13 are required for normal development.

UNIPARENTAL DISOMY (UPD) UPD was first discovered in PWS in 1989, in which studies with molecular polymorphisms showed that two PWS children had inherited two maternal alleles but no paternal allele for chromosome 15 (Fig. 117-2). Subsequent studies showed that maternal UPD is quite common in PWS, occurring in 25% of cases. There is an association of advanced maternal age with UPD in PWS, consistent with maternal nondisjunction and subsequent formation of a trisomic zygote. Since trisomy 15 is lethal during embryogenesis, there is selection for loss of one chromosome 15, which one-third of the time would lead to maternal UPD and hence PWS. UPD also occurs in AS, in which it is paternal in origin (Fig. 117-2) and may be associated with a milder phenotype, but a larger study population is needed to confirm this.

The finding of UPD confirms that the parental origin of 15q11–q13, and hence genomic imprinting, underlies the etiology of PWS and AS. Thus, a second totally normal copy of a maternal chromosome 15 cannot complement the missing paternal chromosome in PWS, indicating that the maternally inherited PWS genes are normally silent, and that the paternally inherited PWS genes are expressed. Likewise, paternal UPD in AS indicates that the paternally inherited AS gene is normally silent, and that it is the maternally inherited allele that is active. Therefore, the absence of expression of the active PWS or AS genes leads to the respective syndrome (by any mechanism in Fig. 117-2).

PATERNAL PWS AND MATERNAL AS GENES In AS, there are about 20% of patients who do not have a deletion, UPD, nor imprinting mutation *(see below)*. Some of these cases are familial. These patients inherit a copy of chromosome 15 from each parent (biparental) and likely have a point mutation (or small DNA rear-

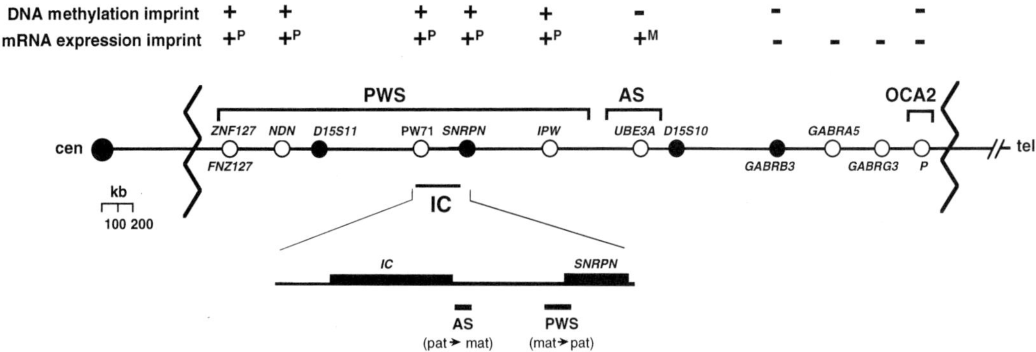

Figure 117-3 Human chromosome 15q11–q13 map. Genetic loci are shown as circles and FISH probes as filled circles. Regions containing the AS and PWS structural genes are indicated above the line, and the region affected by microdeletions in AS and PWS imprinting mutation patients in the expanded segment below (the latter define the imprinting center, IC). Two genes are expressed from the IC, the *SNRPN* gene and *IC* transcript. The shortest region of microdeletion overlap in AS and PWS is shown by bars; these correspond to elements critical for paternal (pat) to maternal (mat) imprint switching in the female germline or maternal to paternal imprint switching in the male germline, respectively. At the top, the presence (+) and absence (–) of imprinted features are shown. The zigzag lines reflect the end points of the common cytogenetic deletion in AS and PWS. P, paternal-only expression; M, maternal-only expression in brain; cen, centromere; tel, telomere.

rangement) in a single, maternally expressed gene (Fig. 117-2). Recently, the *UBE3A* gene (formerly *E6AP*), encoding a ubiquitin-protein ligase thought to be involved in protein degradation pathways, was shown to have mutations in AS patients of this class. Recent studies have shown that the *UBE3A* gene undergoes spatially (tissue-specific) regulated imprinted expression in human and mouse.

In contrast, no PWS patients with the classical phenotype appear to come under this class (Fig. 117-2). This may mean that at least two genes are required for classical PWS (all cases of PWS would then represent a contiguous gene syndrome); mutations in a single gene may therefore only result in a PWS-like syndrome that is presently unrecognized. Consistent with this idea, there are multiple paternally expressed genes in the 15q11–q13 region involved in PWS (Fig. 117-3). Nevertheless, a single major gene has not yet been ruled out.

FAMILIAL CASES RESULTING FROM IMPRINTING MUTATIONS About 5% of AS and PWS patients have been shown to have inherited a copy of chromosome 15 from both the mother and the father, but they have abnormal DNA methylation imprints *(see below)* throughout the imprinted 15q11–q13 region (Fig. 117-2). However, the DNA methylation is typical of the syndrome (uniparental maternal in PWS and uniparental paternal in AS). This suggests that such patients have a mutation in the imprinting process, since the paternally inherited chromosome in PWS patients has maternal DNA methylation, and the maternally inherited chromosome in AS patients has paternal DNA methylation. These AS and PWS patients have the classical clinical phenotype, and about half the cases are familial. The molecular basis of this class of patients is described below.

BALANCED TRANSLOCATIONS IN PWS Three PWS patients have been described with a balanced translocation of 15q11–q13. One patient with classical PWS has a breakpoint in the 5' part of the *SNRPN* gene, implicating this gene as a major PWS gene. Two patients with a PWS-like syndrome (not fulfilling all major clinical criteria of PWS) are associated with a second cluster of breakpoints about 50–150 kb distal of the *SNRPN* gene, and thus other genes may contribute to the PWS phenotype. However, how the translocations lead to the phenotype in this rare class of patients is presently not understood.

MOLECULAR DIAGNOSTICS OF PRADER-WILLI AND ANGELMAN SYNDROMES

FLUORESCENT *IN SITU* HYBRIDIZATION (FISH) FISH, with unique probes from 15q11–q13 (Fig. 117-3), and a centromeric control probe, is the method of choice of cytogenetic diagnostic laboratories to identify large deletions or unbalanced translocations in suspected PWS and AS cases. Probes within at least the PWS and AS critical regions (Fig. 117-3) should be utilized.

MICROSATELLITE ANALYSIS FOR UPD Polymorphic marker analysis, preferably the use of highly informative microsatellites such as $(CA)_n$ markers, using parental and affected-child DNA samples, is commonly used to identify UPD. However, both parental DNA samples are often not available.

DNA METHYLATION ANALYSIS Several genes and DNA markers in 15q11–q13 (*ZNF127, NDN, PW71, SNRPN* [Fig. 117-3]) have been shown to display differential DNA methylation of the paternal and maternal alleles. These differences arise in the male and female germline or are established in early development. The most reliable methylation probe is at *SNRPN*, in which the maternal allele is completely methylated, and the paternal allele is completely unmethylated (Fig. 117-4), in all tested tissues. Clearly, AS samples with only the unmethylated band and PWS samples with only the methylated band can be easily distinguished from one another and from normal controls (or patients with another diagnosis). Methylation at *SNRPN* represents the best single diagnostic tool for these syndromes, since it identifies all PWS and AS patients with a deletion, unbalanced translocation, UPD, or imprinting mutation (it does not detect the biparental class of AS patients), and does not require parental DNA samples. However, DNA methylation is not reliable to distinguish between different classes of PWS and AS patients. Neverthless, DNA methylation detects about 98% of classical PWS patients (deletion, UPD, and imprinting mutations) and 80% of AS patients (deletion, UPD, and imprinting mutations).

PWS AND AS IMPRINTING MUTATIONS Imprinting mutation cases are diagnosed by the absence of a deletion by FISH (with the exception of a *SNRPN* deletion only) and the absence of UPD (tested by polymorphic markers), but with the presence of abnormal DNA methylation using any of the probes that detect differential DNA methylation. About one-half of cases, including

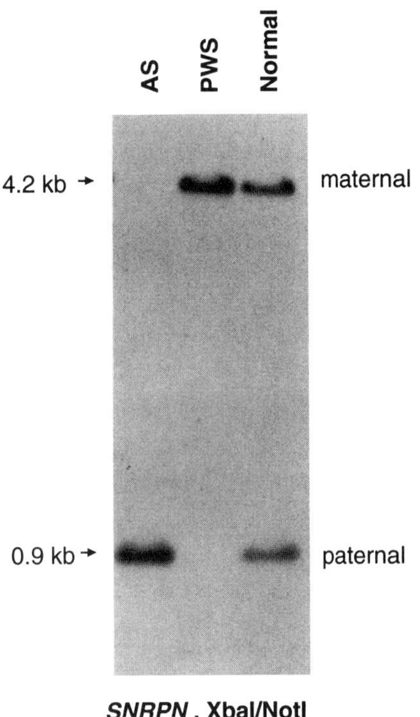

Figure 117-4 Molecular diagnosis by DNA methylation. DNA from peripheral blood leukocytes is digested with *XbaI/NotI* and probed with a *SNRPN* 5' probe. *NotI* does not cut if DNA is methylated (maternal band; PWS UPD patient) but does cut if DNA is unmethylated (paternal; AS UPD patient). PWS and AS patients are easily distinguished from each other and from normal individuals, who show a normal "biparental" pattern.

all familial cases, have a microdeletion overlapping the first exon (PWS) or upstream of the first exon of the *SNRPN* gene (AS). This region is termed the imprinting center (IC), and microdeletions or mutations in the IC are detected by molecular techniques in a research laboratory (Fig. 117-3).

STRUCTURAL GENE MUTATION IN AS Since the *UBE3A* gene has been identified as the AS gene, it is now possible to perform mutation analysis. However, since most cases arise *de novo*, it is likely that most patients will have different mutations in the AS gene. The ease of performing repeated mutation screens on each new case will depend on whether mutations cluster in functional domains of the encoded protein or throughout the fairly large coding region (or in regulatory regions) of the *UBE3A* gene.

GENETIC COUNSELING IN PRADER-WILLI AND ANGELMAN SYNDROMES

DELETIONS AND UPD IN PWS AND AS Essentially, the recurrence risk of a deletion or UPD in extended families is the population risk (1/10,000 to 1/20,000). Nevertheless, in instances of advanced maternal age, the risk for having a child with UPD is significantly larger, though still small, but prenatal screening is possible where there is concern for the risks. The presence of a familial, phenotypically silent balanced translocation in chromosome 15q11–q13 has a risk of meiotic rearrangement or nondisjunction, leading to a deletion of 15q11–q13 or UPD, respectively, and prenatal diagnosis and genetic counseling are recommended in such cases.

IMPRINTING MUTATIONS IN PWS AND AS In those families in which a microdeletion in the IC has been identified, or in which multiple sibs of PWS or AS have already occurred, "at risk" or prenatal diagnosis are options, based on detection of the microdeletion. Since imprinting mutations can be transmitted silently for multiple generations *(see below)*, relatives of the same sex as the transmitting parent have up to a 50% risk for transmitting the mutation silently, whereas offspring of the opposite sex have a risk of up to 50% for a child with the syndrome. In such cases, referral for molecular testing and genetic counseling are strongly recommended (*see* Saitoh et al., 1997, for further discussion of recurrence risks). In cases with no detectable microdeletion or IC mutation, no known recurrence has occurred, and such cases may be sporadic (unpublished data).

OTHER FAMILIAL AS In families with multiple affected AS cases, once an imprinting mutation has been ruled out, it is likely that there is an inherited mutation in the AS gene. Paternal inheritance of this gene will be phenotypically silent, since the paternal AS gene is normally silent, and the AS phenotype will only appear after maternal inheritance. Now that the *UBE3A* gene has been identified as the AS gene, the specific familial mutation can be identified, and "at risk" individuals can be screened. Females carrying the mutation inherited from their father have a 50% recurrence risk. Prenatal testing and counseling are recommended in such cases.

MOLECULAR GENETICS OF PRADER-WILLI AND ANGELMAN SYNDROMES

FEATURES OF IMPRINTING As is evident from the preceding discussion, imprinted genes are characterized by monoallelic expression (paternal or maternal allele only) and differential DNA methylation imprints, whereby the two alleles differ in methylation status. In addition, imprinted chromosome regions show asynchronous DNA replication, in which the two parental alleles appear to replicate at different times in S phase of the cell cycle, in comparison to nonimprinted chromosome regions in which replication is synchronous for the two alleles. Nevertheless, the basis for replication timing asynchrony is unknown, and it may be a consequence rather than a cause of imprinting. Replication timing has been used to specifically identify PWS and AS UPD patients by cytological techniques. The potential role of other factors in imprinting, such as chromatin structure, histone acetylation, and DNA binding proteins, is presently unknown.

The mechanism of imprinting is complex and not completely understood, but the following picture has emerged. Imprinting is set in the germ line, and must be erased and reset (i.e., is reversible) at each generation, specific for the sex of that individual. The first step in imprint erasure and resetting is controlled by the IC, since mutations in this region block resetting of the imprint *(see below)*. The IC signal is then transferred bidirectionally by an unknown mechanism to each imprinted gene in 15q11–q13 (Fig. 117-3). This allows each imprinted gene to set its own germ line (gametic) imprint, based on DNA methylation specific for the male or female germ line. Subsequent to fertilization, some imprinted genes carry the gametic imprint in the body of the gene and undergo modification of the imprint at the promoter, which then locks in the imprinted state and/or determines the allele-specific expression. It is well-known that the presence of DNA methylation blocks transcription, whereas an unmethylated promoter is capable of transcription, depending on tissue-specific factors.

OCULOCUTANEOUS ALBINISM The only clinical feature known to be shared between PWS and AS, in deletion patients, is hypopigmentation of the skin, hair, and eyes, and is thus a result of a nonimprinted gene (the *P* gene). Therefore, at least in deletion patients, AS and PWS represent contiguous gene syndromes in which the clinical features arise because of more than one gene. Some PWS (and AS) patients have albinism (OCA2), at the frequency expected for carriers of OCA2, which arises from inheritance from one parent of a *P* gene mutation coupled with a large deletion of the other allele.

MOUSE MODELS All the identified genes from human chromosome 15q11–q13, including imprinted genes and nonimprinted genes, have homologs in the same respective genetic order in the central part of mouse chromosome 7. The imprint status of these genes is also conserved between humans and mice. These findings suggest that mouse models should be an excellent model of PWS and AS. Mice with radiation-induced deletions of the nonimprinted genes allow assessment of the contribution of such genes to recessive phenotypes in this chromosomal region. Mice with maternal UPD specifically for the PWS/AS homologous region, or with paternal UPD, albeit for a much larger chromosome region that may contain other imprinted genes, have been generated by clever breeding techniques, and these animals have imprinted phenotypes that may provide models of the imprinted PWS and AS phenotypes. For example, the maternal UPD mice die at birth, probably because of the inability to feed, which may mimic the failure to thrive and gavage feeding necessary for newborn PWS infants. Nevertheless, such animals are difficult and expensive to generate, and models based on targeted mutation of the mouse homologs of the specific PWS and AS genes, or the IC elements, may provide more workable models in the future.

IMPRINTING MUTATIONS Perhaps one of the most remarkable findings to come from the study of PWS and AS is that of patients with mutations in the imprinting process. These patients have microdeletions that define an IC, overlapping and upstream from the *SNRPN* gene (Fig. 117-3), as previously discussed. Familial mutations of the IC can transmit silently through many generations, as long as the transmitting sex does not change (Fig. 117-5). Imprinting is a reversible process in which the germline imprint must be erased and reset at each generation; thus, in the male germline, the maternally inherited imprint must be erased and reset as a male imprint, or epigenotype (referring to information that is heritable and alters the phenotype of offspring but is not encoded specifically in the genetic code of DNA), and in the female germline, the paternally inherited imprint must be erased and reset (switched). IC mutations block this resetting of the imprint in the opposite germline, leading to a failure to reset the imprint specific for the sex of that individual.

Thus, when a maternally derived imprinting mutation [represented by M(M)] is transmitted through a male, the maternal epigenotype cannot be reset in his germline to the normal paternal epigenotype (Fig. 117-5A). He therefore transmits a maternal imprint on his paternal chromosome [P(M)] to 50% of his gametes; resulting offspring inheriting the abnormal gametic epigenotype [P(M)] also inherit a normal maternal epigenotype (M) from their mother, and thus they are homozygous for a maternal epigenotype (Fig. 117-5A). This is equivalent to maternal UPD, and hence PWS develops. Likewise, transmission of a paternally derived imprinting mutation [P(P)] through a female results in failure to switch the imprint and inheritance of the abnormal epigenotype [M(P)], along

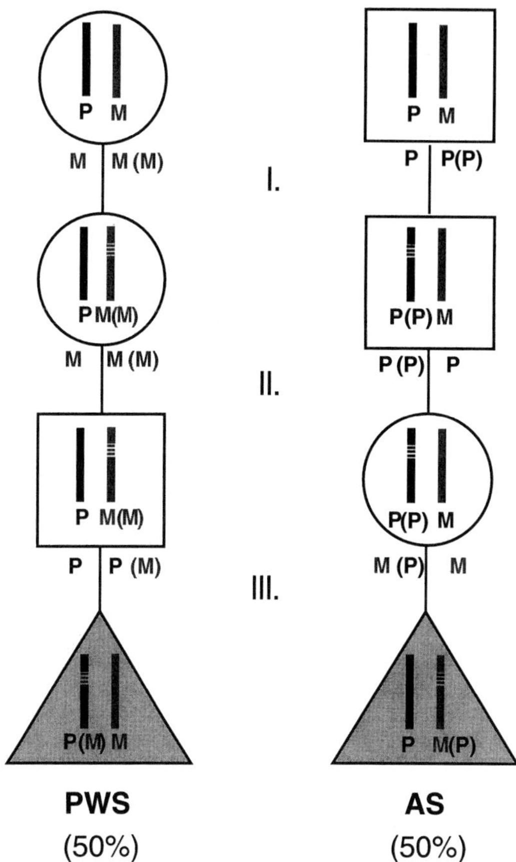

Figure 117-5 Inheritance of imprinting mutations. The inherited chromosome 15 imprint (epigenotype) in somatic cells is shown inside the female (circles) and male (squares) symbols, whereas the germline imprint is shown below these symbols. When an imprinting mutation in the IC arises during maternal meiosis (I, left), a maternal epigenotype (i.e., imprint) is fixed into this chromosome. Females transmit the maternal epigenotype silently (I and II, left), but the IC mutation blocks resetting of the imprint in a male (III, left). Thus, he transmits a maternal epigenotype to 50% of his offspring, who have a "uniparental" maternal epigenotype and hence will have PWS. An analogous pattern occurs for origin and transmission through males of an IC mutation generating a fixed paternal epigenotype, but maternal transmission now gives rise to AS at 50% risk (right).

with a normal paternal imprint (P), and thus the resulting offspring are homozygous for a paternal imprint and develop AS (Fig. 117-5B). In such PWS and AS patients, the mutation has no direct effect in the patient; rather, the mutation exerts its effect in the parental germ line, and it is a consequence of this effect that genetic disease arises in the offspring. This clearly represents a new paradigm as a mechanism of inherited genetic disease.

FUTURE STUDIES

IDENTIFICATION OF THE PWS AND AS GENES The most important immediate research is to identify the gene(s) responsible for clinical features in PWS and to explain the clinical pleiotropy (range of features) of AS in terms of the molecular functions of the *UBE3A* gene. Accurate molecular diagnosis can then follow in those cases in which a gene mutation is a possible mechanism for the syndrome. Identification of the etiological gene will allow subsequent studies of:

1. Developmental expression of the gene, which may lead to insight as to the embryological or postnatal stages at which cellular and hence phenotypic abnormalities arise.
2. Characterization of the protein product of the gene.
3. Development of mouse models in which the function of the mouse homolog of the PWS or AS gene is ablated.
4. Ultimately, the derivation and testing of potential therapeutic approaches to clinical features of the two syndromes.

MECHANISM OF IMPRINTING AND RELATIONSHIP TO OTHER DISORDERS INVOLVING IMPRINTED GENES Imprinting also plays a role in several cancers and other genetic disorders, such as Beckwith-Wiedemann syndrome (BWS; *see* Chapter 116). In particular, many of the same mechanisms, including UPD, specific parental origin chromosome rearrangements and imprinting mutations occur in BWS, suggesting that an understanding of the imprinting and disease mechanisms in PWS and AS may lead to insight in other conditions.

THERAPEUTIC APPROACHES TO PWS AND AS Additional advances may result from clinically based applications (previously discussed), such as melatonin treatment of the sleep disorder in AS and PWS. Recent advances in understanding the genes involved in feeding behavior and obesity, such as the *Ob* gene, may lead to better understanding of the pathway of hyperphagia and obesity in PWS and hence to therapeutic approaches, even though specific mutations in such genes are not present. More important will be the identification of the specific gene products missing in PWS patients, and the protein substrates of the *UBE3A* gene product that are deregulated in AS patients, which may lead to important therapeutic approaches. Finally, an understanding of the mechanism of imprinting, by which genes are silenced or activated as a consequence of their parental origin (set during gametogenesis), may lead to therapeutic approaches based on reactivation of silent imprinted genes or silencing of abnormally expressed imprinted genes in somatic cells.

ACKNOWLEDGMENTS

This chapter is dedicated to the memory of Dr. Harry Angelman. I sincerely thank the AS and PWS families who make this work possible, my friends who work with me as collaborators, as well as Jim Amos-Landgraf and Nancy Rebert for illustrations. Work from the author's laboratory is supported by the NIH #HD31491, March of Dimes Birth Defects Foundation, and the International Human Frontiers of Science Project.

SELECTED REFERENCES

Albrecht U, Sutcliffe JS, Cattanach BM, et al. Imprinted expression of the murine Angelman syndrome gene, *Ube3a*, in hippocampal and Purkinje neurons. Nat Genet 1997;17:75–78.

Angelman H. "Puppet children": a report on three cases. Develop Med Child Neurol 1965;7:681–688.

Boyd SG, Harden A, Patton MA. The EEG in early diagnosis of the Angelman (Happy Puppet) syndrome. Eur J Pediatr 1988;147:508 –513.

Butler MG. Prader-Willi syndrome: current understanding of cause and diagnosis. Am J Med Genet 1990;35:319–332.

Cassidy SB. Prader-Willi syndrome. Curr Prob Pediat 1984;14:1–55.

Cassidy SB. Prader-Willi syndrome. <http://www.hslib.washington.edu/genline/pws.html>. 1996.

Cassidy SB. Uniparental disomy and genomic imprinting as causes of human genetic disease. Environ Mol Mutag 1995;25(Suppl 26):13–20.

Cassidy SB, Beaudet AL, Knoll JMH, et al. Diagnostic testing for Prader-Willi and Angelman syndromes. Report of the ASHG/ACMG Test and Technology Transfer Committee. Am J Hum Genet 1996;58:1085–1088.

Cassidy SB, Ledbetter DH. Prader-Willi syndrome. Neurol Clin 1989; 7:37–54.

Cattanach BM, Barr JA, Evans EP, et al. A candidate mouse model for Prader-Willi syndrome which shows an absence of *Snrpn* expression. Nat Genet 1992;2:270–274.

Christian SL, Bhatt NK, Martin SA, et al. Integrated YAC contig map of the Prader-Willi/Angelman region on chromosome 15q11-q13 with average STS spacing of 35 kb. Genome Res 1998;8:146–157.

Christian SL, Robinson WP, Huang B, et al. Characterization of two proximal deletion breakpoint regions in both Prader-Willi and Angelman syndrome patients. Am J Hum Genet 1995;57:40–48.

Clayton-Smith J, Pembrey ME. Angelman syndrome. J Med Genet 1992;29:412–415.

Conroy JM, Grebe TA, Becker LA, et al. Balanced translocation 46,XY,t(2;15)(q37.2;q11.2) associated with atypical Prader-Willi syndrome. Am J Hum Genet 1997;61:388–394.

Dittrich B, Buiting K, Korn B, et al. Imprint switching on human chromosome 15 may involve alternative transcripts of the *SNRPN* gene. Nat Genet 1996;14:163–170.

Driscoll DJ. Genomic imprinting in humans. In: Friedman T, ed. Molecular Genetic Medicine, ch. 4. New York: Academic, 1994; pp. 37–77.

Dykens EM, Leckman JF, Cassidy SB. Obsessions and compulsions in Prader-Willi syndrome. J Child Psychol 1996;37:995–1002.

Fryburg JS, Breg WR, Lindgren V. Diagnosis of Angelman syndrome in infants. Am J Med Genet 1991;38:58–64.

Glenn CC, Driscoll DJ, Yang TP, Nicholls RD. Genomic imprinting: potential function and mechanisms revealed by Prader-Willi and Angelman syndromes. Molec Hum Reprod 1997;3:321–332.

Glenn CC, Saitoh S, Jong MTC, et al. Gene structure, DNA methylation and imprinted expression of the human *SNRPN* gene. Am J Hum Genet 1996;58:335–346.

Greenberg F, Elder FFB, Ledbetter DH. Neonatal diagnosis of Prader-Willi syndrome and its implications. Am J Med Genet 1987; 28:845–856.

Gunay M, Cassidy SB, Nicholls RD. Prader-Willi and other syndromes associated with mental retardation and obesity. Behaviour Genet (Special issue, Allison D., Faith MS, ed.) 1997;27:307–324.

Holm VA, Cassidy SB, Butler MG, et al. Prader-Willi syndrome: consensus diagnostic criteria. Pediatrics 1993;91:398–402.

Horsthemke B, Maat-Kievit A, Sleegers E, et al. Familial translocations involving 15q11–q13 can give rise to interstitial deletions causing Prader-Willi or Angelman syndrome. J Med Genet 1996;65:133–136.

Kishino T, Lalande M, Wagstaff J. *UBE3A*/E6-AP mutations cause Angelman syndrome. Nat Genet 1997;15:70–73.

Knoll JHM, Nicholls RD, Magenis E, Graham JM, Jr, Lalande M, Latt SA. Angelman and Prader-Willi syndromes share a common chromosome 15 deletion but differ in parental origin of the deletion. Am J Med Genet 1989;32:285–290.

Knoll JHM, Rogan PK, Nicholls RD, Wu B, Korf B, White LM. Allele-specific replication of 15q11-q13 loci: a diagnostic test for detection of uniparental disomy. Am J Hum Genet 1996;59:423–430.

Lee S-T, Nicholls RD, Bundey S, Laxova R, Musarella M, Spritz RA. Mutations of the *P* gene in type II oculocutaneous albinism, Prader-Willi syndrome plus albinism, and "autosomal recessive albinism." New Engl J Med 1994;330:529–534.

MacDonald HR, Wevrick R. The necdin gene is deleted in Prader-Willi syndrome and is imprinted in human and mouse. Hum Molec Genet 1997;6:1873–1878.

Matsuura T, Sutcliffe JS, Fang P, et al. *De novo* truncating mutations in E6-AP ubiquitin-protein ligase gene (*UBE3A*) in Angelman syndrome. Nat Genet 1997;15:74–77.

Mitchell J, Schinzel A, Langlois S, et al. Comparison of phenotype in uniparental disomy and deletion Prader-Willi syndrome: sex specific differences. Am J Med Genet 1996;65:133–136.

Mutirangura A, Jayakumar A, Sutcliffe JS, et al. A complete YAC contig of the Prader-Willi/Angelman chromosome region (15q11–q13) and refined localization of the *SNRPN* gene. Genomics 1993; 18:546–552.

Nakao M, Sutcliffe JS, Durtschi B, Mutirangura A, Ledbetter DH, Beaudet AL. Imprinting analysis of three genes in the Prader-Willi/Angelman region: *SNRPN*, E6-associated protein, and *PAR-2* (*D15S225E*). Hum Mol Genet 1994;3:309–315.

Nicholls RD, Saitoh S, Horsthemke B. Imprinting in Prader-Willi and Angelman syndromes. Trends Genet 1998;14:194–200.

Nicholls RD, Glenn CC, Jong MTC, Saitoh S, Mascari MJ, Driscoll DJ. Molecular pathogenesis of Prader-Willi syndrome. In: Bray GA, ed. The Genetics and Molecular Biology of Obesity. Pennington Center Nutrition Series, vol. V. Baton Rouge: Louisiana State University Press, 1996; pp. 560–577.

Nicholls RD, Gottlieb W, Russell LB, Davda M, Horsthemke B, Rinchik EM. Evaluation of potential models for imprinted and nonimprinted components of human 15q11–q13 syndromes by fine structure homology mapping in the mouse. Proc Natl Acad Sci USA 1993;90: 2050–2054.

Nicholls RD, Knoll JHM, Butler MG, Karam S, Lalande M. Genetic imprinting suggested by maternal heterodisomy in non-deletion Prader-Willi syndrome. Nature 1989;342:281–285.

Prader A, Labhart A, Willi H. Ein syndrom von adipositas, kleinwuchs, kryptorchismus and oligophrenie nach myotonicartigem zustand in neugeborenalter. Schweiz Med Wochenschr 1956;86: 1260,1261.

Rinchik EM, Bultman SJ, Horsthemke B, et al. A gene for the mouse pink-eyed dilution locus and for human type II oculocutaneous albinism. Nature 1993;361:72–76.

Rougeulle C. Glatt H, Lalande M. The Angelman syndrome candidate gene, UBE3A/E6-AP, is imprinted in brain. Nat Genet 1997; 17:14,15.

Saitoh S, Buiting K, Rogan PK, et al. Minimal definition of the imprinting center and fixation of a chromosome 15q11–q13 epigenotype by imprinting mutations. Proc Natl Acad Sci USA 1996;93:7811–7815.

Saitoh S, Cassidy SB, Conroy JM, et al. Clinical spectrum and molecular diagnosis of Angelman and Prader-Willi syndrome imprinting mutation patients. Am J Med Genet 1997;68:195–206.

Saitoh S, Kubota T, Ohta T, et al. Familial Angelman syndrome caused by imprinted submicroscopic deletion encompassing $GABA_A$ receptor β3-subunit gene. Lancet 1992;339:366,367.

Sapienza C. Parental imprinting of genes. Sci Am 1990;263:52–60.

Smeets DFCM, Hamel BCJ, Nelen MR, et al. Prader-Willi syndrome and Angelman syndrome in cousins from a family with a translocation between chromosomes 6 and 15. N Engl J Med 1992;326:807–811.

Spritz RA, Bailin T, Nicholls RD, et al. Hypopigmentation in the Prader-Willi syndrome correlates with *P* gene deletion but not with haplotype of the hemizygous *P* allele. Am J Med Genet 1997;71:57–62.

Vu TH, Hoffman AR. Imprinting of the Angelman syndrome gene, UBE3A, is restricted to brain. Nat Genet 1997;17:12,13.

Wevrick R, Francke U. Diagnostic tests for the Prader-Willi syndrome by SNRPN expression in blood. Lancet 1996;348:1068,1069.

Williams CA, Angelman H, Clayton-Smith J, et al. Angelman syndrome: consensus for diagnostic criteria. Am J Med Genet 1995a;56:237,238.

Williams CA, Zori RT, Hendickson J, et al. Angelman syndrome. Curr Prob Pediatr 1995b;25:216–231.

Williams CA, Zori RT, Stone JW, et al. Maternal origin of 15q11–13 deletions in Angelman syndrome suggests a role for genomic imprinting. Am J Med Genet 1990;35:350–353.

118 Fragile X Syndrome

DAVID L. NELSON

INTRODUCTION

Fragile X syndrome (MIM 30955) is among the most common of human single-gene disorders and is the leading cause of inherited mental retardation, with an estimated frequency of 1/2000 to 1/4000 individuals. It is inherited as an X-linked dominant disorder with reduced penetrance. Males and females can be affected; however, the degree of mental retardation is usually more severe in males.

Fragile X syndrome derives its name from the observation of a folate-sensitive fragile site at Xq27.3 in chromosomes at metaphase prepared from afflicted individuals (Fig. 118-1). This site was initially identified in 1969, although more complete characterization of the parameters of its appearance was not completed until the mid-to-late 1970s. Fragile X syndrome had previously been recognized clinically as Martin-Bell syndrome, after a report of X-linked mental retardation in an English family in 1943.

The defective gene in fragile X syndrome *(FMR1)* was identified by positional cloning in 1991 following efforts to locate the chromosomal anomaly. Both the fragile site and the gene defect derive from expansion and methylation of a trinucleotide repeat (CGG) located in the 5' untranslated region of the *FMR1* mRNA. This was the first of a large number of unstable trinucleotide repeats found to cause human genetic disorders and remains among the best understood for the mutation's effect on gene function.

CLINICAL FEATURES

The association of the fragile X site with families exhibiting X-linked mental retardation allowed the clinical description of the syndrome to be improved. This description is being refined with the advent of DNA-based diagnosis; however, it remains a highly variable phenotype. The syndrome is difficult to diagnose in newborns and the physical features gradually accumulate with age. However, even in fully affected males, the facies are subtle and generally unremarkable to those unfamiliar with the syndrome, especially those in younger patients (Fig. 118-2).

Adult male patients generally exhibit a long and narrow face with moderately increased head circumference (>50th percentile). Prominence of the jaw and forehead with particularly large and mildly dysmorphic ears are typical. Some of the phenotype is reminiscent of a mild connective-tissue disorder, exhibiting hyperextensible joints, high arched palate, pes planus, pectus excavatum, and mitral valve prolapse. Macroorchidism (enlarged testicular volume) is a common finding in postpubescent affected males. Almost 90% of such males exhibit testicular volumes in excess of 25 mL as measured by an orchidometer.

Mental retardation and developmental delay are the most significant clinical features of the fragile X syndrome. Prepubescent males have delayed developmental milestones, and some may display avoidance behavior similar to autism, as well as hyperactivity and attention deficit. The latter two are frequent presenting complaints in boys with fragile X syndrome. Development of speech and language is almost always involved but to variable degrees. While absence of speech is rare, milder communication difficulties are common, including a characteristic jocular, litany-like speech. Mental retardation ranges from profound to borderline with an average IQ in the moderately retarded range. It has been estimated that fragile X syndrome accounts for as much as 20% of all boys with IQ levels between 30 and 55.

Females are usually much less involved compared with affected males. Somatic signs may be absent or mild, although the facies of older females may tend to resemble affected males. The mental retardation, in particular, is less severe with most female patients falling in the mild-to-borderline range. A number of studies suggest increased emotional lability in both affected and carrier females. These manifest as both behavioral and psychiatric abnormalities. While these are highly variable, several studies have identified schizotypal features, depression, social avoidance, anxiety, and shyness among girls and women with IQs in both the normal and affected ranges.

DIAGNOSIS

Patients are typically referred for developmental delay, and because of the relatively mild phenotype in young patients, diagnosis is rarely achieved on clinical grounds alone. Any family with an X-linked pattern of mental retardation should be considered for fragile X testing. Cytogenetic testing for the presence of the fragile site was the only diagnostic test available until the discovery of the gene and mutation. Since the CGG repeat expansion mutation is found in virtually all fragile X patients, the use of DNA testing for diagnosis is highly reliable and has largely supplanted the use of cytogenetic testing for the fragile site. However, because of the prevalence of mental retardation from other cytogenetic abnormalities, it is important to consider a routine karyotype in the evaluation of any case of developmental delay.

MOLECULAR GENETICS

MUTATIONS The vast majority (>99.5%) of fragile X patients carry the same mutation, which is a massive expansion of

From: *Principles of Molecular Medicine* (J. L. Jameson, ed.), ©1998 Humana Press Inc., Totowa, NJ.

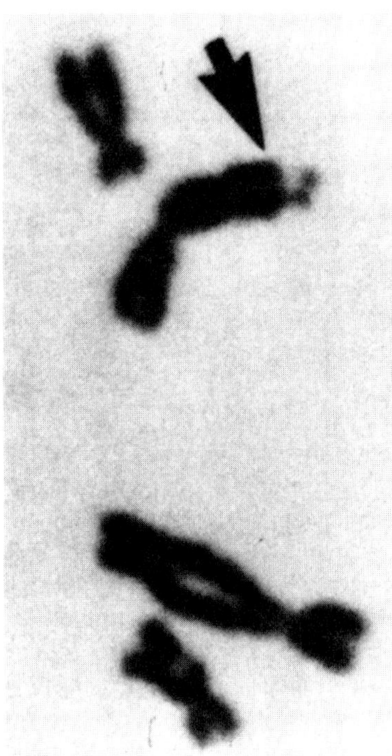

Figure 118-1 Partial karyotype of Geimsa-stained human chromosomes showing the fragile X site (arrow). (Reprinted with permission from JAMA 1994;271:536–542.)

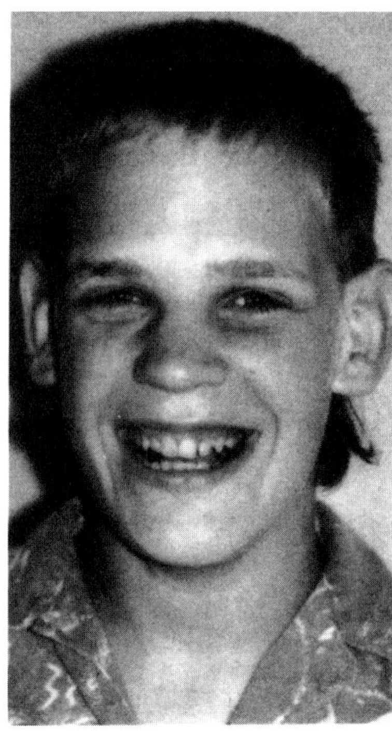

Figure 118-2 Mentally retarded adolescent male with fragile X syndrome. Note long facies with prominent forehead and ears. Typical of most patients, there is no major dysmorphia associated with this syndrome, confounding the clinical diagnosis. (Reprinted with permission from JAMA 1994;271:536–542.)

a trinucleotide repeat (CGG) located in the 5' untranslated region of the *FMR1* gene. This repeat is polymorphic in the human population and outside of fragile X families ranges in length from 5 to as many as 50 triplets. The most common alleles carry either 29 or 30 repeats. Approximately 70% of females are heterozygous at this locus, and normal-sized alleles are transmitted with high fidelity to the next generation. Affected individuals are found to carry more than 200 repeats and typically exhibit repeats in excess of 500. These can range to as many as 2000 and are often mosaic in length, with many different lengths observed in a single sample from an individual. These large numbers of repeats are termed "full mutations" and are usually found to be methylated at C residues within the repeat sequence as well as in the nearby CpG island that marks the gene's promoter. Methylation has been found to correlate with loss of mRNA production, presumably through diminished transcriptional initiation. This results in loss of the product of the *FMR1* gene (FMRP) and the disease. Thus, the expansion mutation in fragile X syndrome leads to loss of function of the *FMR1* gene. Additional loss of function mutations have been identified in the *FMR1* gene, and these are found to confer the same phenotype, reducing the likelihood that other genes are affected by methylation of the region and play a significant role in the phenotype. Mosaicism in the pattern of methylation is seen in some patients, and it is methylation status that most closely correlates with disease severity, although the extent of variation of the mutation among tissues in a single individual complicates such correlation studies, which typically rely on blood leukocytes for DNA testing. There is evidence that translation of mRNAs carrying long (>200) CGG repeats is also diminished, suggesting that large, unmethylated alleles may also confer the disease.

Alleles of a size intermediate between those found in the general population and those in affected individuals have been termed "premutations." These are found in unaffected carriers (both male and female) of the disorder in fragile X families. No instance of expansion has been identified to arise from a normal allele, and premutations appear to be maintained for many generations in fragile X lineages without selective disadvantage. Premutations can range in length from 44 to ~200 repeats and are typically found to be between 70 and 100 repeats. They are not methylated in males, although they, like normal alleles, are subject to methylation associated with X inactivation in females.

Premutations are found to change in size in nearly all transmissions from parent to offspring, yet are usually somatically stable. Thus they exhibit an extremely high mutation frequency. Mutations can take the form of changes within the premutation size range or they can involve massive expansions (transitions) to the disease, causing full mutation (Fig. 118-3). However, these latter events are found exclusively to occur on transmission from mothers to their children, never from fathers to their daughters. This sex-specificity had been recognized in empiric pedigree studies of fragile X families along, with the tendency for the probability of this event to increase in subsequent generations of a fragile X family. The molecular genetic basis for the female transition specificity is as yet unknown. However, as shown in Table 118-1, the increasing likelihood of the disease in a family can be accounted for by the observation of increasing risk of transition to the full mutation with escalating size of premutation in a female carrier, coupled with the tendency for the repeats to increase in size, while transmitted in the premutation size. This unstable character to the CGG repeat explains most of the peculiar (non-Mendelian) inheritance patterns found in fragile X syndrome. Similar phenomena in other human genetic disorders caused by unstable triplet repeats can also explain the deviations from Mendelian inheritance in those diseases as well.

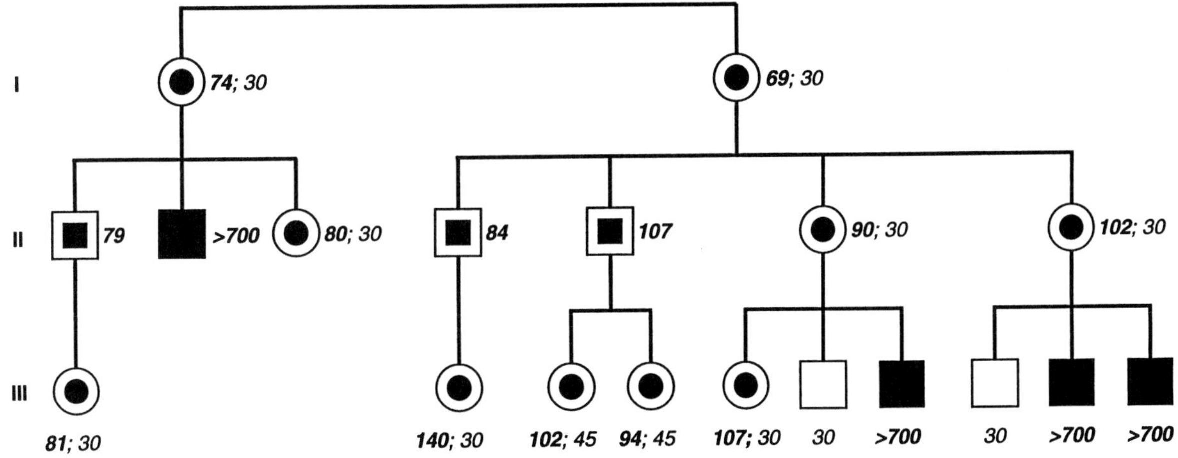

Figure 118-3 Representative fragile X syndrome pedigree. Partially filled circles (female) and squares (male), nonpenetrant carriers; closed squares, penetrant males; open squares, normal males. Numbers by each symbol indicate the number of *FMR1* trinucleotide repeats (bold numbers signify the abnormal allele). Note that the premutation changes when transmitted as evidenced by siblings having unique premutation sizes. (Reprinted with permission from JAMA 1994;271:536–542.)

Table 118-1
Incomplete Penetrance Based on Repeat Length—Risk[a] of Full Expansion on Transmission

Repeat number[b]	*Maternal carrier, %*	*Paternal carrier, %*
<60	<1	0
61–70	17	0
71–80	71	0
81–90	86	0
>91	>99	0

Table reprinted with permission from JAMA 1994;271:536–542.

[a]Risk of having penetrant offspring for fragile X syndrome based on premutation size.

[b]Parental alleles. Risk of the premutation expanding to a full mutation is indicated for maternal or paternal transmission. Actual risk for a penetrant offspring of a carrier female is half the indicated value to reflect segregation of the normal X chromosome, which half the time will be included in the mature ovum. These data from Fu et al., which illustrate the molecular basis of the Sherman paradox, require further investigation before being used as definitive risk assessments during genetic counseling.

Instability of the *FMR1* CGG repeat has been found to increase as the number of repeats is enlarged; however, interrupting AGG triplets have been found to play an important role in maintaining stability of the repeat, both in human pedigrees and in evolutionary time. A threshold of approximately 35 uninterrupted CGG repeats appears to mark the transition from reasonably stable to completely unstable transmissions and explains the observation of stable alleles with longer repeat tracts than some unstable alleles. The *FMR1* gene has conserved the CGG repeats throughout mammalian evolution, suggesting that these have a specific function in the gene. A report of specific binding proteins suggests one possibility for function.

PREVALENCE OF THE PREMUTATION The high incidence of fragile X syndrome, coupled with the rather unusual inheritance pattern of premutation alleles, suggests a very high prevalence of premutations in the general population. Small-scale studies have suggested allele frequencies of 1/500 to 1/600. A recent large study found a carrier frequency for premutations (defined as >55 repeats) of 1/259 women (approximately 1/500 X chromosomes). This finding underscores the impact of this very common genetic disorder.

GENE AND GENE PRODUCTS The *FMR1* gene has been completely sequenced (GenBank accession L29074), and spans 38 kb divided into 17 exons. To date, no other genes have been described in the immediate vicinity. A variety of alternatively spliced transcripts has been observed in human and mouse. These lead to a number of protein isoforms.

The protein product of the *FMR1* gene, FMRP has been found to be present in many adult and fetal tissues, but is concentrated in neurons, particularly those of the hippocampus and in Purkinje cells of the cerebellum. High levels of FMRP are also found in cells of the testis, primarily spermatogonia. These two sites of high-level expression are consistent with the major phenotypic aspects of the disorder.

Within the cell, FMRP appears predominantly cytoplasmic; however, isoforms lacking exon 14 appear to be limited to the nucleus. In the cytoplasm, the protein appears to interact with ribosomes and may form complexes with two or more recently identified proteins of similar amino acid sequence, *FXR1* and *FXR2*. Homologs of all three members of this gene family have been identified from a variety of vertebrates. Each of these three proteins is found to have features of RNA-binding proteins, and RNA binding has been demonstrated in vitro for each. FMRP appears to have a selectivity for certain mRNAs. These features of FMRP begin to suggest a protein involved in mRNA metabolism, perhaps with a role in the regulation of translation. It remains to be discovered how defects in this function might lead to mental retardation.

NEARBY FRAGILE SITES Two additional rare, folate-sensitive fragile sites are found distal to FRAXA, the site in the *FMR1* gene responsible for fragile X syndrome (Fig. 118-4). These are FRAXE and FRAXF, which were both assumed to be FRAXA by cytogenetic testing, and were only distinguished after the development of DNA probes at FRAXA. Each of these sites also results from expansion and methylation of CGG repeats, and FRAXE is clearly associated with a relatively rare form of mental retardation distinguishable from fragile X syndrome. FRAXF appears to cause no abnormalities in individuals carrying expanded repeats. A gene *(FMR2)* whose expression is reduced by FRAXE expansion has been recently identified. This gene is quite large (approximately 500 kb) and is transcribed from the FRAXE CpG island. The gene

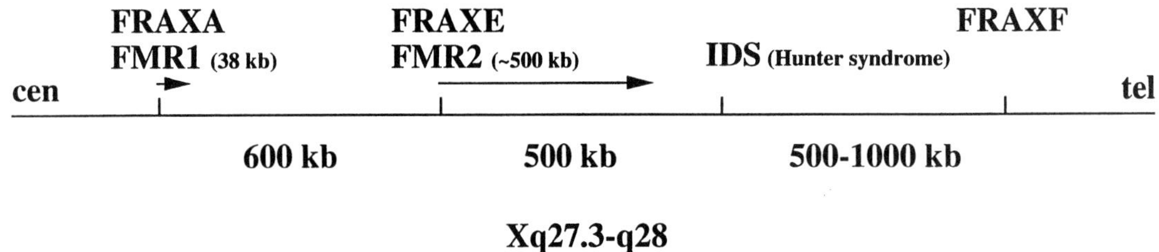

Figure 118-4 Map of the Xq27.3–q28 region. Three fragile sites—FRAXA, FRAXE, and FRAXF—are shown relative to the X chromosome at Xq27.3–q28. The two genes associated with FRAXA and FRAXE are indicated as *FMR1* and *FMR2*, respectively, with their lengths. IDS indicates iduronate sulfatase, the gene defective in Hunter's syndrome. Distances indicated are approximate.

product bears no resemblance to the *FMR1* gene, and its function is not suggested by its sequence, although it shares similarity with transcription factors.

MOLECULAR GENETICS OF CHROMOSOMAL FRAGILE SITES Two additional autosomal folate-sensitive fragile sites have been characterized at the molecular level. These are FRA16A and FRA11B. Each results from an expansion of a polymorphic CGG repeat sequence, with strong similarity to the expansions seen at FRAXA, FRAXE, and FRAXF. Each shows significant methylation in the fully expanded form, suggesting that methylation of expanded CGGs does not require that the repeat be located on the X chromosome. FRA16A, like FRAXF, is not known to be associated with pathology in the expanded form. FRA11B, however, appears to predispose to the loss of the terminal portion of 11q in the gametes of carriers of the fragile site. The resulting offspring develop 11q- or Jacobsen syndrome, a disorder resulting from haploidy for this region of chromosome 11 (11q23–qter). Jacobsen syndrome patients exhibit severe mental retardation and specific dysmorphic features. FRA11B results from expansion of a CGG repeat found in the 5' untranslated region of the proto-oncogene CBL2. No relationship between this fragile site and elevated risk of oncogenesis has been found.

Each of the five fragile sites identified at the molecular level is characterized by expanded and methylated CGG repeats, and each is rare and folate-sensitive. Fragile sites are classified as either rare or common depending on their frequency in the human population, with common sites being homozygous in nearly every person. Rare fragile sites are typically found in less than 1% of individuals. Fragile sites are visualized in metaphase preparations of chromosomes after "induction" or treatment of the cells with a variety of reagents that elicit the sites. In addition to folate, fragile sites can be induced by distamycin-A, BrdU, aphidicolin, and 5-azacytidine. The folate-sensitive sites are the most numerous of the rare fragile sites, but aphidicolin-inducible sites are plentiful among the common sites. There are 21 known folate-sensitive sites, and these can be elicited by a variety of conditions. A culture medium lacking folic acid and thymidine is the simplest method, although inhibitors of folate metabolism such as methotrexate can also be used. High thymidine can also induce these fragile sites at concentrations below those that result in mitotic arrest. These treatments all impinge on the pyrimidine biosynthetic pathway and result in diminished dTTP pools in the cell. The mechanism by which the depletion of dTTP results in a chromosomal abnormality at a CGG repeat is unknown, as is the precise molecular nature of the fragile site itself. It is likely that all folate-sensitive fragile sites will be found to result from CGG repeat expansion. Recent work has described a common aphidicolin-sensitive site on chromosome 3 (FRA3B) as a broad region without specific repetitive sequence elements. However, a gene associated with renal carcinoma, FHIT, has been found to span the region of fragility. It remains to be seen whether specific sequence elements will be found associated with common fragile sites.

MOLECULAR PATHOPHYSIOLOGY

The emerging evidence that *FMR1* plays a role in cytoplasmic mRNA metabolism, possibly in control of translation, is somewhat at odds with the pathophysiology of fragile X syndrome. The disorder has profound consequences on intellect, yet few structural or pathological abnormalities are found. It might be expected that loss of a protein involved in a fundamental process such as translational control would lead to much more widespread anomalies. It may therefore be the case that for most tissues, sufficient redundancy of function is provided by other similar proteins (*FXR1* and *FXR2*, for example), and that it is only in the neurons that absence of *FMR1* is problematic. A knockout mouse model of fragile X syndrome is similarly mildly affected, with very subtle learning defects and enlarged testes. Thus, the very highly conserved *FMR1* protein can be regarded as dispensable for normal growth and structural development (if not normal intellectual development).

MANAGEMENT/TREATMENT

Currently, a variety of educational interventions are employed to treat fragile X children. These can have significant benefits. Pharmacological treatment has yet to be standardized, with trials ongoing of a variety of psychoactive substances, particularly serotonin reuptake inhibitors. Additional understanding of the normal function of the *FMR1* gene may provide suggestions for effective drug intervention. The potential for treating the disease through gene therapy is tempered by the observation of affected females, which suggests strongly that the gene product acts in a cell-autonomous fashion. In females, the random pattern of X-inactivation found in the critical tissue (presumably neurons) affects the intellectual potential of women carrying full mutations. This has significant bearing on the potential for treatment by gene therapy, since this modality would necessitate targeting of neurons and would require a rather high efficiency (50% or higher) to exceed the average number of expressing neurons found in female patients.

FUTURE DIRECTIONS

Of the large number of human genetic disorders known to be caused by expanding trinucleotide repeats, fragile X syndrome is the best characterized with respect to the effect of the mutation on the gene. The challenges that remain, however, are large. They include development of a better understanding of the natural history of the fragile X mutation and improved methods for its detection. With improved tests, the potential for population-based screening for this common mutation will be a reality; however, along with such a scheme comes a significant challenge in providing meaningful information to those at risk. The very dynamic nature of this mutation is confusing to professionals, and this can be quite difficult to convey to individuals at risk. Given the high frequency of the disease and its profound cost to families and society, the demand for population-based screening will be high. It will be vital to develop inexpensive and accurate tests in support of such efforts, along with effective vehicles to convey the information to the public.

Clearly, a large focus on the function of the *FMR1* gene product is required for developing rational treatment strategies. What is the role of *FMR1* in the development of neuronal circuits? What are the consequences of its absence, and how can these be modulated? Despite 5 years of attention to this interesting protein, these investigations remain in their infancy. The added benefit of such studies may be an improved understanding of fundamental cell biological processes, possibly ones integral to learning and memory.

ACKNOWLEDGMENTS

The author wishes to acknowledge his many friends and colleagues for advice and assistance in preparation of this manuscript and to extend thanks to the many fragile X families whose samples and support have aided in the studies described. Figures 118-1 through 118-4 and Table 118-1 are reprinted by permission from JAMA, vol. 271, pp. 536–542, copyright 1994, American Medical Association. Work described in this manuscript was supported in part by a grant from NIH #R01-HD29256.

SELECTED REFERENCES

Ashley CT Jr, Wilkinson KD, Reines D, Warren ST. FMR1 protein contains conserved RNP-family domains and demonstrates selective RNA binding. Science 1993;262:563–566.

Bakker CE, Verheij C, Willemsen R, et al. Fmr1 knockout mice: a model to study fragile X mental retardation. Cell 1994;78:23–33.

Eberhart DE, Malter HE, Feng Y, Warren ST. The fragile X mental retardation protein is a ribonucleoprotein containing both nuclear localization and nuclear export signals. Hum Mol Genet 1996;5:1083–1091.

Eichler EE, Holden JJA, Popovich BW, et al. Length of uninterrupted CGG repeats determines instability in the FMR1 gene. Nat Genet 1994;8:88–94.

Feng Y, Zhang F, Lokey LK, et al. Translational suppression by trinucleotide repeat expansion at FMR1. Science 1995;268:731–734.

Fu YH, Kuhl DPA, Pizzuti A, et al. Variation of the CGG repeat at the fragile X site results in genetic instability: resolution of the Sherman paradox. Cell 1991;67:1047–1058.

Gecz J, Gedeon AK, Sutherland GR, Mulley JC. Identification of the gene FMR2, associated with FRAXE mental retardation. Nat Genet 1996;13:105–108.

Gu Y, Shen Y, Gibbs RA, Nelson DL. Identification of FMR2, a novel gene associated with the FRAXE CCG repeat and CpG island. Nat Genet 1996;13:109–113.

Hansen RS, Canfield TK, Fjeld AD, Mumm S, Laird CD, Gartler SM. A variable domain of delayed replication in FRAXA fragile X chromosomes: X inactivation-like spread of late replication. Proc Natl Sci USA 1997;94:4587–4592.

Hirst MC, Barnicoat A, Flynn G, et al. The identification of a third fragile site, FRAXF in Xq27–28 distal to both FRAXA and FRAXE. Hum Mol Genet 1993;2:197–200.

Jones C, Slijepcevic P, Marsh S, et al. Physical linkage of the fragile site FRA11B and a Jacobsen syndrome chromosome deletion breakpoint in 11q23.3. Hum Mol Genet 1994;3:2123–2130.

Khandjian EW, Corbin F, Woerly S, Rousseau F. The fragile X mental retardation protein is associated with ribosomes. Nat Genet 1996;12:91–93.

Knight SJL, Flannery AV, Hirst MC, et al. Trinucleotide repeat amplification and hypermethylation of a CpG island in FRAXE mental retardation. Cell 1993;74:127–134.

Kooy RF, D'Hooge R, Reyniers E, et al. Transgenic mouse model for the fragile X syndrome. Am J Med Genet 1996;64:241–245.

Lachiewicz AM. Females with fragile X syndrome: a review of the effects of an abnormal FMR1 gene. Mental Retardation and Developmental Disabilities Res Rev 1995;1:292–297.

Lubs HA. A marker X chromosome. Am J Hum Genet 1969;21:231–244.

Lugenbeel KA, Peier AM, Carson NL, Chudley AE, Nelson DL. Intragenic loss of function mutations demonstrate the primary role of FMR1 in fragile X syndrome. Nat Genet 1995;10:483–485.

Martin JP, Bell J. A pedigree of mental defect showing sex-linkage. J Neurol Psychiatry 1943;6:154–157.

Nancarrow JK, Kremer E, Holman K, et al. Implications of FRA16A structure for the mechanism of chromosomal fragile site genesis. Science 1994;264:1938–1941.

Oberlé I, Rousseau F, Heitz D, et al. Instability of a 550-base pair DNA segment and abnormal methylation in fragile X syndrome. Science 1991;252:1097–1102.

Ohta M, Inoue H, Cotticelli MG, et al. The FHIT gene, spanning the chromosome 3p14.2 fragile site and renal carcinoma-associate t(3; 8) breakpoint, is abnormal in digestive tract cancers. Cell 1996;84:587–597.

Parrish JE, Oostra BA, Verkerk AJMH, et al. Isolation of a GCC repeat showing expansion in FRAXF, a fragile site distal to FRAXA and FRAXE. Nat Genet 1994;8:229–235.

Pieretti M, Zhang F, Fu YH, et al. Absence of expression of the FMR-1 gene in fragile X syndrome. Cell 1991;66:817–822.

Richards RI, Holman K, Yu S, Sutherland GR. Fragile X syndrome unstable element, p(CCG)n, and other simple tandem repeat sequences are binding sites for specific nuclear proteins. Hum Mol Genet 1993;2:1429–1435.

Rousseau F, Rouillard P, Morel M-L, Khandjian EW, Morgan K. Prevalence of carriers of premutation-size alleles of the FMR1 gene-and implications for the population genetics of the fragile X syndrome. Am J Hum Genet 1995;57:1006–1018.

Schwemmle S, de Graffe E, Deissler H, et al. Characterization of FMR1 promoter elements by in vivo-footprinting analysis. Am J Hum Genet 1997;60:1354–1362.

Sherman SL, Jacobs PA, Morton NE, et al. Further segregation analysis of the fragile X syndrome with special reference to transmitting males. Hum Genet 1985;69:289–299.

Siomi H, Siomi MC, Nussbaum RL, Dreyfuss G. The protein product of the fragile X gene, FMR1, has characteristics of an RNA-binding protein. Cell 1993;74:291–298.

Sittler A, Devys D, Weber C, Mandel J-L. Alternative splicing of exon 14 determines nuclear or cytoplasmic localisation of FMR1 protein isoforms. Hum Mol Genet 1996;5:95–102.

Sutherland GR. Fragile sites on human chromosomes: demonstration of their dependence on the type of tissue culture medium. Science 1977;197:265,266.

Verkerk AJMH, Pieretti M, Sutcliffe JS, et al. Identification of a gene (FMR-1) containing a CGG repeat coincident with a breakpoint cluster region exhibiting length variation in fragile X syndrome. Cell 1991;65:905–914.

Warren ST. The expanding world of trinucleotide repeats. Science 1996;271:1374,1375.

Wilke CM, Hall BK, Hoge A, Paradee W, Smith DI, Glover TW. FRA3B extends over a broad region and contains a spontaneous HPV16 integration site: direct evidence for the coincidence of viral integration sites and fragile sites. Hum Mol Genet 1996;5:187–195.

Willemsen R, Smits A, Mohkamsing S, et al. Rapid antibody test for diagnosing fragile X syndrome: a validation of the technique. Hum Genet 1997;99:308–311.

Yu S, Pritchard M, Kremer E, et al. Fragile X genotype characterized by an unstable region of DNA. Science 1991;252:1179–1181.

Zhang Y, O'Connor P, Siomi M, et al. The fragile X mental retardation syndrome protein interacts with novel homologs FXR1 and FXR2. EMBO J 1995;14:5358–5366.

119 Down Syndrome

Stylianos E. Antonarakis

BRIEF HISTORICAL NOTE

Down syndrome was first described by Dr. Langdon Down in 1866. The advanced mean maternal age at the time of birth of an individual with Down syndrome was first emphasized in a study by Shuttleworth in 1909. Lejeune, Gautier, and Turpin showed in 1959 that individuals with Down syndrome had a supernumerary small acrocentric chromosome that was subsequently recognized as being chromosome 21. Soon after (1960–1961), cases of trisomy 21 resulting from translocations were described by Polani and Fraccaro. Mosaicism for trisomy 21 was first published by Clarke in 1961. In the same year, some patients were described with partial trisomy 21 and phenotypic characteristics of Down syndrome (Ilbery et al., 1961; Dent et al., 1963; Hall, 1963). The parental and meiotic origin of the extra chromosome 21 was first studied (1970–1980) by cytogenetic heteromorphisms (e.g., de Grouchy 1970) and more recently by DNA polymorphisms (e.g., Antonarakis et al., 1991). The association of recombination rate and abnormal chromosomal segregation was first observed in 1987 (Warren et al.). The human genome project and the identification of genes on chromosome 21 are beginning to provide the tools for understanding the pathophysiology of the diverse phenotypes in Down syndrome. Important landmarks in this process are the descriptions of the first linkage map of chromosome 21 (Warren et al., 1989) and the first physical map using yeast artificial chromosomes (Chumakov et al., 1992).

THE CLINICAL PHENOTYPES OF DOWN SYNDROME

The clinical diagnosis of Down syndrome (DS) (MIM 190685) depends on the presence of a number of different abnormal features that affect many tissues and organs. Table 119-1 contains a partial list of physical characteristics and abnormalities found in DS, and Fig. 119-1 shows an individual with the syndrome. No individual DS patient has all of these features. Furthermore, these features may be present in other syndromes or in otherwise normal individuals. Diagnostic indexes and scoring systems have been developed for accurate diagnosis in patients suspected to have DS. Mental retardation is always present. The mean intelligence quotient (IQ) typically drops from about 80 the first year to approximately 30 the second decade of life. Newborns and infants invariably have hypotonia, which is the most common feature of the phenotype. The pathological, metabolic, and neurochemical changes of Alzheimer disease are present after the third decade in the brains of almost all individuals with DS, who also show a progressive loss of cognitive functions. Congenital heart disease, mainly atrioventricular (AV) canal and ventricular septal defect (VSD) is present in 30–40% of living individuals with DS, while in affected fetuses the estimated presence of AV canal is about 70%. Duodenal stenosis or atresia, imperforated anus, and Hirschsprung disease are present in 1.0–2.5% of DS individuals, frequencies much higher than in the general population. Furthermore, DS patients have a 10–20 times greater risk of developing acute leukemia. Both acute nonlymphoblastic and acute lymphoblastic leukemia may be observed. The most characteristic leukemia of DS is the acute megakaryocytic leukemia (AMKL); it has been estimated that AMKL is 200–400 times more frequent in DS than in the normal population. Another form of abnormal clonal cellular proliferation of white blood cells that is observed in some newborns with DS is the "transient" acute leukemia or "leukemoid reaction." There is spontaneous, complete remission of this blood abnormality. Additional phenotypic findings in trisomy 21 of note include immunologic defects, hematologic alterations, hyperuricemia, thyroid dysfunction and autoimmunity, growth retardation, and sterility in males. The life expectancy of DS patients is reduced, and the causes of death are the congenital malformations (mainly heart defects), infections, and leukemia.

CHROMOSOMAL ABNORMALITIES IN DOWN SYNDROME

Since the discovery of Lejeune in 1959, the phenotype of DS has been associated with trisomy for chromosome 21. Trisomy 21 is the most common autosomal aneuploidy in live births; it occurs with a frequency of 1.03–1.30 per 1000 live births in all ethnic groups. Table 119-2 shows the frequencies at birth of specific chromosomal disorders, including trisomy 21.

The majority of trisomy 21 cases are because of a free supernumerary chromosome 21. For every 1000 individuals with DS, 925 are because of free trisomy 21, 46 to translocation of the supernumerary, 21 to another acrocentric chromosome, and two to other reciprocal translocations (Fig. 119-2). Recognizable mosaicism for a normal and a trisomic cell line accounts for 27 of 1000 individuals with DS.

MATERNAL AGE AND DOWN SYNDROME

It has long been recognized that maternal age is an important determinant of the incidence of DS in newborns. Figure 119-3 shows the increase of the incidence of trisomy 21 in mothers of

From: *Principles of Molecular Medicine* (J. L. Jameson, ed.), ©1998 Humana Press Inc., Totowa, NJ.

Table 119-1
Phenotypic Features of Down Syndrome[a]

	%
Physical characteristics	
Oblique (upslanting) palpebral fissures	80
Loose skin on nape or neck	80
Narrow palate	75
Brachycephaly	75
Hyperflexibility	75
Flat nasal bridge	70
Large gap between 1st and 2nd toes	70
Short, broad hands	65
Short neck	60
Abnormal teeth	60
Epicanthic folds	60
Short 5th finder	60
Open mouth	60
Brushfield spots	55
Furrowed tongue	55
Transverse palmar crease	55
Folded or dysplastic ear	50
Protruding tongue	45
Abnormal dermatoglyphics	85
Skeletal abnormalities	
Incurved 5th finder	55
Pelvic dysplasia (newborns)	70
Atlantoaxial or atlantoccipital instability	15–20
Mental retardation	100
Hypothyroidism	7–17
Neurological features	
Hypotonia	100
Delayed dissolution of early reflexes	80
Alzheimer-like brain pathology (over 35 years of age)	100
Congenital anomalies	
Congenital heat defects (CHD) (of living patients)	30–40
AV canal (of total CHD)	40
VSD (of total CHD)	31
ASD (of total CHD)	9
Fallot's tetralogy (of total CHD)	6
PDA (of total CHD)	9
Gastrointestinal abnormalities	
Duodenal atresia	2.5
Imperforated anus	1.0
Hirschsprung disease	0.6
Infertility in males	100
Leukemia	1.1
AMKL (acute megakaryocytic)	200–400 × normal
AML/ALL	10–20 × normal
Leukemoid reaction (newborn)	0.1

[a]The frequencies of phenotypic features were obtained from numerous sources, and most have been rounded to the nearest 5%. (Majority of data are from Epstein CJ, 1995.)

different ages. The risk remains low, at about 1 in 1500 to 1 in 1000 live births, until age 30 and then increases substantially. For mothers of 35 years of age, the risk is about 1 in 380 live births, at age 40 it is 1 in 110, and at 45 years about 1 in 30. The reason for this strong maternal age effect is presently unknown, and many theories have been formulated to explain this well-documented phenomenon. There is no convincing evidence for a paternal age effect. Molecular analysis has clearly shown that this advanced maternal age effect is associated with errors of maternal meiotic origin and not paternal or mitotic errors; in these latter two categories of errors, the mean maternal age is not different from that of the mean maternal age in Western societies. This finding is against the theory of relaxation of selection in utero that seeks to explain the increased incidence of DS with maternal age by a decrease (in older mothers) in the rate of a spontaneous abortion of aneuploid embryos and fetuses. In addition, there is no maternal age effect in trisomy 21 resulting from translocations. The theory of aging of sperm has not been supported, as no paternal age effect has been shown in paternally derived trisomy 21; however, more data are needed for this category of meiotic errors. Interestingly, more male trisomy 21 individuals than expected have been observed in DS originating from paternal meiotic errors.

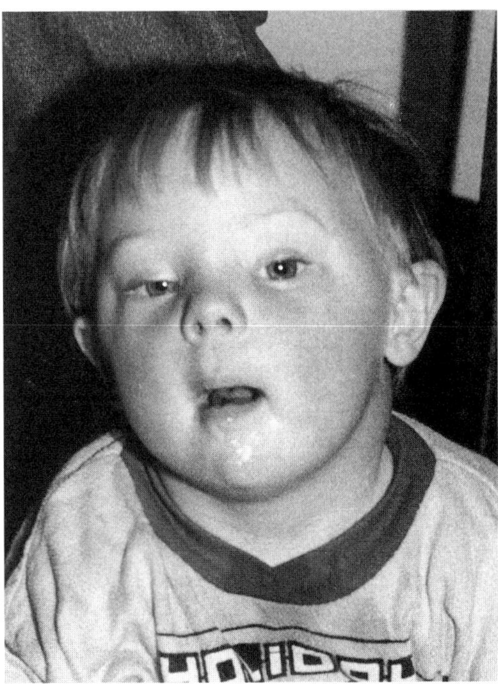

Figure 119-1 Facial photograph of a 2-year-old male with trisomy 21 (Down syndrome).

Many conspectuses with trisomy 21 do not survive to birth. Data from amniocentesis without any further intervention during pregnancy revealed that over 20% of the DS fetuses die *in utero*. Furthermore, data from chorionic villus sampling at approximately 9–10 weeks of gestation indicate that about 20% of DS fetuses die between the 9th to 10th and 16th to 18th week of gestation. The estimate of survival of a DS fetus to term is about 30%.

The production-line hypothesis was advanced by Henderson and Edwards in 1968. Based on mouse studies, they proposed that oocytes with greater number of chiasmata in their chromosomes are formed earlier in embryogenesis and are ovulated earlier in adult life than oocytes with fewer chiasmata. Warren et al. in 1987 first provided evidence that there is a reduced number of crossing-over events in chromosomes 21 that undergo nondisjunction. Further studies from our laboratory and that of Sherman/Hassold have shown that, in maternal meiosis I errors, the number of cases with no detectable crossover is excessive, and the total length of the observed linkage maps of these nondisjoined chromosomes 21 is about half of normal. Thus, it is now clear that there is abnormal (reduced) recombination rate in maternal meiosis I nondisjunction; this abnormality in recombination may have some causative effect in nondisjunction. In maternal meiosis II errors, Lamb et al. (1996) observed increased recombination that was largely restricted to the maximal long arm of chromosome 21.

ORIGIN OF THE EXTRA CHROMOSOME IN TRISOMY 21

FREE TRISOMY 21 The availability of highly informative DNA polymorphic markers has allowed the determination of the parental origin of the extra chromosome 21 in free trisomy 21. Furthermore, DNA markers close to the centromeric region can indicate the stage of meiosis in which the segregation error had occurred. Finally, homozygosity for all markers throughout 21q, including the pericentromeric markers, is interpreted as the result of a mitotic, postzygotic error. Table 119-3 shows the results of two large independent studies of more than 500 families. The conclusions are as follows:

1. Errors in meiosis that result in trisomy 21 were overwhelmingly of maternal origin, as only about 6.5% occurred during spermatogenesis.
2. The majority of errors in maternal meiosis occurred in meiosis I, and the mean maternal age associated with these was 31.2 years. The meiosis I errors accounted for 77.5% of maternal meiotic errors and 68% of all instances of free trisomy 21.
3. Maternal meiosis II errors comprised 22.5% of maternal origin errors and 20% of all cases of free trisomy 21. The mean maternal age in these errors was 32.5 years.
4. In a minority (6.6%) of the total number of families in which there was paternal nondisjunction, there are more meiosis II than meiosis I errors (62% and 38% of paternal meiosis I and II errors, respectively). The mean maternal and paternal ages in this category were similar to the mean reproductive age in Western societies.
5. In about 5.5% of free trisomy 21, the extra chromosome 21 appeared to result from an error in mitosis. In these families, the mean maternal age was around 28 years, which is similar to the mean maternal reproductive age. As expected, there was no preference for which chromosome 21 was duplicated in mitotic errors, and the extra chromosome was equally likely to be derived from either parent.

TRANSLOCATION TRISOMY 21 In all 24 cases examined of *de novo* translocation t(14;21) trisomy 21, the extra chromosome 21 appears to be maternal in origin. In these cases, the mean maternal age was 29.2 years. The most likely mechanism of these events is that the translocation occurs before crossing over in meiosis I and is followed by normal segregation in meiosis I and II.

In the majority (14 of 17 cases) of *de novo* translocation t(21;21) trisomy 21, the abnormal chromosome is an isochromosome (dup21q), rather than the result of a translocation caused by a fusion between two heterologous chromatids. About half of the isochromosomes studied were of paternal and half of maternal origin. The dup21p was probably formed by failure of separation, either of the chromatids in meiosis II or of sister chromatids in early mitosis. Finally, all of the t(21;21) true *de novo* translocations are of maternal origin similar to the t(14;21).

ORIGIN OF THE EXTRA CHROMOSOME IN OTHER TRISOMIES For comparison with trisomy 21, the parental and meiotic origin of other human trisomies are as follows:

1. In trisomy 18, in which more than 150 families were studied, the origin of the extra chromosome 18 is maternal in about 90%. Postzygotic, mitotic errors probably account for about 8% of the cases. Among the maternal meiotic errors, about 34% occur in meiosis I and 66% in meiosis II. The excess of maternal meiosis II errors is in contrast with the data from all the other aneuploidies studied. Increased maternal age is associated with both maternal meiotic errors.
2. In trisomy 16, the most common trisomy at conception but not at birth, because virtually all such fetuses are spontaneously aborted, the origin of the extra chromosome 16 is always maternal. Furthermore, in all cases the error is found

Table 119-2
Chromosomal Abnormalities in 1000 Live Births[a]

All abnormalities	5.71–6.25
Autosomal trisomies	1.23–1.42
Trisomy 21	1.03–1.30
Trisomy 18	0.09–0.12
Trisomy 13	0.05–0.07
Balanced autosomal rearrangements	1.85–1.93
Unbalanced autosomal abnormalities	0.48–0.59
Sex chromosomal abnormalities in phenotypic males	2.55–2.59
XXY	0.92–1.04
XYY	0.90–0.92
Sex chromosomal abnormalities in phenotypic females	1.33–1.51
45,X	0.09–0.13
XXX	0.86–1.04

[a]Numbers have been derived after karyotyping of more than 70,000 consecutive newborns. (Most of the data are from Hook and Hamerton, 1977.)

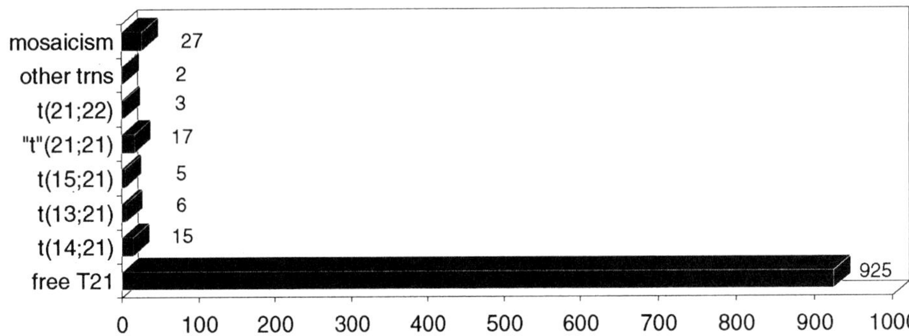

Figure 119-2 Histogram of frequencies of the various chromosomal abnormalities found in Down syndrome. The number of abnormalities per 1000 individuals with Down syndrome is shown. The data are averages from various sources.

in maternal meiosis I. There is increased maternal age associated with trisomy 16.

3. In trisomy 13, the data from about 50 families show that the origin of the extra chromosome 13 was maternal in about 90% of cases. Among maternal errors, the great majority (approximately 90%) occur in maternal meiosis I.
4. The data on a limited number of families with spontaneous abortions with trisomies 14, 15, and 22 indicate that, again, the majority of the errors (87%) occur in maternal meiosis.
5. In XXY (Klinefelter) syndrome, about half of the cases result from paternal and half from maternal meiotic errors. Among the paternal errors, all occur in meiosis I; among the maternal errors, 75% occur in meiosis I and 25% in meiosis II. About 5% of the maternal cases can be attributed to mitotic error. In XXX females, only 10% have received two copies of the paternal X, the remaining 90% have inherited two copies of the maternal X chromosome. Among the maternal origin XXX females, 68% are because of meiosis I and 32% to meiosis II errors.

PRENATAL DIAGNOSIS AND COUNSELING

Programs for prenatal detection of trisomy 21 have been introduced by many public and private health care providers. Chromosomal analysis after amniocentesis or chorionic villus sampling have been done in hundreds of thousands of pregnancies. Amniocentesis is usually carried out at approximately 16 weeks, while chorionic villus sampling is performed at 8–10 weeks of pregnancy. In most health systems, both of these procedures are usually offered to women over 35 years of age because the risk of abortion from the procedure almost equals the risk of trisomy 21. Prenatal detection of trisomy by cytogenetic analysis of the fetus has slightly reduced the number of liveborn with DS, since in the general population only a minority of trisomy 21 individuals are born to mothers older than 35 years of age. Rapid DNA-based methods (either fluorescent *in situ* hybridization [FISH] or DNA polymorphisms or dosage analysis) have been developed to detect trisomy 21 in fetal tissues (after amniocentesis or chorion villus sampling); however, these methods are not in wide use, because they only detect trisomy 21, whereas a karyotype detects all of the other visible chromosomal abnormalities.

Monitoring of all pregnancies using maternal serum alpha fetoprotein (AFP) in combination with chorionic gonadotropin (UCG), inhibin A, and unconjugated estrol (uE3) have provided a way to estimate a woman's risk of having an affected fetus. If the risk exceeds a specified cutoff level (usually 1 in 250), then a karyotypic analysis of fetal cells is indicated. Although this "triple test" is not trisomy 21-specific and has a high false positive rate, it is a valuable tool for the *in utero* detection of trisomy 21. The introduction of this screening test in the United Kingdom and elsewhere had resulted in the in utero detection of more than half of all cases of trisomy 21.

Many efforts are now being directed toward the development of methods to detect aneuploidies in fetal nucleated erythrocytes or other cells in the maternal circulation. No such method has yet been introduced in large-scale clinical trials, because their technology is still in the development stage.

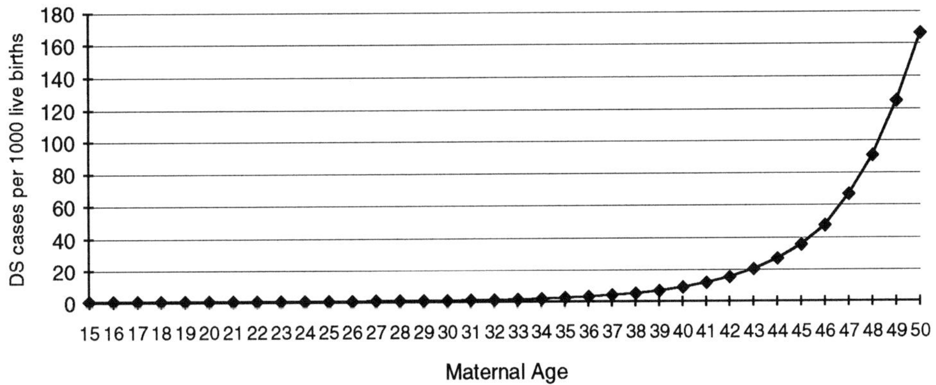

Figure 119-3 Incidence of Down syndrome cases per 1000 live births as a function of maternal age.

Table 119-3
Analysis of the Origin of the Supernumerary Chromosome 21 in 510 Families with Free Trisomy 21 Using DNA Polymorphisms[a]

Error	*N*	*%*	*Mean maternal age (years)*
Maternal meiosis I	347	68.04	31.2
Maternal meiosis II	101	19.80	32.5
Paternal meiosis I	13	2.55	26.4
Paternal meiosis II	21	4.12	27.9
Mitosis	28	5.49	28.4
Maternal chrom duplication	17		27.2
Paternal chrom duplication	11		28.4

[a]Data are from two major studies: Johns Hopkins University (Antonarakis, et al., Nature Genet 1993) and Emory University (Sherman/Hassold) (Lamb et al., 1996).

The counseling of pregnant couples includes the explanation of the incidence of trisomy 21 in different-age mothers, the phenotypes of DS, and the presentation of risks of available diagnostic and screening procedures. Postdiagnostic counseling (after the discovery of a chromosomal abnormality) is necessary. The risk of a couple with one member being a carrier for a Robertsonian or reciprocal chromosome 21 translocation differs according to the translocations and the sex of the carrier parent. This empirically observed risk differs from the theoretical risk based on the meiotic products. Empirical data show that if the mother is a Robertsonian translocation carrier of chromosome 21 and either 13, 14, 15, or 22, the risk for an unbalanced, trisomy 21-affected offspring is about 15%; if the father is the carrier of such a translocation the risk is about 2%. For reciprocal translocations involving chromosome 21, the empirical risk is about 10% for both translocation carriers. The risk of trisomy 21 among the viable offspring of t(21;21) carriers is the expected 100%. The maternal age-independent risk for recurrent trisomy 21 for a couple who already has one child with free trisomy 21 is slightly higher than that of the general population of the same maternal age. This is probably because of germline and/or somatic mosaicism for a trisomy 21 cell line in one of the parents. In a recent study of 22 families with two free trisomy 21 offspring, parental mosaicism has been detected in five cases. It is not known if a predisposition for nondisjunction (other than mosaicism) exists in some families with two or more affected offspring.

CHROMOSOME 21: GENOME MAPPING

In order to understand the pathophysiology of the different phenotypes of trisomy 21, knowledge of the genes that map in chromosome 21 is necessary. The identification and characterization of these genes and the subsequent elucidation of their function may permit the assignment of specific phenotypes to specific gene products. The elucidation of the role of the additional copy of certain genes in specific clinical abnormalities may then open new possibilities for intervention in order to modify the resulting phenotype.

The effort for mapping, cloning, sequencing, and initial characterization of chromosome 21 genes is part of the international human genome project initiative, which is already greatly enhancing the understanding of the molecular pathophysiology of human disorders. Chromosome 21 is the smallest human chromosome. The long arm (21q) is approximately 40 Mb (40 million nucleotides) and makes up about 1.2% of the human genome; the short arm (21p), which is highly homologous to those of the other four acrocentric chromosomes, is around 10–15 Mb. Because complete absence of 21p is not associated with clinical phenotypes, and trisomy 21 resulting from t(21;21), in which 21p is also deleted from the translocated chromosomes, is not different from the free trisomy 21, we do not consider 21p to be as important or contributory to the phenotypes of trisomy 21. The estimated number of genes on 21q is approximately 600–1000. Figure 119-3 shows schematically the different maps that have been developed for chromosome 21. The information from these different maps is integrated in a unifying system, the final goal of which is to decipher the nucleotide sequence of the entire 21q. The different maps are briefly described below.

CHROMOSOMAL BREAKPOINT MAP The breakpoints of naturally occurring chromosomal abnormalities serve as the initial landmarks in the building of maps. A large collection of such abnormal chromosomes has been introduced into rodent-human somatic cell hybrids and used to divide the chromosome in intervals of a few megabases each.

LONG-RANGE RESTRICTION SITE MAP A relatively accurate estimate of the distance in kilobases between landmark cleavage sites of selected restriction endonucleases is provided after restriction analysis. Infrequent cutting enzymes studies, such as *Not*I, are used for the initial "framework" map that provides information about the size of the chromosome. An approximately 37-Mb-long range map of *Not*I restriction sites has been produced for 21q.

LINKAGE MAP At present, the linkage map is perhaps the most medically useful of all chromosomal maps. It consists of polymorphic DNA markers ordered, by recombination frequencies to each other, throughout the entire length of the chromosome. The majority of the polymorphic markers used are because of the normal variation of short sequence repeats and can be detected after PCR amplification. The current linkage map of 21q is the most dense map of all human chromosomes. More than 130 DNA markers have been analyzed and placed on the linkage map; the average genetic distance between adjacent markers is less than 1.5% recombination. The linkage map constructed from male meioses is shorter than that made from female meioses, probably because the meiotic process is different in the two sexes. The female map is usually longer in the proximal half of 21q; however, in the most distal region of 21q, there is an excess of male recombination and therefore a longer male linkage map. The total lengths of the male and female maps are about 55 cM, and 85 cM respectively; the sex-averaged map is 67 cM long. The linkage map of chromosome 21 is an outstanding tool for mapping both Mendelian and complex polygenic traits for the identification of specific chromosomes involved in aneuploidies or malignancies, for the determination of the origin of nondisjunction, and for the determination of the extent of partial trisomies 21.

RADIATION HYBRID MAP When somatic cell hybrids that contain a single chromosome 21 are irradiated and then fused with a rodent cell line, radiation hybrids are produced that carry only small fragments of the human chromosome. By screening a large number of such hybrids for the presence or absence of particular loci, another type of a statistical map can be built up. Neighboring loci are most likely to be present together in these hybrids, while distant loci are separated. The major advantage of radiation hybrid mapping is that there is no need for polymorphic markers; any piece of DNA can be assigned to this map. The radiation hybrid map of chromosome 21 is becoming increasingly important with the addition of expressed sequence tags (ESTs), the short sequences of human cDNA clones.

CLONING OF CHROMOSOME 21 IN OVERLAPPING CLONES The cloning of chromosomal 21 DNA and the identification of a continuous array of overlapping clones (contigs) is an essential step in the characterization of disease-related genes, sequencing of chromosomal DNA, precise mapping of genes, and study of the importance of partial trisomy 21 to the DS phenotypes. Various vectors have been used to clone large fragments of DNA; the most widely used are cosmids, yeast artificial chromosomes (YACs), P1 bacteriophage, P1 artificial chromosomes (PACs), bacterial artificial chromosomes (BACs). An almost continuous array of chromosome 21 YACs has been produced for 21q and now serves as the backbone for the mapping efforts. This contig was composed of 810 YACs and extends from the 21cen to 21qter. There are several areas of noncoverage, with YACs and regions with erroneous order of the mapping objects; this map is therefore in constant improvement. A cosmid contig of a 4-Mb region in the so-called DS critical region *(see below)* has been recently made. Additional smaller cosmid contigs for different regions of 21q have been constructed. All of these maps of overlapping clones are necessary for the identification and characterization of chromosome 21 genes that are involved in various disease phenotypes, including those of DS.

DOWN SYNDROME CRITICAL REGION (DSCR) It has long been recognized that some patients with a clinically recognized DS have only a partial trisomy 21. Many laboratories have therefore collected DNA from patients with (1) phenotypic characteristics of DS and partial trisomy 21, (2) partial trisomy 21 without the phenotypes of DS, and (3) phenotypes of DS without any obvious chromosomal abnormality. The latter group of patients is intriguing, because even after careful and extensive molecular analysis, no chromosome 21 triplication has been found, and yet the phenotypic analysis of these patients fulfills the minimal criteria for the diagnosis of DS. It is possible that these patients have a small triplicated region of chromosome 21 that has yet escaped detection or that abnormalities of few genes on chromosome 21, or elsewhere, result in a phenotype similar to that of DS.

The study of patients with partial trisomy 21 and several phenotypes of DS suggested that there is a region of approximately 4 Mb between DNA markers D21S17 and ETS2 (Fig. 119-4) that, if triplicated, is associated with numerous features of DS, including flat nasal bridge, protruding tongue, high arched or narrow palate, folded ears, short and broad hands, clinodactyly of fifth finger, large gap between first and second toes, joint hyperlaxity, muscular hypotonia, short stature, and mental retardation. This region is termed Down syndrome critical region (DSCR). Extension of the triplication distally to DNA marker BCEI includes additional features of DS, such as oblique eye fissure, epicanthus, Brushfield spots, transverse palmar crease, and several dermatoglyphic signs. In all of these studies, the presence of a phenotypic feature is of importance; its absence is not taken into account, because patients with the full trisomy 21 do not show all of the phenotypic characteristics. The DSCR, which is about 10% of 21q, may contain between 50 and 100 genes (assuming that the gene distribution is the same throughout 21q).

There are, however, three known patients with proximal triplication of chromosome 21 (that does not extend to the DSCR) and several phenotypes of DS, including facial features, microcephaly, short stature, hypotonia, abnormal dermatoglyphics, and mental retardation. This observation argues against a single chromosomal region being responsible for most of the DS characteristics. On the other hand, the conflicting data can be explained by a DSCR as described on distal 21q and an additional partial trisomy 21 syndrome on proximal 21q. More cases are necessary to clarify the contribution of several 21q regions to the phenotypes of DS and the precise mapping of these regions. For the remaining discussion of this chapter, the DSCR definition is for the region between D21S17 to ETS2. The atrioventricular canal, which is a characteristic heart defect in DS, has been mapped to a large 5- to 6-Mb region between D21S267 and MX1.

GENES AND DISORDERS The number of genes on chromosome 21 is estimated to be about 600–1000. The gene density varies according to the chromosomal band. There are, therefore, "gene-rich" and "gene-poor" regions on 21q. Chromosomal bands 21q22.3 and 21q22.1, which do not stain with Giemsa, probably contain the majority of genes of this chromosome. In contrast, the large Giemsa-positive 21q21 band is apparently gene-poor.

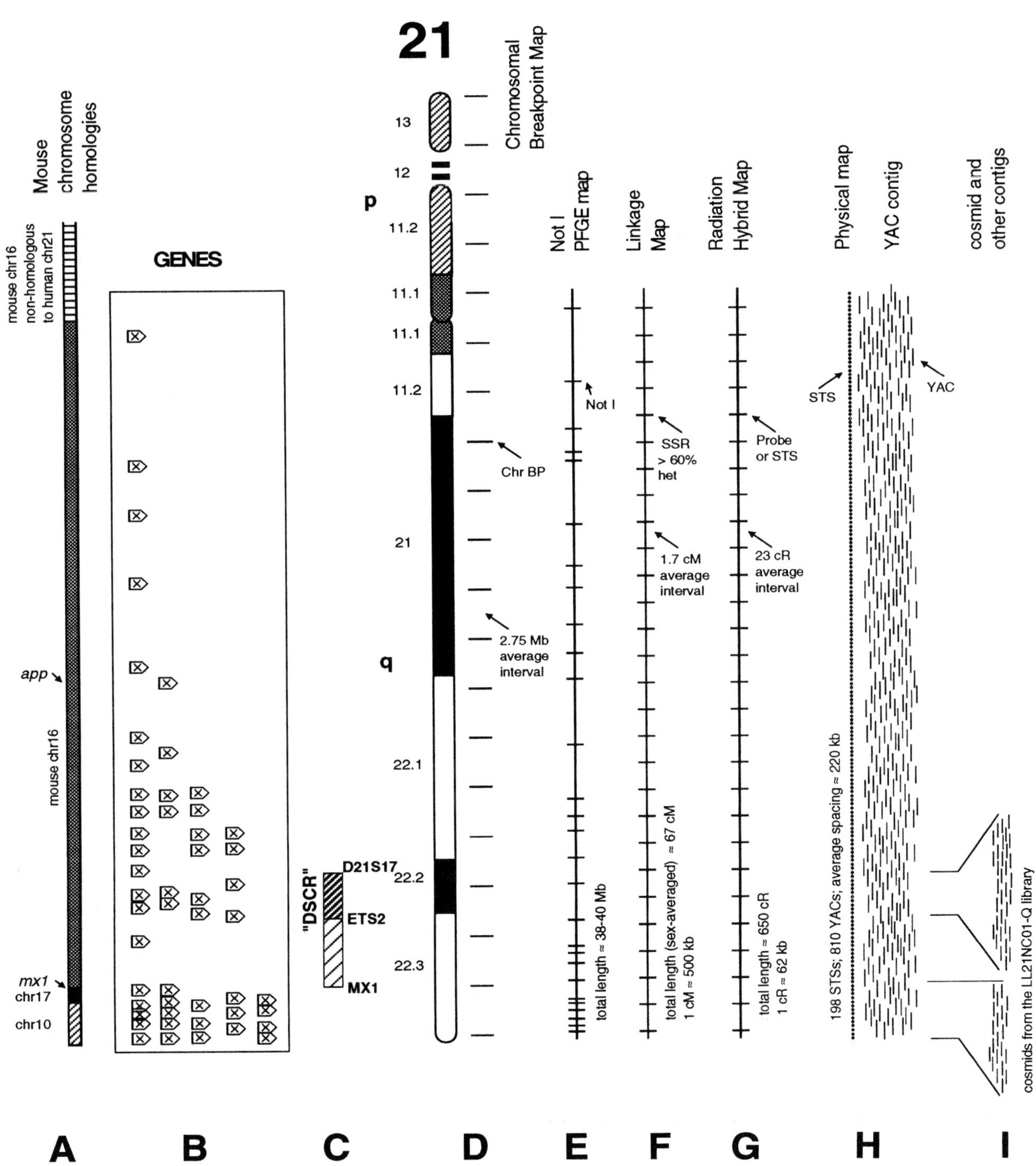

Figure 119-4 Schematic representation of chromosome 21 and several of its maps. **(A)** Human chromosome 21 homologous regions of mouse chromosomes. **(B)** Mapping of the known cloned genes on chromosome 21. **(C)** Down syndrome critical region (DSCR). **(D)** Chromosome 21 breakpoint map. **(E)** Pulsed field gel electrophoresis map of *Not*I restriction fragments. **(F)** Linkage map using highly informative, short sequence repeats, polymorphic markers. **(G)** Radiation hybrid map. **(H)** sequence tagged site (STS) map and yeast artificial chromosome (YAC) contig. **(I)** Cosmid contigs of the DSCR and a portion of chromosomal band 21q22.3.

A total of 54 genes thus far have been described that map on 21q. These represent only 5.4–9% of the total number of genes on 21q, and more information on them can be obtained from the publicly available databases (Genome Database, OMIM, Genbank). The function of some of these genes is known; their protein products belong to various categories, such as proteins involved in cell division, cell signaling and communication, cell structure and motility, metabolism, cell defense, gene/protein expression, and development of the organism. Some genes have been associated with specific disorders such as the APP with a rare form of early onset Alzheimer's disease (MIM 104760), CBS with homocystinuria (MIM 236200), ITGB2 with a leukocyte adhesion deficiency syndrome (MIM 600065), AML1 with translocations involved in acute myeloid leukemia (MIM 151385), PFKL with a form of hemolytic anemia caused by phosphofructokinase deficiency (MIM 171860), SOD1 with one form of amyotrophic lateral sclerosis (MIM 147450), HCS with biotin-responsive multiple carboxylase deficiency (MIM 253270), ENTC with enterokinase deficiency (MIM 226200), and CST6 (cystatin B) with one type of progressive myoclonus epilepsy (MIM 254800). The loci for several monogenic hereditary disorders have been mapped to chromosome 21, such as the autoimmune polyglandular disease syndrome (MIM 240300), one form of manic-depressive illness (MIM 125480), one form of hereditary deafness (MIM 601072), and one form of a platelet disorder. The genes for all of these disorders map outside of the DS critical region, and all but one map in the gene-rich 21q22.3 region.

The following genes map in the so-called DSCR (from D21S17 to ETS2):

1. Carbonyl reductase (CBR) is one of several monomeric, NADPH-dependent oxidoreductases with wide specificity for carbonyl compounds. Lymphoblasts with increased copy number of CBR show increased aldo-, keto-, and quinone reductase activity.
2. SIM2 is homologous to the drosophila single-minded gene. Its protein product is a transcription factor with basic helix-loop-helix motif and two PAS domains. The drosophila sim protein is a master developmental regulator of the fly nervous system midline lineage. The role of three copies of SIM2 in trisomy 21 is under investigation.
3. The gene for the p60 subunit of the human chromatin assembly factor I (CAF1p60) encodes a protein that belongs to the WD-motif family and interacts with other polypeptide subunits to promote assembly of histones to replicating DNA. Its potential role in some phenotypes of DS is also under investigation.
4. The holocarboxylase synthetase (HCS) gene encodes an enzyme that catalyses biotin incorporation in various carboxylases involved in fatty acid synthesis, gluconeogenesis, or amino acid catabolism.
5. The ERG oncogene is related to the ets family of oncogenes. It encodes a nuclear phosphoprotein that binds to purine-rich sequences, and perhaps it is required for maintenance or differentiation of early hematopoietic cells. Translocation of chromosome 21 associated with some forms of myeloid leukemias or Ewing sarcomas show breakpoints within the ERG gene, resulting in abnormal fusion of mRNA transcripts. The role of ERG in some phenotypes of DS is unknown.
6. The gene for G-protein-coupled inwardly rectifying potassium channel (GIRK2) has been also mapped within the DSCR. Its mouse homolog gene is responsible for the weaver mutant mouse. The GIRK2 belongs to a family of proteins that participate in the formation of heteromultimeric channels whose activation is regulated via a G-protein-coupled receptor. The role of GIRK2 in DS is unknown.
7. The gene for the small polypeptide PEP19 that accumulates in the developing cerebellum encodes a cytoplasmic protein containing several motifs common in proteins involved in calcium-dependent signal transduction. It is predominantly expressed in cerebellar Purkinje cells and granule cells of the olfactory bulb.
8. The gene for TPRD that encodes a protein with tetratricopeptide repeat motifs; these domains were found in proteins involved in the regulation of RNA synthesis or mitosis. The involvement of this gene in DS is unknown.

Short sequences of additional genes map in the DSCR and have been obtained as parts of the exon trapping and cDNA selection experiments or the EST collections from various laboratories. The full content of genes in the DSCR and other parts of 21q will soon permit the exploration of the contribution of each gene to the trisomy 21 phenotypes.

THE TRANSCRIPTION/GENE MAP A medically and biologically important map is being developed, in which the mapping objects are sequences from transcripts of chromosome 21 genes. Two main methods, namely exon trapping and cDNA selection, using the cloned material from the physical maps, are now contributing to the development of such a map. More than 1000 partial sequences from chromosome 21 genes have already been identified; these sequences are probably obtained from at least 50% of the genes of this chromosome. In addition, large international efforts to partially sequence hundreds of thousands of human cDNAs from different tissues (ESTs) will soon result in the mapping of many new transcripts to chromosome 21. Finally, future efforts to determine the sequence of the entire 21q will provide the basis for understanding the contribution of chromosome 21 genes in human disease and DS in particular.

MOUSE MODELS FOR TRISOMY 21

The laboratory mouse has attracted attention as a potential model for trisomy 21. Because three copies of many genes are contributing to DS transgenic mice with three or more copies of the mouse homologs of chromosome 21, genes can serve as models for overexpression of selected genes. Transgenic mice with overexpression of genes such as SOD1 or APP or other genes have been made in order to study the contribution of each gene to the phenotype. Furthermore, breeding of transgenic mice with different transgenes will produce strains with more than one overdosed gene. The use of YACs for microinjected material into mouse oocytes will also permit the study of overexpression of several neighboring genes (perhaps all of the DSCR genes) in one transgenic strain.

Human chromosome 21 is homologous to segments of three mouse chromosomes, namely mouse chromosomes 16, 17, and 10, as shown in Fig. 119-4A. The entire DSCR is included in the mouse chromosome 16. A mouse with trisomy 16 (Ts16) was created that exhibited some characteristics of DS; however, its value was limited because Ts16 mice die *in utero*, and mouse chromosome 16 contains a number of genes found on human chromosomes other than 21. A more recent mouse model has been generated using a reciprocal chromosomal translocation. This model, Ts65Dn, contains a partial trisomy 16 that corresponds to human chromosome 21 from marker APP to MX1, which includes all of the DSCR. However, in addition, the Ts65Dn mouse contains a trisomy for the pericentromeric region of mouse chromosome 17 that is not homologous to human chromosome 21. The Ts65Dn mice display a variety of phenotypic abnormalities, including early developmental delay, reduced birth weight, muscular trembling, male sterility, abnormal facies, and impaired performance in the Morris water maze test. The heart defect characteristic of DS has never been observed in liveborn Ts65Dn mice, nor do these mice show the pathology of early-onset Alzheimer's disease. More extensive evaluation of the phenotype of the Ts65Dn mice is needed to further assess the similarity of this mouse model to the human trisomy 21.

TRISOMY: MOLECULAR PATHOPHYSIOLOGY OF INCREASED GENE DOSAGE

Trisomy 21 and all other partial or full trisomies are fascinating disorders in which the phenotypes do not result from abnormal gene products but result from increased (three instead of two) copies of *normal* genes. The different phenotypes of trisomy 21 can therefore be viewed as the result of the increased concentration of gene products of a number of genes that map on chromosome 21. Gene dosage effects for autosomal loci have been described in Drosophila. In addition, overexpression of transgenes in mice cause distinctive phenotypes. For example, mice with an additional copy of the human erythropoietin gene develop polycythemia, a condition of increased number of red blood cells resulting from the stimulatory hematopoietic effect of the increased levels of erythropoietin in mouse.

A duplication of a relatively small region (about 1.5 Mb) on chromosome 17 that includes the PLP22 gene causes Charcot-Marie-Tooth disease type IA, which is a common autosomal-dominant peripheral neuropathy. Overexpression of bmi-1 gene (a member of the polycomb-group gene family) in transgenic mice results in abnormalities of the axial skeleton of the animals. Furthermore, transgenic mice with overexpression or ectopic expression of hox transgenes develop skeletal abnormalities and other malformations. It is therefore conceivable that the increase dose of some chromosome 21 genes trigger directly or indirectly (through products of genes throughout the genome) a pathway that results in a physical abnormality, homeostatic disturbance, altered developmental process, and abnormal cognitive function. It is also conceivable that some but not all genes, when in three copies, result in an abnormal phenotype. There are perhaps hundreds of genes on chromosome 21, a trisomy of which does not have any effect on the phenotype. In contrast, the trisomy 21 of some genes may always be detrimental for the organism and always results in an abnormality (Fig. 119-5A). Furthermore, some phenotypes may be allele-specific (i.e., only the triplication of certain alleles is associated with a phenotype), whereas extra copies of other alleles are compatible with normal development (Fig. 119-5B). Of course, as with many of the Mendelian, monogenic disorders, the phenotype can be modified by the contribution of the protein products of all of the other human genes, as well as by environmental factors.

Gene dosage may be important in a number of gene products. Some illustrative examples from genes in mammals include the following:

1. Receptors and ligands. Increased amounts of ligands or receptors may modify the receptor-mediated cascades. For example, as mentioned above, increased levels of erythropoietin (a ligand for the erythropoietin receptor) lead to increased volume of red blood cells because of stimulation of erythropoiesis. Overexpression of the low-density lipoprotein receptor in transgenic mice prevents diet-induced hypercholesterolemia.

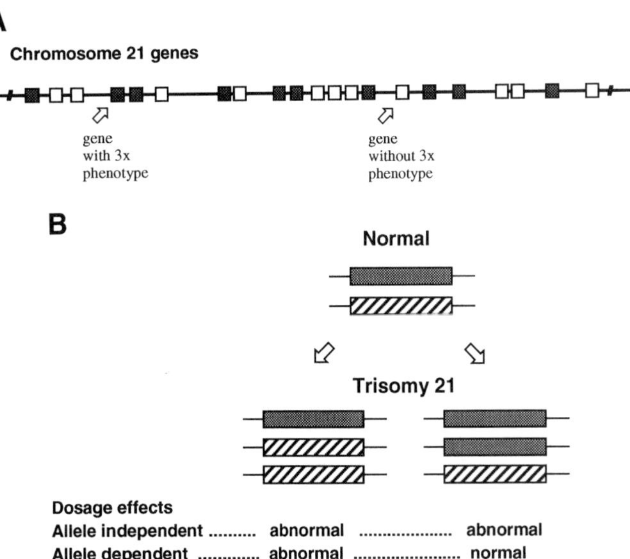

Figure 119-5 (**A**) Schematic representation of the effect of different chromosome 21 genes on the pathophysiology of Down syndrome. Filled squares represent genes, three copies of which contribute to the DS syndrome. Empty squares represent genes that, if trisomic, do not contribute to the DS phenotype. (**B**) Possible effects of trisomy of genes in the pathophysiology of Down syndrome. Examples of allele-independent and allele-dependent dosage effects are shown. In the allele-dependent example, the combination of two stripped and one gray allele contributes to the phenotype; in contrast, the combination of two gray and one stripped allele does not have an effect on the phenotype.

2. Genes important in pattern formation in development. The overexpression or ectopic expression of hox and other development-controlling genes in transgenic mice results in abnormalities of the skeleton and other organs.
3. Enzymes. The overproduction of such proteins involved in key steps of metabolic pathways may result in a recognizable phenotype. A mutant form of alpha$_1$-antitrypsin, which acts as antithrombin III, causes a fatal bleeding disorder from an effective increase of antithrombin III activity by 50%. However, the enzyme levels are usually not tightly regulated, and in general, three copies of genes encoding enzymes are probably not associated with phenotypes of trisomy.
4. Molecules involved in cell–cell interactions. The rate of cellular adhesivity is modified by differences in concentration of the neural cell adhesion molecule (NCAM). A 50% increase in concentration produces a fourfold increase in cell adhesion. This particular alteration may be important for some aspects of morphogenesis and anomalies of trisomy.
5. Subunits of multimeric proteins. Many proteins are composed of a number of subunits, each being a product of a different gene. The number of molecules of each subunit in the multimeric protein is constant and well-regulated. Abnormalities in the function of the multimeric protein can therefore arise by a change in the number of molecules of a particular subunit in the whole complex. This abnormal stoichiometry may result from the extra copy of a certain gene in a trisomy. Imbalance of α- and β-subunits of human hemoglobin leads to different forms of thalassemias (hereditary anemias).

6. Transcription factors. Gene products that regulate the expression of "downstream" genes are perhaps the best candidates for gene-dosage imbalance. Increased concentration of transcriptional regulators may either increase or decrease the expression of genes or alter the temporal or tissue distribution of expression of these genes.

The examples and possibilities listed above are only some alternatives to understanding the relationship of increased gene product and a resulting phenotype. The list can be enriched by other examples of different classes of gene products; furthermore, additional examples come from other model organisms, cellular biology, and transgenic animals.

THE FUTURE

Patients with Down syndrome will greatly benefit from the results of the human genome project, in the identification of all chromosome 21 genes and the elucidation of their function. Products of these genes will be associated with specific phenotypes of the syndrome. Therapeutic interventions based on the molecular pathophysiology of the syndrome will be introduced that may ameliorate or prevent the appearance of certain phenotypes. Better, faster, and more accurate diagnostic methods will be introduced. Further understanding of the molecular and cellular bases of cognitive functions may also lead to prevention or treatment of the mental impairment of this common syndrome.

ACKNOWLEDGMENTS

Research in the author's laboratory on human chromosome 21 and Down syndrome is supported by grants from the Swiss FNRS, the European Union, and funds from the University and Cantonal Hospital of Geneva. I thank all members of the laboratory (past and present) for their ideas, discussion, debates, and planning and execution of experiments, and all the clinical colleagues for their excellent care of patients and families enrolled in our studies. Dr. H. Scott is particularly acknowledged for the critical reading of this manuscript. This chapter is dedicated to all families with Down syndrome members.

SELECTED REFERENCES

Aitken DA, Wallace EM, Crossley JA, et al. Dimeric inhibin A as a marker for Down's syndrome in early pregnancy. N Engl J Med 1996;334:1231–1236.

Antonarakis SE. Human chromosome 21: genome mapping and exploration, circa 1993. Trends Genet 1993;9:142–148.

Antonarakis SE, Avramopoulos D, Blouin JL, Talbot CC, Schinzel AA. Mitotic errors in somatic cells cause trisomy 21 in about 4.5% of cases and are not associated with advanced maternal age. Nat Genet 1993;3:146–150.

Antonarakis SE and the Down Syndrome Collaborative Group. Parental origin of the extra chromosome in trisomy 21 as indicated by analysis of DNA polymorphisms. N Engl J Med 1991;324:872–876.

Chen H, Chrast R, Rossier C, et al.. Cloning of 559 potential exons of genes on human chromosome 21 by exon trapping. Genome Res 1996;6:747–760.

Chumakov I, et al. A continuum of overlapping clones spanning the entire human chromosome 21. Nature 1992;359:380–386.

Delabar JM, Theophile D, Rahmani Z, et al. Molecular mapping of 24 features of Down syndrome on chromosome 21. Eur J Hum Genet 1993;1:114–124.

De la Cruz F, Gerald PS. Trisomy 21 (Down Syndrome): Research Perspectives. Univ Parc Press, 1981.

Epstein CJ. Down syndrome (trisomy 21). In: Scriver CR, Beaudet AL, Sly WS, Valle D, eds. The Metabolic and Molecular Bases of Inherited Disease. New York: McGraw-Hill, 1995; pp. 749–794.

Epstein CJ. Mechanisms of the effects of aneuploidy in mammals. Ann Rev Genet 1988;22:51–75.

Hook EB, Hamerton JL. The frequency of chromosome abnormalities detected in consecutive newborn studies, differences between studies, results by sex and severity of the phenotypic involvement. In: Hook EB, Porter IH, eds. Population Cytogenetics: Studies in Humans. New York: Academic, 1977; pp. 63–79.

Jacobs PA , Hassold TJ. The origin of numerical chromosomal abnormalities. Adv Genet 1995;33:101–133.

Korenberg JR, et al. Down syndrome phenotypes: the consequences of chromosomal imbalance. Proc Natl Acad Sci USA 1994;91: 4997–5001.

Lamb NE, et al. Susceptible chiasmate configurations of chromosome 21 predispose to non-disjunction in both maternal meiosis I and meiosis II. Nature Genet 1996;14:400–405.

Lucente D, Chen HM, Shea D, et al. Localization of 102 exons to a 2.5 Mb region involved in Down syndrome. Hum Mol Genet 1995;4: 1305–1311.

McInnis MG, Chakravarti A, Blaschak J, et al. A linkage map of human chromosome 21: 43 PCR markers at average interval of 2.5 cM. Genomics 1993;16:562–571.

Peterson A, Patil N, Robbins C, Warg L, Cox DR, Myers RM. A transcript map of the Down syndrome critical region on chromosome 21. Hum Mol Genet 1994;3:1735–1742.

Reeves RH, Irving NG, Moran TH, et al. A mouse model for Down syndrome exhibits learning and behaviour deficits. Nat Genet 1995;11: 177–183.

Sherman SL, Petersen MB, Freeman SB, et al. Non-disjunction of chromosome 21 in maternal meiosis I : evidence for a maternal age-dependent mechanism involving reduced recombination. Hum Mol Genet 1994;9:1529–1535.

Warren AC, Chakravarti A, Wong C, et al. Evidence for reduced recombination of a non-disjoined chromosome 21 in Down syndrome. Science 1987;237:652–654.

120 The 22q11 Deletion

DiGeorge and Velocardiofacial Syndrome

DEBORAH A. DRISCOLL AND BEVERLY S. EMANUEL

INTRODUCTION

The association of thymic aplasia with congenital hypoparathyroidism was initially noted by Lobdell in 1959 but was not recognized as a syndrome until 1965, when Dr. Angelo DiGeorge described a group of infants with congenital absence of the thymus and parathyroid glands. Subsequently, facial dysmorphia and cardiac defects, specifically conotruncal malformations, were included in the spectrum of DiGeorge syndrome (DGS) (MIM 188400). Acknowledgment of the phenotypic overlap with velocardiofacial syndrome (VCFS) (MIM 192430) and identification of a common genetic etiology for these disorders has led to further expansion of the phenotype and a better understanding of the physical, cognitive, neurological, and psychiatric disorders that DiGeorge and velocardiofacial patients may develop.

DGS was presumed to be a heterogeneous disorder. However, cytogenetic and molecular studies have shown that deletion of chromosomal region 22q11 is the leading cause of DGS and VCFS. This may result from an unbalanced translocation with monosomy 22pter→q11.2, a cytogenetically visible interstitial deletion of 22q11 [del(22)(q11.21q11.23)] or a submicroscopic deletion. In rare instances, DGS has been associated with other chromosomal abnormalities, in particular, deletions of the short arm of chromosome 10 [del(10)(p13)]. Individual case reports of other chromosomal rearrangements seen in association with DGS include monosomy and trisomy 18q, monosomy 18p, monosomy 12p with trisomy 1q, monosomy 5p, partial trisomy 1q, and duplication 9q. DGS has been associated with exposure to teratogens such as retinoic acid and alcohol, and with maternal diabetes. There have been several reports of cytogenetically normal infants with DGS and renal agenesis born to women with insulin-dependent diabetes. Molecular studies of two of these patients failed to detect a deletion within 22q11.

DGS is believed to arise as a result of abnormal cephalic neural crest cell migration into the third and fourth pharyngeal arches. The neural crest cells populate the pharyngeal pouches that contribute to the development of the bones of the skull, mesenchyme of the face and palate, thymus, and thyroid, and the neuronal constituents of the head and neck. Kirby (1983) demonstrated that removal of the premigratory cardiac neural crest cells in the chick embryo results in cardiac outflow tract anomalies similar to those seen in DGS. The cardiac neural crest cells have also been shown to be important in supporting the development of the glandular derivatives of the pharyngeal arches, lending further support to the hypothesis that this is a disorder of the neural crest cells (Kirby and Bockman, 1984).

DGS was initially considered a rare disorder. However, recent studies suggest that the 22q11 deletion, seen in approximately 90% of DGS patients, may occur as frequently as 1 in 3000–4000 live births. The majority of 22q11 deletions occur as new mutations in the affected individual. However, a deletion may be transmitted in an autosomal-dominant fashion from parent to offspring. The clinical features are highly variable between individuals and within families with the 22q11 deletion, ranging from classic DGS to individuals with mild facial dysmorphia and a history of learning and speech difficulties. Although previously described as two distinct disorders, DGS and VCFS are manifestations of a single disorder, the 22q11 deletion.

CLINICAL FEATURES

DiGEORGE SYNDROME The three classic features of DGS include congenital cardiac defects, immune deficiencies secondary to aplasia or hypoplasia of the thymus, and hypocalcemia resulting from small or absent parathyroid glands. The cardiovascular malformations involve the conotruncal region and include interrupted aortic arch type B, truncus arteriosus, and tetralogy of Fallot. The immunologic deficits are variable. Although some patients may have a profound immunodeficiency requiring thymic transplantation, many patients can maintain reasonable lymphocyte counts and normal proliferative responses to mitogens. Recent studies suggest that patients are at risk for a spectrum of parathyroid gland abnormalities, including latent hypoparathyroidism which may evolve into hypocalcemic hypoparathyroidism during adolescence or early adulthood. Patients with DGS often have dysmorphic facial features, such as hypertelorism, low-set prominent ears, and micrognathia. Since 1965, the spectrum of clinical features associated with DGS has expanded to include cleft palate, cleft lip, renal agenesis, neural tube defects, and hypospadias. Advances in medical and surgical management of children with complex congenital cardiac disease have led to increased survival of newborns and children with DGS. Recent neuropsychological evaluations indicate that these children are at risk for cognitive impairment and neurological and psychiatric problems.

From: *Principles of Molecular Medicine* (J. L. Jameson, ed.), ©1998 Humana Press Inc., Totowa, NJ.

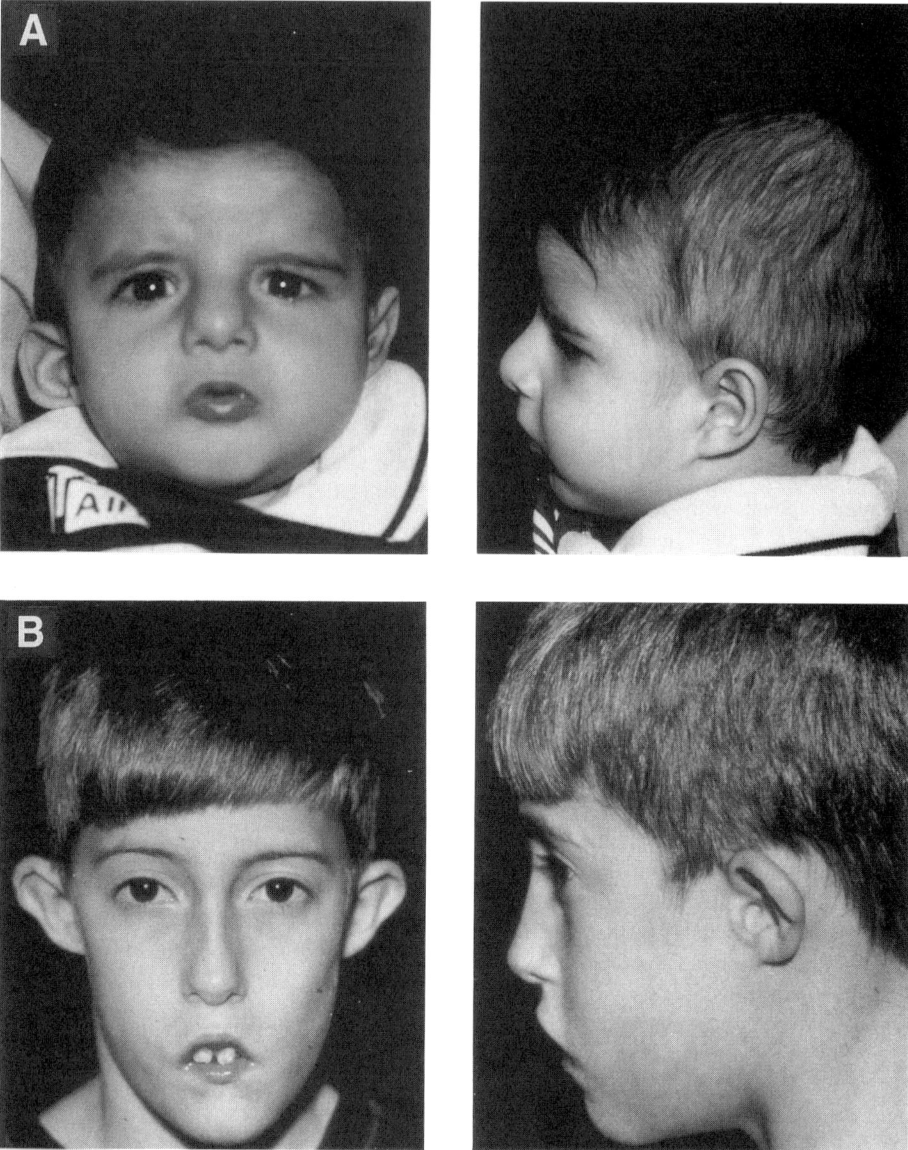

Figure 120-1 Frontal and side views of two patients with the 22q11 deletion syndrome. **(A)** Note prominent nasal root, bulbous nasal tip, protruberant right ear with underdeveloped superior helix in 9-month-old Hispanic male. **(B)** Note prominent nasal root, bulbous nasal tip, malar hypoplasia, long facies, thick superior helices, and protruberant ears in 11-year-old Caucasian male. (Kindly provided by Dr. EH Zackai and DM McDonald-McGinn, MS.)

VELOCARDIOFACIAL SYNDROME The major clinical features in VCFS include palatal abnormalities (cleft palate, submucous cleft palate and velo-pharyngeal insufficiency [VPI]), cardiac defects, learning disabilities, and a characteristic facial appearance. Other features seen less frequently include microcephaly, short stature, slender hands and digits, inguinal and umbilical hernias, and scoliosis. Parents may report a history of nasal regurgitation, feeding difficulties, and failure to thrive. In contrast to DGS, ventricular septal defects are the most frequent cardiac defects in VCFS patients. Characteristic facial features have been described that include a long face, a prominent nose with a bulbous nasal tip and narrow alar base, almond-shaped or narrow palpebral fissures, malar flattening, recessed chin, and malformed prominent ears (Fig. 120-1). However, these features are not always apparent during infancy and childhood.

An early study of clinically diagnosed VCFS children reported a history of developmental delay and mean verbal IQ scores in the dull normal intelligence range to mildly retarded range. More recently, an analysis of the psychoeducational and neurodevelopmental status of a cohort of patients, ages 4–20, with the 22q11 deletion, found similar full-scale IQ scores (mean 73.1 ± 10.1). In contrast, there was a striking difference between verbal and performance IQ scores with 9 of 10 patients demonstrating higher verbal IQ scores. These studies suggest that both males and females with the 22q11 deletion are at risk for nonverbal learning disabilities.

In addition to developmental delay and hypotonia, neural tube defects have been described in a small number of patients. Magnetic resonance imaging (MRI) of the brains of VCFS patients has identified several structural brain abnormalities including a small vermis, small posterior fossa, and small cysts adjacent to the anterior horns, suggesting that neurological findings may not be uncommon. However, these findings did not appear to correlate with developmental, cognitive, or personality disorders. In contrast,

Lynch et al. (1995) described a symptomatic 34-year-old man with VCFS and a 22q11 deletion who presented with progressive gait difficulties, muscle stiffness, dysarthria, and dysmetria suggestive of a neurodegenerative disorder. Cerebellar atrophy was diagnosed by MRI. The significance of these findings will require prospective neurological assessments of deletion-positive patients to determine their risk for developing neurological problems.

Recent studies suggest that individuals with VCFS are at a higher risk than the general population to develop schizophrenia during late adolescence and early adulthood. Additional studies that include a larger sample size will be necessary to determine the relative risk for developing schizophrenia in this population of patients. Molecular studies of families with schizophrenia have suggested linkage to the long arm of chromosome 22, and it has been hypothesized that there may be a schizophrenia-susceptibility gene in this region. However, it remains to be proven whether these two findings indicate the presence of a single locus associated with schizophrenia within the DiGeorge chromosomal region (DGCR) on 22q.

PHENOTYPIC VARIABILITY ASSOCIATED WITH THE 22q11 DELETION SYNDROME There is a wide range of intra- and interfamilial phenotypic variability associated with the 22q11 deletion. While some individuals present with classic findings of DGS, others, including the parents of some individuals, have relatively subtle features such as minor dysmorphic facial features and mild cognitive impairment. Furthermore, the observed differences between patients with DGS and VCFS probably reflects an ascertainment bias. For example, the majority of DGS patients are identified in the neonatal period with a major congenital heart defect, whereas many patients with VCFS are diagnosed in a cleft palate or craniofacial center and remain unrecognized until they reach school age when speech and learning difficulties are evident. DGS and VCFS were previously recognized as two distinct disorders. However, there is significant phenotypic overlap and they share a common etiology. Thus, we and others consider deletion-positive DGS and VCFS patients as having the same disorder, the 22q11 deletion syndrome.

OTHER DISORDERS ASSOCIATED WITH THE 22q11 DELETION The DiGeorge anomaly has been observed in several other syndromes, including CHARGE association, asymmetric crying face syndrome, Kallman syndrome, and Noonan syndrome. However, the 22q11 deletion has not been found to be causally related to these disorders in a significant number of cases. In contrast, deletions of 22q11 have been detected in patients with conotruncal cardiac malformations, conotruncal anomaly face syndrome (CTAFS), and Opitz syndrome. Knowledge of the genetic basis for these disorders has also expanded the spectrum of features associated with DGS and, more specifically, with the 22q11 deletion.

CONOTRUNCAL CARDIAC MALFORMATIONS Several studies have detected 22q11 deletions in patients with isolated and familial forms of congenital cardiac defects, suggesting that the genes in this region play a major role in cardiac development. Goldmuntz et al. (1993) demonstrated that 20–30% of newborns and children ascertained through the cardiology clinic with one of the three most common types of cardiac defects seen in DGS (interrupted aortic arch type B, truncus arteriosus, and tetralogy of Fallot) have deletions within 22q11. Although patients with hypocalcemia and immunodeficiencies were excluded from the study, prospective follow-up of these patients has demonstrated that they eventually manifest subtle dysmorphic facial features and report a history of nasal regurgitation suggestive of velopharyngeal insufficiency or unrecognized palatal problems. Similar findings were noted in the reported familial studies.

CONOTRUNCAL ANOMALY FACE SYNDROME Conotruncal anomaly face syndrome (CTAFS) has striking similarities to DGS and VCFS and is characterized by the presence of conotruncal cardiac defects in association with a characteristic facial appearance. The facial features include ocular hypertelorism, lateral displacement of the inner canthi, flat nasal bridge, small mouth, narrow palpebral fissures, bloated eyelids, and malformed ears. This syndrome has been well characterized in a population of Japanese patients. The finding of 22q11 deletions in CTAFS patients confirmed an earlier suggestion that CTAFS and VCFS are the same entity.

OPITZ/GBBB SYNDROME Recent cytogenetic and molecular studies suggest that Opitz/GBBB syndrome is genetically heterogeneous. However, there appears to be at least one autosomal-dominant locus on chromosome 22q11.2. Opitz/GBBB syndrome is characterized by hypospadias, laryngotracheal anomalies, and hypertelorism. Patients may have other features, including cleft lip and palate, cardiac defects, umbilical and inguinal hernias, cryptorchidism, imperforate anus, and facial dysmorphia such as telecanthus, prominent nasal bridge, or depressed nasal root with anteverted nares. Four patients, including a father and son, with Opitz syndrome with 22q11 deletions have been reported, suggesting that, in some cases, deletions within 22q11 are causally related to Opitz syndrome. Linkage analysis of families with Opitz syndrome provide additional evidence that there is a genetic locus within 22q11 responsible for this disorder as well as a locus on the X chromosome (Xp22). While there are some phenotypic similarities between these disorders, additional studies will be necessary to determine if Opitz syndrome is a genetically distinct disorder from DGS and VCFS.

CYTOGENETIC AND MOLECULAR STUDIES

Cytogenetic studies of patients with DGS provided the initial evidence linking chromosome 22 to DGS. Early reports of DGS patients with unbalanced translocations resulting in the loss of 22pter→q11 and two patients with interstitial deletions of 22q11 suggested that this region of 22 was important in the etiology of DGS. Subsequently, restriction fragment-length polymorphism analysis and DNA dosage studies demonstrated that approximately 90% of cytogenetically normal DGS patients have microdeletions within 22q11. The presence of features common to DGS in patients diagnosed with VCFS prompted investigators to study VCFS patients for evidence of a 22q11 deletion. Cytogenetic studies using high-resolution banding techniques detected interstitial deletions (del[22][q11.21q11.23]) in 20% of VCFS patients. Molecular studies with chromosome 22 probes previously shown to be deleted in patients with DGS demonstrated that the majority of individuals with VCFS have deletions of 22q11. Furthermore, these studies coincided with the increasing utilization of fluorescence *in situ* hybridization (FISH) for the detection of microdeletions and subtle translocations. FISH of metaphase chromosomes using DNA probes from the DiGeorge chromosomal region (DGCR) led to a dramatic increase in the detection of 22q11 deletions in patients with features of DGS, VCFS, CTAFS, and conotruncal cardiac malformations (Fig. 120-2).

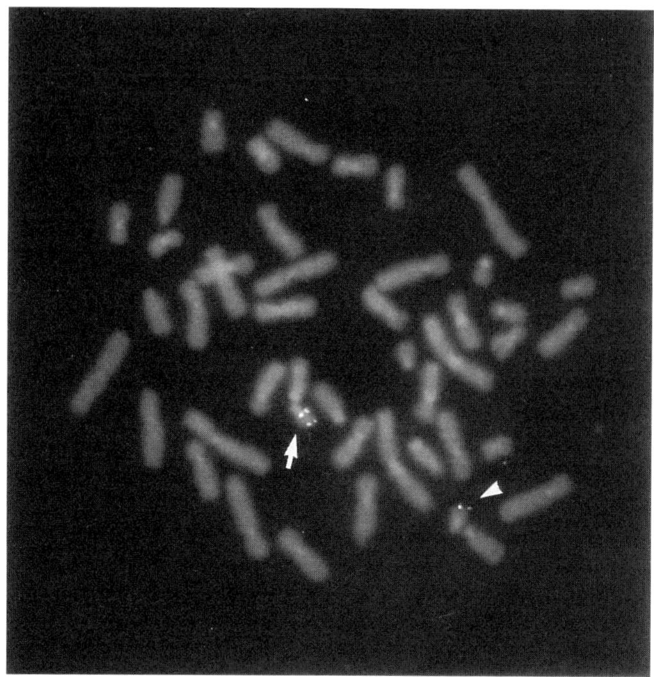

Figure 120-2 FISH. Metaphase chromosomes from a patient with 22q11.2 deletion syndrome hybridized with the probe N25 (D22S75) from the DGCR and control probe cos 82 that marks the distal long arm of 22. A hybridization signal for N25 is seen on only one chromosome 22 (arrow). This is consistent with a deletion on the other 22 (arrowhead).

THE DiGEORGE CHROMOSOMAL REGION The majority of patients have large deletions (1–2Mb) within 22q11; this commonly deleted region is referred to as the DiGeorge chromosomal region (DGCR). Delineation of this region was initially based on the finding of a consistently deleted region within 22q11 in patients with DGS; the minimal region of overlap in the first 14 patients studied spanned the region from D22S75 (N25) through D22S259 (R32). Since then, efforts in several laboratories have been directed toward determining the "minimal critical region" or the smallest region of overlap between patients with unbalanced translocations and interstitial deletions. YAC and cosmid contigs have been constructed across this region to facilitate the identification of candidate genes, and pulsed field gel electrophoresis (PFGE) and translocation breakpoint mapping have been utilized to develop a physical map of the region.

The positioning of DGS/VCFS-associated translocations in this region of 22 has been used to refine the localization of DNA markers within the region and to narrow the "minimal critical region." Many of these translocations serve as landmarks within 22q11 (Fig. 120-3). Initially, the critical region was defined by positioning a balanced 10;22 translocation (GM05878) established from an unaffected father of a child with DGS. Subsequently, an unbalanced 11;22 translocation (GM00980) from a VCFS patient was positioned centromeric to the 10;22 translocation as the distal boundary of the minimal critical region. More recently, we have narrowed the critical region to a 200- to 300-kb segment by positioning the 22q11 breakpoint of an unbalanced 15;22 translocation from a patient with features of DGS and VCFS between locus D22S75(N25) and GM00980. The proximal boundary of the critical region and the commonly deleted region lies between loci D22S427 and D22S36.

Within this "minimal critical region" lies a balanced 2;22 translocation that was initially described by Augusseau in 1986. The patient (ADU) had telecanthus, micrognathia, severe aortic coarctation with a hypoplastic left aortic arch, decreased E rosettes, and mild neonatal hypocalcemia consistent with a diagnosis of partial DGS. Her mother (VDU), who is also a balanced carrier of this translocation, reportedly has features suggestive of VCFS including hypernasal speech, micrognathia, and an inverted T4/T8 ratio. This is the only balanced translocation in the region that is associated with a classical DGS/VCFS phenotype. Budarf et al. (1995) recently cloned this translocation and identified a candidate gene, DGCR3, which is disrupted by the chromosomal rearrangement. Numerous other DGS/VCFS-associated translocations have been localized within the commonly deleted region, distal to the minimal critical region (Fig. 120-3).

PARENTAL ORIGIN OF THE 22q11 DELETION Sporadic 22q11 deletions may be of either maternal or paternal origin. Several investigators have suggested that there may be an excess of maternally-derived *de novo* 22q11 deletions; however, these studies are limited by their small sample size. Furthermore, both maternally and paternally derived DGS/VCFS-associated translocations occur with approximately equal frequency, suggesting that there is not a preferential parental origin associated with DGS and VCFS. Hence, it is unlikely that parental origin accounts for the phenotypic variability seen in association with the 22q11 deletion. This is in contrast to Prader-Willi and Angelman syndromes, where paternal and maternal deletions of chromosome 15q11–13, respectively, are the rule.

CLINICAL AND PRENATAL DIAGNOSIS

Deletions of 22q11 may be detected using high-resolution banding techniques; however, several studies have clearly shown that FISH of metaphase chromosomes using DNA probes from this region of chromosome 22 is the most efficient method for detecting 22q11 deletions. Routine cytogenetic analysis continues to be important for the detection of other chromosomal rearrangements, such as translocations, which may involve chromosomes other than 22. Hence, it is recommended that FISH be used as an adjunct to routine cytogenetic analysis.

At the present time, many commercial and hospital-based laboratories are utilizing FISH with the probes from the DGCR for the clinical and prenatal detection of the 22q11 deletion (Fig. 120-2).

Antenatal detection of the 22q11 deletion by FISH has been successfully performed on cultured amniocytes and chorionic villi obtained from at-risk pregnancies by FISH. Pregnancies considered at high risk include those of deletion-positive parents and those in which ultrasound or echocardiography demonstrates a fetal conotruncal cardiac malformation. Although the recurrence risk for normal parents with a previously affected child is low, parents often request prenatal testing for the deletion to exclude the small possibility of germline mosaicism. Since the size and extent of the deletion do not correlate with the phenotype, the phenotypic outcome cannot be predicted based solely on the presence of a deletion. Fetal imaging techniques, such as ultrasonography and fetal echocardiography, may be used to evaluate the

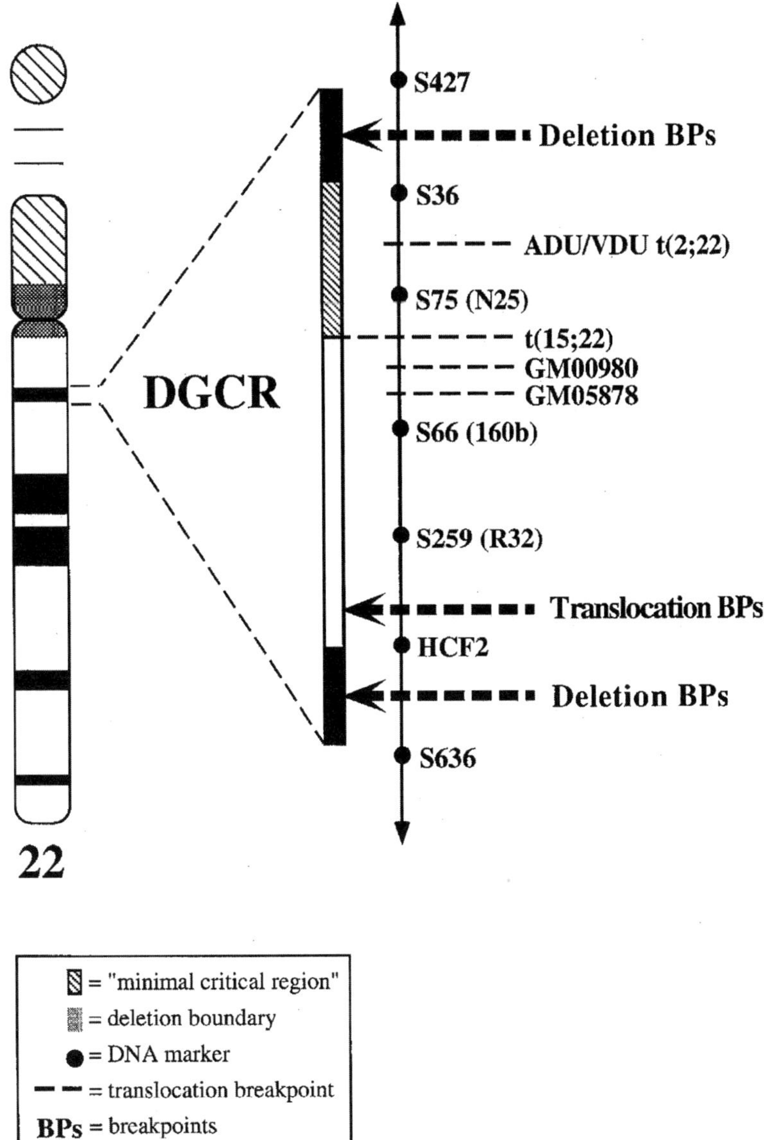

Figure 120-3 Diagram of the DGCR demonstrating the relative positions of several loci and translocations, including ADU/VDU and the t(15;22), GM00980, and GM05878, which have been used to define the minimal critical region. The location of the breakpoints associated with the interstitial deletions or microdeletions and the distal translocations are included. The commonly deleted region or DGCR includes the deletion boundaries and the minimal critical region.

fetus for the presence of a cleft palate and/or cardiac malformation. Subtle congenital anomalies, such as a submucous cleft palate and dysmorphic features, cannot be appreciated by sonography. Fetal sonography and echocardiography are the only available prenatal tests that are helpful when evaluating at-risk pregnancies that are not causally related to an abnormality of 22q11.

MANAGEMENT ISSUES Patients with the 22q11 deletion are ascertained through a variety of medical specialty clinics on the basis of their presenting feature(s). Recognition of which patients are at risk for the deletion is important so that the medical community and the schools can meet their needs. This has been clearly demonstrated in the cardiology clinic where a significant number of deletion-positive patients were ascertained solely by the presence of a conotruncal malformation. Because of the wide range of congenital anomalies, immune, endocrine, speech, neurologic, cognitive, and psychiatric problems that 22q11 deletion patients may develop, we urge clinicians to consider comprehensive evaluations by a team of medical professionals in genetics, cardiology, immunology, endocrine, plastic surgery, speech and hearing, and developmental pediatrics. Because DGS, VCFS, CTAFS, and (in some instances) Opitz/GBBB syndrome share a common etiology, we should consider deletion-positive patients with these disorders as having the 22q11 deletion syndrome. Prospective studies of 22q11 deletion patients will further delineate the range and severity of physical, cognitive, and neuropsychological problems for which these patients are at risk.

Furthermore, identification of a 22q11 deletion enables the clinician to provide the affected patients and their families with a more accurate assessment of their recurrence risk. Although the majority of the 22q11 deletions occur *de novo* only in the affected individual, a deletion may be transmitted in an autosomal-dominant fashion. Hence, we recommend deletion testing of parents of deletion-positive individuals. Because the phenotype is so variable, parents with only minor features and mild cognitive impairment are often undiagnosed until the birth of a more severely affected child. Features that are highly suggestive of a 22q11 deletion in one of the parents include mild facial dysmorphia, history of poor school performance, hypernasal speech, and nasal regurgitation. Deletion-positive parents and children have a 50% chance of transmitting the deletion-bearing chromosome in a subsequent pregnancy.

Presently, it remains difficult to counsel families of nondeleted children with DGS and VCFS unless an etiology such as a translocation or maternal diabetes has been identified. It remains a possibility that these individuals may have a smaller deletion that cannot be detected with the probes currently available or a mutation within one of the genes in the DGCR. Alternatively, there may be more than one chromosomal locus associated with DGS and VCFS.

IDENTIFICATION OF GENES IN THE DiGEORGE CHROMOSOMAL REGION (DGCR)

Two genes, catechol-*O*-methyltransferase *(COMT)* and glycoprotein Ibβ *(GpIbb)*, have been mapped to the DGCR, but distal to the minimal critical region. COMT is important in the metabolism of catecholamines, such as noradrenaline, adrenaline, and dopamine. It has been suggested that it may play a role in the development of the psychiatric disorders associated with the 22q11 deletion syndrome. *GpIbb* is a component of the major platelet receptor for von Willebrand factor. Defects in the receptor result in a rare autosomal-recessive bleeding disorder, Bernard-Soulier syndrome (BSS), which is characterized by excessive bleeding, thrombocytopenia, and very large platelets. A single patient with features of BSS and VCFS with a 22q11 deletion has been described. Haploinsufficiency for this region of 22 unmasked a mutation in the remaining *GpIbb* allele, resulting in manifestations of BSS. Although presumably an infrequent occurrence, this mechanism, unmasking a recessive allele, might explain some of the phenotypic variability seen among patients with 22q11 deletions.

Several genes have been isolated from the DGCR that may play a role in the development of some of the phenotypic features observed in association with deletions of 22q11. The most promising candidate genes lie within the minimal critical region. One of the first novel genes described in the region, N25 cDNA clone, was identified by screening fetal liver and brain libraries with a chromosome specific *Not*I linking clone from the commonly deleted region. The N25 cDNA is expressed in adult skeletal muscle, and studies are in progress to determine its function and developmental expression pattern. *DGCR3* was identified using a positional cloning approach. It was hypothesized that the only balanced translocation associated with a DGS/VCFS phenotype in the DGCR, ADU/VDU [t(2;22)], interrupts a locus critical to DGS. The 2;22 translocation disrupts an open reading frame whose predicted protein product is weakly homologous to rat and mouse androgen receptor sequences at the N-terminal transactivation domain. In addition, it contains a leucine zipper motif, suggesting that it might be a DNA binding protein. Another candidate gene, *DGCR2*, maps 10 kb distal to the ADU/VDU breakpoint, within the minimal critical region, and is deleted in known-deletion patients. This gene is expressed in a variety of human adult and fetal tissues and codes for a potential adhesion receptor, which might mediate specific adhesive interactions resulting in abnormal migration of the neural crest cells or interaction with the branchial arches. By sequence analysis, this gene appears to be homologous to the genes *LAN* and *IDD*. Although these genes are not disrupted by the ADU/VDU translocation, the translocation may separate a locus control region from the coding sequence. The human homolog of the rodent citrate transport protein *(CTP)* gene has been cloned and mapped to the minimal critical region in 22q11. *CTP* is located on the mitochondrial inner membrane and functions as an anion transport protein. However, its role in the 22q11 deletion syndrome remains to be determined. Several groups have isolated a gene *(CLTCL/CLTD/CLH-22)* with significant homology to clatharin heavy chain, a major structural component of coated pits and vesicles. *CLTCL* lies within the minimal critical region and is expressed predominately in adult skeletal muscle. Further studies will be necessary to determine the possible role this gene plays in the 22q11 deletion syndrome.

Several other genes have been identified distal to the minimal critical region, suggesting that they may not be as crucial to the phenotype. Functional and genetic analyses of these genes may determine whether they modify or influence the phenotypic outcome. The novel gene, N41 cDNA, is expressed in human tissue, including heart, liver, brain, and placenta. A zinc finger gene, *ZNF74*, is expressed during mouse embryogenesis as well as in human fetal tissues. A cDNA clone, T10, isolated from a mouse embryo library, encodes a serine and threonine-rich protein with no strong homologs or known function. This gene is expressed during early mouse embryogenesis as well as in human fetal tissue, but is probably not the major gene involved in DGS. Another cDNA, *TUPLE1*, was isolated from a human fetal brain library and a 10.5-day mouse embryo library. *TUPLE1*, also referred to as *HIRA*, encodes a putative transcriptional regulator. Although it has been shown to be deleted in patients with known 22q11 deletions, it does not appear to be deleted nor rearranged in nondeleted patients with DGS, VCFS, or conotruncal cardiac defects. Finally, the gene LZTR-1, was isolated from a fetal brain cDNA library. Sequence analysis demonstrates homology to a leucine-zipper-like transcriptional regulator protein. *LZTR-1* is expressed in fetal brain, heart, liver, kidney, and lung. However, the *LZTR-1* gene is not consistently deleted in DGS patients and does not appear to be rearranged in the nondeleted patients. Thus, it is unlikely to be a good candidate gene for the major features of DGS/VCFS.

Further studies are necessary to understand the role that each of these genes might play in the development of the complex and variable phenotype of the 22q11 deletion syndrome. Additional studies are in progress to determine whether nondeleted patients with DGS/VCFS have mutations within these or other genes in the minimal critical region. To understand the effects of haploinsufficiency of these genes, functional studies and the creation of transgenic or knockout mice will be required. These studies may enable us to determine if these disorders are caused by deficiency of a single gene or loss of several genes within the DGCR.

CONCLUSION

The 22q11 deletion associated with DiGeorge and velocardiofacial syndrome is one example of a microdeletion syndrome. Such syndromes were well-defined clinical entities prior to the identification of a specific chromosomal deletion. The deletion is rarely identified by routine cytogenetic analysis, often requiring high-resolution banding and/or molecular cytogenetic techniques such as FISH. These techniques have led to the detection of deletions in a proportion of patients with the following clinically recognizable syndromes: Prader-Willi and Angelman syndromes (15q), Miller Dieker and Smith Magenis syndromes (17p), Langer-Gideon (8q), WAGR (Wilm's tumor, aniridia, genital abnormalities, and retardation) (11p), Williams syndrome (7q), Alagille syndrome (20p), and Rubenstein-Taybi syndrome (16p). These disorders have been referred to as "contiguous gene deletion syndromes" or, more recently, "microdeletion syndromes." It has been hypothesized that the clinical features result from the deletion of several different genes in close proximity within the same chromosomal segment. The deleted region presumably contains numerous genes, and it is unlikely that all of these genes play a major role in the development of the phenotype associated with these disorders. Some of these disorders may result from haploinsufficiency of a single gene, whereas others may result from the loss of several genes within the deleted segment. As the genes are identified within the segment lost in each of the microdeletion syndromes, additional studies will be necessary to understand their function and role in the pathogenesis of each disorder.

SELECTED REFERENCES

Budarf ML, Collins J, Gong W, et al. Cloning a balanced translocation associated with DiGeorge syndrome and identification of a disrupted candidate gene. Nat Genet 1995;10:269–278.

Burn J, Takao A, Wilson D, et al. Conotruncal anomaly face syndrome is associated with a deletion within chromosome 22. J Med Genet 1993;30:822–824.

Conley ME, Beckwith JB, Mancer JFK, Tenckhoff L. The spectrum of the DiGeorge syndrome. J Pediatr 1979;94:883–890.

Daw SC, Taylor C, Kraman M, et al. A common region of 10p deleted in DiGeorge and velocardiofacial syndromes. Nat Genet 1996;13:458–460.

Demczuk S, Aledo R, Zucman J, et al. Cloning of a balanced translocation breakpoint in the DiGeorge syndrome critical region and isolation of a novel potential adhesion receptor gene in its vicinity. Hum Mol Genet 1995;4:551–558.

Driscoll DA, Budarf ML, Emanuel BS. A genetic etiology for DiGeorge syndrome: consistent deletions and microdeletions of 22q11. Am J Hum Genet 1992;50:924–933.

Driscoll DA, Salvin J, Sellinger B, et al. Prevalence of 22q11 microdeletions in DiGeorge and velocardiofacial syndromes: implications for genetic counselling and prenatal diagnosis. J Med Genet 1993; 30:813–817.

Driscoll DA, Spinner NB, Budarf ML, et al. Deletions and microdeletions of 22q11.2 in velo-cardio-facial syndrome. Am J Med Genet 1992; 44:261–268.

Emanuel BS, Driscoll D, Goldmuntz E, et al. Molecular and phenotypic analysis of the chromosome 22 microdeletion syndromes. In: The Phenotypic Mapping of Down Syndrome and Other Aneuploid Conditions. New York: Wiley-Liss, 1993; pp. 207–224.

Goldmuntz E, Driscoll D, Budarf ML, et al. Microdeletions of chromosomal region 22q11 in patients with congenital conotruncal cardiac defects. J Med Genet 1993;30:807–812.

Gong W, Emanuel BS, Galili N, et al. Structural and mutational analysis of a conserved gene (DGSI) from the minimal DiGeorge syndrome critical region. Hum Mol Genet 1997;6:267–276.

Gottlieb S, Emanuel BS, Driscoll DA, et al. The DiGeorge syndrome minimal critical region contains a goosecoid-like (GSCL) homeobox gene that is expressed early in human development. Am J Hum Genet 1997;60:1194–1201.

Greenberg F. DiGeorge syndrome: an historical review of clinical and cytogenetic features. J Med Genet 1993;30:803–806.

Greenberg F, Elder FFB, Haffner P, Northrup M, Ledbetter DH. Cytogenetic findings in a prospective series of patients with DiGeorge anomaly. Am J Hum Genet 1988;43:605–611.

Halford S, Wadey R, Roberts C, et al. Isolation of a putative transcriptional regulator from the region of 22q11 deleted in DiGeorge syndrome, Shprintzen syndrome and familial congenital heart disease. Hum Mol Genet 1993;2:2099–2107.

Holmes SE, Riazi MA, Gong W, et al. Disruption of the clathrin heavy chain-like gene (CLTCL) associated with features of DGS/VCFS: a balanced (21;22)(p12;q11) translocation. Hum Mol Genet 1997;6: 357–367.

Jaquez M, Driscoll DA, Li M, et al. Unbalanced 15;22 translocation in a patient with manifestations of DiGeorge and velocardiofacial syndrome. Am J Med Genet 1997;70:6–10.

Karayiorgou M, Morris MA, Morrow B, et al. Schizophrenia susceptibility associated with interstitial deletions of chromosome 22q11. Proc Natl Acad Sci USA 1995;92:7612–7616.

Kirby ML, Bockman DL. Neural crest and normal development: a new perspective. Anat Rev 1984;209:1–6.

Kirby ML, Gale TF, Stewart DE. Neural crest cells contribute to aorticopulmonary septation. Science 1983;220:1059–1061.

Lammer EJ, Opitz JM. The DiGeorge anomaly as a developmental field defect. Am J Med Genet 1986;29:113–127.

Lindsay EA, Greenberg F, Shaffer LG, Shapira SK, Scambler PJ, Baldini A. Submicroscopic deletions at 22q11.2: variability of the clinical picture and delineation of a commonly deleted region. Am J Med Genet 1995;56:191–197.

Lindsay EA, Halford S, Wadey R, Scambler PJ, Baldini A. Molecular cytogenetic characterization of the DiGeorge syndrome region using fluorescence in situ hybridization. Genomics 1993;17:403–407.

Lynch DR, McDonald-McGinn DM, Zackai EH, et al. Cerebellar atrophy in a patient with velocardiofacial syndrome. J Med Genet 1995; 32:562,563.

McDonald-McGinn DM, Driscoll DA, Bason L, et al. Autosomal dominant "Optiz" GBBB syndrome due to a 22q11.2 deletion. Am J Med Genet 1995;59:103–113.

Pulver AE, Nestadt G, Goldberg R, et al. Psychotic illness in patients diagnosed with velo-cardio-facial syndrome and their relatives. J Nerv Ment Dis 1994;182:476–478.

Ravnan JB, Chen E, Golabi M, Lebo RV. Chromosome 22q11.2 microdeletions in velocardiofacial syndrome patients with widely variable manifestations. Am J Med Genet 1996;66:250–256.

Scambler PJ, Carey AH, Wyse RKH, et al. Microdeletions within 22q11 associated with sporadic and familial DiGeorge syndrome. Genomics 1991;20:201–206.

Shprintzen RJ, Goldberg RB, Young D, Wolford L. The velo-cardio-facial syndrome: a clinical and genetic analysis. Pediatrics 1981;67:167–172.

Sirotkin H, Morrow B, DasGupta R, et al. Isolation of a new clathrin heavy chain gene with muscle-specific expression from the region commonly deleted in velo-cardio-facial syndrome. Hum Mol Genet 1996;5:617–624.

Wadey R, Daw S, Taylor C, et al. Isolation of a gene encoding an integral membrane protein from the vicinity of a balanced translocation breakpoint associated with DiGeorge syndrome. Hum Mol Genet 1995;4:1027–1033.

Wilson DI, Cross IE, Goodship JA, et al. A prospective cytogenetic study of 36 cases of DiGeorge syndrome. Am J Hum Genet 1992;51:957–963.

121 Orofacial Clefting

JACQUELINE T. HECHT AND SUSAN H. BLANTON

INTRODUCTION

Clefts of the orofacial region are a group of common birth defects that may range from those with little clinical consequence, such as a bifid uvula, to those requiring extensive surgical intervention, such as bilateral cleft lip with palatal involvement. While orofacial clefts often occur as isolated defects, they are also part of over 300 recognized genetic syndromes. In most cases, the underlying etiology is unknown, but it is widely accepted that genetic and nongenetic factors are important. The most common orofacial clefts involve the lips and palate. As with the larger group of orofacial clefts, clefts of these structures most often occur as isolated defects. However, McKusick currently lists cleft lip with or without associated cleft palate (CLP) or only cleft palate (CP) in nearly 100 syndromes each. These do not include the nearly 100 recognized chromosome syndromes.

Whereas the causes of clefting are poorly understood, nonsyndromic cleft lip with or without cleft palate (CL/P) and nonsyndromic cleft palate (CPO) are generally regarded to be distinct conditions. This distinction is based on both population and embryologic studies. Epidemiological and observational studies have demonstrated that CL/P and CPO do not usually segregate together in the same families.

Animal studies have shown that neural crest cells migrate into the region that eventually becomes the facial structures, and these cells play an important role in the skeletal, connective, and dental tissues of facial morphogenesis. The anterior neuropore closes at the fourth gestational week, and there is active growth during the fifth and sixth weeks. Maxillary swellings arise and enlarge through ectomesenchymal proliferation, and these swellings become the anterior portion of the first pharyngeal arch. The medial nasal prominences merge with each other and the bilateral maxillary processes. The upper lip is formed laterally by the maxillary prominences and medially by fused nasal prominences by the end of the sixth week. A defect in any of the developmental steps could lead to a cleft lip.

The primary palate consists of two merged medial nasal prominences called the intermaxillary segment. This segment is made up of two portions, the labial component, which becomes the philtrum and the triangular palatal component of bone that includes four maxillary incisor teeth. The secondary palate includes 90% of the hard and soft palate but does not include the anterior portion that holds the incisor teeth. The palatal shelves originate from swellings on the medial surface of the maxillary prominences that appear during the sixth week and grow downward and lateral to the tongue. Elevation of the palatal processes to a horizontal plane begins during the seventh week, and closure occurs by the ninth week. Closure occurs by fusion and is slightly later in males than females. Clefts of the secondary palate may result from hypoplasia of the shelves, delayed timing of the shelf fusion, interruption of normal fusion, or a problem in programmed cell death.

CL/P and CPO are complex malformations that require a multidisciplinary approach with evaluations by plastic surgery, otolaryngology, genetics, speech pathology, dental, and dietary disciplines. Practitioners representing these disciplines usually comprise the craniofacial teams that provide care for these children. Multiple surgeries are often required for lip and palate repair. Recurrent otitis media is a common complication, often requiring placement of PE tubes, especially when there is palatal involvement. Dental, especially orthodontic, intervention, is required for most of the children, and speech therapy is commonly necessary because of nasal speech patterns. Finally, genetic evaluation and counseling provides information pertaining to correct diagnosis and recurrence risks for future children. The following discussion will focus on some common causes and research pertaining to the etiology of clefting.

From: *Principles of Molecular Medicine* (J. L. Jameson, ed.), ©1998 Humana Press Inc., Totowa, NJ.

NONSYNDROMIC CLEFTING

NONSYNDROMIC CLEFT LIP AND PALATE (CL/P) CL/P occurs in approximately 1/1000 live births, and males are affected approximately twice as frequently as females. CL/P is unilateral in 80% of cases and bilateral in the remaining 20% (Fig. 121-1). The left side is affected in 70% of the unilateral cases; 85% of the bilateral and 70% of the unilateral cases are associated with cleft of the anterior palate.

Etiologic studies of CL/P are complicated by the difficulties in sorting out the inheritance patterns. Familial recurrences are well-documented but do not follow a Mendelian pattern of inheritance. The multifactorial model was developed to explain the familial recurrences, and the recurrence risk estimates used in genetic counseling practice are based on this model. For isolated cases, a recurrence risk of 3–5% for subsequent pregnancies is given, but higher risks of 10% are quoted if there are other affected first-degree relatives. While the multifactorial model has been useful, it has not provided a completely satisfactory explanation for the observed familial cases. Indeed, complex segregation analyses of different populations have suggested a Mendelian contribution with auto-

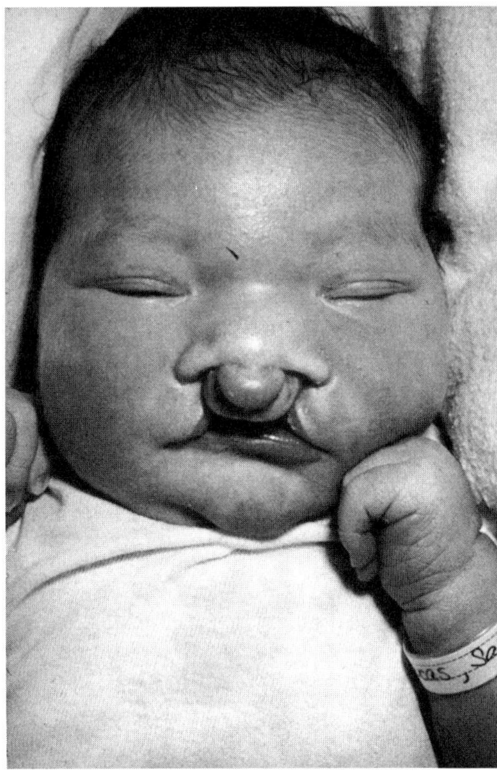

Figure 121-1 Infant with bilateral CL/P.

somal-dominant and/or recessive genes that are influenced by other genes, sex, and environmental factors (Table 121-1). Other studies suggest that oligogenic inheritance with as many as six to eight major genes may play a role in the development of CL/P. Growth factors are an example of multiple interacting genes that may play a role in orofacial clefting and are discussed below. Thus CL/P appears to be a genetically heterogeneous condition with multiple factors impacting the final developmental outcome. Identification of these genetic factors has proven to be a challenge.

Two approaches, association and linkage studies, using candidates genes and random mapped polymorphic markers, have been undertaken to study the genetic basis of CL/P. These approaches have been successfully used to delineate the molecular causes of other multifactorial conditions such as Hirschsprung disease and diabetes. The two statistical methods of studying clefting, linkage and association studies, each has strengths and weaknesses. Linkage testing requires multiplex families, generally with at least three affected offspring, and some assumptions regarding the mode of inheritance must be made. With these criteria fulfilled, it is possible to perform genome-wide screening to look for linkage. In some cases, a single family may be sufficient to establish linkage, although this has not been the case with clefting, as there are generally only a few affected individuals in a pedigree. Association studies, on the other hand, make no assumptions about the mode of inheritance. They require only a single affected individual from a family, but large numbers are required. A control population is also needed, and special attention must be paid to ensuring that the allele frequencies being used are correct. Association studies are looking for a specific allele of a gene to be associated with the disease, so that random testing is not practical, but testing of candidate genes is. Finally, association studies are generally better at detecting modifier loci than a linkage study. Given the apparent complex nature of clefting, it is unlikely that a single method will succeed in elucidating the etiologies of clefting.

Candidate genes have been identified in human and/or murine embryology studies. For example, transforming growth factor-α (TGF-α) is expressed in the pharyngeal pouch and activates epidermal growth factor (EGF/TGFA) receptors. It has been suggested that cell–cell contacts during embryogenesis may be discrete, and sequential events are mediated by growth factor receptor transduction. For this reason, all of the growth factors—such as retinoic acid receptor-α (RAR-α), TGFs, EGF, and so on— are excellent candidates and many of these have been tested. The results of both association and linkage studies are summarized in Table 121-2. Association studies from different populations have suggested that TGF-α plays a role in the development of CL/P. However, two linkage studies have demonstrated that TGF-α does not segregate with the disease phenotype in 20 multigenerational families. TGF-α is now considered to have a modifying effect on the development of CL/P.

Two candidate genes for CL/P, RARA-α and MSX1 (Hox 7), have been identified in murine models. MSX1 knockout mice exhibit craniofacial and tooth abnormalities in addition to cleft palate, and a CL/P gene has been mapped to the mouse chromosomal region containing RAR-α. Association of RAR-α with CL/P has been demonstrated in two population studies but not in a third, and linkage was excluded to RAR-α in ten multigenerational CL/P families. These results suggest that RAR-α does not play a major role in CL/P. MSX1 was excluded in a CLP linkage study, but the results of a recent association study suggest this locus may play a role in CPO.

Linkage studies have suggested there may be CL/P loci on chromosomes 6p, 4p, and 19q. A locus on chromosome 6p was first suggested by Eiberg et al. in 1987, when evidence for linkage to Factor 13A (F13A) at 6p23 was found. Additionally, linkage to F13A was demonstrated in 14 of 21 families from Italy, and chromosomal rearrangements involving 6p in individuals with CL/P have been reported. However, linkage to F13A was not found in 20 US and UK CL/P families, and a subsequent study expanded to include 33 Caucasian CL/P families was not able to confirm linkage to the 6p chromosomal area that spans from F13A to D6S89. A LOD (Log odds) score suggestive of linkage to an anonymous marker, D4S192, was reported in a single large family, and an association study provided evidence for linkage disequilibrium with the same marker. These findings could not be substantiated in 33 multigenerational CL/P families. Finally, linkage has recently been reported to BCL3 on chromosome 19q. Seventeen of thirty-nine families were found to have a posteriori probability of greater than 50% of being linked to this chromosomal region. BCL3 is a proto-oncogene, which was the candidate gene in the immediate chromosomal vicinity. Additional studies need to be performed to determine whether mutations can be identified in BCL3 or whether there is another candidate gene in close proximity to BCL3. The families linked to BCL3 have been excluded from the chromosome 4 and 6 markers, providing additional evidence that CL/P is genetically heterogeneous. A great deal of work remains to be done to identify the genetic loci that contribute to human CL/P. This will entail large numbers of families and populations for linkage and

Table 121-1
Segregation Analyses

Author(s)/year	*Mode inheritance/model*	*Population*
Chung et al., 1974	Multifactorial/AR/major gene	Hawaiian
Chung et al., 1984	Multifactorial/major gene	Chinese
Demanis et al., 1984	Multifactorial/mixed	Caucasian
Chung et al., 1986	AR/major gene	Caucasian
	Multifactorial	Japanese
Marazita et al., 1986	AR/major gene	Caucasian
	Major gene	Chinese
Hecht et al., 1991	AD/major gene	Caucasian
Marazita et al., 1992	AR/major gene	Chinese
Nemana et al., 1992	Major gene	Indian
Ray et al., 1993	AD/coD/major gene	Indian

Table 121-2
Loci Implicated in Development of CL/P Loci

Locus	*Method*	*Results*
TGFA	Association	±
	Linkage	–
RARA	Association	+
	Linkage	–
F13A	Linkage	±
D6S89	Linkage	±
D4S192	Association	+
	Linkage	±
BCL3	Linkage	+

association studies, respectively, in order to have sufficient power to identify the different CL/P loci.

NONSYNDROMIC CLEFT PALATE (CPO) CPO occurs in 0.4/1000 live births, and females are affected more often than males. CPO most commonly occurs sporadically; however, isolated families with multiple affected family members have been reported. A multifactorial model has also been used to describe recurrence of CPO in families. However, segregation analysis has suggested that a major gene explains half the familial recurrence of CPO. It has also been suggested that an oligogenic model with six loci would explain the data. Interestingly, in a large breeding colony of Brittany spaniels, CPO was found to be segregating as an autosomal-recessive disorder.

A chromosomal locus on chromosome 6p has also been implicated in CPO, but has not been confirmed by linkage studies in multigenerational CPO families. Association of TGFA with CPO has been reported in one study. A systematic study of CPO by both association and linkage methods remains to be undertaken.

SYNDROMIC CLEFT LIP AND PALATE (CLP) AND CLEFT PALATE (CP) Some of the several 100 syndromes that feature orofacial clefts have been mapped, and the genes responsible are known in some cases (Table 121-3). Here we discuss a few of the syndromes in which orofacial clefts are a prominent finding.

Van der Woude syndrome (VWS) is a well-described autosomal-dominant condition associated with CLP and/or CP, cleft uvula, hypodontia, and paramedian lower-lip pits. Lip pits are observed in 65–80% of cases, and surgical removal is recommended as these fistulas may communicate with underlying salivary glands, which can produce watery discharge. Not all gene carriers exhibit lip pits or CLP/CP, and family studies suggest that the penetrance is 75–80%. One to three percent of CLP cases are estimated to be VWS. VWS was mapped to chromosome 1q in 1990 with tight linkage to the renin gene. The chromosomal region containing the VWS gene has since been refined to a 4.1-cM region between microsatellite markers D1S245 and D1S414. Linkage of nonsyndromic CL/P and CPO to VWS was excluded using tightly linked markers.

Stickler syndrome (Hereditary Arthro-ophthalmopathy) is an autosomal-dominant condition characterized by flat facies, CP, myopia, retinal detachment, deafness, and epiphyseal abnormalities. Pierre Robin sequence (*see* Sporadic Conditions discussion) may be the presenting diagnosis in infancy. Stickler syndrome demonstrates marked variability, and individuals may inadvertently be misdiagnosed as CPO. Retinal detachments, myopia, and sensorineural deafness are common complications, and annual ophthalmologic and hearing evaluations are suggested. Arthritis occurs in adulthood and may be progressive with advancing age. Mutations in COL2A1 (12q14.3) and COL11A2 (6p21.2) have been identified in individuals with Stickler syndrome. The mutations in COL2A1 produce stop codons that lead to truncated proteins, whereas the characterized COL11A2 mutation causes a change in the splice donor site, resulting in an in-frame exon skipping. The associated phenotype appears to be milder than that observed for COL2A1 mutations; however, only one case has been reported. An autosomal-recessive mutation in COL11A2 has been reported, and the associated phenotype appears to be more severe than the autosomal-dominant form. Other type II collagenopathies, Kniest dysplasia and spondyloepiphyseal dysplasia, also have CP.

An X-linked type of CP (CPX) associated with ankyloglossia (tongue-tie) was first described and characterized in an Icelandic native family and later in a Mennonite native family. Males are affected with CP and tongue-tie, and only rarely will carrier females be similarly affected. Submucous CP and bifid or absent uvula are also found in this condition. The CPX gene was mapped to Xq in a large Icelandic family in 1987 and the map location has been further refined to a 5-cM region within the interval of Xq21.1–q21.31.

CHROMOSOMAL CAUSES OF CLEFTING Velocardial facial syndrome (VCF) or Shprintzen syndrome was first described by Shprintzen et al. in 1978 and is characterized by craniofacial,

Table 121-3
Mapped Clefting Syndromes

MIM	*Syndrome*	*Location*	*Locus*
Cleft lip/palate			
109400	Basal cell nevus syndrome	9q22.3–q31	
129900	EEC syndrome	7q11.2–q21.3	
305400	Faciogenital dysplasia	Xp11.21	FGD1
161200	Nail-Patella syndrome	9q34.1	
263520	Polydactyly with neonatal chondrodystrophy	4q13	
312870	Simpson dysmorphia syndrome	Xcen–q21.3	
313850	Thoracoabdominal syndrome	Xq26.1	
119300	Van der Woude syndrome	1q32–q41	
194190	Wolf-Hirschorn syndrome	4p13.7	
193500	Waardenburg syndrome, Type I	2q235	PAX3
Cleft palate			
101400	Acrocephalosyndactyly type III	7p21.3–p21.2	
301590	Anophthalmos	Xq27–q28	
222600	Diastrophic dysplasia	5q31–17q24.2q33	DTD
211970	Camptomelic dwarfism	17q24.2	SOX9
215150	Chondrodystrophy with sensorineural deafness	6p22–p21.3	COL11A2
154500	Mandibulofacial dysostosis	5q31.3–q32	
311300	Otopalatodigital syndrome	Xq28	
182290	Smith-Magenis syndrome	17p11.2	
309583	Snyder-Robinson syndrome	Xp21	
183900	Spondyloepiphyseal dysplasia, congenita	12q13.11	COL2A1
108300	Stickler syndrome, type 1	12q13.11	COL2A1
184840	Stickler syndrome, type 2	6p22–	COL11A2
303400	X-linked cleft palate	Xq13–q21	
214100	Zellweger syndrome 1	7q11	
170995	Zellweger syndrome-2	1p22–p21	PXMP1
170993	Zellweger syndrome-3	8q21.1	PAF1

cardiac, and palatal abnormalities. It is estimated to be the most common syndrome featuring CP, having a prevalence of 1/5000 live births. The facies are distinctive with malar hypoplasia, prominent nose with a squared nasal root and narrow alar base and CP. Hypotonia, failure to thrive, and short stature are frequent in infancy and childhood. Cardiac anomalies include ventricular septal defect, right aortic arch, tetralogy of fallot, and aberrant left subclavian artery. Robin sequence is occasionally observed. Learning disabilities and impairment are consistent findings. Speech development is delayed and hypernasality is common. Phenotypic findings can overlap with the DiGeorge syndrome, which also includes thymic aplasia/hypoplasia and hypocalcemia.

Most cases of VCF syndrome are sporadic, although familial cases demonstrating autosomal-dominant inheritance have been reported. Cytogenetic abnormalities involving 22q11 are detected in approximately 20% of VCF syndrome patients. Deletion of molecular markers from this chromosomal region have recently been identified in 82% of VCF patients. No difference in the sex of the parent transmitting the chromosomal deletion was found among the patients with deletions and on whom DNA was available suggesting that imprinting does not play a major role in the etiology of this syndrome. Further discussion of VCF can be found in Chapter 120.

Trisomy 13 is a common chromosomal abnormality, with a prevalence of 1/5000 live births. Microcephaly, secondary to the holoprosencephaly spectrum of brain abnormalities, microphthalmia, retinal dysplasia, and polydactyly of the hands and sometimes in the feet are common. CLP is present in about 60–80% of cases. Cardiac abnormalities are identified in 80% of cases and include ventricular septal defect, patent ductus arteriosus, and atrial septal defect. The constellation of phenotypic findings is caused by the presence of an extra chromosome 13, either as a free trisomy or, rarely, as a translocation. The risk of recurrence for trisomy 13 is less than 1% except where maternal age is a factor, which elevates the risk. Translocations are associated with an empiric risk of recurrence of 5–10%, depending on the sex of the parent who is the translocation carrier. Trisomy 13 is generally lethal by 1 year of age with only a few long-term survivors reported.

TERATOGENIC CAUSES OF CLEFTING Fetal Hydantoin syndrome is a constellation of phenotypic findings associated with *in utero* exposure to Dilantin or phenytoin. These findings include unusual facies, digit and nail hypoplasia, and growth and mental deficiencies. CLP is found approximately 11 times more frequently in exposed offspring compared with those not exposed.

Deficiency of folic acid during pregnancy may play an etiologic role in some cases of CL/P and CPO. A recent study has demonstrated that supplementation during pregnancy decreased the birth prevalence of orofacial clefting.

SPORADIC CONDITIONS WITH CLEFTING Pierre Robin sequence is characterized by micrognathia, glossoptosis, and a U-shaped CP. Posterior airway obstruction may occur secondary to the small mandible and tongue obstruction. Hypoplasia of the mandibular area prior to 9 weeks' gestation is postulated to be an initiating defect in this condition. The tongue becomes posteriorly displaced and interferes with the normal movement and fusion of the palatal shelves, causing the large U-shaped cleft compared with the V-shaped palate defect observed in CPO. Deformational processes have also been implicated in some cases.

The etiology and natural history depends on whether there are other associated anomalies or whether it is part of a syndrome as observed in the Stickler syndrome *(see above)*.

Facio-auriculo-vertebral spectrum (Goldenhar/Hemifacial microsomia) is a nonrandom association of anomalies involving the first and second branchial arches. The prevalence is estimated to be 1/3000–5000 live births, and males are affected more often than females. The spectrum includes unilateral hypoplasia malar, maxillary and mandibular regions facial musculature, vertebral and ocular abnormalities, with epibulbar dermoid being the most common eye finding. The clefts most often associated with this spectrum are lateral-like extensions from the corner of the mouth, although CLP and CP have been observed. Unilateral microtia with accessory pits and tags are frequent and may be associated with deafness. The soft palate may show poor resilience and lead to speech problems. Hemivertebrae, most commonly in the cervical spine, are often present, and cardiac and renal anomalies may occur. The etiology is unknown, and there is a very low recurrence risk for other family members.

CONCLUSION

As illustrated, CLP and CP are associated with a wide range of syndromes whose underlying etiologies are diverse. Although not all of the known genes for syndromic forms of CLP and CP have been tested for linkage to the nonsyndromic forms, most of them have been excluded from playing a major role in the development of nonsyndromic CL/P and CPO. Given the complex nature of craniofacial embryology, it is not surprising that many different genes may exert an effect.

SELECTED REFERENCES

Ahmad NN, Ala-Kokko L, Knowlton RG, et al. Stop codon in the procollagen II gene (COL2A1) in a family with the Stickler syndrome (arthro-ophthalmopathy). Proc Natl Acad Sci USA 1991;88: 6624–6627.

Ardinger HH, Buetow KH, Bell GI, Bardach J, VanDemark DR, Murray JC. Association of genetic variation of the transforming growth factor alpha gene with cleft lip and palate. Am J Hum Genet 1989;45: 348–359.

Asada H, Kawamura Y, Maruyama K, et al. Cleft palate and decreased brain gamma-aminobutyric acid in mice lacking the 67-kDa isoform of glutamic acid decarboxylase. Proc Natl Acad Sci USA 1997;94: 6496–6499.

Beiraghi S, Foroud T, Diouhy S, et al. Possible location of a major gene for cleft lip and palate to 4q. Clin Genet 1994;46:255,256.

Blanton SH, Crowder E, Malcolm S, et al. Exclusion of linkage between cleft lip with or without cleft palate and markers on chromosomes 4 and 6. Am J Hum Genet 1996;58:239–241.

Carinci F, Pezzetti F, Scapoli L, et al. Nonsyndromic cleft lip and palate: evidence of linkage to a microsatellite marker on 6p23. Am J Hum Genet 1995;56:337–339.

Carter CO. Genetics of common disorders. Br Med Bull 1969;25:52–57.

Carter CO, Evans K, Coffey R, Fraser Roberts JA, Buck A, Fraser Roberts M. A three generation family study of cleft lip with or without cleft palate. J Med Genet 1982;19:245–261.

Chenevix-Trench G, Jones K, Green A, Martin N. Further evidence for an association between genetic variation in transforming growth factor alpha and cleft lip and palate. Am J Hum Genet 1991;48:1012,1013.

Chenevix-Trench G, Jones K, Green AC, Duffy DL, Martin NG. Cleft lip with or without cleft palate: associations with transforming growth factor alpha and retinoic acid receptor loci. Am J Hum Genet 1992;51:1377–1385.

Chung CS, Ching GHS, Morton NE. A genetic study of cleft lip and palate in Hawaii. II Complex segregation analysis and genetic risks. Am J Human Genet 1974;26:177–188.

Chung CS, Bixler D, Watanabe T, Koguchi H, Fogh-Anderson P. Segregation analysis of cleft lip with or without cleft palate: a comparison of Danish and Japanese data. Am J Hum Genet 1986;39:603–611.

Davies AF, Stephens RJ, Olavesen MG, et al. Evidence of a locus for orofacial clefting on human chromosome 6p24 and STS content map of the region. Hum Mol Genet 1995;4:121–128.

Demenais F, Bonaiti-Pellie C, Briard ML, Feingold J. An epidemiological and genetic study of facial clefting in France. II Segregation analysis. J Med Genet 1984;21:436–440.

Eiberg H, Bixler D, Nielsen LS, Conneally PM, Mohr J. Suggestion of linkage of a major locus for nonsyndromic orofacial cleft with F13A and tentative assignment to chromosome 6. Clin Genet 1987;32: 129–132.

Farrall M, Holder S. Familial recurrence-pattern analysis of cleft lip with or without cleft palate. Am J Hum Genet 1992;50:270–277.

Feng H, Sassani R, Bartlett SP, et al. Evidence from family studies for linkage disequilibrium between TGFA and a gene for nonsyndromic cleft lip with or without cleft palate. Am J Hum Genet 1994;55: 932–936.

Ferguson MW. Palate development: mechanisms and malformations. Isr J Med Sci 1987;23:309–315.

Field LL, Ray AK, Marazita ML. Transforming growth factor alpha: A modifying locus for nonsyndromic cleft lip with or without cleft palate? Eur J Hum Genet 1994;2:159–165.

Fitzpatrick D, Farrell M. An estimation of the number of susceptibility loci for isolated cleft palate. J Craniofac Genet Dev Biol 1993;13: 230–235.

Gorlin RJ. Syndromes of the Head and Neck. New York: Oxford University Press, 1990.

Gorski SM, Adams KJ, Birch PH, Chodirker BN, Greenberg CR, Goodfellow PJ. Linkage analysis of X-linked cleft palate and ankyloglossia in Manitoba Mennonite and British Columbia native kindreds. Hum Genet 1994;94:141–148.

Hanson JW. Risk of the offspring of women treated with hydantoin anticonvulsant with emphasis on the fetal hydantoin syndrome. J Pediat 1989;4:662–668.

Healey SC, Mitchell LE, Chenevix-Trench G. Evidence for an association between non-syndromic cleft lip with or without cleft plate and a gene located on the long arm of chromosome 4. Am J Hum Genet 1994;55:A47.

Hecht JT, Annegers JF. Familial Component of Epilepsy in Cleft Lip and Palate. Ann Arbor, MI: Univer Microfilms Int, 1988.

Hecht JT, Wang Y, Blanton SH, Michels VV, Daiger SP. Cleft lip and palate: no evidence of linkage to transforming growth factor alpha. Am J Hum Genet 1991;49:682–686.

Hecht JT, Wang Y, Connor B, Blanton SH, Daiger SP. Nonsyndromic cleft lip and palate: no evidence of linkage to HLA or factor 13A. Am J Hum Genet 1993;52:1230–1233.

Hecht JT, Yang P, Michels VV, Buetow KH. Complex segregation analysis of nonsyndromic cleft lip and palate. Am J Hum Genet 1992a;49:674–681.

Hecht JT, Wang Y, Blanton SH, Michels VV, Daiger SP. Cleft lip and palate: no evidence of linkage to transforming growth factor alpha. Am J Hum Genet 1991;49:682–686.

Holder SE, Vintiner GM, Farren B, Malcolm S, Winter RM. Confirmation of an association between RFLPs at the transforming growth factor-alpha locus and non-syndromic cleft lip and palate. J Med Genet 1992;29:390–392.

Jara L, Blanco R, Chiffelle I, Palomino H, Carreno H. Evidence for an association between RFLPs at the transforming growth factor alpha (locus) and nonsyndromic cleft lip/palate in a South American population. Am J Hum Genet 1995;56:339–341.

Jones KL. Smith's Recognizable Patterns of Human Malformations, 4th ed. Philadelphia: WB Saunders, 1988.

Juriloff DM, Mah DG. The major locus for multifactorial nonsyndromic cleft lip maps to mouse chromosome 11. Mammalian Genome 1995, 6:63–69.

Lidral A, Basart A, Romitti P, et al. Candidate gene analysis of nonsyndromic cleft lip with or without cleft palate (NS-CL/P) and cleft palate (NS-CPO) in humans. Am J Hum Genet 1995;57(Abstract 58).

Marazita ML, Hu D-N, Spence MA, Liu Y-E, Melnick M. Cleft lip with or without cleft palate in Shanghai, China: evidence for an autosomal major locus. Am J Hum Genet 1992;51:648–653.

Marazita ML, Spence MA, Melnick M. Major gene determinationof liability to cleft lip with or without cleft palate: a multiracial view. J Craniofacial Genet Dev Biol 1986;2:89–97.

Mitchell LE. Transforming growth factor alpha locus and nonsyndromic cleft lip with or without cleft palate: a reappraisal. Genet Epidemiol 1997;14:231–240.

Mitchell LE, Risch N. Mode of inheritance of nonsyndromic cleft lip with or without cleft palate: a reanalysis. Am J Hum Genet 1992;51:323–332.

Moore GE, Ivens A, Chambers J, et al. Linkage of an X-chromosome cleft palate gene. Nature 1987;326:91,92.

Moore K. The Developing Human: Clinically Oriented Embryology, 4th ed. Philadelphia: WB Saunders, 1988.

Morrow B, Goldberg R, Carlson C, et al. Molecular definition of the 22q11 deletions in velo-cardio-facial syndrome. Am J Hum Genet 1995;56:1391–1403.

Murray JC, Nishimura DY, Buetow KH, et al. Linkage of an autosomal dominant clefting syndrome (Van der Woude) to loci on chromosome 1q. Am J Hum Genet 1990;46:486–491.

Nemana LJ, Marazita ML, Melnick M. Genetic analysis of cleft lip with or without cleft papate in madras, India. Am J Med Genet 1992;42:5–9.

Oliver-Padilla, Martinez-Gonzalez. Cleft lip and palate in Puerto Rico: a thirty-three year study. Cleft Palate J 1986;23:48–57.

Online Mendelian Inheritance in Man, OMIM (TM). The Human Genome Data Base Project, Johns Hopkins University, Baltimore, MD. World Wide Web <URL:http//gdbwww.gdb.org/omim/docs/omimtop.html>, 1995.

POSSUM, V4.0. Computer Power Group and The Murdoch Institure for Research into Birth Defects. Melbourne, Australia.

Ray AK, Field LL, Marazita ML. Nonsyndromic cleft lip and palate with or without cleft palate in west Bengal, India: evidence for an autosomal major locus. Am J Hum Genet 1993;52:1006–1011.

Richtsmeier JT, Sack GH JR, Grausz HM, Cork LC. Cleft palate with autosomal recessive transmission in Brittany spaniels. Cleft Palate-Craniofacial J 1994;31:364–371.

Sanford LP, Ormsby I, Gittenberger-de Groot AC, et al. TGFbeta2 knockout mice have multiple developmental defects that are non-overlapping with other TGFbeta knockout phenotypes. Development 1997; 124:2659–2670.

Sassani R, Bartlett SP, Feng H, et al. Association between alleles of the transforming growth factor-alpha locus and the occurrence of cleft lip. Am J Med Genet 1993;45:565–569.

Satokata I, Maas R. MSX1 deficient mice exhibit cleft palate and abnormalities of craniofacial and tooth development. Nat Genet 1994; 6:348–355.

Shiang R, Lidral AC, Ardinger HH, et al. Association of transforming growth factor alpha gene polymorphisms with isolated non-syndromic cleft palate (CPO). Am J Hum Genet 1993;53:836–843.

Shprintzen RJ, Goldberg RJ, Young D, Wolford L. The velo-cardio-facial syndrome: a clinical and genetic analysis. Pediatr 1981;67:167–172.

Spranger J, Winterpacht A, Zabel B. The type II collagenopathies: a spectrum of chondrodysplasias. Eur J Pediatr 1994;153:56–65.

Stein J, Hecht JT, Blanton SH. Exclusion of retinoic acid receptor and a cartilage matrix protein in non-syndromic CL(P) families. J Med Genet 1995a;32:78.

Stein J, Mulliken JB, Stal S, et al. Nonsyndromic cleft lip with or without cleft palate: evidence of linkage to BCL3 in 17 multigenerational families. Am J Hum Genet 1995b;57:257–272.

Stoll C, Qian JF, Feingold J, Sauvage P, May E. Genetic variation in transforming growth factor alpha: possible association of BamH1 polymorphism with bilateral sporadic cleft lip and palate. Am J Hum Genet 1992;50:870,871.

Tolarov M, Harris J. Reduced recurrence of orofacial clefts after periconceptional supplementation with high-dose folic acid and vitamins. Teratology 1995;51:71–78.

Vikkula M, Mariman EC, Lui VCH, et al. Autosomal dominant and recessive osteochondrodysplasias associated with the COL11A2 locus. Cell 1995;80:431–437.

Vintiner GM, Holder SE, Winter RM, Malcolm S. No evidence of linkage between the transforming growth factor-alpha gene in families with apparently autosomal dominant inheritance of cleft lip and palate. J Med Genet 1992;29:393–397.

Wyszynski DF, Mestri N,. McIntosh I, et al. Evidence for an association between markers on chromosome 19q and non-syndromic cleft lip with or without cleft palate in two groups of multiplex families. Hum Genet 1997;1:22–26.

122 Molecular Genetics of Hearing Disorders

WILLIAM J. KIMBERLING

BACKGROUND

Hearing is the result of a mechanical transduction process that translates sound waves into neural signals, which are then interpreted by our minds as language, music, signals of danger, or just plain noise. Hearing is a critical sense for communication, and whenever hearing is impaired, oral communication suffers, and one's quality of life is considerably diminished. The cochlea is the sensory organ responsible for hearing; it is complex and hundreds of genes must be responsible for its development and normal homeostasis. Thus, it is no surprise that hearing loss occurs in a great many different genetic disorders.

The three major parts of the ear are the outer, middle and inner ear. The inner ear develops from the otic placode, whereas the middle and outer ear develop primarily as a result of differentiation of the first and second branchial arches. The inner ear is divided into two parts: the membranous labyrinth (balance) and osseous labyrinth or cochlea (hearing). While both structures share certain features, they are quite different in function. Consequently, each part of the ear must be controlled by different sets of genes, but their effects must be well coordinated in order to produce a single effective hearing organ. As expected, some genes are expressed in more than one part of the ear, whereas others are specific. For example, some hearing loss disorders have vestibular symptoms and others do not; some disorders involve neurosensory hearing loss in combination with conductive loss resulting from external and/or middle ear abnormalities, and others have only a neurosensory component. The clinician must be cognizant of the fact that the ear comprises a set of embryologically related but distinct structures, and that patterns of involvement of the parts of the hearing organ are often important clues in the differential diagnosis of hearing disorders.

Hearing loss disorders are divided into syndromic and nonsyndromic categories, depending on whether there are any associated nonotologic symptoms accompanying the hearing deficit. While most childhood deafness is nonsyndromic, advances in the molecular genetics of the auditory system have occurred more with syndromic disorders because they can be recognized as distinct groups and are more amenable to positional cloning strategies.

Epidemiological studies to determine the magnitude of hereditary vs nongenetic causes of hearing loss are not common, especially when adult-onset hearing impairment is being considered. The role of heredity in causing hearing impairment in children is better defined, and most studies indicate that the overall frequency of deafness in children is about 1/1000. Over one-half of all causes of childhood deafness can be identified as genetic in origin. Information about the role of heredity in adult-onset hearing loss is virtually nonexistent, although one would predict that genes play a major role; the fact that several adult-onset progressive hearing loss genes have been localized supports this hypothesis.

From: *Principles of Molecular Medicine* (J. L. Jameson, ed.), ©1998 Humana Press Inc., Totowa, NJ.

DIAGNOSIS OF HEARING IMPAIRMENT

The diagnosis of hearing impairment is aided by the consideration of a variety of symptoms that permit the subcatergorization of hearing loss disorders into several different groups. The list below gives some of the clinical parameters and tests that are frequently helpful in diagnosing the different forms of hearing impairment:

1. Mode of inheritance (dominant, recessive, x-linked, mitochondrial, not inherited).
2. Age of onset (congenital, early childhood, young adult, and so on).
3. Severity (mild to profound).
4. Ears involved (bilateral vs unilateral or symmetric vs asymmetric).
5. Type of hearing loss (sensorineural, conductive, or mixed).
6. Frequencies involved and audiologic profile (e.g., high frequency, low frequency, U-shaped, and so on).
7. Presence and degree of vestibular deficit.
8. Presence of external-, middle-, or inner-ear malformation.
9. Evaluation for common syndromes: electroretinogram (Usher syndrome), thyroid function and perchlorate discharge test (Pendred syndrome), electrocardiogram (Jervell and Lange-Nielsen syndrome), renal function tests (Alport syndrome).

The audiogram defines the severity of the hearing loss and is an indispensable component to the clinical evaluation of patients and families with hereditary types of hearing impairment. Some families have distinct audiometric patterns, whereas other families show considerable variation in hearing acuity. Examples of selected different audiologic profiles are presented in Figure 122-1. In some disorders, such as Usher Type II, the audiologic profile is quite consistent across families, whereas in other disorders, like Branchio-oto-renal syndrome, the audiological phenotype can vary considerably even between ears of the same person. Hearing can also be assessed using auditory brain-stem responses (ABR)

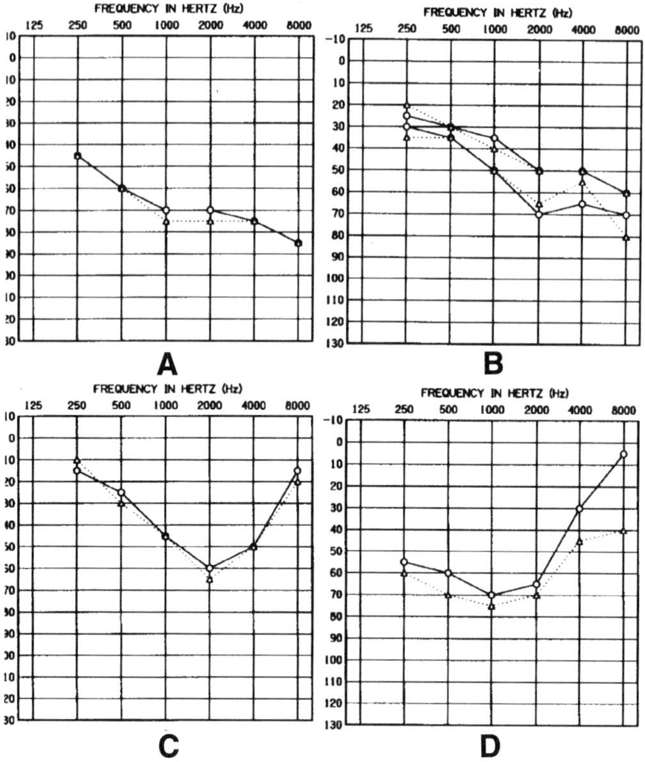

Figure 122-1 This presents examples of different types of audiograms seen in a few hereditary disorders. The circles and triangles indicate the hearing loss observed in right and left ears, respectively. **(A)** Sloping audiogram characteristic of Usher Type II; the hearing loss is mild in the low frequencies and tapers to a severe-to-profound loss in the high frequencies. **(B)** Two audiograms at different ages and illustrates a configuration and progression typical of dominantly inherited high-frequency hearing loss. **(C)** U-shaped audiogram where the loss of hearing acuity is mostly in the middle frequencies. **(D)** Low-frequency type of hearing impairment. Such audiometric configurations are often helpful in diagnosing specific inherited forms of deafness.

and oto-acoustic emissions (OAE). The ABR is useful for separating a central from a peripheral (i.e., cochlear) hearing problem, and the OAE assesses hair cell function. The age at onset and nature of the progression of the hearing loss are also important variables in characterizing a family's phenotype. Some dominant progressive hearing losses involve a specific range of frequencies early in life, and only at older ages are all the frequencies involved. It is frequently necessary to ask for older audiograms to document the type hearing loss at an earlier age. The role of the inner ear for balance is often forgotten by geneticists, and the presence or absence of vestibular symptoms can often be important for the differential diagnosis. For example, Usher syndrome type I has vestibular areflexia, whereas the milder type II does not. Inner-ear malformations are associated with some syndromes and not others. For example, Pendred syndrome often has a Mondini deformity. The audiogram, vestibular studies, and CT of the temporal bone are essential for giving a full description of the hearing loss phenotype.

CLINICAL FEATURES OF DISORDERS WITH HEARING LOSS

NONSYNDROMIC HEARING LOSS Dominant Nonsyndromic Hearing Loss The identification of the genes responsible for nonsyndromic hearing loss has been difficult and slow. The traditional approach to positional cloning for dominantly inherited disorders relies on having large, multigenerational kindreds. When families are large enough, evidence of linkage can be found without having to pool information from several different families, thus avoiding the problem of heterogeneity. Unfortunately, this research strategy is difficult to apply to dominant congenital profound deafness. Congenitally deaf people belong to a separate subculture and will tend to marry other deaf people, thus complicating attempts to follow gene transmission. Because of this phenomenon, the initial focus of localization of nonsyndromic dominant genes has been directed toward dominantly inherited progressive hearing loss. Because of their later age of onset, members of families with progressive hearing loss seldom see themselves as part of the deaf community and do not marry within it. At least 10 dominant hearing loss genes exist. The first gene for nonsyndromic hearing loss, called DFNA1, was localized to chromosome 5q31 (DFNA is used as code for dominant hearing impairment genes and DFNB for recessive genes; the numerals 1, 2, ... are assigned in order of discovery). The first linkage was observed in a large Costa Rican kindred whose members had a rapidly progressing hearing loss with adult onset that initially involved the low frequencies. Replication of this linkage in a second family has not been reported, and so it must be presumed that the gene is uncommon. A second gene was localized to chromosome 13q at or near a nonsyndromic recessive deafness gene (DFNA2). This family had a hearing loss that was evident by 4 years of age. Hearing impairment ranged from 15 to 90 dBHL, and the higher frequencies were more involved than the lower frequencies. The HL was not progressive in most gene carriers. Another dominant progressive hearing loss gene was localized to chromosome 1p32 (DFNA3) in two families, one Indonesian and the other American, both of which showed a progressive loss with onset in the high frequencies. A gene for a progressive hearing loss involving all frequencies was localized to chromosome 19, and a family with high-frequency hearing loss has been linked chromosome 7p15, whereas another with a low-frequency loss was localized to 4p16.3. An up-to-date listing of the new localizations of dominant, recessive, X-linked, and mitochondrial hearing loss genes can be found on the Internet by accessing the Hereditary Hearing Loss Homepage at www.uia.ac.be/u/dnalab/hhh.html . This web site also gives the flanking markers for each linkage as well as the appropriate references citing the original linkage observation.

Recessive Nonsyndrome Hearing Loss Autosomal recessive nonsyndromic hearing impairment is responsible for 80% of all the cases of childhood deafness. Most deaf-by-deaf marriages result in hearing offspring, a phenomenon that underscores the fact that several different loci are involved. The number of genes responsible has been variously estimated as at between 7 and 150. Since the recessive nonsyndromic families cannot be differentiated from each other, few useful pools of families are generated for gene localization research. Despite this problem, significant advances have been made into locating recessive genes responsible for nonsyndromic hearing loss, notably by focusing research efforts on population isolates. Three loci for autosomal-recessive congenital profound nonsyndromic hearing loss have been localized. Two are from consanguineous kindreds from Tunisia: One at 13q13 (DFNB1) and a second at 11q13 (DFNB2) in the region homologous to the mouse shaker-1 gene and close to myosin VIIa, the gene for Usher Type Ib. A third gene (DFNB3) for nonsyndromic recessive congenital deafness has been localized to chro-

Table 122-1
Usher Syndrome Genotype/Phenotype Relationship

	Subtype	*Location*	*Gene*	*Phenotype*[a]
Type I (MIM 276900)	1a	14q		Profound sensory neural hearing loss
	1b	11q	Myosin VIIa	Vestibular areflexia
	1c	11p		
	1d	Unlinked		
Type II (MIM 276901)	2a	1q		Sloping mild-to-profound hearing loss
	2b	Unlinked		Normal vestibular responses
Type III	3	3q		Progressive hearing loss Variable vestibular deficit

[a]All have retinitis pigmentosa.

mosome 17p in an Indonesian population. A congenital-recessive severe-to-profound deafness (DFNB4) found in the Druze population has been mapped to 7q13, and consanguineous families from India were used to identify a locus on chromosome 14q.

X-Linked Hearing Loss X-linked deafness is a special category of deafness because its pattern of inheritance is distinctive. As a specific cause of hearing impairment, X-linkage is not common, accounting for no more that 2% of all cases. The most common form is X-linked deafness with stapes fixation and perilymphatic gusher (DFN3), which has been localized to Xq13–q21.1. The structural defect is an open connection between the cerebrospinal fluid and the perilymph that causes the "gusher" seen in inner-ear surgery. The human gene, Pou3F4, was found to carry mutations that correlate with the gusher phenotype, suggesting that it and DFN3 are the same. Two other X-linked nonsyndromic genes are know to be located at Xq21(15) and Xp21.2.

Mitochondrial Inheritance Defects in the mitochondria affect the cellular respiratory chain and lead to a wide variety of progressive clinical manifestations, namely ataxia, epilepsy, dementia, myopathy, polyneuropathy, retinal pigment anomalies, and cardiomyopathy with conduction anomalies (*see* Chapter 103). Hearing loss is a regular feature and is often the first clinical symptom of many of the mitochondrial disorders. Some mitochondrial disorders involve a full spectrum of disease, whereas others involve only hearing. For example, one family with sensorineural hearing loss of varying severity but with no other pathological feature had a mutation at nucleotide position 7445, which converted the 3' terminal T residue of tRNA-ser to a C and caused a silent alteration to the stop codon. Another mutation close to the same position was reported in association with Leber's hereditary optic neuropathy, pointing to the fact that the mitochondrial mutations do not yet sort into neat diagnostic categories.

Summary Progress has been made in the localization of genes involved in nonsyndromic hearing loss. However, studies of associated symptoms are still lacking. Presence or absence of vestibular defect, existence of inner-ear structural abnormality, brain stem responses, and the results of oto-acoustic emission studies are infrequently reported. As a consequence, it is not yet possible to determine if different hearing loss genes produce slightly different phenotypes. Undoubtedly, as research progresses, clinical studies will be found that will aid in the differentiation of one nonsyndromic type from another.

SYNDROMIC HEARING LOSS There are two syndromes that, because of their high frequency among the congenitally deaf, are especially important to consider when evaluating the deaf patient. These are Usher syndrome and Waardenburg syndrome. Together, these syndromes comprise the largest proportion of identifiable hereditary deafness. It is important to realize that, because of the late diagnosis of the RP for Usher syndrome and the reduced penetrance for Waardenburg syndrome, many patients with either syndrome may initially be considered to have a nonsyndromic hearing loss.

Usher Syndrome Usher syndrome (US) is defined as hearing impairment with retinitis pigmentosa and is estimated to be responsible for about 5% of all of the cases of childhood deafness. It is both clinically and genetically heterogeneous. There are three phenotypic types (Table 122-1). Type I has a congenital profound hearing loss, vestibular areflexia, and retinitis pigmentosa. It has a frequency of 4.4/100,000 people. Type II is milder, showing a stable sloping audiogram (*see* Fig. 122-1A); patients with US II have reasonably good speech and are often helped by hearing aids. Significantly, they have a normal vestibular response. Type III displays a progressive hearing loss and variable vestibular responses. There are at least five, possibly seven, genes responsible for the different types of Usher syndrome. Table 122-1 outlines the relationship between the five known genes and the three phenotypes as they are currently recognized.

The most common types of US are Usher IIa (on chromosome 1q) and Usher Ib (on chromosome 11q). Usher Type III is linked to markers on chromosome 3q and is more common in Finland. In the United States, it was estimated that 88% of all Usher II result from mutations at the USH2a locus on chromosome 1, and the rest were either type III or unlinked to either 1q or 3q markers. Thus, it is likely that many families failing to show linkage to 1q are actually Type III Usher syndrome. However, a very small proportion, between 4 and 6%, are not linked to either the USH2a locus nor to the USH3 locus and may represent a novel type of Usher syndrome Type II.

Usher type I also shows considerable genetic heterogeneity. The first localization was to chromosome 14q. This gene was subsequently found to constitute approximately 20–30% of Usher I patients in a worldwide series of patients. Two other Usher I linkages were found, one to 11q (USH1b) and one on 11p (USH1c). The Usher Ic variant appears to be limited mostly to the French Acadian population of southern Louisiana and has not yet been observed outside of descendants of that population. Usher Ib accounts for 70–80% of the Usher cases seen in a large series from the United States and Europe. Myosin VIIa on human chromosome 11q has been recently been identified as the gene responsible for Usher Ib. Myosin VIIa is coded by a large gene of over 110 kb

Table 122-2
Locations of Nonsyndromic Hearing Loss Genes

Gene ID[a]	*Location*	*Phenotype*
Dominant		
DFNA1	5q31	Low-frequency HL beginning in the second decade progressing to a profound loss involving all frequencies
DFNA2	1p32	Variably late-onset high-frequency HL with variable rates of progression to a severe-to-profound loss
DFNA3	13q	Juvenile-onset high-frequency HL
DFNA4	19q13	Mild HL across all frequencies progressing to a severe-to-profound loss
DFNA5	7p15	Adult-onset high-frequency HL
DFNB6	4p13.6	Adult-onset low-frequency HL
Recessive		
DFNB1	13q	Profound congenital HL
DFNB2	11q	Profound, childhood-onset HL
DFNB3	17p	Profound congenital HL
DFNB4	7q13	Severe-to-profound congenital HL
DFNB5	14q	Profound congenital HL
X-linked		
DFN1	Xq21	Congenital
DFN2	Xp21.2	Profound HL in males; mild-to-moderate HL in female heterozygotes
DFN3	Xq21	Mixed conductive and HL; perilymphatic gusher with stapes fixation

[a]There is not yet a common consensus for locus nomenclature, and the gene ID given here may differ slightly with some reports in the literature.

Table 122-3
Identified Genes Causing Hearing Impairment in Humans

Disorder (MIM no.)	*Inheritance*	*Linkage*	*Gene*
Neural crest/pigmentary			
Waardenburg syndrome Type I (193500)	AD	2q35	PAX3
Waardenburg syndrome Type II (193510)	AD	3p12	MITF
Craniofacial			
Treacher Collins syndrome (154500)	AD	5q13	TCOF1
Crouzon syndrome (123500)	AD	10q25	FGFR2
Collagen disorders			
Alport syndrome (203780)	AR	2q35	COL4A3/4
Alport syndrome (301050)	XL	Xq	COL4A5
Osteogenesis imperfecta (166200)	AD	17q21	COL1A1
Stickler syndrome (108300)	AD	12q12	COL2A1
Stickler syndrome (108300)	AD	6p21.3	COL11A2
Other disorders			
Norries disease (310600)	XL	Xp11.4	NDP
Neurofibromatosis Type II (101000)	AD	22q12.2	NF2
Stapes fixation with gusher (304400)	XL	Xq13	POU3F4

of genomic sequence whose coding region of about 7.5 kb has now been completely sequenced. Forty-nine exons have been identified, and several mutations occurring primarily in the first 14 exons have been observed. The role of Myosin VIIa in the inner ear and the retina has yet to be elucidated.

Waardenburg Syndrome Waardenburg syndrome (WS) is an autosomal-dominant disorder that is recognized by its characteristic signs of pigmentary abnormality in the form of a white forelock, premature graying, and heterochromia iridis (two different colored eyes). About 2% of all children in schools for the deaf have Waardenburg syndrome. Deafness is variable; sometimes it is bilateral, sometimes unilateral, sometimes there is no hearing impairment at all. The syndrome is divided into two types, WS1 and WS2, based on the presence or absence of the dystopia canthorum. WS1 has been shown to be a result of mutations in the PAX3 gene on chromosome 2. The PAX3 gene is a transcription factor and controls the migration of melanocytes from the neural crest. A second gene for WS2 has been localized to chromosome 3 and has been shown to be homologous to microphthalmia in the mouse. This gene, MITF, is also a transcription factor (*see* Chapter 112).

COLLAGEN DISORDERS ASSOCIATED WITH HEARING LOSS

ALPORT SYNDROME Alport syndrome (AS) is glomerular nephritis with high-frequency progressive sensorineural hearing loss (*see* Chapter 68). Most cases of AS are inherited in an X-linked pattern, although both autosomal-dominant and recessive patterns of inheritance have been noted in a few families. Typical of X-linked disorders, males are more severely affected than females. X-linked AS is a result of mutations in the collagen 4α5 gene (COL4A5). Collagen 4α5 is a component of the basement membrane of the glomerulus and the cochlea. Mutations in COL4A5 result in a defective collagen that renders the basement membrane susceptible to lamelation and splitting. Presumably, this process leads to the gradual deterioration of the glomerulus and the cochlea, which accounts for the gradual nature of the disease.

The range and severity of expression of the Alport gene is more variable between families than within, suggesting that different mutations have different clinical effects. For example, some X-linked Alport cases do not have an associated hearing deficit but others do. No correlation between the site of mutation and the presence of hearing deficit has yet been made, but it is tempting to speculate that some parts of the COL4A5 molecule are more critical for hearing impairment than other regions. A recessive form of Alport syndrome with mutations in the COL3A3 and COL3A4 collagen genes has recently been described.

STICKLER SYNDROME Stickler syndrome is a clinically variable disorder associated with arthropathy, ocular symptoms (vitreoretinal degeneration, severe myopia, retinal detachments, and cataracts), hearing impairment, Pierre-Robin sequence, and midface hypoplasia. There is great phenotypic variation both between and within families. Whereas the hearing loss is variable, it seems to involve the high frequencies more often, and no correlation between the hearing loss and degree of orofacial involvement has been noted. Stickler syndrome was found to result from mutations in the COL2A1 gene. The type of COL2A1 mutation may be related to the severity of the Stickler phenotype. Mutations causing premature termination of transcription of the COL2A1 gene are associated with the "typical" Stickler phenotype, which includes hearing loss and facial hypoplasia, while mutations replace glycine codons with codons for bulkier amino acid appear to produce phenotypes of lethal chondrodysplasia or with only ocular problems. About 50% of Stickler syndrome families fail to show linkage to COL2A1, indicating the existence of a second type of Stickler syndrome from a mutation in another gene that may be located on chromosome 6p22–6p21.3.

OSTEOGENESIS IMPERFECTA Osteogenesis Imperfecta refers to several different heritable disorders characterized by bone fragility. Deafness is a frequent feature of both Types I and IV. Type I is a result of mutation in the COL1A1 gene on chromosome 17q21, and Type IV is a result of mutations in the COL1A2 gene on chromosome 7. About 50% of all Type I patients have hearing loss. Type IV (COL1A2) is also associated with hearing loss but only in about 30% of the cases.

CRANIOFACIAL DISORDERS

BRANCHIO-OTO-RENAL SYNDROME Branchio-oto-renal syndrome (BOR) is characterized by renal anomaly, external ear anomaly, and mixed hearing impairment. The hearing impairment can range from none to severe. It may be sensorineural (20%), conductive (30%), or mixed (50%). The hearing loss is quite variable between individuals and even between the ears of the same person. The inner-ear anomalies include malformations of the middle ear, cochlear hypoplasia, a wide internal auditory canal, and malformation of the vestibular system. The gene for BOR has been localized to chromosome 8q, but has not yet been identified.

CROUZON SYNDROME Crouzon syndrome is one of the most distinctive and frequent forms of dominantly inherited craniosynostosis. Fifty-five percent of Crouzon patients have a conductive hearing loss and 13% have atresia of the external auditory canals. Crouzon syndrome has been mapped to chromosome 10q25–26 and found to result from mutations in the fibroblast growth factor receptor-2 gene (*see* Chapter 114).

TREACHER COLLINS SYNDROME (MANDIBULOFACIAL DYSOSTOSIS) Treacher Collins syndrome shows significant craniofacial dysmorphology. The phenotype is characterized by down-slanted palpebral fissures with a coloboma on the outer supraorbital rims, and zygomas give the face a narrow appearance. Cleft palate is seen in about 35% of the cases. The external auricle is often malformed. The ossicles as well as the cochlea and labyrinth have been observed to be absent or hypoplastic. Bilateral hearing loss is seen in over half of the cases. The gene (PTX-2) has been mapped 5q13–5q33.3 near the gene for DFNA1.

OTHER DISORDERS ASSOCIATED WITH HEARING LOSS

PENDRED SYNDROME Pendred Syndrome is an association between deafness and euthyroid goiter (*see* Chapter 50). The hearing loss may be progressive. The cause of the hearing defect is a congenital bilateral malformation of the cochlea of the Mondini type. A patient with multiple congenital anomalies and Pendred syndrome was observed to have a chromosomal abnormality, dup(10p)del(8q), suggesting that a gene for Pendred was on one or the other of these chromosomes.

NEUROFIBROMATOSIS 2 Neurofibromatosis Type 2 (NF2) is an autosomal-dominant disorder characterized by the development of bilateral schwannomas from the vestibular nerves (*see* Chapter 106). Gene carriers often show eighth nerve dysfunction starting in early childhood and is manifest by tinnitus, bilateral hearing loss, and vestibular dysfunction. NF2 is always important to consider in the differential diagnosis of patients with sudden onset hearing loss, especially when unilateral. Gene linkage analysis has localized the NF2 gene to chromosome band 22q2. The NF2 gene has recently been identified and encodes a protein that has a high degree of homology with moesin, ezrin, and radixin, a family of proteins probably responsible for linking the cell membrane with the cytoskeleton. The mechanism by which mutations of this gene act to cause tumor growth is not known.

NORRIES DISEASE Norries Disease (ND) is an X-linked disorder characterized by progressive atrophy of the eyes, mental disturbances, and deafness. It has been mapped to chromosome Xp11.4, and its gene spans 28 kb and consists of three exons. Detailed molecular analyses of genomic deletions in Norrie patients shows that they are heterogeneous, both in size of material deleted and in position of the deletions. It has been hypothesized that, because of homology with known proteins, that norin codes for a protein that regulates neural cell differentiation and proliferation.

MANAGEMENT AND TREATMENT OF HEREDITARY HEARING IMPAIRMENTS

From a genetic perspective, diagnosis is the main problem encountered when dealing with hereditary hearing loss disorders and must be solved before other issues of management can be effectively addressed. Advances in molecular diagnostics will undoubtedly prove to be valuable in this area. Even though a limited number of syndromic genes have been identified so far, it is possible to verify diagnosis for Waardenburg syndrome, one type of Usher syndrome, Alport syndrome, X-linked gusher, and Norries disease. Together, these syndromes constitute a large proportion of patients seen for hearing impairments. With regard to nonsyndrome hearing losses, several linkages have been found, but none of the specific genes responsible have been identified. Improved efficiency in diagnostic screening is certainly to be expected as more genes are identified, and it is reasonable to expect that such screening will become increasingly important in other aspects of management. Early diagnosis is critical for the development of communication skills in children with hearing losses. As more mutations are identified, infants in at-risk families can be diagnosed as early as desired. Early diagnosis may be important with regard to other strategies of intervention. For example, Usher I patients seem to do well with cochlear implants and early diagnosis would be useful in planning patient care that could lead to implant surgery done at a stage of development most effective for enhancing the language skill of Usher patients. Thus, it is expected that, as molecular genetics improves the diagnostic skills for the detection of specific genetic mutations, novel approaches to the treatment of the hearing-impaired will emerge.

SELECTED REFERENCES

Barker DF, Hostikka SL, Zhou J, et al. Identification of mutations in the COL4A5 collagen gene in Alport syndrome. Science 1990;248:1224–1227.

Chen ZY, Battinelli EM, Hendriks RW, et al. Norrie disease gene: characterization of deletions and possible function. Genomics 1993;16: 533–535.

de Kok YJ, van der Maarel SM, Bitner-Glindzicz M, et al. Association between x-linked mixed deafness and mutations in the POU domain gene POU3F4. Science 1995;267:685–688.

Fontaine B, Rouleau GA, Seizinger BR, et al. Molecular genetics of neurofibromatosis 2 and related tumors (acoustic neuroma and meningioma). Ann NY Acad Sci 1991;615:338–343.

Fraser FC, Ling D, Clogg D, Nogrady B. Genetic aspects of the BOR syndrome—branchial fistulas, ear pits, hearing loss, and renal anomalies. Am J Med Genet 1978;2:241–252.

Garretsen TJ, Cremers CW. Clinical and genetic aspects in autosomal dominant inherited osteogenesis imperfecta type I. Ann NY Acad Sci 1991;630:240–248.

Gorlin RJ, Toriello HV, Cohen MM. Hereditary Hearing Loss and Its Syndromes. New York: Oxford University Press, 1995.

Kelsell DP, Dunlop J, Stevens HP, et al. Connexin 26 mutations in hereditary non-syndromic sensorineural deafness. Nature 1997;387:80–83.

Liu XZ, Walsh J, Mburu P, et al. Mutations in the myosin VIIA gene cause non-syndromic recessive deafness. Nat Genet 1997;16:188–190.

Moller CG, Kimberling WJ, Davenport SL, et al. Usher syndrome: an otoneurologic study. Laryngoscope 1989;99:73–79.

Morton NE. Genetic epidemiology of hearing impairment. Ann NY Acad Sci 1991;630:16–31.

Petit C. Genes responsible for human hereditary deafness: a symphony of a thousand. Nat Genet 1996;14:385–391.

Weil D, Blanchard S, Kaplan J, et al. Defective myosin VIIA gene responsible for Usher syndrome type 1B. Nature 1995;374:60,61.

Weil D, Kussel P, Blanchard S, et al. The autosomal recessive isolated deafness, DFNB2, and the Usher 1B syndrome are allelic defects of the myosin-VIIA gene. Nat Genet 1997;16:191–193.

Zlotogora J, Sagi M, Schuper A, Leiba H, Merin S. Variability of Stickler syndrome. Am J Med Genet 1992;42:337–339.

Index

B

C

E

F

G

H

M

N

O

R

T

Y

Z